COMPANION CD-ROM RESOURCES

PHARMACOLOGY TUTORIAL

DORLAND'S AUDIO PRONUNCIATIONS

ANIMATIONS

Anoxic Brain Injury, Anoxia, Oxygen Deprivation, in Infant Meningitis
Neuron Function
Parkinson's Disease
Primary Brain Tumor
Atrial Fibrillation Leading to Stroke, Cerebrovascular Accident (CVA)
Blood Clot Leading to Stroke
Brain Abscess
Brain Anatomy: Cerebral Cortex, Cerebellum, Brainstem
Brain Anatomy: Temporal Lobe, Brainstem, Cerebral Peduncle, Thalamus
Brain Inflammation, Edema of Brain
Brainstem and Respiration
Cerebellar Infarct; Stroke
Displaced Disks; Spine Injury
Quadriplegia; Spinal Cord Injury
Spine Structure
Intubation, Incorrect Placement in Lung
Intubation, Normal; Endotracheal Intubation
Opening an Airway (Emergency)
Pneumonia
Pneumonia, Resolution of
Pulmonary Embolus
Asthma
Primary Lung Tumor
Tuberculosis
Dilutional Anemia
Hemophilia A
Mature Blood Cells
Normal Clotting
Platelet Function
Red Blood Cell Function
Sickle Cell Anemia
Thrombocytopenia
Transfusion Effect
Basophil Function
Eosinophil Function
Lymphocyte Function
Anemia, Cardiovascular Effects
Atrial Fibrillation
Capillary Leak
Congestive Heart Failure
Coronary Oxygenation
Defibrillation
Defibrillation in Ventricular Fibrillation

Heart Monitoring
Normal Cardiopulmonary Physiology
Structure of the Heart
Ventricular Fibrillation
Normal Vascular System
Pulmonary Hypertension
Bleeding Ulcer, Pathophysiology, Symptoms; Hematemesis
Bowel Obstruction, Early Pathophysiology & Symptoms
Colonoscopy
Digestion, Entire Process
Duodenal Ulcer, Pathophysiology, Symptoms
Endotracheal Intubation, in Child, Correct Procedure
Esophageal Intubation
Esophageal Varices, Development
Intubation, Emergency (Brief) (Interactive)
Primary Colon Tumor
Primary Stomach Tumor
Stomach Ulcer
Bile Release in Digestion
Cirrhosis (Pathophysiology), Liver Disease, Esophageal Varices
Gallbladder Physiology
Hepatobiliary Anatomy (Liver, Pancreas)
Laparoscopic Cholecystectomy; Gallbladder Removal
Pancreatic Enzymes in Digestion
Primary Liver Tumor
Primary Pancreas Tumor
Creatinine Formation
Insertion of Foley Catheter (Male and Female)
Nephrostomy
Primary Bladder Tumor
Primary Kidney Tumor
Renal Anatomy and Function
Renal Stone; Kidney Stone; Nephrolithiasis
Urinary Tract Infection, Kidney Infection
Urine Flow
Urine Formation
Ankle Fracture
Dislocation of Bones: Hip, Knee, Shoulder, Elbow
Hip Fracture, Femur Fracture, Femoral Fracture
Primary Bone Tumor
Adrenal Function
Thyroid Gland, Hormone Release
Insulin Function
Breast Cancer Spread, Metastasis
Ovarian Cyst
Primary Breast Tumor
Primary Cervix Tumor
Primary Ovarian Tumor
Primary Uterine Tumor
Primary Prostate Tumor
Anatomy of Eye
Retinal Detachment

INTRODUCTION TO
MEDICAL-
SURGICAL
NURSING

Adrianne Dill Linton, PhD, RN

Associate Professor and Chair
Department of Chronic Nursing Care
The University of Texas Health Science Center
  at San Antonio
School of Nursing
San Antonio, Texas

SAUNDERS

ELSEVIER

SAUNDERS
ELSEVIER

11830 Westline Industrial Drive
St. Louis, Missouri 63146

Vice President, Publishing Director: Sally Schrefer
Executive Publisher: Tom Wilhelm
Managing Editor: Robin Levin Richman
Publishing Services Manager: Deborah L. Vogel
Senior Project Manager: Jodi M. Willard
Design Direction: Teresa McBryan

Printed in the United States of America

Last digit is the print number: 9 8 7 6 5 4 3 2

*Dedicated to the memory of my brother **Michael Lynn Dill** (1950-2006),
whose life was one of service to others.*

ADRIANNE DILL LINTON

Acknowledgments

Writing, editing, illustrating, publishing, and revising *Introduction to Medical-Surgical Nursing* has been an effort involving many outstanding individuals. Grateful thanks to the staff of Elsevier Science, especially to Robin Levin Richman, Managing Editor, Nursing Editorial, for her great effort in seeing this edition through to completion and to Melissa Martin, freelance Developmental Editor, for developing and carrying this edition to publication with great skill and creativity. Other Elsevier supporters include Marie Thomas, Senior Editorial Assistant; Ryan Creed, Associate Developmental Editor; Kathy Mantz, Marketing Manager; Teresa McBryan, Senior Book Designer; Debbie Vogel, Production Services Manager; and Jodi Willard, Senior Project Manager. In addition, I would like to recognize the contributions of Ilze Rader, former Senior Editor, Nursing Books, who got this project off the ground.

I appreciate the patience and skill of the artists and photographers who produced the fine illustrations. They, along with the reviewers, ensured readability, accuracy, and timeliness of the manuscript. During the past decade, students who have used the text have offered suggestions that have been most helpful. Their feedback has always been welcome.

Also, thanks to Tracy Brady, RN, BSN, for her thoughtful input and excellent proofing skills and to Dr. Charles Brady for serving as a resource and consultant.

I wish the best to my colleague Dr. Mary Ann Matteson, who was co-author of the first two editions, as she continues to enjoy her retirement. Dr. Nancy Maebius continues to be a strong force in the development of this text and remains the author of the Study Guide. As an LVN educator, her insights and guidance are vital. I am grateful to the chapter contributors, who ensured accurate and current information, and to the many individuals involved in the development of the ancillary materials.

I must not overlook my family, who remained patient and encouraging as I immersed myself in this process once again. I want to express my appreciation to my husband, Ken, and to my daughter, Leigh, and son-in-law, Paul.

Contributors & Reviewers

CONTRIBUTORS

VICTORIA DITTMAR, MSN, RN
Instructor/Clinical
Department of Acute Nursing Care
The University of Texas Health Science
    Center at San Antonio
School of Nursing
San Antonio, Texas

STEPHANIE ELMS, MSN, RN
Instructor/Clinical
Department of Acute Nursing Care
The University of Texas Health Science
    Center at San Antonio
School of Nursing
San Antonio, Texas

LESLIE GODDARD, RN, PhD, CNRN
Clinical Nurse Specialist, Neuroscience
Methodist Healthcare System
San Antonio, Texas

MARY L. HEYE, BSN, MSN, PhD
Associate Professor
The University of Texas Health Science
    Center at San Antonio
School of Nursing
San Antonio, Texas

LISA HOOTER, RN, MSN, CDE
Staff Development Educator
St. Luke's Baptist Hospital
San Antonio, Texas

JANEAN W. JENKINS, MSN, RN, CNRN, CNS
Methodist Healthcare System
San Antonio, Texas
Clinical Faculty
The University of Texas Health Science
    Center at San Antonio
School of Nursing
San Antonio, Texas

LOUIS K. LINTON, BS, RRT, CPFT
Instructor of Respiratory Therapy (Ret.)
U.S. Army: Respiratory Specialist
    Program
Brooke Army Medical Center
Ft. Sam Houston, Texas

JUDY L. MALTAS, MSN, CCRN
Clinical Assistant Professor
The University of Texas Health Science
    Center at San Antonio
School of Nursing
San Antonio, Texas

MARK A. MEYER, MSN, RN, ACRN
Instructor
University of Texas at Arlington
Arlington, Texas

BARBARA L. OWENS, PhD, RN, OCN
Assistant Professor/Clinical
Department of Acute Nursing Care
The University of Texas Health Science
    Center at San Antonio
School of Nursing
San Antonio, Texas

LINDA PORTER, PhD, RN, MSN, CNAA, MA, LPC, NCC
Assistant Professor
Director, Flexible Process
Department of Chronic Nursing Care
The University of Texas Health Science
    Center at San Antonio
School of Nursing
San Antonio, Texas

KATHLEEN A. REEVES, RN, MSN, C
Clinical Assistant Professor
The University of Texas Health Science
    Center at San Antonio
School of Nursing
San Antonio, Texas

MARK D. SOUCY, MS, APRN, BC
Assistant Professor/Clinical
The University of Texas Health Science
    Center at San Antonio
School of Nursing
San Antonio, Texas

CATHERINE ROBICHAUX, RN, PhD
Assistant Professor/Clinical
The University of Texas Health Science
    Center at San Antonio
School of Nursing
San Antonio, Texas

CHERYL ROSS STAATS, MSN, RN, CS
Associate Professor/Clinical
The University of Texas Health Science
    Center at San Antonio
School of Nursing
San Antonio, Texas

MARY WALKER, MSN, CCRN, CCNS
Clinical Instructor
Department of Chronic Nursing Care
The University of Texas Health Science
    Center at San Antonio
School of Nursing
San Antonio, Texas

STACEY YOUNG-McCAUGHAN, RN, PhD, AOCN
Deputy Director
Congressionally Directed Medical
    Research Programs
Fort Dietrich, Maryland

REVIEWERS

Reviewers for the Third Edition

LINDA C. ARNOLD, RN, BSN
Ivy Tech State College
Bloomington, Indiana

JO-ANN DEAN, RN, BSN, MS
New England Technical Institute
New Britain, Connecticut

SHARON M. ERBE, RN, BSN
Washington-Saratoga-Warren-Hamilton-
  Essex Board of Cooperative Education
  Services
Southern Adirondack Education Center
  Career & Technical School
Hudson Falls, New York

BARBARA C. FAIR, RN, MA
St. Clair County Community College
Port Huron, Michigan

DARLENE D. GATTENS, RN, MN
Alvernia School of Practical Nursing at
  St. Francis Medical Center
Pittsburgh, Pennsylvania

M. SUSAN GRINSLADE, RN, MSN, PhD
Assistant Professor
The University of Texas Health Science
  Center at San Antonio
School of Nursing
San Antonio, Texas

KAREN KATHRYN HAAGENSEN, RNC
Howard College
San Angelo, Texas

BEVERLY F. HALTER, RN, BSN, MSN
Consultant
North Central Baptist Hospital
San Antonio, Texas

PAMELA ROCHELLE HINCKLEY, RN, MSN
Redlands Adult School
Redlands, California

PATRICIA A. KNECHT, RN, MSN
Center for Arts and Technology
Coatesville, Pennsylvania

FRANK LAUREANO, RN, MSN, CNOR
Assistant Professor/Clinical
The University of Texas Health Science
  Center at San Antonio
School of Nursing
San Antonio, Texas

VALERIE I. LEEK, RN, MS, CS
Cumberland County Technical-Education
  Center
Bridgeton, New Jersey

YVONNE B. MEINKET, RN, BS, MEd
Charlotte Vocational Technical Center
Port Charlotte, Florida

LISA D. MORLAN, RN, BSN
Gordon Cooper Technology Center
Shawnee, Oklahoma

LORI MOSELEY, RN
Hill College
Cleburne, Texas

SALLIE NOTO, RN, MS
Career Technology Center School of
  Practical Nursing
Scranton, Pennsylvania

TONI L. PRITCHARD, RN, LPN, ADN
Louisiana Technical College, Lamar Salter
  Campus
Leesville, Louisiana

JULIE S. VERNON, BSN
Tri Country Technical College
Pendleton, South Carolina

KAY YANNACCONE, RN, BS
Central Susquehanna LPN Career Center
Washingtonville, Pennsylvania

Reviewers for the Fourth Edition

KATHLEEN K. GUDGEL, RN, MSN
Instructor, Nursing Programs
Pennsylvania College of Technology
Williamsport, Pennsylvania

NANCY TURNER, MSN, RNC
Associate Professor, Practical Nursing
West Kentucky Community & Technical
  College
Paducah, Kentucky

DAWN R. WARREN, RN, MSN
Assistant Professor, School of Nursing
University of South Dakota
Rapid City, South Dakota

To the Instructor

The first three editions of this text were designed to provide practical and vocational nursing students with accessible, comprehensive coverage of the nursing care of adults with disorders requiring medical, surgical, and psychiatric management. The needs of older adults and residents of nonacute care settings received special attention. The fourth edition has maintained that focus. To keep pace with the rapidly evolving field of nursing, we have added useful and exciting new features, many of which were suggested by instructors and students.

ORGANIZATION

Unit 1 explores patient care concepts, including the health care system, patient care settings, leadership, the nurse-patient relationship, cultural aspects of nursing care, the nurse and the family, health and illness, nutrition, developmental processes, the older patient, and the nursing process and critical thinking. A chapter on legal and ethical issues is new to this edition. **Unit 2** focuses on physiologic responses common to many disorders: inflammation, infection, and immunity; imbalances of fluids and electrolytes; and pain. **Unit 3** covers first aid and emergency care, shock, general care of the surgical patient, and intravenous therapy. The in-depth coverage of topics in Units 2 and 3 provides both a foundation for understanding many disorders and a scientific basis for many aspects of nursing care. This approach is efficient because conditions such as common electrolyte imbalances need not be explained repeatedly in the many situations in which they occur.

Acknowledging the important role the LPN/LVN plays in the care of older adults, **Unit 4** provides comprehensive coverage of four clinical problems (falls, incontinence, confusion, and immobility) as well as end-of-life care. The last of the introductory units, **Unit 5,** takes a broad look at the nursing care of patients with cancer and patients with ostomies. This overview creates a foundation for the student to build on when studying a variety of systems and disorders. **Units 6** through **16** follow a systems approach to medical-surgical disorders. For each system, a thorough nursing assessment, age-related considerations, diagnostic tests and procedures, drug therapy, and other common therapeutic measures are discussed. Although complete assessment data are included, the specific role of the LPN/LVN in data collection for focused assessments is emphasized. Common therapeutic measures are intended not to replace a fundamentals text but, instead, to provide a limited summary or review of key aspects of nursing care.

Specific aspects are covered, including pathophysiology, signs and symptoms, complications, diagnosis, and medical treatment. New to this unit is a separate chapter on HIV/AIDS (Chapter 34).

Unit 17 consists of three chapters that address psychosocial responses to illness, psychiatric disorders, and substance abuse. This unit can eliminate the need for a separate mental health nursing textbook.

KEY FEATURES

Introduction to Medical-Surgical Nursing has been enthusiastically received by both students and instructors. They told us which features were most helpful to them, and we listened.

Accessible Language

The text is straightforward and direct, avoiding the cumbersome third person. What's more, we have continued to improve consistency and to standardize the reading level throughout.

Key Terms with Phonetic Pronunciations

Complex medical, nursing, and scientific words can be tricky to understand and pronounce. A Key Terms list at the beginning of each chapter shows students how to pronounce important terms they may encounter as nurses. All phonetic pronunciations have been reviewed by a specialist in English as a Second Language (ESL). Key terms appear in color in the text and are defined.

Nursing Diagnoses, Goals, and Outcome Criteria

Nursing care is the heart of this text, which is organized according to the steps of the nursing process. For each major disorder covered, nursing diagnoses, goals, outcome criteria, and relevant interventions are presented. The nursing assessment is described, with an emphasis on data collected by the LVN/LPN.

Patient Teaching Plans

Patient and family teaching are emphasized throughout, with teaching plans presented in a special format. The patient teaching plans are intended not to be complete but, rather, to give the student some critical points to emphasize.

Diagnostic Tests and Procedures Tables

Each chapter dealing with a particular body system contains a table detailing specific diagnostic tests and procedures for selected nursing diagnoses.

Pharmacology Capsules

Important drug information, including drug actions, potential drug interactions, adverse effects, and nursing considerations are highlighted in these brief boxes within the text of each chapter.

Nutrition Concepts

A poor diet can affect a patient's health, but failing health can compromise a patient's nutritional status as well. Important nutrition-related topics are spotlighted at appropriate points throughout the text.

Put on Your Thinking Cap!

These questions, which appear in brief boxes throughout the text, invite students to take their reading a step further by thinking critically about the material and applying it to realistic scenarios.

Cultural Coverage

In our increasingly diverse culture, nurses must be comfortable working with patients of every conceivable ethnic and cultural background, religion, lifestyle, and sexual orientation. To help students see the connection between culture and care, a feature called What Does Culture Have to Do With . . . ? appears at relevant points in the chapter text. In addition, an entire chapter (Chapter 6: "Cultural Aspects of Nursing Care") explores transcultural nursing in detail.

Consider the Alternative

Will taking St. John's wort interfere with my amitriptyline? Does echinacea really help prevent colds? Nurses hear these kinds of questions from patients every day. Our Consider the Alternative feature raises nurses' awareness of the herbal remedies, dietary supplements, and complementary and alternative therapies their patients are interested in and may be using.

Key Points

To succeed in the fast-paced world of health care, the nurse must be able to put it all together. Each chapter brings students a few steps closer by summarizing the most important points in a succinct, memorable way.

NEW TO THIS EDITION

The fourth edition has been completely updated to include the latest developments in patient care and to present them in a way that is accessible to students at all levels. As instructors, we know that our students are concerned about preparing for the NCLEX-PN® examination. The following features were developed in response to the latest test plan—which, of course, reflects changes in the practice of nursing itself:

- **Companion CD-ROM**
  Bound with the book, the companion CD-ROM includes an entire Pharmacology Tutorial tied to the text, as well as vivid animations of anatomy/physiology and procedures from ARCHIE-MD.

- **Drug Therapy Tables**
  Promising new prescription drugs are continually entering the marketplace, making this area of nursing practice more complex than ever. The NCLEX-PN® test plan reflects this new reality. Nurses need to be familiar with drug names, dosages, and routes of administration. Each body systems chapter includes a table that summarizes pharmaceutical options accurately and concisely.

- **Multiple-Choice Review Questions**
  These are provided at the end of each chapter for immediate reinforcement of chapter content. Answers are located in Appendix E.

- *New Chapter:* **Legal and Ethical Considerations**
  The latest NCLEX-PN® test plan calls for a higher percentage of questions on legal and ethical issues, many of which fall into a category the plan refers to as "Coordinated Care." Chapter 3, "Legal and Ethical Considerations," is new to this edition. This chapter explores the nurse's increasing responsibilities in areas such as patient confidentiality, informed consent, prevention of medical errors, and documentation.

- **Management and Supervision**
  The test plan also calls for more emphasis on prioritizing and assigning tasks to nurse assistants, patient care technicians, and unlicensed assistive personnel. To help students sort out these sometimes perplexing issues, this edition of *Introduction to Medical-Surgical Nursing* includes Management and Supervision boxes in many chapters.

- **Health Promotion Considerations**
  The NCLEX-PN® test plan calls for a renewed emphasis on health promotion and maintenance. New Health Promotion Considerations boxes highlight wellness and disease prevention topics nurses need to know about.

The following content and features are also new to this edition:

- *New Chapter:* **HIV/AIDS**
  Responsible health care professionals now recognize that HIV/AIDS has many routes of transmission and should not, then, be lumped into the category of sexually transmitted infections. Because of the special threat the disease poses to public health, this edition of *Introduction to Medical-Surgical Nursing* addresses HIV/AIDS in a new, separate chapter (Chapter 34), contributed by an expert in the field.

- *New Appendix:* **Laboratory Reference Values**
  Laboratory reference values presented in this new appendix give students a handy frame of reference for interpreting laboratory results, a task that is new to many of them.

- *New Appendix:* **Helpful Phrases for Communicating in Spanish**
  For the native Spanish-speaking or ESL (English as a Second Language) student, this appendix is a

valuable addition to the textbook. English-speaking students who are not bilingual will find the appendix helpful in learning a few words and phrases to use in communicating with their Spanish-speaking patients.

- **Nursing Care Plans with Critical Thinking Questions**

  Sample nursing care plans illustrate how the text translates into a bedside tool for patient care. Focused critical thinking questions at the end of each care plan allow the student to check his or her understanding of the concepts presented in the chapter and synthesized in the care plan. Answers are given in the Instructor's Resource Manual portion of the Instructor's Electronic Resource.

- **Updated Content Throughout**

  Instructors and students trust *Introduction to Medical-Surgical Nursing* because it has led the way in presenting innovative, accurate, up-to-date content. Here is a sampling of the new content in this edition:
  - Bioterrorism and the nurse's role in disaster management
  - Safety in nursing practice
  - Critical thinking skills and clinical application
  - Expanded coverage of intravenous therapies
  - Increased data collection/assessment content

ANCILLARIES

For the Instructor

- **Instructor's Electronic Resource**
  - Instructor's Resource Manual
  - PowerPoint Presentation (approximately 3300 slides)
  - ExamView Test Bank with NCLEX®-style questions and answers, separate test bank in Word for alternate-format questions, approximately 1400 questions total. Each question in the test bank includes topic, nursing process step, objective, cognitive level, correct answer, rationale, and text page number references
  - Image Collection (all images in the textbook plus supplemental images from other Elsevier sources)
  - Instructor Resources also available online via Evolve
- **Evolve Learning Resources**
  - Instructor's Resources include everything on the Instructor's Electronic Resource plus WebLinks

- **TEACH Online**
  - Lesson Plan Manual based on textbook chapter learning objectives
  - Provides roadmap to link and integrate all parts of the educational package
  - Available for adopters of the textbook

FOR STUDENTS

- *NEW!* **Companion CD-ROM** (bound with the text) includes the following:
  - Pharmacology tutorial
  - Realistic 3-D animations of physiology and procedures from the ARCHIE-MD Patient Simulation Library
  - Audio pronunciations
- **Study Guide**

  Practical and student-friendly, this useful study guide, based on the textbook chapter objectives, is designed to help students master the content presented in the text. It includes the following:
  - Learning Activities (including listing, matching, and labeling exercises) and Multiple-Choice Questions
  - Text page references are included for each question
  - Answers are included in the Instructor's Resource Manual
- **Virtual Clinical Excursions 3.0**

  This interactive workbook and CD-ROM package complements the textbook and guides students through a multi-floor virtual hospital in a true-to-life, hands-on clinical learning experience. Students can collect and analyze data to assist in making nursing diagnoses, planning interventions, prioritizing, and implementing and evaluating care. NCLEX-PN®–style review questions provide immediate testing of clinical knowledge.
- **Evolve Learning Resources**
  - Student Resources include everything on the Companion CD-ROM plus WebLinks

  Contact your local Elsevier sales representative to request a copy of the Instructor's Electronic Resource.

  We welcome suggestions and comments you may have concerning *Introduction to Medical-Surgical Nursing*, fourth edition, and its ancillaries. Please address your comments to the Nursing Editorial Department, Elsevier Inc., 1600 John F. Kennedy Boulevard, Suite 1800, Philadelphia, PA, 19103-2899.

LPN Threads

Introduction to Medical-Surgical Nursing, fourth edition, shares some features and design elements with other Mosby and Saunders LPN textbooks. The purpose of these "LPN Threads" is to make it easier for students and instructors to incorporate multiple books into the fast-paced and demanding LPN curriculum.

The shared features in *Introduction to Medical-Surgical Nursing,* fourth edition, include the following:

- A **reading level evaluation** was performed on every manuscript chapter during the book's development.
- Cover and internal **design similarities.**
- Numbered lists of **Objectives** that begin each chapter.
- **Key Terms** with phonetic pronunciations and page number references at the beginning of each chapter. The key terms are printed in color. An English as a Second Language (ESL) consultant reviewed all pronunciations.
- **Health Promotion Considerations** boxes highlight wellness and disease prevention topics.
- **Management and Supervision** boxes emphasize prioritization of tasks and assignment to nurse assistants, patient care technicians, and unlicensed assistive personnel.
- **Drug Therapy Tables** help familiarize nurses with drug names, dosages, and routes of administration by summarizing pharmaceutical options accurately and concisely.
- **Critical Thinking Questions** throughout the text. Answers to the critical thinking questions are pro-

vided in the Instructor's Resource Manual component of the Instructor's Electronic Resource.

- Bulleted lists of **Key Points** at the end of each chapter.
- **Multiple-Choice Review Questions** at the end of each chapter. For easy access, answers are provided in the textbook.
- A **Complete Bibliography and Reader References** list at the end of the text.
- A **Glossary** at the end of the text.
- An **ExamView Test Bank** with the following categories of information: Topic, Step of the Nursing Process, Objective, Cognitive Level, NCLEX Category of Client Need, Correct Answer, Rationale, and Text Page Reference.
- A **PowerPoint slide presentation** in the Instructor's Electronic Resource.
- **Open-Book Quizzes** in the Instructor's Resource Manual.
- **Study Guide answer keys** in the Instructor's Resource Manual. The Study Guide itself contains text page number references where students can find the answers.
- **Tips for teaching ESL students** in the Instructor's Resource Manual.
- **Study Hints for ESL students** in the Study Guide.

In addition to content and design threads, these LPN/LVN textbooks benefit from the advice and input of the LPN/LVN Advisory Board.

LPN/LVN Advisory Board

To The Student

KEY FEATURES

Designed with the student in mind, *Introduction to Medical-Surgical Nursing*, fourth edition, has a visually appealing and easy-to-use format that will help you master medical-surgical nursing. The **FREE CD-ROM** packaged in your copy of the book contains the following sections: an extensive Pharmacology Tutorial, 3-D animations from ARCHIE-MD, and audio pronunciations that include Key Terms and other term pronunciations.

Following are some of the numerous special features and aids to help you as you study.

Objectives provide an overview of what students will learn from the chapter content.

Key Terms with **phonetic pronunciations** and page number references emphasize and clarify essential terminology.

New! **Chapter 3, Legal and Ethical Considerations,** explores the increasingly complex legal landscape and outlines the nurse's central ethical responsibilities.

Full-Color Design and Illustrations increase effectiveness of key concepts.

Management and Supervision boxes help nurses prioritize tasks and assign them safely and efficiently.

New! **Chapter 34, HIV/AIDS,** addresses rapid advances in the vital field of HIV/AIDS prevention, treatment, and research and describes the nurse's role in caring for the unique needs of HIV/AIDS patients.

Cultural Considerations provide essential knowledge to ensure individualized care of patients.

Nutrition Concepts emphasize the role nutrition plays in disease and nursing care.

Patient Teaching Plans illustrate examples of individualized patient care using the nursing process.

Consider the Alternative boxes increase awareness of nontraditional approaches in today's health care settings.

Pharmacology Capsules alert students to important precautions, interactions, and adverse effects of medications.

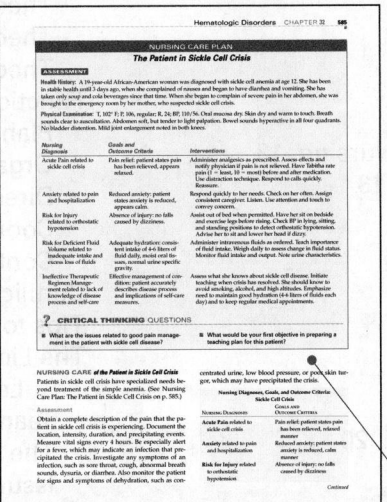

Health Promotion Considerations boxes highlight timely wellness and disease prevention topics.

Drug Therapy tables and Diagnostic Tests and Procedures tables in each systems chapter provide quick references to relevant drugs and tests.

Put on Your Thinking Cap boxes encourage analysis of content for application to clinical situations.

Nursing Care Plans with Critical Thinking Questions at the end of each care plan encourage students to synthesize key concepts. Answers are given in the Instructor's Electronic Resource.

New! **Laboratory Reference Values,** an appendix new to this edition, offers a convenient, accurate summary of lab values commonly referred to in medical-surgical settings.

Key Points reinforce important information in each chapter.

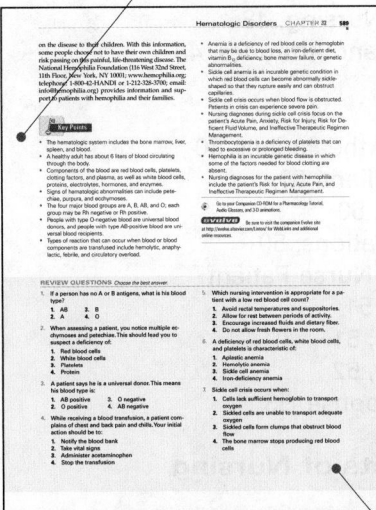

Multiple-Choice Review Questions test knowledge of the chapter content.

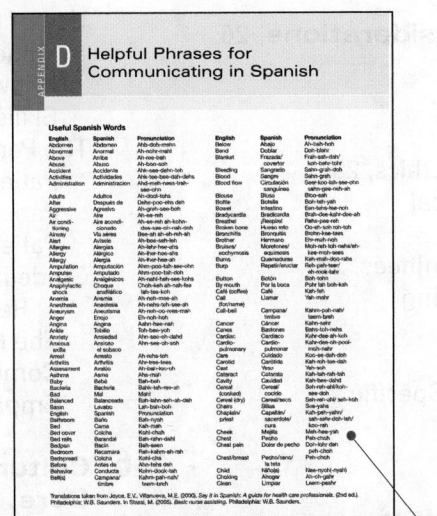

New! **Helpful Phrases for Communicating in Spanish,** an appendix new to this edition, is a valuable resource for ESL students and others who care for Spanish-speaking patients.

FULLY UPDATED STUDY GUIDE

Study guide provides detailed, clear methods to identify the most important material for more efficient learning.

Contents

UNIT **TWO** PHYSIOLOGIC RESPONSES
TO ILLNESS

The Health Care System

evolve http://evolve.elsevier.com/Linton/

Objectives

After reading and studying this chapter, you should be able to:

1. Describe the organization of the health care system in the United States.
2. Describe the focus of public health services.
3. Define the three levels of prevention.
4. Discuss financing of health care in the United States, including Medicare and Medicaid programs.
5. Describe the components of the health care system that provide outpatient and inpatient care and the types of service each provides.
6. Describe the impact of cost-containment measures on the delivery of care.

Key Terms

 Be sure to check out the bonus material on the Companion CD-ROM, including selected audio pronunciations.

capitation (p. 4)
diagnosis-related group (DRG) (p. 4)
extended care (p. 11)
fee-for-service (p. 3)
health maintenance organization (HMO) (p. 1)
long-term care facility (p. 11)
managed care (p. 1)
Medicaid (p. 5)
Medicare (p. 4)
Older Americans Act (p. 9)
preferred provider organization (PPO) (p. 1)
primary prevention (p. 2)
Public Health Service (p. 2)
secondary prevention (p. 3)
skilled nursing facility (p. 11)
tertiary prevention (TĔR-shē-ĕr-ē, p. 3)

In the United States, which is one of the few industrialized nations that does not have a comprehensive national health care program, the health care system is very complex. With an increase in the older adult population and a resulting rise in the numbers of people with chronic illness, costs have risen alarmingly. Government officials, health care providers, and consumers now face the hard issues of deciding who is to receive care, what type of care should be provided, and how to pay for it. Health care reform is a major issue for government officials and the American people, all of whom are interested in the provision of equitable health care to all Americans.

ORGANIZATION OF THE HEALTH CARE SYSTEM

The health care system is made up of the patient, the patient's family, the community, governmental agencies, health care providers, and insurance companies. Nevertheless, many of the health-related services available to individuals are funded with financial assistance from government or private agencies. Unfortunately, not all citizens of the United States are eligible for government funds, and some are unable or unwilling to obtain private insurance. In addition, government funding and private insurance frequently do not cover all the costs of health care. Therefore many people are unable to pay for care and may not receive the services they need. In the United States, about 17% of the population is uninsured. Nineteen percent (48 million) of Americans younger than 65 years and 12% (8.5 million) of children younger than 18 years are uninsured.

Whereas ensuring care for older adults and children is a great concern, young adults actually are the least likely to be covered. Thirty-five percent of young persons ages 19 to 24 are uninsured. By race/ethnicity, the uninsured population includes one in three Hispanics, one in five blacks, and one in seven whites.

In addition to the problem of financing, there is no overall philosophy or plan for health care. Critical care and the treatment of illness receive more attention than health promotion and disease prevention. Standards to ensure quality of care are inadequate, and there is little consumer participation in decision making. There is a lack of coordination of services, and communication among service providers is poor.

The health care system is now dominated by managed care. Managed care is intended to provide comprehensive health care at a reasonable cost through enrollment in a health maintenance organization (HMO), preferred provider organization (PPO), or similar plan that includes incentives to save costs. Managed care has stimulated increased interest in wellness and prevention, increased outpatient and home health care, and increased cost sharing.

ADMINISTRATION

In 1953, the Department of Health, Education and Welfare was established to organize the various health and welfare agencies of the U.S. government. The department became known as the *Department of Health and Human Services (DHHS)* in 1980, when education became a separate department. Today, DHHS programs are administered by the Public Health Service and three human services agencies: Centers for Medicare and Medicare Services, Administration for Children and Families, and the Administration on Aging. The Public Health Service agencies include the National Institutes of Health, the Food and Drug Administration, the Centers for Disease Control and Prevention, the Indian Health Service, Health Resources and Service Administration, Substance Abuse and Mental Health Services Administration, and the Agency for Healthcare Research and Quality. The role of the DHHS is to protect the health of all Americans and to provide essential human services, especially for those who cannot help themselves. The major activities of the Public Health Service Agencies are to:

- Support medical research
- Support research on health care systems, health care quality and cost issues, access to health care and effectiveness of medical treatments
- Ensure the safety of foods and cosmetics
- Ensure the safety and efficacy of drugs and medical devices
- Monitor and prevent disease outbreaks
- Provide health services to American Indians and Alaska Natives
- Provide access to essential health care services for low-income uninsured persons with limited access to health care
- Improve substance abuse prevention, addiction treatment, and mental health services

The Centers for Medicare and Medicaid Services (CMS) administer the services that provide health insurance and prescription drugs for older and disabled Americans. The Health Promotion Considerations box at right describes how nurses can help ensure that patients know how to access this benefit. Medicaid works with state agencies to provide health care for low-income persons, including nearly 22 million children. Through Medicaid, all states offer free or low-cost health insurance to children from low-income families. Read the Health Promotion Considerations box on p. 3 for more information about this program.

The Administration for Children and Families (ACF) directs programs that promote economic and social well-being of children, families, and communities. The ACF administers the Head Start program for pre-school children. The Administration on Aging provides services to enable older adults to remain independent.

 Health Promotion Considerations

Helping Patients Access the Medicare Prescription Drug Benefit

Nurses may be key contacts for patients who have questions about the Medicare prescription drug benefit. Training and educational materials for you and other members of the health care team are available by contacting Medicare at 1-800-MEDICARE or by going to www.cms.hhs.gov/medlearn/drugcoverage.asp. Becoming familiar with the information from Medicare and in this supplement will help you respond accurately to your patient's questions.

You can help the patient and his or her family with the following. Make sure:

- The patient and his or her family and caregivers are aware that the Medicare prescription drug benefit replaces Medicaid drug coverage.
- The patient is aware that Medicare Preferred Drug Plan enrollment is a condition of Medicaid eligibility. If the beneficiary refuses to enroll in a Preferred Drug Plan, he or she may lose all of his or her health care benefits.
- The patient retains and does not throw away any mail from Medicare or Medicaid concerning the drug benefit.
- The patient has received and saves the yellow letter from the Centers for Medicare and Medicaid Services (CMS) that identifies the plan to which he or she has been initially assigned.
- The patient's pharmacy is in the network of the assigned plan.
- The patient's drugs are covered by the assigned plan formulary.
- The patient's prescribing provider is aware of the drugs included in the patient's Part D plan and action is taken, if necessary, to ensure that the patient receives the necessary drugs (either by requesting an exception or by the prescriber writing a new prescription for a drug that is covered by the plan).

Adapted from New York State Department of Health, Office of Medicaid Management, DOH Medicaid Update December 2005, "Medicare Prescription Drug Benefit to Start January 1, 2006," Special Edition, vol. 20, no. 14, www.health.state.ny.us.

Public Health

Public health is concerned with the improvement of the health of communities and aggregates (collections of people) rather than the individual. The main goals of public health intervention are to protect and improve the health of populations at risk in the community and to prevent disease and disability. The focus of public health usually is directed to the levels of prevention traditionally classified as primary, secondary, and tertiary (Box 1-1). See Chapter 8 for prevention behaviors related to the health of individuals.

Primary Prevention. Primary prevention aims to improve health and prevent disease and injury. Examples of health promotion activities include exercise pro-

Health Promotion Considerations

Finding Health Insurance for Children

Every state in the nation has a health insurance program for infants, children, and teens. The insurance is available to children in working families, including families whose members are not U.S. citizens. (Visit www.ask.hrsa.gov to find materials that explain more about children's health insurance and immigration status.)

For little or no cost, this insurance pays for:

- Physician visits
- Prescription drugs
- Hospitalization

Children who do not currently have health insurance are likely to be eligible, even if their parents are working. Each state has different eligibility rules, but in most states, uninsured children 18 years old and younger whose families earn up to $34,100 a year (for a family of four) are eligible. To learn more, visit www.insurekidsnow.gov/states or call 877-KIDS-NOW.

Adapted from U.S. Department of Health and Human Services, www.insurekidsnow.gov, June 2006.

Pharmacology Capsule

The Medicare prescription drug benefit covers insulin and diabetes-testing supplies, such as syringes, needles, gauze, and swabs.

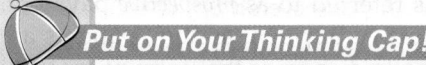

Put on Your Thinking Cap!

You have a friend who has limited income and no health insurance. She is a single mother with two small children. She has been advised to apply for Medicaid, and she asks you to help her. Find out the qualifications for Medicaid and how to make an application. Obtain an application form and complete it. Discuss the implications of the application process for persons with low reading levels, poor vision, poor hearing, no personal transportation, and/or no telephone.

What Does Culture Have to Do with Access to Health Care?

The U.S. Department of Health and Human Services offers Medicare and Medicaid publications in English, Spanish, Chinese, Korean, Russian, Tagalog, and Vietnamese.

grams to improve strength and cardiovascular fitness, campaigns in schools to discourage children from smoking, and efforts to educate people to wear seat belts.

Secondary Prevention. Secondary prevention focuses on early detection and treatment of disease to improve patient outcomes. Papanicolaou ("Pap") smears and

screening mammograms are examples of secondary prevention activities.

Tertiary Prevention. Tertiary prevention aims to prevent disease recurrences or complications. The use of physical therapy to prevent contractures in a stroke patient and teaching proper diet and foot care to a person with diabetes are examples of this third level of prevention activities.

FINANCING

An overview of health care financing is essential in light of the astronomical rise in expenditures. The health care system of the United States is the most expensive in the world. In 2002, $1.6 trillion, equal to 14.9% of our gross domestic product, was spent on health care, compared with 5% in 1960. By 2013, it is projected that total health care expenditures will total $3.6 trillion and will account for 18.4% of the gross domestic product. The largest component of health care costs (32%) is hospital expenditures. Prescription drug expenditures contribute significantly to overall health care costs. After progressively increasing over a period of years, the rate of growth in drug costs has slowed somewhat though it continues to exceed the rate of growth in total health care expenditures.

It has become obvious that measures must be taken to control what is spent on health care. In an effort to contain the rapidly rising costs of health care, the government has established rules and regulations aimed at decreasing costs. *Cost containment* occurs when the rate of increase is controlled rather than costs being reduced. As a result, private spending for health care is growing rapidly. Prescription drugs account for 9.4% of the privately paid costs.

Many different approaches to health care financing are used in the United States. HMOs, PPOs, and governmental agencies all affect the way in which health care is delivered. For the most part, health care systems have operated on a fee-for-service basis. This means that the patient pays a fee to the provider for specific services, after which the patient may seek reimbursement from an insurance company. Although this traditional system of payment is changing, some private-pay insurance options still support fee-for-service activities. Such coverage tends to be costly, typically requires deductions and copayments, and has limits that may not cover actual costs. However, it permits the patient to choose care providers, rather than being assigned to them. Many employers provide group health care insurance for employees. A type of coverage that blends multiple options is the point-of-service (POS) arrangement. Point-of-service includes a variety of options including HMO and PPO participation. Each option has advantages and disadvantages. Enrollees select which option they want to use. When health insurance pays for the health care expenses of members enrolled in health care plans, the payments are called *third-party reimbursements*.

Capitation is a strategy designed to control costs. With capitation, HMOs pay physicians a fixed amount of money each month for each member (patient) enrolled in the plan, regardless of whether or not the physician sees the patient that month. If physician costs are below the payment amount, the physician keeps the difference. However, if costs exceed the payment amount, the physician does not receive additional payment. There are a variety of HMOs that receive capitated payments from enrollees to cover a variety of services, such as preventive care and acute care.

Most health care agencies are funded through government funds or private insurance. Others are funded through out-of-pocket fees-for-service. The major means of government funding are Medicare and Medicaid, which are overseen by the Health Care Financing Administration (HCFA) (Table 1-1). Increasingly, other components of the health care system in addition to HMOs are moving toward capitation. With hospitals offering capitation contracts, new budget-cutting procedures have been implemented.

Medicare

Established in 1965, Medicare is a health insurance program administered by the U.S. government (the Centers for Medicare and Medicaid Services) as part of the Social Security Act. It helps pay for health care for anyone age 65 and older, persons of any age with permanent kidney failure, and individuals younger than 65 who qualify for Social Security disability benefits. Medicare insures more than 42 million older and disabled Americans. A monthly premium is deducted from each worker's paycheck, and the funds are matched by the federal government. Medicare insurance provides two types of coverage. Part A, hospital insurance, helps pay for inpatient care in a hospital or a skilled nursing facility and certain home health services. Part B, medical insurance, helps pay for physician services and other services not covered by Part A. The list of services covered varies from time to time, depending on changing government regulations. Medicare benefits are geared toward acute, short-term care. Coverage in a skilled care facility is usually limited to a period of 100 days, and patient eligibility is based on the need for skilled care services on a daily basis. Medicare does not cover long-term care, such as nursing home care, over an extended period.

Changes in hospital funding in the early 1980s caused hospitals to discharge patients more quickly than ever before. Up to that time, hospitals had billed Medicare for their costs after they were incurred, a process referred to as *retrospective* payment. That system offered little incentive to save money. The system changed in 1983, and since that time hospitals have been advised in advance how much they would be reimbursed for treatment of a patient with a certain condition. This is referred to as *prospective* payment. Under the prospective payment system, patients are grouped according to diagnoses that account for similar amounts of resources, or diagnosis-related groups (DRGs). Under this system, hospitals are reimbursed a flat fee for a specified number of days based on a predetermined fee schedule for a diagnosis. If the patient gets better faster, the hospital makes money. If the patient requires a longer stay, the hospital loses money. This abrupt change in Medicare financing has caused the early discharge of thousands of patients and stim-

Table 1-1	*Comparisons Between Medicare and Medicaid*	
	MEDICARE	**MEDICAID**
Funding	Monthly premium from paycheck; funds matched by federal government	Federal, state, and local taxes
Eligibility	All persons older than 65 years, anyone with permanent kidney failure, plus disabled persons younger than 65 who qualify for Social Security benefits	Needy, low-income, and disabled persons younger than 65 years and their dependent children
How Administered	Federal government	Both federal and state governments
Benefits	Physician services, hospital expenses, home health care, and outpatient services; geared toward acute, short-term care	Same health benefits as Medicare, plus nursing home care

ulated interest in transitional and community-based health care services.

The prospective payment system was originally developed by the federal government for Medicare patients, but it has been adopted by other insurers as well because it rewards cost-effective management of patients. A method for reimbursing hospice care was included in the 1982 revision.

As of January 1, 2006, a new Medicare prescription drug coverage option went into effect. Persons with Medicare Part A and/or Medicare Part B can enroll in the plan by paying a monthly premium. Once a person is enrolled, a $250 deductible must be met after which Medicare typically will pay about half of the individual's annual drug costs. If prescription drugs exceed $3600 in out-of-pocket costs in a year, 95% of the excess is covered by Medicare for the remainder of that year. Persons with limited income and resources may qualify for additional coverage of drug costs.

Medicaid

Like Medicare, Medicaid was established in 1965 as part of the Social Security Act. It is the government insurance program for persons of very low income. Unlike Medicare which is administered only by the federal government, Medicaid is funded by federal, state, and local taxes, and is administered by both federal and state governments on a partnership basis. States develop and operate the Medicaid programs within federal guidelines. Thus, benefits vary from state to state.

Medicaid benefits are provided for needy, low-income, disabled individuals under age 65 and their dependent children. Individuals older than 65 who are below a specified income level may also receive benefits, including services that Medicare does not cover. Services covered by Medicaid include inpatient and outpatient care, maternal and child health care, skilled nursing home care, physicians' fees, medications, laboratory work, radiographs, equipment, and home health care. Medicaid is more likely to cover long-term care than Medicare. Medicaid provides health coverage for nearly 45 million persons.

Many problems have developed related to Medicare and Medicaid because costs have risen much more quickly than anticipated. Some instances of fraud and abuse related to these programs have been reported. The goals of providing comprehensive health care for those over 65 and for the indigent have not yet been achieved.

COMPONENTS OF THE HEALTH CARE SYSTEM

Components of the health care system can be categorized into outpatient (ambulatory) care and inpatient care. Outpatient care is provided for patients who do not need hospitalization. It may involve health promo-

tion and disease prevention, the diagnosis of disease, or the treatment and follow-up of disease processes. Outpatient care settings include physicians' offices, clinics, day surgery centers, adult day care centers for the handicapped or disabled, patients' homes, and hospices.

Inpatient settings include acute care hospitals, transitional and subacute hospitals, emergency rooms, psychiatric hospitals, rehabilitation centers, and long-term care facilities. The number of persons in inpatient settings has decreased as the length of hospitalizations is reduced and as services have shifted to outpatient settings.

Over the past decade, cost-containment measures have resulted in a shift from inpatient care so that more services are offered in outpatient settings. The term *community based care* is sometimes used to describe the variety of services, both inpatient and outpatient, provided to meet the changing needs of patients in various states of health. The term also implies the provision of services based on the needs of individual communities.

OUTPATIENT CARE

Physicians' Offices

Many people, especially older adults, receive their primary medical care in physicians' offices. Older people have more office visits per year than younger people, especially since the enactment of Medicare and Medicaid. The cost of visits to physicians' offices is covered in part by some forms of private health insurance and by Medicare, Part B. Physicians may practice in individual or group settings. Many group practices now are made up of various medical specialties, so that clients may have all of their health care needs dealt with in one location. The focus of medical care traditionally has been on the diagnosis and treatment of specific conditions rather than on health promotion and preventive services. However, medical education has begun to place greater emphasis on health maintenance.

Clinics

Outpatient clinics may be freestanding or associated with community hospitals, teaching hospitals, or public health departments (Fig. 1-1). They usually focus on care for people with chronic illnesses, such as diabetes or heart disease, but people with acute illnesses also may be seen. The primary goal of care in clinics is to diagnose and treat most illness.

Clinics offer many services, including physician services, nursing services, rehabilitative services, prenatal care, well-baby checkups, immunizations, preventive dental and eye care, and laboratory and diagnostic services. In large hospitals, clinics are usually organized according to medical subspecialties, such as urology, neurology, and orthopedics. For many people, especially older adults, specialty clinics can be a problem because older adults have many chronic illnesses and

FIGURE **1-1** Outpatient clinics serve many people in the community.

are seen in many different clinics. This makes the coordination of care more difficult than if the patient were seen in a facility with one set of health care providers.

Health Maintenance Organizations

HMOs provide health care and services through group practice. The principles on which HMOs are based include group practice with prepayment, voluntary enrollment, a combination of hospital and outpatient facilities, an emphasis on health promotion and prevention of illness, and physician responsibility for direction of patient care. The membership fee covers all health care services. Depending on the plan, there may be an additional small charge, called a copayment, for services. The copayment is paid at each visit.

Because HMOs collect only a set fee from clients, they have an interest in promoting health and maintaining wellness. Healthy clients do not need as many services as sick ones and therefore are less expensive to treat. HMOs employ physicians, nurses, and other health care providers and also have a broad group of specialists available for referral. Clients are required to use only the services of the health care providers and hospitals associated with the HMO.

In 1973, the federal government enacted the Health Maintenance Organization Act. Its purpose was to help private agencies develop new methods of health care delivery in an effort to control the accessibility, quality, and cost of health care. This act helped stimulate the development of HMOs throughout the United States. The original HMO in the United States was the Kaiser-Permanente Medical Care Program.

HMOs are considered to be one way to stop rising health care costs and have become very popular in the United States. These organizations are able to provide both inpatient and outpatient care to persons at about the same cost that commercial insurance companies charge for inpatient care only. Costs have been contained as a result of utilization reviews conducted by the HMO, discharge planning, and home or "step-down" care. Utilization review entails looking at how resources are used and how health care money is spent. It is the process of reviewing resource utilization based on an external standard. Utilization reviews have resulted in decreased rates of hospitalization, shorter lengths of stay (by up to 45%), and the promotion of preventive care and wellness.

Ambulatory Surgery Centers (Outpatient or Day Surgery)

An alternative to inpatient surgery is outpatient or day surgery. Increasingly, surgical procedures are being done in ambulatory settings. Ambulatory surgery centers may be located in hospitals, freestanding clinics, health care centers, and physicians' offices. Many procedures such as cataract extraction, hernia repair, tonsillectomy, and the removal of foreign objects that once required hospitalization are now often done in outpatient facilities. Most forms of insurance cover the expenses. In addition, urgent care centers provide 24-hour service for patients with minor injuries or illnesses such as lacerations or influenza.

Ambulatory surgery is less costly and allows people to recover in the familiar surroundings of their own homes. Preoperative assessments and laboratory tests are usually performed on an outpatient basis several days ahead of the procedure, and then the patient reports to the setting early on the morning of surgery. Following recovery from anesthesia, the patient is discharged home, usually the same day.

The primary criticism of outpatient surgery is concern that patients may be at greater risk for postoperative complications in the absence of professional monitoring. This makes the role of the nurse in patient and family teaching a critical one. It also requires that the patient have appropriate support at home.

Home Health Agencies

History of Home Health Care. Home health nursing has a long and distinguished history that began when St. Vincent de Paul organized the Daughters of Charity in 1617. Members went from house to house, bringing food, education, and health care to the sick in their homes. This was one of the first organized groups to provide health education to the poor and to help people help themselves.

In the mid-1800s, William Rathbone, a wealthy English businessman, was impressed with the skill of the nurses who cared for his dying mother at home. Convinced that visiting nurses could help the poor and ill of Liverpool, he organized the first district nursing organization. This experiment was so successful that he opened the first training school for visiting nurses in 1859. Rathbone often is called the Father of the Visiting

Nurses Association because he was the first to employ the district nursing concept.

In the United States, Lillian Wald is considered to be the forerunner of the modern public health nurse. She came from a wealthy family and studied nursing at New York Hospital in 1891. Her experiences teaching bedside nursing to women in the poor sections of New York City had a profound impact on her and led to the founding of the Henry Street Settlement House in 1893. The facility was a place where the poor could come for care and was supported by funds from the wealthy. Lillian Wald believed that all people had the right to direct access to the services of a nurse. She also maintained that nurses should live in the area where their patients lived to gain insight into the complexity of health care problems and their probable causes. Many of Lillian Wald's beliefs about people and nursing find expression today in Nursing's Agenda for Health Care Reform, in which community-based services and access to care are key issues.

Focus of Home Health Care. Home health services are provided to individuals and families in their homes or in assisted living centers to promote, maintain, or restore health or to minimize the effects of illness and disability (Fig. 1-2). As hospitals strive to reduce inpatient days, the demand for professional home health care is rising in all age-groups. One of the fastest growing fields of nursing is home health care. Fewer people are being admitted to hospitals, and they are being discharged sooner with more needs for special care. The necessary services may include medical and dental care, nursing care, physical and occupational therapy, speech therapy, enterostomal therapy, social work, nutrition counseling, transportation, laboratory services, provision of medical equipment and supplies, and the assistance of home health aides and homemakers. Home health care is provided by hospitals, private profit-making and nonprofit agencies, and public agencies, such as public health and social service departments.

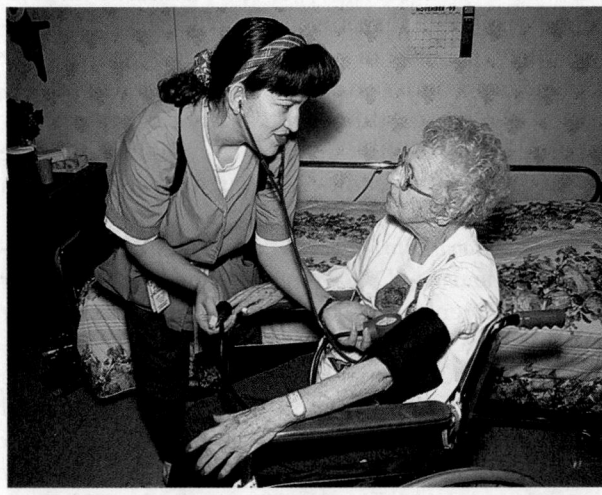

FIGURE 1-2 A nurse takes the blood pressure of a resident in an extended care facility.

Funding of Home Care Services. Home care services may be short term, long term, or intermittent. Services are funded by individual payment, by private insurance, by Medicare, and by Medicaid. To be covered by Medicare, the agencies must adhere to regulations put forth by the federal government. Most nursing services that are paid for by Medicare must be skilled care, with strict governmental guidelines defining the skilled care that must be provided. Regulations vary from state to state but are generally patterned after federal governmental regulations. The registered nurse is the case manager of services provided by health care workers in the home. Federal Medicare regulations for home care identify standard duties of the licensed practical nurse, which include furnishing health services, preparing progress notes, assisting the registered nurse in special procedures, and assisting the patient in learning self-care techniques.

Types of Home Care Agencies. There are several types of home care agencies: voluntary, official, proprietary, and hospital-based agencies. Some agencies specialize in specific care such as intravenous therapy or ventilator management. These include hospital-based, private for-profit, nonprofit, and Medicare-certified agencies.

Voluntary Agencies. Voluntary agencies were the first to deliver nursing care in the home. They were financed by wealthy philanthropists in the community, and their mission was to care for the sick poor. Today the Visiting Nurses Associations are the most common examples of voluntary agencies. These associations are usually governed by a community board of directors that determines service delivery policies and assists with fund-raising. Because board members are drawn from different areas and social strata within the community, services often reflect community needs. Funding for voluntary agencies usually comes from a variety of sources, including Medicare, Medicaid, the United Way, private insurance, endowments, donations, and patients themselves. Once the primary provider of home care services, Visiting Nurses Associations saw their share of the home care market dwindle with the growth of proprietary (for-profit) agencies during the 1990s. However, the 1997 Balanced Budget Act put a limit on the amount of money spent on a patient's home health care regardless of diagnosis or needs. This payment limitation has been a factor in the closing of many home health agencies.

Official Agencies. Official agencies are those supported by tax dollars and are authorized by law to deliver services to a defined area or community. Traditionally, state, regional, and local health departments have been assigned the responsibility of providing health promotion and disease prevention services as well as communicable disease investigation and environmental health protection. The nursing divisions of state, regional, and local health departments are usually tasked with delivering nursing services to populations at risk. In most states, this includes maternal and child services, sexually transmitted infection clinics, tuberculosis surveillance and treatment, and other health services as funds permit.

Thirty years ago, home health services were often delivered by local health departments as well as by voluntary agencies. As the concept of public health became more defined, caring for the sick in the home was no longer seen as a public health role. Gradually, more and more health departments dropped home health services. By the 1980s, competition from proprietary and hospital home health agencies had reduced the number of official home health agencies to a handful.

Proprietary Agencies. Proprietary agencies are organized to make a profit on their operation. They may or may not participate in Medicare, but most do. Proprietary agencies may be owned by individuals or by corporate chains. Often their sources of revenue are private insurance, private-pay clients, Medicare, and Medicaid.

The prospective payment system contributed substantially to the growth of home health care. Much of this growth was in the number of proprietary and hospital-based home health agencies. As noted earlier, the limitations imposed by the Balanced Budget Act (1997) affected the profitability of proprietary agencies, and many have closed.

Hospital-based Agencies. Institution-based home health agencies also increased in number during the 1990s. Hospitals that were losing money under the prospective payment system saw the opportunity to recoup lost profits by opening home health agencies. These agencies are usually governed by the hospital's board of directors. The hospital-based agency usually gets most of its referrals from the hospital itself. Philosophy and policies are usually consistent with those of the parent institution. Some hospital-based agencies closed when profits declined.

Home Health Care Services. There are three primary skilled services in home health care: (1) nursing, (2) physical therapy, and (3) speech therapy. Secondary services include occupational therapy (which may be primary under certain conditions), social work services, and home health aide services. The role of the nurse in home health is discussed in detail in Chapter 2. An overview of other services is provided here.

Physical Therapy. Home health patients recovering from health problems affecting mobility, such as hip fractures and strokes, are common candidates for physical therapy. Physical therapists assess the need for assistive devices such as walkers, wheelchairs, and grab bars and work with patients and their families on therapies to regain strength and mobility. To receive these services in the home, it is necessary for the patient to be homebound.

Speech Therapy. Speech therapists work with patients who have speech or swallowing disorders. A common indication for speech therapy is aphasia. As with all home health services, to receive speech therapy in the home that is reimbursed by Medicare, it is necessary to meet all of the criteria for Medicare.

Occupational Therapy. Patients who have conditions impairing movement of the upper extremities are prime candidates for occupational therapy. People with arthritis or strokes may benefit from assistive devices for dressing and other daily personal care and household activities. Occupational therapists also provide muscle reeducation, splinting, and improved control of fine motor movement. Timely occupational therapy interventions can help the patient become safer and more independent in the home setting.

Social Work Services. Social workers can provide valuable assistance to families trying to manage chronic illness in the home. Typically, social workers work with families to identify problems that arise in managing illness at home and recommend referrals to community resources. They may also provide information about financial assistance and help families with applications for community services such as Meals on Wheels and respite care.

Home Health Aide Services. The home health aide is a valuable member of the home care team. Home health aides provide personal care for the patient in the home, such as bathing, ambulating, transferring, skin care, and oral hygiene. They may also measure and record vital signs and do other basic, nonskilled tasks. Incidental homemaking such as making the bed and straightening the client's room are also common home health aide tasks. General housecleaning, shopping, and laundry are inappropriate for home health aides. Patients qualify for home health services if they already receive one of the three primary skilled services.

Homemaker Services. Homemakers are usually provided by families or state and local assistance programs. Their duties include common household chores such as cooking, light housekeeping, laundry, shopping, and picking up medications.

Enterostomal Therapy. Enterostomal therapists are employed in many large home health agencies. They are specialists in the care of all types of wounds, such as pressure ulcers, surgical wounds, and ostomies. They provide care to patients and consultation to nurses on how to manage wounds. They also have extensive knowledge of skin care products and ostomy appliances.

Other Home Health Care Services. Dietitians, nurse practitioners, or psychologists may deliver services in the home.

Specialty Home Care Services. Prospective payment systems and the use of DRGs have provided a stimulus for the development of specialty home care, especially for pediatric, psychiatric, and terminally ill patients. In addition, insurance companies, faced with the rising costs of intravenous and ventilator therapies in the hospital setting, have recognized the potential cost savings of delivering these therapies in the home. In the past few years, the use of high technology in the home has increased dramatically. Patients using these technologies most commonly are those needing intravenous therapy or those who are ventilator dependent. Pediatric home care and mental health home care are also specialties.

Pediatric Home Care. Since the late 1980s, the number of sick children cared for in the home has increased. This increase is largely the result of advances in technology that have enabled the medical community to save many newborn infants who otherwise would not have survived. These same technological advances have produced the equipment necessary to provide adequate care in the home environment. Small, compact pumps, ventilators, and monitors have enabled children with cancer, respiratory disease, and cerebral palsy to live more normal lives at home.

Pediatric home care provides a better quality of life for young patients, but it also contributes to strain and role overload for parents and other caregivers. Many pediatric home care services are funded by Medicaid and state children's services. Private insurance companies are becoming more interested in funding pediatric home care because of the potential cost savings over hospital treatment.

Mental Health Home Care. Another growing area of home health care is the delivery of mental health services in the home. Nurses in this role have advanced training in psychiatric disorders; they provide medication monitoring and teaching and perform mental status examinations and suicide assessments. They often provide consultation to other home care nurses on mental health problems that arise in patients with nonpsychiatric problems.

Hospice

The hospice concept is a concept of caring that originated in fifteenth-century Europe as the provision of respite and comfort for travelers. Later, this concept was extended to the dying in both hospitals and home settings. Families and hospital personnel collaborated to provide palliative care to dying family members.

During the early part of the twentieth century, the dying experience in the United States gradually shifted from the home to the hospital. Instead of being surrounded by family and friends in familiar settings, the dying found themselves in unfamiliar settings and being largely cared for by strangers. The first hospice in America was established in Connecticut in 1974 and provided both home care and inpatient care. Today, many more freestanding and hospital-based hospices all over the country deliver around-the-clock services to the dying.

Hospice services may be delivered in the home, acute care hospital, or extended care facility. Requirements for admission to hospice care include the following:
- A diagnosis of a terminal illness
- A prognosis of less than 6 months to live
- Informed consent by the patient to elect hospice care
- A physician's order

Hospices provide care for terminally ill patients in the home and other specified facilities. Their purpose is to enable terminally ill patients to live as full a life as possible, with skilled personnel managing the pain, discomfort, and other symptoms associated with the illness. In addition, hospices assist families during the bereavement process. Some hospices are associated with hospitals, whereas others are associated with home health agencies. Most are independent organizations in the community.

Hospice services are provided by the Medicare statute. Under law, hospice services are granted for a total of 210 days. If the patient elects hospice services, he or she must waive the traditional home health services. All the criteria for the home health care benefit must be met except for the homebound requirement. In return, the patient is eligible for the following services:
- Nursing, home health aide, social worker, and therapist visits as determined by the team
- Other services, including pastoral care, dietary counseling, and respite care
- Prescription drugs related to symptom management and pain control
- Durable medical equipment as required

Hospice care is a worthwhile alternative for the terminally ill person that provides a more natural and humane approach to the dying process. The team method is used to meet a variety of physical, psychological, social, and spiritual problems encountered by the terminally ill and their families. A multidisciplinary team of professionals and volunteers contributes collective efforts to provide a better quality of life for the dying and their families.

Adult Day Care Centers

Day care is a structured program designed to provide activities related to health and socialization for selected populations. The activities are most often directed toward older adults and the mentally ill. Day care centers may be associated with hospitals or nursing homes, or they may function independently. Older people benefit from day care services because they can continue to live in the community and have supervision during the day while family members work. The centers provide all kinds of health-related services, health promotion programs, nutritious meals, and social activities. Most services are provided on a sliding scale fee basis or without charge.

Many of the services provided at day care centers are funded through the Older Americans Act, which was originally passed in 1965. The goals of the Older Americans Act are to ensure that older adults have adequate income and suitable housing, physical and mental health services, community services, and the opportunity to pursue meaningful activities.

Mental health services are also offered through day care. People who need counseling, follow-up care after hospitalization, and rehabilitation related to chemical dependence may benefit from day care programs. Most are covered by private insurance for a limited period.

INPATIENT CARE

Hospitals

Hospitals vary greatly in size, shape, and organization throughout the United States. Some are small, 20-bed rural hospitals; some are intermediate-sized community hospitals; and others are large, urban university medical centers. Some hospitals are public and financed by the local, state, or federal government; others are private and owned by churches, businesses, corporations, or charitable organizations. Hospital care accounts for about 40% of personal health care expenditures in the United States. The average hospital charge in 2002 was $17,300, and the average length of stay was 5 days. The predominant sources of payment for hospital services are Medicare (34%), Medicaid (22%), and private insurance (36%). About 5% of all hospitalizations are not covered by any type of insurance.

Among the most frequent reasons for hospitalization are infant delivery, cardiovascular disease, chest pain, pneumonia, and depression. Hospitals are major providers of health and related services to older adults. People ages 65 and older, while comprising only 13% of the U.S. population, account for 36% of all hospital stays. In addition, older people tend to account for more hospital stays than other age-groups (Fig. 1-3).

The DRG system has had a great impact on hospital care and length of stay for patients. Because hospitals receive only a fixed amount of money, physicians are now discharging patients as early as possible to reduce costs. As a result, admissions to nursing homes and the use of home health agencies are increasing to care for people who are not leaving the hospital as fully recovered as those who have had longer hospital stays. Therefore the demand for high-technology services such as respiratory therapy and intravenous therapy at home and in nursing homes is increasing. In addition, many health care providers feel there is now a "revolv-

FIGURE **1-3** A large number of patients in the hospital setting are older adults.

ing door syndrome" with clients: patients return to the hospital for care after discharge because they did not fully recover at home.

Transitional and subacute facilities are intended to provide intermediate levels of care when needed after hospital discharge. Transitional hospitals receive patients with acute but stable conditions who will need a lengthy minimum stay (often 25 days). Examples of patients who might need such a service are those with spinal cord injuries, patients with severe diabetes who have had amputations, and patients who are ventilator dependent. DRG requirements for Medicare patients are waived for transitional care. Some transitional hospitals lease space in acute care hospitals and contract for some of the acute care facility's services, such as laboratory and radiology services.

Subacute care units provide care for patients who need more intensive care than what is usually provided in a skilled nursing facility but who no longer need acute care. When DRG days are used up, patients may be transferred from acute care hospitals to subacute units.

Psychiatric Hospitals. Psychiatric patients may be treated in specialty areas of regular acute care hospitals, or separate hospitals may be designated specifically for mentally ill patients. These facilities provide inpatient and outpatient treatment for individuals with acute psychiatric illnesses, with a focus on helping clients control their behavior or restore their behavior to what it was before entering the hospital.

Psychiatric hospitals may be private, nonprofit organizations that are sponsored by organized churches or may be operated by the local, state, or federal governments. The cost of care is covered by most private insurance companies, but only for 30 to 60 days.

Rehabilitation Centers

The aim of rehabilitation is either to restore individuals to their former level of functioning or to maintain or maximize remaining function (Fig. 1-4). Rehabilitation can and should be carried out in all health care settings by a variety of health care professionals with the active involvement of patients and their families. Most formal rehabilitation centers are located either within the hospital or nursing home or in a freestanding residential institution.

Rehabilitation may focus on physical problems, such as those caused by stroke, spinal cord injury, or amputation, or on mental health problems, such as drug dependency or mental illness. To restore affected persons to their highest level of functioning, the rehabilitation process attempts to meet psychological, social, and physical needs. Therefore the rehabilitation team includes many health professionals, including physicians, nurses, social workers, physical and occupational therapists, and speech therapists. It is very difficult to conduct a rehabilitation program without a team effort.

FIGURE **1-4** A patient is assisted with ambulation in a rehabilitation center.

Long-Term Care Facilities

The term long-term care facility was originally used to describe institutions that were attached to hospitals for the purpose of recovery from acute illness. The term is now used to describe several different kinds of institutions, such as nursing homes, convalescent homes, and some residential institutions, whose primary purpose is to care for people with chronic illnesses and physical impairments. The focus of care is on those who do not need hospitalization but who are unable to care for themselves.

Modern long-term care for older adults and disabled individuals had its beginnings in nursing home care, which dates back at least to the turn of the twentieth century. Ill individuals and older adults who had no families to care for them were housed in publicly funded homes or boarding homes. The care provided was largely custodial and included housing, food, and personal care. These homes were not licensed, and standards were few. Quality depended on the good graces of those providing the care. Later, nursing home care became tied to the medical care system, and the nursing home increasingly became a place for patients needing skilled nursing and social services.

The range of services now available for people requiring some level of assistance is expanding to provide a variety of options. Examples include independent living retirement centers, boarding and personal care homes, assisted living facilities, special care units for dementia patients, intermediate-care nursing homes, and skilled nursing homes. Independent living retirement centers commonly offer levels of care that permit the resident to access the level of care needed at a given point in time. Boarding and personal care homes typically provide a room and meals and, in some cases, minimal assistance and supervision. Residents of these facilities usually come and go as they please. Assisted living facilities permit a high degree of independence but usually have access to limited nursing care. Help with medications and some treatments may be provided. Although residents often have kitchens, some group meals are typically provided. The intermediate-care skilled nursing facility provides care from a licensed nursing staff member, including rehabilitative care for people who have the potential to regain function. Services include medical and nursing care; physical rehabilitation; long-term ventilator care; wound care; pharmaceutical, dietary, and social services; dental care; and activities. Federal regulations require a registered nurse to serve as director of nursing and a licensed nurse to be on duty at least 8 hours a day in an intermediate-care facility. This level of care is also referred to as extended care.

To be admitted to a skilled nursing facility, residents must be in need of nursing care that consists of observation during an acute or unstable phase of an illness, administration of enteral (tube) feedings or intravenous fluids, bowel and bladder retraining (for a limited period), administration of intramuscular or intravenous medications, or changing of sterile dressings. Persons who do not fit into any of these categories are deemed to be in need of custodial care and thus are ineligible for skilled nursing care benefits under Medicare. These facilities must have skilled health professionals available around the clock. The care of patients in these settings requires physician supervision and the services of a registered nurse, physical therapist, or speech therapist.

Key Points

- The health care system is made up of patients, families, the community, governmental agencies, health care providers, and insurance companies.
- Despite a complex health care system, some people in the United States still do not receive the services they need.
- One effect of managed health care is an increasing focus on wellness and prevention.
- The Department of Health and Human Services is charged with organizing the various health and welfare agencies in the federal government.
- The purpose of the Public Health Services are to provide better health services by reviewing health care, providing grants and conducting research, raising public awareness of health problems, operating hospitals for national health problems, providing health science training grants, and publishing vital statistics.
- Financing of health care is a complex system made up of insurance companies, health maintenance organiza-

tions, preferred provider organizations, and governmental systems.

- Medicare is a federal health insurance program that is geared toward acute, short-term care for people ages 65 and older and for disabled people of any age, including those with permanent kidney failure.
- Medicaid provides health care benefits for needy, low-income, and disabled people and their children.
- Cost increases have created stresses in the health care system and have resulted in a variety of approaches to contain costs.
- The health care system includes outpatient and inpatient services.
- Increasingly, more health care, including surgery, is being carried out in ambulatory settings, and the number and length of hospitalizations are decreasing.
- Outpatient services are provided in physicians' offices, clinics, ambulatory (day) surgery facilities, and day care centers.
- Hospice services may be delivered to terminally ill patients who meet certain criteria in their homes, in acute settings, or in extended care facilities.

- Inpatient services are provided in acute care hospitals, in psychiatric hospitals, in rehabilitation centers, and in long-term care facilities.
- Home health care grew rapidly through the 1990s as fewer people were admitted to hospitals and those admitted were being discharged sooner with special needs for health care services.
- The Balanced Budget Act of 1997, which limited the total amount that could be spent on a patient's home health care regardless of diagnosis, resulted in the closure of many home health agencies.
- Long-term care facilities include nursing homes, skilled nursing facilities, and intermediate-care (extended care) facilities.

 Go to your Companion CD-ROM for a Pharmacology Tutorial, Audio Glossary, and 3-D animations.

evolve Be sure to visit the companion Evolve site at http://evolve.elsevier.com/Linton/ for WebLinks and additional online resources.

REVIEW QUESTIONS *Choose the best answer.*

1. One outcome of managed care has been:
   1. Decreased cost sharing
   2. Increased emphasis on inpatient care
   3. Decreased use of home health care
   4. Increased focus on wellness

2. The main goals of the Public Health Services are to protect and improve the health of populations at risk in the community and to:
   1. Control health care costs
   2. Improve Medicare services
   3. Prevent disease and disability
   4. Provide home-based nursing care

3. Medicare coverage includes:
   1. Inpatient care in a hospital or skilled nursing facility
   2. Unlimited nursing home care
   3. No eligibility requirements for skilled nursing care
   4. Private nursing care when needed

4. Criteria for admission to hospice care include the following:
   1. A prognosis of less than 1 year to live
   2. A diagnosis of a terminal illness
   3. Cooperation of the patient's family
   4. Inability to pay for care in a hospital

5. Which of the following has most directly resulted in earlier discharge of patients from hospitals?
   1. Decreased Medicare/Medicaid funding
   2. Balanced Budget Act of 1997
   3. The implementation of DRGs
   4. Improved medical and surgical care

Patient Care Settings

evolve http://evolve.elsevier.com/Linton/

Objectives

After reading and studying this chapter, you should be able to:

1. Describe the role of the nurse in community and home health, rehabilitation, and long-term care settings.
2. Differentiate community health and community-based nursing.
3. Describe the types of specialty care that nurses may provide in home health care.
4. Describe the principles of rehabilitation.
5. List the four levels of disability.
6. Discuss legislation passed to protect the rights of the disabled.
7. Identify the goals of rehabilitation.
8. Name the members of the rehabilitation team.
9. List the types of long-term care facilities.
10. Discuss the effects of institutionalization on the older adult.
11. Describe the principles of nursing care in long-term residential facilities.

Key Terms

 Be sure to check out the bonus material on the Companion CD-ROM, including selected audio pronunciations.

disability (p. 17)
handicap (p. 18)
impairment (p. 17)
rehabilitation (p. 17)

Chapter 1 briefly introduced the most common settings in which health care is delivered. Throughout this book, the care of patients in acute care settings is covered in detail. As the health care system changes, however, licensed practical nurses are finding a variety of opportunities for employment in community, rehabilitation, and long-term care settings. This chapter provides a more complete description of nursing in those settings.

COMMUNITY AND HOME HEALTH NURSING

Community health nursing and home health nursing are specialized areas of nursing practice that are often thought of as being similar. This probably comes from defining community health nursing as anything that occurs outside the hospital setting. These two practice areas, although sharing common historical roots, have significant differences.

COMMUNITY HEALTH NURSING

For both humane and economic reasons, it is better to keep people healthy than to wait until disease or disability occurs. Traditional community health nursing focuses on (1) improving the health status of communities or groups of people (called *aggregates*) through public education, (2) screening for early detection of disease, and (3) providing services for people who need care outside the acute care setting.

Community Health Nursing Roles

The following example demonstrates typical community health nursing roles.

A community health nurse notices a rise in blood pressure, an increase in weight, and a general lack of fitness in members of a senior citizen high-rise in her district. Her assessment shows that there are no recreational facilities nearby, the meals served at the high-rise tend to be high in fat, and there is a general lack of social activity at the facility. On the positive side, a residents' organization exists, although it has never been very active. By working with the residents' organization and a local church, the nurse initiates a group exercise program to improve the strength, cardiovascular fitness, and weight control of the elderly residents. By working with the management of the high-rise and the residents' association, the nurse gets the building manager to serve low-fat, low-cholesterol meals. The nurse also asks a local school of nursing to hold a monthly blood pressure and health education clinic for the residents.

In this example, the community health nurse not only gave direct service to individual clients but also worked with three existing community groups to provide a number of services designed to increase the health of the senior citizen group. Community health nurses often work with many different individuals and groups to create or modify systems of care to improve the health of a defined group. This function requires the nurse to assume a number of roles to accomplish care goals. The roles listed in the example include case finder, care manager, teacher, advocate, and coalition builder. The Management and Supervision box on p. 14 lists many of the

Community Health Nursing Roles

Advocate	Group leader
Caregiver	Health planner
Care manager	Home visitor
Case finder	Occupational health nurse
Clinic nurse	Researcher
Coalition builder	School nurse
Counselor	Supervisor
Epidemiologist	Teacher

roles assumed by the community health nurse. Most of these roles require at least a bachelor's degree in nursing to perform all aspects of the role; however, the LPN is increasingly visible in community health settings.

Community-Based Nursing

The term *community-based nursing* has been used in several contexts but should not be confused with community health nursing. Community-based nursing may be described as deriving health care services based on identified community needs and providing various types of care that meet the needs of citizens at various levels of wellness and illness. In a more general sense, the term is sometimes used to describe the provision of various levels of care in traditional and nontraditional community settings.

HOME HEALTH NURSING

Home health nursing blends direct nursing care and community health nursing. The main difference between home health nursing and traditional public health nursing is that home health nursing provides more direct care to patients. The main difference between home health nursing and nursing in an institution is the increased emphasis on the family and the environment in the home.

Home health nursing requires careful consideration of the family and its role in the care of the ill member. Although giving direct care to an individual is an important part of home health care, a more important nursing role is to teach the patient and family to care for themselves (Fig. 2-1). This important role is similar to that of the rehabilitation nurse, for whom the goal is the independent functioning of the patient and family.

The environment in which home health nursing is practiced is very different from the hospital practice environment. Homes often have only a fraction of the resources of the hospital. Small bedrooms, low beds, inadequate climate control, and limited space are common. Often families are overwhelmed by the task of caring for loved ones. They need instruction not only in the care of the patient but also in how to perform the care within the context of daily family activities in a home that was not designed for that purpose.

FIGURE 2-1 Home health agencies deliver the services of a variety of professionals.

Home health nurses must assess the patient, the family, and the environment and use that information to plan care. Ongoing assessments are critical because the home health nurse often sees the patient more frequently than other care providers and can detect problems early. For example, the observation of weight gain and ankle edema alerts the nurse to possible heart failure in the cardiac patient. Prompt intervention may prevent serious consequences.

To illustrate the importance of assessing the family and the environment, consider the patient who requires wound care. In the home setting, decisions to make include the following: Who can do the care? What does that person need to know? What supplies are needed and where can they be obtained? What is the best way to dispose of soiled dressings? Questions like these require the home health nurse to be resourceful, knowledgeable, skillful, and creative.

Reimbursement Realities in Home Health Nursing

Medicare, though not the sole source of home health care funding, is probably the most important. Reimbursement by the Medicare program depends on documentation that four basic conditions have been met: (1) the physician has determined the need for home care and has made a plan for home care; (2) the patient needs intermittent skilled nursing care, physical or speech-language therapy, or continued occupational therapy; (3) the patient is homebound; and (4) the agency providing the care is Medicare-certified. The number of hours per day and days per week that Medicare will cover are limited. Medicare will not pay for 24-hour-a-day care at home, meals delivered to the home, or personal care given by home health aides if that is the only care needed. The patient may be required to pay a portion of the cost of Medicare-covered medical equipment such as oxygen equipment.

The Physician Must Design or Authorize a Plan of Care. All home care treatment must be authorized by a physician. A plan of care must include pertinent diagnoses, mental status evaluations, identification of the types of services needed, the supplies and equipment ordered, frequency of visits, prognosis, rehabilitation potential, functional limitations, nutritional requirements, medications, and treatments. This plan must also include safety measures to protect against injury and plans for discharge from home care.

In practice, the initial referral usually includes the patient's name, address, and telephone number, the major diagnoses, and a list of medications and treatments—not unlike a physician's orders in a hospital. On the first visit, the admitting nurse usually formulates the plan of care, adding all other required elements. This plan is sent to the physician for review and signature. Because the care provided in the home is predominately *nursing* care, it is not surprising that the nurse has a major role in developing the plan of care.

Care Must Be Skilled, Intermittent, Reasonable, and Necessary. Medicare reimburses nursing care in the home if the care given is "skilled." This means that the care delivered must be the type that only a nurse trained in that care could be expected to do. However, not all the care done by a nurse qualifies as skilled care. Skilled nursing care is discussed further with the types of home health services.

Nursing is one of three primary home health care services considered skilled. The others are physical therapy and speech therapy. Occupational therapy may be considered skilled, depending on the complexity of the patient's problems. Social work and home health aide services are not considered skilled in themselves but may be reimbursed if the patient has qualified for one of the three primary skilled services. These home care services are discussed in more detail later in this chapter.

The preceding definition of skilled care is an interpretation of the Medicare law. Some nursing activities that require the skill of a nurse may not be recognized as skilled under Medicare. Medicare law does not prevent nurses from giving the care they judge necessary. It only defines what care is *reimbursable* under that law.

Medicare reimbursement requires that the nursing visits be intermittent in nature. This means that visits occur periodically and usually do not exceed 28 hours per week. Under normal circumstances, the patient is not seen daily. Situations exist, however, in which daily visits are justified. In these situations, there is usually the need for family members to be trained in daily procedures such as diabetic care or dressing changes. Under these circumstances, Medicare will reimburse daily visits for 2 or 3 weeks. These are considered special cases, and reimbursement depends on clear and accurate documentation of the need for daily visits.

Otherwise, visiting frequency can range from three to four times per week to monthly.

To demonstrate that care is reasonable and necessary, objective clinical evidence clearly justifying the type and frequency of services is required. The nurse must clearly document functional losses and goals for care. Ongoing progress or lack of progress toward treatment goals must be documented. Poor documentation not only jeopardizes patient care but also often results in denial of the agency's claim for payment because the documentation did not prove that the care given was "reasonable and necessary."

The Patient Must Be Homebound. This criterion does not mean that the patient must be bedridden. It does mean, however, that the patient must exert considerable effort to leave the home. Medicare also requires that absences from home be infrequent and of short duration. According to Medicare regulations, if patients are well enough to leave home frequently, they are able to visit a physician's office for treatment and therefore are not in need of home care.

The Home Health Agency Must Be Medicare-Certified. Medicare-certified home health agencies can be located in the telephone directory, by referral from a health care provider or other persons who have used these services, or from a list of Medicare-approved agencies on www.medicare.gov. The list is found under "Home Health Compare." A home health agency can decline to accept a patient if it cannot meet the patient's needs.

Types of Home Health Services

The primary skilled services in home health care are (1) nursing, (2) physical therapy, and (3) speech therapy. Secondary services include occupational therapy (which may be primary under certain conditions), social work services, and home health aide services.

Skilled Nursing. According to Medicare regulations, skilled nursing includes skilled observation and assessment, teaching, and performing skilled procedures.

Skilled Observation and Assessment. The phrase "skilled observation and assessment" implies that the skills of a nurse are required to observe a patient's progress, to assess the importance of signs and symptoms, and to decide on a course of action. For example, good assessment and judgment skills are needed to detect the signs and symptoms of congestive heart failure early enough to prevent rehospitalization.

Teaching. Teaching is considered a skilled task because to do it effectively the nurse must identify the patient's and family's current level of knowledge, discern their learning style, relay information at a pace they can handle, and evaluate the results of the teaching.

Teaching is the most important skill in home care. Much of what is done in the home must be done by the patient and caregiver. Good patient teaching begins in the hospital setting, but newly arrived home care patients may need considerable teaching to manage their care at home. When high-technology therapies are involved, teaching is doubly important.

Families who have difficulty understanding high-technology concepts may be intimidated when answers to their questions are not readily available. Skilled nurses understand this problem and ensure that their teaching is thorough and addresses precisely what the family needs to know to care successfully for their loved one at home. To do this, the nurse must identify the exact nature of the problem. A family member's difficulty in administering an injection may arise from a lack of knowledge of the procedure, a fear of needles, an inability to read the markings on the syringe, or a denial of the disease process. Identifying the specific learning need is critical to successful patient teaching. In teaching high-technology care, it is especially important to keep instructions as simple and specific as possible. Each step in the procedure should be written down and reviewed with the patient. The skill should be demonstrated several times, asking the family caregiver to cue the nurse for each step. After this is done a few times, the caregiver should perform a return demonstration of the skill.

Family caregivers must understand exactly what should be done in an emergency. Any questions about the family's ability to manage their portion of the care should be immediately referred to the home care nurse responsible for establishing the care plan and managing the case.

Performing Skilled Procedures. Skilled procedures include dressing changes, Foley catheter insertions, and venipunctures. However, after certain nursing procedures are taught to the family, they are no longer considered skilled procedures and are not reimbursable under Medicare. For example, injecting insulin is not considered skilled because most diabetics can inject insulin themselves. Teaching how to draw up the insulin and inject it properly, however, is considered skilled because teaching is considered a skilled activity. Once the injection skill is learned, the injection itself is no longer a skilled activity according to the Medicare definition. Also, procedures such as enema administration, unsterile dressing changes, care of small wounds, and administration of eyedrops usually are not considered skilled because they can be performed safely by most people.

Specialty Home Care

In the past few years, the number of high-technology cases in the home has increased dramatically. Most often, patients need intravenous therapy or are ventilator dependent.

Intravenous Therapy. Rising hospital costs and the development of reliable intravenous pumps have stimulated the growth of intravenous therapy in the home. The most common intravenous therapies provided in the home are hydration, antibiotics, pain control, total parenteral nutrition, and chemotherapy. Many different types of intravenous lines may be used. Nurses should be familiar with the devices commonly used in their communities. Chemotherapy drugs are almost always given through central lines.

High-technology therapies add to the complexity of home health care. Home use may be more cost-effective than a hospital stay, but it also significantly increases the risk to the client and the liability of the home health agency. Agency policies and procedures should be current and specific enough to guide the nurse in managing the provision of intravenous therapy in the home. These policies protect not only the agency and the patient but also the nurse.

The successful provision of any high-technology therapy in the home depends on the commitment of everyone involved. Families must be capable of understanding what is required and have the time to participate fully in the patient's care. Nurses delivering this type of care must be thoroughly trained in the procedures and use of equipment involved in these therapies. Agencies must have appropriate staff to provide care at any time if needed, including days, evenings, nights, and weekends. The pharmacy or intravenous therapy company must provide high-quality products and support to both the nurse and the family. Finally, physicians must be closely involved and available to the nurse and family to respond to emergency problems.

The nurse's role in the delivery of high-technology care in the home includes skilled observation and assessment, the ability to perform skilled procedures, and teaching. Skilled observation and assessment in the delivery of intravenous therapy includes determining the adequacy of the home environment and the patient's and family's knowledge regarding care procedures. The intravenous access site must be assessed for signs of swelling and redness. Any side effects of the treatment should be noted, along with the family's level of comfort with performing specific procedures.

Skilled procedures include changing access site dressings and performing venipunctures. Because home care nurses are not instantly available 24 hours a day, some procedures must be taught to the family.

Ventilator Therapy. Ventilator-dependent patients are increasingly being cared for in the home setting. This type of care is complex and should be provided only by nurses and caregivers specifically trained in the use of necessary equipment and procedures. Often the care of ventilator-dependent patients in the home is coordinated by the respiratory therapist. The home care nurse seeing the patient should be aware of policies and procedures followed by the respiratory therapy company, be familiar with respiratory therapy equipment, and be certified in cardiopulmonary resuscitation.

Initial assessment of the home environment includes an assessment of all the factors important in other high-technology therapies, with the addition of an assessment of the electrical and structural condition of the home. This is important to ensure proper functioning of the equipment and necessary backup systems. As with intravenous therapy, committed family members or other caregivers must be available. In this case, the commitment is for around-the-clock observation. Physicians and respiratory therapists must be on call for any problems.

Communication Among Home Health Care Team Members

The importance of the team approach in home health care cannot be overemphasized. Quality home care requires the collaboration of several disciplines. Because these disciplines may provide their services in the home at different times, communication among health care team members is necessary if effective collaboration is to occur. Interdisciplinary communication is accomplished through clear, detailed documentation and case conferences.

Documentation. In any interdisciplinary work, the actions of one discipline often depend on the actions of another. A nursing discovery of an unused walker in the corner of a room may prompt the physical therapist to recommend strengthening exercises and gait training. A social worker's attempts to find funding for a patient's medications may reveal that the patient is fearful of taking pain medications, which can be addressed by the nurse. If these concerns are not communicated, however, they will not be addressed. Most quality-of-care problems in home health care can be attributed to failure to communicate patient care problems. Most of the time, the failure lies with either incomplete documentation or failure to keep the nursing case manager informed.

As mentioned earlier, reimbursement for home health nursing visits depends on clear documentation of the patient's homebound status, the skilled nature of the services provided, and the medical need for the services. Failure to provide such documentation often results in denial of reimbursement by Medicare. Denials of reimbursement have serious consequences for the home health agency and, when excessive, have resulted in agencies going out of business.

Case Conferences. Clear documentation of interdisciplinary case conferences can go a long way toward preventing reimbursement denials based on lack of medical necessity. These conferences often provide detailed information about the complexity of problems that justifies increased visits.

Usually, a home health nurse must report to a patient's case manager who is responsible for admitting the patient, establishing the plan of care, including visit frequencies, and coordinating the efforts of other disciplines. The case manager schedules periodic, formal case conferences in which all disciplines work together to solve clinical problems. The details of these conferences are recorded in the patient's record.

In addition to these regularly scheduled conferences, it is important to keep the case manager informed of any changes in the response of the patient or family to the plan of care. Changes in vital signs, weight, and wound parameters are important physiologic indications for a call to the case manager. A change in the home environment such as an absence of family caregivers, deterioration in sanitation, or signs of patient neglect or abuse should also prompt a call to the case manager.

Communication by the case manager also is important. Field nurses have the right to expect clear and current information regarding recent changes in physicians' orders, current laboratory information, and the availability of documentation by other nurses and disciplines. High-quality patient care cannot be accomplished without meticulous communication from all disciplines involved in the care of the patient.

REHABILITATION

The acute phase of many illnesses is often followed by a prolonged chronic phase. This phase may last from days to years and usually involves the delivery of a number of health care services in a variety of settings, such as rehabilitation centers, long-term care facilities, outpatient facilities, group residential homes, and, increasingly, the patient's own home. Rehabilitation focuses on restoring maximum possible function after illness or injury.

REHABILITATION CONCEPTS

Rehabilitation Is a Process of Restoration

Rehabilitation is the process of restoring an individual to the best possible health and functioning after a physical or mental impairment. The type of assistance provided allows people to care for themselves as much as possible. Inherent in this process is a commitment by the caregiver to provide the care and support that foster the client's independence.

Impairment Is a Disturbance in Functioning

Impairment refers to a disturbance in functioning that may be either physical or psychological. An example of physical impairment is paralysis of an arm or leg as the result of a stroke. Mental impairment such as loss of memory may occur as a result of Alzheimer's disease. In either case, there is a loss of function.

Disability Is a Measurable Loss of Function

The term disability generally refers to a measurable loss of function and is usually delineated to indicate a diminished capacity for work. For example, individuals with an injured back may be classified as 50% disabled, meaning that they are incapable of doing 50% of their job. This type of measurable loss of function allows for specific reductions in work responsibility or may indicate how much compensation a worker may be entitled to receive.

Handicap Is an Inability to Perform Daily Activities

The term handicap means that an individual is not able to perform one or more normal activities of daily living (ADL) because of a mental or physical disability. For example, the person who experienced a stroke may be handicapped in driving a car because of the paralysis.

Remember that disability and handicap are not the same thing. A person can be moderately disabled but still manage to perform routine daily activities. People who were born without arms are often able to perform all essential ADL by using their feet and certain assistive devices. It can be said that, although these people are disabled, they are not handicapped. Impairments and their resulting disabilities may not be reversible, but handicaps often can be prevented or reduced with modifications of the environment and a community attitude that seeks to promote the abilities of the disabled.

LEVELS OF DISABILITY

A disability is often classified by level to determine its impact on an individual's quality of life and appropriate levels of compensation:

- Level I: Slight limitation in one or more ADL, usually able to work
- Level II: Moderate limitation in one or more ADL, able to work but workplace may need modifications
- Level III: Severe limitation in one or more ADL, unable to work
- Level IV: Total disability characterized by nearly complete dependence on others for assistance with ADL, unable to work

GOALS OF REHABILITATION

Rehabilitation aims to return the disabled individual to the highest possible level of functioning. The specific goals are to promote self-care, maximize independence, restore and maintain optimum function, prevent complications, and encourage adaptation. The rehabilitation team must treat the "whole" patient, meaning it must consider not just the patient's physical condition but also the emotional state and the psychological and social needs of both the patient and family.

Return of Function

The goal of return of function includes the restoration of as much function as possible in the traditional ADL, such as bathing, dressing, eating, toileting, and walking. Ideal functioning includes independence in the instrumental activities of daily living (IADL) as well, such as preparing meals, shopping, doing laundry, and using the telephone. The ultimate goal of rehabilitation is to live independently. Full independence implies a return to employment status. Not all patients can be restored to their previous state, but they can learn to adapt to the changes they have experienced. This requires emphasis on abilities rather than disabilities. Instead of focusing on what is lost, the patient and the care providers must focus on what remains.

Prevention of Further Disability

Rehabilitation also involves the prevention of further disability (secondary disability) that may potentially be caused by the patient's primary disability. Examples include prevention of problems in stroke patients such as pneumonia, decubitus ulcers, and limb contractures, which are often caused by lack of mobility. The nurse plays an important role in the prevention of secondary disability.

Rehabilitation is a long-term process requiring the commitment of both the patient and the family. The process is often difficult and marked by periods of progress followed by occasional relapses in functional disability. These relapses can be frustrating to everyone involved and require determination on the part of the family as well as patience and understanding by the nurse. The rehabilitation process can place additional burdens on family members when roles once filled by the disabled family member must be filled by other members. Attention is frequently focused on the disabled member, leaving other family members feeling neglected. Ongoing family problems may intensify during this time, making the rehabilitation process even more difficult.

It is important when caring for a disabled patient to be aware of the attitudes and behaviors of all family members. Often families can be assisted in adjusting to role changes that occur during the rehabilitation process. The more consistently patients and family are involved in the process, the more likely it is that success will occur. Involvement in goal setting and a clear explanation of patient and family roles in daily rehabilitation activities help families understand better the challenges of the process. This gives a sense of control and increases family strength.

LEGISLATION

Public attitudes toward people with disabilities play a significant role in the degree of handicap experienced by the disabled. Lack of knowledge about a disability often causes the public to react negatively to people who appear disabled. Individuals who are blind are sometimes treated as though they are deaf as well. People with conditions such as cerebral palsy that affect speech and muscle control are often treated as though they have decreased intelligence. Employers may be reluctant to hire disabled workers, fearing an increase in insurance rates or negative reactions from their customers (see the Health Promotion Considerations box below).

The federal government has passed laws over the years to protect the rights of the disabled. The first law passed to aid the rehabilitation of World War I veterans was the Vocational Rehabilitation Act of 1920. This law provided job training for injured veterans. The Social Security Act of 1935 provided additional aid to states for both direct relief and vocational rehabilitation. It was the Rehabilitation Act of 1973, however, that provided a comprehensive approach to problems experienced by the disabled. The act not only expanded available resources for vocational training but also defined services to be included in rehabilitation programs. It also began affirmative action programs to assist in the

Health Promotion Considerations

Helping Disabled Patients Understand Their Employment Rights Under ADA

- Nurses and other providers should understand basic laws that affect their patients' well-being even after they leave the health care setting. One of the most important pieces of health care legislation to be passed in recent decades is the Americans with Disabilities Act of 1990.
- Title 1 of the act prohibits private employers with 15 or more employees, state and local governments, employment agencies, and labor unions from discriminating against qualified individuals with disabilities. The areas in which discrimination is prohibited include job application procedures, hiring, firing, advancement, compensation, job training, and other terms, conditions, and privileges of employment.
- An employer is required to accommodate the disability of a qualified applicant or employee if it would not impose an undue hardship on the employer's business. However, an employer is not required to lower quality or production standards to make an accommodation. The employer is also not obligated to provide personal-use items such as glasses and hearing aids.
- Employers may not ask job applicants about the existence, nature, or severity of a disability. They are allowed to ask applicants about their ability to perform specific job functions. A job offer may be made on the condition that the applicant passes a medical examination, but only if the examination is required for all newly hired employees in similar jobs. These medical examinations must be job related and consistent with the employer's business needs. To learn more, visit www.eeoc.gov.

employment of the disabled and prohibited discrimination against the disabled in programs receiving federal funds. In 1990, the Americans with Disabilities Act was passed. This law extended the protection given to the disabled in the public sector by the Rehabilitation Act of 1973 to the private sector as well. It was designed to give the disabled full access to housing, employment, transportation, and communications. As a result of this law, any business endeavor designed to serve the public must ensure that its services are accessible to the disabled. In many cases, this involves the installation of wheelchair ramps, the construction of restrooms that can accommodate wheelchairs, and the provision for communication services for the hard of hearing and speech impaired. Public transportation authorities must ensure that buses, train cars, and concession shops are all accessible to the disabled. Businesses with fewer than 15 employees are currently exempt from many of the law's provisions. This law has prompted significant progress toward improving the quality of life of many disabled people.

THE REHABILITATION TEAM

Nurses who care for disabled clients must consider the whole patient when planning interventions. Difficulties in physical functioning may affect many aspects of a person's life and require the coordinated services of a number of health care professionals in order for the individual to stay well and avoid complications or injuries.

The case of Mr. Thompson, who has had a recent stroke and resulting right-sided paralysis, provides a good example of the types of expertise and the number of services that may be required during rehabilitation.

Mr. Thompson, age 72, suffered a left-sided brain hemorrhage 3 weeks earlier. Because of this, he was unable to speak or use his right arm or leg. He was also incontinent of urine and exhibited some right-sided facial paralysis. After 5 days in the hospital, it was determined that Mr. Thompson's condition had stabilized and he was transferred to a rehabilitation facility to continue the rehabilitation process. At this time, his speech had returned but was slurred and halting. He had minimal movement in his right arm and leg but was still unable to walk or feed himself. The incontinence of urine persisted, and he had several reddened areas on his right hip and coccyx. Before his injury, Mr. Thompson had been living with only his wife of 50 years, who also was in poor health. They had no family living in the state, and she was quite concerned about how she would care for him once he was sent home.

When trying to comprehend all that is involved in helping Mr. Thompson return to full functioning (if that is possible), it is helpful first to imagine a typical day in the Thompson household and to identify all the ADL and IADL competencies required to get through the day. Next, the types of people and services that may be necessary to prevent further injury and to increase functioning should be considered. At a minimum, the rehabilitation team will consist of the patient's spouse, personal physician, rehabilitation physician, and rehabilitation nurse. Other likely members include the physical therapist, who assists the patient in all aspects of mobility from regaining strength and function in the extremities to the use of assistive devices such as crutches and walkers; the occupational therapist, who assists the patient with regaining fine motor skills necessary for dressing, eating, and grooming; the speech therapist, who assists the patient in regaining swallowing or speaking functions; and the social worker, who may assist with coordinating resources for placement in the home or a convalescent facility after discharge. Other members of the team may include a clinical nurse specialist in rehabilitation nursing, a psychologist, a recreational therapist, and a vocational counselor.

The nurse's concern at this time should be that of becoming an effective member of the rehabilitation team. The successful resolution of rehabilitation problems often depends on the ability of health care workers to consider how the individual functions within the family and to work closely with other health professionals toward a common goal. If this goal is to be successful, good communication skills are essential. These entail clear, specific documentation of the patient's functional deficits and abilities and active participation in multidisciplinary conferences to resolve patient problems.

APPROACHES TO REHABILITATION

Perhaps the most important goal of successful rehabilitation of a disabled person is independence. This fact is sometimes forgotten when a caregiver sees the slow, agonizing attempts to move an arm or a leg. The tendency is to do for patients what is difficult for them to accomplish on their own. There are times when patients should be helped to complete a task, especially when they become increasingly frustrated. However, caregivers who intervene too soon encourage dependence and delay rehabilitation. Rehabilitation patients should be cheerfully encouraged to do as much as possible for themselves. Praise for accomplishing a task should be given promptly, and caregivers should reflect continuing optimism about the patient's progress.

Health professionals frequently plan comprehensive programs of rehabilitation without much thought as to how the program will be implemented once the patient returns home. To be effective, the program should commence immediately after an injury and should involve the patient and family from the outset. Failure to involve the family in establishing goals and strategies often produces family dependence, just as doing too many things for the patient produces individual dependence.

Rehabilitation nurses undertake a number of roles, all designed to assist the patient and family in returning to a high level of functioning. These roles include care planner, teacher, caregiver, counselor, coordinator, and advocate.

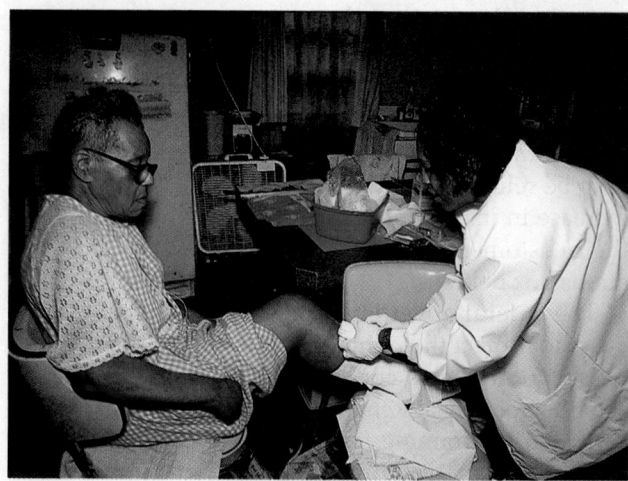

FIGURE **2-2** An important nursing role in home health care is to teach patients to care for themselves.

In the home setting, nurses can best assist patients and families by helping them adjust their activities to accommodate the disability (Fig. 2-2). Even though families may have been taught care routines in a previous setting, routines must often be adapted to the new setting and prioritized differently. In this role, the nurse is an expert caregiver and teacher. Problem-solving sessions often identify ways in which care routines can be adapted to the realities of the home setting. Caregivers may not have thought through changes in sleeping arrangements, how they will transport the patient for follow-up office visits, or how to plan for periodic relief from their caregiver role. Nurses can help families anticipate these predictable stress points and plan realistically for how they will handle them.

Nurses should also be prepared to handle a wide range of patient and family emotions, ranging from extreme optimism to depression. At these times, families need a great deal of support and may need the assistance of outside community support systems. Local support groups can often be very effective in helping families respond appropriately to the stresses of a disabled family member. Professional organizations such as the Association of Rehabilitation Nurses can be an invaluable resource to nurses working in the rehabilitation field.

LONG-TERM CARE

In the United States, 16,500 Medicare or Medicaid-Certified nursing homes provide residential skilled nursing care. The great majority of these are freestanding, with the others being hospital-based. After an acute care hospitalization of at least 3 days, Medicare covers 100 days per event in a skill nursing facility (SNF).

The nursing home population in the United States is about 3.5 million people. Many people think only of older adults in institutional settings when they think of long-term care settings. Long-term care services, however, are required by people of all ages who are temporarily or permanently unable to function independently. Thus long-term care refers to a range of services that address the health, personal care, and social needs of all people who lack some ability necessary for self-care. It may be a surprise to many that a relatively small percentage of older adults live in institutions. Many live with extended families or by themselves. Unfortunately, a significant number of older adults who live alone are poor and live in inadequate housing, often without adequate heat, ventilation, food, or telephones. Eventually, problems with mobility and mental functioning force many older adults into nursing homes.

RISKS FOR INSTITUTIONALIZATION

Government statistics indicate that only 1% of people ages 65 to 74 reside in nursing homes. This figure rises to 6% for ages 75 to 84 and to 20% for those 85 and over. The main reason for institutionalization, however, is not age. The best indicator of who will need nursing home placement is ADL dependency. Only about 12% of those with one or two ADL limitations live in nursing homes, whereas 50% of older adults with five or six ADL limitations reside there. These statistics highlight the fact that if home care services were available to assist older adults in meeting more ADL needs, costly institutionalization could be delayed. Individual characteristics associated with increased risk of nursing home residency include age 85 and older, female gender, African-American race, and reliance on Medicaid.

Other factors bearing on who requires nursing home placement include such things as financial resources, whether the person lives alone or with family, the presence of mental illness, the type of disease process, and the degree of social support.

LEVELS OF CARE

Modern long-term residential care consists of four levels: (1) domiciliary care, (2) sheltered housing, (3) intermediate care, and (4) skilled care. Often one type of facility will offer more than one level of care (usually skilled and intermediate); however, in most states, institutions must have approval for whatever levels of care they plan to provide.

Domiciliary Care

Facilities providing basic room, board, and supervision are sometimes called *domiciliary care facilities*. In this arrangement, 24-hour care is not provided and residents usually come and go as they please.

Sheltered Housing

Similar to domiciliary care facilities, sheltered housing settings have some modification to provide care for frail older adults and usually include community dining facilities. However, 24-hour care is not provided.

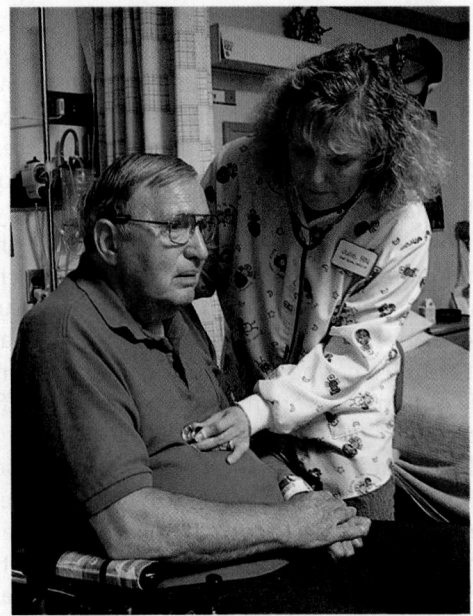

FIGURE 2-3 Patients in skilled-care facilities have access to professional care around-the-clock.

Intermediate Care

Intermediate-care facilities provide custodial care at a level usually associated with nursing homes. Patients at this level often need assistance with two or three ADL (Fig. 2-3). Facilities offering this level of care must have personnel available 24 hours a day. They are not considered by the government to be medical facilities and thus receive no reimbursement under Medicare. Many do, however, receive the bulk of their financing under Medicaid. Federal regulations require a registered nurse to serve as director of nursing and a licensed nurse to be on duty at least 8 hours a day.

Skilled Care

Skilled nursing facilities must have skilled health professionals present around the clock. The care of patients in skilled nursing facilities must be supervised by a physician and requires the services of a registered nurse, physical therapist, or speech therapist.

IMPACT OF RELOCATION

Relocation to a long-term care facility is rarely easy. In the best of circumstances, patients, families, and health professionals anticipate the possible future need for long-term care, set aside funds for that purpose, and make plans that are acceptable to all. When patients cannot make sound decisions for themselves, families seek help from extended family members and professionals in making decisions for long-term care placement. More commonly, however, the situation is quite different. Often a crisis situation precipitates the decision. A sole caregiver may become ill, leaving the care of the disabled older adult to the hands of extended family members who may be either unable or unwilling to continue care. Patients suddenly may become physically or mentally incapable of caring for themselves or making their own decisions. Family members frequently feel guilty for considering institutional care. Few know very much about modern long-term care facilities and have not investigated potential placement.

In this situation, home health nurses, social workers, and other health professionals must work closely with the family to defuse the crisis situation and provide realistic options from which the family may choose. This is a time when families need the utmost support and acceptance. Simply clarifying the situation, affirming the family's caring and concern, and pointing out realistic options will often return a family to effective functioning.

If placement in a long-term care facility is the only logical choice, the patient and family must be prepared for the relocation. Research has shown that the more prepared the patient, the better is the adjustment. Preparation includes providing as much choice as possible for the patient and responding to patient questions and concerns. If possible, choices of facility, room location, types of personal belongings, and room decor are helpful, as are tours of the facility before entering. It also is helpful if professional staff check on the new patient frequently during the first few weeks. Patients should be introduced to other residents with like interests and invited or assisted to participate in appropriate activities.

EFFECTS OF INSTITUTIONALIZATION

The effects of institutionalization are predictable and must be considered in helping the new nursing home resident adjust to the surroundings. Frequently observed effects include depersonalization, indignity, redefinition of "normal," regression, and social withdrawal.

Depersonalization

Depersonalization plays a major part in institutional life. Caregivers often know little of a resident's life history and therefore treat individual residents in light of their diagnosis or dysfunctional behavior patterns. The case study about Herman and Kristina in Box 2-1 illustrates this point.

One way to help see the resident of a long-term care facility as a whole person with past relationships, accomplishments, and interests is to ask family members to bring in photographs. The photographs may have been taken on significant occasions, such as graduation or wedding days or may be simple family pictures that depict the older person's place in the family or community. The photographs can be mounted on poster board or placed on a bulletin board in the resident's room. This effort helps caregivers see more than a frail, weak, older person and can open up conversation that encourages reminiscing, which is a therapeutic means of dealing with one's past life and preparing for death.

Indignity

Indignity is another effect of institutionalization. Routine activities such as toileting and obtaining food and drink must be requested. Sometimes the prompt fulfillment of the request depends on the relationship between the patient and the caregiver. Residents of long-term care facilities may be exposed unnecessar-

---

| Box 2-1 | *Case Study* |

I don't think I truly understood what depersonalization was until I met Herman. Herman and his wife Kristina lived alone in a small house in a northwestern city. Herman was 62 years old and had Alzheimer's disease. I met them while working as a home health nurse. I was asked to look into respite services to help relieve Kristina of the strain of caring for Herman. I remember my first impression of Herman, formed after reading his chart and talking to the staff nurse about his care problems. He was starting to neglect his personal appearance. The staff nurse said he often put soup on the stove for lunch and then went out into the garden to tend his flowers, forgetting about the soup. This and other images of his functioning created in me a picture of an incompetent and helpless old man.

Over a period of weeks, Kristina shared many stories with me about who this man was, what he cared about, how they met, and her deep devotion to her husband of 35 years. Gradually, I was able to see the distorted image I held. In his youth, Herman was an Olympic gold medal skier from Austria who came to this country as a young man. He held several jobs as a ski instructor and repaired ski equipment until he met and married Kristina and moved to the northwestern United States to become owner and manager of a small ski resort. He was tall and muscular with an easy smile and a kind word for everyone. He was admired by many in the community for his skill as a skier and his friendliness. He was a good father and family man who was known as "the rock" because all of his family and friends relied on him for advice and assistance.

Over a period of 5 years, Herman became more and more forgetful, less talkative, and often preoccupied with household tasks that he would start but not complete. He also failed to recognize many of his close friends and, at times, would wander off downtown without knowing why or where he was going. Throughout this, Kristina remained fiercely devoted to Herman, though the strain of the caregiver role was beginning to affect her health. "He cared for us for so many years. Now it is my turn to care for him."

I was surprised at how different was my previous view of Herman. I was seeing him as dependent, helpless, and a burden to his small and frail wife—a view created by my observations of his behavior and what I knew of the Alzheimer's disease process and a view that changed radically once I knew more about Herman. I doubt I will ever minimize the importance of learning about the whole patient.

ily, especially when caregivers enter rooms without knocking. Simple courtesies such as using a person's title and last name, knocking before entering the room, and draping during care activities help the resident maintain dignity. It is useful to think to yourself, "How would I want to be treated if I were weak and frail and could not do the things that I can do for myself now?"

Redefinition of "Normal"

Behaviors that were considered normal at home may be labeled abnormal or be unacceptable in an institution. Watching television at 3 AM, loud singing, or sexual activity may not be tolerated, depending on the residence's rules and routines. Although consideration of others is important, it also is important to give residents of long-term care facilities some flexibility and some measure of control in their daily lives.

Regression

Over time, a resident's physical, mental, and social abilities may be lost because of disuse. If people are left in bed a greater part of the day, it soon becomes impossible for them to walk. If visits from friends and relatives are few, the skill of conversation may also be lost. It is important to encourage independence and social interaction as much as possible. Avoid infantilizing older patients. Although it may be necessary to simplify language and activities for those who are cognitively impaired, avoid baby talk.

Social Withdrawal

If a resident never leaves the nursing home or if family visits are few and include little discussion of the outside world, the institution can become a barrier, cutting off interest and participation in the outside world. If this is allowed to continue, life in the facility becomes, for many patients, their entire world. They tend to withdraw into the boundaries of their own room. Nurses can help by conversing with residents about events inside and outside the nursing home. When you know your patients well, you can bring up news that you expect will be of interest to them. Discussion of current events in small groups can broaden the resident's horizons.

PRINCIPLES OF LONG-TERM RESIDENTIAL CARE

Long-term residential care has been called *custodial care.* This term invokes passive images such as maintenance, warehousing, or waiting to die. Some people have called such facilities "heaven's waiting rooms." Publicized abuses by some nursing homes are at least partly responsible for negative stereotypes of long-term residential care. However, long-term care facilities in general have changed substantially in recent years. Although some continue to provide care of questionable quality, many excellent facilities do exist.

Modern facilities care for residents with a wide array of medical and surgical problems. Not all residents are admitted for permanent stays in the facility. In many communities, the nursing home has become a convalescent hospital for older adults who have recently undergone surgical procedures, such as repair of a fractured hip. These acute cases often strain already limited resources. Many are admitted for short stays that are prompted by care demands that temporarily overwhelm the family. Illness of a family caregiver also can result in temporary admission to the facility. When the home situation has stabilized, these residents often return home. Increasingly, those admitted for long stays are older adults and suffer from mental health problems. In these cases, the family has exhausted most of its physical, emotional, and financial resources and home care is no longer feasible.

 Put on Your Thinking Cap!

If you have a clinical experience in a long-term care facility, interview a resident there. Specifically, ask:
1. What circumstances brought you here to live?
2. What are the benefits and disadvantages of living in this type of facility?
3. What advice would you give to a new resident here?
4. What can nurses do to make it easier for you to adjust to living here?

Discuss the resident's responses in relation to the effects of institutionalization and implications for nurses.

When the resident is admitted to a long-term care facility, the care delivered should be based on three principles: (1) promotion of independence, (2) maintenance of function, and (3) maintenance of autonomy.

Promotion of Independence

Successful relocation to a long-term care facility depends in part on the ability of residents to do things for themselves and on the involvement of families to keep the older adult family member in contact with the outside world. It may be tempting for institutional caregivers to feed residents rather than to spend time encouraging residents to feed themselves. When the workday is a never-ending series of tasks, doing things quickly often takes priority over promoting independence. Watch for this type of behavior, and try to restructure assignments of nursing assistants to reward the promotion of independence. This can be accomplished by setting specific goals for each resident that encourage independent functioning. Then explain to the staff members how their efforts can contribute to the goal. Involvement of staff in this way often produces results.

Maintenance of Function

Often it is loss of function that prevents an older adult from staying at home. Health professionals who are disease-oriented often concentrate on the disease process at the expense of a functional assessment. An incontinent resident may be incorrectly perceived as having a complication of the aging process. This type of thinking fosters an emphasis on maintenance care, leading to efforts to prevent skin breakdown by frequent changes of clothing and linens. A more thorough assessment would begin with the determination of possible causes for the incontinence. A functional assessment explores factors that might be responsible for the incontinence. Immobility may be the basic problem. Questions to ask include the following: Is the resident normally mobile? If so, is there a light in the room that facilitates locating the bathroom? Is the resident able to manage clothing for independent toileting? Are the side rails normally up or down? Viewing this problem as a functional problem may lead to simple solutions such as placing a light in the room at night or a urinal next to the bed. Interventions, whenever possible, should focus on restoring and preserving function.

Maintenance of Autonomy

Most people value control over their lives. Successful relocation to a long-term care facility depends on preserving as much autonomy as possible. Older adults who participate in selecting the facility adjust better than those who have no choice in the matter.

It is also important to allow as much flexibility as possible in establishing a routine for the new resident. Choices in activities, such as when to have a bath or how late to watch television, go a long way toward preserving the autonomy and self-esteem of the older adult resident. As much as possible, encourage the resident to assist in establishing care goals. For example, the frequency and duration of exercise and goals for weight loss or gains require the facility resident's commitment. Mutually established goals are more likely to be achieved than those selected for the resident.

Families also have a role in maintaining autonomy in the older adult. Autonomy depends on knowing one's place in the world and what roles one still holds in the family structure. Families who relate to their older adult members by reinforcing their importance in the family and keeping them up to date on family happenings and decisions reinforce the idea that the older adult remains a valued family member who simply resides at another address.

Put on Your Thinking Cap!

Identify one thing you can do to achieve each of the following: (1) maintain autonomy, (2) maintain function, and (3) promote independence in:
  a. The long-term care facility resident
  b. The hospitalized patient

OTHER PATIENT CARE SETTINGS

The settings addressed in this chapter represent many of those that traditionally employ licensed nurses. Other employment settings include clinics, physicians' offices, schools, adult day care, respite care, and correctional facilities. Each setting presents unique experiences and challenges. In some of these settings, the LPN may be the only licensed nursing professional on site. Therefore it is vital that the nurse's responsibilities be clearly defined and consistent with legal functions.

 Key Points

- The changing health care system has greatly increased the number and types of health care settings.
- Community health nurses work with individuals and groups to improve the health of the entire community.
- The main difference between home health care and public health nursing is that home health care is more focused on providing direct care to patients.
- A major nursing function in home health care is teaching patients and families to care for themselves to promote independent functioning.
- Medicare is a major source of home health care funding.
- To receive Medicare reimbursement for home health care, four conditions must be met: (1) the physician has determined the need for home care and has made a plan for home care, (2) the patient needs intermittent skilled nursing care, or physical or speech-language therapy, or continued occupational therapy, (3) the patient is homebound, and (4) the agency providing the care is Medicare-certified.
- Specialty home care services include high-technology interventions (the provision of intravenous therapy and ventilator therapy), hospice services, pediatric care, and mental health care.
- Rehabilitation is the process of restoring an individual to the best possible health and functioning after a physical or mental impairment and the prevention of further disability.
- Caring for disabled patients requires the coordinated services of a number of health care professionals to help patients stay well and avoid complications or injuries.
- As an effective member of a multidisciplinary rehabilitation team, the nurse is a care planner, teacher, caregiver, counselor, coordinator, and advocate.
- Health care workers must consider the way a disabled individual functions within the family, and the patient and family should be involved from the outset in determining the plan of care.
- Government statistics indicate that only 1% of people ages 65 to 74, 6% of people ages 75 to 84, and 20% of people ages 85 and over reside in nursing homes.
- Dependence in activities of daily living is the best indicator of who will need nursing home placement.

- Modern long-term residential care exists in four levels: (1) domiciliary care, (2) sheltered housing, (3) intermediate care, and (4) skilled care.
- Care delivered in a long-term care residential facility is based on three principles: (1) promotion of independence, (2) maintenance of function, and (3) maintenance of autonomy.

 Go to your Companion CD-ROM for a Pharmacology Tutorial, Audio Glossary, and 3-D animations.

evolve   Be sure to visit the companion Evolve site at http://evolve.elsevier.com/Linton/ for WebLinks and additional online resources.

REVIEW QUESTIONS *Choose the best answer.*

1. A home health nurse performed all the activities listed below with Medicare patients. Which one may *not* be reimbursable?
   1. Used sterile technique to clean and dress a large wound
   2. Took a frail older couple for a short walk to provide exercise
   3. Performed a venipuncture to obtain a blood sample for lab tests
   4. Taught a patient with recently diagnosed diabetes how to inject insulin

2. Which nursing activity might commonly be provided by home health nurses but not by community health nurses?
   1. Conducting health education programs in a senior citizen residence
   2. Assessing the recovery of a postoperative patient at home
   3. Arranging blood pressure screening at a community shopping center
   4. Seeing patients in a clinic to monitor problems related to chronic illness

3. The definition of the term *community-based nursing* is best reflected in which of the following activities?
   1. Meeting with residents of low-income housing to identify their health needs
   2. Telephoning patients at home after discharge from the hospital
   3. Asking nurses to identify the health services most needed in their communities
   4. Developing a hospital-based home health care service

4. Individuals who are unable to feed or dress themselves independently because of a neurological disease are most accurately described as:
   1. Impaired
   2. Disabled
   3. Handicapped
   4. Disadvantaged

5. Which legislation was the first to begin affirmative action programs to protect the disabled from discrimination in employment?
   1. Social Security Act
   2. Americans with Disabilities Act
   3. Rehabilitation Act
   4. Vocational Rehabilitation Act

6. A patient who has suffered a head injury is feeding herself with considerable difficulty. In terms of rehabilitation, what is the most appropriate nursing response?
   1. Offer to feed her so that she will not be embarrassed by her handicap.
   2. Order a liquid diet so that she will not have to use eating utensils.
   3. Point out that the sooner she can feed herself, the sooner she can go home.
   4. Be sure her food is accessible, and compliment her efforts at self-feeding.

7. A nursing home resident has his name neatly printed on the door to his room. The interior of the room is decorated in masculine colors. One wall is covered with pictures of the resident at various occasions in his personal and professional life. In one corner is a leather recliner with a reading lamp and table. This room reflects an effort to:
   1. Avoid depersonalization
   2. Maintain the resident's dignity
   3. Prevent regression
   4. Prevent social withdrawal

Legal and Ethical Considerations

evolve http://evolve.elsevier.com/Linton/

Objectives

After reading and studying this chapter, you should be able to:

1. Define ethics, bioethics, values, morality, moral uncertainty, moral distress, moral outrage, and moral/ethical dilemma.
2. Explain the principles of ethics: autonomy, justice, fidelity, beneficence, nonmaleficence.
3. Explain how values are formed.
4. Explain how values clarification is useful in nursing practice.
5. Discuss the relationship between culture and values.
6. Describe the following philosophical bases for ethics: deontology, utilitarianism, feminist ethics, ethics of care.
7. Describe the steps in processing ethical dilemmas.
8. Describe the role of institutional ethics committees.
9. Explain the role of the LVN/LPN in relation to informed consent.

Key Terms

Be sure to check out the bonus material on the Companion CD-ROM, including selected audio pronunciations.

autonomy (ăh-TĂWN-o-mē, p. 27)
beneficence (be-NEF-i-sens, p. 27)
bioethics (bī-ō-ETH-iks, p. 26)
confidentiality (p. 27)
deontology (dē-on-TOL-o-gē, p. 28)
DNR (do not resuscitate) orders (p. 33)
ethical dilemmas (p. 26)
ethics (p. 26)
ethics of care (p. 28)
ethnocentrism (eth-nō-SEN-tresm, p. 28)
feminist ethics (p. 28)
informed consent (p. 32)
justice (p. 27)
malpractice (p. 31)
morality (p. 26)
moral distress (p. 26)
moral outrage (p. 26)
moral uncertainty (p. 26)
nonmaleficence (non-mă-LEF-i-sens, p. 27)
statutory laws (STĂCH-ū-tor-ē, p. 29)
tort (p. 29)
utilitarian (ū-til-i-TĂR-ē-ăn, p. 28)
values (p. 28)
values clarification (p. 28)
veracity (ve-RĂS-i-tē, p. 27)

Nursing practice is guided by both ethical and legal principles. These topics usually are addressed in fundamentals, but their importance merits a review in this text as we begin to address serious and often complicated medical-surgical and psychiatric conditions.

ETHICS

Ethics deals with values relevant to human conduct. It is concerned with defining what actions are right and wrong and whether the motives and outcomes of those actions are good or bad. If choices were simply two opposite actions with one clearly good and one clearly bad, ethical decision making would be simple, but they are not. Often the choices are shades of gray, not black and white, or a choice must be made between two good or two bad options. **Ethical dilemmas** are perplexing because ethics does not prescribe one right answer. Rather, ethics defines formal processes to explore what is proper conduct. **Bioethics** is concerned with the ethical questions that arise in the context of health care.

The concept of morality is closely related to ethics because moral beliefs provide a foundation for rules of action. Within a society or culture, **morality** is defined by the shared ideas of what is right or good. A situation in which a nurse confronts a moral problem can be described as moral uncertainly, moral/ethical dilemma, moral distress, or moral outrage (Jameton cited in Burkhardt and Nathaniel, 2002). **Moral uncertainty** occurs when the nurse senses that a situation is a moral problem but cannot define it clearly or reach a decision because of uncertainty about the morally correct action. When no one solution seems to be satisfactory because of conflicting morals or ethical principles, an ethical dilemma exists. **Moral distress** occurs when the nurse feels powerless because his or her moral beliefs cannot be followed because of institutional or other barriers. Moral distress is believed to be one reason that some nurses leave nursing, others experience "burnout," and still others seem to stop caring about their patients. When another person in the health care setting acts in a way that the nurse believes is immoral and the nurse feels powerless to intervene, the nurse feels **moral outrage.**

Put on Your Thinking Cap!

Describe a specific patient-care situation in which a nurse is likely to feel moral distress. How might repeated witnessing of similar incidents lead to moral outrage and eventually to job burnout? What can a hospital, clinic, or other institution do to help prevent such burnout?

PRINCIPLES OF ETHICS

The principles of health care ethics are autonomy, justice, fidelity, beneficence, and nonmaleficence (Box 3-1). When facing decisions that have no easy answers, nurses can consider options against each of these principles. Recognition of **autonomy** is inherent in the concept of informed consent and in advance directives. Respect for the rights of persons to make decisions about their own health and health care, such as accepting or refusing blood transfusions or medications, is based on the principle of autonomy. **Beneficence** is another core value in nursing. It incorporates actions to promote good, prevent harm, or remove the patient from harm. To act with beneficence means that the nurse behaves in the patient's best interest. The problem is to define good, recognizing that the definitions of the patient, the family, the nurse, and the physician may differ. An example of preventing harm is reporting a co-worker who is impaired or incompetent. **Justice** is concerned with fairness, equity, and appropriateness of treatment considering what is due to a person. An important aspect of justice is the recognition that goods and services are limited so that giving to some means that others will not receive those goods and/or services. An important role of the government is to devise and implement policies for the fair and equitable distribution of scarce resources. Decisions about who will receive limited resources can be based on various philosophies and might use the criteria of equal distribution; individual need, merit, social contribution, rights, or effort; or serving the greatest good for the greatest number of individuals. The principle of **nonmaleficence** requires that the nurse "do no harm." Of course, there are times when therapeutic interventions are uncomfortable, but the benefits must be judged to justify the discomfort. A patient getting out of bed for the first time after surgery likely will experience some pain, but the benefits of mobilization far outweigh temporary discomfort. Fidelity, or faithfulness, is a commitment to carry through on promises. Such promises may be spoken or implied. Patients in health care settings have the right to expect that staff will be committed to their care and will not abandon them. Another aspect of fidelity is the duty of the nurse to practice within the legal definition of the profession and to remain competent.

Nursing and other professions have sets of ethical principles that are accepted as basic to the profession. These principles may be set forth as a Code of Ethics,

Box 3-1 *Principles of Health Care Ethics*

- The nurse, in all professional relationships, practices with compassion and respect for the inherent dignity, worth, and uniqueness of every individual, unrestricted by considerations of social or economic status, personal attributes, or the nature of health problems.
- The nurse's primary commitment is to the patient, whether an individual, family group, or community.
- The nurse promotes, advocates for, and strives to protect the health, safety, and rights of the patient.
- The nurse is responsible and accountable for individual nursing practice and determines the appropriate delegation of tasks consistent with the nurse's obligation to provide optimum patient care.
- The nurse owes the same duties to self as to others, including the responsibility to preserve integrity and safety, to maintain competence, and to continue personal and professional growth.
- The nurse participates in establishing, maintaining, and improving health care environments and conditions of employment conducive to the provision of quality health care and consistent with the values of the profession through individual and collective action.
- The nurse participates in the advancement of the profession through contributions to practice, education, administration, and knowledge development.
- The nurse collaborates with other health professionals and the public in promoting community, national, and international efforts to meet health needs.
- The profession of nursing, as represented by associations and their members, is responsible for articulating nursing values, for maintaining the integrity of the profession and its practice, and for shaping social policy.

From American Nurses Association: *Code of ethics for nurses with interpretive statements.* Washington, DC, 2001, American Nurses Publishing.

which defines ideals of conduct. Several documents define ethical codes for nurses, but their common themes are responsibility, accountability, advocacy, confidentiality, and veracity. Nurses are accountable to themselves, their patients, their employers, the profession, and society. Adherence to standards of care is one way that nurses demonstrate accountability for their actions. A responsible nurse knows right from wrong and carries out duties in a knowledgeable and careful manner. The **confidentiality** of patient information must be protected. Patients have the right to control who has access to personal information. Nurses must guard against the careless, accidental, or deliberate sharing of private information. **Veracity** (truth) requires that nurses be honest not only with patients but also in documentation and communication with colleagues.

The Code of Ethics for the LPN/LVN as defined by the National Association for Practical Nurse Education and Service is listed in Box 3-2.

Box 3-2   *NAPNES Code of Ethics for LPN/LVNs*

The Licensed Practical/Vocational Nurse Shall:
1. Consider as a basic obligation the conservation of life and the prevention of disease.
2. Promote and protect the physical, mental, emotional and spiritual health of the patient and the family.
3. Fulfill all duties faithfully and efficiently.
4. Function within established legal guidelines.
5. Accept personal responsibility (for his/her acts) and seek to merit the respect and confidence of all members of the health team.
6. Hold in confidence all matters coming to his/her knowledge, in the practice of his/her profession, and in no way and at no time violate this confidence.
7. Give conscientious service and charge just remuneration.
8. Learn and respect the religious and cultural beliefs of his/her patient and of all people.
9. Meet his/her obligation to the patient by keeping abreast of current trends in health care through reading and continuing education.
10. As a citizen of the United States of America, uphold the laws of the land and seek to promote legislation that will meet the health needs of its people.

Reprinted with permission of the National Association for Practical Nurse Education and Service, Alexandria, VA. Copyright © 1999.

VALUES

Values are those beliefs and attitudes that are important to a person and that influence the choices that a person makes on a daily basis. For example, one person may value kindness and honesty, whereas another values financial success and material possessions. Our values affect our choice of friends, mates, and professions.

Values are learned as a result of cultural, social, and personal experiences. The family provides the foundation for values formation. Ideas about children and child-rearing reflect not only how children are valued but also what values will be rewarded. As the child's experiences extend beyond the family, some values are reinforced, some challenged, and some new ones formed through contacts with peers, the church, schools, and the media. Some modes by which values may be acquired include copying role models (modeling), moralizing by authority figures, personal exploration, and experiences that are rewarded or punished. Values that have been identified as essential for professional nurses include altruism, equality, esthetics, freedom, human dignity, justice, and truth (AACN, 1986).

Values Clarification

Professional education is an example of an experience that can profoundly influence a person's values. To help nursing students acquire values of the profession, faculty encourage them to become aware of their personal values and how those values affect their behavior. This is a process of self-discovery called **values clarification**. The value of this process is that a person

learns to make choices from alternatives and to determine whether those choices were made carefully. Values clarification enables nurses not only to understand themselves better but also to understand their patients and to help patients explore what is important to them. Nurses need to be aware of the tendency toward **ethnocentrism**—the belief that one's own culture (and its values) is superior to others.

 What Does Culture Have to Do with Values?

Ethnocentric beliefs about issues such as drug use and sexual orientation can influence a nurse's attitude toward patients so subtly that he or she might not even be aware of it. Professional education and training can assist in the process of values clarification to ensure that the patient receives optimal care regardless of a nurse's personal convictions.

Values Conflicts

The term *values conflict* is used when the values of individuals and/or institutions are different. In this situation, there is a risk that the patient's values may not be recognized or respected. As a nurse, you can recognize values conflicts by being aware of your own values and learning about those of your patients. A positive response to values conflicts is to try to understand the other person's views and to find common ground.

PHILOSOPHICAL BASES FOR ETHICS

Determining what is right or wrong, good or bad is no simple task. The conclusions reached in various situations may vary depending on the philosophy that forms a base for a person's values. Some examples of philosophies that help shape ethical principles are deontology, utilitarianism, feminist ethics, and ethics of care. **Deontology** defines right and wrong on the basis of whether an action meets the criteria of fidelity, veracity, autonomy, beneficence, and justice. The consequences of the action are not considered. A limitation of deontology is apparent when an action represents conflicting values. For example, controlling the activity of a confused person may prevent harm (a good thing!) but also interfere with autonomy (a bad thing?). From a **utilitarian** point of view, the "right" action is that which produces the greatest good for the greatest number of people. The challenge here is to come to agreement as to what the "greatest good" is! Among human beings, there are bound to be differences in opinion as to what constitutes a good outcome. **Feminist ethics** focuses on inequalities among people, particularly on the basis of gender, and places value on relationships. Closely related to feminist ethics is **ethics of care**, a theory that sees care as a "central activity of human behavior and one that deserves special attention in health care" (Potter and Perry, 412). This theorist would ask how particular actions reflect caring. The emphasis

Box 3-3 *Steps in Ethical Decision Making*

- **Step 1** Is this an ethical dilemma? If a review of scientific data does not resolve the question, if the question is perplexing, and if the answer will have profound relevance for several areas of human concern, then an ethical dilemma may exist.
- **Step 2** Gather all of the information relevant to the case. To be sure it is a true dilemma, it will be important to review all pertinent information. Occasionally an overlooked fact may provide quick resolution. At this point, client, family, institutional, and social perspectives are important sources of relevant information.
- **Step 3** Examine and determine your own values on the issues. Values clarification provides a foundation for clarity and for confidence during discussions, which will be necessary for resolution of a dilemma.
- **Step 4** Verbalize the problem. A clear, simple statement of the dilemma may not always be easy, but it is essential for the next step to take place.
- **Step 5** Consider possible sources of action. To respect all sides of an issue, it is helpful to list potential actions, especially when the list will reflect opinions that conflict.
- **Step 6** Negotiate the outcomes. Sometimes courses of action that seem unlikely at the beginning of the process take on a new possibility as they are put to rational and respectful consideration. Negotiation requires a confidence in one's own point of view and a deep respect for the opinions of others.
- **Step 7** Evaluate the action.

From Potter, P.A., Perry, A.G. (2005). *Fundamentals of nursing* (6th ed.). St. Louis: Mosby.

on relationships and patients' stories is quite different from theories that rely on universal principles.

STEPS IN PROCESSING ETHICAL DILEMMAS

Because of the emotional component in many ethical dilemmas, a guide for addressing them is recommended. The initial task is to decide whether the situation actually constitutes an ethical problem. An ethical problem has one or more of the following characteristics (Curtin & Flaherty, 1982 in Potter and Perry, 2005):

- Scientific information alone does not provide the answer.
- The problem is perplexing; that is, the answer is not simple.
- The solution is profoundly relevant to several areas of human concern.

During the data-gathering process, participants need to consider their own values in relation to the problem or issue. Once it is agreed that the problem is an ethical one, the problem must be stated clearly so that all can agree on it. Next, possible courses of action and consequences are outlined. Options should be discussed in an atmosphere of mutual respect until agreement is reached. Action then is taken and the outcome evaluated (Box 3-3).

 Put on Your Thinking Cap!

Give an example of an ethical problem related to patient care that has been in the news recently. How does the issue or situation meet the three-part definition of an ethical problem?

INSTITUTIONAL ETHICS COMMITTEES

Health care providers deal with ethical issues frequently and usually are able to resolve problems with patients, families, and the health care team. Sometimes, however, formal help is needed. Most institutions have committees to process ethical dilemmas. The membership usually is multidisciplinary and seeks input from patients, families, professionals, and administrators. The functions of the ethics committee typically include education, policy recommendation, oversight of policy implementation, and consultation on specific cases.

LEGAL IMPLICATIONS FOR NURSING PRACTICE

The law defines the boundaries of nursing practice. Nurses are obligated to know their functions and limitations to protect both their patients and themselves. A nursing license is granted only to persons who have met specific educational standards and demonstrated the minimal required level of knowledge as assessed by an examination. The state board of nursing can revoke or suspend the license of a nurse who violates the provisions of the licensing statutes. The scope of LVN/LPN practice is outlined in the NCSBN Model Nursing Practice Act (see the Management and Supervision boxes on pp. 30 and 31).

TYPES OF LAW

Laws that guide nursing practice are derived from three types of law: statutory, regulatory, and common law. Laws created by elected legislative bodies, including nurse practice acts, are statutory laws. The legal boundaries of nursing practice in a given state are defined and described in nurse practice acts. Statutory law is classified as either civil or criminal. Criminal laws are concerned with preventing or punishing harm to society, whereas civil laws protect individual rights. A felony is a serious crime, and a misdemeanor is a crime that is less serious. Administrative bodies such as state boards of nursing create regulatory laws in the form of rules and regulations that address the conduct of nurses. Common law is the result of judicial decisions made when individual cases are decided in the courts.

Tort

A civil wrong against a person or property is called a tort. Torts are classified as intentional or unintentional. Examples of intentional torts are assault, battery, invasion of privacy, and defamation of character. Nursing

Management and Supervision

NCSBN Model Nursing Practice Act

Scope of Nursing Practice Boards of Nursing publish standards of nursing care to communicate broad expectations and to guide nurses for safe and effective practice. Professional and specialty organizations may develop more detailed, specific standards intended to promote excellence in clinical practice. According to the National Council of State Boards of Nursing (2005):

- Practice as a licensed practical/vocational nurse means a directed scope of nursing practice, with or without compensation or personal profit, under the direction of the registered nurse, advanced practice registered nurse, licensed physician, or health care provider authorized by the state; is guided by nursing standards established or recognized by the board; and includes, but is not limited to:
  - Collecting data and conducting focused nursing assessments of the health status of individuals. A focused assessment is an appraisal of an individual's status and situation at hand, contributing to comprehensive assessment by the registered nurse, supporting ongoing data collection, and deciding who needs to be informed of the information and when to inform.
  - Planning nursing care episode for individuals with stable conditions.
  - Participating in the development and modification of the comprehensive plan of care for all types of clients.
  - Implementing appropriate aspects of the strategy of care within the client-centered health care plan.
  - Participating in nursing care management through delegating to assistive personnel and assigning to other LPNs/LVNs nursing interventions that may be performed by others and do not conflict with this act.
  - Maintaining safe and effective nursing care rendered directly or indirectly.
  - Promoting a safe and therapeutic environment.
  - Participating in health teaching and counseling to promote, attain, and maintain the optimum health level of clients.
  - Serving as an advocate for the client by communicating and collaborating with other health service personnel.
  - Participating in the evaluation of client responses to interventions.
  - Communicating and collaborating with other health care professionals.
  - Providing input into the development of policies and procedures.
  - Other acts that require education and training as delineated by the board, commensurate with the licensed practical/vocational nurse's experience, continuing education, and demonstrated licensed practical/vocational nurse competencies. Each nurse is accountable for complying with the requirements of this Act; and for the quality of nursing care rendered; and for recognizing limits of knowledge and experience and planning for management of situations beyond the nurse's expertise.

From National Council of State Boards of Nursing. (2005). *Standards of nursing care*. Chicago, IL: Author.

Management and Supervision

Standards of LPN/LVN Responsibilities

The standards that define LPN/LVN responsibilities for nursing practice implementation follow.

The licensed practical/vocational nurse practicing under the direction of a registered nurse, advanced practice registered nurse, licensed physician, or other authorized licensed health care provider:

- Conducts a focused nursing assessment, which is an appraisal of the client's status and situation at hand that contributes to ongoing data collection.
- Plans for episodic nursing care.
- Demonstrates attentiveness and provides client surveillance and monitoring.
- Assists in identification of client needs.
- Seeks clarification of orders when needed.
- Demonstrates attentiveness and provides observation for signs, symptoms, and changes in client condition.
- Assists in the evaluation of the impact of nursing care. Contributes to the evaluation of client care.
- Recognizes client characteristics that may affect the client's health status.
- Obtains orientation/training for competency when encountering new equipment and technology or unfamiliar care situations.
- Implements appropriate aspects of client care in a timely manner:
  - Provides assigned and delegated aspects of client's health care plan.
  - Implements treatments and procedures.
  - Administers medications accurately.
- Documents care provided.
- Communicates relevant and timely client information with other health team members.
  - Client status and progress.
  - Client responses or lack of response to therapies.
  - Significant changes in client condition.
  - Client needs.
- Participates in nursing management:
  - Assigns nursing activities to other licensed practical/vocational nurses.
  - Delegates nursing activities for stable clients to assistive personnel.
  - Observes nursing measures and provides feedback to nursing manager.
  - Observes and communicates outcomes of delegated and assigned activities.
- Takes preventive measures to protect client, others, and self.
- Respects client's rights, concerns, decisions, and dignity (this standard includes respecting the client's concerns regarding end-of-life care).
- Attends to client or family concerns or requests.
- Promotes a safe client environment.
- Maintains appropriate professional boundaries.
- Assumes responsibility for nurse's own decisions and actions.

Reprinted with permission from the National Association for Practical Nurse Education and Service, Alexandria, VA.

Management and Supervision

Standards of LPN/LVN Professional Accountability

Specific standards are detailed that relate to professional accountability, membership on an interdisciplinary health care team, and nursing practice implementation. Standards related to licensed practical/vocational nurse professional accountability include the following:

- Practices within the legal boundaries for practical nursing through the scope of practice authorized in the MNPA and rules governing nursing.
- Demonstrates honesty and integrity in nursing practice.
- Bases nursing decisions on nursing knowledge and skills, the needs of the clients, and the expectations delineated by the board.
- Accepts responsibility for individual nursing actions, competence, decisions, and behavior in the course of practical nursing practice.
- Maintains continued competence through ongoing learning and application of knowledge in the client's interest.

Reprinted with permission from the National Association for Practical Nurse Education and Service, Alexandria, VA.

Management and Supervision

Standards of LPN/LVN as Member of Interdisciplinary Health Care Team

Standards that define the responsibilities of the LPN/LVN as a member of an interdisciplinary health care team include the following:

- Functions as a member of the health care team, contributing to the implementation of an integrated health care plan.
- Respects client property and the property of others.
- Protects confidential information unless obligated by law to disclose the information.

students may be surprised to learn that some nursing actions could be considered torts. For example, assault is a threat of some contact without the patient's consent. If a nurse threatened to restrain or medicate a person against his wishes, the patient could claim assault by the nurse. If the patient is actually touched in an offensive or harmful manner without consent, the nurse could be accused of battery. For both assault and battery, the key issue is whether the patient consented to the action. Patients have the right to be protected against unwanted intrusion into their private affairs. When that right is violated, the patient can claim invasion of privacy. Examples of invasion of privacy could include improper release of medical information or publication of patient photographs. If false information that could damage a person's reputation is released, a charge of defamation of character could be made. If the information is spoken, it is called *slander*; if written, it is called *libel*.

Unintentional torts include negligence and malpractice. Negligent conduct is that which falls below the

Management and Supervision

NAPNES Standards for Nursing Practice

The standards for nursing practice of LPNs/LVNs as defined by the National Association for Practical Nurse Education and Service are (NAPNES, 2005):

- The LPN/LVN provides individual and family-centered nursing care by:
  - Utilizing appropriate knowledge, skills, and abilities.
  - Utilizing principles of the nursing process in meeting specific patient needs in diversified health settings.
  - Maintaining appropriate written documentation and utilizing effective communication skills with patients, families, significant others, and members of the health team.
  - Executing principles of crisis intervention to maintain safety.
  - Providing appropriate education to patients, families, and significant others to promote health, facilitate rehabilitation, and maintain wellness.
  - Serving as a patient advocate to protect patient rights.

Management and Supervision

Professional Responsibilities of the LPN/LVN

The LPN/LVN fulfills the professional responsibilities of the practical/vocational nurse by:

- Applying the ethical principles underlying the profession.
- Following legal requirements.
- Following the policies and procedures of the employing facility.
- Cooperating and collaborating with all members of the health care team to meet the needs of family-centered nursing care.
- Assuming accountability for his/her nursing actions.
- Seeking educational opportunities to improve knowledge and skills.
- Building post-licensure skills to ensure and increase continuing competence.

standard of care. Professional negligence is called **malpractice**. To be found liable for malpractice, the following conditions must be met: the nurse owed a duty to the patient, the nurse did not carry out that duty, the patient was injured, and the injury was caused by the nurse's failure to carry out the duty. Examples of common negligent acts are listed in Box 3-4.

The nurse's best protection against negligence and malpractice is to adhere to standards of care. Other measures are to provide competent care; communicate with other members of the health care team; fully document assessments, interventions, and evaluations; and establish good relations with patients (Potter & Perry, 2005).

Student nurses are held to the same standards of care as are licensed nurses. Students should never

Box 3-4 | *Common Negligence Errors*

- Medication errors that result in injury to patients
- Intravenous therapy errors resulting in infiltrations or phlebitis
- Burns to patients caused by equipment, bathing, or spills of hot liquids and foods
- Falls resulting in injury to patients
- Failure to use aseptic technique where required
- Errors in sponge, instrument, or needle counts in surgical cases
- Failure to give a report or giving an incomplete report to an oncoming shift
- Failure to adequately monitor a patient's condition
- Failure to notify a physician of a significant change in a patient's status

From Potter, P.A., Perry, A.G. (2005). *Fundamentals of nursing* (6th ed.). St. Louis, Mosby.

perform care for which they have not been prepared. When nursing students are employed as nursing assistants, they must perform only tasks that are within the job description of the nursing assistant even if they have acquired additional skills as nursing students. For more information on scope of practice, standards of care, and professional responsibility and accountability for LPN/LVNs, see the Management and Supervision boxes on pp. 30 and 31.

Malpractice Insurance

Health care institutions commonly provide malpractice insurance for nurses they employ. This coverage generally covers legal fees and awards if a nurse is sued for professional negligence or medical malpractice. However, if the act in question occurs outside the place of employment, the agency insurance does not cover the nurse. Therefore nurses need to decide whether to carry personal liability insurance as well. It is wise to seek legal advice regarding this decision (Brostron, 2001).

At times, nurses administer assistance at the scene of accidents. As long as nurses' actions are within accepted standards, Good Samaritan laws protect them from liability. Because state laws vary, nurses should acquaint themselves with the laws in their states of residence (Brostron, 2001).

LEGAL CONSIDERATIONS IN SPECIFIC SITUATIONS

Confidentiality

Nurses have access to volumes of extremely private information that must be protected. Patients have a right to expect that their personal information including medical diagnoses and treatment be kept confidential. Therefore you must protect the privacy of patient records and avoid public discussion of patient information. Never copy or remove any part of a patient's record. If you make notes about patients or write care plans for nursing school assignments, do not include

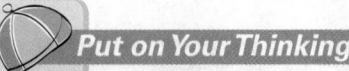 *Put on Your Thinking Cap!*

If a patient's partner accompanies her to an appointment with her obstetrician and calls the clinic later that afternoon to ask a question about the woman's care, can you discuss her medical record with him? Is your answer the same if the man's name is noted in the patient's record as being the father of the child?

identifying information such as the name, initials, or social security number. Such assignments should be shared only with your instructor. The HIPAA laws that went into effect in 2003 have made health care providers acutely aware of the actions needed to protect patient confidentiality. Your employing agency should have written policies for informing patients of their rights and how their health care information can be used (Box 3-5).

Consent

The ethical principle of autonomy mandates that patients have the right to make decisions about their own care and that caregivers should not impose care against the patient's wishes. The term informed consent means that health care providers must provide sufficient information for the patient to make an informed decision. The essential elements of informed consent are patient decision-making capacity, sufficient information, and voluntary agreement.

State law defines who can give consent, including who can give consent for minors or persons who are not capable of making their own decisions. Remember that a confused or sedated person cannot give consent even if that person usually is capable of making deci-

Box 3-5 | *What Does HIPAA Mean for You?*

- You can discuss patient health information with other health care providers who are directly involved in the patient's care.
- You can have patients in a clinic or office register on a "sign in" sheet if no sensitive data are available for others to see.
- With the patient's permission, you can inform clergy that a church member is in the facility.
- You can have patients' names on their rooms.
- You cannot post names with medical diagnoses, surgical procedures, etc. where they can be seen by persons not involved in the patient's care.
- You cannot give health care information to a patient's family or other persons without the patient's permission.
- You can obtain additional information from the Office of Civil Rights at http://www.hhs.gov/ocr/flqs1001.doc .

From Brooke, P.S. (2005). Understanding HIPAA compliance. *LPN 2005, 1*(4), 37-39.

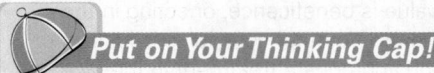

Put on Your Thinking Cap!

What are some reasons a mentally competent person might choose to sign a DNR order in the event that his breathing ceases or his heart stops?

sions. Therefore signatures on consent forms must be obtained before administering preoperative medications. For the patient to have sufficient information for informed consent, the person must have been advised of risks, benefits, alternatives, and consequences of refusing the treatment. A patient has the right to have all questions answered. Consent must be voluntary; there can be no real or implied coercion. That is, the patient must be making the decision freely without fear of retaliation for refusal or because of expectation of some real or implied reward beyond the medical benefit.

In various health care settings, you should know the agency policies regarding the need for signed consent forms. They are required for hospital admission, surgery, some treatments, and research participation. The physician is responsible for obtaining informed consent. Nurses may obtain patient signatures and serve as witnesses to the signature as agency policy permits. If the nurse suspects the patient lacks decision-making capacity or does not fully understand the implications of the consent form, the physician should be contacted and the supervisor notified.

Physician Orders

Legal, appropriate physicians' orders should be carried out. If the nurse believes an order is erroneous or inappropriate, the physician should be contacted for confirmation or correction. If the physician confirms the order and the LVN/LPN still believes it is inappropriate, the nurse should contact the supervisor to intervene. The nurse may share legal responsibility for harm that follows implementation of an inappropriate order. Verbal orders increase the risk for error; follow agency policy regarding these.

DNR (Do Not Resuscitate) Orders

Sometimes a decision is made by the patient or other decision-maker in consultation with the health care team that resuscitation will not be initiated if a patient ceases to breathe or the heart stops. Once such a decision is made, DNR (do not resuscitate) orders should be written, and they should be reviewed regularly in case the patient's status changes. Nurses are encouraged to talk with patients and, if appropriate, with patients' families to help them understand the practical and legal implications of a DNR order. In many states in the absence of a written order, it is assumed that resuscitation is appropriate. "Slow code" orders may be interpreted as below the standard of care.

Short Staffing

When nurses believe staffing is inadequate to provide competent care, the supervisor should be notified. A written protest should be submitted when required to accept an assignment without adequate staffing. Walking out or refusing an assignment could be viewed as patient abandonment. Nurses should know their state regulations and agency policies for such situations. For example, the Texas Nurse Practice Act focuses on the nurse's duty to the patient and emphasizes that "the nurse's duty is not defined by any single event such as clocking in or taking report." Actions that could be interpreted as patient abandonment include sleeping on the job, leaving in the middle of a shift without notifying anyone, failing to show up or complete an agreed assignment in a home setting, and leaving the patient care area and remaining unavailable such that patient safety may be compromised. In some settings, a nurse may be able to invoke "safe harbor" if given an assignment that the nurse believes violates his or her duty to the patient. Safe harbor protects nurses from actions against their license when they notify the supervisor at the time the assignment is made. Again, agency policies and state law must be considered by the individual nurse.

Floating

Nurses are obligated to inform supervisors if they lack skill to care for particular patients. (See the Management and Supervision box below to learn where you can find out more about challenging delegation issues like this one.) Nurses who float to new units

Management and Supervision

The National Council of State Boards of Nursing: A Resource for LPNs

More detailed information about the legal roles and responsibilities of the LPN/LVN are available at the website of the National Council of State Boards of Nursing (www.ncsbn.org) and from individual state licensing bodies. Here's a sampling of what you'll find on the NCSBN site:

- A list of legal requirements for becoming a licensed LPN/LVN, including an NCLEX candidate bulletin and fact sheet
- Complete, current contact information for the board of nursing in your state, including a link to the board's website
- Information about the progress of the NCSBN in developing continued competence assessments for nurses
- The NCSBN's position statements on the issue of working with nursing assistive personnel (NAP), also referred to as unlicensed assistive personnel (UAP)
- A delegation decision-making tree and grid, as well as a concept paper that outlines practical guidelines for delegating responsibilities
- The Five Rights of Delegation

must be oriented to the setting and trained for the new area.

Right to Refuse Treatment

Patients have the right to refuse medical treatment, including life-sustaining care. When patients are not competent to make their own decisions, an effort is made to determine what the person would have wanted. Advance directives help define the patient's wishes. Highly publicized cases like that of Theresa Schiavo have increased public awareness of the importance of making one's wishes known in writing while still able to make decisions. See Chapter 24 for a more complete discussion of legal and ethical issues related to death and dying.

SUMMARY

Patient care is much more than just the management of the effects of illness or injury. The clinical decision-making process must continually screen decisions against the guidelines for ethical conduct. Understanding values, ethics, legal constraints, and the process of resolving ethical dilemmas will facilitate the LVN/LPN in providing care that is not only safe but also ethical.

 Key Points

- Ethics is a system of values for governing human behavior based on morality, motives, and outcomes. In the context of health care, this ethical system is known as *bioethics*.
- Morality is a set of principles, judgments, and beliefs by which a society or culture determines what is right and wrong.
- When moral or ethical principles conflict, an ethical dilemma exists.
- Moral distress occurs when a person feels powerless to follow his or her moral beliefs because of institutional or other barriers. Moral outrage occurs when a person is unable to intervene in an immoral situation.
- Informed consent and advance directives give patients autonomy (self-determination) by allowing them to make their own health care decisions.

- A core nursing value is beneficence, or acting in the patient's best interest. Another core value is justice, or fair, equitable, and appropriate treatment in the face of scarce goods and services.
- The principle of nonmaleficence requires that the nurse not harm the patient, but this idea must weigh the patient's short-term discomfort against long-term treatment goals.
- Fidelity, or faithfulness, is a spoken, written, or implied commitment to provide appropriate, competent patient care within the professional's scope of practice.
- Accountability and responsibility are key aspects of nurses' professional code of ethics. In addition, nurses must provide advocacy for their patients' needs, protect confidentiality of patients' medical records, and maintain veracity (truthfulness) in written and spoken communication with patients and colleagues.
- Values are the beliefs and attitudes that underpin our personal and professional choices. Sometimes our values tend to be ethnocentric, or biased toward our own religious and cultural belief systems.
- Professional education and training can assist in the process of values clarification, which allows us to discover how our values affect our behavior.
- Philosophical frameworks that provide the basis for various ethical belief systems include deontology, utilitarianism, feminist ethics, and ethics of care.
- Ethical problems are complex, cannot be resolved with scientific information alone, and are broadly relevant to other areas of human endeavor.
- Nursing practice is governed by laws that define nurses' functions for their protection and that of their patients.
- Tort law is a specific kind of civil law that classifies violations into intentional and unintentional torts. Malpractice, or professional negligence, is an unintentional tort.
- Informed consent means that a non-sedated adult patient who is sufficiently able to make voluntary decisions is given the information necessary to agree to a procedure or course of treatment.
- A written, legally binding DNR (do not resuscitate) order ensures that a patient will not be resuscitated against his or her wishes.

 Go to your Companion CD-ROM for a Pharmacology Tutorial, Audio Glossary, and 3-D animations.

evolve   Be sure to visit the companion Evolve site at http://evolve.elsevier.com/Linton/ for WebLinks and additional online resources.

REVIEW QUESTIONS *Choose the best answer.*

1. Which of the following is *not* true of ethics in nursing?
   1. It deals with issues of human conduct.
   2. It is concerned with actions, motives, and outcomes.
   3. It prescribes the right answer when an ethical dilemma is present.
   4. It defines processes to explore what constitutes proper conduct.

2. Which of the following is a core nursing value that involves promoting good, preventing harm, and removing the patient from harm?
   1. Malfeasance
   2. Beneficence
   3. Autonomy
   4. Veracity

3. Which of the following is one possible indication that a situation poses an ethical dilemma?
    1. A personal injury attorney has filed a lawsuit.
    2. Scientific information alone does not provide the answer.
    3. Government agencies have been unable to agree on a course of action.
    4. Legislation has been proposed but not enacted into law.

4. Which of the following laws has been enacted primarily to protect patient confidentiality?
    1. Tort law
    2. Do not resuscitate (DNR) orders
    3. Health Insurance Portability and Accountability Act (HIPAA)
    4. Texas Nurse Practice Act

5. Who is able to give legal consent to his or her own treatment?
    1. A 17-year-old honor student who has been accepted to the nursing program at a local college
    2. A recently retired man who is showing unexplained signs of confusion
    3. A known drug user who says she does *not* understand the procedure but trusts the nurse's judgment
    4. A pregnant woman who says she *does* understand the proposed procedure and trusts the nurse's judgment

6. Which of the following statements about do not resuscitate (DNR) orders is true?
    1. The orders should be reviewed regularly in case the patient's status changes.
    2. Even if a written order exists, the physician on call may legally choose to resuscitate a patient if he or she thinks survival is likely.
    3. If a patient is especially ill or is an older adult, the health care team may decide to initiate a "slow code."
    4. The health care institution cannot be held liable for ignoring DNR orders if its staffing falls below a predetermined minimal level.

4 The Leadership Role of the Licensed Practical Nurse

LINDA PORTER

evolve http://evolve.elsevier.com/Linton/

Objectives

After reading and studying this chapter, you should be able to:

1. Differentiate leadership from management.
2. Describe leadership styles.
3. Discuss leadership theories.
4. Discuss management theories.
5. List tips for effective management.
6. Describe the role of the licensed vocational nurse as a team leader.

Key Terms

Be sure to check out the bonus material on the Companion CD-ROM, including selected audio pronunciations.

assignment (p. 41)
autocratic leadership (p. 38)
chaos (p. 36)
delegation (p. 44)
democratic leaders (p. 38)
laissez-faire leadership (lĕs-ā-FĂR, p. 38)
leadership (p. 37)
management (p. 37)
multicratic leaders (p. 39)
participative leadership (păr-tĭs-ĭ-PĀ-tĭv, p. 38)
theory X (p. 39)
theory Y (p. 39)
theory Z (p. 40)
transformational leadership (p. 39)

Licensed practical nurses (LPNs) manage the care of patients in many health care settings in addition to the hospital. In clinics, home health care, and especially in long-term care settings, they typically also manage other care providers. However, the LPN of tomorrow will be expected to have additional skills not only as managers but also as leaders. To move from a focus on tasks for a specific patient to a focus on facilitating the care process, the LPN will need to collaborate with others and influence people and decisions in new ways.

A variety of factors are contributing to this evolution. Formerly, the health care delivery system was predictable in that there was one generally accepted "right way to do things." However, over the past two decades, the system has become increasingly chaotic (disordered) as we embrace the new era of rapid change in infor-

mation and technology and struggle with containing costs. Vicenzi (1997, p. 26) define chaos as "the apparently irregular, unpredictable behavior of deterministic, non-linear systems." In other words, our health care systems are changing quickly and in unique ways as they struggle to provide quality care in an economic manner; however, they are doing so in many creative and varied ways. In chaos there is the opportunity to discover new and more effective ways to provide care. Finding answers to these opportunities will be critical to the survival of our health care organizations and to our patients' well-being. The challenge of finding new ways to provide care is shared by all employees in the organization. Because nurses are so closely involved in the business of health care, that is, in providing the actual care those organizations exist to provide, they are in a critical position to meet this challenge. To find new answers, managed care increasingly demands rapid, coverage specific, decision making at the point of care, expediting cost-efficient care. Consumers of care expect increasingly high-quality care from all care providers. Who better than those who are doing the work to find better ways to do it?

The latest nurse shortage is upon us as well—a situation that often stimulates reevaluation of job responsibilities. Nurses at all levels are being called on to add new skills and functions. Cost-control measures seek to maximize the contribution of each member of the health care team. LPNs bring valuable knowledge and skill to many practice arenas and are positioned to be both leaders and strong collaborative followers in managing and providing care. They are critical players in addressing the increasingly serious nursing shortage. In addition, the increase in long-term residential care required by the growing older adult population has increased the demand for LPNs.

Most long-term care homes are staffed primarily by LPNs and nursing assistants, who provide the bulk of the "hands-on" care. LPNs have traditionally filled leadership or management positions in long-term care facilities, usually as team leaders. Because LPNs are managers of care for the patients to whom they are assigned, it is important that LPNs have a working knowledge of leadership, management, and safe health care delivery. LPNs are assuming more responsible positions such as charge nurses in long-term care facilities and various management roles in other settings. So, we are seeing a shift to LPNs who not only must manage their assigned patients but also must plan, organize, direct, coordinate, and control care provided by others. As changes evolve, LPNs must stay informed of the laws that define their practice in the state where they are employed.

LEADERSHIP VERSUS MANAGEMENT

The terms leadership and management are sometimes used interchangeably, but in fact they have different meanings. Leadership is a broader and more futuristic role, whereas management is more local and task focused. A leader creates a vision that energizes others to follow; a manager is assigned or appointed to the role and focuses on the day-to-day work at hand for the organization. Leadership is a difficult concept to define, but it generally means "guidance" or showing the way to others. Leaders clarify and punctuate unifying values for groups to draw from that, when combined with vision, create a mission for the group to work toward. There are formal leaders (e.g., your boss may be a leader), and there are informal leaders (a person without an official title to whom people listen). Leaders inspire people to strive to accomplish particular goals by doing the right thing. They see beyond the here and now, perhaps beyond the organization's current status, to what might be and are internally driven toward that vision. In contrast, management is the effective use of selected methods to accomplish current organizational goals. Managers are generally driven by external organizational rewards. Management provides the means to achieve the organization's goals by doing the thing right. Managers get things organized so the leader's vision can be achieved. In other words, leadership may be thought of as the inspiration and management may be thought of as the perspiration. Ideally, leadership and management complement and build upon each other.

Both leaders and managers must have certain characteristics to be effective. First, they must be competent. They must have the respect of the people who work with them to accomplish their goals. Second, they must be able to communicate with others. People in leadership and management positions work with other people. Success or failure in interactions depends on their ability to communicate. Finally, leaders and managers must be able to motivate others. They must determine what other people consider important and why they behave as they do. Leaders motivate through values and vision and manage through organizational benefits, such as merit raises and recognition. Use of both leadership and management skills reinforces motivation and enhances positive outcomes for everyone. Some people are motivated by internal forces, such as

Management and Supervision

Characteristics of Leaders and Managers

A good leader and manager:

- Sets realistic goals and works to achieve them
- Seeks new ideas and methods; is willing to try them
- Is a positive thinker
- Is accountable for actions
- Is willing to make decisions even though they involve risks
- Is competent in performing work
- Is an effective communicator
- Is assertive; refuses to be manipulated
- Accepts responsibilities of leadership and delegation
- Is emotionally mature; exercises self-control
- Is committed to providing quality patient care
- Recognizes worth of co-workers and welcomes suggestions; answers their questions
- Is not selfish; is willing to share information with co-workers
- Is able to use self-criticism; gives constructive criticism to others
- Has a sense of humor; is able to laugh at self, never at others
- Is loyal to co-workers
- Is self-confident
- Is never self-satisfied; recognizes the need for continued improvement
- Is a facilitator

Adapted from Corona, D.F. (1982). Followership: The indispensable corollary to leadership. In E.C. Hein & M.J. Nicholson (Eds.), *Contemporary leadership behavior: Selected readings.* Boston: Little, Brown.

altruism, and some are motivated by external forces, such as financial security. Many are motivated in multiple ways. Astute leaders and managers provide multiple motivators.

Good leaders and managers seem to have certain characteristics in common, such as the ability to set realistic goals, the willingness to try out new ideas, and the ability to think positively. The Management and Supervision box above lists the characteristics of good leaders and managers.

LEADERSHIP STYLES

Many different leadership styles are used in various situations. The four basic types of traditional leadership are (1) autocratic, (2) democratic, (3) laissez-faire, and (4) multicratic. As an LPN, you need to understand your predominant style and how to reinforce it or change it, depending on how effective it is in a given situation. You need to understand the styles and approaches of others in these roles. Leadership styles vary according to degrees of freedom and control, the identity of the decision makers, leader activity level, assumption of responsibility, output of the group, efficiency, and the situation

(Table 4-1). Other factors that influence which leadership style will be most effective are the maturity of the group and of the group's leader, the skills of the leader and group members, the cohesiveness of the group, and the predictability of the work to be done. These factors also may determine who the leader should be. The recent application of chaos and quantum theory to leadership suggests a transformational style of leadership in which all members of a group may assume leadership and followership roles in various circumstances based on their unique skills and talents.

AUTOCRATIC LEADERSHIP

Autocratic leadership is also known as *authoritarian, directive,* or *bureaucratic.* Individuals who practice this type of leadership achieve their goals by setting objectives and having them carried out without input or suggestions from others on how to do so. They believe that they have complete authority that should not be questioned. Autocratic leaders do not encourage individual initiative or cooperation among members of the organization; instead, they are task oriented, making decisions independently and issuing orders to those working with them. When an autocratic leader hires an autocratic manager, a power struggle is likely to occur.

Although autocratic leadership does not work well in many situations, in other situations this type of leadership is necessary. For example, during an emergency, one person must take charge because there is no time for group conferences on the best plan of action. Autocratic leadership may also be justified when the leader obviously knows more or has more experience than anyone else in the group. In this situation, group members often need or want someone to tell them what to do and how to do it.

DEMOCRATIC LEADERSHIP

Democratic leaders achieve their goals through the participation of group members by focusing on the individual abilities of each member. People are encouraged to provide input into the problem-solving process, and decisions often are made through group consensus. Everyone in the group is informed of the goals and direction of the organization, so that input has a direct relationship to attaining the goals. Instead of power struggles, democratic leaders turn problems over to the group to manage. The term participative leadership could be seen as a type of democratic leadership. Sources that differentiate the two types describe participative leadership in terms of less freedom for group members, more leader control, and a higher level of responsibility than in the democratic model.

The primary role of the leader is to keep the group headed in the right direction. Democratic leaders lead by suggestion rather than by domination. They persuade and teach rather than rule. Most people who work with a democratic leader have a feeling of satisfaction because they have a part in managing their work situation.

LAISSEZ-FAIRE LEADERSHIP

The opposite of autocratic leadership is laissez-faire leadership. A laissez-faire leader provides little or no directive leadership. Individuals working in this environment are allowed to do anything they want with no direction from administration. Often the result is that people do not know or care about what they are supposed to do, and they may lose all sense of initiative and desire for achievement. The organization then gradually disintegrates into a muddle of confusion. However, laissez-faire leadership may work well with a highly motivated, focused group.

Table 4-1 *Comparison of Traditional Leadership Styles*				
	AUTHORITARIAN	**DEMOCRATIC**	**LAISSEZ-FAIRE**	**MULTICRATIC**
Degree of freedom	Little freedom	Moderate freedom	Much freedom	Little to moderate freedom
Degree of control	High control	Moderate control	No control	Moderate to high control
Decision making	By the leader	By the leader and group	By the group or by no one	By the leader with group input
Leader activity level	High	High	Minimal	High
Assumption of responsibility	Primarily by the leader	Shared	Abdicated	Primarily by the leader
Output of the group	High quantity, good quality	Creative, high quality	Variable, may be poor quality	High quality, high quantity
Efficiency	Very efficient	Less efficient than authoritarian	Inefficient	Efficient

Modified from Tappen, R.M. (1989). *Nursing leadership and management: Concepts and practice* (2nd ed.). Philadelphia: Davis.

MULTICRATIC LEADERSHIP

Multicratic leaders are crosses between autocratic and democratic leaders. They are sometimes called *situational leaders*. They present their own personal views to group members, who provide criticism and comments. The multicratic leader analyzes feedback from the group and then makes all final decisions. Multicratic leaders work well within a group as well as in emergency situations when events need to be handled quickly. The response may not be as quick as it is under autocratic leadership. Group members assist the multicratic leader with setting goals, thereby achieving for themselves a sense of empowerment and control.

TRANSFORMATIONAL LEADERSHIP

Quantum theory tells us that collectively we seek order in our lives and work but that many possibilities for that order exist and that it is not static. In other words, we may deal with the same situation in many different ways, each of which may work; some may work better than others, depending on the context or the people involved. One person cannot see or act on all potential possibilities with equal clarity and skill. Experience, personal values, individual personality, maturity, and education all may influence how one sees a situation as well as what solutions are identified. **Transformational leadership** suggests that, in a well-functioning group that shares a common vision, leadership will flow among the members based on the task or problem at hand and the members' individual skills. Thus all members of the group are both leaders and followers. This style of leadership may not replace reporting lines or formal job responsibilities but it may be very effective in identifying the best option at the moment and in energizing others to take action as they are very involved in the decision-making process.

CLASSIC MANAGEMENT THEORIES

Management theories attempt to explain what motivates people to work. Awareness of management theories helps nurses determine the best management style for their work setting. The classic management theories are labeled *X, Y,* and *Z.* Numerous other types of theories exist. These are briefly described in Table 4-2.

THEORY X

In 1957, Douglas McGregor developed two theories, which he labeled **theory X** and **theory Y**, to explain the nature of people and their relationship to the work environment. Theory X assumes that people in the workplace:

- Find no pleasure in their work
- Dislike responsibility
- Are naturally lazy and prefer to do nothing
- Work mainly for the money
- Work only because they fear being fired
- Are basically childlike and like being told what to do
- Do not want to think for themselves
- Are not capable of making decisions for themselves

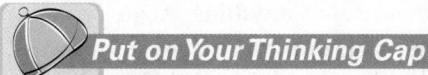

Put on Your Thinking Cap!

Think of a person in your class whom you consider to be a leader. Write down the characteristics that led you to this conclusion. Compare your class leader's characteristics with the identified characteristics in this chapter. Identify the person's leadership style.

Table 4-2 | *Major Leadership Theories*

CLASSIFICATIONS OF THEORIES	CHARACTERISTICS	COMMENTS
Trait	Leaders are those who have specific traits such as the "right" social background, assertiveness, initiative, or charisma. The *great man theory* proposes that leaders are born, not made.	No traits have been identified that are present in all leaders, although they often are above average height and weight, energetic, well educated, self-confident, and have good judgment and interpersonal skills.
Attitudinal	A leader's behavior is shaped by his or her attitude toward employees and production.	The leader may be production-oriented or employee-oriented.
Situational	A leader's effectiveness is affected by the environment and specific situation.	The leader may be described as being the right person in the right place at the right time.
Contemporary	Effective leadership results from the characteristics (traits) of the leader, the leader's attitude, the situation in which leadership is required, and the characteristics of the followers.	Without followers, there would be no leaders. A leader's vision and ability to communicate and move toward that vision is emphasized.

Data from Grossman, S.C., & Valiga, T.M. (2005). *The new leadership challenge: Creating the future of nursing* (2nd ed.). Philadelphia: Davis.

According to theory X, people have these general characteristics and therefore want to be directed and controlled.

Leaders who adhere to the X theory of management usually have an autocratic style.

THEORY Y

According to theory Y, people are dynamic, flexible, and adaptive. It is assumed by believers in this theory that people:

- Are active and enjoy setting their own goals
- Work for rewards other than money, such as doing the job well and working with others in the process
- Are productive because of their own personal goals rather than because of goals set for them
- Are mature and responsible
- Are self-directed
- Accept responsibility
- Care about what they are doing
- Are constantly striving to grow

According to theory Y, people are thought to like their work when they know what is expected of them and when their work gives them satisfaction. Leaders who adhere to the Y theory of management usually have a democratic style.

THEORY Z

Theory Z originated in Japan and describes an organizational philosophy and structure. It grew out of the times when most employees were related to one another and worked together for the good of the company rather than for individual gain. The focus is on participative management based on mutual trust and loyalty.

Employees frequently remain with the same organization for their entire career, learning all areas of its operations and merging their individual success with that of the organization. This form of management involves all workers in every phase of the operation of the company, including planning, organizing, decision making, and problem solving (Fig. 4-1). All members of the

group have similar abilities and status, so they may be rotated to perform different duties. They have complete knowledge and understanding of their organizational objectives and methods of achieving them. It is thought that the theory Z form of management results in greater efficiency and satisfaction among members of the workforce. Leaders with a democratic management style often are able to fit into this type of management.

 Put on Your Thinking Cap!

Situation: You are the charge nurse in a long-term care facility. The nurse manager has asked you to explain the increasing use of disposable items being used on your shift. Explain how you would approach this problem using X, Y, and Z management theories.

FUNCTIONS IN THE MANAGEMENT PROCESS

Management is a problem-oriented process similar to the nursing process. The major functions of management are planning (what is to be done), organizing (how it is to be done), directing (who is to do it), coordinating (who is doing what), and controlling (when and how the task is done).

PLANNING

Planning is the first step in the management process. Planning entails deciding in advance what needs to be done and how to do it. To provide effective care for patients, a good plan for carrying out their care must be developed. Effective planning is as important for individual patient care as it is for a group of patients.

Two important components of planning are *decision making* and *problem solving*. Decision making is the process of selecting one course of action from alternatives. Problem solving is a part of the decision-making process.

The first step in decision making is to identify a problem. Sometimes the problem is quite obvious, but at other times underlying issues make the real problem less obvious. You should go on a "fact-finding mission" to explore all aspects of the situation to identify the real problem. Seek answers to such questions as who, how, when, and why.

Once the real problem has been identified, all possible solutions should be explored. This is a creative process that can involve other people in the health care setting. Often brainstorming sessions are held to obtain input from a variety of sources.

The next step in the decision-making process involves choosing the most desirable action for solving the problem. To select the best solution, you must consider whether the action is likely to accomplish the objectives of the organization. In addition, it is desirable to determine whether the action increases the effective-

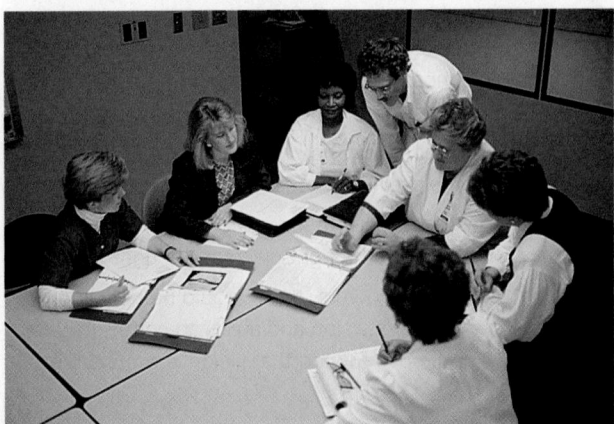

FIGURE **4-1** In the theory Z form of management, workers are involved in every phase of the operation of the organization.

ness and efficiency of the organization and whether it is realistic to try to implement it.

After the decision has been made, it can be implemented. The decision should be communicated to other people who are involved in the organization to gain their support for carrying out the action. The communication should be expressed in such a way that other individuals become supportive of the decision rather than antagonistic toward it. Antagonism and negative feelings can be avoided in many cases when others are involved in the decision-making and problem-solving process from the beginning.

The final step in the decision-making process is to determine how the results will be evaluated. There are many ways to carry out an evaluation. Written tools such as audits or checklists may be used, as may verbal or written feedback from individuals in the organization or from patients who are receiving the care. If the chosen solution to the problem is not satisfactory, another alternative can be selected and tried, followed by another evaluation. The Management and Supervision box below lists the steps in the decision-making process.

ORGANIZING

Organizing is the second step in the management process. When the planning has been completed, there must be a formal structure or organization to ensure that individuals can carry out actions in the most efficient and effective manner possible. Organization also helps develop order, promote cooperation among workers, and foster productivity.

Part of the process of organizing is developing objectives. Objectives help guide the process of planning and organizing. Another part is establishing policies and procedures to provide guidelines for carrying out the objectives. The most qualified people should be assigned to carry out the specific activities and tasks that will best achieve the objectives. To make appropriate staff assignments may involve the development of job

Management and Supervision

Steps in the Decision-Making Process

PROCESS	HOW TO ACCOMPLISH
• Identify a problem	• Go on fact-finding mission: who, how, when, why
• Explore possible solutions	• Involve others: brainstorm
• Choose most desirable action	• Determine whether action is realistic and can achieve organization's objectives
• Implement action	• Communicate decision to others
• Plan evaluation	• Identify how results will be evaluated (audits, feedback, etc.)

descriptions, performance standards, and staffing patterns to provide the best patient care possible.

DIRECTING

The third step of the management process is directing. Directing involves making assignments and directing people to carry out the assignments. It also involves explaining what is to be done, how it is to be done, and why it is to be done.

In nursing, making assignments is related to patient care. Assignments should be made carefully so that the skills of assigned personnel match patient needs. It is important to estimate the difficulty of the task and the time needed to complete the care. Help or additional instruction should be provided whenever necessary.

Only one person should be responsible for making assignments, especially with team nursing. Assignments must be specific, easily understood, and posted where everyone can see them. Staff members should be helped to understand their assignments and the importance of each task.

Directing people to carry out their assignments requires good communication skills and assertive behavior. For directions to be effective, they must be complete and understandable. It is also helpful to give directions in a clear, logical order and to limit the number of directions given at any one time. Providing written directions increases understanding and compliance.

The manner in which directions are given is also important. Usually directions are given in the form of a request, such as "Will you help Mrs. Smith with her bath today?" Requesting an individual to carry out a task encourages cooperation and tends to result in more being accomplished. It implies that the individuals who are giving directions are "working with" people rather than having people "work for" them.

COORDINATING

The fourth step of the management process is coordinating. Coordinating helps pull together various activities to achieve a goal. It ensures that all important activities are being carried out and helps identify overlap, duplication, and omissions. In nursing, coordinating involves personnel and services. You must be sure that proper nursing care is given by the appropriate people.

The coordination process may be carried out within a single nursing unit or among units and departments in a hospital, long-term care facility, or community agency. For example, the nurse may want to be sure that medications are being given by designated team members on a unit.

Coordinating involves skill and experience in problem solving and decision making. It also requires good communication skills and an ability to resolve conflicts within an organization. To be a good coordinator, you should be able to assess what all individuals and groups in the organization are doing and recognize that it is important for all parts of the organization to function effectively for the good of the whole.

CONTROLLING

Controlling or evaluation is the last step in the management process. It is an ongoing process in which the activities of the organization are analyzed to make sure that the plans are being carried out. Both the efficiency and the effectiveness of the organization are evaluated in the controlling process. The purposes of control in nursing service are to determine whether there are enough staff and supplies, whether the operation is economical, and whether the desired objectives have been achieved. Controlling is basically a form of evaluation.

Control has three basic steps:

1. Establishing standards and objectives
2. Measuring performance and comparing the results with the standards
3. Making corrections or adjustments to remedy any deficiencies in the caregiving operations

Continuous Quality Improvement

Quality assurance (QA), *continuous quality improvement* (CQI), and *total quality management* (TQM) are terms that frequently are used in relation to control. Quality assurance measures performance against set standards and expectations and alerts the organization when an action or an outcome falls below the standard. Most agencies have QA committees that set standards for care and evaluate compliance. The American Nurses Association, the American Hospital Association, and the Joint Commission on Accreditation of Healthcare Organizations are organizations that set standards for nursing practice and medical care. Agencies are evaluated to ensure that objectives and standards are being met, and recommendations are made for necessary change. The purpose of CQI is to continually seek new ways to improve nursing practice. CQI is carried out through total quality management and moves the organization to higher performance than QA alone will.

CONFLICT RESOLUTION

Dealing with conflict is an important part of the manager's role. Conflicts arise from differences in many factors such as beliefs, knowledge, opinions, values, personalities, and backgrounds. When a conflict occurs, it creates stress and negative feelings that can adversely affect the work situation. A conflict may be within an individual (intrapersonal conflict), between two or more people (interpersonal conflict), or between individuals and organizations (organizational conflict).

Conflict is a process with four stages:

1. **Frustration:** People believe their goals are being blocked; they feel frustrated. Individuals may become angry or resigned to the situation.
2. **Conceptualization:** Each party formulates a view of the basis for the conflict. Conflicts typically center on perceived differences in facts, goals, how to achieve goals, and the values on which goals are based.
3. **Action:** The conflict leads to various behaviors that may or may not help resolve the conflict.
4. **Outcomes:** Outcome follows the action; goals may be reformulated so they are acceptable to all parties; one party may "win," the other "lose"; emotions may be positive or negative.

There are multiple approaches to conflict resolution. The positive and negative consequences of each are summarized in Table 4-3. Each approach has advantages and disadvantages, so the leader must select the best approach in each situation. To understand how each of these approaches works in a "real" situation, consider the following scenario: You are the charge nurse on a 30-bed unit in a long-term care facility. Nursing assistants (NAs) are assigned to equal numbers of residents in adjacent rooms. During report, one NA, Alice, complains that her assignment is unfair because all but two of her residents require almost total care. She says that all the other NAs have easier assignments. Using various strategies, here are possible solutions:

- *Accommodation:* You shift the care of two residents to other NAs.
- *Collaboration:* You reassess the needs of each group of assigned residents. Recognizing that Alice is correct, you work with the NAs to identify more equitable distribution of assignments to ensure good patient care.
- *Compromise:* You tell Alice that you will alternate NAs assigned to that group of residents.
- *Competition:* You tell Alice that everyone has some residents who require a lot of care and the assignment will stand.
- *Avoidance:* You tell Alice that you have more important things to deal with right now and you go to your office.

For each of these "solutions," think about the positive and negative outcomes. Again, realize that the best solution will vary with the situation. The art of management is to select the best approach for the situation.

TIPS FOR EFFECTIVE MANAGEMENT

Managing health care workers is a complex task. Some strategies you may use to improve your management skills are to (1) take an active approach to planning, avoiding conflict before it happens; (2) have a clear vision, communicate it well, listen and stay focused, (3) emphasize the importance of documentation as a part of management; (4) treat other health care workers or

Table 4-3 | *Modes of Conflict Resolution*

MODE	POSITIVE OUTCOMES	NEGATIVE OUTCOMES	WHEN TO USE
Accommodation	Agreement is reached.	Differences are suppressed; may leave anger or resentment.	You are wrong. The other person really does have a better idea. The issue is more important to the other party than to you. You are outnumbered or outranked.
Collaboration	Generates commitment to work together. Focuses on shared higher goals such as good patient care—not individual immediate needs. Builds understanding and empathy.	Wastes time if used for resolution of trivial issues or issues in which the outcome has already been decided.	To build understanding. To find creative solutions that accommodate higher common goals. To address difficult issues that affect productivity.
Compromise	Can produce mutually acceptable solutions. Both parties have achieved something they wanted.	The compromised solution may not be the best even though it "keeps the peace."	When time pressures require quick solution. When each party is firmly committed to different views. A compromise can produce acceptable outcomes.
Avoidance	Temporarily defuses highly charged, emotional disagreement. Allows both parties to "cool off" until a reasonable approach can be considered.	The conflict is not resolved. Neither party is satisfied.	To deal with trivial issues when more important issues are waiting. To delay a decision until parties are calmer, more information is obtained, etc. When one party's demands cannot possibly be met. When others could resolve the issue more readily.
Competition	Reflects a strong stance to defend important principles, protect vulnerable parties. Person in power takes responsibility for a decision.	Can generate bad feelings. Creates a winner and a loser. May generate behaviors that block the actions of the "winner."	When a quick decision is essential. To implement unpopular, nonnegotiable actions. To defend important principles, individual rights, group welfare.

team members as you would like to be treated yourself; (5) keep confidential information confidential; (6) make employees accountable for their actions and be accountable for yours; and (7) seek help and support from a variety of sources. LPNs frequently are asked to assume responsibilities for the care that other staff members give to patients. You may have nursing assistants, unlicensed assistive personnel, technicians, or other practical nurses reporting to you. Your role is not simply to tell them what to do; you must be both a leader and a manager.

THE LICENSED PRACTICAL NURSE AS A LEADER

TEAM NURSING

Team nursing was introduced during the 1950s when there was a shortage of professional nurses and an abundance of auxiliary nursing staff. The team functions by using the skills and knowledge of the professional nurse to direct the care provided by a diverse staff through group action. All members of the team are expected to have input into the nursing care process by contributing suggestions and sharing ideas.

THE ROLE OF THE TEAM LEADER

The functions of the team leader are to plan, set priorities for, supervise, and evaluate patient care. The role of the team leader traditionally was carried out by a registered nurse (RN) because it was thought that only RNs were prepared to plan nursing interventions, provide supervision, make independent decisions, and evaluate nursing care or the work of team members. However, in many cases, an LPN is assigned to the position of team leader, especially in long-term care settings. In these cases, the job description must differentiate between the practice of an RN team leader and that of an LPN team leader.

Team leaders are responsible for the ongoing collection of data about each patient and for assisting in the determination of appropriate nursing interventions. They must be sure that medical orders and plans are carried out and documented. Team leaders initiate discharge planning, identify referral needs, and facilitate patient education. They are also responsible for keeping care plans current and documenting the nursing care provided. In addition, team leaders are responsible for planning and conducting team conferences and reporting changes to the RN supervisor. An LPN who assumes the position of team leader can help carry out these responsibilities under the supervision and guidance of an RN.

ISSUES RELATED TO TEAM LEADERSHIP

Specific issues such as making assignments and delegation, accident prevention and safety, and accountability concern the team leader.

Making Assignments

You cannot do everything for all patients. To be effective, you must be able to assign tasks to others who are hired to perform them and make sure that those tasks are carried out. An ongoing delegation process by nurses allows nurses to accomplish nursing care for more clients than one individual could provide alone. Before you make assignments or delegate as a team leader, you must consult your nurse practice act. Delegation, as defined by the National Council of State Boards of Nursing (NCSBN) is "the act of transferring to a competent individual the authority to perform a selected nursing task in a selected situation." (*To assign* is to direct an individual to do activities within an authorized scope of practice. Using the verb *assign* in this way is a variation of delegation.) Among nurses working in clinical settings, delegation involves "working through others" and assignment describes "what a person is directed to do" (NCSBN, 2006, p. 20). Assignment describes the distribution of work that each staff member is to accomplish in a given work period. In this book, *delegation* will refer to "working through others" and *assignment* describes what a person is asked to do. Currently, 39 state boards of nursing authorize delegation by RNs; 23

boards authorize delegation by LPNs/LVNs (NCSBN, 2006, p. 6). There is no clear consensus among the states regarding use of delegation. Some states allow RNs only to delegate to unlicensed personnel. In one state, nurses never delegate. Other states allow nurses to delegate to other licensed personnel.

The assignment is used in many work settings by LPN/LVNs. Making assignments involves identifying specific tasks needed to provide care for a specific person. You usually assign the care of several patients to each staff member. Before you can make assignments, you must know what care each patient requires and you must know the strengths and weaknesses of staff members. Assignments are based on patient needs, available staff, job descriptions, scope of practice for licensed nurses, and scope of functions for nursing assistants (NCSBN, 2006, p. 13).

Although LPNs do not have to delegate authority in many states and cannot delegate tasks to unlicensed personnel, they can assist RNs in the management process. Following delegation by an RN to unlicensed personnel, LPNs may assist in the supervision of unlicensed personnel, may assist in training unlicensed personnel, and may verify competencies of unlicensed assistive personnel. In many states, the delegating RN remains accountable for this process, since RNs are accountable for the tasks delegated to unlicensed persons. Delegation is a management tool that RNs (and in some states, LPNs) use at their discretion. Always, when delegating a task, you have a duty to maintain patient safety. Effective delegation requires delegating a clearly identified task, identifying patient needs, empowering the staff person to carry out activities to complete the task, and monitoring staff performance. Delegating tasks is specified in your job description; you are delegating some of your responsibilities, according to your state's nurse practice act. To delegate, you must know the background skill level of the persons to whom you delegate tasks. You must find out what the unlicensed personnel know, delegate appropriately, and document the outcomes.

Essential elements of effective delegation include knowing your state nurse practice act statements on delegation and your institution's policy and procedures manual, knowing the training and background of persons to whom you delegate tasks, deciding which tasks can be safely delegated, and evaluating the patient's response. You must delegate only *tasks* to unlicensed personnel; you may not delegate *nursing processes* to unlicensed personnel. The nursing practice functions of assessment, planning, evaluation, and nursing judgment cannot be delegated. Delegation is specific on each client. An unlicensed person who completes a task for one patient cannot do the same task for all patients. Delegation is also situation specific. You delegate a task for one patient in one situation.

Accident Prevention and Safety

Every health care facility must meet minimum safety regulations established by law in addition to those adopted by the agency to meet its unique needs. All staff members, particularly the team leader, should learn these regulations during orientation to the job. The team leader should know the regulations and be sure that staff members are aware of them. Everyone must understand procedures to follow in case of disasters such as fires, tornadoes, or hurricanes. In addition, everyday safety issues related to handling equipment, using proper procedures, and working with potentially dangerous drugs must constantly be addressed to be sure that knowledge and skills are up to date.

Accountability

Team leaders must demonstrate accountability for their own actions as well as the actions of the staff they are directing. Accountability means that a person is answerable for his or her actions; that is, he or she may be called on to explain or justify them. Team leaders also are legally responsible for all nursing care and documentation. It is the responsibility of the RN team leader to ensure that proper and accurate charting is carried out for all nursing assessments, interventions, and evaluations.

Accountability also involves communicating patient needs to others through both oral and written interactions. A common form of communication is the report given at the end (or beginning) of every shift. The LPN is usually responsible for reporting to the RN in charge but may be only indirectly responsible for the report. Guidelines for clear and complete reporting are as follows:

- Organize the report before beginning.
- Give the patient's room number, name, age (if appropriate), diagnosis, and physician.
- Provide a brief account of each patient's condition, including new or changed orders.
- Refer to vital signs, temperature elevations, intravenous fluids, and intake and output as relevant.
- For patients receiving pain medication, note the drug name, dosage, prescribed frequency, time of last administration, and effectiveness.
- Cover the necessary information for preoperative patients, including the preoperative teaching done, the time of preoperative medications, completion of surgical checklists, and the like.
- Give information about postoperative patients, including the time of arrival from the operating or recovery room, general condition, vital signs, intravenous fluids required (e.g., kind, rate of flow, fluids to follow), dressings, voiding, diet, nature of breathing, coughing, and type, location, and patency of tubes.

The report may be given by means of a tape recording, in a one-to-one discussion with another nurse, as a summary in a group conference, or during walking

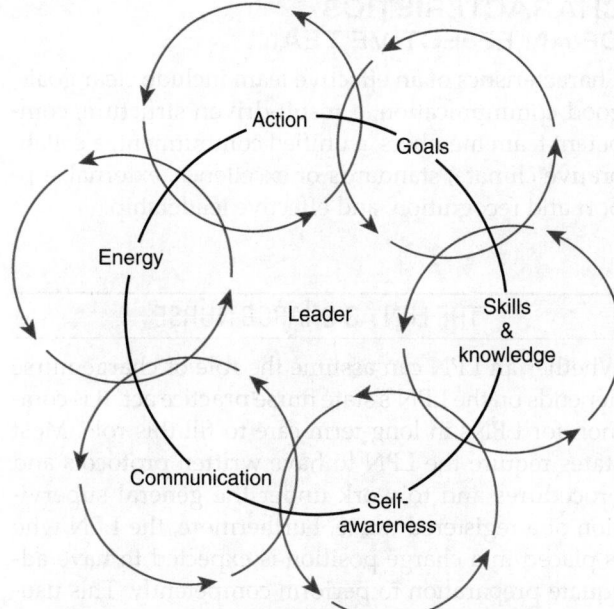

FIGURE **4-2** Components of effective team leadership.

rounds at the bedside. The key to good communication is to be clear, concise, and thorough.

CHARACTERISTICS OF AN EFFECTIVE TEAM LEADER

Effective team leaders must have skills in leadership, management, and supervisory techniques. They should be able to communicate effectively, both orally and in writing. Effective team leaders are able to work well with others and show that they value others' input and suggestions regarding patient care. Figure 4-2 illustrates components of effective team leadership. The leader's possession of these qualities leads to greater satisfaction among the staff and a higher quality of patient care.

To be a good team leader, you must also understand how to build an effective team. A team is more than just a group of people. It is a group of people who need to work together to achieve a goal or task (in this case, delivery of care to patients). Strategies to build an effective team include the following:

- **Establish a clear purpose.** All team members must understand and value their purpose.
- **Listen actively.** Active listening requires genuine interest in understanding another's message, not just waiting for your turn to speak.
- **Be compassionate.** Recognize stress and distress in team members; show genuine concern.
- **Be honest.** Take ownership of your opinions and attitudes; provide constructive feedback.
- **Be flexible.** Recognize that good ideas can come from any team member; invite input and be willing to consider other suggestions and viewpoints.
- **Be committed to conflict resolution.** Resolve to find creative solutions that leave all involved in agreement.

CHARACTERISTICS OF AN EFFECTIVE TEAM

Characteristics of an effective team include clear goals, good communication, a result-driven structure, competent team members, a unified commitment, a collaborative climate, standards of excellence, external support and recognition, and effective leadership.

THE LPN AS CHARGE NURSE

Whether an LPN can assume the role of charge nurse depends on the LPN's state nurse practice act. It is common for LPNs in long-term care to fill this role. Most states require the LPN to have written protocols and procedures and to work under the general supervision of a registered nurse. Furthermore, the LPN who is placed in a charge position is expected to have adequate preparation to perform competently. This usually requires education, training, and/or experience beyond the basic LPN educational program. To function as charge nurse, the LPN should be able to assign patient care, assess patients, delegate or assign tasks (as permitted by state laws), receive and give shift report, and handle common workplace issues.

Key Points

- Licensed practical nurses make up the primary staffing and management of most long-term care homes.
- Leadership is defined as guidance, or showing the way to others.
- Management is defined as the effective use of selected methods to accomplish goals.
- Leaders and managers must be competent, must have the respect of the people they work with, and must be able to motivate others.
- Four basic types of leadership are autocratic, democratic, laissez-faire, and participative.
- Autocratic leaders are authoritarian, meaning they act without input or suggestions from others.

- Democratic leaders achieve their goals through participating, encouraging others to provide input, and making decisions through group consensus.
- Laissez-faire leaders allow group members to do anything they want with no direction from administration.
- Participative leaders have a mixture of autocratic and democratic characteristics, soliciting input from group members but making the final decisions themselves.
- Leadership styles are based on leaders' assumptions about workers' motivations.
- The major functions of management are planning, organizing, coordinating, directing, and controlling.
- Planning, the first step in the management process, involves decision making and problem solving.
- Organizing provides a structure for carrying out the plan.
- Directing involves making assignments and directing people to carry out the assignments.
- Coordinating pulls various activities together to achieve a goal.
- Controlling includes establishing standards, measuring performance by the standards, and making corrections to remedy deficiencies.
- Strategies for conflict resolution include accommodation, compromise, competition, avoidance, and collaboration.
- The most appropriate strategy for conflict resolution depends on the situation.
- Team nursing was designed to use the skills and knowledge of the licensed nurse to direct the care provided by a diverse staff through group action.
- Team leaders conduct ongoing assessments of patients and determine appropriate nursing interventions.
- A good team leader is skilled in leadership, management, and supervisory techniques.
- To build an effective team, the leader must establish a clear purpose; listen actively; be compassionate, honest, and flexible; and be committed to resolution of conflicts.

 Go to your Companion CD-ROM for a Pharmacology Tutorial, Audio Glossary, and 3-D animations.

evolve Be sure to visit the companion Evolve site at http://evolve.elsevier.com/Linton/ for WebLinks and additional online resources.

REVIEW QUESTIONS *Choose the best answer.*

1. An LPN has been offered a position as a charge nurse in a nursing home. How can the nurse best determine the legal limits of practice in this role?
   1. Ask the nursing home administrator what the charge nurse is expected to do.
   2. Review a textbook that discusses the LPN as charge nurse.
   3. Ask other LPNs who have experience as charge nurses.
   4. Contact the state board of nursing.

2. Which leadership style is demonstrated when a charge nurse makes the following statement during report: "I don't care how you organize your work, as long as you finish your assignments on time"?
   1. Autocratic
   2. Democratic
   3. Laissez-faire
   4. Participative

3. A manager who applies the theory Y assumes that people in a work environment:
   1. Find no pleasure in their work
   2. Work mainly for the money
   3. Are mature and responsible
   4. Have similar abilities and status

4. The nursing assistants on your unit complain that the workload is unevenly distributed and ask you to try to find a better way to make assignments. The first step in your decision-making process should be to:
   1. Identify and explore the nature of the problem
   2. List potential solutions to the problem
   3. Tell the nursing assistants to work it out together
   4. Change the way you make their assignments

5. Which direction by the team leader is most likely to encourage cooperation among nursing assistants?
   1. I expect you to pitch in and help each other.
   2. Since you have finished your morning care, go help Mary catch up.
   3. Whoever finishes morning care first can take the first lunch break.
   4. Ed, would you please help Mary by taking vital signs on her newly admitted patient?

6. What is the most important factor an LPN team leader must consider when assigning a task to a nursing assistant?
   1. Institutional policies regarding nursing assistant functions
   2. The background skill level of the nursing assistant
   3. The nursing assistant's willingness to perform the task
   4. State board of nursing regulations related to nursing assistants

Objectives

After reading and studying this chapter, you should be able to:

1. Define the holistic view of nursing.
2. Define the concept of *self*.
3. Discuss the use of self in the practice of nursing.
4. Compare the meaning of the terms *patient* and *client*.
5. List commonly held expectations of patients and families.
6. Describe the meaning of the AHA Patient Care Partnership document.
7. Describe guidelines for nurse-patient relationships.
8. Describe basic components of communication.

Key Terms

Be sure to check out the bonus material on the Companion CD-ROM, including selected audio pronunciations.

action (p. 48)
caring (p. 48)
client (p. 50)
empathy (p. 53)
empower (p. 50)
holism (p. 48)
patient (p. 50)
self (p. 48)
therapeutic relationship (p. 48)
understanding (p. 48)
values (p. 49)

Nursing means caring for persons. **Caring** is a process characterized by understanding, action, and concern. **Understanding** is the ability to listen to and relate to others to perceive their feelings and the meaning of their words. **Action** denotes responding to others with genuineness, compassion, sensitivity, and self-disclosure to promote their well-being.

In the caring process, a therapeutic relationship develops between patients and nurses. Unlike a social relationship, a **therapeutic relationship** is goal-directed and focuses on one individual (the patient). To develop therapeutic relationships, nurses must value and accept patients as unique individuals. In addition, nurses must be aware of themselves as individuals. Knowing how your own attitudes, feelings, and beliefs affect others is vital to effective communication. A nonjudgmental attitude of caring is essential to the practice of nursing.

A HOLISTIC VIEW OF NURSING CARE

Holism is a way of viewing people as whole individuals. According to the holistic theory, people are complex creatures made up of many parts. Each part interacts with the others, and the sum of the parts forms a unified whole. Holistic health care is a system of comprehensive patient care that considers the physical, emotional, social, economic, and spiritual needs of individuals and families. The importance of the family to the individual and the role of the nurse in working with families are discussed in Chapter 7.

Individuals are composed of mind, body, and spirit. It is not possible to care for one part without considering how the other parts are affected. Thus a nursing plan of care must consider physiologic, psychological, sociologic, and spiritual influences (Fig. 5-1). For example, a surgical patient has many physical needs such as pain management, fluid replacement, and wound healing. But these needs reflect only the physical component. The patient also may be frightened about the surgery itself or fearful that he will not be able to return to work. Perhaps he needs education so that he can care for himself after discharge or needs help locating appropriate social services. If the illness is chronic or life-threatening, his spiritual needs may become more prominent.

USE OF THE SELF IN NURSING

Many tools are used in the process of providing nursing care, including stethoscopes, sphygmomanometers, and thermometers; however, there is no more important tool that you bring to each patient encounter than the use of self. **Self** is a term used to describe one's personhood: the knowledge, experience, values, beliefs, perceptions, strengths, and weaknesses that make each individual unique. As a nurse, your attitudes, beliefs, self-esteem, and feelings become a part of the patient's therapeutic environment, just as those of the patient become a part of your environment. With your assistance, individuals and their families may find meaning in their experience and may achieve a harmonious state of health.

VALUES, BELIEFS, AND ATTITUDES

Self-awareness involves knowing one's own values, beliefs, and attitudes. You should be able to answer

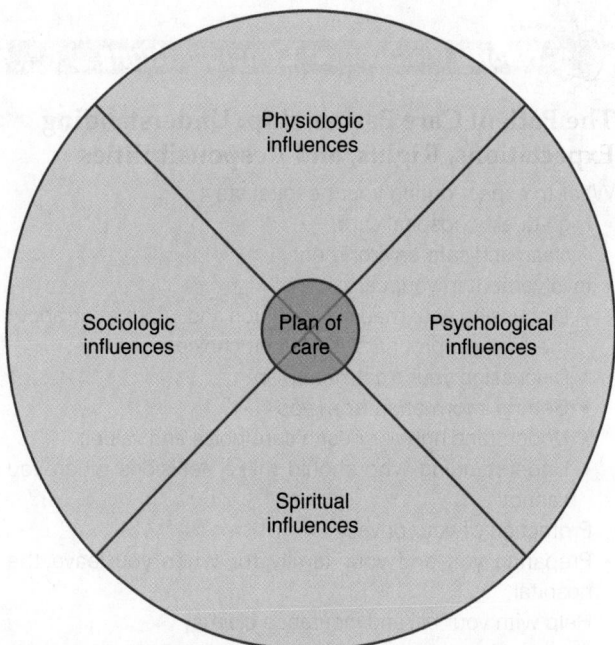

FIGURE **5-1** Physiologic, psychological, sociologic, and spiritual influences on individual behaviors become integrated into a plan of care.

the questions "Who am I?," "What do I believe?," and "What is important to me?" so that you can help others answer those questions. Almost every day, you will encounter situations that require value judgments. You must make certain choices related to patient care, respond to requests for help and guidance, and provide emotional and spiritual support. Your values, attitudes, and beliefs are outwardly expressed in your behavior as you interact with patients.

As discussed in Chapter 3, values can be defined as principles or standards shared by members of a society that determine what is desirable or worthwhile. A value is reflected in the worth you give to an idea or action. A *belief* is a conviction or opinion. *Attitudes* are reactions that flow from values and beliefs. An attitude indicates a feeling toward persons or things. Values and personal beliefs are developed in many ways. They may be acquired from religious education, from examples set by authority figures such as parents and teachers, or from peers. Acquiring values and beliefs is a lifelong process that is affected by one's life experience. As people age, they generally have a fairly fixed set of values, but even older people are able to grow and change.

KNOWLEDGE

Knowledge is a component of self that is acquired through experience or study. The safe practice of nursing depends on one's knowledge base, and nursing education provides a basic understanding of the physical and social sciences. Nurses use their knowledge of biological, psychological, and social sciences

to give the best care possible. This knowledge is often shared with patients, families, and the community to promote health, prevent disease, and cope with illness. Nurses also share their knowledge with colleagues on the health care team. Because knowledge about health care is continually growing and the health care system is changing, you will be challenged to continue to learn and expand your knowledge. For example, there is a greater emphasis on prevention of disease and promotion and maintenance of health than in the past. Nurses not only must be informed about healthy practices but also must act as models of healthy living.

Simply having a collection of facts is not sufficient. As a nursing student, you will be expected to develop your critical thinking skills. Critical thinking enables you to think through problems in an efficient and organized manner. It requires that you seek and use information, not just recite facts. This is essential because real-life situations are seldom as "cut and dried" as they are in textbooks. Because each patient is unique, nursing care must be individualized, and that requires critical thinking. Chapter 12 discusses critical thinking in relation to nursing care.

SKILLS

Nursing is a skill-oriented field. Nursing care involves the use of many skills that require efficiency and safety. A nurse must master the skills required to carry out nursing interventions including the technical skills needed to use sophisticated equipment. Your hands can be instruments of healing when used with compassion, competence, and gentleness. The simple act of giving a bed bath or a backrub can be the best use of self that you offer a suffering patient.

Nurses need *interpersonal skills* to communicate effectively and to establish caring relationships with patients. It is through the caring relationship that you are able to build a therapeutic relationship with the patient. Developing therapeutic nurse-patient relationships requires:

- A humanistic system of values
- Ability to instill faith and hope
- Sensitivity to one's self and to others
- Ability to develop helping, trusting relationships
- Ability to express both positive and negative feelings
- Ability to use problem-solving methods for decision making
- Ability to promote interpersonal teaching and learning
- Ability to provide a supportive, protective, and corrective mental, physical, sociocultural, and spiritual environment
- Ability to assist with meeting human needs
- Ability to allow for the uniqueness of individuals and their experiences

THE PERSPECTIVE OF THE PATIENT

The term patient is used to refer to an individual, a family, a group, or a community. Patients may function in independent, interdependent, and dependent roles. As recipients of nursing care, patients may receive nursing interventions related to disease prevention, health promotion, health maintenance, illness management, and end-of-life care.

PATIENT VERSUS CLIENT

Some nurses use the term *client* rather than *patient*. This term evolved from a general belief or attitude about the nurse-patient relationship. Those who prefer the word client believe it denotes a feeling of partnership or working with someone and that the word *patient* has a connotation of doing to or for someone. The word patient also may imply that an individual is ill. For some nurses, *client* seems to represent a more accurate view of the roles in the nurse-patient relationship because the nurse values patients as individuals, honors their individuality, and helps them achieve the highest level of wellness possible. However, because *patient* also is used and accepted by nurses and other health care professionals, and frequently by older adults as well, *patient* and *client* are used interchangeably. The term *patient* has been used for years and is used frequently in this text in support of the long-established tradition of the nurse-patient relationship. Depending on the context, patients may be referred to as *clients* or *consumers of nursing services*. Client is more commonly used in outpatient settings. Another term, *resident*, is commonly used to refer to persons who reside in long-term care settings.

PATIENTS' RIGHTS

Patients, as participants in nursing care, are entitled to receive quality care in a safe, supportive, and nurturing environment. As the health consumer movement becomes more and more active, greater attention is being paid to the rights of patients. In 1973, the American Hospital Association issued a Patients' Bill of Rights that outlined the rights of hospital patients and incorporated the components of quality care. Recently this document was replaced with a pamphlet that advises patients how they can expect to be treated during hospitalization and what caregivers will need from the patient to provide good care. Key topics of this pamphlet are outlined in the Health Promotion Considerations box above. Nurses are in a position to be certain that many of these rights are respected. One very basic way to help patients feel respected as individuals is to address and refer to them by name at all times. Be careful to pronounce the name correctly, and introduce the patient by name to other health care providers. Never refer to patients by bed number or medical diagnosis.

All patients, no matter what their age or state of mind, deserve to be treated with the same respect. It is

Health Promotion Considerations

The Patient Care Partnership: Understanding Expectations, Rights, and Responsibilities

What to expect during your hospital stay:
- High-quality hospital care
- A clean and safe environment
- Involvement in your care:
  - Discussing your medical condition and information about medically appropriate treatment choices
  - Discussing your treatment plan
  - Getting information from you
  - Understanding your health care goals and values
  - Understanding who should make decisions when you cannot
- Protection of your privacy
- Preparing you and your family for when you leave the hospital
- Help with your bill and insurance claims

Reprinted with permission of the American Hospital Association. Copyright © 2003.

inappropriate for a nurse to call an older patient anything other than Mr. Smith or Mrs. Smith unless the patient has requested it. Terms such as "Pops," "Sweetie," "Gramps," or "Baby" are unprofessional and demeaning to older individuals (Fig. 5-2).

PATIENTS' EXPECTATIONS
Explanation of the Care

The experience of illness and all the changes in a person's life that it precipitates is very stressful. A method that you can use to help reduce patients' stress and anxiety levels is to empower them to participate in their care. To do this, patients must be given the information they need to be active participants. Patients need and are entitled to an explanation of the care to be given so that they know what to expect and what is expected of them. Patients who are knowledgeable about their care are more likely to be active participants who are better satisfied and less anxious. Explanations and teaching often are left to the nurse. Communication should take place in language that patients understand, without talking down to them. Interpreters should be utilized if needed to improve communication. Patients who are not given adequate explanations of what is to be done have been denied their rights as human beings.

With so many technological and medical advances, many options for treatment may be available to the patient. To make informed decisions about their health care choices, patients need to be provided or have access to the knowledge needed. The nurse may be able to help the patient acquire that information by providing a referral to an appropriate source. Health care information and disease prevention guidelines need to be provided in a way that is individualized to their personal characteristics and lifestyles.

FIGURE **5-2** Older people should be treated with the same respect as younger people.

Patients as Partners in Care

As consumers of health care services, most patients no longer are willing to assume a passive role. They not only want to assume more responsibility for their care but also expect to do so. Patients who see themselves as partners in their care are more likely to accept responsibility for their care. Their sense of responsibility may improve compliance with the plan of care, thereby preventing needless complications.

The patient can assume an active role from the point of admission. The initial encounter is your first opportunity to set the tone for a relationship that encourages patient participation. You can help patients understand that their participation is not only wanted but also needed. You should assess patients to determine to what extent they wish to participate in their care. The patient's family also should be encouraged to participate in the care whenever possible.

Some patients are more willing than others to accept the role of partner. Factors that may have an effect on patients' decisions to participate in their care are age, ethnicity, personality, social class, educational level, and previous experiences.

Acceptance of Patient Behaviors

Illness is a stressful event and can cause people to react in unusual ways. In many cases, individuals' behavior is different from what it would be under normal circumstances, and nurses should not take this personally. It is important to patients that nurses and health care providers accept patients' behavior.

For a nurse-patient relationship to be therapeutic, you must be able to see patients' experiences from their perspectives. Encourage patients to share thoughts and feelings freely without fear of being judged. You must be willing to accept unconditionally the patient's values, beliefs, behaviors, and attitudes. Avoid imposing your own values and beliefs on the patient whose values differ from yours. This kind of nurse-patient relationship is a special kind of caring in which the nurse has a high regard for the whole person. It conveys a sense of worth and dignity. Nurses should provide compassionate understanding of their patients' behavior and maintain a therapeutic, accepting environment.

Safety and Security

You have a high degree of responsibility for keeping your patients both physically and psychologically safe while in your care. You must assess a situation quickly, make a decision, and act promptly to solve the problem. A patient needs to feel that a nurse can act quickly and decisively in a crisis to provide the best care possible.

Competence and consistency are two factors that can alleviate stress in patients. Nurses who appear confident and competent help patients feel more secure. In addition, performing nursing procedures consistently can help reduce anxiety and build patients' confidence in the nurse. For example, changing dressings in the same step-by-step manner every time helps patients know what to expect and reassures them of the competence of your care.

GUIDELINES FOR THE NURSE-PATIENT RELATIONSHIP

THE HELPER ROLE

A helping role occurs when one person reaches out to help another. The goal is to help another individual grow, mature, cope, and function. A helping relationship is one in which there is genuine caring and compassion.

The following characteristics are necessary for the nurse to assume a helping role:

- Awareness of self
- Ability to analyze own feelings
- Ability to serve as a model to others
- Desire to help others
- Strong sense of ethics and high principles
- Sense of responsibility

Nurses act as helpers by administering direct care to patients, acting as advocates on their behalf, giving psychosocial support, and providing health education and counseling. As a helper, the nurse strives to establish and maintain a therapeutic relationship. The first step in developing a therapeutic relationship is to build trust. Trust develops as the patient begins to feel safe with the nurse. A feeling of safety comes from knowing that the nurse is honest and open and from gaining confidence in the nurse's skill and knowledge. Nurses may use friendly, informal communication initially as a means of putting the patient at ease, but eventually the conversation must focus back on the patient. One strategy to build a therapeutic relationship is to encourage patients to share personal stories about their lives.

A helper in the professional sense is different from a friend. The term *friend* connotes intimacy or affection. You must transcend the role of friend to take on a caring role that requires the patient's needs to take priority over your own. In this way you can facilitate the health of the patient. There is mutual responsibility between patient and nurse in a partnership that is different from the responsibilities that friends have toward one another. Friendships with patients can interfere with the therapeutic process, but strong, authoritarian approaches can interfere also. Including patients and their families in care planning is an example of shared responsibility.

Therapeutic communication is an art and a skill. It takes time and practice to maintain the focus on the patient with genuine warmth and honesty. Self-disclosure refers to the ability to be open and honest about one's feelings. You should not disclose personal information, however, as you would do in a friendship. Table 5-1 notes some differences between a helping person and a friend.

Touch can be used to show concern, to let the patient know you are present, or to provide comfort. Giving a bedridden patient a backrub before sleep can stimulate circulation, provide a caring moment, and promote relaxation. However, responses to touch differ from person to person. Some people are more comfortable with touching and being touched than others. Some patients may mistake touch as an invitation to intimacy.

COMMUNICATION

Communication skills are essential for carrying out the helper role. Communication is the process of exchanging ideas, beliefs, thoughts, and feelings between two or more people. It involves a message, a sender, and a receiver. The sender gives the message to the receiver.

The two types of communicative behavior are verbal and nonverbal language. Verbal language conveys meanings through words, whereas nonverbal language conveys meanings through symbols and actions other than words. Examples of nonverbal communication are body position, facial expression, gestures, moaning, crying, laughing, and smiling. Observation of nonverbal language is as important to the communication process as listening is to verbal language. Nonverbal language can indicate a person's thoughts and feelings as well as, if not better than, verbal language can. Nonverbal actions can be in conflict (i.e., incongruent) with the content of what is being said and thus can give clues to true feelings. For example, patients may claim that everything is all right but may be slumped over and wringing their hands. An astute nurse should recognize that something is indeed wrong even though patients deny it verbally. Language is influenced by the cultural context in which it is used. To interpret the meaning of what is said or done without consideration of cultural context equals stereotyping.

Communication can be assertive or aggressive. Assertive communication is the ability to express yourself without violating the rights of another person. Aggressive communication does violate the rights of others. Try to express yourself without violating the rights of another person.

Two essential parts of communication are *listening* and *observation*. Listening is an active process that involves trying to understand what is being said. The listener must display genuine interest and concentration to derive meaning from the words. A good listener can provide reassurance, lighten another person's burden, and clarify misunderstandings.

Professional communication refers to the factors that help create a therapeutic relationship. The nurse demonstrates professional communication by practicing common courtesy, introducing himself or herself to patients and their families, addressing patients respectfully by their last name, maintaining privacy and confidentiality, being trustworthy, and being self-directed and self-assured.

Therapeutic communication is a skill that can be learned through study, observation, and practice. It

Table 5-1	*Comparison Between a Nurse as a Helping Person and a Nurse as a Friend*

HELPING PERSON	FRIEND
Responsible to client	Relationship is for friendship or support
Objective of relationship is to meet client's needs	Individuals meet each other's needs
Relationship is goal directed	No plan is involved
Attitude is nonjudgmental	Both individuals express feelings, attitudes, and opinions
Does not attempt to influence client to helper's way of thinking	Friends try to influence each other in discussing issues such as religion, politics, and personal philosophy
Does not keep secrets, and explains in a direct manner the need to work with the treatment team	Friends may keep secrets
Discourages any sexual overtones in relationship	Sexual overtones or a sexual relationship may develop
Interacts with clients in health care settings	Interaction may occur in any setting.
Relationship is time limited	Relationship may continue

requires you to be open, honest, and nonjudgmental. Self-awareness is basic to meaningful interactions. Nurses must actively seek to be cognizant of their own thoughts, feelings, values, beliefs, and behaviors. To do this, they need to self-explore and assess how the following areas may affect their ability to establish a therapeutic nurse-patient relationship:

- Ethnic, cultural, and socioeconomic background
- Attitudes, values, opinions, and beliefs
- Past unresolved experiences that are still emotionally laden
- Physical and psychological strengths and weaknesses

To initiate a therapeutic interaction, focus your attention on the patient and listen carefully. Data that will help obtain a holistic assessment of the patient include the following:

- The patient's age.
- The patient's cultural background.
- The patient's perception of his or her illness.
- The patient's use of direct eye contact.
- The patient's body language. Is it relaxed or tense?
- Quality of the patient's voice. Is it loud or soft?
- The patient's use of gestures.
- The patient's emotional tone (or affect). Is it constant, or does it vary? (For example, does the patient appear sad, happy, or angry?)
- Congruence of the verbal message with the patient's body language. (For example, is the patient smiling while speaking of a happy event?)

Listening is an active element of therapeutic communication. You must listen and attempt to understand what the patient is saying. Tips for effective listening include the following:

- Make sure you hear what is said; focus on the message, clarify if needed.
- Accept your patient's needs and feelings.
- Pay attention to nonverbal communication.
- Obtain feedback of your understanding by verifying what you have heard.

Understanding is the ability to listen to others to perceive their feelings and the meaning of their words. Some techniques used to facilitate communication are listed in Table 5-2. Other suggestions for therapeutic communication are listed in the Health Promotion Considerations box at right.

Processing is the act of reviewing a nurse-patient interaction with a trusted teacher, supervisor, or colleague to evaluate content and themes as well as the techniques that are used. This tool enables the

 What Does Culture Have to Do with Communication?

Culture influences a person's comfort with touch, personal space, and eye contact.

nurse to be critiqued (obtain feedback) and to learn new techniques. Communication is a complex process. "Helping" can occur regardless of one's experience if respect and authenticity are brought to each interaction.

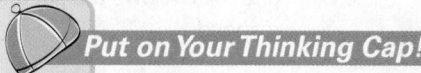 **Put on Your Thinking Cap!**

During your next clinical experience, listen for therapeutic and nontherapeutic communication techniques used by health care providers in interactions with patients. Describe and label three examples. Discuss the impact of each statement on the interaction.

EMPATHETIC RESPONSE

Effective communication requires an empathetic response from a nurse. Empathy is the ability to identify with and understand another person's situation, feelings, and motives. An empathetic response requires compassion, understanding, and good therapeutic communication skills. Empathy differs from *sympathy*. When people sympathize with others, they understand another's feelings but they also become personally involved in the situation. Whatever affects one affects the other. The person who sympathizes can become as distressed as the person getting the sympathy. Empathy, in contrast, is an expression of understanding of another's thoughts and feelings without becoming overly emotionally involved or distressed.

Empathy can be communicated simply through the use of verbal and nonverbal language. You can communicate empathy by telling the patient what to expect, even when the patient is not responsive

 Health Promotion Considerations

Suggestions for Improving Therapeutic Communication

- Use *I statements.* These are sentences that begin with the word *I* and indicate acceptance of responsibility for one's feelings and thoughts (e.g., "I worry less when I know what to expect."). *I statements* generally are better accepted by the patient than y*ou statements* such as, "You ought to try getting more sleep."
- Observe the patient's gestures and nonverbal behavior. All behavior has meaning. Try to understand the meaning in the patient's behavior.
- Use open-ended questions. Stay clear of questions that can be answered with a "yes" or a "no." Instead, try questions like, "Tell me about your surgery," or "What was that like for you?"
- Focus the patient on pertinent issues. For example, "Let's talk about your diabetes medications."

Table 5-2 *Therapeutic and Nontherapeutic Communication Techniques*

TECHNIQUE	DESCRIPTION	EXAMPLE
THERAPEUTIC		
Silence	Waiting attentively while the patient speaks or thinks. Allows the patient to think and respond.	Sitting quietly and expectantly when the patient is speaking or gathering his thoughts. Resisting the urge to fill quiet periods with conversation.
Reflecting	"Mirrors" back to patients what you have heard them say. Provides opportunities for patients to confirm whether they were understood.	"You say you're feeling better since your brother has returned?"
Summarizing	Reviews the subject matter that the client has discussed. Ensures common understanding between nurse and patient.	"So you have decided to have surgery but will delay it until after Christmas."
Restating	Repeats information in your own words so the patient can confirm your interpretation.	"I hear you're concerned about your son."
Clarification	Seeks additional information so you can better understand the patient's meaning.	"Do you mean sad when you say upset?"
Open-ended statement	A question or comment that requires more than a yes or no answer. Indicates interest, but leaves specific details for client to provide.	"Tell me your reactions to your new treatment."
NONTHERAPEUTIC		
Premature advice	Offers advice without first encouraging clients to explore their feelings fully. The problem must be explored carefully and potential actions considered before the patient can make a good decision. You cannot decide what is best for the patient.	"The first thing you need to do is make your teenagers help you more."
Assuming truth of statements rather than checking them out	Accepts information without questioning or clarifying. Misunderstandings can persist.	"It's incredible that your doctor did not tell you when to take this medication."
Commanding	Directing client to do something that creates a power struggle or resistance.	"You must quit smoking immediately."
Communication cut-off	Remark that discourages patient communication. Shows lack of effort to understand.	"Try to think positively."
False reassurance	Inappropriately offers personal opinion that the patient should not be concerned about something. Minimizes the patient's feelings. Can lead to feelings of guilt and anger.	"You shouldn't worry about the new treatment."

or confused. Discussing plans for care, such as treatments or medications, and explaining laboratory studies can provide reassurance to patients who may be frightened. You can also demonstrate your concern to patients and families by sharing your feelings. By sharing feelings, nurses show that they are human and can understand the difficulties of being ill or hospitalized. For example, a nurse might be tearful when

a patient is given bad news or might say "I was nervous when I had surgery too."

You can show sensitivity nonverbally by respecting confidentiality, allowing the expression of feelings, and respecting patients' privacy. The use of touch is an excellent means of communicating empathy. Holding a patient's hand during a period of anxiety or pain can communicate caring and support and, in many cases,

FIGURE **5-3** The judicious use of touch conveys the message that "I care what happens to you, and I will help you in every way I can."

can be more effective than any verbal interaction. The judicious use of touch conveys the message that "I care what happens to you, and I will help you in every way that I can" (Fig. 5-3).

When you respond empathetically, you respond with genuineness, warmth, and sensitivity to promote well-being in the patient. This is the essence of therapeutic communication.

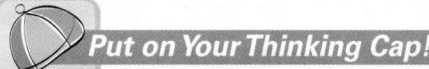

Put on Your Thinking Cap!

Describe three things you did in your last patient contact that demonstrated empathy.

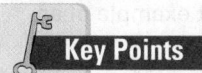

Key Points

- Caring is a process characterized by understanding and action.
- Action is the response to others with genuineness, warmth, sensitivity, and self-disclosure to promote their well-being.
- Holism views people as complex creatures made up of many parts that interact and form a unified whole.
- The nurse incorporates physiologic, psychological, sociologic, and spiritual influences into the plan of care.
- Nurses must have awareness of their own values, beliefs, and attitudes and be willing to accept unconditionally the patient's values, beliefs, and attitudes.
- Nurses use their knowledge of physiology, psychology, and social science disciplines as well as their technical and interpersonal skills to give the best possible care to clients.
- Nurses can reduce patients' stress and anxiety levels by empowering them to participate in their own care and by demonstrating competence and consistency.
- Patients are the recipients of nursing care and are entitled to receive respectful quality care.
- The role of a helper is to assist another to grow, mature, cope, and function.
- Communication is basic to the helper role.
- Empathy, genuineness, warmth, sensitivity, and self-disclosure are essentials of therapeutic communication.
- Empathy is the ability to identify with and understand another person's situation, feelings, and motives.

 Go to your Companion CD-ROM for a Pharmacology Tutorial, Audio Glossary, and 3-D animations.

evolve   Be sure to visit the companion Evolve site at http://evolve.elsevier.com/Linton/ for WebLinks and additional online resources.

REVIEW QUESTIONS *Choose the best answer.*

1. The main difference between social and therapeutic relationships is that therapeutic relationships:
   1. Focus on both the patient and the nurse
   2. Are developed only in inpatient settings
   3. Help the nurse work through personal problems
   4. Exist to meet patient-centered goals

2. You are caring for an older adult who has been chronically ill for several years. The patient has decided not to continue life-sustaining treatment. You believe that life should be maintained at all costs. Which action best reflects acceptance of the patient in a therapeutic relationship?
   1. Ask the patient's family members to try to convince their loved one to continue treatment.
   2. Tell the patient that you believe life is sacred and it is wrong to refuse available treatment.
   3. Tell your nurse manager you cannot continue to care for the patient who refuses treatment.
   4. Plan with the patient ways to maintain quality of life for as long as possible.

3. Within a therapeutic relationship, it is appropriate for you as a nurse to:
   1. Be honest about your feelings
   2. Spend time with the patient in social settings
   3. Try to influence the patient's religious beliefs
   4. Assure the patient that any information shared will be kept secret

4. Which of the following reflects an empathetic response to a patient who is distressed?
   1. Ask the physician to order a sedative.
   2. Tell the patient that the situation could be worse.
   3. Gently touch the patient's arm.
   4. Firmly advise the patient to regain control.

5. "Reactions that flow from beliefs and values" defines:
   1. Ethics
   2. Attitudes
   3. Empathy
   4. Holism

6. Which of the following is the best example of an *open-ended* question?

1. "How many children do you have?"
2. "Describe your usual day."
3. "I see that you take thyroid replacement drugs."
4. "Are you nervous about surgery?"

7. A patient who is scheduled for a biopsy of a lump in her breast says tearfully, "I am so afraid it will be cancer." The nurse replies, "There is no sense worrying about that until you know for sure." This is an example of:

1. Premature advice
2. Commanding
3. False reassurance
4. Assuming truth of statements

Cultural Aspects of Nursing Care

Objectives

After reading and studying this chapter, you should be able to:

1. Describe cultural concepts related to nursing and health care.
2. Identify traditional health habits and beliefs of major ethnic groups in the United States.
3. Explain cultural influences on the interactions of patients and families with the health care system.
4. Discuss cultural considerations in providing culturally sensitive nursing care.
5. Discuss ways in which planning and implementation of nursing interventions can be adapted to a patient's ethnicity.

Key Terms

Be sure to check out the bonus material on the Companion CD-ROM, including selected audio pronunciations.

assimilation (ă-sĭm-ĭ-LĀ-shŭn, p. 66)
cultural diversity (p. 57)
culture (p. 57)
enculturation (ĕn-kŭl-chĕr-Ā-shŭn, p. 57)
ethnic group (p. 58)
subculture (p. 57)
transcultural nursing (p. 57)

Nurses encounter people of many different backgrounds in their practice. The differences may stem from race, ethnicity, language, or religion. Diverse backgrounds affect the ways individuals react to health and illness, hospitalization, and nursing care.

CULTURAL CONCEPTS

CHARACTERISTICS OF CULTURE

Culture is an integrated system of learned values, beliefs, and practices that guides an individual's behavior. Culture includes the arts, beliefs, customs, folk practices, habits, institutions, and all other products of human work and thought created by a people or a group at a particular time. Culture represents the ideas, beliefs, values, and attitudes that a group of people possess. These values and beliefs are the foundation for setting standards and rules of behavior that members of a society consider acceptable and proper. Culture includes learned ways of acting and thinking that are transmitted by group members and that provide solutions for problems. Dietary habits, customs, modes of communication, religion, art, and history are all aspects of culture. Not only does culture affect a person's decisions and actions, but also it affects health care practices.

Cultural diversity is a term used to describe the existence of many cultures in a society. The United States has a rich cultural diversity as a result of the large number of immigrants who have entered the country over the past 200 years. America is sometimes called a "melting pot" because many immigrants have been assimilated into their new society. Today, the term "salad bowl" is often used instead to describe the way in which new arrivals seek to maintain individual differences while acclimating to new surroundings. It is important to value and respect the differences among the various cultural groups within our society, for each group provides unique contributions to art, science, politics, and health care.

Within certain cultures are groups of individuals who share different beliefs, values, and attitudes from those of the dominant culture. These groups are called subcultures. Examples of subcultures in the United States are members of various ethnic groups, such as African Americans, Latinos/Hispanics, Asians, and American Indians (Fig. 6-1); homosexuals; the military; and religious groups such as the Amish and Mormons. Transcultural nursing is the integration of culture into all aspects of nursing care.

Similarities

All cultures share certain basic characteristics: (1) culture is learned; (2) culture is shared; and (3) culture is based on symbols. People *learn* to be a part of a culture as they are growing up, and the learning may continue into adulthood. This process is known as enculturation. Cultural learning is passed down from parent to child to grandchild, affecting the personality development of each generation. People learn what is expected of them and how they should behave, dress, and interact on particular occasions. For example, important life events are celebrated differently in different cultures (Fig. 6-2). Weddings and funerals may be

FIGURE **6-1** Many people living in the United States represent many different subcultures.

FIGURE **6-2** People of various heritages share a culture as they adopt American practices.

quiet, small occasions for introspection, or they may be robust, noisy celebrations with a crowd of people in attendance.

Culture also is *shared*. Cultural beliefs, values, and behaviors are shared among individuals within a particular group. Individual behavior does not reflect a particular culture unless it is manifested by other people in the cultural group. From group behavior, the behavior of individuals can then be predicted.

Culture is based on *symbols*. Symbols represent means of communication, spiritual beliefs, economic interactions, and national origins, among other things. Examples of symbols are language (words), religious artifacts (crucifix, Star of David), money (economic interactions), and flags (national origin). Symbols help convey the beliefs, values, and behaviors of a society or culture.

Differences

Cultural differences may occur among various groups in relation to family, religion, communication, educational background, social class, and economic level. Nurses should be aware of the differences in these areas and recognize how they affect the wellness, illness, and health care practices of their patients.

Family. The family provides a major means for reproducing the population and rearing its children. The family unit is basic to every society. It is mainly through the family that cultural attitudes, values, and behaviors are transmitted.

The family structure may vary among and within cultures. The traditional nuclear family, consisting of a mother, a father, and children, is becoming less of a standard. Single-parent families make up about 20% of all households in the United States. In addition, some cultural groups continue to have extended families living under the same roof (e.g., grandparents, parents, children, and other relatives). Some families have a strong patriarchal (male, father-dominated) structure, whereas others have strong matriarchal (female, mother-dominated) tendencies.

Culture can influence the attitudes and beliefs of families in relation to health care. Behaviors related to health practices, hospitalization, and placement in long-term care facilities can vary among cultures. For example, Latinos and Filipinos are thought to have strong extended family units and family ties, and when a person is hospitalized, family members visit frequently. In addition, Latinos and Filipinos have tended to care for their elders in a home setting rather than placing them in residential facilities. Nurses should become acquainted with the various cultural backgrounds of families and how they influence behavior rather than be judgmental about family behaviors.

Religion. Religious beliefs are culturally determined, and the way individuals fulfill their spiritual needs stems from a lifetime of experience. Religious beliefs and practices can influence perceptions of health and illness, hospitalization, and death and dying. Some patients may observe specific dietary rules, and others may have particular practices regarding dress, modesty, daily living habits, or medical interventions. Religious differences also occur in relation to the observation of the Sabbath, baptism, the sacrament of the sick, and last rites (Table 6-1).

Communication. Communication involves language. Certain cultural or ethnic groups speak different languages, making communication almost impossible without an interpreter. However, there are also subtler forms of miscommunication that can arise because of group differences. The speed with which people speak and their tone and inflections vary according to cultural background.

Nonverbal communication also is culturally based. Personal space, eye contact, gestures, displays of emotions, and the amount and meaning of touch that are acceptable are culturally determined. Some cultures find emotional display more acceptable than others. Some are more comfortable with silence than others.

Educational Background and Economic Level. There are wide differences in educational backgrounds within

Text continued on p. 66.

Table 6-1 | *Religious Beliefs and Practices Affecting Health Care*

RELIGIOUS GROUP	BELIEFS AND PRACTICES
WESTERN RELIGIONS *Judaism* Orthodox Jews and some Conservative Jewish groups	*Care of women:* A woman is considered to be in a ritual state of impurity whenever blood is coming from her uterus, such as during menstrual periods and after the birth of a child. During this time, her husband will not have physical contact with her. When this time is completed, she will bathe herself in a pool called a mikvah. Nurses need to be aware of this practice and be sensitive to the husband and wife because the husband will not touch his wife. He cannot assist her in moving in the bed, so the nurse will have to do this. An Orthodox Jewish man will not touch any woman other than his wife, daughters, and mother.

Dietary rules: (1) Kosher dietary laws include the following: No mixing of milk and meat at a meal; no consumption of food or any derivative thereof from animals not slaughtered in accordance with Jewish law; use of separate cooking utensils for milk and milk products; if a patient requires milk and meat products for a meal, the dairy foods should be served first, followed later by the meat. (2) During Yom Kippur (Day of Atonement), a 24-hour fast is required, but exceptions are made for those who cannot fast because of medical reasons. (3) During Passover, no leavened products are eaten. (4) May say benediction of thanksgiving before meals and grace at the end of the meal. Time and a quiet environment should be provided for this.

Sabbath: Observed from sunset Friday until sunset Saturday. Orthodox law prohibits riding in a car, smoking, turning lights on and off, handling money, and using the television and telephone. Nurses need to be aware of this when caring for observant Jews at home and in the hospital. Medical or surgical treatments should be postponed if possible.

Death: Judaism defines death as occurring when respiration and circulation are irreversibly stopped and no movement is apparent. (1) Euthanasia is strictly forbidden by Orthodox Jews, who advocate the strict use of life-support measures. (2) Prior to death, Jewish faith indicates that visiting of the person by family and friends is a religious duty. The Torah and Psalms may be read and prayers recited. A witness needs to be present when a person prays for health so that if death occurs God will protect the family and the spirit will be committed to God. Extraneous talking and conversation about death are not encouraged unless initiated by the patient or visitors. In Judaism, the belief is that people should have someone with them when the soul leaves the body, so family and/or friends should be allowed to stay with the patients. After death, the body should not be left alone until buried, usually within 24 hours. (3) When death occurs, the body should be untouched for 8 to 30 minutes. Medical personnel should not touch or wash the body but allow only an Orthodox person or the Jewish Burial Society to care for the body. Handling of a corpse on the Sabbath is forbidden to Jewish persons. If need be, the nursing staff may provide routine care of the body, wearing gloves. Water in the room should be emptied, and the family may request that mirrors be covered to symbolize that a death has occurred. (4) Orthodox Jews and some Conservative Jews do not approve of autopsies. If an autopsy must be done, all body parts must remain with the body. (5) For Orthodox Jews, the body must be buried within 24 hours. No flowers are permitted. A fetus must be buried. (6) A 7-day mourning period is required by the immediate family. They must stay at home except for Sabbath worship. (7) Organs or other body parts such as amputated limbs must be made available for burial for Orthodox Jews, because they believe that all of the body must be returned to earth.

Birth control and abortion: Artificial methods of birth control are not encouraged. Vasectomy is not allowed. Abortion may be performed only to save the mother's life.

Organ transplants: Donor organ transplants generally are not permitted by Orthodox Jews but may be allowed with rabbinical consent.

From Black, J.M., & Matassarin-Jacobs, E. (1993). *Luckmann and Sorensen's medical-surgical nursing: A psychophysiologic approach* (4th ed.). Philadelphia: Saunders. Modified from Carson, V.B. (1989). *Spiritual dimensions of nursing practice.* Philadelphia: Saunders.

Continued

Table 6-1 | *Religious Beliefs and Practices Affecting Health Care—cont'd*

RELIGIOUS GROUP	BELIEFS AND PRACTICES
WESTERN RELIGIONS—cont'd *Judaism—cont'd* Orthodox Jews and some Conservative Jewish groups—cont'd	*Shaving:* The beard is regarded as a mark of piety among observant Jews. For the very Orthodox, shaving should not be done with a razor but with scissors or electric razor, because a blade should not contact the skin. *Head coverings:* Orthodox men wear skull caps at all times, and women cover their hair after marriage. Some Orthodox women wear wigs as a mark of piety. Conservative Jews cover their heads only during acts of worship and prayer. *Prayer:* Praying directly to God, including a prayer of confession, is required for Orthodox Jews. Nurses should provide quiet time for prayer.
Reform Jews	*Care of women:* Reform Jews do not observe the rules against touching. *Dietary rules:* Reform Jews usually do not observe kosher dietary restrictions. *Sabbath:* Usually worship in temples on Friday evenings. No strict rules. *Death:* Advocate use of life support without heroic measures. Allow for cremation but suggest that ashes be buried in a Jewish cemetery. *Organ transplants:* Donation or transplantation of organs allowed with permission of a rabbi. *Head coverings:* Generally pray without wearing skullcaps.
Christianity Roman Catholic	*Holy Eucharist:* For patients and health care givers who are to receive communion, abstinence from solid food and alcohol is required for 15 minutes (if possible) prior to reception of the consecrated wafer. Medicine, water, and nonalcoholic drinks are permitted at any time. If a patient is in danger of death, the fast is waived because the reception of the Eucharist at this time is very important. *Anointing of the sick:* The priest uses oil to anoint the forehead and hands and, if desired, the affected area. The rite may be performed on any who are ill and desire it. Patients receiving the sacrament seek complete healing and strength to endure suffering. Prior to 1963, this sacrament was given only to patients at the time of imminent death, so the nurse must be sensitive to the meaning this has for the patient. If possible, the nurse calls a priest before the patient is unconscious but may also call when there is sudden death, because the sacrament may also be given shortly after death. The nurse records on the care plan that this sacrament has been administered. *Dietary habits:* Obligatory fasting is excused during hospitalization. However, if there are no health restrictions, some Catholics may still observe the following guidelines: (1) Anyone 14 years or older must abstain from eating meat on Ash Wednesday and all Fridays during Lent. Some older Catholics may still abstain from meat on all Fridays of the year. (2) In addition to abstinence from meat, persons 21 to 59 years of age must limit themselves to one full meal and two light meals on Ash Wednesday and Good Friday. (3) Eastern Rite Catholics are stricter about fasting and fast more frequently than Western Rite Catholics, so it is important for the nurse to know if a patient is Eastern or Western Catholic. *Death:* Each Roman Catholic should participate in the anointing of the sick as well as Eucharist and penance before death. The body should not be shrouded until after these sacraments are performed. All body parts that retain human quality must be appropriately buried or cremated. *Birth control:* Prohibited except for abstinence or natural family planning. Referral to a priest for questions about this can be of great help. Nurses can teach the techniques of natural family planning if they are familiar with them; otherwise, this should be referred to the physician or to a support group of the church that instructs couples in this method of birth control. Sterilization is prohibited unless there is an overriding medical reason.

From Black, J.M., & Matassarin-Jacobs, E. (1993). *Luckmann and Sorensen's medical-surgical nursing: A psychophysiologic approach* (4th ed.). Philadelphia: Saunders. Modified from Carson, V.B. (1989). *Spiritual dimensions of nursing practice.* Philadelphia: Saunders.

Table 6-1	*Religious Beliefs and Practices Affecting Health Care—cont'd*

RELIGIOUS GROUP	BELIEFS AND PRACTICES
WESTERN RELIGIONS—cont'd *Christianity—cont'd*	
Roman Catholic—cont'd	*Organ transplants:* Donation and transplantation of organs are acceptable as long as the donor is not harmed and is not deprived of life. *Religious objects:* Rosary prayers are said using rosary beads. Medals bearing the images of saints, relics, statues, and scapulars are important objects that may be pinned to a hospital gown or pillow or be at the bedside. Extreme care should be taken not to lose these objects, because they have special meaning to the patient.
Eastern Orthodox	*Holy Eucharist:* The priest is notified if the patient desires this sacrament. *Anointing of the sick:* The priest conducts this in the hospital room. *Dietary habits:* Fasting from meat and dairy products is required on Wednesday and Friday during Lent and on other holy days. Hospital patients are exempt if fasting is detrimental to health. *Special days:* Christmas is celebrated on January 7 and New Year's Day on January 14. This is important to the care of a patient who is hospitalized on these days. *Death:* Last rites are obligatory. This is handled by an ordained priest who is notified by the nurse while the patient is conscious. The Russian Orthodox Church does not encourage autopsy or organ donation. Euthanasia, even for the terminally ill, is discouraged, as is cremation. *Birth control:* This as well as abortion is not permitted.
Protestant Assemblies of God (Pentecostal)	*Holy Communion:* Notify clergy if the patient desires. *Anointing of the sick:* Members believe in divine healing through prayer and the laying on of hands. Clergy is notified if patient or family desires this. *Dietary habits:* Abstinence from alcohol, tobacco, and all illegal drugs is strongly encouraged. *Death:* No special practices. *Other practices:* Faith in God and in the health care providers is encouraged. Members pray for divine intervention in health matters. Nurses should encourage and allow time for prayer. Members may speak in "tongues" during prayer.
Baptist (over 27 different groups in the United States)	*Holy Communion:* Clergy should be notified if the patient desires. *Dietary habits:* Total abstinence from alcohol is expected. *Death:* No general service is provided, but the clergy does minister through counseling, prayer, and Scripture as requested by the patient or family, and the patient is encouraged to believe in Jesus Christ as Savior and Lord. *Other practices:* The Bible is held to be the word of God, so the nurse should either allow quiet time for Scripture reading or offer to read to the patient.
Christian Church (Disciples of Christ)	*Holy Communion:* Open communion is celebrated each Sunday and is a central part of worship services. The nurse notifies the clergy if the patient desires it, or the clergy may suggest it. *Death:* No special practices. *Other practices:* Church elders as well as clergy may be notified to assist with meeting the patient's spiritual needs.
Church of the Brethren	*Holy Communion:* Usually received within church, but clergy will give it in the hospital when requested. *Anointing of the sick:* Practiced for physical healing as well as spiritual uplift and held in high regard by the church. The clergy is notified if the patient or family desires. *Death:* The clergy is notified for counsel and prayer.
Church of the Nazarene	*Holy Communion:* Pastor will administer if the patient wishes. *Dietary habits:* The use of alcohol and tobacco is forbidden. *Death:* Cremation is permitted, and term stillborn infants are buried. *Other practices:* Believe in divine healing but not to the exclusion of medical treatment. Patients may desire quiet time for prayer.

Continued

■

Table 6-1 | *Religious Beliefs and Practices Affecting Health Care—cont'd*

RELIGIOUS GROUP	BELIEFS AND PRACTICES
WESTERN RELIGIONS—cont'd *Christianity—cont'd* *Protestant—cont'd* Episcopal (Anglican)	*Holy Communion:* The priest is notified if the patient wishes to receive this sacrament. *Anointing of the sick:* Priest may administer this rite when death is imminent, but it is not considered mandatory. *Dietary habits:* Some patients may abstain from meat on Fridays. Others may fast before receiving the Eucharist, but fasting is not mandatory. *Death:* No special practices. *Other practices:* Confession of sins to a priest is optional; if the patient desires this, the clergy should be notified.
Lutheran (18 different branches)	*Holy Communion:* Notify the clergy if the patient desires this sacrament. Clergy may also inquire about the patient's desire. *Anointing of the sick:* The patient may request an anointing and blessing from the minister when the prognosis is poor. *Death:* A service of Commendation of the Dying is used at the patient's or family's request.
Mennonite (12 different groups)	*Holy Communion:* Served twice a year, with foot washing as part of ceremony. *Dietary habits:* Abstinence from alcohol is urged for all. *Death:* Prayer is important at time of crisis, so contacting a minister is important. *Other practices:* Women may wear head coverings during hospitalization. Anointing with oil is administered in harmony with James 5:14 when requested.
Methodist (over 20 different groups)	*Holy Communion:* Notify the clergy if a patient requests it prior to surgery or another health crisis. *Anointing of the sick:* If requested, the clergy will come to pray and sprinkle the patient with olive oil. *Death:* Scripture reading and prayer are important at this time. *Other practices:* Donation of one's body or part of the body at death is encouraged.
Presbyterian (10 different groups)	*Holy Communion:* Given when appropriate and convenient, at the hospitalized patient's request. *Death:* Notify a local pastor or elder for prayer and Scripture reading if desired by the family or patient.
Quaker (Friends)	*Holy Communion:* Because Friends have no creed, there is a diversity of personal beliefs, one of which is that outward sacraments are usually not necessary because there is the ministry of the Spirit inwardly in such areas as baptism and communion. *Death:* Believe that the present life is part of God's kingdom and generally have no ceremony as a rite of passage from this life to the next. Personal beliefs and wishes need to be ascertained, and the nurse can then act on the patient's wishes.
Salvation Army	*Holy Communion:* No particular ceremony. *Death:* Notify the local officer in charge of the Army Corps for any soldier (member) who needs assistance. *Other practices:* The Bible is seen as the only rule for one's faith, so the Scriptures should be made available to a patient. The Army has many of its own social welfare centers with hospitals and homes where unwed mothers are cared for and outpatient services provided. No medical or surgical procedures are opposed, except for abortion on demand.
Seventh-Day Adventist	*Holy Communion:* Although this is not required of hospitalized patients, the clergy are notified if the patient desires. *Anointing of the sick:* The clergy are contacted for prayer and anointing with oil.

From Black, J.M., & Matassarin-Jacobs, E. (1993). *Luckmann and Sorensen's medical-surgical nursing: A psychophysiologic approach* (4th ed.). Philadelphia: Saunders. Modified from Carson, V.B. (1989). *Spiritual dimensions of nursing practice*. Philadelphia: Saunders.

Table 6-1 | *Religious Beliefs and Practices Affecting Health Care—cont'd*

RELIGIOUS GROUP	BELIEFS AND PRACTICES
WESTERN RELIGIONS—cont'd *Christianity—cont'd* *Protestant—cont'd* Seventh-Day Adventist—cont'd	*Dietary habits:* Because the body is viewed as the temple of the Holy Spirit, healthy living is essential. Therefore, the use of alcohol, tobacco, coffee, and tea and the promiscuous use of drugs are prohibited. Some are vegetarians, and most avoid pork. *Special days:* The Sabbath is observed on Saturday. *Death:* No special procedures. *Other practices:* Use of hypnotism is opposed by some. Persons of homosexual or lesbian orientation are ministered to in the hope of correction of these practices, which are believed to be wrong. A Bible should always be available for Scripture reading.
United Church of Christ	*Holy Communion:* Clergy are notified if the patient desires to receive this sacrament. *Death:* If the patient desires counsel or prayer, notify the clergy.
Other Christian Science	*Dietary habits:* Because alcohol and tobacco are considered drugs, they are not used. Coffee and tea are often declined. *Death:* Autopsy is usually declined unless required by law. Donation of organs is unlikely but is an individual decision. *Other practices:* Christian Scientists do not normally seek medical care, because they approach health care in a different, primarily spiritual, framework. They commonly use the services of a surgeon to set a bone but decline drugs and, in general, other medical or surgical procedures. Hypnotism and psychotherapy are also declined. Family planning is left to the family. They seek exemption from vaccinations but obey legal requirements (e.g., report infectious diseases and obey public health quarantines). Non-medical care facilities are maintained for those needing nursing assistance in the course of a healing. *The Christian Science Journal* lists available Christian Science nurses. When a Christian Science believer is in the hospital, the nurse should allow and encourage time for prayer and study. Patients may request that a Christian Science practitioner be notified to come.
Jehovah's Witnesses	*Dietary habits:* Use of alcohol and tobacco is discouraged because these harm the physical body. *Death:* Autopsy is a private matter to be decided by the persons involved. Burial and cremation are acceptable. *Birth control and abortion:* Use of birth control is a personal decision. Abortion is opposed based on Exodus 21:22-23. *Organ transplants:* Use of organ transplant is a private decision and if used must be cleansed with a nonblood solution. *Blood transfusions:* Blood transfusions violate God's laws and therefore are not allowed. Patients do respect physicians and will accept alternatives to blood transfusions. These might include use of nonblood plasma expanders, careful surgical techniques to decrease blood loss, use of autologous transfusions, and autotransfusion through use of a heart-lung machine. Nurses should check unconscious patients for Medic Alert cards that state that the person does not want a transfusion. Since Jehovah's Witnesses are prepared to die rather than break God's law, nurses need to be sensitive to the spiritual and the physical needs of the patient.
The Church of Jesus Christ of Latter-Day Saints	*Holy Communion:* A hospitalized patient may desire to have a member of the church priesthood administer this sacrament. *Anointing of the sick:* Mormons frequently are anointed and given a blessing before going to the hospital and after admission by laying on of hands. *Dietary habits:* Abstinence from the use of tobacco; beverages with caffeine such as cola, coffee, and tea; alcohol and other substances considered injurious. Mormons eat meat but encourage the intake of fruits, grains, and herbs. *Death:* Prefer burial of the body. A church elder should be notified to assist the family. If need be, the elder will assist the funeral director in dressing the body in special clothes and give other help as needed.

Continued

▮ Table 6-1 ▮ *Religious Beliefs and Practices Affecting Health Care—cont'd*

RELIGIOUS GROUP	BELIEFS AND PRACTICES
WESTERN RELIGIONS—cont'd **Other—cont'd**	
The Church of Jesus Christ of Latter-Day Saints—cont'd	*Birth control and abortion:* Abortion is opposed except when the life of the mother is in danger. Only natural means of birth control are recommended. Artificial means can be used when the health of the woman is at stake (including emotional health). *Personal care:* Cleanliness is very important to Mormons. A sacred undergarment may be worn at all times by Mormons and should only be removed in emergency situations. *Other practices:* Allowing quiet time for prayer and the reading of the sacred writings is important. The church maintains a welfare system to assist those in need. Families are of great importance, so visiting should be encouraged.
Unitarian Universalist Association	*Death:* Cremation is often preferred to burial. *Other practices:* Use of birth control is advocated as part of responsible parenting. Strong support for a woman's right to choice regarding abortion is maintained. Unitarian Universalists advocate donation of body parts for research and transplants.
Unification Church	*Baptism:* No baptism occurs. *Special days:* Sunday mornings are used to honor Reverend and Mrs. Moon as the true parents, and members get up at 5:00 AM, bow before a picture of the Moons three times, and vow to do what is needed to help the Reverend accomplish his mission on earth. *Death:* They believe that after death one's place of destiny will depend on his or her spirit's quality of life and goodness while on earth. In the afterlife, one will have the same aspirations and feelings as before death. Hell is not a concern, because it will not be a place as heaven grows in size. Persons who leave the Unification Church are warned that Satan may try to possess them. *Other practices:* All marriages must be solemnized by Reverend Moon to be part of the perfect family and have salvation. The church supplies its faithful members with life's necessities. Members may use occult practices to have spiritual and psychic experiences.
Islam	*Dietary habits:* No pork is allowed, or alcoholic beverages. All halal (permissible) meat must be blessed and killed in a special way. This is called zabihah (correctly slaughtered). *Death:* Prior to death, family members ask to be present so that they can read the Koran and pray with the patient. An Imam may come if requested by the patient or family but is not required. Patients must face Mecca and confess their sins and beg forgiveness in the presence of their family. If the family is unavailable, any practicing Muslim can provide support to the patient. After death, Muslims prefer that the family wash, prepare, and place the body in a position facing Mecca. If necessary, the health care providers may perform these procedures as long as they wear gloves. Burial is performed as soon as possible. Cremation is forbidden. Autopsy is also prohibited except for legal reasons, and then no body part is to be removed. Donation of body parts or organs is not allowed, because according to culturally developed law, persons do not own their body. *Abortion and birth control:* Abortion is forbidden, and many conservative Muslims do not encourage the use of contraceptives because this interferes with God's purpose. Others feel that a woman should have only as many children as her husband can afford. Contraception is permitted by Islamic law. *Personal devotions:* At prayer time, washing is required, even by those who are sick. A patient on bedrest may require assistance with this task before prayer. Provision of privacy during prayer is important. *Religious objects:* The Koran must not be touched by anyone ritually unclean, and nothing should be placed on top of it. Some Muslims wear taviz, a black string on which words of the Koran are attached. These should not be removed and must remain dry. Certain items of jewelry such as bangles may have religious significance and should not be removed unnecessarily.

From Black, J.M., & Matassarin-Jacobs, E. (1993). *Luckmann and Sorensen's medical-surgical nursing: A psychophysiologic approach* (4th ed.). Philadelphia: Saunders. Modified from Carson, V.B. (1989). *Spiritual dimensions of nursing practice.* Philadelphia: Saunders.

Table 6-1   *Religious Beliefs and Practices Affecting Health Care—cont'd*

RELIGIOUS GROUP	BELIEFS AND PRACTICES
WESTERN RELIGIONS—cont'd **Islam—cont'd** American Muslim Mission	*Care of women:* Because women are not allowed to sign consent forms or make a decision regarding family planning, the husband needs to be present. Women are very modest and frequently wear clothes that cover all of the body. During a medical examination, the woman's modesty should be respected as much as possible. Muslim women prefer female doctors. For 40 days after giving birth and also during menstruation, a woman is exempt from prayer because this is a time of cleansing for her. *Dietary habits:* In addition to refusing pork, many will not eat traditional black American foods such as corn bread and collard greens. *Death:* The family is contacted before any care of the deceased is performed. There are special procedures for washing and shrouding the body. *Other practices:* Quiet time is necessary to permit prayer. Members are encouraged to use black physicians for health care. Because these patients do not smoke, their request for a nonsmoking roommate should be honored.
EASTERN RELIGIONS **Hinduism**	*Dietary habits:* Some sects are vegetarian, believing meats and intoxicants to be too stimulating to the senses. *Belief about illness:* View illness as a result of misuse of the body or a consequence of sins committed in a previous life. They do not oppose medical treatment, but view its effect as transitory. Believe that praying for health is the lowest form of prayer. *Death:* See death as a union with Brahman (God) achieved through prayers, ritual, purity, self-control, detachment, truth, nonviolence, charity, and compassion toward all creatures. Following death, one will be reborn (reincarnated) into a future life based on the behavior in this life. The record of behavior is called karma. Eventually, the process of rebirth stops, which is called moksha. A priest may be called at the time of death, and may tie a thread around the neck or waist as a blessing. The family washes the body, and it is cremated. *Other practices:* Offer daily worship at a shrine in the home. Daily offering to God, and morning and evening rites. Society is organized into castes, or strata. People are born into a caste, and the caste shapes one's entire life. Hindus practice a discipline of the mind and body, called yoga, to reach God. In the highest state, a meditating yogi does not see, hear, taste, feel, or smell. Beyond good and evil, time and space, the yogi is one with God.
Buddhism	*Death:* Believe that salvation depends on one's own right living. Believe in reincarnation. Can speed the process toward Nirvana, the goal of all humanity's striving, through acts of merit. Meditation, worship, and prayer are some of the acts of merit. Buddhists may drive themselves into more and more ritual or contemplation in the hope that their last moments of consciousness may be filled with thoughts worthy enough to elevate them to a higher existence. Last rights of chanting may be performed at bedside. *Renunciation:* The most important Buddhist feasts. Young boys are taught to despise the world's vanity, and the boy spends a night in a nearby monastery.
Taoism/Confucianism	*General beliefs:* Founded on ethical principles of Confucius. God is not clearly defined as in other religions. Taoism is a mixture of magic and religion. Believe that humans and nature are inseparable, and that if heaven is upset, earth does not prosper. This relationship is described as yang and yin, which are two interplaying forces. When yang and yin are in balance, good occurs. *Death:* The dead are remembered in all festivals. The fate of the dead in the afterworld depends not only on the life they led but also on being properly honored after death. Otherwise they may become demons. Graves are mounds like those dedicated to the gifts of the soil. Graves and houses must be in harmony with the universe, otherwise evil will befall the occupants.

the United States. Approximately 60 million Americans have literacy skills below the eighth grade level. That means that one of every three people has difficulty with reading and writing.

Educational level attained is strongly tied to ethnicity and economic background. School dropout rates appear to be higher among teenagers living in poverty areas. Ethnic groups that are found in large numbers in poverty areas tend to have high dropout rates.

Educational background and economic levels affect the ways in which people perceive the world, health and illness, and the health care system. Teaching about health becomes a challenge because many with low literacy levels have difficulty reading the materials presented and understanding health care jargon. In addition, people from economically deprived backgrounds may live in crowded, unsafe housing and have inadequate diets. Such conditions make health promotion and disease prevention more difficult.

CULTURAL BELIEFS RELATED TO HEALTH AND ILLNESS

Health and illness have different meanings for different people and cultural groups. For some groups, illness is something that is expected as part of life and is out of one's own control. For others, it is believed that illness can be prevented by taking action, such as eating a proper diet, getting exercise, or scheduling regular physical examinations.

Some groups attempt to attach meaning to illness to explain why it occurs. Many beliefs have developed regarding the onset, course, and cure of disease, as well as the process of death and dying. For example, some believe illness is a type of divine punishment. Believers in divine punishment claim that illness is a result of punishment for a sin that an individual has committed. Another belief involves an individual's balance with nature. If a person maintains a proper balance, good health results; if a person is not in harmony with the environment, illness occurs.

The "hot" and "cold" theory is an ancient belief about health and illness that still is held widely in many cultures. According to the hot and cold theory, health and illness are influenced by four humors that regulate body functions. The four humors are phlegm, blood, black bile, and yellow bile. The humors are considered either hot (blood and yellow bile) or cold (phlegm and black bile), and an imbalance between the hot and the cold areas of the body causes illness. Examples of illnesses that are thought to be caused by cold entering the body are earaches, paralysis, stomach cramps, and arthritis. Examples of illnesses thought to be caused by heat include dysentery, sore throats, abscessed teeth, and kidney disease. Illnesses are treated with herbs, potions, and food that are considered to be either hot or cold, depending on their effects on the body.

Many ethnic groups use healers who practice health care outside of the formal health care delivery system.

Patients may visit a folk healer or use folk remedies along with or in place of conventional treatment. Western societies generally believe that illness has a known cause that can be treated or cured if the cause is identified. Western medicine is also focused on risk reduction and prevention. Generally, non-Western societies believe illness is due to supernatural causes, and they have a more holistic approach to illness. Traditional healers employ forms of healing that may be secular, sacred, or both. The variety of healers depends on the number of health cultures. Examples of traditional healers are root doctors, who traditionally practiced among urban African Americans, and *curanderos*, who may be consulted by Latinos. They may be sought when mainstream health care is perceived as being too expensive, inconvenient, or unable to provide relief for the problem at hand. The healers provide psychosocial support and counseling in addition to helping with physiologic problems. They use a variety of potions and plants in their practice.

TRADITIONAL HEALTH HABITS AND BELIEFS OF MAJOR ETHNIC GROUPS IN THE UNITED STATES

Although it is inappropriate to stereotype individual members of any culture or subculture, various ethnic groups in the United States tend to have unique, traditional health-culture beliefs and practices. Great variations in beliefs and practices exist not only between but also within ethnic and subcultural groups. Although individuals vary, in a given ethnic group generally there are some common ideas and practices regarding health promotion and disease prevention, attitudes and behaviors related to illness, and utilization of health care resources. One factor that affects the extent to which an individual maintains traditional practices is the extent of enculturation and assimilation into U.S. society that has occurred. First- or second-generation Americans may have more characteristics associated with their ethnic group than people who have been in the United States for several generations.

Listed next are examples of traditional health care beliefs and practices of selected ethnic groups. Remember that these examples are included to show a range of possible health customs for selected ethnic groups. They cannot be generalized to all members of the ethnic group or subculture.

WHITES (EURO-AMERICANS)

Like other racial/ethnic groups, white Americans are very homogeneous even though most descended from European roots. Nevertheless, it is useful to identify some values and beliefs common to this group of people. Whites generally believe in the work ethic, which values personal achievement, individualism, and competition. Values related to health include individual decision making, personal space, and privacy. Illness is viewed primarily as caused by germs in the environment or, in certain religious groups, by divine punishment. The risk of illness can be reduced by eating a proper diet, getting enough exercise, and allowing for adequate rest. In the treatment of illness, the mind, body, and spirit are thought of as separate. Whites look to science and technology for the treatment of illness.

White Americans often communicate directly and tend to express feelings of pain openly. Although members of this group tend to use the formal health care system for their medical and nursing needs, they may consult spiritual advisers in times of illness. Traditionally, the health care provider has been seen as the manager of care.

AFRICAN AMERICANS

African Americans value family, community, religion, health, and work. In addition to an understanding about germs as a cause of illness, some traditional beliefs attribute illness to divine punishment or to an imbalance among body, mind, and spirit. Prevention of illness is thought to be achieved through eating good food, living right, and keeping the system cleaned out. Communication may be direct or indirect, and expressions of pain during illness may entail varying degrees of stoicism or vocal outcries to God for assistance. African Americans tend to attempt self-care before consulting a health care professional when they are ill. They also may use folk medicine or consult a root doctor or spiritualist for help.

LATINOS/HISPANICS

People whose heritage is rooted in various parts of South or Central America refer to themselves as Latinos or Hispanics. To reduce repetition, the term Latinos will be used in this text. Latinos, particularly those who live in the southwestern United States, are family oriented and value harmony in interpersonal relationships. Traditional beliefs about the cause of illness include magical fright, divine punishment, an imbalance of hot and cold elements in the body, and environmental hazards. Some believe that illness can be prevented through the use of charms, amulets, or crucifixes. Communication is usually indirect; however, expressions of pain are open and direct. Folk health specialists (*curanderos*) and family members may be consulted along with the formal health care system in times of illness.

ASIANS

Asians value self-respect, self-control, respect for elders, family honor, loyalty, and pride. There is an emphasis on holistic health and harmony between the self and the universe. Asians in the United States may favor health care that is provided by herbalists, acupuncturists, and other cultural healers, but many use the formal health care system in times of illness. Communication patterns tend to be indirect, and pain is endured with varying degrees of stoicism.

AMERICAN INDIANS

There is considerable diversity among tribes and groups, so it is important to use caution when making generalizations about American Indians. However, some general characteristics may be noted. American Indians value family, respect for elders, generosity, and cooperation with others. They attempt to live in harmony with nature and have deep respect for the environment. Communication is usually indirect, with a great emphasis on nonverbal cues. Pain is usually dealt with stoically. Traditional health practices emphasize total healing, mental and spiritual renewal, and health maintenance. Ceremonial rituals guided by a medicine man may be used for treating illnesses before structured medical care is sought.

To emphasize once again, the examples given here are intended to convey the wide scope of culturally based practices that may need to be considered when working with individuals from various cultures. The nursing assessment should include gathering information about personal health practices so that the care plan can be individualized.

 Put on Your Thinking Cap!

Considering your own race/ethnicity, identify three cultural beliefs related to health that are held by your family. For example, how are you expected to respond to illness or stress? When do you seek medical care, and what kind of provider do you see? Do you use any complementary or alternative therapies? What activities are believed to promote health or prevent disease?

CULTURAL INFLUENCES ON PATIENT AND FAMILY INTERACTIONS WITH THE HEALTH CARE SYSTEM

In all health care settings, patients of different cultures may exhibit behavior that is not understood by health care providers from other cultures. The culturally different patients may be labeled "complaining," "difficult," "uncooperative," or "noncompliant" when, in reality, they are struggling to adapt to a culture that is foreign to them. Fear of the unknown may result in these behaviors. Culturally competent care is urgently needed. With increasing cultural diversity among all people in the United States, you must consider your patients' cultures and develop culture-specific nursing care.

HOSPITAL HEALTH CARE

The hospital environment is often frightening, even to people who are familiar with it. For individuals who speak different languages, have different eating preferences, and view health and illness differently, adapting to the hospital environment is a formidable task. Admission to the hospital may seem like traveling to a foreign country where an entirely different language is spoken. Hospital personnel become authority figures, and their permission is needed to carry out the most basic activities, such as toileting, eating, and dressing. Patients are stripped of their dignity when they are told to wear hospital gowns that barely cover private parts of the body. Modesty is often ignored, causing humiliation and anxiety.

Not only do people find themselves in a totally new environment, but also they must endure separation from their family and friends. Their support systems topple when strict visiting rules are enforced. In some cultures, families expect to help with the nursing care or at least sit with sick people to keep them company and provide support. Nurses and hospital personnel often are uncomfortable with this infringement on their territory. Language barriers may complicate the process of providing care. Many hospitals have access to professional translation services. When available, the professional translator is recommended because family members and friends may not have the language to correctly convey medical information. Furthermore, information exchanged in the health care setting should be confidential and use of a lay translator may violate this confidentiality.

Culture shock associated with hospitalization occurs in three phases. During the first phase, the patient asks questions regarding the hospital routine and the hospital's expectations of the patient. In the second phase, the patient becomes disenchanted with the whole situation and is frustrated, hostile, and then depressed and withdrawn. In the final phase, the patient begins to adapt to the new environment and is even able to maintain a sense of humor during interactions with others.

COMMUNITY AND HOME HEALTH CARE

Community settings in which culturally different individuals interact with the health care system include physicians' offices, outpatient clinics, community mental health centers, home health care, hospices, and day care centers. As mentioned earlier, individuals who have different cultural backgrounds also may have their own network of health care, such as spiritualists, *curanderos*, or root doctors. A day's assignment in home health care may include visits to Jewish, Hispanic, Filipino, and Anglo-American homes. Community nursing presents examples of cultural diversity that nurses everywhere are experiencing with the expanded need for home health services.

Many ethnic or cultural minorities have difficulty getting through the maze of health care services, either because of language differences or because of negative attitudes toward health care providers based on past experiences. Minority group members whose financial resources are limited frequently are clinic patients who must wait hours for an appointment, only to receive a cursory assessment from the physician or nurse. Their questions about their condition may be left unanswered because of communication barriers, which can affect the ability to follow directions for care. These patients may be labeled "noncompliant" or "difficult," which only perpetuates a cycle of negative attitudes among patients and health care providers alike.

When you enter a patient's home, watch for symbolic objects that may indicate cultural identity. Shrines, religious pictures or statues, and special candles are examples of symbols. Assess your patient's health beliefs and practices that are affected by culture. Patients and their families may have magical, religious, biomedical, or holistic beliefs.

If the patient speaks a different language from yours, sometimes a family member is able to translate. If there is no translator available, you may need to spend extra time demonstrating a procedure to the patient and the family.

LONG-TERM FACILITY HEALTH CARE

The majority of residents in long-term care facilities are white females. Some ethnic groups such as Latinos and Asians are extremely reluctant to admit older relatives to residential care facilities and prefer to provide care at home.

Many residents of such facilities suffer from functional impairments (impaired ability to carry out activities of daily living such as bathing and dressing). Those from different cultural groups have the added strain of communication problems and extreme changes in lifestyle and dietary practices. These differences may contribute to confusion, disability, and incontinence. For example, an older woman who speaks little English may have difficulty asking for help getting to the bathroom or using a bedpan. Because older people tend to have very little time between the urge to void and the actual voiding experience, urinary incontinence can occur when a nurse cannot understand the patient's needs.

CULTURAL EXPRESSIONS AND IMPLICATIONS FOR NURSING CARE

When caring for a patient who is from another religious or ethnic background, you should be sensitive to different cultural attitudes, beliefs, and behaviors. Cultural sensitivity and valuing alternative ways of dealing with health issues as well as spiritual beliefs allow you to individualize care. Avoid labeling patients "difficult" or "uncooperative" because you do not understand their behavior. As a practical nurse, you must be able to accept a wide diversity of beliefs, practices, and ideas about health and illness, including many that are different from your own. The more sensitive you are to cultural differences, the more effective your nursing intervention will be. Failure to provide culturally sensitive care can cause additional stress and prolong the patient's recovery time.

It is important to gather information regarding the cultural background of a patient to provide sensitive care. For example, communication patterns, including the language spoken and the use of touching and gesturing, may differ among patients. Obtain information regarding health beliefs, interpersonal relationships, the role of the family during illness, attitudes toward modesty, expressions of fear and pain, and dietary practices. Remember that reactions to pain differ among cultures; some groups are very stoic and do not complain, whereas other groups cry out with pain much of the time.

Sensitivity to cultural factors that affect behavior comes from cultural awareness. To develop cultural awareness, make a conscious and consistent effort to study different cultural groups and their special cultural background. It is helpful to learn the language of your patients. No matter how different your beliefs are from your patient's beliefs, you must respect each person's values and cultural beliefs and respond in a nonjudgmental way.

THERAPEUTIC RELATIONSHIP

Because all nursing care takes place in the framework of the nurse-patient relationship, an environment of acceptance and respect for the beliefs and behaviors of culturally different patients should be established. For patients to trust the nurse, they must feel safe, respected, and accepted.

Maintain an open and inquiring, respectful attitude regarding cultural differences. Patients of another culture initially may be quiet, polite, conforming, or shy. This behavior may reflect a guarded or cautious response because patients are not sure what is expected of them and how the interaction will go. It is a time to "size up" unfamiliar health care personnel without being too offensive or alarming. A good rule of thumb during an initial encounter with minority patients is to speak softly and in an unhurried manner to put them at ease. When nursing staff members are aggressive and demanding, patients tend to be silently angry and withdrawn. Take the time to sit down with patients and their families, listen to their needs and concerns, and learn how they interact.

Culture serves as a guide to action and beliefs in times of crisis. Illness is a time of crisis. Therefore you need to know the patient's cultural patterns of thinking, feeling, and acting before developing a therapeutic plan of care. Once you understand the lifestyle of the patient, you can tailor the nursing care plan to help the patient get through the crisis. Involve the patient in the care plan, identifying familiar ways of coping with an illness or with any other crisis.

Conflicts between the patient's health practices and beliefs and those of the health care system may arise. However, the cultural values of patients and families must be given full consideration. Patients are not likely to change their cultural values if they do not want to.

Changes in health patterns for many patients often require some major changes in lifestyle. If a patient does not respond well to prescribed changes in health practices or lifestyle, the patient may be labeled "uncooperative." Try to understand each situation from the viewpoint of the patient, family, and community. It is only then that effective modifications in health practices can take place. As a culturally competent nurse, you can respond to diversity with respect based on accurate knowledge, an accepting attitude, and a belief in the value of each individual. Cultural competence involves knowledge about cultural differences and interpersonal skills in adapting care to these differences.

BASIC PHYSIOLOGIC NEEDS

Cultural attitudes may affect patients' perceptions of personal hygiene and the role of the nurse in assisting with caring for basic bodily needs. Some patients may not take baths routinely. Others may be extremely modest about disrobing in front of family and strangers. Show sensitivity to these feelings by knocking before entering the room and asking permission before touching the patient or assisting with personal hygiene.

During the bath, do not remove a patient's charms, crosses, medals, or other objects without permission. These objects usually have special meaning and cultural significance. If the patient wishes, family members may assist with the bath, oral hygiene, bed making, ambulation, or other care giving. The inclusion of significant others in care giving helps alleviate the stress and anxiety associated with entering the hospital environment and helps fulfill cultural expectations for both patients and family members.

Nutrition is an aspect of care affected by culture. Diet is often culturally based, and modifications in diet, to be successful, must take culture into account. An example is recommending corn tortillas instead of flour tortillas because corn tortillas have more nutritional value.

DRUG THERAPY

We are just beginning to understand how ethnicity influences how people react to drugs. Factors that contribute to the differing responses can be categorized as environmental, cultural, and genetic. Environmental factors related to drug absorption, metabolism, and action include diet, smoking, and alcohol use. For example, Japanese diets are typically high in salt, which may make antihypertensive drugs less effective.

Cultural factors can affect drug response by influencing the patient's expectations, adherence to prescribed drugs, and willingness to report problems to the physician. In addition, some culturally based nontraditional remedies can interact with prescribed drugs to increase or decrease their effects.

Perhaps the greatest influence of ethnicity in relation to drug therapy is that liver enzymes are controlled by genetic factors. Liver enzymes determine the rate and extent of drug metabolism. People who metabolize drugs slowly are generally at greater risk for drug toxicity than those who metabolize drugs rapidly. To illustrate, people of Japanese and Chinese descent are more likely to be oversedated by diazepam (Valium) because they metabolize the drug more slowly than people of European descent.

There are numerous other examples of variations in drug effects related to ethnicity. In the treatment of hypertension, when compared with whites, blacks respond better to diuretics and not as well to beta blockers and angiotensin-converting enzyme inhibitors. Also, for unknown reasons, people of Asian and Hispanic descent generally require lower doses of antidepressants than whites.

This information is important for the nurse to know when teaching patients about drugs and monitoring for therapeutic and adverse effects. When a patient is not responding in the way we would expect, ethnicity may explain the difference. The patient may require a change in dosage or a different medication.

PATIENT TEACHING

Communication between the nurse and patients and families of different cultures may be especially difficult in the context of teaching. Patients and their families may not be able to understand health and illness information in English even if they have some command of the language. Much of the language of health and illness is confusing and complicated and contains many new words that have not been heard before.

The first approach with people of other cultures is to be warm, understanding, and patient. It is important to establish a good interpersonal relationship to develop enough trust so that people feel free to ask questions. Many patients and their families nod their heads in agreement with everything that is taught, even though little comprehension is taking place.

Using both oral and written communication can help reinforce what has been taught. Written communication in the native language of patients and families greatly aids in their understanding. Having them demonstrate what they have learned helps confirm that learning has taken place. It may be helpful to seek assistance from staff members who are from the same or similar ethnic backgrounds to facilitate communication. Health care facilities should have a list of interpreters available.

Consider the timing of patient and family teaching in culturally diverse populations. Many cultural groups do not work by the clock and schedules; persons from these groups may not appear for appointments or may come several hours late. Rather than characterizing such individuals as "lazy" or "undisciplined," it would be wiser to carry out patient teaching

informally and spontaneously when the opportunity arises.

In addition to considerations of communication and time, other factors related to cultural uniqueness are important to assess when you are teaching patients. These factors include personal space, social organization (patterns of behavior around life events such as illness or death), environmental control, and biological variations (such as the occurrence of specific diseases in certain ethnic groups).

COMPLEMENTARY AND ALTERNATIVE THERAPIES

Until fairly recently, Western medicine looked at many culturally based preventive and treatment agents and practices as unscientific at best and as dangerous at worst. Growing public interest in the use of "natural" remedies either to replace or to complement Western medicine has gradually forced a reevaluation of the use of such remedies. In 1998, Congress established the National Center for Complementary and Alternative Medicine to formally evaluate these products for safety and effectiveness and to provide a source of information for the public. Research is beginning to support the use of some "folk" treatments and to dispel the value of others. This is a rapidly growing field of study, and you are likely to see an increase in the use of these treatments, either alone or in concert with traditional Western practices.

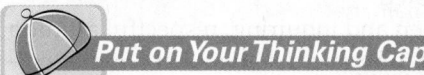

Put on Your Thinking Cap!

Consider how your family reacts to health crises. Identify your family practices related to death. Identify food preferences in your family and discuss health implications. Discuss these culturally related factors with classmates.

Key Points

- Culture is the integrated system of learned values, beliefs, and practices that is characteristic of a society and that guides individual behavior.
- Cultural diversity denotes the existence of many cultures in a society.
- Culture is learned, shared, and based on symbols.
- Cultural differences may occur among various groups in relation to family, religion, communication, educational background, and economic level.
- Health and illness have different meanings for different people and cultural groups; the nurse must be careful not to stereotype people on the basis of their culture.
- When caring for a patient who is from another religious or ethnic background, the nurse should be sensitive to different cultural attitudes, beliefs, and behaviors.

Go to your Companion CD-ROM for a Pharmacology Tutorial, Audio Glossary, and 3-D animations.

evolve   Be sure to visit the companion Evolve site at http://evolve.elsevier.com/Linton/ for WebLinks and additional online resources.

REVIEW QUESTIONS *Choose the best answer.*

1. The process of replacing or giving up values, beliefs, and practices for those of another culture is:
   1. Enculturation
   2. Assimilation
   3. Immigration
   4. Diversification

2. In the United States, Asians and American Indians are said to be subcultures, which means that they:
   1. Share beliefs, values, and attitudes that are different from those of the dominant culture
   2. Are opposed to the basic political structure in the United States
   3. Are highly unlikely to become assimilated into U.S. culture in the future
   4. Believe that their native cultures are superior to the dominant U.S. culture

3. A patient who is a recent Vietnamese immigrant is recovering from abdominal surgery. Four hours after surgery, he has not asked for any pain medication. It would be most appropriate for you to:
   1. Assume that he has a very high level of pain tolerance
   2. Consider that he may be reluctant to report pain
   3. Administer pain medication even if he does not want it
   4. Tell him that suffering is unnecessary when pain medication is ordered

4. In Labor and Delivery, two patients are at the same stage of labor. Ms. L. is lying still with her eyes closed and her breathing controlled. Ms. G. is grasping the side rails and crying out with each contraction. The nursing assistant says, "I don't know why Ms. G. can't be quiet like Ms. L." Your best response is:
   1. "Tell Ms. G. to be quiet because she is disturbing the other patients."
   2. "There is no reason for Ms. G. to be having more pain than Ms. L."
   3. "People like Ms. G. just like to be very dramatic to get a lot of attention."
   4. "Some people believe that pain should be quietly endured; others express it freely."

5. Nurses need to understand culture because:
   1. Care can be based on the patient's culture rather than on individual assessments
   2. All members of an ethnic group have the same beliefs, values, and attitudes
   3. Culture influences beliefs about health and illness and about health practices
   4. Nurses should encourage members of subcultures to adopt the dominant culture

Objectives

After reading and studying this chapter, you should be able to:

1. Describe the concept of family and its relationship to society.
2. Compare various family structures or lifestyles that characterize modern American families.
3. Discuss the family from a developmental perspective.
4. Describe roles and communication patterns within families.
5. Describe adaptive and maladaptive mechanisms used by families to cope with various stressors.
6. Describe the role of the nurse in dealing with families experiencing various stresses.
7. Identify community resources that may help meet the family's needs.

Key Terms

Be sure to check out the bonus material on the Companion CD-ROM, including selected audio pronunciations.

dysfunctional communication (p. 75)
family (p. 72)
functional communication (p. 75)
role (p. 74)

The family is fundamental to human life. Families exist everywhere and have existed since humankind began. The family unit occupies a position between the individual and society, functioning to meet the needs of the individual members and the needs of the society of which it is a part. The family meets individuals' needs in several ways. For the spouse or adult members, it helps stabilize their lives by meeting their affectional, socioeconomic, and sexual needs. For children, the family provides physical and emotional support, directs personality development, and is the main learning context for behaviors, thoughts, and feelings. Among its many functions, of prime importance is the role of providing emotional support and security to its members through love, acceptance, concern, and nurturing.

There are several definitions of a family. A general definition is "two or more persons who are joined together by bonds of sharing and emotional closeness and who identify themselves as being part of the family" (Friedman, 1997, p. 9).

TYPES OF FAMILIES

Families differ in their makeup, interactions, and relationships. Many families today vary from the traditional formula of mother, father, and children. More and more family units are composed of single parents or a combination of spouses and offspring from previous marriages. In addition, friends or partners of the same or opposite sex now are often considered family or extended family.

The major types of families are nuclear, extended, stepparent, single-parent, and nontraditional. The traditional nuclear family is made up of biological or adoptive parents—a mother and father—and their children. The extended family consists of relatives of either spouse who live with the nuclear family. This type of family arrangement was more prevalent in the late 1800s and early to mid-1900s than it is now; however, extended family living arrangements still exist, primarily to meet financial or caregiving needs. The stepparent family, or blended family, is made up of stepparents and their children, most often a mother, her biological children, and a stepfather; however, other variations exist. The single-parent family is characterized by one head of the household, usually a mother or father. The parent may be widowed, divorced, separated, or never married. The nontraditional family takes various forms, including open marriages, communal families, cohabiting couples, group marriages, and gay and lesbian families.

The 2000 Census Bureau data on married couple and unmarried-partner households reported that 52% (54.5 million) of households were maintained by married couples. Another 5.5 million were living together but not married. Most unmarried partner households (6 million) had partners of the opposite sex; however, about 1 in 9 of these had same-sex partners. Almost half of married households included one or more children under the age of 18 years. Children under the age of 18 resided in 40% of opposite-sex partner households. One third of female partner households and one fifth of male partner households included children. There were some differences according to race. Children of racial minorities were twice as likely as Anglo children to live in extended families; blended families were more common for African Americans, American Indians, and Alaskan natives. Six percent of couples in married households are of different races.

FAMILY AND CULTURE

In the United States, there are many variations in cultural patterns among families. Within the family, cultural patterns are transmitted from parent to child. The cultural patterns are related to the ethnic background and class of the family and the attitudes of the parents toward people of other ethnic backgrounds and classes. Cultural values and attitudes influence how a family communicates and interacts, carries out activities of daily living, and views health and health care.

Cultural diversity may occur within ethnic groups and classes, so the best way to assess specific cultural patterns of a family is to get the information from the family itself. It is important to determine the family's values, beliefs, customs, and behaviors that influence health needs, health care practices, and family attitudes toward health and illness, health care providers, and health care systems.

 What Does Culture Have to Do with Families?

Culture influences most aspects of family function including communication, childrearing, and health practices.

FAMILY DEVELOPMENTAL THEORY

FAMILY LIFE CYCLE AND DEVELOPMENTAL TASKS

Every family goes through predictable stages of growth and development, just as individuals do. However, because not all families fit into the traditional nuclear family model, there is variation among stages, depending on the makeup of the family. Responsibilities for growth (developmental tasks) must be met at each developmental stage to meet biological needs, cultural demands, and goals. Traditionally, the five major stages of the family life cycle are beginning families, families with young children, families with adolescents, launching children and moving on, and families in later life (Table 7-1).

Beginning Families

The beginning families stage is also referred to as *married couples* or the *stage of marriage*. The marriage of a couple marks the beginning of a new family in which the couple moves from their families of origin to a new relationship. During this stage, the developmental tasks include establishing a mutually satisfying marriage, working out satisfactory relationships with each spouse's family, and making decisions about parenthood.

Families with Young Children

During the stage when families have young children, the major activities are childbearing and childrearing up to about age 12. The major developmental tasks are setting up a young family as a stable unit (including integrating a new baby into the family), developing parental roles to meet the changing needs of the children as they grow, maintaining a satisfying marital relationship, maintaining and expanding relationships with the extended family by adding parenting and grandparenting roles, socializing the children, and maintaining healthy relationships outside the family.

Families with Adolescents

The stage when families have teenagers is often the most challenging and difficult. As an adolescent moves from being dependent on and controlled by parents to independence and assumption of adult roles, conflicts and turmoil often emerge. The family developmental tasks at this stage are balancing freedom with responsibility as teenagers mature and become increasingly independent, refocusing on the marital relationship, and communicating openly between parents and children.

Launching Children and Moving On

The stage when families are launching young adults and moving on begins when the first child leaves the parental home and ends with the "empty nest," when the last child has left home. This stage can be short or long, depending on the number of children in the family, how many children remain at home after finishing high school or college, and how many children move back into the home after living independently for a while. The parents are generally middle-aged and may feel "sandwiched" between the demands of youth and the needs of their own older family members. It also is a time when they assume the grandparenting role, which requires a change in their roles and self-image. The major family goal is the reorganization of the family into a continuing unit while releasing mature young people into lives of their own. The developmental tasks of this stage include expanding the family circle to include new family members acquired by marriage of children, continuing to renew and readjust in the marital relationship, and assisting aging and ill parents of the husband and wife.

An increasing number of grandparents in the United States live with and have primary responsibility for grandchildren younger than 18 years. The major reasons that grandparents assume the parenting role are substance abuse, incarceration, teen pregnancy, emotional problems, and parental death. For these grandparents, this stage of family development is prolonged.

Table 7-1 *Stages of the Family Life Cycle*

STAGE	DEVELOPMENTAL TASK
Beginning families	Establish mutually satisfying marriage. Work out satisfactory relationship with spouse's family. Make decisions about parenthood.
Families with young children	Set up young family as a stable unit. Develop parental roles to meet changing needs of children. Maintain satisfying marital relationship. Maintain and expand relationships with extended family. Maintain healthy relationships outside the family.
Families with adolescents	Balance freedom with responsibility in teenagers. Refocus on the marital relationship. Communicate openly between parents and children.
Launching children and moving on	Expand family circle to include new family members acquired by marriage of children. Continue to renew and readjust in the marital relationship. Assist aging and ill parents of the husband and wife.
Families in later life	Maintain satisfying living arrangement. Adjust to loss of a spouse. Maintain intergenerational family ties. Continue to make sense of one's existence.

Families in Later Life

The last stage of the family life cycle begins with the retirement of one or both spouses, continues through the loss of one spouse, and ends with the death of the other spouse. In retirement and during the aging process, role modification is necessary and declines in income, self-esteem, status, and health may occur. The family developmental tasks for this stage are maintaining a satisfying living arrangement, adjusting to a reduced income, maintaining the marital relationship, adjusting to the loss of a spouse, maintaining intergenerational family ties, and continuing to make sense of one's existence.

At each stage, working on and maintaining the marital relationship is identified as a developmental task when the family is made up of a married couple. This type of responsibility for growth is an ongoing and never-ending process throughout life.

FAMILY ROLES AND COMMUNICATIONS

FAMILY ROLE STRUCTURE

Each member of the family has a role. A role is how one is expected to behave in a situation or what is expected of a person in a certain position. Culture and social class usually influence how roles are allocated to family members, although greater flexibility of roles has become apparent in recent years. Through these roles, family functions are carried out. Family roles may be performance oriented, such as breadwinner, homemaker, handyman or handywoman, or gardener, or the roles may be emotional, such as leader, nurturer, protector, healer, or rebel. Members may fill more than one role, and any member can satisfactorily fill any role in either category. A healthy family is one in which there is opportunity to shift roles easily from time to time.

In the traditional nuclear family, roles frequently are characterized as formal or informal. Formal roles consist of a limited number of positions in the family that are explicitly defined, such as wife-mother, husband-father, son-brother, and daughter-sister. There are certain role expectations with each of the formal roles, such as wage earner, homemaker, financial manager, cook, and so on, and these roles are usually given to the person with the skills to carry them out. In smaller families, there are fewer people to take on the various roles, so individuals may play several roles at different times. If for some reason a family member is unable to fill a role or roles, another member must step in to keep the family functioning.

Whereas formal roles are explicit roles that each family role structure contains, informal roles are often not as apparent and usually meet the emotional needs of individuals or maintain the family's equilibrium. Informal roles have different requirements that are less likely to be based on age or sex and more likely to be based on the personality attributes of individual members. Effective performance of informal roles can strengthen the performance of the formal roles. Some of the roles enhance the well-being of the family, whereas others can interfere with family functioning.

Common informal roles include encourager (praises others' contributions to the family), harmonizer (mediates differences among other members), initiator-contributor (suggests new ideas and initiates action), blocker (opposes and rejects all ideas), martyr (sacrifices everything for the sake of the family), family scapegoat (problem member of the family), family caretaker (nurtures and cares for other members in need), family go-between (the family "switchboard"—transmits and monitors communication within the family), and family coordinator (organizes and plans family activities). The scapegoat usually assumes or is assigned this role to preserve the family and maintain homeostasis. Scapegoating of a family member generally serves to divert attention from marital conflict between the spouses. The go-between is usually the mother, who monitors all communications and is in charge of settling all disputes. When the conflicts are not resolved, the go-between is often blamed. This type of interaction is sometimes considered dysfunctional because it interferes with direct communication among family members.

Family members assume informal roles through role modeling, having to fill in gaps in family roles, and being reinforced for role behaviors. Parents reward children for fulfilling certain roles, so the children gradually adopt these roles as they are growing up. The children then begin to develop a self-identity based on the roles, which may be either positive or negative, and may continue in these roles throughout their lives.

FAMILY INTERACTION

Family interaction is a unique form of social interaction based on a set of intimate and continuing relationships. It is the sum total of all the family roles being actualized within a family at a given time. Family functions and tasks are carried out through the process of interaction. One of the most important influences on family interaction is the self-esteem of each member. If adult members have adequate self-esteem, they are able to provide the love and nurturing to develop self-esteem, belonging, and acceptance necessary for the growth and development of the children. If they lack self-acceptance and self-respect, it is unlikely that they will be loving spouses or parents. In a healthy family, the members love and respect one another.

FAMILY COMMUNICATION PATTERNS

Within family interactions, certain types of communication patterns develop. Communication refers to the process of exchanging feelings, desires, needs, information, and opinions. Just as individuals have their own distinct style of communication, families also have their unique communication style or pattern. Clear communication is a means of providing a nurturing environment in which family members function well. Conversely, unclear communications may be a major contributor to poor family functioning.

A continual exchange of communication occurs in families. This involves introducing new information, correcting misinformation, problem solving, and having and resolving misunderstandings. The information exchanged may take different routes to reach the receivers. The routes taken depend on the relationships and roles within the family, and these depend on the family power structure, the closeness of relationships, and the popularity of individual members. For example, as noted earlier, many routes of information may go through one person—the go-between, a central member who holds the power and popularity in the family.

Communication in the family may be functional or dysfunctional. However, communication patterns are not totally one way or the other. Rather, they exist on a continuum from functional to dysfunctional, with the patterns of most families falling somewhere in between the polar extremes.

Functional Communication

Functional communication is the clear transmission of a message or information that enables the receiver to understand the intent or meaning of what the sender transmits. Communication in healthy families is a dynamic, two-way process, so that both the sender and the receiver are active participants in the communication. Communication patterns in a functional family demonstrate acceptance of individual differences, openness, honesty, and recognition of the needs and emotions of one another. In addition, the acknowledgment of feelings is essential to healthy family communication. A functional family uses communication to create and maintain mutually beneficial relationships.

Functional patterns of communication include emotional and affective communication. Emotional communication deals with the expression of emotions or feelings, such as anger, hurt, sadness, happiness, affection, and tenderness. A healthy, functional family demonstrates a wide range of emotions and feelings. For family members to be able to enjoy one another, their responses to each other should be fresh and spontaneous rather than controlled, repetitive, and predictable. Affective communication involves verbal messages of caring and nonverbal, physical gestures of touching, caressing, holding, and looking. Physical expressions of affection usually predominate in early childhood and are essential in the development of normal affectional responses. As children grow older, verbal expressions of affection usually predominate.

Families with functional communication patterns value openness, a mutual respect for each other's feelings, thoughts and concerns, spontaneity, and self-disclosure. They usually are able to discuss most personal issues and concerns and resolve conflicts.

Dysfunctional Communication

Dysfunctional communication is the opposite of functional communication. It is an unclear transmission of a message or information that prohibits the receiver from understanding the intent or meaning of what the sender transmits. Low self-esteem of the family members is the prime reason for dysfunctional communications. Communications become confusing, vague, indirect, secretive, and defensive because the individuals lack the ability to appreciate individual differences, thoughts, and feelings of other family members and are unable to deal with conflict. Children growing up in this environment often are unable to recognize and interpret a variety of feelings and experiences.

Dysfunctional patterns of communication may be subtle, and the intent of the communication is not clear. For example, individuals in an interaction may constantly restate their own issues without really listening to others' points of view or acknowledging their needs. Another example is the inability to focus on one issue. Each individual in the interaction rambles from one issue to another instead of resolving any one problem. Or there are unwritten rules about subjects that are allowed for discussion; dysfunctional families have more forbidden subjects than functional families. Sometimes they avoid discussing meaningful issues or expressing feelings by using chitchat—they talk about unimportant daily occurrences rather than the meaningful issues of family life.

Remember that cultural aspects of family communication must be considered when determining whether a family is functional or dysfunctional. Some cultures are more open and communicative, whereas others are less likely to discuss various topics or to show feelings or emotions.

FAMILY COPING

Family coping refers to a positive response that families employ to resolve problems or reduce the stress produced by a problem or event. Family coping processes and strategies enable the family to maintain its necessary functions. Without effective coping and adaptation, family functions cannot be adequately managed.

STRESS AND ADAPTATION

Coping involves the processes of stress and adaptation. The definitions of stress and adaptation are the same for families as they are for individuals. Stress is the response produced by a stressor (or event causing the stress). Adaptation is the process of adjustment to change. How a family adapts to stress and change affects family health and functioning. If adaptation to stress is negative, the family functions less effectively than if the adaptation to stress is positive.

If a family is handling stress poorly or using ineffective adaptive strategies, it may be in crisis. When a family crisis occurs, the stressors are overwhelming and the family is unable to cope and resolve problems. You may be in a position to determine whether a family is in trouble by determining whether the family's problem is being adequately managed by family members, whether a crisis state exists, or whether the current problem is part of a chronic inability to solve problems.

The same strategies for adapting to stress in individuals are used by the family. They include defense mechanisms, coping strategies, and mastery. Defense mechanisms are usual ways of responding to stress. They are usually avoidance behaviors, meaning that people avoid facing problems or stressors. Defense mechanisms are generally considered to be negative responses. Coping strategies are behaviors or efforts used for effective problem solving and are generally considered to be positive responses. Mastery is the end result of using effective coping strategies. Problems are solved competently, and the family functions in a healthy manner.

COPING STRATEGIES

Family coping strategies are actions that families use to respond to stressors. Coping strategies change over time in response to the particular demands or stressors being experienced.

There are several types of coping responses. One effective way that families cope with stress is to deal with the situation causing the problem. It is geared toward altering or eliminating the stressor itself. For example, if a family suddenly becomes homeless because of a major disaster, the family takes steps to find temporary quarters and a new permanent residence. Another way of coping is to attach meaning to a problem. For example, one family may be devastated by becoming homeless, whereas another may find meaning in the situation by saying that at least the family is together and no one was hurt. A third way to cope with stress occurs when families help one another rather than deal with the stressor or situation itself. For example, the family may cope by comforting one another rather than taking action to remedy the situation. The use of many coping strategies is generally more useful than using a single coping mechanism for every stressor, event, or problem.

Coping responses include internal and external coping strategies. Internal coping strategies refer to the ability of the family to pull together and respond to problems as a cohesive unit. Positive family communication patterns are crucial for successful internal coping. External coping strategies refer to the use of social support systems to solve problems. Knowledge of resources in the community and willingness to accept help from outside the family are important for successful external coping. Specific types of internal and external family coping strategies are listed in the Health Promotion Considerations box on p. 77.

FAMILY NURSING CARE

Some general concepts can be used when assessing families and their coping strategies. First, determine what stressors are being experienced by the family, what kinds of coping mechanisms are used, and how well the family is coping with stress. Find out whether the family uses a variety of internal and external cop-

Health Promotion Considerations

Internal and External Family Coping Strategies

Internal Family Coping Strategies

1. Family group reliance: Becoming more reliant on its own resources
2. The use of humor: Relieving anxiety and tension with humor
3. Maintaining cohesiveness: Sharing feelings, thoughts, and experiences to maintain a cohesive family unit
4. Controlling the meaning of the problem: Interpreting events in a positive way
5. Joint family problem solving: All members working together to solve problems
6. Role flexibility: Changing roles as needed
7. Normalizing: Maintaining as normal a life as possible in the face of stressors

External Family Coping Strategies

1. Seeking information: Obtaining information about a situation to maintain control
2. Maintaining active linkages with the community: Participating in clubs or community organizations, using societal resources and information as an adjunct to serve family members' needs
3. Seeking social support: Using informal and formal support systems and support groups
4. Seeking spiritual support: Obtaining spiritual support for coping with stress

From Friedman, M.M. (1992). *Family nursing: Theory and practice* (3rd ed., p. 326). Norwalk, CT: Appleton & Lange.

FIGURE **7-1** Family members need information and reassurance.

ing strategies or whether the stress is too much to cope with and puts the family in crisis. It is important to know how well the family communicates and whether it is a functional or dysfunctional unit.

When assisting families to cope, encourage all family members to be involved in the process. Support or reinforce coping patterns that are or have been successful in the past. Help families learn additional positive coping responses by referring them to resources that can assist them by providing support for both internal and external coping strategies.

ROLE OF THE NURSE

Family members frequently provide support for patients. They also may need a great deal of support themselves during a loved one's illness. Consider the needs of family members, especially in cases in which there is a serious illness or threat of death. Families often need information and reassurance. Providing information can relieve anxiety and fear of the unknown (Fig. 7-1).

It is important to assess the relationships among the patient and other family members. Families can impose a number of burdens, provide considerable

emotional support, or offer a mixed blessing. You should determine whether family members are supportive or detrimental in the recovery process. Also consider the family's influence on individual members as you assess, diagnose, plan, implement, and evaluate nursing care. The inclusion of family members in the client's care and the decision-making process helps maintain the self-esteem of both clients and families.

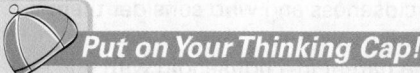
Put on Your Thinking Cap!

Recall a patient whose family was present when you took care of the patient. Discuss how the family member(s) and the patient interacted with each other and how the family member interacted with health care providers. What needs of family member(s) can you identify? How can nurses help meet the needs of families?

COMMUNITY RESOURCES

Referral to community resources can help families cope with health care problems. You should be well acquainted with both informal and formal community resources. Informal resources usually consist of family members or friends who supply long-term support, comfort, and nurturing. Formal resources include community agencies that provide ongoing services.

Information provided through books, magazines, and leaflets can help families learn about an illness or condition, learn what to expect with the disease, know that they are not alone, and deal with the situation. Information also can be provided through community groups, such as support groups, as well as health care providers and social agencies. Formal support systems help by assisting with problems such as home, institutional, and long-term care; finances; transportation; and social support. Many community agencies can help families dealing with stress or those in crisis.

Key Points

- The family unit occupies a position between the individual and society, functioning to meet the needs of the individual members and the needs of the society of which it is a part.
- A family is defined as "two or more persons who are joined together by bonds of sharing and emotional closeness and who identify themselves as being part of the family" (Friedman, 1997, p. 9).
- The major types of families are nuclear, extended, stepparent, single-parent, and nontraditional.
- Cultural values and attitudes influence how a family communicates and interacts, carries out activities of daily living, and views health and health care.
- Traditionally, the five major stages of the family life cycles are beginning families, families with young children, families with adolescents, launching children and moving on, and families in later life.

- Each family member has a role that defines expected behavior in given situations.
- Families have their own unique communication styles or patterns.
- Families, like individuals, use a variant of coping strategies to adapt to stressors.
- The inclusion of family members in a client's care and the decision-making process helps maintain the self-esteem of both clients and families.
- When working with families, the nurse assesses stressors, coping strategies, family communication, and resources.

 Go to your Companion CD-ROM for a Pharmacology Tutorial, Audio Glossary, and 3-D animations.

evolve Be sure to visit the companion Evolve site at http://evolve.elsevier.com/Linton/ for WebLinks and additional online resources.

REVIEW QUESTIONS *Choose the best answer.*

1. The best definition of a family is:
    1. One male and one female parent with children
    2. Two or more individuals who share bonds and emotional closeness and who consider themselves a family
    3. At least one parent in a household with one or more children
    4. A group of individuals related by blood and marriage who make up a single household and share financial resources

2. The Census Bureau reveals the following about households in the United States:
    1. Married couples maintain 90% of all households.
    2. Very few children reside in same-sex partner households.
    3. Children of racial minorities are more likely to live in extended families.
    4. One million couples are living together but not married.

3. What function does scapegoating serve in the family?
    1. Diverts attention from conflict between spouses
    2. Brings attention to the family member who contributes the least
    3. Tests the bonds of loyalty within the family
    4. Motivates children to compete with siblings

4. After a tornado, survivors are being interviewed. A common statement made by the survivors is "We lost everything but each other. This has taught us what is really important in life." This is an example of what type of coping strategy?
    1. Dealing directly with the cause of the problem
    2. Providing comfort to each other
    3. Denying the seriousness of the situation
    4. Attaching meaning to the experience

5. The family of a critically ill patient is comforted by visits from their minister and church members. They pray often for their loved one's recovery. This is an example of an:
    1. Internal family coping strategy
    2. Anticipatory grieving
    3. External family coping strategy
    4. Unrealistic thinking

Objectives

After reading and studying this chapter, you should be able to:

1. Describe the health-illness continuum.
2. Discuss traditional and current views of health and illness.
3. List Maslow's five basic human needs, and explain why they constitute a hierarchy.
4. Explain the four levels of adaptability to stress.
5. Discuss concepts related to health promotion, disease prevention, and health maintenance.
6. Define acute and chronic illness.
7. Discuss illness behavior and the impact of illness on the family.
8. Describe nursing measures for health promotion, health maintenance, and illness.
9. Describe complementary and alternative therapies and the nurse's role in relation to both.

Key Terms

Be sure to check out the bonus material on the Companion CD-ROM, including selected audio pronunciations.

acute illness (p. 85)
alternative therapy (p. 80)
chronic illness (p. 85)
complementary therapy (p. 80)
coping (p. 83)
homeostasis (hō-mē-ō-STĀ-sĭs, p. 84)
primary prevention (p. 84)
secondary prevention (p. 84)
stress (p. 81)
tertiary prevention (TĔR-shē-ĕr-ē, p. 84)

Human beings are complex organisms with interacting biological, psychological, behavioral, emotional, and spiritual systems. Systems within the human body are referred to as the *internal environment.* Systems outside the human body are known as the *external environment.* Health and illness are affected by both the internal and the external environments.

The human body, mind, and spirit are parts of a living system. Human responses to actual or potential health problems include a myriad of reactions, many of them based on thoughts, emotions, and past experiences.

Because of cultural, educational, and social differences, individuals have very different concepts about what constitutes health and illness. People define health and illness according to how they view themselves as human beings and in relation to the surrounding environment. It is important to know how people view health and illness so that you can help them achieve their personal goals for health and wellness.

THE HEALTH-ILLNESS CONTINUUM

TRADITIONAL VIEWS OF HEALTH AND ILLNESS

Traditionally, health and illness have been viewed as separate entities. Either people were healthy or they were sick. Health and illness were seen as **physiologic** phenomena. A typical dictionary definition of health is "soundness, especially of body or mind; freedom from disease or abnormality" (*American Heritage Dictionary*). In 1946, the World Health Organization defined health as "the state of complete physical, mental, and social well-being and not merely the absence of disease or infirmity."

Most definitions of health have not allowed for degrees of health or illness and have failed to reflect the dynamic, ever-changing nature of health. Although the World Health Organization broadened the concept of health from a strictly physiologic state to one that encompasses mental and social well-being, its definition is still seen today as a narrow view of health and illness.

CURRENT VIEWS OF HEALTH AND ILLNESS

Currently, health and illness are viewed as relative states along a continuum. Individuals have neither absolute health nor absolute illness but are in an ever-changing state of being, ranging from peak or high-level wellness to extremely poor health, with death being imminent (Fig. 8-1).

Well-being or lack of well-being for individuals fluctuates along the continuum on a daily basis. Personal and environmental factors contribute to this state of flux. Unique factors within each individual influence how that person responds to external forces.

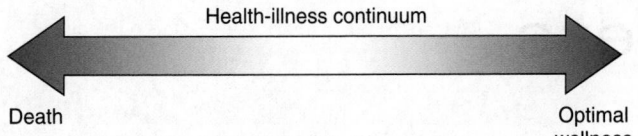

FIGURE **8-1** Common concept of health as a continuum ranging from optimal wellness at one end to illness culminating in death at the other end.

These responses determine how individuals fulfill their needs and reach their highest health potential.

According to Dunn, who first used the expression "high-level wellness," people must accept responsibility for their own wellness and take an active part in improving and maintaining it. Health and illness are relative terms. Each person's state of health integrates factors beyond biological fitness. Personal, psychosocial, and spiritual values and beliefs influence how a person views health and illness.

This current view of health and illness differs from the traditional view, in which health and illness were thought to be completely separate entities. An individual was considered either sick or well, with the focus of treatment on the physiologic aspects of the disease rather than on the person. The emphasis was on curing the disease or injury, not on helping individuals maintain the highest quality of life possible when diseases were not curable. Traditional health care focused on illness rather than on health promotion and disease prevention.

If we keep in mind the dynamic continuum of health and illness, health may be viewed as the ability to express the full range of one's physical and mental potential within one's environment. A healthy person maintains stability and comfort by adapting physically, mentally, emotionally, and socially to internal and external events.

In American culture, disease is regarded as a disruption of biological and/or psychological function. Disease is a condition that can be recognized through objective findings such as fever, the presence of bacteria, or an individual's inability to perform social role tasks. Illness has a broader definition than disease as it incorporates personal, interpersonal, and cultural perceptions of and reactions to disease.

The growing use of complementary and alternative therapies, which are discussed later in this chapter, reflects views of health that may be different from traditional or mainstream views.

BASIC HUMAN NEEDS

Key concepts in health and wellness include homeostasis, adaptation, the dynamic nature of the health-illness continuum, the influence of the internal and external environments, comfort, safety, social relationships, and prevention of disease and disability. To maintain the highest level of health and wellness, people must satisfy basic human needs.

Three broad categories of human needs must be met: (1) physiologic, (2) libidinal (sensual and affectional), and (3) ego developmental. Physiologic needs include oxygen, water, food, elimination, sleep, shelter, safety, and mobility. These needs must be met for individuals to survive. Libidinal needs refer to sensual-sexual and affectional-emotional needs. Sensual-sexual needs encompass the physiologic and psychological aspects of sexuality. Affectional-emotional needs are satisfied through love, security, approval, respect, support, and care. Ego developmental needs refer to needs that must be met to sustain cognitive and perceptual growth and memory development. They are satisfied through education and training and enable individuals to develop motor coordination, independence, self-identity, social skills, communication skills, problem-solving skills, and a moral view.

Abraham Maslow was a psychologist who organized human needs into a hierarchy (Fig. 8-2). Maslow's hierarchy of human needs has five levels: (1) physiologic, (2) safety and security, (3) belonging and love, (4) self-esteem, and (5) self-actualization. A person generally progresses up the hierarchy in an attempt to satisfy needs. Physiologic needs usually must be met before a person progresses to the satisfaction of safety and security needs; safety and security needs must be satisfied before the needs of belonging and love can be met; and so on.

Physiologic needs include the needs for oxygen, fluids, nutrition, life-sustaining environmental temperature, elimination, shelter, rest, and sex. Physiologic needs are the most fundamental because they sustain life. Individuals cannot live without air, water, and food. Once the physical needs are satisfied, *safety needs*, such as security, protection from harm, and freedom

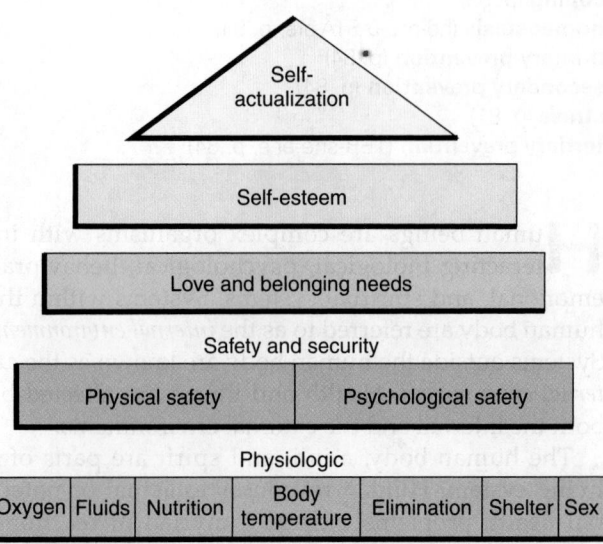

FIGURE **8-2** *Maslow's hierarchy of needs.* Needs must be met in ascending order. For example, safety and security must be achieved before love and belonging needs can be met.

from anxiety and fear, can be addressed. People need order and structure in their lives, and illness or disease can be very disruptive.

Love and belonging needs emerge after safety needs are met. They include feeling loved by one's family and friends and accepted by one's peers and community. Love and belonging are related to self-esteem, which is essential for carrying out health-promoting behaviors. *Self-esteem* means feeling good about oneself and feeling that others hold one in high regard. Individuals with high self-esteem feel confident about themselves and confident that they are appreciated by others. People with low self-esteem may feel helpless and inferior.

Self-actualization, or self-fulfillment, is the highest level of Maslow's hierarchy. Self-actualized people are characterized by the following traits: (1) ability to solve problems, (2) willingness to accept suggestions and criticism from others, (3) broad interests, (4) good communication skills, (5) self-confidence and high self-esteem, (6) maturity, and (7) desire for new experiences and knowledge. Individuals rarely achieve self-actualization; rather, they spend most of their lives attempting to live more fully.

Although the hierarchy of needs is arranged in levels, the individual responds as a unified whole. Therefore the needs cannot be isolated, nor can the focus of care be only on one level. In addition, individuals may move from one level to another under different conditions. However, priorities for nursing care can be based on the level of human needs, so that the physical needs must take priority over those for safety and security.

ADAPTATION TO STRESS

Human beings cannot go through life without stress. Stress is as much a part of life as breathing and eating. Internal and external factors can trigger stress (Table 8-1). Environmental factors, life changes, and physiologic or emotional illness all contribute to stress.

Life changes that cause stress for most people include the following:
- Death of a spouse
- Divorce
- Marital separation from mate
- Detention in jail or other institution
- Death of a close family member
- Major personal injury or illness
- Marriage
- Being fired at work
- Marital reconciliation with mate
- Retirement from work
- Trouble with in-laws
- Change in schools

Table 8-1 | *Stressors*

SOURCES	EXAMPLES
INTERNAL STRESSORS	
Physical	Overexertion or other imposed strains on body system; infections or allergens; physical trauma (e.g., surgery, accident); nutritional deficiency
Psychological	
Intrapsychic conflict	Feeling anger while fearing the consequences of expressing it
Perception of threat from events	Observing an angry person; illness of a loved one
Feelings of inadequacy, dependency, helplessness, powerlessness	Belief that life is impossible without the help and love of a significant other
Boredom	Isolated from friends and/or gratifying life experiences
EXTERNAL STRESSORS	
Interpersonal Relations	
Conflictual relations	Marital conflict; incompatibility at work
Loss of relationship	Death of a loved one
Inability to relate, or so perceived	Language barrier
Socioeconomic	
Economic inadequacies	Unemployment, poor diet, poor housing, little recreation
Climatic extremes	Rain, clouds, little sun
Noxious stimuli	Noise, odors
Sensory deprivation	Isolation from things, people
Political climate	Repressive social system
Ethnic, religious, or national difference	Prejudice based on nationality, race, or creed

From Varcarolis, E.M. (1990). *Foundations of psychiatric mental health nursing* (p. 320). Philadelphia: Saunders.

Life changes can be positive or negative, but they require people to expend energy to adapt to the change. Many studies have found a significant relationship between life changes and the development of physical and mental illness.

Hospitalization is a stressful event for most people. The hospital environment introduces new sights, sounds, smells, and routines into daily life. These changes challenge the patient's autonomy and control. Even people who are sick want to maintain a sense of control over their environment. When they cannot maintain control, powerlessness becomes an additional stressor. While they are sick, people seek control in relation to the following:

- Avoidance of pain and incapacitation
- The immediate hospital environment
- Treatments and procedures
- Relationships with hospital personnel
- Emotional balance
- A satisfactory self-image
- Relationships with family and friends
- Preparing for an uncertain future

THE STRESS RESPONSE

There are two types of stress response: local adaptation and general adaptation. Hans Selye called these responses to stress *syndromes.* Local adaptation syndrome is a short-term, localized response to a specific stressor that restores a body region or body part to homeostasis. Examples of this syndrome are blood clotting, wound healing, pain, and inflammation.

The general adaptation syndrome is a physiologic response of the whole body to stress. Because it involves primarily the autonomic nervous system and the endocrine system, it is often referred to as the *neuroendocrine response.* The general adaptation syndrome consists of three stages: (1) the alarm reaction, (2) the resistance stage, and (3) the exhaustion stage (Fig. 8-3). The alarm reaction causes the body to respond to stress physiologically. Hormone levels, heart rate and cardiac output, respiratory rate, oxygen intake, and mental energy are increased. The pupils are dilated to cover a larger visual field. These reactions together are called the *fight-or-flight response,* which helps the body defend against stressors.

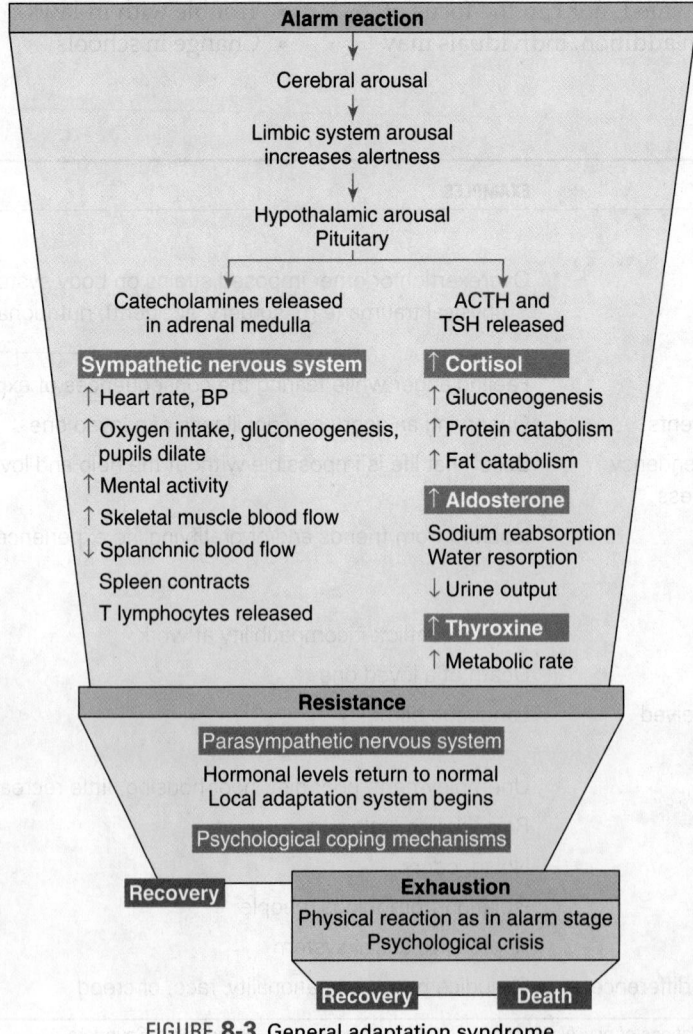

FIGURE **8-3** General adaptation syndrome.

After the initial alarm stage, the body stabilizes and physiologic processes return to normal levels. The resistance stage is characterized by adaptation to the stressor. If the stressor can be overcome or the damage repaired, as in a short-term illness or injury, the body begins to heal. If the stressor is long-term, such as one that accompanies a chronic physical or mental illness, an individual may enter the third stage of adaptation: exhaustion. During the exhaustion stage, the body is drained of energy and can no longer defend itself against the stressor. Death may be the ultimate outcome.

There are many signs and symptoms of stress. Among them are cold hands and feet, tensed muscles, nervous movements, excessive sweating, tooth grinding, headaches, insomnia, and subjective complaints of feeling tense or nervous. When individuals do not cope well with stressors and are unable to adapt, they may withdraw and become depressed. Signs and symptoms of withdrawal and depression are slowed speech; a lowered, hesitant speaking voice; decreased bodily movement; a hunched-over, tired posture; insomnia; and subjective complaints of feeling sad, depressed, or unable to concentrate.

Put on Your Thinking Cap!

Recall a frightening experience. Write down how you felt mentally and physically. Explain your feelings using the general adaptation syndrome (stress response).

COPING

Coping is any behavioral or cognitive activity used to deal with stress. People cope with stress in different ways. They may use problem-solving strategies, which involve identifying the problem, generating alternatives, choosing the best alternative, and applying it to the problem. Lazarus describes the effectiveness of coping as being related to how a person interprets the problem. He explains the daily hassles in life as stressors and the daily uplifts as buffers to daily hassles. For example, some hassles of daily life include "too many things to do" and misplacing things. Uplifts include feeling healthy and getting enough sleep. Hardiness is another concept that influences a person's response to stress. Hardiness encompasses concepts of control, commitment, and ability to handle challenges.

Others may cope with stress by using emotion-focused strategies. Examples of emotion-focused strategies are distancing oneself from the stress-provoking situation or denying its seriousness, self-isolation or withdrawal, blaming oneself or accepting responsibility for the problem, drawing strength from adversity, tension reduction, hostility, fatalism, social support, and faith. Common coping strategies and examples are listed in the Health Promotion Considerations box below.

ADAPTATION

Adaptation to stress is essential to maintaining health. Through adaptation, individuals cope constructively with stressful conditions. Adaptation depends on accurate appraisal of stressful situations and effective coping. Adaptation can lead to physiologic and psychological well-being.

For reasons we do not fully understand, some people adapt better than others to life circumstances. It is generally thought that adaptability is a characteristic that is either inborn or acquired in very early childhood. People who are able to adapt to stress usually live constructively and in relative harmony with others. They view stress as a challenge to be overcome, and they have a sense of control over their lives. Adaptable people demonstrate the ability to rebound in the face of adversity.

Nurses can help patients deal with stress by identifying the patient's usual methods of coping or adapting. These methods rely on internal and external resources. Examples of internal resources are physiologic and psychological responses that occur when one is faced

Health Promotion Considerations

Common Coping Strategies and Examples

COPING STRATEGY	EXAMPLE
Event rehearsal	Mental and verbal preparation for an event or practice of coping strategies
Confrontation	Aggressive seeking of information, anger, refusal of treatments
Distancing or denial	Unwillingness or inability to talk about events; going on as if nothing has happened
Self-control	Stoicism, showing no feelings
Social support	Seeking out family, friends, or others in similar situations
Accepting responsibility	Verbally placing responsibility for situation on self
Faith	Praying, reading religious material, seeking out of clergy or religious guidance
Problem solving	Making plans, verbally outlining what will be done next
Positive reappraisal	Speaking of how situation has fostered growth
Event review	Discussing situations or coping that has occurred

From Ignatavicius, D.D., Workman, M.L., & Mishler, M. (1999). *Medical-surgical nursing: A nursing process approach* (3rd ed., p. 100). Philadelphia: Saunders.

with a stressful situation, such as smoking, drinking alcohol, eating, crying, and exercise. External responses include getting help from family, friends, and service agencies in the community.

HOMEOSTASIS

Homeostasis is a term derived from Greek that describes a tendency of the body to maintain stability of the internal environment. The body adapts to internal and external changes in the environment, adjusts to changes, and maintains equilibrium, or homeostasis. For example, the body adjusts heart rate, blood pressure, respiration, temperature, and hormone secretions to maintain an internal steady state or balance. Continuous adaptation and change in the internal environment are essential for the organism to exist in the external environment.

HEALTH PROMOTION, DISEASE PREVENTION, AND HEALTH MAINTENANCE

Health promotion activities are directed toward maintaining or enhancing well-being as a protection against illness. Through public education, Americans have become increasingly health conscious and many are beginning to take more responsibility for maintaining healthy lifestyles.

The U.S. Department of Health and Human Services has developed a document outlining goals for the year 2010, called *Healthy People 2010. Healthy People 2010* is a national health promotion and disease prevention initiative that aims to increase the quality and years of healthy life and to eliminate health disparities. Twenty-eight focus areas are identified, each with specific objectives and strategies (Box 8-1). Factors being used to measure progress toward meeting the goals and objectives of *Healthy People 2010* are called *leading health indicators* and are shown in Box 8-2.

Specific activities that are generally thought to promote health are as follows:

- Adequate nutrition based on the "pyramid" concept (see Chapter 9). Foods should be eaten in moderation, with an emphasis on complex carbohydrates, followed by fruits and vegetables, proteins and dairy products, and a minimum amount of fats (no more than 30% of calories consumed) and simple sugars. Approximately 20 to 30 grams of dietary fiber should be taken in daily.
- Moderate exercise on a routine schedule. Twenty minutes of walking three times per week is considered ideal.

Put on Your Thinking Cap!

List five ways to promote your own health while you are a nursing student.

Box 8-1 | *Healthy People 2010* Focus Areas

1. Access to quality health services
2. Arthritis, osteoporosis, and chronic back conditions
3. Cancer
4. Chronic kidney disease
5. Diabetes
6. Disability and secondary conditions
7. Educational and community-based programs
8. Environmental health
9. Family planning
10. Food safety
11. Health communication
12. Heart disease and stroke
13. HIV
14. Immunizations and infectious diseases
15. Injury and violence prevention
16. Maternal health, infant health, and child health
17. Medical product safety
18. Mental health and mental disorders
19. Nutrition and overweight
20. Occupational health and safety
21. Oral health
22. Physical activity and fitness
23. Public health infrastructure
24. Respiratory diseases
25. Sexually transmitted infections
26. Substance abuse
27. Tobacco use
28. Vision and hearing

From U.S. Department of Health and Human Services, Public Health Service. (2000). *Healthy People 2010.* Available at http://www.health.gov/healthypeople/ March 6, 2001.

Box 8-2 | *Healthy People 2010* Leading Health Indicators

1. Physical activity
2. Overweight and obesity
3. Tobacco use
4. Substance abuse
5. Responsible sexual behavior
6. Mental health
7. Injury and violence
8. Environmental quality
9. Immunization
10. Access to health care

From U.S. Department of Health and Human Services, Public Health Service. (2000). *Healthy People 2010.* Available at http://www.health.gov/healthypeople/ March 6, 2001.

- Rest, 7 to 8 hours of sleep every 24 hours.
- Healthy lifestyle, especially no smoking and limited consumption of alcohol.
- Balance of work and recreation.

Disease or illness prevention behavior is action taken by individuals to decrease the potential or actual threat of illness and its harmful consequences. The three levels of prevention (primary, secondary, and tertiary) are described in Chapter 1.

THE CONCEPT OF ILLNESS

Illness is a deviation from a healthy state that may occur acutely or as a series of long-term events. Acute and chronic illnesses are experienced and viewed differently.

Acute illness is an illness or disease that has a relatively rapid onset and short duration. The condition usually responds to a specific treatment and ends in full recovery. Examples of acute illnesses are the common cold or influenza, appendicitis, and urinary tract infections.

Chronic illness usually involves permanent impairment or disability and requires long-term rehabilitation and medical or nursing treatment. Examples of chronic illnesses are coronary artery disease, chronic obstructive pulmonary disease, hypothyroidism, and diabetes mellitus. Some chronic illnesses such as rheumatoid arthritis and asthma are characterized by periods of remission and exacerbation. During remissions, the disease seems to go away. During episodes of exacerbation, acute symptoms recur.

ILLNESS BEHAVIOR

Reactions to illness vary among individuals. Some people take action, whereas others may do nothing. Those who take action may seek the help of health care providers, such as physicians, nurses, or dentists; others may seek help from friends or family members. Among some cultures in the United States, people may seek help from folk healers or herbalists. The actions taken by individuals are influenced by the availability and affordability of health care, the individual's perception of the problem, others' perception of the problem, and the failure or success of self-prescribed treatment.

People who take no action may wait to see whether the symptoms go away by themselves. Others may deny that something is wrong and refuse to admit that they are ill. People who take no action may be influenced by the same factors that affect those who take action.

Some individuals take counteraction in response to illness. This means that they engage in activities that should be avoided just to prove to themselves that the symptoms do not exist. For example, a person with symptoms of chronic bronchitis may continue to smoke, regardless of the impaired breathing and coughing that the smoke may cause. Patients who have a history of failure to follow proper health practices or treatment regimens are referred to as "noncompliant." Such behaviors can have harmful effects on health and self-esteem and can lead to death. Because of the judgmental tone of the word "noncompliant," many people prefer to use the term "nonadherence."

The Sick Role

When people become ill, they frequently adopt a "sick role." The sick role allows individuals time to recover from their disease. When they cannot get well on their

Table 8-2	*Sick Role Behaviors*

1. Exemption from normal activities
2. Recognition that the sick person is not responsible for causing the condition
3. Expectation that the sick person wants to get well
4. Obligation to seek competent help

own, others must care for them. They are temporarily exempt from social responsibilities so that they can concentrate on getting well. It is assumed that people who are sick want to get well and therefore should seek the help of health professionals and cooperate with prescribed health care regimens (Table 8-2). However, some people are reluctant to give up the sick role because of the attention they get or because they wish to avoid work.

IMPACT OF ILLNESS ON THE FAMILY

Illness affects not only the individual but also the entire family. An illness may affect the roles of family members, the daily activities carried out, and the family's economic stability.

Three factors influence the effect of illness on the family. The first factor is the identity of the member of the family who is ill. For example, if the head of the household and chief breadwinner is sick, the financial resources may be threatened. If the person who normally cares for the home and children becomes ill, others have to pitch in to help. If an older member of the family becomes ill, grown children may have to provide care. The reversal in the parent-child roles may be difficult for both parents and children.

The second factor influencing the effect of illness on the family is the seriousness and duration of the disease. An acute illness does not produce the long-term effects of a chronic disease. Family members are able to change roles temporarily to manage an acute illness, but during the long duration of a chronic illness, family relationships may become strained.

The third factor is the social and cultural customs of the family. Families of various cultures have different attitudes toward illness, caregiving, and changing family roles.

All of these factors can have an effect on family functioning. Feelings of frustration, anger, and grief must be dealt with so that all members of the family can function at their highest potential while providing care for the sick member. Chapter 7 provides more in-depth coverage of nursing care of families.

IMPLICATIONS FOR NURSING CARE

PREVENT HEALTH PROBLEMS

Nurses can help people engage in healthier lifestyles to prevent disease. Nursing measures are geared toward helping others make informed decisions regarding their health care practices. For example, the nurse can:

- Inform patients of daily activities, such as the proper diet, exercise, and adequate sleep, that help maintain optimal health.
- Inform patients about the diseases for which they are at risk.
- Explain the consequences of the disease for which they are at risk.
- Give patients specific information about how they can reduce their risk for the disease.

When counseling patients and their families, it is important to keep in mind that most health promotion and disease prevention measures require a change in lifestyle. Take into consideration the biophysical, psychological, sociocultural, spiritual, and environmental dimensions of family life and structure and be realistic in your expectations for change.

Put on Your Thinking Cap!

Identify three factors that are threats to your health, and identify ways to deal with each of them.

HELP SATISFY THE PATIENT'S UNMET BASIC HUMAN NEEDS

For people to maintain the highest levels of health and wellness, basic human needs must be met. According to Henderson (1964), "The unique function of the nurse is to assist the individual, sick or well, in the performance of those activities contributing to health or its recovery (or to a peaceful death) that he would perform unaided if he had the necessary strength, will, or knowledge. And to do this in such a way as to help him gain independence as rapidly as possible."

Henderson identified 14 components of basic nursing care. These components include normal breathing, eating and drinking adequately, eliminating body wastes, maintaining desirable posture, sleeping and resting, selecting suitable clothing (dressing and undressing), maintaining normal body temperature, keeping the body clean, avoiding dangers in the environment, communicating with others, worshiping, working to achieve a sense of accomplishment, playing, and learning. These components of basic nursing care are closely related to Maslow's hierarchy of human needs, in that the first eight components address physiologic needs. Other components refer to safety needs, to belonging and love needs, and to self-esteem and self-actualization needs. Henderson's work provides a useful way to identify human needs that must be met for optimum health.

INCREASE ADAPTABILITY

The first step in helping patients increase their adaptability is to determine what the patient perceives as stressful and how stressful it is. One way to assess the degree of stress is to ask patients to name the worst possible stressor and then compare the present stressor with that one. The second step is to assess past methods of coping with stress that have been successful for the patient. It is then helpful to apply past coping strategies to new situations. To assess internal coping strategies, ask, "What kinds of things do you do when you are stressed?" "Do you eat more or less?" "Do you drink alcohol?" "Do you smoke more?" "Do you sleep more or less?" Questions that help determine external coping strategies include, "To whom do you turn when you are feeling stressed?" "Do you talk with others or do you keep things inside?" "Do you contact any professionals such as social workers, nurses, doctors, or social agencies when you have a problem?"

Older persons have particular difficulty coping with stress and adapting to new situations. When any type of stressor occurs, it takes longer and is much harder to get back to their previous level of functioning. Fortunately, people who have lived a long time have experienced many stresses throughout life and generally have developed a wide range of coping mechanisms and skills for adapting to change. Help older patients use past successful coping mechanisms to deal with new stressors. Emphasize strengths rather than limitations.

During hospitalization, you can help patients and families adapt to a difficult situation by helping them cope with the stress of a new environment, illness, and uncertainty. Some patients and families benefit from detailed information about the disease and the hospital procedures; others prefer not to know. Allowing patients to have as much control as possible helps reduce stress. Even people who are very dependent on hospital personnel need to feel that they have some control over their lives. Other measures that may help relieve stress and promote coping and adaptation are biofeedback, progressive muscle relaxation, meditation, and imagery. These strategies generally focus attention inward on the patient's own mind and body and reduce either physical or emotional tension.

FOSTER INDEPENDENCE

In acute illness, recovery often is speedy and people return quickly to their previous lifestyle. However, individuals with chronic illnesses must spend a lifetime managing symptoms. Many older adults have one or more chronic illnesses and may need some type of assistance in their daily lives. The goal is to maintain the highest level of independence possible and prevent further disability. The following tasks have been identified for chronically ill individuals: prevent and manage crises, carry out prescribed regimens, control symptoms, reorder time, adjust to changes in the course of the illness, prevent social isolation, and attempt to normalize social interactions.

Prevent and Manage Crises

When symptoms flare up, a crisis situation may arise. You can help patients and families prevent and control a crisis situation. The patient and family members must learn the signs and symptoms of the onset of a crisis and make a plan for how to deal with the crisis.

Carry Out Prescribed Regimens

Chronically ill individuals may need to take many medications, eat special foods, or restrict some activities. It is very difficult to have a restricted lifestyle day in and day out, especially when symptoms are not apparent. Nursing interventions include teaching patients about the need to carry out regimens, providing moral support and encouragement, and finding ways to make carrying out regimens easier. You can increase patient compliance by forming "alliances" with them so that they understand that they are important participants in developing their own health regimen. Of course, when it comes to lifestyle changes, only the patient can control them.

Manage Symptoms

Chronically ill individuals must learn to manage symptoms to continue desired activities. Gear nursing interventions toward helping patients learn about the pattern of symptoms (typical onset, duration, and severity) and the limits of their ability to control symptoms. Arrange daily routines so that the highest-level activities are carried out when symptoms are lessened or absent and periods of rest are taken when symptoms are most acute.

Reorder Time

People with chronic illness may find they have either too much or too little available time. Forced retirement may increase the amount of free time; conversely, carrying out regimens to manage symptoms may be extremely time-consuming for patients and caregivers. In both situations, the chronically ill and their family members may become frustrated and depressed. The nurse can help patients and caregivers develop a daily schedule that allows time for desired activities while managing the regimens of the chronic illness.

Adjust to Changes in the Course of the Disease

Chronic illnesses often have unpredictable courses, and individuals must learn to live with the ups and downs of the disease. Chronically ill individuals need support if they are to achieve their highest potential.

Prevent Social Isolation

Chronically ill individuals and their families often become socially isolated. The ill person may withdraw from others, or others may feel uncomfortable and withdraw. Support groups are helpful for providing a social outlet with others in the same situation.

Attempt to Normalize Social Interactions

Chronically ill people need to maintain as normal a lifestyle as possible despite having to manage symptoms, adapt to changes in appearance caused by the illness, or use adaptive equipment or prostheses. Encourage them to live as independently as possible in spite of their illness.

It is important to assess the support systems for the chronically ill. Families are the major support systems for persons with chronic illnesses and often provide the day-to-day ongoing care. Formal support systems include social service agencies, health care providers, and community agencies. If family members are unavailable or unable to provide support, formal services may be needed.

HELP FAMILY MEMBERS DEAL WITH THE PATIENT'S ILLNESS

Families provide the bulk of support for the chronically ill, and the burden of caregiving is heavy for them. They must take on more physical work because of the need to assist with activities of daily living, deal with changes in the progress of the disease, cope with feeling psychologically and physically overwhelmed, and adapt to changes in their own social roles and identities as well as those of the ill family member. In some cases, a family caregiver also may have a chronic illness that must be managed, or he or she may develop a physical illness or disability as a result of the burden of caregiving. This is especially true for older caregivers.

Health care providers need to assist patients and their family members in developing a collaborative plan of care. In some cases, relief or respite can be obtained to ease the caregiving responsibility. Many communities have adult day care centers for older adults or persons with particular chronic illnesses. These centers enable both the older or chronically ill individuals and their caregivers to have a more normal lifestyle, with social interaction and structure. Formal support services should be used whenever they are needed to assist families in caring for their chronically ill loved ones.

ASSIST TERMINALLY ILL PATIENTS TO A PEACEFUL DEATH

Unfortunately, everyone must die. Nurses are often the health care providers who have the most intimate relationship with people who are terminally ill. When death comes accidentally or after an acute illness, there is little or no time to prepare for death. But when disease is chronic, patients and families often need to make difficult decisions regarding death.

In today's health care system, with its sophisticated technology, terminally ill patients can be kept alive longer than was ever possible in the past. Issues related to the setting in which the terminally ill are cared for, whether machines for artificial physiologic functioning are used, and when these machines are to be turned off must be faced on a daily basis. More than anyone else, family members have to live with the memory of their loved ones and the events surrounding their death.

Nurses should be supportive of decisions made by patients and families. The dying patients and their loved ones should be informed of the options for care and their consequences. The living will and durable power of attorney for health care are legal documents called *advance directives.* They allow patients to designate, in advance, what treatments they would want in specific situations (living will) or to appoint one person to make treatment decisions when they are not able to make those decisions (durable power of attorney). In 1991, the federal government passed the Patient Self-Determination Act, stating that persons admitted to hospitals and nursing homes must be asked if they want to prepare an advance directive. Open communication and an acknowledgment of different attitudes toward terminal illness and death are extremely important. The nurse should have knowledge of the dying process and the needs of the dying person to provide compassionate care, promote comfort, and make the pain and physical treatment bearable. More detailed information on caring for terminally ill patients is found in Chapter 24.

COMPLEMENTARY AND ALTERNATIVE THERAPIES

This chapter has focused on health and illness as defined by conventional Western medicine. However, Americans are increasingly turning to other therapies in addition to, or along with, conventional medicine. These nontraditional therapies are called *alternative* therapies if they are used in place of conventional medicine. An example of an alternative therapy is the use of relaxation therapy or acupuncture instead of analgesics to treat pain. Nontraditional therapies that are used along with conventional therapies are called *complementary* therapies. For example, a patient with chronic pain might take analgesics but also practice guided imagery.

Conventional and nontraditional medicines are based on differing views of health and illness. Conventional medicine focuses on diseases that are treated by correcting the underlying pathological processes with drugs, surgery, diet, and physical manipulation. Health is viewed primarily as prevention of disease. Most nontraditional therapies are based on the belief that illness is caused by lack of balance or harmony within the individual or between the individual and the environment. Therapy aims to restore balance or harmony, which puts the individual in a position such that healing can occur. Many of the nontraditional therapies have long been used in folk medicine; others have been developed more recently. Examples of complementary and alternative therapies are presented in Table 8-3.

Why is the use of nontraditional therapies becoming more common in the United States? First, many can be self-taught or learned from practitioners whose fees, if any, are typically less than those of medical doctors. Botanicals and other folk remedies are available without medical prescriptions. Second, nontraditional therapies are usually noninvasive. Third, they are part of a holistic approach to health and healing rather than just focusing on the disease or injury. Fourth, many

Table 8-3 · *Types of Complementary and Alternative Therapies*

TYPE	DESCRIPTION	EXAMPLES
Alternative systems of medical practice	Ranges from self-care based on folk principles to organized care using alternative methods	Herbal tea for a cold, acupuncture, traditional Oriental medicine
Mind-body interventions	Uses the power of the mind and the body to affect each other	Psychotherapy, meditation, yoga, prayer, guided imagery, biofeedback, relaxation therapy
Manual healing methods	Uses touch, manipulation of body parts	Osteopathic medicine, massage, chiropractic, reflexology, acupuncture
Bioelectromagnetic applications	Uses electromagnetic fields for their effects on the body	Nerve stimulation, hyperthermia, laser surgery
Herbal medicine	Uses plants and plant products as remedies	Echinacea, ginger, *ginkgo biloba*, ginseng, St. John's wort
Pharmacologic and biologic treatments	Uses drugs, vaccines, etc. that have not yet been approved by the Food and Drug Administration for specified purposes	Antioxidants, chelation, metabolic therapy
Diet, nutrition, and lifestyle changes	Affects biochemical and physiologic processes	Macrobiotic diet, high-dose vitamin therapy

Modified from U.S. Office of Alternative Medicine. (1994). Alternative medicine: Expanding medical horizons (pp. 3-206). Washington, DC: National Institutes of Health. In Black, J.M., Hawks, J.H., & Keene, A.M. (2001). *Medical-surgical nursing: Clinical management for positive outcomes* (6th ed.). Philadelphia: Saunders.

Health Promotion Considerations

Considering Nontraditional Therapies

The role of the nurse in relation to nontraditional remedies and therapies includes:

- In your nursing assessment, always ask about the use of nontraditional remedies and/or therapies: what the patient is using, why, whether it has been helpful, and any negative outcomes.
- Be open-minded about nontraditional therapies as a valid choice by some patients. Learn about these therapies, and try some if you feel comfortable doing so. For example, imagery and relaxation techniques are useful in many situations and have no adverse effects. However, do not attempt to use techniques with patients unless you have been properly instructed in their use. Professional education courses are a good place to learn noninvasive techniques that can be used with many types of patients.
- Teach patients about any adverse effects of nontraditional remedies.
- Be aware of potentially dangerous remedies and those that can interact with prescription drugs that the patient is taking. Among dangerous remedies are the following herbs: sassafras, ephedra, chaparral, borage, calamus ("sweet flag"), comfrey, germander, life root, and pokeroot. See Table 8-4 for examples of drug interactions.
- Caution patients about very expensive therapies, especially if they make outlandish claims.

people have found these therapies to be effective. Fifth, though not always true, people generally believe nontraditional practices are safer than medical and surgical treatment. Sixth, there is a perception that anything labeled "natural" is better.

Only recently have medical and nursing publications begun to include nontraditional therapies. At this time, a relatively small number of nontraditional remedies have been scientifically studied, so we are just beginning to have scientific information to use in discussing these remedies with patients. The Health Promotion Considerations box at left discusses some of the pros and cons of nontraditional therapies.

Key Points

- Because of cultural, educational, spiritual, and social differences, individuals have very different concepts about what constitutes health and illness.
- Western culture views health and illness as relative states along a continuum that fluctuates on a daily basis.
- Disease is a biologic or psychophysiologic malfunction, or both, and illness refers to how a person perceives and responds to not being well.
- To maintain the highest level of health and wellness, people must satisfy basic human needs.
- The three broad categories of human needs are physical, libidinal, and ego developmental.
- Stress is mental or emotional pressure resulting from internal or external causes.
- Coping is any behavioral or cognitive activity used to deal with stress.
- Homeostasis describes a tendency of biologic systems to maintain stability of the internal environment while continuously adjusting to changes necessary for survival.
- Health promotion activities are directed toward maintaining or enhancing well-being as a protection against illness.
- Illness is a deviation from a healthy state that may occur in the form of an acute episode or as a series of long-term events.
- Reactions to illness vary among individuals.
- When people become ill, they often assume a "sick role" that allows them time to recover from their disease.
- The impact of illness on the family depends on which family member is ill, the seriousness of the illness, and the social and cultural customs of the family.
- Nurses help people by striving to prevent disease, helping satisfy patients' unmet basic needs, helping patients increase adaptability, fostering independence, helping family members deal with patients' illnesses, and assisting terminally ill patients to a peaceful death.

Table 8-4   *Examples of Dangerous Herbal Remedy—Drug Interactions*

REMEDY	DRUG	POTENTIAL EFFECT OF INTERACTION
Echinacea	Immunosuppressants	May inhibit immunosuppression
Ginseng	Aspirin	Increased anticoagulation → risk of bleeding
Goldenseal	Antihypertensives	Increased BP
Hawthorn	Cardiac glycosides	Increased effects of glycoside → risk of toxicity
Aloe (oral)	Potassium-wasting diuretics	Increased risk of hypokalemia
Kava-kava	Central nervous system (CNS) depressants	Increased sedation
Garlic	Anticoagulants	Increased anticoagulation → risk of bleeding
Ephedra (ma huang)	Antihypertensives	Increased blood pressure
Valerian	CNS depressants	Increased sedation

From Deglin, J.H., & Vallerand, A.H. (1999). *Davis's drug guide for nurses.* Philadelphia: F.A. Davis.

- Complementary and alternative therapies are often based on holistic beliefs about the nature of health and illness.
- Complementary therapies are employed along with conventional treatment; alternative therapies are used in place of conventional therapies.
- The nurse should be open-minded about complementary and alternative therapies and should learn about them.

 Go to your Companion CD-ROM for a Pharmacology Tutorial, Audio Glossary, and 3-D animations.

evolve Be sure to visit the Companion Evolve site at http://evolve.elsevier.com/Linton/ for WebLinks and additional online resources.

REVIEW QUESTIONS *Choose the best answer.*

1. A cancer patient has decided to treat herself with herbal remedies instead of receiving chemotherapy and radiotherapy. The use of herbal remedies in this situation is an example of:
   1. Complementary therapy
   2. Conventional therapy
   3. Alternative therapy
   4. Allopathic therapy

2. Which statement illustrates why Maslow's basic human needs are presented as a hierarchy?
   1. The sequence in which needs are met is not important.
   2. Each level of need must be satisfied before moving to the next step.
   3. At birth, humans are self-actualized and must learn to meet other needs.
   4. A person can move only upward in a hierarchy, never downward.

3. A clinic patient cut his arm at work 3 days ago. The skin around the wound is red, warm, and swollen. The patient reports that the wound is painful. The patient's signs and symptoms are evidence of:
   1. General adaptation
   2. Defense mechanisms
   3. Local adaptation
   4. Fight-or-flight response

4. Homeostasis is:
   1. The exhaustion stage of the stress response
   2. The use of home remedies in treatment of illness
   3. The ability of a living organism to remain unchanged
   4. A tendency of the body to maintain internal stability

5. A patient who has a chronic disease is in a period of exacerbation. This means:
   1. Symptoms have returned
   2. The disease has been cured
   3. Symptoms will soon reappear
   4. The terminal stage of the disease has begun

6. Nursing interventions that can help patients adapt to stress include the following:
   1. Limit teaching to what the patient needs to know
   2. Do not require that the patient make any decisions
   3. Discourage the use of complementary and alternative therapies
   4. Identify the patient's previously successful coping strategies

7. After receiving a diagnosis of Parkinson's disease, a patient signed up for an educational seminar, joined a community support group, planned home adaptations, and found Internet information sites. What coping strategy is the patient using?
   1. Self-control
   2. Positive reappraisal
   3. Confrontation
   4. Denial

8. Among complementary and alternative therapies, which of the following uses the power of the mind and body to affect each other?
   1. Nerve stimulation
   2. Guided imagery
   3. *Ginkgo biloba*
   4. Metabolic therapy

Nutrition

Objectives

After reading and studying this chapter, you should be able to:

1. Explain the role of the gastrointestinal system in the digestion of food.
2. Describe how food is digested and absorbed.
3. List the functions of each of the six classes of essential nutrients.
4. Define macronutrient and micronutrient.
5. Identify the food sources of proteins, carbohydrates, and fats.
6. Identify the food sources of dietary fiber.
7. List the possible health benefits of dietary fiber.
8. Identify the food sources of each of the vitamins and minerals.
9. Describe the changes in nutrient needs as an individual ages.
10. Differentiate anorexia nervosa, bulimia, and binge eating disorder.
11. Discuss the different types of nutritional support.
12. Identify guidelines for the nutritional assessment.

Key Terms

Be sure to check out the bonus material on the Companion CD-ROM, including selected audio pronunciations.

amino acids (ă-MĔ-nō ĂS-ĭds, p. 103)
basal metabolic rate (BMR) (BĀ-săl mĕt-ă-BŎL-ĭk, p. 93)
calorie (p. 94)
complementary protein (p. 104)
complete protein (p. 103)
incomplete protein (p. 104)
insoluble fibers (ĭn-SŎ-ū-b'l, p. 95)
lipids (LĬ-pĭds, p. 96)
lipoproteins (lĬ-pō-PRŌ-tēns, p. 97)
macronutrients (măk-rō-NŪ-trē-ĕnts, p. 92)
micronutrients (mīk-rō-NŪ-trē-ĕnts, p. 92)
minerals (p. 105)
protein (p. 103)
resting energy expenditure (REE) (p. 93)
saturated fatty acids (p. 96)
triglycerides (trī-gliss-er-īdz, p. 96)
unsaturated fatty acids (p. 96)
vitamins (p. 104)

Nutrition is the cornerstone of the healing process. To support and maintain life or fight disease, the body must be supplied with the proper nutrients.

ANATOMY AND PHYSIOLOGY OF THE GASTROINTESTINAL SYSTEM

The gastrointestinal system (GI tract or "gut") is the long, continuous tube that receives and transports food, absorbs nutrients, and eliminates waste products of digestion. The primary organs that comprise the GI tract are the mouth, pharynx, esophagus, stomach, small intestine, and large intestine. In addition, the liver, gallbladder, and pancreas are called *accessory organs* of the GI tract because they have roles in food digestion even though they are not part of the digestive tract.

DIGESTION AND ABSORPTION

Normally, 92% to 97% of the mixed American diet is digested and absorbed. Most substances such as water, simple sugars, vitamins, minerals, and alcohol are absorbed in their original form. However, other substances such as lipids, proteins, and complex sugars must be converted to simple forms before they are absorbed.

The digestion of food is made possible by hydrolysis, a process through which water splits complex molecules into smaller units. Enzymes along with cofactors such as bile and hydrochloric acid govern the process of hydrolysis. Enzymes help break down food particles to their simplest form so that the nutrients can be absorbed. Enzymes are secreted throughout the intestinal tract, except in the large intestine. Because digestion and absorption already have been completed by the time the food mixture reaches the colon, only water, salt, vitamins, and minerals are absorbed there.

REGULATORS OF GASTROINTESTINAL ACTIVITY

The gastrointestinal system is regulated by (1) neural control and (2) hormone secretion. Neural control is managed by the autonomic nervous system and a nerve network in the gut wall called the *enteric nervous system.* The autonomic nervous system consists of sympathetic and parasympathetic nerve fibers. Parasympathetic nerves generally stimulate digestive activity, whereas sympathetic nerves inhibit activity. A parasympathetic effect that is conveyed by the vagus nerve is the stimulation of acid secretion in the stomach in response to the sight or smell of food. The enteric nervous system receives information from receptors in the gastric mucosa that are sensitive to the acidity of the gastrointestinal tract and the feeling of fullness.

Hormones are secreted into the gastrointestinal tract to help regulate gastric pH, gastric motility, and appetite. They also stimulate the pancreas to secrete insulin and enzymes.

DIGESTIVE PROCESS

Digestion of food occurs in three areas of the gastrointestinal system: (1) the mouth, (2) the stomach, and (3) the small intestine. When food is placed into the mouth, the teeth grind and crush the food into small particles. The food forms into a mass that is moistened and lubricated by saliva. While food is still in the mouth, a secretion containing an enzyme known as *amylase (ptyalin)* begins to digest any starch that is present. The mass, or bolus, is then passed to the pharynx and through the esophagus by the process of swallowing. *Peristalsis* moves the food rapidly through the esophagus into the stomach.

In the stomach, the mass is mixed with gastric secretions. Active chemical digestion is accomplished by the secretion of gastric juice. The stomach produces an average of 2000 to 2500 mL of gastric juice daily. The juice contains hydrochloric acid, enzymes, mucus, and the gastrointestinal hormone *gastrin.* The juice aids in the digestive process by converting the mass to a semiliquid substance called *chyme.*

The stomach is normally emptied in 1 to 4 hours, depending on the amount and kinds of foods eaten. When eaten alone, carbohydrates leave the stomach most rapidly, followed by protein, and then by fat. However, in a mixed diet, emptying of the stomach is prolonged.

Valves (sphincters) located at the entrance (cardiac sphincter) and exit (pyloric sphincter) of the stomach prevent the backflow of the food mass from the stomach into the pharynx and from the duodenum into the stomach. The small intestine is divided into the duodenum, the jejunum, and the ileum. Most of the digestive process is completed in the duodenum, and the jejunum and ileum function mostly in the absorption of nutrients. The remaining chyme is delivered to the large intestine, where water and electrolytes are absorbed, leaving a mass of wastes called *feces.* The fecal mass is stored in the rectum, where it triggers the defecation reflex. When the anal sphincters relax, feces pass out of the body through the anus.

Mechanisms of Absorption

The small intestine is the primary organ of absorption. It is 22 feet long and arranged in folds. The interior surface of the folds is covered with finger-like projections called *villi.* The nutrients are absorbed into the blood through the villa and lymph vessels that support them. Each day, the small intestine absorbs several hundred grams of carbohydrate, 100 grams or more of fat, 50 to 100 grams of amino acids, 50 to 100 grams of ions, and 7 to 8 liters of water.

Absorption is accomplished by the combination of the processes of diffusion and active transport. *Diffusion* involves the movement of particles from an area of higher concentration to an area of lower concentration. *Active transport* requires the input of energy for the movement of particles across a membrane against an energy gradient. This movement requires a carrier protein. The best-known carrier is the *intrinsic factor,* which is responsible for the absorption of vitamin B_{12}.

NUTRIENTS

Food contains many nutrients, including carbohydrates, proteins, lipids, vitamins, minerals, and fluids. Each of these nutrients is digested and absorbed differently. Macronutrients are essential nutrients that have a large minimum daily requirement; they include carbohydrates, lipids, and proteins. Other dietary essentials including vitamins and minerals are called micronutrients because they are required in small quantities.

Carbohydrates

Carbohydrate digestion, as discussed earlier, begins in the mouth where the enzyme amylase is released. When carbohydrates reach the stomach, the activity of amylase is halted when it comes in contact with hydrochloric acid. If the carbohydrates remain in the stomach long enough, the hydrochloric acid reduces most of them to their simplest form. The stomach generally empties into the small intestine before this occurs, so most of the digestion of carbohydrates occurs within the small intestine. In the small intestine, pancreatic amylase is released to continue carbohydrate digestion. After the carbohydrates have been broken down, they pass through the villi into the bloodstream, where they are carried by the portal vein to the liver. From the liver, most of the glucose is transported to the tissues. However, some is stored for later use in the liver in the form of glycogen and in the muscle. Some forms of carbohydrate, particularly fiber, cannot be digested by humans and are excreted unchanged in the feces.

Protein

Digestion of protein does not begin until it reaches the stomach. There proteins are split into smaller molecules. Most protein digestion occurs in the duodenum, not in the stomach. Almost all of the protein is absorbed by the time it reaches the end of the jejunum. Only 1% of ingested protein is found in the feces.

Fat

Digestion of fat also begins in the stomach. Gastric lipase, an enzyme, breaks down the triglycerides that make up fat into fatty acids and glycerol. The major portion of fat digestion takes place in the small intestine. The peristaltic action of the small intestine, along with bile that has been secreted by the liver, breaks down the larger fat globules into smaller particles.

Fluids, Vitamins, and Minerals

Fluids, vitamins, and minerals are absorbed through the intestinal mucosa. Each day about 8 liters of fluid from the body pass back and forth across the membrane of the gut to keep the nutrients in solution. Vitamins and water pass unchanged from the small intestine into the blood by passive diffusion. Mineral absorption is a more active, complex process that takes place in several stages.

FACTORS AFFECTING DIGESTION

Factors that affect the digestion of food include psychological state, bacterial action, and food processing.

Psychological State

The look, smell, and taste of food have an impact on digestion, as does the emotional climate surrounding eating. When humans see, smell, taste, and even think of food, secretions of saliva and gastric juices increase. On the other hand, emotions such as fear, anger, and worry can inhibit peristalsis and depress gastric secretions.

Bacterial Action

The second factor that affects digestion is related to bacterial action in the gastrointestinal tract. The gut is inhabited by about 100 different species of bacteria. A healthy person is not usually disturbed by these bacteria because they dwell in the gastrointestinal tract as normal flora. Bacterial action is most intense in the large intestine. Colonic bacteria are needed to help form vitamin K, vitamin B_{12}, thiamine, and riboflavin. They also produce various gases, acids, and other toxic substances, many of which contribute to the odor of feces.

Food Processing

The last factor that affects digestion is food processing. Cooked foods generally are more digestible than raw foods. The manner in which the food was cooked can also affect digestion. Foods fried at excessive temperatures retard the flow of digestive juices, whereas foods with meat extracts added stimulate digestion. Personal characteristics or allergies may account for differences in the way various people react to certain foods, their preparation, and additives in the foods.

ENERGY

A common definition of *energy* is the capacity to do work. In the context of nutrition, the term refers to the way in which the body makes use of the energy received through the food that is eaten.

ENERGY EXPENDITURE

To understand the concept of energy, it is important to examine energy expenditure. Energy expenditure has three components:

- **Resting energy expenditure (REE):** the energy used to maintain vital body processes. These activities include respiration and circulation, synthesis of organic products, maintenance of body temperature, and movement of ions across membranes. Most of our energy (60% to 75%) is expended in these activities.
- Energy expended in physical activity (EEPA): the energy used to support voluntary activity.
- Thermic effect of food (TEF): the energy used to digest, absorb, and metabolize nutrients, including the synthesis and storage of protein, fat, and carbohydrate.

Measurement of Energy Expenditure

Energy expenditure is measured as the basal metabolic rate (BMR) or the *resting energy expenditure* (REE). These rates are measured when the patient is awake but in a state of complete physical and mental rest. The test must be scheduled several hours after any strenuous exercise or activity. The temperature and environment must be comfortable. The difference between measurements of BMR and REE is that the BMR is measured in the morning after the subject awakens, 10 to 12 hours after the last meal. REE, on the other hand, is measured at any time of day, 3 to 4 hours after the last meal. Factors that can cause the metabolic rate to vary among individuals include body size and composition, periods of growth, secretion of hormones, temperature, the menstrual cycle, and pregnancy.

Body Size and Composition. In terms of body size and composition, the key factors that affect metabolic rate are body surface area and fat-free or lean body mass and body weight. A person with a large body surface area loses more heat by evaporation from the skin, thereby expending more energy. A person with a high proportion of lean body mass to adipose tissue also expends more energy because resting skeletal muscle has a high metabolic rate. Estimates of metabolic rate based on body weight are also thought to be reasonably accurate. Interestingly, even though the ratio of lean mass to fat is generally higher in males, gender does not significantly affect the estimate.

Periods of Growth. The metabolic rate is highest during the first and second years of life—a period of rapid growth. A second, lesser peak occurs during puberty and adolescence.

Hormones. The principal regulators of the metabolic rate are hormones, particularly thyroxine and epinephrine. A person with an underactive thyroid gland does not produce sufficient thyroxine, resulting in a lower metabolic rate. Conversely, a person with an overactive thyroid gland produces too much thyroxine, which increases the metabolic rate. Other hormones that have an effect on the BMR include cortisol, growth hormone, and insulin.

Other Factors. Other factors that affect the BMR are sleep, fever, environmental temperature, the menstrual cycle, and pregnancy. The BMR of a sleeping person is approximately 10% below that of an alert person as a result of muscle relaxation and decreased activity of the sympathetic nervous system. A fever can increase the BMR by about 7% for each degree above 98.6° F. Environmental temperature affects the metabolic rate as well. People who live in very warm climates typically have higher resting energy expenditure than people who live in temperate climates. The BMR rises and falls during the menstrual cycle and remains elevated during pregnancy.

As noted earlier, physical activity can affect the BMR. The expenditure of energy associated with exercise can vary considerably, depending on body size, level of fitness, and amount of muscle mass. Although students might disagree, it has been found that mental activity does not affect energy requirements appreciably.

Eating is another activity that can affect the BMR. The metabolism of protein increases the metabolic rate by about 25% of the total calories consumed. Compare this with the metabolism of carbohydrates and fats, which increase the metabolic rate of total calories consumed by about 5%.

Energy Measurements and Calculations

The *calorie* is the standard unit for measuring energy. A calorie is the amount of heat energy needed to increase the temperature of 1 gm of water at standard temperature by 1° C. A kilocalorie (kcal), which is equal to 1000 calories, is the measurement used most often in nutritional guidelines. Most people refer to a kilocalorie as a Calorie (with a capital "C").

Several methods can be used to measure each component of human energy expenditure. They include direct calorimetry, indirect calorimetry, and doubly labeled water. The measurements obtained in these human studies can be used to calculate the energy required for food digestion and metabolism and for physical activity. Because actual measures require expensive procedures, many equations have been developed to estimate measurements of energy expenditure and requirements based on patient characteristics.

CARBOHYDRATES

DEFINITION AND COMPOSITION OF CARBOHYDRATES

Most of the energy we require is consumed in the form of carbohydrates. These are organic compounds consisting of carbon, hydrogen, and oxygen. All of the sugars and starches that people eat and most types of fibers are carbohydrates. The simplest sugars are monosaccharides, which cannot be hydrolyzed to a simpler form. Monosaccharides can combine to form more complex carbohydrates.

Plants manufacture and store carbohydrates as their chief source of energy. The plants gather carbon dioxide from the air and water from the soil, and with chlorophyll found inside the plant, they use the energy of sunlight to form glucose. When animals consume plants, the glucose furnishes the energy needed to live. Glucose is the main sugar in the blood and the body's basic fuel; it serves as the primary source of energy.

CLASSIFICATION AND FOOD SOURCES OF CARBOHYDRATES

Carbohydrates are classified according to the number of simple sugars or saccharides: (1) monosaccharides, (2) disaccharides, (3) oligosaccharides, and (4) polysaccharides. *Monosaccharides* (one saccharide) are the simplest form of carbohydrate. Examples of monosaccharides are glucose, fructose, and galactose. Major food sources are fruits, vegetables, and honey. *Disaccharides* (two saccharides) contain two monosaccharide molecules. Examples of disaccharides are sucrose, lactose, and maltose. Disaccharides are found in maple or corn syrup (sucrose), milk (lactose), and malt products (maltose). *Oligosaccharides* contain three to ten monosaccharide molecules.

Polysaccharides have 10 to 10,000 or more molecules. Some polysaccharides are soluble (digestible), whereas others are insoluble (indigestible). Starch and glycogen are soluble (digestible) polysaccharides. Starch is found in grains and vegetables, and glycogen is in meat products and seafood. Fibers such as cellulose are usually insoluble (indigestible). Major food sources of cellulose include stalks and leaves of vegetables, outer coverings of fruits and seeds, and beans. Table 9-1 shows the carbohydrate content of certain foods.

CARBOHYDRATE METABOLISM

Carbohydrates are converted to glucose for immediate use by the body's cells and to glycogen for storage. The serum glucose level is maintained within normal limits through the regular intake of nutrients, storage or breakdown of glycogen, glucogenesis, and gluconeogenesis. Normal blood glucose levels are 70 to 100 mg/100 mL under fasting conditions. After a meal, the blood glucose level may rise to 130 mg/100 mL but returns to normal within 2 to 3 hours as some glucose is metabolized and the excess stored in the liver. Eventually the serum glucose level falls, and glycogen in the liver is converted to glucose by the process of glycogenolysis. During long periods of fasting or prolonged exercise, glycogenolysis may not be able to provide sufficient glucose. Then amino acids are converted to glucose in the liver through the process of gluconeogenesis. This process provides additional glucose to meet metabolic demands.

A number of hormones are involved in the regulation of blood glucose levels. They include insulin,

Table 9-1   *Carbohydrate Content of Foods*

SUGAR	CARBOHYDRATE CONTENT (%)	STARCH	CARBOHYDRATE CONTENT (%)
CONCENTRATED SWEETS		**GRAIN PRODUCTS**	
Sugar: Cane, beet, powdered, brown, maple	99.5	Starches: Corn, tapioca, arrowroot	86-88
Candies	70-95	Cereals (dry): Corn, wheat, oat, bran	68-85
Honey (extracted)	82	Flour: Corn, wheat (sifted)	70-80
Syrup: Table blends, molasses	55-75	Popcorn (popped)	77
Jams, jellies, marmalades	70	Cookies: Plain, assorted	71
Carbonated, sweetened beverages	10-12	Crackers, saltines	72
FRUITS		Cakes: Plain, without icing	56
Prunes, apricots, figs (cooked, unsweetened)	12-31	Bread: White, rye, whole wheat	48-52
Bananas, grapes, cherries, apples, pears	15-23	Macaroni, spaghetti, noodles, rice (cooked)	23-30
Fresh: Pineapples, grapefruits, oranges, apricots, strawberries	8-14	Cereals (cooked): Oat, wheat, grits	10-16
MILK		**VEGETABLES**	
Skim	6	Boiled: Corn, white and sweet potatoes, lima beans, dried beans, peas	15-26
Whole	5	Beets, carrots, onions, tomatoes	5-7
		Leafy: Lettuce, asparagus, cabbage, greens, spinach	3-4

From Mahan, L.K., & Escott-Stump, S. (2000). *Krause's food, nutrition, and diet therapy* (10th ed., p. 43). Philadelphia: Saunders.

Table 9-2   *Hormones Involved with the Regulation of Blood Glucose*

HORMONE	SITE OF PRODUCTION	EFFECTS
Insulin	Beta cells of the islets of Langerhans in the pancreas	Increases the rate of glucose utilization for oxidation, glycogenesis, and lipogenesis
Glucagon	Alpha cells in the islets of Langerhans in the pancreas	Raises the amount of glucose in the blood by increasing glycogenolysis and gluconeogenesis; it also stimulates the release of insulin from the pancreas
Epinephrine	Adrenal gland	Causes the breakdown of liver and muscle glycogen to yield blood glucose; also decreases the release of insulin from the pancreas
Glucocorticoids	Adrenal cortex	Stimulates gluconeogenesis, reduces glucose utilization, and increases the rate at which glycogen is converted into glucose
Growth hormone	Anterior pituitary gland	Increases amino acid uptake and protein synthesis by all cells, the uptake of glucose, and the mobilization of fat for energy

glucagon, epinephrine, glucocorticoids, and growth hormone. These hormones and their actions are summarized in Table 9-2.

DIETARY FIBER

Fiber (or roughage) is a group of polysaccharides that act differently from other carbohydrates. They are found only in plant foods and are resistant to human digestive enzymes. Their major digestive role is to help form a soft, firm stool and to aid in the process of elimination.

There are two types of fiber, insoluble and soluble. **Insoluble fibers** include cellulose, hemicellulose, and lignin. They act as sponges to absorb many times their weight in water, swelling up in the intestine. Insoluble fibers help provide a full feeling long after they have been consumed and seem to help normalize intestinal transit time (the time required for food to pass through the GI tract). *Soluble fibers* such as gums and pectin help produce a softer stool but do less to help the passage of food. Soluble fiber prevents or reduces the absorption of certain substances in the bloodstream.

Functions of Carbohydrates in the Body

Each gram of carbohydrate yields about 4 kcal of energy. The functions of carbohydrates, in the form of glucose, are to:

- Serve as a major source of energy to body tissues
- Serve as the sole source of energy for the brain
- Maintain functional integrity of nerve tissue
- Spare fats from being used for metabolism under normal circumstances
- Serve as precursors (basic building blocks) for other physiologic substances.

Lactose remains in the intestines longer than other sugars. It promotes growth of beneficial bacteria, including those that synthesize vitamin K.

Glucuronic acid is a product of glucose metabolism that combines with toxins in the liver and converts them to a form that is readily excreted.

The functions of dietary fiber are to:

- Stimulate salivation and gastric juice secretion
- Promote a sense of gastric fullness
- Slow the rate of digestion and absorption of nutrients
- Normalize transit time through the intestines
- Increase fecal bulk
- Help lower serum cholesterol
- Promote fermentation in the colon

RECOMMENDED DIETARY ALLOWANCE

The ideal daily dietary intake for carbohydrates is not known. However, the dietary guidelines for Americans recommend the selection of fiber-rich fruits, vegetables, and whole grains; foods and beverages prepared with little added sugars or caloric sweeteners; and infrequent consumption of sugar- and starch-containing foods and beverages. Grains include all foods made from wheat, rice, oats, cornmeal, and barley. Of all grains consumed, at least half should be whole grains. Insufficient intake of carbohydrates can lead to ketosis. *Ketosis* is a condition caused by lack of adequate glucose that causes an excessive breakdown of tissue protein, loss of sodium and other cations, and involuntary dehydration. Carbohydrates should make up 45% to 65% of dietary intake.

Several groups have recommended that Americans increase their intake of dietary fiber and that this increase should come from a wide variety of whole-grain products, fruits, vegetables, and legumes. Fiber intake should consist of a 3:1 ratio of soluble to insoluble fiber. The DRIs recommend 21 grams per day for adult females and 30 grams per day for adult males (Institute of Medicine, 2004). The mean fiber intake for adults in the United States is estimated to be about 11 to 13 gm/day, or about 6 gm/1000 kcal. Table 9-3 lists the dietary fiber content of some foods.

Tables 9-4 through 9-9 show the recommended dietary reference intakes (DRIs) for a variety of nutrients.

LIPIDS

Substances that are classified as **lipids** include fats, oils, waxes, and related compounds. Lipids may be solid or liquid forms. A characteristic of all lipids is that they are insoluble in water. Lipids are similar to carbohydrates and contain the same three elements—carbon, hydrogen, and oxygen. Fat metabolism utilizes more oxygen and releases more energy than either carbohydrate or protein metabolism. The structure of lipids also allows them to be stored compactly with little or no water. Proteins and carbohydrates generally require more space for storing the same number of calories.

Triglycerides, also called *neutral fats,* are the most common fat found in foods of both animal and plant origin. Triglycerides consist of three fatty acids attached to a glycerol molecule. These fatty acids vary in length and in degree of saturation of hydrogen atoms, and it is these variations that determine the properties of different fats.

All fats are combinations of **saturated** and **unsaturated fatty acids**. Fats containing mainly saturated fatty acids are described as "highly saturated," whereas fats that are primarily polyunsaturated or monounsaturated are described as "highly unsaturated." Saturated fatty acids are loaded with all the hydrogen atoms they can carry. Fats that are largely saturated come chiefly from animal sources and include butter, milk fat, and the fat in meats; two vegetable oils, coconut and palm oils, also are highly saturated. Highly saturated fats are usually solid at room temperature and keep well.

Unsaturated fatty acids do not have all the hydrogen atoms they can carry. Depending on the number of missing hydrogen atoms, these fatty acids are called either *monounsaturated* (olive, peanut, canola, and avocado oils are largely monounsaturated) or *polyunsaturated* (corn, safflower, and sesame oils). The important dietary unsaturated fats come from plants and fish. They are generally liquid at room temperature and may become rancid quickly because the absence of hydrogen makes the carbon atoms very reactive.

LIPID TRANSPORT AND STORAGE

Most dietary lipids (fats) are absorbed into the lymphatic system through the intestinal mucosa. The exception is certain fatty acids that are absorbed directly into the portal blood. For fat to be digested, it must be emulsified, or pulled into suspension with digestive juices. Bile, a secretion of the liver, is necessary to emulsify fat. Bile is stored in the gallbladder and dis-

Table 9-3 | *Dietary Fiber Content of Foods in Commonly Served Portions*

FOOD GROUP	LOW AMOUNTS (<1 GM)	MODERATE AMOUNTS (1-4 GM)	HIGH AMOUNTS (≥4GM)
Breads (1 slice)	Bagel, white, French	Whole wheat, bran muffin (1)	
Cereals (1 oz)	Rice Krispies, Special K, Cornflakes	Wheaties, Shredded Wheat, Most, Honey Bran	Bran Chex, 40% Bran Flakes, Raisin Bran, Corn Bran, All-Bran, Bran Buds, 100% Bran
Pasta (1 cup)		Macaroni, spaghetti, whole wheat spaghetti	
Rice (½ cup)	White	Brown	
Legumes		Lentils	Lima beans, dried peas, kidney beans, baked beans, navy beans
Vegetables (½ cup cooked unless stated)	Cucumber, lettuce (1 cup), green pepper	Asparagus, green beans, cabbage, cauliflower, potato (without skin, 1), celery, broccoli, Brussels sprouts, carrots, corn, potato (with skin, 1), spinach, peas	NA
Fruits (1 medium unless stated)	Grapes (20), watermelon (1 cup)	Apricots (3), grapefruit (½), peach with skin, pineapple (½ cup), apple without skin, banana, orange, apple with skin, pear with skin, raspberries (½ cup)	NA

From Mahan, L.K., & Escott-Stump, S. (2000). Krause's food, nutrition, and diet therapy (10th ed., p. 40). Philadelphia: Saunders. Adapted with permission from Slavin, J.L. (1987). Dietary fiber: Classification, chemical analyses, and food sources. *Journal of the American Dietetic Association, 87,* 1164. Copyright © The American Dietetic Association.

pensed into the duodenum when fat is present. Once emulsified, fats can be broken down and absorbed.

After absorption, lipids are transported in the bloodstream in packages of lipids wrapped in protein called lipoproteins. Types of lipoproteins include chylomicrons, high-density lipoproteins (HDLs), low-density lipoproteins (LDLs), and very-low-density lipoproteins (VLDLs). Of particular interest in cardiovascular disease are the HDLs and the LDLs. Both lipoproteins carry cholesterol in the bloodstream; however, it appears that the cholesterol found in the LDLs increases the risk of atherosclerosis by contributing to plaque buildup on the artery walls. In contrast, HDL cholesterol seems to have the opposite effect. It appears that the HDLs carry cholesterol from the bloodstream to the liver to be degraded and excreted. The LDLs are sometimes referred to as carrying the "lethal" cholesterol, whereas the HDLs carry the "healthy" cholesterol.

An enzyme converts the lipids into substances that are small enough to pass through the cell walls of adipose (fat) tissue. Once inside the cell, lipids are stored as triglycerides and phospholipids. These fat cells can store up to 95% of their volume as triglycerides, which provides a reserve source of energy.

Most human adipose cells are in the form of white fat, which accumulates in subcutaneous tissue (50%), around the internal organs in the abdominal cavity (45%), and in the intramuscular tissue (5%). Brown fat is much less abundant and is located primarily in the interscapular region and on the back of the neck. The amount of this fat is higher in the neonate and decreases with age, but it can increase with extended exposure to cold.

LIPID METABOLISM

Lipids are a source of energy for most body tissues except the brain, blood cells, skin, and renal medulla. Even when glucose is available, muscle tissue readily uses fatty acids for energy. When the body needs to draw on fat reserves for energy, the fat cells release glycerol and free fatty acids by the process of lipolysis. Few tissues can use glycerol, so the liver picks it up and converts it to triglycerides or glucose. Free fatty acids

Text continued on p. 102.

Table 9-4 | *Dietary Reference Intakes (DRIs): Recommended Intakes for Individuals, Macronutrients*
Food and Nutrition Board, Institute of Medicine, National Academies

LIFE STAGE GROUP	TOTAL WATER[a] (L/day)	CARBOHYDRATE (g/day)	TOTAL FIBER (g/DAY)	FAT (g/day)	LINOLEIC ACID (g/day)	α-LINOLENIC ACID (g/day)	PROTEIN[b] (g/day)
Infants							
0-6 mo	0.7*	60*	ND	31*	4.4*	0.5*	9.1*
7-12 mo	0.8*	95*	ND	30*	4.6*	0.5*	**11.0**[c]
Children							
1-3 y	1.3*	**130**	19*	ND	7*	0.7*	**13**
4-8 y	1.7*	**130**	25*	ND	10*	0.9*	**19**
Males							
9-13 y	2.4*	**130**	31*	ND	12*	1.2*	**34**
14-18 y	3.3*	**130**	38*	ND	16*	1.6*	**52**
19-30 y	3.7*	**130**	38*	ND	17*	1.6*	**56**
31-50 y	3.7*	**130**	38*	ND	17*	1.6*	**56**
51-70 y	3.7*	**130**	30*	ND	14*	1.6*	**56**
> 70 y	3.7*	**130**	30*	ND	14*	1.6*	**56**
Females							
9-13 y	2.1*	**130**	26*	ND	10*	1.0*	**34**
14-18 y	2.3*	**130**	26*	ND	11*	1.1*	**46**
19-30 y	2.7*	**130**	25*	ND	12*	1.1*	**46**
31-50 y	2.7*	**130**	25*	ND	12*	1.1*	**46**
51-70 y	2.7*	**130**	21*	ND	11*	1.1*	**46**
> 70 y	2.7*	**130**	21*	ND	11*	1.1*	**46**
Pregnancy							
14-18 y	3.0*	**175**	28*	ND	13*	1.4*	**71**
19-30 y	3.0*	**175**	28*	ND	13*	1.4*	**71**
31-50 y	3.0*	**175**	28*	ND	13*	1.4*	**71**
Lactation							
14-18 y	3.8*	**210**	29*	ND	13*	1.3*	**71**
19-30 y	3.8*	**210**	29*	ND	13*	1.3*	**71**
31-50 y	3.8*	**210**	29*	ND	13*	1.3*	**71**

NOTE: This table presents Recommended Dietary Allowances (RDAs) in **bold** type and Adequate Intakes (AIs) in ordinary type followed by an asterisk (*). RDAs and AIs may both be used as goals for individual intake. RDAs are set to meet the needs of almost all (97%-98%) individuals in a group. For healthy infants fed human milk, the AI is the mean intake. The AI for other life stage and gender groups is believed to cover the needs of all individuals in the group, but lack of data or uncertainty in the data prevents being able to specify with confidence the percentage of individuals covered by this intake.
[a]*Total* water includes all water contained in food, beverages, and drinking water.
[b]Based on 0.8 g/kg body weight for the reference weight.
[c]Change from 13.5 in prepublication copy due to calculation error.

Table 9-5 | *Dietary Reference Intakes (DRIs): Additional Macronutrient Recommendations*
Food and Nutrition Board, Institute of Medicine, National Academies

MACRONUTRIENT	RECOMMENDATION
Dietary cholesterol	As low as possible while consuming a nutritionally adequate diet
Trans fatty acids	As low as possible while consuming a nutritionally adequate diet
Saturated fatty acids	As low as possible while consuming a nutritionally adequate diet
Added sugars	Limit to no more than 25% of total energy

Table 9-6 *Dietary Reference Intake (DRIs): Estimated Average Requirements for Groups*

Food and Nutrition Board, Institute of Medicine, National Academies

LIFE STAGE GROUP	CHO (g/day)	PROTEIN (g/day)[a]	VIT A (mcg/day)[b]	VIT C (mg/day)	VIT E (mg/day)[c]	THIAMINE (mg/day)	RIBOFLAVIN (mg/day)	NIACIN (mg/day)[d]	VIT B₆ (mg/day)	FOLATE (mcg/day)[e]	VIT B₁₂ (mcg/day)	COPPER (mcg/day)	IODINE (mcg/day)	IRON (mg/day)	MAGNESIUM (mg/day)	MOLYBDENUM (mcg/day)	PHOSPHORUS (mg/day)	SELENIUM (mcg/day)	ZINC (mg/day)
Infants																			
7–12 mo		9*												6.9					2.5
Children																			
1–3 y	100	11	210	13	5	0.4	0.4	5	0.4	120	0.7	260	65	3.0	65	13	380	17	2.5
4–8 y	100	15	275	22	6	0.5	0.5	6	0.5	160	1.0	340	65	4.1	110	17	405	23	4.0
Males																			
9–13 y	100	27	445	39	9	0.7	0.8	9	0.8	250	1.5	540	73	5.9	200	26	1055	35	7.0
14–18 y	100	44	630	63	12	1.0	1.1	12	1.1	330	2.0	685	95	7.7	340	33	1055	45	8.5
19–30 y	100	46	625	75	12	1.0	1.1	12	1.1	320	2.0	700	95	6	330	34	580	45	9.4
31–50 y	100	46	625	75	12	1.0	1.1	12	1.1	320	2.0	700	95	6	350	34	580	45	9.4
51–70 y	100	46	625	75	12	1.0	1.1	12	1.4	320	2.0	700	95	6	350	34	580	45	9.4
>70 y	100	46	625	75	12	1.0	1.1	12	1.4	320	2.0	700	95	6	350	34	580	45	9.4
Females																			
9–13 y	100	28	420	39	9	0.7	0.8	9	0.8	250	1.5	540	73	5.7	200	26	1055	35	7.0
14–18 y	100	38	485	56	12	0.9	0.9	11	1.0	330	2.0	685	95	7.9	300	33	1055	45	7.3
19–30 y	100	38	500	60	12	0.9	0.9	11	1.1	320	2.0	700	95	8.1	255	34	580	45	6.8
31–50 y	100	38	500	60	12	0.9	0.9	11	1.1	320	2.0	700	95	8.1	265	34	580	45	6.8
51–70 y	100	38	500	60	12	0.9	0.9	11	1.3	320	2.0	700	95	5	265	34	580	45	6.8
>70 y	100	38	500	60	12	0.9	0.9	11	1.3	320	2.0	700	95	5	265	34	580	45	6.8
Pregnancy																			
14–18 y	135	50	530	66	12	1.2	1.2	14	1.6	520	2.2	785	160	23	335	40	1055	49	10.5
19–30 y	135	50	550	70	12	1.2	1.2	14	1.6	520	2.2	800	160	22	290	40	580	49	9.5
31–50 y	135	50	550	70	12	1.2	1.2	14	1.6	520	2.2	800	160	22	300	40	580	49	9.5
Lactation																			
14–18 y	160	60	885	96	16	1.2	1.3	13	1.7	450	2.4	985	209	7	300	35	1055	59	10.9
19–30 y	160	60	900	100	16	1.2	1.3	13	1.7	450	2.4	1000	209	6.5	255	36	580	59	10.4
31–50 y	160	60	900	100	16	1.2	1.3	13	1.7	450	2.4	1000	209	6.5	265	36	580	59	10.4

SOURCES: Dietary, Reference Intakes for Calcium, Phosphorous, Magnesium, Vitamin D, and Fluoride (1997); Dietary Reference Intakes for Thiamin, Riboflavin, Niacin, Vitamin B₆, Folate, Vitamin B₁₂, Pantothenic Acid, Biotin, and Choline (1998); Dietary Reference Intakes for Vitamin C, Vitamin E, Selenium, and Carotenoids (2000); Dietary Reference Intakes for Vitamin A, Vitamin K, Arsenic, Boron, Chromium, Copper, Iodine, Iron, Manganese, Molybdenum, Nickel, Silicon, Vanadium, and Zinc (2001), and Dietary Reference Intake for Energy, Carbohydrate, Fiber, Fat, Fatty Acids, Cholesterol, Protein, and Amino Acids (2002). These reports may be accessed via www.nap.edu.

Note: This table presents Estimated Average Requirements (EARs), which serve two purposes: for assessing adequacy of population intakes, and as the basis for calculating Recommended Dietary Allowances (RDAs) for individuals for those nutrients. EARs have not been established for vitamin D, vitamin K, pantothenic acid, biotin, choline, calcium, chromium, fluoride, manganese, or other nutrients not yet evaluated via the DRI process.

[a]For individual at reference weight. (* indicates change from prepublication copy due to calculation error.)

[b]As retinol activity equivalents (RAEs). 1 RAE = 1 mcg retinal, 12 mcg β-carotene, 24 mcg α-carotene, or 24 mcg β-cryptoxanthin. The RAE for dietary provitamin A carotenoids is twofold greater than retinol equivalents (RE), whereas the RAE for preformed vitamin A is the same as RE.

[c]As α-tocopherol. α-Tocopherol includes RRR-α-tocopherol, the only form of α-tocopherol that occurs naturally in foods, and the 2R-stereoisomeric forms of α-tocopherol (RRR-, RSR-, RRS-, and RSS-α-tocopherol) that occur in fortified foods and supplements. It does not include the 2S-stereoisomeric forms of α-tocopherol (SRR-, SSR-, SRS-, and SSS-α-tocopherol), also found in fortified foods and supplements.

[d]As niacin equivalents (NE). 1 mg of niacin = 60 mg of tryptophan.

[e]As dietary folate equivalents (DFE). 1 DFE = 1 mcg food folate = 0.6 mcg of folic acid from fortified food or as a supplement consumed with food = 0.5 mcg of a supplement taken on an empty stomach.

Table 9-7 *Dietary Reference Intakes (DRIs): Recommended Intakes for Individuals, Vitamins*

Food and Nutrition Board, Institute of Medicine, National Academies

LIFE STAGE GROUP	VIT A (mcg/day)[a]	VIT C (mg/day)	VIT D (mcg/day)[b,c]	VIT E (mg/day)[d]	VIT K (mcg/day)	THIAMINE (mg/day)	RIBO-FLAVIN (mg/day)	NIACIN (mg/day)[e]	VIT B6 (mcg/day)	FOLATE (mcg/day)[f]	VIT B12 (mcg/day)	PANTO-THENIC ACID (mg/day)	BIOTIN (mcg/day)	CHOLINE[g] (mg/day)
Infants														
0–6 mo	400*	40*	5*	4*	2.0*	0.2*	0.3*	2*	0.1*	65*	0.4*	1.7*	5*	125*
7–12 mo	500*	50*	5*	5*	2.5*	0.3*	0.4*	4*	0.3*	80*	0.5*	1.8*	6*	150*
Children														
1–3 y	**300**	**15**	5*	**6**	30*	**0.5**	**0.5**	**6**	**0.5**	**150**	**0.9**	2*	8*	200*
4–8 y	**400**	**25**	5*	**7**	55*	**0.6**	**0.6**	**8**	**0.6**	**200**	**1.2**	3*	12*	250*
Males														
9–13 y	**600**	**45**	5*	**11**	60*	**0.9**	**0.9**	**12**	**1.0**	**300**	**1.8**	4*	20*	375*
14–18 y	**900**	**75**	5*	**15**	75*	**1.2**	**1.3**	**16**	**1.3**	**400**	**2.4**	5*	25*	550*
19–30 y	**900**	**90**	5*	**15**	120*	**1.2**	**1.3**	**16**	**1.3**	**400**	**2.4**	5*	30*	550*
31–50 y	**900**	**90**	5*	**15**	120*	**1.2**	**1.3**	**16**	**1.3**	**400**	**2.4**	5*	30*	550*
51–70 y	**900**	**90**	10*	**15**	120*	**1.2**	**1.3**	**16**	**1.7**	**400**	**2.4**[i]	5*	30*	550*
>70 y	**900**	**90**	15*	**15**	120*	**1.2**	**1.3**	**16**	**1.7**	**400**	**2.4**[i]	5*	30*	550*
Females														
9–13 y	**600**	**45**	5*	**11**	60*	**0.9**	**0.9**	**12**	**1.0**	**300**	**1.8**	4*	20*	375*
14–18 y	**700**	**65**	5*	**15**	75*	**1.0**	**1.0**	**14**	**1.2**	**400**[i]	**2.4**	5*	25*	400*
19–30 y	**700**	**75**	5*	**15**	90*	**1.1**	**1.1**	**14**	**1.3**	**400**[i]	**2.4**	5*	30*	425*
31–50 y	**700**	**75**	5*	**15**	90*	**1.1**	**1.1**	**14**	**1.3**	**400**[i]	**2.4**	5*	30*	425*
51–70 y	**700**	**75**	10*	**15**	90*	**1.1**	**1.1**	**14**	**1.5**	**400**	**2.4**[h]	5*	30*	425*
>70 y	**700**	**75**	15*	**15**	90*	**1.1**	**1.1**	**14**	**1.5**	**400**	**2.4**[h]	5*	30*	425*
Pregnancy														
14–18 y	**750**	**80**	5*	**15**	75*	**1.4**	**1.4**	**18**	**1.9**	**600**[j]	**2.6**	6*	30*	450*
19–30 y	**700**	**85**	5*	**15**	90*	**1.4**	**1.4**	**18**	**1.9**	**600**[j]	**2.6**	6*	30*	450*
31–50 y	**700**	**85**	5*	**15**	90*	**1.4**	**1.4**	**18**	**1.9**	**600**[j]	**2.6**	6*	30*	450*
Lactation														
14–18 y	**1200**	**115**	5*	**19**	75*	**1.4**	**1.6**	**17**	**2.0**	**500**	**2.8**	7*	35*	550*
19–30 y	**1300**	**120**	5*	**19**	90*	**1.4**	**1.6**	**17**	**2.0**	**500**	**2.8**	7*	35*	550*
31–50 y	**1300**	**120**	5*	**19**	90*	**1.4**	**1.6**	**17**	**2.0**	**500**	**2.8**	7*	35*	550*

Note: This table (taken from the DRI reports, see *www.nap.edu*) presents Recommended Dietary Allowances (RDAs) in **bold type** and Adequate Intakes (AIs) in ordinary type followed by an asterisk (*). RDAs and AIs may both be used as goals for individual intake. RDAs are set to meet the needs of almost all (97%–98%) individuals in a group. For healthy breastfed infants, the AI is the mean intake. The AI for other life stage and gender groups is believed to cover needs of all individuals in the group, but lack of data or uncertainty in the data prevents being able to specify with confidence the percentage of individuals covered by this intake.

[a] As retinol activity equivalents (RAEs). 1 RAE = 1 mcg retinol, 12 mcg β-carotene, 24 mcg α-carotene, or 24 mcg β-cryptoxanthin. The RAE for dietary provitamin A carotenoids is twofold greater than retinol equivalents (RE), whereas the RAE for preformed vitamin A is the same as RE.

[b] As cholecalciferol. 1 mcg cholecalciferol = 40 IU vitamin D.

[c] In the absence of adequate exposure to sunlight.

[d] As α-tocopherol. α-Tocopherol includes RRR-α-tocopherol, the only form of α-tocopherol that occurs naturally in foods, and the 2*R*-stereoisomeric forms of α-tocopherol (*RRR*-, *RSR*-, *RRS*-, and *RSS*-α-tocopherol) that occur in fortified foods and supplements. It does not include the 2*S*-stereoisomeric forms of α-tocopherol (*SRR*-, *SSR*-, *SRS*-, and *SSS*-α-tocopherol), also found in fortified foods and supplements.

[e] As niacin equivalents (NE). 1 mg of niacin = 60 mg of tryptophan; 0–6 months = preformed niacin (not NE).

[f] As dietary folate equivalents (DFE). 1 DFE = 1 mcg food folate = 0.6 mcg of folic acid from fortified food or as a supplement consumed with food = 0.5 mcg of a supplement taken on an empty stomach.

[g] Although AIs have been set for choline, there are few data to assess whether a dietary supply of choline is needed at all stages of the life cycle, and it may be that the choline requirement can be met by endogenous synthesis at some of these stages.

[h] Because 10% to 30% of older people may malabsorb food-bound B12, it is advisable for those older than 50 years to meet their RDA mainly by consuming foods fortified with B12 or a supplement containing B12.

[i] In view of evidence linking folate intake with neural tube defects in the fetus, it is recommended that all women capable of becoming pregnant consume 400 mcg from supplements or fortified foods in addition to intake of food folate from a varied diet.

[j] It is assumed that women will continue consuming 400 mcg from supplements or fortified food until their pregnancy is confirmed and they enter prenatal care, which ordinarily occurs after the end of the periconceptional period—the critical time for formation of the neural tube.

Table 9-8 *Dietary Reference Intakes (DRIs): Recommended Intakes for Individuals, Elements*

Food and Nutrition Board, Institute of Medicine, National Academies

LIFE STAGE GROUP	CALCIUM (mg/day)	CHRO-MIUM (mcg/day)	COPPER (mcg/day)	FLUO-RIDE (mg/day)	IODINE (mcg/day)	IRON (mg/day)	MAGNE-SIUM (mg/day)	MANGA-NESE (mg/day)	MOLYB-DENUM (mcg/day)	PHOS-PHORUS (mg/day)	SELE-NIUM (mcg/day)	ZINC (MG/day)	POTAS-SIUM (g/day)	SODIUM (g/day)	CHLORIDE (g/d)
Infants															
0–6 mo	210*	0.2*	200*	0.01*	110*	0.27*	30*	0.003*	2*	100*	15*	2*	0.4*	0.12*	0.18*
7–12 mo	270*	5.5*	220*	0.5*	130*	11	75*	0.6*	3*	275*	20*	3	0.7*	0.37*	0.57*
Children															
1–3 y	500*	11*	340	0.7*	90	7	80	1.2*	17	460	20	3	3.0*	1.0*	1.5*
4–8 y	800*	15*	440	1*	90	10	130	1.5*	22	500	30	5	3.8*	1.2*	1.9*
Males															
9–13 y	1300*	25*	700	2*	120	8	240	1.9*	34	1250	40	8	4.5*	1.5*	2.3*
14–18 y	1300*	35*	890	3*	150	11	410	2.2*	43	1250	55	11	4.7*	1.5*	2.3*
19–30 y	1000*	35*	900	4*	150	8	400	2.3*	45	700	55	11	4.7*	1.5*	2.3*
31–50 y	1000*	35*	900	4*	150	8	420	2.3*	45	700	55	11	4.7*	1.5*	2.3*
51–70 y	1200*	30*	900	4*	150	8	420	2.3*	45	700	55	11	4.7*	1.3*	2.0*
>70 y	1200*	30*	900	4*	150	8	420	2.3*	45	700	55	11	4.7*	1.2*	1.8*
Females															
9–13 y	1300*	21*	700	2*	120	8	240	1.6*	34	1250	40	8	4.5*	1.5*	2.3*
14–18 y	1300*	24*	890	3*	150	15	360	1.6*	43	1250	55	9	4.7*	1.5*	2.3*
19–30 y	1000*	25*	900	3*	150	18	310	1.8*	45	700	55	8	4.7*	1.5*	2.3*
31–50 y	1000*	25*	900	3*	150	18	320	1.8*	45	700	55	8	4.7*	1.5*	2.3*
51–70 y	1200*	20*	900	3*	150	8	320	1.8*	45	700	55	8	4.7*	1.3*	2.0*
>70 y	1200*	20*	900	3*	150	8	320	1.8*	45	700	55	8	4.7*	1.2*	1.8*
Pregnancy															
14–18 y	1300*	29*	1000	3*	220	27	400	2.0*	50	1250	60	12	4.7*	1.5*	2.3*
19–30 y	1000*	30*	1000	3*	220	27	350	2.0*	50	700	60	11	4.7*	1.5*	2.3*
31–50 y	1000*	30*	1000	3*	220	27	360	2.0*	50	700	60	11	4.7*	1.5*	2.3*
Lactation															
14–18 y	1300*	44*	1300	3*	290	10	360	2.6*	50	1250	70	13	5.1*	1.5*	2.3*
19–30 y	1000*	45*	1300	3*	290	9	310	2.6*	50	700	70	12	5.1*	1.5*	2.3*
31–50 y	1000*	45*	1300	3*	290	9	320	2.6*	50	700	70	12	5.1*	1.5*	2.3*

SOURCES: Dietary Reference Intakes for Calcium, Phosphorous, Magnesium, Vitamin D, and Fluoride (1997); Dietary Reference Intakes for Thiamin, Riboflavin, Niacin, Vitamin B6, Folate, Vitamin B12, Pantothenic Acid, Biotin, and Choline (1998); Dietary Reference Intakes for Vitamin C, Vitamin E, Selenium, and Carotenoids (2000); Dietary Reference Intakes for Vitamin A, Vitamin K, Arsenic, Boron, Chromium, Copper, Iodine, Iron, Manganese, Molybdenum, Nickel, Silicon, Vanadium, and Zinc (2001); and Dietary Reference Intakes for Water, Potassium, Sodium, Chloride, and Sulfate (2004). These reports may be accessed via *http://www.nap.edu*.

Note: This table presents Recommended Dietary Allowances (RDAs) in **bold type** and Adequate Intakes (AIs) in ordinary type followed by an asterisk (*). RDAs and AIs may both be used as goals for individual intake. RDAs are set to meet the needs of almost all (97%–98%) individuals in a group. For healthy breastfed infants, the AI is the mean intake. The AI for other life stage and gender groups is believed to cover needs of all individuals in the group, but lack of data or uncertainty in the data prevents being able to specify with confidence the percentage of individuals covered by this intake.

Table 9-9 *Dietary Reference Intakes (DRIs): Estimated Energy Requirements (EER) for Men and Women 30 Years of Age[a]*
Food and Nutrition Board, Institute of Medicine, National Academies

HEIGHT (m [in])	PAL[b]	WEIGHT FOR BMI[c] OF 18.5 kg/m^2 (kg [lb])	WEIGHT FOR BMI OF 24.99 kg/m^2 (kg [lb])	EER, MEN[d] (kcal/day)		EER, WOMEN[d] (kcal/day)	
				BMI OF 18.5 kg/m^2	BMI OF 24.99 kg/m^2	BMI OF 18.5 kg/m^2	BMI OF 24.99 kg/m^2
1.50 (59)	Sedentary	41.6 (92)	56.2 (124)	1848	2080	1625	1762
	Low active			2009	2267	1803	1956
	Active			2215	2506	2025	2198
	Very active			2554	2898	2291	2489
1.65 (65)	Sedentary	50.4 (111)	68.0 (150)	2068	2349	1816	1982
	Low active			2254	2566	2016	2202
	Active			2490	2842	2267	2477
	Very active			2880	3296	2567	2807
1.80 (71)	Sedentary	59.9 (132)	81.0 (178)	2301	2635	2015	2211
	Low active			2513	2884	2239	2459
	Active			2782	3200	2519	2769
	Very active			3225	3720	2855	3141

Copyright © 2004 by the National Academy of Sciences. All rights reserved.
[a]For each year below 30, add 7 kcal/day for women and 10 kcal/day for men. For each year above 30, subtract 7 kcal/day for women and 10 kcal/day for men.
[b]PAL = physical activity level.
[c]BMI = body mass index.
[d]Derived from the following regression equations based on doubly labeled water data:
Adult man: EER = 662 − 9.53 × age (y) + PA × (15.91 × wt [kg] + 539.6 × ht [m])
Adult women: EER = 354 − 6.91 × age (y) + PA × (9.36 × wt [kg] + 726 × ht [m])
Where PA refers to coefficient for PAL:
PAL = total energy expenditure ÷ basal energy expenditure
PA = 1.0 if PAL ≥ 1.0 < 1.4 (sedentary)
PA = 1.12 if PAL ≥ 1.4 < 1.6 (low active)
PA = 1.27 if PAL ≥ 1.6 < 1.9 (active)
PA = 1.45 if PAL ≥ 1.9 < 2.5 (very active)

bind to albumin for transportation in the blood and interstitial tissue. Most lipids are carried to the liver for conversion to energy or for use in the synthesis of new triglycerides. The center for lipid metabolism is the liver, which helps regulate lipid levels in the body by the following processes:

- Synthesis of triglycerides and other lipids from fatty acids, carbohydrates, or protein
- Desaturation of fatty acids
- Catabolism (breakdown) of triglycerides for use as energy

If the body relies too heavily on fats for energy, large quantities of fatty acids accumulate in the liver. Through a series of physiologic processes, the liver produces acetoacetic and beta-hydroxybutyric acids, leaving a by-product called *ketone bodies*. The excretion of acetoacetic and beta-hydroxybutyric acids by the kidneys results in excessive loss of bicarbonate. The net effect is lowering of body fluid pH—a condition called *ketoacidosis*.

RECOMMENDED DIETARY ALLOWANCE

The Dietary Reference Intakes recommend that 20% to 35% of the adult diet be composed of fats (Institute of Medicine, 2004). People also should try to eat unsaturated fats rather than saturated fats to minimize the risk of heart disease. Studies have shown

that Americans tend to consume too much fat, which can contribute to the development of cardiovascular disease and diabetes mellitus. Therefore health promotion efforts have centered on teaching people how and why to limit the dietary intake of fat, particularly saturated fat.

FOOD SOURCES OF FAT

Animal products are the major source of saturated fats in the American diet. They include beef, dairy products, and eggs. Interestingly, many manufacturers are making fat-free products such as nonfat milk, cheese, and ice cream. In addition, cattle and pigs are being bred to yield beef and pork lower in saturated fat. Sources of unsaturated fats are vegetable oils, including corn oil, cottonseed oil, and safflower oil. Fruits, vegetables, and cereal grains are relatively low in fat. Refer to Box 9-1 for more sources of dietary fat.

FUNCTIONS OF LIPIDS

The functions of lipids are to (1) store energy, (2) maintain healthy skin and hair, (3) carry fat-soluble vitamins, (4) supply essential fatty acids, and (5) promote satiety. Although carbohydrates are the body's main source of food energy, fats are the most concentrated source, supplying 9 kilocalories per gram, whereas carbohydrates and protein supply only 4 kilocalories per gram.

■

■ **Box 9-1** | *Fat Content of Some Common Foods*

0 Grams of Fat
Most fruits and vegetables
Nonfat milk
Nonfat yogurt
Plain pasta and rice
Angel food cake
Popcorn, air-popped, unbuttered
Soft drinks
Jam, jelly

1-3 Grams of Fat
Popcorn, oil-popped, unbuttered, 1 cup
Low-calorie salad dressing, 1 T
Baked beans, ½ cup
Soup, chicken noodle, canned, 1 cup
Whole wheat bread, 1 slice
Dinner roll, 1
Waffle, frozen, 4-inch, 1
Coleslaw, ½ cup
Flounder or sole, baked, 3 oz
Chicken, without skin, roasted, 3 oz
Tuna, canned in water, 3 oz
Cheese, cottage, 2% fat, ½ cup
Ice milk, soft serve, ½ cup

4-6 Grams of Fat
Low-fat yogurt, 1 cup
Cheese, mozzarella, part skim, 1 oz
Chicken, roasted with skin, 3 oz
Egg, scrambled, 1
Turkey, roasted, 3 oz
Granola, 1 oz
Muffin, bran, 1 small
Pizza, cheese, ¼ of 12-inch pie
Burrito, bean, 1
Brownie, with nuts, 1 small
Margarine or butter, 1 tsp
Popcorn, oil popped, buttered, 1 cup
French dressing, regular, 1 T

7-10 Grams of Fat
Cheese, cheddar, 1 oz
Milk, whole, 1 cup
Bologna, beef, 1 slice
Sausage, 1 patty
Steak, sirloin, broiled, 3 oz
Potatoes, French fried, 10
Chow mein, chicken, 1 cup
Chocolate candy bar, 1 oz
Corn chips, 1 oz
Doughnut, cake type, plain, 1
Mayonnaise, 1 T

15 Grams of Fat
Hot dog, beef, 2 oz
McDonald's Chicken McNuggets, 6 pieces
Peanut butter, 2 T
Pork chop, broiled, 3 oz
Sunflower seeds, dry roasted, ¼ cup
Avocado, ½ medium
Chop suey, beef and pork, 1 cup
Cinnamon roll, 1

20 Grams of Fat
Cheesecake, 1⁄12 cake
Lasagna with meat, 1 medium piece
Macaroni with cheese, homemade, 1 cup
Peanuts, dry roasted, ¼ cup
Ground beef, broiled, 3 oz

25+ Grams of Fat
Polish sausage, 3 oz
Cheeseburger, large
Pie, pecan, ⅛ 9-inch pie
Chicken pot pie, frozen, baked, 1 pie
Quiche, bacon, ⅛ pie

From Mahan, L.K., & Escott-Stump, S. (2000). *Krause's food, nutrition, and diet therapy* (10th ed., p. 44). Philadelphia: Saunders. Data from Healthy Dividends, Rosemont, Ill, National Dairy Council, 1990.

T, Tablespoon; *oz*, ounce; *tsp*, teaspoon.

PROTEINS

DEFINITION AND COMPOSITION OF PROTEINS

Protein is not a single, simple substance but a multitude of thousands of chemical combinations. The basic structure of protein is actually a chain of amino acids that can form many different configurations and can combine with other substances. Like carbohydrates and fats, proteins contain carbon, hydrogen, and oxygen. However, they also contain nitrogen, sulfur, and sometimes other elements such as metals, acids, lipids, and polysaccharides. Simple proteins are those that are made of only amino acids, whereas conjugated proteins are made of amino acids in combination with other substances.

There are 22 common amino acids, and they can be bonded in a variety of ways to form different proteins. The body uses all 22 amino acids, but only nine of them are considered essential amino acids. Each amino acid has a specific, important function. The nine *essential* amino acids must be obtained from the diet. They include cysteine, proline, leucine, isoleucine, valine, tryptophan, phenylalanine, methionine, and histidine. The body can manufacture adequate amounts of the other amino acids from the essential amino acids.

Food proteins can be classified as either complete or incomplete. A complete protein contains all nine essential amino acids in sufficient quantity and ratio for the body's needs. Complete proteins are generally of animal origin and are found in foods such as meat, poultry, fish, milk, cheese, and eggs.

Incomplete proteins are lacking in one or more of the essential amino acids. Incomplete proteins are of plant origin, such as the proteins in grains, legumes, nuts, and seeds. For the body to use protein for functions other than energy, all nine essential amino acids must be present at the same time. When various incomplete proteins are consumed at the same time, the body can use them together to obtain a balance of the essential amino acids. Incomplete proteins consumed together are called complementary proteins.

PROTEIN METABOLISM AND SYNTHESIS

When food containing protein is eaten, the protein is broken down in the small intestine to the constituent amino acids by a process called *deamination*. Deamination produces ammonia, which may be used in synthesis or transported to the liver, where it is converted to urea for excretion. The amino acids are then transported by the blood to the cells, where they can be synthesized into tissue protein, processed to produce ATP, or converted into glucose.

Protein synthesis in the body is controlled by DNA in the cells. DNA essentially provides a form to link up the exact combination of amino acids needed to form a particular protein. It is important to note that if one or more of the essential amino acids are in short supply or not available at all, nonessential amino acids that may be on hand cannot be used to form a protein. That is why it is important to eat a diet that contains all of the essential amino acids, plus enough additional amino acids to allow for synthesis of the nonessential amino acids.

PROTEIN DEFICIENCY

The body cannot store protein, so it needs to be eaten in the diet each day. Nitrogen in the urine is a good indicator of protein levels in the body. If protein intake is inadequate, nitrogen will be conserved by the kidneys, causing the urine nitrogen to be low. When this adaptive process is no longer adequate, evidence of protein deficiency appears. The signs and symptoms include edema, wasting of body tissues, fatty liver, dermatosis (thickening and hardening of the skin), diminished immune response, weakness, and loss of energy.

EVALUATION OF PROTEIN QUALITY

The average American consumes considerably more than the RDA for protein. The assessment of the adequacy of one's protein should include both the quantity and the quality of the protein consumed. The protein content, by weight, of cooked meat, fish, poultry, and milk solids is between 15% and 40%. The protein content of cooked cereals, beans, and lentils ranges from 3% to 10%. Ingesting a diet high in animal protein is not necessary and may be too high in fat. Eating a mixture of foods in a meal, if the quantity is sufficient, tends to provide all of the essential amino acids.

More total protein is required in a vegetable protein diet than in a diet of mixed vegetable and animal proteins because more of the lower-quality protein is needed to meet the minimum requirements for amino acids and nitrogen. Because of their lower digestibility values, vegetable proteins are less available. Box 9-2 gives the protein content of typical foods in the American diet.

Functions of Proteins

The roles of proteins in the body are to:
- Furnish building blocks (amino acids) to build and repair tissue
- Serve as an energy source
- Help form enzymes, hormones, and other body fluids and secretions
- Assist in the transport of fats, fat-soluble vitamins, and other substances
- Help maintain osmolarity of body fluids

RECOMMENDED DIETARY ALLOWANCE

The recommended dietary reference intake for protein is 56 grams/day for males and 46 grams/day for females. Protein should contribute 10% to 35% of the macronutrients in the adult diet (Institute of Medicine, 2004).

VITAMINS

Vitamins are organic compounds that the body needs for normal growth and development. They help regulate metabolic functions within cells; however, only tiny amounts are needed to carry out these functions. Because the body cannot manufacture vitamins, they must be obtained in the diet. As mentioned earlier, vitamins are micronutrients. Most vitamins have multiple forms called *vitamers*. For example, vitamers of vitamin A are retinol, retinal, and retinoic acid.

The use of over-the-counter vitamin supplements is very popular. It is based on the perception that modern diets and processed foods do not provide the daily vitamin requirements. It is important to educate our patients about sources of vitamins, daily needs, and the dangers of excessive vitamin intake. Although scientific evidence is lacking, many manufacturers promote "natural" vitamin supplements as being superior to other supplements. Often "natural" products cost more but really offer no additional benefits. The use of very large doses of vitamins may be appropriate in certain conditions but generally is not thought to be beneficial and may be harmful.

Vitamins are usually designated by letters and are classified into two groups on the basis of solubility:

0-1 Gram
Butter, margarine, 1 tsp
Pear, 1 medium
Cake, 1 piece

2-3 Grams
Milk chocolate, 1 oz
Cereal, refined, 1 oz
Bread, 1 slice
Corn, canned, ½ cup
Chicken noodle soup, 1 cup
French fries, 1 regular serving

4-6 Grams
Cereal, bran, 1 oz
Baked potato, 1 large
Peas, ½ cup

7-8 Grams
Navy beans, cooked, ½ cup
Egg, 1 medium
Cheese, 1 oz
Tuna, 1 oz
Tofu, 3½ oz
Milk, 1 cup

9-10 Grams
Peanuts, roasted, 1 oz
Macaroni and cheese, ¾ cup
Pizza, cheese, ⅛ of a 12-inch pie

12-15 Grams
Taco, 1
Hamburger, 1
Chili with meat, 1 cup

22-26 Grams
Meat, lean, 3 oz
Big Mac, 1

From Mahan, L.K., & Arlin, M. (1992). *Krause's food, nutrition, and diet therapy* (8th ed., p. 67). Philadelphia: Saunders.

(1) fat-soluble vitamins that can be dissolved in fat, and (2) water-soluble vitamins that can be dissolved in water.

FAT-SOLUBLE VITAMINS

Fat-soluble vitamins include vitamins A, D, E, and K. Because they are fat soluble, they are usually absorbed in the body with other lipids. Like lipids, fat-soluble vitamins need bile and pancreatic juices for absorption. After entering the body, fat-soluble vitamins attach to lipoproteins and are transported to the liver. If the amount of a vitamin taken in exceeds the amount needed, the extra amount is stored in the fat cells of the body. As stores build up, the excess vitamins can become toxic. Therefore it is recommended that people *not* take excessive amounts of these vitamins.

WATER-SOLUBLE VITAMINS

Water-soluble vitamins include the B-complex group (thiamine, riboflavin, niacin, B_6, folate, B_{12}, panto-thenic acid, and biotin) and vitamin C (ascorbic acid). Excessive intake of these vitamins is not as dangerous as high intake of fat-soluble vitamins because water-soluble vitamins are readily excreted from the body. Therefore they do not generally accumulate and become toxic. If taken in very large doses, some can have "bad" effects, but such doses are unlikely when food is the major source of these vitamins. However, because water-soluble vitamins are readily excreted, they should be replaced daily.

Most of the water-soluble vitamins are components of essential enzyme systems. Many are involved in the reactions that support energy metabolism. They have an essential role in the metabolic processes of living cells, both plant and animal. Table 9-10 gives more information about the sources and functions of vitamins.

MINERALS

Minerals are another group of micronutrients. They are involved in enzyme regulation, maintenance of acid-base balance and osmotic pressure, and maintenance of nerve and muscular irritability. Doubtless, there are other functions that are not well understood at this time. Because excess minerals are not readily excreted from the body, there is the potential for toxicity if taken in large amounts.

Minerals are classified on the basis of the daily requirement. Macrominerals (calcium, phosphorus, magnesium, sulfur, sodium, chloride, potassium) are required in amounts of 100 mg/day or more. Microminerals, or trace elements, are required in amounts of less than 15 mg/day (iron, zinc, iodine). Minerals that are required in amounts measured in micrograms (selenium, chromium, copper, manganese, molybdenum, boron, cobalt) are called *ultratrace elements*. Minerals are present in the body in ionized forms (sodium, potassium, etc.) or as constituents of organic compounds (phospholipids, hemoglobin, etc.).

Minerals account for 4% to 5% of body weight. Calcium and phosphorus make up about 75% of this amount. The remaining 25% is made up of all the other minerals. Food sources and functions of minerals are presented in Table 9-11.

WATER

Water is the largest component of the body and body tissues and is essential to all life processes in the body. It provides form and structure to cells and tissues; it is essential to the digestion, absorption, and excretion of metabolic and indigestible wastes; it is a transport medium for nutrients and all body substances; it maintains physical and chemical constancy of intracellular and extracellular fluids; and it regulates body temperature through the process of evaporation of perspiration.

Table 9-10 | *Summary of Information on Vitamins*

NAME	SOURCES	COMMENTS
FAT-SOLUBLE VITAMINS		
Vitamin A	Liver, kidney, milk fat, fortified margarine, egg yolk, yellow and dark leafy vegetables, apricots, cantaloupe, peaches.	Essential for normal growth, development, and maintenance of epithelial tissue. Essential to the integrity of night vision. Helps provide for normal bone development and influences normal tooth formation. Toxic in large quantities.
Vitamin D	Vitamin D milk, irradiated foods, some in milk fat, liver, egg yolk, salmon, tuna fish, sardines.	Essential for normal growth and development; important for formation of normal bones and teeth. Influences absorption and metabolism of phosphorus and calcium. Toxic in large quantities.
Vitamin E	Wheat germ, vegetable oils, green leafy vegetables, milk fat, egg yolk, nuts.	Is a strong antioxidant. May help prevent oxidation of unsaturated fatty acids and vitamin A in intestinal tract and body tissues. Protects red blood cells from hemolysis.
Vitamin K	Liver, soybean oil, other vegetable oils, green leafy vegetables, wheat bran. Synthesized in intestinal tract.	Aids in production of prothrombin, a compound required for normal clotting of blood. Toxic in large amounts.
WATER-SOLUBLE VITAMINS		
Thiamine	Pork, liver, organ meats, legumes, whole-grain and enriched cereals and breads, wheat germ, potatoes. Synthesized in intestinal tract.	Aids in removal of CO_2 from alpha-keto acids during oxidation of carbohydrates. Essential for growth, normal appetite, digestion, and healthy nerves.
Riboflavin	Milk and dairy foods, organ meats, green leafy vegetables, enriched cereals and breads, eggs.	Essential for growth. Plays enzymatic role in tissue respiration and acts as a transporter of hydrogen atoms.
Niacin	Fish, liver, meat, poultry, many grains, eggs, peanuts, milk, legumes, enriched grains. Synthesized by intestinal bacteria.	Aids in transfer of hydrogen and acts in metabolism of carbohydrates and amino acids. Involved in glycolysis, fat synthesis, and tissue respiration.
Vitamin B_6	Pork, glandular meats, cereal bran and germ, milk, egg yolk, oatmeal, and legumes. Synthesized by intestinal bacteria.	Aids in the synthesis and breakdown of amino acids and in the synthesis of unsaturated fatty acids from essential fatty acids. Essential for normal growth.
Folate	Green leafy vegetables, organ meats (liver), lean beef, wheat, eggs, fish, dry beans, lentils, cowpeas, asparagus, broccoli, collards, yeast. Synthesized in intestinal tract.	Essential for normal maturation of red blood cells.
Vitamin B_{12}	Liver, kidney, milk and dairy foods, meat, eggs. Vegans require supplement.	Role in metabolism of nervous tissue. Involved with folate metabolism. Related to growth.
Vitamin C (ascorbic acid)	Acerola (West Indian cherry-like fruit), citrus fruit, tomato, melon, peppers, greens, raw cabbage, guava, strawberries, pineapple, potato.	Important in immune responses, wound healing, and allergic reactions. Increases absorption of iron.
Pantothenic acid	Eggs, kidney, liver, salmon, yeast.	Involved in synthesis and breakdown of many compounds; essential for metabolism.
Biotin	Liver, mushrooms, peanuts, yeast, milk, meat, egg yolk, most vegetables, banana, grapefruit, tomato, watermelon, strawberries.	Essential component of enzymes.

Adapted from Mahan, L.K., & Escott-Stump, S. (2000). *Krause's food, nutrition, and diet therapy* (10th ed., pp. 105–106). Philadelphia: Saunders.

The intake of water is controlled by thirst. The sensation of thirst serves as a signal to seek fluids. Water is also ingested through food. The breakdown of food in the body produces water as an end product. Water is lost from the body through the kidneys as urine, through the intestines as part of feces, through the lungs with expired air, and through the skin as evaporated sweat. When an imbalance in the amount of water taken in versus the amount of water lost occurs, various organs in the body, especially the kidneys, compensate by conserving more water and excreting less. The amount of water taken in daily should be equivalent to the amount of water lost.

Table 9-11 | *Minerals in Human Nutrition*

MINERAL	LOCATION IN BODY AND SOME BIOLOGIC FUNCTIONS	FOOD SOURCES
Calcium	99% in bones and teeth. Ionic calcium in body fluids essential for ion transport across cell membranes.	Milk and milk products, sardines, clams, oysters, kale, turnip greens, mustard greens, tofu.
Phosphorus	About 80% in inorganic portion of bones and teeth. Phosphorus is a component of every cell as well as of important metabolites, including DNA, RNA, ATP (high-energy compound), and phospholipids. Important to pH regulation.	Cheese, egg yolk, milk, meat, fish, poultry, whole-grain cereals, legumes, nuts.
Magnesium	About 50% in bone. Remaining 50% is almost entirely inside body cells, with only about 1% in extracellular fluid. Ionic Mg functions as an activator of many enzymes and thus influences almost all processes.	Whole-grain cereals, tofu, nuts, meat, milk, green vegetables, legumes, chocolate.
Sodium	About 30% to 45% in bone. Major cation of extracellular fluid, with only a small amount inside cell. Regulates body fluid osmolarity, pH, and body fluid volume.	Common table salt, seafoods, animal foods, milk, eggs. Abundant in most foods except fruit.
Chloride	Major anion of extracellular fluid, functioning in combination with sodium. Serves as a buffer, enzyme activator; component of gastric hydrochloric acid. Mostly present in extracellular fluid, with less than 15% inside cells.	Common table salt, seafoods, milk, meat, eggs.
Potassium	Major cation of intracellular fluid, with only small amounts in extracellular fluid. Functions in regulating pH and osmolarity and cell membrane transfer. Iron is necessary for carbohydrate and protein metabolism.	Fruits, milk, meat, cereals, vegetables, legumes.
Sulfur	Bulk of dietary sulfur is present in sulfur-containing amino acids needed for synthesis of essential metabolites.	Protein foods such as meat, fish, poultry, eggs, milk, cheese, legumes, nuts.
Iron	About 70% is in hemoglobin; about 26% stored in liver, spleen, and bone. Iron is a component of hemoglobin, important in oxygen transfer.	Liver, meat, egg yolk, legumes, whole or enriched grains, dark green vegetables, dark molasses, shrimp, oysters.
Zinc	Present in most tissues, with higher amounts in liver, voluntary muscle, and bone. Constituent of many enzymes and insulin.	Oysters, shellfish, herring, liver, legumes, milk, wheat bran.
Copper	Found in all body tissues; larger amounts in liver, brain, heart, and kidney.	Liver, shellfish, whole grains, cherries, legumes, kidney, poultry, oysters, chocolate, nuts.
Iodine	Constituent of thyroxine and related compounds synthesized by thyroid gland. Thyroxine functions in control of reactions involving cellular energy.	Iodized table salt, seafoods, water and vegetables in nongoitrous regions.
Manganese	Highest concentration is in bone; also relatively high concentrations in pituitary, liver, pancreas, and gastrointestinal tissue.	Beet greens, blueberries, whole grains, nuts, legumes, fruit, tea.
Fluoride	Present in bone and teeth. In optimal amounts in water and diet, reduces dental caries, and may minimize bone loss.	Drinking water (1 ppm), tea, coffee, rice, soybeans, spinach, gelatin, onions, lettuce.

Adapted from Mahan, L.K., & Escott-Stump, S. (2000). *Krause's food, nutrition, and diet therapy* (10th ed., pp. 147–148). Philadelphia: Saunders.

There is no way the body can store water. It is essential that all living things replenish water daily to maintain health and efficiency. The longest period of time that people can go without water and sustain life is approximately 4 days. Adults generally should take in about 2500 mL, or 2 to 3 quarts, of water per day. More in-depth discussion of fluid balance is provided in Chapter 14.

AGE-RELATED CHANGES

Healthy eating is a lifelong commitment that pays particular benefits in the later years of life. Maintaining a good diet can help middle-aged and older people maintain a high level of function and reduce the risks of chronic disease. Table 9-12 summarizes changes occurring with aging that are relevant to nutrition.

Table 9-12 *Nutrition-Related System Changes in the Older Adult*

SYSTEM	CHANGES
Sensory	Senses of taste, smell, sight, hearing, and touch are diminished. There is a decreased number of taste buds and a decreased sensitivity to sweet and salty tastes. Patient may experience glossodynia (pain in the tongue).
Gastrointestinal	Changes in appetite response contribute to anorexia. Ill-fitting dentures and periodontal disease make eating painful. Decreased salivary secretion decreases the ability to chew and swallow foods. Decreased acid secretion causes an overgrowth of the bacteria of the gut. Lack of intrinsic factor leads to decreased absorption of vitamin B_{12}. There is an increased incidence of gallbladder disease; decreased motility of intestines leads to constipation.
Metabolic	Decreased tolerance to glucose leads to an increase in plasma glucose levels. Basal metabolic rate decreases by 20% due to decrease in lean body mass.
Cardiovascular	Blood vessels become less elastic. Total peripheral resistance increases. There is an increased risk for hypertension.
Renal	Kidney function diminishes, and the acid-base response to metabolic challenges is slowed. There is increased difficulty in handling excessive amounts of protein waste products.
Musculoskeletal	Progressive replacement of lean body mass by fat and connective tissue. Body protein is decreased by 30%–40%. More fat is deposited on the trunk and around the visceral organs. Bone density is diminished, and there is shortening of the spinal column.
Immunocompetence	The immune function declines with age. There is a diminished ability to fight infection.
Psychosocial	Many experience depression as a result of a sense of loss or of loss of loved ones, productivity, a sense of worth, mobility, income, and body image.

ENERGY

Because of the normal decline in metabolism and common decrease in physical activity, energy needs are lower with age. Therefore the older person often reduces the kilocalories taken in per day. This can result in an inadequate intake of other essential nutrients. The recommended daily energy intake for light to moderately active older adults is 30 kcal/kg of body weight. This reflects a reduction of 600 kcal/day for older men and 300 kcal/day for older women. However, lifestyle and health status of older adults vary widely, and these figures may need adjustments for each individual. Nutrients previously discussed in this chapter, including proteins, carbohydrates, lipids, vitamins, minerals, and water, may need adjustment as people age (Table 9-13). For those who are less active, less than the usual recommended amounts of thiamine, riboflavin, and niacin are needed. Nevertheless, many older people take vitamin supplements believing that their diets provide insufficient vitamins and that supplements will provide energy, slow the aging process, and prevent illness.

Psychosocial factors also may lead to poor nutrition in the older person. Depression, cognitive impairment, and loneliness can affect appetite and the intake of food. The term "failure to thrive" has been applied to older adults who are undernourished, depressed, and declining physically and cognitively. Failure to thrive has been attributed to organic and nonorganic factors. This phenomenon is the subject of study to determine how to identify reversible conditions and how best to intervene.

NUTRITIONAL CARE OF THE OLDER ADULT

Dietary Planning

Dietary planning for the older adult is no different from planning for a younger adult. Meals need to be appealing, taking into consideration individual likes and dislikes, and should be tasteful and filling. Planning may be different for older adults with special needs. Some prefer four or five small meals over three large ones. In addition, problems such as difficulty swallowing, dentures that do not fit properly, and arthritis, which makes using utensils uncomfortable, must be considered.

The diet should include all of the food groups. Severely restricted diets such as low-sodium and low-fat diets generally are not advised for older adults. When food is unappetizing, the older person may simply not eat enough to obtain necessary nutrients. The Patient Teaching Plan on p. 109 gives suggestions for teaching older patients about nutrition.

Nutrition Programs

Many community-based programs, administered by both public and private agencies, provide hot, nutritious meals to older adults. The meals are served either in a group setting or in the home. Special regulations and conditions must be met to qualify for these programs.

Nutritional Needs During Prolonged Illness

All people have increased nutritional needs during periods of illness. Older adults with chronic diseases

Table 9-13 *Changes in the Nutritional Requirements for the Older Adult*

NUTRIENT	CHANGES IN NEEDS	SPECIAL PROBLEMS
Protein	Need unchanged (0.8 gm/kg) unless ill. Needs may increase with infection, altered GI function, or chronic diseases that affect metabolism.	Protein-calorie undernutrition may be a special problem for older men who live alone.
Carbohydrate	Need less sugar, more complex carbohydrates. Complex carbohydrates should contribute 55% of calorie intake.	Reduced glucose tolerance, lactose intolerance.
Lipid	Same as younger adult (not more than 30% of the total kilocalories).	Serum cholesterol levels in men tend to peak during middle age and then drop slightly; levels in women continue to rise with increasing age.
Minerals	The needs for trace elements may be reduced owing to decreased lean body mass; calcium intake of 1000–1500 mg/day for postmenopausal women.	Hypertension is common, which results in the need to decrease sodium and increase potassium and magnesium for those taking diuretics.
Vitamins	Vitamin A is sufficient in the older adult owing to stores in the liver; may require vitamin D supplement if patient is not exposed to sunlight; some require vitamin C supplements; vitamin B_6 and folate are maintained with normal diet; vitamin B_{12} may be deficient owing to loss of intrinsic factor.	A maintenance level multivitamin and mineral supplement may be required. Patient must be monitored closely for overdose.
Water	30–35 mL/kg of ideal body weight.	Dehydration is the most common fluid and electrolyte disturbance. Patient must be monitored closely.

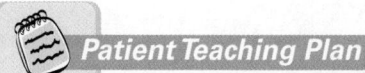 *Patient Teaching Plan*

Nutrition for the Older Patient

In addition to general information about nutritional requirements, you should share the following with the older-adult patient:

- A normal diet typically supplies adequate vitamins; however, a daily multivitamin may be recommended.
- Megadoses (very large doses) of vitamins have not been proven beneficial and can be harmful.
- "Natural vitamins" are more expensive, and there is no evidence that they are better than synthetic vitamins.
- Vitamins do not provide more energy.

such as emphysema and bronchitis, cancer, organic brain disease, cirrhosis, and maldigestion or malabsorption syndromes are at increased risk for protein deficiency and negative nitrogen balance. Individuals at risk need to be watched very carefully for this condition, which can be prevented by increasing nutritional support. Nasogastric tube feedings or parenteral nutrition may be required to meet these increased needs.

Nutritional Care in Institutional Settings

Good nutrition can have a dramatic effect on the physical, mental, and emotional function of your older-adult patients. Nurses in long-term care and home health settings must be especially vigilant in monitoring the nutritional status of older-adult patients. Age-related changes, chronic and acute conditions, cognitive and emotional disorders, medications, and situational factors can contribute to inadequate nutritional intake, digestion, or elimination. Also, patients who are obese have special needs. Excess body weight makes it more difficult to control many chronic conditions and can greatly interfere with activities of daily living. The nutritional needs of older adults in institutional settings may change over a period of time. Therefore periodic reassessment of nutritional status is critical to avoid imposing unnecessary diet restrictions or missing important nutritional needs.

Assisting older-adult patients with meals must be a high priority. How many times have you seen a meal cart with trays that have barely been touched being returned to the kitchen? You should question why patients are not eating and implement nursing measures to improve the situation.

GUIDELINES FOR DIETARY PLANNING

MY PYRAMID

A number of guidelines have been established in the United States to help in planning for optimal nutrition. Until July 1992, the basic four food groups were considered the standard food guide. At that time, the U.S. Department of Agriculture established the food guide pyramid. The food guide pyramid expanded the basic four food groups (milk, meat, fruits and vegetables, and grains) and added a fats, oils, and sweets group. It was intended to show the ideal natural grouping for the way the American public should eat.

More recently, the USDA presented a more personalized science-based food guidance system called MyPyramid (Fig. 9-1, *A*). It incorporates the 2005 USDA Dietary Guidelines for Americans. The new symbol includes a figure climbing the steps of the pyramid to emphasize exercise in addition to nutrition. Colored bands on the pyramid represent the recommended proportions of vegetables (green), grains (orange), fruits (red), milk products (blue), meats and beans (purple), and oils (yellow). An individual can obtain a personalized pyramid by going to http://mypyramid.gov and entering age, gender, and activity level. Figure 9-1, *B*, shows a pyramid for a 59-year-old female who

exercises 30 to 60 min/day and Figure 9-1, *C*, shows a pyramid for a 25-year-old male who exercises more than an hour per day (Combs, 2005). MyPyramid is based on recommendations from the 2005 USDA Dietary Guidelines for Americans.

Food Labeling

With the increase in public awareness of health and nutrition, people have expressed an increased need to be informed about what they are eating. Many more foods are now labeled so that the average person can make determinations about the quality and quantity of the nutrients consumed. Because of the lack of space available on a package label, the table is abbreviated to include essential information to describe the number of nutrients per serving (Fig. 9-2).

Anatomy of MyPyramid

One size doesn't fit all
USDA's new MyPyramid symbolizes a personalized approach to healthy eating and physical activity. The symbol has been designed to be simple. It has been developed to remind consumers to make healthy food choices and to be active every day. The different parts of the symbol are described below.

Activity
Activity is represented by the steps and the person climbing them, as a reminder of the importance of daily physical activity.

Moderation
Moderation is represented by the narrowing of each food group from bottom to top. The wider base stands for foods with little or no solid fats or added sugars. These should be selected more often. The narrower top area stands for foods containing more added sugars and solid fats. The more active you are, the more of these foods can fit into your diet.

Personalization
Personalization is shown by the person on the steps, the slogan, and the URL. Find the kinds and amounts of food to eat each day at MyPyramid.gov.

Proportionality
Proportionality is shown by the different widths of the food group bands. The widths suggest how much food a person should choose from each group. The widths are just a general guide, not exact proportions. Check the Web site for how much is right for you.

Variety
Variety is symbolized by the 6 color bands representing the 5 food groups of the Pyramid and oils. This illustrates that foods from all groups are needed each day for good health.

Gradual Improvement
Gradual improvement is encouraged by the slogan. It suggests that individuals can benefit from taking small steps to improve their diet and lifestyle each day.

MyPyramid.gov
STEPS TO A HEALTHIER YOU

USDA U.S. Department of Agriculture
Center for Nutrition Policy
and Promotion
April 2005 CNPP-16

USDA is an equal opportunity provider and employer.

GRAINS   VEGETABLES   FRUITS   OILS   MILK   MEAT & BEANS

FIGURE **9-1** **A,** FDA MyPyramid. **B,** MyPyramid for a 59-year-old female who exercises 30 to 60 minutes a day. **C,** MyPyramid for a 25-year-old male who exercises more than 1 hour a day.

MyPyramid
STEPS TO A HEALTHIER YOU

B

Based on the information you provided, this is your daily recommended amount from each food group.

GRAINS 6 ounces	VEGETABLES 2 1/2 cups	FRUITS 1 1/2 cups	MILK 3 cups	MEAT & BEANS 5 ounces
Make half your grains whole	**Vary your veggies**	**Focus on fruits**	**Get your calcium-rich foods**	**Go lean with protein**
Aim for at least **3 ounces** of whole grains a day	Aim for these amounts each week:	Eat a variety of fruit	Go low-fat or fat-free when you choose milk, yogurt, or cheese	Choose low-fat or lean meats and poultry
	Dark green veggies = 3 cups	Go easy on fruit juices		Vary your protein routine— choose more fish, beans, peas, nuts, and seeds
	Orange veggies = 2 cups			
	Dry beans & peas = 3 cups			
	Starchy veggies = 3 cups			
	Other veggies = 6 1/2 cups			

Find your balance between food and physical activity

Be physically active for at least **30 minutes** most days of the week.

Know your limits on fats, sugars, and sodium

Your allowance for oils is **5 teaspoons a day.**

Limit extras—solid fats and sugars—to **195 calories a day.**

Your results are based on a 1800 calorie pattern.   Name: _____

This calorie level is only an estimate of your needs. Monitor your body weight to see if you need to adjust your calorie intake.

MyPyramid
STEPS TO A HEALTHIER YOU

C

Based on the information you provided, this is your daily recommended amount from each food group.

GRAINS 10 ounces	VEGETABLES 4 cups	FRUITS 2 1/2 cups	MILK 3 cups	MEAT & BEANS 7 ounces
Make half your grains whole	**Vary your veggies**	**Focus on fruits**	**Get your calcium-rich foods**	**Go lean with protein**
Aim for at least **5 ounces** of whole grains a day	Aim for these amounts each week:	Eat a variety of fruit	Go low-fat or fat-free when you choose milk, yogurt, or cheese	Choose low-fat or lean meats and poultry
	Dark green veggies = 3 cups	Go easy on fruit juices		Vary your protein routine— choose more fish, beans, peas, nuts, and seeds
	Orange veggies = 2 1/2 cups			
	Dry beans & peas = 3 1/2 cups			
	Starchy veggies = 9 cups			
	Other veggies = 10 cups			

Find your balance between food and physical activity

Be physically active for at least **30 minutes** most days of the week.

Know your limits on fats, sugars, and sodium

Your allowance for oils is **10 teaspoons a day.**

Limit extras—solid fats and sugars—to **510 calories a day.**

Your results are based on a 3000 calorie pattern.   Name: _____

This calorie level is only an estimate of your needs. Monitor your body weight to see if you need to adjust your calorie intake.

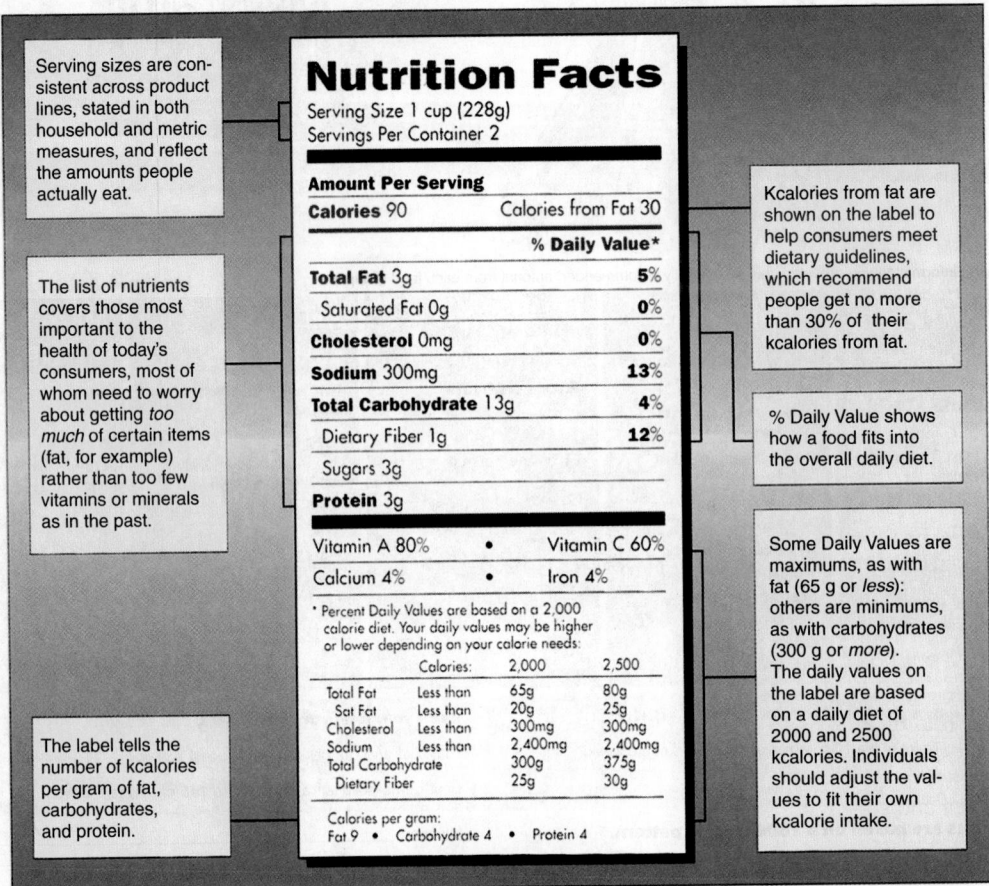

Serving sizes are consistent across product lines, stated in both household and metric measures, and reflect the amounts people actually eat.

The list of nutrients covers those most important to the health of today's consumers, most of whom need to worry about getting *too much* of certain items (fat, for example) rather than too few vitamins or minerals as in the past.

The label tells the number of kcalories per gram of fat, carbohydrates, and protein.

Kcalories from fat are shown on the label to help consumers meet dietary guidelines, which recommend people get no more than 30% of their kcalories from fat.

% Daily Value shows how a food fits into the overall daily diet.

Some Daily Values are maximums, as with fat (65 g or *less*): others are minimums, as with carbohydrates (300 g or *more*). The daily values on the label are based on a daily diet of 2000 and 2500 kcalories. Individuals should adjust the values to fit their own kcalorie intake.

Nutrition Facts

Serving Size 1 cup (228g)
Servings Per Container 2

Amount Per Serving

Calories 90   Calories from Fat 30

% **Daily Value***

Total Fat 3g	5%
Saturated Fat 0g	0%
Cholesterol 0mg	0%
Sodium 300mg	13%
Total Carbohydrate 13g	4%
Dietary Fiber 1g	12%
Sugars 3g	
Protein 3g	

Vitamin A 80%	•	Vitamin C 60%
Calcium 4%	•	Iron 4%

* Percent Daily Values are based on a 2,000 calorie diet. Your daily values may be higher or lower depending on your calorie needs:

		Calories:	2,000	2,500
Total Fat	Less than		65g	80g
Sat Fat	Less than		20g	25g
Cholesterol	Less than		300mg	300mg
Sodium	Less than		2,400mg	2,400mg
Total Carbohydrate			300g	375g
Dietary Fiber			25g	30g

Calories per gram:
Fat 9 • Carbohydrate 4 • Protein 4

FIGURE 9-2 Example of a nutrition label.

NATIONAL GUIDELINES FOR DIET PLANNING

Because of increased public awareness of the importance of health and good nutrition, much research has been done on the connection between nutrition and disease. As a result, many current guidelines are available concerning proper nutrition to maintain health and prevent disease. The task of planning a proper diet that includes recommendations from the various guidelines is sometimes a difficult one. Table 9-14 presents a composite of the dietary guidelines from the Surgeon General's Report on Nutrition and Health (1988) that can be used as a basis for dietary planning.

VEGETARIAN DIETS

Vegetarian diets are not new but have only gradually gained acceptance as a balanced nutritional option. Many Americans who call themselves vegetarians eat all foods except red meat, although some exclude poultry and fish as well. A *lactovegetarian* diet includes milk, cheese, and other dairy products but excludes meat, fish, poultry, and eggs. A *lacto-ovo-vegetarian* diet includes dairy products and eggs but excludes meat,

fish, and poultry. A person who consumes no foods of animal origin is said to be a *vegan*. Only the vegan is at real risk for nutritional deficiencies if the diet is not carefully planned.

There is some evidence that vegetarian diets have distinct health benefits including reduced risks of type 2 diabetes mellitus, breast and colon cancer, and cardiovascular and gallbladder disease. Vegetarians generally consume less protein than nonvegetarians, but most still exceed the RDA for protein.

Adaptations that the vegetarian will need to be aware of include the following:

- Vegans are at risk for megaloblastic anemia resulting from vitamin B_{12} deficiency. Many foods, such as fortified breakfast cereals, can provide adequate B_{12} supplements.
- Vegetarian diets must be planned to assure adequate calcium, iron, zinc, and vitamins B_{12} and D.

NURSING ASSESSMENT OF NUTRITIONAL STATUS

DIETARY HISTORY

The first step in determining the nutritional status of any person is assessment. The areas covered in a nutritional assessment include a dietary history, anthropometric data, laboratory data (if available), and physical examination data. Throughout the assessment interview, observe the patient's physical appearance for signs of malnutrition, obesity, and other factors that may indicate nutritional deficits. The well-nourished person should have shiny and healthy-looking hair, bright and clear eyes, smooth facial skin with good color, smooth lips and tongue, and healthy teeth and gums. Signs of malnutrition include dull, thin, and sparse hair; pale conjunctiva; a swollen or pale face; swollen lips and tongue; teeth with cavities or missing teeth; and bleeding or receding gums.

The diet history includes physical, psychological, social, and medical data that may have an impact on nutritional status. Box 9-3 summarizes information you should obtain in the dietary history. Commonly used tools to collect retrospective ("after the fact") data about dietary patterns include the 24-hour recall and the food frequency record. For a 24-hour recall, ask the patient to recall everything eaten dur-

ing the past 24 hours, usually from the time of awakening until the next morning. Note everything that entered the mouth, including meals, snacks, drinks (especially water), and seasonings (especially salt). The food frequency record uses a list of foods from all food groups to assess how often the patient consumes specific foods. Because neither tool provides perfectly accurate data, it is probably best to use both of them. From these assessments, general dietary deficits and excesses can be determined.

Anthropometric Data

Anthropometric data include height, weight (including weight patterns), and body composition. Height and weight measurements should be performed correctly to complete an accurate assessment of the patient. Box 9-4 gives guidelines on the proper way to perform these measurements.

Body composition is related to the ratio of fat to lean muscle mass. Determining a person's body composi-

---

Box 9-3 | *Dietary History Information*

Economics
Income (frequency and steadiness of employment)
Amount of money for food each week or month, and individual's perception of its adequacy for meeting food needs
Eligibility for food stamps and cost of stamps
Public aid recipient?

Physical Activity
Occupation (type, hours per week, shift, energy expenditure)
Exercise (type, amount, frequency [seasonal?])
Sleep (hours per day [uninterrupted?])
Handicaps

Ethnic or Cultural Background
Influence on eating habits
Religion
Education

Home Life and Meal Patterns
Number in household (eat together?)
Person who does shopping
Person who does cooking
Food storage and cooking facilities (stove, refrigerator)
Type of housing (home, apartment, room, etc.)
Ability to shop and prepare food

Appetite
Good, poor; any changes?
Factors that affect appetite
Taste and smell perception; any changes?

Attitude Toward Food and Eating
Disinterest in food
Irrational ideas about food, eating, and body weight
Parental interest in child's eating

Allergies, Intolerances, or Food Avoidances
Foods avoided and reason why
Length of time of avoidance
Description of problems caused by foods

Dental and Oral Health
Problems with eating
Foods that cannot be eaten
Problems with swallowing, salivation, food sticking

Gastrointestinal
Problems with heartburn, bloating, gas, diarrhea, vomiting, constipation, distention
Frequency of problems
Home remedies
Antacid, laxative, or other drug use

Chronic Disease
Treatment
Length of time of treatment
Dietary modification (physician prescription?, date of modification, education, compliance with diet)

Medication
Vitamin and/or mineral supplements (frequency, type, amount)
Medications (type, amount, frequency, length of time on medication)

Recent Weight Change
Loss or gain
How many pounds, over what length of time?
Intentional or nonvolitional?

Dietary or Nutritional Problems (as Perceived by Patient)

Data from U.S. Department of Agriculture. Retrieved November 28, 2005, from *http://www.health.gov/dietaryguidelines/dga2005/recommendations.htm*.
NOTE: The Dietary Guidelines for Americans 2005 contains additional recommendations for specific populations. The full document is available at *www.healthierus.gov.dietaryguidelines*.

ADEQUATE NUTRIENTS WITHIN CALORIE NEEDS

Consume a variety of nutrient-dense foods and beverages within and among the basic food groups while choosing foods that limit the intake of saturated and trans fat, cholesterol, added sugars, salt, and alcohol.

Meet recommended intakes within energy needs by adopting a balanced eating pattern, such as the U.S. Department of Agriculture (USDA) Food Guide or the Dietary Approaches to Stop Hypertension (DASH) Eating Plan.

WEIGHT MANAGEMENT

To maintain body weight in a healthy range, balance calories from foods and beverages with calories expended.

To prevent gradual weight gain over time, make small decreases in food and beverage calories and increase physical activity.

PHYSICAL ACTIVITY

Engage in regular physical activity and reduce sedentary activities to promote health, psychological well-being, and a healthy body weight.

To reduce the risk of chronic disease in adulthood: Engage in at least 30 minutes of moderate-intensity physical activity, above usual activity, at work or home on most days of the week.

For most people, greater health benefits can be obtained by engaging in physical activity of more vigorous intensity or longer duration.

To help manage body weight and prevent gradual, unhealthy body weight gain in adulthood: Engage in approximately 60 minutes of moderate- to vigorous-intensity activity on most days of the week while not exceeding caloric intake requirements.

To sustain weight loss in adulthood: Participate in at least 60 to 90 minutes of daily moderate-intensity physical activity while not exceeding caloric intake requirements. Some people may need to consult with a health care provider before participating in this level of activity.

Achieve physical fitness by including cardiovascular conditioning, stretching exercises for flexibility, and resistance exercises or calisthenics for muscle strength and endurance.

FOOD GROUPS TO ENCOURAGE

Consume a sufficient amount of fruits and vegetables while staying within energy needs. Two cups of fruit and 2½ cups of vegetables per day are recommended for a reference 2000 calorie intake, with higher or lower amounts depending on the calorie level.

Choose a variety of fruits and vegetables each day. In particular, select from all five vegetable subgroups (dark green, orange, legumes, starchy, vegetables, and other vegetables) several times a week.

Consume 3 or more ounce-equivalents of whole-grain products per day, with the rest of the recommended grains coming from enriched or whole-grain products. In general, at least half the grains should come from whole grains.

Consume 3 cups per day of fat-free or low-fat milk or equivalent milk products.

FATS

Consume less than 10 percent of calories from saturated fatty acids and less than 300 mg/day of cholesterol, and keep *trans* fatty acid consumption as low as possible.

Keep total fat intake between 20 and 35 percent of calories, with most fats coming from sources of polyunsaturated and mono-unsaturated fatty acids, such as fish, nuts, and vegetable oils.

When selecting and preparing meat, poultry, dry beans, and milk or milk products, make choices that are lean, low-fat, or fat-free.

Limit intake of fats and oils high in saturated and/or *trans* fatty acids, and choose products low in such fats and oils.

CARBOHYDRATES

Choose fiber-rich fruits, vegetables, and whole grains often.

Choose and prepare foods and beverages with little added sugars or caloric sweeteners, such as amounts suggested by the USDA Food Guide and the DASH Eating Plan.

Reduce the incidence of dental caries by practicing good oral hygiene and consuming sugar- and starch-containing foods and beverages less frequently.

SODIUM AND POTASSIUM

Consume less than 2300 mg (approximately 1 teaspoon of salt) of sodium per day.

Choose and prepare foods with little salt. At the same time, consume potassium-rich foods, such as fruits and vegetables.

ALCOHOLIC BEVERAGES

Those who choose to drink alcoholic beverages should do so sensibly and in moderation—defined as the consumption of up to one drink per day for women and up to two drinks per day for men.

Alcoholic beverages should not be consumed by some individuals, including those who cannot restrict their alcohol intake, women of childbearing age who may become pregnant, pregnant and lactating women, children and adolescents, individuals taking medications that can interact with alcohol, and those with specific medical conditions.

Alcoholic beverages should be avoided by individuals engaging in activities that require attention, skill, or coordination, such as driving or operating machinery.

FOOD SAFETY

To avoid microbial foodborne illness:

- Clean hands, food contact surfaces, and fruits and vegetables. Meat and poultry should not be washed and rinsed.
- Separate raw, cooked, and ready-to-eat foods while shopping, preparing, or storing foods.
- Cook foods to a safe temperature to kill microorganisms.
- Chill (refrigerate) perishable food promptly and defrost food properly.
- Avoid raw (unpasteurized) milk or any products made from unpasteurized milk, raw or partially cooked eggs or foods containing raw eggs, raw or undercooked meat and poultry, unpasteurized juices, and raw sprouts.

Data from U.S. Department of Agriculture. Retrieved November 28, 2005, from *http://www.health.gov/dietaryguidelines/dga2005/recommendations.htm*.
NOTE: The Dietary Guidelines for Americans 2005 contains additional recommendations for specific populations. The full document is available at *www.healthierus.gov.dietaryguidelines*.

Box 9-4 **Recommendations for the Measurement of Height and Weight**

Height

- Height should be measured without shoes.
- Feet should be together with the heels against the wall or measuring board.
- The subject should stand erect, neither slumped nor stretching, looking straight ahead, without tipping the head up or down. The top of the ear and outer corner of the eye should be in a line parallel to the floor.
- A horizontal bar, a rectangular block of wood, or the top of the stadiometer should be lowered to rest flat on the top of the head.
- Height should be read to the nearest ¼ inch or 0.5 cm.

Weight

- Use a beam balance scale, not a spring scale, whenever possible.
- Periodically calibrate the scale for accuracy, using known weights.
- Weigh the subject in light clothing without shoes.
- Record weight to the nearest ½ lb or 0.2 kg. Measurements above the 90th or below the 10th percentile warrant further evaluation.

tion requires taking several measurements. These measurements include skinfold thickness and hydrostatic weighing. Skinfold thickness is measured by means of calipers that pinch skin over areas of the body that seem to reflect best the fat content of the subcutaneous tissue. These sites include areas over the triceps, over the biceps, below the scapula, above the iliac crest, and on the upper thigh (Fig. 9-3).

Hydrostatic weighing is done underwater. The advantage of weighing underwater is that it provides a good estimate of body density as a person is submerged, indicating the amount of adipose tissue or percentage of body fat. Body mass index (BMI) is a way to evaluate the weight of an adult. BMI is obtained by the following formula (a value of 20 to 25 is optimal):

$$\frac{\text{Patient's weight in kilograms}}{\text{Height in meters} \times \text{Height in meters}}$$

FIGURE **9-3** Skinfold calipers measure in millimeters the thickness of the subcutaneous fat tissue, which gives a rough measurement of adiposity.

Laboratory Data

Laboratory tests that are helpful in assessing nutritional status are serum albumin, total lymphocyte count (TLC), urine creatinine/height index, nitrogen balance, mean corpuscular volume (MCV), and transferrin saturation:

- *Serum albumin:* There are several possible explanations for low serum albumin, including protein depletion. The normal serum albumin level is 3.5 to 5 gm/dL.
- *Total lymphocyte count:* Protein and calorie deficits interfere with immune function, resulting in a low TLC. The normal lymphocyte count is 2500 mm^3. A count of less than 1500 mm^3 is consistent with protein/calorie malnutrition.
- *Urine creatinine/height index:* Expected urine creatinine is based on the patient's height. It provides an evaluation of body muscle mass.
- *Nitrogen balance:* Nitrogen balance exists when nitrogen intake and excretion are equal. A patient who is in a state of starvation will excrete more nitrogen in the urine than consumed, creating a negative nitrogen balance.
- *Mean corpuscular volume:* MCV measures the size of red blood cells (RBCs). With different types of anemia, RBC size varies. Therefore, when anemia is present, MCV helps determine the type of anemia.
- *Transferrin saturation:* Transferrin is a protein that transports iron. Transferrin saturation is normally between 30% and 50%; less than 30% indicates anemia; more than 50% indicates iron overload.

WEIGHT MANAGEMENT AND EATING DISORDERS

Many Americans today are on some form of "diet." People feel an increasing dissatisfaction with their appearance and a constant need to change that appearance. Most people view dieting as deprivation at best and punishment at worst. Changing eating patterns takes motivation, hard work, and a willingness to control behavior over a long period. Most adults have the ability to maintain a constant weight, but to do so, they must maintain consistent eating and exercise patterns on a daily basis. Table 9-15 shows estimated daily energy needs for both genders and all age ranges. Table 9-16 gives MyPyramid recommendations of how those calories should be distributed across the various food groups.

Overweight individuals are considered obese if their weight is 20% or more above ideal body weight. Obesity is associated with coronary artery disease, lipid disorders, and type 2 diabetes mellitus (non–insulin-dependent diabetes mellitus). It is also considered a risk factor for some kinds of cancer and is associated with joint disease, gallstones, and respiratory problems.

The underweight person is one whose weight is 15% to 20% or more below accepted weight standards. This may be caused by an insufficient food intake to meet activity needs, excessive activity, poor absorption and utilization of food consumed, a wasting disease, or psychological or emotional stress.

Eating disorders are fairly common, especially among teenaged girls and young women, and may persist into adulthood. Two eating disorders, anorexia nervosa and bulimia, usually begin in adolescence or early adulthood. A third disorder, binge eating disorder, is not as well documented but represents a significant proportion of people in weight-loss programs.

Table 9-15 *Estimated Daily Calorie Needs*

To determine which food intake pattern to use for an individual, the following chart gives an estimate of individual calorie needs. The calorie range for each age/sex group is based on physical activity level, from sedentary to active.

	CALORIE RANGE		
CHILDREN	**SEDENTARY**	→	**ACTIVE**
2–3 years	1000	→	1400
FEMALE			
4–8 years	1200	→	1800
9–13	1600	→	2200
14–18	1800	→	2400
19–30	2000	→	2400
31–50	1800	→	2200
51+	1600	→	2200
MALES			
4–8 years	1400	→	2000
9–13	1800	→	2600
14–18	2200	→	3200
19–30	2400	→	3000
31–50	2200	→	3000
51+	2000	→	2800

Sedentary means a lifestyle that includes only the light physical activity associated with typical day-to-day life.
Active means a lifestyle that includes physical activity equivalent to walking more than 3 miles per day at 3 to 4 miles per hour, in addition to the light physical activity associated with typical day-to-day life.

These disorders may develop when people attempt to achieve the "perfect" body. Puberty brings with it hormonal changes and the emergence of sexual characteristics. Some teenagers, particularly girls, resist these changes and turn to inappropriate dieting. However, it is too simplistic to say that the desire to be thin is the cause of eating disorders. It is thought that multiple biologic, psychological, sociocultural, and spiritual factors influence the development of these conditions. The most common eating disorders are described here. Management of these conditions requires psychotherapy and specialized nutritional intervention that is beyond the scope of this textbook. Specialty resources should be consulted.

ANOREXIA NERVOSA

Anorexia nervosa is an eating disorder characterized by self-imposed starvation. Certain features are common in individuals with this disorder. They are generally girls in their mid-teens, although young adult women and men sometimes develop the disorder. Often they are high achievers from educated, middle-class families. The young person with anorexia nervosa is frequently a perfectionist who uses food and exercise as a means of controlling the body.

People with anorexia nervosa become obsessed with weight loss and soon develop a distorted body image, seeing themselves as fat even when their weight is much less than average for their height and age. They experience personality changes, depression, and apathy. Death may occur in as many as 20% of those with anorexia nervosa. Psychiatric treatment is usually recommended (see Chapter 55).

BULIMIA

Bulimia is an eating disorder characterized by periods of binge eating followed by purging. This behavior may alternate with periods of fasting as well. The cycle may go something like this: The person may binge several times a week. The episode may last 2 hours or more. The person consumes large amounts of easily ingested kilocalorie-dense foods such as ice cream, candies, cakes, breads, and pastries. The binge often is followed by self-induced vomiting or the use of laxatives, diuretics, or a combination of these.

Bulimia occurs more frequently than anorexia nervosa and is also seen most often in young women. People with bulimia are usually of normal weight or even overweight. Most are aware that their eating patterns are abnormal. They may experience fear of not being able to stop eating and depression, guilt, and remorse after a binge. Clinical signs of bulimia may include tooth erosion, calloused knuckles, stomach lacerations, and esophageal infections from excessive vomiting. Electrolyte imbalances may occur, leading to abnormal heart rhythms and injury to the kidneys. Repeated infections of the bladder and kidney may lead to renal failure.

Table 9-16 *MyPyramid: Food Intake Patterns*

The suggested amounts of food to consume from the basic food groups, subgroups, and oils to meet recommended nutrient intakes at 12 different calorie levels. Nutrient and energy contributions from each group are calculated according to the nutrient-dense forms of foods in each group (e.g., lean meats and fat-free milk). The table also shows the discretionary calorie allowance that can be accommodated within each calorie level, in addition to the suggested amounts of nutrient-dense forms of foods in each group.

DAILY AMOUNT OF FOOD FROM EACH GROUP

CALORIE LEVEL[1]	1000	1200	1400	1600	1800	2000	2200	2400	2600	2800	3000	3200
Fruits[2]	1 cup	1 cup	1.5 cups	1.5 cups	1.5 cups	2 cups	2 cups	2 cups	2 cups	2.5 cups	2.5 cups	2.5 cups
Vegetables[3]	1 cup	1.5 cups	1.5 cups	2 cups	2.5 cups	2.5 cups	3 cups	3 cups	3.5 cups	3.5 cups	4 cups	4 cups
Grains[4]	3 oz-eq	4 oz-eq	5 oz-eq	5 oz-eq	6 oz-eq	6 oz-eq	7 oz-eq	8 oz-eq	9 oz-eq	10 oz-eq	10 oz-eq	10 oz-eq
Meat and Beans[5]	2 oz-eq	3 oz-eq	4 oz-eq	5 oz-eq	5 oz-eq	5.5 oz-eq	6 oz-eq	6.5 oz-eq	6.5 oz-eq	7 oz-eq	7 oz-eq	7 oz-eq
Milk[6]	2 cups	2 cups	2 cups	3 cups	3 cups	3 cups	3 cups	3 cups	3 cups	3 cups	3 cups	3 cups
Oils[7]	3 tsp	4 tsp	4 tsp	5 tsp	5 tsp	6 tsp	6 tsp	7 tsp	8 tsp	8 tsp	10 tsp	11 tsp
Discretionary calorie allowance[8]	165	171	171	132	195	267	290	362	410	426	512	648

VEGETABLE SUBGROUP AMOUNTS ARE PER WEEK (CUPS PER WEEK)

CALORIE LEVEL	1000	1200	1400	1600	1800	2000	2200	2400	2600	2800	3000	3200
Dark green veg	1 c/wk	1.5 c/wk	1.5 c/wk	2 c/wk	3 c/wk	3 c/wk	3 c/wk	3 c/wk	3 c/wk	3 c/wk	3 c/wk	3 c/wk
Orange veg	0.5 c/wk	1 c/wk	1 c/wk	1.5 c/wk	2 c/wk	2 c/wk	2 c/wk	2 c/wk	2.5 c/wk	2.5 c/wk	2.5 c/wk	2.5 c/wk
Legumes	0.5 c/wk	1 c/wk	1 c/wk	2.5 c/wk	3 c/wk	3 c/wk	3 c/wk	3 c/wk	3.5 c/wk	3.5 c/wk	3.5 c/wk	3.5 c/wk
Starchy veg	1.5 c/wk	2.5 c/wk	2.5 c/wk	2.5 c/wk	3 c/wk	3 c/wk	6 c/wk	6 c/wk	7 c/wk	7 c/wk	9 c/wk	9 c/wk
Other veg	3.5 c/wk	4.5 c/wk	4.5 c/wk	5.5 c/wk	6.5 c/wk	6.5 c/wk	7 c/wk	7 c/wk	8.5 c/wk	8.5 c/wk	10 c/wk	10 c/wk

[1]Calorie Levels are set across a wide range to accommodate the needs of different individuals. The attached table "Estimated Daily Calorie Needs" can be used to help assign individuals to the food intake pattern at a particular calorie level.

[2]Fruit Group includes all fresh, frozen, canned, and dried fruits and fruit juices. In general, 1 cup of fruit or 100% fruit juice, or 1/2 cup of dried fruit can be considered as 1 cup from the fruit group.

[3]Vegetable Group includes all fresh, frozen, canned, and dried vegetables and vegetable juices. In general, 1 cup of raw or cooked vegetable or vegetables juice, or 2 cups of raw leafy greens can be considered as 1 cup from the vegetable group.

[4]Grains Group includes all foods made from wheat, rice, oats, cornmeal, barley, such as bread, pasta, oatmeal, breakfast cereals, tortillas, and grits. In general, 1 slice of bread, 1 cup of ready-to-eat cereal, or 1/2 cup of cooked rice, pasta, or cooked cereal can be considered as 1 ounce equivalent from the grains group. At least half of all grains consumed should be whole grains.

[5]Meat & Beans Group in general, 1 ounce of lean meat, poultry, or fish, 1 egg, 1 Tbsp. peanut butter, 1/4 cup cooked dry beans, or 1/2 ounce of nuts or seeds can be considered as 1 ounce equivalent from the meat and beans group.

[6]Milk Group includes all fluid milk products and foods made from milk that retain their calcium content, such as yogurt and cheese. Foods made from milk that have little to no calcium, such as cream cheese, cream, and butter, are not part of the group. Most milk group choices should be fat-free or low-fat. In general, 1 cup of milk or yogurt, 1 1/2 ounces of natural cheese, or 2 ounces of processed cheese can be considered as 1 cup from the milk group.

[7]Oils include fats from many different plants and from fish that are liquid at room temperature, such as canola, corn, olive, soybean, and sunflower oil. Some foods are naturally high in oils, like nuts, olives, some fish, and avocados. Foods that are mainly oil include mayonnaise, certain salad dressings, and soft margarine.

[8]Discretionary Calorie Allowance is the remaining amount of calories in a food intake pattern after accounting for the calories needed for all food groups—using forms of foods that are fat-free or low-fat and with no added sugars.

BINGE EATING DISORDER

Binge eating disorder is characterized by the intake of excessive calories at least twice a week for 6 months. The person eats very rapidly, sometimes consuming as much as 20,000 calories in one sitting. After the binge episode, the person feels guilty, embarrassed, and depressed. Binge eaters are often dieters, and many are overweight.

NUTRITIONAL SUPPORT WITH SUPPLEMENTAL FEEDINGS

The preferred method of meeting nutritional requirements is, of course, through eating a balanced diet. This is not always possible, however, and there are times when a person's nutritional needs cannot be met by oral feeding. At these times, a person's needs must be met with some type of nutritional supplement. These supplements can be formulated using liquid or powdered milk, powdered whole eggs, and powdered egg albumin as concentrated protein sources. Liquid feedings can meet the nutritional requirements of patients who are unable to take solid food. Examples of formulas used for enteral feedings

are Ensure, Compleat, Sustacal, Criticare HN, Pulmocare, Trauma Cal, Travasorb HN, and Travasorb Renal. Table 9-17 summarizes the situations that might require artificial feeding. Nursing care of patients receiving enteral and parenteral feedings is covered in Chapters 9 and 38.

ENTERAL TUBE FEEDINGS

Patients who are unable to take in supplemental liquid feedings orally may require enteral tube feedings. Enteral feedings bypass the mouth and deliver nutrients directly into the stomach or small intestine through inserted tubes. Conditions that interfere with taking in liquids orally include oral surgery, gastrointestinal surgery, dysphagia (difficulty swallowing), unconsciousness, anorexia, or esophageal obstruction. The tubes can be inserted into the stomach, duodenum, or jejunum through the nose or through the abdominal wall (Fig. 9-4).

Enteral tube feedings may cause complications such as nausea or vomiting, diarrhea, gastrointestinal bleeding, aspiration pneumonia, hyperkalemia (excessive serum potassium), hyponatremia (serum sodium deficit), hyperglycemia (elevated blood glucose), or nutritional deficiencies. They are caused either by problems

Table 9-17 *Situations Requiring Artificial Feeding Techniques*

PHYSIOLOGIC PROBLEM	RECOMMENDED FEEDING	CLINICAL SITUATION OR DISORDER
Inability to ingest food	Liquid feedings: whole food or milk-based formula Route of administration: Tube Nasogastric Gastrostomy Jejunostomy Oral	Carcinoma of esophagus or stomach Dental or oral surgery Inflammatory disease of esophagus Coma
Inability to digest food	Chemically defined diet Route of administration: Oral Tube	Pancreatitis Biliary tract disease
Decreased ability or inability to absorb food	Chemically defined diet Route of administration: Oral Tube Peripheral vein nutritional support Total parenteral nutrition	Radiation therapy Sprue Inflammatory bowel disease Short-bowel syndrome Inflammatory bowel disease
Inability to handle colonic residue	Chemically defined diet Route of administration: Oral Tube Peripheral vein nutritional support Total parenteral nutrition	Presurgical preparation Ileostomy, colostomy Draining fistula
Inability to meet nutritional requirements fully with normal foods	Liquid feeding Oral supplement Tube feeding Peripheral vein nutritional support Central vein nutritional supplementation	Major surgery Burns Trauma Extended fever Anorexia of chronic illness Anorexia nervosa

From Mahan, L.K., & Escott-Stump, S. (1996). *Krause's food, nutrition, and diet therapy* (9th ed., p. 426). Philadelphia: Saunders.

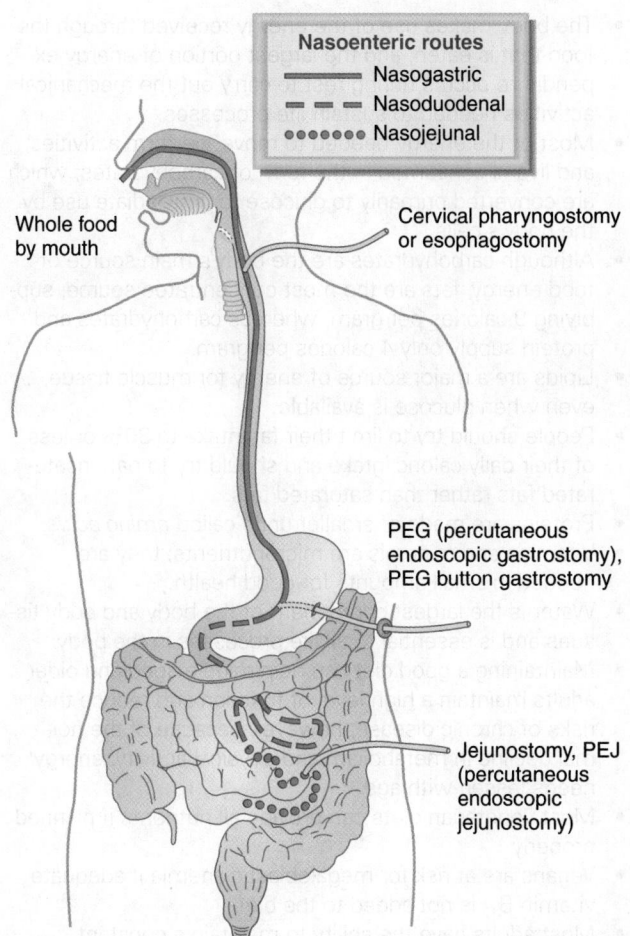

Nasoenteric routes
—— Nasogastric
— — — Nasoduodenal
•••••••• Nasojejunal

Whole food by mouth

Cervical pharyngostomy or esophagostomy

PEG (percutaneous endoscopic gastrostomy), PEG button gastrostomy

Jejunostomy, PEJ (percutaneous endoscopic jejunostomy)

FIGURE **9-4** Diagram of the placement of enteral feeding tubes.

with the liquid supplement or by mechanical difficulties with the tube feeding, such as misplacement of the tube or too rapid administration of the feeding. Dumping syndrome may occur when hypertonic fluid enters the jejunum; water is drawn into the lumen of the intestine to dilute the fluid, causing a drop in circulating blood volume. Tube blockage can occur, most likely caused by viscous formulas with inadequate flushing, crushed medications, and incompatible medications that form clumps.

PARENTERAL NUTRITION

Another method of administering nutrients is through parenteral nutrition. The two major types of parenteral nutrition are (1) peripheral parenteral nutrition (PPN) and (2) central parenteral nutrition (CPN) or total parenteral nutrition (TPN). Peripheral parenteral nutrition is given through the peripheral veins in the arms and legs and may employ a peripheral venous catheter or a peripherally inserted central catheter. CPN or TPN is given through a central vein, usually the superior vena cava. This method is used for nutrition only if the gastrointestinal tract cannot be used; it can be lifesaving.

Peripheral Parenteral Nutrition

Peripheral parenteral nutrition is the standard intravenous therapy, which may be composed of dextrose (5% to 10%), amino acids, vitamins, minerals, and electrolytes. Fat emulsions may be administered peripherally as well. Total nutritional requirements usually are not met with PPN therapy, and at most it supplies 1800 kcal/day. It is used primarily for short-term nutritional support.

Total Parenteral Nutrition

Central parenteral nutrition or TPN feedings are used for patients who are unable to obtain adequate nutrition enterally or with PPN. They are usually debilitated and malnourished, with a weight loss of 10% of the body weight or more. Patients with short-bowel syndrome, bowel fistulas or obstruction, inflammatory bowel disease, or hypermetabolic states in which the gastrointestinal tract is completely or partially unusable benefit from this form of nutritional support.

Total parenteral nutrition can meet the high energy and protein needs of burn patients. It can also be used for cancer patients who have become malnourished as a result of oncologic treatments. Total parenteral nutrition can supply up to 4000 kcal/day. This is possible because the solution is administered through a Hickman or Broviac-type catheter inserted into the superior vena cava, where the hypertonic solution can be diluted rapidly by the large, fast-flowing volume of blood.

Patients who are being fed parenterally should be monitored closely for any signs of complications. Potential complications include pulmonary complications, injury to the veins and arteries surrounding the TPN catheter site, air embolism, infection, electrolyte imbalance, mineral deficiencies, hyperglycemia, and, if treatment is ended suddenly, rebound hypoglycemia.

TRANSITIONAL FEEDING

When patients are ready to be changed from one of these methods to another, they are ready for transitional feeding. Transitional feeding can be from parenteral nutrition to enteral tube feeding or oral intake, from enteral tube feeding to oral formula or food, or a combination of these.

It is important that transitional feeding be done gradually and with specific principles in mind. If patients who have been without adequate food for an extended period are given food too quickly, they may develop nutritional recovery syndrome. This syndrome causes hypophosphatemia (deficiency of phosphates in the blood) from the shift of phosphorus from the plasma into the cells. This shift may also affect potassium as it moves into cells with the glucose during refeeding.

Refeeding of the malnourished patient disrupts the adaptive state of starvation and therefore must proceed slowly with close patient monitoring. The ideal early feeding appears to be moderate in carbohydrates, low in sodium, lactose free, and supplemented with phosphorus and potassium.

When moving from parenteral to oral or enteral feeding, it is important to continue the parenteral feeding. This allows for maintenance of adequate nutrient and fluid intake as tolerance of enteral feedings is assessed. As the patient is able to tolerate the oral or enteral feedings, the parenteral feedings can be tapered off.

When moving from enteral to oral feedings, the patient may complain of a poor appetite. In making this transition, it may be helpful to change the enteral feeding from a continuous drip to an intermittent feeding. In this way the patient has a chance to get hungry between feedings, and desire for food may increase.

Put on Your Thinking Cap!

Interview an older person (a patient, family member, or other acquaintance) about how their eating habits have changed with age. Identify any changes that could lead to inadequate nutrition.

Key Points

- Nutrition is the cornerstone of the healing process. To support and maintain life or fight disease, the body must be supplied with the proper nutrients.
- During the digestive process, enzymes help break down food particles to their simplest form so that the nutrients can be absorbed by the body.
- Regulation of the gastrointestinal system involves neural control and the secretion of hormones.
- Parasympathetic nerves generally stimulate digestive activity, and sympathetic nerves inhibit activity.
- The stomach is normally emptied in 1 to 4 hours, depending on the amount and kinds of foods eaten.
- The primary organ of absorption is the small intestine.
- Fluids, vitamins, and minerals are absorbed through the intestinal mucosa.

- The body makes use of the energy received through the food that is eaten, and the largest portion of energy expenditure occurs during rest to carry out the mechanical activities needed to sustain life processes.
- Most of the energy needed to move, perform activities, and live is consumed in the form of carbohydrates, which are converted primarily to glucose for immediate use by the body's cells.
- Although carbohydrates are the body's main source of food energy, fats are the most concentrated source, supplying 9 calories per gram, whereas carbohydrates and protein supply only 4 calories per gram.
- Lipids are a major source of energy for muscle tissue, even when glucose is available.
- People should try to limit their fat intake to 30% or less of their daily caloric intake and should try to eat unsaturated fats rather than saturated fats.
- Proteins are made of smaller units called *amino acids*.
- Vitamins and minerals are micronutrients; they are needed in small amounts for good health.
- Water is the largest component of the body and body tissues and is essential to all life processes in the body.
- Maintaining a good diet can help middle-aged and older adults maintain a high level of function and reduce the risks of chronic disease; however, because of the normal decline in metabolism and physical activity, energy needs lessen with age.
- Most vegetarian diets can provide all nutrients if planned properly.
- Vegans are at risk for megaloblastic anemia if adequate vitamin B_{12} is not added to the diet.
- Most adults have the ability to maintain a constant weight, but to do so, they must keep up consistent food and exercise patterns on a daily basis.
- Anorexia nervosa, bulimia, and binge eating disorder are eating disorders that often begin in adolescence.
- Eating disorders are thought to be caused by multiple biologic, psychological, sociocultural, and spiritual factors.
- For the patient who cannot take oral feedings, nutritional support may be provided through enteral tube feedings, or peripheral or central catheters.

 Go to your Companion CD-ROM for a Pharmacology Tutorial, Audio Glossary, and 3-D animations.

evolve Be sure to visit the companion Evolve site at http://evolve.elsevier.com/Linton/ for WebLinks and additional online resources.

REVIEW QUESTIONS *Choose the best answer.*

1. Most of the absorption of nutrients occurs in the:
   1. Stomach
   2. Small intestine
   3. Large intestine
   4. Liver

2. Lipase and amylase are examples of:
   1. Macronutrients
   2. Metabolic wastes
   3. Carrier proteins
   4. Digestive enzymes

3. When is the metabolic rate highest?
   1. Infancy
   2. Puberty
   3. Adolescence
   4. Young adult

4. Excess glucose is stored in the liver as:
   1. Monosaccharides
   2. Amino acids
   3. Glycogen
   4. Lactic acid

5. The functions of dietary fiber are to:
   1. Absorb excess gastric acid
   2. Increase the rates of digestion and absorption
   3. Decrease fecal bulk
   4. Help form a soft stool

6. Nutritionists recommend that dietary fats not exceed which percentage of the daily caloric intake?
   1. 10%
   2. 20%
   3. 30%
   4. 40%

7. Which of the following is a water-soluble vitamin?
   1. Vitamin E
   2. Vitamin A
   3. Vitamin C
   4. Vitamin D

8. Factors to consider when planning meals with older adults include the following:
   1. Older people should eliminate all sodium from their diets.
   2. Older people who are less active need fewer calories than they did when younger.
   3. Most older people require megavitamins to meet basic requirements.
   4. A moderately active older woman needs 500 fewer calories daily than when younger.

9. A patient reports that she is lactovegetarian. You know that her diet includes:
   1. Eggs
   2. Fish
   3. Poultry
   4. Milk

10. Complications of total parenteral nutrition include the following:
    1. Vomiting
    2. Air embolism
    3. Hypoglycemia
    4. Aspiration

11. Patients must be changed *gradually* from parenteral nutrition to oral nutrition to prevent nutritional recovery syndrome, which is characterized by:
    1. Hypophosphatemia
    2. Hypocalcemia
    3. Hyponatremia
    4. Hypoglycemia

Developmental Processes

Objectives

After reading and studying this chapter, you should be able to:

1. List the developmental tasks for successful adulthood.
2. Identify the health problems specific to the adult age-groups.
3. Discuss the health care needs of young, middle-aged, and older adults.

Key Terms

Be sure to check out the bonus material on the Companion CD-ROM, including selected audio pronunciations.

biologic age (p. 126)
psychological age (p. 126)
social age (p. 126)

Each stage of life has specific developmental processes that must be undertaken and mastered for a person to go on to the next stage successfully. These developmental processes consist of physical, emotional, social, and psychological changes that present challenges to every living human being. In this chapter, we discuss the developmental processes associated with young adulthood, middle age, and older age.

Major changes in the stages of development in the life cycle have occurred in the past 20 years. Americans are marrying later, having fewer children, and living longer. Certain marker events, such as marriage, childbirth, acquiring a first job, and the departure of young adults from the family home occur in various developmental stages. Despite the recent changes in the life cycle, there are still broad, general stages of adulthood with predictable movement between them. Erik Erikson developed the basis of our view of human growth and development; he introduced the idea that each stage of life is associated with specific developmental tasks (Table 10-1).

YOUNG ADULTHOOD

Young adulthood comes at a time when physical growth ends and social expectations begin. It is considered to occur during a person's 20s, 30s, and 40s; however, these decades are often divided by such terms as

young young adult (ages 20 to 35) and *old young adult* (ages 35 to 45).

Young adulthood is a time for settling down to a job and raising a family and taking on new responsibilities. Most people in this age-group are expected to leave their parents' home and establish their own home. People in their 20s and early 30s begin this process by establishing an intimate, lasting relationship with another person in which the physical satisfaction and psychological security of another are more important than their own. Without the development of an intimate relationship, the young adult can become isolated, lonely, and self-absorbed. In addition, young adults are establishing career goals.

Many young people have extended their education and have prolonged the time in which they continue to live at home; or a job loss, divorce, or other stressor may precipitate a move back home. The entire family then has to adjust to a young adult living at home by redistributing roles and responsibilities, maintaining adequate communication, and reallocating budget and space.

This may be a difficult time for parents, who had expected a new time of freedom and independence in their middle years. It is especially difficult if young grandchildren are included in the package.

DEVELOPMENTAL TASKS

The following developmental tasks must be achieved by young adults:

- Accept self and stabilize self-concept and body image.
- Establish independence from parental home and financial aid.
- Assume responsibilities and independent decision making.
- Become established in a vocation or profession that provides personal satisfaction, economic independence, and a feeling of making a worthwhile contribution to society.
- Learn to appraise and express love responsibly through more than sexual contact.
- Establish an intimate bond with another, either through marriage or with a close friend.
- Establish and maintain a home and manage a time schedule and life stresses.

Table 10-1 | *Erikson's Adult Developmental Tasks*

DEVELOPMENTAL STAGE	DEVELOPMENTAL TASK	NURSING ASSESSMENT DATA
Young adulthood	Intimacy versus isolation	Assess whether the patient has meaningful, intimate relationships. If the patient has no intimate relationships, ask whether he or she has had one or more in the past. Assess other support systems that the patient may have.
Middle adulthood	Generativity versus stagnation	Assess whether the patient is employed. Ask the patient what he or she does for leisure or recreation. If the patient is not employed or has no regular leisure activity, ask the patient what he or she does during a 24-hour day. Assess for signs of depression, such as excessive sleeping and decreased appetite.
Older adulthood	Ego integrity versus despair	Assess what the patient does each day. Ask about the patient's family and other relationships. Ask the patient if he or she feels lonely; if so, assess for signs of depression.

From Ignatavicius, D.D., Workman, M.L., & Mishler, M. (1999). *Medical-surgical nursing: A nursing process approach* (3rd ed., p. 44). Philadelphia: Saunders.

- Find a congenial social and friendship group.
- Decide whether to have a family and carry out tasks of parenting.
- Formulate a meaningful philosophy of life and reassess priorities and values.
- Become involved as a citizen in the community.

It is evident that these developmental tasks focus on marriage, childbearing, and work. However, many young adults are delaying marriage, electing to remain single, or are divorced. It should be clear that a young adult does not have to marry to be well adjusted and achieve the identified developmental tasks.

HEALTH PROBLEMS

Young adults, especially those in their 20s and early 30s, have relatively few health problems. The four major causes of death in the young adult age-group do not result from illness but from accidents and violence: (1) vehicular accidents, (2) other accidents, (3) suicide, and (4) homicide. As young adults progress into their late 30s and early 40s, the primary causes of death are malignancies and heart disease, followed by accidents and infection with the human immunodeficiency virus (HIV).

Typical health problems are related to stress on the job or in social interactions, lifestyle, and childbearing. They include depression; anxiety; complications of pregnancy; cervical and breast cancer; and back, hip, and limb injuries. In the quest for meaningful social relationships and a career that will gain them independence and success, young adults may experience tension and stress and may lack the time to attend to health-promoting activities such as a proper diet and nutrition. They may work hard and party enthusiastically. Meals may be eaten on the run, and the diet may consist primarily of junk foods. The total number of calories needed is less than during adolescence, since the adult has completed physical growth. Smoking and alcohol or drug abuse are common. These practices may have a direct bearing on health in the later years (Table 10-2). Women are advised to begin annual Pap smears beginning at age 18 or when they become sexually active. After three successive normal tests, the interval between tests can be increased (ACS, 2000).

As young adults enter their 30s and early 40s, their focus is directed mainly toward raising a family and furthering their career (Fig. 10-1). It may be a time to reassess their lives and careers, and often major changes are made. Factors that contribute to health problems are stress related to work, marital problems, and stress related to managing a household. Couples who have postponed childbearing may have difficulties with conception and pregnancy.

HEALTH CARE NEEDS

Health care needs are related to promoting optimal health. It is a good idea to have at least one thorough physical examination during the 20s. A physical examination should include tests for sexually transmitted infections, hypertension, and elevated blood lipids. During young adulthood, several types of health screening (mammograms, clinical breast examinations, breast and testicular self-examination, pelvic examinations, and Papanicolaou [Pap] smears) should be initiated and repeated at regular intervals. Monthly

Table 10-2 *Harmful Health Practices, Effects on Health in the Later Years, and Preventive Measures*

HARMFUL HEALTH PRACTICE	POSSIBLE EFFECTS ON HEALTH	PREVENTIVE MEASURES
Lack of physical activity	Diabetes, osteoporosis, heart disease, cancer, obesity, stroke, depression	Increase moderate daily physical activity, and reduce sedentary lifestyle.
Obesity	Heart disease, hypertension, insulin-dependent diabetes mellitus, degenerative joint disease, cancer, stroke, atherosclerosis	Maintain ideal weight; maintain low-cholesterol, low-fat (<30%), nutritious diet with plenty of vegetables, fruits, and grain products.
Cigarette smoking	Heart disease; cancers of the lung, larynx, pharynx, oral cavity, esophagus, pancreas, and bladder; chronic bronchitis and emphysema	Stop smoking, or do not start smoking.
Alcohol and drug abuse	Malnutrition, cirrhosis of the liver, brain damage, mental status changes, homicides, suicides, motor vehicle fatalities	Limit alcohol intake and stop using drugs or do not start; participate in 12-step program for rehabilitation.
Stress	Stress-related conditions such as hypertension and heart disease	Recognize and modify stressors; use a stress management program, such as exercise or biofeedback.

Adapted from U.S. Department of Health and Human Services. *Healthy People 2010* (2nd ed.). *With understanding and improving health and objectives for improving health.* (2 vols.). (2000, Publication No. [PHS] 99-1256). Washington: U.S. Government Printing Office.

FIGURE **10-1** Middle age is a time of relatively good health, with new opportunities and personal freedom for many.

breast self-examination is an option for women beginning in their 20s. A tetanus booster should be given if persons have not received one in the past 10 years. The hepatitis B vaccine is recommended for adults at risk of exposure to blood and body fluids. Routine dental and eye examinations should be scheduled. Young women should have a Pap smear done every 3 years. By age 40, women should begin having annual mammograms and clinical breast examinations. Women may be taught breast self-examination but should be told that it does not replace periodic professional examinations. Young men should be taught to do a testicular examination.

Health counseling in the 20s should focus on health-promoting behaviors. Programs may be established to include topics such as nutrition, exercise and leisure, rest and sleep, human sexuality and family planning, and the effects of smoking, drugs, and alcohol.

In the years between 30 and 45, especially after age 35, young adults should begin to think about the

prevention of chronic illness, particularly cancer and heart disease. They should have periodic physical examinations, usually recommended at ages 30 and 35, and then every 3 years thereafter. The physical examination should include tests for hypertension, anemia, and elevated serum lipids, and a cervical Pap smear for women. It is suggested that people in this age-group examine their skin and mouth periodically for precancerous lesions. Preventive dental checkups and treatment are usually recommended every 6 months to 2 years. The American Cancer Society's recommendations for early detection of certain cancers are found in Chapter 26 and at http://www.cancer.org.

Health promotion and disease prevention programs have a similar focus as those for people in their 20s. Stress management, effective parenting, proper diet and nutrition, exercise, drug and alcohol awareness, and smoking cessation are appropriate topics for health teaching and counseling.

 Put on Your Thinking Cap!

When a young adult is diagnosed with a serious chronic illness, how might developmental tasks be affected?

MIDDLE YEARS

The terms *middle years, middle age,* and *middle adulthood* usually refer to the ages between 45 and 65. However, other factors define middle age, particularly how a person acts and feels. Because life expectancy has increased so dramatically during the past 50 years, middle age is a relatively new concept. Previously, the majority of people did not live past their 40s, and what used to be old age is now middle age. Middle age today has been pushed into the 50s; 50 is now what 40 used to be. A child born in 2003 now has a life expectancy of 77.6 years (74.8 for men, 80.1 for women). A woman who reaches the age of 50 today free of cancer and heart disease can expect to live until she is 91. After reaching their 50th birthday, women can expect to live 40 or more years. A healthy man who is 65 can expect to live until he is 81 (Sheehy, 1995).

More than 40 million Americans, or one fourth of the U.S. population, are considered middle-aged. They earn most of the money, pay most of the taxes, and have most of the power in business and government. Middle age is a time of relatively good health for most. People experience a new personal freedom and enjoy maximum command of themselves and influence over others.

Many people who are in their middle years belong to a group called the "sandwich generation." They may have teenagers and young adults at home and at the same time have ailing, older-adult parents to care for. The fact that most middle-aged Americans today still have a living parent is a great change in family dynamics. People who delayed pregnancy and childbearing may have even younger children at home.

Many of today's middle-aged women work outside the home and have developed important careers. Work and family obligations together may require a balancing act for middle-aged women who are trying to maintain continued involvement both at work and at home. In addition to caring for children, the middle-aged woman is the most likely caregiver to older-adult parents. The result can be a great deal of stress and conflict.

DEVELOPMENTAL TASKS

The following developmental tasks should be accomplished by people in their middle years:

- Discover and develop new satisfaction with a mate or significant other by enjoying mutual activities, providing mutual support, and developing a deeper sense of unity and intimacy.
- Help growing and grown children become happy and responsible adults.
- Balance work and other roles; prepare for retirement.
- Accept role reversal with aging parents; prepare emotionally for the eventual death of living parents.
- Achieve mature social and civic responsibilities and give time and resources to the community.
- Accept and adjust to the physical changes of middle age and establish and maintain a healthy lifestyle.
- Continue to formulate a philosophy of life and grow spiritually.
- Develop satisfying leisure activities.
- Recognize the inevitability of death and prepare for one's own eventual death.

Middle-aged persons who successfully master developmental tasks begin to accept their age and gradually come to value the wisdom gained from living and experience rather than the physical power and strength that accompany youth. Emotional and mental flexibility increase the ability to change and adapt to new situations and to be open to others. It is a time of "mellowing-out," of accepting what life has to offer.

HEALTH PROBLEMS

People in their middle years continue to be relatively healthy, and the same factors that contribute to the deterioration of health habits in the young adult apply to those in middle age. The major cause of death is cardiovascular disease, and the most common health problems, along with cardiovascular disease, are cancer, pulmonary disease, diabetes, obesity, alcoholism, anxiety, depression, and glaucoma. Respiratory conditions are a frequent cause for days absent from work in women; injuries are a frequent cause for men. Bone mass begins to decrease. Women lose calcium from bone tissue after menopause, leading to an increased risk of osteoporosis. Muscle mass is reduced as a result of decreased muscle fiber. In the 40s, changes in vision typically begin. Age-related farsightedness, called *presbyopia*, develops as a result of decreasing elasticity of the lens. The clue to developing presbyopia is that the middle-aged adult begins to hold reading material at a distance to focus on it better. *Presbycusis* (normal loss of hearing acuity associated with aging) may begin to appear. This is an important life stage to focus on prevention. Lifestyle changes yield significant benefits in terms of a longer, healthier life (Geberding quoted by Stobbe, 2005).

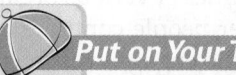 *Put on Your Thinking Cap!*

Suppose a middle-aged adult is diagnosed with a life-threatening illness. What are the effects on family, job, and other roles? How easy do you suppose it is for such a person to concentrate on the needs of treatment?

HEALTH CARE NEEDS

The health care goals for middle-aged people are the same as those for younger adults. They are focused on health promotion and disease prevention to preserve and prolong the period of maximum energy and optimal mental and social activity.

During the middle years, regular assessment of health status is important for maintaining good health. Early diagnosis of illness helps prevent later complications. A complete physical examination is recommended every 3 years and should include routine blood pressure screening and cholesterol and glucose testing.

Women should continue to have an annual mammogram and clinical breast examination. After age 30, a woman who has had three normal Pap test results in a row can decrease the frequency of this test to every 2 or 3 years. Regular breast self-examination may help with early detection of abnormalities but should not replace medical evaluation (ACS, 2005). Women usually enter a perimenopausal period between the ages of 45 and 50. Menopause is preceded by the perimenopausal period (approximately 5 years) during which there is a gradual decrease in estrogen accompanied by a gradual decrease in menstrual flow. The permanent cessation of menstruation typically occurs between the ages of 45 and 55. During the menopausal years, women may experience symptoms such as hot flashes, dizziness, headaches, perspiration, palpitations, water retention, nausea, muscle cramps, fatigue, insomnia, or tingling of the fingers and toes. Many women take estrogen to relieve some of the symptoms of menopause.

Health-promoting activities during middle age are the same as for young adults. The focus is on proper nutrition, exercise, stress management, and the reduction or elimination of smoking, drug use, and alcohol use.

OLDER ADULTS

Age 65 is commonly thought of as the beginning of old age. However, many people in their 60s and older do not consider themselves old, and they continue to live healthy, productive lives. Because people are generally healthy today, people are entering old age in better health than in the past. In America today, 8 in 10 people will live past their 65th birthday. Markers that may be more accurate than chronologic age to define older age include the following: (1) biologic age, (2) psychological age, and (3) social age. *Biologic age* focuses on the functional capabilities of various organ systems in the body. Many older people continue to function well, especially those who engage in exercise and other health-promoting activities, whereas others seem to be prematurely ill and frail. *Psychological age* refers to the behavioral capacity of the person to adapt to changing environmental demands. The older person's ability to remember, learn, and exercise behavioral control is a factor that affects psychological age. *Social age* refers to the roles and habits of a person in relation to other members of society, including such aspects as the person's type of dress, language, and social relationships.

During older age, men and women are required to make many adjustments to physiologic, psychological, and social changes. Declines in bodily function, particularly in vision and hearing, and diminished physical strength and resiliency may have an effect on day-to-day functioning. Psychological changes include a decreased short-term memory, slower performance on cognitive tasks, and longer learning time. Older people retain psychological skills, but those skills usually take

longer to accomplish. Social changes include retirement, a change in living conditions, and loss of spouse and significant others.

Put on Your Thinking Cap!

Consider your own biologic age, psychological age, and social age. Using examples of family, friends, and acquaintances in your life, think of ways that people can act differently in psychological and social ages from their biologic ages.

DEVELOPMENTAL TASKS

The following developmental tasks must be achieved by older adults:

- Recognize the aging process and adjust to decreasing physical strength and health changes.
- Adjust to retirement; adjust living standards to retirement income.
- Establish satisfactory living arrangements as a result of role changes.
- Maintain emotional satisfaction in relationships with spouse, children, grandchildren, and other living relatives.
- Establish an affiliation with members of own age-group; maintain an interest in people outside the family and in the community.
- Maintain maximum level of health; learn to adjust to the loss of physical strength, illness, and one's own mortality.
- Cope with the death of parents, spouse, and friends.
- Learn to combine new dependency needs with the continuing need for independence.

Developmental tasks in older age focus on the redirection of energy and talents to new roles and activities, the acceptance of life with its joys and limitations, and the development of a personal view of death in preparation for this final stage of life.

HEALTH PROBLEMS

The major causes of death in older age are related to chronic illness, specifically cardiovascular disease, cancer, and diabetes mellitus. Accidents, including falls, are the fourth leading cause of death in this age-group. The most common illnesses are arthritis, gastrointestinal problems (peptic ulcer, constipation), acute and chronic respiratory diseases (influenza, pneumonia, emphysema), and gallbladder disease. Benign or malignant enlargement of the prostate is common in older men; breast cancer is common in older women.

HEALTH CARE NEEDS

The health care goals in the older age-group are to manage chronic illnesses and to maintain and prolong the period of optimal physical, mental, and social activity. It is important to help older adults maintain their independence as long as possible in the face of one or more chronic illnesses.

Physical examinations should be done yearly and include the same assessment as indicated for middle-aged adults. Dental examinations and treatment should also be continued into older age. As people age, periodic evaluation and treatment of the feet by a podiatrist are recommended to promote mobility. An influenza vaccination is recommended yearly for persons older than 65 years. A single-dose pneumococcal vaccine is recommended with revaccination every 5 years for people with chronic illnesses. Also, individuals who were vaccinated 5 or more years previously and were younger than age 65 at the time of the first vaccination should have a one-time revaccination.

Health-promoting activities should continue into older age. These activities can increase quality of life and, in many cases, prevent many of the chronic illnesses that accompany the later years. Proper nutrition, especially a low-fat, high-fiber diet with a large amount of complex carbohydrates, helps maintain energy, promote intestinal motility, and decrease susceptibility to some chronic illnesses. Exercise can benefit older adults, even the very old who begin an exercise program for the first time. Walking is the ideal exercise, and 20 to 30 minutes three times a week can help maintain weight, blood pressure, coordination, and mobility and create a positive outlook on life. Older people also can benefit from counseling for alcohol and drug abuse and smoking cessation. It is never too late to improve one's health habits.

Chapter 11 discusses health care issues related to the older adult in greater depth.

Key Points

- Developmental processes are changes that present challenges that must be undertaken and mastered for a person to go on to the next stage successfully.
- Developmental tasks for young adults center on acceptance of self, independence, intimacy, home and time management, social relationships, community involvement, and formulation of a meaningful philosophy of life.
- Health problems of young adults are related to stress on the job or in social interactions, lifestyle, and childbearing.
- Developmental tasks for middle-aged adults focus on interpersonal relationships, guidance of grown children, creation of a pleasant home, balanced roles, care of aging parents, civic responsibilities, adjustment to physical changes, pursuit of satisfying leisure activities, formulation of a life philosophy, and recognition of death's inevitability.
- Health problems of middle-aged adults include cardiovascular disease, cancer, pulmonary disease, diabetes, obesity, alcoholism, anxiety, depression, and glaucoma.
- Developmental tasks for older adults include adjustment to aging and retirement, establishment of satisfactory living arrangements, maintenance of emotional satisfaction in relationships, affiliation with peers, maintenance of maximal level of health, coping with the deaths of others, and learning to combine new dependency needs with the need for independence.
- Health problems for older adults include cardiovascular disease, cancer, diabetes mellitus, accidents, arthritis, gastrointestinal problems, and respiratory diseases.

 Go to your Companion CD-ROM for a Pharmacology Tutorial, Audio Glossary, and 3-D animations.

evolve Be sure to visit the companion Evolve site at http://evolve.elsevier.com/Linton/ for WebLinks and additional online resources.

REVIEW QUESTIONS *Choose the best answer.*

1. An important developmental task of the young adult is to:
   1. Accept role reversal with aging parents
   2. Develop satisfying leisure activities
   3. Establish an intimate bond with another
   4. Achieve mature social and civic responsibilities

2. Which intervention is directed toward reducing the most common cause of death among young adults?
   1. Teach early warning signs of cancer
   2. Encourage cardiovascular fitness
   3. Teach principles of safe sex
   4. Promote safe driving practices

3. The term *sandwich generation* is used to describe:
   1. Young adults who tend to eat on the run, primarily fast food
   2. Middle-aged adults caring for both children and parents
   3. Children who are left to care for themselves in single-parent homes
   4. Older adults who are in transition from independent to assisted living

4. Health promotion activities designed to reduce the major cause of death for middle-aged adults include the following:
   1. Cardiovascular fitness programs
   2. Screening for diabetes mellitus
   3. Driving instruction for older people
   4. Stress management classes

5. A developmental task of older adults is to:
   1. Maintain the pace of middle age despite physical changes
   2. Maintain emotional satisfaction in relationships with others
   3. Decrease one's involvement in social activities
   4. Remain independent regardless of physical and emotional health

6. A leading cause of death among both young adults and older adults is:
   1. Cancer
   2. Accidents
   3. Suicide
   4. Diabetes mellitus

The Older Patient

Objectives

After reading and studying this chapter, you should be able to:

1. Describe the roles of the gerontological nurse.
2. Determine the extent to which selected myths and stereotypes about older adults are factual.
3. Describe biologic and physiologic factors associated with aging.
4. Explain psychosocial factors associated with aging.
5. Describe modifications needed for activities of daily living.
6. Explain why drug dosage adjustments may be needed for older persons.

Key Terms

Be sure to check out the bonus material on the Companion CD-ROM, including selected audio pronunciations.

ageism (ĀJ-ĭz-ĕm, p. 130)
aging (p. 129)
cataract (KĂT-ă-răkt, p. 136)
conduction deafness (kŏn-DŬK-shŭn DĔF-nĕs, p. 135)
gerontological nurse (jĕ-rŏn-tō-LŎJ-ĭ-kăl, p. 130)
gerontology (jĕr-ŏn-TŎL-ō-jē, p. 129)
glaucoma (glăw-KŌ-mă, p. 136)
kyphosis (kī-FO-sĭs, p. 135)
presbycusis (prĕz-bĕ-KŪ-sĭs, p. 135)
presbyopia (prĕz-bĕ-Ō-pē-ă, p. 136)
sensorineural deafness (sĕn-sŏ-rĕ-NŪ-răl DĔF-nĕs, p. 135)

The care of older adults can be an extremely rewarding experience. Armed with the tools of caring, kindness, and knowledge, the nurse is in a position to help older persons maintain health and function often while coping with health threats common to the later years of life. The need for nurses with knowledge about healthy aging and the management of chronic illness will continue to grow as people who reach age 65 can now expect to live into their 80s. Toward the end of life, the medical focus tends to shift from curing to caring. However this should not imply that "nothing can be done," because each stage of life, including the final one, offers opportunities for growth. This chapter provides an overview of the aging process and the needs of older persons.

DEFINITIONS OF OLD AGE

Defining *old age* is not as simple as it might seem. A child or teenager may define "old people" as persons in their 30s, 40s, or 50s, whereas people in their 50s may define old as "at least 10 years older than I am." Age identification consists of much more than just recognition of chronological age.

Most definitions of *old age* refer to having lived for a long time. *Aged* is defined as old or advanced in years. However, aging is defined as the process of growing older or more mature. We all experience the process of aging, but not all of us are old in years, roles, behaviors, health, or physical limitations.

Aging is an ongoing developmental process that begins at conception and ends in death. Most gerontologists agree that old age is not measured in years. Although the age of 65 is commonly used to indicate the onset of old age, this number is clearly arbitrary and a function of social policy.

Gerontology, the study of aging, can be dated to the early 1950s and includes aging research, education, and training activities. Geriatrics is the biomedical science of old age and the application of knowledge related to the biologic, biomedical, behavioral, and social aspects of aging to the prevention, diagnosis, treatment, and care of older persons. The term *geriatrics* was coined in recognition of the similarity to the field of pediatrics. Both gerontology and geriatrics are critical components of a young science with practitioners from many disciplines, including nursing, medicine, dentistry, psychology, anthropology, and political science.

ROLES OF THE GERONTOLOGICAL NURSE

In 1989, 12% of the U.S. population were age 65 and over. By the year 2030, it is predicted that 21.8% of the population will be age 65 and older. By 2020, the median age in the United States is expected to be 40 (versus 33 in 1990), and the older population is expected to reach 52 million. These older adults will need regular primary health care services to help them maintain their health and prevent disabling and life-threatening diseases and conditions. Nurses have always been involved in the care of the aged. However, many nurses need additional education to build a foundation for

| Box 11-1 | *A Young Girl Still Dwells* |

What do you see, Nurse, what do you see?
Are you thinking when you look at me
A crabbed old woman, not very wise,
Uncertain of habit with far away eyes,
Who dribbles her food and makes no reply
When you say in a loud voice, "I do wish you'd try."
Who seems not to notice the things that you do
And forever is losing a stocking or shoe,
Who resisting or not, lets you do as you will
With bathing and feeding, the long day to fill.
Is that what you're thinking is that what you see
Then open your eyes, nurse. You're not looking at me.

Focus on the Family, 1985

quality gerontological nursing care that aims to maximize well-being.

Formal preparation for specialized care of the older adult occurs at the master's degree level, but there are also nursing personnel who have demonstrated competencies as a result of on-the-job training. At least 11 different levels of preparation exist for those providing care to the aged, as shown in the Management and Supervision box on p. 131, and the only consistent credentialing mechanism in the United States is the state licensing examination for registered nurses and licensed vocational or practical nurses. Employment settings for licensed vocational or practical nurses have shifted from traditional hospital-bound positions to a range of community-based long-term care facilities and home health care positions. The shift to more community-based sites should enhance the level of care in these settings.

The term **gerontological nurse** typically refers to professional nurses and advanced-level practitioners, such as nurse practitioners, clinical specialists, and nurses holding national certification in the specialty of gerontological nursing. Laurie Gunter and Camen Estes describe gerontological nursing as a health service that incorporates basic nursing methods and specialized knowledge about the aged to establish conditions within the patient and within the environment that (1) increase healthy behaviors in the aged; (2) minimize and compensate for health-related losses and impairments of aging; (3) provide comfort and sustenance through the distressing and debilitating events of aging, including dying and death; and (4) facilitate the diagnosis, care, and treatment of disease in the aged.

AGEISM—MYTHS AND STEREOTYPES

Are old people more or less highly valued in our society today than they were a century or more ago? This is hard to answer because we have relatively little evidence about the lives of older people in the past. Along with the limited factual information is an abundance of

Health Promotion Considerations

Myths About Aging

Some of the myths associated with old age include nonproductivity, disengagement, inflexibility, senility, inability to learn, retirement being a cause of death, and sexlessness. Myths are a poor substitute for scientific data.

When older people are properly motivated, their intelligence does not wane. In fact, with better organizational skills born of experience, the ability to organize thoughts efficiently may actually improve as one ages. Normal aging does not cause the intelligence quotient (IQ) to plummet, nor do most individuals become senile. Only about 10% of persons older than 65 have dementia, with the greatest incidence after age 85. Cognitive changes in the older person are often a consequence of disease, overmedication, neglect, and despair. Most of these conditions can be reversed.

Old age, like retirement, does not kill, nor does it render older adults sexless. According to researchers Masters and Johnson, sexual activity may continue well into the ninth decade. Saying that older people are not interested in sex is another way of disguising the belief that older people should not be interested in sex. Sexual activity is a healthy expression of life and vitality. However, sexual dysfunction can occur at any age and is usually evidence of some illness or disease process or a result of medication side effects. Knowledge of age-related biologic, physiologic, and psychosocial factors tends to negate many of the stereotypes of aging.

Other myths abound, but one must be shattered forever, and that is that older people are isolated, poor, ill, disabled, and living in long-term care facilities. Most older adults are members of multigenerational units and have extended family and support networks. However, most older adults prefer being independent as long as possible. The majority of older adults are not disabled, and only about 6% of the older population live in long-term care facilities. Although many older persons live in poverty, people older than 65 make up the wealthiest group in today's economy. This collective group leads in buying power and disposable income.

What other myths have you heard about aging?

myths and stereotypes about older persons that have been accepted as reality. Nurses must be knowledgeable about aging to avoid generalizing about older adults.

Ageism is a concept introduced by a well-known gerontologist, Dr. R. N. Butler, in 1969. Ageism is the process of systematic stereotyping and discrimination against people because of their age, most often directed toward older adults. Older people are ridiculed and labeled senile, rigid in thought, asexual, and morally old-fashioned. Ageism allows for separation and denial of the older person's humanness. It also allows those who practice ageism to distance themselves from their own aging. Ageism, like all other prejudices, influences the behavior of its victims. Some older people confront the stereotypes, whereas

Management and Supervision

Levels of Nursing Personnel Involved in Care of the Aged

PRACTITIONER	FUNCTION	EDUCATION PREPARATION
Nursing assistant (also known as patient care assistants [PCAs], nurses' aides [NAs])	Assist professional nurse in patient care tasks	On-the-job training, certified through taking short courses at technical colleges or through in-service training
Licensed practical nurse (LPN) or licensed vocational nurse (LVN)	Assist professional nurse in patient care tasks	Technical college or vocational high school preparation, must pass licensure examination and maintain licensure to practice
Registered nurse (RN)	Practice professional nursing with patients and families in any health care setting	Multiple levels of entry, including (1) associate degree (ADN) in 2-year program, (2) diploma (3-year hospital-based program), (3) baccalaureate degree (BSN) through 4-year university-based program, (4) nursing doctorate (ND) through 4-year program after college degree in another field; state licensure required for all levels of entry
Nurse practitioner (NP) (sometimes also qualified by specialty area, such as *geriatric nurse practitioner* [GNP] or *family nurse practitioner* [FNP])	Expanded nursing role, such as management of chronic disease, prescription of medicines, diagnosis of disease	All are RNs certified jointly by state boards of nursing and medicine; usually have master's degree in nursing
Clinical specialist	Advanced practitioner of nursing, clinical teacher	Individuals with master's degree (MSN, MN) who also are RNs
Nurse scientist	Nurse researcher, nurse educator, or both	Doctor of nursing science (DNSc), or doctor of philosophy (PhD) in nursing or other field (psychology, sociology, physiology, anthropology)

Modified from Matteson, M.A., McConnell, E.S., & Linton, A.D. (1997). *Gerontological nursing: Concepts and practice.* (2nd ed., p. 42). Philadelphia: Saunders.

others deny them with age-inappropriate behaviors (e.g., the 69-year-old who attempts to dress and act young in 3-inch heels and short skirts). Some myths about aging are discussed in the Health Promotion Considerations box on p. 130.

BIOLOGIC AND PHYSIOLOGIC FACTORS IN AGING

The search for immortality and the renewal of youth have captured the imagination of humankind since time began. The ancient Greeks and Romans ascribed immortality to their gods and the few humans who they believed became gods. Magical potions to fend off death have been sought by such diverse cultures as the Chinese, the ancient Hebrews, and the Europeans of the Middle Ages.

The theme of immortality surfaces in nearly every area of human experience. Medical science has made great strides in conquering many ills, but little has been achieved in extending the life span. In modern times, the longest documented human life, recorded in Japan, was 120 years, and most experts believe that the maximal attainable age is approximately 115 to 120 years.

How and why do humans age? Why is individual aging so varied? Which of the many theories of aging are valid? Each of these questions represents a fascinating area for scientific exploration. However, despite intense interest in longevity by so many cultures, scientists do not agree on precisely why or how humans age. Much of what is now known comes from our increasing awareness of the growth in absolute numbers of older people and in the proportion of the population that is old. Knowledge of the underlying mechanisms of aging is critical for the development of a system that considers the special needs and health conditions of an aging population.

THEORIES OF AGING

Proposed theories of aging have ranged from the concept of purely genetic control of aging to the concept of environmental assaults on the organism that result in death (Table 11-1). Most experts now believe that aging is not explainable by a single theory but represents many processes working simultaneously. Therefore several theories may be needed to explain all aging processes.

Most theories of aging can be divided into two general categories: error theories and programming theories. Error theories are based on the belief that the rate of aging is directly related to the organism's rate of living and that external events cause damage to the organism's cells. The damage from all causes accumulates over time, resulting in cellular, molecular, and organ malfunction or errors. Examples of these theories include error, catastrophe, and wear-and-tear theories.

Programming theories are based on the belief that aging is an event that is programmed into the cell itself and is internal to the organism. These theories postulate that aging, like prenatal development and menopause, is the natural and expected result of a purposeful sequence of events written internally into gene structure. Examples of these theories include programmed senescence and immunologic theory. It is important to remember that theories about aging continue to evolve and that no one theory is entirely explanatory or universally accepted.

PHYSIOLOGIC CHANGES IN BODY SYSTEMS

Aging occurs slowly and is a complex and dynamic process involving many internal and external influences. It is a process that affects virtually every system, organ, and cell in the body to varying degrees. With increasing age, the ability to maintain physiologic functions in the face of challenges is reduced.

Consequently, an understanding of the age-related effects on body systems is an integral part of the scientific basis for nursing care of the aged. The effects of aging on principal systems of the body are discussed below. These changes are not universal and may not be characterized as inevitable consequences of aging. It is nevertheless important that nurses be prepared to incorporate goals, plans, and actions related to nutrition, exercise, and behavior modification in providing care to older people with health problems.

Table 11-1	*Selected Theories of Aging*
THEORY	**PROPONENT SCIENTIST (YEAR)**
ERROR THEORIES	
Wear-and-tear theory	Pearl (1924)
Metabolic theory	Pearl (1928)
Somatic mutation theory	Sziliard (1959)
Error catastrophe theory	Orgel (1963)
Free radical theory	Harman (1955)
PROGRAMMING THEORIES	
Collagen theory	Verzar (1957)
Programmed senescence theory	Hayflick (1961)
Cross-linking theory	Bjorkstein (1968)
Immunologic theory	Walford (1969)

Adapted from National Institute on Aging. (1997). *Answers about aging: New pieces to an old puzzle.* Washington, DC: U.S. Department of Health and Human Services.

NERVOUS SYSTEM

Some of the most frequently discussed changes that occur with aging focus on the neural structures. However, it is essential that nurses know that in the absence of disease, most aged people remain alert, with functional intellectual capability, sound judgment, and creativity. Only modest impairments in memory and learning are observed after age 70 in most people who are relatively free from major disease.

Brain size is generally thought to decrease with age, although evidence for this belief is not conclusive. Loss of neurons (brain cells) begins in the early 30s and continues progressively. Nevertheless, functional ability may not be affected significantly because reserve cells are able to compensate. In addition to the reduced number of neurons, other aging changes in the nervous system include decreased conduction speed and diminished activity of the enzymes associated with synaptic transmission. These changes may result in a progressive slowing of responses, problems with short-term memory, and altered learning.

Short-term memory loss is frequently a concern of the aged, although long-term memory may remain intact. Short-term memory is associated with a stimulus input into the neurons and is dependent on adequate tissue oxygenation. The aging brain may be considered to be in a chronic hypoxic state. The deficit in oxygen is related to atherosclerosis as well as decreased cellular respiration. Consequently, the aged person may experience difficulty remembering planned events for the day but may recall young adulthood experiences without difficulty. Momentary lapses in memory such as forgetting a name or misplacing an item are common examples of normal memory changes. People who have more persistent memory problems with otherwise normal cognitive function are said to have mild cognitive impairment (MCI). Forty percent of people who develop MCI will develop Alzheimer's disease within 3 years; others do not progress to more serious impairment.

Various strategies may be used to cope with memory problems. Using mnemonics (stringing together known and unknown information) and rehearsal memory training (repetition) may improve memory performance for some older adults experiencing memory deficits. Further, some research indicates that long-term memory is not affected by chronic cerebral tissue hypoxia but may be attributed to permanent changes in the structure of the neuron. If this is the case, then efforts to improve memory would most likely be managed with medications to prevent permanent neuron changes.

Other neurologic functions that are affected by age-related changes include temperature regulation, pain perception, and tactile sensation. The aged individual usually has a low tolerance for extremes in temperature, which may be related to deterioration in the vascular tone as well as changes in hypothalamic temperature control. Some researchers have found dulling of pain and tactile sensation in older persons, but these results are not consistent. Many diseases and medications might alter sensory perception.

The neurologic changes associated with aging occur gradually; thus the aged person compensates for these changes by modifying behavior. For example, the person may avoid temperature extremes and accomplish tasks at a slower pace. However, stressors such as an illness or an environmental change may overwhelm the person's ability to compensate and may contribute to confusion or disorientation.

RESPIRATORY SYSTEM

Tests of pulmonary physiology have shown a number of age-related alterations. Forced vital capacity, vital capacity, and maximum breathing capacity are thought to decrease progressively with aging. These alterations are related to atrophy and weakening of the respiratory muscles and to an increase in the anteroposterior diameter of the chest as a result of kyphosis, vertebral loss of calcium, and calcification of costal cartilage.

In addition, with aging there is a loss of elastic tissue surrounding alveoli and alterations in pulmonary circulation that result in decreased diffusion across the alveolar-capillary membrane. This physiologic alteration is reflected in arterial oxygen values that decrease progressively throughout aging to approximately 70 to 80 mm Hg by the age of 70.

Pulmonary blood flow in the aged person decreases because of a reduction in cardiac output. Alterations in the pulmonary system associated with aging include a decreased number of capillaries, thickened capillary walls, and fewer capillaries surrounding the alveoli. The changes in the capillaries affect pulmonary diffusion so that gas exchange is impaired. With increasing age, alveolar dead space also occurs.

Despite the physiologic changes associated with aging, the ability of the older adult to maintain adequate oxygenation is not seriously impaired under conditions of health and moderate activity. Problems arise when increased demands are placed on the body as occurs during periods of extreme exertion or respiratory illness. Exertional dyspnea (shortness of breath with exertion) is a frequent complaint with the older adult. The ability to perform prolonged strenuous work decreases with aging.

Lung disease, acute or chronic, poses a threat to the older adult, and pulmonary secretions are handled less effectively. Ciliary action, responsible for the movement of secretions, is compromised because of epithelial atrophy. The cough reflex is frequently diminished as a consequence of altered sensitivity to stimuli and decreased muscle tone. These factors, in concert with impaired gas exchange, are responsible for the devastating effects of respiratory problems in old age.

You are considered to be a patient advocate and should be concerned about environmental pollution and hazards associated with smoking. Assess baseline resting and exertional respiratory rates and pulmonary function test results, as appropriate. Deep-breathing exercises and positioning to facilitate lung expansion and gas exchange are standard components of respiratory care for older adults.

CARDIOVASCULAR SYSTEM

Resistance to blood flow in many organs increases as people age. In the absence of cardiovascular disease, heart size remains unchanged or slightly decreased as a result of shrinkage or loss of myocardial fibrils. Aging results in the development of whitish patches, fibrosis, and sclerosis in the endocardium—the tissue layer that lines the inside of the heart chambers. The heart becomes more rigid, and myocardial contractility is compromised. Coronary blood flow in the aged person may be reduced by as much as 35% because of changes in the vessels. With advancing age, valvular rigidity and incomplete closure of the aortic and pulmonic valves may result in murmurs. Aging heart cells have a decreased capacity to utilize oxygen, which may help explain the aged person's reduced tolerance for physical work.

The blood vessels of the heart and the systemic circulation, particularly the arteries, undergo age-related changes that may begin as early as the teen years. Thickening and calcification of the intimal layer are evident in the coronary arteries and aorta, usually by age 20. Arterial dilation, vessel lengthening, and rigidity are in part due to changes in the structure of collagen. With aging, the pulse tends to increase in force and the pulse pressure widens. By 70 years of age, the systolic blood pressure increases to approximately 150 mm Hg and the diastolic blood pressure to 90 mm Hg for many people. These changes are due in part to decreased baroreceptor reflexes and inelasticity of the vessel walls. Because of the newest guidelines for diagnosis of hypertension, older persons are more likely to be treated for a blood pressure reading that once was considered normal.

Another cardiovascular change related to aging is a decrease in resting cardiac output, which is the amount of blood pumped by the heart each minute. Between ages 25 and 65, resting cardiac output falls 30% to 40%. This reduced cardiac output reflects a decreased heart rate and a decreased stroke volume. Despite the diminished cardiac output, cerebral blood flow is maintained. However, other body systems, such as the liver and kidneys, receive a diminished blood supply. Even with diminished blood supply, the organs maintain adequate function, partly because of reduced functional requirements.

RENAL SYSTEM

The renal system of healthy older adults is functionally adequate; however, in the event of injury, disease, or disability, the additional demands may adversely affect the aging renal system. The aging kidneys are characterized by a decrease in renal function, a decrease in cell mass, and an increase in extracellular fluid. By the seventh decade, the number of nephrons in each kidney is reduced by one half to two thirds, with corresponding changes in the glomeruli. Aging is accompanied by decreases in filtration rate, plasma flow rate, and tubular reabsorption and secretion. Blood urea nitrogen tends to increase. The renal system helps regulate acid-base balance. However, the tubules of the aging kidneys are less able to conserve base and eliminate excess hydrogen ions.

With advancing age, the ability to concentrate or dilute urine is diminished. This is believed to be related to a decreased secretion of antidiuretic hormone by the pituitary or an over-responsiveness of the kidneys to this hormone. Additional changes brought on by aging are noted in the ureters, bladder, and urethra as a result of deterioration in muscle tone. The bladder capacity may be reduced by half, resulting in frequent trips to the bathroom. Further, response to the stretch receptors in the bladder wall that signal the need to void may be delayed until the pressure is high and the bladder almost filled to capacity. This condition results in an urgency to urinate, which may be problematic for older adults with visual and motor limitations. Urge incontinence is a major health concern for older adults. Lax muscle tone may lead to incomplete emptying of the bladder. This residual volume may put the older person at risk for subsequent urinary tract infections. Other types of incontinence may appear as a symptom of upper or lower urinary tract dysfunction. For several of these conditions, conservative behavioral treatment is recommended as the first level of intervention. Behavioral treatments may include scheduled or prompted voiding, environmental adaptation, and pelvic muscle exercises (Kegel exercises). Interventions for incontinence are discussed in Chapter 23.

INTEGUMENTARY SYSTEM

Skin changes caused by aging can be the most distressing to the older person because they are so visible and readily apparent. They serve as a constant reminder that youth is fleeting. Changes related to aging of the skin include dryness, loss of elasticity, wrinkles, uneven pigmentation and brown spots, roughness, looseness, thinness, and the development of various skin lesions.

One of the first signs of aging is the development of wrinkles. Wrinkles occur when the deep layer of the skin loses moisture and elasticity. Tiny creases and folds are formed. The extent and timing of these wrinkles are determined by genetics and sun exposure. Persons in certain ethnic groups with thicker, oilier skin wrinkle at a slower rate and tend to maintain a youthful, wrinkle-free appearance longer. The same is true of older men because of their thicker and oilier skin.

Skin that is exposed to the sun most often, such as the face, hands, and back of the neck, wrinkles quickly. Older people are encouraged to use sunscreens (SPF 15) to prevent excessive dryness and to prevent skin cancer, which is common in women over the age of 50.

Itching related to loss of oils in the skin is a common complaint of older persons. Nurses might suggest to older persons that they take tepid baths, use moisturizers liberally, and avoid overuse of antiperspirants, soaps, perfumes, and hot baths. Furthermore, generalized itching should be reported to the health care provider because it may be a sign of illness such as diabetes, cancer, kidney disease, or liver disease.

Most older people can expect some hair loss, hair thinning, and color changes in the hair and nails. Men tend to grow bald, and women experience thinning of the hair on the head and genitalia. The number of facial and nasal hairs may increase. Gray hair is caused by a slowing of the pigment production in the hair follicles. Graying is determined by genetics and tends to be irreversible. Nails tend to become yellow and thicker. Routine visits to a podiatrist are encouraged for nail trimming and care of corns and calluses.

The most common benign lesions of aging are seborrheic dermatitis, acne, contact dermatitis, drug reactions, pressure ulcers, stasis ulcers, pruritus, herpes zoster, onychomycosis and tinea pedis, and impetigo. Routine skin assessments should be part of the comprehensive nursing assessment for older adults.

GASTROINTESTINAL SYSTEM

Changes in gastrointestinal functions occur with normal aging. Changes in the oral cavity include deterioration in the teeth and a decrease in the functional taste buds. The commonly observed decrease in the secretion of saliva is probably related to medications, inadequate hydration, and illness states rather than being a normal aging change. Saliva tends to become more alkaline as the salivary glands secrete less ptyalin and amylase. The muscles associated with chewing weaken, peristalsis is slower, and the risk of formation of intestinal diverticula increases. These changes tend to interfere with an older person's ability and desire to eat a nutritious meal.

Gastric emptying is slower in older people than in the young. The gastric glands decrease the volume and concentration of hydrochloric acid, intrinsic factor, and pepsin. With advanced age, the amount of calcium absorbed is reduced. Further, some reports indicate that bile tends to be thicker and that the gallbladder empties more slowly.

Collectively, the changes in the gastrointestinal system caused by aging increase the older person's risk for anorexia, bloating, indigestion, gas, pernicious anemia, and diarrhea or constipation. Constipation is one of the most frequent gastrointestinal complaints of older adults. Constipation may result from decreased intestinal motility, altered bacteria flora, a diet low in bulk and roughage, medications, and lack of physical activity. Many experts believe it is not inevitable in older persons and likely is a result of lifestyle and medications rather than a normal age-related change.

Because digestive complaints can be signs of more serious disorders, nurses must assess them completely. Symptoms that may suggest possible illness are decreased appetite, unexplained weight loss, excessive thirst, blood in the stool, or a change in the usual pattern of bowel movements.

You can assist older adults to maintain gastrointestinal function by sharing information about the normal ranges for bowel activity. The usual frequency for a bowel movement may range from as many as three movements per day to as few as one bowel movement every 7 days. Educate older adults about diet, activity, increased fluid intake, and avoidance of laxative abuse.

MUSCULOSKELETAL SYSTEM

Of the multiple changes associated with an aging musculoskeletal system, changes related to mobility are most significant. Many people begin to feel old when they wake up with stiff joints. Other age-related changes include decreases in muscle strength, endurance, range of motion of joints, coordination, bone density, and elasticity and flexibility of connective tissue.

Arthritis is the most prevalent chronic disease in men. However, it is more severe in women and is the leading cause of disability in old age. Osteoarthritis, the most common form of arthritis, is caused by damage to the inside surface of the joint. Age is the primary risk factor for arthritis, with heredity and obesity contributing to its development. The large weight-bearing joints (knees, hips, spine) are most affected. Kyphosis is the term applied to the curvature of the thoracic spine and gives rise to the bent-over appearance of some older adults.

Assess and document range of motion in all joints, signs of inflammation, and complaints of pain associated with mobility. Assess muscle strength bilaterally, and note the typical amount, type, and frequency of exercise. In addition, note a history of falls and whether the person takes hormonal replacement therapy and/or calcium supplementation.

Teach older adults about the benefits of weight-bearing exercises. Instruct them in the benefits of walking, bicycling, and stair climbing to help maintain bone and muscle mass (Fig. 11-1). If necessary, they should use assistive devices for walking and preventing falls. They should avoid too much bed rest because of the detrimental effects of immobility.

SENSORY SYSTEM

Because we depend on our five senses for almost everything we do, any loss of sensory ability can greatly affect our quality of life and general well-being. Sensory changes in the older adult also place them at risk for injury and weaken self-confidence.

Presbycusis is the term for hearing loss associated with old age. Twenty-five percent of older adults over age 69 and as many as half of adults over age 85 are hard of hearing. Older men tend to experience greater hearing loss than women. Many older adults are less able to hear high-pitched sounds and consonants, particularly *ch, f, g, s, sh, t, th,* and *z.* Not all older adults experience this type of loss, and causes other than old age may be involved.

There are basically two types of hearing loss. Conduction deafness is a blockage of the ear canal caused by excessive wax buildup, abnormal structures, or infection. This type of loss may be easily treated. The other type of hearing loss is sensorineural deafness. It results from damage to nerve tissue as a result of exposure to loud noises, disease, and certain drugs. Hearing aids often can provide significant improvement.

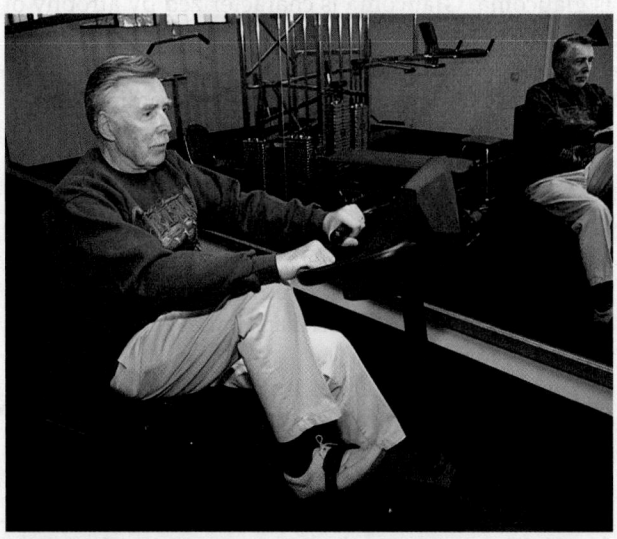

FIGURE **11-1** Regular exercise is an important part of health promotion for the older adult.

Tinnitus, an annoying ringing or buzzing in the ear, is a sensorineural disorder. Some cases of tinnitus can be caused by the use of aspirin, certain antibiotics, or diuretics or by tumors.

Failing eyesight is not an inevitable consequence of age, but several eye diseases are associated with aging. The leading cause of new cases of blindness in older people is age-related macular degeneration, a disease that affects the macula, the part of the eye that is responsible for sharp central vision. Laser surgery may be effective in preventing or delaying visual loss, and older adults should be informed of this as a treatment option.

Another serious eye disorder that occurs with aging is cataract. Cataract is clouding or opacity of the normally transparent lens within the eye. Cataracts are caused by changes in structural lens proteins, by damage to the lens as a result of high levels of blood glucose in people with diabetes, or by other factors.

Cataract is treated by surgical removal of the clouded lens. Surgery is highly successful, and vision is usually restored in 90% to 95% of the cases. An artificial lens usually is placed in the eye after cataract removal. Eyeglasses may be prescribed after surgery to further improve vision.

A less serious age-related vision change is a condition called presbyopia. Presbyopia affects the shape of the lens. The shape of the lens is controlled by muscles in the eye. By changing its shape, the lens allows us to change focus when looking from objects that are near to objects that are far. With age, the lens becomes more rigid and less able to change shape. Consequently, reading and other types of close work become difficult. Presbyopia is easily corrected by reading glasses or bifocal lenses. Further, adapting to changes in lighting is also a function of the lenses. Maintaining bright lighting in the home, particularly in hallways and around walkways, can help prevent falls and other accidents.

The leading cause of blindness in the United States is glaucoma. Glaucoma is characterized by atrophy of the optic nerve usually associated with elevated pressure of the fluid in the eye. Because the optic nerve carries visual impulses from the eye to the brain, damage to it can result in vision loss, which is characterized by progressive "tunnel vision."

At present, glaucoma is not curable but is treatable with drugs or surgery. If glaucoma is detected early and treated effectively, the disease process can be halted or slowed and the remaining eyesight saved. Older adults should receive annual eye examinations and a test for glaucoma.

Disorders of the senses involving taste and smell are called *chemosensory disorders*. More than 10 million Americans are affected by this type of disorder. Most of these disorders occur after age 60 and involve the ability to differentiate scents. Men tend to be more affected than women, and many causes exist. Causes include nasal obstruction, allergies, and the use of certain drugs. Some scientists believe that the decline in smell is due to a decrease in olfactory nerve fibers.

A gradual loss in the number of taste buds begins around 50 to 60 years of age. In spite of this progressive loss, there is little perceptible change in taste sensitivity that can be attributed to increased age alone. Major changes in the ability to taste usually are caused by diseases or the side effects of certain drugs. Dentures, hormonal changes, medications, and changes in chemicals needed to transmit taste are all potential causes of the older person's diminished sense of taste. This loss can affect changes in appetite.

Sensory losses are more than a minor nuisance for older adults. Poor vision and hearing increase a person's risk for falls and other accidents, which are leading causes of death and disability in people over the age of 65. Further, the inability to smell smoke, poisons, or other noxious odors endangers the lives of many older people. Decreased ability to taste food puts the older person at risk for malnutrition and food poisoning. Sensory changes greatly reduce the quality of life. The nurse must assist older adults to control, correct, or compensate for sensory losses. Assessment is, of course, the first step.

To summarize, the physiologic changes associated with aging may reflect more the presence of age-related diseases than aging itself. The interrelationship between the process of normal aging and the effects of age-related disease has not yet been defined universally. Nurse scientists are actively engaged in this process as well as in other scientific endeavors to better understand and provide care to the growing numbers of older adults. Research is rapidly expanding and changing our knowledge of aging. Conditions once thought to be the consequence of normal aging are now known to be the product of disease. Many of the conditions can be prevented or controlled by good health practices and competent nursing care.

PSYCHOSOCIAL FACTORS ASSOCIATED WITH AGING

Psychosocial as well as biologic changes associated with aging should be considered. Older adults show cumulative developmental effects that produce unique personality styles, coping mechanisms, challenges, and growth. Family, friends, and the community are influential in the aging process and can support the individual in adapting to age-related changes (Fig. 11-2).

The fact that a person has survived to old age is one marker of successful adaptation. The survival of large numbers of relatively healthy older people is a new experience for humankind. The vast majority of older people have adapted adequately. These individuals are able to function independently and maintain a sense of well-being. Only about 15% of the aged are unable to function independently and fail to maintain or sustain a sense of well-being.

FIGURE **11-2** Most older adults are active and independent.

Effective adaptation requires the individual to meet environmental and functional needs and to attain some sense of well-being. The achievement of each developmental task of aging requires successful coping and adaptation to changes in the environment. Remember, environment refers to both internal and external realms.

Maturity is defined as an optimal psychological, social, and biologic adaptation achieved at some point during the midlife years, arbitrarily set between 45 and 65 years of age. The years preceding the attainment of maturity are characterized as ascending and accelerating. The years thereafter are regarded as descending and decelerating. It is thought that midlife crisis occurs, in part, when the individual in midlife becomes fully aware of his or her mortality.

Erik Erikson developed one of the first developmental theories in the area of aging. He viewed the entire process of human development as a series of stages a person goes through to develop the ego fully. Erikson described eight stages of ego development from infancy to old age. Each of his stages represents a choice of crises in the ego. A complete discussion of adult developmental tasks is found in Chapter 10.

The final developmental task identified by Erikson is ego-integrity versus despair, which is the one typically associated with old age (late 60s or early 70s and older). The developmental challenge is to review life and gain a feeling of accomplishment and fulfillment. Older adults are expected to be concerned with life in the face of death and to begin to experience the wisdom that they have gained. The opposite of ego-integrity is feelings of despair, in which people feel bitter about their lack of accomplishments in life and tend to regret life as they

have lived it. Many people say that they have more regrets about the things they have not done or the risks they have not taken than the mistakes they have made.

Old age involves much more than a psychological waiting station before death. It represents an important stage of development and coping that occurs between the high points and accomplishments of the midyears and the concerns that are involved as the end of life approaches. Movement toward ego integrity is facilitated when the older person:

- Recognizes and accepts changes in physical and mental capabilities
- Gives up some roles and develops new ones
- Develops new activities that can be carried out successfully with aging
- Develops a different self-concept
- Revises life goals
- Adapts to new lifestyles

In the final stage of development, older persons are faced with a variety of internal and external losses that require coping and adaptation using diminished biologic, psychological, and social resources. The challenge is to maintain performance in the face of adverse circumstances.

COPING AND ADAPTATION

Old age has been described as the season of losses, including loss of roles, statuses, physical abilities, and deep personal losses through the deaths of friends and the disruption of family networks. Loss, whether real, threatened, or imaginary, is a stressor that requires adaptation, flexibility, and resiliency if a person is to cope successfully.

In most respects, older people cope in much the same way as younger people. Differences are largely the result of the different types of stressors experienced. Older people tend to experience more negative and irreversible types of stressors. Given the many losses associated with old age as potential stressors, the older person may cope with these losses with positive or negative adaptation. Positive adaptation might include rational action, perseverance, positive thinking (e.g., the lost loved one is now out of pain), intellectual denial (e.g., "I don't want to think about it now"), restraint, drawing strength from adversity, and humor.

Unfortunately, some older individuals are unable to cope effectively with their losses. Some older people respond to losses by losing their sense of personal identity and fulfillment and suffer from deterioration in self-esteem, an altered self-concept, and a loss of meaningfulness in life. Many older people become seriously depressed and experience additional losses. Many lose motivation for working, playing, and living. Depression resulting from loss is associated with approximately two thirds of the suicides among older people.

FAMILY

With an aging population that needs support and assistance in positive coping and adaptation, kinship networks take on added importance. Most of the older persons in the United States occupy a variety of family roles and come from multigenerational units. It is not uncommon for a person at age 65 to be married, have at least one living adult child, have at least one living brother or sister, be a grandparent, and also be a great-grandparent. The person over age 65 may also be a child of a much older parent. The kinship network may also include cousins, nieces, and nephews. Of all these roles and relationships, marital relations and the relationships between parent and child seem to be most important.

In an era when the old are sometimes referred to as burdens, it is important to recognize that more financial support flows from the old to the young in the family than in the reverse direction. Although family responsibility appears to be an internalized value for most people, it is important to know that more than half of the states have legal statutes that can require children to provide financial support for needy parents. However, what is most needed and most often given is emotional support and help in times of illness and disability. Home health care for the frail older adult is most often given by a spouse or a child. Typically, the caregiver is a daughter. Three out of four caregivers are women, and almost half of these are raising children of their own simultaneously.

The combination of personal limitations, competing roles, and stresses generated by the care recipient's behavior and the physical demands created by various levels of emotional, physical, financial, and family strain places enormous stress on informal caregivers. Caregivers frequently report symptoms of depression, anxiety, helplessness, low morale, and emotional exhaustion. Try to be aware of the stressful impact of caregiving and implement actions to minimize the stresses and burdens on both the caregiver and the care recipient.

In part because of caregiver stress, more than 1 million older persons are abused physically and psychologically or are neglected each year by their caregivers. You are in an excellent position to assess stress, depression, and abuse among caregivers and care recipients and to recommend interventions to alter these conditions. Education for learning and positive adaptive behaviors can assist both caregivers and care recipients. Caregivers who feel knowledgeable, useful, and productive are usually happier, less stressed, and less prone to be abusive. Families must be part of the holistic approach in the assessment and care of the aged.

FUNCTIONAL ASSESSMENT

Assessment has become a key word in gerontology and geriatrics because of its importance in care planning and care delivery. Functional assessment includes acquiring information about activities of daily living as well as environmental, financial, family, economic, and community resources. Functional assessment data are useful during times of health, at the onset of illness, at the beginning of treatment, and following therapeutic interventions. Comparisons across these time points help you plot an individual's functions, which can serve to increase understanding of the older person's problems and the effects of interventions.

Functional assessment is more than a diagnosis. A diagnosis alone cannot tell you how sick an older person is or how much care is needed. For example, a medical diagnosis of coronary artery disease does not tell you whether the older person is independent and the disease is controlled appropriately with medication or is totally dependent on care and currently needing intensive coronary care. For effective gerontological care, functional assessment is the crucial denominator in deciding care needs.

Functional status is more than a measure of activities of daily living. Knowing what activities an individual performs alone, what activities require assistance, and what activities the person is totally unable to perform or to perform safely is essential to define care needs. This information plus a diagnosis helps you to know the cause of self-care problems and whether the problems are amenable to therapeutic intervention.

The older person's database should describe both basic and instrumental activities of daily living. The following areas are generally considered in an assessment of activities of daily living: grooming, bathing, dressing, eating, elimination, and mobility. Instrumental activities of daily living are less important in institutional settings but are essential for a person to continue or to return to independent living. Instrumental activities of daily living generally consider the older adult's ability to prepare a meal, shop for groceries, use the telephone, negotiate transportation, take medications, and maintain housekeeping and laundry tasks.

The Duke Older Americans Research and Services (OARS) Multidimensional Functional Assessment Questionnaire (MFAQ) is one example of a valid and reliable assessment guide for gathering information on the overall personal functional status and service use of adults. The OARS questionnaire has been used mainly with older adults and has two parts. The first part provides for assessment of the older adult in terms of social, economic, mental, and physical health and ability to perform activities of daily living. The second part provides for assessment of the older adult based on the need for 24 rather universal services. A content

Put on Your Thinking Cap!

Discuss the importance of functional assessments of older adults who receive home health care.

Box 11-2 *Content Areas of the OARS Multidimensional Functional Assessment Questionnaire*

Part A: Functional Assessment

Social
Contact with others
Help from family and kin

Economic
Amount of income and adequacy
Home ownership

Mental
Mental and psychiatric status
Mental well-being

Physical
Prescribed medications used
Physical conditions with impairment levels

Activities of Daily Living
Physical and instrumental activities of daily living

Demographics and Administrative
Age, gender, race
Location, length of interview
Information source

Part B: Services

Transportation
Social or recreational
Employment
Sheltered employment
Education
Remedial training
Mental health
Psychotropic drugs
Personal care
Medical care
Supportive devices
Physical therapy
Continuous supervision
Checking
Homemaker
Meal preparation
Legal and protective
Systematic evaluation
Financial
Food, groceries
Housing
Coordination
Information
Referral

Adapted from Older Americans Research and Services. (1978). *Multidimensional functional assessment questionnaire.* Durham, NC: Center for the Study of Aging and Human Development, Duke University Medical Center.

summary is provided in Box 11-2. In most instances, the nursing home Minimum Data Set incorporates all components of a quality functional assessment. This comprehensive assessment tool is valid and reliable and currently used in research.

 Put on Your Thinking Cap!

What functions would an older adult need to manage self-care in the home?

DRUG THERAPY AND AGED ADULTS

ABSORPTION, DISTRIBUTION, METABOLISM, AND EXCRETION

Eighty-eight percent of older persons in the United States who reside in the community use one or more medications. In long-term care facilities, more than 75% receive 4 or more medications and 33% receive 7 to 10 medications. Imagine the potential for errors and drug interactions with so many medications! Age-related changes affect patterns of drug use, consumption of drugs, and actions of medications on target organs (Table 11-2). The most important changes involve body composition, the cardiovascular system, the central nervous system, renal function, tissue sensitivity to drugs, and blood pressure reflex sensitivity. Age-related and disease-related changes in the older

Table 11-2 *Association Between Age-Related Physiologic Changes and Drug Effects*

AGE-RELATED CHANGES	DRUG EFFECTS
Increased body fat	Increased drug storage
Decreased body water	Increased drug/active concentration
Decreased hepatic blood flow	Decreased drug clearance
Decreased lean muscle mass	Increased drug tissue concentration
Decreased renal function	Decreased drug elimination
Decreased serum albumin	Increased free drug concentration

person slow the clearance of drugs, which increases the risk of adverse effects.

With aging there is a reduction in body size, with a decrease in lean body mass and body water content (extracellular volume) and an increase in fat. The serum albumin concentration is lower, which tends to make more free drug available to tissues or to permit more rapid elimination of the drug. A gradual decrease in blood flow to the internal organs in the abdomen reduces drug clearance through the liver or kidney. For example, a water-soluble drug may result in higher blood concentrations of that drug. However, a highly fat-soluble drug might bind to the increased fat in the aged body and may be stored longer before excretion. To illustrate, a 75-year-old woman was misdiagnosed as having progressive brain damage after she developed urinary incontinence, general mental deterioration, and inability to walk. She had taken 5 mg of diazepam (Valium) daily for at least 1 year. Diazepam is a fat-soluble drug that has the potential for increased distribution in tissues and for delayed elimination. After the drug was discontinued, the patient recovered in 3 days.

The liver prepares drugs for elimination in the urine or in feces. Age-related changes that have an impact on the inactivation of drugs by the liver include decreased liver size, reduced hepatic blood flow, and reduced liver enzyme activity on drugs. These changes have the overall effect of increasing drug concentrations in the blood and possibly increasing the amount of time it takes the body to get rid of the drug. Drugs that are eliminated principally in the urine may be given to older persons in reduced doses or less frequently to avoid accumulation and adverse effects.

Older persons tend to respond more vigorously to drugs that act on the central nervous system because of a greater tissue sensitivity and altered physiologic changes, as described earlier. Some of the potential adverse effects are postural imbalance, staggering, uncoordinated movements, respiratory depression, and changes in mental alertness. Drugs such as opiates, diazepam, and nifedipine may cause these effects.

ADVERSE DRUG REACTIONS

Adverse drug reactions are more common in older people partly because they use more drugs, as previously cited. The risk factors for adverse drug reactions are age, sex, race (occurring most frequently in older white females), number of drugs consumed, dosage, duration of treatment, severity of illness, and patient cooperation. Some of the common symptoms and signs of adverse drug reactions in the older person are restlessness, falls, depression, confusion, loss of memory, constipation, and urinary incontinence. Some drugs associated with adverse drug reactions

are listed in Table 11-3. When multiple drugs are prescribed and patients experience unpleasant side effects, they may not follow the prescribed regimen. The use of fewer drugs at lower doses usually increases patient adherence.

Because older adults experience a greater number of drug reactions and interactions than younger people and are believed to be more sensitive to some medications, nurses must monitor their drug regimens carefully. It is helpful to assist the patient in maintaining a record of blood pressure, pulse, respiration, drug effect, and state of alertness in relation to current drug therapy. Such a record could be helpful in making necessary changes. It may be necessary to change a drug, reduce the dosage, or lengthen the intervals between doses to minimize the risk of adverse drug reactions. You are very often in the best position to minimize drug reactions. Baseline and continual assessments should include the following:

- The amount, frequency, and purpose of all medications taken
- The older person's ability and willingness to take recommended medications
- The potential for drug interactions and adverse drug reactions
- The effectiveness of the medication over time
- Whether any of the drugs taken can be discontinued or decreased in dose

Assessment of drug effects and adverse reactions must be documented.

This presentation of adverse drug reactions would not be complete without mentioning the hazards associated with potential drug interactions between over-the-counter medications and prescription medications taken by older adults. Examples might include the use of aspirin, which enhances the effect of an anticoagulant, or the use of large amounts of sodium bicarbonate, which counteracts diuretic actions. Further concern is raised in relation to the possibility of older adults mixing older prescription medications with newer ones and failing to discontinue and discard older prescriptions. Hoarding of medications may be viewed as fu-

Table 11-3 *Drugs Commonly Associated with Adverse Drug Reactions in Older Persons*

DRUG CLASS	EXAMPLE	PROBLEM
Analgesics	Aspirin	Bleeding
Antibiotics	Streptomycin	Nephrotoxicity
Anticoagulants	Warfarin	Hemorrhage
Antidepressants	Amitriptyline	Sedation
Antihypertensives	Verapamil	Hypotension
Antiparkinsonians	Levodopa	Extrapyramidal symptoms, dystonia
Antipsychotics	Haloperidol	Confusion
Diuretics	Diuril	Hypokalemia
Sedatives/hypnotics	Flurazepam	Drowsiness

ture savings by an older adult. Nevertheless, you must learn to recognize the inherent dangers in this situation and teach older adults to review all medications, prescription and over-the-counter, with their primary nurse or other health care providers.

One of the greatest challenges for those working within health care is addressing the physiologic, psychosocial, behavioral, and mental well-being of older adults. Management and care of an aging population affect every sector of the nursing profession. Nurses at all levels of preparation are encouraged to meet this mandate with care, concern, and competence.

Put on Your Thinking Cap!

Recall an older adult who has been discharged from the hospital with some impairments. What instrumental activities of daily living are likely to be affected in that person?

Key Points

- Aging is an ongoing developmental process that begins at conception and ends at death.
- Gerontology is the study of aging.
- Geriatrics is the biomedical science of old age and the application of knowledge related to the biologic, biomedical, behavioral, and social aspects of aging to the prevention, diagnosis, treatment, and care of older persons.
- Gerontological nursing aims to increase healthy behaviors in the aged, minimize and compensate for health-related losses and impairments of aging, provide comfort and sustenance through the events of aging, and facilitate the diagnosis, care, and treatment of disease in the aged.
- Health care providers must recognize myths about the older adult and aging that result in stereotyping and discrimination against older people.
- Aging occurs slowly and is a complex and dynamic process involving many internal and external influences.
- Physiologic changes that are associated with aging may reflect more the presence of age-related diseases than the process of aging itself.
- The older adult shows cumulative developmental effects that produce unique personality styles, coping mechanisms, challenges, and growth, all of which occur in a societal context.
- Age-related changes that contribute to a decreased ability to clear drugs through the liver and renal system place the older adult at risk for adverse drug effects.

 Go to your Companion CD-ROM for a Pharmacology Tutorial, Audio Glossary, and 3-D animations.

evolve   Be sure to visit the companion Evolve site at http://evolve.elsevier.com/Linton/ for WebLinks and additional online resources.

REVIEW QUESTIONS *Choose the best answer.*

1. Which of the following statements about aging is correct?
   1. Many older people continue to enjoy sexual activity.
   2. Older people generally lack family and other support networks.
   3. Almost 50% of people over age 65 have dementia.
   4. 25% of the older population reside in nursing homes.

2. Neurologic changes commonly found in the healthy older adult include the following:
   1. Impaired short-term memory
   2. Inability to learn new material
   3. Decline in intellectual capability
   4. Loss of creative abilities

3. Mr. J. had been a healthy 90-year-old man until he developed pneumonia. While acutely ill with the pneumonia, he showed signs of early heart and renal failure. He became weak, and his tolerance for physical activity declined. Even though the pneumonia resolved, it was several months before he returned to his previous level of functioning. How would you explain this?
   1. At age 90, immune function is severely impaired.
   2. He probably did not seek treatment for his pneumonia soon enough.
   3. Acute illness overwhelmed his already limited cardiac and renal function.
   4. He wanted to continue getting the attention he received when he was acutely ill.

4. When teaching a group of active older people about skin care, you would include the following:
   1. Older skin thickens, which makes sunscreens no longer necessary
   2. Hot baths or showers followed by vigorous towel drying remove dead skin
   3. Generous use of moisturizers and minimal use of soap prevent skin drying
   4. Generalized itching is common and is insignificant for older adults

5. You observe that an older patient's thoracic spine is curved, causing her to bend forward. This condition should be described as:
   1. Patient cannot stand up straight
   2. Patient has kyphosis
   3. Patient leans forward
   4. Patient's spine is crooked

6. A new patient admitted to your long-term care facility has presbycusis. What are the relevant nursing interventions?
   1. Be sure room lighting is adequate.
   2. Lower the pitch of your voice.
   3. Monitor her blood pressure.
   4. Implement body fluid precautions.

7. Which of these statements by older adults reflects movement toward ego integrity?
   1. "Since I cannot drive now, I rarely get out or see other people."
   2. "After my children grew up and my husband died, I just wasn't needed anymore."
   3. "In my day, when you got married, you stayed married, no matter how bad it was."
   4. "I can't run marathons anymore, but I still enjoy a brisk walk around the neighborhood."

8. The home health nurse assesses an older adult's ability to carry out instrumental activities of daily living. These include the following:
   1. Grooming
   2. Bathing
   3. Shopping
   4. Elimination

9. An older postoperative patient is receiving pain medications that depress the central nervous system. Based on your knowledge of drug therapy and aging, what adverse effect is most likely?
   1. Respiratory depression
   2. Difficulty sleeping
   3. Vomiting and diarrhea
   4. Agitation and confusion

10. A clinic patient reports that she bruises very easily. She cut herself this morning, and the wound continues to ooze blood. An assessment of her medication history reveals that she takes the diuretic Diuril and verapamil for hypertension, Maalox for heartburn, and aspirin for arthritis pain. Which drug would you suspect is related to her bleeding?
    1. Diuril
    2. Verapamil
    3. Maalox
    4. Aspirin

12 The Nursing Process and Critical Thinking

Objectives

After reading and studying this chapter, you should be able to:

1. Describe the components of the nursing process.
2. Explain the role of the LPN/LVN in the nursing process.
3. Describe the proper documentation of the nursing process.
4. Describe the relationship of the nursing process with the process of documentation.
5. Explain the relationship between the nursing process and critical thinking.
6. Describe the characteristics of a critical thinker.
7. Describe how critical thinking skills are used in clinical practice.
8. Describe principles of setting priorities for nursing care.

Key Terms

Be sure to check out the bonus material on the Companion CD-ROM, including selected audio pronunciations.

assessment (p. 143)
auscultation (ăw-skul-TĀ-shun, p. 146)
critical thinking (p. 157)
evaluation (p. 143)
implementation (p. 143)
inspection (p. 146)
nursing diagnosis (p. 148)
nursing process (p. 143)
objective data (p. 144)
palpation (p. 146)
percussion (p. 146)
problem-oriented medical record (POMR) (p. 155)
subjective data (p. 144)

The **nursing process** is a systematic method of providing care to patients. It is a problem-solving approach that enables the nurse to provide care in an organized, scientific manner. Specifically, the nurse uses the process to explore the patient's health status, identify actual or potential health care problems, determine the desired outcomes, deliver nursing care, and evaluate the care given. The goal of the nursing process is to prevent, alleviate, or minimize health problems. It enables the nurse to provide care in the areas of health maintenance and promotion, management of acute or chronic illness, and rehabilitation.

The nursing process can be applied in any interaction that involves a nurse and a patient or client. (As noted earlier, the terms *patient* and *client* are used interchangeably in this text.) The patient or client can be defined as an individual, a family, a group, a community, or a society. The process can take place in a variety of settings, including a hospital, community setting, private home, or long-term care facility.

COMPONENTS OF THE NURSING PROCESS

The five components or steps in the nursing process are: (1) assessment (the systematic collection of data relating to patients and their problems), (2) nursing diagnosis (interpretation of the data for problem identification), (3) planning (goals and selected interventions), (4) **implementation** (putting the plan into action), and (5) **evaluation** (assessing the achievement of goals and changing the plan as indicated by current needs). Initially, the steps are followed in sequence—first data collection and assessment, then identification of the problems or nursing diagnoses, followed by planning care, implementation of the plans, and evaluation. However, after the process has begun, it becomes continuous or cyclic. Each phase of the nursing process is dependent on the others, and there is a continuous interaction among the stages as information about the status of the patient changes. Evaluation and revision of the plan of care occur constantly. As problems are alleviated, new problems may arise, requiring new plans and actions. The Management and Supervision box on p. 144 describes the LPN's/LVN's role in relation to the nursing process.

ASSESSMENT

The **assessment** phase of the nursing process involves collecting data about the health status of the patient. A registered nurse must perform the initial admission assessment for each patient; the LPN/LVN collects data through surveillance and monitoring to contribute to the comprehensive assessment and performs focused nursing assessments. A focused nursing assessment is defined as "an appraisal of the client's status and situation at hand that contributes to ongoing data collection" (NCSBN, 2006).

Management and Supervision

The LPN and the Nursing Process

Licensed practical nurses commonly work in settings in which the nursing process is used. Standards of care for registered nurses and LPNs/LVNs define the responsibilities of each in relation to the nursing process (see Chapter 3).

Although the registered nurse has responsibility for developing the nursing process, the licensed practical nurse makes important contributions. Roles for LPNs/LVNs in relation to the nursing process include the following:

1. To contribute to an assessment database for patients by collecting data using a standardized form, performing basic psychosocial assessment, and taking objective measurements of body functions
2. To assist with the development of nursing care plans and the implementation of the established plan of care
3. To perform basic therapeutic and preventive nursing measures
4. To participate in the evaluation of the care given by reporting observed outcomes and making necessary changes according to the results of the evaluation.

The word *data* is the plural of *datum* and means information, especially information organized for analysis or decision making. There are two types of data—subjective and objective. Subjective data consist of information that is reported by the patient and family members in a health history in response to direct questioning or in spontaneous statements. Subjective data usually are documented in the patient's own words and include information such as previous experiences and sensations or emotions that only the patient can describe. Objective data are those that the nurse or other members of the health care team obtain through observation, physical examination, or diagnostic testing. Objective data can be seen or measured; for example, heart rate, wound condition, and laboratory values. Sources of subjective and objective data are the patient, the family and significant others, medical records, and other health care team members.

Subjective Data: The Health History Interview

The health history collects subjective data by interviewing the patient or family members or both. The manner in which the interview is conducted directly affects the accuracy and completeness of the information gained. Communication should be purposeful, orderly, and systematic. Open-ended questions will allow patients to express their thoughts and feelings. Allowing expression of feelings helps establish a better working relationship with patients and families.

To obtain the health history, arrange a quiet, private area to ensure comfort and confidentiality. Explain the purpose of the interview to the patient and family members with the assurance that they can refuse to answer any questions and can add any pertinent information that is helpful. Usually the interview takes no longer than 20 to 30 minutes. Older patients, who may have a complex health history, may require additional time. Also, older patients may tire more easily than younger patients, so that several short interviews may be necessary.

Various approaches to data collection may be used to ensure that the nursing database is as complete as possible. The traditional health history format includes the following data:

1. Biographical data
2. Reason for seeking care, commonly called the "chief complaint"
3. Present health or history of present illness
4. Medical history
5. Family history
6. Review of systems
7. Functional assessment of activities of daily living

Box 12-1 briefly describes each of these components. Another format uses a structured database based on 11 functional health problems developed by Mary Gordon. Other formats include the focused assessment, which is concerned with one very specific problem area such as pain, and the use of Maslow's hierarchy of needs.

When the interview is complete, review the data with the patient or family members to be sure the information gathered is correct. Summarizing the data demonstrates interest in the patient and the patient's needs and strengthens the nurse-patient relationship. As the level of trust increases, the patient may add information that was not included earlier. Subjective data usually are charted as "Patient states . . .". For example, when a patient reports pain, it could be documented: "The patient states 'I have a shooting pain in my left arm.'"

Objective Data

Objective data are obtained through physical examination, diagnostic tests, and patient records. Observation is one of the most important means of data collection. The senses of sight, hearing, smell, and touch are used to collect objective data. For example, a patient's disheveled appearance (sight) on admission may indicate an inability to carry out self-care activities at home. A patient's noisy and labored breathing (hearing) may suggest respiratory problems. A fruity mouth odor (smell) may be a sign of diabetic acidosis. Cold and clammy skin (touch) may signal that a patient is in shock. When recording observational data, write exactly what is observed. Avoid words such as good, bad, better, or worse. For example, "The skin is warm and dry" is preferable to "The skin looks good."

Physical Examination. Physical examination is a systematic way of obtaining comprehensive objective data. It is conducted by the registered nurse. However, some parts of this examination may be performed by the

Box 12-1 | *The Health History*

Biographical Data

Name, address, phone number, age, birth date, birthplace, sex, marital status, race, ethnic origin, occupation, educational level

Source of History

Who furnishes information (patient, family); estimate of reliability of information

Reason for Seeking Care

Chief complaint (put in patient's own words)

History of Present Illness

Events leading up to chief complaint or reason for seeking care:

- Location of symptoms (e.g., pain in the chest radiating to the left arm)
- Character or quality (e.g., burning, sharp, or dull pain; sticky, dark, or coffee grounds–colored emesis)
- Quantity or severity (severity of pain interrupts normal daily activities)
- Timing (onset, duration, frequency); when symptoms appeared; how long they lasted; how often they occurred
- Setting (what was happening when symptoms occurred; what brought it on)
- Aggravating or relieving factors (what makes symptoms worse; what makes them better)
- Associated factors (what other symptoms are related, e.g., urinary frequency and burning associated with fever or chills)
- Client's perception (meaning of symptoms to client; how they affect daily activities)

Past Health

Childhood illnesses
Accidents or injuries
Serious or chronic illnesses
Hospitalizations
Operations
Obstetric history
Immunizations
Last examination date
Allergies
Current medications

Family History

Age, health, and cause of death of blood relatives
Family history of heart disease, high blood pressure, stroke, diabetes, blood disorders, cancer, sickle cell anemia, arthritis, allergies, obesity, alcoholism, mental illness, seizure disorders, kidney disease, and tuberculosis

Review of Systems

Evaluate past and present health state of each body system:

- General overall health state (present weight, weight gain or loss, fatigue, weakness, fever, chills, night sweats)
- Skin (history of skin disease; change in color, pigment, or mole; excessive dryness or moisture; itching; excessive bruising; rash or lesion)
- Hair (recent loss, change in texture; change in shape, color, or brittleness of nails)
- Head (history of head injury, headache, dizziness, or vertigo)
- Eyes (difficulty with vision, including decreased acuity, blurring, blind spots; eye pain; double vision; redness or swelling; watering or discharge; glaucoma or cataracts)
- Ears (earaches, infections, discharge, tinnitus or ringing in the ears)
- Nose and sinuses (discharge, frequent or severe colds, sinus pain, nasal obstruction, nosebleeds, allergies or hay fever, change in sense of smell)
- Mouth and throat (mouth pain, frequent sore throat, bleeding gums, toothache, difficulty swallowing, hoarseness, altered taste)
- Neck (pain, limitation of movement, lumps or swelling, enlarged or tender nodes, goiter)
- Gastrointestinal (history of abdominal diseases, e.g., ulcer, liver or gallbladder, jaundice, appendicitis, colitis; appetite; food intolerance; difficulty swallowing; heartburn; indigestion; abdominal pain; nausea and vomiting; vomiting blood; flatulence; type and frequency of bowel movement; rectal conditions, e.g., hemorrhoids, fistula)
- Breast (pain, lump, nipple discharge, rash, history of breast disease or surgery)
- Axilla (tenderness, lump or swelling, rash)
- Musculoskeletal system (history of arthritis, gout, back pain or disk disease; pain, stiffness or swelling of joints; deformity; limitation of motion; noise with joint motion; muscle pain, cramps, or weakness; problems with gait or coordination; back pain, stiffness, or limitation of motion)
- Neurologic system (history of seizure disorder, stroke, fainting, or blackouts; weakness, tic, or tremor; paralysis or coordination problems; numbness or tingling; cognitive disorder; nervousness, mood changes, depression, or history of mental illness)
- Respiratory system (lung diseases, e.g., asthma, emphysema, bronchitis, pneumonia, tuberculosis; chest pain with breathing; wheezing or noisy breathing; shortness of breath; cough; sputum; hemoptysis or coughing up blood)
- Cardiovascular (chest pain, heart palpitation, cyanosis, dyspnea on exertion, orthopnea, nocturia, edema, heart murmur, hypertension, coronary artery disease, anemia)
- Peripheral vascular (coldness, numbness and tingling of extremities; swelling of legs; discoloration of hands or feet; varicose veins; intermittent claudication or pain in legs on exertion; thrombophlebitis; leg ulcers)
- Endocrine system (history of diabetes or diabetic symptoms, or thyroid disease; intolerance to heat and cold; change in skin pigmentation or texture; excessive sweating; relationship between appetite and weight; abnormal hair distribution; nervousness; tremors)

Continued

Box 12-1   *The Health History—cont'd*

Review of Systems—cont'd
- Urinary system (history of kidney disease, kidney stones, or urinary tract infections; frequency of urination; urgency; nocturia or number of times person awakens at night to urinate, painful or difficult urination; oliguria or polyuria; color of urine, e.g., cloudy, bloody, straw-colored; incontinence; pain in the flank, groin, supra-pubic region, or lower back)
- Male genital system (penile or testicular pain; penile discharge; sores or lesions; lumps; hernia)

- Female genital system (menstrual history, e.g., age at menarche, last menstrual period, cycle and duration, amenorrhea [absence of periods], or menometrorrhagia [bleeding between periods]; premenstrual pain or dysmenorrhea [menstrual pain]; vaginal itching; discharge and its characteristics; age at menopause; menopausal signs or symptoms; postmenopausal bleeding)

Functional Assessment
Self-care ability, including bathing, dressing, grooming, toileting, and transfer from bed to chair.

Adapted from Jarvis, C. (1999). Physical examination and health assessment, (3rd ed., pp. 79-84). Philadelphia: Saunders.

LPN/LVN. Sometimes a complete head-to-toe examination is conducted, whereas at other times only one or two systems may be examined, as warranted by the patient's symptoms. For example, when a patient is in acute respiratory distress, only the respiratory and cardiovascular systems might be examined initially. This is called a *focused assessment*. A complete examination would be delayed until the patient's breathing improves. Although some aspects of the physical examination require advanced training, an overview of the complete physical examination process is presented here.

There are four methods of examination: (1) inspection, (2) palpation, (3) percussion, and (4) auscultation.

Inspection. Inspection is purposeful observation of the person as a whole and then systematically from head to toe (Fig. 12-1). The observation begins as soon as you meet the patient and continues throughout the examination.

Palpation. Palpation uses the sense of touch to assess various parts of the body and helps confirm findings that are noted on inspection. The hands, especially the fingertips, are used to assess skin texture, moisture, and temperature, or the presence of swelling, lumps, masses, tenderness, or pain (Fig. 12-2). Warm your hands before palpating the patient. When examining

the abdomen, palpation should be light at first for surface characteristics and then deeper for abdominal contents. If any tender areas are noted, they should be palpated last. Deep palpation is usually done only by nurses with advanced skills.

Percussion. Percussion is tapping on the skin to assess the underlying tissues. The chest and abdomen are the most common areas for percussion. Short, sharp strokes elicit sounds and subtle vibrations that are characteristic of underlying organs and certain conditions. The sounds, called "notes," are described as *resonant* (heard over normal lung tissue), *hyperresonant* (heard over the lungs of a person with emphysema), *tympany* (heard over air-filled organs such as the stomach), *dull* (heard over a dense organ like the liver), and *flat* (heard over structures with no air such as bone or muscle). To percuss, place one hand flat on the skin over the area to be assessed. Use the tip of the middle finger of your other hand to lightly tap the middle finger of the hand that rests on the patient (Figs. 12-3 and 12-4). Tap two times just behind the nail bed before moving on to the next area.

Auscultation. Auscultation is listening to sounds produced by the body, such as heart, lung, and intestinal sounds. Auscultation is performed with a stetho-

FIGURE **12-1** Inspection.

FIGURE **12-2** Palpation.

FIGURE **12-3** The stationary hand in percussion.

FIGURE **12-4** The striking hand in percussion.

scope (Fig. 12-5). Some stethoscopes have a single end piece, whereas others have two: a bell and a diaphragm. The diaphragm is best for listening to high-pitched sounds such as the lung and bowel sounds and normal heart sounds. The bell is best for listening to low-pitched sounds such as heart murmurs. The earpieces should fit snugly and point forward to the nose. The room should be quiet so that an accurate assessment of sounds can be made. The diaphragm of the stethoscope is most frequently used for assessment. Warm the diaphragm by rubbing it against your palm, and then place it lightly over the area that is being assessed. If the area is hairy, you may hear a crackling sound, which could be misinterpreted as abnormal breath sounds. To minimize the problem, press the stethoscope more firmly against the chest or wet the hair with a damp cloth before examination.

The physical examination includes assessment of general appearance, height and weight, vital signs, and body systems. The LVN/LPN collects data for the RN, who finalizes the assessment. Box 12-2 presents an overview of the content of a complete physical examination.

Diagnostic Tests. Examples of common diagnostic tests are radiographic studies (x-rays), electrocardiograms (ECGs), magnetic resonance imaging (MRI) scans, computed tomography (CT) scans, positron emission tomography (PET) scans, ultrasound studies, laboratory blood and urine testing, and wound cultures. The information from these tests can be helpful in identifying general areas in which a patient might have a health care problem or in validating a nursing diagnosis. Relevant diagnostic tests are addressed with each body system throughout this text.

Patient Records. Patient records provide a valuable source of information regarding the medical history and illness patterns. They can confirm the subjective data and history that the patient and family provide.

When documenting data collected during the assessment phase, record exactly what was heard, seen,

FIGURE **12-5** Auscultation.

felt, or smelled. All documentation should be complete and factual because the data provide the foundation for making the nursing diagnoses and your documentation communicates your findings to other care providers. After the data are collected, the information must be organized into meaningful and usable clusters. Baseline data also are used to assess the patient's progress or lack of progress over time.

NURSING DIAGNOSIS

The nursing diagnosis is derived from data gathered during the assessment. A nursing diagnosis is different from a medical diagnosis. The medical diagnosis focuses on the etiology (cause) of the dysfunction of a specific organ or system. In contrast, the nursing diagnosis focuses on the patient's physical, psychological, and social responses to a health problem or potential health problem. Nursing diagnoses provide a basis for planning nursing interventions that can help prevent, minimize, or alleviate the problem. Although the RN formulates nursing diagnoses, the LPN/LVN is expected to assist with the identification of patient needs and the implementation of the plan of care after the nursing diagnoses are made.

The concept of nursing diagnosis has been discussed for many years. In 1973, the National Conference Group

---

Box 12-2 *The Physical Examination*

Physical Appearance
Age, sex, level of consciousness, skin color, facial features, no signs of acute distress

Body Structure
Stature, nutrition (normal weight for height and body build), symmetry, posture, body build (normal proportions), obvious physical deformities

Mobility
Gait, range of motion, no involuntary movement

Behavior
Facial expression, mood and affect, speech, dress, personal hygiene, hair, and makeup

Measurements
Height, weight, vital signs

Skin, Hair, and Nails
Skin (color, general pigmentation, widespread color change, temperature, moisture, texture, thickness, edema, mobility and turgor, hygiene, vascularity or bruising, lesions)
Hair (color, texture, distribution, scalp lesions)
Nails (shape and contour, consistency, color)

Head and Neck
Head (size and shape of skull, symmetry, expression of face)
Neck (symmetry, range of motion, lymph nodes)

Eyes
Central visual acuity, near and far vision, peripheral vision, extraocular muscle function (parallel alignment, nystagmus), external eye structures (eyebrows, eyelids and lashes, eyeballs, conjunctiva and sclera, lacrimal apparatus, cornea, lens, iris and pupils)

Ears
External ear (size and shape, skin condition, tenderness, the external auditory meatus), external canal, tympanic membrane, hearing acuity, vestibular apparatus

Nose, Mouth, and Throat
Nose (external nose, nasal cavity, sinus area)
Mouth (lips, teeth and gums, tongue, buccal mucosa, palate)
Throat (tonsils)

Breasts and Regional Lymphatics
General appearance, skin, lymphatic drainage areas, nipple, axilla

Thorax and Lungs
Posterior chest (symmetric expansion, fremitus [palpable vibration], lung fields, breath sounds)
Anterior chest (shape and configuration of chest wall, level of consciousness, skin color and condition, quality of respirations, symmetric chest expansion, forced expiratory time [number of seconds to exhale])

Heart and Neck Vessels
Carotid artery pulse, jugular venous pulse, jugular venous pressure, anterior chest inspection, cardiac rate and rhythm, heart sounds, murmurs

Abdomen
Inspection (contour, symmetry, umbilicus, skin, pulsation or movement, hair distribution)
Palpation (surface and deep areas, liver edge, spleen, kidneys)
Percussion (general tympany, liver span, splenic dullness)
Auscultation (bowel sounds, vascular sounds)

Peripheral Vascular System
Pulses, capillary refill, skin color and temperature, edema, pain

Musculoskeletal System
Joint (size, contour, swelling, warmth, range of motion, crepitus)
Muscles (tone, strength, size)

Neurologic System
Cranial nerves, motor system (muscles, cerebellar function), sensory system (pain, temperature, light touch, vibration, position), reflexes (stretch or deep tendon reflexes, superficial reflexes)

Female Genitalia
External genitalia (skin color, hair distribution, labia majora, labia minora, clitoris, urethral opening, vaginal opening, perineum)
Internal genitalia (cervix, vagina)

Anus, Rectum, and Prostate
Perianal area, anus, rectum, stool

on the Classification of Nursing Diagnosis began meeting to develop standardized nursing diagnoses to be used in all health care settings. The group, now known as the North American Nursing Diagnosis Association (NANDA), met to develop and revise nursing diagnoses. Table 12-1 shows a list of accepted nursing diagnoses. Nursing diagnoses are written in a format, called PES, developed by NANDA. *P* stands for the *problem*, *E* stands for the *etiology* or cause of the problem, and *S* stands for the *signs* and *symptoms* of the problem. Only actual problems require signs and symptoms; potential problems do not list them. The PES format helps make the general nursing diagnosis fit a specific patient care problem. The following example shows the application of the general nursing diagnosis "Impaired Skin Integrity" to a specific patient situation. For a female older adult who has developed a 2-cm pressure ulcer on her sacrum because she is bedridden and immobilized, the nursing diagnosis would be written in the following manner: Impaired Skin Integrity *(P)* related to immobility *(E)* as evidenced by 2-cm pressure ulcer on sacrum *(S)*. The problem *(P)* or nursing diagnosis is "Impaired Skin Integrity," the etiology *(E)* or cause is "immobility," and the signs or symptoms *(S)* are "2-cm pressure ulcer on sacrum."

Although NANDA is continually working to define new nursing diagnoses and to standardize nursing diagnoses, they still are not universally used and accepted. However, nurses must work together to de-velop the most appropriate diagnoses to reflect current nursing practice. Some references identify collaborative problems as well as nursing diagnoses. Collaborative problems require intervention by multiple members of the health care team. The format for nursing diagnoses in this book states only the problem and the etiology to avoid repetitious lists of signs and symptoms. In an actual patient care plan, you would include the patient's specific signs and symptoms.

PLANNING

The planning phase of the nursing process involves the development of a nursing care plan for the patient based on the nursing diagnoses. Nursing care plans are a form of communication with other health care professionals to ensure continuity of care, to prevent complications, and to provide for health teaching and discharge planning. Like the other steps of the nursing process, the comprehensive plan of care is initiated and finalized by the RN. The LPN/LVN may be involved in planning episodic nursing care. In some settings, especially long-term care, LPNs/LVNs may construct a plan for the approval of the RN.

The steps in planning nursing care are to (1) determine priorities from the list of nursing diagnoses, (2) set long-term and short-term goals to determine outcomes of care, (3) develop objectives to reach the goals, and (4) write nursing orders to direct care to meet the goals. Priorities are established according to

Table 12-1 | *Approved Nursing Diagnoses, North American Nursing Diagnosis Association, 2005*

Activity Intolerance	Conflict, Decisional (specify)	Family Processes: Alcoholism,
Activity Intolerance, Risk for	Conflict, Parental Role	Dysfunctional
Adjustment, Impaired	Confusion, Acute	Family Processes, Interrupted
Airway Clearance, Ineffective	Confusion, Chronic	Family Processes, Readiness for
Allergy Response, Latex	Constipation	Enhanced
Allergy Response, Latex, Risk for	Constipation, Perceived	Fatigue
Anxiety	Constipation, Risk for	Fear
Anxiety, Death	Coping, Ineffective	Fluid Balance, Readiness for
Aspiration, Risk for	Coping, Readiness for Enhanced	Enhanced
Attachment, Impaired Parent/Infant/	Coping, Community, Ineffective	Fluid Volume, Deficient
Child, Risk for	Coping, Community, Readiness for	Fluid Volume, Excess
Autonomic Dysreflexia	Enhanced	Fluid Volume, Deficient, Risk for
Autonomic Dysreflexia, Risk for	Coping, Defensive	Fluid Volume, Imbalanced, Risk for
Body Image, Disturbed	Coping, Family, Compromised	Gas Exchange, Impaired
Body Temperature, Imbalanced, Risk	Coping, Family, Disabled	Grieving, Anticipatory
for	Coping, Family, Readiness for	Grieving, Dysfunctional
Bowel Incontinence	Enhanced	Grieving, Dysfunctional, Risk for
Breastfeeding, Effective	Denial, Ineffective	Growth and Development, Delayed
Breastfeeding, Ineffective	Dentition, Impaired	Growth, Disproportionate, Risk for
Breastfeeding, Interrupted	Development, Delayed, Risk for	Health Maintenance, Ineffective
Breathing Pattern, Ineffective	Diarrhea	Health-Seeking Behaviors
Cardiac Output, Decreased	Disuse Syndrome, Risk for	Home Maintenance, Impaired
Caregiver Role Strain	Diversional Activity, Deficient	Hopelessness
Caregiver Role Strain, Risk for	Energy Field, Disturbed	Hyperthermia
Comfort, Impaired	Environmental Interpretation Syn-	Hypothermia
Communication, Verbal, Impaired	drome, Impaired	Identity, Personal, Disturbed
Communication, Readiness for	Failure to Thrive, Adult	Incontinence, Urinary, Functional
Enhanced	Falls, Risk for	Incontinence, Urinary, Reflex

Continued

Table 12-1 | *Approved Nursing Diagnoses, North American Nursing Diagnosis Association, 2005 —cont'd*

Incontinence, Urinary, Stress	Peripheral Neurovascular Dysfunc-	Sorrow, Chronic
Incontinence, Urinary, Total	tion, Risk for	Spiritual Distress
Incontinence, Urinary, Urge	Poisoning, Risk for	Spiritual Distress, Risk for
Incontinence, Urinary, Urge, Risk for	Post-Trauma Syndrome	Spiritual Well-Being, Readiness for
Infant Behavior, Disorganized	Post-Trauma Syndrome, Risk for	Enhanced
Infant Behavior, Disorganized,	Powerlessness	Sudden Infant Death Syndrome,
Risk for	Powerlessness, Risk for	Risk for
Infant Behavior, Organized, Readi-	Protection, Ineffective	Suffocation, Risk for
ness for Enhanced	Rape-Trauma Syndrome	Suicide, Risk for
Infant Feeding Pattern, Ineffective	Rape-Trauma Syndrome: Compound	Surgical Recovery, Delayed
Infection, Risk for	Reaction	Swallowing, Impaired
Injury, Risk for	Rape-Trauma Syndrome: Silent	Therapeutic Regimen Management,
Injury, Perioperative Positioning,	Reaction	Effective
Risk for	Religiosity, Impaired	Therapeutic Regimen Management,
Intracranial Adaptive Capacity,	Religiosity, Readiness for Enhanced	Ineffective
Decreased	Religiosity, Risk for Impaired	Therapeutic Regimen Management,
Knowledge, Deficient	Relocation Stress Syndrome	Community, Ineffective
Knowledge of (Specify), Readiness	Relocation Stress Syndrome, Risk for	Therapeutic Regimen Management,
for Enhanced	Role Performance, Ineffective	Family, Ineffective
Lifestyle, Sedentary	Self-Care Deficit, Bathing/Hygiene	Therapeutic Regimen Management,
Loneliness, Risk for	Self-Care Deficit, Dressing/Grooming	Readiness for Enhanced
Memory, Impaired	Self-Care Deficit, Feeding	Thermoregulation, Ineffective
Mobility, Bed, Impaired	Self-Care Deficit, Toileting	Thought Processes, Disturbed
Mobility, Physical, Impaired	Self-Concept, Readiness for	Tissue Integrity, Impaired
Mobility, Wheelchair, Impaired	Enhanced	Tissue Perfusion, Ineffective
Nausea	Self-Esteem, Chronic Low	Transfer Ability, Impaired
Neglect, Unilateral	Self-Esteem, Situational Low	Trauma, Risk for
Noncompliance	Self-esteem, Situational Low,	Urinary Elimination, Readiness for
Nutrition, Readiness for Enhanced	Risk for	Enhanced
Nutrition, Less Than Body Require-	Self-Mutilation	Urinary Elimination, Impaired
ments, Imbalanced	Self-Mutilation, Risk for	Urinary Retention
Nutrition: More Than Body Require-	Sensory Perception, Disturbed	Ventilation, Spontaneous, Impaired
ments, Imbalanced	Sexual Dysfunction	Ventilatory Weaning Response,
Nutrition: More Than Body Require-	Sexuality Pattern, Ineffective	Dysfunctional
ments, Risk for Imbalanced	Skin Integrity, Impaired	Violence, Other-Directed, Risk for
Oral Mucous Membrane, Impaired	Skin Integrity, Impaired, Risk for	Violence, Self-Directed, Risk for
Pain, Acute	Sleep Deprivation	Walking, Impaired
Pain, Chronic	Sleep Pattern, Disturbed	Wandering
Parenting, Readiness for Enhanced	Sleep, Readiness for Enhanced	
Parenting, Impaired	Social Interaction, Impaired	
Parenting, Impaired, Risk for	Social Isolation	

the most immediate needs of the patient. They usually are based on Maslow's hierarchy of needs and on what the patient perceives as important. For example, you should focus on decreased cardiac output (a physiologic need) before addressing disturbed body image (a self-esteem need).

Goals may be short-term or long-term, meaning that some may be achievable immediately, whereas others will take a longer period of time. Goals should be stated in terms of patient outcomes. To continue with our example of the patient with impaired skin integrity, the goal could be stated as "Pressure ulcer over sacrum will be healed within 2 weeks." A classification system for outcomes can be used. The system, called Nursing Outcome Classification (NOC), includes outcomes such as Tissue Integrity: Skin and Mucous Membranes; Wound Healing: Primary Intention; and Urinary Continence. Each of the nursing-sensitive out-

comes (outcomes amenable to nursing intervention) is labeled, is defined, and includes criteria for assessing the status of the outcome over time.

Nursing orders are the actions or interventions prescribed to help achieve the stated goals and objectives. Nursing orders should include a specific description (what, where, when, how much, and how long) of how the order should be carried out. For example, "Keep off sacrum to promote healing; turn side to side q 2 hr. Get OOB [out of bed] twice a day; begin ambulating as tolerated." The Nursing Interventions Classification (NIC) is a standardized list of nursing interventions. An NIC intervention consists of a label name, definition, specific nursing activities, and background readings. Development of NIC interventions is ongoing and currently includes nearly 500 interventions divided into 7 domains and 30 classes. To use NIC interventions, the nurse selects the appropriate activities for a

PATIENT	HEALTH TEAM MEMBERS	HEALTH CARE AGENCY
Consumer involvement	Standardized, organized care	Supported by Joint Commission on Accreditation of Healthcare Organizations
Patient education	Improved communication	Supported by third-party payers
Mutual goal setting	Reflection of current practice	Integration of quality improvement, utilization management, and risk management
Increased patient satisfaction	Increased staff satisfaction, educational tool for students and new graduates	Improved communication Decreased length of stay Better competitive position Decreased costs Availability of data for evaluating care

From Ignatavicius, D.D., & Hausman, K.A. (1995). *Clinical pathways for collaborative practice* (Table 1-2, p. 11). Philadelphia: Saunders.

specific intervention based on individual patient data. Examples of intervention labels are: Pressure Management, Pressure Ulcer Care, Skin Surveillance, Preparation for Childbirth, Fall Prevention, and Incision Site Care. Depending on the situation, additional activities might be added. An example of a nursing care plan using NANDA, NIC, and NOC is shown on p. 152.

INTERVENTION (IMPLEMENTATION)

Implementation is the actual performance of the nursing interventions in the plan of care. The interventions are coordinated with other members of the health care team and include direct patient care, health teaching, or carrying out ordered medical treatments such as medications or dressing changes. Nurses provide care to achieve established goals of care and then communicate the nursing interventions by documentation and report. Some interventions are unplanned because the nurse must respond to crises that demand immediate attention. Thus the care plan must be flexible and reflect changes in the patient's health care needs.

EVALUATION

Evaluation is an ongoing process that enables you to determine what progress the patient has made in meeting the goals for care. The outcome criteria provide objective measures for determining the effects of care. Using the previous example of impaired skin integrity, the outcome criteria could be "intact skin" and "absence of redness over bony prominences." Actual outcomes then are compared with expected outcomes of patient care to determine whether the goals have been met, partially met, or not met. If met, the goal was achieved. If not met, the goal was not achieved and reassessment is necessary. The plan of care should be reexamined and modified where necessary. Ongoing evaluation is a tool for quality improvement. In the patient care sections of this text, evaluation is not discussed separately.

Evaluation not only is important in individual patient care, but it also provides data regarding the qual-

ity of care in a health care institution. Quality assurance audits are conducted by individual health care agencies as well by as the Joint Commission on Accreditation of Healthcare Organizations, an organization that requires systematic review of hospitals and other health care organizations. Areas evaluated include the standards of nursing care used, the quality and effectiveness of nursing care, and the organization of the patient care system. Nursing audits are conducted by examining patient records as one method of gathering information to evaluate nursing performance. The American Nurses Association Standards of Care are used as a measure to determine whether nurses have carried out the nursing process as documented in the patient records.

Clinical Pathways

Clinical pathways are used in some health care facilities. They are standard care plans developed to set daily care priorities, schedule achievement of outcomes, and reduce length of hospital stays. They include patient outcomes and timelines for the sequence of interventions. Clinical pathways are collaborative and comprehensive in that they are jointly developed by all members of the health care team and they cover many aspects of care rather than just nursing interventions. The benefits of clinical pathways for patients, health team members, and health care agencies are summarized in Box 12-3. The use of clinical pathways is controversial. There are concerns about the potential for legal liability when there are deviations from pathways (even when justified). Research still is needed to determine their value. A sample clinical pathway is presented in Box 12-4. However, the nursing process will be used to provide the framework for nursing care throughout this text.

Concept Maps

Concept maps are visual plans of care that illustrate the relationships between and among pathophysiology, signs and symptoms, nursing diagnoses, and collaborative interventions. They are used primarily

Text continued on p. 155.

NURSING CARE PLAN

Plan of Care for Mrs. C.

CASE STUDY

Mrs. C., a 38-year-old woman, is married and has two adult stepchildren. She maintains a healthy lifestyle and has no family history of cancer. She performs breast self-exams routinely and has never identified a lump or any unusual finding during her monthly exam. Mrs. C. works full time as a magazine publisher. One day at work as she was going down a flight of stairs, her high heel caught on the rung of the step and she fell to the next landing. She received multiple bruises, including one in the chest area where she hit a metal railing. Ignoring her injuries because she was embarrassed about the fall, she continued to work throughout the day. That evening she told her family about her fall at work. Everyone was concerned, but she downplayed the incident since she was still more embarrassed about falling than concerned about the injuries she sustained.

Subsequently, Mrs. C. experienced localized pain in her left breast. The pain started out as a dull ache and did not improve over time. For several days Mrs. C. was aware of the breast pain but disregarded it as simply being a bruise resulting from the accident. The pain gradually became worse, and ultimately, Mrs. C. could feel a lump in her breast at the site of the pain. She finally went to a doctor 2 months after her fall. Upon examination, the doctor recommended a biopsy of the lump in her breast. The biopsy was done a week later and confirmed the presence of a malignant tumor. Mrs. C. had a radical mastectomy of the left breast several days later.

Mr. C. was at the hospital during the surgery but left for work after Mrs. C. entered postanesthesia recovery. After work Mr. C., an alcoholic, decided to go to the bar for a few drinks. He phoned Mrs. C. from the bar and told her he would call her again once he reached home. Mrs. C. was concerned about her husband driving home from the bar and worried a great deal about this during the evening. Several hours later he phoned her from home. While talking to her he "passed out" on the other end, and she could not disconnect from him. This upset Mrs. C. because she knew he was not dealing well with the mastectomy. She needed his support to deal with her recovery, and he needed her to help him cope with her surgery. Mrs. C. relied on the nursing staff for support with accepting her body image changes and also for emotional support. The staff located Reach for Recovery, a breast cancer support group, to help Mrs. C. through this difficult time in her life. The plan of care provides a summary of the information in this case showing the linkages among NANDA, NOC, and NIC.

Nursing Diagnosis	Goals and Outcome Criteria	Interventions
Disturbed Body Image	**Body Image**	**Body Image Enhancement**
Defining Characteristics	**Indicators**	**Nursing Activities**
Nonverbal response to actual or perceived change in structure and/or function; verbalization of feelings that reflect an altered view of one's body in appearance, structure, or function	Congruence between body reality, body ideal, and body presentation	Assist patient to discuss changes caused by illness or surgery
	Description of affected body part	Assist patient to separate physical appearance from feelings of personal worth
	Willingness to touch affected body part	Assist patient to discuss stressors affecting body image after surgery
	Satisfaction with body appearance	Monitor frequency of statements of self-criticism
Objective: Missing body part; not touching body part; not looking at body part	Adjustment to changes in physical appearance	Monitor whether patient can look at the changed body part
	Adjustment to changes in health status	Monitor for statements that identify body image perceptions concerned with body shape and body weight
Subjective: Negative feelings about body; fear of rejection or of reaction by others	Willingness to use strategies to enhance appearance and function	Determine patient's and family's perception of the alteration in body image versus reality
		Determine if a change in body image has contributed to increased social isolation
		Assist patient to identify actions that will enhance appearance
Related Factors		Facilitate contact with individuals with similar changes in body image
Surgery; illness treatment		Identify support groups available to patient

? **CRITICAL THINKING** QUESTIONS

■ Do you believe it is as important to collect data about a patient's emotional state as it is to collect data about his or her physical state? Explain your answer.

■ Which of the approved NANDA nursing diagnoses on pp. 149 and 150 indicate a need for emotional support of a patient who is distressed about a diagnosis of cancer?

From Johnson, M., et al. (2001). *Nursing diagnoses, outcomes, & interventions: NANDA, NOC and NIC linkages.* St. Louis: Mosby.

Box 12-4   *Clinical Pathway for Hepatic Cirrhosis (Without Variceal Bleeding)*

ICD-9 CODE 571.5 NURSING DIAGNOSIS/ COLLABORATIVE PROBLEM	ELOS 3 DAYS EXPECTED OUTCOME (THE PATIENT IS EXPECTED TO...)	MET/ NOT MET REASON	DATE/INITIAL
Fluid volume excess (ascites)	Have a decrease in extra-vascular and intra-abdominal fluid as evidenced by decreased abdominal girth and decreased peripheral edema.		
Potential for/actual chronic confusion	Be oriented to time, place, and person.		
Potential for major complications (esophageal varices, renal failure, advanced encephalopathy)	Not experience bleeding; have renal function tests at or near baseline; have intact neurologic function.		

ASPECT OF CARE	DATE _____ DAY 1	DATE _____ DAY 2	DATE _____ DAY 3
Assessment	Measure vital signs q 4 hr if stable. Systems assessment with focus on breath sounds, abdomen, and skin. Assess mental state q 8 hr. Observe for bruisability or frank bleeding. Measure abdominal girth daily.	Same as day 1	Same as day 2
Teaching	Orient to hospital and unit. Review clinical pathway/ plan of care with patient and family. Review diagnosis, including etiology and expected treatment.	Reinforce relationship of alcohol consumption to cirrhosis. Review discharge instruc-tions regarding: • Drug therapy (diuretics, H_2-receptor antagonist) • Avoidance of medi-cations other than prescribed • Diet therapy • Rest • Alcohol abstinence • Fluid restriction	Reinforce discharge instructions from day 2.
Consults	Respiratory therapist Alcohol counselor Social worker	N/A	N/A

Continued

Box 12-4   *Clinical Pathway for Hepatic Cirrhosis (Without Variceal Bleeding)—cont'd*

ASPECT OF CARE	DATE _____ DAY 1	DATE _____ DAY 2	DATE _____ DAY 3
Laboratory Tests	Complete blood cell count, aspartate aminotransferase, alanine aminotransferase, lactate dehydrogenase, alkaline phosphatase, bilirubin, serum proteins, ammonia, prothrombin time, electrolytes Urine studies for urobilinogen Stool for urobilinogen	N/A	Transaminases, prothrombin time, complete blood cell count, ammonia
Other Tests	Chest x-ray Electrocardiography Abdominal x-ray/computed tomography of abdomen	N/A	N/A
Medications	Diuretics as needed, such as Lasix by IV push or PO Zantac, 150 mg twice daily MVI daily Antacids PRN, such as Riopan or Amphojel Lactulose for increased ammonia levels Neomycin for increased ammonia level IV albumin if low serum albumin	Same as day 1	Same as day 2
Treatments/Interventions	Oxygen PRN for dyspnea Paracentesis if needed for comfort Daily weight Input and output q 8 hr Fluid restriction to 1500 mL/day Skin care for dryness and jaundice	Oxygen PRN Daily weight Input and output Fluid restriction Skin care	Same as day 2
Nutrition	High-protein, low-to-moderate-fat, high-carbohydrate diet (Low-protein diet if ammonia level increased)	Same as day 1	Same as day 2
Lines/Tubes/Monitors	IV at 50 mL/hr, then convert to saline loc	Saline loc	D/C saline loc

| Box 12-4 | *Clinical Pathway for Hepatic Cirrhosis (Without Variceal Bleeding)—cont'd* |

ASPECT OF CARE	DATE _____ DAY 1	DATE _____ DAY 2	DATE _____ DAY 3
Mobility/Self-Care	Put up in chair twice daily. Keep head of bed elevated to promote breathing comfort. Keep feet elevated while patient is out of bed. Assist with ADL as needed.	Walk in room with supervision. Raise head of bed. Keep feet elevated when out of bed. Assist with ADL.	Same as day 2
Discharge Planning	Assess home environment and available support systems. Determine need for placement in long-term care facility or other supervised environment.	If discharged to home, make arrangements with home health services to follow patient. If discharged to long-term care facility or other facility, make transportation and admission arrangements, if not done.	Arrange for follow-up appointment with physician as specified.

From Ignatavicius, D.D., & Hausman, K.A. (1995). *Clinical pathways for collaborative practice* (pp. 180-182). Philadelphia: Saunders.
ICD, International classification of diseases; *ELOS,* expected length of stay; *MVI,* multivitamin; *PRN,* as needed; *IV,* intravenous; *PO,* orally; *ADL,* activities of daily living.

as learning tools to develop comprehensive plans of care. An example of a concept map for a patient with hypertension is provided (Fig. 12-6).

NURSING DOCUMENTATION

Documentation is an important component of the nursing process. Patient assessments and observations and all nursing interventions should be charted as a permanent part of the patient's medical record, which is a legal record. Documentation helps achieve continuity of care because it provides for communication among caregivers and is a record of the patient's progress. In addition, documentation provides a legal record of care provided and a means to verify services rendered for insurance payments.

The following should be documented:
- All treatments and care given, including medications
- Diagnostic procedures performed at the bedside, on the unit, or inside or outside the facility
- The patient's reaction to therapeutic and diagnostic procedures
- Observations of the patient
- Subjective and objective signs and symptoms experienced by the patient
- Evidence of changes in the patient's physical, psychosocial, and spiritual needs and status
- Any unusual incidents such as falls or injuries that occur during the patient's stay in the health care facility

Documentation should be factual, current, complete, organized, and accurate. With paper charts, each page should have the patient's name and the date and time should be noted for each entry. Writing should be legible, using proper grammar, punctuation, and spelling. Fill all spaces, leaving no empty lines. Chart as soon after care is given as possible (never before care). Observations should be stated objectively, describing only what was seen, heard, felt, or smelled. Direct quotations from the patient regarding symptoms are very appropriate. Each time an entry is made, sign with your full name and title. Use only permanent ink, and make no erasures. If you make an error in charting, cross out the entry and write "error" or "mistaken entry," followed by your initials. Increasingly, patient records are entered and maintained in computerized charting systems. Some systems allow documentation at the patient's bedside. Nurses' notes may be composed by selecting from a menu of options related to the plan of care. Advantages of computerized charting include standardization of patient data, ease of retrieving data, and convenient storage. One disadvantage is the risk of information access by unauthorized persons.

DOCUMENTATION FORMATS

Various formats are used for the documentation of patient care, including nurses' notes, flow sheets, and problem-oriented medical records (POMR). Nurses' notes traditionally consisted of pages of narrative recordings containing assessment data, interventions carried out by the nurse, and evaluation data collected.

FIGURE **12-6** Hypertension concept map. The concept map is a visual plan that shows the relationships among parts of the plan. (Concept Map by Elaine Bishop Kennedy, EdD, RN.)

Flow sheets may be graphs of vital signs or tables in which nurses may check or initial boxes indicating activities or care provided.

Examples of charting approaches include focus charting (using key words such as action or response to organize charting); source-oriented charting (charting on separate sheets for different health care workers, such as physical therapy on one page and nurses on another); multidisciplinary charting (charting by different disciplines on the same page); charting by exception (CBE; charting narrative notes only when there is a change in the patient's condition); and computerized patient records (CPR; nurses' notes are recorded on computers). Health care facilities may combine one or more of these methods.

The POMR is a method of record keeping that focuses on patient problems rather than on medical diagnoses. This method is popular in many clinical areas because it provides an excellent means of communication among the various disciplines that are providing care. Each health care provider involved in the care of the patient charts on the same progress notes in the same format. The data from the history, physical examination, diagnostic tests, and medical diagnoses provide a foundation for problems formulated in the POMR. The problem list consists of active, inactive, potential, and resolved problems. The charting is done in a SOAPIER format. SOAPIER is an acronym for the components of the charting:

S *Subjective* information, or how the patient perceives the problem

O *Objective* information, or what the nurse observes about the patient

A *Assessment*, or why the patient has the problem

P *Plan*, or how the intervention is to be carried out

I *Intervention*, or what specific care is given

E *Evaluation*, or how effective was the plan or intervention

R *Revision*, or what changes should be made in the original plan of care

In many cases, the SOAPE form is used, omitting the intervention and revision sections. The intervention is closely related to the plan and can be a reiteration of the plan; a revision can be made in the plan by simply revising the original SOAPE notes.

An example of a SOAPE note using our previous example is as follows:

S Feels weak; does "not have the energy to move around"

O Does not turn self in bed; 2-cm stage 2 pressure ulcer on sacrum

A Pressure ulcer on sacrum related to immobility

P Turn from side to side q 2 hr. Get out of bed at least twice a day. Begin ambulating as tolerated.

E Turned q 2 hr. OOB twice a day, taking 6 small steps to and from bed. Pressure ulcer healing; now 1.5 cm.

Another common format is PIE charting, which includes the problem, intervention, and evaluation. An example might be:

P Risk for impaired skin integrity related to unrelieved pressure on sacrum.

I Patient informed of need to shift positions and increase ambulation to relieve pressure on sa-

crum. Assisted to reposition hourly, and to get out of bed twice.

E Patient is repositioning herself with occasional prompting. Walked for two 10-minute periods today.

A large amount of time is spent charting and keeping records, and many facilities are transforming their record keeping into more time-saving methods of documentation, such as computerized nursing care plans and nurses' notes. Nevertheless, regardless of the format, the essential data should always be recorded systematically and must be individualized for each patient.

Put on Your Thinking Cap!

Agree with some classmates to observe 5 minutes of the local television news on a specific date and time and to watch a specific channel. Using objective language, document your observations of the speaker(s). Compare your description with that of classmates. If they have differences, discuss possible explanations.

CRITICAL THINKING

Critical thinking is defined as "reflective and reasonable thinking that is focused on deciding what to believe or do" (Ennis, 1985, p. 45). Although more sophisticated definitions exist, this one is appropriate for our purposes. You will hear a lot about critical thinking during your nursing education. Because you spend a lot of time reading and learning facts, you may assume that critical thinking is just learning many facts. Although facts are indeed important, nursing deals with people in states of change in an environment that is constantly evolving. You will forget many of the facts you learn this year, but if you become a critical thinker, you will always have the tools to seek and apply knowledge. This example illustrates the pitfalls of trying to use facts without thinking critically: A student assigned to a patient on the first day after abdominal surgery outlines detailed plans (from a textbook care plan) for ways to promote urination. Definitely important! However, the patient had a Foley catheter. With critical thinking skills, the student would have based plans on actual patient data so that the plan of care would have been appropriate.

RELATIONSHIP OF CRITICAL THINKING TO THE NURSING PROCESS

Why do you need both critical thinking and nursing process? The nursing process is a framework for developing, implementing, and evaluating a plan of care. It spells out the patient's needs and problems, the goals for care, interventions to achieve goals, and how goal achievement will be assessed.

If you have seen a well-written nursing process, you can see how it can be used to guide care. It tells you exactly what to do, right? Unfortunately, it's not that simple. Suppose the patient's care plan says he is to be assisted to take a shower for the first time since surgery as part of the plan to promote increasing independence in self-care. However, when you assist the patient out of bed, he becomes dizzy and nauseated. What do you do now? This is a simple situation that can be used to illustrate how critical thinking is used in nursing. Table 12-2 carries this situation through and reflects the steps of the nursing process along with the critical thinking that occurs at each step. One point to notice is that the nursing process does not flow smoothly from one step

Table 12-2 | *Analysis of Critical Thinking in a Clinical Situation*

Situation: You are assigned to care for Mr. A. today. It is his second postoperative day. One goal for the day is to promote independence in self-care. The nursing care plan notes that you should assist the patient with a shower.

The following table reflects a possible sequence of events when you attempt to implement the plan of care. The steps of the nursing process and the critical thinking skills are identified to illustrate how they are used and interact in a common situation.

SEQUENCE OF EVENTS	NURSING PROCESS STEPS	CRITICAL THINKING TOOLS
When you help Mr. A. stand at the bedside, he becomes dizzy and says he is nauseated. You ease him back into bed knowing that he is at risk for falling. Because Mr. A. is nauseated, you anticipate vomiting and reach for an emesis basin.	Intervention Assessment Intervention Planning Intervention	Inference: drawing conclusions Evaluation: assessing possibilities
You collect additional information immediately after Mr. A. lies down. His skin is pale, cool, and moist. His pulse is 110 and faint, and his blood pressure is 90 mm Hg/60 mm Hg. When asked how he feels, he replies: "I feel better lying down."	Assessment	Interpretation: clarifying the meaning of events
Knowing that dizziness is associated with hypotension and that the supine position improves blood flow to the brain, you advise him to remain flat in bed for the time being.	Diagnosis Intervention	Inference: drawing conclusions
You reassess Mr. A. after a few minutes in the supine position. His skin is pink and warm, his pulse rate is 84 and full, and his blood pressure is 114 mm Hg/74 mm Hg.	Assessment	Interpretation: clarifying meaning of data
What do you do now? The care plan said you were supposed to get him up for a shower. You ask yourself what has just happened. You consider a drop in blood pressure related to drug effects, immobility, or dehydration.	Planning	Inference: deriving alternatives Interpretation: clarifying meaning of events
You consider your options: Try again to get him up; give him a bed bath; let him rest for a while and see how he feels later; exercise his legs before helping him stand; notify the physician. These are all possibilities.	Planning	Inference: deriving alternatives Analysis: examining ideas
How do you choose one option? Think about the possible outcomes (positive and negative) of each action.	Planning	Inference: drawing conclusions
Choose the option that would seem to be safe for the patient without delaying his recovery.	Intervention	
You think the patient should remain in bed today. However, as a novice nurse, you are a bit unsure of yourself, so you explain the situation to the charge nurse and request feedback. The charge nurse suggests that you wait and try again later.	Planning	Self-regulation: recognizing need to make changes, reconsidering conclusions
After half an hour, Mr. A.'s vital signs are stable. You place a chair in the shower, exercise his legs, and then slowly get him up. He tolerates standing without dizziness. You assist him with morning care in the shower chair. You document the events.	Assessment Intervention Evaluation	Interpretation: clarifying meaning of data Inference: deriving alternatives

to the next, but often moves back and forth between steps. This common scenario illustrates the many decision-making points that can occur in handling a fairly routine nursing situation. Notice that critical thinking was used to determine focused assessments needed, interventions to be implemented, and evaluation data to collect. The nursing process is a sequence of steps that should be based on critical thinking. That is why your faculty may discourage you from using standardized care plans for patient care. Ready-made care plans bypass the vital experience of thinking through each step so that the care plan is specific and individualized for your patient.

CHARACTERISTICS OF A CRITICAL THINKER

In the situation just described, you (the nurse) demonstrated various characteristics of a critical thinker. Those characteristics include the following:

- *Curiosity:* The desire not just to know but also to understand how and why to apply knowledge
- *Systematic thinking:* Uses an organized approach to problem solving rather than knee-jerk responses
- *Analytical:* Applies knowledge from various disciplines, approaches a problem by examining the parts and seeing how they fit together
- *Open-minded:* Willing to consider various alternatives
- *Self-confident:* Sense of assurance that the problem-solving process produces a good conclusion/plan
- *Maturity:* Recognition that many variables are at work in patient situations and sometimes the best plans do not work (back to the drawing board!!)
- *Truth-seeking:* Eager to know, asking questions, seeking answers, reevaluates "common knowledge"

CRITICAL THINKING TOOLS

Just as the critical thinker has certain characteristics, the critical thinker also uses specific tools. These include the following:

- *Interpretation:* Clarifying meaning of events, data
- *Analysis:* Examining ideas, breaking down into components
- *Evaluation:* Assessing possibilities, opinions, usual practices
- *Inference:* Deriving alternatives, drawing conclusions
- *Explanation:* Presenting arguments for views, decisions; justifying
- *Self-regulation:* Reconsidering conclusions, recognizing need to make changes

Throughout this text, you will find exercises labeled "Put on your THINKING CAP." As you encounter these, your first reaction may be to try to find the answer in the chapter. What you will find is that the content provides only the knowledge *base* to answer the question, not the answer itself. A trick question, you say. Not at all. The purpose is to help you develop the essential skills for *critical thinking*.

In closing, the nursing process is a tool—a roadmap for planning and providing care. It is critical thinking that makes the nursing process scientifically sound, appropriate, flexible, and individualized.

Key Points

- The nursing process is a problem-solving approach that enables the nurse to provide care in an organized, scientific manner.
- The comprehensive nursing assessment and plan of care are developed by the registered nurse.
- The LPN/LVN assists with data collection, identifying patient needs, planning care, and evaluating the outcomes of care.
- The steps of the nursing process are assessment, nursing diagnosis, planning, implementation, and evaluation.
- Assessment involves collection of subjective and objective data about the client or patient from the client, family, significant others, medical records, and other care providers.
- The interview is used to obtain an objective picture of the patient's personal and family health history.
- The physical examination uses inspection, auscultation, palpation, and percussion to collect objective data about the patient.
- The nursing diagnosis is a statement of an actual or potential health problem derived from the assessment.
- Nursing diagnoses differ from medical diagnoses in that nursing diagnoses focus on the response of the whole person to the medical problem.
- The parts of a NANDA diagnosis are the label, definition of the diagnosis, defining characteristics (signs and symptoms), and related (causative or associated) factors.
- The planning phase of the nursing process involves the development of a nursing care plan for the patient based on the nursing diagnoses.
- The Nursing Outcomes Classification includes standardized outcomes that serve as criteria to judge the results of nursing interventions.
- Planning includes priority setting, goal statements, and nursing interventions to achieve the goals.
- NIC interventions are standardized interventions, each including a label name, definition, list of nursing activities, and background readings.
- Implementation refers to the actual performance of the nursing interventions identified in the plan of care.
- Evaluation is an ongoing process in which the nurse uses outcome criteria to determine what progress has been made toward meeting the goals.
- The value of using systems such as NANDA, NIC, and NOC is that they standardize language that describes what nurses do.
- Documentation of data collected, interventions, and evaluation data is an essential aspect of nursing care.

- Clinical pathways are standardized, interdisciplinary plans of care that specify the sequence and timing of interventions.
- Critical thinking is defined as "reflective and reasonable thinking that is focused on deciding what to believe or do" (Ennis, 1985, p. 45).
- Critical thinking makes the nursing process appropriate, scientifically sound, flexible, and individualized.
- Critical thinking skills include interpretation, analysis, evaluation, inference, explanation, and self-regulation.

- A critical thinker is curious, open-minded, a systematic thinker, analytical, truth seeking, and has self-confidence and maturity.

Go to your Companion CD-ROM for a Pharmacology Tutorial, Audio Glossary, and 3-D animations.

evolve Be sure to visit the companion Evolve site at http://evolve.elsevier.com/Linton/ for WebLinks and additional online resources.

REVIEW QUESTIONS *Choose the best answer.*

1. An example of subjective data is:
   1. Lung sounds clear to auscultation
   2. Urine clear, light yellow
   3. Heart rate 90 bpm and regular
   4. Headache and sensitivity to light

2. "Patient states pain in his neck began when he was wrestling with his brother. The pain radiates across his right shoulder and worsens with movement of the right arm." This is an example of:
   1. Biographical data
   2. Chief complaint
   3. Family history
   4. Review of systems

3. Percussion is used primarily to assess the:
   1. Chest
   2. Skin
   3. Joints
   4. Cranium

4. Which of the following is a complete, correctly stated NANDA diagnosis?
   1. Disturbed body image as a result of surgical scars, as evidenced by crying and concealing scars
   2. Decreased cardiac output related to excessive blood loss
   3. Noncompliance related to refusal to take medications as evidenced by high blood pressure
   4. Diabetes mellitus related to obesity as evidenced by high serum glucose

5. Which goal is most complete and measurable?
   1. Patient will demonstrate clean wound dressing change before discharge.
   2. Patient will know how to care for wound before leaving the hospital.
   3. Patient will take care of wound himself when he goes home.
   4. Patient will understand the principles of medical asepsis to use during dressing changes.

6. The nurse's responsibility for documentation includes:
   1. Record names of all visitors
   2. Document all medical interventions
   3. Never chart care in advance
   4. Carefully erase errors completely

7. Which of the following skills is used in critical thinking?
   1. Copy
   2. Recite
   3. Memorize
   4. Analyze

8. A characteristic of a critical thinker is:
   1. Self-controlled
   2. Self-confident
   3. Self-centered
   4. Self-righteous

9. According to the American Nurses Association Standards of Care, the nurse evaluates the client's progress toward attainment of outcomes. What measurement criterion is used for this standard?
   1. Revisions in diagnoses, outcomes, and the plan of care are documented.
   2. Interventions are consistent with the established plan of care.
   3. Plan is developed with the client, significant others, and health care providers, when appropriate.
   4. Outcomes are realistic in relation to the client's present and potential capabilities.

13 Inflammation, Infection, and Immunity

evolve   http://evolve.elsevier.com/Linton/

Objectives

After reading and studying this chapter, you should be able to:

1. Describe physical and chemical barriers.
2. Describe how inflammatory changes act as bodily defense mechanisms.
3. Identify the signs and symptoms of inflammation.
4. Discuss the process of repair and healing.
5. Differentiate infection from inflammation.
6. Discuss the actions of commonly found infectious agents.
7. Describe the ways that infections are transmitted.
8. Identify the signs and symptoms of infection.
9. Compare community-acquired and nosocomial infections.
10. Discuss the nursing care of patients with infections.
11. Describe the Centers for Disease Control and Prevention (CDC) Standard Precautions guidelines for infection control.
12. Describe the CDC isolation guidelines for Airborne, Droplet, and Contact (Transmission-Based) Precautions.
13. Describe the immune response.
14. Identify the organs involved in immunity.
15. Compare natural and acquired immunity.
16. Differentiate between humoral (antibody-mediated) and cell-mediated immunity.
17. Describe the nursing care of patients with immunodeficiency and of those with allergies.
18. Describe the process of autoimmunity.

Key Terms

Be sure to check out the bonus material on the Companion CD-ROM, including selected audio pronunciations.

allergen (ĂL-ĕr-jĕn, p. 177)
antibodies (ĂN-tĭ-bŏ-dēs, p. 174)
antigen (ĂN-tĭ-jĕn, p. 174)
autoimmunity (ăw-tō-ĭ-MŪ-nĭ-tē, p. 178)
bacteria (p. 164)
communicable disease (kŏ-MŪ-nĭ-kă-b'l dĭ-ZĔZ, p. 167)
contamination (p. 166)
fungi (FŬN-jī, p. 165)
health care–associated infection (p. 168)
immunity (ĭ-MŪN-ĭ-tē, p. 173)
immunodeficiency (ĭm-ū-nō-dĕ-FĬSH-ĕn-sē, p. 176)
infection (p. 164)

inflammation (ĭn-flă-MĀ-shŭn, p. 162)
medical asepsis (ă-SĔP-sĭs, p. 169)
nosocomial infection (nō-sō-KŌ-mē-ăl ĭn-FĔK-shŭn, p. 168)
surgical asepsis (SŬR-jĕ-kăl ă-SĔP-sĭs, p. 170)
virus (VĪ-rŭs, p. 165)

Suppose you were being attacked. How would you defend yourself? Perhaps you would shout or in some other way sound an alarm. You might even call for reinforcements to help you fight off the attacker, telling them the most direct route to your location. You would probably surround yourself with some sort of barrier either to shield yourself from further harm or to keep the attacker in the area so that he or she would not escape and harm someone else. Then, after the battle was over, you would likely enlist the help of some friends to clean up the debris and return your situation to normal.

It is quite remarkable to realize that, at a cellular level, the human body is protected in much the same way. The body relies on many effective barriers to protect itself from injury and disease. However, if these barriers are compromised, several sophisticated processes are triggered to isolate and eliminate the offender. In this chapter, how the body defends itself from injury and disease, what happens when defenses fail, and how good nursing care helps the processes are described.

PHYSICAL AND CHEMICAL BARRIERS

The skin and mucous membranes are the body's first line of defense. They act as a protective covering and secrete substances that inhibit the growth of microorganisms. The sweat glands secrete lysozyme, an antimicrobial enzyme. Sebaceous glands secrete sebum, which has antimicrobial and antifungal properties. Acidic secretions from the skin and the mucosa of the gastrointestinal and genitourinary systems inhibit the growth of many pathogenic organisms. Secretions from the mammary glands and the respiratory and gastrointestinal tracts contain the antibody *immunoglobulin A*, as well as cleanup phagocytes. In addition, skin and mucous membrane surfaces are colonized by "normal" bacterial flora, which prevent pathogens (disease-causing organisms) from gaining access to the body. The cilia in the respiratory tract, the motility of the gastrointestinal tract, and the sloughing of dead skin cells all work to distribute and remove microorganisms, preventing their overgrowth and invasion.

The second line of defense involves two processes: phagocytosis and inflammation. Phagocytosis helps rid the body of invading microorganisms and debris. White blood cells (leukocytes) are colorless blood cells that have the ability to phagocytose (ingest) bacteria that can cause infection when they invade the body. Two types of leukocytes, neutrophils and monocytes, are especially suited for this purpose. Neutrophils fight bacterial infections. Monocytes circulate in the blood for about 1 day before they enter tissue, where they are called *macrophages*, and ingest many foreign antigens. Eosinophils fight parasitic infections and increase during allergic reactions. Basophils initiate the inflammatory response and release histamine. Measuring the number of these cells gives an indication of the severity of infection in the body. B lymphocytes produce antibodies, and T lymphocytes increase the body's immune response. Therefore lymphocyte counts provide a measure of immune function. A more complete description of blood and components of the immune system may be found in Chapters 32 and 33 (Hematology and Immunology).

Reticuloendothelial cells are found in the blood, connective tissue, liver, spleen, bone marrow, and lymph nodes. Some reticuloendothelial cells protect the body by digesting and absorbing foreign material, such as old red blood cells, bacteria, and colloidal particles. These cells may also be called *tissue macrophages.*

THE INFLAMMATORY PROCESS

The inflammatory process is a series of cellular changes that signal the body's response to injury or infection. Although infection is a common cause of inflammation, this complex phenomenon may be caused by trauma from (1) physical agents (excessive sunlight, x-rays), (2) chemical stimuli (insect venom, other chemicals), and (3) biologic agents (bacteria, viruses).

The word inflammation means literally "the fire within." This descriptive phrase illustrates the four classic manifestations of inflammation: (1) rubor (redness), (2) calor (heat), (3) tumor (swelling), and (4) dolor (pain). It is helpful to think about the appearance of a bee sting and recall the redness, warmth, swelling, and pain that it produces. These signs are the direct result of several related actions that occur when the inflammatory process is initiated. The actions involve hemodynamic changes, increased permeability of membranes, chemical mediators, and hormonal factors.

ACTIONS IN THE INFLAMMATORY PROCESS

Hemodynamic Changes

The first actions of the inflammatory process are the hemodynamic changes. The body initially responds to an injury or infection with dilation of the capillary bed. This dilation brings increased blood flow to the area. The increase in blood flow is responsible for the characteristic warmth and redness at the site of inflammation.

Increased Permeability

The second action is an increased capillary permeability (Fig. 13-1). After the increased blood flow brings leukocytes into the area, chemical mediators cause leukocytes to line the small blood vessel walls near the inflammatory site. This process is called *pavementing.* Gradually these cells pass through the vessel walls and inhabit the inflamed area. These cells, largely neutrophils and monocytes, are drawn to the site of injury or infection, where they ingest and carry away bacteria and other foreign substances (phagocytosis) (Fig. 13-2). The permeability of these vessels causes protein-rich fluid to flow through the vessel walls into the interstitial space. Some red blood cells may pass through into this area as well. This collection of fluid is responsible for the swelling that is noted when the inflammation site is close to the surface of the skin. This swelling may also produce pain.

Chemical Mediators

The hemodynamic changes and vascular permeability occur with the help of several chemical mediators, including prostaglandins, histamine, and leukotrienes. These powerful substances are found in various body tissues and are liberated during the inflammatory process. Cytokines and eicosanoids, described in Chapter 33, cause blood and blood vessel changes. The kinin system produces bradykinin, which also mediates blood vessel dilation and permeability. It also produces pain, another classic sign of inflammation. Other mediators include the complement system, which is especially important in immunologically mediated reactions involving antigen-antibody complexes. These reactions cause a massive release of histamine and other substances that produce marked vasodilation, vascular permeability, and smooth muscle contraction. These cellular changes produce the classic signs of anaphylactic shock: hypotension, swelling, and bronchoconstriction.

Anti-Inflammation

Cortisol, a hormone produced by the adrenal cortex, is an anti-inflammatory substance that slows the release of histamine, stabilizes lysosomal membranes, and prevents the influx of leukocytes. The end result of these actions is to impede the inflammatory process. By limiting the inflammatory process, cortisol protects

FIGURE **13-1** The inflammatory response after tissue injury.

the body from the effects of excessive or prolonged inflammation. Drugs (such as corticosteroids) that mimic the action of cortisol are often used in the treatment of inflammatory conditions.

SIGNS AND SYMPTOMS OF INFLAMMATION

The signs and symptoms of inflammation vary depending on whether the reaction is local or systemic. Local inflammation generally produces the classic signs of heat, swelling, redness, and pain, all of which result in loss of function.

Systemic inflammation produces somewhat different reactions. Swelling, redness, and local warmth may not be visible; however, signs of the effects of the chemical mediators may be recognized in other ways. Fever is a common sign of systemic inflamma-

tion, probably caused by pyrogens (fever-producing substances) or by defense mechanisms that are liberated during phagocytosis, or by bacterial endotoxins, antigen-antibody complexes, and certain viruses. Other symptoms of systemic inflammation include headache, muscle aches, chills, and sweating.

Leukocytosis is another sign of systemic inflammation. This is a defensive reaction that provides abundant white blood cells for the inflammatory response. If infection is not present, inflammatory leukocytosis disappears within a few hours.

WOUND HEALING

Repair and regeneration of tissue are set in motion from the very beginning of the inflammatory process. The speed at which this **process** takes place depends on the type of tissue injured, the severity of

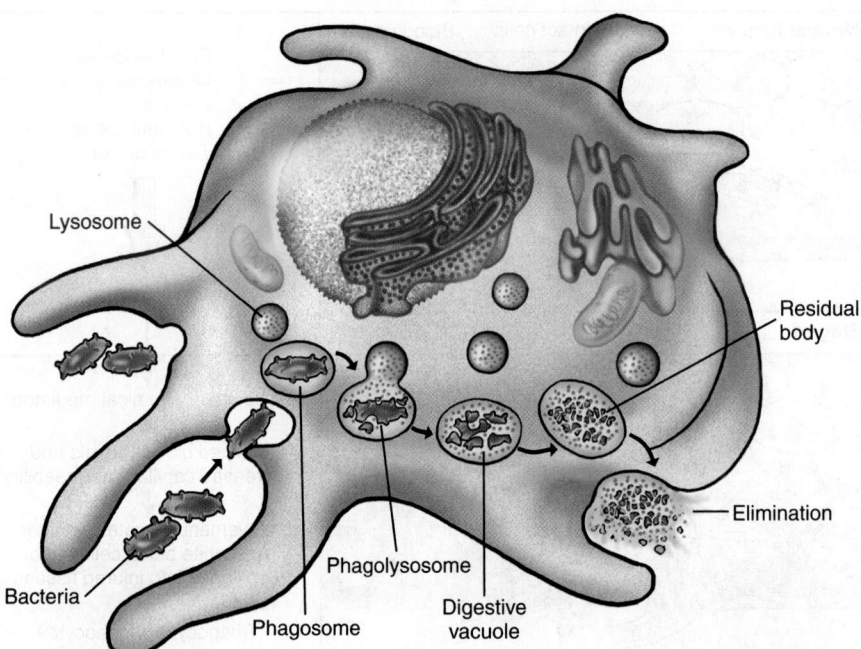

FIGURE **13-2** Phagocytosis. (1) Macrophages migrate to an inflammatory site by chemotaxis. (2) Macrophages engulf the microorganisms. A phagosome or phagocytic vacuole forms around the microorganisms. (3) Lysosomes attach to the phagosome and release their enzymes, which destroy the microorganisms.

the wound, the presence of infection, and the health of the host. At the outset, macrophage cells are produced to clean up inflammatory debris. Fibroblasts begin the repair process by laying down elastin and collagen at the edges of the wound; these substances gradually migrate to the base, forming granulation tissue. Epithelial cells migrate over the wound and under the scab (usually formed of dried blood and fibroblasts). After a few days, the scab falls off. Damaged cells are replaced by new cells of their own composition by the process of regeneration. Some tissue regenerates well, whereas other tissue must undergo repair, which may involve the replacement of injured cells with connective tissue that will eventually create a scar. In fact, both types of tissue repair occur in most wounds.

The age and general health of the person affect how rapidly the regeneration and repair processes occur. The healing process can be delayed in the older person as a result of decreased tissue elasticity and decreased blood supply. Deficiencies of vitamin C, zinc, and other important vitamins and minerals can also delay the regeneration and repair processes.

Occasionally a wound becomes infected or ulcerated, resulting in tissue loss. Granulation tissue and capillary buds form at the margins of the wound, and it is eventually filled with granulation tissue. Sometimes the wound bed is too large for the granulation tissue to fill. In this case, the wound is cleaned and débrided in an effort to enhance healing. When infection

is no longer present, the wound is sutured closed. This is called *delayed primary closure.*

INFECTION

Infection is a process involving the invasion of body tissues by microorganisms, the multiplication of the invading organisms, and the subsequent tissue damage. Infection is different from inflammation in that inflammation is a nonspecific reaction by the body to tissue injury, whereas infection refers to a specific process that causes tissue injury. Infection nearly always results in inflammation, but inflammation may be caused by processes other than infection. Inflammation precedes infection. Infection is usually the end result of the invasion by organisms. Infection may be caused by a wide variety of microorganisms.

INFECTIOUS AGENTS

The major infectious agents are bacteria, viruses, fungi, protozoa, rickettsiae, helminths, and mycoplasmas.

Bacteria

Bacteria are one-celled microorganisms capable of multiplying rapidly within a susceptible host. Among the factors that protect these organisms from phagocytosis are a rigid cell wall and a gelatinous capsule. Bacteria are classified as either gram positive or gram negative, depending on their ability to take up and retain a violet-colored solution called Gram stain. Gram-positive bacteria retain the stain, whereas gram-negative bacteria can be decolorized and counterstained pink.

Bacteria are also classified according to shape. Round bacteria are called *cocci;* they are further classified according to how they group or cluster together. Groups of two are called *diplococci,* and clusters of cocci are called *staphylococci.* Chains of these microorganisms are called *streptococci.*

Rod-shaped organisms, called *bacilli,* may be further subdivided into fusiform (with tapered ends) or spirochetes (spirals).

Bacteria may also be classified according to their ability to grow in the presence of oxygen. Those that do are classified as *aerobes;* those that do not are labeled *anaerobes.*

These classifications have a very important purpose. Each classification highlights a characteristic of a microorganism that is considered in the design of an antimicrobial drug to kill or retard the growth of the organism. For example, gram-positive bacteria have a thick polypeptide and peptidoglycan covering that absorbs Gram stain. Antibiotics synthesized to fight these microorganisms interfere with the formation of that covering, causing the cell wall to be destroyed. Similarly, other antibiotics rely on the ability of a bacterial cell to take up oxygen to produce its effects.

The staining process aids in the identification of the organisms. The Gram stain differentiates bacteria into two major categories: gram positive and gram negative. The acid-fast stain is used to identify bacteria such as *Mycobacterium tuberculosis.* Immunofluorescent stains reveal complexes composed of various antigens (bacteria, viruses, fungi, protozoa) and antibodies when exposed to ultraviolet light.

Viruses

Viruses are very small microorganisms that cause significant morbidity (disease) in humans. Viruses cause a variety of illnesses, ranging from the common cold to acquired immunodeficiency syndrome (AIDS). Many childhood illnesses (e.g., measles, chickenpox) as well as several forms of hepatitis are caused by viruses. These microorganisms cannot be seen with ordinary microscopes but are visible with electron microscopy. They contain a strand of genetic material and are surrounded by a protein capsule but have no cell wall. Viruses cannot replicate on their own; they depend on the resources of the host cell.

Viruses produce their damage by stimulating the antigen-antibody response in the tissues that causes inflammation and cell destruction. Because replication of the virus occurs within the host cell, it is seldom possible to kill the virus without harming the host cell. This explains why there are relatively few antiviral drugs available. Current antiviral drugs suppress viral reproduction or growth so that they decrease the severity

or duration of the infection, but they are not curative. Prevention (immunizations, hygiene) is still the best way to combat viral illness.

Fungi

Fungi are vegetable-like organisms that exist by feeding on organic matter. Mushrooms and molds are examples of fungal organisms. A few species of fungi are capable of producing disease in humans. Ringworm (tinea corporis) and athlete's foot (tinea pedis) are two examples. Many of these infections are superficial skin infections that rarely produce serious illness. Systemic fungal infections caused by *Cryptococcus* and *Aspergillus* species, however, can be life-threatening. Patients who have conditions that affect their immune system (e.g., HIV) are at especially high risk of acquiring opportunistic fungal infections. Fungal infections are called *mycoses.* Because fungi tend to form spores that are resistant to many antiseptics and disinfectants, they are difficult to treat. Both systemic and topical antimycotic drugs are used to treat fungal infections.

Protozoa

Protozoa make up a large group of one-celled organisms. Ones that produce disease in humans include the *Plasmodium* species (malaria), *Entamoeba histolytica* (amoebic dysentery), *Giardia lamblia* (giardiasis, characterized by diarrhea), and *Trypanosoma gambiense* (sleeping sickness). Infections are often spread by food or water that is contaminated by human or animal feces. *Pneumocystis jiroveci* is another protozoal infection that was relatively rare before the onset of the HIV/AIDS epidemic. Lowered immunity with HIV infection is responsible for the dramatic rise in pneumocystic pneumonia.

Rickettsiae

Rickettsiae are microorganisms that are between bacteria and viruses in size. They may appear as rods, cocci, or pleomorphic (varied) shapes. These organisms multiply in the cells of animal hosts, such as rats and squirrels, and are transmitted to humans through the bites of fleas and ticks. Diseases produced by these microorganisms include Rocky Mountain spotted fever and typhus. Diseases caused by rickettsiae tend to be more prevalent in areas in which sanitation is poor and rodent and insect populations are not well controlled.

Helminths

Helminths are worms. These parasites are found in soil and water and are generally transmitted from hand to mouth. Infections occur commonly in the gastrointestinal tract and may produce mild abdominal pain and bloating, or they may be asymptomatic. Pinworms are most common, especially in children, and often produce rectal irritation. Tapeworms can be found in the gastrointestinal tract. Weight loss and abdominal pain and bloating may be early signs and symptoms. Hookworms often enter an individual through the soles of the feet and migrate throughout the body. Symptoms initially may be respiratory, but these parasites can also produce abdominal pain, diarrhea, and anemia.

Mycoplasmas

Mycoplasmas are gram-negative, multishaped organisms without cell walls that are responsible for several infections in humans. They are sometimes called *pleuropneumonia-like organisms.* Mycoplasma infections are responsible for primary atypical pneumonia and have been linked to Reiter's syndrome, a multisystem inflammatory disease that may be associated with urethritis, conjunctivitis, and pharyngitis. Infections are usually found in the upper respiratory tract and most often affect children and young adults. Mycoplasma infections respond well to erythromycin.

TRANSMISSION OF INFECTION

Infection is possible only when several factors are present. These factors must occur in sequence for human infectious disease to occur. They include (1) a causative agent, (2) a reservoir, (3) a portal of exit, (4) a mode of transfer, (5) a portal of entry, and (6) a susceptible host. This is referred to as the *chain of infection.*

Causative Agent

Causative agents are the microorganisms (e.g., bacteria, viruses, protozoa) that are present in sufficient number and virulence to damage human tissue.

Reservoir

Areas in which organisms can pool and reproduce are called *reservoirs.* Reservoirs may be human or animal tissues as well as any substance such as soil or animal feces in which microorganisms can pool and multiply. When a reservoir of microorganisms occurs in the tissues of human, the human is called a *host.*

Portal of Exit

Portal of exit refers to the route by which the infectious agent leaves one host and travels to another. A common route is the gastrointestinal tract, through which bacteria or viruses may escape an infected host. The nose and mouth also are common portals of exit for organisms spread by droplet contamination through sneezing or coughing. Fecal-oral transmission also occurs; hepatitis A virus is acquired by ingesting the virus in water contaminated with feces or by direct fecal-oral transmission.

Mode of Transfer

Mode of transfer refers to the means by which a microorganism is transported to a host. Person-to-person transfer may take place in either a direct or an indirect manner. *Direct contact* refers to the transfer of microorganisms directly, as occurs in sexually transmitted infections. *Indirect contact* occurs when pathogens are spread through droplets expelled during a sneeze or a cough or through inanimate objects (e.g., eating utensils on which microorganisms can be transported [fomites]).

Common vehicle transmission occurs when water, food, blood, or air currents contaminated with a pathogen are shared by a number of people. Air currents, for example, are often the common vehicle for transmission of *Legionella,* the organism responsible for Legionnaire's disease. Vector transmission occurs when microorganisms are transported into a host by a living organism such as a fly or mosquito. Fomites are any items that have been touched or cross-contaminated by the host, such as bed linen, side rails, or hygiene items.

Portal of Entry

Portals of entry are the doorways or pathways into the host. Flu and cold viruses often enter the body through the mucous membranes of the nose and mouth. Other portals of entry often accessed by bacteria are the gastrointestinal tract and the urethra. Open wounds, intravenous access devices, urinary catheters, and drains also can be portals of entry for bacteria.

Susceptible Host

To produce tissue damage, microorganisms must become implanted into a susceptible host. Not all people exposed to disease-producing microorganisms become ill. Populations adequately immunized against rubella, for example, are not susceptible to measles. Similarly, individuals who have had chickenpox have developed immunity to the virus and, if exposed a second time, do not become ill.

SIGNS AND SYMPTOMS OF INFECTION

Once an individual becomes infected with a pathogen, symptoms may or may not be apparent. Often there is a period of subclinical infection or an incubation period during which there are few, if any, symptoms. During this period, asymptomatic persons may be more contagious than those who are exhibiting symptoms. This is true of people infected with such viruses as measles and many cold viruses. Persons recently infected with HIV may feel well but are highly contagious. Persons who have illnesses such as tuberculosis may remain relatively well. Still other persons may remain contagious throughout their convalescence. Asymptomatic carriers, such as patients recovering from typhoid, may go back to their communities and inadvertently infect others.

Symptoms of *localized infections,* such as bacterial infection of a wound, are essentially the symptoms of inflammation: redness, pain, warmth, and swelling. In addition, pus may form.

Patients with *generalized infections* may not show all the signs that are apparent in localized infections. Redness, for example, may not be visible. Pain may be moderate to severe, depending on the location of the infection. Swelling of infected tissues may produce symptoms ranging from mild to severe, depending on its location. Swelling in a large organ, such as the liver, may produce a dull ache, whereas swelling in a small structure, such as an infected appendix, may produce severe discomfort. Warmth is generally expressed as fever in a generalized infection as pyrogens are produced as part of the inflammatory process. Other symptoms that often are present in generalized infections include malaise, anorexia, and prostration.

In some cases, infections in the extremities such as the hands or feet exhibit a faint red line as infection extends upward along the lymphatic channels. Lymph nodes in this chain also are swollen and tender. Prompt antibiotic treatment is necessary in these cases.

TYPES OF INFECTIONS

Two types of infections are (1) community acquired and (2) health care–associated.

Community-Acquired Infections

Community-acquired infections are acquired in day-to-day contact with the public. Many viral infections are pervasive in society and occur at predictable times of the year. Childhood illnesses are common in September when children take to school all the new viruses they were exposed to during the summer. This sharing of microorganisms is made easier when 20 to 40 children occupy the same classroom. During the fall and winter, people share more indoor activities, thus increasing the likelihood that they will share microorganisms with one another.

Poverty, low immunization rates, overcrowding, unsanitary living conditions, and resistant strains of pathogens are at least partially responsible for the increase in infectious diseases that were once well controlled. The recent resurgence of tuberculosis is an example. This increase was attributed to poverty, the HIV/AIDS epidemic, an increase in the number of infected immigrants, declining public health resources, and the emergence of strains of bacteria that are resistant to multiple drugs. Effective treatment now requires at least two drugs to which a particular tuberculosis bacillus is susceptible.

Foodborne illness is a common community-acquired infectious disease. It is more common in the summer, when picnics and hot weather bring the possibility of food poisoning from *Staphylococcus* and *Salmonella* organisms. Periodic outbreaks of hepatitis A are possible at any time of the year and are the result of poor hygiene by food handlers.

Sexually transmitted infections such as gonorrhea, syphilis, and HIV also are spread into the community. These diseases and many others are required to be reported to public health authorities. The reports are important because they facilitate disease control, make possible the evaluation of control programs, and keep track of emerging disease patterns.

Certain communicable diseases must be reported to state health departments. State laws vary regarding which diseases must be reported. A list of reportable diseases is given in Box 13-1.

Prevention and Control. Prevention and control of communicable diseases are possible in a number of ways. Some childhood infectious diseases can be prevented by ensuring childhood immunizations. Indifference toward childhood immunizations has resulted in the re-emergence of several childhood diseases that were once well controlled. Although state laws that require certain

---

Box 13-1 | *Common Reportable Diseases*

Acquired immunodeficiency syndrome/HIV infection	Mumps
Amebiasis	Pertussis (whooping cough)
Anthrax	Plague
Aseptic meningitis	Poliomyelitis
Botulism	Psittacosis
Brucellosis	Rabies
Chancroid	Rheumatic fever
Cholera	Rocky Mountain spotted fever
Diphtheria	Rubella (German measles)
Encephalitis	Salmonellosis
Gonorrhea	Shigellosis
Granuloma inguinale	Syphilis
Hansen's disease (leprosy)	Tetanus
Hepatitis (all types)	Toxic shock syndrome
Legionellosis	Trichinosis
Leptospirosis	Tuberculosis
Lyme disease	Tularemia
Lymphogranuloma venereum	Typhoid fever
Malaria	Typhus
Measles (rubeola)	Yellow fever
Meningococcal infections	

immunizations before a child starts school have improved the picture somewhat, large groups of children from 2 to 5 years of age remain susceptible to serious illness. In addition, repeat vaccinations of older schoolchildren may be required to prevent illnesses such as measles. Adult immunizations also help prevent and control communicable diseases.

Although the solutions to this problem defy easy answers, at least part of the problem includes barriers in the health care system that result in missed opportunities to immunize those who are most susceptible. Barriers include such factors as rigid fee schedules; giving immunizations only during regular working hours, Monday through Friday; and giving immunizations only at official, fixed sites such as health departments. It is important for health professionals to take advantage of all possible opportunities to immunize. Schools, physicians' offices, shopping malls, and neighborhood health fairs are places where large numbers of children and parents may present themselves for immunization.

Transmission of infectious agents can be interrupted in a number of ways. First, education of food handlers regarding the importance of hand washing and proper food handling and refrigeration techniques decreases the spread of foodborne disease. Second, diseases such as tuberculosis can be detected through screening and treated early to prevent their spread. Isolation separates the infected individual from the public, thereby breaking the chain of infection. Other examples of measures aimed at interrupting transmission include control of vectors (spraying for mosquitos), administration of antimicrobials to children exposed to *Neisseria* meningitis, and the prompt treatment of streptococcal pharyngitis (strep throat). Sanitation of water supplies helps prevent the occurrence of waterborne diseases. Cooking meat, eggs, and poultry until well done kills bacteria that can cause serious illness and, in some cases, death.

Personal measures to control the spread of communicable disease include the use of personal barriers such as condoms and proper hygiene, especially hand washing. Deciding to stay home when symptoms of an infectious disease are present also can help break the chain of infection.

Health Care–Associated Infections

Health care–associated (nosocomial) infections are an important cause of increased morbidity, prolonged hospitalization, and higher health care costs. These infections occur within a health care facility and may affect both the patient and the health care worker. These infections are much more serious than those acquired in the community because strains of bacteria in the hospital are usually more virulent and often are resistant to antibiotics. In addition, the patient's resistance is already compromised from the disorder that led to hospitalization.

A growing number of pathogenic bacteria that are no longer susceptible to previously effective antibiotics are found in hospital patients. Vancomycin-resistant enterococcus (VRE) is one example; the incidence of vancomycin resistance in patients with nosocomial enterococcal infection is rapidly increasing. The Centers for Disease Control and Prevention (CDC) has emphasized the importance of the careful use of antibiotics and infection control measures in preventing the spread of VRE. In health care agencies where the use of antibiotics has increased, an increase in bacterial resistance is also found. Antibiotics alter the body's normal flora so that resistant strains of enterococci replace susceptible strains. To prevent VRE infection, the CDC has recommended the following guidelines for limiting patient-to-patient transmission:

- Place VRE-infected patients in a single room or in a room with other VRE patients.
- If the patient must be transported from the room, take precautions to minimize the risk of transmission of microorganisms to other people and to prevent contamination of the environment and equipment.
- Wear clean, nonsterile gloves while in the room because organisms can extensively contaminate surfaces such as doorknobs and side rails (fomites).
- Wear a gown when you anticipate substantial contact with the patient or surfaces in the room or if you anticipate contact with urine, stool, or wound drainage.
- Remove gloves and gown before leaving the patient's room, and wash your hands immediately with an antiseptic soap or a waterless antiseptic agent.
- After removing your gown and gloves and washing your hands, make sure that your hands and clothing do not touch surfaces, such as curtains or doorknobs, that may be contaminated.
- Use separate thermometers and stethoscopes for VRE-infected patients.
- Make sure that all patient care equipment used with VRE-infected patients is carefully disinfected.

Bacteria employ a variety of mechanisms to develop resistant strains. Bacterial cells normally develop mutations. Because antibiotics suppress normal forms of the bacteria, the mutations have opportunity to grow. Chromosomal mutation also permits some bacteria to produce enzymes that deactivate the antibiotic. Some bacteria are able to alter their metabolic cycles to avoid destruction by antibiotics. Finally, mutation alters bacterial cell membranes, making antibiotic penetration more difficult. Newer antibiotics are then developed to counteract the most resistant strains. As these antibiotics in turn become more frequently used, resistance again develops and the cycle is repeated. This cycle can be slowed by the practice of culturing wound drainage fluid, collecting urine and blood for laboratory analysis, and identifying specific pathogens and their sensitivities to specific antibiotics. This practice allows more specific therapy to be administered and delays the onset of resistant strains. Efforts also are made to limit the use of antibiotics that are effective against resistant strains. This practice provides fewer opportunities for the development of strains resistant to the drug.

Nosocomial infections are more serious for the hospitalized patient who may have low resistance. These infections also have been exposed to many antibiotics so they are more likely to resist therapy. Patients with compromised immune systems are much more susceptible to hospital-acquired infections. These groups include patients with AIDS and cancer patients who are receiving chemotherapy. Common sites for nosocomial infections in hospitalized patients include surgical wounds, the urinary tract, and the respiratory tract. Occasionally a patient who has had a urinary catheter inserted develops a urinary tract infection because of improper technique during insertion. The risk for this infection can be reduced by using proper techniques for catheter insertion and care for indwelling catheters. Health care workers are also at higher risk for hospital-acquired infections. Hepatitis B, for example, may be transmitted through needle punctures. Small, open wounds on the upper extremities may come in contact with resistant strains of *Staphylococcus* or *Pseudomonas* and become infected. In addition, health care workers and patients have developed Legionnaire's disease when *Legionella* was spread through the facility on air currents from air conditioning systems that became contaminated with infected water.

Iatrogenic infections are caused by the treatment given the patient. For example, iatrogenic infections may be caused by giving immunosuppressive drugs to prevent rejection of a transplanted organ, resulting in an infection. Another form of iatrogenic infection can be caused by the treatment of a primary infection. Antibiotic therapy for one microorganism can cause the overgrowth of a second microorganism that can also cause illness. The term for this process is *superinfection*. It is especially common with treatment using broad-spectrum antibiotics. An example of this phenomenon is the occurrence of a bowel infection after treatment with oral broad-spectrum antibiotics. The organism *Clostridium difficile* resides in the gastrointestinal tract of many individuals. It is kept in check by the normal bacterial flora of the gastrointestinal tract. Broad-spectrum antibiotics can kill enough of the normal flora to allow *C. difficile* to grow out of control, producing severe colitis and diarrhea.

CARE OF PATIENTS WITH INFECTION

Just as controls must be instituted to stop the spread of infections acquired in the community, so must there be a process to keep hospitalized patients from acquiring a nosocomial infection. The key to preventing the spread of infection is good medical and surgical asepsis.

MEDICAL ASEPSIS

Medical asepsis means limiting the spread of microorganisms as much as possible. This is often called *clean technique* and refers to practices such as changing bed linen, sanitizing bedpans, using individual medication cups for each patient and for each medication administration, and frequent hand washing.

Hand Washing

The most basic and effective method of preventing cross-contamination is hand washing (Fig. 13-3). Soiled hands are the primary mode of transmission of nosocomial infections. Although everyone agrees in principle with the need for frequent hand washing, problems arise when nurses are busy. For example, suppose a nurse is passing medications and is asked by a patient with pulmonary secretions to hand her the box of tissues. At the same time, the patient's roommate asks the nurse to fill her water glass. After doing this, the nurse hurries out of the room to assist a physician with a procedure. This example illustrates how a chain of infection begins. Unless the nurse interrupts the chain with good hand-washing technique, infection is easily spread from one patient to another.

Good hand-washing technique includes the use of running water, soap, and friction. The lathered hands should be rubbed together for at least 15 seconds, and longer if the nurse works in a high-risk area. The use of antimicrobial soaps is also recommended when working with patients who are more susceptible to infection, such as premature infants or immunocompromised patients.

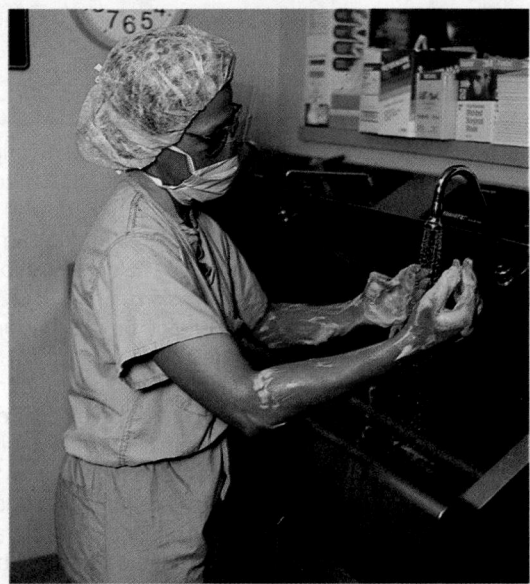

FIGURE **13-3** Hand washing is the most basic and effective way to prevent cross-contamination.

SURGICAL ASEPSIS

Surgical asepsis, or *sterile technique*, refers to the elimination of microorganisms from any object that comes in contact with the patient. This practice includes care techniques that prevent unsterile surfaces from coming in contact with the patient, such as during dressing changes.

STANDARD PRECAUTIONS

A set of infection control guidelines has been developed for hospitals and other health care agencies by the Hospital Infection Control Practices Advisory Committee (HICPAC) and the CDC. Previously the terms *Universal Precautions, Body Substance Isolation Precautions,* and *Disease-Specific Isolation Precautions* were in use. The current guidelines, called *Standard Precautions,* combine the major features of Universal Precautions and Body Substance Isolation Precautions. Standard Precautions are used for the care of all patients in hospitals regardless of their isolation status. All patients who previously required category- and disease-specific precautions are now covered under Standard Precautions. Another change from the previous (1983) CDC guidelines combined the old categories of Isolation Precautions (strict isolation, contact isolation, respiratory isolation, tuberculosis isolation, enteric precautions, and drainage/secretion precautions) and the old disease-specific precautions into *Transmission-Based Precautions.*

Use Standard Precautions when you perform procedures in which you will have contact with a patient's blood, body fluids, secretions (except sweat), excretions, broken skin, and mucous membranes. In addition, use Standard Precautions when you have contact with materials that are soiled or contaminated with body fluids or blood. Use Standard Precautions with all patients, no matter what their diagnosis or infectious status may be. Guidelines for the use of Standard Precautions are listed in Box 13-2.

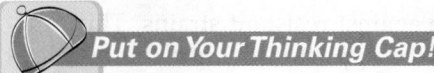
Put on Your Thinking Cap!

For one clinical day, note everything you did that represents the use of Standard Precautions.

TRANSMISSION-BASED (ISOLATION) PRECAUTIONS

To prevent the spread of infection in a health care facility, infected patients are sometimes isolated from other patients. Precautions and examples of illnesses requiring Transmission-Based Precautions are listed in Box 13-3. The extent of the isolation depends on the type of infection. Patients infected with highly virulent microorganisms that are spread easily by air or direct contact require strict precautions. Microorganisms that are less easily spread require less stringent precautions. The Transmission-Based Precautions were developed to reduce the risk of airborne, droplet, and contact transmission in hospitals. Guidelines for using Transmission-Based Precautions are listed in Box 13-4.

Airborne Precautions

Use Airborne Precautions when caring for patients who have diseases that are spread through the air. Examples of diseases that are spread through the air are tuberculosis, varicella (chickenpox), and rubeola (measles). Respiratory protection, provided by wearing properly fitted high-efficiency particulate air (HEPA) filter respirators or N95 respirators, is indicated when entering the room of patients with tuberculosis. A private room is required. Also recommended is a ventilation sys-

---

Box 13-2 | *Guidelines for Use of Standard Precautions*

These precautions are to be used for the care of all patients.
Wash hands immediately after touching blood, body fluids, secretions, excretions, and contaminated objects, even if gloves were worn.
Wash hands between tasks and procedures on the same patient to prevent cross-contamination of different body sites.
Wear gloves when touching blood, body fluids, secretions, and contaminated objects. Put on clean gloves before touching mucous membranes and nonintact skin.
Change gloves after each patient contact, before touching noncontaminated items and environmental surfaces. If patient is allergic to latex, use only non-latex gloves.
Wear masks, eye protection, or face shields to protect mucous membranes of the eyes, nose, and mouth during procedures that are likely to generate splashes of blood, body fluids, secretions, or excretions.
Wear gowns during procedures that are likely to result in splashes of blood, body fluids, secretions, or excretions.
Handle patient care equipment soiled with blood, body fluids, secretions, and excretions so that skin and mucous membrane exposures, contamination of clothing, and transfer of microorganisms to other settings are prevented.
Place needles and sharp instruments in puncture-resistant containers for disposal to prevent injuries from needles or other sharp items. Do not recap or bend needles or remove them from the syringe.
Perform mouth-to-mouth resuscitation using mouthpieces or other ventilation devices.

Data from *CDC Isolation Guidelines, 1996.* (1996). Atlanta: U.S. Centers for Disease Control and Prevention.

tem that prevents contaminated air from being vented outside the room. In addition, patients with infections spread by airborne transmission must wear surgical masks when leaving their rooms. Surgical masks filter expired air; respirators such as the HEPA filter respirator and the N95 respirator filter inspired air.

Droplet Precautions

Use Droplet Precautions when taking care of patients with infections that are spread by droplets or dust particles containing the infectious agent. Droplets are spread primarily during coughing, sneezing, or talking and during certain procedures such as suctioning and bronchoscopy. Because droplets usually travel only about 3 feet before falling from the air, special air handling and ventilation are not required to prevent droplet transmission, as is the case with Airborne Precautions. The door to the room may be left open. Diseases transmitted by droplets include rubella, mumps, diphtheria, and influenza. Patients should be placed in private rooms. Wear a surgical mask when you are within 3 feet of the patient to protect yourself from contaminated droplets.

Contact Precautions

Use Contact Precautions when you are caring for patients who are infected by microorganisms that are transmitted by direct (skin-to-skin) or indirect contact with contaminated equipment. Needles, dressings, stethoscopes, bed rails, and doorknobs may become contaminated. The patient is placed in a private room. Wear gloves when entering the infected patient's room; before leaving the patient's room, remove your gloves and wash your hands. Wear a gown if your clothing will come in contact with the patient, contaminated equipment, or environmental surfaces in the patient's room. A gown is also recommended if the patient is incontinent or has wound drainage. Remove the gown before leaving the patient's room. In addition, use dedicated equipment when treating patients with multidrug-resistant organisms. Contact Precautions are used for conditions such as gastrointestinal, respiratory,

---

Box 13-3 *Types of Precautions and Patients with Whom Precautions Must Be Used*

Standard Precautions
Use Standard Precautions for the care of all patients.

Airborne Precautions
In addition to Standard Precautions, use Airborne Precautions for patients known or suspected to have serious illnesses transmitted by airborne droplet nuclei. Examples of such illnesses include the following:
  Measles
  Varicella (including disseminated zoster)
  Tuberculosis

Droplet Precautions
In addition to Standard Precautions, use Droplet Precautions for patients known or suspected to have serious illnesses transmitted by large-particle droplets. Examples of such illnesses include the following:
  Invasive *Haemophilus influenzae* type b disease, including meningitis, pneumonia, epiglottitis, and sepsis
  Invasive *Neisseria meningitidis* disease, including meningitis, pneumonia, and sepsis
  Other serious bacterial respiratory infections spread by droplet transmission, including:
  Diphtheria (pharyngeal)
  Mycoplasma pneumoniae
  Pertussis
  Pneumonic plague
  Streptococcal (group A) pharyngitis, pneumonia, or scarlet fever in infants and young children
  Serious viral infections spread by droplet transmission, including:
  Adenovirus
  Influenza
  Mumps
  Parvovirus B19
  Rubella

Contact Precautions
In addition to Standard Precautions, use Contact Precautions for patients known or suspected to have serious illnesses easily transmitted by direct patient contact or by contact with items in the patient's environment. The following are examples of such illnesses:
  Gastrointestinal, respiratory, skin, or wound infections or colonization with multidrug-resistant bacteria judged by the infection control program, based on current state, regional, or national recommendations, to be of special clinical and epidemiological significance
  Enteric infections with a prolonged environmental survival, including:
  Clostridium difficile
  For diapered or incontinent patients:
  Enterohemorrhagic *Escherichia coli* 0157:H7, *Shigella*, hepatitis A, or rotavirus
  Respiratory syncytial virus, parainfluenza virus, or enteroviral infections in infants and young children
  Skin infections that are highly contagious or that may occur on dry skin, including:
  Diphtheria (cutaneous)
  Herpes simplex virus (neonatal or mucocutaneous)
  Impetigo
  Major (noncontained) abscesses, cellulitis, or decubitus
  Pediculosis
  Scabies
  Staphylococcal furunculosis in infants and young children
  Herpes zoster (disseminated or in the immunocompromised host)
  Viral/hemorrhagic conjunctivitis
  Viral hemorrhagic infections

Data from *CDC Isolation Guidelines, 1996.* (1996). Atlanta: U.S. Centers for Disease Control and Prevention.

Box 13-4 | *Guidelines for Use of Transmission-Based Precautions*

Airborne Precautions

Use Airborne Precautions with patients who have microorganisms transmitted by droplet nuclei smaller than 5 microns. Patients with tuberculosis, measles (rubeola), and chickenpox (varicella) are in this category.

Patient Placement. Place the patient in a private room with negative air pressure of 6 to 12 air changes per hour. Keep the patient in the room with the door closed. When a private room is not available, place the patient in a room with a patient who has the same microorganism, but with no other infection (cohort).

Respiratory Protection. Wear respiratory protection when entering the room of patients with tuberculosis. If susceptible persons must enter the room of patients with rubeola or varicella, they should wear respiratory protection.

Patient Transport. Limit patient to essential transport only. If patient must be transported, place a surgical mask on the patient.

Droplets Precautions

Use Droplet Precautions for patients infected with microorganisms that are larger than 5 microns that are spread by coughing, sneezing, talking, or the performance of procedures. Patients with diphtheria, rubella, streptococcal pharyngitis, pneumonia, and mumps are in this category.

Patient Placement. Place the patient in a private room or with a cohort if a private room is not available. The door may remain open, and special air handling and ventilation are not necessary.

Mask. Wear a mask when working within 3 feet of the patient; many hospitals require wearing a mask to enter the room.

Patient Transport. Limit the transport of patients to essential trips only. If transport of the patient is necessary, minimize patient spread of droplets by masking the patient.

Contact Precautions

Use Contact Precautions for patients with microorganisms that can be transmitted by direct contact with the patient (hand or skin-to-skin contact) or indirect contact (touching surfaces or environmental items). Patients with multidrug-resistant organisms, major wound infections, *Shigella*, herpes simplex, and scabies are in this category.

Patient Placement. Place the patient in a private room or with a cohort.

Gloves and Hand Washing. Wear clean gloves when entering the room. Change gloves after contact with infective material. Remove gloves before leaving the patient's room, and wash hands immediately.

Gown. Wear a gown into the room if you think your clothing will have contact with the patient or environmental surfaces or if the patient is incontinent or has diarrhea. Remove the gown before leaving the patient's room.

Patient Transport. Limit the transport of patients to essential trips only. If the patient must be transported, make sure precautions are implemented to reduce transmission of microorganisms.

Patient Care Equipment. Dedicate the use of equipment to a single patient to avoid sharing between patients. If you must use common equipment, clean and disinfect it before use for another patient.

Data from *CDC Isolation Guidelines, 1996.* (1996). Atlanta: U.S. Centers for Disease Control and Prevention.

skin, or wound infections with multiple antimicrobial-resistant microorganisms such as VRE and methicillin-resistant *Staphylococcus aureus* (MRSA). Contagious skin diseases, such as impetigo and scabies, as well as respiratory syncytial virus represent conditions requiring Contact Precautions. Clinical conditions, potential pathogens, and recommended precautions are listed in Box 13-3.

BIOTERRORISM

So far, we have been discussing infection as a communicable disease that is assumed to be transmitted by unintentional or careless exposure to a pathogen. However, a special situation called *bioterrorism* is the intentional use of microorganisms to cause death or disease. Methods used to spread agents of bioterrorism are varied and might include powders, aerosols, or contamination of food or water. Among the pathogens considered potential biologic weapons are those that cause anthrax, botulism, plague, smallpox, tularemia, and Ebola. In addition to pathogens, bioterrorists may use toxins such as ricin, chemicals such as sarin, and radioactive material released in small explosions ("dirty bombs"). Nurses should be aware of their employing agency's plans for dealing with public exposure to bioterrorism agents including decontamination procedures and personal protective equipment and procedures (The Bioterrorism Institute, 2005).

IMMUNOCOMPROMISED PATIENTS

Immunocompromised patients have decreased immunity to infection and are at increased risk for bacterial, fungal, parasitic, and viral infections. Patients receiving chemotherapy and other patients with low white blood cell counts are at increased risk of infection. Leukemia and aplastic anemia are two examples of disorders that cause low white blood cell counts. The use of Standard Precautions for all patients and of Transmission-Based Precautions for specific situations should reduce the risk of acquiring infections from other persons and from the environment. See Chapter 33 for a discussion of precautions to be used with immunocompromised patients.

NURSING CARE *of Patients with Infections*

Patients with generalized infections easily become dehydrated because of fever and anorexia. Urge the patient to consume adequate fluids, especially water. Fluid intake should be at least 2 liters per day to replace fluids lost through perspiration. Fluid intake is also important in the transportation of nutrients to the cells to fight infection. Nutrition is very important. Encourage patients to consume a high-protein, high-vitamin diet. Vitamin C is important for wound healing and in the prevention of future infections. The patient with a poor appetite may benefit from a consultation with a dietitian.

If a patient's infection requires isolation, remember that effective isolation techniques may also isolate the patient from normal human contact. You may be tempted to hasten your work to minimize your chance of becoming infected. Forced seclusion can cause patients, particularly children, to feel lonely, rejected, and depressed. Engage the patient in conversation while giving direct care. Discussing subjects other than the patient's disease may lessen the feeling of being unclean or rejected. Encourage the patient to move about as much as possible to increase stimulation.

Under the current CDC guidelines, some infections and conditions fall into two categories because the microorganisms are transmitted in more than one way. For example, chickenpox can spread through both the airborne and contact routes. Both Airborne Precautions and Contact Precautions are followed.

Laboratory tests used to screen patients for infection include the following:

- White blood cell count—increased in infection
- Erythrocyte sedimentation rate—elevated with inflammation
- Iron level—decreased in chronic infection
- Cultures of urine, blood, wound, sputum, and throat—infectious microorganisms are found in the culture
- White cell differential count (neutrophils, lymphocytes, monocytes, and eosinophils)—increased; used to help differentiate causes of infection

Examples of nursing diagnoses for patients with infections or who are vulnerable to infections include Risk for Infection, Risk for Injury, Impaired Tissue Integrity, Social Isolation, and Disturbed Body Image. Ineffective Therapeutic Regimen Management is another related nursing diagnosis. The primary goals in caring for patients with infection are recovery from the infection and prevention of the spread of infection to others.

Antibiotic drug therapy is the cornerstone of treatment for many infections. Early hospital discharges mean that patients are frequently discharged on a regimen of oral antibiotics. Many people stop taking antibiotics once they begin to feel better. This permits surviving organisms, which may be resistant, to thrive, possibly causing a recurrence of illness. Therefore caution patients not to stop taking the medication when

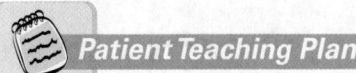

Patient Teaching Plan

Hyperbaric Oxygen Therapy

- Do not smoke for several hours before and after treatment to decrease lung irritation.
- You can prevent pressure buildup in the ears by swallowing.
- You must wear 100% cotton clothing in the hyperbaric oxygen chamber to prevent static electricity.

they start feeling better. They should continue their antibiotics until the entire course has been completed or until their physician specifically orders them to stop taking the medication. The emergence of antibiotic resistance is one important reason why antibiotic therapy for bacterial infections may fail. Increasingly, bacteria are becoming resistant, often because of the widespread or inappropriate use of antibiotics, which leads to the killing of susceptible bacteria and allows more resistant strains to multiply.

Hyperbaric oxygen therapy is an intervention that is used to treat infection. Breathing 100% oxygen at higher-than-atmospheric pressure in a closed chamber increases the amount of dissolved oxygen transported in plasma. The oxygen-rich environment improves leukocyte phagocytic activity and kills anaerobic bacteria. See the Patient Teaching Plan above.

During hyperbaric oxygen therapy, the patient must be monitored for the following complications: ear or sinus pain (from pressure buildup), respiratory problems (as a result of oxygen toxicity), seizures (a central nervous system symptom of oxygen toxicity), and bradycardia (reflex response to oxygen toxicity).

Earlier hospital discharges mean that substantial therapy may continue in the home after discharge. Home health care is frequently ordered for infected patients for a number of reasons. The patient has fewer opportunities to acquire a nosocomial infection, there are fewer opportunities for infection to be spread to other hospitalized patients, and patients often do better in their own surroundings. If therapy is to be continued at home, teach the patient and other family members how to manage the remaining part of the care. Close coordination between the hospital nurse and the home health nurse is important to ensure good continuity of care. Guidelines for infection control in the home are given in the Patient Teaching Plan on p. 174.

IMMUNITY

The immune system is the body's defense network against infection. **Immunity** provides the body with resistance to invading organisms and enables it to fight off invaders once they have gained access. The body is constantly exposed to microorganisms capable of causing

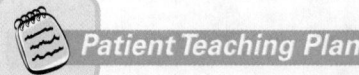

Infection Control in the Home

Infection control in the home setting is based on Standard Precautions. In the home, adapt the guidelines to the equipment and supplies available:

• *Equipment:* List for the family the activities that require the use of gloves, and identify the proper gloves to use. Instruct caregivers to use an apron if clothing is likely to become contaminated and to wear gloves to change dressings.

• *Hand Washing:* Demonstrate good hand-washing technique to all household members. Tell family members that hand washing is the most important action they can take to prevent the spread of infection, and inform them when hand washing is appropriate.

• *Sharps Disposal:* If a sharps container is not available, tell the family to use a puncture-resistant container such as a detergent bottle or coffee can with the lid securely taped.

• *Bandages and Linens:* Instruct household members to seal soiled dressings tightly in a plastic bag and dispose of dressings in the trash bag. Clothing and linens with body fluids should be stored in a plastic bag until they are laundered, at which time they should be washed in water as hot as the fabric will tolerate. One cup of bleach is added to the detergent in each load.

• *Spills:* Instruct household members to wash contaminated surfaces with detergent and water and then wash the surfaces with a freshly made solution of 1:10 household bleach. Disposable towels should be used.

• *Dishes:* Leftover portions of uneaten food should not be saved. Soiled dishes should be washed in detergent and hot water immediately after use.

---

disease. If the immune system is intact and functioning properly, it is able to provide adequate protection from most infections and diseases in a healthy individual. When the immune system is not functioning properly, the potential for overwhelming infection exists. Many factors can compromise the immune system, such as disease states, congenital defects, aging, stress, and therapeutic interventions (e.g., drugs, radiation therapy). Understanding the normal immune response and common immune system disorders will help you assess patients at risk for infection and provide appropriate interventions.

Any substance that is capable of stimulating a response from the immune system is called an **antigen**. In most cases the antigen is foreign to the body, and the body recognizes the antigen because it is different from itself (nonself). Antigens can be microorganisms (bacteria, viruses, fungi, parasites), abnormal or mutated body cells, transplanted cells (from blood transfusions, organ transplants), noninfectious substances from the environment (pollens, insect venom, foods), or foreign molecules from drugs such as penicillin. When healthy, the body protects what it recognizes

as self and attempts to destroy that which is nonself. Tissue that is normally recognized as self may be seen as nonself by the immune system if the tissue undergoes change (mutation), is in an abnormal location, or changes structure. Once the body recognizes a substance as an antigen, natural and acquired defenses are put into action to destroy the invader and prevent disease.

Antibodies, also known as *immunoglobulins*, are proteins that are created in response to specific antigens. The formation and function of antibodies are discussed in the "Antibody-Mediated (Immediate) Immunity" section of this chapter, p. 175.

INNATE (NATURAL) VERSUS ACQUIRED IMMUNITY

Innate (natural) immunity is present in the body at birth and is not dependent on a specific immune response or previous contact with an infectious agent. It may be specific to a species, a race, or an individual. For instance, humans are not as susceptible to distemper as dogs and cats are. Factors such as nutritional status, stress, and environment may influence natural immunity. Nonspecific defense mechanisms that include physical and chemical barriers to infection, phagocytosis (the process of enveloping and destroying foreign matter), and the inflammatory process contribute to natural immunity.

An individual develops acquired immunity after birth as a result of the body's natural immune responses to antigens. Acquired immunity depends on the proper development and functioning of B and T lymphocytes, which are white blood cells that fight infection.

Active acquired immunity is developed after direct contact with an antigen through illness or vaccination. Vaccinations may be prepared by three methods: (1) using dead organisms that can no longer cause disease, as in the diphtheria and pertussis vaccines; (2) destroying bacterial toxins that act as antigens, as in the tetanus toxoid vaccine; and (3) altering the structure of live organisms so that they are unable to cause disease yet maintain their antigenic properties to prevent many viral diseases, such as measles and poliomyelitis vaccines. Once the body has been exposed to an antigen through illness or vaccination, antibodies develop and retain memory for the antigen. If the body is exposed to the same antigen later, the antibodies can react quickly to fight off disease.

When people are injected with immune globulin or antiserum (made from human or animal blood) that contains antibodies to a specific agent, such as for the emergency treatment of snakebite, rabies, or exposure to hepatitis, they receive antibodies or lymphocytes that were produced by another individual. This type of immunity, called *passive acquired immunity*, is temporary and is the kind of immunity newborns receive from their mothers through the placenta or through ingestion of breast milk (especially colostrum).

Both natural and acquired immunity are necessary for a healthy individual to have protection from disease. Innate and acquired immunity are discussed further in Chapter 33.

CELLS AND ORGANS INVOLVED IN IMMUNITY

A variety of cells work together to provide the body with an adequate defense against injury or disease. Leukocytes (white blood cells) play a key role in immune responses to infectious organisms and other antigens. There are two categories of white blood cells: granulocytes and nongranulocytes. Blood cells involved in immune disorders are described in Chapter 32.

Although all parts of the body work together as a whole to resist and fight off disease, several organs are vital to a functional immune system. They include the thymus, bone marrow, lymph nodes, spleen, and liver (Fig. 13-4). The thymus and bone marrow participate in the formation and maturation of immune system cells. Located throughout the body, the lymph nodes attack antigens and debris in the interstitial fluid and produce and circulate lymphocytes. The spleen acts as a filter to remove dead cells, debris, and foreign molecules from the blood. The liver filters the blood and plays a part in the production of specific immunoglobulins and other chemicals involved in the immune response.

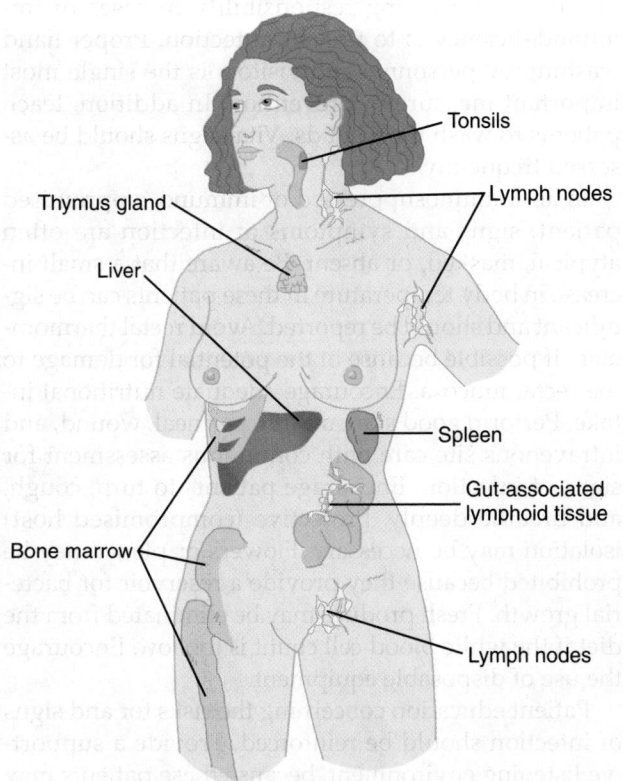

FIGURE **13-4** Organs involved in immunity.

Tonsils

Lymph nodes

Thymus gland

Liver

Spleen

Gut-associated lymphoid tissue

Bone marrow

Lymph nodes

NONSPECIFIC DEFENSES AGAINST INFECTION

Innate (natural) immunity is present at birth and consists of physical and chemical barriers to invasion of the body as well as processes and substances that protect and repair tissues and stimulate the body to fight off disease. Physical and chemical barriers, inflammation, and phagocytosis are nonspecific defenses against infection.

Other nonspecific defenses against infection that protect the body include complement, pyrogen, and interferon. Complement is a series of proteins that enhance the inflammatory process and the immune response. Chemotaxis, phagocytosis, and the activity of antibodies are stimulated by complement. Pyrogen (an eicosanoid) is a substance released in inflammation that causes body temperature to increase. Fever is thought to inhibit the growth of pathogens and slow enzymatic reactions that occur in infectious processes. Another substance, interferon, is produced in viral infections and acts to inhibit the replication of viruses. Interferon (a cytokine) also affects the function of T lymphocytes and is used in the treatment of selected malignancies. Eicosanoids and cytokines are discussed in Chapter 33.

SPECIFIC DEFENSES AGAINST INFECTION—THE IMMUNE RESPONSE

The immune response is the process by which antigens are recognized as foreign, processed, and destroyed. The two types of immune responses, antibody-mediated (immediate or humoral) and cell-mediated, function interdependently to provide the immune response.

ANTIBODY-MEDIATED (IMMEDIATE) IMMUNITY

Antibody-mediated (humoral) immunity is immediate. This first-line defense involves B lymphocytes and the production of antibodies in response to specific antigens. The humoral immune response is initiated when an antigen binds to a special receptor on a B lymphocyte. This results in the production of antibodies that seek out and "stick to" specific antigens in the body. This combination forms antigen-antibody complexes, which are then targeted for cleanup by neutrophils and macrophages. Formation of these complexes activates complement and intensifies T-lymphocyte activity. Because circulating antibodies bind with antigens as soon as they are recognized, the chemical process is triggered immediately.

Antibodies (immunoglobulins) are divided into five classes: IgG, IgM, IgA, IgE, and IgD. IgG is the most abundant immunoglobulin; it crosses the placenta to provide passive immunity for the newborn. IgE is important in allergic reactions and in parasitic infections.

CELL-MEDIATED (DELAYED) IMMUNITY

Cell-mediated immunity is a delayed response to injury or infection. Cellular immunity is delayed because of the time needed for the migration of T cells and for the production of substances that enhance the immune response and influence the destruction of antigens.

T cells include helper cells, suppressor cells, and killer cells. Helper T cells enhance humoral immunity; suppressor T cells help "turn off" the humoral response. Disease may occur when the normal ratio of helper to suppressor cells (2:1) is altered. In AIDS, for instance, the number of helper T cells is diminished. When the number of suppressor T cells is too high, infections, allergy, or immune disease develop. Killer T cells directly destroy antigens.

Cellular immunity fights most viral or bacterial infections and hinders the growth of malignant cells. This process also launches an attack on transplanted tissue or organs in the body.

IMMUNODEFICIENCY

ETIOLOGY AND RISK FACTORS

When the body's self-defenses against foreign invasion fail to function normally, a state of immunodeficiency (immunosuppression) exists. In this state, known as an *immunocompromised* or *immunosuppressed state*, the body is unable to launch an adequate immune response and is at great risk for infection. The primary clinical clue to immunodeficiency, whatever the cause, is the tendency to develop recurrent infections. Immunodeficiencies can be congenital or, more commonly, acquired, and can result from problems with humoral immunity, cell-mediated immunity, vital mediators such as complement, or the process of phagocytosis.

In congenital immunodeficiencies, some part of the immune system fails to develop properly. The result is a defect in the B or T lymphocytes, phagocytes, or complement.

Acquired immunodeficiencies result from factors outside the immune system that render a previously functional immune system inadequate. Some causes of acquired deficiencies are infections, malignancies, autoimmune diseases (systemic lupus erythematosus, rheumatoid arthritis), chronic diseases (diabetes mellitus, renal disease), drugs, aging, stress, and malnutrition.

Stress, whether physical or emotional, alters the body's response to disease. Although the mechanism is not fully understood, the release of hormones plays a part. Stressors include such things as serious illness, job loss, and divorce; even noise and cold play a part.

The nutritional state of the patient also affects immunity. The malnourished patient is much more susceptible to infection, especially when a protein deficiency exists. People with chronic conditions such as diabetes and renal disease may become debilitated and unable to fully resist infection. Trauma victims, especially those with burns, have diminished immune responses. Many malignant disorders alter the functioning of the immune system. Infectious diseases also cause immunodeficiencies, especially acute viral infections.

Many treatments and interventions aimed at helping patients cause immunodeficiency. Medications often place patients at risk for infection—corticosteroids, antineoplastic drugs (used to treat cancer), and immunosuppressive drugs (used for transplant recipients) are a few.

Surgery, anesthesia, and irradiation for cancer also can alter immune function. In addition, invasive procedures such as urinary catheterization and venipuncture for intravenous therapy or blood work bypass the patient's first line of defense. In the hospitalized patient, all of these factors come into play—disease, stress, nutritional alterations, medications, and invasive procedures all set the patient up for infection.

MEDICAL TREATMENT

Congenital immunodeficiencies usually are treated with replacement therapy of the deficient immune component. Bone marrow transplants or fetal thymus tissue transplants may be used in some cases. Treating an acquired immunodeficiency entails correcting the underlying condition that is causing the problem, such as reducing stressors, correcting malnutrition, and discontinuing medications that alter immunity.

NURSING CARE *of the Immunosuppressed Patient*

The primary nursing responsibility in cases of immunodeficiency is to prevent infection. Proper hand washing by personnel and visitors is the single most important measure in prevention. In addition, teach patients to wash their hands. Vital signs should be assessed frequently.

In an immunosuppressed or immunocompromised patient, signs and symptoms of infection are often atypical, masked, or absent. Be aware that a small increase in body temperature in these patients can be significant and should be reported. Avoid rectal thermometers if possible because of the potential for damage to the rectal mucosa. Encourage adequate nutritional intake. Perform good skin, mouth, perineal, wound, and intravenous site care with continuous assessment for signs of infection. Encourage patients to turn, cough, and breathe deeply. Protective (compromised host) isolation may be necessary. Flowers or plants may be prohibited because they provide a reservoir for bacterial growth. Fresh produce may be eliminated from the diet if the white blood cell count is too low. Encourage the use of disposable equipment.

Patient education concerning the risks for and signs of infection should be reinforced. Provide a supportive listening environment, because these patients may have anxiety as well as a high stress level and often feelings of powerlessness are overwhelming.

HYPERSENSITIVITY AND ALLERGY

ETIOLOGY AND RISK FACTORS

The term *allergy* (or *hypersensitivity*) describes an atypical immune response that is activated by a foreign substance that normally is inoffensive. Although immune responses usually are beneficial, hypersensitivity can be harmful, even deadly. It is estimated that 20% to 25% of the U.S. population suffer from allergies of some sort, with allergic rhinitis (hay fever) and asthma occurring most often. Other allergic disorders include allergic contact dermatitis, angioedema (localized swelling), dermatitis, anaphylaxis (severe allergic reaction), gastrointestinal allergies, and urticaria (hives). The tendency to develop an allergy is inherited, although the type of allergy may vary. Someone who is prone to allergies may be referred to as *atopic*. Hypersensitivity as an immune disorder is discussed in Chapter 33.

An antigen that causes a hypersensitive reaction is called an **allergen.** Any substance can act as an allergen to a susceptible person, but some of the more common ones are house dust, animal dander, pollens, molds, foods, pharmacologic agents, cigarette smoke, feathers, and insect venoms. Table 13-1 lists common allergens.

The allergic response begins with sensitization. The first encounter with a specific allergen results in only a small amount of antibody production. With subsequent exposure, however, the body steps up its defense by producing large amounts of antibodies, which circulate in the bloodstream and travel to the affected tissues. This triggers the release of histamine and other chemical agents. Neutrophils arrive at the scene to engulf and destroy the antigens. A cascade of reactions occur that produce the symptoms typical of an allergic response, although they vary according to the area affected. Local manifestations of allergic reactions include urticaria, pruritus, conjunctivitis, rhinitis, laryngeal edema, bronchospasm, dysrhythmia, gastrointestinal cramps and malabsorption, and angioedema.

MEDICAL TREATMENT

The medical treatment of allergic patients varies depending on the specific allergy. In general, antihistamines are used to reduce the symptoms caused by histamine release. Many people suffer side effects from antihistamines, such as dry mouth, nausea, blurred vision, dizziness, and drowsiness. For asthma sufferers, bronchodilators, corticosteroids, or both may be prescribed to improve air movement and decrease inflammation in the lungs; oxygen and breathing treatments may also be ordered. Besides antihistamines, topical lotions and ointments may be prescribed to relieve itching associated with urticaria, atopic dermatitis, or allergic contact dermatitis.

Long-term medical treatment of allergies involves testing to determine specific allergens. Testing is performed by injecting small amounts of allergen under the skin (intradermally) or by pricking the surface of the patient's skin and monitoring for the degree of wheal-and-flare reaction. After the specific agents have been identified, the patient may be desensitized by injections of minute quantities of the allergen, with the dosage gradually increased over a prolonged period of time. Desensitization is aimed at increasing tolerance to the offending agent and decreasing the severity of the allergic response.

NURSING CARE *of the Patient with Allergies*

When dealing with the hospitalized allergic patient, the most important nursing intervention is to document all allergies, the symptoms they cause, and any treatment currently used. Allergies should be posted on the front of the patient's chart, on all medication records, on the nursing care plan, and on a patient identification band. Never administer any drug to which the patient reports a previous allergic reaction.

Alert the pharmacy and dietary departments to drug and food allergies. Notify the physician of any allergies that may determine which medications to avoid. For instance, a patient who is allergic to shellfish should not receive drugs containing iodine because an anaphylactic reaction may result. Make sure that patients who have been taking allergy medication, such as inhaler treatments, continue taking these medications when admitted to the hospital. A growing number of patients, as well as health care providers, are reporting latex allergies, necessitating the use of non-latex gloves.

Patient education is important for all patients with allergies. This includes knowledge of specific allergens, limiting exposure to or avoiding allergens, the proper use of medications such as inhaled bronchodilators, and the actions and side effects of drugs. Patients who are at risk for life-threatening (anaphylactic) reactions

Table 13-1 | *Common Allergies and Their Causes*

ALLERGIC REACTION	STIMULUS
Asthma	Pollens, dust, molds, cigarette smoke, air pollutants, animal dander
Allergic rhinitis	Pollens, dust, molds, animal dander
Anaphylaxis	Antibiotics (penicillin) Insect venom (bee, wasp stings) Blood transfusions
Urticaria (hives)	Foods, drugs
Atopic dermatitis (eczema)	Soaps, cosmetics, chemicals, fabrics
Allergic contact dermatitis	Plants (poison ivy) Metals (nickel) Chemicals, cosmetics Latex gloves
Gastrointestinal allergies	Foods, drugs

should wear a medical alert bracelet that identifies their allergy. Individuals with insect sting allergies should obtain an emergency sting kit and be taught how to self-inject epinephrine. This kit should be kept readily available at all times.

Nurses should avoid the overuse of perfumes and scented cosmetics while working with patients. Live plants and flowers should not be allowed in the allergic patient's room.

ANAPHYLAXIS

ETIOLOGY AND RISK FACTORS

When an allergen enters the bloodstream, an allergic reaction called *anaphylaxis* can occur throughout the body within minutes. Anaphylaxis is a life-threatening situation that can quickly deteriorate into shock, coma, and death. Histamine released in anaphylaxis causes bronchospasm, vasodilation, and increased capillary permeability throughout the body, which causes fluid to leave the circulation and enter the tissues, causing shock from hypovolemia. Signs and symptoms of anaphylaxis include anxiety, wheezing and difficulty breathing, cyanosis (bluish skin color), hives, facial edema, arthralgia (joint pain), and hypotension (low blood pressure).

Anaphylaxis is an emergency situation, and the patient's life depends on rapid intervention. The most common cause of anaphylaxis is the use of antibiotics, especially penicillin. Other causes include the use of medicines or serum from animal sources, insect venom (especially from bees and wasps), iodinated radioactive contrast media, local anesthetic, and blood products.

MEDICAL TREATMENT

In anaphylaxis, oxygen is given in addition to intravenous epinephrine, aminophylline, diphenhydramine, and corticosteroids. Other drugs that might be given are dopamine to raise the patient's blood pressure and a nebulized bronchodilator to relax the bronchi and improve ventilation.

NURSING CARE *of the Patient with Anaphylaxis*

The best care is to prevent anaphylaxis whenever possible by obtaining a history of allergies and taking precautions to protect the patient from substances (often drugs) that may trigger this reaction. However, when anaphylaxis occurs, prompt recognition is vital because it is a life-threatening situation. In some settings, nurses may have protocols for administering subcutaneous epinephrine in the event of severe allergic reactions. Nursing interventions are aimed at minimizing the patient's anxiety and, once medical care is initiated, administering prescribed drugs including oxygen and monitoring intravenous fluids. Monitor respirations, color, heart rate, and oxygen saturation until the patient is fully recovered.

AUTOIMMUNE DISEASES

ETIOLOGY AND RISK FACTORS

The body's ability to determine self from nonself is called *tolerance*. When tolerance is disrupted, the immune system reacts against and destroys its own tissues. This breakdown in tolerance and subsequent damage to self is termed **autoimmunity**. An autoimmune process may be initiated when there is injury to tissues, infection, or malignancy. The exact causes and pathology of most autoimmune diseases are poorly understood, but many of these disorders cause severe illness and death.

Genetic factors appear to be involved because autoimmune diseases tend to be familial. Some autoimmune disorders have apparent causes, such as drug-induced anemia or a low platelet count (thrombocytopenia). Infection often is present before the onset of an autoimmune disease, leading to the conclusion that the disease results as a complication (sequela) of the infection. Autoimmune diseases cause injury in three ways: (1) by the effect of antibodies on cell surfaces; (2) through the deposit of antigen-antibody complexes (particularly in capillaries, joints, and renal tissue), and (3) through the action of sensitized T cells.

Autoimmunity can involve any tissue or organ system. In multiple sclerosis, the white matter of the brain and spinal cord is affected and the myelin sheath that protects nerve fibers is destroyed. Rheumatoid arthritis affects the lining of the joints. In type 1 diabetes mellitus, the pancreatic cells that secrete insulin are attacked. Table 13-2 lists some of the more common autoimmune disorders and the tissues they affect. Probably the most familiar of the autoimmune disorders is systemic lupus erythematosus, which affects multiple organs.

MEDICAL TREATMENT

Medical interventions vary depending on the specific autoimmune disease and the tissues affected, as well as the symptoms. In general, corticosteroids and nonsteroidal anti-inflammatory drugs (NSAIDs) are used to treat inflammation. Immunosuppressive therapies may be tried to moderate the autoimmune response.

NURSING CARE *of the Patient with an Autoimmune Disorder*

Although nursing interventions vary according to the specific disorder, many nursing diagnoses apply to patients with an autoimmune disease. They include Risk for Activity Intolerance, Anxiety, Impaired Skin Integrity, Ineffective Breathing Pattern, Impaired Gas Exchange, Deficient Knowledge, Chronic Pain, Fear, Fatigue, Self-Care Deficit, Ineffective Coping, Risk for Infection, and Imbalanced Nutrition: Less Than Body Requirements. Adequate rest, maintenance of optimal hydration and nutritional status, and prevention

Table 13-2 *Autoimmune Disorders and Their Targets*

DISORDER	TISSUE AFFECTED
ENDOCRINE SYSTEM	
Hyperthyroidism (Graves' disease)	Thyroid
Autoimmune thyroiditis	Thyroid
Insulin-dependent diabetes mellitus	Pancreas
Addison's disease	Adrenal gland
CENTRAL NERVOUS SYSTEM	
Multiple sclerosis	Brain and spinal cord
Myasthenia gravis	Neuromuscular junctions
CARDIOVASCULAR SYSTEM	
Rheumatic fever	Heart
Cardiomyopathy	Heart
GASTROINTESTINAL SYSTEM	
Ulcerative colitis	Colon
Crohn's disease	Ileum
CONNECTIVE TISSUE	
Rheumatoid arthritis	Joints
Systemic lupus erythematosus	Multiple tissues
Scleroderma	Multiple tissues
HEMATOLOGIC SYSTEM	
Autoimmune hemolytic anemia	Red blood cells
Autoimmune thrombocytopenic purpura	Platelets
Idiopathic neutropenia	Neutrophils
Idiopathic lymphopenia	Lymphocytes
RESPIRATORY AND RENAL SYSTEMS	
Goodpasture's syndrome	Lung, kidney
SKIN	
Pemphigus vulgaris	Skin
Psoriasis	Skin

Adapted from McCance, K.L., & Huether, S.E. (1994). *Pathophysiology: The biologic basis for disease in adults and children* (2nd ed., pp. 270-271). St. Louis: Mosby.

of infection are vital in preventing complications in these patients. In addition, a supportive, caring atmosphere is important to enhance the patient's coping skills and promote emotional health. Specific autoimmune disorders are addressed with appropriate systems in this textbook.

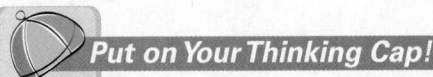

Put on Your Thinking Cap!

In your clinical site, locate everything you would need if a patient had an anaphylactic reaction to a drug. What procedure should you use to alert other personnel?

Key Points

- Physical and chemical barriers that shield the body from disease or injury include the skin, the mucous membranes, and various blood cells.
- Many types of leukocytes, especially neutrophils and monocytes, act as nature's cleanup mechanism by migrating to infected or inflamed areas and engulfing and destroying antigens through a process known as *phagocytosis.*
- Reticuloendothelial cells, or tissue macrophages, found in the blood, connective tissue, liver, spleen, bone marrow, and lymph nodes, protect the body by digesting and absorbing foreign material such as old red blood cells, bacteria, and colloidal particles.
- The four classic signs of inflammation are rubor (redness), calor (heat), tumor (swelling), and dolor (pain).
- Wound healing begins at the same time that the inflammatory process begins.
- The process of wound healing includes the production of macrophage cells to clean up inflammatory debris, the initiation of the repair process by fibroblasts, the formation of capillaries to provide circulation and nutrients to the new tissue, and the migration of epithelial cells under the scab to form a scar.
- Age and general health affect how rapidly wound healing occurs. Older adults heal more slowly as a result of a decreased blood supply to the tissues, a decrease in tissue elasticity, and poor or inadequate nutrition.
- The major infectious agents are bacteria, viruses, fungi, protozoa, rickettsiae, helminths, and mycoplasmas.
- Infection, or the invasion of the body by microorganisms, is possible only when a causative agent, a reservoir, a portal of exit, a mode of transfer, a portal of entry, and a susceptible host are present.
- Signs and symptoms of generalized infection are moderate to severe pain, swelling, fever, malaise, anorexia, and prostration.
- Two types of infections are (1) community-acquired infections, acquired through daily contact with the public, and (2) health care–associated, or nosocomial, infections.
- The most basic and effective method of preventing cross-contamination is hand washing with adequate friction.
- The Centers for Disease Control and Prevention recommends the use of Standard Precautions for all patients, especially those cared for in settings in which exposure to blood is common.
- The immune system is the body's defense network against infection; it provides the body with resistance to invading organisms and enables it to fight off invaders once they have gained access.
- Antigens are substances that stimulate a response from the immune system. Antibodies, also known as *immunoglobulins,* are proteins that are created in response to specific antigens.
- Innate (natural) immunity is present in the body at birth, whereas acquired immunity develops after birth as a result of the body's immune responses to antigens.
- Acquired immunity depends on the proper development of B and T lymphocytes, which are white blood cells that fight infection.

- Body organs that are vital to a functional immune system include the thymus, bone marrow, lymph nodes, spleen, and liver.
- The two types of immunity—antibody-mediated (humoral) and cell-mediated—function interdependently to provide the immune response.
- Immunodeficiency occurs when the body is unable to launch an adequate immune response, resulting in risk for infection.
- When a normally inoffensive foreign substance stimulates an atypical immune response, allergy or hyper-

sensitivity occurs; if anaphylaxis occurs, it is a crisis situation.
- Autoimmunity occurs when the body fails to recognize itself and the immune system reacts by destroying the body's own tissues.

 Go to your Companion CD-ROM for a Pharmacology Tutorial, Audio Glossary, and 3-D animations.

evolve   Be sure to visit the companion Evolve site at http://evolve.elsevier.com/Linton/ for WebLinks and additional online resources.

REVIEW QUESTIONS *Choose the best answer.*

1. A condition in which the body's immune system destroys its own tissues is:
   1. Immunodeficiency
   2. Nosocomial infection
   3. Autoimmunity
   4. Inflammation

2. Bacteria that reside on the skin but do not cause infection serve what purpose?
   1. They stimulate the development of antibodies against pathogens.
   2. They prevent pathogens from gaining access to the body.
   3. They secrete sebum, which inhibits the growth of microorganisms.
   4. They phagocytose pathogenic bacteria that invade the body.

3. The classic signs of inflammation are redness, heat, swelling, and:
   1. Pain
   2. Drainage
   3. Fever
   4. Pus

4. In the first phase of the inflammatory process, capillary permeability increases. What purpose does this serve?
   1. Reduces pain in the inflamed tissue by diluting bradykinin
   2. Draws excess fluid out of inflamed tissue to reduce swelling
   3. Allows monocytes and neutrophils to pass into the inflamed tissue
   4. Counteracts bronchoconstriction in antigen-antibody reactions

5. Why are there numerous antibacterial drugs but relatively few antiviral drugs?
   1. Viruses have a more advanced ability to develop resistance to drugs.
   2. It is more profitable to make antibacterial drugs because only a few viruses exist.
   3. Very few chemicals have been developed that are capable of killing viruses.
   4. The virus lives inside the host cell, and drugs that harm viruses often harm host cells too.

6. The last factor in the chain of infection is the:
   1. Portal of entry
   2. Reservoir
   3. Susceptible host
   4. Mode of transfer

7. Characteristics of the incubation period of the infectious process include the following:
   1. The infected person is often very contagious
   2. Signs and symptoms are most severe
   3. Usually a high fever is present but no other symptoms
   4. The patient is in the recovery phase of the infection

8. An example of a hospital-borne infection is:
   1. Gonorrhea
   2. Hepatitis A
   3. Tuberculosis
   4. Vancomycin-resistant *Enterococcus*

9. Which of the following measures helps prevent the development of bacterial resistance?
   1. All infections are promptly treated with broad-spectrum antibiotics.
   2. Antibiotic selection is based on results of culture and sensitivity tests.
   3. Antibiotics are discontinued as soon as symptoms resolve.
   4. Antibiotics are prescribed only for life-threatening infections.

10. The primary mode of transmission of nosocomial infections is:
    1. Soiled caregiver hands
    2. Direct contact between patients
    3. Organisms brought in by visitors
    4. Faulty sterilization procedures

11. Which statement is true regarding the need to use Standard Precautions?
    1. Standard Precautions are required only when caring for patients who have open wounds.
    2. You should use Standard Precautions any time you have contact with a patient's blood or other body fluids.
    3. You have to use Standard Precautions only when caring for patients with tuberculosis, hepatitis, or HIV infection.
    4. It is necessary to use Standard Precautions only when caring for patients who are highly susceptible to infection.

12. The advantage of using HEPA filter respirators rather than surgical masks is that:
    1. Surgical masks are too expensive for routine use
    2. HEPA filter respirators protect the caregiver by filtering inspired air
    3. Surgical masks protect the caregiver against tuberculosis but not other infections
    4. HEPA filter respirators protect the patient but not the caregiver

13. After vaccination for measles, a person will not become ill if exposed to the measles virus. The patient's ability to resist the measles virus is called:
    1. Innate immunity
    2. Nonspecific defense mechanism
    3. Active acquired immunity
    4. Passive acquired immunity

14. The rejection of transplanted organs is the result of:
    1. Passive acquired immunity
    2. Antibody-mediated immunity
    3. Cell-mediated immunity
    4. Innate immunity

15. Nursing care of the immunosuppressed patient should include the following:
    1. Taking rectal temperatures every 4 hours to detect low-grade fever
    2. Encouraging fresh fruits and vegetables to increase vitamin intake
    3. Encouraging the family to bring in live plants to increase oxygen in the room
    4. Emphasizing the need for good hand washing by patients, visitors, and staff

CHAPTER 14

Fluids and Electrolytes

evolve http://evolve.elsevier.com/Linton/

Objectives

After reading and studying this chapter, you should be able to:

1. Describe the extracellular and intracellular fluid compartments.
2. Describe the composition of the extracellular and intracellular body fluid compartments.
3. Discuss the mechanisms of fluid transport and fluid balance.
4. Identify the causes, signs and symptoms, and treatment of fluid imbalances.
5. Describe the major functions of all of the major electrolytes—sodium, potassium, calcium, magnesium, and chloride.
6. Identify the causes, signs and symptoms, and treatment of electrolyte imbalances.
7. List data to be collected in assessing fluid and electrolyte status.
8. Discuss the medical treatment and nursing management of persons with fluid and electrolyte imbalances.
9. Explain why older persons are at increased risk for fluid and electrolyte imbalances.
10. List the four types of acid-base imbalances.
11. Identify the major causes of each acid-base imbalance.
12. Explain the management of acid-base imbalances.

Key Terms

Be sure to check out the bonus material on the Companion CD-ROM, including selected audio pronunciations.

acid (p. 196)
acid-base balance (p. 196)
active transport (p. 184)
base (p. 196)
diffusion (dĭ-FŬ-zhŭn, p. 184)
electrolyte (ē-LĔK-trō-līt, p. 183)
extracellular fluid (ēks-tră-SĔL-ū-lăr, p. 182)
filtration (fĭl-TRĀ-shŭn, p. 184)
fluid volume deficit (p. 191)
fluid volume excess (p. 191)
homeostasis (hō-mē-ō-STĀ-sĭs, p. 182)
intracellular fluid (ĭn-tră-SĔL-ū-lăr, p. 182)
osmolality (ŏz-mō-LĂL-ĭ-tē, p. 184)
osmolarity (oz-mō-LĂR-ĭ-tē, p. 185)
osmosis (ŏz-mō-sĭs, p. 184)
selectively permeable membrane (sĭ-LĔK-tĭv-lē PĔR-mē-ă-b'l MĔM-brăn, p. 184)

Many disease processes and medical interventions pose actual or potential threats to patients' fluid and electrolyte balances. Therefore nurses must understand the basic principles of fluid and electrolyte balance to maintain balance and to detect and correct imbalances.

HOMEOSTASIS

Approximately 50% to 60% of the human body is composed of water. To maintain internal balance, the body must be able to regulate the fluids within it. The tendency to maintain relatively constant conditions as in the fluid compartments is called homeostasis. All organs and structures of the body are involved in the maintenance of homeostasis.

Homeostasis is necessary for cells to be able to carry out their work. Body fluids are in constant motion, maintaining healthy living conditions for body cells. The process of homeostasis involves the delivery of essential elements such as oxygen and glucose to the cells and the removal of wastes such as carbon dioxide from the cells. When the body does not maintain homeostasis, the cells cannot function properly, and illness results.

BODY FLUID COMPARTMENTS

Body fluids are classified as intracellular or extracellular, depending on their location. Intracellular fluid is fluid within a cell, and extracellular fluid is fluid outside the cell. Most of the body's fluids are found within the cell.

Extracellular fluids are found in the blood vessels in the form of plasma or serum (called *intravascular fluid*); in the fluid surrounding the cells (called *interstitial fluid*), including lymph fluid; and elsewhere such as in digestive secretions, sweat, and cerebrospinal fluid. Extracellular fluid is mainly responsible for the transport of nutrients and wastes throughout the body. The distribution of total body fluids varies among adult males, adult females, and infants (Table 14-1).

Table 14-1	*Total Body Fluids*		
	ADULT MALE (% TBF)	ADULT FEMALE (% TBF)	INFANT (% TBF)
Intracellular	40	36	40
Extracellular	20	18	35
Total body fluids	**60**	**54**	**75**

TBF, Total body fluids.

COMPOSITION OF BODY FLUIDS

WATER

Water makes up the largest portion of the body weight. The percentage of body weight that is water is affected by age, sex, and amount of body fat. A person's percent of body water usually decreases with advancing age. Females have a lower percentage of body water than males throughout the adult years because women have more fat than men and fat cells contain less water than other cells. Obese people have a lower percentage of body water because of their increased number of fat cells.

SOLUTES

In addition to water, body fluids contain solutes (dissolved substances) such as electrolytes and nonelectrolytes.

Electrolytes

An **electrolyte** is defined as a substance that develops an electrical charge when dissolved in water. Examples of electrolytes are sodium, potassium, calcium, chloride, bicarbonate, and magnesium. When these substances are dissolved in water, they break up into small particles called *ions,* which have either a positive (+) or a negative (−) charge. Ions that have a positive electrical charge are called *cations.* Examples of cations are sodium (Na^+), potassium (K^+), calcium (Ca^{2+}), and magnesium (Mg^{2+}). Ions that have a negative charge are called *anions.* Examples of anions are chloride (Cl^-), bicarbonate (HCO_3^-), and phosphate (HPO_4^-).

Electrolytes maintain a balance between positive and negative charges. For every positively charged cation, there is a negatively charged anion. In every fluid compartment of the body, the cations and anions combine to balance one another. This process keeps the body in homeostasis.

The concentration of an electrolyte in a solution or body fluid compartment is measured in milliequivalents per liter (mEq/L). Milliequivalents indicate the chemical activity or combining power of ions. Hydrogen is used as a standard for comparing chemical activities of electrolytes. One milliequivalent of an electrolyte has the same chemical combining power as 1 mEq of hydrogen.

Electrolytes can move from one fluid compartment to another. However, the normal concentration of specific electrolytes is different in the two compartments (Table 14-2).

Sodium. Sodium (Na^+) is the most abundant electrolyte in the body and the primary electrolyte in the extracellular fluid. It plays a major role in the regulation of body fluid volumes, muscular activity, nerve impulse conduction, and acid-base balance.

Potassium. Potassium (K^+) is found mainly in the intracellular fluid and is the major intracellular cation. Because it is so abundant within the cell, it plays an important role in maintaining fluid osmolarity and volume within the cell. Potassium is essential for normal membrane excitability—a critical factor in the transmission of nerve impulses. It also is needed for protein synthesis, for the synthesis and breakdown of glycogen, and to maintain plasma acid-base balance.

Chloride. Chloride (Cl^-) is an extracellular anion that is usually bound with other ions, especially sodium or potassium. Its major functions are to regulate osmotic pressure between fluid compartments and to assist in regulating acid-base balance.

Calcium. Calcium (Ca^{2+}) is usually combined with phosphorus to form the mineral salts of the bones and teeth. Of the total calcium in the body, 99% is concentrated in the bones and teeth and 1% is in the extracellular fluid. Calcium is ingested through the diet and absorbed through the intestine.

In addition to maintaining strong teeth and bones, calcium promotes normal transmission of nerve impulses and helps regulate normal muscle contraction and relaxation. Constant regulation of calcium levels takes place in the body. If the serum calcium level falls, additional calcium is absorbed in the intestine, reabsorbed through the kidneys, or taken from the bones. If more calcium is needed in the bones, it is taken from the bloodstream and also reabsorbed through the kidneys.

Magnesium. Magnesium (Mg^{2+}) is a cation that is found in bone (50% to 60%), intracellular fluid (39% to 49%), and extracellular fluid (1%). After potassium, magnesium is the most abundant cation in intracellular fluid, so it is vital to cellular function. It plays a role in the metabolism of carbohydrates and proteins, the storage and use of intracellular energy, and neural transmission. Magnesium is important in the functioning of the heart, nerves, and muscles.

About 30% to 40% of magnesium ingested through the diet is absorbed, mainly through the small intestine. Magnesium is excreted through the kidneys, and the rate of excretion is regulated by sodium and calcium excretion, extracellular fluid volume, and parathyroid hormone.

Table **14-2** *Electrolyte Composition of Extracellular and Intracellular Fluids*

ELECTROLYTE	EXTRACELLULAR FLUID (mEq/L)	INTRACELLULAR FLUID (mEq/L)
Sodium (Na^+)	130-145	14
Potassium (K^+)	3.5-5.1	140
Chloride (Cl^-)	98-107	4-6
Bicarbonate (HCO_3^-)	24	12
Calcium (Ca^{2+})	5	1-8
Magnesium (Mg^{2+})	1.5-2.5	6-30
Phosphate ($HPOO_4^-$)	2	40-95

Nonelectrolytes

Although most of the solutes in the body are electrolytes, other substances are dissolved in the body fluids as well. Examples are urea, protein, glucose, creatinine, and bilirubin. These solutes do not carry an electrical charge and are measured in milligrams per deciliter (mg/dL).

TRANSPORT OF WATER AND ELECTROLYTES

MEMBRANES

The fluid compartments of the body are separated by selectively permeable membranes that control movement of water and certain solutes. Selective permeability maintains the unique composition of each compartment of the body while allowing for the transport of nutrients and wastes to and from cells. For example, selectively permeable membranes surround cells to separate fluid in the cells from fluid in the tissues. Some solutes cross membranes more easily than others. Small molecules and water move freely across membranes, whereas larger molecules such as protein move less readily.

TRANSPORT PROCESSES

Water and solutes are transported between intracellular and extracellular fluid compartments by one or more of the following processes: (1) diffusion, (2) active transport, (3) filtration, and (4) osmosis.

Diffusion

Diffusion is the random movement of particles in all directions. The natural tendency is for a substance to move from an area of higher concentration to an area of lower concentration. One example is the movement of oxygen from the alveoli to the pulmonary capillaries. The concentration of oxygen in the alveoli is greater than in the capillaries; therefore oxygen diffuses into the capillaries and is transported through the bloodstream to other parts of the body. The term *facilitated*

diffusion is used when a carrier protein transports the molecules through membranes toward an area of lower concentration.

Active Transport

Carrier proteins can transport substances from an area of lower concentration to an area of equal or greater concentration. This process, which requires expenditure of energy, is called active transport. Many solutes, such as sodium, potassium, glucose, and hydrogen, are actively transported across cell membranes. An example is the sodium pump. The concentration of sodium is highest in extracellular fluid. Therefore excess sodium cannot leave the cell by diffusion. Active transport "pumps" the excess sodium out of the cell into the extracellular fluid.

Filtration

Filtration is the transfer of water and solutes through a membrane from an area of high pressure to an area of low pressure. This pressure is known as *hydraulic pressure* and is a combination of pressures from the force of gravity on the fluid and the pumping action of the heart. Filtration is a necessary process for moving fluid out of the capillaries into the tissues and for filtering plasma through the kidneys.

Osmosis

Osmosis is the movement of water across a membrane from a less concentrated solution to a more concentrated solution. It involves the movement of water only, but sometimes the force of movement across the membrane carries some solutes along. If a fluid compartment has less water and more sodium, water from another compartment moves to the more concentrated compartment by osmosis to create a better fluid balance.

OSMOLALITY

Osmolality refers to the concentration of a solution determined by the number of dissolved particles per kilogram of water. A higher osmolality means that there is a higher concentration of salt, or any other solute, in the water because the solution contains less water. Osmolality controls water movement and distribution in body fluid compartments by regulating the concentration of fluid in each compartment. When solutes such as electrolytes are added to water, the volume is expanded to include both the water and the solutes.

The osmolality of intracellular fluid and extracellular fluid tends to equalize because of the constant shifting of water. A change in osmolality of intracellular fluid affects the osmolality of extracellular fluid, and vice versa. The osmolality of intracellular fluid is maintained primarily by potassium, and the osmolality of the extracellular fluid is maintained primarily by sodium. The normal range of osmolality of the body fluids is between 280 and 294 milliosmoles per kilogram (mOsm/kg). You will see the term osmolarity also used to refer to the concentration of particles in body water. Osmolarity refers to the concentration of particles per liter of solution. For the study of body fluids, it is more practical to measure liters of fluid than kilograms. Therefore you will see clinical studies of fluids using the term *osmolarity* rather than osmolality.

REGULATORY MECHANISMS

Regulation of fluid balance requires the constant adjustment of fluid volume, distribution, and composition. This process is accomplished by the kidneys and circulatory system, which are influenced by the sympathetic nervous system, specific hormones, and the thirst center.

KIDNEYS

The kidneys are the main regulators of fluid balance. They control extracellular fluid by adjusting the concentration of specific electrolytes, the osmolality of body fluids, the volume of extracellular fluid, blood volume, and pH. Kidney function is delicately controlled by hormones and other coordinating mechanisms (see Chapter 40 for a review of renal structure and function).

The nephron is the functioning unit of the kidney. Each nephron is made up of a glomerulus and tubules. The glomerulus is the filtering portion of the nephron, and the tubule is responsible for secretion and reabsorption. The nephrons conduct the work of the kidney through the processes of filtration, reabsorption, and secretion.

Filtration

A primary activity of the kidney is filtration. Blood plasma entering the kidney via the renal artery is delivered to the glomerulus. About 20% of the plasma is filtered into the glomerular capsule. This fluid is called *filtrate*. Most of the remaining plasma leaves the kidney through the renal vein. The filtrate then moves through the tubules, where it is transformed into urine by the processes of tubular reabsorption and secretion.

Tubular Reabsorption

Tubular reabsorption is a process by which most of the glomerular filtrate is returned to the circulation. Water and selected solutes move from the tubules into the capillaries. Waste products remain in the tubules for excretion, whereas most water and sodium are reabsorbed into the bloodstream. Tubular reabsorption is important for adjusting the volume and composition of the filtrate and for preventing excessive fluid loss through the kidneys.

Tubular Secretion

Tubular secretion is the last phase in the work of the kidneys. During this phase, the filtrate is transformed into urine. Various substances, among them drugs, hydrogen ions, potassium ions, creatinine, and histamine, pass from the blood into the tubules. This process eliminates some excess substances to maintain fluid and electrolyte balance, as well as metabolic waste products.

HORMONES

Hormones that have a major effect on fluid volume and balance are renin, aldosterone, antidiuretic hormone, and atrial natriuretic factor. *Renin* is a hormone that is secreted when blood volume or blood pressure falls. Renin activates angiotensinogen, a substance secreted by the liver, to form angiotensin I. Angiotensin-converting enzyme then converts angiotensin I to angiotensin II. Angiotensin II is a potent vasoconstrictor that also stimulates the release of aldosterone with subsequent sodium and water retention.

Aldosterone is released by the adrenal glands in response to the hormone renin. Aldosterone acts on the kidney tubules to increase the reabsorption of sodium and decrease the reabsorption of potassium. Because the retention of sodium causes water retention, aldosterone acts as a volume regulator. The release of aldosterone from the adrenal gland is stimulated by many factors, including increased potassium levels and decreased sodium levels in the blood.

Antidiuretic hormone (ADH) is produced by the hypothalamus and is secreted into the general circulation by the posterior pituitary gland. It causes the capillaries to reabsorb more water, so that urine is more concentrated and less volume is excreted. An increase in plasma osmolality (plasma is more concentrated) stimulates the release of ADH into the bloodstream to replenish needed fluid in the body. Other factors that stimulate the release of ADH are related to stress situations such as hypotension, pain, surgery, and the use of certain medications.

Atrial natriuretic factor (ANF) is a hormone released by the atria in response to stretching of the atria by increased blood volume. ANF stimulates excretion of sodium and water by the kidneys, decreased synthesis of renin, decreased release of aldosterone, and vasodilation. The effect of these actions is to reduce blood volume and to lower blood pressure.

THIRST

An additional regulatory mechanism is thirst, which regulates fluid intake. Increased plasma osmolality stimulates osmoreceptors in the hypothalamus to trigger the sensation of thirst. In other words, more sodium and less water in the body make a person thirsty. Additional fluids are consumed, and the kidneys conserve water until plasma osmolality returns to normal.

Table 14-3 | *24-Hour Intake and Output of Body Fluids*

FLUID GAINS	AMOUNT (mL)	FLUID LOSSES	AMOUNT (mL)
Liquids	1000	Lungs	400
Food (solid)	1200	Skin	400
H$_2$O of oxidation	300	Kidneys (urine)	1500
Daily total intake	**2500**	Intestines (feces)	200
		Daily total output	**2500**

FLUID GAINS AND LOSSES

In a healthy adult, the 24-hour fluid intake and output are approximately equal (Table 14-3). Fluids are gained by drinking and eating and are lost through the kidneys, skin, lungs, and gastrointestinal tract. The usual adult urine volume is between 1 and 2 liters per day (L/day), or 1 milliliter per kilogram of body weight per hour. In the kidneys, water loss varies largely with the amount of solute excreted and with the level of antidiuretic hormone.

Water and electrolyte (Na$^+$, Cl$^-$, K$^+$) losses through the skin occur by sweating. Water loss through the lungs occurs by evaporation at a rate of 300 to 400 mL/day. In a hot, dry environment, water loss via the skin and lungs increases. In the gastrointestinal tract, the usual loss of fluid is about 100 to 200 mL/day. The bulk of fluid secreted into the GI tract is reabsorbed in the small intestine. Figure 14-1 diagrams the regulation of body fluid volume.

AGE-RELATED CHANGES AFFECTING FLUID BALANCE

Multiple factors place the older person at risk for fluid and electrolyte imbalances. The aging kidney is slower to adjust to changes in acid-base, fluid, and electrolyte balance. The older adult often has a reduced sense of thirst and therefore may be in a state of chronic dehydration because of inadequate fluid intake. Total body water declines with age, with the greatest loss being from the intracellular fluid compartment. Therefore an older person has limited reserves with which to maintain fluid balance when abnormal losses occur.

You must monitor fluid status in the older person and be alert to the consequences of imbalances, including disorientation, confusion, constipation, and falls resulting from postural hypotension. The health history may reveal many chronic conditions, such as heart failure and renal insufficiency, which are more common among older adults and place them at risk for fluid and electrolyte imbalances. Drugs such as antihypertensives, diuretics, and antacids used to treat these and other conditions can also contribute to imbalances. In addition, chronic conditions that affect mobility or mental status may interfere with adequate fluid intake. Some of the contributors to acute fluid deficits are trauma, infection, fever, influenza or cold,

and drug therapies (diuretics, antidepressants, sedatives). In addition to the general assessment data, it is especially important to evaluate fluid intake patterns, medications, mental status, and recent weight loss.

Components of the physical examination are described later in this chapter. Note that skin turgor is a less reliable indicator of fluid status in older persons than in younger individuals because there is normally some loss of skin elasticity with increased age. It is better to assess turgor on the sternum or forehead for better accuracy in the older person. Serum electrolytes should be the same for all adults, so any abnormalities of such in the older person should be investigated.

Unless contraindicated, fluid requirements for older adults, based on ideal body weight, are 30 mL/kg in persons ages 55 to 65 years and 25 mL/kg in persons ages 65 years and older. Using these guidelines, a 60-year-old person who weighs 150 lb (68.1 kg) would need 2000 mL of fluid daily. A person the same weight at age 70 would require 1700 mL of fluid per day for adequate hydration. Fluid intake should be increased gradually in the older adult because the heart and kidneys adapt more slowly to changes in fluid volume. An individual with cardiac or renal disease sometimes has fluid restrictions because of fluid retention.

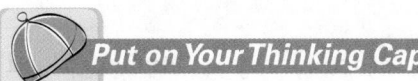

Put on Your Thinking Cap!

Measure your fluid intake and output for 24 hours. If they are not equal, list possible explanations for the difference.

ASSESSMENT OF FLUID AND ELECTROLYTE BALANCE

ASSESSMENT

Health History

Obtain a complete health history to determine whether patients have any conditions that may contribute to fluid or electrolyte imbalances. Examples of conditions that have great potential for disrupting fluid balance are vomiting, diarrhea, kidney diseases, diabetes, salicylate poisoning, burns, congestive heart failure, cerebral injuries, ulcerative colitis, and hormonal imbalances. Other risk factors include the intake of drugs such as diuretics and cathartics and

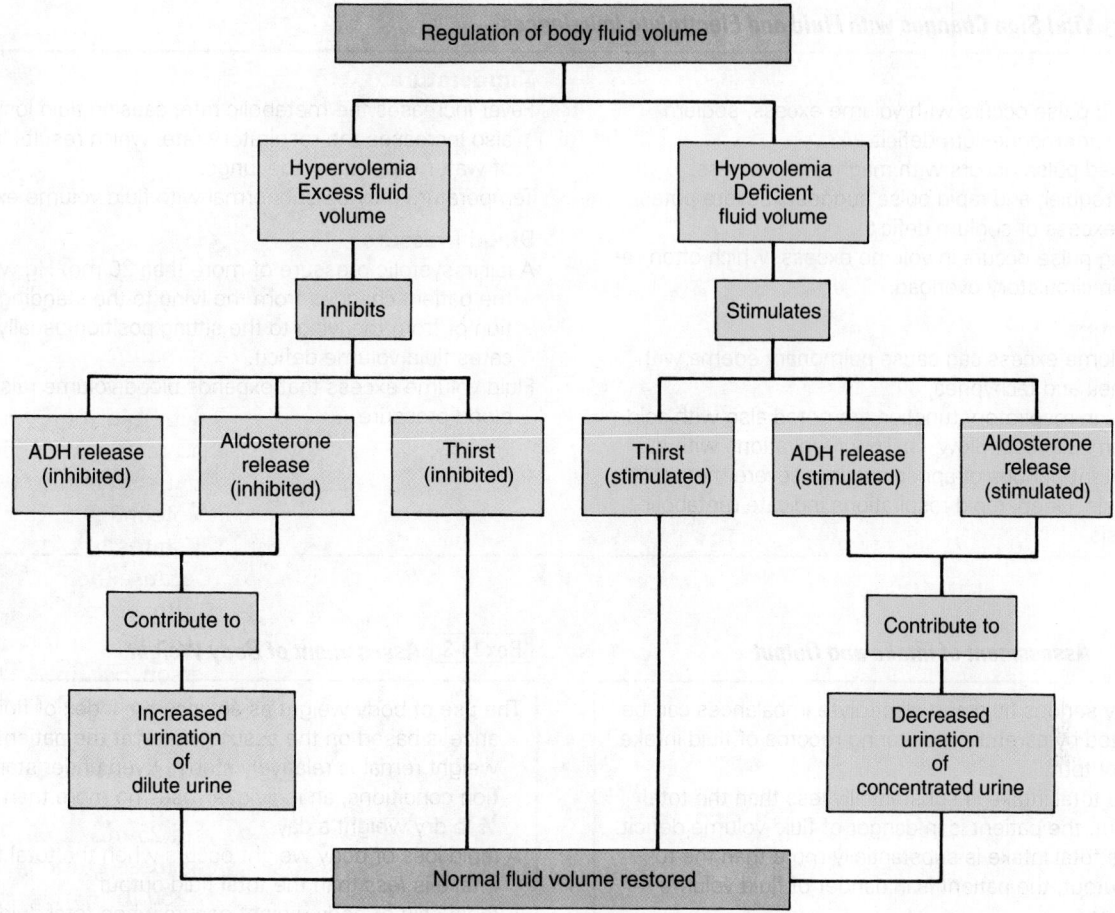

FIGURE 14-1 Regulation of body fluid volume depends on aldosterone, antidiuretic hormone (ADH), and thirst.

medical interventions such as gastric suctioning. Anticipate fluid and electrolyte imbalances in patients who are at risk. Patient complaints of fatigue, palpitations, dizziness, edema, muscle weakness or cramps, dyspnea, and confusion are examples of signs and symptoms that may be associated with fluid imbalances. Because electrolyte disturbances produce nonspecific symptoms, they can be confirmed only with laboratory tests.

Vital Signs

Assessment of pulse, respiration, temperature, and blood pressure can detect indicators of changes in both fluid and electrolyte balance, as shown in Box 14-1. Body temperature variations can be associated with fluid volume excess or deficit. Also, fever poses a risk of water and electrolyte loss associated with sweating and an increased metabolic rate. The pulse rate and quality may change in response to blood volume alterations. Because electrolytes affect the conduction of impulses, electrolyte changes can affect heart rate and rhythm. Blood pressure is directly related to blood volume. Respirations are minimally affected by electrolyte changes. However, rapid respirations increase water loss. Also, fluid volume excess can lead to heart failure and pulmonary edema with shortness of breath. Mea-

suring blood pressure with the patient lying, sitting, and standing can detect positional differences that may reflect inadequate blood volume.

Intake and Output

An accurate record of intake and output is essential to determine whether the patient's intake is equal to output. All fluids entering or leaving the body should be noted, as explained in Box 14-2. A changing urine output may reflect attempts by the kidneys to maintain or restore balance, or it may reflect a problem that causes fluid disturbances. In addition to urine volume, urine characteristics also give clues to fluid balance. Clear, pale urine in a healthy person suggests the excretion of excess water, whereas darker, concentrated urine indicates the kidneys are retaining water.

Body Weight

Measurement of body weight is a good indicator of fluid loss or retention (Box 14-3). Remember that 1 liter of fluid weighs 2.2 lb. Therefore retention of 1 liter of fluid is reflected as a weight gain of 2.2 lb (1 kg). A patient can accumulate up to 10 lb (4.5 kg) of fluid before pitting edema is evident. You should weigh the patient daily on the same scale, at the same time of day, and wearing the same type of clothing.

Box 14-1 | *Vital Sign Changes with Fluid and Electrolyte Imbalances*

Pulse

Increased pulse occurs with volume excess, sodium excess, or magnesium deficit.

Decreased pulse occurs with magnesium excess.

Weak, irregular, and rapid pulse suggests severe potassium excess or sodium deficit.

Bounding pulse occurs in volume excess, which often results in circulatory overload.

Respiration

Fluid volume excess can cause pulmonary edema with dyspnea and tachypnea.

Changes in respiratory function are noted also with acid-base imbalances. Slow, shallow respirations with intermittent periods of apnea occur in severe metabolic alkalosis. Deep, rapid respirations indicate metabolic acidosis.

Temperature

Fever increases the metabolic rate, causing fluid loss. It also increases the respiratory rate, which results in loss of water vapor from the lungs.

Temperature may be subnormal with fluid volume excess.

Blood Pressure

A fall in systolic pressure of more than 20 mm Hg when the patient changes from the lying to the standing position or from the lying to the sitting position usually indicates fluid volume deficit.

Fluid volume excess that expands blood volume raises the blood pressure.

Box 14-2 | *Assessment of Intake and Output*

- Many serious fluid and electrolyte imbalances can be averted by carefully monitoring records of fluid intake and output.
- If the total intake is substantially less than the total output, the patient is in danger of fluid volume deficit.
- If the total intake is substantially more than the total output, the patient is in danger of fluid volume excess.
- Intake should include all fluids taken into the body: oral fluids, foods that are liquid at room temperature, intravenous fluids, subcutaneous fluids, fluids instilled into drainage tubes or irrigants, tube feeding solutions, water given through feeding tubes, and enema solutions.
- Output measures include urine, vomitus, diarrhea, drainage from fistulas, drainage from suction machines, excessive perspiration, and drainage from excisions; normal adult urine output is 40 to 80 mL/hr.

Box 14-3 | *Assessment of Body Weight*

The use of body weight as an accurate index of fluid balance is based on the assumption that the patient's dry weight remains relatively stable. Even under starvation conditions, an individual loses no more than $\frac{1}{3}$ to $\frac{1}{2}$ lb dry weight a day.

A rapid loss of body weight occurs when the total fluid intake is *less* than the total fluid output.

A rapid gain of body weight occurs when total fluid intake is *more* than the total fluid output.

	MILD	MODERATE	SEVERE
Rapid loss	2%	5%	8% = deficit
Rapid gain	2%	5%	8% = excess

Rapid gain or loss of 1 kg (2.2 lb) of body weight is approximately equivalent to the gain or loss of 1 liter of fluid.

Skin

Skin Characteristics. Skin color, moisture, turgor, and temperature all reflect fluid balance. Dry, flushed skin is associated with dehydration. Pale, cool, clammy skin is associated with the severe fluid volume deficit that occurs with shock. Moist, edematous tissue may be seen with fluid volume excess.

Facial Characteristics. The patient who is severely dehydrated usually has a pinched, drawn facial expression. Soft eyeballs and sunken eyes accompany a severe fluid volume deficit. Puffy eyelids and fuller cheeks suggest fluid volume excess.

Skin Turgor. Skin turgor is best measured by pinching the skin over the sternum, the inner aspects of the thighs, or the forehead. In patients who are dehydrated, skin flattens more slowly after the pinch is released. The term *tenting* is sometimes used to describe skin that does not flatten promptly after being gently pinched into a tent shape. The skin of older people generally has a slower return to normal, so it is inappropriate to assume a fluid deficit based only on poor skin turgor in the older person.

Edema. Edema reflects water and sodium retention, which can result from excessive reabsorption or inadequate secretion of sodium, as may occur with kidney failure. Inspect and palpate the skin for edema. Test for edema by pressing the skin that lies over the tibia, fibula, sacrum, or sternum. Edema is described as *pitting* if a depression remains in the tissue after pressure is applied with a fingertip. Pitting edema is evaluated on a four-point scale, ranging from 1+ edema (barely detectable pit) to 4+ edema (deep and persistent pit that is approximately 1 inch or 2.54 cm deep).

Box 14-4 **ASSESSMENT of Fluid and Electrolyte Status**

Health History

Present Illness:
Vomiting, diarrhea, burns, head injury

Past Medical History:
Renal or cardiac disease, diabetes, inflammatory bowel disease, adrenal or thyroid disease

Current Drugs:
Such as diuretics, salicylates, antacids, potassium supplements

Family History:
Diabetes, cardiac disease

Review of Systems:
Fatigue, palpitations, dizziness, edema, dyspnea, confusion

Functional Assessment:
Change in activity tolerance, mental alertness

Physical Examination

General Survey:
Alertness, orientation, posture

Vital Signs:
Pulse rate/rhythm; respiratory rate/pattern; blood pressure in lying, sitting, and standing positions; temperature

Weight:
Present compared with usual

Skin:
Color, moisture, turgor, temperature

Facial Characteristics:
Expression, firmness of eyeballs, edema of eyelids or cheeks

Edema:
Presence, location, pitting or brawny

Mucous Membranes:
Tongue turgor, moisture of the oral cavity

Veins:
Jugular vein distention, hand vein emptying and refilling time

Edema can be so severe that pitting is not possible. The tissue becomes so full that fluid cannot be displaced. When edematous tissue feels hard, it is referred to as *brawny edema*. After a radical mastectomy, brawny edema commonly occurs because the removal of axillary nodes allows fluid to accumulate in the affected arm.

Mucous Membranes

Tongue Turgor. In a normal person, the tongue has one longitudinal furrow. A person with fluid volume deficit has additional longitudinal furrows, and the tongue is smaller, as a result of fluid loss. Sodium excess causes the tongue to appear red and swollen.

Moisture of the Oral Cavity. A dry mouth may be the result of fluid volume deficit or mouth breathing. Normally, there is a pool of saliva in the area where the cheek and the gum meet. Dryness in this area usually indicates a true fluid volume deficit. However, dry mouth is a common side effect of many medications.

Veins

The appearance of the jugular veins in the neck and the veins in the hands can suggest either a fluid volume deficit or a fluid volume excess.

Neck Vein Distention. Distention of the jugular veins can indicate fluid volume excess. Inspect the neck veins for fluid volume excess by having the patient recline with the head of the bed elevated at a 30- to 45-degree angle. If the jugular veins can be seen more than 3 cm above the sternal angle, then fluid volume excess most likely is present.

Fluid volume deficit may be detected by examining the jugular neck veins with the patient lying down. If no distention occurs, then fluid volume deficit most likely is present.

Hand Veins. Observation of hand veins also can be helpful in evaluating the patient's fluid volume. First elevate the hands and then note how long it takes for the veins to empty. Veins usually empty in 3 to 5 seconds. Next place the hands in a dependent position and note how long it takes for the veins to fill. Veins usually fill in 3 to 5 seconds. If the volume is decreased, veins take longer than 3 to 5 seconds to fill. When the fluid volume is increased, veins take longer than 3 to 5 seconds to empty. The nursing assessment of fluid and electrolyte status is summarized in Box 14-4.

DIAGNOSTIC TESTS AND PROCEDURES

A variety of laboratory tests may be performed to assess fluid and electrolyte status and to determine whether they are within the normal range (Table 14-4).

Urine Studies

Urine pH. The kidneys can change the acidity or alkalinity of the urine by excreting hydrogen (H^+) ions. Urine pH is a measure of hydrogen ions in the urine. It is useful for determining whether the kidneys are responding appropriately to metabolic acid-base imbalances. The normal range is 4.5 to 8.0; however, fresh urine is usually acidic (about 6.0). Urine tends to be most acidic in the morning (after a fast) and more alkaline after meals. Diet is a factor in that a person who consumes large amounts of citrus fruits and vegetables tends to have alkaline urine, whereas a person who eats a lot of meat tends to have acidic urine. A urine specimen that is not tested within 4 hours of collection may become alkaline. Therefore urine pH should be measured within 1

Table 14-4 | *Normal Values Related to Fluid and Electrolyte Balance*

URINE		BLOOD	
Urine pH	4.5-8	Arterial blood pH	7.35-7.45
Urine specific gravity	1.010-1.025	Serum osmolality	280-294 mOsm/kg
Urine osmolality	250-900 mOsm/kg H₂O	Serum sodium	136-145 mEq/L
Urine sodium	75-200 mEq/L or 27-287 mmol/24 hr	Serum potassium	3.5-5.1 mEq/L
Urine potassium	25-123 mEq/24 hr	Serum chloride	98-107 mEq/L
Urine chloride	110-250 mEq/24 hr	Serum phosphorus	2.7-4.5 mg/dL
Urine phosphorus	0.4-1.3 g/24 hr	Serum magnesium	1.5-2.5 mEq/L
Urine magnesium	6.0-8.5 mEq/24 hr	Serum calcium	9.0-11.0 mEq/L
		Serum creatinine	0.6-1.5 mg/dL
		Serum bicarbonate	
		Arterial	21-28 mEq/L
		Venous	22-29 mEq/L

From Jaffe, M.S., & McVan, B.F. (1997). *Davis's laboratory and diagnostic handbook.* Philadelphia: Davis; Jacobs, D.S., DeMott, W.R., Grady, H.J., Horvat, R.T., Huestis, D.W., & Kasten, B.L. (1996). *Laboratory test handbook.* Hudson (Cleveland): Lexi-Comp, Inc.; and Heitz, U.E., & Horne, M.M. (2001). *Fluid, electrolyte, and acid-base balance.* St. Louis: Mosby.

to 2 hours of collection. If the specimen cannot be tested promptly, it should be refrigerated.

Urine Specific Gravity. Urine specific gravity (SpG) is a measure of urine concentration. In most instances, normal urine specific gravity is between 1.010 and 1.025 in adults.

Specific gravity is a good indicator of fluid balance. A high specific gravity indicates that the urine is highly concentrated, usually as a result of fluid volume deficit. A low specific gravity indicates that the urine contains a large amount of water in relation to solutes, usually as a result of fluid volume excess. The specific gravity also reflects renal function. If the kidneys are not functioning properly, they may fail to concentrate or dilute urine as needed to maintain extracellular fluid balance. The presence of x-ray dyes, glucose, or protein in the urine can cause an increased specific gravity that may be misleading; that is, the patient may not really have a fluid volume deficit. As people age, their kidneys are less efficient at conserving water by concentrating urine. Therefore the older person may produce relatively dilute urine (low or normal specific gravity) even when he or she is dehydrated.

Urine Osmolality. Osmolality measures the number of dissolved particles in a solution. This provides a more precise measurement of the kidney's ability to concentrate urine than does the specific gravity. The normal urine osmolality range is 250 to 900 mOsm/kg H₂O. For the most accurate interpretation, a serum osmolality should be done simultaneously.

Dilute urine has a low osmolality and generally reflects renal excretion of excess water. Low osmolality also is apparent when kidneys are unable to conserve water by concentrating urine. Concentrated urine has a high osmolality and generally indicates renal conservation of water. It also can be present when the kid-

neys are failing, because the volume of urine secreted declines.

Urine Creatinine Clearance. Urine creatinine clearance tests are used to detect glomerular damage in the kidney. A 24-hour specimen is required. The patient is instructed to void, discard the specimen, record the time, and start collecting all urine thereafter for 24 hours. The specimen must be refrigerated.

During the specimen collection period, the patient should maintain good hydration, should not engage in vigorous exercise, and should avoid high-protein foods, coffee, tea, and cola drinks. Be aware that many drugs, including cephalosporin antibiotics, can alter test results. For best interpretation, serum creatinine clearance should be done as well. Also, the laboratory needs to know the patient's height, weight, and age. The normal creatinine clearance for adult males is 85 to 125 mL/min/1.73 m² of body surface area; for females, it is 75 to 115 mL/min/1.73 m² of body surface area. The range decreases with age.

Urine Sodium. Urine sodium reflects sodium intake and fluid volume status. When the intake of sodium is high, the kidneys will increase the excretion of sodium in the urine. When large amounts of fluids are taken in or sodium intake is restricted, the urine is more dilute, so the urine sodium falls. The urinary excretion of sodium is normally highest during the day. The normal urine sodium is 75 to 200 mEq/L. If collected over a period of 24 hours, the normal range is 27 to 287 mmol/24 hr.

Urine Potassium. Urine potassium is a measure of renal tubular function. A 24-hour specimen is most meaningful because the urinary excretion of potassium is highest at night and lowest during the day. Therefore a random sample would not truly represent function of the renal tubules. The normal value is 25 to 123 mmol/24 hr.

Blood Studies

Serum Hematocrit. The hematocrit is the percentage of blood volume that is composed of red blood cells. An increased hematocrit is seen with fluid volume deficit and dehydration because the blood is more concentrated. A low hematocrit is consistent with fluid volume excess because of dilution. The normal range for hematocrit is 40% to 54% for adult men and 38% to 47% for adult women.

Serum Creatinine. Creatinine is a metabolic waste product. The serum level is a better indicator of renal function than the blood urea nitrogen. A high level of creatinine in the blood indicates poor renal function. The normal range is 0.6 to 1.5 mg/dL. Even small changes in the serum creatinine can be significant.

Blood Urea Nitrogen. Blood urea nitrogen (BUN) provides a measure of renal function. Normal is 8 to 20 mg/dL. A high BUN is associated with fluid volume deficit and possibly impaired renal function; conversely, a low BUN is associated with fluid volume excess.

Serum Osmolality. Serum osmolality is a measure of blood concentration. High serum osmolality is related to a fluid volume deficit, and low serum osmolality is related to fluid volume excess. The normal range is 280 to 294 mOsm/kg.

Serum Albumin. Albumin is a plasma protein that helps maintain blood volume by creating colloid osmotic pressure. The normal range for serum albumin is 3.5 to 5.5 g/dL. Low serum albumin allows water to shift into the interstitial compartment, which reduces blood volume and creates edema.

Serum Electrolytes. Normal values for serum sodium, potassium, chloride, and calcium are shown in Table 14-4.

FLUID IMBALANCES

FLUID VOLUME DEFICITS

A fluid volume deficit occurs when there is less water than normal in the body. There are two types of fluid volume deficits: isotonic extracellular fluid deficit (hypovolemia) and hypertonic extracellular fluid deficit (dehydration). A fluid volume deficit may result from decreased intake, abnormal fluid losses, or both. Examples of abnormal fluid losses are the loss of water as a result of excessive bleeding, severe vomiting and diarrhea, and severe burns.

The signs and symptoms of fluid volume deficit vary depending on how suddenly the deficit develops and how severe it is. Symptoms are not as apparent with deficits that are mild and have a gradual onset, but the symptoms are quite dramatic when the loss is severe and the onset is abrupt. In general, the body attempts to compensate for fluid volume deficits by decreasing urine output. The heart rate increases in an effort to maintain blood flow to body tissues. The blood pressure may fall because of the reduced blood volume.

Treatment varies somewhat according to the cause of a fluid volume deficit and the severity of symptoms. Nursing care should be based on appropriate nursing diagnoses, which might include the following:

- **Deficient Fluid Volume, Risk for Deficient Fluid Volume** related to inadequate fluid intake, excessive fluid loss, high blood glucose, inadequate antidiuretic hormone production or effect, high fever, altered capillary permeability
- **Acute Confusion** related to decreased cerebral tissue perfusion
- **Constipation** related to excessive reabsorption of water from stool in the colon
- **Fatigue** related to decreased blood volume, decreased tissue perfusion
- **Hyperthermia** related to infectious process, decreased fluid volume
- **Risk for Injury** related to decreased level of consciousness
- **Risk for Impaired Skin Integrity** related to poor tissue turgor
- **Ineffective Tissue Perfusion** related to decreased cardiac output secondary to decreased blood volume

The characteristics, causes, assessment findings, treatment, and nursing care for each type of fluid volume deficit are outlined in Table 14-5.

FLUID VOLUME EXCESSES

An increase in body water is called fluid volume excess. The two types of fluid volume excess are extracellular fluid excess (isotonic fluid excess) and intracellular water excess (hypotonic fluid excess). Fluid volume excess may result from renal or cardiac failure with retention of fluid, increased production of antidiuretic hormone or aldosterone, overload with isotonic intravenous fluids, or the administration of dextrose 5% in water (D_5W) after surgery or trauma. The body attempts to compensate for fluid volume excess by increasing the filtration and excretion of sodium and water by the kidneys and decreasing the production of antidiuretic hormone.

As with fluid volume deficit, the severity of the symptoms in fluid volume excess depends on how quickly the condition develops. Severe fluid volume excess can cause or aggravate heart failure and pulmonary edema.

Nursing care varies somewhat according to the cause of a fluid volume excess and the severity of symptoms. Care should be based on appropriate nursing diagnoses, which might include the following:

- **Excess Fluid Volume** related to fluid retention, excess or hypotonic intravenous fluid administration
- **Acute Confusion, Disturbed Thought Processes** related to cerebral edema
- **Activity Intolerance, Impaired Gas Exchange** related to pulmonary edema

Table 14-5 | *Fluid Volume Deficit*

	ISOTONIC EXTRACELLULAR FLUID DEFICIT (HYPOVOLEMIA)	HYPERTONIC EXTRACELLULAR FLUID DEFICIT (DEHYDRATION)
DEFINITION	Deficiency of both water and relative electrolytes	Deficiency of water without electrolyte deficiency
ETIOLOGY	Decreased fluid intake related to inability to obtain or ingest fluids Excessive fluid loss related to vomiting, diarrhea Shifting of fluid into interstitial space (third spacing) related to increased capillary permeability)	Increased water loss related to blood glucose as in uncontrolled diabetes mellitus, inadequate ADH production or renal response to ADH, high fever, excessive sweating Decreased fluid intake with continued intake of electrolytes, as with concentrated tube feedings
ASSESSMENT FINDINGS		
Blood pressure	Hypotension	Hypotension
Pulse	Weak, rapid	Weak, rapid
Respirations	Rapid	Rapid
Temperature	Decreased	Increased
Weight	Loss	Loss
Tissue turgor	Normal or edema	Poor
Mucous membranes	Moist	Dry
Blood cells	Hgb, Hct, RBCs increased	Hgb, Hct, RBCs increased
Urine output	Decreased	Decreased or increased
Thirst	Normal	Thirsty
TREATMENT	Correct underlying cause; replace water and electrolytes.	Correct underlying cause; replace water.
NURSING CARE	Give antiemetics, antidiarrheals as ordered. Document effects. Give oral and intravenous fluids as ordered. Protect edematous tissue with third spacing. Assist with rising and ambulating if patient is dizzy. Keep hourly records of intake and output: expect intake to exceed output at first. Be alert for fluid excess (rising pulse and blood pressure, dyspnea) caused by excessive fluid replacement.	Monitor blood glucose if patient has diabetes. Give oral and intravenous fluids as ordered. Give hypoglycemics, ADH, antipyretics as ordered. Assist with oral hygiene. Assist with rising and ambulating if patient is dizzy. Keep hourly records of intake and output: expect intake to exceed output at first. Be alert for fluid excess (rising pulse and blood pressure, dyspnea) caused by excessive fluid replacement.

ADH, Antidiuretic hormone; *Hgb,* hemoglobin; *Hct,* hematocrit; *RBCs,* red blood cells.

- **Risk for Injury** related to decreased level of consciousness
- **Risk for Impaired Skin Integrity** related to edema
- **Ineffective Tissue Perfusion** related to reduced cardiac output with heart failure

The causes, assessment findings, treatment, and nursing care of the patient with fluid volume excess are outlined in Table 14-6.

ELECTROLYTE IMBALANCES

The two electrolytes that cause the majority of problems when there is an imbalance are sodium (Na^+) and potassium (K^+).

HYPONATREMIA (SODIUM DEFICIT)

Hyponatremia is lower than normal sodium in the blood serum. It can be an actual deficiency of sodium or an increase in body water that dilutes the sodium excessively. Causes include excessive intake of water without sodium; excessive loss of sodium, as with vomiting, diarrhea, or diaphoresis with only water replacement; the use of distilled water to irrigate body cavities; and excessive secretion of antidiuretic hormone (ADH). Increased antidiuretic hormone secretion is associated with severe stress, some head injuries, and a condition called *syndrome of inappropriate antidiuretic hormone secretion (SIADH)*. Other disorders that put the patient at risk for hyponatremia include congestive heart failure, liver cirrhosis, and nephrotic syndrome.

Table 14-6 | *Fluid Volume Excess*

	EXTRACELLULAR FLUID EXCESS (ISOTONIC FLUID EXCESS)	INTRACELLULAR WATER EXCESS (HYPOTONIC FLUID EXCESS)
DEFINITION	Excess of both water and electrolytes. Major symptoms are due to increased blood volume.	Excess of body water without excess electrolytes. Major symptoms are due to cerebral edema.
ETIOLOGY	Retention of water and electrolytes related to kidney disease; overload with isotonic IV fluids.	Overhydration in presence of renal failure; administration of D_5W after surgery or trauma.
ASSESSMENT FINDINGS		
Blood pressure	Increased	Increased systolic
Pulse	Bounding, increased rate	Decreased rate
Respirations	Increased rate, crackles, dyspnea	Increased rate
Weight	Gain	Gain
Edema	Extremities: dependent, pitting Puffy eyelids	Cerebral
Neck veins	Distended	Normal
Mucous membranes	Moist	Moist
Blood	Hgb, Hct, RBCs decreased by dilution	Hgb, Hct, RBCs normal or decreased
Mental status	Irritability, confusion, lethargy	Irritability, confusion, lethargy
Hand vein engorgement	Present	Absent
Pupils	Sluggish response to light with cerebral edema	Sluggish response to light with cerebral edema
TREATMENT	Correct underlying cause. Restrict water and sodium intake. Give diuretics to promote fluid elimination, digitalis to improve cardiac output. Consider renal dialysis if kidney failure is a factor.	Correct underlying cause. Restrict water intake. Give intravenous oral fluids with electrolytes. Give demeclocycline (Declomycin) to decrease kidney response to ADH.
NURSING CARE	Give drugs and IV fluids as ordered. Monitor for excess diuresis. Explain and enforce fluid restriction. Offer ice chips; use small fluid containers, let patient help design plan for fluid intake. If patient not confused, allow to swish fluids in mouth and spit out without swallowing. Explain salt restriction; obtain dietary consult for teaching (Box 14-5). Protect edematous tissue: turn and reposition q 2 hr. Inspect for signs of skin breakdown. If dyspneic: elevate head of bed 30 degrees or for comfort, loosen restrictive clothing, oxygen as ordered.	Give drugs and IV fluids as ordered. Explain and enforce fluid restriction. Offer ice chips, provide oral hygiene, serve only fluids allowed with meal trays, let patient design plan for fluid intake. If patient not confused, allow to swish fluids in mouth and spit out without swallowing. If confused, take safety precautions: side rails up, bed in low position, call light in reach, check often. Seizure precautions per agency policy.

D_5W, dextrose 5% in water; *Hgb,* hemoglobin; *Hct,* hematocrit; *RBCs,* red blood cells; *ADH,* antidiuretic hormone; *IV,* intravenous.

Sodium normally holds water in the extracellular compartment. When serum sodium is low, water can enter cells more freely. This shift of fluids is most significant in relation to brain cells. The accumulation of fluid in brain cells produces the most important physiologic effects of hyponatremia.

Assessment

If hyponatremia is suspected or the patient is at risk, monitor for signs and symptoms, which include headache, muscle weakness, fatigue, apathy, confusion, abdominal cramps, and orthostatic hypotension. Take blood pressures with the patient lying or sitting and then standing to determine whether there is a signifi-

cant drop. A drop in systolic blood pressure of more than 20 mm Hg indicates orthostatic hypotension.

Medical Treatment

The usual treatment for hyponatremia is restriction of fluids while the kidneys excrete excess water. Intravenous normal saline or Ringer's lactate may be ordered. If sodium falls below 115 mEq/L, hypertonic sodium may be ordered. The diuretic furosemide (Lasix) may be ordered because of its ability to promote water loss that exceeds the sodium loss. If the patient has SIADH, drugs such as demeclocycline and lithium that antagonize antidiuretic hormone may be ordered. A balanced diet usually provides adequate sodium, but patients with moderate or severe hyponatremia may need sodium replacement therapy.

NURSING CARE

You can help prevent hyponatremia in patients with feeding tubes by using normal saline rather than water for irrigation. For patients with hyponatremia, administer prescribed medications and intravenous fluids and monitor the response to these. Measure fluid intake and output, and assess mental status. If the patient is confused, take safety measures to prevent injury. If the patient who has hyponatremia has low blood pressure or postural hypotension, assess the need for assistance with ambulation.

HYPERNATREMIA (SODIUM EXCESS)

Hypernatremia refers to a higher-than-normal concentration of sodium in the blood. It is a very serious imbalance that can lead to death if not corrected. Hypernatremia can occur alone or in combination with extracellular fluid volume deficit. The high level of sodium in the serum and other extracellular fluids causes water to shift out of the cells. This creates a condition of cellular dehydration. Hypernatremia occurs when there is excessive loss of water or excessive retention of sodium. Some causes of hypernatremia are vomiting, diarrhea, diaphoresis (profuse sweating), and insufficient antidiuretic hormone. Signs and symptoms of hypernatremia are thirst, a flushed skin, dry mucous membranes, a low urine output, restlessness, an increased heart rate, convulsions, and postural hypotension.

Medical Treatment

Medical intervention focuses on oral or intravenous replacement of water to restore balance. The aim is to restore the fluid balance slowly to prevent cerebral edema resulting from excessive dilution of extracellular fluid. If the patient has an extracellular fluid volume deficit as well, intravenous fluids with decreasing amounts of sodium may be ordered. A low-sodium diet is often prescribed.

NURSING CARE

Encourage patients with hypernatremia to drink water for hydration. Closely monitor the infusion of intravenous fluids, especially when the patient's cardiac or renal function is abnormal. Patient education is important. Teach the patient with hypernatremia to track daily intake and output and to recognize the signs and symptoms of fluid retention or depletion. Advise patients accordingly if any dietary restrictions are part of the treatment. If a low-sodium diet is prescribed, patients should avoid foods that are high in sodium (Na^+): ketchup, monosodium glutamate (Accent), mustard, pickles, olives, ham, most canned foods, artificial sweeteners, laxatives, cough medications, and some antacids. A selection of foods high and low in so-

dium is found in Box 14-5. Salt substitutes can be used if potassium (K^+) intake is not restricted, because salt substitutes contain significant potassium.

HYPOKALEMIA (POTASSIUM DEFICIT)

Hypokalemia is low serum potassium. Causes include vomiting, diarrhea, nasogastric suction, inadequate dietary intake of potassium, diabetic acidosis, excessive aldosterone secretion, and drugs such as potassium-wasting diuretics and corticosteroids. Because potassium is necessary for normal cellular function, deficiencies may result in gastrointestinal, renal, cardiovascular, and neurologic disturbances. Most important is the effect on myocardial cells, which tends to cause abnormal, potentially fatal, heart rhythms.

Box 14-5 | **Common Food Sources of Sodium**

Foods High in Sodium (Approximately 250 mg per Serving)

Grains
Cold cereal, 1 oz
Corn chips, 14 chips
Instant hot cereal, ½ cup
Potato chips, 14 chips

Cheeses
Natural cheese, 1 oz
Processed cheese, 1 oz
Creamed cheese, ½ cup

Meats
Sausage, 1 oz
Luncheon meats, 1 oz
Frankfurters, 1 oz
Cooked bacon, 2 slices
Ham, 1 oz

Convenience Foods
Pizza, 2 to 3 slices
Pot pies, 8 oz
Ravioli, canned, 8 oz
Soups (canned or dehydrated), 1 cup

Foods Low in Sodium (Less Than 50 mg per Serving)

Fruits and Vegetables
Fresh fruits or canned, ½ cup
Fresh, frozen, ½ cup

Grains
Unsalted pastas, ½ cup
Oatmeal, cooked, 1 cup
Popcorn (unsalted), 1 oz
Puffed rice, 1 cup
Shredded wheat, 1 biscuit

Meats
Fresh meat, 1 oz
Fresh chicken, 1 oz
Fresh fish, 1 oz

Data from Laquarta, I., & Gerlach, M. (1990). *Nutrition in clinical nursing.* Albany, NY: Delmar Publishers; Burtis, G., et al. (1988). *Applied nutrition and diet therapy.* Philadelphia: Saunders; and Black, J.M., & Matassarin-Jacobs, E. (1997). Medical-surgical nursing: Clinical management for continuity of care (5th ed., p. 288). Philadelphia: Saunders.

Signs and symptoms of hypokalemia are anorexia, abdominal distention, vomiting, diarrhea, muscle cramps, weakness, dysrhythmias (abnormal cardiac rhythms), postural hypotension, dyspnea, shallow respirations, confusion, depression, polyuria (excessive urination), and nocturia.

Medical Treatment

Potassium replacement by the intravenous or oral route may be prescribed.

NURSING CARE

Assessment consists of monitoring at-risk patients for decreased bowel sounds, a weak and irregular pulse, decreased reflexes, and decreased muscle tone. It is especially important to monitor the heart rate and rhythm of patients taking digitalis, because hypokalemia increases the risk of digitalis toxicity. Cardiac monitors may be used to detect dysrhythmias.

Administer oral potassium supplements as prescribed. Give them with a full glass of water or fruit juice to avoid gastrointestinal irritation. Instruct patients to sip slowly. Encourage dietary sources of potassium, particularly fruits and vegetables, such as bananas and oranges or orange juice. A chart of foods high and low in potassium is found in Box 14-6.

Administer intravenous potassium as ordered. Potassium is *always* diluted and never given in concentrated form. Ideally, it is administered through a central venous catheter, otherwise the potassium may not be adequately diluted by blood before it reaches the heart. Monitor the infusion site because potassium salts can cause inflammation of the veins. Potassium is *never* given by intravenous push.

Check the patient's urine output before starting an intravenous infusion of potassium. When the urine output is low, intravenous fluids without potassium may be given until the urine output is acceptable, and then fluids with potassium are started. If you were to administer the intravenous potassium before normal urinary output was restored, the patient could develop hyperkalemia. Urinary output should be no less than 30 mL/hr. If it is less than 30 mL/hr for 2 consecutive hours, alert the physician, who may order a stop of the infusion.

Pharmacology Capsule

Potassium is always diluted before intravenous administration. Rapid infusion of potassium can cause cardiac arrest.

Box 14-6 | *Common Food Sources of Potassium*

Foods High in Potassium (Average 7 mEq per Serving)	Beverages
Vegetables (½ cup cooked or 1 cup raw)	Brewed coffee
Artichokes	Tomato juice
Broccoli	Vegetable juice cocktail, unsalted
Brussels sprouts	
Cabbage	**Foods Low in Potassium (Average 3 mEq per Serving)**
Carrots	**Vegetables**
Celery	Corn, ⅓ cup
Collards	Sweet potato, yams, ¼ cup
Cucumber	Lima beans, ⅓ cup
Mushrooms	French fried potatoes, 10
Spinach	**Fruit**
Tomatoes	Apple, 1 small
Fruits	Apple juice, ½ cup
Apricots, fresh, 4 medium	Applesauce, ½ cup
Apricots, canned, 4 halves	Blueberries, ¾ cup
Apricots, dried, 7 halves	Cranberries, 1¼ cup
Banana, 7 inches	**Beverages**
Cantaloupe, ¼ small	Coffee, instant
Guava, 1 medium	Cola
Honeydew melon, ⅛ medium	Cranberry juice cocktail, ⅓ cup
Nectarine, ½	Ginger ale
Orange, 1 small	Noncarbonated soft drinks
Prunes, 3 medium	Root beer
Strawberries, 1¼ cup	Lemon-lime soda
Tangerines, 2 medium	
Watermelon, 1¼ cup	

Data from Mahan, K.L., & Arlin, M. (1992). *Food, nutrition and diet therapy* (8th ed.). Philadelphia: Saunders; and Black, J.M., & Matassarin-Jacobs, E. (1997). *Medical-surgical nursing: Clinical management for continuity of care* (5th ed., p. 313). Philadelphia: Saunders.

HYPERKALEMIA (POTASSIUM EXCESS)

Hyperkalemia is high serum potassium. Potassium is plentiful in common foods, so it is easy for people on normal diets to take in adequate amounts. However, the kidneys do not readily conserve potassium, so continuous replacement is necessary. Patients at risk for hyperkalemia are those with decreased renal function, people in metabolic acidosis, and people taking potassium supplements. Also, patients who have had severe traumatic injuries may develop hyperkalemia because of the loss of potassium from damaged cells into the extracellular fluid.

Hyperkalemia is a serious imbalance because of the potential for life-threatening dysrhythmias. Elevated potassium typically causes first bradycardia, and then tachycardia. There is a risk of cardiac arrest. In the gastrointestinal system, hyperkalemia can cause explosive diarrhea and vomiting. Neuromuscular effects are muscle cramps and weakness and paresthesia (a tingling sensation). Other signs and symptoms of hyperkalemia include irritability, anxiety, abdominal cramps, and decreased urine output.

Medical Treatment

Hyperkalemia is treated by correcting the underlying causes and restricting potassium intake. Polystyrene sulfonate (Kayexalate), a drug that can be given orally or rectally, promotes excretion of excess potassium through the intestinal tract. Intravenous calcium gluconate may be given to decrease the effects of potassium on the myocardium. Temporary effects may be obtained by the intravenous administration of insulin and glucose or sodium bicarbonate to promote the shifting of potassium into the cells.

NURSING CARE

Patients with low urine output or those taking potassium-sparing diuretics must be monitored carefully for signs and symptoms of hyperkalemia because decreased renal function can cause hyperkalemia. Patients receiving potassium supplements, especially intravenously, warrant special attention. Carefully monitor the flow rate of intravenous fluids, which should not exceed 10 mEq/hr through peripheral veins. Even when extreme hypokalemia is being treated, no more than 40 mEq/hr should be given and *only* with constant cardiac monitoring. Examine the infusion site because potassium is very irritating to subcutaneous tissues. Extravasation can cause serious tissue damage.

Screen the results of laboratory studies. Because serum potassium levels greater than 5.0 mEq/L can cause cardiac arrest, immediately report the results to the physician and anticipate an order for the patient to be placed on cardiac monitoring.

Teach patients who take potassium supplements to look for signs and symptoms of abnormal potassium levels and to understand why frequent blood tests are required to monitor potassium levels.

CHLORIDE IMBALANCE

Because chloride is usually bound to other electrolytes, chloride imbalances accompany other electrolyte imbalances. High serum chloride, known as *hyperchloremia*, usually is associated with metabolic acidosis. Low serum chloride, known as *hypochloremia,* usually occurs when sodium is lost, because chloride is most frequently bound with sodium. Hypochloremia may be caused by vomiting and uncontrolled diabetes.

CALCIUM IMBALANCE

Calcium in the blood is regulated by the parathyroid glands, which secrete parathyroid hormone (PTH). A low serum level of calcium (hypocalcemia) stimulates PTH secretion. PTH enhances calcium retention and phosphate excretion by the kidneys, promotes calcium absorption in the intestines, and can mobilize calcium from the bones to raise the serum level. Hypocalcemia results from diarrhea, inadequate dietary intake of calcium or vitamin D, and multiple blood transfusions (banked blood contains citrates that bind to calcium), in addition to some diseases including hypoparathyroidism. Hypercalcemia occurs with increased serum levels of calcium. Causes of hypercalcemia include a high calcium or vitamin D intake, hyperparathyroidism, and immobility that causes stores of calcium in the bones to enter the bloodstream. It is also a complication of certain types of cancer.

MAGNESIUM IMBALANCE

A lower-than-normal concentration of magnesium in the bloodstream is known as *hypomagnesemia.* Hypomagnesemia results from decreased gastrointestinal absorption or excessive gastrointestinal loss, usually from vomiting and diarrhea, or from increased urinary loss. Hypomagnesemia often is associated with hypocalcemia and hypokalemia.

A higher-than-normal concentration of magnesium in the bloodstream is known as *hypermagnesemia.* It occurs most often with the excessive use of magnesium-containing medications or intravenous solutions in patients with renal failure or preeclampsia of pregnancy.

ACID-BASE DISTURBANCES

Acid-base balance refers to homeostasis of the hydrogen ion (H^+) concentration in the body fluids. A solution containing a higher number of hydrogen ions is an acid, and a solution containing a lower number of hydrogen ions is an *alkaline* or base. The symbol used to indicate hydrogen ion concentration is pH. pH is reported on a scale of 1 to 14, with 1 to 6.9 being acidic, 7 being neutral, and 7.1 to 14 being alkaline.

The hydrogen ion concentration in extracellular fluid is indicated by the pH of the blood. The normal pH of blood is between 7.35 and 7.45, which is slightly alkaline. The normal acid-base balance is maintained by three primary, complex mechanisms: (1) buffers, (2) respiratory control of carbon dioxide (CO_2), and (3) renal regulation of bicarbonate (HCO_3^-). The principal buffers in renal tubular fluid are the carbonic acid/bicarbonate system, ammonia, and phosphate. Other substances that function as buffers are proteins and hemoglobin. Buffer systems comprise a weak acid and a salt. To maintain body fluids in the normal pH range, the blood buffers circulate throughout the body in pairs, acting as sponges to soak up hydrogen ions. One of the buffers takes away a hydrogen ion if a fluid is too acid, and one of the buffers gives an ion if the fluid is too alkaline.

The lungs and kidneys are the next line of defense after the blood buffers for maintaining acid-base balance. The lungs are primarily responsible for the regulation of carbon dioxide in the blood, which is controlled by the rate and depth of respirations. Carbonic acid in the alveolar capillaries breaks down into water and carbon dioxide, which is eliminated through exhalation. Deep, rapid breathing eliminates excess carbon dioxide, thereby reducing extracellular fluid acidity. Shallow, slow respirations reduce the loss of carbon dioxide, thereby increasing extracellular acidity. If the pH of the blood becomes too high or too low, the respiratory center in the brain sends signals to the lungs to increase or decrease respirations to "blow off" or retain the appropriate amount of carbon dioxide.

The kidneys act as the metabolic regulators of pH by excreting acids or bases as needed. Renal regulation of bicarbonate and excretion of hydrogen ions are the chief means of regulating acid-base balance through the kidneys. Bicarbonate is a major acid buffer in the blood, and it is through the kidneys that bicarbonate is reabsorbed and produced.

If the regulatory mechanisms fail, acid-base imbalances occur. The four major types of acid-base imbalances are (1) respiratory acidosis, (2) respiratory alkalosis, (3) metabolic acidosis, and (4) metabolic alkalosis.

ASSESSMENT OF ACID-BASE STATUS

Health History

Note any history of renal, endocrine, or respiratory disease. A history of diabetes mellitus is especially important because acidosis is a complication of diabetes. Assess the patient for symptoms of acid-base imbalance, which could include very deep and/or rapid respirations, anxiety, confusion, dizziness, lightheadedness, seizures, and change in weight. List any medications the patient is taking.

Physical Examination

Observe the patient's general appearance in terms of responsiveness. Look for signs of anxiety or other distress. Take the vital signs, and weigh the patient. Pay special attention to the rate, depth, and rhythm of respiration. Test muscle strength and sensory function in the extremities. Evaluate mental status.

In addition to collecting data during the nursing assessment, as described in Box 14-7, note the results of arterial blood gas measurements (Table 14-7).

RESPIRATORY ACIDOSIS

Respiratory acidosis occurs when the respiratory system fails to eliminate the appropriate amount of carbon dioxide to maintain the normal acid-base balance. Carbon dioxide is retained, with a resultant accumulation of carbonic acid and a decrease in blood pH. The body responds to respiratory acidosis by stimulating respirations to eliminate excess carbon dioxide. If that mechanism cannot restore balance, renal compensation begins. The kidneys attempt to help by reabsorbing more bicarbonate to balance the amount of carbonic acid in the blood.

Acute respiratory acidosis is caused by respiratory diseases such as pneumonia, drug overdose, head injury, chest wall injury, obesity, asphyxiation, drowning, or acute respiratory failure. People with chronic pulmonary disease may have elevated carbon dioxide levels but a normal pH as a result of renal compensation. Common clinical signs and symptoms include rapid heart rate, headache, sweating, lethargy, and confusion.

Medical Treatment

Interventions for respiratory acidosis are geared toward improving ventilation, which in turn restores the partial pressure of carbon dioxide in arterial blood ($Paco_2$) to normal. Underlying respiratory conditions are treated to eliminate the cause of respiratory acidosis. Antibiotics, bronchodilators, and specific breathing treatments such as intermittent positive-pressure breathing, inspiratory and/or expiratory positive airway pressure, and continuous positive airway pressure may be prescribed.

Box 14-7   *ASSESSMENT of Acid-Base Balance*

Health History
Signs and Symptoms:
Dyspnea, anxiety, confusion, dizziness, seizures, changes in weight, muscle weakness, abnormal sensations (numbness, tingling)
Medical Conditions:
Diabetes mellitus, adrenal disorders, cardiac disorders, renal failure, respiratory impairment
Current Medications

Physical Examination
Height and Weight:
Compared with previous measurements
Vital Signs:
Pulse rate and rhythm; respiratory rate, depth, and rhythm
Neurologic Function:
Muscle strength, sensation in extremities, mental status

Measures of Oyxgenation
Arterial blood gases

Table 14-7 | *Arterial Blood Gas Values with Uncompensated Respiratory and Metabolic Acidosis and Alkalosis*

CONDITION	CAUSE	pH	HCO$_3^-$	Paco$_2$
Respiratory acidosis	Hypoventilation	↓	Normal	↑
Respiratory alkalosis	Hyperventilation	↑	Normal	↓
Metabolic acidosis	Diabetic ketoacidosis	↓	↓	Normal
	Lactic acidosis			
	Diarrhea			
	Renal insufficiency			
Metabolic alkalosis	Vomiting	↑	↑	Normal
	HCO$_3^-$ retention			
	Volume depletion			
	K$^+$ depletion			

In some cases, intubation and mechanical ventilation are necessary (see Chapter 30).

NURSING CARE

Assessment

The most accurate method of assessing for respiratory acidosis is the measurement of the Paco$_2$ level in arterial blood. The Paco$_2$ directly reflects the degree of respiratory dysfunction. In addition, patients should be observed for signs of respiratory distress, including restlessness, anxiety, confusion, and tachycardia. Frequently note the rate, depth, and rhythm of respirations. Respiratory rate and depth vary with the situation. For example, the patient with a head injury or drug overdose may have slow respirations that contribute to carbon dioxide retention. The patient with pneumonia may have rapid respirations in an effort to eliminate carbon dioxide that has accumulated as a result of impaired gas exchange. Assess level of consciousness, including orientation to person, place, and time, to detect changes in mental status.

Intervention

Encourage fluid intake to loosen secretions and keep mucous membranes moist. Position patients with the head elevated 30 degrees to promote comfort and ensure optimal gas exchange. Monitor confused patients frequently, and attempt to anticipate their needs. Because confused patients may fall as they try to get to the bathroom, they should be assisted to the bathroom every 2 hours, especially if fluids are increased. Constant reassurance and reorientation are helpful.

RESPIRATORY ALKALOSIS

Respiratory alkalosis is marked by low Paco$_2$ with a resultant rise in pH. The most common cause of respiratory alkalosis is hyperventilation. Hyperventilation is characterized by rapid or deep respirations that cause excessive amounts of carbon dioxide to be eliminated

through the lungs. When the body fluids become alkaline, ionized extracellular calcium decreases and the patient has symptoms of hypocalcemia.

One cause of hyperventilation leading to respiratory alkalosis is anxiety. Other causes are conditions that result in decreased oxygen in the blood, such as pneumonia, adult respiratory distress syndrome, anemia, severe blood loss resulting from trauma, and congestive heart failure. Fever, pain, drugs (aspirin overdose), head trauma, and gram-negative septicemia also may contribute to respiratory alkalosis. The body attempts to compensate for respiratory alkalosis by eliminating excess bicarbonate through the kidneys. Clinical signs and symptoms include increased respiratory and heart rates, an anxious appearance, irritability, dizziness, lightheadedness, muscle weakness, and tingling or numbness of the fingers. In extreme respiratory alkalosis, confusion, fainting, and seizures may occur. Assessment of the rate and depth of respirations is the key observation for this condition.

Medical Treatment

The major goal of therapy is to treat the underlying cause of the condition. Sedation may be ordered for the anxious patient.

NURSING CARE

Assessment

The general assessment of patients with acid-base imbalances was described earlier in the chapter. With respiratory alkalosis, a description of respiratory status is especially important.

Intervention

In addition to giving sedatives as ordered, reassure the patient to relieve anxiety. Encourage the patient to breathe slowly, which will retain carbon dioxide in the body. Breathing slowly into a paper bag raises the Paco$_2$ because the patient rebreathes exhaled carbon dioxide. When breathing stabilizes, allow the patient to have uninterrupted rest because hyperventilation can result in fatigue.

METABOLIC ACIDOSIS

Metabolic acidosis occurs when the body retains too many hydrogen ions or loses too many bicarbonate ions. With too much acid and too little base, the pH of the blood falls. Metabolic acidosis leads to hyperventilation because the lungs try to compensate by blowing off carbon dioxide and lowering $Paco_2$ levels, which raises the pH.

Causes of metabolic acidosis are starvation, dehydration, diarrhea, shock, renal failure, and diabetic ketoacidosis. Signs and symptoms vary according to the underlying cause and the severity of the acid-base disturbance. However, patients may experience changing levels of consciousness, ranging from fatigue and confusion to stupor and coma, headache, vomiting and diarrhea, anorexia, muscle weakness, and cardiac dysrhythmias.

Medical Treatment

The primary intervention for metabolic acidosis is treatment of the underlying disorder. Mechanical ventilation may be necessary, especially in patients who are comatose. Once corrective measures have been initiated, an intravenous infusion of sodium bicarbonate might be ordered, based on arterial blood gas results.

NURSING CARE

Assessment

Assessment of the patient in metabolic acidosis should focus on vital signs, mental status, and neurologic status.

Intervention

Nursing care is geared toward emergency measures to restore acid-base balance. Administer drugs and intravenous fluids as prescribed. Reassure and orient confused patients.

METABOLIC ALKALOSIS

Metabolic alkalosis is the opposite of metabolic acidosis. It results from an increase in bicarbonate levels or a loss of hydrogen ions. Loss of hydrogen ions may be caused by prolonged nasogastric suctioning, excessive vomiting, diuretics, and electrolyte disturbances. Retention of bicarbonate may result from the administration of bicarbonate or massive blood transfusions.

Clinical signs and symptoms may include headache; irritability; lethargy; changes in level of consciousness; confusion; changes in heart rate; slow, shallow respirations with periods of apnea; nausea and vomiting; hyperactive reflexes; and numbness of the extremities.

Medical Treatment

As with other acid-base imbalances, treatment depends on the underlying cause and severity of the condition.

NURSING CARE

Assessment

Take vital signs and daily weight measurements of the patient, and monitor heart rate, respirations, and fluid gains and losses. Keep accurate intake and output records, including the amount of fluid removed by suction. Assess motor function and sensation in the extremities, and monitor laboratory values, especially pH and serum bicarbonate levels.

Intervention

To prevent metabolic alkalosis, use isotonic saline solutions rather than water for irrigating nasogastric tubes, because the use of water for irrigation can result in a loss of electrolytes. Provide reassurance and comfort measures to promote safety and well-being.

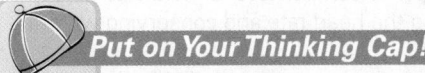
Put on Your Thinking Cap!

Recall a patient who either had or was at risk for fluid and electrolyte imbalances.
1. What assessment data should have been collected?
2. Identify factors that placed the patient at risk.
3. Identify measures to treat or prevent the imbalances.

Key Points

- Approximately 50% to 60% of the human body is composed of water. To maintain homeostasis, the body must be able to regulate the fluids within it.
- The process of homeostasis involves delivery of nutrients and oxygen to the cells and removal of wastes, including carbon dioxide, from the cells.
- Body fluids are classified on the basis of location in body compartments: (1) intracellular fluid (fluid within the cell) and (2) extracellular fluid (fluid outside the cell). Most of the body's fluids are found within the cell.
- Extracellular fluid is mainly responsible for the transport of nutrients and wastes throughout the body.
- Electrolytes, which are substances that develop an electrical charge when dissolved in water, maintain a balance between positive and negative charges to keep the body in homeostasis.
- Total body water decreases in older adults, with the greatest decline in intracellular fluid.
- The fluid compartments of the body are separated by selectively permeable membranes that control movement of water and certain solutes.
- Water and solutes move between intracellular and extracellular fluid compartments by one or more of the following processes: (1) diffusion, (2) active transport, (3) filtration, and (4) osmosis.

- The kidneys are the primary regulators of fluid balance in the body, and the nephrons conduct the work of the kidneys through the processes of filtration, reabsorption, and secretion.
- Hormones that have a major effect on fluid balance include renin, aldosterone, antidiuretic hormone (ADH), and atrial natriuretic factor (ANF).
- Renin is secreted when blood volume or blood pressure falls. It stimulates release of aldosterone and helps produce angiotensin I, which is converted to angiotensin II—a potent vasoconstrictor.
- Aldosterone is secreted by the adrenal glands and promotes sodium retention. Antidiuretic hormone, produced by the hypothalamus and secreted by the posterior pituitary gland, promotes water retention.
- ANF is secreted when stretch receptors in atria detect an increase in blood volume. It promotes excretion of water and sodium, decreases renin synthesis, inhibits release of aldosterone and ADH, and causes vasodilation.
- The thirst center creates a desire to drink fluids when extracellular fluid becomes concentrated.
- In a healthy adult, the 24-hour fluid intake and output are approximately equal.
- The body attempts to compensate for fluid volume deficits by increasing the heart rate and conserving water in the kidneys.
- The body attempts to compensate for fluid volume excess by increasing urine output.
- The kidneys are the primary regulators of electrolytes in the blood.

- Two electrolytes that cause the majority of problems when there is an imbalance are sodium (Na^+) and potassium (K^+).
- Change in body weight is a good indicator of fluid loss or retention.
- Edema reflects sodium retention, which can result from excessive reabsorption or inadequate secretion because of failing kidney function.
- Potassium excess or deficit can lead to life-threatening cardiac dysrhythmias.
- Because older adults often have a reduced thirst sensation and may not conserve water efficiently, they are at risk for fluid volume deficit.
- Acid-base balance is the homeostasis of the hydrogen ion (H^+) concentration in the body fluids.
- Mechanisms that maintain acid-base balance are blood buffers, respiratory control of carbon dioxide, and renal regulation of bicarbonate (HCO_3^-).
- Acid-base imbalances occur when an imbalance in the functioning of the lungs, kidneys, or both exists. The four major acid-base imbalances are (1) respiratory acidosis, (2) respiratory alkalosis, (3) metabolic acidosis, and (4) metabolic alkalosis.

 Go to your Companion CD-ROM for a Pharmacology Tutorial, Audio Glossary, and 3-D animations.

evolve Be sure to visit the companion Evolve site at http://evolve.elsevier.com/Linton/ for WebLinks and additional online resources.

REVIEW QUESTIONS *Choose the best answer.*

1. Fluid surrounding the cells is called:
   1. Intracellular
   2. Lymph
   3. Intravascular
   4. Interstitial

2. The largest portion of a person's body weight is contributed by:
   1. Water
   2. Fat
   3. Bone
   4. Muscle

3. Anions include the following:
   1. Sodium
   2. Calcium
   3. Chloride
   4. Magnesium

4. The movement of water across a membrane from a less concentrated solution to a more concentrated solution defines:
   1. Diffusion
   2. Osmosis
   3. Filtration
   4. Active transport

5. A hormone with physiologic effects that decrease blood pressure is:
   1. Antidiuretic hormone
   2. Renin
   3. Aldosterone
   4. Atrial natriuretic factor

6. Which of the following statements best describes the risk of fluid and electrolyte imbalances in the older adult?
   1. Most older adults can maintain fluid and electrolyte balance just as well as younger adults.
   2. Older adults have limited reserves to maintain fluid balance when abnormal losses occur.
   3. Body water increases with age, putting the older adult at risk for fluid volume excess.
   4. The amount of extracellular fluid declines, leaving the patient with reduced fluid stores.

7. A patient is receiving diuretics to eliminate excess fluid that has been retained in body tissues. In 2 days the patient lost 4.4 lbs (2 kg) in body weight. This represents how much fluid loss?
   1. 1 liter
   2. 2 liters
   3. 3 liters
   4. 4.4 liters

8. You gently pinch the skin over a patient's sternum. The skin does not flatten right away, leading you to suspect:

   1. Recent weight loss
   2. History of excessive sun exposure
   3. Dehydration
   4. Need for increased diuretics

9. Fluid volume excess can be classified as intracellular or:

   1. Extracellular
   2. Intravascular
   3. Interstitial
   4. Extravascular

10. When a patient has a potassium imbalance, which of the following nursing assessments is most important?

    1. Auscultate bowel sounds.
    2. Evaluate muscle strength.
    3. Monitor heart rate and rhythm.
    4. Assess reflexes.

11. Which answer lists in correct order the mechanisms that maintain acid-base balance?

    1. Renal regulation, respiratory regulation, buffers
    2. Buffers, respiratory regulation, renal regulation
    3. Buffers, renal regulation, respiratory regulation
    4. Respiratory regulation, buffers, renal regulation

12. What is the physiologic function of deep, rapid respirations in metabolic acidosis?

    1. Eliminates excess carbon dioxide that is formed in the presence of acidosis
    2. Raises the Pao_2, which reduces the pH of the blood
    3. Supplies additional oxygen needed because of the increased metabolic rate
    4. Reduces $Paco_2$, resulting in a rise in blood pH and correction of acidosis

CHAPTER 15

Pain Management

MARY L. HEYE AND KATHLEEN A. REEVES

evolve   http://evolve.elsevier.com/Linton/

Objectives

After reading and studying this chapter, you should be able to:

1. Define pain.
2. Explain the physiologic basis for pain.
3. Identify situations in which patients are likely to experience pain.
4. Explain the relationships between past pain experiences, anticipation, culture, anxiety, or activity and a patient's response to pain.
5. Identify differences in the duration of pain and patient responses to acute and chronic pain.
6. Explain the special needs of the older adult patient with pain.
7. List the data to be collected in assessing pain.
8. Describe interventions used in the management of pain.
9. Describe the nursing care of patients receiving opioid and nonopioid analgesics for pain.
10. List the factors that should be considered when pain is not relieved with analgesic medications.

Key Terms

Be sure to check out the bonus material on the Companion CD-ROM, including selected audio pronunciations.

acute pain (p. 205)
addiction (p. 217)
analgesia (ăn-ăl-JĒ-zē-ă, p. 204)
analgesic (ăn-ăl-JĒ-zik, p. 202)
anesthesia (ăn-es-THĒ-zē-ă, p. 204)
chronic pain (p. 205)
nociceptor (nō-sē-SEP-ter, p. 203)
pain (p. 202)
pain threshold (p. 204)
pain tolerance (p. 204)
physical dependence (p. 217)
tolerance (p. 217)

Pain is one of the most complex experiences to understand and treat. It is also the most common problem that nurses encounter. Research about pain, analgesics (drugs that relieve pain), and the mind-body influence is just beginning to filter down to nursing practice. Still, many questions about pain remain unanswered.

Pain is influenced by many variables: the individual experiencing it, the cause of the pain, and the environment. Pain may arise from a new source, from an old injury, or from nerve injury. Sometimes the cause is unknown. Pain relief rests primarily with the nurse, who must assess the patient and implement appropriate interventions.

Nurses have many categories of pain-relieving interventions to choose from, yet they frequently administer only analgesics. Most nurses believe that pain is easily managed with analgesic drugs. Patients, however, often report that pain remains moderate to severe despite these medications. Research indicates that nurses fail to assess pain, tend to undermedicate for pain, and have inadequate knowledge of pain relief measures. Because of these findings, the Joint Commission on Accreditation of Healthcare Organizations published standards for the management of pain for all patients. Health care facilities are expected to comply with these standards. These include (1) recognizing the right of patients to appropriate assessment and management of pain, (2) performing pain assessments, (3) recording results of assessment and follow-up, (4) teaching patients about effective pain management, and (5) addressing needs for pain and symptom management at discharge.

The purpose of this chapter is to enable the nurse to understand pain and provide the most effective interventions for pain relief.

DEFINITION OF PAIN

Pain is defined in many ways. The International Association for the Study of Pain defines it as an unpleasant sensory and emotional experience associated with actual or potential tissue damage. McCaffery, a nurse and leader in the pain management field, has a more useful definition for nurses. She says, "Pain is whatever the person experiencing it says it is and exists whenever he says it does."

PHYSIOLOGY OF PAIN

Pain consists of various sensory experiences such as experiences of time and space, emotions, and cognition. The perception of pain involves afferent pathways, the central nervous system, and efferent pathways. Afferent pathways are nerves that carry messages to the brain for interpretation. Efferent (or descending) pathways are nerves that carry messages away from the brain to the rest of the body via the spinal cord.

Afferent pathways are activated by pain receptors called nociceptors. These pain receptors are unevenly distributed in muscles, tendons, subcutaneous tissue, and the skin. This may explain why parts of the body are more sensitive to pain than other parts. Pain receptors are sensitive to chemical changes, temperature, mechanical stimuli, and tissue damage. Some receptors are sensitive to more than one type of stimulus. Pain receptors are unable to adapt to repeated stimuli and thus continue to react until the stimuli are removed.

When pain receptors are stimulated, impulses are transmitted to the spinal cord. The impulses then travel up the spinal cord to the brain. In the brain, the cortex interprets the impulses as pain and identifies the location and qualities of the pain. Other structures involved in the interpretation of pain signals activate the stress response and produce the unpleasant qualities associated with pain, such as fear. Once pain is transmitted to the spinal cord and brain, the descending pathway is activated and several substances like endorphins, serotonin, norepinephrine, gamma-amino butyric acid (GABA), and enkephalins are released that can inhibit pain transmission to the spinal cord.

Endorphins and enkephalins are the body's natural opioid-like substances that block the transmission of painful impulses to the brain. Differences in the amount of endorphins in individuals may explain why some people seem to experience more pain than others. Research suggests that prolonged stress and pain, as well as the prolonged use of morphine and alcohol, decrease endorphin levels. Factors that increase endorphin levels include brief stress and pain, laughter, exercise, acupuncture, transcutaneous electrical nerve stimulation (TENS), massive trauma, and sexual activity.

GATE-CONTROL THEORY

Although many theories have been proposed to explain pain, none fully describe the pain experience. One of the best known theories is Melzack and Wall's gate-control theory. It assumes that the pain experience reflects both physical and psychosocial factors. Painful impulses are transmitted to the spinal cord through small-diameter nerve fibers in the afferent pathway. When these small-diameter fibers are stimulated, the gating mechanism opens in the spinal cord, which permits the transmission of impulses from the spinal cord to the brain. Consequently the patient perceives pain. Factors that cause the gate to open include tissue damage, a monotonous environment, and fear of pain. These small-diameter fibers end in the spinal cord along with large-diameter fibers. The stimulation of large-diameter fibers can close the gate and interfere

with impulse transmission between the spinal cord and the brain. This causes diminished pain perception. Large-diameter nerve fibers are stimulated by cutaneous (skin) stimulation through massage, position change, and heat or cold applications. Sensory input such as distraction, guided imagery, and preparatory information also may close the gate. Figure 15-1 shows the structures and mechanisms associated with the gate-control theory.

FACTORS INFLUENCING RESPONSE TO PAIN

Consider the following example: Miss Smith and Mrs. Johnson are roommates in Room 200. Miss Smith, age 19, underwent a cholecystectomy the previous day, as

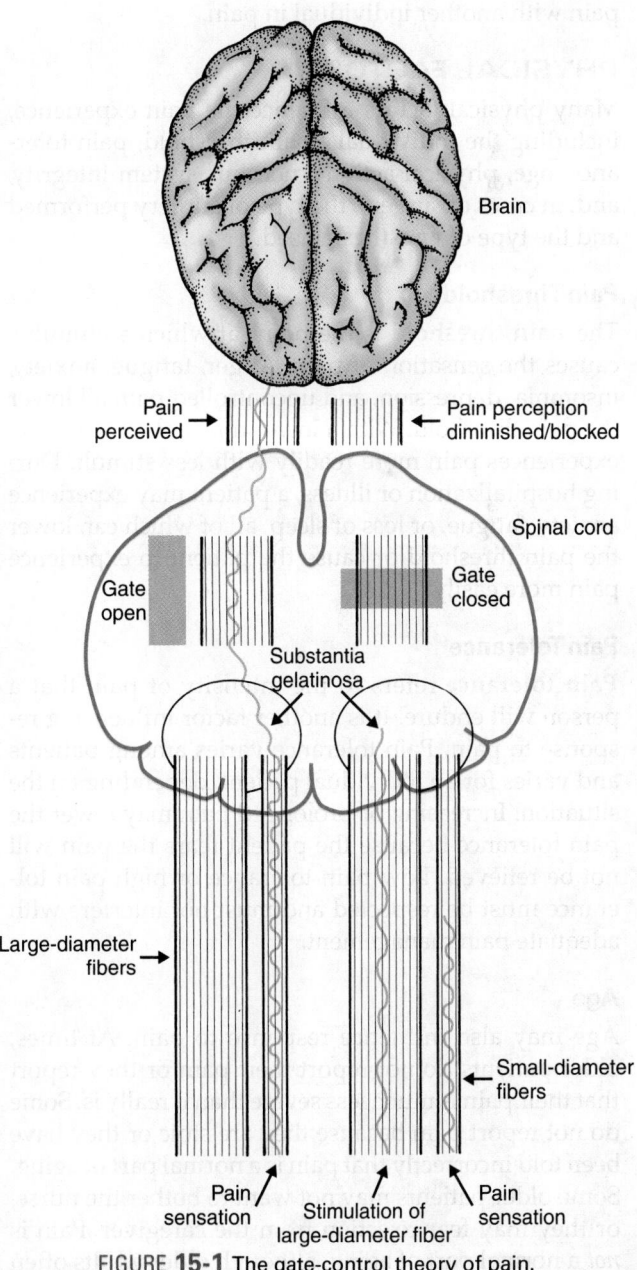

FIGURE **15-1** The gate-control theory of pain.

did Mrs. Johnson, age 67. The nurses discussed the difference in behavior of each patient: "Miss Smith constantly wants more pain medication. She moans and groans all the time. She won't even turn, cough, or breathe deeply for more than 10 seconds. She always rates her pain a 9 or a 10 on the pain scale. On the other hand, look at Mrs. Johnson. She's already ambulating. She rarely rates her pain as more than a 5 or a 6 on the pain scale. She usually just complains of aching, and she sure doesn't ask for as much pain medication as Miss Smith. You'd never guess they had undergone the same procedure."

This example illustrates that although people may have the same injury or insult (in this case, surgery), they may respond differently. This is because many physical and psychosocial factors affect the response to pain. It is important for health professionals to be nonjudgmental and to avoid comparing one individual in pain with another individual in pain.

PHYSICAL FACTORS

Many physical factors influence the pain experience, including the individual's pain threshold, pain tolerance, age, physical activity, nervous system integrity, and, in cases of surgery, the type of surgery performed and the type of anesthesia used.

Pain Threshold

The pain threshold is the point at which a stimulus causes the sensation of pain. Anger, fatigue, anxiety, insomnia, depression, and uncontrolled pain all lower the pain threshold. With a lower threshold, the person experiences pain more readily with less stimuli. During hospitalization or illness, a patient may experience anxiety, fatigue, or loss of sleep, all of which can lower the pain threshold or cause the patient to experience pain more easily.

Pain Tolerance

Pain tolerance refers to the intensity of pain that a person will endure. It is another factor influencing response to pain. Pain tolerance varies among patients and varies for an individual patient, depending on the situation. Increasing or prolonged pain may lower the pain tolerance because the patient fears the pain will not be relieved. Low pain tolerance or high pain tolerance must be respected and must not interfere with adequate pain management.

Age

Age may also influence response to pain. At times, older patients do not report their pain or they report that their pain is much less severe than it really is. Some do not report pain because they are stoic or they have been told incorrectly that pain is a normal part of aging. Some older patients may not want to bother the nurse, or they may fear rejection from the caregiver. Pain is *not* a normal part of aging, although older adults often suffer from chronic conditions such as arthritis, cancer, and bone fractures that are associated with pain.

Physical Activity and Nervous System Integrity

Physical activity and the integrity of the nervous system also can influence the reaction to pain. Physical activity may aggravate or precipitate pain. However, with some patients, physical activity may be used to relieve pain. Because pain is perceived and interpreted within the nervous system, the integrity of the system affects the response to pain. For example, patients with diabetic neuropathy may lose sensation in the extremities and may not feel pain there.

Surgery and Anesthesia

In surgical patients, the type of surgery performed and the type of anesthesia used can influence the response to pain. Surgery on the upper abdominal region of the body is thought to be the most painful type because of the numerous tissues traumatized during the procedure. Within this group are cardiac, pulmonary, gastric, and gallbladder procedures. The type of anesthetic agent used can influence postoperative pain. For example, ketamine has analgesic properties. Some anesthetic agents injected at the operative site may prolong analgesia for 12 to 24 hours after surgery. When these types of agents are used, patients may experience much less pain after surgery than those who do not receive these anesthetic agents.

Surgery or invasive procedures may be performed to relieve pain that is severely debilitating. Rhizotomy and cordotomy are surgical procedures that cut or destroy selected nerve tissue to interrupt the pain pathway. These operations intentionally leave the patient with some neurologic deficit, which may pose a risk for injury. The patient may be unaware that a body area is painful and may not protect that area from harm. Pain relief from these procedures may not be permanent because nerve tissue regenerates. Nerve blocks are procedures that involve destruction or anesthesia of a nerve root with injection of a chemical to achieve pain relief in a specific body area. Drugs are injected to block the transmission of pain signals. For example, intercostal (between the ribs) anesthetic nerve blocks may be performed with cardiac operations to reduce postoperative pain in the thoracic area. Acupuncture is another invasive technique that produces anesthesia or analgesia. It is an ancient Chinese practice in which tiny needles are inserted into the skin or subcutaneous tissues at specific points on the body. This technique may be used to relieve acute and chronic pain such as headache, menstrual cramps, and low back pain.

PSYCHOLOGICAL FACTORS

Along with physical factors, several psychological factors can influence the response to pain, including culture, religion, past experiences with pain, anxiety, and situational factors.

Culture and Ethnicity

Although studies have been conducted to determine the effect of culture and ethnicity on people's reaction to pain, it is critical to avoid making judgments based on how you think a person should react or behave. Some persons may deny pain, remain calm and unemotional, or withdraw. Other persons may cry, moan and groan, and involve their families in the painful experience. Be aware of the different ways of expressing pain, and respect individual variations in the response to pain.

Religious Beliefs

Religious beliefs also may have an impact on reaction to pain. Some patients may pray and believe that divine intervention will help them endure the pain. Others may view pain as a punishment for sins. Some individuals believe that suffering is required before pain relief can be obtained.

Past Experiences and Anxiety

Past experiences and anxiety may affect a person's response to current pain. A person may have developed positive coping strategies to deal with previous painful experiences. If, however, previous coping strategies were unsuccessful, the patient may be very anxious and overwhelmed by another painful experience.

Situational Factors

Finally, situational factors may influence response to pain. If the pain is associated with a serious illness such as cancer, the pain may have a greater impact on mood and activity than if the pain were associated with a less serious condition. The pain associated with childbirth is relatively short-lived and usually results in a beautiful outcome, whereas cancer pain may be chronic and increasing and may be associated with progression of the disease and death.

What Does Culture Have to Do with Pain?

The way a person behaves in response to pain is, in part, determined by cultural norms. Therefore people from some cultures quietly endure pain, whereas people from other cultures loudly express their pain. As nurses, we must accept each response and assess and intervene to promote maximum comfort.

RESPONSES TO PAIN

AUTONOMIC NERVOUS SYSTEM

The pain signal is interpreted by the brain as a stressor. The autonomic nervous system activates the fight-or-flight response, and certain physiologic responses are initiated. Box 15-1 indicates some of the responses that occur and the associated effects. The patient in pain may

---

| Box 15-1 | *Autonomic Nervous System Responses to Pain* |

Sympathetic Nervous System Responses
↑ Blood pressure
↑ Pulse rate
↑ Respiratory rate
Dilated pupils
Perspiration
Pallor

Parasympathetic Nervous System Responses
Constipation
Urinary retention

---

exhibit these physiologic responses, along with behaviors such as grimacing, moaning, and verbalizing pain, or withdrawing. The nervous system responses are measured by an increased heart rate, respiratory rate, and blood pressure. These are predictable responses to acute pain; however, the pain behavior will vary from individual to individual. Acute pain and chronic pain elicit different kinds of responses. Table 15-1 lists some differences between acute pain and chronic pain.

ACUTE PAIN

Most pain experienced in the hospital is acute pain. Acute pain follows the normal pathway for pain from nociceptor activation to the brain and may be called *nociceptive pain*. Examples are postoperative pain from incisions, renal colic pain from kidney stones, bone fractures, and pain in childbirth. Acute pain is temporary, and its cause is known and treatable. It serves as a warning of tissue damage and subsides when healing takes place. Nurses observe behavioral and physiologic signs of acute pain when the patient guards or rubs a body part, wrinkles the brow, bites the lip, and has changes in the heart rate, blood pressure, and respiratory rate. These responses may be absent or lessened in chronic pain.

CHRONIC PAIN

Chronic pain is usually defined as pain that persists or recurs for more than 3 to 6 months; it may last a lifetime. Chronic pain may also be nociceptive; however, most chronic pain is called *neuropathic pain* because it follows an abnormal pathway for pain. This is a new term that encompasses some puzzling and challenging pain syndromes classified as chronic pain. Neuropathic pain results from nerve damage resulting from a wide variety of anatomic and physiologic conditions and underlying diseases. It includes unusual sensations such as burning, shooting pain, and abnormal sensations that occur when there is no painful stimulus present.

The cause of the pain may be unknown. Treatment may or may not be helpful in relieving the pain. There are several types of chronic pain. Some classes of chronic pain and examples are shown in Table 15-2.

Table 15-1 | *Differences in Acute Pain and Chronic Pain*

CHARACTERISTIC	ACUTE	CHRONIC
Time	Limited, short duration	Lasts 3-6 months, longer duration
Purpose	Sign of tissue injury	No purpose
Verbal	Reports pain, focuses on pain	No report of pain unless questioned
Behavioral	Restless, thrashing, rubbing body part, pacing, grimacing, and other facial expressions of pain	Tired-looking, minimal facial expression, quiet, sleeps, rests, attention on other things
Physiologic	Increased heart rate, blood pressure, respiratory rate	Normal heart rate, blood pressure, respiratory rate
Interventions	Responds to analgesics	Less responsive to analgesics
	Standard doses effective	Higher doses needed for pain relief
	Parenteral or oral route used	Oral route preferred
	Additional drugs (adjuvant) seldom needed to manage pain	Additional drugs often needed to manage pain

Table 15-2 | *Chronic Pain*

CLASS	EXAMPLES
Acute pain: recurrent episodes	Neuralgia (herpes zoster) Migraine headaches Sickle cell crisis
Chronic malignant	Cancer pain syndromes
Chronic nonmalignant or benign	Low back pain Rheumatoid arthritis Phantom limb pain

Chronic pain is associated with a variety of diagnoses, including cancer, arthritis, peripheral vascular diseases, and traumatic injuries.

Chronic nonmalignant or benign pain is pain that cannot be explained or that persists after healing has taken place. It usually occurs daily and is not life-threatening. Treatments may or may not be successful in relieving the pain. *Intractable pain* is another term used to describe pain that cannot be relieved and has no known effective treatment.

Many conditions common in older adults may be associated with chronic pain. Phantom limb pain, in which the patient still feels sensations and pain in the amputated limb, is an example of chronic benign pain and neuropathic pain. It can be extremely debilitating if it is not recognized and treated early. It may occur in any related body part that has been amputated or traumatized, for example, amputation of the breast or leg. A number of therapies may be used to reduce this type of pain (e.g., analgesic opioids, antidepressants, nerve block, surgical revision, and physical therapy).

Chronic malignant pain or cancer-related pain may be considered acute and chronic pain. Cancer pain may be chronic pain if it lasts longer than 3 to 6 months. Cancer may also cause the development of new pain when the cancer causes pressure or damage to tissue or nerves. This would be acute pain. Pain related to cancer can be very complex because it may include a variety of pain problems that can be nociceptive and/or neuropathic in nature.

Chronic pain is poorly understood, and new and challenging pain syndromes are currently being identified and classified. Among the treatments that are being tried for chronic pain are surgically implanted stimulators in the spinal cord or brain that can block pain impulses.

COMPARISON OF ACUTE PAIN AND CHRONIC PAIN

In contrast to acute pain, which warns of tissue damage and trauma, chronic pain serves no useful purpose. It can have a debilitating and destructive effect on a person's life. Chronic pain can lead to depression, marital difficulties, loss of self-esteem, immobility, and isolation. The patient in chronic pain often does not report pain and shows little facial expression or few physical signs of pain. When pain is chronic, adaptation may occur. The sympathetic nervous system adapts. The heart rate, blood pressure, and respiratory rate may not be elevated, and the patient may rest, sleep, or turn attention to other activities despite severe pain.

The nurse may underestimate the severity of the pain or undermedicate a patient with chronic pain. Nursing assessment of pain is essential to identify (1) the type and amount of pain, (2) whether the pain is chronic or acute, and (3) whether the patient has both acute pain and chronic pain at the same time. When the patient reports pain but shows no physical symptoms, this does not mean there is no pain. It may simply mean that the patient has learned other ways to deal with the pain or that the patient may be taking medications that block the response of the sympathetic nervous system to pain.

NURSING CARE *of the Patient in Pain*

Pain management continues to be a challenge for every nurse. Every individual experiences pain differently and reacts to pain with a variety of physiologic and behavioral responses. Based on an accurate assessment of pain, the physician prescribes treatment and the nurse provides nonpharmacologic and pharmacologic measures together to provide pain relief. The nurse plays a key role by assessing, intervening, and evaluating the patient in pain. Figure 15-2 shows the variety of interventions you can use to relieve pain.

Assessment

Assessment is the first step in pain management. Assessment of pain should be done on admission and on a regular basis. Anticipate pain as a result of procedures, surgery, or progression of a disease. A pain assessment done with vital signs is called the *fifth vital sign*. Accurately record the data, and compare with previous information. This permits evaluation of the pattern of pain or the effectiveness of an intervention.

It can be difficult to assess pain in some patients, especially older adults. Visual, speech, hearing, and motor impairments may limit the ability of older patients to communicate pain or to use scales to rate pain. Patients with cognitive impairment may be unable to report pain or recall pain sensations. Pain can also cause confusion, irritation, and depression in older adults. Consider these aspects when assessing the older adult.

When the patient cannot communicate verbally, he or she may be able to point to or direct your attention to a location on a body chart or pain intensity scale. You may also have to use family observations and patient behaviors to assess pain and pain relief in this type of situation. When the patient cannot report pain, the nurse may have to perform a different assessment that includes observing for usual or unusual behaviors that may indicate pain. These behaviors are not specific to pain, so other causes of discomfort should be assessed, too, such as impaction or bladder infection.

The six steps in pain assessment are listed in Box 15-2 and are discussed in the following sections.

Accept the Patient's Report

The first step in pain assessment is to establish rapport with the patient and accept what the patient says about the pain. When possible, all information about pain should be obtained directly from the patient. The person in pain is the only authority on the pain; no one else can really know what the pain feels like. Accept the report in a nonjudgmental and caring manner. Obtain

| Box 15-2 | *Six Steps in Pain Assessment* |

1. Accept the patient's report
2. Determine the status of the pain
3. Describe the pain:
   a. Location
   b. Quality
   c. Intensity
   d. Aggravating and alleviating factors
4. Examine the site
5. Identify coping methods
6. Record assessment, interventions, and evaluation of interventions

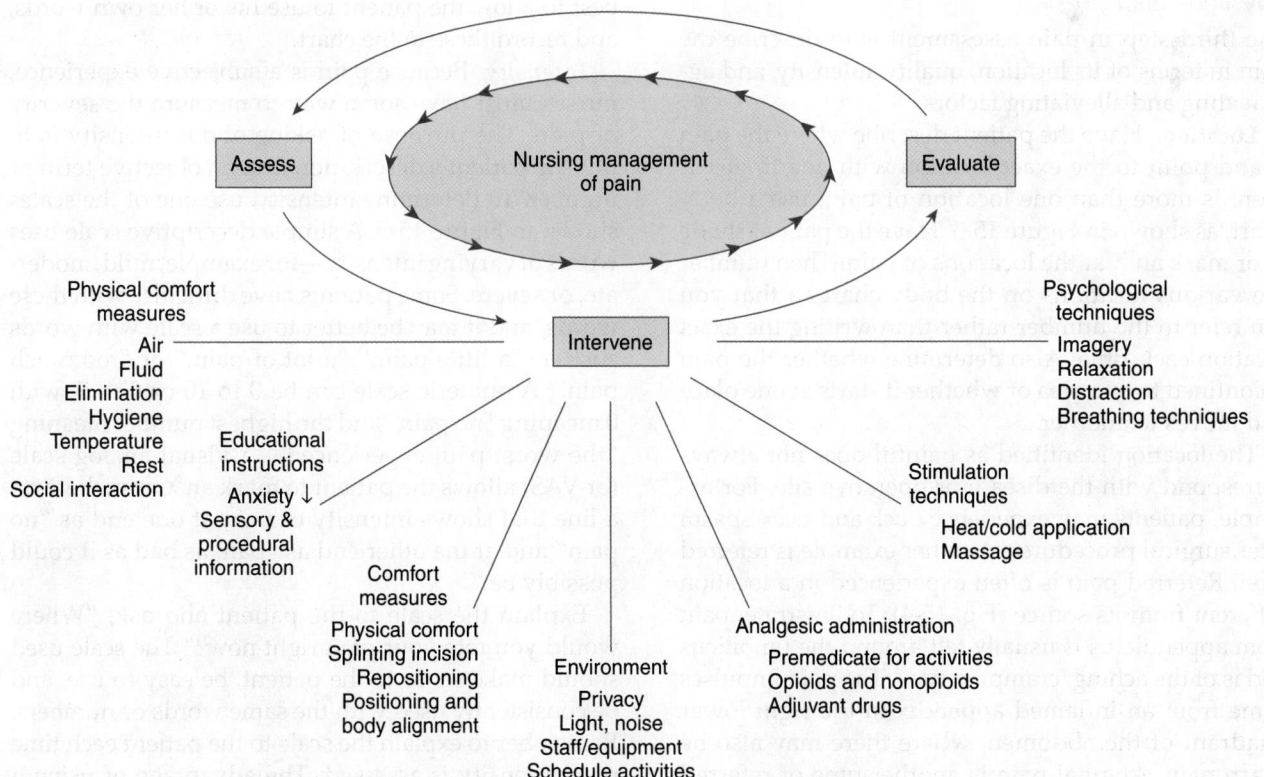

FIGURE **15-2** Nursing management of pain.

specific details about the pain, and respond positively that action will be taken to relieve the pain.

The assessment of pain requires excellent therapeutic communication skills. Important attitudes are conveyed through verbal and nonverbal behaviors. Listen patiently without interruption, use eye contact, touch the patient, and repeat and clarify information in an unhurried manner to establish trust and obtain information. Do not compare one patient's report of pain with another's report, because pain is an individual experience.

Determine the Status of the Pain

The second step in pain assessment is to determine whether the pain is a new occurrence or has been experienced before. Ask the patient if he or she has had this pain before and whether it was diagnosed by a physician. On the basis of the patient's responses and history, decide whether the pain is chronic in nature or acute pain that needs immediate treatment. For example, a patient who is recovering from a prostatectomy may suddenly have chest pain. The patient identifies this discomfort as the typical angina pain for which he has taken medication in the past. A similar patient with chest pain and no previous cardiac history should be seen by a physician immediately because this is a new pain that the patient has not had before. Although both patients need to be evaluated by a physician, an accurate nursing assessment is essential to determine the difference between these two types of pain and consequently the action to be taken.

Describe the Pain

The third step in pain assessment is to describe the pain in terms of its location, quality, intensity, and aggravating and alleviating factors.

Location. Have the patient describe where the pain is and point to the exact location with one finger. If there is more than one location of pain, use a body chart, as shown in Figure 15-3. Have the patient shade in or mark an X at the locations of pain. Then number the various locations on the body chart so that you can refer to the number rather than writing the exact location each time. Also determine whether the pain is confined to one area or whether it starts at one place and moves to another.

The location identified as painful does not always correspond with the disease or operative site. For example, patients may experience back and neck spasm after surgical procedures. Another example is referred pain. Referred pain is often experienced in a location different from its source (Fig. 15-4). To illustrate, pain from appendicitis is usually felt around the umbilicus and is of the aching, cramping type. The pain impulses come from an inflamed appendix in the right lower quadrant of the abdomen, where there may also be sharp pain. Anginal pain is another type of referred

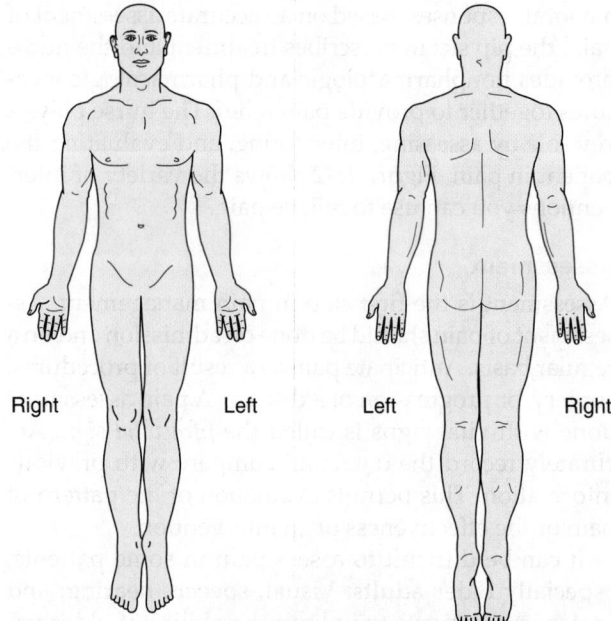

FIGURE **15-3** Body chart.

pain. It is caused by lack of blood flow to the heart muscle and may be experienced as pain in the jaw, arm, and neck as well as in the chest.

Quality. Ask the patient, "What words do you use to describe your pain?" or "What would you do to me to have me feel the pain you have?" If the patient has difficulty describing the pain, suggest words. Commonly used words are sharp, dull, cramping, aching, gnawing, burning, heavy, tender, and throbbing. However, it is best to allow the patient to use his or her own words, and record these in the chart.

Intensity. Because pain is a subjective experience, nurses must have some way to measure the severity of pain. The purpose of asking about intensity is to put the patient's description into an objective term or number. To determine intensity, use one of the scales shown in Figure 15-5. A simple descriptive scale uses words of varying intensity—for example, mild, moderate, or severe. Some patients have difficulty with these words, and it may be better to use a scale with words such as "a little pain," "a lot of pain," or "too much pain." A numeric scale can be 0 to 10 or 0 to 5, with 0 meaning "no pain" and the highest number meaning "the worst pain experienced." A visual analog scale (or VAS) allows the patient to mark an X anywhere on a line that shows intensity of pain at one end as "no pain" and at the other end as "pain as bad as it could possibly be."

Explain the scale to the patient and ask, "Where would you rate your pain right now?" The scale used should make sense to the patient, be easy to use, and be consistently used with the same words or numbers. Remember to explain the scale to the patient each time pain intensity is assessed. The advantage of using a

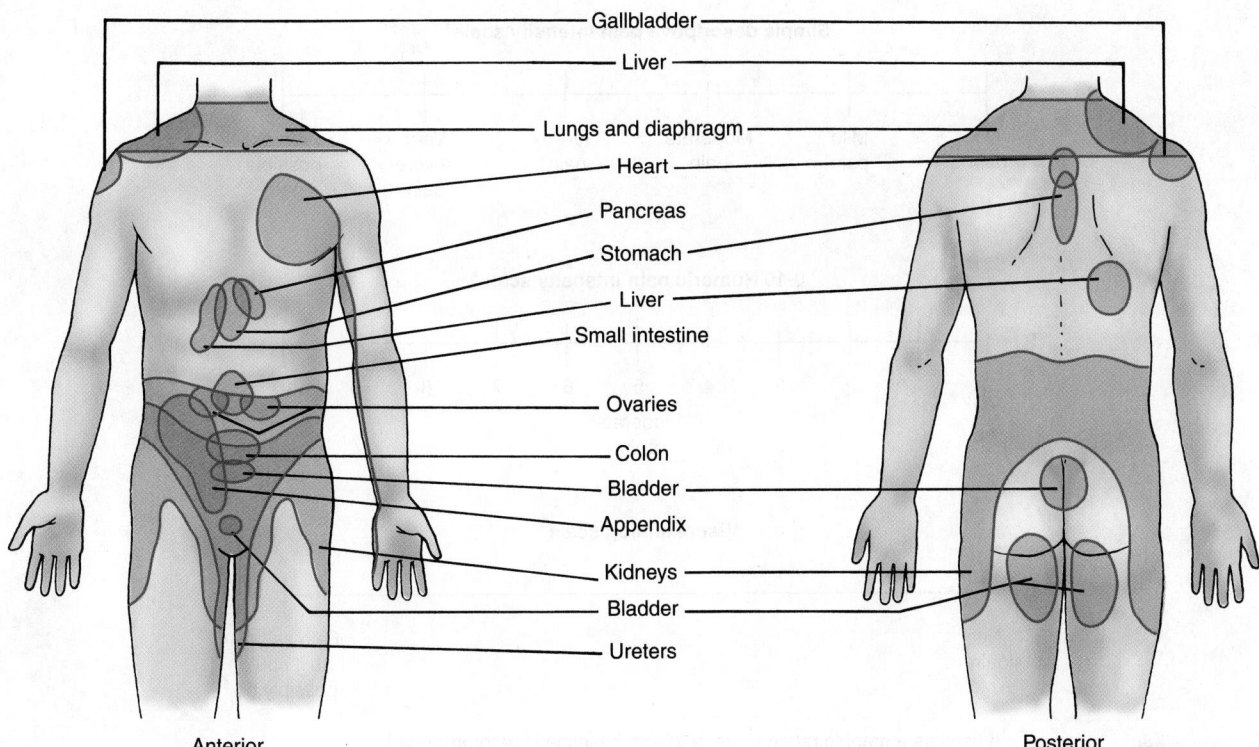

FIGURE **15-4** Anterior and posterior referred pain sites.

scale is that it provides a personal measure of the patient's pain and allows evaluation of pain relief using a consistent measure. A scale that is meaningful to the patient and that can be used repeatedly requires less effort for the patient in pain.

For example, a 42-year-old man with multiple fractures in the right arm used the numeric scale from 0 to 10 for rating pain. The patient complained of throbbing in his right arm and a backache. He rated the intensity of both pains at 7 on the scale at 8 PM. The nurse applied heat to the lower back as ordered, massaged his back, and administered 10 mg of morphine intramuscularly. At 9 PM, the patient rated the intensity of both pains at 2 and stated that the pain was slowly going away. The nurse recorded this information and identified that the interventions were effective in relieving the pain because the pain intensity had decreased from 7 to 2 on the 0-to-10 scale. The nurse also noted that she would reassess the patient's pain every 2 hours. Some hospital policies set a number or "comfort goal" that automatically triggers pain intervention. For example, any pain rating 4 or above on the pain scale requires a nursing intervention for pain relief because research has shown that a pain rating of 4 or above interferes with function and recovery.

Aggravating and Alleviating Factors. Ask if any event or activity causes the pain or makes it better or worse. Ask, "What were you doing when the pain occurred?" Aggravating factors are those that make the pain worse. Certain positions, temperatures, or times of day or night may cause the pain to be more severe. Similarly, alleviating factors might include specific positions, application of heat, cold, or menthol, or physical activities that reduce pain in specific areas.

Patients can usually identify factors that aggravate or reduce pain and what specific pain relief methods have worked in the past. For example, four patients having abdominal surgery may have arthritic shoulder pain and have four different methods of reducing the pain. The first patient obtained relief with elevation and rest of the right arm. The second applied an analgesic balm, a menthol ointment. The third patient used a heating pad on the area, and the fourth increased the anti-inflammatory drug dose as prescribed by the physician.

Examine the Site of the Pain

The fourth step in the assessment of pain is to examine the location that the patient states is painful. Assess the area for heat, redness, swelling, tenderness, abnormal position, or other factors that may be causing local irritation.

Patients may identify a location of pain that is not expected as part of their medical problem. This pain location may be due to a complication or an injury that was sustained during a procedure or hospitalization. For example, one patient who had undergone orthopedic surgery on the ankle had also sustained a large burn on his back at some time during the procedure. When the nurse examined the pain location, the burn was discovered.

¹If used as a graphic rating scale, a 10-cm baseline is recommended.
²A 10-cm baseline is recommended for VAS scales.

FIGURE **15-5** Examples of pain intensity scales. **A,** Simple descriptive pain intensity scale. **B,** 0-10 numeric pain intensity scale. **C,** Visual analog scale (VAS).

Another example is a patient who had undergone abdominal surgery and complained of pain in the right calf. Examination of the right calf revealed a red, firm, tender area that was reported to the physician and diagnosed as thrombophlebitis. When the exact location of the pain was examined, the correct cause of the pain could be identified.

Identify Coping Methods

The fifth step in pain assessment is to identify the patient's coping methods. People develop coping methods to increase control over pain or to relieve pain. Nurses should become aware of the methods patients use to cope with pain and should support the coping method. Some patients actively deal with pain. For example, they may complain and get up and move around or do some other activity. Some patients cope by staying quiet, praying, sleeping, or withdrawing.

Nurses must emphasize to patients and their families that their cooperation and information are critical to achieving pain relief. Some patients expect nurses to know that they are experiencing pain and to know what to do about it. Confirm how the patient copes with pain by discussing observations of the patient's behavior with him or her. You can also suggest other coping methods that could be used to relieve pain (e.g., changing positions, imagery, distraction). Pain in older adults, especially those with cognitive deficits, can be

---

Box 15-3 | *Evaluating Pain in Cognitively Impaired Older Adults and Observing Pain Behaviors*

- Ask the patient about pain first. Many patients who appear cognitively impaired may be able to answer yes/no questions about pain or complete a simple descriptive or numeric pain intensity scale.
- Ask family members and caregivers what particular behaviors indicate pain for the patient.
- Review the medical record to identify a past history of pain or diagnoses that are associated with pain.
- Examine the patient physically to identify potential sources of pain or common problems causing pain.
- Observe behaviors that may indicate pain for the patient. Observe the behaviors at rest and with activity. Note if the behaviors change or improve when pain medication is administered. Assess, intervene, and evaluate behaviors again after intervention.

difficult to evaluate. Boxes 15-3 and 15-4 offer guidelines for evaluating pain in cognitively impaired older adults and list common pain behaviors that are likely to be observed in such patients.

Document Assessment Findings and Evaluate Interventions

The sixth and last step in the pain assessment is to record the information in the patient's chart so that this information can be conveyed to nurses on other shifts and to other health professionals. Record the location,

Box 15-4 | Common Pain Behaviors in Cognitively Impaired Older Adults

Facial Expression
Frown, grimace, rapid blinking, wince, clenched teeth, narrowed eyes

Sounds
Sighing, moaning, groaning, calling out, noisy breathing, cursing during movement

Body Movement
Rigid, tense body posture, fidgeting, pacing, gait changes, rocking, rubbing affected area

Changes in Interactions with Others
Aggressive, striking out, resisting care, withdrawn, decreased social interactions

Changes in Activity Patterns or Routines
Refusing food, appetite changes, sleep or rest pattern changes, increased wandering

Mental Status Changes
Crying, increased confusion, irritability, or distress

quality, and intensity of the pain, related factors, and how the patient copes with pain. Document the interventions provided and their effectiveness. Include the intensity of the pain after the intervention. If the nursing intervention was not effective in relieving the pain or reducing pain to an acceptable comfort goal, record what was done about the pain.

You may also use the following diagnoses to identify other problems that often accompany pain:

- Activity Intolerance
- Anxiety
- Disturbed Sleep Pattern
- Fatigue
- Self-Care Deficit

 Put on Your Thinking Cap!

Think of one of your patients who had pain. Discuss with your classmates how you knew that the patient had pain. Compare and contrast how different patients expressed pain, the interventions that were being used for pain control, and the effectiveness of the interventions.

Nursing Diagnoses, Goals, and Outcome Criteria: Patients in Pain

NURSING DIAGNOSES	GOALS AND OUTCOME CRITERIA
Potential or actual **Acute Pain** related to surgery	Pain relief: Patient states pain is relieved, has relaxed manner
Chronic Pain related to arthritic joint inflammation	Pain reduction or relief: Patient states pain is lessened or relieved, has relaxed manner

Table 15-3 | Nonpharmacologic Interventions

INTERVENTION	COMMENTS
PHYSICAL Heat, cold, massage, transcutaneous electrical nerve stimulation (TENS)	Increase pain threshold, reduce muscle spasm, and decrease congestion in injured area. Effective in reducing pain and improving physical function. Techniques require skilled personnel and special equipment. May be useful as adjuncts to drug therapy.
PSYCHOLOGICAL **Relaxation** Jaw relaxation Progressive muscle relaxation	Effective in reducing mild to moderate pain and as an adjunct to analgesic drugs for severe pain.
Simple imagery	Use when patients express an interest in relaxation. Requires 3-5 minutes of staff time for instructions.
Music	Both patient-preferred and "easy listening" music are effective in reducing mild to moderate pain.
Imagery	Effective for reduction of mild to moderate pain. Requires skilled personnel.
Educational Instruction	Effective for reduction of pain. Should include sensory and procedural information and be aimed at reducing activity-related pain. Requires 5-15 minutes of staff time.

Adapted from Acute Pain Management Guidelines Panel. (1992). *Acute pain management: Operative and medical procedures and trauma. Clinical practice guidelines* (AHCPR Publication No. 92-0032). Rockville, MD: Agency for Health Care Policy and Research, Public Health Service, U.S. Department of Health and Human Services.

Interventions

Nonpharmacologic Interventions

Nonpharmacologic interventions are those that do not employ drugs. They include a wide range of physical and psychological interventions for pain relief (Table 15-3). Physical interventions usually involve comfort measures, adjusting the patient's environment, and cutaneous application techniques such as heat or cold. Psychological interventions include unconditionally accepting the patient's pain report and providing information about pain, analgesics, and procedures or psychological strategies such as relaxation and imagery. These types of interventions should be used along with analgesics to obtain optimal pain relief.

Physical Interventions

Physical Comfort Measures. These nursing interventions focus on the patient and the environment. Comfort may increase pain tolerance and the patient may experience less pain. Because adequate air, food and fluid, elimination, mobility, hygiene, temperature, and rest and sleep are essential to comfort, monitor these areas for potential problems. For example, patients who are sleep deprived or fatigued may have increased pain. Therefore providing for uninterrupted sleep and periods of rest can enhance pain relief.

For some patients in pain, progressive exercise or immobility may be prescribed as a treatment for pain. The patient with an injury or incision should be moved carefully so that further trauma is avoided. Turning the patient carefully from side to side or supporting an affected extremity during activity can reduce pain. Usually the patient can describe which movements or positions increase or decrease the pain.

Administer analgesic medications before painful experiences to reduce the pain intensity and anxiety associated with the event. Aggressively treat pain, nausea, vomiting, appetite suppression, constipation, and other problems. Assist and teach patients how to splint abdominal and thoracic wounds to minimize pain when deep breathing, coughing, and ambulating. A change of bed linen and sheets free of wrinkles can be refreshing and reduce irritation of the skin. Apply ointment to cracked lips, and provide ice chips for a dry mouth. Any tubes or equipment attached to the patient should be secure but should not produce tension on the skin. Correct body alignment and frequent changes of position will relieve monotony, increase circulation, and prevent muscle contractures and spasms, which aggravate pain.

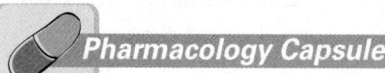

Pharmacology Capsule

Analgesics should be administered before painful activities to reduce the pain and anxiety associated with these events.

Environmental Control. Each patient has individual preferences that affect comfort. Some patients prefer an active environment in which they can be distracted from pain. Listening to tapes or music, watching television, working with the hands, walking around, or visiting with others allows a person to focus attention on stimuli other than the pain sensation. On the other hand, lights, noise, and constant activity of the hospital environment often cause sensory overload for the patient in pain. This can increase pain. When this occurs, coordinate with staff to promote a quiet environment with nonglaring lights and scheduled rest and activity periods that meet the patient's needs.

Stimulation Techniques. Stimulation of the skin and underlying tissues relieves pain. Various types of skin or cutaneous stimulation can be applied, and each has variable effects. These techniques are not curative; rather, they can decrease the intensity of pain or change the sensation so that it is more acceptable.

The exact mechanism for pain relief is unknown, but it is thought that superficial stimulation may block the transmission of pain impulses to the brain. Applications of heat, cold, massage, and TENS are examples of cutaneous stimulation. These interventions tend to be most effective for mild to moderate pain, well-localized pain, and acute and chronic pain. The effects of these therapies last as long as or slightly longer than the application.

The physician may prescribe the application of heat or cold for pain. Heat or cold is used to reduce muscle spasm and decrease congestion or swelling in an injured area. Either therapy may be applied to the painful site, at a location beyond the site, between the site and the brain, or on the opposite side of the body. These therapies should be applied intermittently, not continuously. Heat and cold may be alternated. Both therapies should be applied at a temperature that is comfortable for the patient, and the patient's skin and circulation should be monitored frequently.

Cold may be applied with ice packs or cooling pads to decrease initial tissue injury and swelling (e.g., with musculoskeletal sprains or orthopedic procedures). Cold is contraindicated for patients with peripheral vascular disease or heart disease because it may cause further vasoconstriction of blood vessels and thus decrease circulation. Cold application should be limited to 15 minutes per session to avoid tissue injury or frostbite.

Moist or dry heat can be applied with heating pads, hot-water bottles, towels, gel packs, or warm tub baths or showers. Superficial heat has been shown to be effective for gastrointestinal cramps and muscle and joint pain. Treatment should be limited to 30 minutes to avoid tissue injury. Heat should not be applied to a site of malignancy, to areas of decreased sensation or circulation, or to patients who cannot communicate their discomfort.

Massage involves rubbing, kneading, manipulating, and applying pressure and friction to the body. Rubbing or massaging an area is a natural response when one has an injury or ache. Massage may be used to promote relaxation and relieve muscle cramps. Massage is commonly applied to the back, neck, and large leg muscles; however, massage of the hands and feet is more easily performed and perhaps more effective. Massage should not be applied to areas with injury, phlebitis, or skin lesions or to patients with bleeding problems.

Cold, heat, and massage are easy to apply, inexpensive, effective, and simple for the patient or family to learn. For each therapy, the nurse should evaluate whether the method or location of application is effective, and monitor for any side effects.

Compared with the therapies just mentioned, TENS is much more expensive and less widely available. It requires a physician's order, and often the physical therapy department handles the equipment. The therapy involves external electrical stimulation of the skin and underlying tissues through electrodes attached to a small unit that the patient can carry around. The electrodes are placed over, above, or below painful sites and attached to a battery-operated device that delivers low-voltage electrical currents. The electrical current is adjusted through a dial on the unit. The patient should feel a mild tingling or vibrating or prickly sensation over the area of application. Nursing responsibilities with TENS include the following:

1. Apply electrodes in the correct locations and with good contact with the skin.
2. Check that all connections are secure, from skin electrodes to unit.
3. Adjust the current to the prescribed level and/or the patient's level of comfort.
4. Document and evaluate pain relief.

The major disadvantage of TENS is irritation of the skin under the electrodes. The electrodes should be changed daily, the sites rotated, and the skin inspected. Figure 15-6 shows the application of electrodes and a TENS unit.

Psychological Interventions

Anxiety Reduction. Anxiety, fear of the unknown, and feelings of loss of control may be directly related to the level of pain experienced. The patient who is anxious and uncertain will tend to rate pain high. If the nurse can increase the predictability and control of painful stimuli, pain may be reduced. An important aspect of relieving anxiety associated with pain is the relationship between the nurse and the patient. The nurse can be with the patient, assure the patient that everything possible is being done, and provide timely and appropriate interventions for pain relief.

Several strategies are used to decrease anxiety and increase control. Telling the patient about events and providing descriptions of the sensations or feelings

FIGURE **15-6** Application of a TENS unit.

that may accompany the event can reduce anxiety. However, some patients may prefer not to know this information, and their wishes should be respected. Allowing the patient to choose physical comfort measures and the time for treatments or to rearrange items in the room also provides control.

Preoperative teaching should include skills to help patients cope with their pain, such as breathing, relaxation, or imagery techniques. Providing strategies to help the patient cope with pain and anxiety also provides the patient with a sense of control. The Health Promotion Considerations box on p. 214 describes a sample relaxation exercise, one of the psychological interventions used for pain relief.

Distraction. Distraction refers to focusing on stimuli other than pain. Distraction may help the patient gain a sense of control as well as increase pain tolerance, decrease pain intensity, and alter the quality of pain, but it does not eliminate pain. Because the pain is not eliminated, the patient will usually need analgesics and other methods of pain relief. A patient using distraction may not appear or behave as if in pain, which may cause other people to doubt that the pain exists. After a patient has used a distraction technique, he or she may once again focus on the pain and experience a heightened awareness of pain.

Distraction techniques are often most helpful with mild to moderate pain or during brief periods of pain associated with painful procedures such as dressing changes, intramuscular injections, and venipunctures. Examples of distraction methods include rhythmic breathing, listening to music, laughing, counting, watching television, reading, exercising, resting, talking on the phone, and visiting with others. Older adults may find reminiscing (relating past experiences) to be an effective distraction technique. It is helpful to include several distraction techniques in the plan of care so that the patient can choose the methods most effective for his or her individual pain relief.

Relaxation. Patients should be aware that relaxation is one of the options for pain relief. Patients may already know this technique or may be taught relaxation techniques. Be aware that the patient is using relaxation, know the rationale for using relaxation, and know the effects of relaxation.

Relaxation is a cognitive approach to pain management. It is a self-hypnotic technique that may, but does not always, produce the relaxation response. The relaxation response counteracts the stress response. It is characterized by decreased muscle tension, a decreased heart rate, decreased respiratory rate, and normal or decreased blood pressure. Relaxation decreases mental stress and physical tension; this is helpful because pain is often accompanied by increased anxiety and muscle tension. Relaxation is more effective for mild to moderate pain than for severe pain.

Rhythmic breathing is a relaxation technique that focuses on just breathing, as described in the Health

Health Promotion Considerations

Sample Relaxation Exercise: Slow, Rhythmic Breathing

1. Breathe in slowly and deeply.
2. As you breathe out slowly, feel yourself beginning to relax; feel the tension leaving your body.
3. Now breathe in and out slowly and regularly at whatever rate is comfortable for you. You may wish to try abdominal breathing. If you do not know how to do abdominal breathing, ask your nurse for help.
4. To help you focus on your breathing and to breathe slowly and rhythmically, do the following:
   a. Breathe in as you say silently to yourself, "in, two, three."
   b. Breathe out as you say silently to yourself, "out, two, three."
   c. Each time you breathe out, say silently to yourself a word such as "peace" or "relax."
5. You may imagine that you are doing this in a position and a place you have found very calming and relaxing, such as lying on a beach in the sun.
6. Do steps 1 through 4 only once, or repeat steps 3 and 4 for up to 20 minutes.
7. End with a slow, deep breath. As you breathe out, say to yourself, "I feel alert and relaxed."

Additional Points

If you intend to do this for more than a few seconds, try to get into a comfortable position in a quite environment. You may close your eyes or focus on an object. This technique has the advantage of being very adaptable in that it may be used for only a few seconds or for up to 20 minutes.

Adapted from McCaffery, M., & Beebe, A. (1989). *Pain: Clinical manual for nursing practice*. St. Louis: Mosby.

Promotion Considerations box above. Relaxation techniques that focus on total body relaxation require the patient's active participation. Each part of the body is deliberately relaxed, usually in an orderly sequence such as head to toe or vice versa. Relaxation often involves breathing exercises combined with other methods to promote freedom from anxiety and muscle tension. Methods may include yoga, meditation, and music.

The patient may be taught relaxation through coaching by the nurse, the use of a script, or an audiotaped relaxation exercise. Emphasize to patients that the use of relaxation does not indicate that the pain is thought to be psychological or that the patient must substitute relaxation for analgesics. Relaxation is a technique to be used in addition to analgesics to enhance pain control and reduce anxiety that contributes to pain.

Imagery. Imagery is another cognitive approach to pain control that encourages physical and mental relaxation. Imagery uses a person's imagination to help control pain. Besides promoting relaxation, imagery may be used for distraction or may help the patient imagine pain relief.

Patients are asked to describe the quality of pain they are experiencing. On the basis of this description, imagery can be used to modify the patient's experience. For example, if the pain is described as "burning," an image of something cool may help reduce pain intensity. As with relaxation, the use of imagery does not mean that medical personnel view the pain as imaginary. In both relaxation and imagery, a script or a prerecorded tape may be used to guide the patient through the experiences. Encourage the patient to practice relaxation or imagery, or both, to evaluate their potential effectiveness.

Consider the Alternative

Massage and relaxation with music or imagery are examples of complementary therapies that can be used with analgesics to obtain optimal pain relief.

Pharmacologic Interventions

Drug therapy continues to be the mainstay of pain management. Although the physician orders specific analgesics, it is the nurse's responsibility to assess the pain, to decide which analgesic and how much to administer, and to evaluate the drug's effectiveness.

When administering analgesics, keep in mind that it is critical to use a preventive approach to pain management. When pain is predictable, such as with postoperative pain and cancer pain, analgesics are more effective when given around the clock (ATC) rather than as needed (PRN). An ATC schedule maintains therapeutic blood levels of the analgesics. With a PRN schedule, the patient may have frequent periods of unrelieved pain and may also have more significant and frequent side effects such as sedation. Even when a physician orders analgesics PRN, the analgesics can be given on an ATC schedule. The ATC schedule is usually based on how long the drug lasts; thus when the order reads every 3 to 4 hours, the analgesic should be administered every 3 to 4 hours to maintain pain relief. Of course, you should assess the patient's pain before the analgesic is administered. The duration of analgesic effect varies among patients.

When pain is unpredictable, it may be appropriate to administer analgesics on a PRN basis. In these situations, instruct the patient to request medication as soon as the pain begins rather than waiting for the pain to become more severe. Patients often report that they wait to call for analgesics, thinking that the pain will decrease with time. Unfortunately, waiting often results in pain reaching an intensity level that is difficult to control.

The three categories of drugs that are used to relieve pain are (1) nonopioid analgesics, (2) opioid analgesics, and (3) adjuvant drugs. Figure 15-7 shows how these categories of drugs are used by themselves or in combination to relieve mild, moderate, and severe pain.

FIGURE **15-7** The World Health Organization three-step analgesic ladder.

Nonopioid Analgesics. Nonopioid analgesics include aspirin, acetaminophen, and nonsteroidal anti-inflammatory drugs (NSAIDs) such as ibuprofen. The nonopioids are generally the initial treatment choice for mild pain. These analgesics may also be combined with opioids to control moderate to severe pain.

Nonopioid analgesics act mostly on the peripheral nervous system and are used for pains such as arthritic pain, backache, headache, dysmenorrhea, postoperative pain, cancer pain, and bone pain. Nonopioids may have antipyretic (fever-reducing), analgesic (pain-reducing), and/or anti-inflammatory (inflammation-reducing) properties. This range of actions makes them especially useful for many conditions.

Most of the nonopioids are oral preparations, but a few are available for rectal administration. A parenteral NSAID, ketorolac (Toradol), also is available. It is generally used for the short-term management of postoperative pain. Approximately 30 mg of ketorolac given intramuscularly provides the same amount of pain relief as 12 mg of morphine or 100 mg of meperidine (Demerol) given intramuscularly. Ketorolac has a longer duration of action than many of the opioid analgesics and, like other NSAIDs, can cause nausea and possibly bleeding.

The nonopioids, unlike the opioids, have a ceiling effect on analgesia. This means that, beyond a certain dosage, improved analgesia will not occur. However, these drugs do have side effects, including stomach irritation, fluid retention, and an increased bleeding time. Therefore they are usually not recommended for patients with liver or kidney disorders, thrombocytopenia, or neutropenia. (Thrombocytopenia is a deficiency of platelets in the blood. Neutropenia is a decreased percentage of neutrophils, the white blood cells that respond to inflammation.) Some nonopioids should be used cautiously in patients with congestive heart failure or hypertension because they cause fluid retention, which may aggravate these conditions. Because nonopioids have many side effects, you should assess the patient's history and present condition before administering prescribed analgesics. Some patients have better pain relief with certain types of nonopioids compared with others. It is important to ask which nonopioids work best to relieve their pain.

Table 15-4 identifies commonly used NSAIDs and some considerations to keep in mind when administering these drugs. Older adults may be more sensitive to NSAIDs and may experience more side effects. Carefully monitor each patient's reaction to the analgesic. Older adults especially should be monitored for signs of increased bleeding time, gastrointestinal irritation, and unusual drug reactions such as confusion, constipation, and headaches. Experts agree that some drugs should be avoided in older adults because of the high risk of side effects—for example, propoxyphene, meperidine, indomethacin, ketorolac, and promethazine.

Many nurses forget to administer nonopioids because they fail to recognize the importance of using these drugs for the types of mild to moderate pain mentioned previously. The nonopioids can be administered along with opioids and may be as effective as lower doses of opioids. For instance, 650 mg of aspirin or acetaminophen taken orally provides the same amount of analgesia as 32 mg of codeine or 50 mg of meperidine taken orally. Nonopioids tend to block pain transmission peripherally, whereas opioids block pain transmission in the central nervous system. It is advantageous to administer both for pain relief.

Table 15-4 | *Nonopioid Analgesics: Commonly Used NSAIDs*

DRUGS	COMMENTS
ORAL NSAIDs	
Acetaminophen	Lacks the peripheral anti-inflammatory activity of other NSAIDs
Aspirin*	The standard against which other NSAIDs are compared. Inhibits platelet aggregation; may cause postoperative bleeding
Choline magnesium (Trilisate)	May have minimal antiplatelet activity; also available as trisalicylate oral liquid
Fenoprofen calcium (Nalfon)	
Ibuprofen (Motrin, others)	Available in several brand-name formulations and as a generic product; also available as oral suspension
Ketoprofen (Orudis)	
Magnesium salicylate	Many brands and generic forms available
Naproxen (Naprosyn)	Also available as oral liquid
Naproxen sodium (Anaprox)	
Salsalate (Disalcid, others)	May have minimal antiplatelet activity
Sodium salicylate	Available in generic form from several distributors
PARENTERAL NSAIDs	
Ketorolac	IM administration not to exceed 5 days

Adapted from Acute Pain Management Guidelines Panel. (1992). *Acute pain management: Operative and medical procedures and trauma. Clinical practice guidelines* (AHCPR Publication No. 92-0032). Rockville, MD: Agency for Health Care Policy and Research, Public Health Service, U.S. Department of Health and Human Services.
*Contraindicated in the presence of fever or other evidence of viral illness.
NSAIDs, Nonsteroidal anti-inflammatory drugs; *IM*, intramuscular.
MNSD9Only the NSAIDs listed in the table have been approved by the U.S. Food and Drug Administration for use as simple analgesics, but clinical experience has also been gained with other drugs as well.

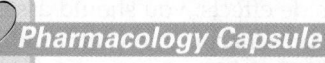

Pharmacology Capsule

The adverse effects of nonopioid analgesics include stomach irritation, fluid retention, and increased bleeding time.

Opioid Analgesics. Opioid analgesics are generally used for moderate to severe acute pain, chronic cancer pain, and some other types of pain. The opioids vary in potency and duration of action.

There are currently two types of opioid analgesics:
- **Opioid agonists.** Examples include codeine, methadone (Dolophine), hydromorphone (Dilaudid), meperidine (Demerol), morphine, and fentanyl.
- **Opioid agonist-antagonists.** Examples include buprenorphine (Buprenex), nalbuphine (Nubain), butorphanol (Stadol), and pentazocine (Talwin).

Both types of opioids relieve pain at the level of the central nervous system. Agonist drugs fit into receptor sites on the cell to "turn on" the site and produce the drug effect. Antagonists are drugs that block drug effects at the receptor sites. Opioid agonists bind to opioid receptors to produce analgesia, but they also bind to other receptors to produce unwanted side effects such as decreased respiration, drowsiness, and nausea. Opioid agonist-antagonists are drugs designed to produce analgesia and also to block certain side effects. The agonist-antagonists block some of the effects of the pure opioid agonists in much the same way that nal-

oxone (Narcan) acts to block or reverse the effects of opioids. Drugs classified as agonist-antagonists (e.g., pentazocine, nalbuphine, buprenorphine) produce analgesia, but they can also block the effects of opioids such as morphine or meperidine if the patient has been receiving these drugs. Thus a patient receiving pure opioid agonists for pain relief should not be given opioid agonist-antagonists because they may block analgesia, precipitate withdrawal symptoms, and increase pain. For example, if a patient has been receiving morphine intramuscularly for several days, it would not be advisable to administer nalbuphine (Nubain) because it may block some of the analgesic effects of morphine.

Older adults are generally more sensitive to the analgesic effects of opioids because of delayed excretion and slower metabolism. Also, side effects may be more pronounced in older adults. Thus the recommended adult dose should be reduced 25% to 50% initially and then titrated (adjusted) for optimum pain control with minimal side effects. Some older adults are small and thin and weigh less than 100 pounds. In this case, charts with recommended opioid doses for adults and children weighing less than 50 kg or less than 110 pounds are available. Table 15-5 provides guidelines for dosing opioids.

It is important to refer to an equianalgesic (approximately equal analgesia) table when changing to a new opioid or a different route. Table 15-5 is such a table, showing approximately equianalgesic oral and parenteral doses. The information in the table helps

| Table 15-5 | *Opioid Analgesics: Starting Oral Dose Commonly Used for Severe Pain* | | | |

| NAME | EQUIANALGESIC DOSE (MG) | | | STARTING ORAL DOSE ADULTS (mg) |
	ORAL	PARENTERAL*		
Morphine	30	10		15-30
Hydromorphone (Dilaudid)	7.5	1.5		4-8
Fentanyl	—	0.1		—
Methadone (Dolophine)	10	5		5-10

From American Pain Society. (2003). *Principles of analgesic use in the treatment of acute pain and cancer pain.* (5th ed., p. 14). Glenview, IL, The Society.
*These are standard intramuscular doses for acute pain in adults. Equianalgesic doses should be based on the opioid characteristics, and patient characteristics such as age, weight, liver and renal function, and reaction to the drug.

estimate the new dose, which should then be modified based on the specific patient reaction and drug. An equianalgesic table shows that oral doses are two to six times larger than parenteral doses of the same drug to achieve the same effect. This is because oral opioids must pass through the liver after absorption, which reduces the amount of medication absorbed. Therefore larger doses of oral opioids must be ordered to provide the same amount of analgesia as parenteral opioids. For example, a patient receives 10 mg of morphine intramuscularly for pain relief and the order is changed to oral morphine. To receive an equianalgesic dose of morphine, the patient should be given 30 mg of morphine orally.

Meperidine or Demerol continues to be used for moderate to severe pain. Clinical practice guidelines state that meperidine may cause central nervous system toxicity. You should be aware that one of the products of meperidine metabolism is normeperidine, which is a central nervous system stimulant. When this metabolite accumulates in the body, the patient may exhibit anxiety, twitching, tremors, muscle jerking, and generalized seizures. This opioid is contraindicated for long-term administration, specifically over 48 hours, and for diminished renal function. Because many older adults have decreased renal function, meperidine should be avoided.

Pharmacology Capsule

Older adults are more sensitive to opioid analgesics and should be monitored frequently for side effects.

Misconceptions About Opioid Analgesics. When discussing opioid analgesics, it is critical to review a few terms that are often misunderstood, resulting in undertreatment of pain. Patients, families, nurses, and physicians have misconceptions about addiction; therefore the term must be defined and differentiated from the terms tolerance and physical dependence. Box 15-5 contains information about these terms. When patients take opioids over a period of time for pain, tolerance and physical dependency may occur. The patient who is tolerant requires higher doses of a

drug to achieve an analgesic effect. The patient who is physically dependent on an opioid will experience unpleasant withdrawal symptoms when the opioid is stopped. Both tolerance and physical dependence are normal responses to continued opioid administration for pain relief; they do not lead to a craving for the drug for its mind-altering effects. Fear of addiction is greatly exaggerated, and addiction rarely occurs (<1%) in patients taking opioids for pain relief. Remind patients that pain relief is an important goal and they should not worry about addiction. Most patients simply stop taking opioids when the pain stops.

Routes of Administration. The opioids can be administered through various routes, depending on the needs of the patient. If tolerated, the oral route is preferred, especially for patients with chronic pain. Oral opioids can control severe pain when given in adequate dosages.

The intramuscular route may be used to administer opioids for breakthrough pain, that is, pain that occurs between regularly scheduled doses of pain medication. Breakthrough pain would require immediate-acting or short-acting analgesic medication such as morphine. Consider the drug being administered when selecting

| Box 15-5 | *Characteristics of Tolerance, Physical Dependence, and Addiction* |

Tolerance
Physiologic changes that occur from repeated doses of opioids.
Result: Higher doses are needed to achieve pain relief.

Physical Dependence
Physiologic changes that occur from repeated doses of opioids.
Result: Withdrawal symptoms (e.g., irritability, chills, sweating, nausea) may occur if the opioid is stopped abruptly.

Addiction
Psychological dependence characterized by continued craving for opioid for other than pain relief.
Result: Compulsive and continued use for psychic effects despite harm.
NOTE: Risk of addiction is not a concern in treating acute or cancer pain.

appropriate needle-gauge size and administration site for intramuscular medication. For example, to administer 10 mg of morphine intramuscularly, use at least a 1.5- to 2.5-inch needle to reach the muscle, depending on the patient's size. Some drugs such as Demerol are more irritating to muscle tissue and should be administered deep into the muscle with the Z-track method. You can use the ventrogluteal, dorsogluteal, and vastus lateralis muscles. The intramuscular route is impractical for repeated injections. Absorption is often unpredictable with intramuscular injections, particularly in older adults, who have reduced muscle mass. This route is also painful. An accessible and appropriate site for the intramuscular injection of analgesics is the ventral gluteal muscle, especially in older adults.

A limited number of opioids, such as morphine, hydromorphone, and oxymorphone, may be administered rectally. This route is useful when the patient is nauseated or has difficulty swallowing.

Opioids may also be administered sublingually (under the tongue). Intermittent bolus injections, continuous infusions, or patient-controlled analgesia (PCA) are methods of administering medications subcutaneously. These methods may be used in patients in whom the oral and rectal routes cannot be used and who also have poor intravenous access.

The intravenous route is another method of administering opioids. Intravenous PCA is commonly used postoperatively. With PCA, the patient is able to self-administer doses of analgesics to control pain. Opioids, when administered intravenously, have a rapid onset but shorter duration of action than when given by any other route. Although the registered nurse is usually responsible for the PCA, the practical nurse may be responsible for monitoring the patient's response and the effectiveness of the medication. Side effects should be reported to the registered nurse.

Opioids can be administered also via the spinal route epidurally (in the epidural space) or intrathecally (in the subarachnoid space). The epidural or intrathecal route may be selected in patients with postoperative pain and chronic cancer pain. The practical nurse

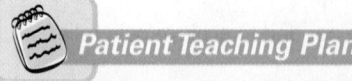

Patient Teaching Plan

Patient-Controlled Analgesia (PCA)

* Safety features: The pump has a delay feature and a lockout interval that prevents the patient from receiving more than the prescribed amount of medication. Only the patient should push the PCA button.
* Patient instruction: Press the PCA button when pain begins to return; then put it down and wait 10-15 minutes to evaluate pain relief. If pain returns, push the PCA button again and repeat the process until the pain is relieved.
* If pain is not relieved: Notify the RN, who can recommend changes in the opioid, bolus amount, or lockout interval to the physician to achieve satisfactory pain relief.

may participate in monitoring the patient. Side effects such as itching, hypotension, nausea, urinary retention, sedation, and respiratory depression may occur more frequently in patients receiving opioids epidurally or intrathecally than by other routes of administration. The older adult who has received a spinal opioid infusion is at increased risk for respiratory depression. If anesthetics such as bupivacaine are used with spinal opioids, the nurse must be alert for the side effects of sensory loss and motor weakness. Side effects, as well as any adverse effects, should be reported promptly. A sedation assessment scale should be used with patients receiving spinal opioid infusions. Sedation is usually seen before signs of respiratory depression.

Other routes of administration of opioids also are available. Liquid morphine may be administered sublingually. Duragesic or fentanyl transdermal patches are used to treat cancer and chronic pain by producing constant delivery of the opioids for 72 hours through the skin surface. Intranasal butorphanol is available and may be used preoperatively for sedation and postoperatively for analgesia. Package inserts should be reviewed for doses, precautions, and administration guidelines.

Side Effects. Regardless of the route of administration, opioid analgesics have specific side effects. A common side effect is constipation. Tolerance for this side effect does not develop. Assess the patient for abdominal distention, cramping, and abdominal pain. Stool softeners and laxatives, along with increased fluid intake, exercise, and bulk-containing foods, may prevent this side effect.

Opioids may also cause nausea, with or without vomiting. Some patients develop a tolerance for nausea but may require antiemetic therapy until tolerance develops. At times, the order may need to be changed to a different opioid to relieve this problem.

Sedation is another side effect that may occur initially with opioids, but it usually subsides in a few days. In patients who have had unrelieved pain for some time and have been sleep deprived, the control of pain may allow the patient to rest, which may be misinterpreted as sedation. When sedation is noted, however, the dose of the opioid may need to be titrated to a level that does not cause sedation but does provide pain relief. Box 15-6 illustrates a sedation scale. Be aware that drugs such as promethazine (Phenergan), which are sometimes ordered to be given with opioids, may also contribute to sedation. Promethazine does not potentiate or increase the analgesic effects of opioids but does potentiate sedation, respiratory depression, and hypotension. If sedated, the patient may benefit from having separate orders for the opioid and for the promethazine. Work with the physician and ordered drug(s) to reduce sedation to a rating of 1-2 on the scale and achieve the most effective pain relief.

Respiratory depression can occur but does not occur as frequently as commonly thought. If a patient is easily arousable, it is highly unlikely that respiratory depression has occurred. If severe respiratory depression occurs (fewer than 6-8 respirations a minute) and stimulation does not awaken the patient, this is an emergency. Stay with the patient and call for help. The RN may administer naloxone (Narcan) intravenously if prescribed to reverse the opioid.

Other side effects may be noted with the use of opioid analgesics. These include confusion, hypotension (especially orthostatic), dizziness, itching, and urinary retention. Nonopioid analgesics given with opioids may allow a decrease in the opioid dose to one that maintains pain control with fewer opioid side effects.

Placebos. Placebos are inactive substances (e.g., saline) used in research or clinical practice to determine the effects of a legitimate drug or treatment. Placebos are appropriately used in studies in which patients consent to participate in the study. Many professional health care organizations take the position that placebos should not be used to assess or manage pain. Nurses have an ethical obligation to ensure that patients are not deceived

and that institutional policies related to placebos are followed.

Adjuvant Analgesics and Medications. Drugs that are not usually classified as analgesics may relieve pain in certain situations. For instance, a patient who has undergone back surgery may complain more about

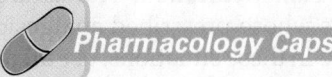

Pharmacology Capsule

The adverse effects of opioid analgesics include constipation, nausea, sedation, respiratory depression, confusion, hypotension, dizziness, itching, and urinary retention.

Put on Your Thinking Cap!

Ask five people (patients, friends, strangers) what helps when they have pain. Compile a list with your classmates, and sort the treatment measures into pharmacologic and nonpharmacologic. Include home remedies and herbal remedies.

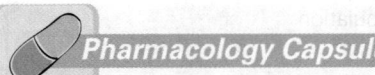

Pharmacology Capsule

Oral analgesics are preferred for the treatment of chronic pain.

Consider the Alternative

Patients who have migraines may be taking feverfew, an herbal supplement, for headache prevention. There is no evidence of effectiveness in treating other conditions. Advise patients that feverfew can increase the risk of bleeding in patients taking aspirin, warfarin, or heparin.

Box 15-6 | *Sedation Scale*

S	Sleeping but easy to arouse when called or stimulated
1	Awake and alert
2	Slightly drowsy but easily aroused
3	Frequently drowsy, arousable but drifts off to sleep during conversation—alert the RN
4	Somnolent, minimal or no response to physical stimulation—emergency

Table 15-6 | *Adjuvant Analgesics and Medications*

DRUG CLASSIFICATON	TYPE OF PAIN OR PROBLEM ASSOCIATED WITH PAIN
ANTIDEPRESSANTS	Neuropathic pain; dull, aching pain
Amitriptyline (Elavil)	Pain associated with herpes zoster (shingles)
Doxepin (Sinequan)	Sleep disturbances
MUSCLE RELAXANTS	Muscle spasms and anxiety
Methocarbamol (Robaxin)	
Cyclobenzaprine (Flexeril)	
BENZODIAZEPINES	Muscle spasms and anxiety
Alprazolam (Xanax)	
Lorazepam (Ativan)	
ANTIHISTAMINES	Nausea, anxiety
Hydroxyzine (Vistaril, Atarax)	
CORTICOSTEROIDS	Spinal cord or nerve compression; bone pain
Prednisone (Deltasone)	
Dexamethasone (Decadron)	
ANTICONVULSANTS/ ANTIEPILEPTICS	Neuropathic pain, stabbing pain
Carbamazepine (Tegretol)	Trigeminal neuralgia
Phenytoin (Dilantin)	Pain associated with herpes zoster (shingles)
Gabapentin (Neurontin)	Other nerve pain
LOCAL ANESTHETICS/ ANTIDYSRHYTHMICS	Postherpetic neuralgia, diabetic neuropathy, other chronic pain conditions
Lidocaine	
Mexiletine	
MISCELLANEOUS	Pain from spinal cord injury, phantom limb pain, peripheral nerve injuries
Clonidine	
PSYCHOSTIMULANTS	Analgesic effect, cancer pain
Dextroamphetamines (Dexedrine)	
Methylphenidate (Ritalin)	

muscle spasms than incisional pain. A muscle relaxant may be more effective in relieving pain than an opioid alone. Specific pain syndromes, especially neuropathic pain syndromes, may be controlled with drugs other than the commonly known analgesics. Table 15-6 lists adjuvant drugs and the conditions they effectively treat.

Problem Solving with Pain Medication. Nurses are often faced with patients whose prescribed analgesic drugs do not relieve pain. In these situations, use all of the information presented here. Ask questions about the analgesic drug and the "five rights" (right dose,

right patient, right time, right route, right analgesic) to determine why the patient is not getting adequate pain relief. Box 15-7 provides a nursing plan of care checklist. Box 15-8 describes a method for problem solving when analgesic drugs do not provide effective pain relief.

The administration of analgesics is simply one intervention in the nursing care of a patient in pain. Nurses should provide many interventions along with analgesics to relieve pain. The Management and Supervision box on p. 221 also includes the expected patient outcomes and guidelines for nursing care.

Box 15-7 | *Southwest Texas Methodist Hospital Nursing Plan of Care: Pain*

NURSING DIAGNOSIS/PATIENT PROBLEM

Pain (Acute/Chronic) related to:
Date/Initials
_____ Disease processes/illness
_____ Surgery
_____ Injury/trauma
_____ Diagnostic procedures
_____ _____
_____ _____

As evidenced by:
_____ Verbalization of pain/discomfort
_____ Verbalization of spasms (specify bladder,
           back, muscle) _____
           _____
_____ Facial grimacing
_____ Tense body posture
_____ Rubbing/guarding of body parts
_____ Inability to concentrate
_____ Increased vital signs
_____ Restlessness/difficulty sleeping
_____ Crying, moaning
_____ Withdrawal
_____ Change in appetite
_____ Decreased activity
_____ _____
_____ _____

Standard of Care/Expected Outcome
Patient will verbalize/demonstrate minimal discomfort or
   absence of pain AEB:
_____ Statements of pain relief and effectiveness of
           pain medications and/or other interventions
_____ Decreased need for pain medication
_____ Relaxed facial expression and body part
_____ Increase in voluntary movement, ambulation, and ADL
_____ Increased ability to concentrate
_____ Stable vital signs
_____ Statements or demonstrations of coping behaviors
           and/or factors that reduce or eliminate
           discomfort or pain
_____ Able to sleep/rest
_____ Increased appetite
_____ _____
_____ _____

STANDARDS OF PRACTICE/GUIDELINES FOR CARE

_____ Accept patient's level/tolerance of pain
_____ Assess pain characteristics to include
           location, intensity, duration, type,
           precipitating factors
_____ Provide the patient with prescribed medication
           as ordered
_____ Provide and teach alternative methods of pain
           relief based on individual needs and/or
           physician orders:
_____ Positioning
_____ Back rub
_____ Massage
_____ Application of heat
_____ Application of cold
_____ Diversion/distraction
_____ Relaxation/imagery
_____ Exercise/ambulation
_____ Range of motion
_____ Other:
_____ Consults: _____
           _____

_____ Teach patient and/or significant other pain
           management strategies:
           _____ Use of PCA
           _____ Medications

_____ Explain procedures to decrease/relieve anxiety
_____ Validate patient's understanding/coping
_____ Evaluate effectiveness of interventions and
           reintervene as necessary

From Southwest Texas Methodist Hospital, San Antonio, TX.
ADL, Activities of daily living; *AEB,* as evidenced by; *PCA,* patient-controlled analgesia.

Box 15-8 *Problem Solving with Pain Medication*

When the analgesic medication prescribed for pain is not effective in relieving pain, the nurse should take the following steps to solve the problem:

1. Check the analgesic order.
   a. **Right dose:** Is the dose prescribed a recommended starting dose for analgesia, or is the dose prescribed less? If a dose range of medication is prescribed, has the maximum dose been administered? If the order states morphine 10-20 mg IM PRN for pain, and 10 mg morphine is ineffective for pain relief, has 20 mg been administered? *Solution:* Adjust the dose up as ordered until pain is relieved without serious side effects or minimal side effects.
   b. **Right patient:** Is the patient experiencing side effects of the analgesic at the present dose? Can the patient tolerate the increase in dose with few side effects?
   c. **Right time:** What is the onset, peak, and duration of the analgesic? Is the analgesic administered around-the-clock based on the duration or properties of the drug? *Solution:* Evaluate pain intensity periodically to see if correct timing of drug is more effective in relieving pain.

If the patient's pain is still not relieved, the following steps should be taken:

2. Consider an alternative prescription.
   a. **Right patient:** What is the diagnosis or source of pain, and what analgesic is most effective for this type of pain? What are patient characteristics to consider (e.g., age, liver or renal problems, NPO status)?
   b. **Right route:** Which route is most appropriate for the patient's condition, severity of pain, and medication prescribed (e.g., IV, IM, PO, or topical administration)?
   c. **Right analgesic:** Which analgesic or adjuvant drug is best for this type of pain? Which analgesic has proven effective for the patient in the past or in a similar condition? Can the opioid or nonopioid prescribed be switched to another drug in the class that may provide more effective pain relief? Have both opioids and nonopioids been prescribed to increase pain relief?
   d. **Right dose:** Has the dose of opioid been titrated up or adjusted to a higher dose to reduce the pain? Has the patient been receiving opioids over time and requires increased doses of opioids to control pain because of the development of tolerance? If switching opioid drugs, is the correct equianalgesic dose calculated to make sure you have the approximate same level of analgesia?
   e. **Right time:** What is the time interval at which the analgesic should be administered or evaluated given its duration of action and patient?

3. Collaborate with patient, other nurses, pharmacist, and family.
   a. Collect information.
   b. Establish credibility with facts about the patient, analgesics, and written references (articles or drug guides).
   c. Anticipate questions.
   d. Be assertive and keep trying.
   e. Always use other nursing interventions in addition to the analgesic to relieve pain.

Adapted from Walker, M., & Wong, D. (1991). A battle plan for patients in pain. Copyright © 1991 *American Journal of Nursing, 91*(6):32-36. Used with permission. All rights reserved.

IM, Intramuscularly; *PRN*, as needed; *NPO*, nothing by mouth; *IV*, intravenously; *PO*, orally.

Management and Supervision

Delegation of Pain Assessment

Pain assessment is one of the most important responsibilities for which the nurse is accountable. According to the American Pain Society, half of all hospitalized patients experience moderate to severe pain during the last days of their lives. Of the 70% of cancer patients with significant pain, fewer than half receive adequate relief. Pain may also be caused by postoperative wounds, sickle cell disease, arthritis, and many other conditions.

Pain assessment cannot be delegated to an unlicensed person. However, it is essential that unlicensed personnel understand the importance of informing the nurse of any reports of pain from the patient. Although a licensed practitioner with prescribing authority is ultimately responsible for adjusting dosages, both the LPN and the RN must be able to assess the patient's pain to implement range dose orders. Working within their scope of practice and adhering to applicable organizational policy, nurses must draw on their knowledge, skills, abilities, and experience to execute the pain management plan. They must be aware of the following:

- The medication to be administered
- Dosage and route of administration
- Potential interactions with other medications
- Time to onset and peak effect
- Duration of action
- Potential side effects

If the patient experiences an unacceptable level of pain or has troublesome side effects, the nurse should document the finding and report it to the prescriber so that appropriate pharmacologic or nonpharmacologic interventions can be implemented. Ideally, the patient will take part in achieving safe, effective pain management. Good communication among all members of the health care team is essential to ensure the patient's optimal comfort and well-being.

Key Points

- Pain is the most common problem that nurses encounter.
- "Pain is an unpleasant sensory and emotional experience associated with actual or potential tissue damage" (International Association for the Study of Pain).
- When pain receptors are stimulated, impulses are transmitted to the spinal cord and then to the brain, where the cortex interprets the signals as pain.
- Endorphins are natural opioid-like substances that block the transmission of painful impulses to the brain.
- According to the gate-control theory, stimulation of large-diameter fibers in the spinal cord interferes with the transmission of painful impulses to the brain.
- Physical factors that influence the pain experience are pain threshold, pain tolerance, age, physical activity, nervous system integrity, and, in surgical patients, the type of surgery and anesthesia.
- Psychological factors that influence the pain experience include culture, religion, past experiences with pain, anxiety, and situational factors.
- Based on the duration and cause, pain is classified as acute, chronic, chronic benign (nonmalignant), and chronic malignant pain (cancer-related pain).
- Most chronic pain is neuropathic because of nerve damage.
- Assessment is the first step in pain management.
- Pain can be described in terms of location, quality, intensity, and aggravating and alleviating factors.

- It is essential to document assessment findings and the effects of pain interventions.
- Nursing diagnoses for the patient in pain may include Acute Pain, Chronic Pain, Activity Intolerance, Anxiety, Fatigue, Self-Care Deficit, and Disturbed Sleep Pattern.
- Examples of nonpharmacologic interventions are comfort measures, control of environmental factors, stimulation techniques, and measures to reduce anxiety.
- Predictable pain is best controlled by around-the-clock (ATC) analgesics rather than as-needed (PRN) medication.
- The categories of drugs used to relieve pain are nonopioid analgesics, opioid analgesics, and adjuvant drugs.
- Fear of addiction to opioids is greatly exaggerated. Addiction rarely occurs when opioids are taken for pain relief.
- Placebos are inactive substances such as saline that are used as a control to determine the effects of a legitimate drug or treatment.
- Most professional health care organizations take the position that placebos should not be used to assess or manage pain.
- Opioid side effects to monitor and treat include constipation, nausea, sedation, and respiratory depression.

 Go to your Companion CD-ROM for a Pharmacology Tutorial, Audio Glossary, and 3-D animations.

evolve Be sure to visit the companion Evolve site at http://evolve.elsevier.com/Linton/ for WebLinks and additional online resources.

REVIEW QUESTIONS *Choose the best answer.*

1. Pain is best defined by the:

   1. Patient
   2. Nurse
   3. Physician
   4. Physiologist

2. When you cut your finger, which of the following represents the steps involved in your experiencing pain?

   1. Afferent pathways activate nociceptors, which transmit information to the spinal cord for interpretation.
   2. Nociceptors are stimulated, and afferent pathways send impulses to the spinal cord and then to the brain.
   3. Efferent pathways stimulate nociceptors, which transmit impulses to the brain.
   4. The brain stimulates nociceptors, which trigger efferent pathways to send impulses to the spinal cord.

3. Mr. A. and Mr. B. both had back surgery yesterday. Mr. A. has used his PCA regularly. He says that he is "pretty comfortable," and he sleeps most of the time. Mr. B. has used the maximum analgesic permitted by his PCA and has required additional analgesic twice while continuing to complain of some discomfort. Of the following, which is the most likely explanation for the difference in the pain experience of these two patients?

   1. Mr. B. is a complainer who is seeking attention.
   2. Mr. B. has higher pain tolerance than Mr. A.
   3. Mr. B. has a lower pain threshold than Mr. A.
   4. Mr. B. is more anxious, which has raised his pain threshold.

4. Autonomic nervous system responses to pain include the following:

   1. Decreased respiratory rate
   2. Flushing
   3. Urinary frequency
   4. Constipation

5. A patient says she has pain whenever she bends over. Which aspect of the pain assessment is she describing?
   1. Location
   2. Alleviating factor
   3. Quality
   4. Aggravating factor

6. A frail, older adult patient who is being cared for by her family at home says she finds a heating pad soothing to stiff joints. What patient/family teaching is needed for safe and effective heat therapy?
   1. "It is more effective to use the heating pad continuously rather than intermittently."
   2. "Do not apply heat to any area that lacks normal sensation or circulation."
   3. "Set the heating pad at the highest temperature that the patient can tolerate."
   4. "Heat application is not a safe or effective strategy for pain management."

7. Which statement correctly describes a nonpharmacologic approach to pain control?
   1. Imagery is the use of the patient's imagination to help control pain.
   2. Distraction is most effective in the management of chronic pain.
   3. Relaxation therapy requires that the nurse must be able to hypnotize the patient.
   4. Patient education is usually all that is needed to reduce anxiety.

8. Nonopioid analgesics must be used cautiously in patients with hypertension because they cause:
   1. Peripheral vasoconstriction
   2. Potassium loss
   3. Sleep disturbances
   4. Fluid retention

9. You should question an NSAID order for a patient who is also taking:
   1. Antibiotics
   2. Decongestants
   3. Anticoagulants
   4. Hormone replacements

10. When patients take opioid analgesics, the nurse must assess for:
    1. Diarrhea
    2. Deficient fluid volume
    3. Respiratory depression
    4. Urinary incontinence

16 First Aid, Emergency Care, and Disaster Management

evolve http://evolve.elsevier.com/Linton/

Objectives

After reading and studying this chapter, you should be able to:

1. List the principles of emergency and first aid care.
2. List the steps of the initial assessment and interventions for the person requiring emergency care.
3. Describe the components of the nursing assessment of the person requiring emergency care.
4. Outline the steps of the nursing process for emergency or first aid treatment of victims of cardiopulmonary arrest, choking, shock, hemorrhage, traumatic injury, burns, heat or cold exposure, poisoning, bites, and stings.
5. Discuss the roles of nurses and nursing students in relation to bioterrorism and natural disasters.
6. Explain the legal implications of administering first aid in emergency situations.

Key Terms

Be sure to check out the bonus material on the Companion CD-ROM, including selected audio pronunciations.

avulsion (ă-VUL-shun, p. 232)
cardiac tamponade (KĂR-dē-ăk tăm-pon-ĀD, p. 233)
cardiopulmonary arrest (kăr-dē-ō-PUL-mō-ner-ē, p. 225)
epistaxis (ep-i-STĀK-sis, p. 230)
evisceration (e-vis-er-Ā-shun, p. 234)
flail chest (flāl, p. 233)
hemorrhage (HEM-or-ij, p. 230)
hemothorax (hē-mō-THŌ-răks, p. 233)
hyperthermia (hī-per-THER-mē-ă, p. 236)
hypothermia (hī-pō-THER-mē-ă, p. 236)
pneumothorax (nū-mō-THŌ-răks, p. 233)
poison (p. 236)
respiratory arrest (RES-pi-ră-tō-rē, p. 225)
shock (p. 230)
sprain (p. 231)
strain (p. 231)

In the inpatient setting, the nurse is often the first on the scene when accidents or emergencies occur. Nurses also need to be prepared to act in emergency situations in homes and other community settings. Prompt intervention can make a dramatic difference in patient outcomes. Knowledge of first aid can make the difference between life and death in many situations. This chapter addresses first aid interventions for common emergencies. Some emergency conditions that re-

quire further medical attention are covered in greater detail elsewhere in this book.

GENERAL PRINCIPLES OF EMERGENCY CARE

When accidents or emergencies occur, the victim and any observers are often understandably frightened. It can be very reassuring to them to know that a nurse is present, but you must remember a cardinal rule: remain calm! Victims react to emergencies in various ways, from stunned silence to hysteria. Although your priority is to preserve life and minimize effects of injuries, the manner in which you conduct yourself also can soothe and reassure the victim.

The nursing process is used in emergencies just as it is in other nursing situations. The important difference is that assessment and intervention must be done very quickly and very efficiently to identify and treat priority needs immediately.

Assessment begins when approaching the victim. Try to determine the nature of the emergency; that is, was the injury caused by an automobile accident, a fall, a diving accident, or an electrocution? Also, look for any hazards to the victim and the rescuer. For example, is the victim in a burning vehicle or lying in the middle of the highway? Failure to recognize such dangers may result in injuries to the rescuer and additional injuries to the victim.

The primary survey looks for life-threatening injuries and intervenes immediately in the following sequence:

1. Assess the ABCs: airway, breathing, circulation.
2. Initiate cardiopulmonary resuscitation or rescue breathing as needed.
3. Look for uncontrolled bleeding, identify the source, and apply pressure to the source.
4. Systematically assess for injuries from the head to the feet, and immobilize spine, limbs, or both as indicated.
5. Look for a medical alert tag—usually a necklace or a bracelet.

After the primary survey, once again go back through a systematic head-to-toe inspection to detect significant changes and other findings that might have been missed initially.

GUIDELINES FOR FIRST AID TREATMENT

General guidelines for first aid treatment of emergency patients are the following:

1. Splint injured parts in the position they are found.
2. Prevent chilling, but do not add excessive heat.
3. Do not remove penetrating objects.
4. Do not try to give anything by mouth to an unconscious person or to one with potentially serious injuries.
5. Stay with the injured person until medical care or transportation arrives.

NURSING ASSESSMENT IN EMERGENCIES

Patient emergencies can occur in every setting. Sometimes nurses observe the events and know what has happened, but at other times, evidence at the scene is needed to determine the circumstances. It is difficult to intervene appropriately in emergencies that cannot be immediately understood. Be prepared to do a quick assessment and then act promptly to provide appropriate care that may save a life. The health history and physical examination are presented separately here but, in fact, may be done almost simultaneously in emergencies.

HEALTH HISTORY

If the victim is able to speak or a witness is available, obtain a brief health history of the victim. Data collection is limited in emergency situations and should include the chief complaint, the treatment given, and the relevant medical history.

Chief Complaint

Determine the nature of the problem, the signs and symptoms, and the circumstances under which the injury or illness occurred. If the victim is or has been unconscious, note the length of time unconscious if possible.

Medical Treatment

Determine whether any treatment has been given and, if so, what effect the treatment had. In the event of an injury, note whether the victim has been moved.

Past Medical History

If possible, determine known health problems including diabetes and cardiac or pulmonary disease, which may provide important clues to the immediate problem or influence the care provided. Check for a medical alert tag, which may provide essential information if the patient cannot. If possible, identify current medications and known allergies. Note any evidence of alcohol or other drugs.

Pharmacology Capsule

The medical alert tag can provide clues about medical emergencies and alert rescuers to known allergies and chronic conditions.

PHYSICAL EXAMINATION

Begin collecting objective data as soon as the victim is seen, and quickly determine whether the patient is responsive. The first assessment priorities must be the ABCs: airway, breathing, and circulation. Watch the victim's chest for rhythmic breathing, and listen near the patient's mouth and nose for air movement. Palpate the carotid and peripheral pulses. Once the adequacy of respiration and circulation has been established, assess for uncontrolled bleeding and shock. If there is no evidence of uncontrolled bleeding or shock, the next step is a systematic head-to-toe assessment. At each step, look for obvious injury, bleeding, swelling, bruising, and drainage. Note circulation, mobility, sensation, and alignment of the entire body. Also note skin color, warmth, and temperature at each step.

The systematic assessment begins with inspection of the head. Speak to the victim and evaluate the response to determine level of consciousness (alert, disoriented, unresponsive). Evaluate comprehension by asking the patient to follow simple commands such as opening and closing the eyes. Inspect the eyes to assess pupil size, equality, and reaction to light. Ask the alert victim about neck pain or stiffness and the ability to swallow. Inspect the chest for symmetry of the chest wall movement. Next assess respiratory effort, dyspnea, and abnormal sounds associated with respirations. Examine the contour of the abdomen to detect distention. Use light palpation to detect areas of pain or tenderness. Inspect the extremities for deformity or injury, and evaluate movement. Then assess peripheral pulses and warmth and sensation in the extremities. Box 16-1 demonstrates the assessment of the patient requiring first aid or emergency care.

SPECIFIC EMERGENCIES

CARDIOPULMONARY ARREST

When the heart stops beating, a person is in cardiac arrest. When respirations cease, the person is in respiratory, or pulmonary, arrest. Cardiopulmonary arrest is the absence of a heartbeat and respirations. The cardiac and respiratory systems are so dependent on each other that when one fails, the other quickly fails as well.

Nerve tissue is so susceptible to hypoxia (low levels of oxygen) that in most circumstances the brain cells begin to die after 4 minutes without oxygen. Unless circulation and oxygenation are restored very quickly

Box 16-1 *ASSESSMENT of the Patient Who Requires First Aid or Emergency Care*

Health History

Chief Complaint:
Nature of illness or injury, signs and symptoms, circumstances of illness or injury, how long unconscious

Treatment:
What has been done, effects, whether moved after injury

Past Medical History:
Current health problems, current medications, allergies

Physical Examination

ABCs:
Airway, breathing, circulation

Skin:
Color, temperature, obvious injury

Head:
Level of consciousness

Eyes:
Opening, pupil size, equality, response to light

Neck:
Stiffness, pain, ability to swallow

Chest:
Symmetry of movement, dyspnea, respiratory rate and effort

Abdomen:
Contour, rigidity, distention, pain, tenderness

Extremities:
Deformity, movement, sensation, peripheral pulses

after cardiopulmonary arrest, permanent brain damage results. Prompt recognition and treatment of cardiopulmonary arrest can maintain the oxygen supply to the brain until circulation and respiration are restored.

Cardiopulmonary resuscitation (CPR) can be part of basic life support or advanced life support. Basic life support is the immediate care given to maintain oxygenation of the brain until advanced medical support is available. This chapter focuses on basic life support given outside of the health care setting. Key points only are emphasized here, but literature published by the American Heart Association or the American Red Cross provides additional, more specific information. Advanced life support is discussed in Chapter 35.

Causes. Among the causes of cardiopulmonary arrest are myocardial infarction, heart failure, electrocution, drowning, drug overdose, anaphylaxis, and asphyxiation.

Signs and Symptoms. Victims of cardiopulmonary arrest collapse and quickly lose consciousness. They have no pulse or respiration.

Nursing Assessment. In cardiopulmonary arrest, assessment and interventions are quickly interwoven. The steps of CPR therefore include assessment and intervention and are presented in sequence below. Only CPR for adults is addressed here.

Nursing Diagnoses, Goals, and Outcome Criteria: Cardiopulmonary Arrest

NURSING DIAGNOSES	GOALS AND OUTCOME CRITERIA
Ineffective Tissue Perfusion related to cessation of heartbeat	Adequate oxygenation until heartbeat and respirations are restored: improving skin color, palpable pulse, spontaneous respirations
Decreased Cardiac Output related to cessation of heartbeat	
Ineffective Breathing Pattern related to inadequate or absent respirations	

Interventions. Refer to the latest American Heart Association guidelines for CPR because the guidelines are revised at intervals. 2006 Guidelines simplified the process for lay rescuers.

The steps outlined here are for adult victims when health care providers are the rescuers (AHA, 2006).

1. Establish that the victim does not respond. Activate emergency response system. If you are alone, get an AED if available. NOTE: The procedure is different for a drowning victim. In this case, if you are alone, provide 5 cycles of CPR before leaving to call for emergency assistance.
2. Open the airway using the head-tilt chin lift unless a neck injury is suspected.
   a. For a head-tilt chin lift:
      i. Place your palm on the victim's forehead and push to tilt the head back (Figure 16-1, A).
      ii. Place two fingers of your other hand under the lower jaw near the chin to bring the chin forward (Figure 16-1, B).
   b. With possible neck injury, use the jaw thrust method to open the airway (Figure 16-2).
3. Look, listen, and feel for breathing for 5 to 10 seconds. If not breathing:
   a. Use the hand on the victim's forehead to pinch the nostrils closed.
   b. Take a normal breath and seal your mouth around the victim's mouth.
   c. Blow into the victim's mouth for 1 second while watching for the chest to rise.
   d. If the chest does not rise, reposition the head and chin and attempt again to ventilate the victim.
   e. NOTE: Various masks and airways are available to avoid direct mouth-to-mouth contact. These should be available in health care settings but may not be on hand in community settings. For that reason, some health care providers routinely carry disposable masks.
4. Check carotid pulse for 5 to 10 seconds.
   a. If no pulse, start CPR.
      i. Kneel or stand at the victim's side.
      ii. Expose the victim's chest.

FIGURE **16-2** To open the airway when a neck injury is suspected, lift the lower jaw with both hands.

FIGURE **16-3** The proper place for compression is located at the level of the nipple line.

FIGURE **16-1 A,** To open the airway when no neck injury is suspected, apply pressure to the victim's forehead with one hand and use the other hand to lift the chin forward. **B,** To ventilate the victim, pinch the victim's nostrils shut, take a deep breath, seal your mouth over the victim's, and breathe into the victim's mouth.

iii. Place the heel of one hand in the center of the sternum between the nipples.
iv. Place the other hand on top of the first.
v. Keeping your arms straight, lean over the victim so that your shoulders are directly over your hands (Figure 16-3).
vi. Compress hard and deep (1.5 to 2 inches).
vii. Compress 100 times per minute.
viii. Allow the chest to recoil completely after each compression.
ix. Minimize interruptions of compressions.
x. In the absence of an advanced airway (e.g., endotracheal tube, laryngeal mask airway, esophageal-tracheal Combitube), maintain a compression-ventilation ratio of 30:2 with either one or two rescuers.

xi. If an advanced airway is put in place, continue compressions at a rate of 100 per minute without pausing for ventilations, which are done at a rate of 8 to 10 per minute.
b. If pulse is present:
i. Continue giving 1 breath every 5 to 6 seconds
ii. Recheck pulse every 2 minutes.
5. If an automatic external defibrillator (AED) is available at the scene:
a. The AED should be placed beside the victim next to the rescuer who will use it.
b. Turn the power on (some units turn on automatically when you open the case).
c. Place electrodes on the victim's bare chest: one on the upper right side of the chest below the collarbone, the other to the left of the left nipple several inches below the left armpit.
d. Be certain no one is touching the victim while the AED analyzes the victim's heart rhythm.
e. If the AED advises a shock, loudly state "clear," meaning that no one should be touching the victim while the shock is delivered.

Table 16-1 | *Summary of Lay Rescuer CPR Maneuvers for Infants, Children, and Adults (Newborn Information Not Included)*

MANEUVER	ADULT: 8 YEARS AND OLDER	CHILD: 1 TO 8 YEARS	INFANT: UNDER 1 YEAR OF AGE
Airway	Head tilt–chin lift (suspected neck injury, use jaw thrust)		
Breathing Initial	2 breaths at 1 sec/breath	2 breaths at 1 sec/breath	2 breaths at 1 sec/ breath
HCP: Rescue breathing without chest compressions	10 to 12 breaths/min	12 to 20 breaths/min	12 to 20 breaths/min
HCP: Rescue breaths for CPR with advanced airway	8 to 10 breaths/min	8 to 10 breaths/min	8 to 10 breaths/min
Foreign-body airway obstruction	Abdominal thrusts	Abdominal thrusts	Back slaps and chest thrusts
Circulation HCP: Pulse check (≤10 sec)	Carotid	Carotid or femoral	Brachial or femoral
Compression landmarks	In center of chest, between nipples	In center of chest, between nipples	Just below nipple line (lower half of sternum)
Compression method Push hard and fast Allow complete recoil	Heel of one hand, other hand on top	Heel of one hand or as for adults	2 or 3 fingers
Compression depth	1½ to 2 inches	Approximately one-third to one-half the depth of the chest	
Compression rate	Approximately 100/min	Approximately 100/min	Approximately 100/min
Compression-ventilation ratio	30:2	1 rescuer: 30:2 2 rescuers: 15:2	1 rescuer: 30:2 2 rescuers: 15:2
Defibrillation AED	Use adult pads. Do not use child pads.	Use AED after 5 cycles of CPR (out of hospital). Use pediatric system for child 1 to 8 years if available. If not, use adult AED and pads. HCP: For sudden collapse (out of hospital) or in-hospital arrest use AED as soon as available.	No recommendation for infants <1 year of age

Data from American Health Association (2006): Highlights of the 2005 American Heart Association Guidelines for cardiopulmonary resuscitation and emergency cardiovascular care. *Currents in Emergency Cardiovascular Care, 16*(4), 15.

f. Press the button to shock the victim.

g. Immediately after the shock, resume CPR beginning with chest compressions. Do not take time to check for a pulse.

h. Every 2 minutes, the AED will advise you to repeat the analysis and shock if needed.

Two-Rescuer CPR. If two trained people are present to perform CPR, one rescuer initiates CPR while the second rescuer activates the emergency response and gets an AED. The second rescuer ventilates the victim with 8 to 10 breaths per minute. The rescuers should swap roles about every 2 minutes to avoid compressor tiring. The switch should occur in less than 5 seconds.

Recovery Position. The unresponsive victim who is breathing should be log-rolled to one side (the *recovery position*) if no cervical trauma is suspected.

The steps are summarized in Table 16-1. Note that there are differences for the lay person and the health care provider.

Documentation. When emergency assistance arrives, provide information about the victim and the incident, including time that elapsed, interventions performed,

and victim response. Identify yourself, and tell how you can be reached if additional information is needed.

CHOKING OR AIRWAY OBSTRUCTION

Choking is airway obstruction caused by a foreign body that enters the airway.

Assessment. The initial response when a person appears to be choking depends on the severity of the airway obstruction.

Mild Airway Obstruction. If the victim has good air exchange, is responsive, and can cough forcefully, do not interfere.

1. Encourage the victim's efforts to breathe and cough.

2. If symptoms persist, activate the emergency response system.

Severe Airway Obstruction. Signs of severe airway obstruction are poor/no air exchange, poor/no cough, high-pitched noise or no noise on inhalation, respiratory distress, cyanosis, inability to speak, inability to move air, and clutching the neck (the universal choking sign depicted in Figure 16-4).

FIGURE **16-4** The universal choking sign.

FIGURE **16-5 A,** The Heimlich maneuver for the conscious choking victim. **B,** The Heimlich maneuver for the unconscious choking victim.

Nursing Diagnoses, Goals, and Outcome Criteria: Choking	
NURSING DIAGNOSES	GOALS AND OUTCOME CRITERIA
Ineffective Airway Clearance related to inability to expel an aspirated foreign object	Patent airway with normal respirations: expulsion of foreign object, audible respirations, improving skin color, decreased coughing, reduced anxiety, normal pulse
Risk for Suffocation related to aspirated foreign object	

Interventions. When these signs are present and the victim is conscious:

1. Ask whether the victim is choking. If he or she nods and cannot speak, activate the emergency response system.
2. If the victim is standing or sitting:
   a. Stand or kneel behind the individual.
   b. Wrap your arms around the victim's waist (see Figure 16-5, A).
   c. Make a fist and place the thumb side of the fist against the abdomen well below the sternum and slightly above the umbilicus.
   d. Place your other hand over your fist and press against the abdomen with a quick upward movement.
   e. Repeat this movement until the obstruction is removed or the victim loses consciousness.
3. If the victim is responsive and is lying down:
   a. Perform abdominal thrusts with the victim lying down (Figure 16-5, B).
4. If a responsive choking victim is pregnant or obese:
   a. Do not attempt abdominal thrusts.
   b. Stand behind the victim.
   c. Reach around the victim with your arms under the victim's axillae.
   d. Position your hands on the victim's upper chest and deliver firm thrusts.

If the choking victim becomes unconscious:

1. Activate the emergency response system.
2. Open the airway and inspect for an object that could be causing the obstruction.
3. Remove any visible object.
4. Begin CPR.
5. Each time you prepare to give breaths, open the victim's mouth wide and look for the object.
6. If you see an object, remove it. If not, continue CPR.
7. If the obstruction is relieved, you should see chest movement with breaths and feel air movement. The next steps are to:
   a. Provide 2 breaths.
   b. Check for a pulse.
   c. If the victim has no pulse and is not breathing, perform chest compressions and attach the AED if available.
   d. If the victim has a pulse but is not breathing, resume rescue breathing and check for a pulse every 2 minutes.
   e. If the victim has a pulse and is breathing, turn the individual on one side (the recovery position) and monitor until emergency personnel arrive.

Complications from Abdominal Thrusts. Because of the risk for damage to internal organs, a person who has received abdominal thrusts should subsequently be examined by a health care provider.

Prevention. Most choking deaths could be prevented if people would do the following:

1. Cut food into small pieces, eat slowly, and chew food thoroughly before swallowing.
2. Not laugh and talk while chewing and swallowing.
3. Perform the Heimlich maneuver promptly when a person is in distress because of an obstructed airway.

SHOCK

Shock results from acute circulatory failure caused by inadequate blood volume, heart failure, overwhelming infection, severe allergic reactions, or extreme pain or fright. Because of the complexity of the topic, shock is covered in detail in Chapter 19.

HEMORRHAGE

Hemorrhage is the loss of a large amount of blood. The loss of more than 1 liter (L) of blood in an adult may lead to hypovolemic shock. Continued uncontrolled bleeding, of course, results in death. Bleeding may be external or internal. Internal bleeding is suspected if a trauma victim shows signs of shock but no external bleeding is evident.

Assessment. Assess for signs and symptoms of hemorrhage, which may include obvious bleeding; cool, sweaty, pale skin; thready pulse; rapid respirations; and decreasing alertness. The victim who is bleeding internally also may have abdominal distention, pain, hematemesis, or dyspnea, depending on the site of the bleeding.

Nursing Diagnoses, Goals, and Outcome Criteria: Hemorrhage

NURSING DIAGNOSES	GOALS AND OUTCOME CRITERIA
Decreased Cardiac Output related to hypovolemia	Increased cardiac output: pulse and blood pressure within normal range, skin warm and dry, no visible bleeding
Fear related to possible impending death	Decreased fear: patient appears more relaxed, states is less fearful

Interventions. The immediate treatment for external bleeding is direct, continuous pressure. Ideally, a sterile dressing is placed over the wound. If sterile supplies are unavailable, use a clean cloth. Elevate and immobilize the injured part (unless fracture is suspected). Elevation decreases blood flow to the area; immobilization prevents dislodging of clots that have formed. After bleeding stops, secure a large dressing, if available, over the wound. Reinforce the dressing but do not change it.

If direct wound pressure and elevation fail to control bleeding, apply indirect pressure, that is, pressure to the main artery that supplies the area (Fig. 16-6).

FIGURE **16-6** Major arterial pressure points.

The use of a tourniquet to control severe bleeding in an extremity is controversial. Tourniquets that are inappropriately placed or left in place too long may result in unnecessary amputations. Therefore they should be applied only by people with advanced training in first aid. Some sources do not recommend it under any circumstances. Others indicate it should be used only as a last resort when a limb is mangled, crushed, or amputated. The least dangerous tourniquet is a pneumatic one, such as a blood pressure cuff, that allows control of pressure. If a blood pressure cuff is used, inflate the cuff above the victim's systolic blood pressure. If the victim's blood pressure cannot be measured, the cuff should be inflated until the bleeding stops. Once the cuff is inflated, only a physician should remove it. When a victim with a tourniquet is transferred, it is critical for the receiving caregiver to know that a tourniquet is in place.

Epistaxis. One type of bleeding that requires special intervention is epistaxis (nosebleed). Blood may come from the anterior or the posterior portion of the nose. Most anterior nosebleeds respond to pressure. Instruct the patient to sit down and lean the head *forward.* Pinch the nostrils of the patient shut for at least 10 minutes (Fig. 16-7). In most cases, this stops the bleeding. Af-

FIGURE **16-7** Epistaxis may be controlled by having the patient sit up and lean forward slightly. Then pinch the patient's nostrils.

terward, advise the patient not to blow or pick at the nose for several hours. Continued bleeding or bleeding from the posterior area of the nose requires medical treatment (see Chapter 53).

TRAUMATIC INJURY

Traumatic injuries result from a variety of events. Sports injuries, motor vehicle accidents, falls, and acts of violence often require emergency treatment at the scene of the injury.

Fractures

A fracture is a break in a bone that may be described as simple or compound, open or closed, complete or incomplete. A simple (closed) fracture does not break the skin. A compound (open) fracture is one in which the ends of the broken bone protrude through the skin. In a complete fracture, the broken ends are separated. The bone ends in an incomplete fracture are not separated. (See Chapter 42 for a discussion of other types of fractures.)

Assessment. Assess the victim of traumatic injury for signs and symptoms of fractures. The primary symptom is pain, although some people, especially older adults, do not always have severe pain with fractures. Numbness and tingling may be present as a result of injury to nerves and blood vessels. Objective signs of fracture include deformity, swelling, discoloration, decreased function, and bone fragments protruding through the skin. Suspected fractures should be treated as such until they are ruled out by the physician.

Nursing Diagnoses, Goals, and Outcome Criteria: Fractures. The primary nursing diagnosis for the emergency treatment of the person with a suspected fracture is **Risk for Trauma** related to movement of unstable

fractures. The goal is reduced risk for trauma, and the outcome criterion is stabilization of the fractured bone.

Interventions. The key to emergency management of fractures is immobilization. Immobilize the injured part, including the joints above and below the injury, to avoid further trauma to the bone and surrounding soft tissue. Do not attempt to straighten a broken bone. Instead, splint the bone in the position in which it was found, with as little movement as possible. Boards, sticks, magazines, and strips of cloth can all be used to immobilize an injured limb. A cool pack may be applied to reduce swelling.

Severe bleeding may be present with compound fractures. In such cases, apply direct pressure to the artery above the injury. Give the victim nothing by mouth, and seek transportation to a medical care facility as soon as possible.

Strains and Sprains

Strains are injuries to muscles or to the tendons that attach muscles to bones, or to both. **Sprains** are injuries to ligaments. Ligaments are bands of tissue that hold bones in position in the joints. These injuries are painful, and swelling may be present. Emergency treatment for both of these injuries is immobilization, elevation, and application of a cool pack. The victim should see a physician for further evaluation.

Head Injury

Head injury is not always apparent immediately after an accident. It should be suspected with any type of blow to the head or any unexplained loss of consciousness. A critical complication of head injury is increased intracranial pressure caused by bleeding or swelling associated with trauma. Increased intracranial pressure progressively impairs brain function and may lead to cessation of breathing.

Older adults are at special risk for head injuries because they are more likely to have sensory deficits, unstable gait, or circulatory disorders. Head injury in an older person may be overlooked if a state of confusion is attributed to age without determining the person's usual level of mental function.

Assessment. When head injury is suspected, assessment includes inspection and palpation of the head and evaluation for signs and symptoms of increased intracranial pressure. Signs of increased intracranial pressure are the following:

- Change in behavior, agitation, confusion
- Decreasing level of consciousness
- Pupil dilation or constriction, inequality, slow response or no response to light
- Impaired sensory or motor function
- Increasing blood pressure with widening pulse pressure
- Decreasing pulse and respiratory rates
- Projectile vomiting

Be alert for the leakage of cerebrospinal fluid that occurs with basilar skull fractures. Cerebrospinal fluid leakage is usually seen as clear, colorless fluid draining from the nose or ear. If the fluid drains onto a white cloth, it appears as a yellowish stain. If there is blood in the fluid, it produces a pink "halo" around the yellow center.

Nursing Diagnoses, Goals, and Outcome Criteria: Head Injury

NURSING DIAGNOSES	GOALS AND OUTCOME CRITERIA
Ineffective Breathing Pattern related to neurologic trauma	Effective breathing pattern: normal respiratory rate and depth, normal pulse
Risk for Injury related to increasing intracranial pressure, improper movement after spinal fracture	Decreased risk for injury: prompt recognition of rising intracranial pressure (altered mental function, unequal pupils, abnormal response of pupils to light), secure immobilization of spine

Interventions. The victim of a head injury must be assessed by a physician as soon as possible. Because head injuries often accompany spinal injuries, always treat the victim as if there is a spinal injury until it is ruled out. This is especially important when the victim is unconscious or when no history can be obtained. Immobilize the neck and keep the victim flat with proper alignment of the neck and head. A backboard should be used for transporting the victim.

Even if the head injury seems to be minor, the physician may admit the victim to the hospital for observation as a precaution. This is because bleeding and swelling are sometimes so slow that signs and symptoms of increased intracranial pressure may not appear until hours or even weeks after the initial injury. (See Chapter 27 for detailed neurologic assessment and care of the hospitalized patient with a head injury.)

Neck and Spinal Injuries

Suspect neck and spinal injuries along with head injuries, especially if the victim has had a diving or motor vehicle accident. Do not move the victim during the initial assessment unless absolutely necessary. Improper movement of the patient with a spinal injury may damage the spinal cord, causing permanent paralysis. After a diving injury, the neck and back should be immobilized while removing the victim from the water.

Assessment. When a victim has a neck or spinal injury, first assess the victim's breathing and circulation and then begin resuscitation if needed. Remember to use the jaw-thrust method to open the airway! Then assess the victim's movement and sensation in all extremities.

Nursing Diagnosis, Goal, and Outcome Criteria: Neck/Spinal Injury. The priority nursing diagnosis for the person with a neck or spinal injury is **Risk for Trauma** related to improper movement of the fractured spine. The goal is decreased risk of additional injury. Outcome criteria include continuous immobilization of the spine and transport for medical care.

Interventions. Immediately summon an expert emergency team when neck or spinal injury is suspected. A professional team has the equipment and the expertise to immobilize and transport the victim properly. In remote or life-threatening settings, the victim may have to be moved. If so, a rolled towel or article of clothing can be used as a collar to support the neck. The victim can then be moved by log-rolling to one side and then rolling back onto a board, keeping the spine as straight as possible. Throughout the movement, one rescuer supports the head while two others support the shoulders, hips, and legs.

Eye Injury

Eye conditions that warrant immediate attention include presence of foreign bodies, chemical contact, perforation of the globe, and eyelid trauma.

Assessment. After an injury of the eye, inspect the patient's eyelid for trauma and the eye itself for redness, foreign bodies, or penetrating objects. To inspect for foreign bodies, evert the eyelids (Fig. 16-8, *A* and *B*). If the eye has been exposed to an irritant, attempt to determine what the substance is.

Nursing Diagnosis, Goal, and Outcome Criteria: Eye Injury. The primary nursing diagnosis is **Risk for Injury** related to foreign body, direct trauma, or exposure to harmful substances. The goal is to minimize injury to the eye. Outcome criteria, depending on the nature of the injury, may be removal of a foreign body or chemical or protection of the eye from further damage while medical attention is being obtained (Table 16-2).

Ear Trauma

The position and structure of the external ear make it vulnerable to traumatic injury. The most serious injury to the external ear is avulsion. Avulsion means that all or part of the auricle is torn loose.

Assessment. Assess the extent of the injury; note whether any tissue is fully separated and also the severity of bleeding. If necessary, apply direct pressure to the site of the injury to control bleeding.

Nursing Diagnosis, Goal, and Outcome Criteria: Ear Injury. If bleeding is under control, the priority nursing diagnosis for a traumatic injury to the auricle is **Impaired Tissue Integrity** related to trauma. The goal is to preserve the tissue to maximize successful repair. Outcome criteria for successful interventions are recovery and protection of avulsed tissue.

Interventions. If the injured part is actually separated, reattachment may be possible. Retrieve the tissue, wrap it in plastic, keep it cool, and transport it with the victim.

Table 16-2	*Interventions for Specific Eye Injuries*
TYPE OF INJURY	**EMERGENCY INTERVENTION**
Foreign bodies	If not embedded: remove by irrigation or by gently touching the object with the corner of a clean cloth or gauze pad or a moistened cotton-tipped applicator. Embedded foreign bodies: should be removed only by a physician.
Chemical contact	Immediately flush the eye for 30 minutes. Sterile normal saline or water is ideal, but tap water may be used. Direct the irrigating fluid to flow from the inner canthus to the outer canthus of the eye. Even if the flushing seems to relieve all symptoms, the patient should see a physician to assess the eye for injury.
Perforation of the globe	Do not attempt to remove an object that has perforated the eye! You could cause greater harm. Instead, limit movement of the object and the eye and transport the victim for immediate medical care. Protect the injured eye by covering it with a shield that does not touch the object. An inverted paper cup can be taped over the eye. Patch the unaffected eye as well because the eyes move together. This limits movement in both eyes. Tell the patient why both eyes need to be covered.
Eyelid trauma	Seek medical evaluation because injury of the globe as well as the lid is always possible. Do not apply direct pressure to a bleeding eyelid. If the globe has been injured, pressure could cause greater harm. Apply a loose dressing and transport the victim for medical care.

A

B

FIGURE **16-8** Eversion of the upper eyelid for inspection. **A,** Gently hold a cotton-tipped applicator against the closed lid and lift the lashes up. **B,** Use your thumb to evert the lid over the applicator and hold the lashes against the bony orbit.

Chest Injury

Injuries to the chest can result in serious impairment of respiratory function. Chest injuries are described as open or closed. The most critical injuries are open pneumothorax, flail chest, massive hemothorax, and cardiac tamponade. Any injury at or below the nipple line may cause both chest and abdominal injuries.

Assessment. Assessment of respiratory status always takes first priority when the victim has sustained a chest injury. Note the rate and character of the victim's respirations, skin color, pulse rate and rhythm, symmetry of the chest wall movement, and the presence of any apparent injuries to the chest. Signs and symptoms of chest injuries that impair respirations are dyspnea, tachycardia, restlessness, cyanosis, asymmetric or other abnormal chest wall movement, and abnormal sounds associated with breathing. Note the patient's mental state and level of consciousness (Fig 16-9).

Nursing Diagnosis, Goal, and Outcome Criteria: Chest Injury. For the patient with a chest injury, the priority nursing diagnosis is **Impaired Gas Exchange** related to altered anatomic structure. The goal is adequate oxygenation, and the outcome criteria are absence of dyspnea, normal pulse and respiratory rates, and normal skin color.

Interventions. Interventions for emergency management of specific injuries are briefly described in Table 16-3. (See "Care of the Patient with a Chest Wound" in Chapter 30 for a more detailed discussion.)

Abdominal Injury

Assessment. Assess the abdomen for evidence of injury. In addition to asking the patient about abdominal symptoms, inspect the abdomen for abnormalities. Suspect internal abdominal injuries when the patient complains of abdominal pain or the abdomen shows

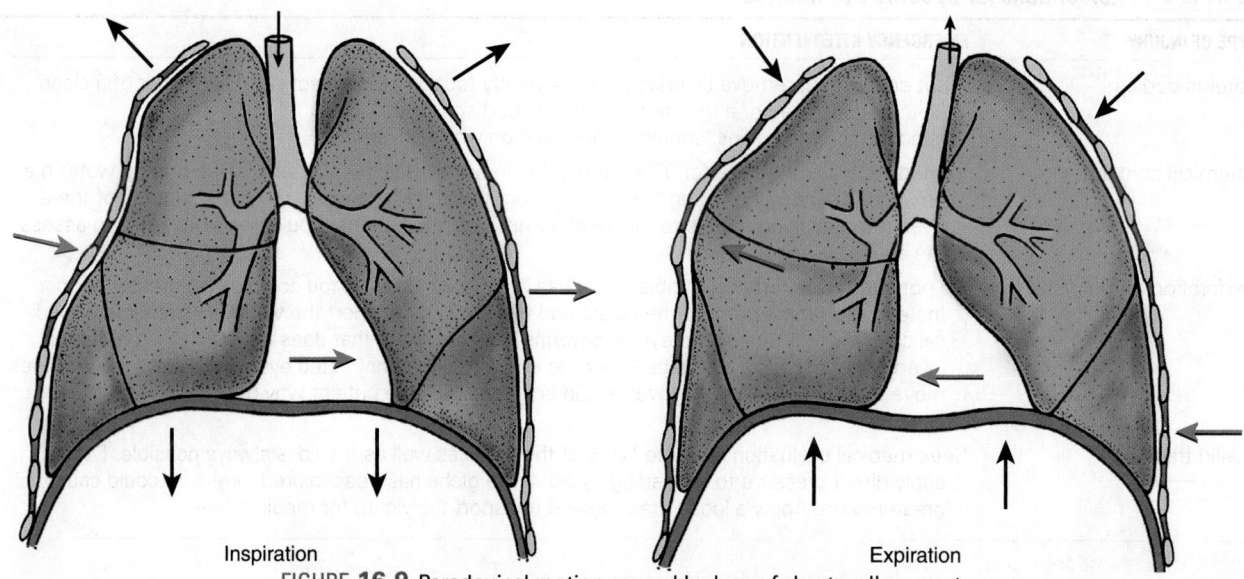

Inspiration   Expiration

FIGURE **16-9** Paradoxical motion caused by loss of chest wall support.

evidence of trauma or distention. The protrusion of internal organs through a wound is called **evisceration.** Eviscerated organs are subject to trauma and drying.

Nursing Diagnoses, Goals, and Outcome Criteria: Abdominal Injury

NURSING DIAGNOSES	GOALS AND OUTCOME CRITERIA
Impaired Tissue Integrity related to mechanical destruction	Protection of injured tissue: proper covering of wound to maintain moisture and warmth
Risk for Infection related to break in skin, possible injury to intestinal tract	Decreased risk of infection: wound protected from contamination

Interventions. Possible internal injuries require medical evaluation. Give the patient nothing by mouth while preparing for transport. Do not attempt to replace eviscerated organs in the abdomen, because this may cause additional harm. Cover eviscerated organs with some material such as plastic wrap or foil to conserve moisture and warmth. A saline-soaked sterile dressing is ideal but is not likely to be available on the scene of an accident. Cover the wound with a clean cloth, and seek transportation to a hospital.

Traumatic Amputation

If body tissue has been partially or completely detached, reattachment is possible. If supplies are available, clean the wound surfaces with sterile water or saline and place the tissue in its normal position. Ideally, a body part that is completely detached should be wrapped in sterile gauze moistened with sterile saline, placed in a watertight container such as a resealable plastic bag, and placed in an iced saline bath. The tis-

sue should not be frozen or placed in contact with ice. Amputated extremities may be healthy enough for reattachment for 4 to 6 hours, whereas digits (fingers and toes) may be viable as long as 8 hours.

BURNS

Care of the burn patient is discussed in detail in Chapter 50. This chapter addresses only emergency measures for burn care. When a burn accident occurs, the immediate concern is to stop the burning process. A victim whose clothing is burning should be told to drop to the ground and roll to extinguish the flames. Smother the flames with coats or blankets, or extinguish the flames with water. Remove burning materials from the victim.

Assessment. First determine the type of burn that has occurred. If the victim has had a flame burn or has been in a closed, smoke-filled area, begin with assessment of respirations. Then determine the extent and depth of the burns. Inspect the skin for color, blisters, and tissue destruction. Superficial burns are typically pink or red and painful. Deeper burns may be red, white, or black and may destroy not only the skin but also the underlying tissues. The deepest burns are not painful because nerves have been destroyed. However, because the depth of a burn often is not uniform, patients with deep burns can still have pain. Determining the extent of the body surface area injured is very important. (See guides for assessing the extent of burn injury in Chapter 50.)

Electrical burns are difficult to assess initially because the full extent of tissue damage may not be apparent for several days. In the event of chemical burns, note and immediately remove any remaining chemical.

Interventions. It is critical to ensure a patent airway and respirations for burn victims. If the burns have been caused by flames, fumes, or chemicals, the victim may have inhaled substances that cause respiratory

Table 16-3 | *Emergency Interventions for Chest Wounds*

TYPE OF INJURY	EMERGENCY INTERVENTION
Pneumothorax: An open chest wound penetrates the pleural cavity, allowing air to enter, which collapses lung on affected side. *Signs and symptoms:* Dyspnea, asymmetric chest wall movement, "sucking" sound as air moves in and out of wound with respirations.	1. Apply vented dressing: sealed on three sides so air can escape, but not enter the wound. *OR* 2. Apply airtight dressing. *IF* patient's condition worsens, suspect tension pneumothorax and loosen the dressing.
Flail chest: Several adjacent ribs are broken in more than one place, causing a loss of support in the affected section of the chest wall. *Signs and symptoms:* The affected section moves inward on inspiration and outward on expiration. This abnormal chest wall movement, called *paradoxical motion*, impairs gas exchange (Fig. 16-9).	Provide support for the injured area. Hold or tape a small pad or pillow over the injury to splint the ribs.
Hemothorax: Accumulation of blood in the pleural cavity; causes the lung or lungs to collapse. *Signs and symptoms:* Increasing respiratory or circulatory failure.	Cannot be diagnosed directly or treated by the first aid care provider. The victim requires prompt treatment in a medical facility.
Cardiac tamponade: Presence of blood in the pericardial sac; causes decreased cardiac output. *Signs and symptoms:* Increasing respiratory or circulatory failure.	Cannot be diagnosed directly or treated by the first aid care provider. The victim requires prompt treatment in a medical facility.

Table 16-4 | *Emergency Interventions for Burns*

TYPE OF BURN	EMERGENCY INTERVENTION
Minor, superficial	Immerse the injured body part in cool water for 2 to 5 minutes. Applying butter to the burn is contraindicated. Medical care usually is not required.
Sunburn	Topical preparations with benzocaine may be soothing. Many people believe that aloe vera is very effective in treating minor burns, but this treatment is still being studied. Children and older adults with extensive sunburn may require hospitalization for dehydration.
Extensive burns	Cover burns with a clean, dry dressing or cloth. Do not apply medications or absorbent materials. Wrap burned fingers and toes separately to prevent sticking together. Have the victim transported for medical care immediately.
Chemical burns	Remove contaminated clothing. Thoroughly dust powdered chemicals from the skin, and then flush with water for 30 minutes. If the dry chemical is not removed before flushing, the water may cause the chemical to become caustic, resulting in additional injury. Flush liquid chemicals from the skin with running water for at least 30 minutes. Apply a dressing or covering, and have the victim transported for medical care.

impairment. Rescue breathing, if needed, is described under Cardiopulmonary Arrest. Other interventions are addressed in Table 16-4 for each of the major types of burns.

Nursing Diagnoses, Goals, and Outcome Criteria: Burns

Depending on the severity and type of the burn, nursing diagnoses and goals for the burn victim immediately after the injury may include the following:

NURSING DIAGNOSES	GOALS AND OUTCOME CRITERIA
Impaired Gas Exchange related to inhalation or thermal injury, edema of airway tissues	Improved gas exchange: normal pulse and respiratory rates; no dyspnea, confusion, or cyanosis; normal arterial blood gases
Impaired Skin or **Tissue Integrity,** or both, related to thermal destruction, chemical injury	Limited extent of injury: no additional damage after initial burn, skin surfaces protected and free of burning materials
Acute Pain related to thermal injury	Reduced pain: victim calmer, states pain is lessened

HEAT AND COLD EXPOSURE

Extreme heat or cold may have local or systemic effects. A number of mechanisms work to maintain body temperature within a fairly narrow range. If the body temperature rises or falls excessively, vital functions begin to fail. Infants and older adults are less able to adapt to temperature extremes than other people. This places them at greater risk for excessive alterations in body temperature.

Hyperthermia

Excessive heat exposure may cause hyperthermia, a condition in which body temperature rises above 37.2° C (99° F). Heat edema and heat cramps are mild degrees of hyperthermia. These mild forms of hyperthermia can usually be treated by moving the individual into a cool place and providing fluids with electrolytes such as sports drinks. Salt tables are not generally recommended. Heat exhaustion and heat stroke are more serious. Treatment details are presented in Table 16-5. See also the Patient Teaching Plan below.

Hypothermia

Hypothermia is a decrease in body core temperature below 35° C (95° F). It may be caused by prolonged exposure to cold, extremely cold temperatures, or immersion in cold water. Hypothermia causes depression of vital functions, and if it is not corrected, death results from cardiac dysrhythmias. Hypothermia is classified on the basis of core body temperature as mild (32° to 35° C), moderate (28° to 32° C) or severe (<28° C). In the mild stage, the patient shivers in an effort to generate body heat. Blood vessels in the extremities are constricted, and performing complex motor tasks is impaired. Persons in moderate hypothermia appear dazed and have poor motor coordination, slurred speech, and violent shivering. They may behave irrationally. Severe hypothermia is characterized by waves of shivering, rigid muscles, and pale skin. The pulse rate is slow, and the pupils are dilated.

Older adults are susceptible to hypothermia because of loss of subcutaneous fat, diminished circulation, and reduced neural control over circulation. They are unable to conserve heat effectively. It has been found that confusion in some older people is the result of hypothermia.

Table 16-5 addresses treatment of systemic responses to heat and cold exposure and local cold injuries. Local thermal injuries were discussed previously under Burns.

POISONING

A poison is any substance that, in small quantities, is capable of causing illness or harm after ingestion, inhalation, injection, or contact with the skin. Large quantities of most chemicals, including all medications, can act as poisons. Even common drugs such as aspirin, acetaminophen, and vitamins can be poisonous if taken in excessive amounts.

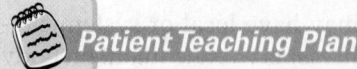

Prevention of Heat Exhaustion

* Avoid strenuous activities outdoors when it is very hot.
* Increase fluid intake to replace excessive fluid loss.
* When working in hot, humid weather, take frequent rest breaks.

Carbon Monoxide Poisoning

Carbon monoxide is an odorless, invisible gas emitted by automobile engines, gas stoves and furnaces, and burning charcoal and other combustible materials. When carbon monoxide is inhaled, it enters the bloodstream and promptly binds with hemoglobin. Carbon monoxide binds to hemoglobin much more readily than oxygen. Therefore it soon occupies many of the sites on the hemoglobin needed to transport oxygen to the cells. The patient becomes hypoxemic and can die.

Assessment. Assess for early signs and symptoms of carbon monoxide poisoning, which include headache and shortness of breath with mild exertion. Dizziness, nausea, vomiting, and mental changes appear next. As the amount of carbon monoxide in the bloodstream rises, the victim loses consciousness and develops cardiac and respiratory irregularities. A victim usually dies when the carbon monoxide bound with hemoglobin exceeds 70%. Although a cherry-red skin color is a clear indicator of carbon monoxide poisoning, skin color often is found to be pale or bluish with reddish mucous membranes.

Nursing Diagnosis, Goal, and Outcome Criteria: Carbon Monoxide Poisoning. The primary nursing diagnosis for the victim of carbon monoxide poisoning is **Impaired Gas Exchange** related to carbon monoxide poisoning. The goal of nursing care for the emergency treatment of the victim of carbon monoxide poisoning is normal oxygenation. Criteria for evaluating the effects of nursing interventions are regular pulse with a rate of 60 to 100 beats per minute, regular respirations with a rate of 12 to 20 per minute, and alert mental state.

Interventions. Immediately move the victim of carbon monoxide poisoning to fresh air. If the person is not breathing, start rescue breathing. Seek emergency medical assistance immediately. Give the victim oxygen as soon as it is available. At the hospital the patient may be placed in a hyperbaric oxygen chamber. A hyperbaric chamber uses pressure to force oxygen into the blood and tissues. See the Patient Teaching Plan below for ways to prevent carbon monoxide poisoning.

Drug or Chemical Poisoning

Poisoning by drugs or chemicals can result from accumulation, excessive dosage, drug interactions, or ingestion of inappropriate substances.

Prevention of Carbon Monoxide Poisoning

* Keep gas furnaces and stoves in proper repair.
* Burners that use gas must be vented to the outside.
* Do not use charcoal or wood-burning devices in a closed area without ventilation.
* Never let an automobile engine run in a closed garage.
* Use a carbon monoxide alarm device.

Table 16-5 | *Emergency Interventions for Heat and Cold Exposure*

TYPE OF EXPOSURE/INJURY	EMERGENCY INTERVENTION
HEAT EXHAUSTION Caused by excessive fluid loss when exposed to high environmental temperature and humidity. Rising body temperature and metabolic rate increase oxygen demand. Cardiac output and heart rate first increase, then fall. Loss of fluids causes hypovolemia (low blood volume) and electrolyte imbalances. *Signs and symptoms:* Dizziness, headache, muscle cramps, nausea and vomiting, and collapse. Skin is usually pale and damp. Elevated rectal temperature; may be as high as 41.1° C (106° F).	Move the person to cooler environment, preferably one that is air-conditioned, and loosen clothing. Splash cool water on the skin. If the victim is alert, offer fluids such as commercially prepared electrolyte drinks, if available.
HEAT STROKE Body core temperature of 41.1° C (106° F) or greater. Temperature regulating mechanisms in the brain fail. Heart, kidneys, and central nervous system functions are depressed. The victim is unable to sweat and will die if the temperature is not lowered. Usually associated with strenuous activity in hot, humid weather. *Signs and symptoms:* Similar to heat exhaustion at first: dizziness, weakness, nausea. As the condition worsens, the skin becomes red, hot, and dry. *Perspiration is noticeably absent.* If the condition is not reversed, the victim may collapse and have seizures. The body temperature may reach as high as 43.3° C (110° F).	It is critical to cool the person quickly. Immediate transport for medical care is recommended. Anyone who cannot be transported immediately should be moved into the shade or to an air-conditioned area if possible. Apply wet, cool towels to the trunk and the extremities, and place ice packs on the forehead and axillae. If a tub is available, the victim can be placed in a cool bath. Continue cooling measures until the body temperature falls below 38.3° C (101° F).
FROSTNIP AND FROSTBITE Frostnip: mild tissue damage caused by cold. Frostbite: more serious cold injury. Blood vessels in the skin and the extremities constrict when exposed to extreme cold. Blood clots form, and circulation to the affected areas decreases. Cells die because of lack of oxygen and nutrients and because of formation of crystals that cause them to swell and rupture. Nose, cheeks, fingers, and toes are affected most often *Signs and symptoms:* Pain at first; then tingling, followed by numbness.	Immediate treatment of mild cold injury: rapid rewarming. For example, have the patient place cold hands in his axillae or between his thighs. More serious cold injuries: patients should be transported for medical treatment as soon as possible. If transport is delayed, seek a setting where warm water is available. *Do not attempt to thaw the tissue unless warmth can be maintained.* Frostbitten extremities are best rewarmed by immersion in a warm water bath of 37.7° to 40.5° C (100° to 105° F). Handle affected areas very gently to avoid additional tissue trauma. Do not rub, massage, or apply cold to the tissue. As tissue warms, the skin turns bright pink and blisters. Rewarming is very painful. If the procedure is done in a medical facility, analgesics will be ordered before rewarming. After warming the extremities, pat dry and wrap in sterile dressings. Wrap each finger or toe separately to prevent injured tissues from sticking together. Immobilize and elevate affected parts. With severe or deep frostbite, thawed tissue dies and eventually has to be surgically débrided (removed).
HYPOTHERMIA Rectal temperature lower than 35° C (95° F). *Signs and symptoms:* Mild hypothermia: shivering and impaired performance. Progressive chilling; decreasing heart and respiratory rates and blood pressure. Irregular heart and breathing patterns; cardiopulmonary arrest if not treated.	Mild hypothermia: Wrap victim in warm, dry clothing and blankets. Severe hypothermia: Transport immediately for treatment. Must be rewarmed aggressively, but gradually, because too rapid rewarming sends lactic acid and cold blood from the extremities to the heart, possibly triggering cardiac dysrhythmias. Warm the torso first. It may be wrapped in blankets or immersed in tepid water. Once the rectal temperature reaches 35° C (95° F), turn attention to warming the extremities also. Internal rewarming (warmed oxygen and intravenous fluids, peritoneal lavage, and extracorporeal blood warming) may be ordered in a medical facility.

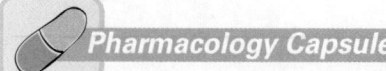

Pharmacology Capsule

Diuretics and anticholinergics increase the risk of heat stroke by affecting the body's heat-reducing defenses.

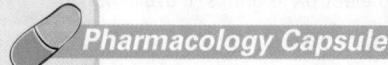

Pharmacology Capsule

Common drugs such as aspirin, acetaminophen, and vitamins can be poisonous if taken in excessive amounts.

Assessment. In situations that suggest poisoning, collect data about relevant signs and symptoms. The signs and symptoms vary with the type of poison. The history is an important part of the assessment of a poisoning victim and should include the following:

1. Name of the drug or chemical involved. If the victim cannot provide the information, look for clues and save the container.
2. Amount of substance consumed.
3. Length of time since the substance was taken.
4. Last food consumed: amount, time.
5. Signs and symptoms that may be caused by poisons.
6. Victim's age and approximate weight.
7. Other medications, drugs, or alcohol ingested.

Nursing Diagnosis, Goal, and Outcome Criterion: Drug or Chemical Poisoning. The primary nursing diagnosis for the victim of drug or chemical poisoning is **Risk for Injury** related to poison. The general goal of nursing intervention for a poisoning victim is decreased or minimized risk for injury caused by the poisoning agent. The criterion for evaluating successful intervention for drug or chemical poisoning is the absence of ill effects from the substance.

Interventions. In the event of poisoning, The American Association of Poison Control Centers (2006) recommends that you immediately call your poison center. It is helpful to have the product container with you because specific interventions depend on knowing exactly what poison was consumed. The poison center staff person will ask about the condition, age, and weight of the individual; exactly when the poisoning occurred; and your name and telephone number. Whereas some poisonings can be treated at home, others require treatment by a physician or in a hospital.

In years past, syrup of ipecac was commonly used to induce vomiting after ingestion of poisons. However, the benefits of this drug are questionable, and it has significant contraindications and adverse effects. Under limited circumstances, the poison center or an emergency department physician may recommend its use. Vomiting is specifically contraindicated if the victim is already vomiting, the victim is unconscious or having seizures, or the substance ingested was a caustic substance or a petroleum product. Treatment

of poisoning in an emergency facility may be treated with activated charcoal, total bowel lavage, and/or cathartics. Activated charcoal is useful because it binds to many poisons, thus preventing their absorption. Bowel lavage and cathartics cause rapid transit of the poison through the intestinal track for elimination.

Food Poisoning

Food poisoning is caused by ingesting contaminated food. Contaminants can be bacteria, chemicals, or natural toxins. Bacteria most often associated with food poisoning are *Clostridium botulinum, Staphylococcus aureus, Clostridium perfringens,* and *Salmonella* (Table 16-6).

Assessment. Victims of food poisoning often recognize the relationship between their symptoms and the ingestion of food. The most common symptoms of food poisoning are nausea, vomiting, abdominal cramps, and diarrhea. Botulism caused by *C. botulinum* has neurotoxic effects, including difficulty breathing, seeing, and swallowing. An important clue that food poisoning is causing the victim's symptoms is that all who consumed a certain food become ill. To assist in identifying poisons, the nurse should collect samples of stool or vomited materials for possible laboratory analysis.

Nursing Diagnosis, Goal, and Outcome Criterion: Food Poisoning. The primary nursing diagnosis for the victim of food poisoning is **Risk for Injury** related to poisoning. The specific type of injury depends on the action of the contaminant. In general, the treatment of food poisoning aims to identify the poison and decrease the symptoms. The goal of nursing care for the victim of food poisoning is the absence or reduction of ill effects from the poison. The criterion for evaluating the effects of intervention for food poisoning is diminished symptoms (e.g., decreased pain, respiratory rate of 12 to 20, depending on the poison).

Interventions. Medical care is necessary if symptoms are severe or persistent, especially in children and older adults. The physician may order antiemetics and antidiarrheals, but sometimes vomiting and diarrhea are allowed to continue within limits to eliminate the offending substances. Intravenous fluids may be prescribed with severe vomiting and diarrhea. Patients with botulism may require ventilatory support.

Prevention. Most cases of food poisoning can be attributed to improper storage or preparation of perishable foods. People need to be taught the importance of cleanliness when handling and cooking food and the correct way to prepare food for storage.

Pharmacology Capsule

Many drugs and chemicals have antidotes. Antidotes are substances that block or reverse the effects of other substances. If the poisonous substance is known, an antidote may be ordered.

Table 16-6   *Food Poisoning*

ORGANISM	SOURCE	SIGNS AND SYMPTOMS	TREATMENT	PREVENTION
Clostridium botulinum	Improper home canning	Onset 18-36 hr after ingestion: nausea and vomiting, headache, dry throat and mouth, dysphagia, diplopia 4-5 days after ingestion: descending paralysis affecting speech, breathing, and swallowing Can be fatal	Gastric lavage, IV fluids, trivalent botulism antitoxin (ABE), mechanical ventilation if needed	Discard food containers that are swollen or have broken seals Spores are not destroyed by boiling Do not depend on taste or odor to detect *C. botulinum*
Staphylococcus aureus	Poor hygiene of food handlers; inadequate refrigeration of food, especially milk products and mayonnaise	Onset within 6 hr: weakness, nausea and vomiting, diarrhea, abdominal cramps Rarely fatal	IV fluids, antiemetics, sedation	Proper refrigeration of food Good hygiene
Clostridium perfringens	Improper canning; inadequately cooked meat or poultry	Onset 6-12 hr after ingestion: abdominal cramps, diarrhea	Antidiarrheals	Thorough cooking
Salmonella	Contaminated food; undercooked meat, eggs	Abdominal cramps, diarrhea, nausea and vomiting	Antidiarrheals, antiemetics, IV fluids	Thorough washing and cooking

IV, Intravenous.

Bites and Stings

Snakes, ticks, bees, wasps, household pets, and even humans are capable of causing serious harm by their bites or stings. The most serious effects of bites are anaphylactic shock, infection, and tissue destruction.

Assessment. In the assessment, the nurse should try to determine the type of bite the patient has received. Inspect the bite wound to identify the characteristics of the actual bite site and any changes in surrounding tissue. Ask the patient about any symptoms that developed after the bite, such as pain, edema, numbness, tingling, nausea, fever, dizziness, and dyspnea.

Nursing Diagnoses, Goals, and Outcome Criteria: Bites and Stings

NURSING DIAGNOSES	GOALS AND OUTCOME CRITERIA
Risk for Infection related to break in skin by bite of human, animal, or insect	Reduced risk for infection: clean wound
Risk for Injury related to exposure to allergens or toxins	Reduced risk for injury: absence of dyspnea, absence of specific toxic effects

Interventions. See Table 16-7 for interventions related to bites. The Patient Teaching Plans on pp. 241 and 243 discuss insect bite allergy and Lyme disease.

ACTS OF BIOTERRORISM

In the past decade, numerous events including the bombing of the World Trade Center have made us aware that we are vulnerable to attacks using various means. Bioterrorism is the deliberate release of pathogens to kill and injure people. The biologic agents most likely to be used in terrorism attacks are anthrax, botulism, plague, smallpox, and tularemia. Because these agents are easily spread, they have the potential to cause many deaths. Imagine the public panic that might follow an outbreak of smallpox! A major problem in the United States is lack of experience in recognizing and treating these infections. Basic information about the biologic agents most likely to be used as bioterrorism weapons is provided in Table 16-8.

In the event of an outbreak of disease related to bioterrorism, health care providers must know how to protect themselves and others. Health care facilities should have readily available information on resources including the local health department and the Centers for Disease Control and Prevention (CDC). Staff should know where to obtain personal protective equipment and what types of precautions (e.g., patient isolation) should be taken. Staff who are exposed should obtain prophylactic therapy if appropriate. Persons with weakened immune systems should not provide direct care for affected individuals.

Table 16-7 *Interventions for Specific Bites*

TYPE OF BITE	EFFECTS	INTERVENTIONS
Snake	Venom that is injected through the fangs into the victim may affect the nervous system or the blood and blood vessels. Venom that affects the nervous system is *neurotoxic* and can cause nausea, vomiting, dizziness, tachycardia, muscle twitching, respiratory distress. *Local effects:* Discoloration, pain, mild to severe edema. Bites of poisonous snakes usually leave two distinct fang marks, although a finger or a toe may be pierced by only one fang.	Seek medical care immediately. A description of the snake (shape of head, color) assists in identification, which may affect treatment. To limit absorption of venom, immobilize the part where the bite is located and keep it at or below the level of the heart. Try to keep the patient still. Wipe the wound. If available, a suction cup can be applied to aspirate the wound. Antivenom may be given to counteract the effects of the venom. Some tissue around the bite often becomes necrotic and must be removed surgically. *No longer recommended* (risks outweigh benefits): Tourniquet, ice, incision and suction.
Insect bite or sting	*Common reactions:* Local itching, edema, and erythema. People who have serious allergies react with systemic symptoms of urticaria (hives), edema, and possibly fatal anaphylaxis. Characteristics of anaphylaxis are difficulty breathing and a drop in blood volume and blood pressure. If the process is not reversed, the victim quickly loses consciousness and dies (see Chapter 33).	Especially anticipate anaphylaxis in victims who develop systemic symptoms rapidly. *Mild reactions:* Calamine lotion or a paste of baking soda or meat tenderizer is soothing. *Severe allergic responses:* The patient with severe allergies should be taken to a medical facility. Epinephrine (subcutaneous), diphenhydramine chloride (Benadryl), aminophylline, and hydrocortisone may be administered after a bite or sting to prevent anaphylaxis. *Prevention:* People who are severely allergic to insect venom should carry emergency epinephrine that can be given subcutaneously after a bite or sting to prevent anaphylaxis. Only the honeybee leaves its stinger, which continues to inject venom into the victim. Immediately remove the stinger with a scraping motion rather than by grasping and pulling on it. Pinching the stinger to grasp it injects more venom.
Animal	All animal bites should be taken seriously because of the risk of wound infections and rabies. Rabies is an infection of the central nervous system that is almost always fatal.	Clean the wound thoroughly; apply a bulky dressing. Advise the patient to have a tetanus booster if immunizations are not current. Patient should see a physician for antibiotic therapy. Follow local protocol to assess whether animal has rabies. If the animal shows signs of rabies or cannot be located, the victim will be given a prophylactic (preventive) rabies vaccine in five doses over a 1-month period. If the victim was bitten on the face or head, the virus may reach the central nervous system more quickly. Therefore treatment may be started before the disease is confirmed in the animal.
Human	Human bites are potentially very dangerous because of the risk of infection. The most common site is the hand or fingers, caused by hitting a person in the mouth.	Clean thoroughly, and apply a dressing. Advise the victim to seek medical attention for antibiotic therapy.
Tick	Tick bites require attention because ticks carry organisms that cause Lyme disease and Rocky Mountain spotted fever.	When a tick is discovered, remove it promptly. *CDC recommendation:* Grasp the tick near the skin with tweezers and use a firm, steady motion to remove the tick. After tick removal, inspect to see if it is intact (no part remaining in the victim's skin). Wash the site with soap and water; apply antiseptic.

Table 16-7 | *Interventions for Specific Bites —cont'd*

TYPE OF BITE	EFFECTS	INTERVENTIONS
Tick *(cont'd)*	*Lyme disease:* *Early localized stage:* Flu-like symptoms with or without a ring-shaped reddened area around the bite ("bull's-eye lesion"). *Early disseminated stage:* Fatigue, anorexia, vomiting, neurologic symptoms. *Late disseminated stage:* Joint (Lyme "arthritis") and muscle involvement, progressive neurologic symptoms ("arthritis"). *Rocky Mountain spotted fever:* *Symptoms:* Appear 3 to 10 days after the bite: chills, fever, headache, pain behind the eyes, joint and muscle pain, and a rash that begins on the wrists and ankles and spreads to the extremities, the trunk, and sometimes the face. Can be fatal if not treated.	*Lyme disease:* Tell patient to notify the physician if flu-like symptoms or a "bull's-eye lesion" develops in next 7 to 10 days. *Diagnosis:* Skin biopsy to detect the causative organism, *Borrelia burgdorferi*. A blood test can detect antibodies about 2 months after onset of the infection. *Treatment:* Early localized or disseminated stages: doxycycline or amoxicillin. *Lyme "arthritis" and neurologic symptoms:* Penicillin, cephalosporin, or chloramphenicol. *Rocky Mountain spotted fever treatment:* Tetracycline and chloramphenicol.
Spider bites	Most spider bites cause only local irritation.	For any bite, wash the site and apply a cool compress. Transport the victim for medical care if bite was by black widow or brown recluse.
Black widow	Venom is neurotoxic; causes pain, nausea and vomiting, fever, weakness, muscle cramps, headache. *More serious effects:* Respiratory distress, hypertension, seizures, and shock.	*Black widow* is shiny black with red hourglass on abdomen. Antivenin is available for black widow spider bites. *Not recommended:* Constricting bands.
Brown recluse	Bite not especially painful, area usually swells within a few hours. Initially, a bluish ring appears around the bite. Later it is surrounded by a white ring with a red "halo." Some people experience nausea and vomiting, fever, and joint pain. Severe cardiac, renal, and neurologic reactions are uncommon. In 3 to 4 days after a bite, the affected tissue becomes necrotic.	*Brown recluse* is light brown with a fiddle-shaped mark on the thorax. Medical attention should be sought for these bites. There is no specific antivenin to counteract the venom of the brown recluse. Eventually the tissue sloughs off or needs to be débrided. The injury can be so extensive that reconstructive surgery is needed.

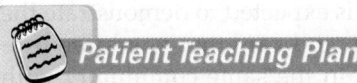 *Patient Teaching Plan*

Insect Bite Allergy

People who are very sensitive to venom should be taught how to avoid and treat bites. The teaching plan should include the following:

- Always wear a medical alert tag stating "Allergic to insect bites."
- Obtain an emergency allergy treatment kit. Learn to use it. Teach a family member to use it. Carry it with you at all times.
- Avoid perfumes, hair spray, and bright colors when working outside. Insects are drawn to strong scents and bright colors.
- Wear long pants and sleeves, shoes and socks, and gloves when gardening.
- Keep the car windows closed when driving.
- Consider desensitizing injections if recommended by a physician. These injections gradually reduce sensitivity to venom.
- Use an insect repellant containing DEET.

DISASTER PLANNING

A challenge for the health care system is to be ready for natural disasters that often occur with short warning. Organizations such as the American Red Cross and the Salvation Army that are experienced in handling these situations quickly move in to help. However, a call for nurse volunteers usually follows. Regardless of the area of clinical expertise, there is certain to be a way each nurse can contribute. The Red Cross offers courses in disaster training for nurses and nursing students. With appropriate supervision, nursing students can assist with many services in disaster situations.

Table 16-8 | *Biologic Agents Most Likely to be Used as Bioterrorism Weapons*

BIOLOGIC AGENT	CHARACTERISTICS	TREATMENTS AND OUTCOMES
Anthrax	After exposure, symptoms may appear in 7-42 days. Three types: 1. Skin (cutaneous): painless lesion begins as small sore and then blisters, ulcerates, and blackens. 2. Lungs (inhalation): sore throat, mild fever, muscle aches, cough, shortness of breath. 3. Digestive tract (gastrointestinal): nausea, anorexia, bloody diarrhea, severe stomach pain.	Antibiotic treatment with fluoroquinolones used for prevention following exposure (along with vaccine). Antibiotics alone for infection. Cutaneous: usually responds to antibiotics. Gastrointestinal: fatal in 25%-50% of cases. Inhalation: fatal in about half of all cases.
Botulism	Toxins are ingested in foods. Onset of symptoms 6 hours to 2 weeks after ingestion. Causes progressive paralysis with double vision, drooping eyelids, slurred speech, dry mouth. Progresses downward to arms, chest, and legs. Can paralyze muscles of respiration.	Centers for Disease Control and Prevention stock antitoxin, which can reduce severity of symptoms if given early. Most people recover after weeks to months of supportive care.
Pneumonic Plague	Normally spread by rodents but can be spread in an aerosol form, and then transmitted from one person to another. Causes fever, weakness, rapidly developing pneumonia, shortness of breath, cough.	Prompt antibiotic therapy (within 24 hours after onset of symptoms) may be effective in prevention after exposure. Antibiotics include tetracyclines, chloramphenicol, streptomycin, and gentamicin.
Smallpox	Caused by a virus transmitted from person to person. Onset of symptoms 10-12 days after exposure includes high fever and pain. Rash with small papules progresses to pustules and then to scabs.	Can be prevented with vaccine, but that is not routinely given now in the United States. There is no specific treatment. Among infected persons who have not been vaccinated, 25%-30% die.
Tularemia	In nature, is carried by rodents and rabbits. As a weapon, can be made into an aerosol or dispersed in food or water. Onset of symptoms usually 3-5 days after exposure. Manifestations: sudden fever, chills, headache, diarrhea, muscle aches, joint pain, dry cough, progressive weakness.	Antibiotics usually are effective. Efforts to have a vaccine approved are underway.

Data from Henderson, D.A. (1998). *Bioterrorism as a public threat.* Retrieved January 28, 2006, from *http://www.cdc.gov/ncidod/eid/vol4no3/hendrsn. htm.* Centers for Disease Control and Prevention. (2004). Emergency preparedness and response. Retrieved January 28, 2006, from *http://www.bt.cdc. gov/agentlist-category.asp.*

When Hurricane Katrina struck the gulf states, local nurses, nursing faculty, and nursing students were indispensable in providing care to persons affected and displaced by the storm. The competencies for nurses in relation to emergency and disaster preparedness are listed in Box 16-2. See the Health Promotion Considerations box on p. 244 for a review of how HIPAA law applies during disaster response situations.

Internet resources for emergency preparedness information include the following:

- U.S. Department of Health and Human Services, Office of Emergency Preparedness. http://ndms .dhhs.gov
- Federal Emergency Management Agency (FEMA). www.fema.gov
- Centers for Disease Control and Prevention. www .cdc.gov

LEGAL ASPECTS OF EMERGENCY CARE

Although we do not ordinarily treat people without their permission, in emergencies they may be unable to consent to care. In such cases, treatment can be provided under the assumption (called the *emergency doctrine*) that the patient would have consented if able.

In the first aid treatment of emergencies outside the hospital, the nurse is expected to demonstrate the same skill, knowledge, and care that would be provided by other nurses in the same community with the same credentials. Good Samaritan laws in most states limit liability and provide protection against malpractice claims when health care providers render first aid at the scene of an emergency. Although many Samaritan laws cover nurses, not all do. It is important to remember that these laws do not protect the nurse in the event of gross negligence or willful misconduct.

Be aware that situations involving legal matters may depend on evidence at the scene of the injury. Remember that clothing and other materials may provide important information and should not be discarded. Victims requiring first aid have the same rights to privacy and confidentiality as those treated in health care facilities. Do not disclose to the public any information about the victim's condition or treatment. In cases involving possible criminal activity, preserving all evidence such as soiled or damaged clothing and body fluids may be critical.

Box 16-2   *Emergency and Disaster Preparedness: Core Competencies for Nurses*

- Describe the agency's role in responding to a range of emergencies that might arise.
- Describe the chain of command in emergency response.
- Identify and locate the agency's emergency response plan (or the pertinent portion of it).
- Describe emergency response functions or roles, and demonstrate them in regularly performed drills.
- Demonstrate the use of equipment (including personal protective equipment) and the skills required in emergency response during regular drills.
- Demonstrate the correct operation of all equipment used for emergency communication.
- Describe communication roles in emergency response.
- Identify the limits of your own knowledge, skills, and authority, and identify key system resources for referring matters that exceed these limits.
- Apply creative problem-solving skills and flexible thinking to the situation, within the confines of your role, and evaluate the effectiveness of all actions taken.
- Recognize deviations from the norm that might indicate an emergency, and describe appropriate action.
- Participate in continuing education to maintain up-to-date knowledge in relevant areas.
- Participate in evaluating every drill or response, and identify necessary changes to the plan.

Additional competencies specific to nurses with managerial or leadership responsibilities are:
- Ensure that there is a written plan for major categories of emergencies.
- Ensure that all parts of the emergency plan are practiced regularly.
- Ensure that identified gaps in knowledge or skills are filled.

From Gebbie, K.M., & Qureshi, K. (2002). Emergency and disaster preparedness: Core competencies for nurses. Copyright © 2002. *American Journal of Nursing,* *102*(1), 46-51. Used with permission. All rights reserved.

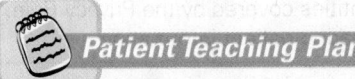 **Patient Teaching Plan**

Lyme Disease

Untreated Lyme disease, transmitted by the deer tick, can have serious chronic effects on the brain, eyes, joints, muscles, heart, blood vessels, lungs, skin, liver, spleen, stomach, and intestines. Adherence to the following guidelines can reduce the risk of contracting Lyme disease:

- After engaging in outdoor activities, inspect body folds and hairy areas for ticks. If ticks are removed within 36 hours, the odds of getting Lyme disease are greatly reduced.
- If you have a tick bite and develop flu-like symptoms within 7 to 10 days, seek medical care. Antibiotic therapy can arrest Lyme disease at this early stage.
- The vaccine, LYMErix, which has been recommended for people who are at high risk, has been linked with activating an incurable form of autoimmune arthritis. Discuss risks and benefits with your physician.

 Put on Your Thinking Cap!

You are traveling with your spouse when a van in front of you swerves, runs off the road, and rolls over. You summon help on your cellular phone and then stop to help. You find the following: Mr. A., in the driver's seat, complains of severe chest pain from striking the steering wheel; Mrs. B., lying on the ground, has an open compound fracture that is bleeding heavily; Teenager C., in the back seat, complains of severe neck pain; Teenager D., beside the van, has blood streaming from her nose and a cut on her forehead; and Grandmother E. is wandering around in a dazed state with her hands to her head. Fill in the table below to show the type of injury you think each may have sustained, assessment and interventions for each injury, and the sequence of your interventions. Compare your completed table with your classmates', and reach agreement on the best answers.

Victim	Type of Injury	Priority	Assessment	Interventions
Mr. A.	_____	_____	_____	_____
Mrs. B.	_____	_____	_____	_____
Teen C.	_____	_____	_____	_____
Teen D.	_____	_____	_____	_____
Grandmother E.	_____	_____	_____	_____

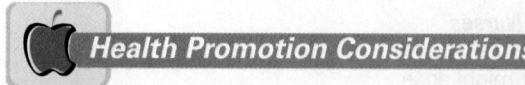

Health Promotion Considerations

HIPAA Privacy and Disclosures in Emergency Situations

The HIPAA Privacy Rule allows patient information to be shared to assist in disaster relief efforts, such as those that occurred after Hurricane Katrina. Providers and health plans covered by the HIPAA Privacy Rule can share patient information in all the following ways.

Treatment
Health care providers can share patient information as necessary to provide treatment. Treatment includes:
- Sharing information with other providers (including hospitals and clinics)
- Referring patients for treatment (including linking patients with available providers in areas where the patients have relocated)
- Coordinating patient care with others (such as emergency relief workers or others that can help in finding patients appropriate health services)

Notification
Health care providers can share patient information as necessary to identify, locate and notify family members, guardians, or other persons responsible for the individual's care or the individual's location, general condition, or death. Thus, when necessary, the hospital may notify the police, the press, or the public at large to the extent necessary to help locate, identify or otherwise notify family members and others as to the location and general condition of their loved ones.

Imminent Danger
Providers can share patient information with anyone as necessary to prevent or lessen a serious and imminent threat to the health and safety of a person or the public, consistent with applicable law and the provider's standards of ethical conduct.

Facility Directory
Health care facilities maintaining a directory of patients can tell people who call or ask about individuals whether the individual is at the facility, their location in the facility, and general condition.

Of course, the HIPAA Privacy Rule does not apply to disclosures if they are not made by entities covered by the Privacy Rule. Thus, for instance, the HIPAA Privacy Rule does not restrict the American Red Cross from sharing patient information.

Source: www.hhs.gov/ocr/hipaa.

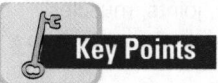

Key Points

- Knowledge of first aid can make the difference between life and death in many situations.
- The cardinal rule in emergency situations is: Remain calm!
- The primary survey includes evaluation of airway, breathing, and circulation.
- Look for medical alert tags, which may give some clues about the patient's health status.
- Critical interventions that may be needed are CPR or rescue breathing; application of pressure to control bleeding; head-to-toe inspection; and immobilization of injured spine/limbs.
- Because brain cells begin to die after 4 minutes without oxygen, treatment of cardiopulmonary arrest must begin immediately.
- The universal sign of choking is grabbing the throat with one or both hands.
- The Heimlich maneuver uses pressure on the diaphragm to force air and obstructions out of the airway.
- Shock results from acute circulatory failure as a result of inadequate blood volume, heart failure, overwhelming infection, severe allergic reactions, and extreme pain or fright.
- The immediate treatment for external bleeding is direct, continuous pressure.
- Tourniquets are controversial but may be used to control bleeding as a last resort.
- For epistaxis, the patient should be told to sit down and lean forward; then pinch the nostrils shut for at least 10 minutes.

- The key to emergency management of fractures is immobilization.
- Sprains and strains are treated initially with immobilization, elevation, and cool packs.
- Assess for increased intracranial pressure with any head injury.
- Improper movement of the patient with a spinal injury may damage the spinal cord, causing permanent paralysis.
- Only a physician removes foreign bodies embedded in the eye.
- When tissue is actually torn from the body, it should be retrieved, wrapped in saline-moistened gauze, placed in a plastic bag, kept cool, and transported with the patient for possible reattachment.
- When there is a chest injury, assessment of respiratory status always takes first priority.
- Open chest wounds that penetrate the pleural cavity allow air to enter (pneumothorax), causing the lung on the affected side to collapse.
- Cover eviscerated organs with some material such as plastic or foil to conserve moisture and warmth; do not attempt to replace the organs in the abdomen.
- The first concern with burns is to stop the burning process and then to ensure a patent airway and respirations.
- Cover large burns with clean, dry dressings, and transport the victim to a care facility immediately.
- Extreme heat or cold can have serious local or potentially fatal systemic effects.
- People with heat stroke will die if the body temperature is not lowered quickly.

- Perspiration is noticeably absent with heat stroke.
- Victims of severe hypothermia must be rewarmed gradually to prevent triggering cardiac dysrhythmias.
- A hyperbaric oxygen chamber may be used to treat carbon monoxide poisoning.
- Instructions about treatment of poisoning can be obtained from the Poison Control Center; instructions also may be found on product labels.
- In the event of poisoning, the first action is to call the local Poison Control Center for expert guidance.
- The most serious effects of bites and stings are anaphylactic shock, infection, and tissue destruction.
- Lyme disease, transmitted by tick bites, can lead to chronic cardiac, neuromuscular, and musculoskeletal disorders.
- Among the agents used as bioterrorism weapons are anthrax, botulism, pneumonic plague, smallpox, and tularemia.

- HIPPA privacy rules allow patient information to be shared to assist in disaster relief efforts.
- The emergency doctrine assumes that people would give consent for treatment of life-threatening conditions if they were able.
- Good Samaritan laws do not protect nurses against gross negligence or willful misconduct.

 Go to your Companion CD-ROM for a Pharmacology Tutorial, Audio Glossary, and 3-D animations.

evolve   Be sure to visit the companion Evolve site at http://evolve.elsevier.com/Linton/ for WebLinks and additional online resources.

REVIEW QUESTIONS *Choose the best answer.*

1. After determining that an accident victim is breathing and has a pulse, you should next assess for:
   1. Bleeding
   2. Spinal injury
   3. Fractures
   4. Chest injury

2. Circulation must be restored within 4 minutes of cardiopulmonary arrest because:
   1. Irreversible kidney failure develops
   2. The blood begins to coagulate
   3. The lungs fill with fluid
   4. Brain cells begin to die

3. When performing CPR, the correct ratio of compressions to ventilations when there is no advanced airway is 30 to _____.
   1. 1
   2. 2
   3. 3
   4. 4

4. The Heimlich maneuver is used to:
   1. Close an open chest wound
   2. Dislodge a foreign body from the airway
   3. Correctly align the ends of a fractured bone
   4. Restore circulation after cardiopulmonary arrest

5. What first aid treatment is most appropriate for a fractured leg?
   1. Immobilize the leg in the position in which you found it.
   2. Gently straighten the leg and immobilize it.
   3. Apply a tourniquet above the fracture if bleeding is present.
   4. Elevate the injured part above the level of the victim's heart.

6. Your assessment of a person who has sustained a head injury reveals the following: headache, decreasing blood pressure, increasing respiratory rate, unequal pupils. Which finding would cause you to suspect increased intracranial pressure?
   1. Headache
   2. Decreasing blood pressure
   3. Increasing respiratory rate
   4. Unequal pupils

7. While at a picnic on the lake, a person catches his clothing on fire while trying to start a charcoal fire. You should first:
   1. Tell him to run and jump in the lake
   2. Try to extinguish the flames with your hands
   3. Tell him to drop to the ground and roll
   4. Run to a telephone to call for help

8. A high school football player collapses during practice on a hot, humid day. He is breathing but not responding verbally. His skin is hot, red, and dry. You should:
   1. Have him go take a cool shower
   2. Call for EMS and apply cool, wet towels
   3. Notify his parents to take him to the hospital
   4. Encourage him to take sips of ice cold liquids

9. The patient with hypothermia must be *gradually* rewarmed to prevent:
   1. Pain in the extremities
   2. Formation of blood clots
   3. Fingers from sticking together
   4. Cardiac dysrhythmias

10. You notice a peculiar ring-shaped, reddened area on the leg of a child in the immunization clinic. When asked about it, the mother stated that she had removed a tick from that area last week. What should you do?
   1. Suspect early Lyme disease and refer the child for medical treatment.
   2. Advise the mother to apply antibiotic ointment to the lesion daily.
   3. Recognize the bite of a black widow spider and apply a constrictive band.
   4. Contact the physician for an order for brown recluse spider antivenin.

Objectives

After reading and studying this chapter, you should be able to:

1. State the purpose of each type of surgery: diagnostic, exploratory, curative, palliative, and cosmetic.
2. List data to be included in the nursing assessment of the preoperative patient.
3. Assist in identifying the nursing diagnoses, goals and outcome criteria, and interventions during the preoperative phase of the surgical experience.
4. Outline a preoperative teaching plan.
5. List the responsibilities of each member of the surgical team.
6. Explain the nursing implications of each type of anesthesia.
7. Explain how the nurse can help prevent postoperative complications.
8. List data to be included in the nursing assessment of the postoperative patient.
9. Identify nursing diagnoses, goals and outcome criteria, and interventions for the postoperative patient.
10. Explain patient needs to be considered in discharge planning.

Key Terms

Be sure to check out the bonus material on the Companion CD-ROM, including selected audio pronunciations.

anesthesiologist (ăn-es-thē-zē-OL-ō-jist, p. 258)
anesthetic (ăn-es-THET-ik, p. 258)
cosmetic surgery (p. 247)
curative surgery (p. 247)
dehiscence (dē-HIS-ens, p. 263)
diagnostic surgery (p. 246)
evisceration (e-vis-er-Ā-shun, p. 263)
exploratory surgery (p. 246)
hypothermia (hī-pō-THER-mē-ă, p. 260)
nurse anesthetist (p. 258)
palliative surgery (PĂL-ē-ă-tiv, p. 247)
sanguineous (săng-GWIN-ē-us, p. 270)
serosanguineous (se-rō-săng-GWIN-ē-us, p. 270)
serous (SĒ-rus, p. 270)

Surgical treatments have been attempted since early times, but until fairly recently surgery was considered the last resort, to be used only when more conservative measures had failed. However, twentieth century advances brought antibiotics, safe anesthesia, refined surgical techniques, and improved diagnosis and treatment of illness and injury. Through these advances surgery became safer, and now it is almost commonplace (Fig. 17-1).

Surgical procedures are performed in physicians' offices, clinics, ambulatory surgery centers, and full-service hospitals. Over recent years, cost control measures resulted in a tremendous shift toward ambulatory surgery centers for many procedures. In all of these settings, nurses play important roles. Nurses who care for patients before, during, and after surgery are called *perioperative nurses.* They admit surgical patients, do initial assessments and prepare them for surgery, assist in the procedures, and provide postoperative care. Because hospital stays for surgical procedures have shortened dramatically and many procedures are done in ambulatory settings, nurses now provide (or teach patients and families to provide) much postoperative care in the home. The importance of good patient and family education cannot be overemphasized.

PURPOSES OF SURGERY

Surgery may be done for a variety of reasons. Surgical procedures classified by purpose include diagnostic, exploratory, curative, palliative, and cosmetic.

Diagnostic surgery involves the removal and study of tissue to make an accurate diagnosis. An example is a biopsy of a skin lesion or a lump in breast tissue.

Exploratory surgery is a more extensive procedure than a biopsy. It usually requires opening a body cavity to diagnose and to find out the extent of a disease process. A common example is an exploratory laparotomy, in which the abdomen is opened to find the cause of unexplained pain. Some exploratory surgery can be done using specialized scopes inserted into the body through small incisions.

Curative surgery is done to remove diseased tissue or to correct defects. The term *ablation* refers to removal of tissue. Removal of an inflamed appendix, for example, is curative for appendicitis. Defects that can be corrected include cleft lip, arthritic joints, and hernias. The repair of damaged tissue is a reconstructive procedure,

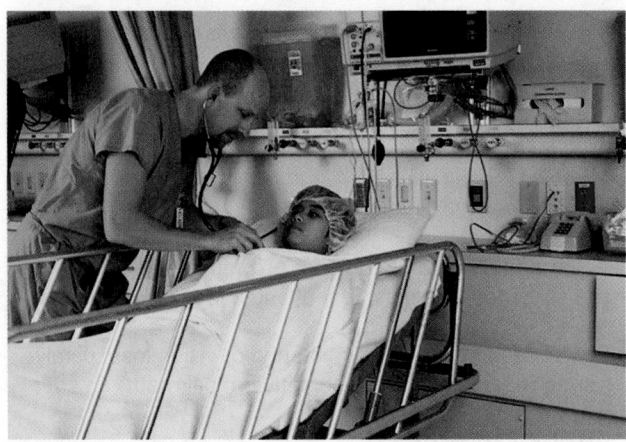

FIGURE **17-1** The nurse provides continuity of care for the surgical patient. This patient will see the same nurse again after surgery.

whereas a constructive procedure repairs congenitally malformed structures.

Palliative surgery relieves symptoms or improves function without correcting the basic problem. For example, palliative surgery may be done just to remove a malignant tumor obstructing the intestine even though the cancer is widespread elsewhere in the body.

Cosmetic surgery can be done to correct serious defects that affect appearance, but it is often done simply because the patient wants to change a physical feature. Common cosmetic procedures are performed to change the shape of facial features, remove wrinkles, flatten the abdomen, and change the size or shape of the breasts.

VARIABLES AFFECTING SURGICAL OUTCOMES

Among the variables that must be considered when caring for surgical patients are age, nutritional status, fluid and electrolyte balance, medical diagnoses, drugs, and habits.

AGE

Health care providers and older adults themselves often believe that surgery is dangerous for older people. This is unfortunate, because modern surgical techniques can restore many lost functions and often greatly improve the patient's quality of life. It is true that people over age 70 who are frail or have cardiovascular disease or diabetes are at greater risk for surgical complications. Hospitalization and surgery may disrupt control of chronic conditions, leading to impaired healing and recovery. However, older adults who are in good health are likely to do just as well in surgery as younger people.

As a general rule, inactivity is not good for anyone. It is especially bad for the older person, who takes longer to regain strength. One other important consideration is that older people may respond differently to

drugs because of age-related changes in liver and kidney function and drug interactions.

Surgical risks for the older adult can be greatly reduced if chronic conditions are well controlled, drug therapy is carefully evaluated, and the patient is well hydrated and nourished before surgery. For that reason, emergency procedures carry greater risks for older patients than scheduled procedures.

NUTRITIONAL STATUS

Patients who are overweight or underweight present special problems. The patient who is malnourished is at risk for poor wound healing and infection. Obese patients are generally in surgery longer and are more likely to have postoperative respiratory and wound complications. Effective deep-breathing exercises are limited by the excess weight. Because adipose tissue has poor blood supply, the healing process is slower. The obese patient also may take longer to recover from anesthesia because the drug tends to remain longer in adipose tissue.

FLUID BALANCE

Fluid and electrolyte status can have a significant bearing on the outcome of surgery. Adequate fluids are necessary to maintain blood volume and urine output. However, excess body fluid can overload the heart, aggravating the stress of surgery. Sudden changes in fluid volume are especially dangerous for the older patient who cannot adapt as efficiently as a younger person. Electrolyte imbalances also may predispose the patient to dangerous cardiac dysrhythmias. Physicians usually order laboratory tests to measure serum electrolytes before surgery. Fluid and electrolyte imbalances can then be corrected preoperatively.

MEDICAL DIAGNOSES

A number of medical conditions increase surgical risks or require special attention in the perioperative period. Patients with bleeding disorders are at risk for excessive bleeding and must be closely monitored. People with heart disease are at risk for cardiac complications related to anesthesia and the stress of surgery. Chronic respiratory disease increases the risk of pulmonary complications as a result of anesthesia or hypoventilation. A patient who has liver disease may have impaired wound healing and may experience drug toxicity arising from the inability to metabolize drugs effectively. Patients with diabetes mellitus also heal more slowly and are at greater risk for infection. In addition, the control of chronic conditions may be disrupted by surgery, which may mandate adjustments in therapy. Also, patients who undergo surgery in life-threatening situations are at greater risk of complications.

DRUGS

Many drugs, such as those listed in the Drug Therapy table on p. 249, have the potential to interact with anesthetic agents. Serious adverse effects may result. The effects of surgery or additional drugs may require dosage adjustments in drugs the patient had been taking routinely.

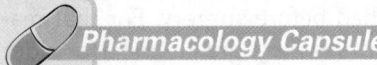

Pharmacology Capsule

Drugs that should be held or modified before surgery include anticoagulants, NSAIDs, aspirin, and herbal products including ginkgo and ginseng.

HABITS

Habits that alert the nurse to the possibility of specific perioperative complications are smoking and alcohol use. Smoking increases the risk of pulmonary complications because secretions are more copious and tenacious and ciliary activity is less effective. Alcohol interacts with many drugs. In addition, patients who use alcohol excessively may need a higher dose of anesthetic agent because of increased drug tolerance. If liver damage has occurred, the metabolism of drugs, including anesthetic agents, can be impaired. In addition, patients with liver disease are at increased risk for bleeding.

THE PREOPERATIVE PHASE

PREOPERATIVE NURSING CARE

The preoperative phase begins when a decision is made to perform a surgical procedure. It ends when the patient enters the operating room. During the preoperative phase the goals of nursing care are to inform the patient of what to expect, reduce patient anxiety, and decrease the risk of complications during and after surgery.

Assessment

When nonemergency surgery is scheduled, a thorough assessment is made that starts with the patient's health history and physical examination. Although not responsible for total patient assessment as described here, the LPN/LVN often assists by collecting specific, relevant data. This is usually done before admission to the nursing care unit. Laboratory studies of blood and urine, blood grouping and crossmatching, chest radiography, pulmonary function tests, and electrocardiography (ECG) may be done. Often these and other procedures are done on an outpatient basis before admission.

Most surgical facilities have standardized forms for assessing the newly admitted patient. The nursing assessment should obtain important data needed to plan preoperative, intraoperative, and postoperative care. It also provides baseline data for monitoring the patient's status. Box 17-1 shows the elements of assessment for

---

Box 17-1 | **ASSESSMENT of the Preoperative Patient**

Health History
Identifying Data:
Age, marital status
History of Present Illness:
Problem being treated surgically
Past Medical History:
Acute and chronic conditions, previous hospitalizations and surgeries, allergies, recent and current medications
Review of Systems:
Disabilities and limitations: hearing or vision loss, paralysis, stiffness, weakness, cognitive impairment; any current health deviations
Functional Assessment:
Occupation, roles, responsibilities, diet and fluid intake, exercise, tobacco and alcohol use, sources of stress and support, coping strategies, expectations of surgery

Physical Examination
General Survey:
Emotional state, ability to communicate, response to directions
Height and Weight

Vital Signs

Skin:
Color, lesions, bruises, warmth, turgor, moisture
Thorax:
Respiratory pattern and effort, breath sounds, apical pulse
Abdomen:
Distention, scars, bowel sounds
Extremities:
Color, hair distribution, lesions, deformities, range of motion, crepitus, pain, weakness
Prostheses:
Hearing aids, eyeglasses, contact lenses, dentures, artificial limbs, other devices

---

the preoperative patient. For outpatient surgery, it is especially important to obtain some information in advance because the time available for a comprehensive assessment will be limited.

Health History

Identifying Data. Record identifying data, including the patient's age.

History of Present Illness. Describe the problem that is being treated surgically.

Past Medical History. Include acute and chronic conditions, hospitalizations, surgeries, allergies, and drug history. Record all chronic health problems such as diabetes, heart failure, pulmonary disease, or kidney disease.

Document any known allergies (food, drug, tape, chemical) according to agency policy. Place an allergy alert bracelet on the patient's wrist if there are any allergies. A number of drugs are routinely given to surgical patients. During and immediately after sur-

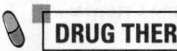

DRUG THERAPY | *Drug Interactions with General Anesthetic Agents*

DRUGS	EFFECTS OF INTERACTION	NURSING IMPLICATIONS
DRUGS THAT INCREASE EFFECTS OF GENERAL ANESTHETICS		
Some antibiotics: bacitracin, aminoglycosides, polymyxin B	Excessive muscle relaxation	Assess motor function Monitor respirations
Antihypertensives	Hypotension	Monitor blood pressure
Catecholamines: dopamine, epinephrine	Cardiac dysrhythmias	Monitor heart rate and rhythm
Central nervous system (CNS) depressants: alcohol, antianxiety agents, anticonvulsants, antihistamines, antidepressants, antipsychotics, barbiturates, opioid analgesics, sedative-hypnotics	Excessive CNS depression	Monitor blood pressure, level of consciousness, respirations, and blood pressure
Corticosteroids	Hypotension	Monitor blood pressure
Monoamine oxidase (MAO) inhibitors; isoniazid, procarbazine	CNS depression	Monitor respirations and blood pressure
Muscle relaxants: succinylcholine, tubocurarine	Excessive skeletal muscle relaxation	Assess motor activity
DRUGS THAT DECREASE EFFECTS OF GENERAL ANESTHESIA		
Alcohol	Patients with history of chronic alcohol intake develop tolerance to alcohol and require more general anesthesia	Monitor vital signs and alertness
Atropine	Given to reduce risk of reflex bradycardia with some anesthetics	Monitor pulse
DRUGS THAT INCREASE EFFECTS OF LOCAL ANESTHETIC AGENTS		
Cardiac depressants: general anesthetic agents, propranolol (Inderal)	Hypotension and dysrhythmias	Monitor blood pressure and pulse
CNS depressants	Excessive CNS depression	Monitor respirations and blood pressure
Epinephrine	Prolongs effects of local anesthetic agents	Protect anesthetized tissue
Succinylcholine (Anectine)	Risk of apnea	Monitor respirations
DRUGS THAT INCREASE EFFECTS OF NEUROMUSCULAR BLOCKING AGENTS		
Aminoglycoside antibiotics Potassium-wasting diuretics General anesthetics Local anesthetics MAO inhibitors Opioid analgesics Antidysrhythmics: procainamide and quinidine	For all drugs in this category: Additive respiratory depression, prolonged muscle relaxation	For all drugs in this category: Monitor respirations and assess muscle activity
DRUGS THAT DECREASE EFFECTS OF SUCCINYLCHOLINE		
Anticholinesterase drugs (e.g., neostigmine)	Respiratory depression	Monitor respirations

Data from Abrams, A.C. (2001). *Clinical drug therapy* (6th ed.). Philadelphia: Lippincott.

gery, the patient is unable to report allergies, so if an emergency should arise, any allergies can be determined promptly by checking the patient's allergy alert bracelet.

Compile a complete list of medications and complementary and alternative therapies the patient is taking or has recently taken. Knowledge of the patient's

Pharmacology Capsule

Long-term drug therapy with agents such as anticoagulants and hypoglycemics may require dosage adjustments before and after surgery.

drug history enables you to anticipate possible effects of drug interactions.

Review of Systems

Collect data about each body system, noting any abnormalities. Record any disabilities or limitations. Include the presence of acute problems, for example, a cold or a bout of diarrhea that could necessitate delay of a surgical procedure. In addition to the conditions identified in the past medical history, document problems that may be significant during the surgical experience, such as vision or hearing loss, partial paralysis or joint stiffness, weakness, or cognitive impairment.

Functional Assessment

Describe the patient's usual activity pattern, including occupation, roles, and responsibilities. Determine the usual diet and fluid intake as well as the use of tobacco and alcohol. Note exercise and rest patterns. Ask about sources of stress and support, usual ways of coping, and specific fears or concerns about this surgery. Although some anxiety is normal, be alert for indications of excessive anxiety (e.g., tearfulness, trembling, tachycardia).

Physical Examination

Throughout the physical examination, be alert to the patient's emotional state, ability to communicate, and ability to understand directions.

Height and Weight. Measure height and weight. Unless the patient is very ill or malnourished, the admission weight provides a goal weight to be maintained after surgery.

Vital Signs. Vital signs measured shortly after admission provide a baseline for evaluating readings after surgery. If the patient's pulse and blood pressure are slightly higher than expected on admission, it may be due to anxiety. After allowing the patient to rest, retake the vital signs. If they remain abnormal, notify the physician.

Skin. Inspect the skin for color, lesions, and bruises. Palpate to determine texture, warmth, turgor, and moisture.

Thorax. Observe the patient's respiratory rate, pattern, and effort. Auscultate lungs to assess breath sounds. Assess the apical heartbeat for rate and rhythm.

Abdomen. Inspect the abdomen for distention and scars, and auscultate bowel sounds.

Extremities. Inspect the extremities for skin color, hair distribution, lesions, and deformities. Assess range of motion while listening for crepitus and noting pain or weakness.

Prostheses. Note the presence of any prosthetic devices, including hearing aids, contact lenses, eyeglasses, dentures, artificial limbs, or other devices used to maintain appearance or function.

More specific diagnoses and goals are made based on individual patient data and specific surgical procedures.

Nursing Diagnoses, Goals, and Outcome Criteria: Preoperative Nursing Goals

Some of the nursing diagnoses and goals that might be made during the preoperative phase are:

NURSING DIAGNOSES	GOALS AND OUTCOME CRITERIA
Anxiety related to uncertain outcome of surgery, anticipated pain, potential disfigurement, or loss of function	Patient's anxiety is reduced: patient calm, states anxiety reduced
Deficient Knowledge related to the surgical experience	Patient understands the surgical experience: patient describes preoperative and postoperative routines, what to expect

Interventions

Anxiety

Most patients are somewhat anxious about surgery. Determine the presence and the level of anxiety, the contributing factors, and the need for intervention. It is especially important to find out the patient's previous experiences, if any, with hospitalization and surgery. If a patient admitted for heart surgery had an acquaintance who died after similar surgery, the patient might understandably be frightened. However, a person whose previous experiences have been positive is more likely to expect this procedure to go well. If it seems that the patient is excessively nervous or fearful about the surgery, report this to the surgeon or to the anesthesia personnel. Extreme fear is associated with surgical complications, so it should be controlled with preoperative medication and other therapeutic interventions. Sometimes surgery is postponed until anxiety is reduced.

Deficient Knowledge

Patient teaching may be done in the physician's office, the clinic, during the preadmission workup, or after admission to the hospital. Ideally, it is not left until shortly before surgery, when many activities are scheduled and the patient may be distracted. A cost-saving trend is to admit patients very early in the morning on the day of surgery. In this case, the burden of preoperative teaching rests heavily on the physician, the office nurse, the admission nurse, or the clinic nurse.

Preoperative teaching should include the patient and those who will be with the patient during the recovery period. An attentive family member or companion can reinforce instructions and help reassure the patient. Telling the patient and family or friends what to expect in the immediate postoperative phase can prevent unnecessary stress. An appropriate teaching plan is based on an assessment of what the patient already knows, wants to know, and needs to know (Fig. 17-2). Verbal instructions should be supplemented with written material.

FIGURE **17-2** Preoperative teaching prepares the patient for the surgical experience.

Teaching Methods. The teaching methods selected depend on the situation. Direct patient teaching by the nurse is probably used most often. This has advantages in that the teaching plan can be individualized and the patient can ask questions freely. The main disadvantage of one-to-one instruction is that it is time-consuming.

Some hospitals have group classes for all preoperative patients. The main advantage of group classes is economy of time. Also, some people like talking to others who are having similar procedures. Group classes have several disadvantages. It may be difficult to schedule times that are accessible to multiple patients before admission. Some patients are less likely to ask questions or express fears in a group setting. Also, information presented to mixed groups of patients is necessarily rather general.

Books, pamphlets, audiotapes, and videotapes are available for patient use. Whatever approach is used for patient teaching, it may be supplemented with these audiovisual materials. Ideally, they are used along with other teaching strategies. Provide the materials for the patient's use, and return later to answer questions and assess understanding of the material.

Unfortunately, many patient teaching materials are appropriate only for a limited audience. The reading level may be above the patient's ability, or too many technical terms may be used. We sometimes forget how we felt the first time we encountered medical terminology. In the United States many people do not speak or read English well enough to learn from these materials. So, although audiovisual materials can be very helpful, do not depend on them completely for patient teaching.

Preparation for Surgery

Preparation of the patient for surgery starts before or shortly after admission. Patients admitted for emergency surgery may not have the benefit of preoperative teaching.

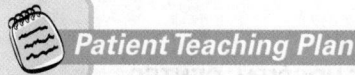
Patient Teaching Plan

Preoperative Patient

The nurse determines how much detail is appropriate for each patient. Most people need basic information and simple explanations without technical details. The family will probably want to know the expected time of surgery, where to wait for the patient, and how they will be informed when the procedure is over. The teaching plan should include an orientation to the unit and the following:

• In preparation for surgery, you will have specific treatments based on the specific surgical procedure, agency protocols, and physician's orders.
• In the postanesthesia care unit (commonly called the *PACU* or *recovery room*):
  • You may have tubes, dressings, or equipment in place.
  • Nurses will take your pulse and blood pressure often and perform other procedures specific to your surgery.
  • You will be asked to deep breathe, cough, turn, and exercise your legs to help you eliminate your anesthetic and to prevent complications.
  • You may be asked to respond to various commands, depending on your surgery.
  • You need to report pain so that measures can be taken to provide pain relief.

Informed Consent

Before surgery, a patient must sign a legal document called a *consent form* (Fig. 17-3). It states that the patient has been informed about the procedure to be done, the alternative treatments, and the risks involved and that the patient agrees to the procedure. Written consent is intended to protect the patient from unwanted procedures. It also protects the health care facility and caregivers. It is the physician's responsibility to explain the procedure and risks to the patient, but the nurse may obtain and witness the patient's signature on the form if agency policy allows. If the patient has questions or seems to be in doubt, contact the physician.

Because the consent form is a legal document, the patient must be fully alert and aware of what it contains when signing it. If the patient is a minor, a parent or guardian must sign the form. The age at which a person is considered an adult varies from state to state. Know the law in the state in which you practice.

A patient who is confused, mentally incompetent, or under the influence of drugs cannot give informed consent. For that reason, the consent form is always signed before the patient is given preoperative medications.

The patient should sign the consent form in the presence of a witness who also signs the form. The witness's signature confirms that the patient was observed signing the form. The consent form becomes part of the patient's record.

NORTHWEST HOSPITAL CENTER

REQUEST AND AUTHORIZATION FOR MEDICAL AND/OR SURGICAL TREATMENT

1. I HEREBY REQUEST AND AUTHORIZE DR._____ AND/OR HIS ASSOCIATES AND WHOMEVER THEY MAY DESIGNATE AS THEIR ASSISTANTS, TO ADMINISTER SUCH TREATMENT AS IS NECESSARY, AND TO PERFORM THE FOLLOWING OPERATION_____

    _____AND SUCH ADDITIONAL OPERATIONS OR PROCEDURES AS ARE CONSIDERED NECESSARY ON THE BASIS OF CONDITIONS THAT MAY BE REVEALED DURING THE COURSE OF SAID OPERATION OR TREATMENT.

2. I REQUEST AND AUTHORIZE THE ADMINISTRATION OF SUCH ANESTHETICS AND/OR OTHER MEDICATIONS AS ARE NECESSARY.

3. FINAL DISPOSITION OF ANY TISSUES OR PARTS SURGICALLY REMOVED IS TO BE HANDLED IN ACCORDANCE WITH THE CUSTOMARY PRACTICES OF THE HOSPITAL.

4. REASONS WHY THE ABOVE NAMED SURGERY AND/OR TREATMENT IS CONSIDERED NECESSARY, ITS ADVANTAGES, PROBABILITY OF SUCCESS, POSSIBLE COMPLICATIONS, AND RISKS, AS WELL AS POSSIBLE ALTERNATIVE MODES OF TREATMENT WERE EXPLAINED TO ME BY DR._____.

5. I AM AWARE THAT THE PRACTICE OF MEDICINE AND SURGERY IS NOT AN EXACT SCIENCE AND I ACKNOWLEDGE THAT NO GUARANTEES HAVE BEEN MADE TO ME CONCERNING THE RESULTS OF THE OPERATION OR PROCEDURE.

6. I HEREBY ACKNOWLEDGE THAT I HAVE READ AND FULLY UNDERSTAND THE ABOVE REQUEST AND AUTHORIZATION FOR MEDICAL AND/OR SURGICAL TREATMENT.

DATE:_____

TIME: _____

SIGNED: _____
Patient

OR: _____
Legal representative

WITNESS _____

Relationship (if any) _____

/PL/2736N
702/1019-E-R-5/90   40-1331

FIGURE **17-3** Surgical consent form.

Preparation of the Digestive Tract

The extent of bowel preparation, if any, depends on the type of anesthesia and the type of surgery planned. For surgery on the abdomen or the digestive tract, laxatives and enemas are generally given to empty the bowel.

Sometimes patients are instructed to do this at home before being admitted to the hospital.

Bowel cleansing serves three purposes. First, it reduces the risk of contamination from fecal matter during the operation. Second, it helps prevent postoperative distention until normal bowel function returns. Third, it avoids constipation and straining in the postoperative period. Straining can create pressure on the surgical wound. Surgery may be canceled if bowel preparation is inadequate.

Food and Fluid Restriction

Even if bowel cleansing is not ordered, ingestion by mouth of fluids and foods is restricted for a specific period of time. The evening meal before the day of surgery may be restricted to fluids. Traditionally, adult patients were given nothing by mouth (nil per os, NPO) from midnight before the scheduled surgery. This was thought to reduce the risk of vomiting and aspiration during or after anesthesia. In 1999, the American Society of Anesthesiologists recommended shorter minimum fasting times depending on the type of food and liquid taken (Table 17-1). If a patient routinely takes an oral medication that is considered essential, it may be ordered early on the morning of surgery with a few sips of water or given parenterally.

Skin Preparation

When an incision is made in the skin, microorganisms can enter the wound. Skin preparation is intended to reduce the number of organisms near the incision site. It usually includes scrubbing and removing hair from a wide margin around the planned surgical site (Fig. 17-4). The exact skin preparation is ordered by the physician or outlined in a procedure manual.

A typical procedure requires the patient (if able) to shower and wash with an antiseptic soap the evening before the surgery and again the next morning. The perioperative nurse or operating room technician scrubs the operative site shortly before surgery. If the patient's skin is very hairy or if the hair might interfere with the surgical procedure, it can be removed by clipping with electrical surgical clippers, using a depilatory cream, or shaving. Shaving was once routine, but current thinking is that shaving causes tiny nicks in the skin that shelter organisms. Therefore shaving, if done, is often delayed until shortly before surgery to allow less time for organisms to multiply. If a depilatory cream is to be used, test for allergy before applying it to the patient's skin.

Dress and Grooming

On the morning of surgery, provide a clean gown and instruct the patient to remove all undergarments unless agency policy dictates otherwise. Jewelry should be removed. If a ring cannot be removed or the patient refuses to remove it, it can be secured in accordance with agency policy. Because jewelry often has considerable sentimental as well as monetary value, handle it carefully. The patient may leave jewelry with a relative or friend. It should not be left at the bedside or accepted by the nurse for safekeeping. Most hospitals have a process for valuables to be collected, signed for, and stored in a safe until the patient asks for them to be returned. Document the disposition of jewelry and dentures in the patient's chart.

Braid or secure long hair with a rubber band. Remove hairpins or clips. Provide a cap to cover the hair. Traditionally, dentures have been removed and placed in a denture cup and stored in a safe place. Many anesthesiologists and nurse anesthetists today prefer that dentures be left in. Institutional policies should be specific about this.

Remove nail polish to permit assessment of nail beds for circulation and to permit use of a pulse oximeter. If the patient has acrylic nails, consult with the anesthesiologist or perioperative nurse about the need to remove them. At least one acrylic nail is usually removed so the pulse oximeter can be used. Makeup, including mascara, is also removed.

A patient identification band must be in place on the patient's wrist on admission. Other wristbands are placed to indicate allergies and blood type. Before surgery, check to be sure all bands are in place. Allergies must be clearly identified on a wristband and in the patient's chart because the anesthetized patient cannot report them to the surgical staff.

Prostheses

Prostheses are usually removed, marked, and secured before surgery to prevent them from being lost or damaged and to prevent them from causing injury during anesthesia. Be sure that the devices are returned to the patient as soon as possible after surgery. If the patient is very stressed at having to go to surgery without the

---

Table 17-1   *Preoperative Fasting Recommendations* of the American Society of Anesthesiologists*

LIQUID AND FOOD INTAKE	MINIMUM FASTING PERIOD (hr)
Clear liquids (e.g., water, clear tea, black coffee, carbonated beverages, and fruit juice without pulp)	2
Breast milk	4
Nonhuman milk, including infant formula	6
Light meal (e.g., toast and clear liquids)	6
Regular or heavy meal (may include fried or fatty food, meat)	8

From Practice guidelines for preoperative fasting and the use of pharmacologic agents to reduce the risk of pulmonary aspiration: Application to healthy patients undergoing elective procedures: A report by the American Society of Anesthesiologists Task Force on Preoperative Fasting. (1999). *Anesthesiology, 90,* 896.
*For healthy patients of all ages undergoing elective surgery (excluding women in labor).

Head surgery

Unilateral chest surgery

Thoracoabdominal surgery

Abdominal surgery

Forearm, elbow, or hand surgery

Gynecologic surgery

Genitourinary surgery

Hip surgery

Thigh and leg surgery

Foot/lower leg surgery

Ankle, foot, or toe surgery

FIGURE 17-4 Skin preparation of common surgical sites.

prosthesis, consult with the perioperative nurses about making an exception to the rule. A patient who is hard of hearing and does not have a hearing aid may be anxious or unable to cooperate with postoperative care; therefore hearing aids often are left in place for surgery.

Preoperative Medications

Physicians' orders for the surgical patient often include a preoperative medication to be given shortly before the patient is transported to surgery or when the patient is in a holding area. If the drug is ordered "on call," operating room personnel will notify you concerning when it should be given. If the exact time of surgery is known, the order may specify that the drug be given at a certain time.

Preoperative medication may include an opioid to decrease anxiety and promote sedation, an antiemetic to control nausea and vomiting, and an anticholinergic drug to decrease secretions. Examples are listed in the Drug Therapy table below and on p. 256.

Preoperative medications must be given at the time they are ordered because they interact with the anes-

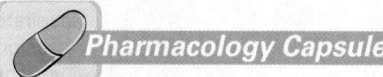

Pharmacology Capsule

Preoperative medications usually consist of a combination of an antianxiety agent, sedative-hypnotic, opioid analgesic, antiemetic, and anticholinergic drug.

DRUG THERAPY | *Preoperative Medications*

DRUG	USE/ACTION	SIDE EFFECTS	NURSING INTERVENTIONS
TRANQUILIZERS			
Chlorpromazine (Thorazine)	Anticholinergic Sedative Antiemetic	Hypotension, dizziness and fainting with parenteral administration Dry mouth, blurred vision, urinary retention, constipation Extrapyramidal symptoms: akathisia, parkinsonism, dystonias	Keep patient in bed after parenteral administration Intramuscular (IM) dose: inject slowly, deeply; massage site Contraindicated with severe central nervous system (CNS) depression Monitor blood pressure Take safety measures for drowsiness
Diazepam (Valium)	CNS depressant Skeletal muscle relaxation	Intravenous (IV) route: respiratory depression, dysrhythmias, thrombophlebitis Drowsiness, ataxia, orthostatic hypotension, headache, blurred vision, confusion	Do not mix parenteral form with other drugs IM injection in deep deltoid site; IV route should use large vein Monitor pulse and respirations Contraindicated with acute narrow angle glaucoma or acute alcohol intoxication Keep in bed after parenteral administration
Hydroxyzine hydrochloride (Vistaril, Atarax)	CNS depressant Anticholinergic	Tissue damage with IM route Drowsiness, dry mouth, pain at injection site, dizziness, ataxia	IM dose should be given deep in large muscle mass using Z technique Maintain oral hygiene Take safety measures for drowsiness
Promethazine hydrochloride (Phenergan)	Sedative Antihistamine Anticholinergic Antiemetic	Drowsiness, disorientation, hypotension, confusion Fainting in older adults Dry mouth, urinary retention, thickening of bronchial secretions Paradoxical reaction: excitation	IM dose must be deep IV dose given through IV infusion tube Contraindicated with CNS depression, acute asthma attack Monitor pulse and blood pressure Maintain oral hygiene Take safety precautions for drowsiness
OPIOID ANALGESICS			
Meperidine hydrochloride (Demerol)	Analgesic Decreases response to CO_2 Decreases gastrointestinal (GI) secretions	Sedation, nausea, vomiting, lightheadedness, dizziness, sweating, constipation Respiratory depression with overdose Tolerance and physical dependence with repeated use	Slow parenteral injection Monitor pulse, blood pressure, and respirations Withhold if respiratory rate less than 12/min Take safety precautions for drowsiness Contraindicated with monoamine oxidase (MAO) inhibitors

Continued

DRUG THERAPY *Preoperative Medications—cont'd*

DRUG	USE/ACTION	SIDE EFFECTS	NURSING INTERVENTIONS
OPIOID ANALGESICS—cont'd			
Morphine sulfate (MS Contin, Duramorph)	Analgesic Decreases response to increased CO_2 Decreases GI secretions	Circulatory collapse, cardiac arrest with rapid IV administration Dizziness, hypotension, nausea and vomiting Respiratory depression Occasional: sedation, vomiting, flushing, urinary retention	Administer parenteral forms slowly; rotate sites Dose should be reduced in older adults Monitor respirations and blood pressure Take safety precautions if drowsy Contraindicated with surgical anastomosis, after biliary tract surgery
ANTICHOLINERGICS			
Atropine sulfate Glycopyrrolate (Robinul)	Decreases secretions Decreases GI and urinary motility Mydriatic Reduces salivation, respiratory and GI secretions	Dry mouth, decreased sweating, constipation, blurred vision, drowsiness, urinary retention Tachycardia, palpitations, tachypnea with overdose	Oral hygiene Monitor vital signs; record bowel movements and urine output Take safety precautions if drowsy Numerous contraindications
SEDATIVES AND HYPNOTICS			
Pentobarbital (Nembutal) Secobarbital (Seconal)	Produces sedation	Drowsiness, sedation, lethargy, irritability, nausea, anorexia, muscle aches and pain, gastric distress Severe CNS depression with overdose Tolerance/dependence with prolonged use	Deep IM injection in large muscle Monitor vital signs before and after IV administration Administer IV at prescribed rate Take safety precautions if drowsy Dosage should be reduced for older adults Monitor pulse, blood pressure, and respirations
Chloral hydrate (Noctec)	CNS depression	Occasional nausea, vomiting, flatulence, diarrhea, disorientation Somnolence, confusion, respiratory depression, coma with overdose	Monitor pulse, blood pressure, and respirations

thetic agent. For safety reasons, ask the patient to void immediately before the preoperative medication is given. Tell the patient that the medications will cause drowsiness and dry mouth. Raise side rails, place the call bell within reach, and instruct the patient to remain in bed.

Preoperative Checklist

Most agencies have a preoperative checklist that must be completed and signed before the patient leaves the unit. Check to be sure that all laboratory and radiology reports are with the chart; that jewelry, prostheses, and nail polish have been removed; that the patient has voided; that premedication has been given; that vital

Pharmacology Capsule

Because preoperative medications have a sedative effect, the surgical consent form must be signed before medications are given. After the medications are given, instruct the patient to remain in bed to prevent falls.

Put on Your Thinking Cap!

What observations would lead you to think a patient is excessively anxious before surgery? What are some interventions that might reduce the patient's anxiety?

signs have been recorded; and that the consent form has been signed (Fig. 17-5).

THE INTRAOPERATIVE PHASE

Operating room personnel transfer the patient from the nursing unit to the surgical suite. They assist the patient onto a gurney (wheeled stretcher) and take the patient and the chart to the surgical area.

The patient may be taken directly to an operating room or may go to a holding room first. In the holding room, skin preparation may be done and intravenous fluids started, if these procedures were not done earlier.

Preoperative checklist			
Allergies:	Date of surgery:_____		Addressograph plate
CLINICAL DATA:	**Yes**	**No**	**Comments**
Authorization for surgical treatment completed			
Height and weight charted			
History and physical			
Chest x-ray			
ECG report			
Urine report			
Blood glucose within acceptable range (50-300 mg/dL)			
Hematocrit within acceptable range (30-50 mL/dL)			
Potassium within acceptable range (3.5-5.0 mEq/L)			
Unacceptable test results reported to physician	Time	By	
CLIENT PREPARATION	**Yes**	**No**	**Comments**
Jewelry removed			
Hairpiece, wig, hairpins, barrettes, beads, rubber bands removed			
Loose teeth or caps noted			
Dentures removed			
Artificial eye, contact lenses, glasses removed			
Any prosthetic appliance removed			
Voided or catheterized–I&O sheet on chart			
Identification bracelet in place			
Parenteral fluids patent and infusing at _____ mL/h			
B/P, T.P.R. charted			
Premedication given as ordered			
Side rails up–care data and care plan on chart			
Is client on isolation? If so, what type?			
COMMUNICATION ASSESSMENT	**Normal**	**Abnormal**	**Comments**
Vision			
Hearing			
Mental			
Speech			
Other			
Patient's preferred name:			
NURSE TO NURSE REFERRAL			

Limb for burial _____ Yes _____ No   at _____ Funeral home

FIGURE 17-5 The preoperative checklist must be completed before the patient goes to surgery.

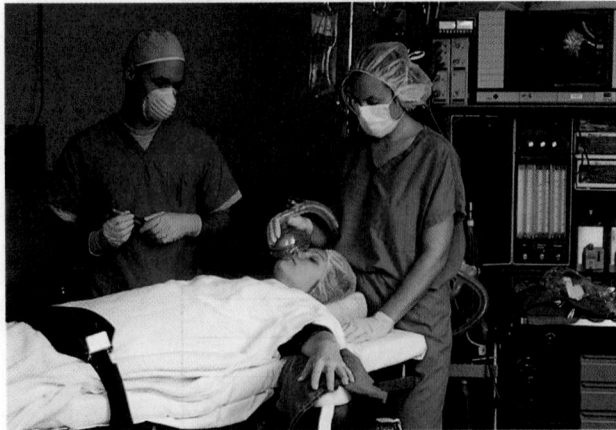

FIGURE 17-6 The nurse ensures the patient's safety on the operating table.

In some settings, preoperative medications are not given until the patient is received in the holding area. The patient who has been told earlier what to expect will feel more secure in the surgical area.

When moved into the operating room, the patient can expect to see many pieces of equipment, bright lights, and various people. The patient is helped to move to the operating room table and positioned in a specific way for the type of surgery being done. Safety straps are applied carefully because there is a risk of impaired circulation or nerve damage caused by pressure. Comfort and alignment are confirmed while the patient is awake (Fig. 17-6). The anesthetic agent is then administered and is maintained throughout the procedure. The guidelines to eliminate surgery on the wrong site are detailed in Box 17-2.

THE SURGICAL TEAM

On arrival in the surgical suite, the patient is greeted by the nurse, the physician, the anesthesiologist, or the nurse anesthetist. A number of people participate in the intraoperative period. They include the following:

- The surgeon who actually performs the procedure.
- An assistant surgeon, a nurse first assistant, or a physician assistant, who assists the surgeon in the procedure.
- The registered nurse who circulates. This nurse is responsible for assessing the patient, planning intraoperative nursing care, functioning as patient advocate, and maintaining patient safety. This person is in charge of the operating room. Responsibilities include setting up the room, monitoring aseptic technique, assisting in positioning and monitoring the patient, preparing the skin, providing needed supplies and equipment, and documenting nursing care (Fig. 17-7).
- A registered nurse first assistant (RNFA) works collaboratively with the surgeon and has advanced training for specific duties such as suturing and handling tissue with instruments.

Box 17-2 | *Guidelines to Eliminate Wrong Site Surgery*

The following guidelines are supported by both the Association of Operating Room Nurses and the American College of Surgeons.

1. Verify that the correct patient is being taken to the operating room. This verification can be made with the patient or the patient's designated representative if the patient is underage or unable to answer for him/herself.
2. Verify that the correct procedure is on the operating room schedule.
3. Verify with the patient or the patient's designated representative the procedure that is expected to be performed, as well as the location of the operation.
4. Confirm the consent form with the patient or the patient's designated representative.
5. In the case of a bilateral organ, limb, or anatomic site (e.g., hernia), the surgeon and patient should agree and the operating surgeon should mark the site prior to giving the patient narcotics, sedation, or anesthesia.
6. If the patient is scheduled for multiple procedures that will be performed by multiple surgeons, all the items on the checklist must be verified for each procedure that is planned to be performed.
7. Conduct a final verification process with members of the surgical team to confirm the correct patient, procedure, and surgical site.
8. Ensure that all relevant records and imaging studies are in the operating room.
9. If any verification process fails to identify the correct site, all activities should be halted until verification is accurate.
10. In the event of a life- or limb-threatening situation, not all of these steps may be followed.

Reprinted with permission from AORN, www.aorn.org. Copyright © 2003, AORN, Inc. 2170 South Parker Road, Suite 300, Denver, CO 80231.

- A registered nurse, LPN, or surgical technician, who scrubs and handles instruments within the sterile field during the procedure.
- The anesthesia care provider (ACP) can be a nurse anesthetist or anesthesiologist. The ACP administers anesthetics and monitors the patient's status throughout the procedure. A **nurse anesthetist** is a registered nurse with special training in anesthesia. An **anesthesiologist** is a physician who specializes in anesthesia.
- Other technical personnel with specialized jobs. For example, a perfusionist operates the heart bypass machine during open heart surgery.

ANESTHESIA

Although surgery has been done since prehistoric times, anesthesia has been used only for approximately 150 years. **Anesthetic** agents are used to alter sensation so that surgical procedures can be done painlessly and safely. Agents used for anesthesia include local and general anesthetics.

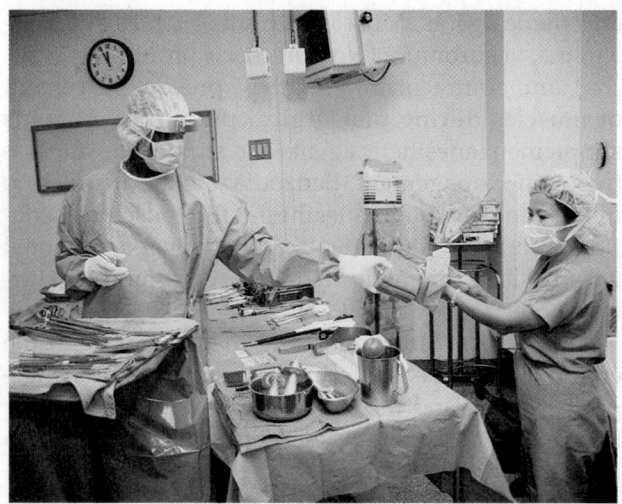
FIGURE **17-7** The nurse sets up the operating room.

Local and Regional Anesthesia

Regional anesthesia is achieved by using local anesthetics that block the conduction of nerve impulses in a specific area. These anesthetics do not cause the patient to lose consciousness. For some procedures, intravenous sedatives are given in addition to the local anesthetic.

Examples of local anesthetics are lidocaine hydrochloride (Xylocaine), bupivacaine hydrochloride (Marcaine HCl), tetracaine (Pontocaine), and ropivacaine (Naropin). They are commonly used for dental procedures, eye surgery, cosmetic surgery on the face, repair of lacerations, childbirth, and other procedures in which general anesthesia is not needed or desired by the patient. Local anesthetics are often the agents of choice for older adult patients because of other medical conditions.

Local anesthetics may be administered topically, by local infiltration, and by nerve-blocking techniques. Topical anesthetics are applied directly to the area to be anesthetized. For local infiltration, the anesthetic agent is injected into and under the skin around the area of treatment. A nerve block is done by injecting an anesthetic agent around a nerve to block the transmission of impulses. Epidural anesthesia and subarachnoid anesthesia are examples of regional nerve blocks. Both are achieved by injecting the anesthetic agent into the area around the spinal nerves. Motor and sensory functions are blocked below the level of the anesthetic administration. This anesthesia is especially useful for surgical procedures on the lower abdomen and legs. The level of anesthesia is controlled by the amount of the drug injected and the position of the patient on the operating table.

As a rule, spinal and epidural anesthesia pose less risk for respiratory, cardiac, and gastrointestinal complications than general anesthesia. If the level of spinal or epidural anesthesia rises higher than intended, there is a risk of respiratory and cardiovascular depression.

One complication of spinal anesthesia is postspinal headache. It is caused by the leaking of cerebrospinal fluid at the puncture site. Postspinal headache can be severe and may last for several weeks. It is relieved by lying flat. It is more common in women, especially postpartum women. Keeping the patient flat for a specified period of time after spinal anesthesia may reduce the risk of headache. The nurse should always check the postoperative orders, however, for any positioning or activity restrictions. Forcing fluids in the postoperative period, if allowed, may help.

Severe spinal headache is sometimes treated by injecting a small amount of the patient's blood into the epidural space at the site of the previous subarachnoid puncture. The blood clots, forming a "blood patch" that prevents further leaking. The procedure can be repeated if it is unsuccessful the first time. A successful patch relieves the headache immediately. Postanesthesia headache should not occur with epidural anesthesia.

As the effect of a regional anesthetic wears off, the patient often reports that the affected limbs feel numb and heavy. You should reassure the patient that this is normal and that movement and sensation gradually return to normal. It is vital to do passive range-of-motion exercises until mobility returns, to prevent thrombus (clot) formation. Typically, motor function returns before sensory function. At that time, the patient is susceptible to injury resulting from trauma or pressure because movement is possible but pain is not perceived.

Complications of local anesthesia include toxic effects caused by overdose, local tissue damage, and allergic responses. Initial signs and symptoms of toxic effects are excitement and central nervous system stimulation, followed by depression of the central nervous system and the cardiovascular system. Local tissue effects may be inflammation and edema. Abscesses and necrosis sometimes develop at the injection site. This is thought to be caused by poor technique rather than by the anesthetic agent.

Preanesthetic Agents

Before receiving anesthesia, the patient may be given preanesthetic agents, which can include antianxiety agents, sedative-hypnotics, anticholinergics, and opioid analgesics. Preanesthetic medications reduce anxiety without causing excessive drowsiness, induce perioperative amnesia, and reduce the amount of anesthesia required. In addition, they reduce the risk of some adverse effects of anesthetic agents, effects such as salivation, bradycardia, coughing, and vomiting.

General Anesthesia

General anesthesia acts on the central nervous system (CNS), causing loss of consciousness, sensation, reflexes, pain perception, and memory. Combinations of drugs are used to achieve these effects without excessive CNS depression. This use of multiple drugs, referred to as *balanced anesthesia,* allows lower dosages of each drug, which reduces the risks of adverse effects. General anesthetic agents are most often given by inhalation or intravenous infusion. Although the intramuscular and rectal routes can be used to administer anesthetic agents, the use of those routes is uncommon.

Near the end of procedures done under general anesthesia, the anesthetist or anesthesiologist administers drugs to reverse the effects of the anesthetic. When the procedure is completed, a member of the surgical team escorts the patient to the postanesthesia care unit, where careful monitoring can be done until the patient recovers from the anesthesia.

Inhalation Agents. Inhalation agents include isoflurane (Forane), sevoflurane (Ultane), enflurane (Ethrane), desflurane (Suprane), methoxyflurane (Penthrane), and nitrous oxide. For most procedures using inhalation agents, the patient is first induced with a short-acting intravenous agent that causes rapid loss of consciousness. Then an endotracheal tube is inserted into the patient's trachea to permit administration of the maintenance inhalation anesthesia and to control mechanical ventilation. A cuff on the endotracheal tube is inflated to prevent leakage during mechanical ventilation and aspiration of gastric contents while the patient is unconscious (Fig. 17-8).

Intravenous Agents. Intravenous agents include thiopental sodium (Pentothal), methohexital sodium (Brevital Sodium), propofol (Diprivan), midazolam (Versed), etomidate (Amidate), sufentanil (Sufenta), alfentanil (Alfenta), fentanyl (Duragesic), droperidol (Inapsine), and ketamine hydrochloride (Ketalar).

Other Agents. Muscle relaxants, opioids, benzodiazepines, and antiemetics are often given with the anesthetic agents. Muscle relaxants such as succinylcholine, vecuronium (Norcuron), rocuronium (Zemuron), and cisatracurium (Nimbex) prevent movement of muscles during the surgical procedure. Opioids supplement anesthetic agents and support postoperative pain management. Benzodiazepines are used to induce and maintain anesthesia, for conscious sedation, and to sedate patients during local or regional anesthesia. Antiemetics help prevent vomiting during surgery.

Complications. Inhalation anesthetic agents and the endotracheal tube itself can cause irritation of the respiratory tract and the larynx. Individual agents may have the potential to cause serious adverse effects such as cardiac dysrhythmias, seizures, liver damage, nausea and vomiting, and death.

Malignant Hyperthermia

Malignant hyperthermia is a rare but life-threatening complication that occurs in response to certain drugs. Susceptibility to this response is inherited. It may occur when succinylcholine is used with some general anesthetic agents. It is characterized by increasing body temperature and metabolic rate, tachycardia, hypotension, cyanosis, and muscle rigidity. When malignant hyperthermia occurs, the surgery is interrupted and measures are taken to cool the patient (e.g., with iced intravenous solutions and/or ice packs). One hundred percent oxygen is administered, and the patient is given dantrolene sodium, furosemide (Lasix), mannitol, sodium bicarbonate, and diuretics.

Hypothermia

Hypothermia refers to a condition in which the body temperature is lower than normal. For some surgical procedures, the body temperature is deliberately lowered to reduce the metabolic rate and the need for oxygen. Cooling or freezing of a local area to block pain impulses is called *cryoanesthesia.*

Conscious Sedation

Conscious sedation employs intravenous drugs to reduce pain intensity or awareness without loss of reflexes. It is used with some diagnostic and therapeutic procedures, including cardiac catheterization and endoscopy. Only patients who meet specific psychological and physiologic criteria are candidates for conscious sedation. Registered nurses with specialized training may administer the drugs used for conscious sedation. During the procedure, the patient's vital signs, oxygen saturation, airway, level of consciousness, and electrocardiogram must be closely monitored. Documentation must include assessment data, interventions such as oxygen therapy, and the time, dosage, route, and effects of all drugs administered. Complications include respiratory depression and apnea, hypotension, excessive sedation approaching that of general anesthesia, and agitation and combativeness.

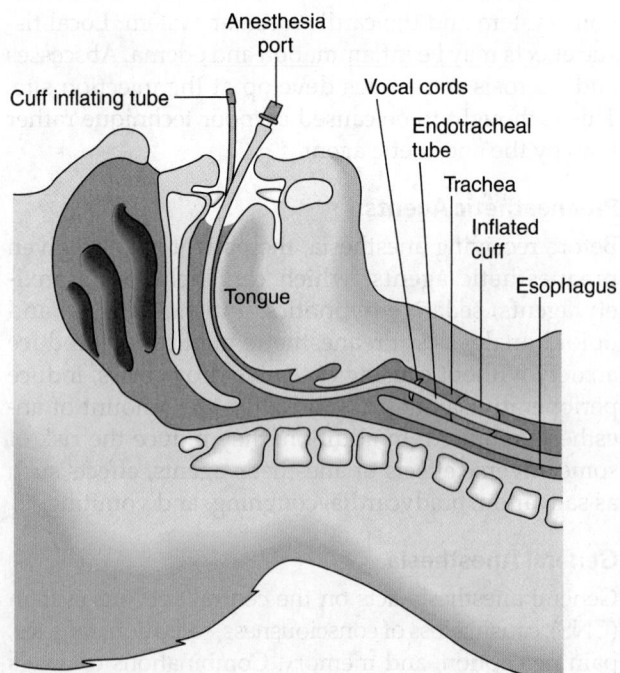

Anesthesia port

Cuff inflating tube

Vocal cords

Endotracheal tube

Trachea

Inflated cuff

Esophagus

Tongue

FIGURE **17-8** Inhalation anesthetic is given through an endotracheal tube.

After procedures using conscious sedation, the patient may be discharged home with a responsible person when the following conditions are met: stable vital signs, patent airway, intact motor function and reflexes, satisfactory surgical site, no nausea or vomiting, and the patient is alert and able to void.

INTRAOPERATIVE NURSING CARE

Intraoperative nursing care is a specialty and is beyond the scope of this chapter. Only potential nursing diagnoses and goals are listed here.

Nursing Diagnoses, Goals, and Outcome Criteria: Intraoperative Nursing Care

NURSING DIAGNOSES	GOALS AND OUTCOME CRITERIA
Risk for Injury related to the effects of anesthesia, positioning, use of restraints	Absence of physical injury: complete recovery from anesthesia, no pressure or traumatic tissue damage associated with positioning or restraints
Impaired Gas Exchange related to the effect of anesthesia and immobility	Adequate gas exchange: normal arterial blood gases
Decreased Cardiac Output related to drug effects or blood loss	Adequate cardiac output: heart rate and blood pressure consistent with patient norms
Risk for Deficient Fluid Volume related to blood loss, insensible loss of water, NPO status	Normal fluid volume: balanced intake and output, pulse and blood pressure consistent with patient norms

THE POSTOPERATIVE PHASE

When the surgical procedure is completed, the patient is usually transferred to the postanesthesia care unit (PACU or "recovery room") or the critical care unit before returning to the nursing unit. Exceptions are patients who have undergone minor procedures with only local anesthesia.

SURGICAL COMPLICATIONS

The postoperative patient is at risk for a number of complications. These complications may be related to the surgical procedure itself, to the drugs used before and during the procedure, or to immobility during and after the procedure. The types of postoperative complications vary depending on the length of time elapsed since the surgical procedure. For example, shock and hypoxia are most likely to occur in the immediate recovery period. Wound infection, however, does not appear until several days after surgery. Complications in the immediate and later postoperative periods are described in Table 17-2. Prevention, recognition, and nursing implications are discussed in the section on nursing care.

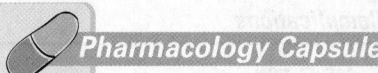

Pharmacology Capsule

Opioid analgesics given before the effects of general anesthesia wear off may cause a drop in blood pressure and slow respirations.

Shock

Shock is most likely to occur as an effect of anesthesia or loss of blood. If opioid analgesics are given before the anesthesia wears off, they may contribute to a drop in blood pressure.

Shock may also result from low blood volume (hypovolemic shock). Bleeding is an obvious cause of low blood volume, but other factors may contribute as well. Dehydration without adequate fluid replacement or fluid losses through wounds and suction can explain low blood volume.

There is growing interest in "bloodless" surgical procedures. These procedures employ a variety of strategies to reduce the need for blood replacement necessitated by excessive blood loss. Such strategies include drug therapy to stimulate production of red blood cells; the use of gamma-knife radiosurgery, electrocautery, and laser beam coagulation; and the collection and reinfusion of the patient's own blood during the procedure.

Hypoxia

Hypoxia refers to inadequate oxygenation of body tissues. The patient is at risk for hypoxia in the immediate postoperative phase for several reasons. First, general anesthetics depress respirations, so that the patient's breathing efforts may be inadequate initially. Second, when the patient is unconscious, the tongue may fall back and block the airway. Third, anesthesia depresses the cough and swallowing reflexes. Until these reflexes return, vomitus and saliva can enter the airway. A fourth reason that hypoxia may occur in the immediate postoperative period is the risk of laryngospasm or bronchospasm. Spasm of the larynx or bronchi narrows the airway and obstructs airflow.

Injury

Immediately after surgery, the patient is at risk for injury because of the decreased level of consciousness associated with general anesthesia or other sedatives. If regional anesthesia was used, the affected body part may be injured because it lacks sensation.

Pharmacology Capsule

Regional anesthesia blocks sensation and movement, so the affected body part is at risk for injury.

Table 17-2 *Surgical Complications*

COMPLICATIONS	PREVENTION	TREATMENT
Shock	Assess wound dressing Report excessive drainage or bleeding Monitor vital signs q 15 min until stable Note early changes in vital signs Report tachycardia, tachypnea, hypotension Monitor input and output Keep intravenous fluid rate on schedule Assess respirations before giving opioids	Fluid or blood replacement Vasopressors (drugs to raise blood pressure) as ordered Additional surgery may be needed to control bleeding
Hypoxia	Keep airway in place until patient awakens Position unconscious patient on side, if not contraindicated Suction as necessary Monitor vital signs q 15 min until stable Encourage deep breathing	Position to promote effective ventilation Suction as necessary Administer oxygen Encourage deep breathing and coughing
Impaired wound healing Dehiscence Evisceration Infection	Adequate fluids and nutrition Splint incision during activity, coughing and deep breathing Good hand washing; sterile or clean technique for wound care as appropriate	Cover open wound with sterile dressing If organs protrude, saturate the dressing with normal saline and cover wet dressing with dry, sterile dressing; notify physician Keep patient still and quiet with knees flexed Anticipate return to surgery; withhold opioids until consent form signed
Inadequate oxygenation Pneumonia Atelectasis	Change position at least q 2 hr Assist to cough and deep breathe hourly Incentive spirometry	Rest Oxygen and antibiotics as ordered
Digestive disturbances Nausea and vomiting	Withhold oral fluids until nausea subsides Give antiemetics to prevent vomiting as soon as nausea is reported	Antiemetic drugs as ordered
Altered elimination Urine retention	Provide privacy; offer warm bedpan; position comfortably; take to bathroom or bedside commode chair if allowed; pour warm water over the perineum; let tap water run	Catheterization as ordered
Kidney failure	Promptly report urine output of less 30 mL/hr	
Abdominal distention	Nothing by mouth until bowel sounds return	Use rectal tube, heat to abdomen, bisacodyl suppositories as ordered Position on right side Nasogastric intubation with suction as ordered
"Gas" pains	Encourage ambulation as allowed	Ambulate frequently when permitted
Constipation	Encourage fluids, food, and ambulation as ordered; use stool softeners as ordered	Laxatives or enemas, or both, as ordered
Thrombophlebitis	Avoid pressure on blood vessels Leg exercises q 1-2 hr Early, frequent ambulation as ordered Elastic or automatic compression stockings	Bedrest Anticoagulant therapy as ordered
Fluid and electrolyte imbalances	Monitor intravenous fluid rate Provide a variety of oral fluids when permitted Treat vomiting Recognize signs of imbalances (see Chapter 14)	Give intravenous fluids as ordered Encourage oral intake when allowed

Pharmacology Capsule

General anesthetics and opioid analgesics depress respirations.

Pneumonia and Atelectasis

Drug effects and immobility place the surgical patient at risk for pneumonia and atelectasis. Patients who are most prone to these complications are older adults, the obese, those with chronic pulmonary disease, and those who have undergone chest or abdominal surgery. General anesthetics and opioid analgesics depress respiratory function. Anticholinergics cause pulmonary secretions to be drier and thicker.

Immobility limits lung expansion and allows fluids to pool in the lungs. Fluid provides a medium for infectious organisms to grow. An infection of the lungs associated with immobility is called *hypostatic pneumonia.*

As secretions accumulate, they begin to block off branches of the respiratory tree. When gases can no longer enter or leave the affected alveoli, they collapse. *Atelectasis* is the term used to describe collapse of a portion or all of a lung. Because atelectasis impairs the exchange of gases, it can be very serious.

WOUND COMPLICATIONS

Complications in wound healing include dehiscence, evisceration, and infection. All are, to some extent, preventable.

Dehiscence and Evisceration

Dehiscence is the reopening of the surgical wound. It involves one or more layers of tissue. Dehiscence is most likely to happen when strain on the suture line is excessive. Factors that increase the risk of dehiscence include wound infection, malnutrition, obesity, dehydration, and extensive abdominal wounds or injuries. Dehiscence is most likely to occur between the 5th and 12th postoperative days. Evisceration is the term used when body organs protrude through the open wound. Dehiscence and evisceration are illustrated in Figure 17-9.

Infection

The risk of wound infection is greatest in cases of traumatic injuries, wounds that were not treated promptly, and wounds that were infected before surgery.

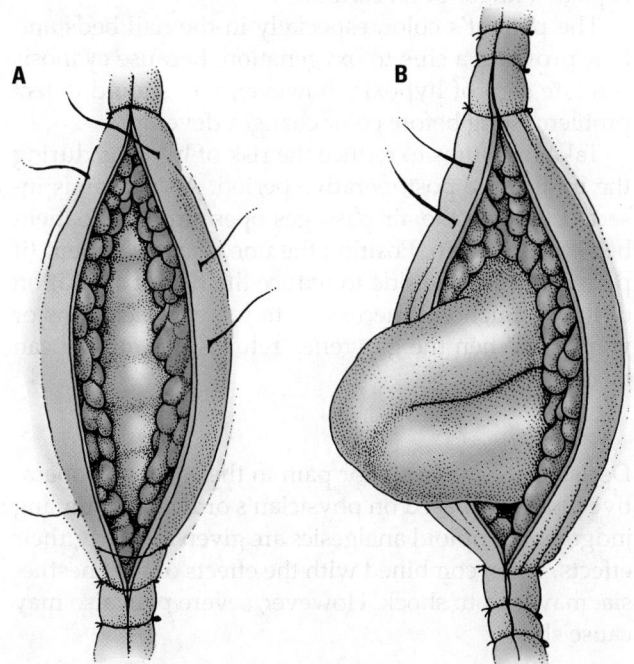

Dehiscence   Evisceration
FIGURE 17-9 Complications of wound healing. **A,** Dehiscence. **B,** Evisceration.

GASTROINTESTINAL DISTURBANCES

The primary gastrointestinal problems that follow surgery are nausea, vomiting, impaired peristalsis, and constipation. Nausea and vomiting are most common in the early postoperative period. Causative factors include anesthesia, pain, opioids, decreased peristalsis, and resuming oral intake too soon.

Factors that cause peristalsis to be impaired after surgery include anesthesia, immobility, opioid analgesics, and handling of the bowel during surgery. Patients who develop metabolic imbalances, respiratory problems, or shock are also at risk for gastrointestinal disturbances.

The effects of slowed peristalsis can be mild or severe. Gas normally forms in the digestive tract. When peristalsis is slow, the gas builds up and causes cramping pain and distention. Mild effects are generally experienced as gas pains that typically occur on the second or third postoperative day. Constipation is also related to slow peristalsis.

If peristalsis stops completely, the patient is said to have a paralytic ileus. The patient with a paralytic ileus has abdominal distention that may be severe enough to impair lung expansion and decrease blood return from the legs, causing cardiac output to fall. Distention also causes strain on an abdominal incision.

URINARY RETENTION AND RENAL FAILURE

With urinary retention, the kidneys produce urine but the patient is unable to empty the bladder. Urinary retention can be caused by the effects of anesthesia or opioids, trauma to the urinary tract, or anxiety about voiding. Urine output may also be decreased because of dehydration or blood loss.

With kidney failure, the kidneys are unable to produce enough urine to remove wastes from the body. Urine output falls dangerously low.

THROMBOPHLEBITIS

The risk of hemorrhage and shock decreases after the immediate postoperative period. A more common circulatory problem in the later period is thrombophlebitis. Thrombophlebitis is the inflammation of veins with the formation of blood clots. It occurs most often in the legs after a period of immobility. Patients who have very lengthy surgical procedures or who must be immobilized are most likely to develop thrombophlebitis.

Clots that cling to the walls of blood vessels are called *thrombi.* Thrombi that break loose and flow with the blood are called *emboli.* Emboli formed in the legs

Put on Your Thinking Cap!

Use the "Stress Response" discussed in Chapter 8 to explain the signs and symptoms of deficient fluid volume during the immediate postoperative period.

are most likely to pass through the heart and lodge in the pulmonary circulation. If they are large enough to seriously impair pulmonary blood flow, the patient develops severe respiratory distress and may even die.

IMMEDIATE POSTOPERATIVE NURSING CARE *in the PACU*

Assessment

When the patient is admitted to the postanesthesia care unit (PACU), determine the medical diagnosis and the surgical procedure. Promptly assess the patient's status (level of consciousness, vital signs) and inspect the wound or dressing. Check and set up equipment, such as suction devices, oxygen, urinary drainage, and intravenous lines, as needed. When the patient returns to the nursing unit, a more complete assessment will be done.

Nursing Diagnoses, Goals, and Outcome Criteria: Immediate Postoperative Care

Depending on the specific surgical procedure, nursing diagnoses and goals for the patient immediately after surgery may include the following:

NURSING DIAGNOSES	GOALS AND OUTCOME CRITERIA
Decreased Cardiac Output related to excessive loss of blood and other body fluids or the effects of drugs	Normal cardiac output: pulse and blood pressure consistent with patient norms, normal skin color
Ineffective Breathing Pattern and/or **Ineffective Airway Clearance** related to effects of anesthetic agents or pain	Adequate oxygenation: respiratory rate, effort, and pattern consistent with patient norms; normal arterial blood gases; breath sounds clear
Acute Pain related to tissue trauma or to positioning during surgical procedures	Decreased pain: relaxed expression, patient statement of pain relief
Disturbed Thought Processes related to the effects of anesthetic agents	Normal thought processes: absence of confusion; orientation to person and place
Risk for Injury related to decreased level of consciousness or loss of sensation and movement as effect of anesthesia	Patient remains safe during recovery period: no falls, bruises, trauma when under effects of anesthesia

Interventions

Decreased Cardiac Output

Be alert to the possibility of shock. To detect impending shock, the patient's vital signs are monitored every 5 to 15 minutes in the PACU. Signs and symptoms of impending shock include a rapid, thready pulse; restlessness; decreasing blood pressure; and decreasing urine output. Use the patient's preoperative vital signs to evaluate whether postoperative vital signs are

normal. An increasing pulse usually precedes a fall in blood pressure. Monitor intravenous fluid intake and urinary output. When blood volume is low (hypovolemia), the kidneys reduce urine production. Continuous cardiac monitoring is often done to identify early signs of hypovolemia or potentially dangerous changes in cardiac rhythm.

Measures to reduce the risk of shock include prompt recognition and treatment of bleeding, replacement of lost fluids, and the cautious use of opioid analgesics. Frequently inspect wound dressings and drains for the color and amount of drainage. The amount of bleeding expected varies with different surgical procedures.

An open intravenous route must be maintained during the early postoperative period. This permits the infusion of fluids, blood, and emergency medications if needed. Therefore check the venipuncture site to be sure the fluid is infusing properly. The intravenous fluid infusion rate is ordered by the physician, but the nurse regulates the rate. If the rate falls behind, the patient may not receive adequate fluids to replace losses during surgery. If given too rapidly, intravenous fluids can overload the circulatory system, causing heart failure.

Ineffective Breathing Pattern

To detect early signs of hypoxia in the PACU, monitor the patient's respiratory status. Assess respiratory depth, rate, and effort. Listen for abnormal breath sounds that suggest breathing difficulty. Also be alert for changes in the pulse rate because an increasing pulse rate is often an early indicator of poor oxygenation. An oximeter is used to monitor the oxygenation of the blood. The oximeter is a device with a wire that clips to a finger or an earlobe.

The patient's color, especially in the nail beds and lips, provides a clue to oxygenation. Because cyanosis is a late sign of hypoxia, however, you should detect problems long before color changes develop.

Take measures to reduce the risk of hypoxia during the immediate postoperative period. An airway is inserted to keep the air passages open until the patient begins to awaken. Position the unconscious patient (if permitted) on one side to reduce the risk of aspiration of fluids. Suction if necessary to remove secretions or vomitus. When the gag reflex returns, the airway can be removed.

Acute Pain

Decisions to medicate for pain in the early postoperative phase are based on physician's orders and nursing judgment. If opioid analgesics are given too early, their effects, when combined with the effects of the anesthesia, may lead to shock. However, severe pain also may cause shock.

Disturbed Thought Processes

As patients begin to regain consciousness, they may move around and touch dressings and drains. Tell them where they are, that the surgery is over, and what is happening. Simple explanations and gentle reminders are often sufficient to calm and reassure them. The amnesic effects of drugs used in surgery may cause the patient to forget what was said, making it necessary to repeat information.

Risk for Injury

Patients who have had local anesthesia may be sent to the PACU postoperatively, or they may be returned directly to the nursing unit or the ambulatory surgery unit. In the immediate postoperative period they are usually drowsy because preoperative and intraoperative sedatives typically have been given.

When regional block anesthesia is used, remember that sensation in that area is impaired. Take care, therefore, to prevent injury to the anesthetized body region.

After spinal anesthesia, the patient regains the ability to move the legs before sensation returns. Chart the times that the patient regains both movement and sensation. Assess the bladder for distention because the patient is unable to feel pressure. Patients may be kept flat for a specific period of time in the belief that it may help prevent spinal headache.

The Patient's Family

The time between the patient's leaving the nursing unit and returning can be 3 or 4 hours, even for relatively simple procedures. This may seem like a very long time for family and friends who are waiting. Most hospitals have some system for communicating the patient's sta-

---

NURSING CARE PLAN

The Postoperative Patient

ASSESSMENT

Health History: 27-year-old Susan Matthews was admitted for a hysterectomy and surgical excision of endometriosis implants. She is a secretary, married, and the mother of a 3-year-old child. Is 1 day post-surgery. Complains of moderate abdominal and incisional pain. Has been out of bed three times since surgery. Ambulated well with assistance. Foley catheter removed 3 hours ago. Has not voided since. Intravenous fluids infusing at 100 mL/hr. No nausea, but nothing by mouth (NPO) until noon, when 550 mL of clear liquids was taken and retained.

Physical Examination: Alert and oriented. Vital signs: temperature 99.4° F orally; pulse 90, respirations 16, blood pressure 130/86. (Admission vital signs were temperature 99° F orally; pulse 94, respiration 20, blood pressure 126/82.) Breath sounds diminished in lower lobes. Abdomen soft. No bladder distention. Wound covered with dry dressing. Bowel sounds present but hypoactive.

Nursing Diagnosis	Goals and Outcome Criteria	Interventions
Acute Pain related to tissue trauma	Patient will report pain relief and appear more relaxed.	Assess nature, location, and severity of pain. Evaluate effectiveness of patient-controlled analgesia. Assure patient that opioids can be taken safely for acute pain for a limited time. Assist to change positions at least q 2 hr. Give back rub. Coach in relaxation exercises and mental imagery. Assess anxiety, and explore causes. Be available. Reassure.
Impaired Tissue Integrity related to surgical incision	Patient's wound edges will remain clean and closed until discharge.	Check dressing hourly for bleeding first 24 hours, then twice each shift. Report bleeding to physician. Protect wound by supporting during respiratory exercises. Treat nausea promptly.
Risk for Infection related to break in skin, invasive devices, and procedures	Patient will remain free of infection, as evidenced by oral temperature less than 100° F, decreasing redness of incision, no purulent drainage, clear breath sounds, no dysuria, no phlebitis.	Monitor vital signs q 4 hr. Report increasing temperature. Assess wound for increasing redness, edema, or drainage each shift. Inspect for purulent drainage. Exercise good hand washing. Aseptic technique for wound care. Monitor and encourage fluid intake. Collect specimens for culture if ordered. Teach patient how to care for wound after discharge.
Impaired Gas Exchange related to stasis of pulmonary secretions	Patient's breath sounds will remain clear and respiratory rate will be between 12 and 20 without dyspnea.	Help patient support incision and turn, cough, and deep breathe or use incentive spirometry at least q 2 hr. Teach to take 10 deep breaths each hour. Auscultate breath sounds for crackles or atelectasis q 2 hr. Encourage fluid intake.
Urinary Retention related to effects of anesthesia	Patient's urine output will be approximately equal to fluid intake; no bladder distention.	Measure all fluid intake and output. Palpate for distended bladder q 2 hr. Provide privacy and try to stimulate voiding. Catheterize using sterile technique as ordered if patient is unable to void.

Continued

NURSING CARE PLAN

The Postoperative Patient—cont'd

Nursing Diagnosis	Goals and Outcome Criteria	Interventions
Constipation related to effects of drugs, immobility, bowel manipulation during surgery	Patient will have bowel sounds and pass flatus before discharge.	Assess bowel sounds and ask patient to report passage of flatus ("gas"). Count and document gurgles per minute. Encourage frequent ambulation as allowed. Position the patient on the right side. Report distention.
Risk for Deficient Fluid Volume related to wound drainage, NPO status	Patient's fluid intake and output will be approximately equal; serum electrolytes will remain within normal limits.	Measure fluid intake and output. Assess fluid status: tissue turgor, mucous membranes, pulse quality. Administer antiemetics promptly for nausea or vomiting. Offer fluids as prescribed.
Impaired Physical Mobility related to weakness, tissue trauma	Patient will gradually increase activity and assume more self-care.	Assist out of bed until patient can do so alone. Teach patient importance of ambulation to promote healing and prevent complications.
Disturbed Body Image related to abdominal wound	Patient will state any concerns about appearance of wound.	Observe patient's reaction to the incision. Ask if there are any questions or concerns. Answer questions honestly or refer to surgeon. Tell the patient the incision will fade and the edema will diminish.
Deficient Knowledge related to postoperative routines	Patient will correctly describe postoperative routines and self-care during hospitalization and after discharge. Patient will identify complications that should be reported to the physician.	Reinforce physician's instructions for wound care and activity limitations. Encourage consideration of adaptations needed in work or home roles and responsibilities. Stress need for good nutrition. Explain any drugs being prescribed: dosage, schedule, side effects, and adverse effects that should be reported to the physician. Include husband in teaching.

? CRITICAL THINKING QUESTIONS

■ In addition to your desire to make sure the patient is comfortable, why is it necessary to collect data about postoperative pain?

■ Members of the health care team often repeat and reinforce one another's instructions when talking to the patient. Explain at least three reasons it's important to do so.

tus to those who wait. These visitors are usually relieved to know when the patient is in the recovery room. Many surgeons take time to speak with the family shortly after the surgery is completed. When problems arise, it is thoughtful to offer visitors privacy and the services of a patient representative or a spiritual counselor.

Discharge from the Postanesthesia Care Unit

The patient's progress in the PACU is carefully monitored. Several systems of scoring have been used to determine when recovery is adequate and the patient can be transferred. In general, the patient can be moved from the recovery room when the following conditions are met:
1. Vital signs are stable.
2. Respiratory and circulatory functions are adequate.
3. The patient has minimal pain.
4. The patient is awake or can be wakened easily.
5. Complications are absent or are under control.
6. The gag reflex is present.

Most patients remain in the PACU for 1 to 2 hours, although the time varies considerably. Patients who are unstable or who need very close observation may be transferred to a critical care unit.

POSTOPERATIVE NURSING CARE on the Nursing Unit

When the patient is transferred to the nursing unit, the PACU nurse reports on the patient to the nurse who will be caring for that patient. Several people are usually necessary to move the patient safely from the gurney to the bed. Be careful to prevent pulling or dislodging tubes and to prevent a shearing force on the skin. Hang intravenous fluids, and set at the ordered rate. Connect nasogastric suction tubes to suction equipment. Identify and arrange drains to avoid obstruction. Safety precautions include raising the side rails, lowering the bed, placing the call bell within reach, and instructing the patient not to get up without assistance (see Nursing Care Plan: The Postoperative Patient on pp. 265 and above).

Assessment

Health History

Review the patient's preoperative assessment (outlined in Box 17-1), noting long-term conditions, disabilities, prostheses, drugs, and allergies. When the patient is able to respond, ask about significant symptoms, including pain, nausea, and altered sensations, as explained in Box 17-3.

Physical Examination

Vital Signs. Take vital signs and compare the results with the preoperative readings. Note the respiratory rate, depth, and effort. Take the pulse, noting rate, rhythm, and quality. Record the blood pressure. Measurements are usually repeated every 15 minutes until the vital signs stabilize.

Neurologic Status. The assessment of neurologic status includes level of consciousness and pupil size, equality, and reaction to light. Evaluate sensation in affected body areas. Note spontaneous movements and the patient's ability to move affected parts on command. For example, when a cast has been applied to a fractured arm, test the patient's ability to move the fingers.

Integument. Inspect the skin color and palpate for temperature. Inspect the surgical area. If the wound is visible, assess the incision for intactness of the wound margins, drainage, and excessive redness or swelling. If a dressing covers the incision, inspect the dressing for bleeding or other drainage. If closed drains are in place, observe the amount and appearance of the drainage (Table 17-3).

Thorax. Observe chest expansion with respirations. Chest movement should be symmetric. Auscultate for breath sounds to detect atelectasis, crackles, and wheezes.

Heart. Take the apical pulse if the peripheral pulse is weak or irregular or if the patient has heart disease.

Abdomen. Inspect the abdomen for distention and auscultate for bowel sounds. Light palpation also may be done to assess bowel and bladder distention and tenderness. Check the patency of gastrointestinal tubes.

Extremities. Assess the color and capillary refill of nail beds and the presence and quality of peripheral pulses in affected extremities. Note the presence of edema or excessive warmth or redness. Simultaneously assess the color and temperature of both arms or both legs to detect differences. Dorsiflex the foot to assess for pain in the calf, a finding called a *positive Homans' sign*. A positive Homans' sign is suggestive of thrombophlebitis; however, its value is in question. It may be negative even in the presence of thrombophlebitis.

Box 17-3   ASSESSMENT of the Postoperative Patient

Health History
Reason for surgery, name of procedure, medical diagnosis, disabilities, prostheses, drugs, allergies
Presence of pain, nausea, altered sensations

Physical Examination
Vital Signs
Neurologic Status:
Level of consciousness; pupil size, equality, response to light; sensation; spontaneous movement, response to commands
Integument:
Color, temperature, incision or dressing appearance, amount and appearance of drainage
Thorax:
Chest expansion, symmetry, breath sounds
Heart:
Apical pulse
Abdomen:
Contour, bowel sounds, bladder distention, tenderness
Extremities:
Color, capillary refill, pulses, edema, warmth, redness, Homans' sign

---

Nursing Diagnoses, Goals, and Outcome Criteria: Postoperative Nursing Care

Once the immediate postoperative phase has passed, the type of potential complications changes somewhat. The risks of shock and hypoxia lessen. The nurse's attention turns toward other nursing diagnoses and goals, which are detailed in this chart.

NURSING DIAGNOSES	GOALS AND OUTCOME CRITERIA
Acute Pain related to tissue trauma	Reduced pain: relaxed expression, patient statement of pain reduction or relief
Impaired Tissue Integrity related to poor wound healing	Normal wound healing: intact wound margins
Risk for Infection related to break in skin or invasive devices and procedures	Absence of infection: minimal redness, clear drainage, no purulence; no fever
Impaired Gas Exchange related to stasis of pulmonary secretions, thrombosis, or emboli	Adequate oxygenation: respiratory rate and effort consistent with patient norms; normal arterial blood gases. Absence of thrombophlebitis: no redness or swelling in legs; negative Homans' sign
Urinary Retention related to the effects of anesthesia or restricted position	Normal bladder emptying: urine output approximately equal to fluid intake; no bladder distention
Constipation related to the effects of drugs, immobility, or bowel manipulation during surgery	Normal bowel function: bowel sounds present, passage of flatus
Risk for Deficient Fluid Volume related to wound drainage, inadequate intake, vomiting, or gastrointestinal decompression	Normal hydration: approximately equal fluid intake and output, normal serum electrolytes, pulse and blood pressure consistent with patient norms

Continued

Table 17-3 | *Expected Drainage from Tubes and Catheters*

SUBSTANCE	DAILY AMOUNT	COLOR	ODOR	CONSISTENCY
Indwelling catheter: Urine	500-700 mL 1-2 days postoperative; 1500-2500 mL thereafter	Clear, yellow	Ammonia	Watery
Nasogastric tube: Gastric contents	Up to 1500 mL/day	Pale, yellow-green Bloody after gastrointestinal surgery	Sour	Watery
Hemovac: Wound drainage	Variable with procedure	Variable with procedure Usually sero-sanguineous	Same as wound dressing	Variable
T-Tube: Bile	500 mL	Bright yellow to dark green	Acid	Thick

From Lewis, S.M., Heitkemper, M.M., & Dirksen, S.R. (2004). *Medical-surgical nursing* (6th ed.). St. Louis: Mosby.

Imbalanced Nutrition: Less Than Body Requirements related to nausea and vomiting or medical restriction of intake

Adequate nutrition for metabolic demands: retention of oral food and fluids, stable body weight

Impaired Physical Mobility related to weakness, tissue trauma, or medical activity restrictions

Improved physical mobility: gradual increase in mobility to maximal level

Disturbed Body Image related to change in body appearance and function

Adaptation to changes in body image: patient looks at and touches affected area, patient verbalizes acceptance of physical changes

Interventions

Acute Pain

Pain is expected in the early postoperative phase. Pain receptors are stimulated because tissues are cut and stretched during surgery. Muscle spasms in the area around the incision add to the patient's discomfort. The pain is usually most severe during the first 48 hours after surgery. During that time, an intravenous opioid analgesic such as morphine is most appropriate. Patient-controlled analgesia (PCA) may be used to provide prompt relief of pain and to maintain a more stable blood level of the drug. PCA is discussed in Chapter 15. By the third postoperative day, most patients need less medication for pain relief. The dosage or frequency may be reduced, or the order may be changed to an oral analgesic such as acetaminophen with codeine on a PRN basis.

When postoperative patients complain of pain, determine the exact nature of the complaint. Where is the pain located? It is easy to assume that the pain is incisional when in fact the patient may have a headache or a backache. Chest pain, leg pain, or gas pain requires additional assessment and interventions. How severe is the pain? Ask the patient to rate the severity of the pain on a scale of 1 to 10, with 1 being mild pain and 10 being the worst pain imaginable. This provides a system for evaluating response to comfort measures.

During the first few days after surgery, promptly medicate the patient for pain. Pain is controlled better if it is treated before it becomes severe. Some physicians will order routine (rather than PRN) analgesics for the first 24 to 36 hours. This maintains consistent therapeutic blood levels of the analgesic and reduces episodes of acute pain. Pain medication can also be given before activities that normally cause pain. Some patients are afraid that they will become addicted to opioids. Assure them that the short-term use of opioids for acute pain relief generally has not been associated with addiction.

A patient whose pain is controlled adequately is better able to participate in the exercises necessary to prevent postoperative complications. Schedule turning, coughing, deep breathing, and even walking to take advantage of periods when the patient is most comfortable. Of course, a medicated patient must be closely supervised when out of bed.

Although drugs are the mainstay of pain management in the early postoperative phase, other nursing measures can be used to help reduce pain. Position changes and backrubs can be very soothing. Relaxation exercises and mental imagery are often very effective alone or in combination with other nursing measures.

One source of discomfort in the postoperative patient is singultus, commonly known as *hiccups*. Hiccups are caused by intermittent spasms of the diaphragm. They are uncomfortable and may put stress on the incision, disrupt rest, and interfere with the intake of food and fluids. If hiccups persist, notify the physician.

Anxiety seems to intensify discomfort. Measures to decrease anxiety may therefore enhance the effects of pain relief measures. Recognize when the patient is tense and try to discover the source of the anxiety.

Patients need to feel safe and need reassurance about what is happening to them.

Pain management in older adults can pose special challenges. The older patient may be stoic, reluctant to request analgesics, and fearful of addiction and overdose. Nurses, fearing greater risk of adverse effects or believing that the older person experiences less pain, may fail to treat the older person adequately. Good management of postoperative pain in the older person can often be attained with nonsteroidal anti-inflammatory drugs or acetaminophen in combination with opioids at somewhat reduced dosages. The rule of thumb with opioids is to start with a low dose and gradually increase it. Drugs that are more likely to have adverse effects in the older person are meperidine (Demerol) and long-acting benzodiazepines like diazepam (Valium). Well-prepared patients, regardless of age, can participate in pain management by describing and rating their pain, informing the nurse of the effects of treatment, and using patient-controlled analgesia when appropriate.

The management of pain in cognitively impaired older adults is especially difficult. You may have to rely on your observations of patient behavior or family perceptions to recognize pain. Inappropriate behaviors such as pulling at tubes, striking out, and yelling may be manifestations of pain. Some impaired older adults can use pediatric pain rating scales, which provide you with some measure of pain intensity. After procedures that are known to be painful, pain should be assumed and analgesics given in combination with other comfort measures.

Impaired Tissue Integrity

Various techniques are used to close the wound after surgery. The patient's incision may be closed with su-

tures, staples, or tape as shown in Figure 17-10. When the patient returns to the nursing unit, a dressing probably covers the wound. After some procedures such as rectal, vaginal, nasal, or ear surgery, the operative site may be packed with gauze. In some situations, wounds are left open and covered with a dressing.

In healthy people, surgical wounds begin to heal immediately. By the third or fourth day, the healing is stronger. Although the wound appears to be healed after about 10 days, complete healing may take as long as a year.

Clean sutured incisions heal by first *(primary)* intention. Because the wound edges are closed, tissue bonds with little scarring. An infected wound is left open to heal from the bottom up. This is called *healing by secondary intention*. Some sources refer to healing by *tertiary intention*. This term may be used when the wound is initially left open and later closed. Figure 17-11 illustrates these three types of healing.

The physician usually does the first dressing change, inspects the wound, and orders specific wound care. For the first 24 hours, check the dressing hourly for bleeding or drainage. If dressings become saturated, reinforce them using aseptic technique. Depending on physician preference and agency policy, reinforcement may be done several ways. One method is simply to place dry dressings over the wet ones. Another method is to remove bulky outer layers of the wet dressing and replace them with dry dressings. After the first 24 hours, check the dressing once or twice each shift. Bleeding should be minimal and should stop within a few hours after the wound is closed. Report continued or excessive bleeding to the physician.

Some wounds have drains in a "stab" wound close to the incision (Fig. 17-12). Drains remove fluids from

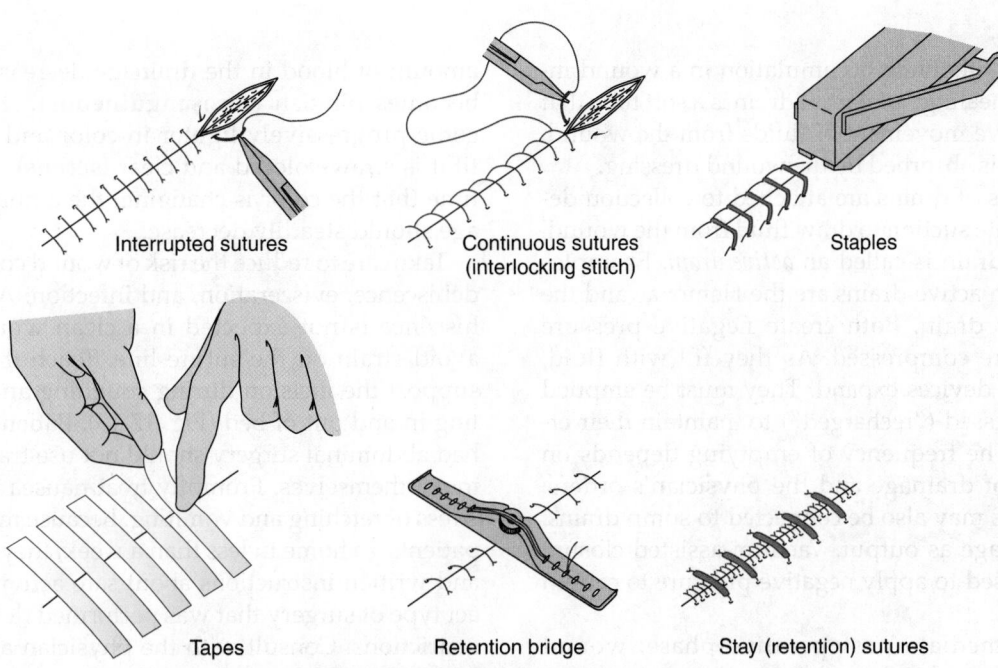

FIGURE **17-10** Methods of wound closure.

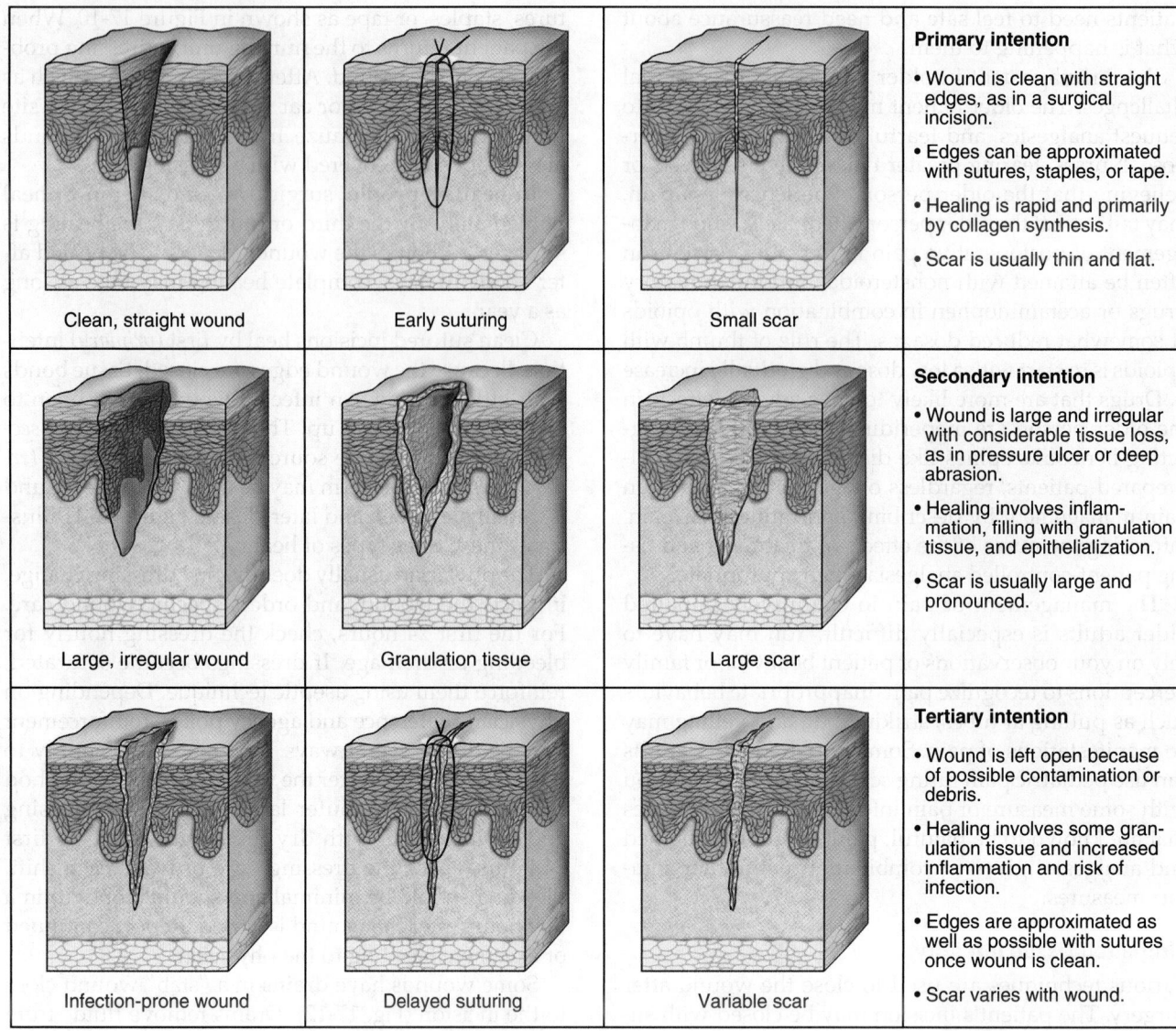

			Primary intention
Clean, straight wound	Early suturing	Small scar	• Wound is clean with straight edges, as in a surgical incision. • Edges can be approximated with sutures, staples, or tape. • Healing is rapid and primarily by collagen synthesis. • Scar is usually thin and flat.
Large, irregular wound	Granulation tissue	Large scar	**Secondary intention** • Wound is large and irregular with considerable tissue loss, as in pressure ulcer or deep abrasion. • Healing involves inflammation, filling with granulation tissue, and epithelialization. • Scar is usually large and pronounced.
Infection-prone wound	Delayed suturing	Variable scar	**Tertiary intention** • Wound is left open because of possible contamination or debris. • Healing involves some granulation tissue and increased inflammation and risk of infection. • Edges are approximated as well as possible with sutures once wound is clean. • Scar varies with wound.

FIGURE **17-11** Wound healing.

the operative site. Fluid accumulation in a wound interferes with healing. A Penrose drain is a soft tube that permits passive movement of fluids from the wound. The drainage is absorbed by the wound dressing.

Other types of drains are attached to collection devices that create suction to draw fluid from the wound. This type of drain is called an *active drain.* Examples of low-suction active drains are the Hemovac and the Jackson-Pratt drain. Both create negative pressure when they are compressed. As they fill with fluid, the collection devices expand. They must be emptied and recompressed ("recharged") to maintain their effectiveness. The frequency of emptying depends on the amount of drainage and the physician's orders. Wound drains may also be connected to sump drains. Record drainage as output. Vacuum-assisted closure devices are used to apply negative pressure to certain open wounds.

In the immediate postoperative phase, wound drainage is often bright red (sanguineous). As the amount of blood in the drainage decreases, the fluid becomes pinkish (serosanguineous). It should become progressively lighter in color and thinner until it is straw-colored and clear (serous). At the same time that the color is changing, the amount of drainage should steadily decrease.

Take care to reduce the risk of wound complications: dehiscence, evisceration, and infection. Although dehiscence is not expected in a clean wound, always avoid strain on the suture line. Teach the patient to support the incision during coughing and when getting in and out of bed (Fig. 17-13). Patients who have had abdominal surgery should not use trapeze bars to move themselves. Promptly treat nausea to avoid the stress of retching and vomiting. Because many surgical patients go home in less than a week, they need verbal and written instructions about safe activities. The exact type of surgery that was performed determines the restrictions. Consult with the physician about correct instructions.

A

B

C

D

FIGURE **17-12** Types of surgical drains used to remove fluid from wounds. Passive or gravity drains include the Penrose drain (**A**) and the T-tube (**B**). Drains that work by creating negative pressure when the receptacle is compressed are the Jackson-Pratt drain (**C**) and the Hemovac (**D**).

FIGURE **17-13** Splinting supports the incision during coughing.

Wounds that are healing normally are unlikely to undergo dehiscence. If infection develops under surgical sutures, the sutures dissolve too soon. Fluid accumulates in the wound, and the wound dehisces. A sudden increase in wound drainage may precede wound dehiscence. When the suture line ruptures, the patient may feel like the wound is "pulling apart."

If dehiscence occurs, keep the patient in bed and in a position to decrease strain on the wound and decrease the risk of evisceration. For example, the patient with an abdominal wound should be in semi-Fowler's position with the knees flexed. If dehiscence or evisceration occurs, the usual practice is to cover the wound with sterile dressings saturated with normal saline and to notify the physician. The saline is thought to prevent damage from drying of the exposed organs. Some are concerned, however, that moisture increases the risk of wound contamination by promoting bacterial movement through the dressings. Covering the saline-soaked gauze with a dry dressing may prevent this complication. After inspecting the wound, the physician may order an abdominal binder. Anticipate a possible return to surgery, and do not administer opioid analgesics until surgical consent is obtained. Infected wounds may be allowed to heal by secondary intention.

Risk for Infection

Continuously assess the patient for indications of infection. Signs and symptoms of wound infection usually do not develop until the third to fifth day after the operation. They may appear as late as a week after surgery. The classic signs and symptoms of wound infection include pain, fever, redness, swelling, and purulent drainage. Surgical pain should decrease as the days go by. Continued or increasing pain suggests the possibility of infection. A low-grade fever is common during the first 2 postoperative days because of the normal inflammation stage of healing. If the temperature is higher than 38° C (100.4° F) or lasts more than 2 days, however, it may be due to infection. Early signs of infection are sometimes hard to detect in older surgical patients because they typically do not develop high fevers even with serious infections. Some redness is expected at the wound suture line and around the sutures or staples. Increasing redness or redness that spreads to surrounding tissue is not normal.

Prevention of wound infection requires decreasing the exposure to microorganisms and maintaining the patient's resistance to infection. Good hand washing, the use of sterile or clean gloves (as appropriate), aseptic dressing changes, and diligent wound care prevent the introduction of infectious organisms. Good hydration and nutrition support the patient's healing and resistance to infection.

If infection is suspected, a culture of any drainage may identify the infectious organism or organisms. The antibiotics that are most likely to be effective can then be prescribed. While awaiting results of the culture and sensitivity tests, the physician often orders a broad-spectrum antibiotic. Collect the culture specimen before antibiotic therapy is begun. Various cleansing procedures may also be ordered. The patient may need to be isolated from other patients to prevent transfer of the organisms. The presence of highly contagious organisms such as methicillin-resistant *Staphylococcus aureus* requires patient isolation.

Because infection may develop after the patient is discharged, patient teaching should include signs and symptoms of infection that should be reported to the physician. The patient also should know whether the wound requires any special treatment. If wound care is needed at home, make sure the patient or a family member is able to do it before the patient leaves the hospital.

Impaired Gas Exchange

Document the patient's respiratory status every hour for the first 24 hours and once or twice a shift after that. Signs and symptoms of pneumonia include dyspnea, fatigue, fever, cough, purulent or bloody sputum, and "wet" breath sounds. When gas exchange is impaired, as with pneumonia or atelectasis, the pulse rate generally increases. Breath sounds are absent in areas of atelectasis.

The most important nursing measures to prevent pneumonia and atelectasis are frequent position changes and coughing and deep-breathing exercises. Initially, assist the patient to turn at least every 2 hours. Patients often are assisted out of bed on the day of sur-

gery. They are usually ambulated several times daily, beginning on the second day. Early ambulation has been found to reduce the respiratory complications of surgery greatly.

Deep breathing inflates the lungs fully, and coughing removes secretions. Help the patient cough and deep breathe every hour. Instruct the patient to take in a deep breath through the nose and gradually blow out through the mouth. After taking several deep breaths, a cough should be attempted to bring up secretions.

The incentive spirometer is a device used to promote lung expansion (Fig. 17-14). It consists of a tube through which air is inhaled and a cylinder containing a ball. The ball rises in the cylinder as the patient inhales through the tube. The more air taken in, the higher the ball moves. Markings on the cylinder indicate the volume of air taken in. This gives the patient a measurable goal to work for while using the spirometer.

Deep breathing and coughing are painful for the patient who has had abdominal or chest surgery. To

FIGURE **17-14** The incentive spirometer is used to promote lung expansion. Shown are **A,** a volume displacement incentive spirometer and **B,** a volume incentive spirometer.

reduce discomfort, coordinate the exercises with analgesics and splint the incision. The patient can splint by holding a pillow firmly over the surgical area while coughing.

It is best to teach turning, deep breathing, coughing, and use of the incentive spirometer before surgery. A patient in pain or drowsy from anesthesia is not in the best condition for learning. There are a few instances in which coughing is contraindicated. They include surgeries for hernias and cataracts, as well as brain surgery.

If the patient develops pneumonia, it is treated with rest, oxygen, and antibiotics. Care of the patient with pneumonia is discussed in Chapter 30.

Another factor that may cause severe, sometimes fatal, respiratory complications is pulmonary embolism. Pulmonary emboli usually arise from thrombi that develop in veins, especially the veins of the legs and pelvis. Measures to prevent thrombophlebitis and related pulmonary emboli include leg exercises, early ambulation, and frequent position changes within the limits of any restrictions imposed by the physician (Fig. 17-15). Antiembolic stockings may be ordered. Signs and symptoms that alert the nurse to possible pulmonary embolism are dyspnea, tachypnea, chest pain, and hemoptysis. If the embolus is very large, the patient may become cyanotic and go into shock. Emboli may be treated with heparin, thrombolytic agents, or both.

Urinary Retention

Carefully monitor urinary output after surgery. In the first 24 hours, urinary output is typically reduced because of the stress response. Be aware, however, of the possibilities of urine retention or kidney failure in the early postoperative phase. Monitor urinary function by measuring intake and output and by checking for bladder distention. If the patient does not void within 6 to 8 hours, catheterization is usually done to empty the bladder.

Pharmacology Capsule

Anesthesia, anticholinergics, and opioid analgesics can contribute to urinary retention.

Patients who have had perineal or abdominal surgery are most likely to have difficulty voiding. They often have indwelling catheters inserted before or during surgery. The patient with a urine retention problem usually reports feelings of fullness and pressure over the lower abdomen. Some patients are unable to void at all. When a patient passes small amounts of urine frequently without feeling relief of the fullness, suspect retention with overflow. The bladder releases just enough urine to reduce the pressure but without complete emptying. Gentle palpation of the lower

FIGURE 17-15 Postoperative leg exercises promote venous return.

abdomen usually reveals the smooth, rounded, full bladder.

If the patient is unable to void, catheterization is necessary. Because catheterization can cause urinary infection, it should be done only if other interventions fail. Interventions must take the physician's activity orders into consideration. The patient should be provided privacy while attempting to void. The toilet is preferred if the patient can go to the bathroom. If a bedpan has to be used, raise the head of the bed, if permitted, to create a normal position for voiding. Men who need to stand to void should be assisted to do so if not contraindicated.

Sensory stimuli help some people overcome difficulty voiding. The sound of running water or the sensation of warm water poured over the perineum or hands may encourage voiding. Use a measured amount of the water so it can be subtracted from the urine output.

If all independent measures fail, a physician's order is required for catheterization. There is usually an "as necessary" order to empty the bladder with a catheter if the patient does not void within 6 to 8 hours after surgery.

Some agencies have policies that limit the amount of urine that can be drained from a full bladder at one time. These limits are usually 750 to 1000 mL. After the removal of the allowed amount of urine, the catheter may be clamped for a specified period of time before the bladder is drained again. This procedure is referred to as *bladder decompression.* Research in this area has raised some question as to whether draining the bladder completely is, in fact, dangerous.

If the patient has to be catheterized several times, the physician may order the insertion of an indwelling catheter. Catheterization and the care of the patient with a catheter are discussed in Chapter 40.

If there are no signs of bladder distention but little or no urine output, the patient may be in kidney failure. The minimum urine output is considered to be 30 mL/hr. Failure to produce at least 30 mL/hr should be reported promptly to the physician. The diagnosis and treatment of kidney failure are discussed in Chapter 40.

Constipation

Gastrointestinal function is disrupted by surgery. Postoperatively, inspect and palpate for abdominal distention and auscultate for bowel sounds. Document the passage of flatus and the first bowel movement. The patient may not realize the significance of passing flatus and may wonder why it should be reported. Explain that passing flatus means the digestive tract is beginning to function again. Most patients pass flatus about 48 hours postoperatively.

Early, frequent ambulation is the best way to prevent gastrointestinal discomfort. The intake of oral fluids and ingestion of a normal diet also help stimulate peristalsis. Oral intake is usually withheld, however, until bowel sounds return (normally 24-48 hours after surgery).

Measures to promote the passage of flatus may be ordered, including early ambulation, insertion of a rectal tube for 20 minutes every 2 to 3 hours, application of heat to the abdomen, positioning the patient prone or on the right side, and insertion of bisacodyl suppositories.

If gastrointestinal function does not resume, the patient has a paralytic ileus, manifested by abdominal pain, distention, tenderness, and absence of bowel sounds. Other signs and symptoms of paralytic ileus are nausea, vomiting, and not passing flatus or feces.

Severe abdominal distention develops if normal bowel activity does not resume within a few days. In that case, a nasogastric tube may be ordered to permit decompression of the intestines. If the surgical procedure is one that often causes gastrointestinal problems, the nasogastric tube may be inserted during surgery to prevent problems.

The patient should have a bowel movement within a few days after resuming the intake of solid foods. Sometimes a suppository or an enema is necessary to stimulate emptying of the bowel.

Deficient Fluid Volume and Imbalanced Nutrition: Less Than Body Requirements

Depending on the type of surgery done, fluid and nutrition needs are met in a variety of ways. Some patients are given regular diets the evening of surgery. Others receive nothing by mouth for several days. Most patients return from the PACU with intravenous infusions. Patients are traditionally given clear liquids at first and then full liquids. If liquids are retained, the diet is advanced to include soft foods and then regular foods. Physiologically, there is no reason to delay the introduction of solids once gastrointestinal function has returned and a few oral liquids are retained, but this practice persists in many settings.

When the patient is able to tolerate liquids well, the intravenous infusion usually is discontinued unless it is needed for the administration of medication. Monitor the flow rate and the patient response. Nursing care of the patient receiving intravenous fluids is discussed in Chapter 18.

To promote healing, the patient's diet must provide adequate carbohydrates, protein, zinc, iron, folate, and vitamins C, B_6, and B_{12}. Alternative methods of feeding may be ordered if the patient is unable to resume oral intake for a long time. These methods are discussed in Chapter 38.

Fluid intake and output are usually measured for several days after surgery. In addition, laboratory studies of serum electrolytes often are ordered.

Nausea and vomiting interfere with the intake of food and fluids and can cause considerable fluid loss. Antiemetics (drugs used to control nausea and vomiting) usually are ordered as necessary. General nursing measures for the patient with nausea and vomiting are discussed in Chapter 38.

Pharmacology Capsule

Antiemetic drugs control postoperative nausea and vomiting.

Impaired Physical Mobility

After general anesthesia and invasive surgical procedures, patients are usually weak and tire quickly. The physician prescribes measures to increase the patient's activity level—progressive ambulation in most cases.

Assist the patient out of bed the first few times until it is evident the patient can safely get up alone. Help the patient sit on the bedside, press the feet on the floor, stand, and then walk increasingly greater distances. Monitor for weakness and dizziness associated with orthostatic hypotension. Emphasize the physical benefits of early ambulation to the patient.

Disturbed Body Image

The effects of surgery (scars, loss of body organs, altered physical functions) can be very traumatic. A sense of loss can be demonstrated by anger, depression, or even denial. The nurse should understand and accept these responses. Nursing care of the grieving patient is discussed in detail in Chapter 24. Surgery can also produce positive changes in body image when it improves appearance or function or relieves symptoms.

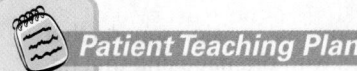

Postoperative Patient

Patient teaching in the postoperative phase emphasizes recovery from the surgical experience and preparation for return to maximum possible function. Discharge planning should be started when the patient is admitted for surgery and revised as needed during the course of hospitalization. Topics to include in the discharge teaching plan are the following:

- Take your prescribed drugs as directed, but notify the physician if you have adverse effects (specify drug, dosage, schedule, and side and adverse effects).
- Wound care: You will need to continue your wound care as I have demonstrated. Notify your physician if you have symptoms of infection (fever, increasing redness, swelling, pain at the incision site).
- When regular activities can be resumed, do not lift anything heavier than specified by your physician.
- If you need assistance, available community services include—(specify services for patient needs).
- If the physician advises specific fluids and nutritional requirements, you need to follow this special diet or take prescribed amounts of fluids.
- You will need some specialized equipment and supplies. (Tell the patient how to obtain and use assistive devices, special equipment, and supplies.)
- Can you identify any adaptations that will be needed in your home environment before you are discharged?
- It is important to keep medical appointments to be sure you are healing properly.

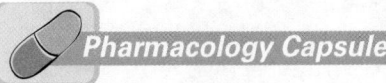

Discharge teaching includes information about drug therapy.

Put on Your Thinking Cap!

Observe the room of a recent postoperative patient and identify four ways the environment can be modified to promote safety.

Key Points

- Surgical procedures classified by purpose are diagnostic, exploratory, curative, palliative, and cosmetic.
- Variables that affect surgical outcomes are age, nutritional status, fluid and electrolyte balance, medical diagnoses, drugs, and habits such as use of tobacco and alcohol.
- The phases of the surgical experience are preoperative, intraoperative, and postoperative.
- Nursing measures to reduce patient anxiety and increase knowledge about the surgical experience may actually decrease complications.
- Preoperative teaching should include surgical preparation; what to expect in the surgical suite and postanesthesia care unit (PACU); what tubes, dressings, or equipment may be in place after surgery; and how patient participation can promote recovery.
- Before surgery, the patient or legal guardian must sign a legal consent form. Consent from the patient must be obtained *before* preoperative medications are given.
- Preparation for surgery may involve bowel cleansing, food and fluid restriction, skin scrubbing and hair removal, securing and covering hair, and administering preoperative medications as ordered. Clothing, jewelry, nail polish, and prostheses are usually removed.
- After preoperative medications are given, the patient should remain in bed.
- The surgical team consists of nurses who circulate, nurses who scrub, a registered nurse first assistant, one or more surgeons, an anesthesiologist or a nurse anesthetist, and other technical personnel.
- Several types of drugs are used for general anesthesia; combined drug effects induce unconsciousness, alter sensation, and prevent movement so that surgical procedures can be done painlessly and safely.
- The nursing diagnoses in the intraoperative phase may include Risk for Injury, Impaired Gas Exchange, Decreased Cardiac Output, and Risk for Deficient Fluid Volume.
- Postoperative surgical complications may include shock, hypoxia, wound infection, wound dehiscence and evisceration, injury, pneumonia, atelectasis, nausea and vomiting, impaired peristalsis, urinary retention, renal failure, and thrombophlebitis.
- Nursing diagnoses in the immediate postoperative period are Decreased Cardiac Output, Ineffective Breathing Pattern, Acute Pain, Disturbed Thought Processes, and Risk for Injury.
- Inform visitors where to wait and how they will be informed of the patient's status.

- Nursing diagnoses after recovery from anesthesia may include Acute Pain, Impaired Tissue Integrity, Risk for Infection, Impaired Gas Exchange, Urinary Retention, Constipation, Risk for Deficient Fluid Volume, Imbalanced Nutrition: Less Than Body Requirements, Impaired Physical Mobility, and Disturbed Body Image.
- Patient teaching for discharge emphasizes drug therapy, wound care, activity limitations, fluid and nutrition needs, equipment and supplies needed, adaptation of the home environment, and the importance of follow-up care.

 Go to your Companion CD-ROM for a Pharmacology Tutorial, Audio Glossary, and 3-D animations.

evolve   Be sure to visit the companion Evolve site at http://evolve.elsevier.com/Linton/ for WebLinks and additional online resources.

REVIEW QUESTIONS *Choose the best answer.*

1. An older adult relative who is scheduled for a surgical procedure expresses fear that he is too old for surgery and asks what you think. Your response should be based on knowledge that:
   1. Older adults are twice as likely to have surgical complications as younger people
   2. An older adult in good health is likely to do just as well in surgery as a younger person
   3. For most older adults, the risks of surgery are too great to justify any possible benefits
   4. Older adults who have chronic health problems are poor candidates for surgery

2. If you obtain a patient's signature on a surgical consent form, your responsibility includes:
   1. Explaining the surgical procedure to the patient
   2. Obtaining the signature before the patient is given sedatives
   3. Informing the patient of possible risks associated with the procedure
   4. Assessing which alternative options the patient has explored

3. Why is it especially important to assess the affected extremities of a patient who is recovering from regional anesthesia?
   1. Regional anesthesia can impair blood flow to the extremities, causing gangrene.
   2. The patient cannot move the extremities despite feelings of pain or pressure.
   3. The extremities are susceptible to injury because movement returns before sensation.
   4. The effects of regional anesthesia may persist for several weeks.

4. One complication that is most likely to occur during the immediate postoperative period is:
   1. Wound infection
   2. Pneumonia
   3. Shock
   4. Thrombophlebitis

5. In a PACU, a patient's vital signs are as follows: Temperature 98° F, pulse 66 and regular, respirations 14, BP 100/56. What other information do you need to evaluate these vital signs?
   1. Medications given during surgery
   2. Length of time under general anesthesia
   3. Whether the patient is having pain
   4. Patient's preoperative vital signs

6. A patient with an abdominal incision reports that his dressing is soaked with drainage and that he felt a pulling sensation when getting out of bed. On inspection, you find that the wound margins have separated. You should:
   1. Lower the head of the bed and have the patient lie flat
   2. Gently reapply the surgical dressing and call the physician
   3. Administer a dose of prescribed opioid analgesic for pain
   4. Apply saline-soaked gauze and cover with a sterile, dry dressing

7. After surgery, a patient voids 20 to 30 mL of urine at frequent intervals. You should suspect:
   1. Urinary retention with overflow
   2. Damage to the bladder during surgery
   3. Fluid volume excess
   4. Kidney failure

8. During report, you learn that your postoperative patient has a paralytic ileus. You would expect:
   1. The patient will not be able to walk
   2. A nasogastric tube and suction may be in place
   3. To monitor breath sounds every 2 hours
   4. The patient will be limited to a liquid diet

Objectives

After reading and studying this chapter, you should be able to:

1. List the indications for intravenous fluid therapy.
2. Describe the types of fluids used for intravenous fluid therapy.
3. Describe the types of venous access devices and other equipment used for intravenous therapy.
4. Given the prescribed hourly flow rate, calculate the correct drop rate for an intravenous fluid.
5. Explain the causes, signs and symptoms, and nursing implications of the complications of intravenous fluid or drug therapy.
6. Explain the nursing responsibilities when a patient is receiving intravenous therapy.

Key Terms

Be sure to check out the bonus material on the Companion CD-ROM, including selected audio pronunciations.

cannula (KĂN-ū-lă, p. 278)
embolism (EM-bō-liz-um, p. 288)
embolus (*pl.* Emboli) (EM-bō-lus, EM-bō-lī, p. 287)
extravasation (eks-trăv-ă-SĀ-shun, p. 285)
hypertonic (hī-per-TON-ik, p. 277)
hypotonic (hī-pō-TON-ik, p. 277)
infiltration (in-fil-TRĀ-shun, p. 285)
isotonic (ī-sō-TON-ik, p. 277)
phlebitis (fle-BĪ-tis, p. 287)
solution (p. 277)
thrombus (*pl.* Thrombi) (THROM-bus, THROM-bī, p. 288)
tonicity (tō-NIS-i-tē, p. 277)

Intravenous therapy is the administration of fluids directly into a vein. Most hospitalized patients receive some form of intravenous therapy. Home infusion of intravenous products has become common as well.

INDICATIONS FOR INTRAVENOUS THERAPY

Intravenous therapy is used to administer drugs, fluids (including nutrients), and blood or blood components. Intravenous administration of drugs may be ordered when a rapid drug effect is needed, when the drug is not available in an oral form, or when the patient is unable to take drugs by mouth. The intravenous route is also recommended when a drug must be maintained at a certain level in the blood.

In addition to drugs, intravenous fluids can provide water, electrolytes, amino acids, lipids, vitamins, and glucose. Intravenous lines may also be used to provide continuous venous access for intermittent drug administration and emergency drug administration.

Whole blood and blood components are also given intravenously. Blood components include packed red blood cells, frozen red blood cells, platelets, and plasma proteins. Blood transfusions are discussed in Chapter 32.

TYPES OF INTRAVENOUS FLUIDS

By definition, a fluid is any liquid or gas. A **solution** is a liquid containing one or more dissolved substances. The terms *fluid* and *solution* are often used interchangeably in relation to intravenous therapy. Fluids that contain water and electrolytes are referred to as *crystalloids*; fluids containing blood and blood components are called *colloids*.

TONICITY

Fluids can be classified by tonicity, a measure of the concentration of electrolytes in the fluid. The normal concentration of electrolytes in body fluids is about 285 milliequivalents per liter (mEq/L). Solutions that have the same concentration as body fluids are called isotonic. When the concentration of a solution is greater than 300 mEq/L, the solution is said to be hypertonic. Hypotonic solutions have a concentration of less than 280 mEq/L. The tonicity of fluids is important because it affects blood volume. Fluid that is hypertonic draws and retains water in the circulation, increasing the blood volume. Hypotonic fluid allows water to shift out of the capillaries into body tissues, resulting in decreased blood volume.

COMPONENTS

Many types of fluids are available for intravenous use. The physician selects the appropriate fluid to meet the patient's needs. The most commonly used intravenous solutions are specific combinations of water, sugar (in the form of dextrose), sodium chloride, and other electrolytes.

In most intravenous solutions, dextrose is the only source of calories. The patient receives 34 calories for each 1% of dextrose in a liter of fluid; thus 1 liter of 5% dextrose provides 170 calories ($34 \times 5 = 170$). Dextrose fluids given in a peripheral vein are 2.5%, 5.0%, or 10.0% dextrose. Fluids infused into a larger (central) vein may have a much higher percentage of dextrose.

Sodium chloride solutions also are commonly used. An isotonic solution is 0.9% sodium chloride and is called *normal saline*. It is used to supply balanced amounts of water and sodium chloride. A hypotonic solution of 0.45% sodium chloride may be ordered if the patient's body fluids are concentrated owing to excessive water loss. More concentrated hypertonic solutions are needed when the patient has had excessive losses of both sodium and chloride.

Dextrose, sodium chloride, and other electrolytes are available in numerous combinations. Some commonly used electrolyte solutions are Plasma-Lyte and lactated Ringer's solution. Dextrose 5% in Ringer's is a combined dextrose and electrolyte solution.

When a patient needs long-term or aggressive intravenous therapy for nutrition, total parenteral nutrition may be indicated. A catheter is placed in a large vein, usually the subclavian, for administering total parenteral nutrition fluids. These fluids provide dextrose, water, amino acids, electrolytes, vitamins, and minerals. Fat emulsions can also be given intravenously. Total parenteral nutrition is discussed in greater detail in Chapter 9.

VENOUS ACCESS DEVICES

Intravenous fluid is delivered by various types of venous access devices (Fig. 18-1). These include needles, over-the-needle catheters, inside-needle catheters (rarely used), subcutaneous infusion ports, and subcutaneously implanted pumps. The term cannula can be used to describe both a needle and a catheter. Cannula size is based on the inside diameter and is expressed as a *gauge*. The smaller the gauge, the larger is the inside diameter of the cannula. Therefore a 14-gauge cannula is larger than a 22-gauge cannula.

The intravenous administration of fluids requires placement of the venous access device into a peripheral or central vein. Peripheral veins are those located in the extremities (and in the scalp of an infant). They are used for short-term therapy, when a patient has healthy veins, and when relatively nonirritating fluids are given.

Central veins, large vessels located nearer the heart, are used when long-term therapy is required, when the patient has poor peripheral veins, and when irritating fluids are to be administered. Central lines are inserted into the subclavian or jugular vein or into the superior vena cava. The line may be placed in the subclavian vein through a surgical incision, inserted into a peripheral vein and advanced to the desired location, or inserted through a skin incision and tunneled under the skin and into the large vessel. Devices placed through a cutdown incision are referred to as *percutaneous catheters*. The central line threaded through a peripheral vein is called a *peripherally inserted central catheter* (*PICC*). Examples of central venous tunneled catheters are the Hickman, Broviac, Groshong, Hickman-Broviac, Raaf, and the implanted venous access ports. Figure 18-2 shows common peripheral infusion sites for intravenous fluids.

A port is a device with a central catheter that is surgically implanted in the subcutaneous tissue. It consists of a venous catheter and a port through which fluids can be injected, but it has no external parts (Fig. 18-3, *A*). The catheter is inserted into a central vein, and the port, which has a rubber septum, can be felt under the skin. A specialized needle that does not damage the septum is used to puncture the skin and deliver fluid and medications through the port and into the catheter (Fig. 18-3, *B*). A port requires less care and is less restrictive than other access devices, but it does require a needle puncture for each infusion.

For therapy over a period of days to weeks, the percutaneous catheter or midline catheter is preferred. Tunneled catheters and implanted ports are more appropriate for long-term use.

NEEDLES

One type of needle used is a winged ("butterfly") infusion needle, a short needle with two plastic wings that are held during insertion. A winged infusion needle is useful in infants when a scalp vein is used for intravenous therapy. It is also used at times in adults who have very poor or small veins, for one-time therapy, to

A

B

| Hydraulic filter | Flash back chamber | Catheter hub | Catheter | Introducer needle |

FIGURE **18-1** Venous access devices. **A,** Winged infusion needles. **B,** Catheter.

draw blood samples, and for therapy of short duration (less than 24 hours).

To reduce the risk of bloodborne injuries acquired through needlesticks, various devices have been developed. One style has a self-sheathing stylet that retracts into a rigid chamber at the catheter hub after insertion. Others use Luer-Lok connections rather than diaphragms that must be punctured with a needle (Fig. 18-4). Concern about bloodborne pathogens has led to the development of various devices to reduce the risk of needlesticks. Among the products that make venipunctures safer for the nurse are systems that cover the needle after it has been used.

CATHETERS

A catheter is a small plastic tube that fits over or inside a needle. After insertion into the vein, the needle is withdrawn, leaving the catheter in the vein. The tubing that will deliver the fluid is then connected to the plastic catheter, which remains in the vein. Catheters are less likely than needles to puncture the vein once they are in place. They come in a variety of lengths. Short catheters are only ¾ to 2 inches in length. Midlength catheters are designed for therapy of 2 to 4 weeks. Midlength catheters are inserted near the antecubital region of the arm and advanced 3 to 10 inches. Nurses generally insert only short (¾- to 2-inch) catheters unless they receive special training.

A central catheter that can be inserted by trained nurses is the PICC (Fig. 18-5). The PICC is inserted into a vein in the antecubital space and advanced into the axillary, subclavian, or brachiocephalic vein or the superior vena cava. Advantages of the PICC over other central catheters include easier insertion, cost savings, and less risk of pneumothorax, hemothorax, infection, or air embolism. Compared with peripheral cannulas, PICCs can be left in place longer, do not restrict arm movement, and are less traumatic to the vein.

Tunneled catheters are inserted only by the physician. An incision is made at the entrance site, a tunnel created in the subcutaneous tissues, and the catheter threaded through the tunnel and into the subclavian vein. Scar formation of a small section of the tunneled catheter holds it in place after a week or two. However, some surgeons leave sutures in place as long as they do not create inflammation. Some special catheters may

FIGURE **18-2** Common peripheral intravenous infusion sites.

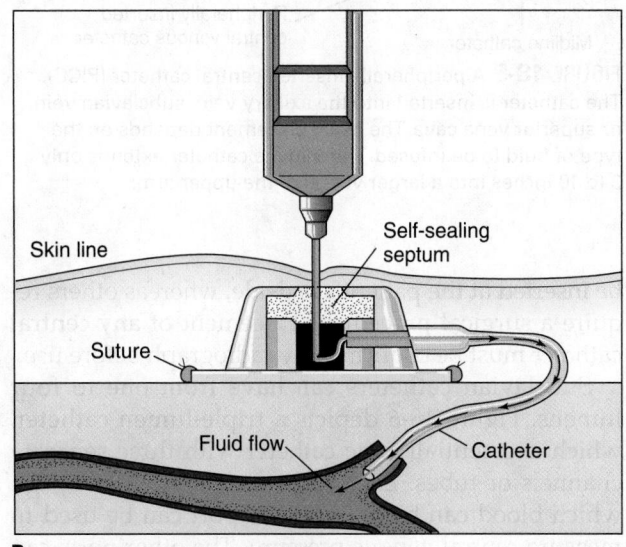

FIGURE **18-3** **A,** An implantable port in place. The entire unit is under the skin. **B,** Injection of medication into the port.

FIGURE **18-4** Needleless system.

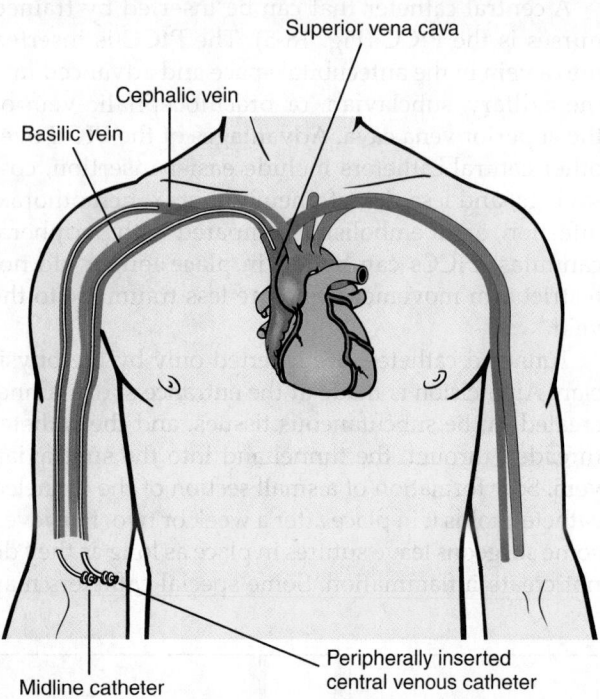

FIGURE **18-5** A peripherally inserted central catheter (PICC). The catheter is inserted into the axillary vein, subclavian vein, or superior vena cava. The exact placement depends on the type of fluid to be infused. The midline catheter extends only 3 to 10 inches into a larger vessel of the upper arm.

Labels on figure 18-5: Superior vena cava, Cephalic vein, Basilic vein, Midline catheter, Peripherally inserted central venous catheter

FIGURE **18-6** A triple-lumen catheter.

be inserted at the patient's bedside, whereas others require a surgical procedure. Placement of any central catheter must be confirmed by radiograph before use.

Subclavian catheters can have from one to four lumens. Figure 18-6 depicts a triple-lumen catheter, which is essentially one catheter with three separate channels or tubes. Each catheter has a port through which blood can be drawn. One port can be used to measure central venous pressure. The other ports can be used to give drugs, fluids, or blood.

IMPLANTED DEVICES

Some devices can be implanted to allow immediate access to a vein without repeated, painful venipunctures. They include infusion ports, described earlier, pumps that are implanted under the skin, and external infusion pumps. Infusion ports consist of a catheter and a chamber into which fluids can be injected directly into a vein or an artery. They are also used for intraspinal infusions. The chamber is easily felt directly under the skin. Infusion pumps are filled using a special needle that is inserted through the skin into the port. They dispense the fluid into the vein at a very slow rate. The rate of infusion is sometimes affected by body temperature, with fever increasing the delivery rate. The infusion rate of some infusion pumps can be set electronically by passing a wand over the pump. Infusion pumps are often used to administer chemotherapy drugs for cancer.

INTERMITTENT INFUSION DEVICES

Many patients need intravenous medications at specific intervals, such as every 4 or every 6 hours. Such drugs are often "piggybacked"; that is, the drug is given through an injection port in the tubing of a continuous infusion. An option for the patient who does not need continuous intravenous therapy is a latex resealable lock, sometimes called a *heparin lock.*

Pharmacology Capsule

A drug given "piggyback" is administered through the tubing of a continuous infusion using the injection port that is closest to the fluid bag. The injection port closer to the patient is used for IV push medications. If the patient does not need continuous fluids, a resealable latex lock can be used to give the medication.

A resealable lock is a short cannula with an attached injection port. It is taped in place, and medications are injected when needed through the port. It may be called a heparin lock because it may be flushed with a dilute heparin solution after each use to keep clots from forming and blocking the catheter. Although research suggests that flushing with normal saline may be just as effective as, and less expensive than, using heparin, the use of heparin persists in some settings. One concern about the use of heparin is that it prolongs the time required for blood to clot, whereas saline does not. You must know the agency's procedure for flushing these devices and exactly what the licensed practical nurse is permitted to do. Any intravenous cannula (needle or catheter) can be converted to intermittent administration by attaching a resealable cap or an extension with a cap.

INITIATION OF INTRAVENOUS THERAPY

Nurse practice acts and agency policies determine which nurses can perform venipunctures, administer intravenous fluids, and give intravenous medications by various routes.

EQUIPMENT

To start intravenous fluids, gather the equipment needed to start the infusion: cannula (needle or catheter), tourniquet, alcohol swabs, skin cleansing solution, tape, dressing supplies, gloves, tubing, solution container, a pole to suspend the container, and possibly an infusion pump. The size of the cannula depends on the patient's condition and the type of fluid to be administered. For patients with multiple trauma or those facing transplantation or heart surgery, a 14- or 16-gauge cannula is appropriate. Other surgical patients and those receiving blood require an 18- or 20-gauge cannula. A 22-gauge is appropriate for most adults receiving crystalloid fluids in ordinary circumstances. Smaller-gauge

cannulas can be used in children, in adults with small veins, and for administration of most other nonirritating fluids. Read the product literature to identify any special requirements such as a filter or special tubing. Obtain the prescribed solution or drug using the "five rights": right solution or drug, right dose or strength, right patient, right route, and right time. Attach tubing to the solution container, fill the drip chamber halfway, and allow some fluid to run through the tubing until the tubing is completely filled with fluid and there are no air bubbles in the tubing.

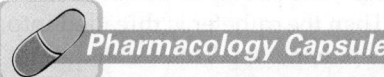
Pharmacology Capsule

The intravenous administration of nitroglycerin, blood, or fat emulsions requires special administration sets.

SITE SELECTION

Select the venipuncture site for the infusion. The site chosen should be the least restrictive (i.e., not over a joint or on the hand). It should have a large vein that is in good condition. A soft, straight vein is best. Avoid veins that are hard and bumpy, bruised, swollen, near previously infected areas, or close to a recently discontinued site. A transilluminator or portable ultrasound can facilitate locating a vein. The preferred site is usually the patient's nondominant arm. Begin with the most distal veins, and then move proximally as needed. Venipuncture should not be done in an arm that has impaired circulation or poor lymphatic drainage, as in a patient who has had a radical mastectomy. Also, do not use an arm that has been affected by a stroke. Although veins on the legs are accessible, they are not normally used in adults.

Put on Your Thinking Cap!

Why should you use the most distal site to start an intravenous infusion?

PROCEDURE

Wash your hands thoroughly, and explain the procedure to the patient. Apply a tourniquet above the venipuncture site to distend the vein. The tourniquet should be flat, should be at least ½ inch wide, should not obstruct arterial blood flow, and should be used on only one patient. A blood pressure cuff inflated just above the patient's diastolic pressure makes an excellent tourniquet and is less traumatic for fragile skin. After locating an appropriate vein, temporarily remove the tourniquet. Vigorously cleanse the venipuncture site in a circular pattern, first with alcohol and then with a recommended solution. Recommended cleansing solutions include 1%

to 2% tincture of iodine, iodophor (povidone-iodine), 70% isopropyl alcohol, and chlorhexidine. If the patient is allergic to iodine, cleanse with alcohol only. Allow the site to air dry after each cleansing step. Do not blow on the site or fan it. Reapply the tourniquet.

Perform the venipuncture using Standard Precautions. Carefully insert the cannula through the skin and guide it into the vein in the direction of blood flow. If the first attempt is unsuccessful, select another site, change cannulas, and try again. After two unsuccessful attempts, call a more experienced nurse to start the infusion. When using the most common cannula, the catheter over needle, the needle is threaded only ¼ inch into the vein. Then the catheter is threaded into the vein as the needle is removed. This technique reduces the risk of trauma to the vein. After threading the cannula into the vein, connect it to the infusion tubing and tape it securely but without restricting circulation. Be careful not to contaminate the open hub of the cannula. Do not apply tape to the site where the cannula enters the skin.

In accordance with your agency procedures, dress the site with a clear occlusive dressing that allows inspection of the insertion site or with a sterile gauze pad. On peripheral sites, gauze dressings are changed every 48 hours and occlusive dressings every 3 to 7 days. Dressings on central lines are changed every 48 hours. Some agencies may use antimicrobial barrier patches that fit around the cannula and under the dressing. The application of antibiotic ointment to the insertion site is controversial. Antibiotic ointments without antifungals have been associated with *Candida* infections.

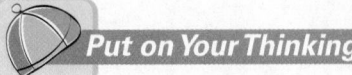

Put on Your Thinking Cap!

What's wrong with this picture? A nurse preparing to start an IV tears strips of tape and sticks them on the edge of the overbed table. The nurse cleanses the site with alcohol and iodophor and blows on the site to hasten drying.

Pain

Venipuncture and cannula placement are painful. Clinicians are seeking measures to reduce the discomfort without making the procedure more difficult. Drugs that have been used to decrease the pain of venipuncture include intradermal lidocaine (Xylocaine), transdermal lidocaine, and prilocaine (EMLA cream). There are some disadvantages to each of these. Intradermal lidocaine may cause vasospasm, allergic reactions, and anaphylaxis. Both lidocaine and EMLA cream must be applied and covered with an occlusive dressing for 60 minutes to be effective. Another option is ionto-

phoresis of lidocaine, a noninvasive system that uses an electrical current to deliver lidocaine to the skin and takes effect in about 10 minutes. Again, there is a risk of reaction to the lidocaine. Intradermal injection of normal saline alongside the vein also produces anesthesia. The Intravenous Nurses Society does not recommend lidocaine or normal saline for this purpose.

DOCUMENTATION

Place a piece of tape on the site dressing with the date and time that the cannula was inserted as well as the length and gauge of the cannula and your initials. Label every bag of fluid and tubing with the date and time that it was hung and the fluid's expiration date.

MAINTENANCE OF INTRAVENOUS THERAPY

The physician orders the type of fluid and the rate at which it is to be given. The nurse is responsible for maintaining the correct rate of flow and for monitoring the patient's response to the infusion. The Management and Supervision box below discusses the LPN/LVN's role in initiating intravenous therapy.

Intravenous fluids can be allowed to flow by gravity or can be regulated by an electronic infusion control device. When gravity flow is used, the rate must be adjusted with the roller clamp or screw clamp on the tubing. The clamp should be positioned on the upper third of the tubing. The slide clamp should *not* be used to set the rate; it is not reliable!

Check the infusion rate hourly even if an infusion control device is used. If the fluid is running too slowly, adjust the flow rate. Do not attempt to "catch up" by administering extra fluid rapidly. If the fluid is running too quickly, slow the rate and assess the patient for signs of fluid volume excess.

If the patient is ambulatory, attach the fluid container to a pole with wheels. Tell the patient to protect the infusion by keeping the solution container above the infusion site and by avoiding pulling on the tubing or applying pressure to the infusion site.

Management and Supervision

Initiation of Intravenous Therapy

Depending on state practice acts, LPNs/LVNs with appropriate training may be able to initiate and monitor intravenous therapy. These responsibilities cannot be delegated to unlicensed assistive personnel (UAP). However, UAPs should be told how to protect the infusion while assisting the patient with basic care.

FACTORS AFFECTING INFUSION RATE

Even after the infusion rate is set, many factors can alter that rate. The main determinants of the infusion rate are the following:

- The height of the fluid container over the patient's heart. When the container is raised, the fluid flows faster. Lowering the container causes the fluid to run more slowly. The optimal height is 30 to 36 inches above the patient.
- The volume of fluid in the container. A full container causes the fluid to run faster. As the container empties, the rate slows down.
- Viscosity of the fluid. Thin fluids such as normal saline flow more quickly than thick fluids such as blood.
- Cannula diameter. Fluid flows more quickly through a large cannula than through a small cannula.
- Venting of the fluid container. Soft plastic bags collapse as they empty, but glass containers and rigid plastic containers cannot do that. Therefore rigid containers must be vented to allow air to enter as fluid leaves. Without proper venting, the fluid does not flow.
- Position of the extremity. With peripheral lines, certain movements or positions may interfere with the flow of fluid. If that happens, the extremity may need to be splinted with an arm board to limit movement, or the patient may be advised to avoid certain movements or positions.

CALCULATING THE INFUSION RATE

You should know how to calculate infusion rates even if infusion control devices are used routinely. To calculate the infusion rate, first determine (1) how much fluid to give each hour and (2) how many drops equal 1 mL in the delivery set used (called the *drop factor*).

The physician's order specifies the amount of fluid to be administered in a specific period of time. The instructions on the delivery set package state how many drops equal 1 mL using that set. Standard delivery sets (sometimes called *macrodrip sets*) deliver 10, 12, 15, or 20 drops per milliliter. Microdrip sets deliver 50 or 60 drops per milliliter. They are used in children and when small volumes of fluid are being given.

Once the infusion rate per minute is known, use the roller clamp or screw clamp on a gravity infusion to adjust the flow rate until the correct number of drops per minute is infusing. Recheck the rate hourly. Com-

mon practice is to put a timed tape on the fluid container that shows where the fluid level should be each hour. This allows a quick assessment of whether the fluid is running on schedule.

INFUSION CONTROL DEVICES

Electronic infusion control devices maintain an infusion rate set by the nurse. The most commonly used types also have alarms that sound when the fluid bag is empty, when there is air in the line, or when there is resistance to infusion. A variety of infusion control devices are available (Fig. 18-7). Ambulatory pumps are available that allow the patient to resume normal activities. You must become familiar with the type used in your work setting. Infusion control devices save time and should prevent accidental delivery of large amounts of fluid. They do not excuse you, however, from monitoring the flow rate at intervals and assessing the catheter or needle insertion site. Box 18-1 gives step-by-step instructions for calculating the flow rate.

INTRAVENOUS INFUSION OF MEDICATIONS

Agency policies usually dictate what medications the nurse may give by piggyback or by direct injection through a cannula into the vein (intravenous push). Many states do not permit licensed practical nurses to give medications by intravenous push. When giving such medications, you must know how to dilute the medication and the correct rate of infusion. Improper administration of intravenous medications can be extremely dangerous. For example, potassium is NEVER

FIGURE 18-7 An electronic infusion pump.

Put on Your Thinking Cap!

A patient is to receive an antibiotic intravenously in 100 mL of IV fluid. Directions are to administer the drug over 30 to 60 minutes. Drop factor: 10 drops/mL. Calculate the minimum and maximum allowable flow rates.

given by direct injection because of the risk of potentially fatal cardiac dysrhythmias. You also must be aware that some medications and intravenous solutions are incompatible; that is, they cannot be given together.

CHANGING VENOUS ACCESS DEVICES AND ADMINISTRATION SETS

Short peripheral cannulas and the tubing are usually changed every 48 to 72 hours in accordance with standards of the Intravenous Nurses Society. If complications occur with 72-hour intervals, the interval should be limited to 48 hours.

Administration sets for continuous peripheral and central infusions are usually changed every 72 hours. PICC lines should be changed every 6 weeks. Tunneled catheters and ports can be left in place for years. Tubing that is used to administer blood, total parenteral nutrition, or lipids must be changed every 24 hours. An intravenous fluid container should not be used for more than 24 hours. Agency policies are generally quite specific about the schedule.

TERMINATION OF INTRAVENOUS THERAPY

To discontinue intravenous therapy with needles or short catheters, put on gloves, stop the flow of fluid, loosen or remove the tape and dressing, gently press a dry gauze pad over the site, and remove the cannula

---

Box 18-1 | *Sample Flow-Rate Calculation*

Physician's Order

1000 mL 5% dextrose in 0.45% normal saline every 8 hours. Delivery set: 20 drops = 1 mL.

Step 1 Calculate how many milliliters should be given in 1 hour. Divide the total number of milliliters to be given by the prescribed number of hours.

$$1000 \text{ mL} \div 8 \text{ hr} = 125 \text{ mL/hr}$$

Step 2 Calculate how many drops should be given in 1 hour. Multiply the number of milliliters to be given each hour times the number of drops in 1 mL using the specific delivery set.

$$125 \text{ mL} \times 20 = 2500 \text{ drops/hr}$$

Step 3 Calculate how many drops should be given in 1 minute. Divide the number of drops per hour by 60 to find out how many drops should be given in 1 minute.

$$2500 \text{ drops} \div 60 \text{ min} = 41.6, \text{ or } 42 \text{ drops/min}$$

Some people prefer to use a formula to calculate the drop rate. The formula is:

(Fluid volume to be infused) × (Number of drops per mL with selected infusion set) ÷ Time (min) = drops per minute.

---

keeping the hub parallel to the skin. Dispose of the needle or catheter according to Standard Precautions guidelines. Elevate the extremity and apply pressure to the puncture site with a sterile gauze pad for 2 or 3 minutes to prevent bleeding; then secure the gauze with tape. Record the appearance of the site, the condition of the catheter, and how the patient tolerated the procedure. Removal of midlength and long catheters requires special training.

PRECAUTIONS

When performing a venipuncture or handling used needles or catheters, always be aware of the risk of exposure to bloodborne pathogens. The most serious pathogens that can be transmitted by this route are the human immunodeficiency virus and hepatitis B virus.

A number of products for venipuncture and intravenous therapy that reduce the risk of needle punctures or other exposure to blood are available. Every nurse should be familiar with the agency needle puncture and body fluid exposure guidelines. In the event of an accidental needlestick, most policies require blood specimens to be drawn from the nurse and the patient to test for bloodborne infections. Drug therapy may be advised if the patient has an infectious disease. Documentation of the incident and the health status of the nurse at the time of the exposure may be very important if the nurse becomes ill as a result of the exposure.

COMPLICATIONS OF INTRAVENOUS THERAPY

Intravenous therapy is so widely used that it is easy to take its safety for granted. Several potential complications of intravenous therapy can be very serious, however. Complications include tissue trauma, infiltration, inflammation, infection, fluid volume excess, bleeding, and embolism. Each of these is discussed in detail under Nursing Care During Intravenous Therapy on p. 285.

THE OLDER PATIENT AND INTRAVENOUS THERAPY

The older patient requires special consideration during intravenous therapy. Key points include the following:

- Anchor the vein with the thumb of your non-dominant hand to hold it in place during venipuncture.
- When performing the venipuncture, you may be able to distend the vessel by simply pressing the vein. If a tourniquet is needed, protect fragile skin by wrapping a washcloth under the tourniquet or using a blood pressure cuff inflated just above the patient's diastolic pressure.

- Special adhesives or dressings may be needed to prevent damage to the skin. A skin polymer solution can be applied to protect the skin from adhesives.
- If the hand or arm is secured to an armboard, the armboard must be padded; apply another piece of tape or gauze to the back of the tape to avoid direct contact of the adhesive with the skin.
- Because older people have less subcutaneous tissue, infiltrated fluid may drain away from the cannula insertion site. For example, if the hand is elevated, fluid may collect in the elbow area.
- If the patient is confused or restless, protect the infusion site and tubing with a commercial securement device or conceal the site under long sleeves.
- If a soft wrist immobilizer is justified, secure the immobilizer to the armboard and then secure the arm with the infusion to the armboard.
- Never apply an immobilizer *over* an infusion site; the immobilizer must be *below* the site.
- Confusion during acute illness is common. Reassure the confused patient, use a calm and gentle approach, and frequently reinforce instructions.
- With dementia patients, distraction may take their attention away from the IV. Keeping the infusion equipment out of sight may reduce attempts to handle it.
- Monitoring for fluid volume excess is especially important because older people often have less efficient cardiac and renal function.

NURSING CARE *During Intravenous Therapy*
Assessment

When a patient is receiving intravenous therapy, frequent assessment is needed to ensure that the correct fluid is infusing at the correct rate and that the patient is not suffering any complications from this therapy (see Nursing Care Plan: The Patient Receiving Intravenous Therapy on p. 286).

Check the physician's order to be sure the correct intravenous solution is infusing. Determine the prescribed rate of flow, and assess the actual flow rate. Inspect the infusion site for edema, pallor or redness, bleeding, and drainage. Palpate the infusion site for edema and warmth or coolness. Ask the patient if the infusion site is painful.

Many people believe that the infusion is not infiltrating if blood flows into the tubing when the fluid container is lowered. This is not an accurate sign because blood may return even when fluid is escaping into the tissue. It is interesting to note that the lack of blood return does not necessarily mean the needle is out of the vein either. Therefore this time-honored test for needle placement is not reliable. Inspection and palpation of the infusion site remain the best means of evaluating for infiltration.

Take the patient's vital signs and compare the readings with previous findings to detect increased pulse and blood pressure. Measure and record the fluid intake and output, and auscultate the patient's lungs for crackles.

Nursing Diagnoses, Goals, and Outcome Criteria: Intravenous Therapy

When a patient is receiving intravenous therapy, nursing diagnoses address the risk for complications, the need for assistance with activities of daily living, and the need for patient teaching. Specific nursing diagnoses and related goals are the following:

NURSING DIAGNOSES	GOALS AND OUTCOME CRITERIA
Risk for Injury related to trauma, infiltration, inflammation	Absence of trauma, inflammation, infiltration: no bruising, bleeding, edema, pallor, redness, or drainage at infusion site
Risk for Infection related to disruption of skin integrity or presence of a cannula in a vein	Absence of infection: normal body temperature, no purulent drainage or redness at venipuncture site
Fluid Volume Excess related to rapid fluid infusion	Normal fluid volume: fluid output approximately equal to intake, no dyspnea or edema
Decreased Cardiac Output related to blood loss through disrupted intravenous line	Normal cardiac output: pulse and blood pressure within normal limits, skin warm and dry, tubing connection intact
Ineffective Tissue Perfusion related to obstruction of blood flow by an embolus	Unobstructed blood flow: normal skin color and warmth in extremities
Self-Care Deficit (bathing/hygiene, dressing/grooming, feeding, toileting) related to restricted movement of infusion site and connection to fluid delivery system	Patient's performance of self-care activities: activities completed without disruption of intravenous therapy therapy

Interventions
Risk for Injury

Trauma. The insertion of a cannula is traumatic to the skin and underlying tissues. Tape may irritate or tear the skin. Use gentle technique when performing the venipuncture, and anchor the cannula to reduce tissue trauma. Apply a commercial site protector, if available, to shield the intravenous site.

Infiltration. Infiltration is the collection of infused fluid in tissue surrounding the cannula. The term extravasation is often used interchangeably with infiltration, but extravasation specifically refers to leakage of fluid from a blood vessel. Infiltration can be caused by leakage at the point where the cannula enters the

NURSING CARE PLAN
The Patient Receiving Intravenous Therapy

ASSESSMENT

Health History: Gary Edwin, age 67, was admitted for nausea and vomiting of 3 days' duration. He reported fluid intake of only water and cola for the previous 2 days and complained of dizziness and fatigue. Intravenous fluids were begun at 150 mL/hr via a 21-gauge cannula.

Physical Examination: Lethargic but oriented. Vital signs: blood pressure, 96/58; pulse, 102; respirations, 22; temperature, 101.6° F orally. Mucous membranes dry and sticky. Urine dark yellow. Intravenous infusion site: no swelling or redness.

Nursing Diagnosis	Goals and Outcome Criteria	Interventions
Risk for Injury related to the trauma, infiltration	The patient will experience minimal trauma, as evidenced by absence of bruising, bleeding, swelling.	Use gentle technique to start the infusion. Inspect the infusion site for swelling and bleeding. Palpate for warmth or coolness. Anchor the tubing securely. Exercise caution to prevent movement of the cannula. Stop the infusion if there are signs of infiltration (swelling near infusion site, pain, slow infusion rate), and restart it.
Risk for Infection related to disruption of skin integrity, presence of cannula in vein	The patient will remain free of infection at infusion site, as evidenced by absence of redness, swelling, edema, or drainage.	Use strict aseptic technique when starting the infusion and handling the site. Assess for signs of inflammation and infection: redness, swelling, warmth, purulent drainage, fever. Report signs to physician. Administer antibiotics, and apply warm compress to inflamed site as ordered.
Fluid Volume Excess related to rapid fluid infusion	The patient's fluid status will be normal, as evidenced by normal vital signs and fluid intake approximately equal to output.	Monitor rate of fluid infusion and maintain correct rate of flow. Measure all fluid intake and output. Assess for signs and symptoms of fluid volume excess (hypervolemia): increasing blood pressure, bounding pulse, dyspnea. If patient is hypervolemic, slow infusion rate, elevate patient's head, and notify physician.
Decreased Cardiac Output related to blood loss	The patient will have no bleeding at infusion or tubing connections.	Check connections to be sure they are secure. Tape tubing to prevent accidental disconnection.
Ineffective Tissue Perfusion related to obstruction of blood flow by embolus	The patient will maintain normal circulation, as evidenced by usual skin color and absence of respiratory distress.	Do not irrigate obstructed cannula. Aspirate gently or administer thrombolytic if permitted per agency protocol. Assess and report any signs of respiratory distress.
Self-Care Deficit (bathing/hygiene, dressing/grooming, feeding, toileting) related to restricted movement of infusion site and connection to fluid delivery system	The patient will accomplish self-care activities without disruption of intravenous therapy.	Provide assistance with meals, hygiene, dressing, and toileting as needed. Provide gown that unfastens at the shoulder. Assure the patient that he can move with the infusion.
Deficient Knowledge of management of intravenous therapy	The patient will demonstrate ability to protect and manage the infusion.	Tell the patient the purpose of the infusion and what symptoms should be reported: pain, bleeding, swelling. Assure the patient that movement is possible with the infusion as long as it is protected and the tubing is not disconnected.

? CRITICAL THINKING QUESTIONS

- Why is it important to tell the patient the purpose of the infusion and possible symptoms?

- What type of aseptic technique should be used in this situation in the initiation, maintenance, and discontinuance of intravenous infusion? Explain your answer.

vein or by puncture of a second site in the vein by the cannula. Drugs that are especially toxic to subcutaneous tissues are called *vesicants*. Common vesicants are vasopressors, potassium chloride, and antineoplastic agents.

Frequently assess for signs and symptoms of infiltration. When the infusion is infiltrated, the patient may report pain or a burning sensation in the area. On inspection, the site may be pale and puffy. If a lot of fluid is in the tissue, it may feel hard and cool. When there is evidence of infiltration, stop the infusion and restart it in a different vein; otherwise the patient may not be receiving the drug or fluid as intended. Tissue that is edematous with infiltrated fluid is fragile, so handle it gently. Elevate the affected arm on a pillow to promote reabsorption of excess fluid.

Because many medications harm subcutaneous tissue, the physician should be notified if a solution containing a vesicant infiltrates. When administering vesicants, it is especially important to select a large, soft vein. Use the smallest appropriate cannula, ensure cannula placement before giving the vesicant, and flush the cannula after the vesicant is given.

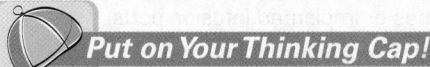

Put on Your Thinking Cap!

A patient complains of pain at an IV insertion site. The site feels cool and is slightly swollen. When the IV fluid container is lowered, blood flows back into the tubing. Do you think the infusion is infiltrated? What should you do?

Risk for Infection

Inflammation of the vein is called **phlebitis**. With intravenous fluid therapy, phlebitis may be due to irritation by the cannula or by medications. Redness, swelling, warmth, and tenderness near the insertion site suggest phlebitis. In addition, an infected site may have purulent drainage and the patient might have a fever. The inflammation may be mild or severe and carries the possibility of the formation of blood clots in the vein (thrombophlebitis).

Infection of a venipuncture site can be caused by contamination of the site itself, by the intravenous fluid, or by the tubing used to deliver the fluid. The infected site is red and warm and may have purulent drainage.

To reduce the risk of inflammation and infection, use strict aseptic technique when starting and handling intravenous infusions. Agency policy describes specific site care, including the frequency of dressing changes.

If the infusion site appears to be inflamed or infected, stop the infusion and restart it in another site. If agency policy permits, a warm compress can be applied to the inflamed site. If there is evidence of infection, notify the physician. Antibiotic therapy may be ordered.

Pharmacology Capsule

Drugs that are toxic to body tissues are called *vesicants*. They can cause phlebitis or tissue necrosis.

Fluid Volume Excess

The patient's blood volume may increase excessively when fluid is delivered directly into the bloodstream. This is most likely to happen when large volumes of fluid are infused, especially in patients who have impaired renal or cardiac function.

Signs and symptoms of fluid volume excess include rising blood pressure, bounding pulse, and edema. Severe fluid volume excess produces congestive heart failure and pulmonary edema (discussed in Chapter 35).

The risk of fluid volume excess is reduced by controlling the rate of fluid infusion. If the infusion falls behind schedule, correct the rate as noted previously but do not increase it to make up for the slow infusion. Normally, fluid intake and output are approximately equal. When the heart or kidneys are unable to handle excess blood volume, heart failure may develop. Young children and older adults must be monitored closely for fluid volume excess because they do not adapt to fluid changes as readily as a young adult. If indications of fluid volume excess (increasing blood pressure, bounding pulse, dyspnea) appear, slow the infusion rate, elevate the patient's head, and notify the physician.

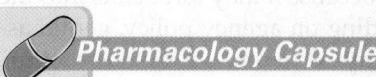

Pharmacology Capsule

Rapid intravenous administration of drugs or fluids may cause fluid volume excess, leading to heart failure.

Decreased Cardiac Output

Bleeding may occur if the cannula is moved excessively after insertion. Even more serious bleeding is possible if the tubing becomes disconnected from the cannula, allowing blood to flow freely from the vein.

To prevent bleeding, make sure all connections in the infusion set are secure. Tape tubing so that it cannot be pulled loose easily. Protect the infusion site and tubing when the patient moves. If a large amount of blood is lost, take the patient's vital signs and notify the physician. Institute emergency measures if the patient is in shock.

Ineffective Tissue Perfusion

An **embolus** (*pl.* emboli) is an unattached blood clot or other substance in the circulatory system. An embolus can have serious, even life-threatening, effects if it lodges and obstructs blood flow in a critical blood vessel. The obstruction created by a trapped embolus is called an **embolism.**

With intravenous therapy, there are risks of emboli from blood clots, air, and broken catheters. A blood clot or **thrombus** (*pl.* **thrombi**) can develop in intravenous needles or catheters. Air can enter the bloodstream if the infusion system is opened. As little as 10 mL of air can cause serious complications. The risk of air embolism with peripheral lines has been greatly reduced by the use of plastic rather than glass fluid containers. The danger is greatest with central venous lines such as the subclavian, Hickman-Broviac, and triple-lumen catheters. If a port is disconnected, air may be drawn into the bloodstream. The patient experiences shortness of breath, hypotension, and possibly shock and cardiac arrest.

A rare occurrence is a catheter embolus. This occurs when a piece of the catheter breaks off in the vein. Broken catheters may be due to defects in the catheter, reintroduction of the needle into the catheter, accidental cutting with scissors, and pulling catheters through needles.

Chest discomfort may be due to a catheter embolism and should be reported to the physician immediately. If a catheter breaks in a peripheral vein, keep the patient quiet with the head elevated. Notify the physician. A radiograph will be ordered to locate the broken catheter, usually in the right ventricle or pulmonary artery. The fragment may be removed with a snare that is passed through the femoral vein.

When the cannula seems to be obstructed, blood clots may have formed in it. Irrigation of the cannula is not recommended because it may force clots into the bloodstream. Depending on agency policy, gentle aspiration may be attempted to remove the obstruction. Alteplase (t-PA) may be ordered to dissolve clots that are obstructing the cannula.

Exercise extra caution to prevent an air embolism when a patient has a central line. The infusion set must remain closed. When hanging new bags of fluid, clamp the catheter port to prevent air entering the bloodstream. When a central catheter is inserted or removed, instruct the patient to take a deep breath and bear down. This helps prevent air entering the bloodstream. If air accidentally enters the line, close the leak immediately. Turn the patient on the left side with the head lowered. This position traps the air in the right atrium, where it can be absorbed gradually. Air in the bloodstream is an emergency situation in which cardiac arrest is possible, so close monitoring is vital. Immediately notify the physician, and keep the emergency supply cart close at hand. One hundred percent oxygen with a nonrebreather mask may be ordered.

Self-Care Deficit

Provide assistance as needed with eating, dressing, toileting, and hygiene. Dressing may be easier if the patient is provided with a gown or shirt that unfastens at the shoulder. These garments are simpler to remove than garments that must be removed over the arm. Some patients are fearful of moving with an intravenous infusion. Explain what restrictions, if any, are needed to protect the infusion. If a commercial intravenous shield is available, consider using one to reduce the risk of trauma at the insertion site.

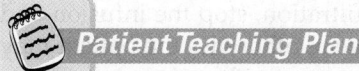
Patient Teaching Plan

Intravenous Therapy in the Home

When intravenous therapy is ordered outside the acute care setting, explain what will be done and why. Teaching should begin well before discharge so that the patient's ability to do the care can be assessed. With long-term therapy, it is especially important to teach the patient (and family, if appropriate) the following:

* Infusion site care
* Proper administration of fluids or drugs
* Signs that should be reported to the physician or home health nurse
* How to flush infusion ports if appropriate
* Care of central lines or implanted infusion ports

Details depend on the situation.

Key Points

* Intravenous therapy is used to administer drugs, fluids including nutrients, and blood or blood products.
* The terms *fluid* and *solution* are used interchangeably in relation to intravenous therapy.
* Tonicity is a measure of the concentration of electrolytes in a fluid.
* Hypertonic intravenous solutions tend to increase blood volume, whereas hypotonic intravenous solutions tend to decrease blood volume.
* A patient receives 34 calories for each 1% of dextrose in a liter of fluid.
* Devices used to deliver intravenous fluids include needles, over-the-needle catheters, inside-needle catheters, subcutaneous infusion ports, and subcutaneously implanted pumps.
* Central veins are large veins located nearer the heart that are used for long-term therapy, when the patient has poor peripheral veins, and when irritating fluids are administered.
* Peripheral veins in the extremities and scalp are used for short-term therapy, when a patient has healthy veins, and when relatively nonirritating fluids are given.
* Nurse practice acts and agency policies govern who can perform venipuncture, administer intravenous fluids, and give intravenous medications.
* Cannula size is selected based on the patient's condition and the type of fluid to be administered.
* Use the "five rights" when administering intravenous fluids as well as drugs.

- Cannulas and tubing are usually changed every 48 hours in accordance with standards of the Intravenous Nurses Society.
- On the site dressing, record the date and time that the cannula was inserted, the length and gauge of the cannula, and your initials.
- When an infusion flows by gravity, the rate is influenced by the height of the fluid container, fluid volume in the container, fluid viscosity, cannula diameter, venting of the fluid container, and position of the extremity.
- If your state permits you to give drugs per IV push, you must know how to dilute the medication, the correct rate of infusion, and whether the drug is compatible with the infusing fluid!
- Use Standard Precautions when starting infusions, providing site care, and discontinuing infusions.
- Complications of intravenous therapy are tissue trauma, infiltration, inflammation, infection, fluid volume excess, bleeding, and embolism.

- Monitor for fluid volume excess in the older person who is receiving intravenous fluids.
- When a cannula appears to be obstructed, irrigation is not recommended because you may force blood clots into the bloodstream.
- With central lines, take precautions to prevent air entering the line, which can cause an air embolism—a potentially fatal complication.

 Go to your Companion CD-ROM for a Pharmacology Tutorial, Audio Glossary, and 3-D animations.

evolve   Be sure to visit the companion Evolve site at http://evolve.elsevier.com/Linton/ for WebLinks and additional online resources.

REVIEW QUESTIONS *Choose the best answer.*

1. Which intravenous cannula is largest?
   1. 12-gauge
   2. 14-gauge
   3. 18-gauge
   4. 22-gauge

2. The tonicity of an IV solution of 0.45% sodium chloride is:
   1. Isotonic
   2. Hypotonic
   3. Hypertonic
   4. Concentrated

3. A patient is to receive 1000 mL of IV fluid every 8 hours at a rate of 34 drops/min. If the infusion has slowed so that he has received only 700 mL near the end of one 8-hour shift, the correct action is to:
   1. Quickly infuse an additional 300 mL before the end of your shift
   2. Increase the infusion rate to deliver an additional 300 mL over the next shift
   3. Notify the physician to determine what action should be taken
   4. Reset the infusion rate at 34 drops/min to continue the infusion

4. An older patient is receiving intravenous fluids to treat dehydration. When she complains of shortness of breath, your assessment reveals a 20-point increase in her systolic blood pressure and a heart rate of 100. You should suspect:
   1. Shock caused by deficient fluid volume
   2. Anxiety associated with hospitalization
   3. Fluid volume excess related to fluid overload
   4. Renal failure caused by circulatory collapse

5. The greatest danger of irrigating an obstructed intravenous line is:
   1. Embolism
   2. Trauma to the blood vessel
   3. Rupture of the cannula
   4. Infusion site irritation

19 Shock

CATHERINE ROBICHAUX

evolve http://evolve.elsevier.com/Linton/

Objectives

After reading and studying this chapter, you should be able to:

1. List the types of shock.
2. Describe the pathophysiology of each type of shock.
3. List the signs and symptoms of each stage of shock.
4. Explain the first aid emergency treatment of shock outside the medical facility.
5. Identify general medical and nursing interventions for shock.
6. Explain the rationale for medical/surgical treatment of shock.
7. Assist in developing care plans for patients in each type of shock.

Key Terms

Be sure to check out the bonus material on the Companion CD-ROM, including selected audio pronunciations.

ischemia (is-KĒ-mē-ă, p. 293)
metabolic acidosis (met-ă-BOL-ik ăs-I-DŌ-sis, p. 293)
multiple organ dysfunction syndrome (MODS) (p. 300)
sepsis (SEP-sis, p. 300)
shock (p. 290)
systemic inflammatory response syndrome (SIRS) (p. 298)

DEFINITION OF SHOCK

Shock is a syndrome characterized by inadequate tissue perfusion resulting in impaired cellular metabolism. Inadequate tissue perfusion deprives cells of essential oxygen and nutrients, forcing cells to rely on anaerobic (without oxygen) metabolism. As a result, less energy is produced and lactic acid, a by-product of anaerobic metabolism, causes tissue acidosis and subsequent organ dysfunction. There are a number of types of shock, each with a different cause that will require specific interventions. Although some aspects of treatment may be appropriate for treating the effects of all types of shock, patient responses will vary, thus requiring continual and astute nursing assessments and prompt interventions.

TYPES OF SHOCK

Shock begins when the cardiovascular system fails to function adequately because of an alteration in at least one of four vital components: circulating blood volume, myocardial contractility, blood flow, or vascular resistance (McKinley, 2005). Types of shock include hypovolemic (inadequate circulating blood volume), cardiogenic (decreased myocardial contractility), obstructive or extracardiac obstructive (inadequate circulatory blood flow caused by a physical impairment or obstruction), and distributive (decreased vascular resistance).

HYPOVOLEMIC SHOCK

Hypovolemic shock occurs when the circulating blood volume is inadequate to maintain the supply of oxygen and nutrients to body tissues. Intravascular or circulating volume deficits can occur from external or internal losses. Blood volume falls when there is excessive blood or fluid loss, inadequate fluid intake, or a shift of plasma from the blood vessels into body tissues or organs. Some causes of blood or fluid loss are hemorrhage, severe diarrhea or vomiting, and excessive perspiration. Excessive shift of plasma can occur with pathologic states, including burns, peritonitis, and intestinal obstruction.

CARDIOGENIC SHOCK

Cardiogenic shock occurs when the heart fails as a pump. A decrease in myocardial contractility results in decreased cardiac output and impaired tissue perfusion. This type of shock is one of the most difficult to treat and usually results when diseased coronary arteries cannot meet the demand of the working myocardial cells, such as occurs in acute myocardial infarction. Other causes include conditions that result in ineffective myocardial cell function such as dysrhythmias, cardiomyopathy, myocarditis, valvular disease, and structural disorders.

OBSTRUCTIVE SHOCK

Obstructive shock is also known as *extracardiac obstructive shock* and occurs when there is a physical impairment to adequate circulating blood flow. Obstruction of the heart or great vessels either blocks venous return to the right side of the heart or prevents effective pumping action. Some causes of obstructive shock include the following: tension pneumothorax, pericardial tamponade, pulmonary embolus, abdominal distention, and aortic dissection.

DISTRIBUTIVE SHOCK

In distributive shock, the problem is not loss of blood but excessive dilation of blood vessels or decreased vascular resistance causing the blood to be improperly distributed. To demonstrate this point, imagine pouring 5 mL of water into a test tube and another 5 mL into a mixing bowl. The water would nearly fill the test tube, exerting even pressure against the walls of the tube. The water in the mixing bowl, however, might just barely cover the bottom of the bowl. The diameter of the mixing bowl is so large that the water exerts pressure primarily against the container bottom. This is similar to what happens in the vascular system when the diameter enlarges. Fluid pools in the dependent areas of the body and is not returned to the arterial circulation to supply critical cellular metabolic needs. Distributive shock can be complicated by increased capillary permeability, which permits plasma to leak into the interstitial compartment, thereby decreasing intravascular blood volume. The three types of distributive shock are anaphylactic, septic, and neurogenic.

Anaphylactic Shock

Anaphylactic shock occurs when a person has a severe allergic reaction that results in the release of chemicals that dilate blood vessels and increase capillary permeability. Fluid leaks out of the capillaries into the tissues. Pooling of blood in peripheral tissues and the shift of fluid out of the capillaries cause venous return and cardiac output to fall. In addition, the allergic reaction causes constriction of the bronchi and airway obstruction. People can be allergic to many substances including drugs, vaccines, contrast media, insect bites and stings, foods and food additives, pet dander, molds, and pollens. The onset of anaphylaxis is typically sudden and dramatic after exposure to a substance to which the patient has developed antibodies.

Septic Shock

Sepsis is a systemic inflammatory response to a documented or suspected infection. Sepsis can progress to septic shock, which is hypotension unresponsive to fluid resuscitation along with signs of inadequate tissue perfusion such as metabolic acidosis, acute encephalopathy, oliguria, and/or coagulation disorders. Septic shock develops when pathogenic organisms (e.g., bacteria, fungi, viruses, rickettsiae) release toxic substances that cause blood vessels to dilate, thereby decreasing vascular resistance and increasing capillary permeability. The increased permeability results in leakage of plasma proteins and reduced intravascular volume, preload, and cardiac output

that contributes to inadequate tissue perfusion and oxygenation.

Neurogenic Shock

Neurogenic shock occurs when a disruption in the nervous system affects the vasomotor center in the medulla. Normally, the vasomotor center initiates sympathetic stimulation of nerve fibers that travel down the spinal cord and out to the periphery where they cause the smooth muscles of the blood vessels to vasoconstrict. In neurogenic shock, disturbances that disrupt sympathetic nerve impulses result in vasodilation or loss of vascular resistance. The patient will have signs and symptoms similar to those just described in the distributive shock syndromes, including pooling of blood in peripheral tissues with subsequent decreased venous return and cardiac output. Bradycardia with hypotension from decreased sympathetic stimulation is also common. Causes of neurogenic shock include, among others, injury or disease of the upper spinal cord, spinal anesthesia, and depression of the vasomotor center from certain drugs.

EFFECTS OF SHOCK ON BODY SYSTEMS AND FUNCTIONS

- **Respiratory system:** tissue hypoxia and anoxia, respiratory failure, acute respiratory distress syndrome (ARDS)
- **Acid-base balance:** metabolic acidosis
- **Cardiovascular system:** myocardial depression, disseminated intravascular coagulation (DIC) (widespread clotting caused by sluggish flow of acidic blood combined with bacterial endotoxins or clotting factors released by destruction of red blood cells [RBCs])
- **Neuroendocrine system:** release of catecholamines (epinephrine and norepinephrine), mineralocorticoids (aldosterone and desoxycorticosterone), glucocorticoids (hydrocortisone), and antidiuretic hormone; decreased level of consciousness when cerebral blood flow falls
- **Immune system:** depressed immune response
- **Gastrointestinal system:** decreased peristalsis, ischemia of intestinal submucosa, impaired liver function
- **Renal system:** reduced glomerular filtration, inadequate renal perfusion, tubular necrosis, renal ischemia

STAGES OF SHOCK

Patient response to shock is individualized; however, a continuum consisting of three stages has been identified: (1) early, reversible, and compensatory;

(2) intermediate or progressive; and (3) refractory or irreversible. Although there is no clear-cut division between the stages, they appear to occur regardless of the type of shock experienced.

EARLY, REVERSIBLE, AND COMPENSATORY STAGE

The compensatory stage of shock begins when the continued reduction in cardiac output triggers a set of neural, endocrine, and chemical compensatory mechanisms in an effort to overcome the consequences of anaerobic metabolism and maintain blood flow to vital organs. During this stage of shock, the following events may occur:

1. Activation of baroreceptors in the carotid arteries and the aorta stimulate the sympathetic nervous system.
2. Sympathetic stimulation causes increased heart rate, constriction of peripheral blood vessels, and reduced blood flow to the kidneys, lungs, muscles, skin, and gastrointestinal (GI) tract.
3. Decreasing renal blood flow triggers the release of renin and a sequence of events that produce angiotensin II, a potent vasoconstrictor.
4. The adrenal cortex secretes aldosterone, which promotes sodium retention by the kidneys.
5. Antidiuretic hormone is released by the posterior pituitary, resulting in additional retention of water by the kidneys.
6. Falling blood pH and increasing arterial carbon dioxide are detected by chemoreceptors in the carotid arteries, which stimulate the respiratory center. Increased respiratory rate and depth help eliminate excess carbon dioxide and normalize the blood pH.

During this stage, the following symptoms may be found on assessment although shock may be reversed with minimal morbidity if appropriate interventions are initiated (Tierney & Messina, 2003):

- **Mental status:** irritability, restlessness
- **Blood pressure:** normal or slightly decreased, decreasing pulse pressure, orthostatic hypotension
- **Pulse:** increased rate; may be thready (as a result of vasoconstriction) or bounding (caused by vasodilation); decreased rate (bradycardia) may be present in neurogenic shock due to loss of sympathetic stimulation
- **Respirations:** increased rate and depth
- **Urine output:** decreased
- **Skin:** cool and pale; *exception:* warm and dry with septic shock
- **Abdomen:** decreased bowel sounds
- **Blood glucose:** increased
- **Other:** thirst

Table 19-1 summarizes the compensatory mechanisms activated in the first stage of shock.

INTERMEDIATE OR PROGRESSIVE STAGE

If the cause of shock is not corrected or if compensatory mechanisms continue without reversing the shock, the patient enters the intermediate or progressive stage. Although the neural, endocrine, and chemical compensatory mechanisms worked together in the early stage, they now begin to function independently and in opposition. In the intermediate or progressive stage of shock, the systemic circulation continues to vasoconstrict in the attempt to maintain blood flow to vital organs. The decrease in peripheral blood flow,

Table 19-1	Compensatory Mechanisms in Shock	
MECHANISM	**RESPONSE**	**BENEFITS**
Baroreceptors activate SNS.	Increased heart rate.	Speeds up delivery of oxygen and nutrients to tissues.
	Peripheral vasoconstriction.	Shunts blood to vital organs, helps maintain BP.
	Constriction of renal arteries.	Activates renin-angiotensin-aldosterone system.
	Renin-angiotensin-aldosterone system activated. Angiotensin is a potent vasoconstrictor.	Vasoconstriction shunts blood to vital organs and helps maintain BP.
	Aldosterone causes the kidneys to retain sodium, which induces ADH secretion and water retention.	Fluid retention increases blood volume by decreasing urine output.
Chemoreceptors in the carotid arteries respond to acidic blood pH and increased arterial carbon dioxide by stimulating the respiratory center.	Increased respiratory rate and depth.	This helps eliminate the excess carbon dioxide and normalize the blood pH. Takes in additional oxygen.

SNS, Sympathetic nervous system; *BP*, blood pressure; *ADH*, antidiuretic hormone.

however, leads to weak or absent pulses and ischemia of the extremities. As intravascular blood volume decreases, the blood becomes more viscous or thick, causing clumping of red blood cells, platelets, and proteins. Deprived of adequate oxygen, cells resort to anaerobic metabolism, which produces lactic acid; this results in metabolic acidosis, which has a depressant effect on myocardial cells. Typical assessment findings are as follows:

- **Mental status:** listlessness, confusion
- **Blood pressure:** decreased; narrow pulse pressure
- **Pulse:** weak and thready, tachycardia, dysrhythmias
- **Respirations:** increased rate, deep, crackles present on auscultation
- **Temperature:** subnormal, except with septic shock
- **Urine output:** decreased; possible renal failure
- **Skin:** cold, pale, clammy, slow capillary refill, cyanosis
- **Other:** dry mouth, thirst, sluggish pupillary response, peripheral edema, muscle weakness

Aggressive interventions are necessary in this stage of shock to prevent the development of multiple organ dysfunction syndrome (MODS).

IRREVERSIBLE (REFRACTORY) STAGE

The final stage of shock is marked by irreversible changes in vital organs as compensatory mechanisms fail. Tissue perfusion deteriorates, as blood remains pooled in the capillary bed where sluggish flow is further compromised by clumping and the formation of clots. Coronary artery perfusion is reduced, causing ischemia and dysrhythmias. Cerebral ischemia occurs as a result of the decrease in cerebral blood flow. Death is imminent. Even patients who are resuscitated during this stage often die within a week or two from MODS. Assessment findings in the irreversible stage include the following:

- **Mental status:** loss of consciousness
- **Blood pressure:** systolic continues to fall; diastolic approaches zero
- **Pulse:** progressive slowing, irregular
- **Respirations:** slow, shallow, irregular
- **Urine output:** minimal
- **Skin:** cold, clammy, cyanosis

DIAGNOSIS

A diagnosis of shock is based on the history and physical examination. Tests and procedures that help establish the type of shock, the stage, and the cause include blood and urine studies, measurement of hemodynamic pressures, chest radiograph, ECG and continuous cardiac monitoring, pulse oximetry and arterial blood gases, and urine output.

FIRST AID FOR SHOCK OUTSIDE THE MEDICAL FACILITY

Treatment that is provided to patients in shock before medical care is available can have a significant impact on the chances of survival. The *Healthy People 2010* objectives (2000) have identified the necessity for both increasing public awareness of how and whom to call for emergency assistance and providing education concerning initial lifesaving procedures to be followed until the arrival of emergency responders. Box 19-1 describes emergency first aid for the patient in shock.

GENERAL MEDICAL TREATMENT

General medical interventions for the patient in shock are directed toward maintaining perfusion of vital organs until the cause is found and treated. Care is directed toward correcting or reversing the altered circulatory component(s) including blood volume, myocardial contractility, blood flow, and vascular resistance in addition to improving oxygen delivery to the cells. Interventions to increase oxygen delivery and a combination of fluid, pharmacologic, and

---

Box 19-1   **ASSESSMENT and First Aid for the Patient in Shock**

Data Collection
Pulse:
Rapid and weak, "thready"
Respirations:
Air hunger initially, then increased rate; shallow
Blood Pressure:
Stable initially, then decreased
Skin:
Cool and moist at first; diaphoresis; later, cyanosis of lips and nail beds
Mental Status:
Restless, then listless; confused; unconscious
Thirst:
Increased

Interventions
- Summon medical assistance.
- Establish/maintain patent airway.
- Control external bleeding with direct pressure or pressure dressing.
- Maintain blood flow to the brain.
- Keep still and quiet.
- Position flat; legs may be elevated unless the shock is caused by heart failure, the head or neck is bleeding, injury is possible, intracranial pressure is increased, or the patient has dyspnea.
- Protect the patient from cold but do not overheat (victim should not shiver or perspire).
- Even if the patient complains of thirst, withhold oral fluids in case surgical intervention is needed.
- Tell the patient what is being done, that someone will stay with him or her, and that help is coming.

mechanical therapies are implemented to maintain tissue perfusion.

OXYGENATION

Brain cells begin to die after 4 minutes without oxygen and oxygen consumption increases as delivery decreases in shock, resulting in a poor patient prognosis. Consequently, current general medical treatment also includes interventions to increase oxygen delivery such as increasing arterial oxygen saturation, hemoglobin, and cardiac output. Supplemental oxygen may be used, or mechanical ventilation may be necessary. Paralytics, sedatives, and analgesics may be ordered to decrease oxygen requirements.

FLUID REPLACEMENT

Except for cardiogenic shock, all types of shock require significant fluid volume replacement. Normal saline is usually administered initially. Subsequent fluids may include various crystalloids and colloids, depending on the situation. Crystalloids provide replacement water and electrolytes for all fluid compartments. Colloids, on the other hand, remain in the vascular system and draw fluid into the bloodstream. Colloids are especially important when large amounts of plasma proteins have been lost. The hemorrhaging patient will require blood to replace deficient hemoglobin. Fluid needs of the patient in cardiogenic shock are determined based on individual patient assessments.

Patient response must be closely monitored during fluid replacement to ensure adequate but not excessive replacement. Fluid replacement is best determined by monitoring pulmonary artery wedge pressure, cardiac output, and urine output. Generally, volume replacement continues until a mean arterial pressure of 60 mm Hg or greater is attained and there is evidence of adequate tissue perfusion. Once sufficient fluids have been administered, an inotropic agent may be ordered to increase myocardial contractility.

PHARMACOLOGIC THERAPY

Pharmacologic interventions for the patient in shock are based on manipulation of the cardiac dynamics: contractility, preload, afterload, and heart rate. Although no one drug will provide nutrients and oxygen to the cells, several agents assist in manipulation of the four circulatory components. The Drug Therapy table below and on p. 295 lists agents that improve the availability of these vital components.

DRUG THERAPY | *Medications Commonly Used In Shock*

DRUG	ACTION	TYPE OF SHOCK	INDICATIONS	SIDE EFFECTS	NURSING INTERVENTIONS
Dopamine (action is dose dependent)	Positive inotropic (lower dose) Vasopressors (higher dose)	Cardiogenic	↑ Myocardial contractility ↑ Afterload ↑ BP when not caused by hypovolemia	↑ HR, dysrhythmias ↑ Myocardial O_2 consumption (MVO_2) Nausea, vomiting	Monitor BP at least q 15 min Administer with IV pump Should be tapered gradually If IV infiltrates, may cause tissue ischemia and sloughing
Dobutamine	Positive inotropic	Cardiogenic with severe systolic dysfunction Septic with normal cardiac output (CO) that is not meeting metabolic demands	↑ BP in low CO states	↑ HR, dysrhythmias ↑ MVO_2 Headache, tremors, nausea	Monitor BP at least q 15 min Administer with IV pump Should be tapered gradually
Norepinephrine	Vasopressor; some inotropic effects	Cardiogenic after MI Septic (increases vascular resistance)	↑ Afterload ↑ BP refractory to other drugs	↑ MVO_2 Dysrhythmias Severe nausea	Monitor BP at least q 15 min Administer with IV pump Should be tapered gradually If IV infiltrates, may cause sloughing

Adapted from Sole, M.L., Klein, D., & Moseley, M. (2005). *Introduction to critical care nursing* (4th ed., pp. 281-282). St. Louis: Saunders.
BP, Blood pressure; *HR,* heart rate; *IV,* intravenous; *MI,* myocardial infarction; *SVR,* stroke volume response.

DRUG THERAPY | *Medications Commonly Used In Shock—cont'd*

DRUG	ACTION	TYPE OF SHOCK	INDICATIONS	SIDE EFFECTS	NURSING INTERVENTIONS
Epinephrine	Vasopressor	Cardiogenic combined with afterload reduction	↑ HR, BP	Chest pain Dysrhythmias Tremors Headache	Monitor BP at least q 15 min Monitor for HR >110
	Bronchodilator	Anaphylactic	Bronchodilation		Monitor for dyspnea, pulmonary edema
Nitroglycerin	Venodilator	Cardiogenic	↓ Preload Pump failure	Headache Hypotension Bradycardia	Monitor BP at least q 15 min Administer with IV pump Should be tapered gradually Use glass or nonabsorbable container and special IV tubing
Nitroprusside	Vasodilator	Cardiogenic with ↑ SVR	↓ Preload and afterload	Myocardial ischemia Hypotension Nausea	Monitor BP at least q 15 min Administer with IV pump Should be tapered gradually Protect from light Monitor patient for cyanide toxicity (tinnitus, hyperreflexia, seizures)
Vasopressin	Vasoconstrictor	Cardiogenic Septic	↑ BP ↑ SVR ↑ Myocardial contractility BP unresponsive to catecholamines	Diaphoresis Tremors Nausea, vomiting ↓ CO Bradycardia	Monitor BP at least q 15 min Administer with IV pump

MECHANICAL MANAGEMENT

The management of shock may also include the use of mechanical devices that assist in the restoration of cellular perfusion (Figures 19-1 and 19-2). These devices are listed in Table 19-2.

SPECIFIC COLLABORATIVE TREATMENT FOR EACH TYPE OF SHOCK

NURSING CARE *of the Patient in Shock*
Assessment

Assessment of the patient who is at risk for shock should include continuous monitoring of cardiac rate and rhythm; blood pressure; body temperature; hemodynamic values; respiratory rate, rhythm, and depth; and arterial blood gases. In the routine nursing assessment, observe the color of the skin and palpate skin

Put on Your Thinking Cap!

Three patients are in the emergency department. All are in the compensatory stage of shock. Patient A is in hypovolemic shock. Patient B is in cardiogenic shock. Patient C is in septic shock.

1. What assessment finding would you expect in Patient C, but not Patient A or Patient B?
2. For which patient(s) would colloid intravenous fluids be contraindicated? Why?
3. Which patient would you expect to have a history of:
    a. Coronary artery disease
    b. Severe vomiting and diarrhea
    c. Urinary tract infection

FIGURE **19-1** MAST garment. **A,** Compartments allow compression of the legs and the abdomen. **B,** Garment in place. Compartments are inflated with a foot pump.

warmth and moisture. Note pupil size, equality, and response to light. Describe the patient's level of consciousness and response to commands, and assess reflexes. Auscultate heart, lung, and bowel sounds. Observe the movement of the chest wall with respirations. Inspect and palpate the abdomen for distention. Palpate for bladder distention, and note the appearance of urine and the hourly output. Inspect the extremities for color and palpate for peripheral pulses and edema. Inspect intravenous infusion sites for pallor, swelling, or coolness that suggests extravasation.

Nursing Diagnoses, Goals, and Outcome Criteria: Shock (General)	
NURSING DIAGNOSES	GOALS AND OUTCOME CRITERIA
Ineffective Tissue Perfusion related to failing cardiac pump, hypovolemia, or inadequate venous return	Normal tissue perfusion: urine output at least 1.0 mL/kg/hr, patient alert and oriented, normal heart rate and rhythm, normal blood pressure, active bowel sounds, extremities warm with palpable pulses
Decreased Cardiac Output related to hypovolemia, peripheral vasodilation, myocardial disorders	Normal cardiac output: normal hemodynamic values, vital signs consistent with patient norms, mental alertness

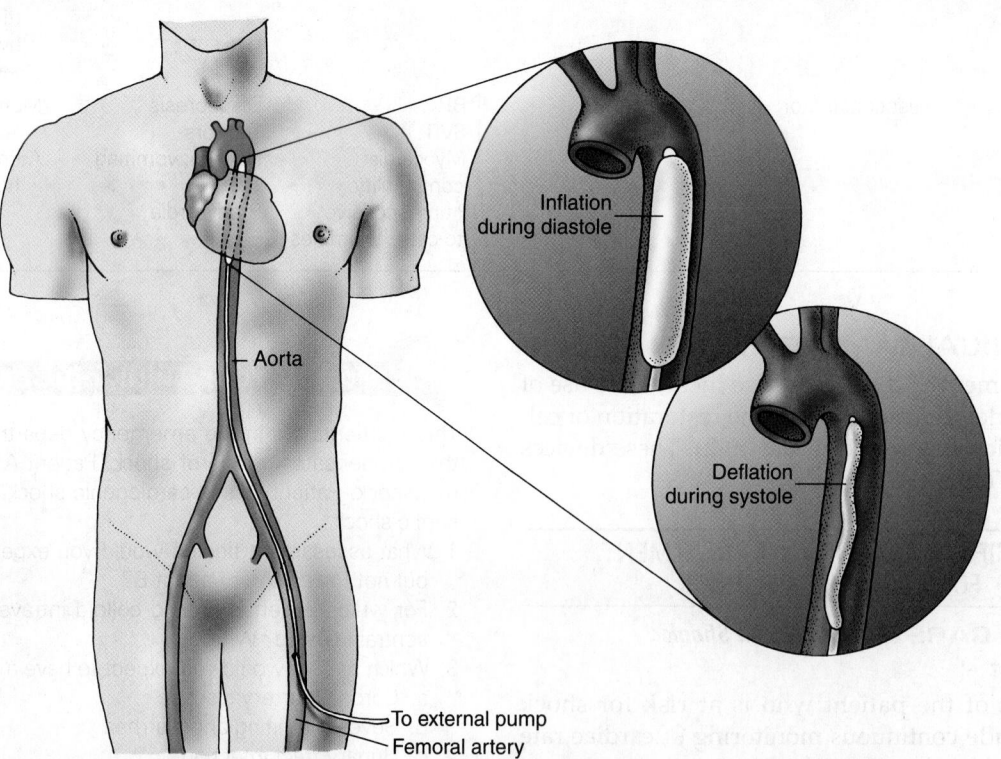

FIGURE **19-2** Intra-aortic balloon pump (IABP). An IABP is inserted into the femoral artery and advanced into the ascending aorta. The catheter is connected to an external pump that inflates the balloon during diastole and deflates it during systole.

Table 19-2 *Mechanical Devices Used in the Treatment of Shock*

DEVICE	DESCRIPTION	PURPOSE
Medical antishock trousers (MAST garment (see Fig. 19-1)	Trousers with inflatable chambers for each leg and the abdomen. Most often used outside hospital for massive blood or fluid loss. *Use is controversial because of possible restriction of lung expansion and accumulation of lactic acid in extremities.*	When chambers are inflated, blood vessels are compressed. Impedes blood flow to raise blood pressure and improve perfusion of vital organs. May reduce leakage of fluid into tissues of legs.
Intra-aortic balloon pump (IABP) (see Fig. 19-2)	A balloon-tipped catheter is inserted into the descending thoracic aorta. The balloon inflates during diastole and deflates just before systole.	Reduces preload with cardiogenic shock. Heart pumps more efficiently; increases cardiac output.
External counterpulsation device	Air- or water-filled devices are applied to the legs. A pump applies pressure during diastole and relieves pressure during systole.	Reduces preload with cardiogenic shock. Heart pumps more efficiently; increases cardiac output.
Ventricular assist devices (VAD)	Various devices include pulsatile and nonpulsatile pumps, external and implantable devices.	Decreases myocardial workload and oxygen demand. Supports circulation until the heart recovers or is replaced.
Extracorporeal membrane oxygenation (ECMO)	Blood is removed from the inferior vena cava, oxygenated, and returned via the femoral artery.	Used for short-term stabilization.

Disturbed Thought Processes related to inadequate cerebral perfusion, metabolic acidosis	Normal thought processes: patient alert and oriented, responds to commands appropriately, behaves appropriately
Deficient Fluid Volume related to hemorrhage, inadequate fluid intake, excessive fluid loss	Normal fluid balance: vital signs consistent with patient norms, capillary refill in 3 to 5 seconds
Anxiety related to hypoxia, life-threatening situation	Reduced anxiety: patient calm, states is less anxious
Risk for Injury related to confusion, adverse effects of drugs, invasive treatments	Absence of injury: no trauma
Risk for Infection related to trauma, invasive therapeutic procedures	Absence of infection: body temperature within normal range, normal WBC count
Compromised Family Coping related to anxiety, uncertainty of patient's outcome	Effective coping: family members are supportive of the patient and each other and indicate that they have adequate resources to cope with present situation

Nursing Diagnosis

The primary nursing diagnosis for all patients in shock is Ineffective Tissue Perfusion. This diagnosis may be related to alteration(s) in circulating blood volume, myocardial contractility, blood flow, or vascular resistance.

Interventions
Ineffective Tissue Perfusion

Your continuous assessment must include all body systems because shock, if not corrected, eventually results in failure of all major organs. Specific organ failures are addressed here under other nursing diagnoses.

Decreased Cardiac Output

Administer intravenous fluids as ordered, and assess for both fluid volume deficit and excess. With cardiogenic shock, it is especially important to monitor hemodynamic parameters. Administer inotropic and antidysrhythmic agents as ordered. Continuous cardiac monitoring enables you to assess the effectiveness of these drugs. You can reduce oxygen requirements by handling the patient gently and coordinating care to allow for rest. Maintain adequate body heat to prevent shivering, which also increases metabolic (and circulatory) demands. Fever may be treated with acetaminophen or nonsteroidal anti-inflammatory drugs. In some situations, a tepid sponge bath or a cooling blanket is ordered.

Disturbed Thought Processes and Anxiety

As patients progress through the stages of shock, they may be anxious, then confused and disoriented, and

 Consider the Alternative

Prayer and religious objects are comforting to many patients.

finally unconscious. For the anxious patient, you must remain calm and give simple explanations of what is being done. Remember that the intensive care environment is foreign and frightening to most people. As much as possible, protect the patient from constant, excessive noise and light.

Protect confused patients from harm. Repeat orientation, instructions, and reassurance often. In the presence of unconscious patients, remember that they may hear even when they cannot respond. Continue to speak to the patient, and beware of negative comments in the patient's presence.

Deficient Fluid Volume

Monitor for hypovolemia (tachycardia, hypotension, tachypnea, decreased urine output, decreased central venous pressure and pulmonary artery pressure). Administer intravenous fluids cautiously while assessing output of urine. Notify the physician if urine output falls below 0.5 mL/kg/hr because low urine output may signal inadequate fluid replacement and/or renal failure. Assess for fluid overload, especially with renal impairment and with intravenous colloids. Signs and symptoms of overload include full, bounding pulse; dilute urine; increased respiratory rate; abnormal lung sounds; dyspnea; and edema.

Risk for Injury

In addition to the risk for injury related to changes in consciousness, the patient in shock can be harmed by the therapeutic measures being used. For example, antidysrhythmics can depress cardiac activity, anticoagulants can permit excessive bleeding, and extravasation of vasopressors (drugs that raise blood pressure by vasoconstriction) can cause local tissue necrosis. Therefore you must closely monitor the patient for both therapeutic and adverse effects of drugs used to treat the patient in shock.

Because of poor peripheral tissue perfusion and the need to minimize activity, the patient in shock is at high risk for complications of immobility. Institute measures to prevent prolonged pressure on susceptible sites. Pressure ulcers can develop very rapidly. Also, personal hygiene may be limited by the patient's tolerance of such activity. A partial bath and gentle range of motion may be done if the patient is stable enough. Mouth care provides some comfort and helps prevent cracking of the lips and dryness of the oral mucosa. Apply water-soluble lubricant to the lips, and moisten the mouth with normal saline.

Risk for Infection

Intravenous lines, indwelling urinary catheters, chest tubes, airways, ventricular assist devices, and other equipment all provide avenues for infection in the patient in shock. The risk of infection is greatest in very young, very old, and immunocompromised patients.

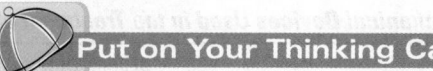

Put on Your Thinking Cap!

Why would a vasopressor be harmful to surrounding tissues if it leaked out of the vein?

To reduce the risk of infection, wash your hands thoroughly between patients. Follow agency guidelines for care of intravenous and urinary catheters. Use aseptic technique when inserting these devices, caring for insertion sites, and providing wound care. Monitor for signs of infection (elevated body temperature and white blood cell [WBC] count; redness, swelling, and warmth of wounds and tube insertion sites; purulent drainage; abnormal breath sounds; and yellow or green sputum). When antibiotics are ordered, administer them on schedule to maintain a therapeutic blood level.

What Does Culture Have to Do with Shock?

A Japanese or Vietnamese family would expect to participate in patient care or to remain at the bedside. Extended families may gather to be near the patient and to support one another. In Mexico, important decisions may be deferred to male relatives in traditional families. In Italy, a fatal prognosis would not be discussed by patients and families before death. In many cultures, rituals related to illness and death are very important to the patient and the family.

Compromised Family Coping

The patient in shock often has one or more family members present. Members of the health care team should be sensitive to the needs of the family for information and support. You can explain the nursing care and encourage them to ask questions. Offer the services of a counselor or patient representative. Table 19-3 summarizes interventions for each type of shock.

SYSTEMIC INFLAMMATORY RESPONSE SYNDROME (SIRS)

Inflammation is a normal response to tissue injury. However, in certain clinical situations, generalized inflammation occurs that threatens vital organs. This state is called systemic inflammatory response syndrome, or SIRS. In addition to shock, some of the conditions that can lead to SIRS are multiple transfusions, massive tissue injury, burns, and pancreatitis.

The effects of SIRS are damage to the endothelium of blood vessels and a hypermetabolic state. Damaged endothelium increases capillary permeability, allowing fluid to leak into body tissues. Hypotension, microemboli, and shunting of blood flow compromise

Table 19-3 | *Interventions for Each Type of Shock*

TYPE OF SHOCK AND ETIOLOGY	INTERVENTIONS	DRUGS/ACTIONS
HYPOVOLEMIC		
Blood loss: trauma, gastrointestinal bleeding, ruptured blood vessel, DIC	Direct pressure. Surgical repair. Replacement of whole blood, blood components, plasma expanders. Crystalloid fluid replacement. Autotransfusion (patient's own blood is collected and administered) in some circumstances. Pneumatic antishock (MAST) garment is controversial.	N/A
Plasma loss	Intravenous fluids. Albumin, fresh frozen plasma, hetastarch, dextran.	Low-dose inotropics.
Crystalloid loss	Intravenous fluids and electrolytes as indicated.	N/A
CARDIOGENIC		
Myocardial and valvular disease or injury	Hemodynamic monitoring. Intravenous fluids. Intra-aortic balloon pump. Surgery for valve disorders. External counterpulsation. Cardiac transplantation.	Inotropics/cardiotonics to improve myocardial contractility. Vasodilators to improve myocardial blood flow. Diuretics to decrease blood volume and reduce workload of the heart.
OBSTRUCTIVE		
External pressure on the heart:		
Pericardial tamponade	Pericardiocentesis, surgical repair.	N/A
Ascites	Paracentesis	N/A
Massive pulmonary embolism		Thrombolytics to dissolve blood clots or anticoagulants to prevent clot formation.
Tension pneumothorax	Air removed with needle or chest tube.	N/A
Cardiac dysrhythmias	Cardiac pacing, cardiopulmonary resuscitation.	Antidysrhythmics to restore normal cardiac rhythm.
DISTRIBUTIVE		
Excessive vasodilation; decreased peripheral resistance		
Anaphylactic		
Allergy to food, drugs, chemicals, insect bites or stings	Maintain airway. Endotracheal intubation or tracheostomy if needed. Ice pack to injection or sting site. Gastric lavage for ingested antigens. Isotonic intravenous fluids.	Epinephrine and xanthines for bronchospasm. Epinephrine also increases the cardiac rate and strength of contraction. H_1 receptor blockers (antihistamines) to block antigen-antibody response. Corticosteroids to reduce inflammatory antigen-antibody response. Vasopressors to constrict peripheral blood vessels and raise blood pressure.
Septic		
Infection, usually gram negative	Culture and sensitivity tests to identify site of infection, causative agent, and effective antimicrobials. Intravenous fluids: normal saline. Maintain body temperature in normal range.	Antimicrobials (e.g., vancomycin) if suspected gram positive. Penicillin or cephalosporin and aminoglycoside if suspected gram negative. Cardiotonics/inotropics to improve cardiac output. Vasopressors to raise blood pressure. Monoclonal antibodies to inhibit endotoxins. Heparin, clotting factors, blood product to treat DIC.
Neurogenic		
Spinal cord injury, spinal anesthesia	Flat with legs elevated 45 degrees. Intravenous normal saline.	Atropine for bradycardia. Vasopressors to raise blood pressure and improve cardiac output.
Pain, emotional distress (vasovagal response)	Recumbent position.	Analgesics for pain. Atropine for bradycardia.

Adapted from Black, J.M., Hawks, J.H., & Keene, A.M. (2001). *Medical-surgical nursing: Clinical management for positive outcomes* (6th ed., pp. 2249-2250). Philadelphia: Saunders.
DIC, Disseminated intravascular coagulation.

organ perfusion. The hypermetabolic state is characterized by increased serum glucose, which eventually depletes carbohydrate, fat, and protein stores.

A diagnosis of SIRS is made when a patient manifests two or more of the following:

- Temperature less than 97° F (36° C) or more than 100.4° F (38° C)
- Heart rate more than 90 bpm
- Respiratory rate more than 20/min, or $Paco_2$ less than 32 mm Hg.
- WBC count less than 4000 cells/mm^3 or more than 12,000 cells/mm^3, or more than 10% immature (band) neutrophils

Manifestations of SIRS range from mild to severe. The term sepsis is used when a patient has SIRS with a confirmed infection. With advanced SIRS and failure of more than one organ, deterioration of the cardiac, pulmonary, renal, and central nervous systems, liver, pancreas, and GI tract occurs. Thrombocytopenia may develop and progress to disseminated intravascular coagulation. If three or more organs fail, the prognosis is very poor.

When more than one organ begins to fail as a result of SIRS, the patient is said to have multiple organ dysfunction syndrome (MODS). As various organs are affected, the patient shows signs of failure specific to the organs affected.

MEDICAL TREATMENT AND NURSING INTERVENTIONS

Detailed care of the patient with SIRS and MODS is beyond the scope of this text. The patient is critically ill and requires critical care nursing. The goals of medical and nursing care for SIRS and MODS are to prevent and treat infection, maintain tissue oxygenation, provide nutritional and metabolic support, and support individual failing organs.

Prevent and Treat Infection

Monitor potential infection sites, and assess for signs and symptoms of infection. Maintain strict asepsis with invasive procedures and equipment. Exercise scrupulous hand washing. Administer antimicrobials as ordered. Administer enteral feedings as ordered to enhance perfusion of the GI tract.

Maintain Tissue Oxygenation

Administer sedatives and analgesics as ordered to reduce oxygen requirements. Monitor the patient on mechanical ventilation. Administer drugs to improve cardiac output and tissue perfusion as ordered. Plan care to minimize physical demands on patient.

Provide Nutritional and Metabolic Support

Provide enteral or parenteral nutrition as ordered (see the Nutrition Concepts box above). Monitor blood glucose and weight.

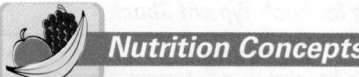

Nutrition Concepts

1. Hypermetabolism in shock causes protein-calorie malnutrition.
2. Early enteral feeding for all patients unable to consume adequate calories orally is thought to both prevent and treat shock; improve perfusion of the GI tract; and reduce the movement of bacteria through the intestinal wall into the bloodstream.
3. Nutritional status of the patient in shock is assessed by monitoring serum protein, nitrogen balance, and blood urea nitrogen (BUN), serum glucose, and serum electrolytes.

Support Failing Organs

Examples of measures to support failing organs could include mechanical ventilation for respiratory distress syndrome and replacement therapy for renal failure.

Key Points

- Shock is a state of acute circulatory failure and impaired tissue perfusion.
- Untreated shock progresses to systemic inflammatory response syndrome and then to multiple organ dysfunction syndrome or death.
- The types of shock are hypovolemic, cardiogenic, obstructive, and distributive.
- Hypovolemic shock results from inadequate circulating blood volume.
- Cardiogenic shock occurs when the heart fails as a pump.
- Obstructive shock occurs when there is physical impairment of adequate circulating blood flow.
- Distributive shock results from the excessive dilation of blood vessels or decreased vascular resistance that causes blood to be improperly distributed.
- The three types of distributive shock are anaphylactic, septic, and neurogenic.
- Compensatory responses to shock represent neurologic, endocrine, and chemical stimulation intended to maintain blood flow to vital organs.
- In the progressive stage of shock, continued vasoconstriction deprives the extremities of blood, blood thickens, and cells must resort to anaerobic metabolism that leads to acidosis.
- The final stage of shock is marked by irreversible changes in vital organs; death is imminent.
- Because brain cells begin to die within 4 minutes without oxygen, a priority in the first aid treatment of shock is to maintain blood flow to the brain.
- Positioning of the patient depends on the type of shock identified and is somewhat controversial.
- Except for cardiogenic shock, all types of shock require significant fluid volume replacement.
- Normal saline usually is administered first, followed by various colloids and crystalloids.

- Notify the physician if urine output falls below 0.5 mL/kg/hr.
- Assessment of the patient in shock includes monitoring of vital signs, hemodynamic values, respiratory status, and arterial blood gases.
- General nursing diagnoses for the patient in shock include Ineffective Tissue Perfusion, Decreased Cardiac Output, Disturbed Thought Processes, Anxiety, Deficient Fluid Volume, Risk for Injury, Risk for Infection, and Compromised Family Coping.
- Systemic inflammatory response syndrome (SIRS) is generalized inflammation that damages the lining of blood vessels and creates a hypermetabolic state.
- Failure of more than one organ as a result of SIRS is called *multiple organ dysfunction syndrome (MODS);*

failure of three or more organs presents a very poor prognosis.
- The goals of care with SIRS and MODS are to prevent and treat infection, maintain tissue oxygenation, provide nutritional and metabolic support, and support individual failing organs.

 Go to your Companion CD-ROM for a Pharmacology Tutorial, Audio Glossary, and 3-D animations.

evolve   Be sure to visit the companion Evolve site at http://evolve.elsevier.com/Linton/ for WebLinks and additional online resources.

REVIEW QUESTIONS *Choose the best answer.*

1. A patient with peritonitis is at greatest risk for which type of shock?
   1. Cardiogenic
   2. Anaphylactic
   3. Neurogenic
   4. Hypovolemic

2. The basic cause of distributive shock is:
   1. Blood or fluid loss
   2. Dilation of blood vessels
   3. An antigen-antibody reaction
   4. Failure of the heart as a pump

3. A patient in anaphylactic shock has massive edema. What would explain this?
   1. Increased capillary permeability
   2. Pooling of blood in dependent parts of the body
   3. Retention of excess water by the kidneys
   4. Overproduction of antidiuretic hormone

4. What do anaphylactic shock, septic shock, and neurogenic shock all have in common?
   1. Infection
   2. Allergic reactions
   3. Vasodilation
   4. Heart failure

5. Which acid-base disturbance would you anticipate in the intermediate/progressive stage of shock?
   1. Metabolic alkalosis
   2. Respiratory alkalosis
   3. Metabolic acidosis
   4. Respiratory acidosis

6. The best indicator of cerebral perfusion is:
   1. Presence of reflexes
   2. Level of consciousness
   3. Emotional state
   4. Mean arterial pressure

7. When patients have lost large amounts of plasma proteins, which fluid is most appropriate for restoring blood volume?
   1. Packed red blood cells
   2. Crystalloid fluids
   3. Normal saline
   4. Colloids

8. The majority of cases of cardiogenic shock are caused by:
   1. Pancreatitis
   2. Anaphylaxis
   3. Acute myocardial infarction
   4. Gastrointestinal bleeding

9. A patient in shock has been given blood, crystalloids, and osmotic fluids. Your assessment reveals: P = 80, bounding, regular; R = 30; BP = 140/86, dyspnea, and crackles throughout lung fields. You should suspect:
   1. Sepsis
   2. Multiple organ failure
   3. Pneumonia
   4. Circulatory overload

10. Providing early enteral feedings for those patients unable to consume adequate calories orally:
    1. May assist in both preventing and treating shock
    2. Is always contraindicated in septic shock
    3. Assists the movement of bacteria through the intestinal wall
    4. Interferes with perfusion of the gastrointestinal tract

CHAPTER 20 Falls

evolve http://evolve.elsevier.com/Linton/

Objectives

After reading and studying this chapter, you should be able to:

1. Define falls.
2. Give the incidence of falls.
3. Describe factors that increase the risk of falls.
4. Discuss the relationship between restraint use and falls, types of restraints, and regulations for restraint use.
5. Describe fall prevention techniques.
6. Describe nursing interventions to use when a fall occurs.

Key Terms

Be sure to check out the bonus material on the Companion CD-ROM, including selected audio pronunciations.

chemical restraint (p. 304)
extrinsic factors (ĕks-TRĬN-sĭk, p. 302)
fall (p. 302)
intrinsic factors (ĭn-TRĬN-sĭk, p. 302)
Omnibus Budget Reconciliation Act (OBRA) (p. 304)
physical restraint (p. 304)

If you were to ask several people whether they had fallen in the past 6 months, the chances are that many would say "yes." The chances are even better that those who had fallen, particularly the young and healthy ones, had not sustained a significant injury. Although falls do not necessarily result in serious physical injuries or death, many older people who have fallen become less confident in their ability to function independently. Those who fear falling tend to restrict their physical and social activities, become more dependent, and have an increased need for long-term care. In addition, caregivers tend to restrict older persons' activity out of concern that ill or frail people who have been weakened from sickness, hospitalization, or aging may fall and injure themselves.

DEFINITION OF FALLS

Definitions of falls vary from "unexpected displacement" to "an unintentional change in position" to "inadvertent events in which the subject comes to rest unintentionally on the ground." A useful definition that seems more descriptive of an actual **fall** is "a circumstance in which one unintentionally falls to the ground or hits an object such as a chair or stair."

INCIDENCE AND RISK FACTORS

Although falls and fall-related injuries occur at every age, the greater severity of injuries in old age, combined with longer recovery periods, makes a fall a particularly serious threat to the health and functioning of older people. One in three persons age 65 or older falls in a given year. There appears to be a steady increase in the number of falls among those ages 75 and older. Older women residing in community and long-term care facilities appear to be at higher risk of falling than older men. However, older men are more likely to fall in a hospital setting.

The risk of injury from falls is highest in people over age 65, and falls are the most frequent cause of accidental injury and death among older adults. Older adults constitute only 12% to 13% of the total U.S. population; however, they account for 72% of total deaths due to falls. The rate of death from falls increases from 5 in 100,000 for persons between ages 45 and 64 to 200 in 100,000 for those older than 85.

The U.S. Public Health Service has estimated that two thirds of the deaths due to falls are preventable. Potentially avoidable environmental factors cause 40% to 50% of fatal falls. Adequate medical evaluation and treatment for underlying medical conditions could probably prevent most of the remaining 50% to 60% of fatal falls, according to the Public Health Service.

Older adults are at particular risk for accidents because changes that commonly occur with aging increase their risk for injury. In addition, older people are more likely to have poorer clinical outcomes after accidents. Falls occur because of two major factors: (1) intrinsic factors, or factors related to the functioning of the individual, such as the aging process or physical illness; and (2) extrinsic factors, or environmental factors. Intrinsic factors enhance the possibility of falling, whereas extrinsic factors enhance the opportunity to fall.

Intrinsic factors related to falls include age-related sensory changes such as reduced vision and hearing; age-related changes in posture and gait; confusion or depression; lack of exercise, leading to weakness and decline in physical vigor; multiple medications related to the increased incidence of chronic illness in older adults; psychotropic medications; acute infections; diseases affecting the central nervous system that may affect balance by causing dizziness and gait disorders; and overestimation of abilities.

Extrinsic factors may differ according to setting. For example, potential hazards in the home environment include low-lying and poorly visible tables, trailing electrical wires, pets, steep and unlit stairs, loose carpeting, unsafe walking aids, and inconvenient bathroom or kitchen arrangements. Falls occurring in the institutional setting as a result of various environmental factors are often related to changes in position, such as transferring to and from a bed or chair, toileting procedures, and unstable and defective equipment (nonfunctioning brake locks on wheelchairs), wet or excessively waxed floors, and improper placement of food trays in the hallway. Falls often occur during periods of high activity when staff persons are busy. In addition, falls may result from imposed immobility. Patients may be confined to a bed or chair or be physically restrained, resulting in weakness or problems with balance.

Injury-causing falls are more likely to occur in long-term care facilities than in the community. Among community-dwelling older persons, about 30% fall every year, compared with 50% of those living in residential care facilities. However, in about 75% of all reported falls, no injuries occur. Contusions, cuts, or lacerations occur in about 25% to 30% of all reported falls, and deep tissue damage or concussion occurs in about 5%. Fractures occur in about 1% to 5% of all reported falls.

In most cases, falls occur because of multiple factors. The following are some of the factors known to increase the risk of falling:

- A history of previous falls (see Nursing Care Plan: The Patient with a History of Falls below)
- Osteoporosis (especially white women over age 75)
- Hemiparesis (weakness or paralysis of one side of the body) related to a prior stroke
- Sensory impairment (vision or hearing deficits)

NURSING CARE PLAN

The Patient with a History of Falls

ASSESSMENT

Health History: A 75-year-old woman resides in a long-term care facility because of chronic health problems, including emphysema, dementia, and a history of several falls at home. She has sustained several fractures as a result of these falls in the past. The nursing staff has used several methods to prevent her from falling, such as restraints, sedation, and sitters, but she continues to have problems. When she is restrained, she becomes very agitated and the staff is unable to calm her without administering sedatives.

Physical Examination: Vital signs: blood pressure, 144/76; pulse, 90; respiration, 22; oral temperature, 97° F. Height, 5'1"; weight, 98 lb. Her skin is warm and dry. Wheezing is noted on expiration. The patient is not oriented to time and place; she is oriented to person.

Nursing Diagnosis	Goals and Outcome Criteria	Interventions
Risk for Injury related to confusion	Patient will remain free from fall-related injury.	Approach patient in a calm manner. Assess patient and environment for possible hazards. Remove environmental hazards. Orient patient frequently to person, place, and time. Keep bed at lowest level; keep wheelchair brakes on. Have patient wear glasses or hearing aid when appropriate. Have someone familiar stay with patient to monitor as frequently as possible. Provide restraints only as a last resort to maintain safety; use type that is least restrictive; monitor frequently while restraint is on patient; remove at least q 2 hr for 10 minutes for range-of-motion exercises, toileting, nourishment, and restorative activities. Get patient up and out of room as tolerated.

? **CRITICAL THINKING** QUESTIONS

- How could glasses and a hearing aid reduce the risk of falls?

- When you are in a clinical site, examine a patient's room to identify some possible hazards in this patient's environment that might contribute to falls.

- Diminished muscle strength, balance, and reaction time
- Diabetes with peripheral neuropathies (decreased circulation and feeling in the lower extremities) and poor healing
- Falls associated with loss of consciousness or on a hard surface
- Multiple medications

 Put on Your Thinking Cap!

Assess one of your patients in the clinical setting to identify intrinsic and extrinsic risk factors for falling. Develop nursing interventions to prevent falls in this specific situation.

RESTRAINTS

Restraints are frequently used to prevent falls. Restraints restrict individuals' movement and are classified as either *physical* or *chemical*. Physical restraints consist of vest, waist, wrist, or ankle ties. Wrist and ankle restraints may be made of soft material or leather. Anything that restricts movement, such as geriatric chairs or side rails, is considered a physical restraint. If patients are able to apply or release a safety device themselves, it is not considered a restraint. A chemical restraint is usually a psychotropic medication that is given to subdue agitated or confused patients.

PHYSICAL RESTRAINTS

Older patients, particularly those who are confused, are more likely to be physically restrained than younger patients, probably because they are thought to be at greater risk of falling. The most common reasons given for using "protective" restraints with older patients in hospitals or long-term care facilities are (1) to protect the patient or others from harm or to prevent tampering with medical devices (e.g., feeding tube, catheter); (2) to prevent falls from the bed or chair; and (3) to prevent wandering. The most common incidents precipitating the use of restraints involve attempts to get out of bed or resistance to treatment while confused or disoriented.

Restraints seldom eliminate the risk of injury, however, and may actually cause or worsen problems. Patients are often able to untie their restraints and wriggle out of them, resulting in falls from wheelchairs and beds. In addition, accidental strangulation can occur when some forms of physical restraint, particularly a restraint vest, are used. The Food and Drug Administration has reported at least 100 restraint-related deaths each year. Nurses have long been taught to raise side rails so that vulnerable patients will either stay in bed or call for help. The wisdom of using side rails is now in question. Patients have been injured, sometimes fatally, after crawling over side rails or becoming trapped

between side rail bars or between side rails and the mattress. A study of patients who had fallen out of bed revealed that 41% had raised side rails. Half rails may be safer than full rails.

Restraints may have damaging psychological effects on older patients. Patients may experience anger, discomfort, resistance, and fear in response to physical restraint. Other behaviors noted include poor self-image, growing dependency, increased confusion and disorientation, regressive behavior, and withdrawal.

Because the use of physical restraints can have so many negative effects, policies for use and alternatives have been developed. The Omnibus Budget Reconciliation Act (OBRA) of 1987 was enacted to protect patients from unnecessary restraint in long-term care facilities. The law specifies that residents of such facilities have the right to be free from any physical restraints imposed and any psychotropic drug administered for the purposes of discipline or convenience and not required to treat residents' medical symptoms. In addition, a physician's order is required for restraint use and the order must specify the duration and the circumstances under which the restraint may be used. When OBRA regulations were enacted, health care providers predicted a surge of fall-related injuries. Although the number of falls did rise, most of those incidents did not result in serious injury. In fact, the most serious injuries occurred among patients who were restrained.

According to OBRA regulations, the only people who are candidates for restraints are those who:

- Have a history of severe falls or are at extremely high risk of taking a fall that is *life-threatening*
- Are neurologically, orthopedically, or muscularly impaired and need postural support for safety or comfort, or both
- Experience any of a number of mental dysfunctions that may cause them to be a *serious hazard* to themselves, objects, or others
- Have medical symptoms that are life-threatening, and a restraint is used *temporarily* to provide necessary treatment

If a physical restraint is used, the least restrictive device is best. For example, use a mitt rather than a wrist restraint that limits movement. Check the patient frequently, at least every 15 to 30 minutes. A patient who is agitated or combative must be monitored continuously. Make sure that the patient's condition is good and that the restraint is used properly and is providing adequate protection and comfort without impeding circulation or breathing. Remove and release physical restraints *every 2 hours* for 10 minutes to provide for range of motion, toileting, nourishment, and restorative activities such as physical therapy, ambulation, and mental stimulation.

Identify patients at risk for restraint so that you can try alternatives. Several alternatives to physical restraint include physical therapy, sitting and talking with patients for short periods of time, and asking staff to be responsible for wanderers in small blocks of time. Box 20-1 lists more alternatives to physical restraint. In addition, patients, family members, or both should be involved in the decision to use or not to use physical restraint. Special units for the care of persons with dementia typically have safe walking areas so that wanderers can move about freely without fear of leaving the premises.

 Put on Your Thinking Cap!

When visiting a patient in the clinical setting, observe the methods used as alternatives to physical restraint. Are there other steps that could be taken?

CHEMICAL RESTRAINTS

The same guidelines that apply to the use of physical restraints apply to chemical restraints. Never use psychotropic drugs for the purposes of discipline or convenience. Use them only when there is a danger of self-injury or injury to others. The administration of a psychotropic drug requires a physician's written order that specifies the duration and circumstance under which the medication is to be used.

Among the most commonly prescribed psychotropic drugs are antidepressants, sedatives/hypnotics (e.g., benzodiazepines), and antipsychotic drugs. All have the potential for causing serious adverse effects, such as greater confusion, agitation, and an increased number of falls in older persons. Many of these drugs can cause orthostatic hypotension, which also may result in falls.

Other drugs that increase the risk of falls because of orthostatic hypotension are some of the antihypertensives and diuretics, both commonly used by older persons.

Avoid the use of psychotropic drugs if at all possible. The same alternatives to physical restraints apply to chemical restraints (see Box 20-1).

NURSING ASSESSMENT AND INTERVENTION

FALL PREVENTION

The most important intervention for falls is prevention. The best prevention is education of patients and caregivers about ways to prevent falls. Prevention is aimed toward minimizing both the intrinsic and the extrinsic factors causing falls and the potential for injury.

The first step in preventing falls and injury is to determine who is at greatest risk. People who are at greatest risk for falls and injury are those who have fallen before and those who have multiple intrinsic risk factors. Table 20-1 lists intrinsic risk factors for falling and possible interventions.

Fall prevention strategies are carried out in the home and institutional environments (Fig. 20-1). Effective interventions need to be individualized to consider the specific factors that create a fall risk for

---

Box 20-1 | Alternatives to Physical Restraint

1. Provide general comfort measures.
2. Position with pillows, recliners, etc.
3. Change forms of treatment contributing to restraint use; e.g., substitute oral feedings for intravenous or nasogastric tubes, and remove catheters or external urinary drains.
4. Provide companionship and supervision by involving staff, family, friends, or volunteers, especially at night.
5. Use therapeutic touch when appropriate.
6. Distract attention with television, radio, tape player, or other activities.
7. Use a circular or semicircular room arrangement around nursing station for maximal visibility.
8. Redesign furniture; e.g., lower beds or put mattress on floor, or remove wheels from furniture.
9. Manipulate environment to provide easy access to nurse and equipment; e.g., call bell accessible, bedside commode accessible, bed rails in down position, adequate lighting.
10. Provide a policy for a restraint-free environment that is supported by administration and staff.

Data from Strumpf, N.E., Evans, L.K., & Schwartz, D. (1991). Physical restraint of the elderly. In W.C. Chenitz, J.T. Stone, & S.A. Salisbury (Eds.), *Clinical gerontological nursing* (pp. 329-344). Philadelphia: Saunders.

FIGURE **20-1** NASA has developed a walker that allows patients to ambulate safely and securely as they regain the ability to walk after a traumatic injury or receive physical therapy for a degenerative disease. A unique harness supports the patient's body weight without restricting hip movement.

Table 20-1 | *Intrinsic Risk Factors for Falling and Possible Interventions*

RISK FACTORS	INTERVENTIONS
IMPAIRED VISION	
Reduced visual acuity	Be sure individual wears glasses, if appropriate. Keep glasses clean. Encourage regular eye examinations.
Impaired dark adaptation	Maintain adequate lighting; reduce glare from shiny floors, and allow time to adjust to light levels (e.g., as patient moves from a dark room to outside). Use a night-light in bedroom and bathroom.
IMPAIRED HEARING	
Impacted cerumen (earwax)	Remove earwax.
Presbycusis	Speak slowly; use low voice; decrease background noise. Encourage use of hearing aid.
BALANCE AND GAIT PROBLEMS	
Musculoskeletal disorders	Encourage balance and gait training and muscle-strengthening exercises.
Balance disorders	Encourage balance exercises. Provide and educate in use of assistive devices.
Peripheral neuropathy	Encourage patient to use correctly sized footwear with firm soles.
FOOT DISORDERS	Trim toenails. Encourage patient to wear appropriate footwear.
CARDIOVASCULAR DISEASE	
Postural hypotension	Encourage dorsiflexion exercises. Use pressure-graded stockings. Elevate head of bed. Teach individual to get up from chair or bed slowly. Individual should avoid tipping head backward.
NEUROLOGIC DISEASE	
Stroke	Place call bell in visual field and within reach of unaffected arm. Anticipate needs for toileting, dressing, eating, and bathing. Assist with transfer. Provide passive range-of-motion exercises to improve functional ability.

Data from Chenitz, W.C., Kussman, H.L., & Stone, J.T. (1991). Preventing falls. In W.C. Chenitz, J.T. Stone, & S.A. Salisbury (Eds.), *Clinical gerontological nursing* (p. 316). Philadelphia: Saunders.

the individual patient. Fall prevention guidelines for the home are listed in the Patient Teaching Plan on p. 307, and those for use in institutional settings are listed in Box 20-2. Finally, the Health Promotion Considerations box on p. 307 gives general tips for preventing falls.

REDUCING FALL-RELATED INJURIES

Some falls will occur no matter what precautions are taken. In some societies, falls are viewed as indicators of greater activity and independence. Health care providers accept an increased number of falls as an inevitable risk that is outweighed by the benefits of physical activity and rehabilitation. The use of hip protectors is one strategy that accepts the risk of falling but aims to decrease the severity of fall-related injuries. Research has shown a decease in hip fractures when the protectors are worn. However, many patients who might benefit decline to wear them, citing discomfort and not liking the way they look. Others disagree with the health care provider's assessment of their fall risk. Individuals at risk for falling also can be taught how to fall in a way that reduces the risk for hip injury. The patient is less likely to sustain a fracture if he or she can rotate forward or backward to avoid falling sideways. Measures to prevent osteoporosis may reduce the risk of fractures associated with falls. These measures are discussed in Chapter 42.

WHEN A FALL OCCURS

When a fall occurs in a hospital or long-term care facility, determine the circumstances of the fall and any injuries sustained. Document the fall according to the agency protocol. Note what the patient was doing at the time of the fall, the patient's mental and emotional status, and environmental factors that may have contributed to the fall. When the cause of the fall is determined, take steps to remove or correct the cause. Have the patient begin ambulating as soon after the fall as possible and at least several times a day to prevent the hazards of bedrest and to restore confidence. It is tempting to apply restraints after a fall, but avoid the use of restraints at all costs.

Dealing with falls in the home requires the cooperation of the person who is at risk, the family, and possibly neighbors. A plan of action for when a fall occurs should include information about getting up and seeking help.

 Put on Your Thinking Cap!

Practice the methods for getting up after a fall described in the Patient Teaching Plan on p. 308. Consider the limitations on patients with restricted movements. Which methods would work best for patients you have seen?

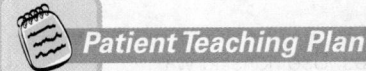

Patient Teaching Plan

Fall Prevention Guidelines for the Home: Instructions for the Client

Lights and Lighting

1. Eyes tire quickly in improper lighting. Illuminate reading material or the object worked on. Illuminate steps, entranceways, and rooms before entering. Use 70- or 100-watt bulbs, not 60-watt bulbs.
2. Avoid glaring light caused by highly polished floors or large expanses of uncovered glass. Use sunglasses to avoid the glare of highway driving, but use light tints or photoray lenses.
3. Allow more time to adjust to changes in light levels. When going from a dark to a light room or vice versa, allow a minute or two for the eyes to accommodate to the change in light before proceeding.
4. Dirty glasses or outgrown prescription lenses inhibit vision. Keep glasses clean. Have regular eye examinations to identify changes and get new glasses when needed. If possible, do not use bifocals when walking because you cannot see the ground clearly.
5. Ability to see up, down, and sideways decreases with age. Observe the "lay of the land"; learn to look ahead at the ground to spot and avoid hazards such as cracks in the sidewalks. Use canes, walking sticks, and walkers that are prescribed.
6. At night, keep a night-light on in your bedroom and bathroom. When getting out of bed at night, put the light on and wait a minute or two for the eyes to adjust before getting up. Have a telephone in the bedroom so you don't have to get out of bed to answer the phone. Before you go out in the evening or late afternoon, turn a light on for your return.

Activity

1. Get up from a chair slowly.
2. When getting out of bed, sit up and then wait a minute or two. Move to the side of the bed and wait another minute. Stand after sitting for a few minutes.
3. If you are dizzy, sit down immediately. Sit on a step or a chair, or ease yourself to the sidewalk if you are outdoors.

4. Avoid tipping the head backward (extending the neck). Activities to avoid (because they extend the neck) are washing windows, hanging clothes, and getting things from high shelves.
5. Use shelves at eye level. Avoid rapid turning of the head.
6. If weather is rainy and windy, avoid going out.
7. Use alcohol and tranquilizers with caution.
8. Exercise programs keep bodies limber. Consult your physician and then enroll in a senior exercise program.
9. Shoes and slippers should be flat and rubber-soled. Avoid clothing such as long robes and loose-fitting garments that may catch on furniture or doorknobs.

Around the House

1. Avoid scatter rugs and small bathroom mats that can slide. Repair loose, torn, wrinkled, or worn carpet.
2. Avoid slick, high polish on floors.
3. Put things in easy reach, and avoid reaching to high shelves.
4. Use nonskid treads on stairs and nonskid mats in tub.
5. You may wish to install a grab rail in the bath, in the shower, and also by the toilet.
6. Install handrails on both sides of the stairs. Paint stair edge in bright contrasting color.
7. Remove door thresholds.
8. Remove low-lying objects, such as coffee tables and extension cords.
9. Wipe up spills immediately.
10. Watch for pets underfoot and scattered pet food.
11. Check for even, nonglare lighting in every room, with easily accessible light switches.
12. Avoid floor coverings with complex patterns.
13. Avoid clutter in living areas.
14. Select furniture that provides stability and support, such as chairs with arms.
15. Check walking aids routinely, such as rubber tips on canes and screws on walkers.

From Chenitz, W.C., Stone, J.T., & Salisbury, S.A. (Eds.). (1991). *Clinical gerontological nursing* (p. 310). Philadelphia: Saunders.

Health Promotion Considerations

Strategies for Preventing Falls

In summary, basic strategies for reducing all types of falls include the following:

- Increase physical activities that enhance and maintain muscular strength, endurance, balance, and flexibility.
- Increase regular, moderate physical exercise.
- Reduce visual impairments.
- Teach and encourage proper use of aids for ambulation (cane, walker).
- Increase provider review of prescribed and over-the-counter medications.
- Increase provider screening and referral for alcohol and drug problems.
- Modify the environment to reduce or eliminate factors that can cause falls or to minimize injury if a fall occurs.

Box 20-2 | *Fall Prevention Techniques Used in Hospitals and Long-Term Care Facilities*

Patient Oriented
1. Encourage exercise to strengthen muscles and prevent weakness.
2. Use electronic alarm devices, such as Bed-Check or Ambularm.

Medications
1. Note hypnotic or sedative drugs given at night, especially to elderly or postoperative patients.
2. Avoid giving diuretics and laxatives at night.

Activities of Daily Living
1. Assist patient to void q 4 hr.
2. Check for proper slippers and footwear (nonskid footwear).
3. Keep patient's belongings close to bed.
4. Provide rehabilitation training to improve functional ability.

Environment Oriented
1. Relocate patients with high fall risk to rooms close to nurses' station or in hallway.
2. Place nurse call light system within reach (e.g., pinned to pillow).
3. Teach patient and family about use of call light system, bed controls, bathroom facility, and movable furniture.
4. Use bed rails judiciously; half rails best.
5. Keep bed in low position (ideally 14"-20" above the floor, including the mattress).
6. Keep room light on, illumination bright and even.
7. Place TV controls within reach.
8. Keep rooms and hallways free of clutter.
9. Carpet all hard surfaces. Use nonskid wax.
10. Clean up spills, including urine.
11. Lock all equipment with wheels.
12. Keep equipment on one side of hallway.
13. Maintain equipment in good repair.
14. Place night-light in rooms.
15. Place safety (grab) bars in bathroom and hall.
16. Install higher-seated lounge chairs and toilets, or use bedside commodes. Remove wheels from bedside commodes. Place safety posters in room to encourage patients to ask for help.

Patient Education
1. Hand out safety brochure to patient and family on admission.
2. Teach patient about safety and equipment; proper use of assistive devices.
3. Encourage patient to request help.
4. Encourage use of bathroom and corridor handrails.
5. Teach transfer from bed to chair.

Nursing Assessment
1. Perform assessment at admission and throughout hospital stay.
2. Assign safety risk.
3. Make frequent rounds/checks/observations.

Other
1. Monitor falls, watch for trends, and conduct in-service training when trend emerges.
2. Have staff move slowly around ambulatory, unsteady patients.

Adapted from Chenitz, W.C., Kussman, H.L., & Stone, J.T. (1991). Preventing falls. In W.C. Chenitz, J.T. Stone, & S.A. Salisbury (Eds.), *Clinical gerontological nursing* (pp. 309-328). Philadelphia: Saunders.

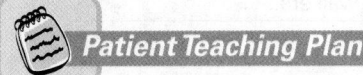 *Patient Teaching Plan*

Methods for Getting Up After a Fall: Instructions for the Patient

The Roll
1. Roll onto your right side.
2. Bend the right knee.
3. Lever upward to the kneeling position by pressing down on the right forearm.
4. Reach out with the left arm to a nearby chair or bed.
5. With a twist of the trunk, pull yourself into a sitting position.
6. Sit on the chair or bed to recover.

The Crawl
1. Roll to a prone position.
2. Get up on all fours.
3. Crawl to a sturdy couch, chair, or bed and place your hands on it.

4. Bring one foot forward, putting the foot flat on the floor.
5. Pull yourself up to a standing position.
6. Sit on the chair or bed to recover.

The Shuffle
1. Pull yourself to a sitting position on the floor.
2. Shuffle on the buttocks to a nearby piece of furniture.
3. Pull yourself up onto your knees directly in front of the item of furniture.
4. Stand up.

The Stair Shuffle
1. Pull yourself to a sitting position on the floor.
2. Shuffle on the buttocks to the stairs.
3. Gradually move up and backward to a stair height suitable for standing.
4. Grab onto the handrail and pull up.

Data from Chenitz, W.C., Kussman, H.L., & Stone, J.T. (1991). Preventing falls. In W.C. Chenitz, J.T. Stone, & S.A. Salisbury (Eds.), *Clinical gerontological nursing* (pp. 321-322). Philadelphia: Saunders.

There are several ways to get up after a fall in the home, as shown in the Patient Teaching Plan on p. 308. These techniques should be practiced by the potential faller to ensure confidence in managing the problem. If none of the methods is possible, a person who is at risk for falling would be wise to have a call system to obtain help from others. Devices worn around the neck that can send signals to a control center are very effective and provide a feeling of well-being for the potential faller. In addition, having a person or agency call every day can provide reassurance.

Key Points

- The risk of injury from falls is highest in people over age 65, and falls are the most frequent cause of accidental injury and death among older adults.
- The U.S. Public Health Service estimates that two thirds of the deaths due to falls are preventable.
- Falls occur in older adults because of intrinsic factors, or factors related to the functioning of the individual, such as the aging process or physical illness, and extrinsic factors, or environmental factors.
- In an institutional setting, falls often occur during periods of high activity when the staff are busy.
- In about 75% of all reported falls, no injuries occur; fractures occur in about 1% to 5% of all reported falls.
- People who are at greatest risk for falls and injury are those who have fallen before and those who have multiple intrinsic risk factors.
- Older patients, particularly those who are confused, are more likely to be physically restrained than younger

patients, probably because they are thought to be at greater risk of falling.
- Restraints seldom eliminate the risk of injury and may actually cause or worsen problems.
- The Omnibus Budget Reconciliation Act (OBRA) of 1987 was enacted to protect patients from unnecessary restraint in long-term care facilities.
- A physician's order is required for restraint use, and the order must specify the duration of use and the circumstances under which the restraint may be used.
- Alternatives to using physical restraint include physical therapy, sitting and talking with patients for short periods of time, and asking staff to be responsible for wanderers in small blocks of time.
- Special care units for persons with dementia allow residents to wander in a safe environment.
- The most important intervention for falls is prevention, and the first step in preventing falls and injury is to determine who is at greatest risk.
- When a fall occurs in a hospital or long-term care facility, nurses should assess the circumstances of the fall and any injuries sustained and report the fall according to the protocol of the institution.
- When the cause of a fall is determined, steps should be taken to remove or correct the cause.
- Because most people who fall have multiple risk factors, fall prevention usually requires individualized care plans.
- Remove restraints for at least 10 minutes every 2 hours.

 Go to your Companion CD-ROM for a Pharmacology Tutorial, Audio Glossary, and 3-D animations.

evolve   Be sure to visit the companion Evolve site at http://evolve.elsevier.com/Linton/ for WebLinks and additional online resources.

REVIEW QUESTIONS *Choose the best answer.*

1. Of all falls among older adults, what percentage results in serious injury such as concussions or fractures?
   1. Less than 10%
   2. 25%
   3. 40%
   4. 65%

2. Of the following, which is the strongest predictor of falling among residents of an assisted living facility?
   1. A history of falling
   2. A diagnosis of heart disease
   3. Recent weight loss
   4. Urinary incontinence

3. Which statement is true regarding the use of restraints?
   1. Anything that restricts movement and cannot be released by the patient is a restraint.
   2. Restraints greatly reduce the risk of injury.
   3. Side rails have been found to be the safest means of preventing falls.
   4. Restraints must be removed once each shift for exercise and to assess skin and circulation.

4. Psychotropic drugs used to control agitation may contribute to falls because they often cause:
   1. Hallucinations and delusions
   2. Constipation
   3. Orthostatic hypotension
   4. Insomnia

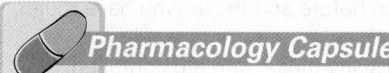 http://evolve.elsevier.com/Linton/

Objectives

After reading and studying this chapter, you should be able to:

1. Describe common problems associated with immobility.
2. Discuss the impact of exercise and positioning on preventing complications related to immobility.
3. Identify the risk factors for pressure ulcers.
4. Describe the stages of pressure ulcers.
5. Describe methods of preventing and treating pressure ulcers.
6. Discuss the effects of immobility on respiratory status, nutrition, and elimination.

Key Terms

Be sure to check out the bonus material on the Companion CD-ROM, including selected audio pronunciations.

active exercise (p. 312)
contracture (kŏn-TRĂK-chŭr, p. 314)
erythema (ĕr-ĭ-THĒ-mă, p. 315)
immobility (p. 310)
isometric exercise (ī-sō-MĔT-rĭk, p. 314)
passive exercise (p. 312)
pressure ulcer (ŬL-sĕr, p. 314)
range-of-motion exercise (p. 313)
shearing forces (p. 315)

Immobility (the inability to move) is a restriction imposed on all or part of the body. People become immobilized for various reasons, including physical factors such as joint disease, paralysis, or pain and psychological factors such as depression or fear. Sometimes immobilization is beneficial. Therapeutic reasons for immobility include (1) to obtain relief from pain and prevent further injury of a part, as in a fractured bone; (2) to reduce the workload of the heart in a cardiac condition; (3) to promote healing and repair; and (4) to reverse the effects of gravity, as in abdominal hernias and prolapsed organs.

Immobility can have a profound impact on both the mind and the body. Psychosocial effects may include depression, fear, anxiety, social withdrawal, apathy, loss of financial and personal independence, and a feeling that one's life has no meaning. Almost every body system can be affected by immobility, depending on the extent and time of immobilization.

The physiologic effects of immobility are described in Table 21-1.

Common aging changes, combined with common medical conditions, place the older adult at risk for immobility and its consequences. Examples of physical changes with age are decreased flexibility and strength and changes in posture and gait. In addition, older adults typically have one or more chronic illnesses that increase the likelihood of immobilization. Examples of such medical conditions are arthritis, stroke, Parkinson's disease, cardiovascular disease, anemia, pulmonary disease, and foot deformities. Pain associated with chronic disease such as arthritis also may be a factor leading to immobility in older adults. Drugs that cause drowsiness, hypotension, vertigo, or loss of sensory function can affect mobility as well.

Pharmacology Capsule

Drugs that cause drowsiness, hypotension, vertigo, or loss of sensory function can impair mobility.

Psychosocial changes that can impair mobility include depression, dementia, bereavement, lack of motivation, fear of falling, isolation, and loss of friends. The older person's environment also can promote or hinder mobility. An unsafe home setting, hospitalization, or institutionalization, for example, may be associated with reduced activity. The older person who is hospitalized may quickly become debilitated and dependent as a result of the combined effects of inactivity, pain, drugs, various therapies such as bed rest or traction, and an unfamiliar environment.

The impact of immobilization on an individual depends on the duration, degree, and type of mobility limitation. Immobility begins a vicious cycle that can lead to an ever-increasing loss of independence for patients. As they become less able to move, they become more dependent. As they become more dependent, they are less able to care for themselves, which in turn leads to an increasing number of adverse effects from immobility.

Whatever the reason for resting a part or all of the body, measures must be taken to manage the adverse

| Table 21-1 | *Consequences of Immobility of Body Systems* |

BODY SYSTEM	CONSEQUENCES
Musculoskeletal	Thickening of joint capsule; loss of smoothness of cartilage surface; decreased flexibility of connective tissues; changes similar to osteoarthritis—joint contractures, demineralization of bone, bone loss; atrophy and shortening of muscle; decrease in muscle strength; decreased muscle oxidative capacity; decline in aerobic capacity
Pulmonary	Arterial oxygen desaturation; increased hypostatic pooling; increased risk of atelectasis and infection
Cardiovascular	Decreased cardiac output and stroke volume; increased peripheral resistance; net loss of total body water and total blood volume
Integumentary	Pressure ulcers
Gastrointestinal	General weakening of muscles, causing altered colonic motility, constipation
Urinary	Increased nitrogen, phosphorus, total sulfur, sodium, potassium, and calcium excretion; renal insufficiency; decreased glomerular filtration rate; loss of ability to concentrate urine; lower creatinine clearance
Metabolic	Decreased basal metabolic rate; increased storage of fat or carbohydrate; negative nitrogen and calcium metabolic balance due to decreased protein and calcium intake; decreased glucose tolerance; metabolic alkalosis
Sensory	Decreased sensory stimulation (kinesthetic, visual, auditory, tactile); decreased social interaction; changes in affect, cognition, and perception

Modified from Chenitz, W.C., Stone, J.T., & Salisbury, S.A. (1991). *Clinical gerontological nursing* (p. 234). Philadelphia: Saunders.

 Health Promotion Considerations

Promoting Independence in Self-Care

Regaining independence in self-care activities requires the collaboration of the physical and occupational therapist, nurse, patient, and family. A rehabilitation plan is designed for the patient by the physical, occupational, and speech therapists, which is then implemented by the nursing staff and family. The plan is developed after thorough assessment of the patient's mobility and motor skills. Rehabilitation seeks to help patients relearn lost skills and compensate for temporary or permanent losses.

As mobility improves and each new skill is demonstrated, the patient practices with ongoing support and encouragement from the nursing staff and family. Families need to be incorporated into all teaching so that they understand how to support independence rather than dependence. Providing extra time for activities is essential. Most motivated patients with moderate impairments can relearn the skills needed for basic activities of daily living.

Assistive devices play a major role in regaining self-care independence because accomplishing basic tasks with limited mobility or impaired motor skills is both challenging and frustrating. A wide variety of devices exist to assist patients with eating and dressing, and the nurse can help the patient and family think of simple modifications that can promote independence, such as slip-on shoes, Velcro closures, loose pullover shirts, and elastic-waisted pants. Patients are encouraged to dress in simple workout-type clothes rather than pajamas and gowns as soon as active rehabilitation is started.

Adapted from Phipps, W., Monahan, F., Sands, J., Marek, J., & Neighbors, M. (2003). *Medical-surgical nursing: Health and illness perspectives* (7th ed.), St. Louis: Mosby.

effects of immobility. You can prevent the vicious cycle of events from the beginning by helping patients maintain normal functioning as much as possible and for as long as possible (see Nursing Care Plan: Preventing Hazards of Immobility on p. 312). Once patients begin to suffer the ill effects of immobility, therapeutic interventions must be implemented immediately. The health care team must work together to develop a plan of care that includes preventive and therapeutic measures that address individual patients' needs. Remember that the patient and family are central members of the health care team. If able, they should participate in care planning. The Health Promotion Considerations box above discusses how the family and the health care team can collaborate to support patients' self-care as they regain their independence.

NURSING ASSESSMENT AND INTERVENTION

A thorough assessment of the patients' needs and limitations is essential to planning interventions. Data collected by the licensed practical nurse make an important contribution to the assessment. Physicians may write specific orders related to immobility, or it may be up to the nurse to carry out independent measures

NURSING CARE PLAN

Preventing Hazards of Immobility

ASSESSMENT

Health History: A 90-year-old retired general lives alone in the assisted living section of a senior retirement community. He has multiple medical conditions and has become increasingly frail. He has fallen three times, with the last fall resulting in a serious knee injury. While recovering from this injury, he has been instructed to use a walker or wheelchair and to avoid full weight bearing. Therefore he was moved to the nursing home area until he can again care for himself. In the nursing home, he has been irritable and insists on caring for himself. He attempts to transfer himself without assistance by bearing weight on one leg. On several occasions he has been unable to delay urination until he could get help. He eats very little other than toast at breakfast and is drinking little fluid.

Physical Examination: Blood pressure, 94/52; pulse, 88; respirations, 18. Height 5'10"; weight 140 lb. Muscle atrophy and weakness in all extremities. Reddened areas noted on elbows and sacrum. Urine dark with strong odor.

Nursing Diagnosis	Goals and Outcome Criteria	Interventions
Risk for Falls related to weakness	The patient will remain safe from falls during his recovery.	Ask patient to request help with transferring. Arrange room for easy movement in wheelchair. Assist with active range-of-motion exercises for unaffected limbs. Suggest possible physical therapy referral to strengthen upper body and weight-bearing leg.
Risk for Infection (Urinary) related to low fluid intake and concentrated urine	The patient's daily fluid intake will be at least 1200 mL. The patient's urine will be clear and light in color.	Explain the need to increase fluid intake to prevent urinary tract infections. Determine preferred liquids and make them available. Instruct CNA to offer 3 ounces of fluids hourly while the patient is awake and to record intake. Report foul urine odor.
Risk for Impaired Skin Integrity related to prolonged pressure while sitting.	Patient's skin will remain intact throughout the recovery period.	Obtain pressure-reducing pad for wheelchair. Teach patient to shift weight every 15 minutes. Plan periods of bed rest to prevent constant pressure on sacrum. Keep sacral area clean and dry.
Ineffective Coping related to loss of independence.	The patient will adapt to temporary dependence by participating in efforts to enhance his recovery and prevent complications of immobility. The patient will resume self-care activities by discharge to his home.	Explain the benefits of rehabilitation activities in relation to regaining independence. Encourage self-care within limitations. Compliment efforts.

? **CRITICAL THINKING** QUESTIONS

■ How do age-related changes increase the risk of complications of immobility?

■ Why is it important to consider both physical and emotional needs of the patient with reduced mobility?

to prevent the side effects of immobility. Nursing interventions include promoting exercise, adequate respiratory status, adequate food and fluid intake, proper elimination, and maintaining proper positioning and skin integrity (Box 21-1).

EXERCISE

Exercise is the best medicine for immobility. Exercise can be done anywhere. A well individual of any age can walk, participate in aerobic exercises, swim, engage in sports activities, garden, or do housework. Those who are ill or disabled usually can engage in some form of exercise regardless of the severity of their disease. For example, patients with fractures can tighten and relax

muscles in an immobilized extremity; debilitated patients can gradually increase their range of movement, number of movements, or resistance against movement; and patients in pain can move slowly and smoothly while breathing deeply to ease pain and anxiety.

Exercises may be **active** (performed by the patients themselves), or **passive** (movement of the patient's body performed by the therapist or nurse without assistance from the patient). Active and passive exercises may be done with the patient lying in bed, sitting in a chair, or standing upright. The exercises do not have to be done as a separate part of care. They can easily be carried out while giving other care, such as during a bed bath or other activities. Examples of bed and chair

Box 21-1 | Case Study: Immobility

Mrs. Smith is an 84-year-old woman who has resided in an intermediate care facility for 2 years. She was admitted to the facility because she had been living at home alone and had become unable to shop and cook for herself or to dress herself after sustaining a broken wrist as a result of a fall. She was incontinent of urine and was mildly confused.

Mrs. Smith had previously been quite active in the community, but in the residential home she remained confined to her room and was not interested in interacting with other people. Her daughter visited her two or three times a week.

Because Mrs. Smith preferred to stay in bed or in a chair most of the time, the nurses and other members of the interdisciplinary team were concerned about the consequences of her immobility. She had fallen many times, usually on the way to the dining room to eat. It had reached the point where she stayed in a wheelchair most of the time because she had become too weak to walk.

The team held a case conference and identified problems associated with her immobility: (1) continued falling, (2) incontinence, and (3) isolation and perhaps depression. They formulated a plan to get her up and moving while at the same time avoiding falls. Every day the nurse walked with

Mrs. Smith three times a day. The first week they walked around the bed. The second week they walked to the door and back. The third week they walked a few feet outside the door to her room. As the weeks progressed, Mrs. Smith was able to walk to the dining room at the end of the hall without falling. The nurses encouraged the in-bed and in-chair exercises to further build up her strength.

Eventually, Mrs. Smith was able to walk to the bathroom independently. The nurses worked with her to develop a regular schedule of toileting so that the number of "accidents" decreased. Because she was slightly confused and disoriented, the nurses provided gentle reminders for her to go to the bathroom. After a meal, they would guide her back to her room to use the bathroom. At other times they would stop by her room, look in, and suggest that she go to the bathroom.

With all of the increased activity, Mrs. Smith became more outgoing and involved in activities. She sat with the same group at meals and developed friendships with others around her. The nurses found that taking small steps with a walking program can have many benefits for a person of any age in any condition.

 Health Promotion Considerations

Sample Exercises

IN-BED EXERCISES

Deep breathing (slow inhalation and full exhalation)

Neck rolls (neck forward flex, backward extend, lateral flex, rotate)

Knee to chest (on back or side, bring one knee to chest, wrap arms around, hold and breathe, straighten leg slowly)

Pelvic tilts (on back, knees bent, feet flat, tuck in tummy, relax)

Bridging (on back, feet flat on bed, raise hips, lower slowly)

Head raising in prone and supine positions

Unilateral leg lifts

Foot dorsiflexion

Rolling

Prone lying

Arms straight over head of bed in supine position

Arms out to sides, palms up, in supine position

Hands behind head, elbows bent

Hands at lower back

IN-CHAIR EXERCISES

Deep breathing

Head rolls (neck forward flex, backward extend, lateral flex, rotate)

Knee to chest

Head to knees

Shoulder rolls (forward and back)

Weight shifts (hip to hip)

Hands on head, elbows out and in, lateral trunk flex-extension, trunk rotation

Leg lifts

Ankle rotation and dorsiflexion

Ankle on knee (external hip rotation, put ankle on opposite knee and lower the bent leg)

Push down on legs as if to stand, lean forward, bear weight

From Giduz, B.H., Snow, T.L., Wildman, D.L., & McConnell, E.S. (1986). *Geriatric first aid kit* (p. 5). Chapel Hill, NC: Program on Aging, University of North Carolina.

exercises are listed in the Health Promotion Considerations box above.

Range-of-Motion Exercises

Range-of-motion exercises are effective in preventing some disabilities of the musculoskeletal system as well as other systems. Each of the joints of the body has a

range of motion—that is, the limits to which the joint may be moved. Muscular activity maintains range of motion by allowing the joint to remain flexible and functional. When there is little or no movement of a joint, its structures change. Normal muscle tissue is replaced by fibrous tissue. Muscles shorten and lose their elasticity. Shortening of muscles and tendons is called a contracture. A contracture can severely and permanently limit joint movement.

The purpose of range-of-motion exercises is to put each joint that is at risk for loss of motion through its full range of motion to the highest degree possible. The major motions are rotation, flexion, extension, abduction, and adduction. The exercises may be active or passive. Range-of-motion exercises should be initiated very early in immobile patients to prevent contractures.

Isometric Exercises

Isometric exercises maintain muscle tone without moving the joint. In these exercises, the muscle is contracted and held in that position for several seconds. The muscle is then relaxed for a few seconds and contracted again. This type of exercise is especially helpful in maintaining muscle strength after a fracture.

POSITIONING

Proper positioning in a bed or chair is extremely important for preventing many of the side effects of immobility. Change the position of the patient *at least every 2 hours* to prevent undue pressure on the skin. Maintain joints in their functional positions so that they are not abnormally flexed or extended. Use foot boards, splints, and bed boards to maintain proper positioning for patients lying in bed. Foot boards keep the feet at right angles to the legs so that footdrop is avoided. Splinting the limbs keeps them straight. Using a bed board prevents curvature of the spine. In addition, placing a firm splint in the hands keeps the fingers from drawing up into a tight fist. Avoid positioning the patient with the knees and hips flexed. Picture how people look while standing and try to achieve that position while they are lying down.

SKIN INTEGRITY

Pressure ulcers are localized areas of tissue necrosis (tissue death) that develop when soft tissue is compressed between a bony prominence and an external surface or when pressure occurs in combination with shearing force and/or friction. Pressure points are areas over bony prominences such as the elbows, hips, shoulders, and sacrum (Fig. 21-1). The most frequent sites of skin breakdown are the sacrum (35%), ischial tuberosities

Management and Supervision

Preventing Complications of Immobility

CNAs need to understand how important turning, positioning, and hydration are to prevent complications of immobility. In addition, turning and properly positioning the patient relieves pressure on sensitive or painful areas, such as decubitus ulcers.

Monitor care to be sure patients are being repositioned on schedule, and that fluids are being provided. Ask CNAs to report constipation, incontinence, or diarrhea if it occurs so that comfort measures can be provided, skin care interventions initiated, or additional fluids administered. Pain, pressure sores, emotional confusion or depression, and other problems should be reported as well. Effective delegation requires open lines of communication among all members of the health care team.

FIGURE **21-1** Possible locations of pressure ulcers.

(16%), heels (11%), trochanters (7%), ankles (3%), and scapulae (2%). The National Pressure Ulcer Advisory Panel prefers the term *pressure ulcers* for what are commonly called "bed sores," "decubitus ulcers," or "decubiti." The word *decubitus* means "lying down," and an ulcer is a lesion produced by the sloughing of necrotic, inflammatory tissue (Fig. 21-2). Thus a decubitus ulcer is an open wound that is associated with lying in bed. However, skin breakdown can just as easily develop in patients who are sitting for a long period of time, as a result of pressure against blood vessels.

Development of Pressure Ulcers

An area of erythema (redness) is the beginning of a pressure ulcer and a sign that capillaries in the area have become congested because of impaired blood flow. Erythema can occur within an hour or two in a person with healthy skin and adequate circulation. It is even more likely to develop and to progress rapidly to an ulcerated stage in persons who are malnourished, obese, aged, or suffering from circulatory disease.

Factors in addition to immobility that contribute to the development of pressure ulcers are shearing forces, chemical irritants such as urine, sedation, and poor nutrition. Shearing forces exert a downward and forward pressure on tissues underlying the skin. Shearing action occurs when a patient slumps down while sitting in bed or in a chair; it also can occur when boosting a patient up in bed.

FIGURE **21-2** Stage IV pressure ulcer, with full-thickness involvement of all soft tissue.

Pressure ulcers are expensive to treat, result in longer hospital stays, increase the likelihood of placement in a long-term care facility, and increase mortality. Therefore it is important to prevent their development whenever possible. *Nursing care is a major factor in pressure ulcer prevention.*

Preventing Pressure Ulcers

The first step in prevention of pressure ulcers is to identify patients who are at risk for developing them. The Norton scale is a useful instrument for identifying those at risk (Fig. 21-3). The scores for all five categories are added. If the total score is greater than 14, there is little risk of pressure ulcer development. If the score is less than 14, there is significant risk for pressure ulcer development. Any patient with a score of less than 14 needs a formal pressure ulcer prevention program started as soon as the risk is recognized. The skin of "at risk" patients should be assessed and documented every day.

A pressure ulcer prevention protocol consists of the following:

1. In accordance with a *written* schedule, reposition the bed patient *at least* every 2 hours (more often if redness persists).
2. To reduce the risk of pressure ulcers, position patients so that they are not resting on pressure points of the skin.
3. Teach wheelchair patients to shift their weight every 15 minutes if able. Patients who cannot do this should be repositioned at least hourly.
4. Keep bed linens dry, smooth, and free of wrinkles.
5. Gently cleanse the skin when soiled and at regular intervals, using warm water and a mild cleansing agent.
6. Use moisturizers, lubricants, protective films, barriers, and dressings to reduce friction and shearing.
7. Avoid friction when moving patients to prevent damage to the uppermost layers of the skin.
8. When the patient is in bed, keep the head lowered as much as possible to reduce shearing force caused by sliding down in bed.
9. Use a special mattress or bed designed to reduce pressure, such as an egg crate–type foam (mini-

NORTON SCALE

		PHYSICAL CONDITION		MENTAL CONDITION		ACTIVITY		MOBILITY		INCONTINENT		
		Good	4	Alert	4	Ambulant	4	Full	4	Not	4	
		Fair	3	Apathetic	3	Walk/help	3	Slightly limited	3	Occasional	3	
		Poor	2	Confused	2	Chairbound	2	Very limited	2	Usually/urine	2	TOTAL
		Very bad	1	Stupor	1	Bedrest	1	Immobile	1	Doubly	1	SCORE
Name	Date											

FIGURE **21-3** Norton scale for identification of those at risk for the development of pressure ulcers.

mum 2 inches thick), static air, alternating air, gel, fluidized air, or water mattress (Fig. 21-4).

10. Apply sheepskin boots to prevent shearing forces to the feet, and use pillows or wedges to prevent heel pressure.

11. Protect the skin from moisture (e.g., absorbent pads or briefs for incontinence).

12. Institute measures that enhance patient mobility, such as installing trapeze bars.

13. Instruct the patient and family about risk factors and strategies for preventing pressure ulcers.

Remember that the best preventive measure is frequent position change. Massage is *not* recommended for pressure points. Any kind of massage around or on a reddened area of skin can damage fragile capillaries. In addition, rubber rings should *not* be used to elevate heels or sacral areas. Rings cause a concentrated area of pressure that puts patients at higher risk for developing pressure ulcers. *Remember: No massage on reddened skin, and no rings!* One other important factor that must be considered is the patient's nutritional status. Adequate nutrients are essential to maintain or restore skin integrity.

A

B

FIGURE **21-4** Specialty beds prevent pressure on bony prominences. **A,** KinAir III beds provide controlled air suspension. **B,** FluidAir Elite beds use airflow and bead fluidization. Both are covered with tough GORE-TEX fabric that is waterproof and serves as a barrier to bacteria. (Courtesy Kinetic Concepts, Inc., San Antonio, TX.)

If pressure ulcers develop despite all preventive measures, assess the stage and describe it precisely. Proper documentation helps evaluate the effectiveness of treatment and progress toward healing and repair. It is especially important to document skin condition and the presence of pressure ulcers on admission to a health care facility.

Stages of Pressure Ulcers

Pressure ulcers are classified into six stages. Figure 21-5 illustrates stages I to IV.

Suspected Deep Tissue Injury. Damage to underlying soft tissue causes purple or maroon discoloration or a blood-filled blister.

Stage I. The major characteristic of stage I is erythema (redness) that does not blanch when pressed. Before stage I begins, a finger pressed on a reddened area causes temporary blanching (whiteness at the point of pressure), followed by a return of the erythema when the finger is removed. In stage I, the redness does not fade when the finger is removed. The color ranges from red to the dusky blue called *cyanosis.* The area of pressure is irregular and ill-defined and reflects the shape of the object creating the pressure or the bony prominence underlying the skin. Pain and tenderness may be present, with swelling and hardening of the tissue and associated heat. At this stage, there is little destruction of tissue and the condition is reversible.

Stage II. In stage II, there is some skin loss in the epidermis and dermis. A shallow ulcer develops and appears blistered, cracked, or abraded (scraped). The ulcer is surrounded by a broad, irregular, and painful reddened area that is warmer than normal.

Stage III. Stage III is characterized by full-thickness skin loss involving damage or necrosis of the dermis and subcutaneous tissue. There is a crater-like sore with a distinct outer margin formed as the epidermis thickens and rolls over the edge toward the ulcer base. The wound may be infected, and it is usually open and draining, with a loss of fluid and protein. The patient may have fever, dehydration, anemia, and leukocytosis (increased white blood cells in the blood).

Stage IV. In stage IV, there is full-thickness skin loss with extensive destruction of the deeper underlying muscle and possibly of the bone tissue. The ulcer is usually extensively infected and may appear black, with exudation, foul odor, and purulent drainage.

Unstageable. In this stage, slough or eschar covers the base of a full-thickness ulcer. The true stage cannot be determined until at least part of the wound base can be examined.

Treatment

The first step in treating pressure ulcers is to continue all preventive measures. A pressure ulcer cannot heal unless measures are taken to relieve the pressure that initially caused it. Numerous treatments are used to promote wound healing. These treatments vary from

Stage I

Epidermis
Dermis
Subcutaneous fat
Muscle
Bone

Non-blanching erythema
of intact skin; the heralding
lesion of skin ulceration

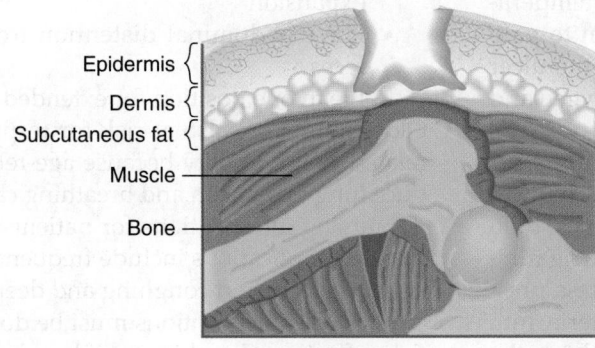

Stage II

Epidermis
Dermis
Subcutaneous fat
Muscle
Bone

Partial-thickness skin loss
involving epidermis and/or
dermis. The ulcer is superficial
and presents clinically as an
abrasion, blister, or shallow
crater.

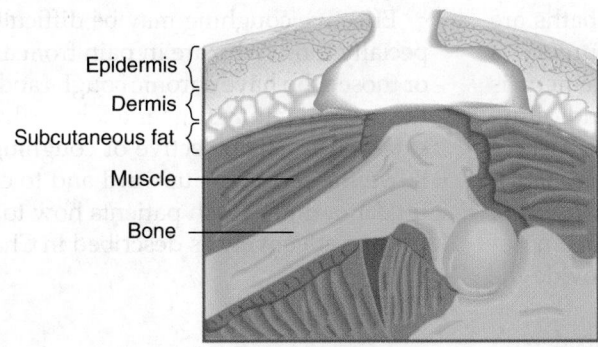

Stage III

Epidermis
Dermis
Subcutaneous fat
Muscle
Bone

Full-thickness skin loss
involving damage or necrosis
of subcutaneous tissue, which
may extend down to, but not
through, the underlying fascia.
The ulcer presents clinically as
a deep crater with or without
undermining of adjacent tissue.

Stage IV

Epidermis
Dermis
Subcutaneous fat
Muscle
Bone

Full-thickness skin loss with
extensive destruction, tissue
necrosis, or damage to muscle,
bone, or supporting structures
(e.g., tendon, joint capsule, etc.)

FIGURE 21-5 Classification of pressure ulcers.

institution to institution because research has not yet shown one method of treatment to be the best.

In general, stages I and II pressure ulcers should be cleaned with mild soap and water or normal saline. Avoid using pastes, creams, ointments, and powder because they may promote infection in the ulcer. Also avoid using alcohol, antiseptics, disinfectants, topical and oral antibiotics, and massage because their effectiveness has not been proved and they may actually cause harm. The use of a heat lamp is not recommended because a rise in temperature increases the metabolic demands of the tissue and places additional stress on the affected area.

The most effective dressing for a stage I or II pressure ulcer is one that provides a moist environment and maintains a temperature close to body temperature. All wound covers should allow oxygen to pass through. Wound healing is enhanced when the ulcer and surrounding tissues can freely take up oxygen and eliminate carbon dioxide.

Stages III and IV pressure ulcers require more extensive treatment and supportive care. Mechanical devices used for irrigation include spray bottles, bulb and piston syringes, and other specialized irrigating devices including a Water Pik. Note that excess pressure can cause trauma and may force bacteria into the wound. The Water Pik should be used only on the lowest setting. Débridement of necrotic tissue is usually necessary to promote granulation of new, healthy tissue. Wet-to-dry dressings and whirlpool baths are used for small amounts of débridement. Surgery is preferred for very advanced cases. Débridement is sufficient when the ulcer bed appears pink, indicating healthy granulation tissue. Supportive care consists of measures to treat anemia, dehydration, protein depletion, and infection. Nutritional intervention consists of oral supplements high in protein and vitamins, nasogastric feedings, or parenteral nutrition to provide the additional nutrients necessary for healing.

Stages II, III, and IV are normally colonized with bacteria. Good wound care usually prevents the bacteria from causing a clinical infection. Topical broad-spectrum antibiotics may be ordered if the wound fails to heal despite good care. If there is evidence of widespread infection, systemic antibiotics are indicated.

In addition to preventive measures, three major principles of wound management should be followed in the treatment of pressure ulcers:

1. Keep the area clean.
2. Promote the formation of granulation tissue by removing debris and dead tissue.
3. Ensure adequate nutritional intake for wound healing.

RESPIRATORY STATUS

Oxygen and carbon dioxide are exchanged in the thin, moist mucous membrane that lines the airway passages and the alveoli. Most healthy people take about six to eight deep, sighing breaths every hour. Sighs help keep the lungs expanded and move secretions upward along the air passages. When a person remains immobile or does not take deep breaths, thick secretions can accumulate and pool in the lower respiratory structures. These secretions interfere with the normal exchange of gases, can cause areas of the lung to collapse (atelectasis), and provide an environment for growth of pathogens. A lung infection associated with immobility is called *hypostatic pneumonia.*

Individuals who are at risk for impaired gas exchange related to immobility include those who:

- Are given drugs that depress respirations, such as general anesthetic agents, narcotics, or sedatives
- Have tight binders or bandages that limit chest expansion
- Have abdominal distention from gas, fluid, or feces
- Lie in one position for extended periods of time

Older adults are also at risk for respiratory problems related to immobility because age-related changes reduce lung expansion and breathing capacity.

Nursing interventions for patients at risk for respiratory complications include frequent turning and position changes and coughing and deep-breathing exercises. These interventions must be done every 2 hours to be effective. Coughing and deep-breathing exercises are done at the same time to allow for periods of rest and to obtain the best results.

Effective coughing may be difficult for patients, especially those who are in pain from a surgical incision or those who have chronic coughs and are worried that the coughing may trigger a long, exhaustive coughing experience. The objective of coughing is to gradually move the secretions upward and to cough them out a little at a time. Teach patients how to cough and deep breathe effectively as described in Chapter 17.

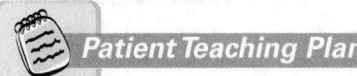

Patient Teaching Plan

Coughing and Deep Breathing

- Coughing and deep breathing are most effective in a sitting position.
- Support your abdomen to minimize discomfort while coughing and deep breathing (especially if you have a surgical incision and sutures).
- Avoid a very large, explosive cough that can be painful or cause exhaustion.
- To breathe deeply, expand the lower chest and use the abdominal muscles and diaphragm.
- Concentrate on exhaling slowly while pursing your lips.
- Focus on how much air you can exhale rather than the force with which you exhale it.
- The most effective technique for clearing secretions from the lower parts of the air passages is to take a single deep breath and follow it with three consecutive coughs, trying to clear all the air from the lungs with each cough.

To evaluate the effectiveness of nursing interventions, monitor the patient's respiratory status. Count the respiratory rate, observe the respiratory effort and chest movement, and listen for crackles in the lung fields.

FOOD AND FLUID INTAKE

In relation to food and fluid intake, the most common problem associated with immobility is *anorexia* (loss of appetite). Factors that contribute to anorexia are worry, depression, anxiety about dependence on others, and decreased metabolic needs resulting from inactivity. *Hypoproteinemia* (protein deficiency) can develop in immobilized patients.

Immobilized patients also may have inadequate fluid intake. Getting up for a drink of water may be too difficult and time-consuming for inactive individuals, or they may not think to drink liquids regularly. Older people are particularly prone to becoming dehydrated from an inadequate fluid intake, resulting in complications such as confusion, constipation, or urinary tract infection.

Keep accurate records of patients' dietary and fluid intakes. Small, frequent meals may be more acceptable than three large meals for patients with anorexia. Dietary supplements that are high in protein content also may be encouraged. Offer fluids, even small sips of water, juice, or other liquids, at least every hour. Fluids need to be within reach so that patients may have easy access to them if they are able to drink without help. Encourage family members to offer fluids while they are visiting.

ELIMINATION

Constipation

One of the most common disorders associated with inactivity and immobility is constipation. Factors that contribute to constipation in the immobile patient include changes in the usual routine and environment, inability to defecate on a bedpan because of embarrassment or discomfort, and weakened muscle tone. Also, many medications cause constipation by slowing intestinal motility. Constipated individuals may strain to defecate, causing an increase in intra-abdominal pressure. This is called the *Valsalva maneuver* or vasovagal reflex, and it can lead to cardiovascular alterations and even to lightheadedness and fainting. The vasovagal reflex can be especially problematic in older persons, whose circulation may be somewhat impaired.

Confused patients may ignore the normal urge to have a bowel movement. If the impulse is ignored for a considerable time, the natural urge to defecate can diminish and eventually disappear.

Long-standing constipation can result in a fecal impaction. *Fecal impaction* is the presence of hardened or puttylike feces in the rectum and sigmoid colon. If the condition is not relieved, intestinal obstruction can occur. Symptoms of a fecal impaction include painful defecation, a feeling of fullness in the rectum, abdominal distention, and sometimes cramps and watery stool. The presence of diarrhea does not mean that a fecal impaction has been removed, because the liquid fecal material may flow around the hardened mass.

When an impaction develops, the mass of feces must be broken up with a gloved finger (a physician's order usually is needed). Before digital removal of the mass, it may be helpful to give an oil retention enema to soften the mass. In addition, an analgesic may be given 1 hour before digital removal of an impaction.

Inactivity, medications, decreased fluid intake, and lack of adequate fiber in the diet all contribute to constipation. A vicious cycle may begin when immobility promotes inactivity, decreased fluid intake, and poor appetite. Patients become weaker, more immobile, and less likely to eat and drink adequately. Encouraging proper foods with adequate roughage, fluids, and as much activity as possible can help prevent or relieve constipation. Whenever possible, patients should use a bedside commode or be taken to the bathroom to defecate rather than trying to use a bedpan. Laxatives should be used sparingly; however, stool softeners may be helpful if the stools are hard and difficult to pass. Patients with long-established laxative dependence may require continued laxative therapy during the period of immobility.

Urinary Incontinence

The urinary system functions best when the body is upright. Urine flows from the kidney downward, drawn by the pull of gravity. When the body is in a reclining position, the kidney must force urine into the ureters against the pull of gravity. Urine is continually being formed in the kidney, but the peristaltic action of the ureters is not strong enough to maintain a constant flow of urine. If the body remains in a supine (lying down) position for even a few days, the flow becomes sluggish and the urine pools. This sets the stage for the development of a urinary tract infection.

Lying in bed also can cause loss of control of the urinary sphincter muscles and result in incontinence. Without the downward pressure of the full bladder against the sphincter muscles, there is less awareness of the need to void. The result can be bladder distention with an overflow or a dribbling of urine that the patient cannot control.

Older persons who have problems with mobility may have functional incontinence because they are unable to respond to the urge to void in time. The bladder is usually fuller when the urge to void occurs, so there is

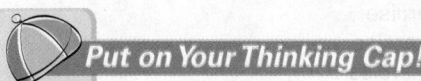

Put on Your Thinking Cap!

With pencil and paper in hand, note the time. Now, sit perfectly still for 10 minutes. At the end of that time, note what sensations and thoughts you experienced. When the time was up, what was the first thing you did? Discuss what a nurse could have done to make you more comfortable. Compare your experience with that of a patient who is immobilized.

less time to get to the bathroom. In addition, their bodies may not be able to move quickly enough because of the slowed reflexes and responses associated with older age or infirmities associated with chronic illness.

The most effective way to prevent urinary incontinence associated with immobility is to set up a toileting program. Patients should have scheduled toiletings with adjustments in schedule based on the patients' voiding patterns. If voiding patterns cannot be assessed, patients should at the very least be taken to the bathroom or commode or offered a bedpan every 2 hours during the waking hours. Some individuals restrict fluids at certain times of the day, especially after dinner and through the night to avoid nighttime incontinence. However, studies have been inconclusive regarding the effectiveness of limiting fluids. Incontinence is covered in greater detail in Chapter 23.

 Put on Your Thinking Cap!

Observe a person during class, church, a movie, or other situation where people are expected to stay seated. Note the number of movements by that person in a 5-minute period. Identify the therapeutic value of those motions.

 Key Points

- The psychological effects of immobility may include depression, fear, anxiety, social withdrawal, apathy, loss of financial and personal independence, and lack of meaningful existence.
- Some of the most problematic physiologic side effects of immobility are pressure ulcers, respiratory problems, impaired nutrition, constipation, and urinary tract infection and incontinence.
- Exercise is the best medicine for immobility.
- Exercises may be active (performed by the patient) or passive (movement of the patient's body performed by the therapist or nurse without assistance from the patient).

- Pressure ulcers are expensive to treat, result in longer hospital stays, increase the likelihood of placement in a residential care facility, and increase mortality.
- Good nursing care is a major factor in pressure ulcer prevention.
- The best preventive measure for pressure ulcers is frequent position changes.
- The major principles of pressure ulcer wound management are the following: (1) clean the area, (2) promote the formation of granulation tissue, and (3) ensure adequate nutritional intake for wound healing.
- Especially in older adults, immobility can contribute to respiratory problems, including impaired gas exchange, atelectasis, and hypostatic pneumonia.
- Factors that contribute to respiratory complications of immobility include drugs that depress respirations; tight binders or bandages that limit chest expansion; abdominal distention from gas, fluid, or feces; and lying in one position for extended periods of time.
- Nursing interventions for patients at risk for respiratory complications include frequent turning and position changes and encouraging coughing and deep-breathing exercises.
- The most common problem associated with immobility in relation to nutrition is anorexia (loss of appetite).
- Immobility causes constipation by causing a change in the usual routine and environment, an inability to defecate on a bedpan because of embarrassment or discomfort, and a weakening of muscle tone.
- Immobility can promote a loss of control of the urinary sphincter muscles, resulting in incontinence.
- The most effective way to prevent urinary incontinence associated with immobility is to set up a toileting program.
- Urinary stasis increases the risk of urinary tract infections.

 Go to your Companion CD-ROM for a Pharmacology Tutorial, Audio Glossary, and 3-D animations.

evolve   Be sure to visit the companion Evolve site at http://evolve.elsevier.com/Linton/ for WebLinks and additional online resources.

REVIEW QUESTIONS *Choose the best answer.*

1. A patient who sustained a head injury has not regained consciousness. The nurse moves the patient's joints through their normal movements twice a day. This intervention is called:

   1. Isometric exercise
   2. Active exercise
   3. Passive exercise
   4. Isotonic exercise

2. The home health nurse is teaching family members how to move a patient up in bed by using a draw sheet to prevent:

   1. Tissue trauma from shearing force
   2. Strain on the caregiver
   3. Disturbing the bed linens
   4. Extension contractures of the spine

3. The nursing care plan for an immobilized patient includes the following interventions. Which one is specifically intended to maintain skin integrity?

   1. Keep joints in functional positions.
   2. Reposition patient at least every 2 hours.
   3. Perform range-of-motion exercises twice daily.
   4. Give at least eight 8-ounce glasses of fluids each day.

4. During a bed bath, you observe a reddened area over the sacrum. You should:

   1. Document erythema and instruct nursing assistants to keep the patient off his back
   2. Gently massage the reddened area with skin lotion to provide protective moisture

3. Place a round inflatable cushion under the patient's buttocks to relieve pressure on the sacrum
4. Position the patient on one side and use a heat lamp to stimulate circulation to the area

5. Instructions in effective coughing for the patient after abdominal surgery should include the following:
    1. Try not to use the abdominal muscles during coughing and deep-breathing exercises
    2. Assume a comfortable side-lying position to reduce strain on the incision
    3. Exhale as forcefully and as long as you can
    4. Take one deep breath and then cough three times, trying to clear all air from the lungs

6. A postoperative patient reports that she was straining to have a bowel movement when she became lightheaded. You should suspect:
    1. The Valsalva maneuver
    2. Internal hemorrhage
    3. Dehydration
    4. Wound dehiscence

7. What is the effect of immobility on the urinary tract?
    1. Decreased urine production by the kidneys
    2. Pooling of urine in the urinary system
    3. Increased blood flow to kidneys
    4. Increased bladder sensitivity to fullness

Objectives

After reading and studying this chapter, you should be able to:

1. Define delirium and dementia.
2. Identify the causes of acute confusion.
3. Explain the differences between delirium and dementia.
4. Discuss nursing assessment and interventions related to delirium and dementia.

Key Terms

 Be sure to check out the bonus material on the Companion CD-ROM, including selected audio pronunciations.

delirium (dĕ-LĬR-ē-ŭm, p. 322)
dementia (dĕ-MĔN-shē-ă, p. 322)

Confusion is a symptom experienced by various patients under varying circumstances. Older people sometimes experience confusion as a first symptom of disease. People of all ages may experience confusion under certain circumstances such as high fever, critical illness, or recovery from anesthesia. Confusion may be acute, transient, or permanent. It has many causes and names and can be very difficult to manage.

The symptoms associated with confusion can be divided into two categories: (1) acute confusional states, or delirium, and (2) chronic confusion, or dementia. **Delirium** is a short-term confusional state that has a sudden onset and is typically reversible. It is more prevalent in children and older adults. **Dementia** is a syndrome that is chronic and rarely reversible. It is characterized by impairment in memory and accompanied by many other cognitive deficits. Dementia is most prevalent in older adults. Delirium and dementia have been called *organic brain syndrome, acute brain syndrome, chronic brain syndrome, senile dementia,* and *senility.*

DELIRIUM

Delirium is characterized by disturbances in consciousness that impair a person's awareness of the environment. People with delirium may have difficulty focusing or paying attention, so that they are easily distracted. It may be difficult to engage people with delirium in a conversation, and questions often must be repeated several times. Impaired recent memory is common, along with disorientation and language problems. Speech may be slurred and disjointed, with aimless repetitions. Individuals may misinterpret what is going on in the environment and may develop delusional thinking and experience hallucinations. For example, they may think that the banging of a door is a gunshot and may develop the delusion that someone is trying to steal from them. There can be a disturbance in the sleep-wake cycle. A delirious person may alternate between hyperactivity and hypoactivity. The level of consciousness may fluctuate from drowsiness to stupor or coma. At the other extreme, the individual may be very alert and agitated. Other symptoms include anxiety, depression, irritability, anger, apathy, or euphoria. Acute confusion begins abruptly and usually lasts a short period of time, perhaps as long as a week but rarely more than a month. However, if the underlying cause is not identified and treated, delirium can become a permanent condition, especially in older adults. The symptoms tend to fluctuate and often become worse at night.

Examples of factors that can contribute to delirium are listed in Box 22-1.

DEMENTIA

Dementia is characterized by impaired intellectual function, problem-solving ability, judgment, memory, and orientation and by inappropriate behavior, as shown in Box 22-2. There are several types of dementia with various causes and symptoms. Some examples are Alzheimer's disease, vascular dementia, Pick's disease, Huntington's disease, and Creutzfeldt-Jakob disease. Some people who have Parkinson's disease develop dementia as well. Other conditions that are associated with dementia include normal pressure hydrocephalus, subdural hematoma, brain tumors, neurosyphilis, and acquired immunodeficiency syndrome (AIDS). Dementia is not a disease itself but a clinical syndrome, a collection of symptoms that can occur with many types of diseases. The two most prevalent types of dementia are Alzheimer's disease (AD) and vascular dementia. The cause of AD is unknown, but characteristic changes in the brain include deposits of

Box 22-1 | *Systemic and Central Nervous System Causes of Delirium*

SYSTEMIC CAUSES		CENTRAL NERVOUS SYSTEM CAUSES	
Cardiovascular disease	Metabolic	Infections	Vascular
Congestive heart failure	Electrolyte and fluid	Meningitis	Transient ischemic
Dysrhythmias	imbalance	Encephalitis	attack
Cardiac infarction	Hepatic, renal, or	Septic emboli	Stroke
Hypovolemia	pulmonary failure	Neurosyphilis	Chronic subdural
Aortic stenosis	Diabetes, hyperthyroid-	Brain abscess	hematoma
Infections	ism, hypothyroidism,	Neoplasm	Vasculitis
Pneumonia	or other endocrine	Primary intracranial	Arteriosclerosis
Urinary tract infections	disorder	Metastatic	Hypertensive
Bacteremia	Nutritional deficiencies	Trauma	encephalopathy
Septicemia	Hypothermia and heat	Subdural hematoma	Subarachnoid
Medications	stroke	Extradural hematoma	hemorrhage
Alcohol	Neoplasm	Contusion	Seizure
Amphetamines	Postoperative state		Ictal and postictal
Analgesics	Poisons		states
Anticholinergics	Heavy metals		
Antidepressants	Solvents		
Antihistamines	Pesticides		
Antiparkinsonian agents	Carbon monoxide		
Cimetidine	Trauma		
Diuretics	Head injury		
Neuroleptics	Burns		
Sedatives/hypnotics	Hip fracture		

From Zisook, S., & Braff, D.L. (1986). Delirium: Recognition and management in the older patient. *Geriatrics, 41*(6), 67-78.

amyloid (a protein), neurofibrillary tangles (tangled microtubules in neurons), and a deficiency of acetylcholine (a chemical that transmits signals in the brain). These changes affect the structure and function of the neurons in the brain. Vascular dementia results from damage to brain cells caused by inadequate blood supply. Patients with vascular dementia often have had a series of small strokes that cause progressive damage.

What Does Culture Have to Do with Dementia?

Caregivers from lower socioeconomic families are more likely to be caring for older parents at an earlier age when the caregiver is employed or still has children at home.

NURSING CARE

Assessment

The first step in collecting data about a confusional state is to observe the patient's behavior and to collect data about orientation, memory, and sleep habits. Family members may be able to provide helpful information if the patient cannot. Ask when the symptoms of confusion started and whether the confusion is constant or intermittent. List any known acute or chronic illnesses and all medications the patient has been taking (including home remedies and over-the-counter drugs). Drugs that most often cause confusion include anticholinergics, digoxin, H_2-receptor blockers, benzodiazepines,

nonsteroidal anti-inflammatory drugs, and many anti-dysrhythmic and antihypertensive drugs.

These assessment data help the physician determine whether the patient is suffering from delirium or dementia. Some major differences between the clinical features of delirium and dementia are described in Table 22-1. Nursing care of delirium and dementia are addressed separately even though they have some common interventions. For tips on helping CNAs provide nursing care for patients with delirium and dementia, see the Management and Supervision box on p. 324.

Nursing Diagnoses, Goals, and Outcome Criteria: Delirium

NURSING DIAGNOSES	GOALS AND OUTCOME CRITERIA
Disturbed Thought Processes related to drugs, infection, dehydration, unfamiliar setting, sensory overload or deprivation, etc.	Improved thought processes: orientation to person, place, and time; calm, no combative behavior
Disturbed Sleep Pattern related to agitation, mood alterations, drug effects	Restoration of patient's usual sleep pattern: fewer nighttime awakenings, patient reports feeling rested
Risk for Injury related to agitation, disorientation, unfamiliar setting	Safety maintained: absence of injury

---

Box 22-2 *Diagnostic and Statistical Manual of Mental Disorders, Fourth Edition (DSM-IV-TR) Criteria for Dementia*

A. The development of multiple cognitive deficits manifested by both:
1. Memory impairment (impaired ability to learn new information or to recall previously learned information)
2. One (or more) of the following cognitive disturbances:
   a. Aphasia (language disturbance)
   b. Apraxia (impaired ability to carry out motor activities despite intact motor function)
   c. Agnosia (failure to recognize or identify objects despite intact sensory function)
   d. Disturbance in executive functioning (i.e., planning, organizing, sequencing, abstracting)
B. The cognitive deficits in criteria A1 and A2 each cause significant impairment in social or occupational functioning and represent a significant decline from a previous level of functioning.
C. The deficits do not occur exclusively during the course of delirium.

Features of Specific Dementias
Dementia of the Alzheimer's Type
The course is characterized by gradual onset and continuing cognitive decline.

   The cognitive deficits in criteria A1 and A2 are not due to any of the following:
1. Other central nervous system conditions that cause progressive deficits in memory and cognition (e.g., cerebrovascular disease, Parkinson's disease, Huntington's disease, subdural hematoma, normal-pressure hydrocephalus, brain tumor)

2. Systemic conditions that are known to cause dementia (e.g., hypothyroidism, vitamin B_{12} or folic acid deficiency, niacin deficiency, hypercalcemia, neurosyphilis, human immunodeficiency virus [HIV] infection)
3. Substance-induced conditions

Dementia Due to Other General Medical Conditions
There is evidence from the history, physical examination, or laboratory findings that the disturbance is the direct physiologic consequence of one of the following medical conditions: dementia due to HIV disease, dementia due to head trauma, dementia due to Parkinson's disease, dementia due to Huntington's disease, dementia due to Pick's disease, dementia due to Creutzfeldt-Jakob disease, dementia due to normal-pressure hydrocephalus, etc.

Vascular Dementia
Focal neurologic signs and symptoms (e.g., exaggeration of deep tendon reflexes, extensor plantar response, pseudobulbar palsy, gait abnormalities, weakness of an extremity) or laboratory evidence indicative of cerebrovascular disease (e.g., multiple infarctions involving cortex and underlying white matter) that is judged to be etiologically related to the disturbance.

Substance-Induced Persisting Dementia
There is evidence from the history, physical examination, or laboratory findings that the deficits are etiologically related to the persisting effects of substance use (e.g., a drug of abuse, a medication).

Modified with permission from American Psychiatric Association. (2000). *Diagnostic and statistical manual of mental disorders* (4th ed., Text Revision). Washington, DC: Author.

Management and Supervision

Working with Dementia Patients

Working with dementia patients can be frustrating for CNAs. The best thing the LPN/LVN can do is model good interactions with patients. Also, explain to CNAs that:
- Rudeness and uncooperative behavior are symptoms of dementia that are best managed with kindness and patience.
- Because dementia patients have memory impairments, information and instructions may have to be repeated at intervals.
- When patients resist care, let the licensed nurse know and try a different approach later.

Interventions: Delirium

When managing delirium, the physician focuses on identifying and treating the cause of the problem. During an episode of confusion, you should focus your attention on supporting the patient to provide safety and comfort and to reduce anxiety (see Nursing Care Plan: The Patient with Delirium on p. 325). Nursing care can be more effective than drugs in managing confusion.

Disturbed Thought Processes

Patients with delirium often need hospitalization. If possible, the patient should be in a private room with continuous supervision. Keep the room quiet and uncluttered to avoid agitation caused by extraneous stimuli. Lighting should be soft and diffuse to avoid shadows that may be misinterpreted and add to the patient's fears. Familiar objects such as pictures, a clock, and a large calendar placed in the room can help orient the patient to time and person (Fig. 22-1). Patients who normally wear hearing aids and glasses should be encouraged to use them.

Communication with a confused patient should be simple and direct. Anyone dealing with a delirious patient should be calm, warm, and reassuring. It is helpful if the same personnel are assigned to care for the patient. Avoid sudden movements and handle the patient gently during procedures or turning.

Patients with delirium may have frightening hallucinations that cause them to strike out, cry, or scream. The best response is to orient the patient to the reality of being sick and hospitalized and to explain that the hallucinations are not real even though they seem to be. You might say, "You are sick in the hospital, and

Table 22-1   *Clinical Features in Delirium and Dementia*

FEATURE	DELIRIUM	DEMENTIA
Duration	Few weeks to 3 months	In progress at least 1-2 years
Paranoid states	Prominent while cognitive impairment is mild or variable	More consistent with degree of impairment; less prominent paranoia
Fluctuations	Marked contrasts in levels of awareness	Not seen in such contrast; progressive decline
Persecutory delusions	Ordered and cohesive	Vague, random, contradictory
General intellectual powers	Preserved during lucid intervals	Consistent loss and decline
Affect	Intermittent fear, perplexity, or bewilderment	Flat or indifferent affect
Perceptual disturbances	Hallucinations often disturbing and very clearly defined	Hallucinations vague, fleeting, ill-defined; in many cases difficult to make a clear judgment that they exist

From Chenitz, W.C., Stone, J.T., & Salisbury, S.A. (Eds.). (1991). *Clinical gerontological nursing* (p. 485). Philadelphia: Saunders.

NURSING CARE PLAN

The Patient with Delirium

ASSESSMENT

Health History: An 81-year-old man was admitted for hip replacement surgery 2 days ago. Before his surgery he lived alone and cared for himself. He was active, alert, and independent. However, since his surgery he has been confused and at times combative with the nurses. His physician believes that he is suffering from delirium related to the anesthesia from surgery and that it should resolve within a few days.

Physical Examination: Blood pressure, 165/95; pulse, 98 with slight irregularity; respiration, 20; temperature, 97.4° F measured orally. Height, 5'7"; weight, 178 lb. Alert, disoriented to time, place, and sometimes person; combative. Awakens during the night. Dark circles around eyes. Refuses food or fluids.

Nursing Diagnosis	Goals and Outcome Criteria	Interventions
Disturbed Thought Processes related to anesthesia during surgery	The patient will have improved thought processes, as evidenced by orientation to time, place, and person and absence of combative behavior.	Place in a private room with minimal stimuli, soft lighting. Request a family member to stay with patient. Maintain consistency with the nursing staff caring for the patient. Approach and communicate with the patient in a calm, reassuring manner. Have patient use hearing aid or glasses if used previously. Reorient patient frequently and consistently. Place familiar objects in the room: pictures, clock, calendar.
Disturbed Sleep Pattern related to agitation and mood alterations	The patient will have adequate sleep and rest, as evidenced by fewer awakenings during the night, absence of dark circles around the eyes, and no complaints of fatigue.	Provide a back rub or offer milk at bedtime. Engage in soothing conversation to relax the patient. Plan activities for long periods (at least 2-4 hours) of uninterrupted sleep.
Imbalanced Nutrition: Less Than Body Requirements related to confused state and poor food intake	The patient will have adequate fluid and food intake, as evidenced by eating meals as offered and maintaining normal body weight.	Assist the patient with meals. Offer small, light meals more frequently. Ask a family member to stay with the patient during meals.

? CRITICAL THINKING QUESTIONS

- Assuming that the patient's delirium is indeed related to the anesthetic, explain how the patient's age might have played a role in his current state.

- The patient's daughter, who lives out of town, arrives for a visit. She is distressed by her father's behavior. What information would be helpful to her?

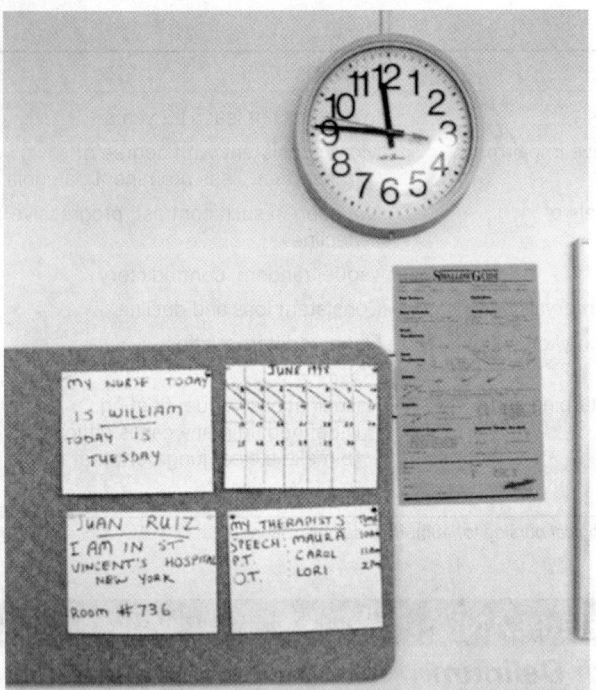

FIGURE **22-1** A clock and calendar may help orient a patient with delirium; however, they must be in a place where they can be seen easily. In addition, patients with sensory impairments should wear their glasses and/or hearing aids, if possible.

FIGURE **22-2** The presence of a family member may help calm a confused patient.

what you are seeing is part of the illness." Hallucinating patients in a delirious state need one-to-one nursing observation and repeated verbal reorientation. They need to be assured that the medical and nursing staff are helping them and keeping them safe.

Frequent orientation to the surroundings and the situation is important for patients with delirium. Orienting phrases such as "here in the hospital" or "now that it is evening" can be woven into the conversation. Keep choices to a minimum. Simple, direct statements ("Now it is time to take your bath") are better than questions ("When would you like to take a bath?"). All communication and nursing care should be carried out in a way that conveys respect and preserves the patient's dignity.

Disturbed Sleep Pattern

Sleep deprivation can cause or contribute to disorientation and confusion. Nursing measures such as giving a back rub, providing a glass of warm milk, and having a soothing conversation may help the patient relax and fall asleep. Schedule medications or treatments at times that do not interrupt nighttime sleep. The presence of a family member may help calm an agitated and confused patient (Fig. 22-2).

Risk for Injury

The patient with delirium may pull on tubes, try to get out of bed unassisted, or attempt to leave the setting. It can be challenging to protect the patient from harm without imposing excessive restrictions. Avoid using physical restraints, which tend to increase anxiety and

agitation in confused patients and often result in injuries. Rather, ask a family member to remain with the patient or assign a staff member to do so. Use common sense. Position tubes out of sight. Put the bed in low position. Postpone activities that are flexible. If there is no reason that confused patients need to stay in bed, try having them sit in chairs or even "visit" the nurses' station in a wheelchair. Avoid arguing with delirious patients. Gently explain what you are doing and why. Try to elicit their cooperation.

These nursing diagnoses are only a few that might apply to the patient with delirium. Depending on the situation, there will be different priorities.

Nursing Diagnoses, Goals, and Outcome Criteria: Dementia

NURSING DIAGNOSES	GOALS AND OUTCOME CRITERIA
Self-Care Deficit related to impaired thinking, sensory and motor dysfunction	Maximum possible independence in ADL: patient participation in bathing, grooming, feeding, toileting with assistance as needed
Imbalanced Nutrition: Less than Body Requirements related to difficulty with self-feeding, inattention	Adequate nutrition: stable weight (within 5 lb. of ideal)
Disturbed Sleep Pattern related to neurologic changes, altered perceptions	Adequate sleep: patient rests at night and remains physically active and awake during the day
Risk for Injury related to poor judgment, physical decline, sensorimotor changes	Absence of injuries: patient has no falls, suffers no bruises, cuts, fractures
Disturbed Thought Processes/Impaired Verbal Communication related to memory loss, altered perception, impaired judgment, anxiety, etc.	Cooperative behavior: patient calm, no combative behavior, no dangerous behavior Effective communication: patient needs are recognized by caregiver

Interventions: Dementia

Most people with dementia suffer from chronic, debilitating illnesses with little hope for recovery. The goal for patients with dementia is to maintain the highest level of functioning possible as their abilities gradually diminish (see Nursing Care Plan: The Patient with Dementia on p. 328).

Self-Care Deficit

As with patients with delirium, the first priority for patients with dementia is to meet their basic needs. Adequate nutrition, fluid and electrolyte balance, sleep, elimination, and hygiene must be maintained. Patients with dementia have varying levels of competence when it comes to carrying out these functions. Determine the patient's level of functioning, and then provide whatever assistance is needed. Patients may be able to participate in self-care if you break down tasks into individual steps to be done one at a time. For example, instead of instructing patients to get dressed, first direct them to put on underclothes, then socks, pants, shirts, belt, and shoes. Allow time for the patient to complete each step before giving another direction. Praise completion of each task.

Dementia patients may be incontinent of urine and feces. Frequent, routine toileting helps prevent incontinence episodes. Document stools, and be alert for signs of constipation (straining, abdominal distention, poor appetite, passage of liquid stool). Avoid laxatives if possible; instead, high-fiber foods in the diet are more effective for promoting regular bowel movements. If constipation cannot be managed with diet, fluids, and exercise, a bulk-forming stool softener may be needed. However, bulk-forming softeners can actually cause impaction if the patient cannot take adequate fluids.

Imbalanced Nutrition: Less Than Body Requirements

People with dementia may eventually need help with eating. Assistance with meals may mean cutting food or total feeding. Foods that can be managed with a single utensil may facilitate self-feeding. Finger foods high in protein and carbohydrates allow patients to feed themselves more easily. Small, frequent meals are less confusing to the patients. Remove distractions from the eating area. Group meals may be helpful because patients often imitate behaviors of others. Offer fluids frequently during the day.

Disturbed Sleep Pattern

Sleep and awakening are often reversed in dementia patients. It is helpful to try to keep them awake during the day and get them to sleep at night. Tests and treatments can be scheduled during the morning and early afternoon to allow the patients time to wind down by bedtime. Some caregivers have found that a quiet hour in the afternoon with soft music playing promotes sleep at night. Patients who awaken during the night and become confused and agitated should be reassured in a soft, soothing manner to avoid precipitating extreme agitation and loss of control.

Risk for Injury

A safe, structured environment is essential for a person with dementia. Nothing should be left around that could harm the patient. Falls and injuries may be prevented with careful observation, muscle strengthening, and a fall prevention program.

Disturbed Thought Processes/Impaired Verbal Communication

Communication usually becomes increasingly difficult. Patients with dementia are disoriented, and their thinking ability is impaired. They are confused by what is going on around them. Communication should be simple and direct. Patients must be approached gently, calmly, and quietly. They tend to copy the behavior of people around them, so a caregiver who is anxious or upset can easily convey these feelings to a patient. Nonverbal communication is extremely important. Look for cues from patients' actions and facial expressions because they frequently are not able to express their needs verbally. When patients resist activities such as bathing or dressing, avoid confrontations. Confrontations only provoke agitation and possible violence; it is better to come back at another time. A consistent schedule of care given by the same caregivers provides security for a dementia patient.

Whereas constant reality orientation is helpful for the patient with delirium, such orientation is not effective for the patient with dementia. Clocks, calendars, constant mention of the date and time, and other such orientation reminders used to be a staple of care for demented patients. However, it is now thought that reality orientation tends to agitate people with dementia by pointing out to them their forgetfulness and confusion. It is better to assist them in a nonconfrontational manner and redirect activities without constantly reminding them of their deficits.

Put on Your Thinking Cap!

A patient's daughter is distressed because her mother does not seem to recognize her at times. What could you say to help the daughter? What suggestions could you give her to promote communication with her mother?

GUIDELINES FOR WORKING WITH DEMENTIA PATIENTS

It is helpful to keep in mind two important concepts when taking care of patients with dementia: (1) they usually forget things relatively quickly, and (2) they are usually unable to learn new things. For example, if persons with dementia start to become very rest-

NURSING CARE PLAN

The Patient with Dementia

ASSESSMENT

Health History: A 75-year-old woman is admitted to a long-term care facility by her daughter because she has been unsafe living alone at home. Her daughter reports that the patient has been in good health, but during the past 5 years she has gradually had more and more problems with her memory, and during the past year, she has resisted taking a bath or changing her clothes. Lately she has had times when she has not even known her daughter. At times she has been unable to find the bathroom and has been incontinent of urine. She often forgets to eat, and when she does eat, prefers only junk foods. Recently she has begun "wandering." She was found at a local park not knowing who she was or where she lived. Her physician has diagnosed probable Alzheimer's disease.

Physical Examination: Blood pressure, 170/95; pulse, 88; respiration, 22; temperature, 98.2° F. Height, 5'3"; weight, 126 lb. Inability to bathe and dress self. Disoriented to time, place, and person.

Nursing Diagnosis	Goals and Outcome Criteria	Interventions
Self-Care Deficit related to impaired thinking, sensory and motor dysfunction	The patient will perform activities of daily living (ADL) as independently as possible, as evidenced by participation in bathing and dressing with the assistance of the nurse as needed.	Assess the patient's ability to perform own ADL. Allow the patient to perform as many of own ADL as possible. Remain with the patient while she performs ADL to maintain safety. Work out a routine toileting schedule and encourage patient to go to bathroom at regular intervals.
Imbalanced Nutrition: Less Than Body Requirements related to difficulty with self-feeding, inattention	The patient will maintain adequate nutrition, as evidenced by keeping within 5 lb of ideal weight.	Cut the food into small portions. Offer finger foods. Offer foods high in protein and carbohydrates. Offer small, frequent meals and snacks. Offer fluids frequently. Stay with the patient while eating.
Disturbed Sleep Pattern related to neurologic changes, altered perceptions	Patient will have adequate sleep, as evidenced by quiet restfulness at night and remaining physically active and awake during the day.	Try to keep her awake during the day and encourage sleep only at night. Minimize activities late in the day to allow her to "wind down" by bedtime. Have a quiet hour in the evening with soft music. If she awakens during the night and becomes confused or agitated, reassure in a soft, soothing manner to avoid precipitating extreme agitation and loss of control. Try gently stroking and singing to her. Provide a comfort object if she has one (e.g., blanket, doll).
Risk for Injury related to poor judgment, physical decline, sensorimotor changes	Absence of injuries: patient has no falls, suffers no bruises, cuts, fractures.	Provide a safe environment: no clutter, no medications or dangerous chemicals within reach. Avoid use of restraints. Provide opportunities for safe, supervised walking. Monitor exits to prevent wandering from the premises.
Disturbed Thought Processes/Impaired Verbal Communication related to memory loss, altered perception, impaired judgment, anxiety	The patient will remain calm, free of combative behavior, as evidenced by a calm, cooperative manner during times when nursing care is performed.	Speak to patient in a calm, reassuring manner. Avoid confrontations with patient. Break tasks down into individual steps to be done one at a time. Provide consistency in nursing care. Attempt to understand what patient is communicating verbally and nonverbally.

? CRITICAL THINKING QUESTIONS

- Why is it important to stay with the resident while she completes ADLs and while she feeds herself?

- What strategies might you use to minimize incidents of urinary incontinence in the resident who has dementia?

less, anxious, or agitated and are becoming more so by the minute, it may be effective to divert their attention somewhere else. They may be gently guided to another activity, and usually within a relatively short period of time they will forget what was bothering them in the first place and focus on the new ac-

tivity (Fig. 22-3). Sometimes agitation indicates pain, hunger, stress, fear, or the need for toileting. Investigate whether any of these problems are present. Take advantage of the fact that patients with dementia are usually slow or unable to learn new things. For example, putting new locks on the doors in new

FIGURE **22-3** It is best to calmly divert the attention of confused, agitated patients somewhere else by gently guiding them to another activity.

places may prevent wandering patients from opening exit doors. You can be very creative in the care of dementia patients by using these two concepts as a basis for their care.

One approach that can also guide care for dementia patients is the Cognitive Developmental Approach (CDA). The CDA adapts interventions based on the patient's cognitive abilities. It is thought to reduce patient stress and frustration by eliminating unrealistic expectations and allowing the patient to do as much as he or she is able. Some principles derived from the CDA that you can apply include the following:

- Accept that the patient with dementia may no longer be able to make adult decisions and behave as a healthy adult would. Offer limited choices to simplify decision making.
- Adapt the environment to the patient rather than trying to adapt the patient to the environment. For example, create a safe environment for wandering instead of trying to keep the patient from wandering.
- Encourage self-care at whatever level the patient can function. If the patient can eat independently with his hands but not with utensils, provide finger foods.
- Recognize irrational fears such as fear of the bathtub and arrange alternative ways to give personal care.
- Accept that, in advanced dementia, patient behaviors and thinking are not typical of a healthy

adult. Some strategies that work with children often work with dementia patients also.

- Recognize that the patient deserves to be treated with dignity regardless of abilities or behaviors. Even the most impaired patient can probably sense compassion in a caregiver.

Key Points

- The two major types of confusion are (1) acute confusional states, or delirium, and (2) chronic confusion, or dementia.
- Older adults are the most susceptible to confusion associated with delirium or dementia.
- Delirium is a short-term confusional state that usually develops over a short period of time and is often reversible.
- Delirium is characterized by disturbances in attention, thinking, perception, orientation, short-term memory, and sleep.
- Delirium is usually caused by some underlying illness such as neurologic, pulmonary, or cardiovascular disease or conditions such as infection, dehydration, and overmedication.
- Dementia is chronic and rarely reversible.
- Dementia is characterized by inappropriate behavior and impairment of intellectual function, problem-solving ability, judgment, memory, and orientation.
- Dementia is not a disease entity itself but a clinical syndrome, a collection of symptoms that may be part of the profile of many diseases, including Alzheimer's disease, vascular dementia, Huntington's disease, and Parkinson's disease.
- The first step in assessing a confusional state is to observe the patient's behavior and to evaluate orientation, memory, and sleep habits.
- Try to determine how long the symptoms of confusion have been present and how and when they started.
- In caring for a patient with delirium, provide safety and comfort and provide frequent orientation to the surroundings and the situation.
- The goal for patients with dementia is to maintain the highest level of functioning possible as their abilities gradually diminish.
- A safe, structured environment is essential for patients with dementia, and tasks should be broken down into individual steps that can be performed one at a time.
- When patients with dementia resist activities such as bathing or dressing, it is best to avoid confrontations and divert their attention elsewhere.
- The Cognitive Developmental Approach adapts interventions to the patient's cognitive level.

 Go to your Companion CD-ROM for a Pharmacology Tutorial, Audio Glossary, and 3-D animations.

evolve Be sure to visit the companion Evolve site at http://evolve.elsevier.com/Linton/ for WebLinks and additional online resources.

REVIEW QUESTIONS *Choose the best answer.*

1. What is the primary difference between delirium and dementia?

   1. Delirium is typically reversible; dementia is rarely reversible.
   2. Agitation is constant with delirium but intermittent with dementia.
   3. The onset of delirium is gradual; the onset of dementia is typically rapid.
   4. Delirium usually lasts only a few minutes; dementia lasts weeks to months.

2. A confused patient repeatedly cries out for her daughter in the middle of the night. What is the best intervention?

   1. Check to see if she has an order for a sedative.
   2. Call her daughter and ask her to come see her mother.
   3. Calmly tell her where she is and that her daughter is not here.
   4. Tell her she needs to be quiet because she is disturbing other patients.

3. A patient with Alzheimer's disease wanders away from the table during meals, leaving most of his food uneaten. What should you do?

   1. Consult with the dietitian about providing finger foods.
   2. Restrain the patient in his seat during meals.
   3. Tell him he must sit down and finish his meal.
   4. Ask another patient to try to keep him at the table.

4. Which message is most appropriate for the patient with dementia?

   1. "You need to be dressed for church in 30 minutes."
   2. "Put your arm in the sleeve of your shirt."
   3. "Put your shirt on."
   4. "What would you like to wear today?"

5. A new nurse on the Alzheimer's special care unit repeatedly asks patients what time it is and if they know where they are. What information should you share with her?

   1. If a patient cannot answer the questions correctly, wait 5 minutes and ask again.
   2. Consistently tell patients the time, date, and place to keep them oriented.
   3. Frequent attempts at orientation tend to agitate Alzheimer's patients.
   4. Have the patient repeat the date, time, and place after you say them.

6. If you applied principles of the Cognitive Developmental Approach to care of a dementia patient, you would:

   1. Consistently follow very specific interventions for dementia patients
   2. Have the patient confront irrational fears so they can be overcome
   3. Insist that the patient behave as a mature adult at all times
   4. Adapt your expectations and interventions to the patient's abilities

CHAPTER

23 Incontinence

evolve http://evolve.elsevier.com/Linton/

Objectives

After reading and studying this chapter, you should be able to:

1. Identify the types of urinary and fecal incontinence.
2. Explain the pathophysiology and treatment of specific types of incontinence.
3. Identify common therapeutic measures used for the incontinent patient.
4. List nursing assessment data needed to assist in the evaluation and treatment of incontinence.
5. Assist in developing a nursing care plan for the patient with incontinence.

Key Terms

Be sure to check out the bonus material on the Companion CD-ROM, including selected audio pronunciations.

anorectal incontinence (ā-nō-RĚK-tăl ĭn-KŎN-tĭ-nĕns, p. 346)

Credé's technique (krā-DĀZ, p. 338)

detrusor overactivity (p. 337)

fecal incontinence (p. 331)

functional incontinence (p. 339)

micturition (mĭk-tū-RĬSH-ŭn, p. 331)

neurogenic bladder (nū-rō-JĔN-ĭk, p. 337)

neurogenic incontinence (p. 346)

overflow incontinence (fecal) (p. 345)

overflow incontinence (urine) (p. 337)

stress incontinence (p. 339)

symptomatic incontinence (p. 346)

transient incontinence (TRĂN-zē-ĕnt, p. 337)

urge incontinence (p. 337)

urinary incontinence (p. 331)

void (p. 331)

*I*ncontinence is the term used to describe the involuntary passage of urine (urinary incontinence) or feces (fecal incontinence). Many conditions and situations can cause either temporary or permanent incontinence. Incontinence deserves special attention because of the toll it takes on the individual. The person who is troubled by incontinence faces physical, psychosocial, and financial burdens. The management of incontinence in patient care settings also requires many hours of nursing care.

The goals of treatment for the incontinent person include restoration or improvement of control for treatable incontinence, management of irreversible incontinence, and prevention of complications.

URINARY INCONTINENCE: PREVALENCE AND COSTS

Statistics on urinary incontinence vary greatly depending on the gender, age, type of incontinence, and place of residence (community vs. institution) of persons studied. Exact figures are difficult to obtain because people often do not report the problem to health care providers. General surveys of adults have found that 5% to 25% note leakage at least once a week and 5% to 15% experience it daily or most of the time. Among U.S. women who live in the community, 15% to 50% are affected by urinary incontinence with 7% to 10% having severe leakage. Although urinary incontinence is twice as common among women compared with men, 17% of men over the age of 60 also have this condition. Among men who have had a radical prostatectomy, as many as 30% have some degree of incontinence.

The cost of managing the incontinence in the United States is estimated to be more than $15 billion each year. Health care providers need to recognize the economic and personal value of treating incontinence aggressively. Nurses play an important role in educating people about the need for evaluation and treatment. Even though it is more common in older people, urinary incontinence should not be considered a normal age-related change. It often can be improved or cured, no matter how old the patient is.

PHYSIOLOGY OF URINATION

The passage of urine is called *urination* or micturition. Nurses and physicians commonly refer to the process of urinating as voiding. For that reason, the terms void and *voiding* are used in this chapter.

Normal controlled voiding requires healthy bladder muscle (detrusor muscle), a patent (open) urethra, normal transmission of nerve impulses, and mental alertness. Alterations in any of these factors may result in incontinence.

The urinary bladder receives urine continuously from the kidneys. The function of the bladder is to store urine until it can be eliminated. The walls of the bladder are muscular and capable of stretching. When 200 to 250 mL of urine collects in the bladder, stretch and tension receptors are stimulated. The bladder contracts, and the internal sphincter relaxes. A message is sent to the brain, making the person aware of the need to void. Because the act of voiding is normally voluntary, it can be delayed until an appropriate time. Then the external sphincter can be relaxed, permitting urine to flow out through the urethra (Fig. 23-1).

There is, of course, a limit to the amount of urine the bladder can hold. When the limit is exceeded, pressure causes the bladder to contract and force urine out involuntarily. If the bladder cannot be emptied, urine backs up into the kidneys (a condition called *hydronephrosis*) and can cause kidney damage.

DIAGNOSTIC TESTS AND PROCEDURES

The presence and specific type of urinary incontinence are diagnosed based on the patient's history, physical examination, and various diagnostic tests and procedures. Diagnostic studies may include laboratory tests, measurement of urine volumes, imaging procedures, endoscopy, stress tests, and urodynamic studies. Other helpful tools are voiding diaries and wet pad counts or weights. The results help define the type of incontinence, which in turn guides treatment decisions.

LABORATORY TESTS

A clean-catch urinalysis with culture and sensitivity testing is usually ordered to assess for infection. The specimen is studied for bacteria, red blood cells, white blood cells, and glucose. If the patient cannot cooperate with the clean-catch procedure, catheterization may be necessary. A blood sample may be collected to measure blood urea nitrogen, creatinine, glucose, and calcium.

POSTVOID RESIDUAL

It is useful to know whether the patient is emptying the bladder completely. The amount of urine remaining in the bladder after voiding is called the *postvoid residual* (PVR). Several methods are used to determine the PVR. One method is to catheterize the patient immediately after voiding and measure the amount of urine obtained by catheterization. A second method is to use an ultrasound device to estimate the amount of urine remaining in the bladder after voiding. Some physicians estimate PVR by abdominal palpation and percussion. Normally less than 50 mL of urine remains after voiding. An amount greater than 199 mL reflects inadequate emptying.

Imaging Procedures

Imaging procedures such as computed tomography or magnetic resonance imaging may be ordered to create images of the urinary structures. Imaging procedures for the urinary tract are discussed in Chapter 40.

Urodynamic Testing

Urodynamic procedures assess the neuromuscular function of the lower urinary tract. These tests are indicated when the cause of incontinence cannot be determined by simpler means.

UROFLOWMETRY

Uroflowmetry measures voiding duration and the amount and rate of urine voided. The patient voids into the funnel of the flowmeter. Sometimes serial measurements are made over 2 to 3 days. The patient is advised to void before defecating and not to allow stool or bathroom tissue to enter the funnel. The patient's position for each voiding is recorded. Fluid intake is measured during the testing period. Additional urodynamic tests are discussed in Chapter 40.

CYSTOMETRY

Cystometry is used to evaluate the neuromuscular function of the bladder. Signed consent is obtained before beginning the procedure. The patient voids into a flowmeter, after which a catheter is inserted and the postvoid residual is measured. Fluid or air, or both, are

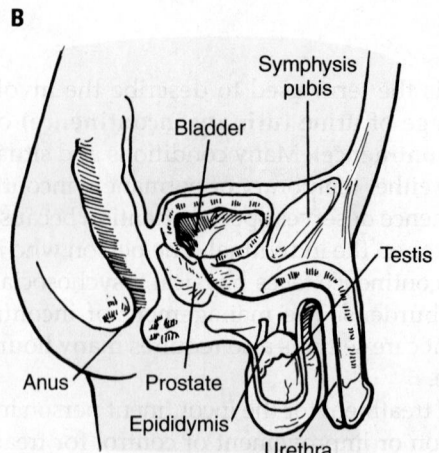

FIGURE **23-1** The bladder, urethra, and adjacent structures. **A,** Female. **B,** Male.

instilled into the bladder, and the patient's sensations and bladder response are determined. The bladder is filled until the patient feels uncomfortable or it is apparent that the patient is unable to sense the pressure. The bladder is then drained, or the patient is permitted to void. The physician may administer a drug that stimulates bladder tone and repeat the test. After the test, the patient should force fluids if not contraindicated. The nurse advises the patient to report difficulty voiding or signs of infection (fever, burning during urination, chills, pain, blood in the urine).

PROVOCATIVE STRESS TESTING

Provocative stress testing is done to detect involuntary passage of urine when abdominal pressure increases. The patient may be positioned in a standing or lithotomy position. The physician encourages the patient to relax and then to cough vigorously. The examiner observes for urine loss during coughing.

CYSTOSCOPY

Cystoscopy is covered in more detail in Chapter 40. In brief, a scope is inserted through the urethra to visualize the urethra and bladder. Signed consent is required, and the procedure may be done under local or general anesthesia. Postprocedure care includes monitoring urine output and encouraging fluid ingestion (if not contraindicated). The patient is advised to report difficulty voiding, continued blood in the urine (it is normally pink-tinged at first), and fever, chills, or pain, which may indicate infection.

COMMON THERAPEUTIC MEASURES

Depending on the type of urinary incontinence, a number of therapeutic measures may be prescribed. These are generally classified as behavioral, pharmacologic, or surgical treatments. Despite the variety of treatments available, many people do not seek medical care for the condition. Some individuals manage with common-sense practices such as limiting trips, restricting fluids, and avoiding activities that induce leakage. Unfortunately, these strategies can have negative consequences such as inadequate fluid intake and giving up social and recreational activities.

BEHAVIORAL INTERVENTIONS

Behavioral interventions include bladder training or retraining, habit training, prompted voiding, and pelvic muscle exercises. These techniques are low risk and are often effective in decreasing the frequency of incontinent episodes.

Bladder Training

Bladder retraining uses patient education, scheduled toileting, and positive reinforcement. The teaching plan includes information about normal urinary anatomy and physiology and the bladder retraining program. With scheduled voiding, the patient is encouraged to delay voiding and void only at scheduled times. Initially, voiding is usually scheduled every 2 to 3 hours while the patient is awake. The length of time between voidings is gradually increased. If the patient voids ahead of schedule, the next voiding may be rescheduled at the prescribed interval. Another approach is to ignore the unscheduled voiding and have the patient void again at the previously scheduled time. The patient's efforts and improvement are positively reinforced throughout the treatment period, which usually lasts several months.

Habit Training

Habit training is also called *timed voiding*. It is similar to bladder training in that the patient is encouraged to void at scheduled intervals. The difference is that the patient is not advised to resist the urge and delay voiding. The voiding schedule is based on the patient's usual pattern.

Prompted Voiding

Prompted voiding is often used with habit training for people who are dependent or cognitively impaired. The caregiver checks the patient for wetness at regular intervals and asks the patient to state whether wet or dry. The caregiver then encourages the patient to try to use the toilet. The caregiver praises the patient for trying to use the toilet and for remaining dry. This process is intended to help the patient recognize incontinence and to ask caregivers for help with toileting.

Pelvic Muscle Rehabilitation

Pelvic muscle rehabilitation aims to strengthen the pelvic floor and includes pelvic muscle exercises, with or without biofeedback, pelvic floor electrical stimulation, and vaginal weight training. Pelvic muscle exercises, commonly called *Kegel exercises*, are described in the Patient Teaching Plan on p. 334. They actively exercise the pubococcygeus muscle, which helps close the urethra and strengthen muscles of the pelvic floor.

Biofeedback may be used in conjunction with other pelvic muscle exercises. Electronic or mechanical sensors are used to help the patient isolate the appropriate pelvic muscles to contract while keeping the abdominal muscles relaxed. Electrical stimulation of the muscles of the pelvic floor can also be employed to cause muscle contraction along with Kegel exercises.

Sometimes vaginal weights ("cones") are used with pelvic muscle training in women. The cones are ceramic devices of various weights that are inserted into the vagina. The patient begins with the lightest cone, inserts it, and tries to retain it for up to 15 minutes twice daily. When the lightest cone is successfully retained, the heavier cones are then used in succession.

Pelvic Muscle (Kegel) Exercises

- Uncontrolled loss of urine is commonly caused by weakness in the perineal muscles that normally control urination.
- Strengthening perineal muscles, which are located around the vagina and the rectum, can improve urinary control.
- To identify the correct muscles that you need to exercise, practice tightening the perineal muscles as if you were trying to control the passage of intestinal gas. Try to hold the contraction for a count of 3, and then relax for a count of 3.
- Your goal is to work up to 3 sets of 10 repeats, done three to four times each day or as recommended by your physician.
- You may notice improvement in urinary control after 3 weeks; however, it may take 6 to 8 weeks before you notice improvement.
- Continue the exercises indefinitely to maintain control.
- You can do these exercises anywhere: at your desk, while driving, standing in line at the grocery store. No one can tell!

Urge Suppression. Patients with urge incontinence may find the following strategy helpful (Miller, 2000):

- If you have the urge to void, stop what you are doing. Sit down or stand quietly.
- Quickly squeeze the pelvic floor muscles several times without resting between squeezes.
- Take a few deep breaths and try to relax except for the pelvic floor muscles.
- Try to suppress the urge to void.
- Wait until the urge passes.
- While continuing to squeeze the pelvic floor muscles, walk to the bathroom at a normal pace.

REFLEX TRAINING

Reflex training is sometimes employed by people with spinal cord injury. This technique uses the Valsalva maneuver with rectal stretching to force urine from the bladder. The Valsalva maneuver is performed by taking a deep breath, holding it, and bearing down. At the same time, the rectum is stretched by inserting a gloved finger into the rectum and pulling toward the back. This creates pressure on the urinary sphincter and relaxes the pelvic floor, allowing urine to flow. Patients who use this method of emptying the bladder should be checked for residual volume at times. Ideally, the residual volume will be less than 100 mL. Patients who learn to use this method successfully may no longer need catheterization.

DRUG THERAPY

Drug therapy, primarily with anticholinergics, may be used to treat stress and urge incontinence. Other clas-sifications of drugs that might be used include smooth muscle relaxants, calcium channel blockers, tricyclic antidepressant agents, nonsteroidal anti-inflammatory drugs, alpha-adrenergic agonists, and estrogen. Examples of these drugs, their side effects, and nursing considerations are presented in the Drug Therapy table on pages 335 and 336. Contigen is one of several materials that may be injected into the tissues around the urethra. The substance adds bulk to the bladder neck, thereby increasing resistance to urine outflow. This procedure, called *periurethral bulking*, is helpful in certain situations for both men and women. The long-term effects of Contigen injection are still being studied. Postmenopausal women with urge or stress incontinence may obtain improvement using intravaginal estrogen cream or tablets.

In addition to drugs used to control incontinence, a variety of creams and sprays are available to coat and protect the skin of the perineum and buttocks of the incontinent patient. A light dusting powder can be used to absorb moisture. Cornstarch is not recommended because it promotes the development of yeast infections. Do not use talc and lotion together on the same area because the combination creates an abrasive paste.

URINE COLLECTION DEVICES

External Devices

External urine collection devices are useful for males. These latex sheaths, sometimes called *condom catheters* or *Texas catheters*, drain urine into a bag that is usually secured to the leg. These are quite effective in maintaining dryness, but the adhesive may cause skin irritation on the penis. The directions for applying a condom catheter must be followed carefully. *Make sure the patient and all caregivers know not to encircle the penis with tape.* To do so can restrict circulation. Elastic tape should be used and wrapped in a spiral pattern. There is no external device for women in common use at this time, although several are being tested.

Indwelling Catheters

An indwelling catheter may be ordered to control urinary incontinence. This is usually done when all other measures have failed and skin integrity is endangered. A catheter may also be needed temporarily if urine is coming in contact with a wound. Care of the patient with an indwelling catheter is covered in Chapter 40.

Intermittent Self-Catheterization

Some patients are quite successful at using intermittent self-catheterization. Of course, this requires dexterity, adequate vision, and ability and motivation to learn. Clean technique rather than sterile is usually taught for use in the home setting. Initially the bladder is drained every 4 hours. If more than 500 mL of urine is obtained, the time interval is shortened. If less than 200 mL is obtained, the time is extended. Most people produce more urine at certain times of the day.

DRUG THERAPY | *Drugs Used to Treat Urinary Incontinence*

DRUG	USE	ACTION	NURSING INTERVENTIONS
CHOLINERGICS			
Bethanechol chloride (Urecholine)	Atonic bladder (overflow incontinence)	Bladder contraction	Common side effects: sweating, flushing, GI distress, headache, visual disturbances Toxicity: nausea, dyspnea, irregular pulse, headache Antidote: atropine Contraindications: bladder or intestinal obstruction, asthma, hyperthyroidism, ulcer, cardiac disease, parkinsonism Works quickly: 15-30 min after SC route, 1 hr after PO route; be sure bedpan or toilet is accessible **Warning**: dosages are very different for SC and PO administration
ANTICHOLINERGICS			
Propantheline bromide (Pro-Banthine)	Urge incontinence	Bladder relaxation and sphincter contraction Delayed desire to void	Common side effects: constipation, dry mouth, blurred vision (pupil dilation), fatigue, tachycardia Contraindications: glaucoma, severe coronary artery disease, some GI disorders Use cautiously in older adults
ANTISPASMODICS			
Oxybutynin chloride (Ditropan) Tolterodine (Detrol)	Urge incontinence	Bladder relaxation Increased bladder capacity Delayed urge to void	Side effects: (less with tolterodine) dry mouth, constipation, tachycardia, drowsiness, urinary retention, insomnia, blurred vision Give 1 hour before meals; provide oral care; potentiates other CNS depressants
ALPHA-ADRENERGICS			
Ephedrine	Stress incontinence Enuresis (with atropine)	Sphincter contraction	Common side effects: cardiac dysrhythmias, nervousness, palpitations Contraindications: Severe hypotension, narrow-angle glaucoma Older adults are more likely to have hallucinations, convulsions, CNS depression, insomnia, and urinary retention
ALPHA-ADRENERGIC BLOCKERS			
Prazosin hydrochloride (Minipress) Phenoxybenzamine hydrochloride (Dibenzyline)	Overflow incontinence	Relaxation of internal sphincter	Side effects: postural hypotension (especially in older adults), tachycardia, headache, dizziness, nasal congestion After the first dose, the patient should lie down for 2 hr to prevent fainting; elastic stockings may help During dosage adjustments, monitor blood pressure; most side effects decrease over time
BETA-ADRENERGIC BLOCKERS			
Propranolol hydrochloride (Inderal)	Stress incontinence	Improved sphincter tone	Side effects: cardiac depression Contraindications: asthma
COLLAGEN			
Glutaraldehyde cross-linked collagen (Contigen)	Stress incontinence	Adds bulk to sphincter to increase resistance to urine	Injected around urethra by physician Monitor voiding and assess bladder for distention

GI, Gastrointestinal; *SC,* subcutaneous; *PO,* by mouth; *CNS,* central nervous system.

Continued

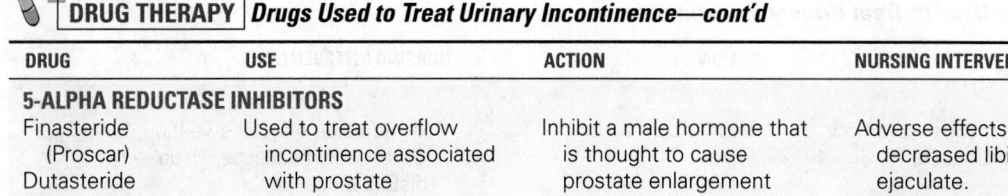

DRUG THERAPY *Drugs Used to Treat Urinary Incontinence—cont'd*

DRUG	USE	ACTION	NURSING INTERVENTIONS
5-ALPHA REDUCTASE INHIBITORS			
Finasteride (Proscar) Dutasteride (Avodart)	Used to treat overflow incontinence associated with prostate enlargement	Inhibit a male hormone that is thought to cause prostate enlargement Shrinking the enlarged prostate allows urine to flow through the urethra more easily	Adverse effects include impotence, decreased libido, decreased volume of ejaculate. Inform patients that pregnant women and women who may become pregnant should not come in contact with this drug or the semen of a man taking the drug

Individual schedules can be adjusted to accommodate this variation.

GARMENTS AND PADS FOR INCONTINENCE

A variety of incontinence products are available that help maintain dryness. Disposable briefs and pads are found in most pharmacies and grocery stores. Some older women wear perineal pads to absorb urine. "Geri pads" are used in some nursing homes. These are washable waterproof briefs with absorbent cotton liners. Another style has a stretchy brief with a perineal pouch through which absorbent pads can be changed. The best product is one that draws urine away from the skin through a liner that remains dry. These products do not, however, protect the skin against feces.

Those who discourage the use of incontinence briefs and pads say it encourages patients to void in their clothing. This may be true at times, but there is a place for these items. It may give a person the confidence to be socially active without the risk of having an embarrassing accident. When trying to restore control, it is best to use briefs that can be removed easily for toileting. For patients who are unlikely to ever be continent, these products may be an acceptable management tool.

For the immobile patient, an absorbent pad with a waterproof backing may be used instead of briefs. These pads can also be placed under the buttocks of a bedridden patient wearing briefs in case leakage occurs. One factor to remember is that multiple layers of padding interfere with special beds or mattresses designed to prevent decubitus ulcers. Some paper pads stick to the skin and become lumpy when wet. The patient should never be placed directly on a plastic surface because this keeps the skin wet from perspiration as well as urine.

PENILE CLAMP

The penile clamp is a device that is applied to the penis. It compresses the urethra, preventing the passage of urine. To prevent circulatory impairment and pressure sores, the clamp must be removed and repositioned frequently. Use of the penile clamp is controversial (Fig. 23-2).

FIGURE **23-2** A penile clamp used for urinary incontinence.

PELVIC ORGAN SUPPORT DEVICES

A *pessary* is a device that is inserted into the vagina to hold the pelvic organs in place. It is sometimes used as a tool to treat incontinence in women with relaxation of pelvic structures. A doughnut-shaped pessary exerts pressure on the vaginal wall, lifting the uterus and holding it in the pelvis. When incontinence occurs because the bladder prolapses into the vagina, other types of pessaries may be used to support the urethra as well. Pessaries are generally recommended for patients who are awaiting surgical treatment or those for whom surgery is contraindicated. Within 24 hours after pessary placement, the patient must be reexamined to ensure proper placement and to rule out urinary obstruction. The device must then be removed periodically for cleansing and replacement as needed. *Be sure to document that the patient has a pessary, so it will not be forgotten.*

For women with stress incontinence, a bladder-neck support prosthesis may be helpful. When the Silastic device is fitted into the vagina, it supports the area where the urethra connects to the bladder, thereby reducing the incidence of involuntary urine loss.

SURGICAL TREATMENT

Surgical intervention may be recommended for some conditions that cause urinary incontinence. Specific surgical procedures may be done to remove obstructions, treat severe detrusor overactivity, implant an artificial sphincter, reposition the sphincter unit, improve perineal support, and inject substances that increase urethral compression (mentioned with drug therapy). Electrostimulation is the use of electrodes that stimulate the pelvic floor muscles. Electrodes can be surgically implanted in the vagina or rectum. Surgical procedures most often used for stress urinary incontinence in women are retropubic urethropexies and pubovaginal slings. A sling procedure for men creates a support system for the urethra so that it does not open inappropriately. Nursing care of the patient undergoing surgery on the urinary tract is described in Chapter 40.

The artificial sphincter illustrated in Figure 23-3 consists of an inflatable cuff, a reservoir of fluid that fills the cuff, and a pump. The cuff is positioned around the urethra or bladder neck. The reservoir is placed in the abdomen and the pump in the scrotum or labia. Fluid fills the cuff, applying pressure to the urethra to prevent urine passage. To void, the patient compresses the pump, which deflates the cuff by transferring fluid from the cuff to the reservoir and allowing urine to pass through the urethra.

TYPES OF URINARY INCONTINENCE

There are several proposed classifications of the types of urinary incontinence. This chapter divides them into four basic types: urge, overflow, stress, and functional (Table 23-1). It is possible for a patient to have more than one type at the same time (mixed incontinence). Urinary incontinence may be transient or persistent. Transient incontinence is caused by reversible conditions and is often corrected by treatment of the underlying problem.

URGE INCONTINENCE
Description

Urge incontinence is the involuntary loss of urine shortly after a strong, abrupt urge to urinate. It most often results from an overactive detrusor (bladder)

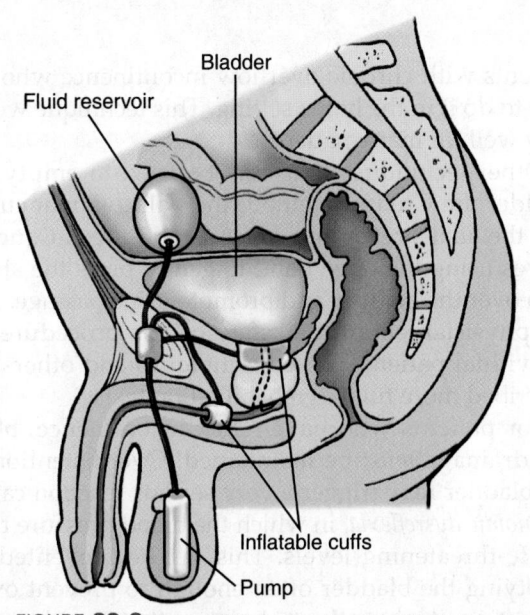

FIGURE **23-3** An artificial urinary sphincter in place.

Bladder

Fluid reservoir

Inflatable cuffs

Pump

muscle. When a specific cause cannot be identified, the condition is referred to as *idiopathic urge incontinence*. When urge incontinence is associated with neurologic disorders such as stroke, multiple sclerosis, and spinal cord lesions, it is classified as neurogenic detrusor overactivity. Detrusor overactivity is the most common cause of incontinence in older adults. Some patients with urge incontinence have involuntary urethral relaxation in addition to abnormal detrusor activity. Urinary tract infection and fecal impaction sometimes cause temporary urge incontinence.

Management

Treatment of urge incontinence is aimed at correcting the cause, if possible: antibiotics for infection, removal of impaction. When the problem is not related to reversible conditions, behavioral techniques, drug therapy, or surgical intervention may be employed. Bladder training with scheduled voiding and positive reinforcement may be effective. Pelvic muscle exercises may be prescribed to supplement bladder training. Anticholinergics and antispasmodics are the drugs most commonly used for urge incontinence. Be aware that anticholinergics may cause confusion and agitation that could be mistaken for dementia in the older patient. Tolterodine (Detrol) is an antispasmodic that is effective in many people, particularly those with overactive bladder. It generally has fewer side effects than the anticholinergics. If behavioral techniques, drugs, or both do not work, some surgical procedures may be recommended.

OVERFLOW INCONTINENCE
Description

Overflow incontinence is the involuntary loss of urine associated with an overdistended bladder. Small amounts of urine are lost either continuously or at frequent intervals. In addition to passing out through the urethra, urine may flow out of the bladder back into the ureters and kidneys and cause hydronephrosis—a condition that can damage the kidneys. Patients who have normal sensation usually feel uncomfortable because of bladder distention. Factors that contribute to overflow incontinence are obstruction to urine flow, an underactive detrusor muscle, or impaired transmission of nerve impulses. In addition, some females have overflow incontinence after anti-incontinence surgery.

These patients are not aware of bladder fullness, and the bladder may become overdistended. Urinary retention with overflow is also fairly common after general anesthesia or childbirth or after removal of an indwelling catheter. Drugs that may cause retention include antihistamines, epinephrine, anticholinergics, and theophylline, as shown in the Drug Therapy table on p. 339. Neurogenic bladder is retention with overflow that is caused by neurologic dysfunction associated with spinal cord injury, radical pelvic surgery, or radiation cystitis. It may be referred to as reflex incontinence.

Table 23-1 *Types of Urinary Incontinence*

TYPE	DESCRIPTION	CAUSES	NURSING CARE	TREATMENT
Urge	Loss of urine that usually follows a strong desire to void	Nervous system disorders Urinary tract infection Bladder obstruction	Scheduled toileting Limit fluids 2 hr before bedtime Administer drugs as ordered to control bladder contractions (see Drug Therapy table on pp. 335-336) Keep incontinence record	Behavior modification Drug therapy: anticholinergics Surgical procedures to increase bladder capacity or decrease bladder contractions
Overflow	Loss of urine associated with a full bladder Frequent voiding Volume usually small	Urethral obstruction Disorders of bladder, nerves, or muscles Spinal cord injury Postanesthesia	Catheterize as ordered; teach self-catheterization as appropriate Administer drugs as ordered to stimulate the bladder and relax the internal sphincter (see Drug Therapy table on pp. 335-336)	Surgery to relieve obstruction Drug therapy to stimulate the bladder and relax the sphincters Catheterization
	Reflex incontinence: loss of urine due to reflexive contraction	Spinal cord injury Radiation cystitis	Cutaneous triggers; teach stimulation techniques	Catheterize as necessary
Stress	Loss of urine during physical exertion	Relaxation of pelvic floor muscles Urethral trauma Sphincter injury	Teach Kegel exercises Advise patient to void frequently Administer drugs as ordered to stimulate sphincter (see Drug Therapy table on pp. 335-336)	Surgical correction Bladder suspension Artificial sphincter Drug therapy to improve sphincter contraction
Functional	Bladder functions normally but subject voids inappropriately	Dementia Head injury Cerebrovascular accident (stroke)	Scheduled toileting Reinforce appropriate behavior Remove environmental barriers	
Total	Loss of urine when other types of incontinence have been ruled out	May be unclear; possibly neurologic, or bladder sphincter injury	Timed voiding Incontinence briefs	Catheterization

Management

The medical treatment of overflow incontinence depends on the cause. The physician may prescribe drugs to stimulate the bladder (bethanechol chloride) and relax the internal sphincter (e.g., prazosin). A common reason for obstruction in males is prostate enlargement. Surgical removal of all or part of the gland often restores normal bladder emptying. Another surgical procedure that may be indicated when the sphincter is obstructing the outflow of urine is a sphincterotomy, in which an incision is made in the sphincter.

In some cases, intermittent or indwelling catheterization is necessary. Postoperative and postpartum patients may require intermittent catheterization once or twice before normal bladder function returns. The indwelling catheter is considered the measure of last resort in the management of overflow incontinence. Self-catheterization using clean technique may be taught to

patients with chronic overflow incontinence who are able to do it in the home setting. This technique works very well for many patients.

Other techniques that may be used to empty the bladder are Credé's method, the Valsalva maneuver, and the anal stretch maneuver. **Credé's technique** involves using the open hand to gently press the abdomen over the bladder and promote urine passage. Ask the physician about the safety of this procedure for individual patients. These techniques and others are described more fully in rehabilitation texts.

For patients who have reflex incontinence, bladder drainage *must* be maintained! Overdistention of the bladder may trigger a very serious reaction called *autonomic dysreflexia*, in which the blood pressure rises to life-threatening levels. This can be prevented by emptying the bladder often enough to prevent overdistention. Among the techniques that may be used

DRUG THERAPY | *Drugs That Cause Urinary Retention or Incontinence*

CLASS	EXAMPLE
URINARY RETENTION	
Anticholinergics	Atropine sulfate
Antihistamines	Diphenhydramine hydrochloride (Benadryl)
Sympathomimetics	Epinephrine hydrochloride (Adrenal chloride)
Xanthine	Theophylline (Theo-Dur)
INCONTINENCE	
Alpha-adrenergic blockers	Prazosin hydrochloride (Minipress)
Anticholinergics	Atropine sulfate
Antihistamines	Diphenhydramine hydrochloride (Benadryl)
Antiparkinson agents	Levodopa (Dopar), trihexyphenidyl hydrochloride (Artane)
Antipsychotics	Chlorpromazine (Thorazine)
High-ceiling diuretics	Furosemide (Lasix)
Opiate agonists	Morphine sulfate (Epimorph)
Sedatives or hypnotics	Phenobarbital sodium (Luminal sodium), diazepam (Valium)
Sympathomimetics	Phenylephrine hydrochloride (Neo-Synephrine), isoproterenol hydrochloride (Isuprel)

to stimulate bladder emptying in patients with reflex incontinence are cutaneous triggering methods, which include tapping the suprapubic area and stroking the inner thigh. These techniques and others are more fully described in texts on rehabilitation. Credé's method is *not* used for patients with reflex incontinence. Chapter 29 discusses care of the patient with spinal cord injury in detail.

STRESS INCONTINENCE
Description
Stress incontinence is the involuntary loss of small amounts of urine during physical activity that increases abdominal pressure. Coughing, laughing, sneezing, and lifting are examples of activities that often result in urine loss. In women it is usually caused by relaxation of the pelvic floor muscles and the urethrovesical juncture as a result of pregnancy, childbirth, obesity, and aging. Urethral trauma, sphincter injury, congenital sphincter weakness, urinary infection, neurologic disorders, and stress can cause stress incontinence in both men and women. It may occur after prostatectomy or radiation therapy.

Management
Sometimes stress incontinence is successfully treated with behavioral methods such as scheduled voiding and pelvic muscle exercises (see Nursing Care Plan: The Patient with Stress Incontinence on page 340). In addition, the patient is advised to maintain a fluid intake of at least 2000 mL/day. Fluids that have a diuretic effect (tea, coffee, cola) should be avoided. Alpha-adrenergic drugs such as pseudoephedrine HCl (Sudafed) may be prescribed to increase bladder outlet resistance. Oral or topical estrogen may be given to strengthen the

bladder outlet in postmenopausal women. The most common surgical interventions now are retropubic urethropexies, pubovaginal slings, and collagen injections. These procedures have largely replaced anterior colporrhaphy and needle suspension.

FUNCTIONAL INCONTINENCE
Description
Functional incontinence is the term used when a person voids inappropriately because of inability to get to the toilet or to manage the mechanics of toileting. The problem can be related to confusion, immobility, or barriers in the environment.

Management
The treatment of functional incontinence depends on the cause. The environment should be arranged to permit independent toileting. Assistive devices that enable the immobile patient to void appropriately are provided. The confused patient may respond well to scheduled or timed voiding and efforts to improve orientation to toilet facilities. In long-term care facilities, it is important to promote the attitude that incontinence can usually be improved even in physically and cognitively impaired patients.

NURSING CARE *of the Patient with Urinary Incontinence*
Assessment
Health History
Your data collection helps determine the type of incontinence, the possible causes, and the patient's response to treatment.

Chief Complaint. A thorough description of the chief complaint is essential. Ask whether the patient is aware

NURSING CARE PLAN

The Patient with Stress Incontinence

ASSESSMENT

Health History: Mrs. Seigel is an 80-year-old resident in a long-term care facility. She complains of having trouble "holding my urine." She is unable to control urination if she strains, coughs, or laughs. She is the mother of five children, all born at home. She reports no other physical complaints except for arthritis in her hips and knees and hypertension. Her medications are acetaminophen, 325 mg q.i.d., and hydrochlorothiazide, 25 mg/day. Fear of losing control of her urine has caused her to avoid leaving her room except for meals. She is wearing perineal pads to keep her clothing dry.

Physical Examination: Vital signs: temperature, 98° F orally; pulse, 72; respiration, 16; blood pressure, 130/86. Height, 5'3"; weight, 179 lb. Heart and breath sounds normal. Abdomen obese and soft. No bladder distention. Faint urine odor present. Rises with some difficulty. Walks slowly with walker. Limited range of motion in knees and hips.

Nursing Diagnosis	Goals and Outcome Criteria	Interventions
Stress Urinary Incontinence related to weak pelvic muscles and high intra-abdominal pressure	Improved urinary control: patient will report fewer incidents of stress incontinence.	Explain to the patient how weak perineal muscles cause stress incontinence. Instruct her how to do Kegel perineal exercises: contract the perineal muscles and hold the contraction for 10 sec; repeat the contraction three more times; repeat the set of four contractions four times a day. Advise the patient to empty her bladder every 2 hr while awake. Encourage intake of normal amounts of fluid but discourage liquids with diuretic effects: coffee, tea, and alcohol. Explain that obesity increases intra-abdominal pressure and contributes to stress incontinence. Explore interest in weight loss and refer to dietitian.
Risk for Impaired Skin Integrity related to prolonged contact of urine with skin	Reduced risk of skin breakdown: skin kept clean and dry; remains intact and free of excessive redness.	Inspect the perineal area and buttocks and report signs of irritation: redness, breaks in the skin. Apply skin protectants as ordered or per agency protocol. Teach the patient the importance of good perineal care to remove urine from the skin. Encourage her to cleanse the area with mild soap, rinse, and gently dry twice daily. Perineal pads or other incontinence pads should be changed promptly if they are wet.
Social Isolation related to fear of embarrassment due to incontinence	Decreased social isolation: patient resumes usual social activities	Identify activities that patient would like to resume. Discuss strategies to decrease embarrassment about incontinent episodes: (1) empty bladder before leaving room; (2) wear perineal pads or special incontinence pads to absorb urine and protect clothing and furniture. Avoid any comments that could humiliate the patient, such as references to "diapers," and avoid discussing her problem in front of others.

? CRITICAL THINKING QUESTIONS

■ What are the possible contributing factors to stress incontinence in this resident?

■ How would you teach the resident the importance of perineal care?

---

of the need to void and is able to hold the urine once the need is felt. Determine the pattern of incontinent voiding, urine volume, and related symptoms.

Pattern. Ask the patient how often incontinent episodes occur and whether they are associated with any particular activities, such as sneezing or laughing. A voiding diary is a helpful tool in identifying the pattern of urinary incontinence. Many patients are able to keep their own diaries. If the patient is unable to maintain an accurate record, you or another caregiver must do it.

Volume. If a patient is incontinent, measurements of urine can only be estimated, but the patient can probably describe the amount voided as being large, mod-

erate, or small. If pads or briefs are used, record the number used and the degree of saturation. Weighing wet pads and subtracting the dry weight of the pad is more precise but not very practical in the home setting. When the patient resides in the long-term care facility or a hospital, measure and record the amount of urine passed with continent voiding as well.

Related Symptoms. Ask whether the patient has had dysuria (painful voiding), pain in the suprapubic area (the lower abdomen where the bladder is located), or polyuria (large urine volume).

Past Medical History. Past problems that might be related to incontinence include urologic, gynecologic, neurologic, and endocrine conditions. Specifically ask if the patient has diabetes mellitus. People who have diabetes may develop neurologic problems that affect the bladder. Also, if their diabetes is poorly controlled, they may produce large volumes of urine that quickly fill the bladder.

Document all abdominal disorders, surgeries, and trauma. Record the number of pregnancies and types of deliveries. Inquire about current and recent medications because many drugs can affect kidney or bladder function. Drugs that might contribute to urinary incontinence are high-ceiling (loop) diuretics, major tranquilizers, antihistamines, decongestants, some sedatives or hypnotics, and antiparkinsonian drugs. Anticholinergics, which are used to treat some types of incontinence, could actually cause overflow incontinence. Other drugs that can disrupt normal voiding are epinephrine, theophylline, isoproterenol, and prazosin.

Pharmacology Capsule

When urinary incontinence develops suddenly, check the patient's drug profile for drugs known to contribute to incontinence.

Review of Systems. The review of systems may detect clues to conditions that contribute to incontinence. For example, the patient with severe arthritis in the hands or severely impaired vision may have difficulty managing toileting independently. Constipation is a common problem that can contribute to incontinence.

Functional Assessment. A description of the patient's usual activities and habits provides clues about possible contributing factors and about the impact of incontinence on the individual. Of special interest in relation to incontinence are usual fluid intake and consumption of alcohol.

Physical Examination

The physical examination begins with the measurement of vital signs and height and weight. Be alert for fever, tachycardia, and weight gain. Note the patient's level of awareness and appropriateness of responses. Inspect the skin for edema.

Sometimes incontinence is first recognized when you detect an odor of urine during the examination or when providing care. When examining the incontinent patient, palpate the abdomen for masses, tenderness, fullness, or distention. A distended bladder or abdominal distention associated with constipation is an important finding. Examination of the male genitalia includes inspection for abnormalities and for skin irritation. Inspect the female perineum for redness or irritation. The physician or nurse practitioner performs a pelvic examination on the female patient to assess for

prolapse of abdominal organs and to evaluate perineal muscle tone. A rectal examination is done to determine sensation, sphincter tone, and presence of fecal impaction. In males, the prostate is palpated for contour and consistency.

Assessment of the patient with urinary incontinence is outlined in Box 23-1. In addition, the environment must be assessed, including toilet accessibility, grab bars, lighting, and availability of toileting options (urinals, commode chairs).

Nursing Diagnoses, Goals, and Outcome Criteria: Urinary Incontinence	
Nursing diagnoses and goals for the patient with urinary incontinence may include the following:	
NURSING DIAGNOSES	GOALS AND OUTCOME CRITERIA
Deficient Knowledge of causes of incontinence and corrective measures	Patient understands condition and management: accurately describes and participates in treatment plan
Functional Urinary Incontinence related to physical, cognitive, or environmental barriers	Continent voiding with appropriate support: decreased episodes of incontinent voiding
Reflex Urinary Incontinence related to neurologic impairment	Adequate management of irreversible incontinence: bladder emptying accomplished with minimal involuntary leakage
Stress Urinary Incontinence related to weak pelvic structures, increased intra-abdominal pressure	Improved control of urine flow: decreased episodes of involuntary voiding when under stress
Total Urinary Incontinence related to neurologic dysfunction	Adequate management of irreversible incontinence to prevent spillage: bladder emptying accomplished with minimal involuntary leakage
Urge Urinary Incontinence related to decreased bladder capacity or bladder spasms	Ability to hold increasing volume of urine: time between voiding increases without leakage
Social Isolation related to fear of embarrassment	Decreased social isolation: patient participates in usual social activities
Situational Low Self-Esteem related to loss of control over voiding	Improved self-esteem: patient demonstrates positive self-image (confidence, pride in appearance)
Risk for Impaired Skin Integrity related to the presence of urine on the skin	Reduced risk of skin breakdown: skin kept clean, dry, and free of urine or feces
Risk for Infection related to chronic bladder distention or catheterization	Absence of urinary tract infection: normal body temperature and white blood cell count

Health History

Chief Complaint:
Pattern of continent and incontinent voiding, behaviors or activities associated with incontinent voiding, amount of urine passed with continent and incontinent voiding, awareness of need to void, ability to hold urine once aware of need to void, dysuria

Past Medical History:
Urologic, gynecologic, neurologic, and endocrine problems; abdominal operations, trauma, disorders; mental confusion; current and recent medications

Review of Systems:
Disorders that might contribute to incontinence: diabetes mellitus, cerebrovascular accident, paralysis

Functional Assessment:
Usual activities, fluid intake, alcohol consumption

Physical Examination

Vital Signs:
Fever, tachycardia

Height and Weight:
Weight gain

Level of Consciousness:
Orientation

Odor of Urine

Abdomen:
Masses, tenderness, fullness, or distention

Male Genitalia:
Abnormalities of foreskin, glans penis, perineal skin

Female Genitalia:
Redness, irritation

Rectal Examination:
Sensation, sphincter tone, fecal impaction

Interventions

Deficient Knowledge

Patient and caregiver education are key elements in the management of urinary incontinence. Often you must overcome the assumption that the condition is not treatable, especially in frail older adults. Emphasize that improvement or correction is possible for most people. Sometimes the incontinent patient is very discouraged and reluctant to try retraining techniques. Be positive, be encouraging, and praise attempts and successes. Many people believe that patients will be more motivated if they are dressed in street clothes and are not wearing incontinence garments.

In the teaching plan, include an overview of normal urination, an explanation of the type of incontinence the patient is experiencing, and detailed explanations of the prescribed treatment. Supplement verbal information with written material. Tell the patient that improvement takes time and not to expect immediate results. Praise the patient's interest in working toward

continence, participation in the treatment plan, and successful voiding. Specific methods for improving continence were discussed earlier. The appropriate methods for managing various types of incontinence are emphasized in the next section.

Incontinence

Nursing interventions for various types of incontinence overlap. Therefore interventions are discussed in general terms here. Table 23-1 summarizes the treatments for each type of incontinence.

Bladder Training or Retraining

Bladder training or retraining may be recommended for stress and urge incontinence. Teach the patient (and caregiver, if appropriate) the basic principles of bladder training. Establish a schedule for voiding every 2 to 3 hours. The patient is not usually asked to get up during the night, so pads or an external collection device may be needed during sleep. Emphasize the importance of the patient trying to delay voiding until the scheduled time. Praise the patient's efforts, and encourage the caregiver to do so as well.

Habit Training

If habit training is prescribed, you may initiate an incontinence record to help establish the schedule for timed voiding (Fig. 23-4). You or other caregivers must then remind the patient to try to void at the scheduled times. It might be argued that the caregiver, rather than the patient, is being trained. This is true to some extent, but in many cases the patient is able to take responsibility for toileting on the prescribed schedule and remain continent.

If the patient has difficulty voiding at the scheduled time, try to stimulate voiding. To promote voiding, establish a comfortable position for the patient, ensure privacy, and use specific stimuli. Stimuli that may encourage voiding include stroking the inner thigh, pouring warm water over the perineum, running water in the lavatory or tub, and drinking water while on the toilet.

Fluid intake may be spaced at 2-hour intervals to provide regular filling of the bladder. Nighttime wetness can be reduced by limiting fluids after 7 PM. Patients or their caregivers sometimes decrease fluid intake excessively to reduce urinary incontinence. This makes it harder to schedule toileting and can lead to other problems (urinary tract infection, urinary calculi). Most references recommend 1500 to 3000 mL of fluid daily unless contraindicated. If a patient has cardiovascular or renal disease, consult the physician about the ideal fluid intake. Gradually increase the fluid intake for older patients, because they often do not adapt well to rapid changes in blood volume.

Social Isolation

The person with urinary incontinence may curtail social activities out of fear of having embarrassing acci-

INCONTINENCE MONITORING RECORD

INSTRUCTIONS: EACH TIME THE PATIENT IS CHECKED:
1) Mark *one* of the circles in the BLADDER section at the hour closest to the time the patient is checked.
2) Make an X in the BOWEL section if the patient has had an incontinent or normal bowel movement.

◔ = Incontinent, small amount	∅ = Dry	X = Incontinent BOWEL
● = Incontinent, large amount	⊿ = Voided correctly	X = Normal BOWEL

PATIENT NAME _____   ROOM # _____   DATE _____

	BLADDER			BOWEL			
	INCONTINENT OF URINE	DRY	VOIDED CORRECTLY	INCONTINENT X	NORMAL X	INITIALS	COMMENTS
12 am	◔ ●	○	△ cc ____				
1	◔ ●	○	△ cc ____				
2	◔ ●	○	△ cc ____				
3	◔ ●	○	△ cc ____				
4	◔ ●	○	△ cc ____				
5	◔ ●	○	△ cc ____				
6	◔ ●	○	△ cc ____				
7	◔ ●	○	△ cc ____				
8	◔ ●	○	△ cc ____				
9	◔ ●	○	△ cc ____				
10	◔ ●	○	△ cc ____				
11	◔ ●	○	△ cc ____				
12 pm	◔ ●	○	△ cc ____				
1	◔ ●	○	△ cc ____				
2	◔ ●	○	△ cc ____				
3	◔ ●	○	△ cc ____				
4	◔ ●	○	△ cc ____				
5	◔ ●	○	△ cc ____				
6	◔ ●	○	△ cc ____				
7	◔ ●	○	△ cc ____				
8	◔ ●	○	△ cc ____				
9	◔ ●	○	△ cc ____				
10	◔ ●	○	△ cc ____				
11	◔ ●	○	△ cc ____				
TOTALS:							

C 1984

FIGURE 23-4 An incontinence record.

dents. Also, access to toilets in public places is often limited, so patients who cannot delay voiding may be afraid to venture far from home. If continence is unlikely or not yet established, a variety of incontinence products are available that may permit the patient to venture out without fear of wetness or odor. Specially designed pads and undergarments as well as some external urine collection devices may be used. As was mentioned earlier, external collection devices are more readily available and more satisfactory for men than for women. The patient also can be encouraged to maintain the voiding schedule during the social outing. If the patient has an incontinent episode, be careful not to show disapproval.

Situational Low Self-Esteem

The ability to control elimination is an important childhood accomplishment. Adults who become incontinent may be so embarrassed that they are reluctant to tell anyone about it. Nurses often discover that a newly admitted patient has concealed incontinence from family and physicians. Some older people do not seek help for incontinence because they think it is caused by old age and cannot be corrected.

You can help patients learn to manage incontinence and see that it is not a barrier to achieving a full life. Your attitude toward the patient and toward incontinence influences how the patient deals with the change in body function. Caregivers must be committed to efforts to help patients avoid incontinence. The following situation should not be allowed to happen:

> A stroke patient in a long-term care facility calls out, "I need to go to the bathroom!" A busy nursing staff member rushes by, pats her on the hand, and says, "That's all right. You have a diaper on. Go ahead and pee."

Encourage the patient to attend to dress and grooming to promote a more positive self-image. The patient who takes an active role in carrying out the treatment plan may feel less helpless and better able to cope with incontinence. Advise caregivers not to refer to incontinence pads and undergarments as "diapers" because of that term's association with infants.

Risk for Impaired Skin Integrity

A major problem for the incontinent patient is the risk of skin breakdown. Urine and feces, if left in contact with the skin, cause a rash. Continuous moisture causes the skin to lose its oily protective barrier. Skin breakdown may follow. The key to preventing breakdown is to keep the skin clean, dry, and free of urine or feces. If a patient is incontinent and unable to report voiding, check hourly for wetness. Immediately remove wet garments and linens. Wash the skin with mild soap and warm water, rinse, and gently pat dry. Inspect the genitals, perineum, thighs, and buttocks for redness and skin breakdown. Apply protective creams as ordered or according to agency policy. If breakdown does occur, notify the registered nurse or physician and provide treatment as ordered or according to agency policy.

Risk for Infection

The patient who is incontinent of urine is at risk for urinary tract infection and urinary calculi (stones). These complications are most likely to occur in patients who retain urine and in those who restrict their fluids. Retained urine is a good medium for bacterial growth, and the overstretched bladder wall is susceptible to infection. Patients may restrict fluid intake to try to reduce the frequency of incontinence. Concentrated urine is a risk factor for infections and calculi. Patients with indwelling catheters are at even greater risk for urinary tract infections.

To reduce the risk of urinary tract infection, have the patient empty the bladder as scheduled, provide adequate fluids, and use strict aseptic technique during catheterization. Also, keep the perineal area clean. Encourage the intake of 1500 to 3000 mL of fluid daily unless contraindicated. Details of catheter care are covered in Chapter 40.

FECAL INCONTINENCE

Fecal incontinence is less common than urinary incontinence, but it can be very distressing for patients who are affected by it. Fecal incontinence is usually related to anal sphincter dysfunction caused by anal surgery, trauma during childbirth, Crohn's disease affecting the anus, or diabetic neuropathy. Some patients experience temporary incontinence with severe diarrhea because they do not have time to reach the toilet. Incontinent diarrhea may also be present with fecal impaction. Diminished muscle strength associated with aging also may be a factor.

PHYSIOLOGY OF DEFECATION

The structures that maintain bowel control are the internal and external sphincters and the puborectal muscle. The muscles of the pelvic floor and the external sphincter are under voluntary control (Fig. 23-5). The bowel has its own nerve network that stimulates peristalsis when it is distended. Therefore disorders of the

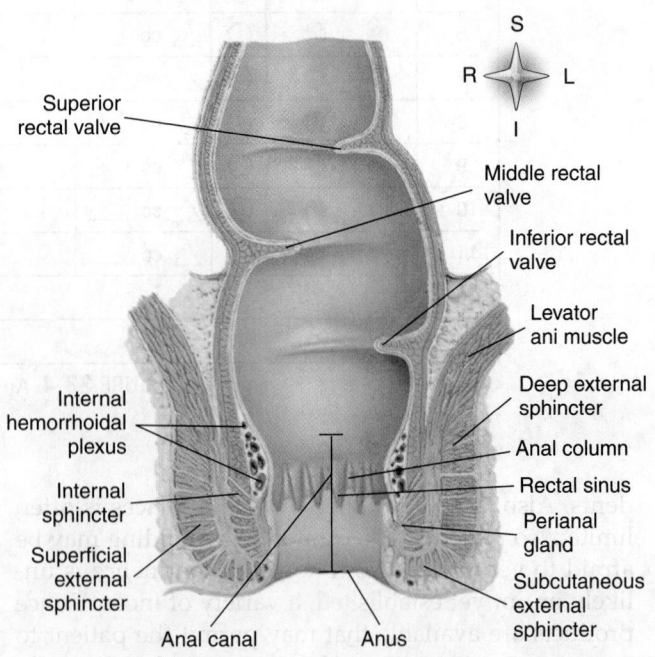

FIGURE **23-5** The anal sphincters and musculature.

central nervous system and spinal cord do not impair bowel control as much as they do bladder control.

The fecal mass enters the rectum by mass movement. The presence of feces in the rectum creates a desire to defecate. Defecation occurs when the anal sphincter relaxes and the rectum contracts. Tightening of the diaphragm and abdominal muscles promotes defecation by increasing pressure in the abdomen. If defecation does not occur soon after this pressure is felt, the sensation of needing to defecate soon fades. People who often ignore or delay defecation tend to become constipated.

DIAGNOSTIC TESTS AND PROCEDURES

Evaluation of fecal incontinence may include assessment of rectal sphincter tone, laboratory examination of a stool specimen for blood or pathogens, and endoscopic or radiologic procedures to detect underlying problems. Diagnostic tests and procedures for the gastrointestinal system are presented in detail in Chapter 38.

COMMON THERAPEUTIC MEASURES

ENEMAS

Enemas may be necessary to stimulate emptying of the bowel in the patient who is prone to impaction. Various types of enemas and nursing considerations are discussed in Chapter 38. In general, frequent use of large-volume enemas is not advised because it overstretches the bowel and may contribute to loss of muscle tone. Sometimes, however, enemas are necessary. The patient with poor rectal sphincter tone may have difficulty retaining enema solutions. An adapter can be placed on the enema tubing and inserted into the anus. The nipple-like adapter helps the patient retain the solution.

POUCHES

Plastic pouches, much like ostomy bags, may be applied to the perianal area and held in place with adhesive. They are helpful for patients who have frequent stools. Because they are bulky and uncomfortable, usually they are not used on ambulatory patients. Another disadvantage is the skin irritation caused by the adhesive. When the pouch is changed, always provide meticulous skin care. An alternative to the pouch is an adult incontinent brief or (for bed patients) linen protectors.

DRUG THERAPY

Types of drugs employed to prevent or treat fecal incontinence include laxatives, stool softeners, and antidiarrheal drugs depending on the cause of the incontinence. If the patient has had fecal impactions,

 Put on Your Thinking Cap!

When would a patient with fecal incontinence need laxatives?

laxatives or stool softeners are appropriate. Antidiarrheal drugs are appropriate if diarrhea is causing the problem. These drugs are discussed in Chapter 38.

BIOFEEDBACK

Patients who are motivated and able to follow directions and whose external anal sphincter is capable of responding to rectal distention may achieve bowel control with biofeedback. A balloon is inserted into the rectum and inflated. A manometer creates a tracing of the normal response of the sphincter to rectal pressure. The patient tries to consciously reproduce the pattern by contracting the muscles that delay defecation. The size of the balloon is progressively decreased to help the patient recognize and respond to the amount of rectal distention expected with normal stool volume. Biofeedback has been effective for many patients but has not proved useful for patients with fecal incontinence associated with diabetes, spinal cord injury, rectal trauma, or radiation injury. Pelvic muscle strengthening exercise as described with urinary incontinence may be helpful.

DIETARY CHANGES

Some foods can contribute to fecal incontinence. For example, chocolate, coffee, tea, and other caffeinated beverages all stimulate the anal sphincters to relax. Raw fruits, fruit juices (especially prune and grape juice), raw vegetables, cabbage, sweets, alcohol, and highly spicy foods stimulate stool production. The patient can be advised to avoid these foods and to consume more foods that thicken the stool. These include bananas, rice, bread, potatoes, cheese, yogurt, oatmeal, oat bran, boiled milk, and pasta. Until fecal incontinence is corrected, the patient may also wish to avoid foods that cause odor and gas. Odor-causing foods include cabbage family vegetables, beans, garlic, eggs, fish, and turnips. Gas-producing foods include beans, beer, carbonated beverages, cucumbers, cabbage, broccoli, dairy products, and corn.

TYPES OF FECAL INCONTINENCE

The four types of fecal incontinence are overflow, anorectal, neurogenic, and symptomatic. Table 23-2 summarizes the features of each type.

OVERFLOW INCONTINENCE
Description

Fecal overflow incontinence is caused by constipation in which the rectum is constantly distended. The fecal

| Table 23-2 | *Types of Fecal Incontinence* |

TYPE	DESCRIPTION	CAUSES	NURSING CARE
Overflow	Uncontrolled, frequent passage of small, semisoft stools Fecal impaction may be present	Constipation in which entire colon is full of fecal matter	Administer laxatives and enemas as ordered Increase fluids and fiber as appropriate
Anorectal	Uncontrolled passage of stool several times a day	Weak pelvic muscles Loss of anal reflexes Poor rectal sphincter tone Rectal prolapse	Teach Kegel exercises Prepare for surgery, if planned
Neurogenic	Formed stools are passed after meals Usually seen in dementia patients	Gastrocolic reflex stimulates defecation Patient does not delay until appropriate time	Scheduled toileting
Symptomatic	Incontinent stools, usually diarrhea Not related to other types of fecal incontinence	Colon or rectal disease	Comfort measures; skin care Prepare for diagnostic tests and procedures

mass backs up until the entire colon is full. There may or may not be a fecal impaction. The patient passes semisolid stools frequently. This condition may be related to a long-standing dependence on laxatives or enemas.

Medical Treatment

Medical management of fecal overflow incontinence is concerned with immediate relief of the constipation and long-term control of the problem. The first step is to cleanse the colon. Phosphate enemas and suppositories may be ordered to empty the rectum. Daily enemas for 7 to 10 days are then needed to empty the entire colon. Instead of the enemas, the physician may order oral laxatives such as bisacodyl or mannitol. If hard masses of stool are present, they can be softened with oil retention enemas and then removed digitally.

Once the colon has been cleansed, regular evacuation is essential. Increased fluids and fiber may be helpful, but some patients need regular aids to elimination. The physician may order enemas or suppositories twice a week or daily laxatives. For older patients, senna or lactulose is preferred by many geriatric specialists. Mineral oil should be avoided because it interferes with absorption of fat-soluble vitamins and because it may be aspirated, causing lipid pneumonia.

NEUROGENIC INCONTINENCE
Description

Many people report having a bowel movement shortly after the first meal of the day. This is caused by the gastrocolic reflex. When food enters the stomach, it stimulates activity throughout the digestive tract and causes the movement of the fecal mass into the rectum. Patients who do not voluntarily delay defecation are said to have neurogenic incontinence. This occurs most often in patients with dementia. These

patients usually have one or two formed stools daily after meals.

Medical Treatment

Neurogenic incontinence is usually treated with scheduled toileting based on the patient's usual time of defecation. If this is not successful, some physicians order a constipating drug (e.g., codeine) each morning and a laxative (e.g., senna, milk of magnesia) each night. This routine results in a controlled bowel movement each morning and avoids later accidents. It does not, however, correct the underlying problem.

SYMPTOMATIC INCONTINENCE
Description

Symptomatic incontinence is the result of colorectal disease. These patients usually have incontinence with diarrhea. Blood or mucus may be seen in the stool.

Medical Treatment

When a patient has symptomatic incontinence, medical care should be sought to identify and treat the cause.

ANORECTAL INCONTINENCE
Description

Anorectal incontinence is associated with nerve damage that causes the muscles of the pelvic floor to be weak. There may be rectal abnormalities, including loss of anal reflex and loss of anal sphincter tone. Patients typically have several incontinent stools a day.

Medical Treatment

Anorectal incontinence is treated with pelvic muscle exercises and sometimes biofeedback. If these techniques are ineffective, surgical repair of the anal sphincter may be advised.

NURSING CARE *of the Patient with Fecal Incontinence*

Assessment

The data you collect can contribute to a thorough nursing assessment that can help diagnose the type and cause of fecal incontinence and guide the selection of treatment.

Health History

Chief Complaint. When a patient has fecal incontinence, determine the usual bowel pattern, changes, stool characteristics, and related symptoms such as pain or cramping.

Bowel Pattern. Bowel patterns are usually well established in the adult. The frequency of bowel movements may range from several times daily to several times a week. Document the patient's usual frequency of bowel movements. In relation to incontinent episodes, ask if the patient is aware of the need to defecate. For dementia patients, a caregiver may be able to detect clues that the patient is about to have a bowel movement. If the patient is confused, initiate a record of times and circumstances when defecation occurs.

Characteristics of Stools. Describe the consistency, color, and constituents of the patient's stools. Terms used to describe consistency include liquid, watery, pasty, tarry, semiformed, formed, and hard. Most of these terms are self-explanatory. Tarry is used to describe stools that are shiny, sticky, and black. Stool is normally brown in color. Abnormal colors are black, red, green, and white. Abnormal stool constituents might include blood, mucus, or undigested food.

Past Medical History. Document chronic illnesses, past acute illnesses, and surgeries or trauma to the abdomen or rectum. Neurologic conditions, including stroke, spinal cord injury, and dementia, are significant. List recent and current medications and all allergies. It is especially important to determine the use of laxatives, enemas, or suppositories. Because these are often purchased without a prescription, the patient may not mention them when reporting medications. Record the obstetric history, including the number of pregnancies, types of deliveries, and complications of childbirth.

Review of Systems. The review of systems identifies problems that may be related to fecal incontinence such as motor, sensory, or cognitive impairments.

Functional Assessment. The functional assessment focuses on habits that may be related to bowel function, including diet, fluid intake, and exercise or activity pattern. Determine whether the patient has the mobility and dexterity to manage toileting independently. Recent travel to other countries may be significant, because travelers sometimes acquire uncommon intestinal infections.

Physical Examination

Inspect and palpate the abdomen for distention and auscultate for bowel sounds. Inspect the perianal area for irritation or breakdown. The physician or nurse practitioner may perform a rectal examination and test the strength of the rectal sphincter.

Assessment of the patient with fecal incontinence is outlined in Box 23-2.

Nursing Diagnoses, Goals, and Outcome Criteria: Fecal Incontinence

Nursing diagnoses and goals for the patient with fecal incontinence may include the following:

NURSING DIAGNOSES	GOALS AND OUTCOME CRITERIA
Bowel Incontinence related to impaction, cognitive impairment, neurologic impairment, environmental barriers, or impaired mobility	Controlled bowel elimination: regular voluntary bowel evacuation of soft, formed stool
Impaired Skin Integrity related to contact of feces with skin	Normal skin integrity: no redness or skin breakdown
Situational Low Self-Esteem related to loss of control over elimination	Improved self-esteem: patient's comments and behavior reflect a positive view of self (confidence, takes pride in appearance)

Interventions

Bowel Incontinence

Continued monitoring is an essential part of the nurse's role in caring for the patient with incontinence. Documentation of the patient's usual bowel pattern provides a guideline for scheduled elimination and for setting realistic goals. To establish a bowel program, take the patient to the toilet at the usual time of defecation, commonly 30 minutes after eating. If suppositories or enemas are ordered, administer them and document the results.

When enemas or laxatives are prescribed on a routine basis for overflow incontinence, caregivers often fear creating laxative or enema dependency. For these patients, however, normal bowel function may not be a realistic goal. They may do better with a program that promotes regular bowel evacuation. It is far better than the miserable process of emptying a full colon every few weeks.

Explain normal bowel physiology and interventions for incontinence to the patient. Advise the patient to consume adequate fluids and fiber to prevent constipation and impaction. A fluid intake of at least 1500 mL/day is recommended if not contraindicated. Increase fluids gradually in the older patient because fluid overload can lead to heart failure. Work with the dietitian to teach the patient that fresh fruits and vegetables provide bulk and fiber that keep the stool moist and soft. Encourage ambulation if the patient is able to walk. If perineal exercises are prescribed, advise the patient to practice contracting the muscles that control defecation.

Box 23-2 | ASSESSMENT of Patients with Fecal Incontinence

Health History

Chief Complaint:
Bowel pattern changes, stool characteristics (consistency, color, constituents), awareness of need to defecate, symptoms associated with passage of incontinent stool

Past Medical History:
Chronic illnesses, past acute illnesses, abdominal or rectal trauma or surgery, abdominal radiotherapy, recent and current medications, dementia, allergies

Review of Systems:
Motor, sensory, or cognitive dysfunction that could affect continence

Functional Assessment:
Diet, fluid intake, exercise or activity pattern, foreign travel

Physical Examination

Abdomen:
Distention, bowel sounds

Perianal Area:
Irritation, breakdown

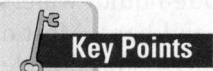 **Put on Your Thinking Cap!**

Four of the patients you have cared for in the past week have had diagnoses of "urinary incontinence." Mrs. A., age 55, was admitted for treatment of her asthma. She has five adult children and often baby-sits for two toddlers. She says she loses a small amount of urine when she coughs or picks up a toddler.

Mr. B., age 72, had a prostatectomy 2 weeks ago. His catheter has been removed, but he was readmitted with a severe urinary tract infection. He complains of constant dribbling of urine that requires wearing incontinence pads. His bladder is not palpable.

Mrs. C., age 25, had an appendectomy. The afternoon of the procedure, she voided 25 to 60 mL of urine at frequent intervals. Her bladder was distended, and she complained of a constant urge to void.

Mr. D., age 85, was admitted with pneumonia. He has a diagnosis of moderate dementia. On two occasions, he was found out of bed and there was urine on the floor. On another occasion, he urinated in the wastebasket.

Decide which type of incontinence each patient probably had, and fill in the chart with the probable cause(s) for the specific patient, the recommended treatment, and the appropriate nursing interventions for each patient in relation to incontinence.

Patient	Type of Incontinence	Probable Cause	Treatment	Nursing Care
Mrs. A.	_____	_____	_____	_____
Mr. B.	_____	_____	_____	_____
Mrs. C.	_____	_____	_____	_____
Mr. D.	_____	_____	_____	_____

The contraction should be held up to 10 seconds and repeated several times each day.

Impaired Skin Integrity

After each incontinent stool, cleanse the patient's perianal area thoroughly. Apply protective creams or ointments as ordered or per agency policy. Incontinence undergarments may be needed to prevent soiling and embarrassment, but they must be checked frequently so that stool does not remain in contact with the skin. Fecal pouches may be used, but the adhesive and plastic can irritate the skin, so good skin care is still a priority.

Situational Low Self-Esteem

Loss of bowel control can be devastating for the patient. Express understanding of the patient's distress, and encourage the patient to strive for as much improvement as possible. Praise the patient for participation in the treatment program and for decreased frequency of incontinent stools. Encourage the patient to practice good grooming and to resume social activities. Help patients coordinate their social schedule with their bowel programs.

Key Points

- Incontinence is the inability to control the passage of urine or feces.
- Normal controlled voiding requires healthy bladder muscle, a patent urethra, normal transmission of nerve impulses, and mental alertness.
- Data collection relevant to urinary incontinence includes recording the voiding pattern, urine volume, associated signs and symptoms, medications, past medical history, and physical findings.
- The types of urinary incontinence are transient, urge, stress, overflow (including reflex), functional, and total.
- Transient incontinence is caused by reversible conditions and is often corrected by treatment of the underlying problem.
- Urge incontinence, involuntary loss of urine after a strong urge to void, may be corrected by treating the cause with behavior modification and drug therapy.
- Overflow incontinence, involuntary loss of urine associated with a full bladder, may be corrected by treating the cause (e.g., enlarged prostate) or by using drugs that stimulate the bladder and relax the internal sphincter.
- Reflex incontinence is one type of overflow incontinence.
- Stress incontinence, the involuntary loss of urine during physical exertion, may be improved by strengthening the perineal muscles, by surgical intervention, or by placement of an artificial sphincter.
- Functional incontinence is inappropriate voiding despite normal urinary function.
- Assessment of fecal incontinence includes recording the usual bowel pattern, stool characteristics, related symp-

toms, activity, diet, fluid intake, medications, and use of aids to help elimination as well as performing an abdominal assessment.

- Types of fecal incontinence include overflow, anorectal, neurogenic, and symptomatic.
- Fecal overflow incontinence is caused by constipation in which the rectum is constantly distended and is treated by relieving the constipation and preventing future episodes.
- Anorectal incontinence is caused by abnormalities in the pelvic muscle, anus, or rectum and may require pelvic floor muscle exercises or surgery.
- Neurogenic incontinence is automatic defecation seen in people (e.g., patients with dementia) who do not voluntarily delay defecation; it may be corrected by scheduled toileting.
- Symptomatic incontinence results from colorectal disease and requires correction of the basic problem.

- Nursing care of the patient who is incontinent may address measures to correct the specific type of incontinence, to maintain skin integrity, to improve situational low self-esteem, and to improve knowledge of management.
- Techniques to restore bladder control include bladder retraining using scheduled toileting, Credé's technique for emptying the bladder, Kegel exercises to strengthen pelvic floor muscles, and reflex training.
- Bowel training may be accomplished by scheduled toileting, stimulation techniques, or both.

 Go to your Companion CD-ROM for a Pharmacology Tutorial, Audio Glossary, and 3-D animations.

evolve Be sure to visit the companion Evolve site at http://evolve.elsevier.com/Linton/ for WebLinks and additional online resources.

REVIEW QUESTIONS *Choose the best answer.*

1. Which of the following diagnostic tests/procedures is done under anesthesia and requires signed consent?
   1. Cystometry
   2. Postvoid residual
   3. Uroflowmetry
   4. Cystoscopy

2. Habit training is being used to treat a patient with urinary incontinence. What will you instruct the nursing assistant to do?
   1. Check the patient for wetness every 2 hours and ask the patient to state whether wet or dry.
   2. Encourage the patient to void every 2 hours on a schedule based on the patient's usual pattern.
   3. Encourage the patient to delay voiding and to void only at scheduled times.
   4. Have the patient practice interrupting urine flow by contracting perineal muscles.

3. Patient teaching for performing pelvic muscle exercises includes:
   1. Contract perineal muscles for 30 seconds, then relax for 30 seconds
   2. Anticipate improvement within 1 week after starting exercises
   3. To do these exercises correctly, you must be in a sitting position
   4. You will need to continue the exercises indefinitely to maintain control

4. How does intermittent self-catheterization in the home setting differ from that in an institution?
   1. Clean technique may be used at home but not in a hospital.
   2. Sterile technique must be used regardless of the setting.
   3. Clean technique may be used anywhere as long as the patient performs the procedure.
   4. Clean technique can be used in long-term care facilities because patients live there.

5. Care of the patient with a pessary includes:
   1. Evaluation of placement position within 1 week after insertion
   2. Documentation of pessary placement so it will not be forgotten
   3. Monitoring for signs of bowel obstruction
   4. Removal for cleansing each time perineal care is done

6. Which of the following is true of urge incontinence?
   1. A strong, abrupt urge to urinate occurs shortly before involuntary urine loss.
   2. Urge incontinence is often caused by anticholinergic drugs.
   3. It commonly occurs in patients who have fecal impactions.
   4. The bladder overfills so that small amounts of urine are passed to relieve pressure.

7. The most serious complication of reflex incontinence is:
   1. Urinary tract infection
   2. Skin breakdown
   3. Autonomic dysreflexia
   4. Bladder rupture

8. Which type of urinary incontinence is sometimes caused by antihistamines or anticholinergic drugs?
   1. Urge   3. Overflow
   2. Reflex   4. Stress

9. Patient teaching related to stress incontinence should include the following:
   1. It is usually caused by relaxation of the pelvic floor muscles
   2. Limit fluid intake to 1000 mL a day
   3. Fluids containing caffeine stimulate contraction of perineal muscles
   4. The only effective treatment for stress incontinence is surgical repair

10. Patients with fecal incontinence should be advised to avoid:
    1. Bananas
    2. Alcohol
    3. Pasta
    4. Cheese

11. A bedridden patient with no history of fecal incontinence has been involuntarily passing liquid stools for 2 days. You should suspect:
    1. The gastrocolic reflex is being stimulated
    2. The patient is too confused to control defecation
    3. The patient may have a fecal impaction
    4. The pelvic muscle floor has been injured

24 Loss, Death, and End-of-Life Care

CHERYL ROSS STAATS

evolve http://evolve.elsevier.com/Linton/

Objectives

After reading and studying this chapter, you should be able to:

1. Describe beliefs and practices related to death and dying.
2. Describe responses of patients and their families to terminal illness and death.
3. Identify nursing diagnoses that are appropriate for the terminally ill.
4. Identify nursing goals that are appropriate for the terminally ill.
5. Identify nursing interventions to meet the needs of terminally ill and dying patients.
6. Discuss the needs of the terminally ill patient's significant others.
7. Discuss the ways nurses can intervene to meet the needs of the terminally ill patient's significant others.
8. Explore the responses of the nurse who works with the terminally ill.
9. Explore the needs of the nurse who works with terminally ill patients.
10. Identify issues related to caring for the dying patient, including advance directives, do-not-resuscitate decisions, brain death, organ donations, and pronouncement of death.

Key Terms

Be sure to check out the bonus material on the Companion CD-ROM, including selected audio pronunciations.

advance directive (p. 362)
algor mortis (ĂL-gŏr MŎR-tĭs, p. 358)
autopsy (ĂW-tŏp-sē, p. 360)
cerebral death (sĕ-RĒ-brăl, p. 358)
denial (p. 354)
grief (p. 352)
livor mortis (LĪ-vŏr MŎR-tĭs, p. 358)
loss (p. 352)
palliative care (PĂL-ē-ā-tĭv, p. 351)
rigor mortis (RĬG-ŏr MŎR-tĭs, p. 358)
shroud (p. 362)

A time to be born and a time to die...
Ecclesiastes 3:2

Throughout history, life and death have intrigued humankind. Artists, writers, philosophers, scientists, religious leaders, and ordinary people have pon-

dered the meaning of life and death. Yet human mortality and the death experience have not been a priority in American society. The culture of the United States tends to be youth and beauty oriented, generally approaching the life cycle in an unrealistic way. Death is a real part of life, just as birth and aging are.

The concepts of death and dying were rarely studied before the 1960s. Many times patients who were not expected to survive were placed in isolated hospital areas and given less than quality care. Many patients who were dying went without appropriate care and technically could have been termed abandoned by the medical profession. Family members, church associates, or both were usually the care providers.

Today, with the reality of the "graying of America" and the increasing number of persons with acquired immunodeficiency syndrome (AIDS), the aging process, terminal illness, and dying are not viewed as the taboo topics they once were. The specialized needs of the dying and the terminally ill are no longer ignored, nor are they denied. The processes associated with dying and death are researched by scientists, health care professionals, theologians, and lay persons. Information concerning death and dying can be found in popular as well as professional literature and is openly discussed.

A **palliative care** movement is aimed toward providing care rather than toward curing treatments. The trend toward palliative care is refocusing health care toward allowing natural death in a pain- and symptom-controlled environment with psychosocial support. Palliative care can take place outside the traditional hospital setting. The environment may be in an institutional setting, in a community setting, or in the home.

This chapter presents information concerning the death process in persons for whom death is imminent. The grieving process for the dying person and the person's friends and family is presented, with a special emphasis on nursing care.

CONCEPT OF LOSS

Death, like birth, is a natural part of the life cycle. Death favors no age, social, religious, economic, or racial groups. It is inevitable for everyone. People in general experience similar feelings and thoughts related to loss, whether the loss is real or potential.

Loss may be defined as a real or potential absence of someone or something that is valued. Real losses occur when something actually happens so that valued people or possessions are no longer available. Potential losses relate to an individual's perceptions of what *might* occur if a valued person or object were lost permanently. Anxiety, fear, and grief are common with both real and potential losses. An example of a potential loss is a 45-year-old woman, pregnant for the first time, who is concerned that her infant may be born with congenital disabilities.

TYPES OF LOSSES

Loss is experienced in many ways. Changes in self-image, developmental changes, loss of possessions, and loss of significant others are common types of loss.

Change in Self-Image

In addition to a perception of self, within each individual's life ideas about personal worth, usefulness, roles, and beliefs are created. Each aspect of the person may be subject to change. Some change is planned. Some change is beyond the individual's control. Situations that lead to a perceived change in body image, such as pregnancy, hair loss, disability, or radical surgery, can alter a person's self-concept. New parenthood and forced retirement often lead to lifestyle changes. These changes include uncertainty about roles, functions, and usual patterns of productivity. The uncertainties and insecurities in role changes result in perceived loss in terms of former roles.

Developmental Changes

Within the life cycle, changes or milestones take place. Insecurities, fears, and feelings of loss result. During infancy and childhood, parents experience a loss of control over their children as children gain independence and self-control. Examples of increasingly independent function are weaning, toileting, walking, talking, and attending school.

As maturation progresses, additional changes take place. As they grow into adulthood, individuals may relate loss to changes in routines that were previously secure and dependable. These changes include moving away from parents, getting a job, and a general loss of dependence and innocence.

Multiple losses can occur throughout the life span. Frequently the losses associated with old age happen rapidly. Age-related physical and body function changes, as well as a return to dependence, lead many individuals to a loss of self-concept in addition to the developmental loss. Dying and death at any age challenge the individual with multiple, successive losses.

Loss of Possessions

Loss of valued possessions may affect the individual. Generally, a possession has a perceived value to the owner and its value may not be readily apparent to others. An object may be irreplaceable because of the memories associated with it, or it may be valuable from a monetary standpoint. Loss of an appointment calendar may be as tragic as the loss of a family heirloom. The loss of a pet can affect the owner as significantly as the loss of a family member. For older persons, the loss of a lifetime's accumulation of possessions through placement into housing for older adults can be devastating. When a significant object is lost or left behind, the individual loses a part of his or her identity.

Loss of Significant Others

Loss of significant others occurs through death but may also occur through separation, growth of children, change of residence, divorce, or lack of communication.

Separation from significant others may be related to actual distance, or it may be emotional in nature. Children leaving their parents to go to school or to start their own families can produce feelings of loss for all concerned. Placement of a family member in an institution for long-term care or acute care can lead to prolonged separation and feelings of loss.

Emotional aspects of loss of significant others may be related to a lack of fulfillment of expected roles. Feelings of disappointment for persons who have remained unmarried or who have not had children can lead to perceptions of loss. Communication breakdowns or barriers can divide significant others as completely as changing their place of residence.

The loss of a loved one through death is a permanent loss. In nonindustrialized societies, death is looked on as a natural, normal event. In American society, death is frequently seen as a negative and unacceptable event. This society values preserving and prolonging life. Americans expect to live into old age, even if old age is not considered as attractive as youth.

A death by accident or by unexpected illness is related to a specific situation. Loss that occurs during normal development, such as children leaving home or the retirement and death of aging friends and family members, can be anticipated and possibly prepared for.

No matter who or what is lost, those left behind react to the event. Not all people react in the same fashion to similar situations.

GRIEF

Grief is a normal, natural response to a loss. It is an emotional reaction that is necessary to maintain quality in both emotional and physical well-being. The grieving process involves a total individual experience associated with thoughts, feelings, and behaviors. The grief process is usually most profound when the loss experienced is death. In particular, grieving during a death loss is a complex and intense emotional experience.

In conjunction with grief, significant others who survive respond to the loss of the loved one through bereavement. Bereavement is the individualized response to the loss of a significant person.

Working through the grief process helps the dying person and the significant others adapt to the loss. Grief that is helpful or that assists the person in accepting the reality of death is called *adaptive grief.* Grief that is prolonged, unresolved, or disruptive to the person who experiences it may be termed *maladaptive* or *dysfunctional grief.*

Adaptive grief is a healthy response. It may be associated with grieving before a death actually occurs or when the reality that death is inevitable is known. This adaptive response is termed *anticipatory grief.* Anticipatory grief is usually related to a loss or death. It may be a healthy or an unhealthy response to the grief process. Both the patient and the family members can experience anticipatory grieving. After an actual loss or a death occurs, the grief is considered to be reactive. That is, with reactive grief the loss has already happened.

Grief that is delayed or exaggerated may be identified as dysfunctional. Dysfunctional grieving may relate to a real loss or a perceived loss. It may occur in the absence of anticipatory grief, when grief is not resolved from a prior experience, or when the expression of grief is blocked in some way. Within dysfunctional grief, feelings and behaviors may become exaggerated and disruptive to a person's typical lifestyle.

Specific behaviors are associated with dysfunctional grief. Many times there are expressions of distress at the loss. Unresolved issues may be identified and past experiences reviewed. Emotions such as anger, sadness, guilt, and denial may be present in all types of grief. Some people have difficulty expressing these feelings. The person experiencing grief may show signs of changes in eating, sleeping, and other activities of daily living.

THE GRIEVING PROCESS

People experiencing the inevitability of death, the final loss, are in need of caregivers who are knowledgeable about personal attitudes that affect the experience. The attitudes of the dying person, those of the significant others, and the nurse's own attitudes affect the death experience.

You must be able to understand various aspects of the dying person's life to provide appropriate care. An adequate understanding of cultural, religious, familial, and developmental influences is beneficial in focusing on the dying person's needs, wants, and fears. Although there may be influences from culture, religion, family, and stages of development, the uniqueness of each person causes responses to vary.

Culture, religious beliefs, and age affect a person's understanding of and reaction to death or loss. Frequently, beliefs and attitudes are interrelated between culture and religion. The American work ethic is closely related to the Protestant ethic, which emphasizes independence, self-reliance, hard work, and rugged individualism. With these attitudes, many people believe that privacy is imperative. Death and dying tend to be private matters shared only with significant others. Often feelings are repressed or internalized. People who believe in "toughing it out" or "being strong" may not express themselves when they have experienced a tragic loss.

Some cultural groups, such as African Americans and Latinos, may express their feelings more easily. In some predominantly African-American churches, expressing emotions plays an important role. Kinship tends to be very strong within the Latino culture. Family members, both immediate and extended, provide support for one another. Expressing feelings of loss is encouraged and accepted easily.

Religious beliefs influence a person's reaction to loss and death. Most religious groups have common practices related to dying and death. Practices and beliefs vary from group to group regarding dying and the care of the body after death. Specific information should be obtained from the family concerning religious preferences.

Family beliefs and practices and family members' stages of development are responsible for attitudes surrounding death and dying. Past experience with facing the death of a loved one provides a frame of reference for members of the family. The past abilities of persons to adapt and accept losses can help them adapt to the death of a loved one.

The age or stage of development affects a person's reactions to death and dying. Through experience with other losses, a generalized acceptance of dying can take place. Maturity contributes toward understanding and accepting death. Table 24-1 identifies some common age-related attitudes associated with death.

Children have a different understanding of loss and death from adults. Some adults believe that children should be protected from the pain associated with the death of a loved one. Often, however, children who are "protected" may feel abandoned, frightened, and alone with their feelings. A child who loses a loved one to death may regress or be delayed in emotional development until the grief can be resolved.

Adults generally become experienced in accepting the inevitability of death. During adulthood, people must come to terms with the death of their parents and other older family members. Coping with the death of one's parents is often identified as a developmental crisis. During adulthood, people have to confront their own mortality.

Table 24-1 | *Age-Related Beliefs About Death*

AGE RANGE	BELIEFS
Infancy to 5 years (preschool)	Little or no understanding of death Death is temporary and reversible, like sleep
6 to 9 years (school age)	Death is final Own death can be avoided Death is related to violence Wishing or hoping for death can make it happen
10 to 12 years (preadolescent)	Death is an inevitable end to life Grasps own mortality by discussing fear of death or life after death Expresses feelings of death based on adult attitudes
13 to 18 years (adolescent)	Afraid of prolonged death May act out defiance for death through dangerous or self-destructive acts Has a philosophical or religious approach to death Seldom thinks about death
19 to 45 years (young adulthood)	Cultural and religious beliefs influence attitudes Death is seen as a future event
45 to 65 years (middle adulthood)	Accepts own mortality as inevitable Faces death of parents and peers May experience death anxiety
65 years and older (older adulthood)	Afraid of prolonged health problems Faces death of family members and peers Sees death as inevitable Examines death as it relates to various meanings, such as freedom from discomfort

For older adults, the impact from the death of a spouse is profound. Older adults may also outlive their children. Loss of one's child at any age is an especially traumatic event. With the increase in the older population, it stands to reason that the majority of deaths are among older adults. What seems to be an increase in health problems for widowed persons during the first year of widowhood has been reported. Older adults make up the largest group of people needing health care services, so it is imperative that nurses be sensitive to their individual needs concerning loss.

STAGES OF GRIEVING

Many researchers have identified stages of grief. Among them are Kübler-Ross, Martocchio, and Rando.

Kübler-Ross

One of the most prominent and popular authors is Elisabeth Kübler-Ross, who in 1969 identified five stages of grieving. The five stages are denial, anger, bargaining, depression, and acceptance. The stages represent a series of responses to an anticipated or actual loss. Kübler-Ross identified specific behaviors for each stage.

Denial. The person refuses to acknowledge the loss and may put forth a cheerful appearance to prolong the denial of the loss. **Denial** serves to protect the patient, family, or both from the reality of the loss.

Anger. The patient or family members may become angry or outraged with situations. The anger and resentment may be a result of a comparison between their sadness and the happiness of others. The anger may be directed toward the nurse, the staff, or the institution, as well as toward significant others.

Bargaining. In the bargaining stage, the person wishes for more time to avoid the loss. The individual may express feelings that the loss is occurring as a punishment for past actions and may try to bargain with a higher power to gain time.

Depression. The patient may speak openly or may withdraw from feelings concerning past losses. The patient needs to review his or her life. In this stage, the person realizes that the loss is final and that the situation cannot be altered.

Acceptance. The patient identifies the loss as inevitable and may want to make plans. Acceptance can involve peaceful acknowledgment of the loss. There is a sense of inner resolution of the loss.

• • •

The stages may alternate with the individual and the situation. Not all people experience all stages, and there is no predictable timetable for the stages to occur.

Martocchio

In 1985, Martocchio presented five clusters of grief. These five clusters are shock and disbelief; yearning and protest; anguish, disorganization, and despair; identification in bereavement; and reorganization and restoration.

Shock and Disbelief. Persons may feel numb. Feelings of anger, sadness, or guilt may be expressed. Denial may be present.

Yearning and Protest. Anger may be directed toward God, health care providers, survivors, and even the deceased for dying. Surviving loved ones may withdraw into themselves, not wishing to share their feelings.

Anguish, Disorganization, and Despair. There may be a decreased interest in the future. Decision making is difficult. Survivors may express a general lack of purpose for living. Crying at this stage is common.

Identification in Bereavement. Behaviors unique to the deceased such as habits, traits, or goals may be imitated by the survivors.

Reorganization and Restoration. Grieving does not simply stop all at once. Typical patterns of life gradually return. No timetable can be set for the process of grieving. Some people seem to recover from grief quickly, whereas others may experience recurrent grief throughout their lives.

Rando

Phases of the grief response were refined in 1993 by T.A. Rando. The three phases of responses that were identified include avoidance, confrontation, and accommodation.

Avoidance. Individuals respond to grief with denial, shock, and disbelief regarding the loss.

Confrontation. Feelings are intense and charged with great emotion. Individuals face the loss, and experience emotional upheaval.

Accommodation. There is a beginning of emotional healing. The intensity of grief gradually subsides. Individuals learn to deal with the loss.

• • •

A comparison of Kübler-Ross's stages of grief, Martocchio's clusters of grief, and Rando's phases of grieving is found in Table 24-2.

COMMON SIGNS AND SYMPTOMS OF GRIEF

Common signs and symptoms of grief are shared by the terminally ill person and those who lose a significant other. Knowledge of the signs and symptoms allows you to better communicate with everyone involved.

Physical symptoms are experienced during the grief process. The physical symptoms are a reaction to stress. Some symptoms include tightness in the chest, sensations of shortness of breath, suffocation, generalized weakness, intense tightening in the abdomen, and emptiness or churning in the stomach. These symptoms may fluctuate throughout the grief process. Generally, they may occur with the initial acknowledgment of death as the outcome. The patient and the family members may experience the symptoms of a stress reaction.

You should be aware that the stress reaction is a very real experience. Nursing intervention may be needed to assist a person in regaining a sense of physical function.

Awareness of Terminal Illness

Awareness of terminal illness and impending death affects the dying person and the family emotionally and physiologically. Strauss and Glaser (1970) have identified three states of awareness: closed awareness, mutual pretense, and open awareness.

Closed Awareness. When closed awareness occurs, the family and the patient recognize that the patient is ill. They may not understand the severity of the illness. There is a lack of awareness related to impending death.

Mutual Pretense. With mutual pretense, the patient, the loved ones, and the care providers know of the terminal prognosis. No one discusses the issue openly, and people may make every effort to avoid the subject. Frequently the patient avoids the subject to protect the family and the caregivers from discomfort.

Open Awareness. Most health care providers prefer open awareness in most situations. With open awareness, the patient and others involved freely discuss the impending death. The discussions may be difficult, but they allow the patient and the family to become comfortable with the topic. The patient can participate in making final arrangements for personal business. Open awareness is not necessarily appropriate for all people. Some people are unable to cope emotionally with an open, honest discussion of death.

Generally, honesty is the best choice in dealing with death. Often ethical dilemmas occur over whether to "tell" the patient about the terminal illness and impending death. At times the physician may decide not to tell the patient about the expected outcome of the illness or disease, frequently opting to discuss the patient's condition with family members. The decision may be the physician's alone, or it may be based on family wishes. Usually the patient knows the prognosis even if he or she is not told directly. If such is the case, the patient may feel distrustful and suspicious of the care providers and the family based on a breach in confidentiality. This suspicion can be a source of great discomfort for the patient.

Honesty in most cases provides patients with the opportunity to accept their fate. Through understanding of the illness and participation in their own care, patients can work through and take control of their grief.

| **Table 24-2** | ***Comparison of Stages of Grieving*** |

KÜBLER-ROSS (1969)	MARTOCCHIO (1985)	RANDO (1993)
Denial	Shock and disbelief	Avoidance
Anger	Yearning and protest	
Bargaining	Anguish, disorganization, and despair	Confrontation
Depression	Identification in bereavement	
Acceptance	Reorganization and restoration	Accommodation

> ### What Does Culture Have to Do with Grief?
>
> Culture strongly influences the way people handle grief. For example, traditional Vietnamese value stoicism, traditional Mexicans express grief openly, and traditional Swedes accept quiet or open grief. Traditional widows in Greece wear black for the rest of their lives.

FEARS ASSOCIATED WITH TERMINAL ILLNESS AND DEATH

Fear is a typical feeling associated with dying. The nurse is frequently called on to deal with the dying person's fears. Three specific fears associated with dying are fear of pain, fear of loneliness, and fear of meaninglessness.

Fear of Pain

There is a tendency to associate death with pain. Common sayings such as "on pain of death" or "a violent death" have colored the way we perceive death. A dying person who has lost a loved one to a painful death may expect the same type of experience. Therefore many people assume that pain always accompanies death.

Physiologically, there is no absolute indication that death is always painful. Psychologically, pain may occur based on the anxieties and separations related to the loss through dying.

Terminally ill patients who do experience physical pain should have medication available. The patient and family need assurance that medication will be given promptly when it is needed. Patients can participate in their own pain relief by discussing pain relief measures and their effects. Most patients want their pain relieved without the side effects of grogginess or sleepiness. Pain relief measures such as medication need not deprive the patient of the ability to interact with others.

Prevention of pain and relief from discomfort should be handled with compassion. Pain control must be consistent. It is necessary to provide constant relief rather than to wait until the pain is unbearable and then try to relieve it. Addiction to opioids is of little concern when dealing with the terminally ill patient. When death is inevitable, nursing interventions are aimed at maintaining comfort rather than promoting wellness. Pain management is discussed in Chapter 15.

Pharmacology Capsule

The terminally ill patient should not be denied pain relief measures. Pain relief is best achieved by scheduled administration of analgesics rather than administration only as necessary.

> ### What Does Culture Have to Do with Pain?
>
> Culture influences how patients respond to pain. Some readily report pain, whereas others try to be stoic. Assess all patients for pain and explain how it can be reduced or relieved to improve quality of life.

Fear of Loneliness

Most terminally ill and dying people do not want to be alone. Many are afraid that they will be abandoned by loved ones who cannot cope with imminent death. Dying patients typically want someone whom they know and trust to stay with them. It may be a loved one or a caregiver. The simple presence of someone provides support and comfort. Neither words nor actions are necessary unless the patient requires something. Holding hands, touching, and listening are quality nursing responses. Simply providing companionship allows the dying person a sense of security.

Fear of Meaninglessness

During the dying process most people review their lives. They review their intentions during life, examining actions and expressing regrets about what might have been. Patients need to look at positive aspects of their lives. Relatives can help patients review their lives. The worth of the dying person needs to be confirmed.

You can assist patients and their families by pointing out the positive qualities of the patient's life. Prayers, thoughts, and feelings may provide comfort for the patient. While remaining nonjudgmental during interventions, you can respect and accept the practices and rituals associated with the patient's life review.

CLINICAL SIGNS OF IMPENDING DEATH

Death occurs when all vital organs and systems cease to function. During the death process, systems and organs slow and lose their ability to maintain life. There is a general loss of muscle tone, a decrease in the cardiovascular system, a decrease in respiratory function, and a decrease in sensory abilities. All systems are involved. Table 24-3 lists the systems and the associated clinical signs of impending death.

LOSS OF MUSCLE TONE

The muscular system weakens gradually. Body movements are slowed. Facial muscles lose tone, and the jaw may sag. Speech may be difficult because of decreased muscle coordination. Swallowing becomes increasingly difficult, and the gag reflex is eventually lost. The functions of the gastrointestinal and the genitourinary systems slow down. Peristalsis diminishes, which can lead to constipation, gas accumulation, distention, and nausea. Pain medications may enhance the gastro-

Table 24-3 *Physical Manifestations of Approaching Death*

	MANIFESTATION
Hearing	Is usually last sense to disappear *Remember that comatose patients may still be able to hear.*
Touch	Decrease of sensation Decrease of pain and touch perception
Taste	Decreases as illness progresses
Smell	Decreases with disease progression Related to loss of taste
Sight	Blurring of vision Sinking and glazing of eyes Blinking stops, and eyelids remain half-opened
Skin	Mottling on hands and feet Cold, clammy skin High fever due to improper functioning of thermo-regulator in the brain or dehydration "Wax-like" skin appearance very near death
Respiration	Breathing becomes rapid and deep with periods of apnea (Cheyne-Stokes breathing) Becomes irregular, gradually slowing down to terminal gasps (may be described as "guppy breathing") Grunting and noisy tachypnea (death rattle) is common *Families need to be reassured that those symptoms do not signal emotional/physical distress.*
Urinary tract	Becomes incontinent of urine or unable to excrete/pass urine
Bowel	Slowing of digestive tract and possible cessation of function (may be enhanced by pain medications) Accumulation of gas, distention, and nausea due to diminished peristalsis Loss of sphincter control may produce incontinence May have a bowel movement when death is imminent
Muscle tone	Sagging of jaw due to loss of tone of the facial muscles Speaking may be difficult due to decreased muscle coordination Swallowing can become more difficult; therefore taking food, fluids, and medications by mouth becomes harder and harder Loss of gag reflex Jerking movements may be seen in patients on large amounts of opioids (myoclonic jerking)
Circulation changes	Slowing and weakening of pulse Blood pressure drops

intestinal slowing. Loss of sphincter control may produce fecal and urinary incontinence.

CIRCULATORY AND RESPIRATORY CHANGES

Vital signs provide valuable information related to cardiovascular and respiratory changes that precede death. The pulse slows and weakens. Blood pressure drops. Temperature may be elevated. Respirations may be rapid, shallow, and irregular, or they may be very slow. Breathing may sound wet and noisy. The noisy, wet-sounding respirations, termed the *death rattle*, are a response based on mouth breathing and accumulation of mucus in the upper airways. Cheyne-Stokes respirations are irregular with periods of apnea and develop as a person nears death.

Decreased circulation causes the skin to become fragile. The extremities become mottled and cyanotic. The skin feels cool to the touch, first in the feet and legs, then progressing to the hands and arms. It is important to remember that the patient may feel warm because of an elevated temperature.

SENSORY CHANGES

Sensation decreases. Sensory changes include decreasing pain and touch perception, blurred vision, and decreasing sense of taste and smell. The blink reflex is lost eventually, and the patient appears to stare. Lubrication of the eyes with liquid tears may be ordered by the physician.

The sense of touch decreases first in the lower extremities in response to circulatory changes. Hearing is commonly believed to be the last sense to remain intact during the death process. You should assume that the patient can hear and understand. Speaking slowly and clearly may increase the patient's understanding. You must explain to the patient's family and visitors that the patient may still be able to hear. Family members should be encouraged to talk to the patient.

During the death process, the body gradually relaxes until all function ends. Generally, the respirations cease first. The heart stops beating within a few minutes. The physician is responsible for ordering discontinuation of life support if it is in use. The physician is also responsible for pronouncement of death in most situations.

In 1968, a committee of the Harvard Medical School faculty developed the Harvard Criteria for determining a permanently nonfunctioning brain. The criteria deal with specific functions that must be evaluated before a physician can determine death. According to the Harvard Criteria, the following must occur:

1. Unresponsiveness to external stimulation that would normally be painful
2. A complete absence of spontaneous movement and breathing
3. A total lack of reflexes that are normally found on a neurologic examination, particularly the reaction of the pupils to light
4. A flat electroencephalogram (EEG) for 24 hours, which indicates that there is no electrical activity in the brain
5. The lack of circulation to the brain for 24 hours as identified by technology

Usually the first three criteria are enough for a pronouncement of death. The EEG and other technology are generally used when life support equipment is in use. The Harvard Committee recommended that if the final two criteria are used, the tests be repeated 24 hours later.

Another definition associated with the diagnosis of death is cerebral or brain death. Cerebral death occurs when the cerebral cortex stops functioning or is irreversibly destroyed. The cerebral cortex or the higher brain is responsible for voluntary movement and actions as well as for thought. Many people believe that cerebral cortex function *is* the individual.

Since technology has been developed that assists in supporting life, many controversies have arisen. Questions and discussions have developed around whether cerebral or brain death occurs when the whole brain (cortex and brainstem) ceases activity or when cortical function alone stops. In 1995, the Quality Standards Subcommittee of the American Academy of Neurology recommended diagnostic criteria guidelines for clinical diagnosis of brain death in adults. The criteria include coma or unresponsiveness, absence of brainstem reflexes, and apnea as three findings in brain death: Specific assessments by a physician are required to validate each of the criteria.

Currently, legal and medical standards require that all brain function must cease for brain death to be pronounced and life support to be disconnected by the physician. Diagnosis of brain death is of particular importance when organ donation is an option.

In some states under specific circumstances, registered nurses are legally permitted to pronounce death. Policies and procedures may vary from state to state, among boards of nurse examiners for registered nurses in each state, and among institutions as well.

PHYSICAL CHANGES AFTER DEATH

After death, many changes take place in the body rapidly. After body functions cease, decomposition takes place. Three specific changes are rigor mortis, algor mortis, and livor mortis.

Immediately after death, some involuntary jerking movements may take place. Within 2 to 4 hours, the body stiffens, a condition referred to as rigor mortis. Rigor mortis is caused by chemical changes within the body's cells that prevent muscle relaxation. It is usually fully developed in 6 to 12 hours and will disappear with the decomposition process within 36 hours.

After death, the body begins to cool. This is known as algor mortis. Body temperature falls until it reaches the environmental temperature in approximately 24 hours. As the body cools, the skin tends to lose elasticity and can be broken easily.

The breakdown of red blood cells after death causes a discoloration in the skin, which is called livor mortis. The skin may appear bruised with reddish purple discoloration. Generally, the blood settles in the dependent parts of the body. Livor mortis usually occurs within 30 minutes to 2 hours.

Decomposition of the body happens faster in warmer temperatures or environments because of bacterial growth. To slow decomposition, the body must be kept cool. Embalming reverses the process of decomposition by replacing the body's fluids with chemicals that prevent further growth of the bacteria that cause decomposition.

NURSING CARE *of Terminally Ill and Dying Patients*

Nursing care of terminally ill and dying patients deals with the psychological and physical aspects of care. Nursing care focuses on the grieving process as well as the physical changes that are associated with dying. The patient and the family need to be the focus of nursing care. Respect, dignity, and comfort are important for the patient and for the family. In addition, nurses and other care providers must recognize their own needs when dealing with grief and dying.

Assessment

Assessment of the terminally ill or dying patient varies with the patient's condition. In general, the assessment is limited to essential data.

The nurse documents the specific event or change that brought the patient into the health care facility. The patient's medical diagnoses, medication profile, and allergies are recorded. If the patient is alert, briefly review the body systems to detect important signs and symptoms. Document discomfort such as pain or nausea for prompt intervention.

The functional assessment of activities of daily living elicits information about the patient's abilities, food and fluid intake, patterns of sleep and rest, and response to the stress of terminal illness. Determine how the patient (if able to communicate) and family are coping. You can draw inferences about the stage of grief and the coping mechanisms based on statements reflecting sorrow, anger, guilt, or denial.

The physical assessment is abbreviated and detects changes that accompany terminal illness. The frequency of assessment depends on the patient's stability but is done at least every 8 hours. As changes occur, documentation is done more frequently.

Neurologic assessment is especially important and includes level of consciousness, reflexes, and pupil responses. Evaluation of vital signs, skin color, and temperature indicates changes in circulation. Monitor the respiratory status and describe the character and pattern of respirations and the characteristics of breath sounds. Renal and gastrointestinal functions are assessed by monitoring nutritional and fluid intake, urinary output, and bowel function. Skin condition must also be monitored, as skin becomes very fragile and may break down. Detailed assessment of the immobile patient is covered in Chapter 21.

To reemphasize, it is important to be sensitive and not to impose repeated, unnecessary assessments on the dying patient. If health history data are available in the chart, you can use that resource rather than tiring the patient with an interview. However, it is important to check on the patient frequently so the patient does not feel abandoned.

Nursing Diagnoses, Goals, and Outcome Criteria: Terminally Ill and Dying Patients

The nursing care plan for the grieving patient must be individualized depending on individual patient data. Below is an example of nursing diagnoses, goals, and outcome criteria frequently used during the process of grieving. Discussion of other diagnoses follows.

Nursing Diagnoses	Goals and Outcome Criteria
Grieving related to an actual or perceived loss	Resolution of grief: patient expresses feelings related to grief, progresses through stages of grief resolution
Anticipatory Grieving related to terminal illness	Resolution of grief: patient acknowledges impending loss, demonstrates behaviors that reflect progress in grief resolution
Dysfunctional Grieving related to the inability to adapt to the loss	Resolution of grief: patient verbalizes feelings related to grief process, begins to move toward resolution of grief

Additional diagnoses for the dying patient and family may be Acute Pain, Fear, Impaired Skin Integrity, Imbalanced Nutrition: Less Than Body Requirements, Ineffective Airway Clearance, Spiritual Distress, Hopelessness, Powerlessness, and Ineffective Coping or Disabled Family Coping. Refer to Chapter 21 for specific nursing diagnoses and interventions for the immobile patient and to Chapter 15 for pain management.

The general nursing diagnosis of Grieving deals with the normal grieving that a person experiences after a loss. It involves psychosocial and physiologic reactions to a loss. Outcome criteria, nursing interventions, and the evaluation of goals center on the patient's abilities to express and share feelings of grief with others.

Resolution of grief is the primary goal for diagnoses of Anticipatory Grieving and Dysfunctional Grieving. Goals and interventions are similar to these two types of grieving, and therefore they are addressed together. Specific goals are formulated for the stage of the grief process or the specific feelings expressed by the patient. Examples of goals for Anticipatory Grieving and Dysfunctional Grieving are patient expression of feelings related to grief, acknowledgment of the impending loss, and demonstration of behaviors that reflect progress in grief resolution.

Evaluation of patient-centered goals focuses on specific coping skills learned and expressed by the patient or the significant others. Outcome criteria for goal achievement include verbalization of specific feelings related to the grief process, expression that the loss is real, and identification of specific progress in the resolution of grief. The criteria are evaluated based on the behaviors and verbalizations of the patient or the significant others.

Interventions

Nurses need to be aware of how grief affects them personally. The nurse who is responsible for the care of terminally ill or dying patients is not immune to feelings of loss. It is common for nurses to feel helpless and powerless when dealing with death. Your feelings of sorrow, guilt, and frustration need to be expressed. Also, remember there are many interventions that help ease physical and emotional suffering. It is necessary to recognize and acknowledge what you can and cannot control. The basic recognition of your own feelings allows an openness with the patient and family in exchanging feelings. You must realize that it is okay to cry with the patient or family during the grief process. It is okay to be human.

Priority interventions for Anticipatory Grieving and Dysfunctional Grieving must focus on providing an environment that allows the patient to express feelings. Open discussion of feelings helps the patient and family work toward resolution of the grief process. The patient should be free to express feelings of anger, fear, or guilt without judgment on the part of the nurse. The patient and family need to know that the grief reaction is normal. Respect for the patient's privacy and need or desire to talk (or not to talk) is important. Honesty in answering questions and giving information is essential.

Families and patients need encouragement to continue their usual activities as much as possible. They need to discuss their activities and maintain some control over their lives. At times, it helps to discuss what can and cannot change.

Grieving relatives, friends, and significant others can provide emotional support for one another. Health care providers need to be sensitive to the importance of significant others who are not necessarily relatives. Resources such as community counseling and local support may assist some people in working through their grief. Generally, simply allowing the involved people to express their feelings helps resolve the grief.

It is useful to identify the stage of grief (denial, anger, bargaining, depression, acceptance) that the person is experiencing. Awareness of the stage permits the nurse to react according to individual needs. Respect for the person's right to privacy, right to have emotions, and right to talk when he or she chooses is necessary for developing the nurse-patient relationship. Assistance with planning for the future or for the funeral may be needed based on the patient's or family's coping abilities.

Anger is a common and normal response to grief. It is important to understand that the grieving person cannot be forced to accept the loss. You need to acknowledge and encourage the expression of feelings but at the same time realize how difficult it is to come to terms with grief. Nurses are sometimes the target of the anger and must understand what is happening and not react on a personal level.

Feelings of hopelessness and powerlessness are common in terminal illness and during grief. Encourage realistic hope within the limits of the situation.

The patient and the family should be allowed to identify and to deal with what is within their control and to recognize what is beyond their control. Patient-identified goals can be encouraged to restore some sense of power.

During terminal illness and after death, physical care is important. Nursing care during the last stages of life involves comfort measures and physical maintenance care.

Meeting the patient's physiologic needs and needs for safety are the priorities. Physical requirements for oxygen, nutrition, pain relief, mobility, elimination, and skin care remain throughout the life cycle. Physical care should be maintained and monitored. People who are dying deserve and require the same physical care as people who are expected to recover.

CARE OF THE BODY AFTER DEATH

After death, the body must be prepared for transfer to the morgue or the funeral home. Nurses are responsible for the care and preparation of the body. Dignity and privacy for the deceased and the family must be maintained. Table 24-4 identifies nursing management in preparation of the body for family viewing after death.

Legal and moral issues may affect the care required for the disposition of the body. In certain instances an autopsy may be required. An autopsy is a postmortem examination of the deceased. An autopsy may be requested by the next of kin, suggested by the physician, or required by law. Consent for an autopsy must be signed before the procedure can be performed unless the law requires that the procedure be performed.

Table 24-4 *Preparation of the Body for Family Viewing After Death*

TOPIC	NURSING MANAGEMENT
Autopsy	Identification band remains on the body. Contact medical examiner/coroner if required. Consent form signed by next of kin if autopsy is requested. Follow legal requirements and agency policy.
Positioning	Place body in supine position with arms at sides or hands folded across the abdomen. Place small pillow under the head/shoulders. Close eyelids gently, hold for a few minutes, or apply moist cotton balls as needed. Close mouth. Place a rolled towel under the chin, as needed. Follow agency policy.
Hygiene	Wash soiled areas of the body. Apply a clean gown. Place linen savers under the buttocks. Comb hair. Apply clean top linens and cover body to shoulder level. Follow agency policy.
Personal effects	Insert dentures gently. Do not force. If dentures cannot be inserted, place in denture container marked with appropriate identification. Secure with tape jewelry that cannot be removed easily. Inventory all valuables and possessions with the family, the funeral director, or the medical examiner/coroner staff. Clearly document the disposition of possessions. Follow agency policy.

Each state has its own laws regarding autopsy. Under the law in most states, an autopsy is required if a person expires by suicide, homicide, within 24 hours of admission to a health care facility, or from unknown causes. In such cases, the coroner or the medical examiner must be notified.

During an autopsy, organ specimens and samples may be removed for examination. Body parts that are removed are either disposed of or preserved for burial, depending on the situation and the family's wishes. Signs of an autopsy are not apparent after embalming.

Typically, the family wants to view the body before it is transported to the mortuary or the morgue. It is important to make the environment as comfortable for the family as possible. It is your responsibility to prepare the body for viewing before the transfer.

Normally, after death you will place the body in the supine position with the arms at the sides or with the hands across the abdomen. Identification bands should remain in place. A single pillow is placed under the head and shoulders to prevent discoloration of the face from pooling of the blood. Large, overstuffed pillows should be avoided.

Gently holding the eyelids closed for a few seconds helps them remain closed. If the eyelids do not remain closed after a few seconds, the application of moist cotton balls for a few minutes may help.

Dentures may be inserted gently to maintain the normal facial appearance. If the dentures cannot be inserted easily, do not force them. Dentures that are not in place should be stored in a denture container, marked with identification, and sent with the body to the mortuary. The mouth should be closed. A rolled towel placed under the chin helps hold the mouth closed.

What Does Culture Have to Do with Care After Death?

Cultural practices related to care of the body after death must be respected. Examples of traditional practices include the following:

- Greece: Body is washed by a relative or older woman.
- Roman Catholics: Body should not be shrouded until sacraments have been performed.
- Orthodox Jews: Dying person is not left. Body is not left alone between death and burial, which must occur within 24 hours. Body is not be touched for up to 30 minutes after death. Only designated Orthodox persons or Jewish Burial Service care for the body.

Areas of the body that are soiled should be washed. Linen savers are placed under the buttocks to absorb urine or feces that may be released as the sphincters relax. A clean gown is applied, and the hair is combed.

Tubes that are present in the body may be removed unless an autopsy is required. Some agencies require that tubes remain in place or that they be trimmed to approximately 1 inch and taped in place. It is important to review state and agency requirements.

Jewelry is generally removed except for the wedding band, which may be taped to the finger. If rings cannot be removed easily, they should be taped in place. An inventory of the deceased's possessions and valuables is done with the family. Each valuable is listed and signed for by the family. If no family is available, the inventory of valuables is listed and signed for by the funeral home director. The disposition of possessions is documented in the medical record.

| **Table 24-5** | *Preparation of the Body for Transfer* |

TOPIC	NURSING MANAGEMENT
Body identification	Identification band remains on the body. Apply additional identification tags to the wrist, ankle, or toe per agency policy. Place additional identification on the outside of the shroud. Communicable disease identification should be listed both on the body and outside of the shroud. Follow agency policy.
Autopsy	Tubes and medical appliances frequently are left as originally placed in accordance with agency policy and legal requirements. Follow agency policy.
Positioning	Place body in supine position with arms at sides or hands folded across the abdomen. Wrists and ankles may be bound following agency policy. Remove gown. Apply shroud. Follow agency policy.
Personal effects	Inventory all valuables and possessions with the family, the funeral director, or the medical examiner/coroner staff. Clearly package and document the disposition of possessions. Follow agency policy.
Transport	Transport via stretcher to the morgue following agency policy. Assist with transfer of the body to the mortician's stretcher for transport.

After the positioning and preparation of the body, straighten the top linens and pull them up to the shoulder level. The family may view the body after preparation is complete.

Often the family needs the nurse's emotional support while viewing the body. If only one family member is present, it is wise to accompany the person who is viewing the body. Close the door to allow for privacy. The family should be allowed as much time as desired.

When the family leaves, apply additional identification tags to the wrist and ankle or toe of the deceased. The gown is removed, and the body may be wrapped in a shroud. The shroud may be a large square or rectangle of cloth or plastic material. An identification tag is placed on the outside of the shroud. Additional identification markings may be required if the deceased had a communicable disease. The body is then transported to the morgue or removed by the mortician. Agency policy regarding the transport of a body from the room may vary. Some agencies require that all patient doors be closed before transport and that service elevators be used. Table 24-5 lists the nursing management for preparation of the body for transfer.

ISSUES RELATED TO TERMINAL ILLNESS AND DEATH

Patients and families struggle with many emotional decisions during the terminal illness and dying experience. The decisions often focus on physical and emotional comfort. Many people decide that the outcomes should be based on their own wishes. The decisions may involve the choice for an advance directive, medical power of attorney, living wills, organ donations, and resuscitation (Fig. 24-1).

ORGAN DONATION

Organ donation may be made by any person who is legally competent. Any body part or the entire body may be donated. The decision to donate organs or to provide anatomic gifts may be made by a person before death. The decision to donate organs may be made by immediate family members after death.

Some people carry donor cards. Some states allow for organ donation to be marked on drivers' licenses. The names of agencies that handle organ donation will vary by locale. Some common names for such an agency might be the *organ bank, organ-sharing network,* and *organ-sharing alliance.* Organ donation follows specific legal guidelines. Legal requirements and facility policy for organ donation must be followed. The physician should be notified immediately when organ donation is intended because some tissues must be used within hours after death.

CARDIOPULMONARY RESUSCITATION

In the past 30 years, cardiopulmonary resuscitation (CPR) has become common practice in health care. Patients who suffered respiratory or cardiac arrest have been given CPR unless a do-not-resuscitate (DNR) order was given by the physician. Often patients and families have had no choice as to whether CPR was used.

In recent years, much has been written concerning the right to die and the right to choose. Many people believe that the patient or the patient's family has the right to decide whether CPR will be used. It is no longer the sole decision of the physician.

In 1991, the Omnibus Budget Reconciliation Act of 1990 became effective. An important part of OBRA 1990 was the *Patient Self-Determination Act.* This act requires that all institutions that participate with Medicare must provide written information to patients concerning their rights to accept or refuse treatment. The information must explain the patient's right to initiate advance directives. Advance directives are written statements of a person's wishes regarding medical care. The first advance directive was developed by the Euthanasia Education Council in 1974. It was called the *Living Will.*

Most states have replaced the idea of living wills with natural death acts. Within many of these acts are specific aspects related to the individual's wishes and durable powers of attorney for health care. Directives to physicians may be included. Under the natural death acts, an individual can tell the physician exactly what is desired. Each state will have its own unique requirements and rules for the use of advance directives. Special forms for durable power of attorney, medical power of attorney, and directives for physicians, family members, or surrogates can be obtained from local medical associations and the Internet. Specific details as to withholding or withdrawing treatments must be included. What is to be done and what is not to be done must be included in very clear terms.

A person may write a durable power of attorney or directive to physicians without special forms. Verbal directives may be given to physicians with specific instructions in the presence of two witnesses. Attorneys and notaries are not necessarily required.

In the event that the person is not capable of communicating his or her wishes, the family and the physician can agree on what measures will or will not be taken. The physician should document the family's decision.

Several different types of CPR decisions can be made. Complete and total heroic measures, which may include CPR, medications, and mechanical ventilation, can be referred to as a *full code.* Some people choose variations of the full code. A *chemical code* involves the use of medications for resuscitation without the use of CPR. A *"no code"* or a *DNR* order allows the person to die without the interference of technology.

Another option is the durable power of attorney for health care or medical power of attorney. This document allows individuals to select someone to make health care decisions for them if they are unable to do

FLORIDA LIVING WILL

Declaration made this _____ day of _____, _____,
    (day)   *(month)*   *(year)*

I, _____, willfully and voluntarily make known
my desire that my dying not be artificially prolonged under the circumstances set
forth below, and I do hereby declare that:

If at any time I am incapacitated and
    __ I have a terminal condition, or
    __ I have an end-stage condition, or
    __ I am in a persistent vegetative state

and if my attending or treating physician and another consulting physician have
determined that there is no reasonable medical probability of my recovery from
such condition, I direct that life-prolonging procedures be withheld or withdrawn
when the application of such procedures would serve only to prolong artificially
the process of dying, and that I be permitted to die naturally with only the administration of medication or the performance of any medical procedure deemed necessary to provide me with comfort care or to alleviate pain.

It is my intention that this declaration be honored by my family and physician as
the final expression of my legal right to refuse medical or surgical treatment and to
accept the consequences for such refusal.

In the event that I have been determined to be unable to provide express and
informed consent regarding the withholding, withdrawal, or continuation of life-
prolonging procedures, I wish to designate, as my surrogate to carry out the provisions of this declaration:

Name: _____
Address: _____
_____ Zip code: _____
Phone: _____

I wish to designate the following person as my alternate surrogate, to carry out
the provisions of this declaration should my surrogate be unwilling or unable to act
on my behalf:

Name: _____
Address: _____
_____ Zip code: _____
Phone: _____

Additional instructions (optional): _____

I understand the full import of this declaration, and I am emotionally and mentally
competent to make this declaration.

Signed: _____

Witness 1:
    Signed: _____
    Address: _____
Witness 2:
    Signed: _____
    Address: _____

A

FIGURE **24-1** Sample advance directive. **A,** Florida Living Will. (Copyright © National Hospice
and Palliative Care Organization. All rights reserved. Reproduction and distribution by an organization or organized group without the written permission of the National Hospice and Palliative Care Organization is expressly forbidden. For more information, contact our website at
www.caringinfo.org).

Continued

FLORIDA DESIGNATION OF HEALTH CARE SURROGATE

Name: _____

(Last)   (First)   (Middle initial)

In the event that I have been determined to be incapacitated to provide informed consent for medical treatment and surgical and diagnostic procedures, I wish to designate as my surrogate for health care decisions:

Name: _____
Address: _____
_____ Zip code: _____
Phone: _____

If my surrogate is unwilling or unable to perform his or her duties, I wish to designate as my alternate surrogate:

Name: _____
Address: _____
_____ Zip code: _____
Phone: _____

I fully understand that this designation will permit my designee to make health care decisions and to provide, withhold, or withdraw consent on my behalf; to apply for public benefits to defray the cost of health care; and to authorize my admission to or transfer from a health care facility.

Additional instructions (optional):

I further affirm that this designation is not being made as a condition of treatment or admission to a health care facility. I will notify and send a copy of this document to the following persons other than my surrogate so they may know who my surrogate is:

Name: _____
Address: _____
Name: _____
Address: _____

Signed: _____
Date: _____

Witness 1:
  Signed: _____
  Address: _____

Witness 2:
  Signed: _____
  Address: _____

B

FIGURE **24-1** cont'd. Sample advance directive. **B,** Florida Designation of Health Care Surrogate.

so for themselves. This power of attorney can be used only if the physician certifies in writing that the person is incapable of making decisions. Until the physician does this, the individual remains in control of his or her own decisions.

In addition to advance directives, another initiative has been put into place. This document is called *Five Wishes.*™ Figure 24-2 shows the first page of this document. The organization Aging with Dignity (www.agingwithdignity.org) developed *Five Wishes*™ to promote better care for individuals and families facing the end of life. This document focuses on a patient's needs and includes personal, medical, spiritual, and emotional needs. Currently, 38 states and the District of Columbia legally recognize the *Five Wishes*™ document as binding.

The *Five Wishes*™ document specifies how the family and the health care team are expected to treat the patient. It includes the following:

- The name of the person to make decisions for health care if the patient cannot do it
- The type of medical care that the patient wants or does not want
- The amount of comfort the patient wants

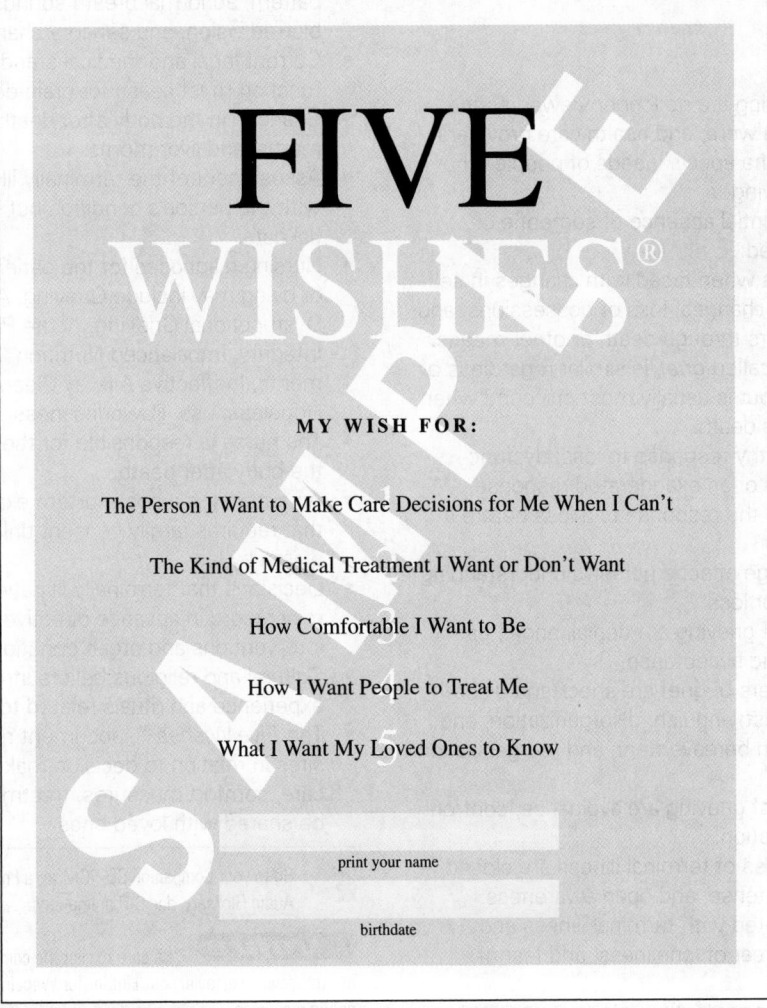

FIGURE **24-2** The *Five Wishes*™ document (www.agingwithdignity.org) helps patients communicate their wishes to their families and to members of the health care team. Written in language that is easily understood by those outside the medical and legal professions, the document helps people discuss and make reasoned decisions about issues that are often difficult to face. This is the first page of the 12-page document that allows individuals to express their wishes on various issues. (Copyright © AGING WITH DIGNITY, P. O. Box 1661, Tallahassee, FL 32302; www.agingwithdignity.org.)

 Put on Your Thinking Cap!

1. Write down the customs and rituals that are followed in your family in relation to deaths: care of the body, viewing, wake, spiritual counselors, services, burial or cremation, types of memorials, support for survivors.
2. Discuss your answers with others in your clinical group.
3. Consider how you reacted to others' customs and rituals. Recognize the importance of your customs and rituals to you, and appreciate the need to be accepting of different practices. Do not assume that your patients will handle death the same way you do.

- How the patient wants to be treated
- What information the patient wants the loved ones to know

You need to be aware of legal issues and the wishes of the patient. Advance directives and organ donor information should be located in the medical record and identified on the Kardex or the nursing care plan. All caregivers responsible for the patient need to know the patient's wishes.

SUMMARY

Terminal illness and dying are very personal events that affect the patient, the family, and the caregivers. Grief is experienced by everyone differently but with similar patterns of behavior. The dying process and death require specific physical, emotional, spiritual, and legal nursing interventions. Caring for the terminally ill and dying is a challenging and rewarding experience.

Key Points

- Terminal illness and dying are no longer viewed as the taboo topics they once were, and health care providers are more sensitive to the special needs of people who are terminally ill and dying.
- Loss is the real or potential absence of someone or something that is valued.
- People experience loss when faced with changes in self-image, developmental changes, loss of possessions, and loss of significant others through death or other means.
- The response to loss, called *grief,* is similar regardless of the nature of the loss but is usually most profound when the loss experienced is death.
- Adaptive grief is a healthy response to loss; dysfunctional grief is a delayed or an exaggerated response.
- Anticipatory grieving is the response to a loss before it happens.
- Culture, religion, and age affect a person's understanding and reaction to death or loss.
- Kübler-Ross's stages of grieving are denial, anger, bargaining, depression, and acceptance.
- Martocchio's five clusters of grief are shock and disbelief; yearning and protest; anguish, disorganization, and despair; identification in bereavement; and reorganization and restoration.
- Rando's three phases of grieving are avoidance, confrontation, and accommodation.
- The stages of awareness of terminal illness are closed awareness, mutual pretense, and open awareness.
- Common fears associated with terminal illness and dying are fear of pain, fear of loneliness, and fear of meaninglessness.
- Clinical signs of impending death are loss of muscle tone, bradycardia, hypotension, abnormal respiratory pattern, abnormal breath sounds, cyanosis, cool skin, blurred vision, and sensory changes.
- Current legal and medical standards require that all brain function must cease for brain death to be pronounced.
- Changes in the body after death are rigor mortis, algor mortis, and livor mortis.
- Assessment of the terminally ill or dying person varies with the person's condition but is often limited to essential data.
- Nursing diagnoses for the patient who is terminally ill or dying may include Grieving, Anticipatory Grieving, Dysfunctional Grieving, Acute Pain, Fear, Impaired Skin Integrity, Imbalanced Nutrition: Less Than Body Requirements, Ineffective Airway Clearance, Spiritual Distress, Hopelessness, Powerlessness, and Ineffective Coping.
- The nurse is responsible for the care and preparation of the body after death.
- An autopsy is a postmortem examination of the body that requires family consent unless the procedure is required by law.
- Decisions that terminally ill patients and their families may record in advance directives include desired medical interventions and organ donations.
- Cultural and religious beliefs strongly influence the grief experience and rituals related to death.
- The *Five Wishes*™, document records the patient's desires in relation to decision-making authority, medical care, comfort measures, treatments, and information to be shared with loved ones.

 Go to your Companion CD-ROM for a Pharmacology Tutorial, Audio Glossary, and 3-D animations.

evolve   Be sure to visit the companion Evolve site at http://evolve.elsevier.com/Linton/ for WebLinks and additional online resources.

REVIEW QUESTIONS *Choose the best answer.*

1. The focus of palliative care is:
   1. Finding alternative methods of treatment of disease
   2. Providing supportive care while allowing natural death
   3. Delaying death as long as possible by any means
   4. Hastening death when there is no hope for a cure

2. An example of a loss related to a change in self-image is:
   1. The first child in a family begins school
   2. Love letters are destroyed in a house fire
   3. An adult child accepts a job in another country
   4. A patient's hair falls out due to chemotherapy

3. When a patient was diagnosed with a terminal illness, his wife began to grieve. Her grief is an example of:
   1. Dysfunctional grief
   2. Anticipatory grief
   3. Reactive grief
   4. Exaggerated grief

4. Ms. A. has been diagnosed with terminal lung cancer. She tells the nurse, "If God will just let me live to see my children finish school, I will never smoke another cigarette." This illustrates which stage of grief according to Kübler-Ross?
   1. Denial   3. Bargaining
   2. Anger   4. Depression

5. Martocchio defines the last cluster of grief as:
   1. Yearning and protest
   2. Anguish, disorganization, and despair
   3. Confrontation and avoidance
   4. Reorganization and restoration

6. Rando describes emotional healing as:
   1. Acceptance
   2. Avoidance
   3. Confrontation
   4. Accommodation

7. Which principle should guide health care providers when a terminally ill person has pain?
   1. Relief of pain must be a priority.
   2. Use caution to prevent addiction.
   3. Keep the patient heavily sedated.
   4. Medicate only when pain is severe.

8. During the last few days of Ms. B.'s life, family members visited her and talked about shared happy memories and how much Ms. B. meant to them. How might this be helpful to Ms. B.?
   1. This would probably benefit the visitors more than Ms. B.
   2. Reviewing her life can help Ms. B. find meaning in her life.
   3. Visitors will keep Ms. B. from focusing on her impending death.
   4. Ms. B. will pretend to feel better in the presence of her visitors.

9. The assessment of a dying patient reveals irregular respirations with periods of apnea. This observation should be documented as:
   1. Intermittent breathing
   2. Decreasing respirations
   3. Cheyne-Stokes respirations
   4. Ineffective airway clearance

10. As Mr. C. nears death, his wife says, "I wish I could do something for him." What could the nurse tell her?
    1. It may be comforting if you will talk to him slowly and clearly.
    2. Unfortunately, there is nothing that you can do at this point.
    3. He probably cannot hear you but may be able to feel your touch.
    4. It is just a matter of time now. Why don't you take a break?

11. A new nursing assistant leaves the room in tears the first time one of her patients dies. What should the nurse say to her?
    1. Get back in there and take care of your patient.
    2. It hurts to lose a patient, but you will get used to it.
    3. You really can't get so emotionally involved with patients.
    4. It is normal for you to feel sad. How can I help you?

25 The Patient with Cancer

BARBARA OWENS*

evolve   http://evolve.elsevier.com/Linton/

Objectives

After reading and studying this chapter, you should be able to:

1. Explain the differences between benign and malignant tumors.
2. List the most common sites of cancer in men and women.
3. Describe measures to reduce the risk of cancer.
4. Define terms used to name and classify cancer.
5. List nursing responsibilities in the care of patients having diagnostic tests to detect possible cancer.
6. Explain the nursing care of patients undergoing each type of cancer therapy: surgery, radiation, chemotherapy, and biotherapy.
7. Assist in developing a nursing care plan for the terminally ill patient with cancer and the patient's family.

Key Terms

Be sure to check out the bonus material on the Companion CD-ROM, including selected audio pronunciations.

adjuvant (ĂJ-ă-vănt, p. 376)
alopecia (ăl-ō-PĒ-shē-ă, p. 378)
alternative therapy (p. 383)
antineoplastic (ăn-tĭ-nē-ō-PLĂS-tĭk, p. 378)
benign (bĕ-NĪN, p. 369)
biotherapy (p. 381)
carcinogen (kăr-SĬN-ō-jĕn, p. 370)
chemotherapy (kĕ-mō-THĔR-ă-pē, p. 378)
complementary therapy (p. 383)
extravasation (ĕks-TRĂV-ă-zā-shŭn, p.381)
Gray (Gy) (p. 376)
malignant (mă-LĬG-nănt, p. 369)
metastasis (mĕ-TĂS-tă-sĭs, p. 370)
neoadjuvant (ne-ō-ĂJ-ă-vănt, p. 376)
neoplasm (NĒ-ō-plăzm, p. 369)
neutropenia (nū-trō-PĒ-nē-ă, p. 382)
radiotherapy (p. 376)
xerostomia (ZĒ-rō-stō-mē-ăh, p. 378)

*We would like to thank Leslie Smetzer, Jan Booth, and Kathy Henye, members of the San Antonio chapter of the Oncology Nursing Society, who contributed their expertise to update this chapter.

WHY STUDY CANCER?

Specific cancers are discussed with every body system in this book. Why, then, is a separate chapter devoted to the subject? The American Cancer Society defines cancer as a large group of diseases characterized by uncontrolled growth and spread of abnormal cells. More than 200 diseases are classified as cancer. They share some common characteristics, progress in similar ways, and respond to similar types of treatments. To reduce repetition throughout the text, this chapter addresses the common features of those diseases known as cancer.

Health statistics often group all types of cancer together. Not surprisingly, cancer is listed as the second most common cause of death in the United States. Almost everyone has been touched by cancer. It is estimated that one in three Americans will have cancer at some time. The most common sites of cancer in men and in women are shown in Figure 25-1. Because so many die of cancer, many people assume that a diagnosis of cancer is a death sentence. In reality, more than 9 million Americans who have a history of cancer are alive today.

Some cancers can be prevented by avoidance of causative agents. Early diagnosis has been found to make a significant difference in survival with many types of cancer, and advances in treatment have prolonged the lives of many cancer patients.

Nurses use their teaching and assessment skills in the prevention and detection of cancer. They also care for patients undergoing diagnostic procedures and treatments for cancer. In almost any specialty, nurses work with patients who are being treated for cancer.

WHAT IS CANCER?

NORMAL BODY CELLS

A normal cell has the following characteristics:
- A distinct, recognizable appearance typical of all cells from a particular tissue ("tissue of origin"); has a single small nucleus
- The ability to perform a specific function when mature
- The production of substances that hold cells from the same type of tissue closely together

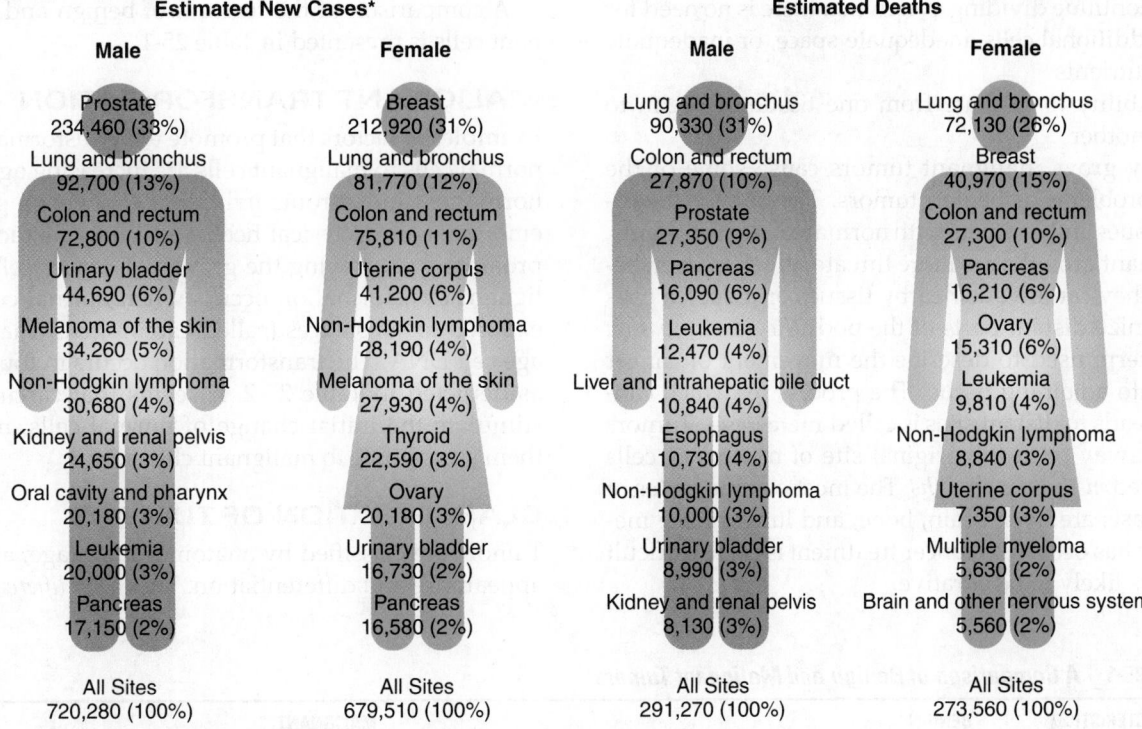

Estimated New Cases*

Male	Female
Prostate 234,460 (33%)	Breast 212,920 (31%)
Lung and bronchus 92,700 (13%)	Lung and bronchus 81,770 (12%)
Colon and rectum 72,800 (10%)	Colon and rectum 75,810 (11%)
Urinary bladder 44,690 (6%)	Uterine corpus 41,200 (6%)
Melanoma of the skin 34,260 (5%)	Non-Hodgkin lymphoma 28,190 (4%)
Non-Hodgkin lymphoma 30,680 (4%)	Melanoma of the skin 27,930 (4%)
Kidney and renal pelvis 24,650 (3%)	Thyroid 22,590 (3%)
Oral cavity and pharynx 20,180 (3%)	Ovary 20,180 (3%)
Leukemia 20,000 (3%)	Urinary bladder 16,730 (2%)
Pancreas 17,150 (2%)	Pancreas 16,580 (2%)
All Sites 720,280 (100%)	All Sites 679,510 (100%)

Estimated Deaths

Male	Female
Lung and bronchus 90,330 (31%)	Lung and bronchus 72,130 (26%)
Colon and rectum 27,870 (10%)	Breast 40,970 (15%)
Prostate 27,350 (9%)	Colon and rectum 27,300 (10%)
Pancreas 16,090 (6%)	Pancreas 16,210 (6%)
Leukemia 12,470 (4%)	Ovary 15,310 (6%)
Liver and intrahepatic bile duct 10,840 (4%)	Leukemia 9,810 (4%)
Esophagus 10,730 (4%)	Non-Hodgkin lymphoma 8,840 (3%)
Non-Hodgkin lymphoma 10,000 (3%)	Uterine corpus 7,350 (3%)
Urinary bladder 8,990 (3%)	Multiple myeloma 5,630 (2%)
Kidney and renal pelvis 8,130 (3%)	Brain and other nervous system 5,560 (2%)
All Sites 291,270 (100%)	All Sites 273,560 (100%)

*Excludes basal and squamous cell skin cancers and in situ carcinoma except urinary bladder.
Note: Percentages may not total 100% due to rounding.

©2006, American Cancer Society, Inc., Surveillance Research

FIGURE **25-1** 2006 American Cancer Society estimates: Leading sites of new cancer cases and deaths.

- The ability to recognize other cells and identify the other cells' tissue of origin
- Reproduce in a controlled manner to produce additional identical cells only as needed for growth and replacement
- Cell division inhibited by inadequate space or insufficient nutrients (see the Nutrition Concepts box at right).
- Remain in their tissue of origin (except for blood cells, which migrate)

Cells that reproduce abnormally and in an uncontrolled manner form **neoplasms** or tumors. Such cells may be benign or malignant.

BENIGN TUMORS

Benign tumors are relatively harmless, primarily because they do not spread to other parts of the body. Benign tumors present problems, however, if they create pressure on or obstruct body organs. Because of this, surgical removal of benign tumors is often recommended.

MALIGNANT TUMORS

The presence of **malignant** cells is the basis for a diagnosis of cancer. Characteristics of cancer cells are the following:

- Change in appearance from normal cells of tissue of origin (said to be *undifferentiated* if tissue of origin cannot be determined); large nucleus or multiple nuclei

Nutrition Concepts

1. Thirty-five percent of all cancers are believed to be related to diet:
   - Diets high in salt-cured, smoked, and nitrate-cured foods are associated with esophageal and stomach cancers.
   - Obesity is associated with cancers of the colon, breast, prostate, gallbladder, ovary, and uterus.
   - Cancers of the breast, colon, and prostate may be associated with high-fat diets.
   - High alcohol intake is associated with cancers of the oral cavity, larynx, esophagus, liver, colon, and breast.
2. To *reduce the risk* of cancer, the American Cancer Society recommends the following:
   - Fruits and vegetables: five or more servings each day.
   - Grains, rice, pasta, beans: several servings each day.
   - Fats: limit consumption.
   - Physical activity: at least moderate activity 30 min or more on most days; maintain healthy weight.
   - Alcohol: none or limited.

- Inability to properly perform function of tissue of origin; may assume functions of other cells
- Cells not readily recognized by other cells
- May have abnormal proteins (called *tumor markers*) on cell surface
- Random, disorganized, uncontrolled growth pattern

- Continue dividing even when there is no need for additional cells, inadequate space, or inadequate nutrients
- Ability to migrate from one tissue or organ to another

As they grow, malignant tumors cause some of the same problems as benign tumors. They press on normal tissues and compete with normal cells for nutrients. Malignant growths are more threatening, however, because they can invade nearby tissues or disperse cells to colonize distant parts of the body. *Regional invasion* is the term used to describe the movement of cancer cells into adjoining tissue. The process by which cancer spreads to distant sites is called metastasis. Tumors found away from the original site of malignant cells are called *metastatic growths.* The most common sites of metastasis are liver, brain, bone, and lungs. Once metastasis has occurred, cancer treatment is more difficult and less likely to be curative.

A comparison of the features of benign and malignant cells is presented in Table 25-1.

MALIGNANT TRANSFORMATION

Examples of factors that promote the transformation of normal cells to malignant cells are increasing age, diet, hormones, and chronic irritation. A person's general emotional and physical health also may be factors in promoting or slowing the growth of cancer cells. Malignant transformation occurs when normal cells are exposed to substances (called carcinogens) that damage cell DNA. The transformation occurs in four steps as depicted in Table 25-2. It seems that carcinogens stimulate the initial change of normal cells, making them susceptible to malignant changes.

CLASSIFICATION OF TUMORS

Tumors are classified by anatomic site, stage, and cell appearance and differentiation. The term *differentiation*

Table 25-1   *A Comparison of Benign and Malignant Tumors*

CHARACTERISTIC	BENIGN	MALIGNANT
Growth rate	Usually slow	Usually rapid, but may be slow
Growth mode	Enlarges and expands	Invades surrounding tissue
Cell structure and differentiation	Cells closely resemble those of tissue of origin	Tissue of origin not readily identifiable
Recurrence after removal	Unlikely	Common
Metastasis	No	Yes
Tissue destruction	Usually none unless compression or obstruction occurs	Can cause necrosis, ulceration, perforation, tissue sloughing; effects can be fatal

Table 25-2   *Steps in Transformation of Normal Cells to Malignant Cells*

STEP	PROCESS	EFFECTS ON CELLS AND TISSUE
Initiation	DNA exposed to a carcinogen Irreversible changes occur in DNA	Cell appears somewhat abnormal Continues to function normally
Promotion	Sufficient exposure to an agent (a *promoter*) to encourage or enhance cell growth	Latent period before increased growth forms tumors (early detection period)
Progression	Accelerated growth rate Enhanced invasiveness Altered appearance and biochemical activity	Tumor development Cells mutate so that they are not all identical and have differing sensitivities to treatment
Metastasis	Tumor develops internal blood vessels Tumor cells extend into normal tissue by producing enzymes that dissolve substances that hold normal cells together Tumor penetrates capillaries, other body structures, and cavities Tumor cells are transported throughout the body; most destroyed by body's defenses Tumor cells are trapped in capillary bed and form a fibrin meshwork that prevents detection by immune system Enzymes dissolve lining of blood vessels; cells invade surrounding tissue Cells attempt to establish blood supply to support development of metastatic colony	Transformed cells relocate by direct extension, invasion, establishment of remote sites

refers to how different cells are from their parent cells ("tissue of origin"). When it is difficult to recognize the original type of tissue from which tumor cells came, they are described as "poorly differentiated cells." When cells are "well-differentiated," the tissue of origin is recognizable.

Anatomic Site

The suffix *-oma* means "tumor." Technically, a tumor is a swelling. The word is most commonly used, however, to refer to a malignant or benign neoplasm. Tumors are named according to the type of tissue from which they developed originally. These names are summarized in Table 25-3.

Additional prefixes may be used to designate the exact type of malignant tissue. For example, a sarcoma could be an osteosarcoma or a chondrosarcoma. An osteosarcoma is a tumor of the bone, whereas a chondrosarcoma is a cartilage tumor. Many other combinations of terms are used to describe tumors precisely by origin and location.

Staging System for Cancer

Because cancers tend to grow and spread in predictable ways, their progress can be described in stages. There are specific stages for all types of cancer. Staging is done at the time of diagnosis and at intervals during

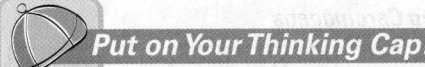
Put on Your Thinking Cap!

You are assigned to care for a patient who has cancer. The cancer has been staged T4, N3, M1. How would you interpret this information?

and after treatment. Such staging is helpful in planning treatments and in predicting long-term survival.

One method of describing the extent of cancer is shown in Table 25-4. A second, more specific system is the TNM staging system (Table 25-5), which specifies the status of the primary tumor, regional lymph nodes, and distant metastases. In the TNM system, *T* refers to the tumor, *N* to regional lymph nodes, and *M* to distant metastases. To illustrate, a patient whose primary tumor has grown and spread to regional lymph nodes but not to distant sites would be staged *T2, N1, M0*.

RISK FACTORS

A single, specific cause of cancer has not been identified. Both genetic and environmental factors appear to increase the risk for development of cancer. Changes in genetic information of a normal cell can cause alterations that lead to malignancies. Cancer-causing agents, called *carcinogens*, include a variety of chemicals, radiation, and viruses. Box 25-1 shows a partial list of carcinogens. Carcinogens such as cigarette smoke, asbestos, and nitrites are commonly found in the environment. Drugs that may act as carcinogens include

Table 25-3 | Tumor Names by Anatomic Site

TYPE OF TUMOR BY ANATOMIC SITE	TISSUE OF ORIGIN
BENIGN TUMOR	
Fibroma	Fibrous connective tissue
Lipoma	Fat tissue
Leiomyomas	Smooth muscle tissue
MALIGNANT TUMOR	
Carcinoma	Skin; glands; linings of digestive, urinary, and respiratory tracts
Sarcoma	Bone, muscle, other connective tissue
Melanoma	Pigment cells in the skin
Leukemia and lymphoma	Blood-forming tissues: lymphoid tissue, plasma cells, and bone marrow

Table 25-4 | Staging Classification for Cancer

STAGE	DESCRIPTION
Stage I	The malignant cells are confined to the tissue of origin. There is no invasion of other tissues.
Stage II	There is limited spread of the cancer in the local area, usually to nearby lymph nodes.
Stage III	The tumor is larger or has spread from the site of origin into nearby tissues, or both. Regional lymph nodes are likely to be involved.
Stage IV	The cancer has metastasized to distant parts of the body.

Table 25-5 | The TNM Staging System for Cancer

T = PRIMARY TUMOR	N = REGIONAL LYMPH NODES	M = DISTANT METASTASIS
T0 — no sign of tumor after treatment	N0 — no regional lymph nodes involved	M0 — no distant metastasis
Tis — malignancy in epithelial tissue but not basement membrane	N1 — minimal regional lymph node involvement	M1 —distant metastasis present
T1 —minimal size and extension	N2 —increased involvement of regional lymph nodes	
T2, T3 — progressively increasing size and extension	N3 —extensive involvement of regional lymph nodes	
T4 —large size and extension		

Box 25-1 | *Common Carcinogens*

Viruses	**Hormones**
Chemicals	Synthetic estrogens
Tar	Androgenic anabolic
Soot	steroids
Asphalt	
Aniline dyes	**Immunosuppressants**
Hydrocarbons	Antimetabolites
Crude paraffin oils	Corticosteroids
Nickel	Alkylating agents
Arsenic	Antilymphocyte serum
Benzene	**Cytotoxic Drugs**
Cadmium	Phenylalanine mustard
	Cyclophosphamide
Physical Agents	
Radiation	
Asbestos	
Tobacco smoke	

diethylstilbestrol, androgenic steroids, and high-dose unopposed synthetic estrogens.

Other factors thought to be associated with cancer development are increasing age, heredity, and hormones. Cancers that appear at a higher rate than expected in one family are called *familial cancers*. In these situations, no single genes have been identified to explain the frequency. Hereditary cancers, on the other hand, have clearly predictable patterns of inheritance based on a single gene. For people with family histories of familial or hereditary cancers, genetic counseling can direct the person to appropriate screening and lifestyle changes and serve as a basis for making decisions about reproductive options.

 Pharmacology Capsule

Some drugs are carcinogenic, meaning they can cause cancer. Examples are diethylstilbestrol, androgenic steroids, high-dose unopposed synthetic estrogens, and some antineoplastic drugs used to treat cancer.

SEVEN WARNING SIGNS

The signs and symptoms of cancer vary with the location and severity of the disease. The American Cancer Society has identified seven warning signs that are associated with many common types of cancer (see the Health Promotion Considerations box above). They can serve to guide the nurse and the public in identifying signs and symptoms that require medical evaluation. The first letters of the warning signs spell out CAUTION, making it easier to remember them.

PREVENTION AND EARLY DETECTION

A number of things can be done to reduce the risk of development of cancer or to detect it in the early stages. They include (1) general measures to promote health,

 Health Promotion Considerations

Warning Signs of Cancer

Change in bowel or bladder habits
A sore that does not heal
Unusual bleeding or discharge
Thickening or lump in a breast or elsewhere
Indigestion or difficulty swallowing
Obvious change in a wart or a mole
Nagging cough or hoarseness

(2) avoidance of known carcinogens, (3) identification of high-risk people, and (4) cancer screening.

Health Promotion

Many behaviors associated with good health may reduce the risk of some cancers. The recommended diet is low in fat, calories, and preservatives and high in fiber with at least five servings of various fruits and vegetables daily. Alcoholic beverages and foods that are salt-cured, smoked, or nitrite-preserved should be taken in limited quantities. Appropriate calorie intake to maintain or attain normal body weight is also important because obesity is a risk factor for some cancers. A balanced program of activity and rest with stress management may enable the body to resist diseases, including cancer.

Avoidance of Carcinogens

Some specific carcinogens were mentioned earlier. They include cigarette smoke, alcohol, intercourse with multiple partners, a variety of chemicals and drugs, and even excessive sun exposure. Public education has focused attention on carcinogens, and people are becoming more aware of the need to avoid them.

For example, smoking tobacco has long been known as a risk factor for cancers of the lung, bladder, head and neck, mouth, and stomach. Only in the past few years, however, have anti-smoking programs had a real impact on tobacco use. The fact that 1 million people quit smoking each year demonstrates that public education is making a difference. On a broader scale, legal restrictions on public smoking are reducing the exposure of nonsmokers to so-called "second-hand smoke."

A harmful effect associated with use of smokeless tobacco is the increased risk of oral cancers. Alcohol consumption also increases the risk of cancers of the mouth, head and neck, and stomach. Many industrial products are recognized as carcinogens as well. Their use is regulated by the Occupational Safety and Health Administration's guidelines for the safety of workers and consumers. Unprotected sun exposure is a risk factor for skin cancers including the most deadly type—melanoma. Increased awareness of the dangers of excessive sun exposure has boosted the use of sunscreens.

Identification of High-Risk People

Identifying people at risk for development of specific cancers serves several purposes. It helps researchers and health care providers recognize factors that may contribute to the development of various cancers Also, people who are known to fall into high-risk categories can be monitored closely to detect cancer early. Examples of people at risk for specific cancers are those with familial rectal polyposis, those with family histories of breast cancer, and those with Down syndrome, who are at increased risk for leukemia. In addition, people with high-risk behaviors and certain racial and ethnic groups have increased risk of specific cancers.

What Does Culture Have to Do with Cancer?

Of all racial and ethnic groups, African-American men have the highest rates of prostate, colon and rectum, and lung and bronchus cancers and are most likely to die of those cancers. Although white women have the highest rates of breast cancer, African-American women are more likely to die from breast cancer. Nurses should encourage African Americans to participate in screenings and to seek early treatment for warning signs of cancer.

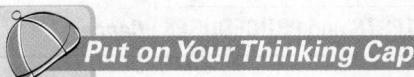

Put on Your Thinking Cap!

1. What are possible reasons that minorities in the United States have higher rates of several types of cancer and are more likely to die from cancer?
2. How can you use your knowledge of culture to intervene?

Screening for Cancer

When cancer does occur, early diagnosis and treatment often increase the chance of cure. Public education should emphasize the following:

- The value of early detection and treatment
- The seven warning signs of cancer
- How to do self-examinations (breast, skin, testicular)
- The importance of periodic examinations for common cancers

The American Cancer Society recommends specific examinations or procedures to detect cancers of the colon, prostate, cervix, endometrium, and breast. The recommendations are summarized in Table 25-6.

Table 25-6   *American Cancer Society Recommendations for Early Cancer Detection in Asymptomatic People*

SITE	GENDER	AGE	RECOMMENDATION
Breast	F	20-39	Clinical breast exam by health professional every 3 yr Monthly self breast exam
		40 and older	Annual mammogram Annual clinical breast exam by health professional Monthly self breast exam
Colon and rectum	M & F	50 and older	Fecal occult blood test every year and flexible sigmoidoscopy every 5 yr *or* colonoscopy every 10 yr *or* double-contrast barium enema every 5-10 yr MNSD9People at moderate or high risk should discuss appropriate testing schedule with physician
Prostate	M	50 and older with life expectancy of at least 10 yr High-risk younger men (start at age 45 for African-Americans)	Annual prostate-specific antigen and digital rectal exam
Uterus (cervix)	F	18 and older who are sexually active	Annual pelvic exam and Pap test (frequency may be decreased after normal findings for 3 or more years)
Uterus (endometrium)	F	Women at high risk	Endometrial biopsy at onset of menopause
Cancer-related checkup	M & F	20 and older	Checkup every 3 yr: thyroid, oral cavity, skin, lymph nodes, testes, ovaries; health counseling

From American Cancer Society. (2000). *Summary of American Cancer Society recommendations for the early detection of cancer in asymptomatic people.* Retrieved June 10, 2001, from http://www.cancer.org/.

DIAGNOSTIC TESTS and PROCEDURES   *Cancer*

TEST/PROCEDURE	EXAMPLES OF USES
TISSUE EXAMINATION	
Specimens of body fluids, secretions, or tissues are obtained and examined microscopically to detect the presence of malignant cells.	Papanicolaou test detects cancer cells in cervical smear. Examination of body fluids from digestive and respiratory tracts for presence of cancer cells.
Fluids and secretions can be obtained by swabs or smears, by venipuncture, or by withdrawal of fluids from body structures.	Blood cells examined to diagnose leukemias and lymphomas.
Tissue samples are obtained by biopsy (the removal of cells from living tissue). Specimen may be entire growth, sample cut from the growth, or cells drawn from the growth with a needle.	Biopsy: samples can be taken from any accessible growth. Tissue is examined for cancer cells.
IMAGING STUDIES	
Plain Radiographs	
Images produced result from the different absorption rates of different tissues. Calcium in bones absorbs x-rays the most; therefore bones look white on the radiograph. Fat and other soft tissues absorb less and look gray. Air absorbs least, and therefore lungs look black.	Chest radiographs detect changes in lung tissue and bones. Can reveal organ size, position, abnormal structures/shapes. Mammography detects potentially malignant breast calcifications before they can be felt.
Contrast Radiographs	
Use contrast media given orally or intravenously to outline hollow organs. Shadows of abnormal structures can be visualized.	Used primarily to detect cancers of the digestive and urinary tracts.
Computed Tomography (CT Scan)	
Provides cross-sectional, three-dimensional views of body tissue (Fig. 25-2). Details much clearer than radiographs. Can be done plain or with contrast media.	Used to detect cancers of the head and trunk, spine, joints, and soft tissue. Also useful in staging bronchogenic and gastrointestinal tumors.
Positron Emission Tomography (PET)	
A nuclear scan that reveals patterns of tissue metabolism. Two intravenous lines are started: one to deliver an isotope, another to draw blood samples.	Used to detect solid tumors in the brain and breast and to assess the effects of cancer treatment.
Magnetic Resonance Imaging (MRI)	
Used radiofrequency waves in the presence of a strong magnetic field. Energy changes are measured and converted to computer images. Does not expose patient to radiation.	Used to detect cancers of the central nervous system, spinal column, neck, bones, joints, lungs, kidneys, and others.
Radionuclide Scans	
Radionuclides are radioactive substances that are taken up by specific body tissues. The patient is given a radionuclide, usually intravenously, and is then scanned to study the pattern of uptake of the radionuclide in target tissues. The radionuclide accumulates in target tissue, with greater uptake in abnormal tissue.	Used to detect tissue abnormalities. For example, technetium tagged with phosphorus is used for bone scans because technetium is absorbed in increased amounts in bone tissue where abnormal activity or increased metabolism is evident. Other radionuclides are used to detect cancers of the thyroid, liver, lung, and breast as well as lymphoma and melanoma.
ENDOSCOPIC PROCEDURES	
Lighted tubes are inserted into hollow organs or body cavities to visualize and take specimens of suspicious tissue for examination.	Examples: Bronchoscopy: bronchi Colonoscopy: colon Cystoscopy: urinary bladder Laparoscopy: abdominal cavity

DIAGNOSIS OF CANCER

The health history and physical examination often provide the first clues to the presence of cancer. Diagnostic procedures may be used when cancer is suspected, when high-risk people are screened, or when determining the extent of known disease. Diagnostic procedures rely on tissue examinations, imaging studies, endoscopic procedures, and laboratory tests. Combinations of procedures may be indicated for cancers that are difficult to locate or to determine whether there is more than one site. It is important to note that many laboratory tests are nonspecific for cancer. Abnormal laboratory results can have many causes, but combined with other data, they assist in the diagnostic process. Also, the same diagnostic tests and procedures may be used during and after cancer treatment to assess treatment effectiveness. The Diagnostic Tests and Procedures table above presents examples of tests and procedures that might be employed in the diagnostic process.

DIAGNOSTIC TESTS and PROCEDURES   *Cancer—cont'd*

TEST/PROCEDURE	EXAMPLES OF USES

LABORATORY TESTS

Oncofetal Antigens

Oncofetal antigens are substances found on fetal cells and the surface of cancer cells. They are called *tumor markers* because elevations are associated with certain cancers. Can be elevated by nonmalignant conditions also. Often used to monitor response to cancer treatments. If treatment is successfully destroying the cancer, the antigen level goes down.

Note that elevated oncofetal antigens can have causes other than cancer. For example, oncofetal antigens may be elevated with cirrhosis of the liver and ulcerative colitis.

The following are examples of oncofetal antigens and the types of cancers they are associated with:

Carcinoembryonic antigen (CEA): digestive tract, breast; also elevated in heavy smokers

Alpha-fetoprotein (AFP): liver, testicle

CA-50: gastrointestinal tract, biliary tract, pancreas, transitional cell carcinoma, non–small cell lung cancer

CA-125: ovary, breast, cervix, colon, endometrium, fallopian tube, gastrointestinal tract, liver, lung, lymphoma, non-Hodgkin's lymphoma, pancreas

Prostate-specific antigen (PSA): prostate

CA-19-9: pancreas, liver, lung, colon, rectum

Pancreatic oncofetal antigen: pancreas and lung

CA 15-3: breast, liver, lung, prostate

BTA: urinary bladder

Human chorionic gonadotropin (HCG): testicle

Other

Other laboratory studies of body fluids do not specifically diagnose cancer but may suggest possible malignancies.

Examples of other useful laboratory tests are:

Serum alkaline phosphatase: elevated with metastatic bone cancer, hyperparathyroidism

Serum acid phosphatase: elevated with metastatic bone cancer, hairy cell leukemia, prostate cancer

Serum and urine calcium: elevated with bladder, breast, kidney, lung, endocrine cancer, leukemia, lymphoma

Thyroid antithyroglobulin antibody: elevated with thyroid cancer

MNSD 9 Elevations can be caused by numerous other, nonmalignant conditions.

FIGURE 25-2 Computed tomography provides cross-sectional, three-dimensional views of body tissue. This upper-abdominal CT scan shows a blood vessel tumor (hemangioma) in the liver. (Courtesy National Institutes of Health.)

MEDICAL TREATMENT OF CANCER

Methods of treating cancer include surgery, radiotherapy, chemotherapy, biotherapy, transplantation of bone marrow and hematopoietic stem cells, and hormone therapy. Various complementary therapies may be employed as well. One treatment or a combination may be recommended, depending on the type and location of the cancer.

SURGERY

Surgery is done in the majority of patients to diagnose and stage the cancer, relieve symptoms, maintain function, effect a cure, or reconstruct affected structures. Although not common, surgery is sometimes done prophylactically in people who are at very high risk for development of specific cancers. For example, those with familial polyposis may have a portion of the colon removed to prevent colon cancer. Surgery is commonly used in the treatment of cancer, often in combination with other therapies. Surgery for cancer may be extensive or simple. A thorough preoperative diagnostic evaluation enables the surgeon to plan the most appropriate procedure.

Surgery is most likely to be curative when tumors are detected early, are slow growing, are confined to one area, and do not invade vital body structures. Surrounding tissues, including lymph glands, are often removed to eliminate malignant cells that have escaped the tumor mass. When surgery is extensive, it is often referred to as a *radical procedure.*

The preoperative and postoperative care of the surgical cancer patient varies with the specific surgery.

General care of the surgical patient is detailed in Chapter 17. Specific surgeries are discussed in individual chapters. After surgery, other therapies may be recommended. The recommended treatment is based on the type of cancer, its location, the staging, and the extent of metastasis. The surgeon often consults with a radiologist and an oncologist (a physician who specializes in treating patients who have cancer) to determine the best therapy.

Adjuvant and neoadjuvant therapies are relatively recent approaches to cancer treatment. Adjuvant therapy may be used when a patient has had surgery or radiotherapy and is free of signs of disease but has a high likelihood of recurrence. Such patients may be given chemotherapy to eradicate any remaining undetected cells. Adjuvant therapy is often used in the treatment of breast cancer. Neoadjuvant therapy uses chemotherapy to reduce the extent of the tumor before surgery or radiotherapy.

RADIOTHERAPY

Radiotherapy is the use of ionizing radiation in the treatment of disease. The unit of measure for radiation doses is now the Gray. Formerly, the *rad* was the unit of measure. One Gray (Gy) equals one hundred rads. Radiation is used to treat cancer because malignant cells are more sensitive than are normal cells to radiation. Radiation has immediate and delayed effects on cells. The immediate effect is cell death due to damage to the cell membrane. The delayed effect is alteration of DNA, which impairs the cell's ability to reproduce. Types of cancer cells vary in their sensitivity to radiation. A tumor is considered *radiosensitive* if it can be destroyed by radiation at a dose that is tolerated by surrounding normal tissue.

Radiotherapy may be given internally or externally. Internal radiation requires the introduction of the radioactive substance into the body. External radiation is given by way of a beam directed at the tumor.

Caregiver Safety

If you understand radiation, you can work with it safely. The amount of radiation received by those who come in contact with the patient depends on the time of exposure, the distance from the radiation source, and the amount of shielding between the caregiver and the source. The less time spent near the source, the less exposure is incurred. Doubling the distance from the source decreases the exposure to one fourth. When the distance from the source is tripled, the exposure is reduced to one ninth (Fig. 25-3). Unless direct care is being given, remain at least 6 feet away from the source. Effective shielding depends on the type of rays being emitted. In general, the denser the material composing the shield, the better protection it provides. Therefore lead is more protective than concrete or wood. Because shielding is awkward and cannot provide complete protection during patient care, many agencies rely more on time and distance to limit exposure.

External Radiation

Procedure. With external radiation therapy, the source of the radioactivity is located outside the body. A special type of x-ray machine is used to deliver a beam of radiation to the area being treated. Beams may be directed from several different angles to provide the greatest dose to the tumor and minimal exposure of other tissues. The number of treatments given is based on the radiation oncologist's recommendation. It is not unusual for a patient to be treated five times a week

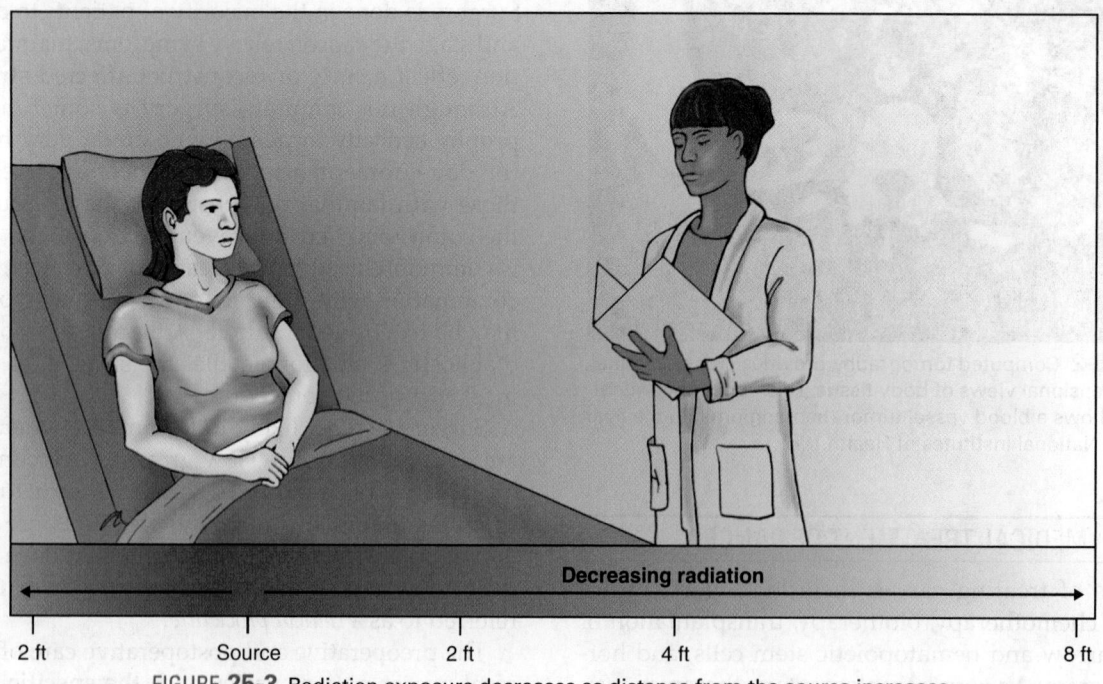

Decreasing radiation

| 2 ft | Source | 2 ft | 4 ft | 8 ft |

FIGURE **25-3** Radiation exposure decreases as distance from the source increases.

for 2 to 8 weeks. A variation of this therapy is intraoperative radiation therapy (IORT), a technique in which the tumor or tumor bed is radiated directly during surgery.

Patient Preparation. Before the first radiation treatment, the patient goes through a treatment simulation, which includes CT scanning, to determine the exact location to be treated. The patient is positioned in various ways while radiographs are taken. The radiation therapist then marks the skin over the area to be treated. The markings are usually made with waterproof ink; however, tiny permanent marking are sometimes made. The markings must remain visible throughout the course of radiation. Instruct the patient not to remove the markings until given permission by the physician. For the actual treatments, various devices are used to shield healthy tissue.

Internal Radiation

Internal radiation involves the introduction of a radiation source into the body. Sources of radiation used for therapy include radioactive forms of iodine, phosphorus, radium, iridium, radon, and cesium. The source may be either sealed or unsealed. In general, patients being treated with internal radiation emit radiation and *do* pose a threat to others until the source is removed or excreted. An exception is the patient who has small radioactive beads permanently implanted to treat localized prostate cancer or inoperable lung cancer.

Sealed-Source Radiation. Sealed-source radiation is inserted into the body in a sealed container. One example of sealed-source radiation is cesium, which is contained in a sealed applicator that is inserted into body cavities to treat cancer of the mouth, tongue, vagina, and cervix. Sealed-source radiation also may be placed in threads, beads, needles, or seeds and implanted into body tissues or may be enclosed in a mold and applied externally. The radiologist determines how long the source is left in place. The patient's body fluids are not radioactive and neither are objects touched by the patient radioactive because the radiation source is closed. Because radiation is emitted from the source while it is in the patient, however, the following safety measures are necessary in most cases to protect all visitors and nurses from excessive exposure to radiation:

1. The patient is placed in a private room, preferably one that is lined with lead.
2. A sign is placed on the door to the patient's room indicating that the room is a radiation area. A standard sign is usually available for this purpose (Fig. 25-4).
3. Anyone who might enter the room for any reason is informed of the proper precautions to be taken. People younger than 18 years and any pregnant woman should not enter the room. This restriction applies to staff as well as others. Exposure to radiation is potentially harmful to a fetus.

Caution

Radioactive Area

FIGURE **25-4** The radiation sign alerts others to the dangers of radiation.

4. The amount of radiation exposure is reduced by limiting time spent in the room and by working as far as possible from the radiation source. Institutional policies prescribe the time restrictions with implants. Nursing personnel who spend the most time with the patient should wear film badges to monitor their radiation exposure.
5. Work must be organized efficiently. For most patients, care can be provided in a total of 30 minutes each shift. Portable lead shields can be used to provide some protection. Lead aprons do not provide adequate protection in this situation.
6. Recognize that sealed sources can be dislodged accidentally. The placement of the source is selected to exert the direct effects of radiation on the area being treated. Specific positions may be ordered for the patient to decrease the risk of displacing the source. Check bedpans and linens for any dislodged source before disposal. If the source moves out of position, immediately notify the physician and the radiation safety personnel. If the source comes out of the patient's body, *do not touch it with bare hands.* Forceps and a lead container (called a *pig*) that are routinely placed in the room are used to retrieve and contain the source.

Unsealed-Source Radiation. When unsealed sources are used, there are some additional considerations. Because body fluids may be contaminated, you must wear gloves when working with the patient. Contaminated fluids, dressings, and the like may require special care, as outlined in the agency policy. Disposable utensils are recommended. Equipment used in the room may need to be checked for radioactivity before it can be removed from the room. The radiologist can advise the staff on specific precautions and how long they are necessary.

Side Effects

The ideal radiation treatment destroys the tumor with the least harm to surrounding cells. Because cells that regenerate rapidly are more susceptible to radiation, both cancer cells and some normal cells may be harmed. Normal cells that are most sensitive to radiation include those of the hair follicle, bone marrow, lining of the digestive and urinary tracts, ovaries, testes, and lymph tissue. Radiation damage to these cells explains many of the side effects of the therapy. Depending on the area being irradiated, the following side effects may occur: bone marrow suppression, alopecia (hair loss), anorexia, dry mouth, nausea and vomiting, diarrhea, and inflammation of the esophagus (esophagitis), lungs (pneumonitis), and bladder (cystitis). Regardless of the site treated, radiation therapy commonly causes skin changes and fatigue. Side effects are usually not evident until at least a week after treatments are started. These side effects are slow to start and slow to subside Some people tolerate therapy well, whereas others become very ill. Factors that influence the severity of side effects include the area being treated, total and daily radiation doses, volume of tissue treated, method of treatment, and individual factors.

Bone Marrow Suppression. In healthy people, the bone marrow produces red blood cells, white blood cells, and platelets. Depending on the treatment site, total area irradiated, and daily radiation dose, radiation treatment can suppress the production of these cells. Anemia results from a deficiency of red blood cells. Without adequate white blood cells, the patient's ability to resist infection is reduced. Without adequate platelets, the patient is at risk for bruising and bleeding. Bone marrow suppression is most common among patients whose treatment area involves a large area of bone.

Blood counts are usually ordered every other week during radiation therapy, depending on the treatment area, to detect excessive bone marrow suppression. If blood counts are too low, transfusions may be required. The radiation treatments may have to be temporarily stopped until the bone marrow recovers. White blood cell and platelet counts usually recover in 2 to 6 weeks. When radiation treatments are in combination with chemotherapy treatments, there is a greater chance of bone marrow suppression. Growth factors for white and red blood cells can be used to help the blood cell counts recover sooner.

Alopecia. Because the cells in the hair follicles are very sensitive to radiation, radiation of the head often produces partial or complete alopecia (loss of hair). Whether the hair grows back depends on the radiation dosage. If the hair does grow back, it may be different in color or texture than it was before treatment.

Anorexia. Anorexia is a loss of appetite. Factors that may cause the patient undergoing radiation therapy

to have anorexia include inflammation of the mouth and tongue, altered taste perception, and nausea. Anorexia is a significant problem because it can lead to inadequate nutrition and weight loss. It is especially problematic for patients being treated for cancer of the esophagus, stomach, neck, or head. Depression may contribute to anorexia in the patient undergoing radiation therapy.

Dry Mouth. Dry mouth, called xerostomia, is a special problem with radiation of the head and neck. The production of saliva decreases, putting the patient at risk for infections of the teeth and gums. Diseased teeth are often extracted before radiation of the head or neck because the risk of osteoradionecrosis is so great. Osteoradionecrosis is destruction of bone caused by radiation. It is a debilitating complication of head and neck radiation. Medication is available that can help protect the salivary glands as well as any mucus-producing tissue. These medications are called *radio-protectors* and are given before radiation treatment on a daily basis or as ordered by the physician.

Effects on Reproduction. Radiation is potentially harmful to reproductive cells as well as to the developing fetus and embryo. Therefore radiotherapy is not recommended during pregnancy and patients are advised to avoid becoming pregnant during the therapy.

The major side effects of radiation are summarized in Table 25-7.

CHEMOTHERAPY

Chemotherapy is the use of chemical agents in the treatment of disease. Chemical agents specifically used to treat cancer are called antineoplastic or *anticancer drugs*. The terms *chemotherapy, anticancer,* and *antineoplastic drugs* are used interchangeably in this chapter, just as they are in common practice. These drugs act by destroying rapidly dividing cells and may be used alone or in combination with other forms of treatment. In some cases, chemotherapy is curative. In other circumstances, it may reduce the number of cancer cells, causing symptoms to decrease and often prolonging life.

Types of Antineoplastic Drugs

Types of antineoplastic drugs now commonly used in chemotherapy include cytotoxic agents, hormones and hormone antagonists, biologic response modifiers, and radio-immunotherapy. Various types of cancer are sensitive to different drugs or drug combinations. Combinations are sometimes used to attack cells at different stages of development. Drugs that are effective only during a particular phase of cell development are said to be *cell-cycle phase-specific*. Drugs that are effective during any phase of cell development are said to be *cell-cycle phase-nonspecific*. Table 25-8 gives examples of drugs used in chemotherapy and the cancers for which they are used. A new class of drugs that is being studied for cancer treatment is called *angiogenesis in-*

Table 25-7 | *Side Effects of Radiation Therapy and Nursing Implications*

SITE	SIDE EFFECTS	NURSING IMPLICATIONS
Skin	Erythema (redness), desquamation (peeling), permanent darkening	Skin is easily injured. Avoid exposure to sun, trauma, harsh chemicals, or soaps. Until therapy is completed, no lotions or topical medications should be applied. Do not remove markings.
Scalp	Partial or complete alopecia (hair loss); may be permanent	New hair may be different color and texture. Cover scalp with wig, cap, or scarf if patient desires. Refer to American Cancer Society for free hairpieces and help with styling and care.
Digestive tract	Anorexia, inflammation and dryness of the mouth, decreased or altered sense of taste	Small, frequent feedings. Respect patient preferences. Frequent oral hygiene. Suggest artificial saliva. Monitor weight to assess nutritional state.
	Dental caries	Encourage dental care. Mouth care per protocol.
	Painful swallowing	Antacids and viscous lidocaine as ordered.
	Nausea, vomiting	Antiemetics as ordered. Monitor intake.
	Diarrhea	Antidiarrheals as ordered. Perianal care.
Urinary tract	Cystitis	Increase fluid intake.
	Contracted bladder	Have patient empty bladder often.
	Crystalluria	Keep intake and output records.
Bone marrow	Suppressed production of red blood cells, white blood cells, and platelets	Schedule activities to prevent overtiring. Protect from infection. Protect from injury. Watch for excessive bruising or bleeding. Check results of blood tests. Report fever. Use soft toothbrush, electric razor.
Lungs	Pneumonitis	Encourage coughing and deep breathing to prevent pneumonia. Use humidifier if ordered. Protect from respiratory infections.
Reproductive organs	Harm to embryo or fetus; sterility, impotence	Patient advised not to become pregnant during therapy or for specified time afterward. Physician may counsel male patient about banking sperm.

hibitors. These agents prevent the development of new blood vessels in tumors so that they cannot grow. Angiogenesis inhibitors will not eliminate tumors but are expected to be safe enough for continuous use because they are less toxic than current drugs.

Chemotherapy is administered by a physician or a nurse who has had specialized education. Some drugs may be given in an outpatient setting, and others must be given in an inpatient setting. The route may be oral, intramuscular, intravenous, intracavity, or intrathecal. *Intracavity* means the drug is instilled into a body cavity such as the bladder. *Intrathecal* chemotherapy is given in the subarachnoid space.

Chemoembolization is a technique in which the drug is injected directly into an artery supplying the tumor. Chemoembolization has been used in the treatment of metastatic liver cancer. The goal of this approach is to stop liver tumors from growing or cause them to shrink; shrinkage occurs in about two thirds of cases treated. This benefit on average lasts 10 to 14 months (sirweb.org/April 17, 2005).

Side Effects

Like radiotherapy, antineoplastic drugs act on both normal cells and malignant cells. The major systemic side effects of antineoplastic drugs are the same as those of radiation: bone marrow suppression, nausea and vomiting, and alopecia. Depending on the specific antineoplastic agent, the patient is also at risk for toxic effects to the heart, lungs, nerve tissue, kidneys, and bladder. These problems and related nursing interventions are discussed in Nursing Care of the Patient Who Has Cancer on pages 385 and 386 and are summarized in Table 25-9.

Although bone marrow suppression is the most *dangerous* side effect, nausea and vomiting are likely to be the most distressing. Antineoplastic drugs simultaneously irritate the lining of the digestive tract and stimulate the vomiting center in the brain. Some agents, especially doxorubicin (Adriamycin), have

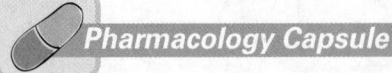
Pharmacology Capsule

The most dangerous adverse effect of antineoplastic drugs used in chemotherapy is bone marrow suppression.

Table 25-8 | *Examples of Drugs Used to Treat Cancer*

CYTOTOXIC DRUGS

Mitotic Inhibitors (Plant Alkaloids)
Docetaxel (Taxotere)
Paclitaxel (Taxol)
Vinblastine (Velban)
Vincristine (Oncovin)
Vinorelbine (Navelbine)

Alkylating Agents
Busulfan (Myleran)
Carboplatin (Paraplatin)
Carmustine (BCNU)
Chlorambucil (Leukeran)
Cisplatin (Platinol)
Cyclophosphamide (Cytoxan)
Ifosfamide (Ifex)
Lomustine (CCNU)
Mechlorethamine hydrochloride (Mustargen)
Melphalan (Alkeran)
Streptozocin (Zanosar)
Temozolomide (Temodar)

Antitumor Antibiotics
Bleomycin (Blenoxane)
Dactinomycin (Cosmegen)
Daunorubicin (Cerubidine, and others)
Doxorubicin (Adriamycin)
Epirubicin (Ellence)
Idarubicin hydrochloride (Idamycin)
Mitomycin (Mutamycin)
Mitoxantrone (Novantrone)
Plicamycin (Mithramycin)
Valrubicin (Valstar)

Antimetabolites
Folic Acid Analog
   Methotrexate (Folex)
Pyrimidine Analogs
   Capecitabine (Cytosar-U, and others)
   Cytarabine (Cytosar-U)
   Fluorouracil (Adrucil)
   Floxuridine (FUDR)
   Gemcitabine (Gemzar)
Purine Analogs
   Fludarabine (Fludara)
   Mercaptopurine (Purinethol)
   Pentostatin (Nipent)
   Thioguanine (Thioguanine)

Topoisomerase Inhibitors
Etoposide (Etopophos, VePesid, and others)
Irinotecan (Camptosar)
Teniposide (Vumon)
Topotecan (Hycamtin)

Miscellaneous
Altretamine (Hexalen)
Asparaginase (Elspar)
Dacarbazine (DTIC-Dome)
Hydroxyurea (Hydrea)
Pegaspargase (Oncaspar)
Mitotane (Lysodren)
Procarbazine (Matulane)

HORMONES AND HORMONE ANTAGONISTS

Androgens
Fluoxymesterone (Halotestin)
Testosterone (generic only)
Testolactone (Teslac)

Gonadotropic-Releasing Hormone Analogs
Leuprolide (Lupron)
Goserelin (Zoladex)

Androgen Receptor Blockers
Flutamide (Eulexin)
Bicalutamide (Casodex)
Nilutamide (Nilandron)

Estrogens
Diethylstilbestrol diphosphate (Stilphostrol)
Ethinyl estradiol (Estinyl)

Estrogen Mustard
Estramustine (Emcyt)

Antiestrogens
Tamoxifen (Nolvadex)
Raloxifene (Evista)
Toremifene (Fareston)

Progestins
Medroxyprogesterone acetate (Depo-Provera)
Megestrol acetate (Megace)

Aromatase Inhibitors
Anastrozole (Arimidex)
Letrozole (Femara)
Exemestane (Aromasin)

Glucocorticoid
Prednisone (Deltasone, and others)

BIOLOGIC RESPONSE MODIFIERS (IMMUNOSTIMULANTS)
Monoclonal Antibodies
Trastuzumab (Herceptin), Breast cancer
Rituximab (Rituxan), Non-Hodgkin's lymphoma
Tositumomab (Zevalin), Non-Hodgkin's lymphoma
Alemtuzumab (Campath), Chronic lymphocytic leukemia

Interferons
Interferon alfa-2a (Roferon-A)
Interferon alfa-2b (Intron A)
Interferon alfa-n3 (Alferon N)
Interferon beta-1a (Avonex)
Interferon beta-1b (Betaseron)
Interferon gamma-1b (Actimmune)

Interleukins
Aldesleukin/Interleukin-2 (Proleukin)
Oprelvekin/Interleukin 11 (Neumega)

Vaccines
BCG vaccine (TheraCys, and others)

Colony-Stimulating Factors
Erythropoietin (Procrit, Epogen)
Darbepoetin alfa/Erythrocytes–(Aranesp)
Filgrastim (G-CSF, Neupogen)
Sargramostim (GM-CSF, Leukine)
Interleukin-3
Macrophage CSF
Pegfilgrastim (Neulasta)

Other
Levamisole (Ergamisol)

Table 25-9 | *Side Effects of Antineoplastic Therapy and Nursing Implications*

SITE	SIDE EFFECTS	IMPLICATIONS
Bone marrow	Suppressed production of red blood cells, white blood cells, and platelets	Monitor blood test results. Balance activity and rest. Prevent overtiring and stress. Protect from infection. Report fever. Watch for excessive bruising or bleeding. Apply pressure to injection sites. Avoid rectal temperatures if white blood cell count is low. Use soft toothbrush and electric razor.
Digestive tract	Nausea and vomiting	Give antiemetics as ordered. Assess for dehydration. No fluids with meals. Pleasant environment. Respect food preferences.
	Anorexia	Small, frequent feedings. Frequent oral hygiene. Monitor weight. Give supplements as ordered.
	Xerostomia	Increase fluid intake. Recommend artificial saliva, sugarless gum or hard candy, ice chips. Moisten dry food.
	Stomatitis	Encourage dental care. Mouth care as ordered or per protocol. Assess for lesions.
	Diarrhea	Antidiarrheals as ordered. Perianal care.
	Constipation	Encourage fluids and high-fiber foods and exercise as tolerated. Give laxatives, stool softeners, enemas as ordered.
Heart	Cardiomyopathy Heart failure	Monitor for dyspnea, edema, increasing pulse pressure. Request electrocardiograms as ordered.
Lungs	Inflammation, fibrosis	Encourage turning, coughing, and deep breathing to prevent pneumonia. Use humidifier as ordered. Elevate head if dyspneic. Protect from respiratory infections. Monitor activity tolerance.
Nerve tissue	Numbness, tingling, loss of deep tendon reflexes.	Assess sensation. Protect affected areas from injury.
Scalp	Alopecia	Cover scalp with hairpiece, scarf, turban if patient wishes. Refer to American Cancer Society for free hairpieces and help with grooming.
Veins	Phlebitis at infusion site	Possible necrosis of surrounding tissue with extravasation. Monitor infusion carefully. Protect infusion site. Report signs of extravasation immediately.
Reproductive cells	Harm to developing embryo or fetus. Sterility, impotence with some agents.	Pregnancy discouraged while on therapy and for specified period thereafter. Physician may discuss banking sperm with male patients.

toxic effects on the heart that may lead to heart failure. Bleomycin (Blenoxane) causes pulmonary inflammation and fibrosis that usually reverse after the therapy is completed. Vinblastine (Velban) and vincristine (Oncovin) are neurotoxic, with effects manifested most often by numbness and tingling of extremities, paralytic ileus, and loss of deep tendon reflexes. Hypersensitivity reactions can occur with paclitaxel (Taxol) and most other chemotherapeutic agents. Like radiation, antineoplastic drugs are hazardous to reproductive cells, and some cause erectile dysfunction and sterility.

Antineoplastic agents also can cause very serious tissue injury to the vein during administration. If the agent leaks out of the vein, surrounding tissue destruction may occur. When **extravasation** is suspected, im-

mediately stop the infusion. Various interventions may be used by the physician or clinical nurse specialist in an effort to limit the harm caused by the agent.

Pharmacology Capsule

Tissue destruction can result from a group of intravenous antineoplastic agents classified as vesicants. Extravasation is leakage of these IV agents into surrounding tissues.

BIOTHERAPY

Agents that work by affecting biologic processes (referred to as **biotherapy**) include hematopoietic growth factors, biologic response modifiers (BRMs), and monoclonal antibodies. Hematopoietic growth factors (see Table 25-8 for list) are colony-stimulating factors (CSFs). Because antineoplastic agents suppress the bone marrow, colony-stimulating factors may be used to stimulate the bone marrow to produce platelets, red blood cells, and white blood cells in patients on chemotherapy. This reduces the risk of infection by shortening the period of neutropenia, which occurs when white blood cells are low, associated with chemotherapy, as well as anemia and thrombocytopenia. Chapters 32 and 33 provide additional information about CSFs. With CSFs, higher doses of chemotherapy can be given for longer periods of time.

Surgery, radiotherapy, and chemotherapy work by destroying malignant cells and thereby reduce the size of the tumor. It is hoped that the body's natural defenses will then destroy the remaining malignant cells. Therapy using BRMs is intended to boost the body's existing defenses. BRMs act directly on malignant cells or stimulate the immune system to act against them. Such therapy is most effective if the immune system is functioning adequately. A skin test may be performed to evaluate the immune response before therapy is started. Examples of BRMs are interferons and interleukins.

Pharmacology Capsule

Biologic response modifiers boost the body's natural defenses to combat malignant cells.

Because the effectiveness of BRM therapy for cancer is still being studied, it is not usually the first line of treatment. The most common side effects are extreme fatigue, headache, muscle aches, chills, and fever. Side effects are more common in older people and in people who are dehydrated, anemic, and malnourished. Previous cardiac, neurologic, gastrointestinal, hepatic, or renal disease also increases the risk of side effects. Table 25-10 outlines side effects of BRM therapy. The patient should be told to report a rash, blister, or pain at the injection site or a fever.

Monoclonal antibodies (MoAbs) are specific for proteins on the surface of certain cancer cells. The use of MoAbs in both the diagnosis and treatment of cancer is the subject of numerous studies.

BONE MARROW AND STEM CELL TRANSPLANTATION

Bone marrow transplantation is most often used after treatment of leukemia and lymphoma with chemotherapy and/or radiation that destroys the patient's bone marrow. Stem cell transplantation can be used to treat the destruction of the bone marrow caused by the chemotherapy and radiotherapy. Transplantation of bone marrow or peripheral blood stem cells is done to restore the blood manufacturing cells. If a patient donates his or her own stem cells or bone marrow before therapy, it is classified as an *autologous transplant*. If a patient receives cells from a sibling or other relative, it is classified as an *allogeneic transplant*; if the cells are donated from an unrelated donor, it is classified as a *matched unrelated donor (MUD) transplant*. See Chapter 33 for additional discussion of CSFs and bone marrow and stem cell transplants.

HORMONE THERAPY

Because some tumors are affected by hormones, various treatments may be used to suppress natural hormone

---

Table 25-10 | *Common Side Effects of Biologic Response Modifiers and Nursing Implications*

SITE	SIDE EFFECTS	NURSING IMPLICATIONS
Generalized	Flu-like symptoms: fever, chills, muscle aches, severe fatigue, malaise, headaches, tachycardia	Side effects may mask signs and symptoms of infection, so assess carefully. Give acetaminophen as ordered (meperidine is sometimes ordered for severe chills). Help patient plan for adequate rest.
Heart	Serious dysrhythmias, myocardial infarction	Monitor heart rate and rhythm. Report abnormal findings.
Capillaries	Increased permeability, pulmonary and dependent edema, hypotension	Assess for edema. Monitor blood pressure. Have patient change positions slowly; avoid prolonged standing, hot baths, and showers. For hypotension, give colloids or vasopressors as ordered.
Bronchi and lungs	Anaphylaxis with bronchial constriction Pulmonary edema	Note signs of allergy: rash, wheezing, itching. For anaphylaxis, give epinephrine or diphenhydramine as ordered. Maintain airway. Assess lungs for crackles. Position for comfort (head elevated).

MNSD: Many other side effects occur with individual biologic response modifiers. They include nausea, diarrhea, anorexia, weight loss, skin redness or rash, pruritus, desquamation, bone pain, renal toxicity, anemia, thrombocytopenia, leukopenia, leukocytosis, altered mental status, and liver toxicity. The nurse should identify the specific effects and implications for the specific agents the patient is receiving.

secretion, block hormone actions, or provide supplemental hormones. For example, hormones may be used to block the male sex hormones in the treatment of prostate cancer and female hormones in the treatment of breast cancer.

Consider the Alternative

Alternative Therapies

The American Cancer Society identifies some complementary therapies that can help relieve symptoms or side effects, ease pain, and increase enjoyment of life. These include the following:

- Aromatherapy
- Art therapy
- Biofeedback
- Massage therapy
- Music therapy
- Prayer, spiritual practices
- T'ai chi
- Yoga

COMPLEMENTARY AND ALTERNATIVE THERAPIES

Some patients choose to use nontraditional treatments such as relaxation techniques, guided imagery, music, meditation, herbal remedies, and acupuncture. If a nontraditional therapy is used with conventional treatment, it is called **complementary therapy**. The term **alternative therapy** is used if the patient uses nontraditional therapy in place of traditional treatment. Research is being conducted by the National Center for Complementary and Alternative Medicine in the National Institutes of Health to determine the therapeutic value of nontraditional therapies.

Many patients with cancer or other chronic conditions use alternative therapies including herbal remedies, and many are "secretive" about their use. It is important for patients to report all herbal products used to their physician and to consider their use carefully. Generally, there are very few clinical trials evaluating the true safety and efficacy of these products. Also, some affect the action of prescribed medications.

UNPROVEN METHODS OF CANCER TREATMENT

Studies have found that 6% to 9% of patients with cancer admit to using some questionable method of cancer treatment. The American Cancer Society discourages the use of treatments that have not been studied and found to be safe and effective. Alternative therapies can be harmful in themselves and may delay treatment with potentially effective conventional therapies. A partial list of treatments considered unproven with regard to safety and effectiveness is presented in Box 25-2. You can direct patients to the American Cancer Society for further information about questionable

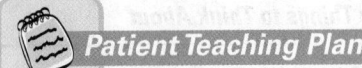

Patient Teaching Plan

Herbal Therapy

- Just because a product is "natural" does not mean it is safe.
- Before taking herbal products, discuss their use with your physician.
- Try to research the product thoroughly to learn as much as you can about it.
- Use products with a single component or ingredient (additional ingredients add to the potential toxicity).
- Use products from a reputable manufacturer. Ensure that the label has the manufacturer's address and expiration date.
- Look for products that have a DIN (drug identification number). The DIN guarantees that the specified medicinal components will be present. For example: Tanacet 125(r) guarantees that an exact amount of tanacet, the medicinal component of feverfew, is present and that the product is quality controlled.

therapies. Special considerations about the use of herbs as therapy can be found in Box 25-3.

NURSING CARE of the Patient Who Has Cancer

When working with people who have cancer, it is easy to focus on the cancer and forget the person. There are many things we can do to help the person who has cancer (see Nursing Care Plan: The Patient with Cancer on pp. 385 and 386) that can significantly affect the person's quality of life. Assessment of the patient who has cancer

| Box 25-2 | **Unproven Methods of Cancer Management** |

- Antineoplastons
- Contreras methods
- Dimethyl sulfoxide (DMSO)
- Electronic devices
- Fresh cell therapy
- Gerson method
- Greek cancer cure
- Hoxsey method/Bio-Medical Center
- Hydrogen peroxide and other "hyperoxygenation" therapies
- Immunoaugmentative therapy
- Iscador
- Kelley malignancy index and ecology therapy
- Laetrile
- Livingston-Wheeler therapy
- Macrobiotic diets
- Metabolic therapy of Harold W. Manner, Ph.D.
- "Psychic surgery"
- Questionable cancer practices in Tijuana and other Mexican border clinics
- Questionable "nutritional" therapies
- Revici method

From American Cancer Society. (1993). *Questionable methods of cancer treatment* (p.15). Atlanta, GA: Author.

Box 25-3   *Herbs: A Few Things to Think About*

The following are common problems with herb use:

- The quantity and quality of any medicinal components in an herbal product can vary considerably. Herbal products are not regulated by the Food and Drug Administration (safety and effectiveness do not have to be demonstrated before these products are marketed).
- No legal standards are applied to their growing conditions, harvesting, processing, or packaging. The possibilities of poor quality, adulteration, contamination and varying strengths must be kept in mind when evaluating them (e.g., they could be sprayed with pesticides, grown in contaminated soil). The country of origin where the herb is grown is often not known (frequently grown outside the United States).
- If the product label has whole plant listed, the amount of active medicinal/chemical agent in the product is not known and can vary considerably. This can make dosing difficult/inaccurate. If the label indicates the chemical in total weight, this can be considered a specific amount of that product. See information about DIN on p. 383.
- Finding herbs in the wild can be dangerous. For example, wild parsley looks very similar to poison water hemlock; poisonous mushrooms are (virtually) indistinguishable from edible ones.
- Many herbs interfere with prescription medications (e.g., some herbs can cause thinning of the blood, which can increase the risk of bleeding for patients on Coumadin/anticoagulation).
- Some natural products such as thymus are derived from animal sources and could be contaminated by prions, which can cause Creutzfeldt-Jakob disease (the human equivalent of mad cow disease). Another example: products that contain thyroid can alter the body's natural balance of thyroid hormone.
- Some herbal products decrease the risk of cancer; others may *increase* the risk of cancer or increase cancer growth. The Oncology Nursing Forum (2004) has a four-part series online for access about herbs and natural products at:
  - *Herbs or Natural Products That Decrease Cancer Growth: Part One of a Four-Part Series*
  - *Herbs or Natural Products That Increase Cancer Growth or Recurrence: Part Two of a Four-Part Series*
  - *Herbs or Natural Products That Protect Against Cancer Growth: Part Three of a Four-Part Series*
  - *Herbs or Natural Products That May Cause Cancer and Harm: Part Four of a Four-Part Series*
- Other Internet resources concerning herbs are:
  - FDA/CFSAN: Article on Herbal Products: Dangerous Combinations
  - Herbal Health Products: What You Should Know—familydoctor.org
  - The website for the American Cancer Society also provides information on this topic (www.nccam.nih.gov/ accessed April 17, 2005).

Consider the Alternative

Myth and Truth About Herbs

Myth: Herbs are natural products and therefore are safe.
Truth: Many have serious side effects, including liver toxicity, even death.
Plants are composed of many different chemicals—some medicinal, others poisonous.

is discussed along with nursing care for each phase of illness: diagnostic phase, treatment phase, rehabilitation, and recurrence of terminal illness.

THE DIAGNOSTIC PHASE

People who develop one of the common signs of cancer are often aware of how serious the condition might be. Out of fear, some ignore the signs until the disease is advanced. When people seek evaluation of the signs, they are likely to be very worried. Patients often say that just "not knowing" is the hardest part. They go through tests and procedures, some uncomfortable, and then wait for the final word. Cancer is often what they fear most.

Assessment

When a patient is having diagnostic procedures related to an actual or a potential diagnosis of cancer, collect data needed for the planning and provision of care.

Health History

Chief Complaint. Begin with the chief complaint. The patient may complain of pain, lesions, lumps, or changes in some body function. Elicit a complete description of the problem and the related signs and symptoms.

Past Medical History. Document chronic illnesses, serious injuries, surgeries, and hospitalizations.

Family History. Inquire about the incidence of cancer and other serious diseases in the patient's immediate family.

Review of Systems. In the review of systems, record any of the following signs and symptoms, if present: pain, lumps, fatigue, activity intolerance, lesions of the skin or mucous membranes, easy bruising or bleeding, headache, vision or hearing disturbances, hoarseness, cough, dyspnea, hemoptysis, loss of appetite, difficulty swallowing, digestive disturbances, blood in the urine or stool, and change in bowel pattern.

NURSING CARE PLAN

The Patient with Cancer

ASSESSMENT

Health History: Mr. Silas Wilson is a 63-year-old African-American man who was recently diagnosed with lung cancer that is being treated with radiotherapy and chemotherapy. He reports a chronic, nonproductive cough but denies dyspnea or hemoptysis. He states that he has been fatigued and weak since starting his therapy. He has had mild nausea, anorexia, and occasional diarrhea. He complains of dry mouth and is having some dysphagia. The skin over the area being radiated is tender. He is married, is the father of three grown children, and is an insurance salesman. He smoked one pack of cigarettes a day for 30 years, having quit smoking in 1996. He continues to work part time and expresses concern about his financial situation. He states he has excellent insurance coverage.

Physical Examination: Height, 5'9", weight, 175 lb. Vital signs: pulse, 72; respirations, 18; blood pressure, 176/92; temperature, 98° F (oral). Alert and oriented but does not initiate conversation. Dry mucous membranes and cracked lips. Skin on upper chest and neck is more darkly pigmented. Central venous catheter in place; insertion site free of swelling or drainage. Respirations are not labored, and breath sounds are clear throughout lung fields. Abdomen is soft and bowel sounds present. Extremities are warm with strong peripheral pulses. No edema. Unable to distinguish warm and cold or sharp and dull sensations in lower legs.

Nursing Diagnosis	Goals and Outcome Criteria	Interventions
Anxiety related to effects of treatment of uncertain outcomes	Patient will experience reduced anxiety as evidenced by patient statements and by more relaxed behavior.	Encourage patient to talk about his illness and his feelings about it. Listen attentively, and use touch to convey concern. Help patient identify sources of anxiety and strategies to deal with it, such as teaching, counseling, spiritual guidance, and support groups.
Ineffective Coping related to multiple stressors	Patient will identify stressors and strategies to deal with them to improve coping.	Help patient set priorities during therapy. Provide information about management of therapy side effects. Encourage self-care as much as possible. Emphasize his strength. Teach relaxation techniques. Refer to American Cancer Society for information about support services in the community.
Deficient Knowledge of the prescribed therapy, effects, and precautions	Patient will correctly describe his disease, treatment, the effects of therapy, and the precautions needed.	Determine what the patient already knows and what additional information he wants. Reinforce pretreatment teaching. Remind him not to wash off skin markings until radiologist gives permission. Do not apply lotion to irritated skin. Recommend cotton clothing over irritated skin. Provide information about specific drugs used in his chemotherapy. Refer to Cancer Information service (1-800-4CANCER) if interested.
Risk for Injury related to side effects of therapy	Patient will have no injuries related to therapy, as evidenced by absence of bleeding, dyspnea, skin lesions, or bruises.	Monitor for excessive bruising or prolonged bleeding, edema, dyspnea, impaired sensation. Report blood in stool, urine, or sputum. Handle gently. Apply pressure for 5 minutes after venipunctures or injections. Instruct to use a soft toothbrush and an electric razor. Protect feet and legs from trauma. Inspect daily for injury. Advise to wear shoes whenever out of bed.
Risk for Infection related to decreased white blood cells, venous access devices	Patient will remain free of infection, as evidenced by normal body temperature and absence of swelling or warmth at central line insertion site.	Advise patient to avoid crowds and people with infection. Report fever, foul wound drainage, or confusion to physician promptly. Teach patient proper care of central venous catheter, and have him return demonstration.
Imbalanced Nutrition: Less Than Body Requirements related to anorexia and nausea	Patient will maintain adequate nutrition, as evidenced by body weight within 10 lb of usual (180 lb).	Emphasize the importance of good nutrition. Request a dietary consult. Consider frequent feedings. Respect preferences and aversions. Suggest soft diet eaten slowly for dysphagia. Tell the patient not to drink alcohol while receiving chemotherapy. Advise not to drink fluids with meals and to decrease intake of sweets and fatty foods. Create a pleasant environment without offensive odors. Suggest mild exercise before meals and rest afterward. Give ordered antiemetics as necessary.

Continued

NURSING CARE PLAN

The Patient with Cancer—cont'd

Nursing Diagnosis	Goals and Outcome Criteria	Interventions
Impaired oral mucous membrane related to decreased salivation, inflammation	Patient will report successful management of dry mouth, and oral mucous membranes will be intact.	Tell patient to do frequent, gentle mouth care. Recommend artificial saliva for dryness. Encourage increased fluids, sugarless gum or candies, and ice chips. Suggest moistening food before eating. When the mouth is inflamed, avoid acidic, salty, or spicy foods.
Fatigue related to anemia, effects of cancer	Patient will report adaptations in lifestyle that reduce fatigue.	Assess patient's need for assistance and schedule activities to conserve energy.
Interrupted Family Processes related to illness and therapy	Patient and family will discuss need to alter roles and relationships during treatment.	Include the family in patient teaching. Encourage them to plan with the patient for accomplishment of family tasks and responsibilities. Acknowledge family stress and fears. Refer to sources of help as needed. Ask the social worker to assist with financial arrangements.

? CRITICAL THINKING QUESTIONS

- How could you find out what the patient already knows about his disease and what he wants to know?

- How might the patient's emotional reaction to the diagnosis of cancer affect his prognosis or treatment?

Functional Assessment. Describe the patient's diet, use of alcohol and tobacco, safe sex practices, activity, and sleep routines. Document the occupation, and describe a usual day. Assess health practices, including frequency of breast self-examination, testicular examination, and medical checkups. Identify the patient's concerns about living conditions and/or location. Ask about sources of stress and of support and usual coping strategies.

Physical Examination

The physical examination begins with measurement of vital signs, height, and weight. Note whether there has been a change in weight. Inspect the face, scalp, and oral mucosa for lesions. Palpate the neck for enlarged lymph nodes. Throughout the examination, inspect the skin for color, lesions, edema, and bruising. Auscultate breath sounds, and observe respiratory effort. Inspect the breasts for symmetry, dimpling, and abnormal skin color, and palpate for lumps or thickened areas. Inspect the abdomen for distention, auscultate for bowel sounds, and palpate for masses. Inspect the genitalia for lesions. Palpate the scrotum for descended testicles and, if present, for testicular lumps.

Nursing Diagnoses, Goals, and Outcome Criteria: Diagnostic Phase

NURSING DIAGNOSES	GOALS AND OUTCOME CRITERIA
Ineffective Denial related to fear of diagnosis of cancer	Acceptance of need for medical evaluation and treatment: patient seeks medical evaluation and treatment
Anxiety related to threat of or change in health status	Reduced anxiety: patient states anxiety reduced, demonstrates calm manner
Deficient Knowledge of diagnostic tests and procedures	Knowledge of tests and procedures: patient correctly describes tests and follows directions in relation to tests

Interventions
Ineffective Denial

When people detect possible signs or symptoms of cancer, they may be so anxious that they cannot deal with their fears. Instead, they deny the seriousness of the situation and do not seek medical care. Such delays may allow the disease to progress, making treatment more difficult and less likely to be successful. Encourage people to learn the warning signs of cancer and to report them promptly. Emphasize that these signs may be caused by conditions other than cancer, but medical evaluation is needed for a correct diagnosis. Stress the fact that many cancers are curable, especially in the early stages.

Anxiety

During the diagnostic phase, the patient needs encouragement, support, and honest information. Be careful to remain hopeful yet not give false reassurance ("I'm sure it will not be cancer."). Clichés are not helpful either ("Everything has a purpose."). It *is* helpful to recognize what the patient seems to be feeling ("You seem to be very worried."). Information about tests and procedures allows the patient to prepare mentally.

Remember that patients who are being evaluated for cancer are under stress. They may show this stress through anger, irritability, fear, or depression. All of these reactions are normal under the circumstances and should be accepted with understanding (Fig. 25-5).

The physician reports findings to the patient and informs the patient of the diagnosis. In the past, it was not uncommon for the diagnosis of cancer to be kept from the patient. Now most patients are told of their diagnoses. This change has come about because patients are better informed, cancer treatment has improved the odds of survival, and the patient's right to know is recognized. Nevertheless, you should know what the patient has been told, to avoid giving the patient conflicting messages. At times, you may need to help patients communicate their needs and questions to the physician.

Once a diagnosis of cancer has been made, the patient needs support to adapt to the situation. Even at this phase of the illness, the patient may show various responses related to grief. Responses could include denial, shock and disbelief, anger, depression, bargaining, and acceptance. It is useful to understand and recognize how to help the grieving patient. Chapter 24 discusses nursing care of the grieving patient.

Patients struggle to adjust to the knowledge that they have cancer. For many, this is the first time they have seriously considered the possibility of their own deaths. They are typically preoccupied with what will happen to them.

People have different ways of coping with a diagnosis of cancer. Poor coping is sometimes related to lack of information about the disease and its treatment. In that case, the oncology clinical nurse specialist may be consulted to provide patient education. Some coping styles are more effective than others. Weisman's research, cited in Dodd et al. (1993), found that patients who had the most difficulty were those who tended to try not to think about the situation, passively accepted treatment, lacked personal support, and tended to expect the worst. Patients who handled the stress of cancer better usually confronted problems directly, wanted to be well informed, had personal support, and were optimistic.

In the diagnostic phase of cancer care, patients typically use their usual methods of dealing with stress. When coping is not effective, a referral to a psychiatric clinical nurse specialist or a mental health counselor may be in order.

Deficient Knowledge

Tell the patient about diagnostic procedures, including preparation, what the procedure is like, and any specific postprocedure care.

THE TREATMENT PHASE

Assessment

During the treatment phase, specific assessments depend on the type and site of cancer and the prescribed treatment. Information obtained in the initial assessment provides baseline data. Frequently and systematically collect data to determine changes related to the disease process and for effects and side effects of therapy. Areas of ongoing data collection are presented here.

Health History

Note the patient's diagnosis and treatment plan. Take the past medical history to reveal other acute and chronic conditions that require attention during cancer therapy. Obtain a complete drug profile, and record allergies prominently. Review the systems to detect significant symptoms related to cancer or the treatment, including fatigue, weakness, headache, sore or dry mouth, dyspnea, palpitations, altered taste sensations, nausea, diarrhea, constipation, blood in stools, change in urinary frequency, hematuria or dysuria, sexual dysfunction, numbness, and tingling sensations. In the functional assessment, determine the effects of the illness and therapy on the patient's daily functioning. Explore the patient's knowledge, fears, concerns, and coping strategies. Also explore adaptations made by the patient and family during this phase.

Physical Examination

Note the patient's general appearance, level of consciousness, posture, and gait. Be alert for clues to the patient's mental and emotional state (e.g., eye contact, mannerisms, tone of voice). Measure weight and vital signs and compare with previous measurements. Assess the skin for lesions and bruises. Inspect the scalp for hair loss. Inspect the oral mucous membranes for lesions and inflammation. Observe the patient's

FIGURE 25-5 Listening and touching convey acceptance and caring.

respiratory effort and auscultate the lung fields for atelectasis or abnormal breath sounds. Inspect the abdomen for distention, and auscultate bowel sounds. Inspect and palpate the extremities for color, edema, and peripheral pulses. Test reflexes and sensation in the extremities.

Assessment of the patient with cancer during the treatment phase is summarized in Box 25-4.

Interventions

Anxiety

The thought of having surgery or of receiving cancer therapy may be very frightening to the patient. Suspect anxiety when a patient seems tense, apprehensive, or helpless. The patient may have poor eye contact, increased pulse and respirations, perspiration, and trembling. Tactfully share your observations, and offer the patient an opportunity to talk. Encourage the patient to express feelings and identify the source of the anxiety. Listening and touch can be very effective in reducing anxiety. Recognize the need for patient teaching or for referrals.

Ineffective Coping

The patient may need help in setting priorities and in coping with the side effects of therapy. Strategies to promote coping include teaching, encouraging self-care within the patient's limitations, treating physical signs and symptoms, emphasizing abilities, coaching in relaxation strategies, and encouraging the use of coping strategies that have been effective in the past.

Support groups may be most effective at this phase. People who have been through the same treatments as the patient can be especially informative and supportive. The local chapter of the American Cancer Society can provide information about services in the patient's community. Some agencies can arrange transportation for therapy and medical care. The Reach for Recovery program trains women who have had mastectomies to counsel others in adapting to their losses. Groups are also available to help patients with ostomies resulting from cancer of the colon, bladder, or larynx.

When a patient must be isolated physically (as when receiving internal radiotherapy), it is difficult to provide emotional support. Remember to check on the patient frequently. Intercom conversations let the patient know he or she has not been forgotten.

Risk for Injury

The patient may exhibit various signs and symptoms of tissue injury associated with cancer therapy. Specific nursing measures are described as follows for some of the injurious effects of cancer therapy.

Pneumonitis and Pulmonary Fibrosis. Encourage patients with pneumonitis to do coughing and deep-breathing exercises to reduce the risk of pneumonia. Protect the patient from exposure to people who have upper respiratory infections. If the patient has dyspnea, elevate the head and schedule care to allow adequate rest and avoid exhaustion.

Cardiac Toxicity. Patients receiving doxorubicin (Adriamycin) may show signs of heart failure, so moni-

---

| Box 25-4 | **ASSESSMENT of the Patient with Cancer in the Treatment Phase** |

Health History

Chief Complaint:
Diagnosis, prominent symptoms related to disease or treatment

Past Medical History:
Acute and chronic conditions, previous surgeries and hospitalizations, drug profile, allergies

Review of Systems:
Fatigue, weakness, headache, sore mouth, dyspnea, palpitations, altered taste sensations, nausea and vomiting, diarrhea, constipation, blood in stools or urine, urinary frequency, dysuria, numbness or tingling sensations, sexual dysfunction

Functional Assessment:
Effects of illness and treatment on functioning, patient knowledge and concerns, stresses and coping strategies, family adaptation

Physical Examination

General Survey:
Level of consciousness, posture and gait, eye contact, mannerisms, tone of voice

Height and Weight:
Present and previous weight

Vital Signs:
Present and previous readings, fever, tachypnea, tachycardia, hypotension, hypertension

Skin:
Lesions, bruises, darkened or irritated areas

Scalp:
Hair loss

Mouth:
Condition of mucous membranes, dryness

Thorax:
Respiratory effort, breath sounds

Abdomen:
Distention, bowel sounds

Extremities:
Color, edema, peripheral pulses, reflexes, sensation

tor for dyspnea, increasing pulse pressure, and edema. Notify the registered nurse promptly if these signs occur. Care of the patient with heart failure is covered in Chapter 35.

Neurotoxicity. The patient who has neurotoxic effects of chemotherapy has special needs as well. Extremities that lack normal sensation are prone to injury and must be protected.

Cystitis and Diarrhea. If the abdomen or lower back is irradiated, encourage the patient to increase fluid intake and empty the bladder often because of the risk of cystitis. Assessments of tissue turgor and mucous membrane moisture help detect dehydration. Diarrhea may require the administration of antidiarrheal drugs and special perianal care.

Thrombocytopenia. Both radiation and chemotherapy can suppress the production of platelets. When a patient has a low platelet count (thrombocytopenia), the blood does not clot promptly. Gentle handling is necessary to avoid trauma and bruising. Invasive procedures, including rectal temperatures, should be minimized. After venipunctures or injections, apply pressure for 5 minutes to control oozing. Instruct the patient to use a soft toothbrush and an electric razor to prevent trauma to the oral tissues or the skin.

Immediately report any blood in the stool, urine, or sputum to the physician. Signs and symptoms of internal bleeding include increased pulse and respirations, restlessness, pallor, decreased urine output, and falling blood pressure (a late sign).

Anemia. Anemia is less common than thrombocytopenia but should be anticipated approximately 3 months after therapy with cisplatin. Therefore those patients should have hemoglobin and hematocrit testing done after treatment. Anemia is treated with packed red blood cells and erythropoietin (epoetin alfa). A diet high in iron is recommended. Tell the patient to report palpitations, pallor, and excessive fatigue to the physician.

Reproductive Cells. Because of the potential for harm to the developing embryo or fetus, women are usually advised not to become pregnant within 2 years of chemotherapy or while receiving radiotherapy. Female patients of childbearing age should discuss specific guidelines with their physicians. Because sperm production is reduced, male patients are counseled about the advisability of banking sperm before beginning therapy with certain drugs.

Risk for Infection

Patients with low white blood cell counts due to radiation or chemotherapy must be protected from infection. They should avoid crowds and close contact with others who have infectious diseases. Promptly report any signs of infection (elevated temperature, foul wound drainage, confusion).

If the white blood cell count is very low, compromised host precautions (or neutropenic precautions)

may be needed to protect the patient. Such precautions include a private room and strict hand washing by all who enter the room. Fresh flowers, fruits, and vegetables are not allowed in the room because they harbor organisms. Additional details on compromised host precautions are presented in Chapters 13 and 33.

Patients who receive chemotherapy may have a venous access device implanted to permit frequent intravenous access without repeated venipunctures. An access device also delivers the antineoplastic agent into a large vein with turbulent blood flow. This decreases the local tissue injury caused by the drug. The venous access device presents a potential portal for infection. Most agencies have standard procedures for care of the device. Because the device usually remains in place for the entire treatment period, the patient or a helper must know how to care for it at home. Care of venous access devices is discussed in Chapter 18.

Imbalanced Nutrition: Less Than Body Requirements

Anorexia is common with cancer therapy, but maintaining good nutrition is essential. The patient is advised to eat a high-protein, high-calorie diet. Small, frequent feedings are sometimes easier to take than three large meals a day. Light exercise before meals may stimulate the appetite. If patients have specific food preferences and aversions, they should be respected. Many patients find that red meat and some other foods taste bitter when on chemotherapy. Use of plastic utensils may decrease the bitter taste. Nutritional supplements (e.g., Carnation Instant Breakfast, Ensure, Sustacal), enteral feedings, or both may be ordered if the patient has excessive weight loss. See the Nutrition Concepts box below.

 Nutrition Concepts

1. Impaired nutrition in patients with cancer can result from the disease itself or from the various treatment modalities, such as chemotherapy and radiation.
2. Cancer cachexia is a complex metabolic problem characterized by weight loss, anemia, and abnormalities in fat, protein, and carbohydrate metabolism.
3. The goals of nutritional care for patients with cancer are to prevent or correct nutritional deficiencies and to minimize weight loss.
4. Interventions for common problems associated with cancer therapy (nausea and vomiting, food aversions, anorexia, dry mouth, diarrhea, constipation) should be geared toward individual needs.
5. Immunotherapy indirectly affects nutrition by causing fatigue, chills, fever, and flu-like symptoms, which may affect appetite.
6. Diets for cancer patients must be individualized depending on their baseline nutritional status, symptoms, and therapy side effects.
7. If oral intake is inadequate, enteral tube feedings or parenteral nutrition is considered.

Be familiar with the specific antineoplastic agents so that the patient can be advised of any specific food restrictions. For example, patients taking procarbazine (Matulane) may have severe hypertensive reactions if they consume foods containing tyramine while on this drug. Foods rich in tyramine include aged cheeses, bananas, beer, beverages containing caffeine, yogurt, and liver. Alcohol should not be consumed if the patient is taking procarbazine.

Persistent nausea and vomiting can lead to dehydration and malnutrition. Various combinations of antiemetics and sedatives can be tried as ordered to obtain relief, as shown in the Drug Therapy table below. Newer antiemetics such as palonosetron (Aloxi), dolasetron (Anzemet), ondansetron (Zofran), and granisetron (Kytril) have greatly improved the management of nausea and vomiting associated with chemotherapy and have fewer side effects.

Contrary to common belief, not all patients with cancer have problems with weight loss. Patients with breast cancer and with Hodgkin's disease often are nauseated but actually gain weight during therapy possibly because they eat often to settle their stomachs. The important point for the nurse is to assess and treat each patient individually.

While antineoplastic drugs are being administered, sedatives are sometimes ordered so the patient can sleep. Nursing measures to manage nausea and vom-

iting are detailed in Chapter 38. Additional suggestions from the National Cancer Institute (1987) are the following:

1. Don't drink fluids with meals.
2. Decrease intake of sweets and fatty foods.
3. Eat food at room temperature.
4. Eat slowly and chew well.
5. Drink clear, cool, unsweetened liquids.
6. Avoid offensive odors.
7. Rest after eating.

Impaired Oral Mucous Membrane

A number of measures are helpful when the patient has xerostomia (dry mouth). Try frequent, gentle mouth care and offer artificial saliva to increase comfort. Several commercial products on the market moisten the mouth. Various protocols for mouth care can be used. For example, the patient can rinse the mouth with normal saline, a solution of 1 tablespoon of hydrogen peroxide in a glass of water, or a solution of $\frac{1}{2}$ teaspoon of bicarbonate of soda in a glass of water. Encourage the patient to increase fluid intake, chew sugarless gum or candies, suck on ice chips, and moisten dry food before eating. Lemon and glycerin swabs are no longer recommended because lemon juice dehydrates oral tissues and glycerin provides a medium for bacterial growth.

Mucositis is inflammation of the mucosa and may extend from the mouth and affect the entire intestinal

DRUG THERAPY *Antiemetics Used with Cancer Therapy*

CLASSIFICATION	SPECIFIC DRUGS	SIDE EFFECTS
Phenothiazines	Prochlorperazine maleate (Compazine) Chlorpromazine hydrochloride (Thorazine) Thiethylperazine maleate (Torecan) Promethazine hydrochloride (Phenergan) Perphenazine hydrochloride (Trilafon) Fluphenazine hydrochloride (Prolixin)	Sedation, hypotension, extrapyramidal symptoms
Antihistamines	Diphenhydramine (Benadryl) Hydroxyzine hydrochloride (Vistaril) Cyclizine hydrochloride (Marezine) Meclizine hydrochloride (Bonine, Antivert) Dimenhydrinate (Dramamine)	Sedation, dry mouth, constipation
Butyrophenones	Droperidol (Inapsine) Haloperidol lactate (Haldol)	Extrapyramidal symptoms, sedation, hypotension
Corticosteroid	Dexamethasone (Decadron)	Fluid retention
Hypnotics or sedatives	Diazepam (Valium)	Sedation, ataxia
	Lorazepam (Ativan)	Amnesia, sedation, dizziness
Cannabinoids	Dronabinol (Marinol)	Visual hallucinations, somnolence, ataxia, hypotension
5-HT₃ Blockers	Ondansetron hydrochloride (Zofran)	Constipation, diarrhea, headache
	Granisetron (Kytril)	Headache, constipation, somnolence, diarrhea, asthenia, fever, taste disorders
	Dolasetron (Anzemet)	Headache, bradycardia
	Palonosetron (Aloxi)	Headache, constipation, diarrhea, dizziness
Miscellaneous	Metoclopramide hydrochloride (Reglan)	Sedation, diarrhea, dizziness, extrapyramidal symptoms
	Aprepitant (Emend)	Abdominal pain, fatigue, dehydration, dizziness

tract. It is a painful condition that can interfere with adequate food intake. The patient who has stomatitis should continue mouth care as prescribed, eat soft foods, and avoid foods that are acidic, salty, or spicy. A soft-bristled or foam toothbrush should be used. Normal saline alone or with sodium bicarbonate makes a soothing mouthwash and should be used at least four times a day.

Constipation

Some patients are constipated while on cancer therapy because of reduced activity, opioid analgesics, and the effects of some antineoplastic agents. Monitor the patient's bowel movements to detect constipation. The physician may prescribe a high-fiber diet, stool softeners, laxatives, and phosphate or biphosphate enemas to prevent or treat constipation.

Fatigue

Fatigue is a common symptom in the patient with cancer. In addition, side effects of therapy may cause the patient to tire easily. Assess the patient's need for assistance, and schedule activities to conserve energy. Encourage the patient to prioritize activities and ask others to assume less important ones. Daily naps and mild exercise may be helpful.

Disturbed Body Image

The effects of cancer and cancer treatments can alter physical appearance and function. For example, patients receiving chemotherapy may have hair loss. Surgical interventions may result in visible scars, altered functioning, loss of body structures, and ostomies.

Be sensitive to the patient's concern about hair loss. At first, the patient may just note extra hair in the brush or comb. Later, the hair often comes out in clumps. Hair loss may be partial or complete. Typically, hair begins to grow back soon after the completion of chemotherapy and 4 to 6 months after the completion of radiotherapy. It is not unusual for the new hair to be a different color or texture. After large doses of radiation to the head, hair in the treated area may not return. Although some patients take this in stride, others may wish to use wigs, scarves, or hats to cover the head. Some insurance companies cover the price of wigs; others do not. The American Cancer Society loans wigs to patients free of charge. The society also sponsors the "Look Good...Feel Better" program to assist patients in looking their best during therapy.

Whereas hair usually grows back, other effects of cancer treatment are often permanent. Patients need time and support to incorporate those changes into their body images and to regain a healthy self-concept.

Dysfunctional Grieving

Treatment of cancer often results in temporary or permanent changes in body appearance or function. Changes or losses often trigger a grief response. The patient may be sad or tearful or verbalize feelings about the loss. Listen in an accepting way that lets the patient know the feelings are understood. Behaviors that suggest that the patient is beginning to accept the loss or change include talking about the loss and looking at or touching the affected part. Support the patient as needed, and provide practical information about adapting to the loss. Participation in a support group may help the patient learn new coping strategies and begin to resolve the grief process.

Interrupted Family Processes

While undergoing treatment for cancer, the patient may be concerned with meeting responsibilities at home and at work. Some treatments extend over many months and make it difficult to maintain one's usual activities. Side effects of the treatment may make the patient feel tired and discouraged. Family and friends need to understand what the patient is going through and what they can do to help. Encourage them to remain involved with the patient. Family members may need some help themselves to handle their responses to the patient's illness.

Financial concerns may be very serious for the patient and family. Obtain a social work consultation if necessary to assist them with insurance and disability claims and financial assistance referrals.

Ineffective Therapeutic Regimen Management

A pretreatment teaching plan informs the patient of what the prescribed therapy involves and what the experience will be like. Know what the physician has told the patient and reinforce that teaching. One source of information is the National Cancer Institute's Cancer Information Service (CIS). Booklets on cancer, cancer therapy, and coping can be obtained by calling CIS at 1-800-4CANCER. A variety of materials are available from the American Cancer Society that can be accessed by calling 1-800-227-2345, or at the Internet address http://www.cancer.org.

Chemotherapy. If chemotherapy is prescribed, the teaching plan includes a description of the drugs to be administered, the potential side effects, and related precautions. Provide written information to supplement the verbal teaching. Explore what the patient has heard about chemotherapy and correct any misconceptions. Many patients have heard horror stories about drug side effects, especially nausea and vomiting. Inform the patient of measures that can be taken that usually make the side effects more tolerable. Key teaching points for the patient who is receiving chemotherapy or radiation therapy are summarized in the Patient Teaching Plans on page 392.

RECOVERY AND REHABILITATION

If the outcome of treatment appears to be a cure, the patient and family are usually overjoyed. Some patients, however, become excessively concerned with

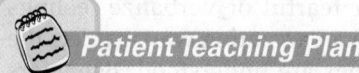

External Radiation Therapy

- Having the treatment is much like having a radiograph (x-ray). You are positioned on a table, and the machine is adjusted to direct the beam appropriately. During the treatment, you are alone in the room, but closed-circuit television permits the staff to see you. In addition, two-way intercom allows you and the therapist to talk as needed during the procedure.
- The treatment is not painful. In fact, there are no sensations at all related to the radiation. The machine that houses the radiation is controlled by a radiotherapist. You will hear whirring or clicking sounds as the machine operates.
- These treatments do not cause you to be radioactive. The radioactive material remains in the machine. Only the rays emitted by the material come in contact with you. When the machine is turned off, there is no radiation exposure.
- The skin markings made by the therapist are used to direct the radiation to the treatment site. Do not wash the marks off until the physician gives permission.
- Skin over the area being treated may become irritated. Irritated skin should be kept clean and dry, but do not apply lotions. Cotton clothing may feel more comfortable over irritated skin. Antiperspirants should not be applied to a treatment site, but cornstarch can be used to absorb moisture. Special lotions are available from your radiation nurse or physician, who will instruct you how and when to use them.

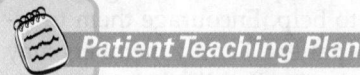

Internal Radiation Therapy

- The radioactive material is given orally, injected into a vein, or implanted by a physician.
- You are placed in a private room for a specified period of time for the treatment.
- Visitors and staff are restricted in the amount of time they can spend in your room, to limit their exposure to radiation. They also will maintain some distance from you when they are in the room.
- If a sealed source is to be placed in a body cavity, you may be required to maintain a certain position to keep the source positioned correctly.

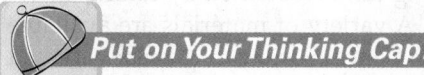

You are assigned to two patients who are being treated for cancer. One is receiving external radiation; the other is receiving chemotherapy.

1. Identify nursing diagnoses that might appear in the care plans of *both* of these patients.
2. Identify one adverse effect that occurs with radiation but not with chemotherapy.
3. Identify one adverse effect that occurs with chemotherapy but not with radiation.

their bodies, constantly monitoring for new evidence of cancer. Periodic checkups are essential but may be dreaded because the patient realizes that complete or permanent recovery cannot be guaranteed. If any signs of a possible recurrence appear, patients are understandably concerned.

As patients recover from the effects of cancer and cancer therapy, rehabilitation may be needed to restore them to the highest possible level of functioning.

TERMINAL ILLNESS

Although increasing numbers of people are surviving cancer, it is still the second leading cause of death. If treatment is unsuccessful, the patient eventually begins to decline. Patients need to know what resources are available to them and their families. The oncology clinical nurse specialist is an excellent resource person for the patient. Provide information about home health care, hospice, and voluntary and charitable organizations whose services might be needed. For patients who wish to die at home, hospice provides the support and teaching needed for this to be honored. The focus of hospice is to keep the patient's symptoms, especially pain, under control during the final period of the illness. In addition, hospice staff provide bereavement care after the patient's death.

To work effectively with these patients, you must be aware of your own feelings about dying. You can help the terminal patient in many ways. Continue to be attentive and accepting. New nurses often fear that patients will ask them questions they cannot answer. It is alright to admit you do not know, but acknowledge the patient's concerns. Listening carefully is more important than talking. Guide patients to claim their accomplishments and find peace with their failures. Terminally ill patients should remember that although they are going to die eventually, they are living now and can still have some pleasure. Chapter 24 discusses care of the dying patient in more detail.

People with terminal cancer often express fear of having great pain as the disease progresses. Although cancer is usually painless in the early stages, advanced disease often causes pain. Cancer pain can be caused by pressure on nerves, interference with circulation, obstruction of hollow structures (e.g., ureter, bowel, bronchi), and local tissue destruction.

General medical and nursing measures for the management of pain are discussed in Chapter 15. An especially good resource is the Agency for Healthcare

Table 25-11   Oncologic Emergencies

EMERGENCY	RISK FACTORS	SIGNS AND SYMPTOMS	TREATMENT	NURSING CARE
Hypercalcemia	Multiple myeloma, metastatic bone cancer; cancer of lung, breast, or kidney; prolonged immobility	Fatigue, confusion, weakness, constipation, polyuria, hypertension, tachycardia, poor muscle tone. If untreated, renal failure, coma, cardiac dysrhythmias, or death can occur.	IV normal saline and furosemide (Lasix). Drugs to promote excretion of calcium: plicamycin, calcitonin, etidronate disodium.	Monitor fluid status. Give IV fluids and drugs as ordered. Record intake and output.
Syndrome of inappropriate antidiuretic hormone	Thoracic or mediastinal tumors, thymoma, lymphomas, pancreatic cancer, cyclophosphamide (Cytoxan) or vincristine (Oncovin) therapy	Water intoxication and dilutional hyponatremia due to water retention: nausea and vomiting, anorexia, weakness. Lethargy at first, followed by confusion, psychosis, loss of deep tendon reflexes, seizures, coma, and death.	Fluids restricted to 500 mL/day. Demeclocycline (Declomycin). IV fluids and diuretics administered only in late stage.	Explain and enforce fluid restriction. Monitor vital signs. Keep intake and output records. Do not give demeclocycline with food or dairy products.
Disseminated intravascular coagulation	Septicemia, transfusion reaction. Some drugs: vincristine, methotrexate, mercaptopurine, prednisone, asparaginase	Normal clotting process is exaggerated, which depletes clotting factors. Early signs: petechiae, ecchymoses, prolonged bleeding from venipuncture. Late signs: signs of vascular obstruction, tachycardia, dyspnea, gastrointestinal bleeding, heart failure, and shock.	Platelets, fresh frozen plasma, other blood components. Heparin may be prescribed.	Avoid trauma. Handle gently. Give blood products and heparin as ordered. Monitor vital signs. Look for bleeding.
Superior vena cava syndrome	Breast or lung cancer, lymphoma, Kaposi's sarcoma, or metastatic testicular cancer that puts pressure on the superior vena cava	Redness and edema of face, conjunctiva; distended neck and thoracic veins; dyspnea, cough, tachypnea, tachycardia, cyanosis progressing to increased intracranial pressure.	Radiation therapy, diuretics, steroids.	Give medications as ordered. Elevate head and arms but not legs. Tell patient not to bend forward. Reassure patient that symptoms usually subside in 2-3 days.
Spinal cord compression	Lung and breast cancers, lymphomas	Tumor in epidural space presses on spinal cord, causing intense pain, weakness, altered sensation in arms or legs, impaired bowel and bladder function.	High-dose radiation, corticosteroids, surgery to relieve pressure.	Give analgesics as ordered. Assess for full bladder, constipation. Do neurologic checks on affected extremities.

From Gribben, M.E. (1990). Could you detect these oncological crises? *RN, 53*(6), 36-42. Copyright © 1990 by Medical Economics Publishing, Montvale, N.J.
IV, Intravenous.

Research and Quality (AHRQ—formerly AHCPR) publication on management of cancer pain. A variety of approaches should be tried to keep the patient as comfortable as possible. With severe, chronic pain, it is appropriate to medicate the patient at fixed intervals rather than on request. The patient may have pain at specific times or during certain activities despite the routine analgesic. This is referred to as *breakthrough pain.* If that happens, there may be an order for the additional PRN use of a short-acting drug with a rapid onset of action. Do not withhold ordered opioids out of concern about causing addiction. Analgesics that may be ordered include long-acting opioids (morphine sulfate [MS Contin, Roxanol], fentanyl patches) that may be supplemented with short-acting opioids for breakthrough pain. Combinations of drugs, including opioids, a stimulant, and an antiemetic, may be effective for the patient with cancer. These "cocktails," although not used as much as they once were, often control pain when given regularly without causing excessive sedation. Advise the physician if pain control is not achieved.

ONCOLOGIC EMERGENCIES

In the patient with cancer, conditions sometimes develop that require emergency intervention as a result of the disease process or the therapy. Some of the conditions requiring prompt recognition and action are hypercalcemia, syndrome of inappropriate antidiuretic hormone, disseminated intravascular coagulation, superior vena cava syndrome, and spinal cord compression. Characteristics of these conditions and related interventions are outlined in Table 25-11.

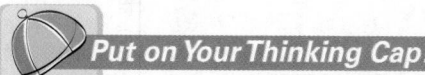

Put on Your Thinking Cap!

A patient who is receiving outpatient chemotherapy for cancer tells you he is using natural vitamins and herbal products to help combat his cancer. He says, "They are all natural products, so they can't be harmful, right?"
1. How should you answer him?
2. What should you advise him to do?

Key Points

- Cancer is the second most common cause of death in the United States.
- Early diagnosis and treatment increase the chances of survival with many types of cancer.

- The risk of developing certain types of cancers, and dying from some cancers, varies with race and ethnicity.
- Cells that reproduce abnormally and in an uncontrolled manner form neoplasms that can be benign or malignant.
- Benign neoplasms do not spread to other parts of the body, whereas malignant neoplasms invade nearby tissues and can form metastases in distant parts of the body.
- Tumors are classified by anatomic site, cell appearance and differentiation, and staging.
- Carcinogens are factors that appear to increase the risk for development of cancer.
- The seven warning signs of cancer are change in bowel or bladder habits, a sore that does not heal, unusual bleeding or discharge, thickening or a lump, indigestion or difficulty swallowing, obvious change in a mole or wart, and a nagging cough or hoarseness.
- A diagnosis of cancer is based on tissue studies, laboratory tests, endoscopic examinations, and radiologic and imaging procedures.
- Surgery is a common treatment for malignant tumors.
- Internal or external radiotherapy is used to treat cancer because malignant cells are more sensitive than are normal cells to radiation.
- Chemotherapy is the use of chemical agents in the treatment of disease.
- Radiotherapy and chemotherapy have serious side and adverse effects, including bone marrow suppression, anorexia, alopecia, nausea and vomiting, and local inflammation.
- Patients who receive internal radiation emit rays that can be harmful to others.
- Biologic response modifiers act directly on malignant cells and promote the body's natural defenses against cancer.
- Patients who have suspected or confirmed cancer are under great stress and may respond with anger, irritability, fear, denial, or depression.
- In addition to helping with specific physical problems, nursing care of the patient with cancer addresses Anxiety, Risk for Injury, Deficient Knowledge, Ineffective Coping, Imbalanced Nutrition: Less Than Body Requirements, Risk for Infection, and Ineffective Therapeutic Regimen Management.

 Go to your Companion CD-ROM for a Pharmacology Tutorial, Audio Glossary, and 3-D animations.

evolve Be sure to visit the companion Evolve site at http://evolve.elsevier.com/Linton/ for WebLinks and additional online resources.

REVIEW QUESTIONS *Choose the best answer.*

1. Benign and malignant tumors are alike in that *both:*
   1. Press on normal tissues and compete with normal cells for nutrients
   2. Usually grow very rapidly
   3. Invade nearby tissues or disperse cells to colonize distant parts of the body
   4. Contain cells that closely resemble the tissue of origin

2. A carcinogen is a:
   1. Drug that is used in the chemotherapeutic treatment of cancer
   2. Cell or group of cells that is undergoing abnormal reproduction
   3. Chemical, viral, or radioactive substance that can cause cancer
   4. Substance that helps the body resist the development of cancer cells

3. Dietary recommendations to reduce the risk of some cancers include the following:
   1. No dairy products or red meat; green, leafy vegetables; low calories
   2. High fiber; variety of fruits and vegetables; low fat and calories
   3. Fish and poultry as primary protein source; high fiber; no alcohol
   4. Limited smoked and nitrate-preserved foods; low fiber and calories

4. A patient's blood level of the oncofetal antigen CA-125 has continued to rise during 6 months of chemotherapy for ovarian cancer. What is the most likely explanation?
   1. The chemotherapy is effectively destroying the cancer cells.
   2. The patient is having an adverse response to the chemotherapy.
   3. The cancer is continuing to grow despite chemotherapy.
   4. The patient's immune system has been strengthened.

5. When working with a patient who has an internal radiation source, safety precautions include the following:
   1. Always wear a lead apron when providing direct care to the patient with internal radiation
   2. If the radiation source comes out of the patient's body, wear gloves to pick it up
   3. When not providing direct care, stay at least 3 feet away from the source
   4. No pregnant visitors or staff should enter the patient's room

6. Adverse effects of radiation therapy commonly affect the bone marrow, hair follicles, and gastrointestinal tract. What makes these tissues especially sensitive to the effects of radiation?
   1. They have inadequate defenses against harmful substances.
   2. These tissues attract radioactive substances.
   3. These tissues have very poor circulation.
   4. They regenerate rapidly.

7. What is the rationale for giving colony-stimulating factors (CSFs) to patients on chemotherapy?
   1. CSFs stimulate the production of white blood cells by the bone marrow.
   2. With CSFs, the dosage of chemotherapy drugs can be reduced.
   3. CSFs reduce the risk of anemia that commonly occurs with chemotherapy.
   4. CSFs eliminate the need for bone marrow or stem cell transplantation.

8. The most dangerous adverse effect of antineoplastic drugs used in chemotherapy is:
   1. Gastrointestinal bleeding
   2. Increased intracranial pressure
   3. Bone marrow suppression
   4. Nausea and vomiting

9. The action of biologic response modifiers (BRMs) is to:
   1. Treat mental depression that is common during cancer treatment
   2. Promote the body's natural defenses against cancer cells
   3. Immunize patients against some types of cancer
   4. Prevent the spread of cancer cells before metastasis occurs

10. Three patients at a urology clinic received diagnoses of prostate cancer. All were in an early stage and had similar expectations of cure. Mr. A. asked many questions and started planning his work schedule around his treatments. Mr. B. stalked out of the office and slammed the door, saying he would rather die than give up sex. Mr. C. was stunned and seemed unable to take in any more information at that time. Which of these patients' responses would be considered "normal" in this situation?
    1. Mr. A.'s
    2. Mr. B.'s
    3. Mr. C.'s
    4. They are all normal reactions to grief.

Objectives

After reading and studying this chapter, you should be able to:

1. List the indications for ostomy surgery to divert urine or feces.
2. Describe nursing interventions to prepare the patient for ostomy surgery.
3. Explain the types of procedures used for fecal diversion.
4. Assist in developing a nursing process to plan care for the patient with each of the following types of fecal diversion: ileostomy, continent ileostomy, ileoanal reservoir, and colostomy.
5. Explain the types of procedures done for urinary diversion.
6. Assist in developing a nursing care plan for the patient with each of the following types of urinary diversion: ureterostomy, ileal conduit, and continent internal reservoir.
7. Discuss content to be included in teaching patients to learn to live with ostomies.

Key Terms

Be sure to check out the bonus material on the Companion CD-ROM, including selected audio pronunciations.

anastomosis (ă-năs-tŏ-MŌ-sĭs, p. 398)
colostomy (kŏ-LŎS-tŏ-mē, p. 404)
continent (p. 401)
ileostomy (ĭl-ē-ŎS-tŏ-mē, p. 397)
nephrostomy (nĕ-FRŎS-tŏ-mē, p. 413)
ostomy (ŎS-tŏ-mē, p. 396)
prolapse (PRŌ-lăps, p. 405)
stoma (STŌ-mă, p. 396)
ureterostomy (ū-rē-tĕr-ŎS-tŏ-mē, p. 409)
vesicostomy (vĕs-ĭ-KŎS-tŏ-mē, p. 413)

Ostomy is the term used to describe the surgical creation of an artificial opening into a body cavity. The site of the opening on the skin is called a **stoma**. An **ostomy** in the digestive tract may be a gastrostomy, jejunostomy, duodenostomy, ileostomy, or colostomy. The gastrostomy is used for long-term feedings and is discussed in Chapter 9. Jejunostomies, duodenostomies, ileostomies, and colostomies are created to drain fecal matter from the intestines. Examples of stomas in the urinary tract are the ureterostomy, ileal or colonic conduit, cystostomy, vesicostomy, and continent

internal reservoir. Ostomies of the urinary tract drain urine from the kidney, ureters, or bladder. Ostomies are sometimes described as means of urinary or fecal diversion. The term *ostomate* refers to a person who has an ostomy. Many people, however, prefer to be thought of as individuals with ostomies rather than as ostomates. This chapter describes the care of patients with ostomies created to pass urine or feces.

INDICATIONS AND PREPARATION FOR OSTOMY SURGERY

Ostomy surgery is done for a number of reasons. A temporary ostomy may be indicated after surgery or trauma or when there is severe inflammation or infection. The ostomy bypasses the affected portion of the bowel or urinary tract, giving it time to heal. Permanent ostomies are usually necessitated by cancer of the bladder or colon or severe inflammatory bowel disease. Pouches are external appliances that are used with most ostomies to collect drainage. Whether ostomies are temporary or permanent, patients require considerable assistance and support to learn to manage them.

Ideally, the patient is prepared for the ostomy before surgery. The physician informs the patient of the need for the ostomy, what it is, and whether it will be temporary or permanent. Sometimes the procedure is done in emergency situations, as when treating acute bowel obstruction or trauma. In these situations, the ostomy may come as a great shock to the patient.

An important resource for both the nurse and the patient is the enterostomal therapist (ET). The ET is a registered nurse who has special training in stoma care. The ET may be a certified ostomy care nurse (COCN) or a certified wound ostomy continence nurse (CWOCN). The ET is often an appropriate person to assess and teach the ostomy patient. This does not, however, relieve the staff nurse of all teaching responsibility. The staff follows up and reinforces the instructions of the ET. In settings in which specialists are not available, the responsibility for teaching may fall primarily on the staff nurse.

The exact placement of the stoma is very important. The ET often consults with the surgeon regarding the ideal site. Two factors must be considered: secure pouch placement and ease of self-care. To provide a good seal, the site must not be too close to the umbilicus, bony prominences, scars, folds, or creases. If the pouch does not fit smoothly around the stoma, liquid stool or urine may leak around it. The stoma is placed below the waistline if possible. If it can be placed within the margins of the rectus muscle, the muscle will help prevent peristomal hernias. The stoma must also be placed where it can be seen and touched by the patient. A patient cannot learn to care for a stoma that is located where it cannot be seen.

 What Does Culture Have to Do with Colon Cancer?

In the United States, African Americans have the highest rates of colon and rectal cancers, which commonly are treated with ostomies. Therefore nurses should counsel African-American patients about the importance of periodic screening. Emphasize that early detection and treatment improve chances of cure.

NURSING CARE *of the Patient Having Ostomy Surgery*

General preoperative nursing care is discussed in detail in Chapter 17. This section emphasizes only those aspects that are unique to the patient with an ostomy.

Assessment

Before ostomy surgery, you should be especially concerned with determining the patient's expectations, understanding of the procedure, information desired, and fears. The health history reveals the reason for the procedure. The medical history documents other acute and chronic conditions that will require management before and after surgery. Note drug therapy and allergies. During the physical examination, expect to see a mark on the abdominal skin where the stoma will be created. See Chapter 17 for other details of the preoperative assessment.

Nursing Diagnoses, Goals, and Outcome Criteria: Ostomy Surgery: Preoperative Phase

The nursing diagnoses and goals that require particular attention are:

NURSING DIAGNOSES	GOALS AND OUTCOME CRITERIA
Anxiety related to perceived threat to self-image, anticipated changes in body appearance and function	Reduced anxiety: patient states anxiety is reduced; relaxed manner
Deficient Knowledge of what to expect after surgery in relation to the stoma	Patient understanding of postoperative routines and procedures in relation to ostomy care: patient describes routines correctly and participates in postoperative care

Interventions
Anxiety

Be accepting of the patient's anxiety and try to help the patient identify exactly what his or her concerns are. Some patients may be concerned about appearance and others about how their jobs or family lives might be disrupted. Encourage patients to talk and to use coping strategies that have been effective in the past. Because moderate or severe anxiety interferes with learning, try to reduce anxiety before teaching.

Deficient Knowledge

Basic aspects of ostomy care should be taught before surgery. Let the patient's responses and questions guide you as to how much detail is appropriate. Remember, however, that preoperative teaching usually requires repetition and reinforcement after surgery.

In addition to the ET, an important resource is a volunteer from an organization like the American Cancer Society or the United Ostomy Association. Volunteers are people with ostomies who have been trained to counsel other patients about adjustment to their ostomies. Their personal experiences in everyday ostomy management can make them very effective role models. Another good reason for using these volunteers is that the patient has a chance to see a well-groomed, active person who is living fully with an ostomy. When a patient is referred to an ostomy group (with the patient's permission, of course), the organization tries to send a volunteer who is similar in age, gender, and occupation.

FECAL DIVERSION

Intestinal ostomies divert fecal matter through a surgically created opening. Although the various types of ostomies have much in common, there are also differences that should be noted. The characteristics of the fecal material vary with the location of the ostomy and influence the type of care needed. Normally, the colon absorbs water from the fecal mass as it moves toward the rectum so that it becomes progressively more solid. When the mass is diverted from the colon, it may be liquid, semisolid, or formed depending on the section of the colon where the ostomy is created. Fecal matter in the ileum is liquid. The closer the ostomy is to the rectum, the more formed the fecal matter will be.

Before fecal diversion, a low-fiber diet may be prescribed for several days. Antibiotics may be given to reduce the bacterial flora in the intestines. Cathartics and laxatives are usually ordered to empty the digestive tract.

ILEOSTOMY

An **ileostomy** is an opening in the ileum. The ileum is the distal portion of the small intestine that empties into the large intestine. An ileostomy is necessary when the entire colon must be bypassed or removed. Conditions that require colon bypass include congenital defects, cancer, inflammatory bowel disease, bowel trauma, and familial conditions such as multiple polyposis. Multiple polyposis is characterized by the presence of many polyps in the colon. Because these polyps often become malignant, removal of the colon may be recommended.

Procedure

A surgical incision is made in the abdomen, and a loop or the end of the ileum is brought out through a second abdominal incision. The edges of the loop or the end of the ileal segment are everted and sutured to the abdominal skin to create a stoma. Loops may be supported with a device such as a rod or bridge instead of being sutured to the skin. Even though the patient is allowed nothing by mouth before surgery, digestive secretions quickly begin to drain from the stoma. The physician applies a temporary plastic pouch or a fluffy dressing in the operating room. The pouch collects fecal drainage to keep it from contaminating the surgical incision and to protect surrounding skin. The plain ileostomy frequently or intermittently drains liquid to pasty stool, so the patient will always have to wear a pouch. The Kock pouch creates a reservoir for the liquid stool so that it can be drained at intervals. The ileal J pouch–anal anastomosis essentially creates a new rectum from the terminal ileum. This procedure allows for nearly normal bowel evacuation. The patient may have a temporary ileostomy while the pouch heals. Laparoscopic procedures are under development and may eventually lead to more rapid postoperative recovery.

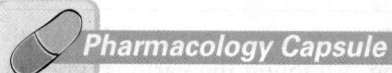

Pharmacology Capsule

Ileostomy patients are usually not given timed-release capsules or enteric-coated tablets because they are likely to be eliminated before they can dissolve and be absorbed.

POSTOPERATIVE NURSING CARE of the
Patient with an Ileostomy

The immediate postoperative care of the patient with an ileostomy is like that of most other patients having abdominal surgery. The patient has a nasogastric tube attached to low intermittent suction. Intravenous fluids are ordered for several days, after which oral intake is gradually increased.

General care of the surgical patient is covered in Chapter 17. This section emphasizes only the special needs of the ileostomy patient beyond the immediate recovery period.

Assessment
Health History

After surgery, document significant symptoms such as pain, anorexia, nausea, vomiting, weakness, thirst, and muscle cramps in the review of systems. The functional assessment reveals how the patient is reacting to the surgery and how he or she thinks it will affect usual functioning. Also determine what stressors the patient perceives, usual coping strategies, and sources of support. Assess the patient's understanding of ileostomy care.

Physical Examination

Begin the physical examination with observation of the patient's general status: level of consciousness, orientation, posture, and expression. Take vital signs and weight and compare with preoperative findings. Assess the skin for color, warmth, and turgor. Inspect the oral tissues for moisture. Observe respiratory effort, and auscultate breath sounds. Assess the abdomen for distention and bowel sounds.

Inspect the stoma for color and bleeding. A new intestinal stoma should be beefy red. When healed, it should be rose red, somewhat darker than the color of the oral mucosa. A very pale, bluish, or black stoma has impaired circulation and MUST be reported to the registered nurse or the physician immediately.

Swelling of the stoma is expected initially, after which it shrinks over a period of 6 to 8 weeks. Inspect the base of the stoma for redness, skin breakdown, and purulent drainage. A small amount of bleeding around the base of a new stoma is not unusual. In fact, it may be a positive sign indicating an adequate blood supply. If edema occurs later, it is probably due to pressure created by an improperly fitting collection device. Ileostomy drainage begins 24 to 48 hours after surgery. Note the characteristics of draining fluid or fecal matter. The presence of some blood and mucus in the drainage is normal at first.

Assess urine appearance and volume. Palpate the extremities for warmth and peripheral pulses. Observe for neuromuscular symptoms such as trembling, twitching, or cramping.

General postoperative assessment of the patient with an ostomy is summarized in Box 26-1.

Nursing Diagnoses, Goals, and Outcome Criteria: Ileostomy

Nursing diagnoses and goals common to most postoperative patients (Acute Pain, Ineffective Airway Clearance, Risk for Infection, Ineffective Tissue Perfusion, and Urinary Retention) are covered in Chapter 17. Additional diagnoses specific to the ileostomy patient in the immediate postoperative phase are the following:

NURSING DIAGNOSES	GOALS AND OUTCOME CRITERIA
Risk for Deficient Fluid Volume related to nothing by mouth status, nasogastric suction, passage of liquid stool	Normal fluid balance: pulse and blood pressure consistent with patient norms, moist mucous membranes, urine output approximately equal to fluid intake

Impaired Skin Integrity related to adhesive, fecal drainage

Normal skin integrity: skin intact with minimal redness around stoma

Disturbed Body Image related to presence of stoma, altered body function

Adjustment to change in body image: patient makes positive statements about ability to adapt; learns and takes over ostomy care

Sexual Dysfunction and/ or Ineffective Sexuality Pattern related to altered body structure and function or reactions to those changes

Fulfilling sexual expression: patient reports satisfying sexual expression, makes adaptations as necessary

Ineffective Therapeutic Regimen Management related to lack of understanding of self-care with ostomy, failure to accept ostomy, lack of resources for proper care

Patient effectively manages ostomy: patient accepts responsibility for self-care, demonstrates proper care of ostomy, obtains necessary supplies

Interventions

Risk for Deficient Fluid Volume

The loss of fluids and electrolytes through nasogastric suction and the passage of liquid stool can lead to deficient fluid volume and electrolyte imbalances. Administer intravenous fluids as ordered, with careful monitoring of hydration status. Keep accurate intake and output records. Measure output from all sources, including urine, gastric contents, and fecal drainage. Closely monitor serum electrolytes, and be alert for signs and symptoms of imbalances: changes in mental status (confusion, anxiety), changes in neuromuscular status (twitching, trembling, weakness), poor tissue turgor, edema, and dry mucous membranes.

When the patient resumes oral intake, advise a daily fluid intake of 2 to 3 liters. During hot weather or illness, additional fluids may be required. It is best to consume a variety of fluids, rather than plain water, to obtain electrolytes. The loss of bicarbonate in ileostomy drainage can result in metabolic acidosis. To prevent this, the physician may order bicarbonate replacement.

Impaired Skin Integrity

Check the pouch hourly at first to detect leakage. When the pouch is emptied or changed, try to keep fecal matter from contaminating the primary incision. Clean the skin around the stoma gently but thoroughly. Maintaining skin integrity is an ongoing problem for the patient with an intestinal ostomy. The presence of fecal matter on the skin provides a medium for bacterial, fungal, and yeast infections. In addition, the materials used to hold the pouch securely can cause traumatic injuries and allergic responses.

A protective barrier must be maintained to prevent skin breakdown. A plastic pouch is used to collect fecal drainage. A good pouch is one that protects the skin, contains wastes and gas, is odor proof, permits freedom of movement, provides security for the patient, and is not noticeable. Many kinds of pouches are available, as seen in Figure 26-1, but the features are basically the same. Some type of adhesive is needed to secure the pouch around the stoma. The pouch has an opening at the bottom that allows for emptying and rinsing. Some have gas filters that allow gas to escape while minimizing odor. There are reusable and disposable pouches, including one that is even flushable for easy disposal. The ET is a good resource person to help the patient find the right appliance.

Periodically (about every 3-5 days), remove the appliance for thorough cleansing of the skin surrounding

---

Box 26-1 | *POSTOPERATIVE ASSESSMENT of the Patient with an Ostomy*

Health History

Chief Complaint and History of Present Illness:
Type of ostomy procedure done and reason

Past Medical History:
Acute and chronic conditions, prescribed drugs, allergies

Review of Systems:
Pain, anorexia, nausea, vomiting, abdominal cramping or pain, weakness, thirst, muscle cramps

Functional Assessment:
Response to surgery, anticipated effects on lifestyle, sources of stress and support, usual coping strategies

Physical Examination

General Survey:
Level of consciousness, orientation, posture, expression

Skin:
Color, warmth, turgor

Mouth:
Moisture

Thorax:
Respiratory effort, breath sounds

Abdomen:
Distention, bowel sounds

Stoma:
Color, bleeding, edema; condition of skin at base of stoma

Characteristics of Drainage:
Amount, color, odor, blood, mucus

Extremities:
Warmth, peripheral pulses

Neuromuscular:
Trembling, twitching, cramping

FIGURE **26-1** Supplies needed to pouch an ostomy may include a pouch with an attached or separate skin barrier, a pouch closure device, skin barrier, paste, and adhesive remover.

the stoma. Gently peel the adhesive off the skin. Rough handling and frequent changes contribute to skin breakdown. Commercial adhesive removers are available if needed. After removing the adhesive, wash the stoma and the area around it with water. If soap is used, it should be nonoily and must be rinsed off thoroughly. Then pat the skin dry. The patient may be surprised to find that the stoma itself has no sensation, but the surrounding skin may be tender.

A protective barrier must be applied before the pouch can be replaced. Skin sealants that come in the form of gels, wipes, sprays, liquids, and roll-ons may be applied to the skin. Sealants protect the skin; they do not hold the pouch in place. Next, apply a skin barrier. Commonly used skin barriers include powders, pastes, wafers, and washers. If the skin around the stoma is broken, ostomy powder may be applied followed by a special coating material or hydrocolloid dressing. Dust away excess powder before the wafer is applied. Wafers and washers may be precut or may have to be cut to fit around the stoma. The opening should be no more than ⅛ inch (some experts favor 1/16 inch) larger than the stoma because a larger opening permits more fecal mat-

ter to come in contact with the skin. If a paste is used, apply it around the stoma or on the cut edge of the wafer. Place the wafer over the stoma and press down. Some pouching systems have the pouch attached to the wafer. Other systems consist of a wafer that is placed around the stoma and a pouch that adheres to the wafer. Some patients have an uneven skin surface around the stoma, making it difficult to create a seal. In that case, a caulking material such as NuHope Barrier Strips can be applied around the stoma to create a smooth surface. After the pouch is securely placed, clamp it. Initially, the pouch opening will probably need to be custom cut. As the stoma heals and shrinks, precut appliances may work well. Custom-cut pouches can be ordered for stomas of unusual size or shape. Patients whose barriers quickly erode and those with very convex stomas can obtain special barriers to maintain good fit. Once the stoma heals, some patients will prefer to cleanse the peristomal skin in the shower.

Disturbed Body Image

Establishment of bowel control is an important developmental task of childhood. The patient who has an ileostomy is no longer able to control the passage of fecal matter and must learn to manage bowel elimination in a new way. This can be very distressing to the adult who fears spillage and exposure.

Inability to control odor associated with passage of gas through the stoma is another concern for the patient with an intestinal ostomy. The characteristic odor of stool is generally considered unpleasant. Because the ostomy patient may have fecal matter draining intermittently, the source of odor is almost always present.

Assure the patient that odor is normal when the pouch is being changed or emptied but that it can be controlled at other times. Causes of odor include certain foods and poor hygiene. Foods that produce gas or stimulate bowel activity are most likely to contribute to odor problems. These generally include spicy foods, onions, garlic, some vegetables like cabbage and beans, and high-fiber foods like whole grains and fresh fruits and vegetables. Reactions to specific foods depend on the individual. Therefore advise the patient to delete and reintroduce various foods to find those that are most troublesome. Because flatus is usually evident several hours after eating gas-forming foods, the patient can eat those foods selectively at times when flatus would not be embarrassing.

Good hygiene also helps control odor. Reusable collection pouches should be washed with soap and water. Rinsing with a vinegar solution neutralizes odors that cling to the pouch. Odor-proof pouches and commercial pouch deodorizers are available as well.

Sexual Dysfunction and/or Ineffective Sexuality Pattern

One area that often worries patients with ostomies is sexuality. Encourage patients to ask questions about how the ostomy might affect sexual function or behavior. Patients may feel unattractive or fear rejection by their partner. Some men have erectile dysfunction or disruption of emission, especially if they have had nerve damage associated with perineal surgery. The surgeon and the ET counsel these men about options, which may include penile implants. Other patients have problems because of psychological factors, which may improve with counseling.

Some practical suggestions may help the patient resume sexual activity. The pouch should be emptied and taped down before sexual intercourse. Pouch covers are available to conceal the appliance and its contents. The partner wearing the pouch should experiment with positions that are most comfortable. Female patients should know that ostomy surgery does not interfere with pregnancy or delivery.

Ineffective Therapeutic Regimen Management

After surgery, some teaching should be included every time stoma care is done. At first, you may simply tell the patient what is being done and why. Then encourage the patient to take over more and more of the procedure. Have the patient demonstrate and practice as much as possible before discharge.

Some patients adjust more easily than others to an ostomy. A first step in accepting the stoma is looking at it. Note when the patient begins to watch stoma care. Encourage, but do not force, patients to participate in the care. If a patient does not begin to show some interest in learning self-care after a few days, consider supportive resources such as the ET or an ostomy

club volunteer. You may feel frustrated if patients seem unwilling to learn self-care. Be sensitive to the patient's feelings. An ostomy requires adjustments in body image and self-concept. Patients also have a grief response to this type of surgery. Chapter 24 explores nursing interventions to help the patient cope with feelings of loss.

Put on Your Thinking Cap!

Locate a resource in the area where you live that provides information for people with ostomies. Share this with classmates.

CONTINENT (POUCH) ILEOSTOMY

The continent ileostomy has an internal pouch created from a loop of ileum for storing fecal matter. The advantage of this type of ileostomy is that the patient does not have continuous drainage and so does not have to wear a pouch.

Not all patients are candidates for the continent ileostomy. It cannot be done for people who cannot drain the pouch or for those who do not have enough ileum for the valve to be constructed. People with ulcerative colitis are candidates for the continent ileostomy, but patients with Crohn's disease usually are not eligible.

Procedure

To create a continent ileostomy, a loop of the ileum is sutured together and then opened. A portion of the

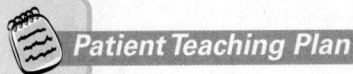
Patient Teaching Plan

Ostomy Surgery

The nurse, ET, or both must help the patient plan for discharge. General topics to include in the teaching plan after ostomy surgery are outlined here. Specifics must be individualized to the patient and the surgical procedure.

- Stoma and skin care: recommended procedure and supplies
- Appliances: list of supplies needed, where to purchase
- Irrigation (if appropriate) or drainage: frequency, procedure, supplies

Other helpful points include the following:

- You can bathe or shower with your appliance in place because the pouch and the seal are waterproof.
- You can wear regular clothing, but avoid direct pressure over stoma.
- You will learn to recognize foods that cause excess gas or odor, so these can be avoided.
- Maintain a fluid intake of at least 2000 mL daily.
- Avoid heavy lifting and strenuous activities at first; there are usually no restrictions after approximately 3 months; ask your physician about specific activities and contact sports.

- Adaptations for sexual activity can include concealing the pouch and experimenting with positions.
- Contact your physician or the ET if you observe skin breakdown, prolapse (bulging out) of the stoma, or obstruction (output absent or markedly decreased).
- Resources for information about living with an ostomy include the American Cancer Society, United Ostomy Associations of America, Crohn's and Colitis Foundations of America, and home health agencies.
- If you enjoy traveling, you can continue doing that. Tips on traveling include the following:
  - Take adequate supplies.
  - If flying, keep the supplies in a hand-carried bag. This could avoid problems if luggage is lost or delayed.
  - Include sealable plastic bags to dispose of used supplies.
  - Exercise caution with new foods that may cause diarrhea or gas.
  - If visiting a country where drinking the water is not advised, do not irrigate a colostomy with the water.
- Provide written care instructions and some temporary supplies when the patient is discharged.

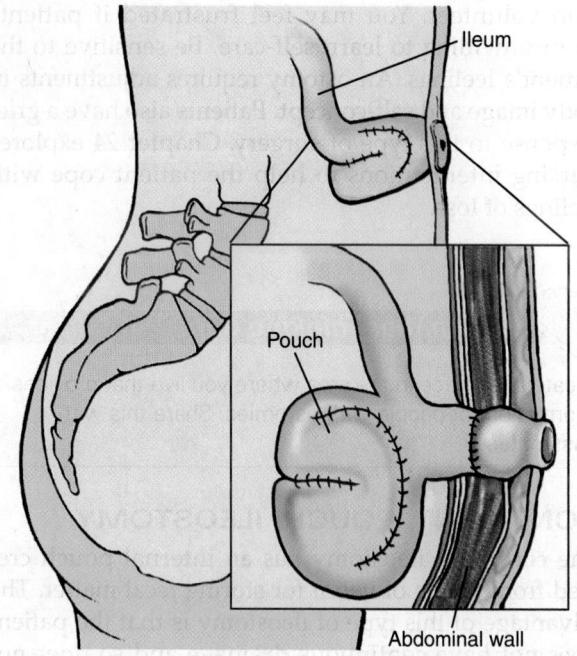

FIGURE 26-2 Continent ileostomy (Kock pouch). The pouch to hold fecal matter is created from a loop of ileum folded back on itself.

distal end of the ileum is inverted within itself to create a nipple valve. The valve prevents the leakage of fluid from the pouch. The looped section of the ileum is then closed, leaving a pouch capable of expanding and storing fecal matter. The distal end of the ileum is brought through the abdominal wall and sutured into place to create a stoma (Fig. 26-2). During surgery, a catheter is placed through the stoma into the pouch and sutured in place. The catheter is connected to low intermittent suction to keep the pouch empty. This prevents stress on the suture lines while the pouch heals.

POSTOPERATIVE NURSING CARE *of the* *Patient with a Continent Ileostomy*

In general, postoperative nursing care is like that described for the patient with an ileostomy. This section provides information on additional nursing measures that are specific to the patient with a continent ileostomy.

Assessment

Postoperative assessment of the patient who has a continent ileostomy is essentially the same as that of the patient with an ileostomy. When the patient has a continent ileostomy, it is especially important to assess for continuous drainage because obstruction of the catheter may occur. Absence of drainage or patient complaints of a feeling of fullness in the pouch suggest obstruction. The drainage from the catheter is bloody at first and then brownish.

Nursing Diagnoses, Goals, and Outcome Criteria: Continent Ileostomy

Nursing diagnoses and goals in addition to those previously listed are the following:

NURSING DIAGNOSES	GOALS AND OUTCOME CRITERIA
Risk for Injury related to obstruction of the pouch drainage	Absence of injury: patient's pouch drains readily
Deficient Knowledge of technique for draining pouch and caring for stoma and pouch	Patient understands pouch and stoma care: patient demonstrates proper pouch drainage and stoma care

Interventions

Risk for Injury

In the initial postoperative period, the patient is given only intravenous fluids. This allows the bowel to heal and peristalsis to resume. The catheter is removed after several days, and the pouch is drained at intervals. At first, the pouch can hold only 70 to 100 mL of fluid. Later, it can hold as much as 600 mL. For the first 2 weeks, the pouch is drained every 3 to 4 hours. Over the next 2 weeks, the interval is lengthened to every 5 hours. Eventually, the patient will need to drain the pouch only two to four times a day. As the patient's body adapts to the ileostomy, the drainage gradually becomes thicker and the color of normal stool.

Deficient Knowledge

Key points in draining the continent ileostomy are as follows:

1. Have the patient sit or lie down for the procedure.
2. Gather supplies: lubricant, No. 28 catheter, drape, basin, irrigating syringe, irrigating solution, gauze dressing.
3. Lubricate the catheter and insert it gently into the stoma.
4. Resistance will be felt when the catheter reaches the nipple valve (approximately 2 inches past the stoma). Instruct the patient to bear down and then roll the catheter between your fingers and advance it into the pouch.
5. As soon as the catheter is in the pouch, gas and fecal matter begin to be expelled. Drainage usually continues for approximately 10 minutes and produces a total volume of 50 to 200 mL.
6. If the drainage is too thick, instill 30 mL of normal saline as ordered. Gently aspirate. Do not do this unless necessary because it may cause dislocation of the nipple.
7. When drainage stops, quickly remove the catheter.
8. Place a gauze dressing over the stoma to absorb any secretions.

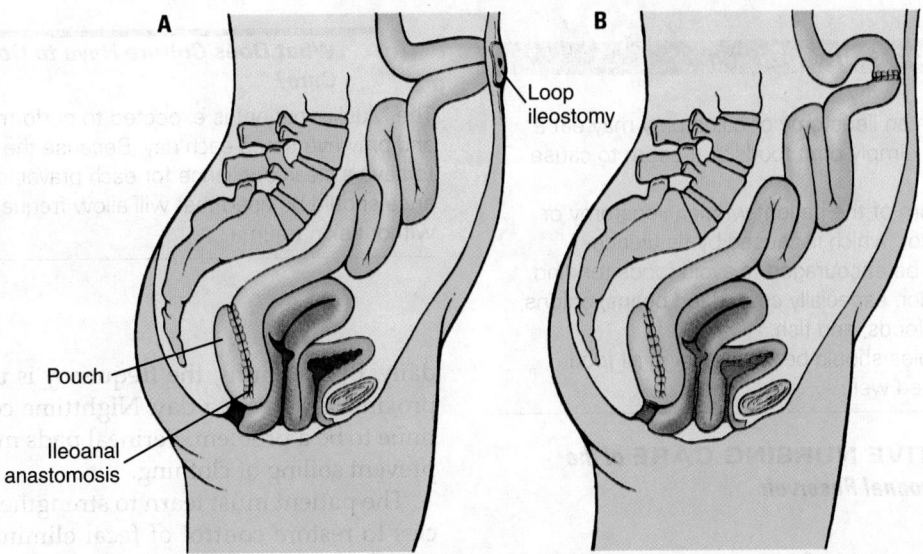

FIGURE 26-3 Creation of an ileoanal reservoir. **A,** Stage 1: The colon is removed, a temporary loop ileostomy is created, and an ileoanal reservoir is formed. The reservoir may be "J" or "S" shaped depending on the technique used. **B,** Stage 2: After the reservoir heals (usually several months), the temporary loop ileostomy is reversed and stool drains into the reservoir for storage until it is eliminated through the rectum.

9. Measure, describe, and discard the drainage.
10. Instruct the patient in how to perform this procedure as soon as possible.
11. Advise the patient to wear a medical alert bracelet at all times that states he or she has a continent diversion that must be drained.

See the Health Promotion Considerations box below and the Nutrition Concepts box on p. 404 for a review of dietary considerations for patients with continent ileostomies.

ILEOANAL RESERVOIR

An ileoanal reservoir is somewhat like the pouch ileostomy except that fecal matter is stored and then eliminated through the rectum. It is an alternative to an ostomy and information about it is included in this chapter because the patient has a temporary ileostomy and the nursing care is similar to that of the ostomy patient.

Procedure

The ileoanal reservoir requires a complex set of surgical procedures that are done in two stages. In the first stage, the colon is removed and an internal pouch that is created from the ileum is attached to the anorectal canal. A temporary ileostomy commonly is made to allow the reservoir to heal. Approximately 2 months later, barium radiographs are taken to be sure that the reservoir is intact. If the reservoir does not leak, the ileostomy is closed (Fig. 26-3). The procedure is not recommended for patients with Crohn's disease or poor rectal sphincter control.

Complications

The major complications of the ileoanal reservoir are small bowel obstruction, leaking of suture lines leading to peritonitis, and inflammation of the reservoir.

Obstruction. Scar tissue or strictures may cause obstruction. Signs and symptoms of small bowel obstruction are abdominal distention, nausea and vomiting, decreased bowel sounds, and a change in bowel pattern.

Peritonitis. If fecal matter leaks through the suture lines of the reservoir into the abdominal cavity, abscesses or peritonitis can develop. Signs and symptoms are increased pulse, respirations, and temperature; rigid abdomen and abdominal pain; and elevated white blood cell count.

Inflammation. Inflammation of the reservoir may be manifested by bloody diarrhea, anorexia, and pain.

Health Promotion Considerations

Dietary Considerations for the Patient with a Continent Ileostomy

Patients with a continent ileostomy will have some dietary restrictions, and it is helpful to request a postoperative dietary consult. The diet is intended to avoid excess gas, maintain a soft stool, and avoid obstruction of the catheter. Be sure patients know they should avoid the following foods:

- Coffee, alcohol, and gas-forming foods (initially)
- Skins, seeds, and nuts (including corn, olives, peas)
- Pineapple, berries, fresh fruit (initially)
- Milk products if they cause excessive gas

Nutrition Concepts

1. The patient with an ileostomy or colostomy may eat a normal diet and simply omit foods that seem to cause problems.
2. The main concern of the patient with an ileostomy or colostomy is odor, which is caused by flatulence.
3. Patients should be encouraged to avoid foods tending to cause bad odor, especially corn, dried beans, onions, cabbage, spicy foods, and fish.
4. Fibrous vegetables should be avoided, and all food should be chewed well.

POSTOPERATIVE NURSING CARE *of the Patient with an Ileoanal Reservoir*

Assessment

The nursing assessment after surgery to create an ileoanal reservoir is the same as for the patient with an ileostomy. In addition, assess for rectal drainage and condition of the perianal skin.

Nursing Diagnoses, Goals, and Outcome Criteria: Ileoanal Reservoir

In addition to the nursing diagnoses and goals for the patient with an ileostomy, the following diagnoses may be appropriate for the patient with an ileoanal reservoir:

NURSING DIAGNOSES	GOALS AND OUTCOME CRITERIA
Risk for Impaired Skin Integrity related to frequent passage of liquid stool through the rectum	Healthy skin: intact skin without excessive redness around the rectum and the perianal area
Bowel Incontinence related to inability to control passage of frequent liquid stools	Control of bowel elimination: decreasing number of incontinent episodes
Risk for Injury related to possible small bowel obstruction, leaking of reservoir suture line, inflammation of reservoir	Absence of signs and symptoms of obstruction, suture leakage, or reservoir inflammation: no fever, abdominal pain or distention, bloody stools

Interventions

Risk for Impaired Skin Integrity

After the first surgical procedure, the patient's skin around the ileostomy stoma and in the perianal area needs special care. Ileostomy care is covered earlier in this chapter. Until the reservoir is well healed, liquid discharge may be expelled without warning. Thorough, gentle cleansing and protective creams help prevent skin breakdown.

Bowel Incontinence

Initially, the patient may have as many as 20 stools a day. After a week, the number decreases to 8 to 10

What Does Culture Have to Do with Stoma Care?

The Muslim patient is expected to perform a washing ritual and pray five times each day. Because the patient will need to have a clean appliance for each prayer, a two-piece appliance should be used that will allow frequent pouch changes without skin trauma.

daily. By 6 months, the frequency is usually only approximately 4 to 6 a day. Nighttime control may continue to be a problem. Perineal pads may be needed to prevent soiling of clothing.

The patient must learn to strengthen perineal muscles to restore control of fecal elimination. A recommended exercise is to tighten the anus, count to 10, and relax. This should be repeated five to six times, four times daily. Also, drugs can be prescribed to decrease the frequency of stools and to make them less watery.

Advise patients to avoid fatty foods at first. There are no absolute restrictions. The patient learns through trial and error how his or her body handles specific foods. Caffeine and fresh fruits and vegetables tend to cause loose, frequent stools. Pasta, boiled rice, and low-fat cheese tend to produce thicker stools.

Risk for Injury

Be alert for signs and symptoms of bowel obstruction (abdominal distention, pain, no stool passage), peritonitis (pain, fever), and inflammation (pain, bloody stools), which should be reported to the physician. If obstruction occurs, the patient is given intravenous fluids and nothing by mouth. A nasogastric tube is inserted to decompress the bowel. If the obstruction is caused by adhesions (scar tissue), surgery may be necessary to release the restriction.

Sometimes a stricture or narrowing develops at the site where the ileum is joined to the rectum. This is most likely to happen in the fourth week after surgery. The physician may be able to stretch the tissue manually and relieve the obstruction. If an abscess or peritonitis develops, the infection is treated with antibiotics. Intravenous fluids are ordered, and a nasogastric tube is inserted for decompression of the bowel. Surgery may be necessary to drain abscesses and repair the leaking suture line.

If the inner lining of the reservoir becomes inflamed or infected, the physician may do a proctoscopic examination to identify the cause. The condition may be treated with metronidazole (Flagyl) and steroids given orally.

COLOSTOMY

A **colostomy** is an opening in the colon through which fecal matter is eliminated. The location of the colostomy affects the characteristics of the fecal drainage: the closer to the rectum, the more formed the stool.

Procedure

A colostomy is performed by bringing a loop or an end of the intestine through the abdominal wall and creating a stoma for the passage of fecal matter. The location of the stoma depends on the portion of the intestine removed. Colostomies are classified by location in the colon. Therefore there are ascending, transverse, descending, and sigmoid colostomies (Fig. 26-4). An ascending colostomy passes relatively liquid material. The drainage from a transverse colostomy is liquid to semisolid. A descending or sigmoid colostomy passes softly formed stool. The colostomy begins to function on the third to fifth postoperative day.

A colostomy may be temporary or permanent. A temporary colostomy is done to allow healing of the intestine after surgery or in certain disease states. Because the intestine below the colostomy is intact, the temporary colostomy may have two stomas. The stoma that drains fecal matter from the intestine is the proximal stoma. The distal stoma opens into the portion of the colon connected to the rectum. This is called a *double-barreled colostomy*. Sometimes the opening of the distal portion is brought through another location on the abdominal wall, creating a fistula through which mucus drains. An end colostomy with a Hartmann pouch for the distal segment is now more common than the double-barreled colostomy. A Hartmann pouch is created by closing the distal bowel and leaving it in place. The patient with a Hartmann pouch passes mucus through the rectum.

When it is necessary to remove a large part of the colon or the rectum, a permanent colostomy is made. Sometimes the colostomy is created in two stages. The patient returns from the first procedure with a loop of intestine protruding from an abdominal wound. The loop is held in place by a rod or a bridge. Later, the surgeon cuts the loop to create the stoma.

The main long-term complications of colostomy are **prolapse** and stenosis. A prolapsed stoma protrudes farther out than usual. It is caused by increased abdominal pressure, as can occur with coughing or sneezing. Other contributing factors might include an abdominal opening that is too large or a poorly attached stoma. Stenosis is the narrowing of the abdominal opening around the base of the stoma. If severe, stenosis blocks the passage of feces. Additional complications are associated with poor blood supply to the stoma, leading to necrosis and peristomal hernia. Peristomal hernia can limit bowel function, causing constipation,

The **ascending colostomy** is done for right-sided tumors.

The **transverse (double-barreled) colostomy** is often used in such emergencies as intestinal obstruction or perforation because it can be created quickly. There are two stomas. The proximal one, closest to the small intestine, drains feces. The distal stoma drains mucus.

The **descending colostomy** is done for left-sided tumors.

The **sigmoid colostomy** is done for rectal tumors.

FIGURE 26-4 Colostomy location depends on the reason for the surgery and, in the case of cancer, the location of tissue that must be removed.

strangulation of the bowel, and poor results from colostomy irrigation.

POSTOPERATIVE NURSING CARE of the
Patient with a Colostomy
Assessment

The postoperative care of the patient with a colostomy is essentially the same as that for the patient with an ileostomy.

Nursing Diagnoses, Goals, and Outcome Criteria: Colostomy

In addition to the nursing diagnoses and goals already identified, the following may also apply to the patient with a colostomy:

Nursing Diagnoses	Goals and Outcome Criteria
Ineffective Therapeutic Regimen Management related to lack of knowledge of irrigation procedure (if ordered), lack of confidence, failure to accept colostomy, lack of resources	Patient manages colostomy effectively: patient demonstrates irrigation (if ordered) and other ostomy care correctly; uses resources as needed
Risk for Injury related to prolapse or stenosis	Absence of signs of prolapse: no protrusion of stoma. Patent stoma with lumen of adequate diameter: regular elimination of feces through stoma

Interventions

Most aspects of care are the same as those discussed in relation to the patient with an ileostomy. A few points specific to the patient with a colostomy are presented here (see also Nursing Care Plan: The Patient with a Colostomy on p. 407).

Ineffective Therapeutic Regimen Management

In the past, people with sigmoid colostomies were taught to irrigate them daily to maintain regular, controlled elimination. This procedure is no longer routinely recommended. Many patients have regular bowel movements without irrigation. Others are unlikely to establish controlled elimination and may find the procedure not worth the trouble. Patients who have liquid stools do not benefit from irrigation because they drain fecal matter continuously. Irrigation is unlikely to establish control if the patient has diarrhea when under stress, has had radiotherapy, has a poor prognosis, or has a history of inflammatory bowel disease.

Irrigation can cause complications. The tube used to introduce irrigating fluid can perforate the bowel. A perforated bowel permits fecal matter to flow into the abdominal cavity, causing peritonitis, a very serious infection. The risk of perforation can be reduced greatly by using a cone-tipped catheter. Other complications are caused by the type, amount, or temperature of the solution used. Plain tap water may cause fluid and electrolyte imbalances if used repeatedly or in large amounts. If too much solution is used or if it is too cold, the patient may experience cramping, nausea, and dizziness. The physician should be advised if weakness occurs after irrigation even after the amount and temperature of the solution are adjusted.

If irrigations are indicated, you or the ET may perform them initially. The goal, however, is for the patient or significant other to learn to do the procedure, so an explanation of the process must be provided.

The following are key points to remember when irrigating a colostomy:

1. Have the patient select the time of day that is most convenient. The procedure should be done at approximately the same time every day. The entire process takes 45 minutes to 1 hour.
2. Have the patient sit on or in front of the toilet if possible. If the patient cannot get out of bed, the procedure can be done while the patient is in bed.
3. Remove the old pouch and apply an irrigating sleeve. This device opens at the top so that the tubing can be inserted into the stoma, and it opens at the bottom so that fecal matter can drain into the toilet.
4. Pour 500 to 1000 mL of lukewarm irrigating solution into an enema fluid container and hold it at the level of the patient's shoulder. Initially, 500 mL is used, but adults eventually increase the fluid to 1000 mL.
5. Clear the air from the tubing, lubricate the tubing, and insert it gently 2 to 4 inches into the stoma. The direction to insert the tubing can be assessed by first inserting a gloved, lubricated finger into the stoma. Do not use force! If a cone-tipped catheter is used, the catheter can be inserted only approximately 1 inch. This reduces the risk of perforation.
6. Allow the solution to flow slowly into the stoma. If the patient has cramping, slow down or stop the flow for a few minutes. Remove the catheter after the solution has been administered.
7. If the solution does not drain promptly, close the bottom of the sleeve so that the patient can carry out other activities. Complete emptying may take 20 to 30 minutes.
8. When elimination is complete, remove, wash, and dry the sleeve.
9. Measure the stoma before applying a new pouch, especially in the first 4-6 weeks, because the stoma size will change as healing occurs. The opening in the skin barrier should be just slightly larger than the stoma.
10. Apply a clean pouch if additional drainage usually occurs during the day. Some patients need only a small dressing or a stoma cap.

NURSING CARE PLAN

The Patient with a Colostomy

ASSESSMENT

Health History: Mr. Chin is a 47-year-old Asian American who had a bowel resection and permanent colostomy in the descending colon to remove a malignant tumor. He is 3 days postsurgery. He has been receiving intravenous morphine by patient-controlled analgesia and reports adequate pain control. He has had no nausea or vomiting but has a nasogastric tube attached to low suction. He is allowed nothing by mouth (NPO) and is receiving intravenous fluids at 150 mL per hour. He participates in turning, coughing, deep breathing, and using incentive spirometry every 2 hours. He has discussed his fear of cancer with the nurse, stating that his mother died of stomach cancer.

Physical Examination: Vital signs: temperature, 100° F orally; pulse, 92; respiration, 20; blood pressure, 118/64. The patient is alert and oriented. His skin is warm and dry with good turgor. Oral mucous membranes are moist. Breath sounds are clear to auscultation. The abdomen is soft, and bowel sounds are present in all four quadrants. The stoma is beefy red and edematous. A temporary drainage device is in place, and the collection pouch has approximately 100 mL of greenish brown liquid stool. Extremities are warm with palpable peripheral pulses. No muscle twitching or cramps are noted.

Nursing Diagnosis	Goals and Outcome Criteria	Interventions
Risk for Deficient Fluid Volume related to NPO status, nasogastric suction, passage of liquid stool	Patient will maintain normal fluid balance, as evidenced by pulse and blood pressure consistent with patient's baseline, moist mucous membranes, and approximately equal fluid intake and output.	Monitor for signs of hypovolemia: tachycardia, hypotension, decreasing urine output, dry mucous membranes. Keep accurate intake and output (urine, liquid stool, gastric fluid) records. Monitor for signs of electrolyte imbalances: confusion, anxiety, twitching, trembling, muscle weakness, cardiac dysrhythmias. Give intravenous fluids as ordered, monitoring rate of flow carefully.
Impaired Skin Integrity related to stoma adhesive, fecal drainage	Skin at the base of the stoma will be healed by time of discharge.	Check pouch hourly to detect leakage. When pouch is removed for emptying, prevent fecal matter from contaminating incision. When changing appliance, gently remove adhesive. Cleanse skin around stoma with soap and water, rinse, and pat dry. Apply a protective skin barrier before replacing pouch. If washers or wafers are used, make the opening not more than ⅛ inch larger than the stoma. Report rash or skin breakdown.
Disturbed Body Image related to presence of stoma, altered body function	Patient will adapt to colostomy as evidenced by self-care and ability to resume normal activities.	Provide an opportunity for patient to share his thoughts about colostomy. Identify specific concerns such as activity limitations, stoma care, odor control, and impact on sexuality. Provide information. Be accepting of patient's feelings. Encourage him to attend to grooming and appearance. Offer to have a volunteer from American Cancer Society or United Ostomy Association visit him. Advise of services of enterostomal therapist, mental health counselor, and spiritual counselor if patient desires.
Ineffective Therapeutic Regimen Management related to lack of understanding of self-care with ostomy, lack of resources, failure to accept ostomy	Patient will manage therapeutic regimen effectively: patient demonstrates proper ostomy care, uses available resources, resumes valued activities with adaptations as needed.	During stoma care in early postoperative period, tell patient what is being done and why. When patient begins to watch procedure, gradually encourage him to participate and then to take over care. Recognize patient's need to grieve and that patient may use denial as a coping mechanism. Develop a teaching plan that includes skin care, pouches, diet, fluids, irrigation if appropriate, activity, sexuality, complications, tips on traveling, and resources.

? CRITICAL THINKING QUESTIONS

- What would be some behaviors that indicate the patient is beginning to accept the permanent colostomy?

- Why might a patient with a new colostomy experience grief?

11. Rectal suppositories can be inserted into a colostomy stoma to stimulate evacuation.
12. Patients who have double-barreled colostomies can be given rectal medications through the distal stoma.

Risk for Injury

Be alert for indications of colostomy complications. Although a prolapsed stoma may look frightening, it is not usually serious. There is no reason for immediate action if it continues to drain feces. It can usually be gently put back in place by the surgeon or ET. If the prolapse is severe or causes fecal obstruction, surgical repair is indicated.

Inform the physician if the ostomy is not draining properly. The surgeon may be able to dilate the stoma and enlarge the opening. If dilation is not successful, surgery may be needed.

What Does Culture Have to Do with Ostomies?

Consider how culturally based individual variables can affect how a person adapts to an ostomy. Culture shapes values related to body image, self-esteem, independence, sexuality, and hygiene.

URINARY DIVERSION

The most common types of urinary diversion are ileal conduits and continent internal reservoirs. Other diversions include cutaneous ureterostomy, colonic (sigmoid) conduit, cystostomy, vesicostomy, and nephrostomy (Fig. 26-5). Ureterosigmoidostomy and ureteroileosigmoidostomy are not performed as commonly now as in the past; however, you may encounter patients who have had them.

Urinary diversion may be temporary or permanent. Permanent urinary diversion is necessary when the bladder is congenitally absent or removed because of

Anastomosis

Anastomosis

Ileal conduit

Colon conduit

Ureterosigmoidostomy

Removed bladder

Stoma is on surface

Cutaneous ureterostomy
(One stoma or two)

Continent internal
ileal reservoir

FIGURE **26-5** Types of urinary diversion.

malignancy or trauma or when extensive pelvic malignancy obstructs urine flow. Temporary diversion may be used when there is obstruction to urine flow, as might be caused by a urinary calculus, or to permit healing of the ureters or bladder.

Preparation of the patient for ostomy surgery is discussed at the beginning of this chapter. Postoperative care after each type of diversion is discussed separately.

CUTANEOUS URETEROSTOMY

A cutaneous ureterostomy is created when one or both ureters are brought out through an opening in the abdomen or flank. Often the two ureters are joined surgically so that only one stoma is needed. In some situations, a stoma is created from each ureter.

A ureterostomy stoma is much smaller than an intestinal stoma. Immediately after surgery, the urinary stoma is pink, but it quickly fades to a lighter color. Because there is no reservoir to hold it, urine drains from the stoma continuously. A pouch is needed to collect the urine and protect the skin.

Complications

Complications experienced by patients with cutaneous ureterostomies include stenosis and urinary tract infections. Stenosis is a narrowing of the opening that interferes with the flow of urine. If the obstruction is not relieved, urine backs up in the kidney. The kidney may become swollen with urine, a condition called *hydronephrosis,* which leads to serious kidney damage. The kidneys can also be damaged by urinary tract infections.

POSTOPERATIVE NURSING CARE *of the Patient with a Cutaneous Ureterostomy*

Assessment
Health History

The preoperative health history may be used to determine the reason for ureterostomy as well as pertinent past medical history, drug profile, and allergies. In the postoperative period, the review of systems should include questions about the presence of flank or abdominal pain, fatigue, malaise, and chills. Also determine the patient's response to the ostomy, knowledge about it, and readiness to learn.

Physical Examination

Begin the physical examination with a survey of the patient's general state. Take vital signs and compare with preoperative readings. Observe respiratory effort and auscultate breath sounds. Assess the abdomen for distention and bowel sounds. Inspect the stoma. It is usually much smaller than an intestinal stoma and lighter in color. Document the amount, appearance, and odor of the urine. Some blood in the urine is normal at first, but it should gradually clear. Ureterostomy drainage should not contain mucus.

Nursing Diagnoses, Goals, and Outcome Criteria: Cutaneous Ureterostomy

In addition to the common diagnoses and goals for postoperative patients (see Chapter 17), the following diagnoses may apply to the patient who has a cutaneous ureterostomy:

NURSING DIAGNOSES	GOALS AND OUTCOME CRITERIA
Impaired Skin Integrity related to contact of urine with skin	Normal skin around stoma: healed stoma base without redness or edema
Risk for Infection related to contamination of stoma	Absence of infection: no fever or foul urine odor
Risk for Injury related to obstruction of urine flow	Unobstructed urine flow: urine output approximately equal to fluid intake
Disturbed Body Image related to presence of stoma, altered body function	Adjustment in body image: patient acknowledges stoma, shows increasing interest in self-care, resumes previous sexual activity
Self-Care Deficit related to management of ostomy	Patient understands self-care with an ostomy: patient demonstrates proper techniques of ostomy care and describes self-care with an ostomy

Interventions
Impaired Skin Integrity

After a ureterostomy, the patient has a ureteral catheter for a week or two. The catheter is attached to a collection device. Once the catheter is removed, an appliance is needed to collect urine drainage. A variety of pouches are available (see Fig. 26-1). Some have antireflux valves to prevent the flow of urine back into the stoma. A skin barrier product can be used around the stoma for protection. Karaya products are used for intestinal ostomies but not for urinary drainage because urine breaks down the product. Belts can be worn with some appliances to hold them in place. Some pouches can be connected to a leg bag for urine collection.

The pouch is usually cleaned once or twice daily. It is changed every 4 to 6 days or when it leaks because frequent changes are irritating to the surrounding skin. When it is changed, gently remove any adhesive. A gauze pad, tampon, or tissue may be placed at the opening of the stoma to absorb urine. Pouch changes are usually done in the morning when urine production is lowest. Steps in the application of a urinary pouch are illustrated in Figure 26-6. Wash the peristomal area with water and pat dry. If soap is used, it should be nonoily and rinsed off thoroughly. If there are crystals present, a gauze pad saturated in a dilute vinegar solution can be used to dissolve them. Urinary stoma problems are summarized in Table 26-1.

Risk for Infection

The stoma serves as a portal for pathogens to enter the urinary tract, causing infection. Urinary tract infections

Table 26-1 *Problems Associated with Urinary Stomas*

PROBLEM	CAUSE	ASSESSMENT/INTERVENTION
Stomal laceration	Pouch opening too small Pouch not positioned correctly	Enlarge pouch opening Reposition pouch Monitor healing
Peristomal laceration	Improperly fitting pouch Improper pouch removal technique	Evaluate pouch fit with patient in sitting, lying, and standing positions. Check fit of belt. Consider need for adhesive removers and/or specialized pouching systems
Bleeding	Trauma	Apply cool cloth Cleanse gently
Crystal formation	Urinary tract infection; stasis	Treat infection, acidify urine; apply vinegar compress to stoma during dressing change Put 1-2 oz of vinegar solution in pouch 20 min bid; then rinse Use vinyl or plastic pouch rather than rubber
Stenosis	Scar formation	Dilation by or under physician's direction
Skin irritation	Skin barrier or wafer too small	Adjust size of skin barrier or wafer to cover skin around stoma
	Leaking appliance	Check belt; if too tight, can break seal Replace appliance PRN
	Hair follicle inflammation	Use topical antimicrobial powder and skin barrier powder Cover lesions with non-stick dressing and cover with barrier before applying pouching system Use adhesive remover; remove sealants gently After skin returns to normal, shave or cut hair around stoma
	Perspiration under pouch	Dry skin well Apply protective barrier Apply powder to skin under pouch Use a soft pouch cover
	Allergy to pouching products	Spot test other brands to find one that does not cause irritation
	Candida ("yeast") infection	Dry well Apply nystatin powder as ordered Cover with sealant
Hernia/prolapse	Muscle weakness Increased intraabdominal pressure	Surgical repair
Wart-like lesions	Excessive peristomal wetness	Reduce pouch opening size or acquire custom-cut system to reduce moisture on skin May require débridement by physician
Odor	Urinary tract infection Appliance soiled or leaking	Treat infection Check seal; change appliance Deodorant tablets PRN

can have serious consequences, including kidney damage and septicemia. Pouch care is treated as a clean rather than sterile procedure because the stoma is not sterile. Still, you should take care to avoid introducing organisms to the area.

Yeast infections that sometimes develop around the stoma are characterized by a skin rash surrounding the stoma. These are usually treated with nystatin powder applied under the skin barrier.

Risk for Injury

If urine does not flow readily, suspect obstruction and notify the registered nurse or the surgeon immediately.

Disturbed Body Image

Adjustment to a stoma can be very difficult. The patient may be afraid of leakage and odor and may feel disfigured. Demonstrate acceptance of the patient and care for the stoma in a matter-of-fact manner. Also express understanding of the patient's feelings. Encourage the patient to groom and dress normally. If odor is a problem, the pouch can be soaked in vinegar water for 20 to 30 minutes. Odor-proof pouches also should be recommended. Learning to care for the ureterostomy boosts the patient's self-confidence and may help restore a more positive body image.

Patients with ostomies commonly experience grief in response to the loss of normal function and perceived disfigurement. This may be exhibited as denial, shock, anger, bargaining, or depression. Chapter 24 offers guidance for dealing with the patient who is grieving.

The change in body image may affect the patient's sexuality. Provide opportunities for patients with an ostomy to ask questions or discuss how the ostomy might affect sexual function or behavior. Patients may

FIGURE 26-6 Procedure for applying pouch. **A,** Gather supplies: pouch, ostomy belt, skin barrier, stoma template, gauze pads, pouch clamp or rubber band, safety pin, and clean gloves. Wash hands and put on gloves. **B,** After removing the old pouch and cleaning the area around the stoma, place a gauze square over the stoma to absorb the drainage. **C,** Use a stoma template to measure the size of the stoma, and then cut an opening the same size as the stoma into the skin barrier and adhesive. **D,** Remove the backing from the adhesive of the new pouch. **E,** Place the opening in the new pouch over the stoma and gently press into place with the pouch drain pointed toward the floor. **F,** Connect the drain to the tubing, or close the drain if appropriate. Secure the tubing to sheets or according to agency policy.

feel unattractive or fear rejection by their partners. People who have had radical perineal surgeries may have physical barriers to sexual performance; other patients have problems because of psychological factors.

The same practical suggestions identified for the patient with an intestinal ostomy may be useful to the patient with a urinary ostomy. The pouch should be emptied before sexual intercourse. Pouch covers are available to conceal the appliance and its contents. The partner wearing the pouch should experiment with positions that are most comfortable. Female patients should know that ostomy surgery does not interfere with pregnancy or delivery.

Self-Care Deficit

Many aspects of teaching the patient with a ureterostomy are the same as those identified for the patient with an ileostomy. The topics to include in the teaching plan are ostomy care, pouches, diet, fluids, activity, sexuality, complications, and resources. See the teaching plan in the section on Ileostomy on p. 401.

From the early postoperative period, try to help the patient learn independent ostomy care. At first, patient teaching may take place each time stoma care is done by simply telling the patient what is being done and why. Encourage the patient to participate and gradually assume more responsibility for the care. Practice builds confidence and provides the patient with the opportunity to identify problems while you are available to help.

Some people adapt more readily to the stoma than others, but you must be sensitive to their feelings and encourage them in a kind way. A volunteer from the American Cancer Society or the United Ostomy Association can be especially helpful as a role model to the patient with a new ostomy. With the patient's and the physician's approval, the agency can be contacted about sending a volunteer to visit the patient.

The nurse, ET, or both must help the patient plan for discharge. Provide written care instructions. The patient needs a list of supplies and places where they can be purchased. In addition, send some temporary supplies home with the patient. Also provide information and make referrals as needed for resources such as home health care and community organizations.

In general, normal activities can be resumed within 3 months, but specific directions should be obtained from the physician or ET. Because the pouch and seal are waterproof, the patient can bathe or shower with the appliance in place. Regular clothing can be worn but should not apply pressure to the stoma. Pouches can be attached to a collection device at night to permit continuous drainage.

Patients with an ostomy who enjoy traveling are encouraged to continue to do so. When traveling, patients are advised to take adequate supplies, including sealable plastic bags to dispose of used materials. If the patient is flying, his or her supplies should be kept in a hand-carried bag to avoid problems if luggage is lost or delayed. On a long flight, a leg bag attached to the pouch may be beneficial in case the patient must remain seated because of turbulence.

ILEAL CONDUIT

The ileal conduit is the most common type of urinary diversion. Other names for the ileal conduit are ureteroileostomy, ureteroileocutaneous anastomosis, ileal loop, and Bricker procedure.

Procedure

The ileal conduit is a urinary drainage system made out of a portion of small intestine. A 6- to 8-inch segment of ileum is first removed. The remaining ends of the ileum are then anastomosed (joined) to restore bowel function. The ureters are cut from the bladder and attached to the ileal segment at an angle to prevent reflux. One end of the ileal segment is sutured closed. The other end of the ileal segment is brought through an abdominal incision and sutured to create a stoma for urine drainage. A similar procedure that uses a segment of large intestine is called a *colonic* or *sigmoid conduit*. The stoma of an ileal or colonic conduit is bright red because it is intestinal mucosa.

Complications

During the postoperative period, the patient is at risk for a number of complications. Complications related to the surgical procedure include leakage of the anastomosed ureters and intestinal segments, ureteral obstruction, and separation of the stoma from surrounding skin.

Other problems include wound infection, necrosis of the stoma, and paralytic ileus. The stoma may become necrotic if the blood supply in the resected segment is inadequate. If the stoma turns gray or black, circulation is impaired; the physician should be notified at once.

Complications that may occur in the later postoperative period are infection, crystal formation, and calculi (stones). The patient may also have problems with the stoma, including retraction, prolapse, or hernia.

POSTOPERATIVE NURSING CARE *of the Patient with an Ileal Conduit*

Nursing care of the patient who has an ileal conduit is essentially the same as that for the patient with an ileostomy. There are a few special points to make about the ileal conduit. This patient will have a nasogastric tube attached to suction to prevent abdominal distention and stress on the resected portion of the ileum while it heals. The patient is allowed nothing by mouth and is given intravenous fluids until bowel sounds return. A temporary ileus (absence of bowel activity) is expected after bowel resection. A ureteral catheter or stent may be in place to drain urine. If one is present, output is monitored because obstruction can occur. Mucus is normally present in drainage from a conduit because it is produced by the lining of the bowel segment. All patients with ileal conduits are advised to attach the pouch to a collection device during the night.

CONTINENT INTERNAL RESERVOIRS

All of the methods of urinary diversion already discussed permit urine to flow steadily through a stoma. Newer procedures have been developed that allow for the storage and controlled drainage of urine. An example of these, called *continent internal reservoirs*, is the Kock pouch. An even more recent development is the ileum neobladder, which eliminates the need for a stoma. The neobladder is an internal urinary reservoir constructed using a resected segment of the colon that is attached to the urethra. Urine drains into the reservoir and is eliminated through the urethra instead of a stoma. The neobladder is used more in men than in women. Continence varies with the neobladder, so an artificial urinary sphincter is sometimes implanted. Another option for patients who cannot achieve continence with the neobladder is intermittent self-catheterization. Even though the procedure is well received by patients, some surgeons are reluctant to spare the urethra with bladder cancer, fearing the urethra could be a site for recurrent cancer.

The Kock pouch is constructed with a segment of ileum. The ureters are implanted in one side of the ileum segment. A nipple valve is constructed from the other side and attached to the skin, where a stoma is created. The valve prevents urine from flowing from the reservoir. A catheter is used to drain the reservoir at 4- to 6-hour intervals.

The Indiana pouch is similar to the Kock pouch except that it is made of a portion of the terminal ileum and the ascending colon. This reservoir is larger than that of the Kock pouch. The Indiana pouch is also drained with a catheter every 4 to 6 hours.

Complications

Complications of the continent pouches are incontinence, difficult catheterization, and urinary reflux leading to pyelonephritis, obstruction, and bacteriuria.

POSTOPERATIVE NURSING CARE *of the Patient with a Kock or Indiana Pouch*

Immediately after surgery, the patient may have a Penrose drain to remove fluid from the operative site and a clear tube in place for continuous urine drainage. Irrigations may be ordered to remove clots and mucus. When the tube is removed, the pouch may be drained every 2 to 3 hours at first. Later, the patient may need to drain the pouch only every 4 to 6 hours during the day and once during the night. If the pouch functions properly, the patient does not have to wear an external appliance. A small gauze dressing may be placed over the stoma to absorb mucus drainage. Advise the patient to wear a medical alert bracelet that identifies the presence of a continent device that needs intubation to drain.

URETEROSIGMOIDOSTOMY AND URETEROILEOSIGMOIDOSTOMY

Ureterosigmoidostomy and ureteroileosigmoidostomy are not done as often now as in the past. You may care for patients, however, who have had these diversions for some time and have adapted well to them. In a ureterosigmoidostomy, the ureters are implanted into the sigmoid colon. Urine drains into the colon and is eliminated through the rectum. For a ureteroileosigmoidostomy, a segment of the ileum is anastomosed to the sigmoid and the ureters implanted into that part of the ileum. Neither procedure provides continence, and both present problems with kidney infections and urinary calculi (stones). Additional complications are caused by the colon's absorption of electrolytes from the urine. Patients are at risk for deficits in potassium and bicarbonate and for excesses in sodium, chloride, and hydrogen. These imbalances may lead to metabolic acidosis.

VESICOSTOMY

Vesicostomy or cystostomy is an opening into the urinary bladder. There are several types. Some are drained continuously through a catheter; others have a nipple valve and are drained at intervals.

NEPHROSTOMY

A nephrostomy tube diverts urine directly from the kidney through a tube that exits through the skin. This device may be used as a temporary or permanent method of urinary diversion. Conditions that may be treated with these tubes are discussed in Chapter 40.

 Key Points

- An ostomy is an artificial opening into a body cavity; a stoma is the site of the opening on the skin.
- Ostomy surgery may be done to bypass a section of the digestive or urinary tract either temporarily or permanently.

- An important resource for nurses and ostomy patients is the enterostomal therapist nurse. These nurses have specialized training in ostomy management and may be a certified ostomy care nurse (COCN) or a certified wound ostomy continence nurse (CWOCN).
- Before ostomy surgery, determine the patient's expectations, understanding of the procedure, information desired, and fears.
- Intestinal ostomies include the ileostomy, the continent ileostomy, the ileoanal reservoir, and the colostomy.
- The characteristics of fecal material depend on the location of the ostomy: liquid stool drains from the ileum, and softly formed stool drains from the descending colon.
- The new intestinal stoma should be beefy red, and a small amount of bleeding around the base is not unusual.
- Postoperative nursing care after intestinal ostomy surgery addresses Risk for Deficient Fluid Volume, Impaired Skin Integrity, Disturbed Body Image, Sexual Dysfunction, and Ineffective Therapeutic Regimen Management.
- Protective barriers are applied around the stoma to fill creases and create a seal, and a pouch is secured over the stoma with adhesive to collect fecal drainage.
- Elimination of gas-forming foods and good hygiene can help control odor associated with an intestinal ostomy.
- The continent pouch ileostomy and the ileoanal reservoir both store fecal matter, but the continent ileostomy is drained periodically with a catheter, whereas the ileoanal reservoir allows fecal elimination through the rectum.
- Routine colostomy irrigations are no longer recommended.
- The most common types of urinary diversion are ileal conduit and continent internal reservoirs; other urinary diversions are cutaneous ureterostomy and colonic conduit.
- A urinary stoma is pink immediately after surgery but quickly fades to a light color.
- Ureterostomies and ileal conduits drain urine continuously, so collection pouches are needed and meticulous skin care must be provided.
- A continent internal reservoir allows for storage and controlled drainage of urine.
- Complications of urinary stomas include urinary infections, obstruction of urine flow, and skin breakdown.

 Go to your Companion CD-ROM for a Pharmacology Tutorial, Audio Glossary, and 3-D animations.

evolve   Be sure to visit the companion Evolve site at http://evolve.elsevier.com/Linton/ for WebLinks and additional online resources.

REVIEW QUESTIONS *Choose the best answer.*

1. An example of a surgically created opening that drains fecal matter from the intestines is a/an:

    1. Gastrostomy
    2. Ileostomy
    3. Ileal conduit
    4. Vesicostomy

2. Which of the intestinal stoma sites will produce the most formed stool?

    1. Jejunostomy
    2. Duodenostomy
    3. Ileostomy
    4. Colostomy

3. The nurse is inspecting a new intestinal stoma on the first postoperative day. The stoma should be:

    1. Beefy red
    2. Rose red
    3. Pale pink
    4. White

4. What is the main reason that a patient with an ileostomy is at risk for fluid and electrolyte imbalances?

    1. There is a significant loss of blood during the surgical procedure.
    2. Patients with ileostomies often have anorexia, nausea, and vomiting.
    3. Fluid normally reabsorbed in the colon is lost through the ileostomy.
    4. Fluid intake will be restricted until the stoma heals completely.

5. Aspects of stoma care include the following:

    1. Remove the drainage appliance daily to cleanse skin around the stoma
    2. Wash the stoma and surrounding skin with a moisturizing soap
    3. Vigorously rub the skin surrounding the stoma to stimulate circulation and healing
    4. Cut the opening on the wafer no more than $\frac{1}{8}$ inch larger than the stoma.

6. When teaching a new colostomy patient how to control odor, the nurse provides list of foods that commonly cause gas. The patient says, "You mean I can't eat any of these foods?" The most appropriate reply is:

    1. Gradually try one at a time to see how you tolerate them
    2. That is correct. You can never eat any of these foods again
    3. Because flatus production is unpredictable, you never know what will happen if you eat these foods
    4. It would be better if you took vitamins instead of eating fresh fruits and vegetables

7. A good strategy for helping patients adjust to a stoma and learn how to do self-care is to:

    1. Shield the stoma from the patient's sight until he or she asks to see it
    2. Tell the patient, "If you don't do your stoma care, no one will do it for you"
    3. Encourage patients to participate in care once they start looking at the stoma
    4. Teach a family member how to do the care in the presence of the patient

8. In a patient with a new continent ileostomy, which assessment finding most suggests an obstruction?

    1. Bloody drainage from the catheter in the stoma
    2. Patient complaint of pain in the incision area
    3. Absence of drainage from the stoma catheter
    4. Abdominal distention and hypoactive bowel sounds

9. Which type of urinary diversion does not require the patient to wear a pouch?

    1. Cutaneous ureterostomy
    2. Ileal conduit
    3. Kock pouch
    4. Ureteroileostomy

10. The main advantage of the ileum neobladder is that:

    1. The patient does not have a stoma for urine drainage
    2. Urinary continence is always maintained
    3. Urine is eliminated through the rectum
    4. The neobladder has to be drained only once a day

27 Neurologic Disorders

LESLIE GODDARD

evolve http://evolve.elsevier.com/Linton/

Objectives

After reading and studying this chapter, you should be able to:

1. Identify common neurologic changes in the older person and the implication of these for nursing care.
2. Describe the diagnostic tests and procedures used to evaluate neurologic function and the nursing responsibilities associated with each.
3. Identify the uses, side effects, and nursing interventions associated with common drug therapies employed in patients with neurologic disorders.
4. Describe the signs and symptoms associated with increased intracranial pressure and the medical therapies used in treatment.
5. List the components of the nursing assessment of the patient with a neurologic disorder.
6. Describe the pathophysiology, signs and symptoms, complications, and medical or surgical treatment for patients with selected neurologic disorders.
7. Assist in developing a nursing care plan for the patient with a neurologic disorder.

Key Terms

Be sure to check out the bonus material on the Companion CD-ROM, including selected audio pronunciations.

aura (ĂW-ră, p. 436)
automations (ăw-TŎM-ăh-shŭn, p. 436)
contralateral (kŏn-tră-LĂT-ĕr-ăl, p. 426)
decerebrate (dĕ-SĔR-ē-brăt, p. 433)
decorticate (dē-KŎR-tĭ-kăt, p. 433)
encephalitis (ĕn-sĕf-ă-LĪ-tĭs, p. 444)
hemiparesis (hĕm-ē-pă-RĒ-sĭs, p. 433)
hemiplegia (hĕm-ē-PLĒ-jă, p. 433)
intracranial pressure (ICP) (ĭn-trăh-KRĀ-nē-ăl, p. 421)
ipsilateral (ĭp-sĭ-LĂT-ĕr-ăl, p. 425)
neuralgia (nū-RĂL-jă, p. 456)
neurotransmitter (nū-rō-trăns-MĬ-tĕr, p. 416)
paresthesias (păr-ĕs-THĒ-zē-ă, p. 444)
postictal (pōst-ĬK-tĕl, p. 437)
seizure (SĒ-zhŭr, p. 435)

Neurologic disease and injury present some of the greatest challenges in health care today. Nurses face the challenge of caring for neurologic patients during the acute and rehabilitation phases of recovery from injuries and diseases. The long-term effects of many neurologic disorders are frequently devastating to both the patient and the family. An important aspect of care is assisting the patient and family to adjust physically and emotionally to the alterations that often result from neurologic dysfunction.

ANATOMY AND PHYSIOLOGY OF THE NERVOUS SYSTEM

In this age of computers, it may be helpful to think of the nervous system as an elaborate control system. The system coordinates and regulates all bodily functions. It receives and interprets information from the external environment and initiates responses to the received information.

The functional unit of the nervous system is the neuron (nerve cell), which conducts electrical impulses within the nervous system. The main cell body has branches called *axons* and *dendrites* (Fig. 27-1). Axons conduct impulses away from the cell body, and dendrites convey impulses toward the cell body. Many axons and dendrites are covered with a material called *myelin*, which enhances conduction along nerve fibers. Myelin gives the axons a white appearance (white matter), whereas cell bodies without myelin are gray (gray matter).

Neurons are classified according to their particular functions. Those that transmit information from distal parts of the body or environment toward the central nervous system (CNS) are sensory neurons, also known as *afferent* ("bearing toward") *neurons*. Motor information is carried from the CNS to the periphery by motor neurons, also known as *efferent* ("bearing away from") *neurons*. There are interneurons, which are like relay stations between sensory and motor neurons.

Coordinated, organized function is a result of a well-integrated system of impulse transmission. When the end of a dendrite is stimulated, a series of electrochemical events are initiated. At the point of stimulation, sodium and potassium ions are exchanged, resulting in a process called *depolarization*. This process continues down the dendrite to the axon, until the ions return to their resting state. This return to the resting state is known as *repolarization*.

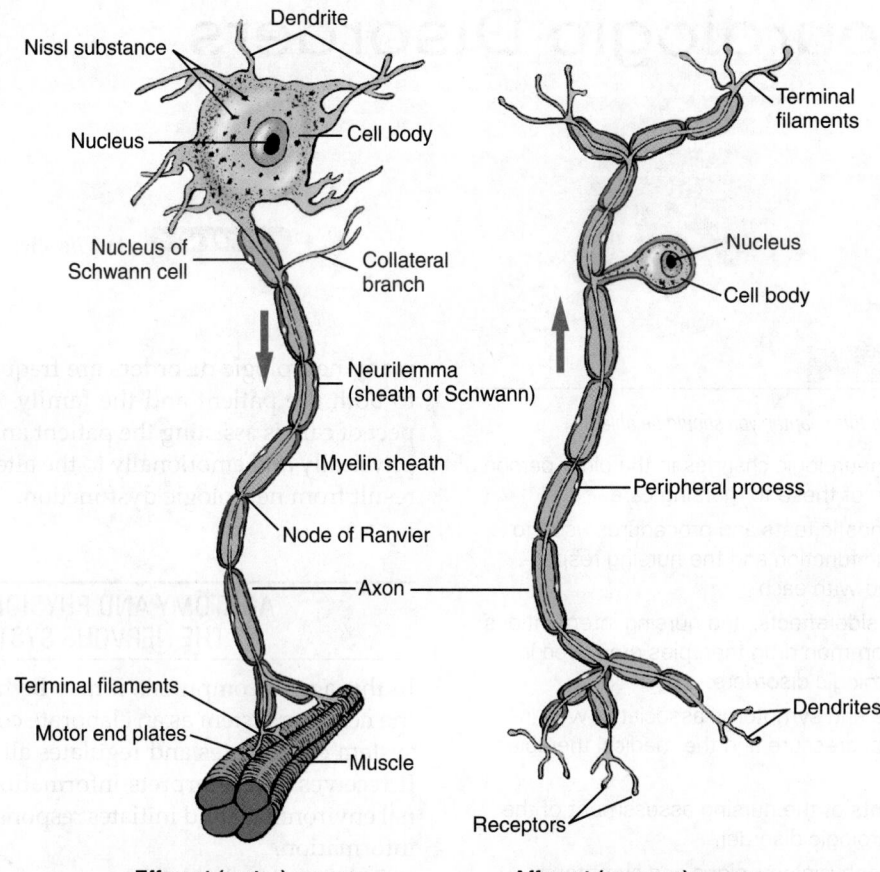

FIGURE 27-1 A neuron (nerve cell). The dendrites receive incoming messages. The axons convey outgoing signals. Diagram of a motor neuron and a sensory neuron. *Arrows* indicate the direction of impulse conduction.

Impulses must be able to pass from one neuron to another across the neural synapse—the space between the axons of one neuron and the dendrites of the next neuron. When an impulse reaches the end of its axon, a biochemical messenger called a **neurotransmitter** is released. Common neurotransmitters are acetylcholine, norepinephrine, epinephrine, and dopamine. The neurotransmitter crosses the synapse to the neighboring dendrite, where it stimulates an electrical impulse. The process of depolarization then continues down the length of the nerve cells.

Structurally, the nervous system is divided into two main parts: (1) the central nervous system (CNS), made up of the brain and spinal cord; and (2) the peripheral nervous system, which comprises all the nerves of the peripheral parts of the body, including both spinal and cranial nerves. The brain is divided into the cerebrum, cerebellum, and brainstem (Fig. 27-2). The cerebrum is composed of left and right hemispheres, which are subdivided into specific lobes. The thalamus, hypothalamus, and basal ganglia are other important structures identified in the cerebrum. Box 27-1 lists the functions of the major parts of the brain.

Cerebrospinal fluid (CSF) is composed primarily of water, glucose, sodium chloride, and protein. It is produced in the ventricles of the brain in the arachnoid granulations. CSF circulates within the subarachnoid space, the ventricles, and the central canal of the spinal cord (Fig. 27-3). The fluid is reabsorbed in the arachnoid villi. The CSF acts as a shock absorber for the brain and spinal cord. If excess fluid forms or if fluid is not normally reabsorbed, pressure within the ventricular system increases.

The spinal cord extends from the border of the first cervical vertebra (C1) to the level of the second lumbar vertebra (L2). Thirty-one pairs of spinal nerve roots exit from the spinal cord, each consisting of a posterior sensory (afferent) root and anterior motor (efferent) root (Fig. 27-4). These nerve roots, along with the 12 cranial nerves, make up the peripheral nervous system.

Part of the peripheral nervous system, known as the *autonomic nervous system,* helps maintain homeostasis for the body. The autonomic nervous system controls the involuntary activities of the viscera, including smooth muscles, cardiac muscle, and glands. The two major subdivisions of the autonomic nervous system are the *sympathetic nervous system* and the *parasympathetic nervous system.*

Stress triggers the sympathetic nervous system to increase the secretion of epinephrine and norepinephrine. These neurotransmitters increase heart rate and constrict peripheral blood vessels, causing the blood

Box 27-1   *Functions of the Major Parts of the Brain*

Brainstem and Diencephalon

Control awareness or alertness through reticular activating system, composed of fibers scattered throughout the midbrain, pons, and medulla.

Medulla

Links higher brain centers to other parts of the body through spinal cord. Controls muscles of respiration through respiratory reflex center. Controls heartbeat (to some extent) through cardiac reflex center. Constricts blood vessels to raise blood pressure through vasomotor reflex center. Is point of origin for some cranial nerves.

Pons

Relays messages from medulla to higher centers in brain. Is reflex center for some cranial nerves.

Cerebellum

Coordinates movement, balance, posture, and spatial orientation.

Hypothalamus

Controls pituitary. Controls appetite, sleep, and some emotions. Controls much activity of autonomic nervous system.

Forebrain (Cerebrum)

Controls higher functions and activities: conscious mental processes, sensations, emotions, and voluntary movements.

Frontal Lobe

Controls voluntary muscle movements, verbal and written speech.

Parietal Lobe

Contains sensory reception areas to interpret pain, touch, temperature, distances, sizes, and shapes.

Temporal Lobe

Contains auditory center for hearing and understanding spoken language. Contains olfactory center for smell.

Occipital Lobe

Contains visual center for seeing and reading.

Data from Jacob, S.W., & Francone, C.A. (1989). *Elements of anatomy and physiology* (2nd ed.). Philadelphia: Saunders.

FIGURE 27-2 Structures of the brain (coronal section).

Superior sagittal sinus

Lateral ventricle

Foramen of Monro

Choroid plexus (fourth ventricle)

Foramen of Magendie

Aqueduct of Sylvius

Arachnoid villi

Subarachnoid space

Choroid plexus (third ventricle)

Cisterna magna

Foramen of Luschka

FIGURE 27-3 Cerebrospinal fluid circulation. Cerebrospinal fluid is produced by the choroid plexus in the lateral ventricles and flows around the brain and spinal cord in the subarachnoid space until it reaches the arachnoid villi, from which it is absorbed into the venous circulation. *Arrows* indicate the major pathway of cerebrospinal fluid flow.

pressure to rise. This reaction to stress is called the "fight or flight" response. The sympathetic nervous system is also referred to as the *thoracolumbar system*.

Conversely, the parasympathetic nervous system mediates a rest response. Stimulation of this system results in decreased heart rate and blood pressure. The parasympathetic nervous system is also known as the *craniosacral system*. Specific effects of the stimulation of the sympathetic and parasympathetic nervous systems are outlined in Table 27-1.

AGE-RELATED CHANGES

With normal aging, the number of nerve cells decreases. Brain weight is reduced, and the ventricles increase in size. An aging pigment called *lipofuscin* is deposited in nerve cells, along with *amyloid*, a type of protein. Increased plaques and tangled fibers are found in nerve tissue. These changes are associated with Alzheimer's disease but also are seen in the brains of people who have no symptoms of dementia. Fortunately, there are many more nerve cells present than are needed for normal function. Therefore most older people retain normal cognition and function despite the decreasing number of nerve cells.

The physical examination reveals some neurologic changes typical of aging. The pupil of the eye is often smaller and may respond to light more slowly. When asked to track (follow with the eyes) a moving object, the older person's eye movements may be jerky rather than smooth. Reflexes are usually intact except for the Achilles tendon jerk, which is often absent.

Older people often demonstrate some changes in functional abilities as well. Reaction time increases with aging, especially for complex reactions. Tremors in the head, face, and hands are common. Some older people develop dizziness and problems with balance, but these are not considered normal age-related changes.

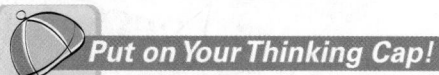

Put on Your Thinking Cap!

Identify three implications for nursing care related to normal neurologic changes that occur with age.

PATHOPHYSIOLOGY OF NEUROLOGIC DISEASES

Potential causes of neurologic disorders include developmental and genetic disorders, trauma, infections and inflammation, neoplasms, degenerative processes, vascular disorders, and metabolic and endocrine disorders.

- **Developmental and genetic disorders.** Developmental disorders include structural problems such as hydrocephalus. An example of a genetic disorder is Huntington's disease.
- **Trauma.** Central nervous system injuries resulting from trauma can be life-threatening or severely disabling. Physical trauma to the nervous system may follow accidental injury, violent crime, or chemical injury caused by drugs, alcohol, or other harmful substances.
- **Infections and inflammation.** Meningitis and encephalitis are examples of disease states that

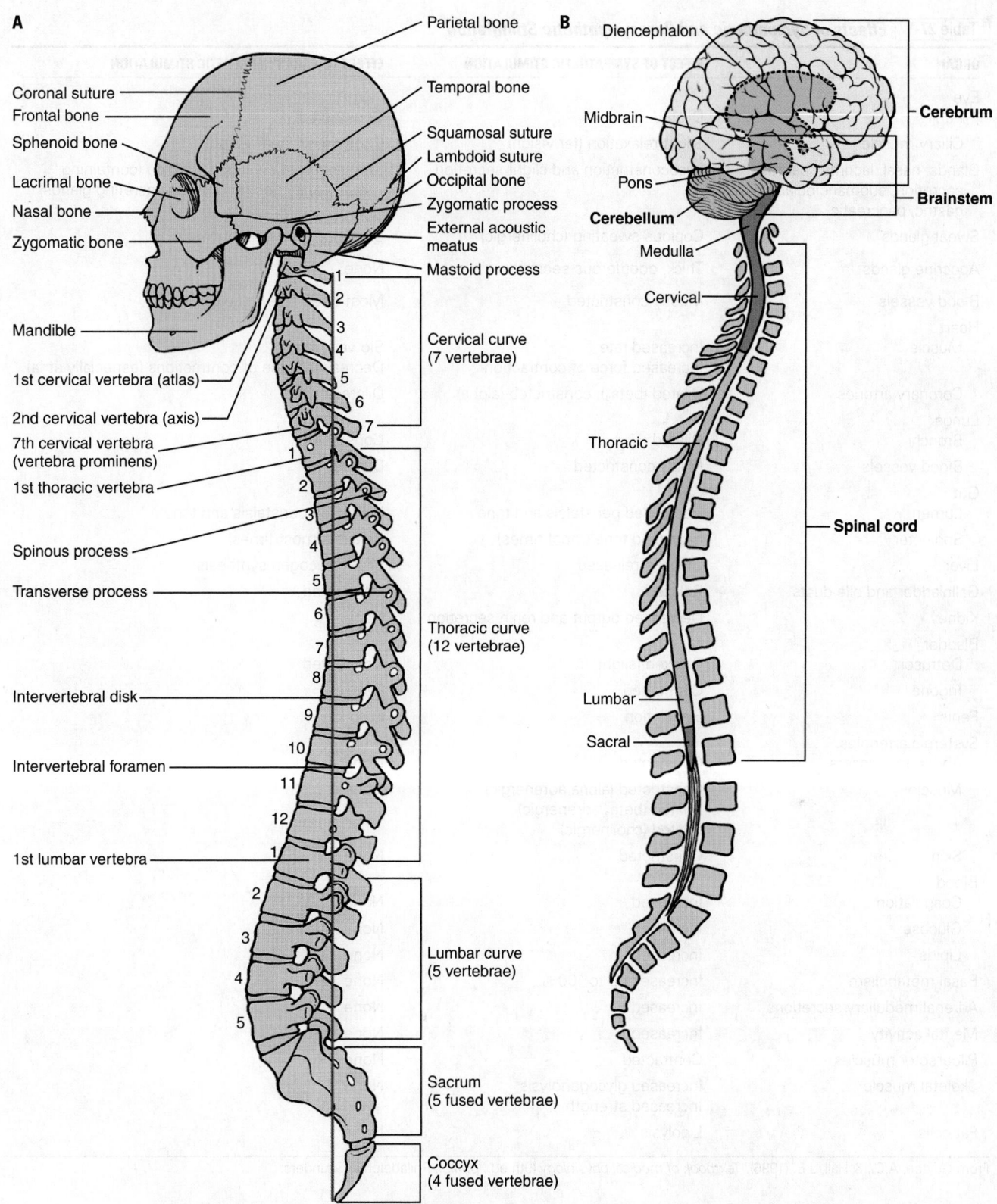

A, Parietal bone
Coronal suture
Frontal bone
Sphenoid bone
Lacrimal bone
Nasal bone
Zygomatic bone
Mandible
1st cervical vertebra (atlas)
2nd cervical vertebra (axis)
7th cervical vertebra (vertebra prominens)
1st thoracic vertebra
Spinous process
Transverse process
Intervertebral disk
Intervertebral foramen
1st lumbar vertebra

Temporal bone
Squamosal suture
Lambdoid suture
Occipital bone
Zygomatic process
External acoustic meatus
Mastoid process
Cervical curve (7 vertebrae)
Thoracic curve (12 vertebrae)
Lumbar curve (5 vertebrae)
Sacrum (5 fused vertebrae)
Coccyx (4 fused vertebrae)

B, Diencephalon
Midbrain
Pons
Cerebellum
Medulla
Cervical
Thoracic
Lumbar
Sacral

Cerebrum
Brainstem
Spinal cord

FIGURE 27-4 **A,** Bony structure of the skull and vertebral column. **B,** Lateral view of the central nervous system, showing its main divisions.

Table 27-1 *Effects of Sympathetic and Parasympathetic Stimulation*

ORGAN	EFFECT OF SYMPATHETIC STIMULATION	EFFECT OF PARASYMPATHETIC STIMULATION
Eye		
Pupil	Dilated	Constricted
Ciliary muscle	Slight relaxation (far vision)	Constricted (near vision)
Glands: nasal, lacrimal, parotid secretion, submandibular, gastric, pancreatic	Vasoconstriction and slight secretion	Stimulation of copious secretion (containing many enzymes for enzyme-secreting glands)
Sweat glands	Copious sweating (cholinergic)	Sweating on palms of hands
Apocrine glands	Thick, odoriferous secretion	None
Blood vessels	Mostly constricted	Most often little or no effect
Heart		
Muscle	Increased rate Increased force of contraction	Slowed rate Decreased force of contractions (especially atria)
Coronary arteries	Dilated (beta$_2$), constricted (alpha)	Dilated
Lungs		
Bronchi	Dilated	Constricted
Blood vessels	Mildly constricted	Dilated
Gut		
Lumen	Decreased peristalsis and tone	Increased peristalsis and tone
Sphincter	Increased tone (most times)	Relaxed (most times)
Liver	Glucose released	Slight glycogen synthesis
Gallbladder and bile ducts	Relaxed	Contracted
Kidney	Decreased output and renin secretion	None
Bladder		
Detrusor	Relaxed (slight)	Contracted
Trigone	Contracted	Relaxed
Penis	Ejaculation	Erection
Systemic arterioles		
Abdominal viscera	Constricted	None
Muscle	Constricted (alpha adrenergic) Dilated (beta$_2$ adrenergic) Dilated (cholinergic)	None
Skin	Constricted	None
Blood		
Coagulation	Increased	None
Glucose	Increased	None
Lipids	Increased	None
Basal metabolism	Increased up to 100%	None
Adrenal medullary secretions	Increased	None
Mental activity	Increased	None
Piloerector muscles	Contracted	None
Skeletal muscle	Increased glycogenolysis Increased strength	None
Fat cells	Lipolysis	None

From Guyton, A.C., & Hall, J.E. (1996). *Textbook of medical physiology* (9th ed., p.775). Philadelphia: Saunders.

cause inflammation of meningeal and brain tissue, respectively. Causative agents may be viruses or bacteria and may be transmitted by a variety of vectors and routes.

- **Neoplasms.** Central nervous system tumors may be primary or metastatic in origin. Although considerable progress has been made in treating these tumors, definitive therapy is often difficult to achieve, depending on the cell type involved in the tumor and the degree of invasion of surrounding tissue.

- **Degenerative processes.** The primary degenerative disease of the brain is Alzheimer's disease, a progressive condition that begins with memory loss and eventually results in severe mental and physical deterioration. Alzheimer's disease is discussed in Chapter 22. Other degenerative disorders are multiple sclerosis, Parkinson's syndrome, amyotrophic lateral sclerosis, and Huntington's disease.

- **Vascular disorders.** Any factor that interferes with blood flow to nervous tissue can lead to cell death, with resulting loss of function. Nerve tissue is so sensitive to hypoxia that cells begin to die after being deprived of oxygen for 4 minutes. Neurologic disorders associated with impaired blood flow include cerebrovascular accident (see Chapter 28) and multi-infarct dementia. Vascular abnormalities, including aneurysms and arteriovenous malformations, can rupture or prevent the delivery of adequate oxygen to affected tissue.
- **Metabolic and endocrine disorders.** The brain depends on constant supplies of glucose and other nutrients. Disturbances in glucose metabolism and electrolyte imbalances can lead to deterioration in thought processes and level of consciousness. Neurologic dysfunction can also result from accumulation of toxins, as in poisoning, renal failure, and liver failure.

NURSING ASSESSMENT OF NEUROLOGIC FUNCTION

A number of diagnostic tests may be done to evaluate and diagnose neurologic problems. However, any evaluation begins with an accurate assessment, which may be initiated by the nurse. The LPN/LVN assists with the assessment by collecting relevant data. Much of the assessment requires simply observing the patient and then recording the findings.

Health History

The general nursing assessment of the patient with a neurologic disorder is described here. Throughout the assessment, the patient's speech, behavior, coordination, alertness, and comprehension should be noted. More sophisticated assessments are discussed in the Diagnostic Tests and Procedures section, beginning on p. 423.

Chief Complaint and History of Present Illness. An initial portion of the neurologic assessment includes an investigation of the health history of the patient, particularly as it relates to the chief complaint. Document the event that prompted the patient to seek medical attention. Describe any injuries. If the patient has pain, note the onset, severity, location, and duration.

Past Medical History. Past neurologic disorders and pertinent signs and symptoms are vital pieces of information. Ask about a history of head injury, seizures, diabetes mellitus, hypertension, heart disease, and cancer. Record dates and types of immunizations, including influenza. List current medications. Record

current drugs and highlight allergies according to agency policy.

Pharmacology Capsule

Many drugs stimulate or depress the CNS.

Family History. Questions about the presence of neurologic disease or other diseases in the immediate family may elicit valuable information about risk factors, such as those for stroke or neuromuscular diseases. Therefore ask whether any immediate family members have had heart disease, stroke, diabetes mellitus, cancer, seizure disorders, muscular dystrophy, or Huntington's disease.

Review of Systems. Important signs and symptoms to be documented in reviewing the system are fatigue or weakness, headache, dizziness, vertigo, changes in vision or hearing, tinnitus, drainage from the ears or nose, dysphagia, neck pain or stiffness, vomiting, problems with bladder or bowel function, sexual dysfunction, fainting, blackouts, tremors, paralysis, incoordination, numbness or tingling, memory problems, and mood changes.

Functional Assessment. Document whether present symptoms interfere with the patient's usual activities and occupation. Explore sources of stress, usual coping strategies, and sources of support.

Physical Examination

A complete physical examination, including the neurologic examination, should be done when the patient is stable. A neurologic assessment provides baseline data to compare with ongoing assessments and serves as the basis for developing the nursing care plan. Four major components of a routine neurologic examination that provide valuable information regarding the overall integrity of the CNS are level of consciousness, pupillary evaluation, neuromuscular response, and vital signs. You must look at the trends in the patient's neurologic status. A single finding considered in isolation may not provide a true picture of the patient's status. For example, one elevated blood pressure reading may not be significant, but continuing increases may be associated with increased intracranial pressure (ICP).

Basic Neurologic Examination

Level of Consciousness. The most accurate and reliable indicator of neurologic status is level of consciousness. Evaluate patients for orientation to person, place, and time by asking them to state their names, where they are, and what time it is. It is important to consider the degree of stimulation required to evoke a response from the patient. If the patient responds only to vigorous physical stimulation, then consciousness is more impaired than if the patient immediately responds to a verbal greeting. Consider patient behavior in response to stimulation.

Does the patient respond pleasantly, or is he or she combative, agitated, or lethargic? All these observations provide additional information regarding mental status.

Some of the common terms used to describe altered levels of consciousness are *somnolence, lethargy, stupor, semicoma,* and *coma.* Somnolence is unnatural drowsiness or sleepiness. Lethargy also is used to describe excessive drowsiness. Stupor suggests decreased responsiveness accompanied by lack of spontaneous motor activity. If a patient is in a stupor (stuporous) but can be aroused, the term *semicomatose* is used. A patient who cannot be aroused even by powerful stimuli is said to be in a coma, or comatose.

Because the terms just mentioned related to altered levels of consciousness are open to interpretation, it is clearer to describe the patient's response to specific stimuli. Always begin with the mildest stimuli and stop when a response is elicited. The mildest stimulus is simply approaching the patient. This can be followed in order with verbal stimuli, with tactile stimuli (shaking the shoulder gently), and finally with painful stimuli. Appropriate methods of applying painful stimuli include applying pressure on the nail bed using an object such as a pen or pinching the trapezius muscle firmly between the thumb and forefinger and twisting.

Pupillary Evaluation. The second major component of the neurologic assessment is the pupillary evaluation. To evaluate the pupils, assess and compare their size, shape, and reactivity. Pupils are normally about 3 mm in size, round, and react briskly to light. Changes in equality or reactivity from one assessment to the next may indicate neurologic deterioration.

Neuromuscular Response. Assessment of neuromuscular response provides a means of evaluating cerebral and spinal cord function. All electrical impulses responsible for eliciting motor responses are initiated in the frontal lobe of the cerebral cortex. The impulses travel down the brainstem into the spinal cord. Motor spinal nerve roots then stimulate muscle movement. Additional techniques for assessing specific neuromuscular responses are found in Table 29-5.

Vital Signs. Monitoring pulse, respirations, and blood pressure provides highly reliable information regarding neurologic well-being. However, changes in vital signs are late indicators of deterioration. The significance of these values is discussed in detail in the Increased Intracranial Pressure section on p. 432. Elevated temperature may be associated with infection or with impaired thermoregulation.

General Physical Examination. Once the neurologic assessment is done, complete the remaining physical examination. If possible, measure height and weight. Throughout the examination, inspect the skin for lesions and color change and palpate for temperature. Assess hydration status by evaluating tissue turgor and moisture of mucous membranes. Inspect the head for

---

Box 27-2 | ASSESSMENT of the Patient with a Neurologic Disorder

Health History

Chief Complaint and History of Present Illness:
Event requiring medical attention

Past Medical History:
Head injury, seizures, other neurologic disorders, other diseases (diabetes mellitus, hypertension, heart disease, cancer), dates of immunizations, current medications, allergies

Family History:
Stroke, neuromuscular diseases, heart disease, diabetes mellitus, cancer, seizures

Review of Systems:
Fatigue, weakness, headache, dizziness, vertigo, changes in vision or hearing, tinnitus, drainage from nose or ears, dysphagia, neck pain or stiffness, vomiting, bladder or bowel dysfunction, fainting, blackouts, tremors, paralysis, incoordination, numbness or tingling, memory problems, mood changes

Functional Assessment:
Usual occupation and activities, impact on life, changes in sexuality, changes in activities of daily living, sources of stress, usual coping strategies, sources of support

Physical Examination
INITIAL
Level of Consciousness:
Response to stimulation

Pupils:
Size, shape, response to light, equality

Neuromuscular Status:
Voluntary movement, reflexes

Vital Signs:
Blood pressure, pulse, respirations, temperature

IF/WHEN STABLE:

Height and Weight

Skin:
Lesions, injuries, turgor

Head:
Lesions, injuries, masses, swelling

Oral Cavity:
Moisture

Thorax:
Respiratory effort, breath sounds

Abdomen:
Distention, bowel sounds

Extremities:
Injuries, abnormal positions

lesions, and palpate for masses or swelling. Observe respiratory effort, and auscultate breath sounds. Inspect the abdomen, auscultate bowel sounds, and palpate for bowel and bladder distention. Inspect the extremities for injuries or abnormal positions. Assessment of motor and sensory function is detailed in Chapter 29.

Assessment of the patient with a neurologic disorder is summarized in Box 27-2.

DIAGNOSTIC TESTS AND PROCEDURES

Once an initial evaluation and history have been obtained, more detailed diagnostic tests and procedures are often indicated (see the Diagnostic Tests and Procedures table below).

Advanced Neurologic Examination

Baseline and serial examinations are critical in the evaluation of the patient with a neurologic disorder. Cranial nerve function, coordination and balance, neuromuscular function, and reflexes are those components that can assist the practitioner in localizing the area of injury or disease and in developing a plan of care relevant to the individual patient. Figure 27-5 is an example of a flow sheet used to record the findings on periodic neurologic assessments.

Cranial Nerves. Various motor and sensory functions are mediated by the cranial nerves. The cranial nerves enter and exit the brain rather than the spinal cord. The primary function of the cranial nerve is to control sensory and motor activities of

DIAGNOSTIC TESTS and PROCEDURES | *Neurologic Disorders*

TEST/PURPOSE	PATIENT PREPARATION	POSTPROCEDURE NURSE CARE
LUMBAR PUNCTURE Used to diagnose infections and other CNS disorders. CSF pressure is measured. A CSF sample is taken for analysis.	Informed consent is required. Tell the patient a fluid sample will be taken from the spinal column. Have the patient void to reduce the discomfort of a full bladder. Support the patient on one side in a knee-to-chest position during the procedure (see Fig. 27-8).	The risk of headache may be reduced by lying flat for a specific period after the procedure. Encourage oral fluids. Assess for numbness, tingling, or pain in the extremities, CSF or bleeding from the puncture site, and changes in vital signs. Promptly deliver labeled specimens to the lab. The puncture site is covered with a small bandage.
ELECTROENCEPHALOGRAPHY (EEG) Used to detect seizure activity by monitoring electrical activity in the brain.	Explain that electrodes will be applied to the scalp; patient will not feel any electrical shocks. Shampoo hair before EEG. Withhold medications (anticonvulsants, sedatives, stimulants, tranquilizers) and caffeine for up to 48 hours before EEG as ordered.	Help patient shampoo hair to remove electrode paste.
ELECTROMYOGRAPHY (EMG) Useful in diagnosing neuromuscular abnormalities such as ALS, peripheral neuropathy, myasthenia gravis, and carpal tunnel syndrome.	Signed consent is required. Tell patient procedure takes 1-2 hours. No caffeine or smoking for 3 hours before EMG.	Inspect the sites of needle electrode placement. Patient may be instructed to return within 5 days to have blood drawn for enzyme tests (AST, CK, LD).
IMAGING STUDIES **Brain Scan** Depicts pattern of distribution of a radioactive isotope that has been injected IV. Used to diagnose brain abscesses, tumors, contusions, vascular occlusions or hemorrhage, and hematomas.	Informed consent required. Contraindicated during pregnancy. KCl is given several hours before the procedure. Tell patient that scan is painless and that radiation exposure is minimal. An isotope will be injected, and the patient will lie on a stretcher while the scanner moves over the head. The scan will be repeated an hour later.	Encourage oral fluids to promote elimination of the isotope.

CNS, Central nervous system; *CSF*, cerebrospinal fluid; *ALS*, amyotrophic lateral sclerosis; *AST*, aspartate aminotransferase; *CK*, creatine kinase; *LD*, lactic dehydrogenase; *IV*, intravenously; *KCl*, potassium chloride; *NPO*, nothing by mouth; *EEG*, electroencephalogram; *EMG*, electromyelogram.

Continued

DIAGNOSTIC TESTS and PROCEDURES | *Neurologic Disorders—cont'd*

TEST/PURPOSE	PATIENT PREPARATION	POSTPROCEDURE NURSE CARE
Cerebral Angiography Uses computer-based images taken after injection of contrast medium to assess abnormalities in cerebral, carotid, and vertebral blood vessels.	Informed consent required. Inform radiologist if allergic to contrast media, shellfish, or iodine. Remove any metal from head area. Tell patient a "dye" will be injected and radiographs taken as the patient lies on a stretcher. When medium is injected, patient may feel flushed, warm, and nauseated and report a salty taste.	Apply pressure to puncture site, and monitor for bleeding. Bed rest may be ordered for specified period. Extremity used to inject contrast medium may be immobilized for a specified period of time; assess circulation and neurologic function. Allergic response to contrast medium causes hives, nausea, swollen salivary glands. Treat with antihistamines as ordered.
Computed Tomography (CT) Shows intracranial structures. Used to diagnose tumors, inflammation, edema, hematomas, and infarctions. Distinguishes normal from clotted blood. May be done along with angiography.	Patient may be NPO 4-8 hours before scan if contrast medium is planned; can take prescribed meds and diabetic diet. Patient must lie still on a stretcher that fits into a doughnut-shaped frame that moves around the head. A mechanical sound can be heard. Procedure is painless and takes 15-20 minutes. Give sedatives as ordered for patients who cannot stay still.	No special aftercare needed. Observe patient who receives contrast medium for a delayed allergic reaction.
MAGNETIC RESONANCE IMAGING (MRI) **Magnetic Resonance Angiogram (MRA)** Creates images of intracranial structures without radiation.	Tell patient he or she will lie on a stretcher that passes into a tubular structure. Loud drumming noises will be heard while imager is in use. No special preparation is required. Sedation may be ordered for confused patients or those who are claustrophobic. Open MRI may be available for claustrophobic patients. Patients with some metal implants cannot be exposed to MRI because magnet can cause metal to move in the body. Special oxygen equipment, ventilators, and infusion pumps must be used.	No special aftercare needed.
Pneumoencephalography Uses injected gas by lumbar puncture and radiography to provide outline of the cerebral ventricles and cisterns. Used to diagnose masses, congenital abnormalities, cysts, and atrophy of cerebral and cerebellar cortex.	Informed consent required. Remove metal objects from head area. Support patient during lumbar puncture.	Perform neurologic checks per agency protocol. Keep patient flat and logroll for up to 48 hours as ordered. Inspect puncture site for CSF leakage or bleeding. Encourage oral fluids if permitted.
BLOOD FLOW STUDIES **Doppler Flow** Uses ultrasound to assess carotid blood flow. Can be used with a duplex scanner to detect plaques in blood vessels.	Signed consent required. Inform patient that test is painless and not to smoke for 30 minutes before test. Patient will need to lie supine while instrument is moved over the neck area.	No special aftercare needed unless activity restrictions are ordered.

MISSION HOSPITAL
REGIONAL MEDICAL CENTER

ADULT NEURO FLOW SHEET

			TIME
			0700 0800 0900 1000 1100 1200 1300 1400 1500 1600 1700 1800 1900 2000 2100 2200 2300 2400 0100 0200 0300 0400 0500 0600

GLASGOW COMA SCALE		Eyes open	
		Best motor	
		Best verbal	
		TOTAL	
VOLUNTARY MOTOR	Right	Upper extremity	
		Lower extremity	
	Left	Upper extremity	
		Lower extremity	
CRANIAL NERVES	PUPILS	Right	Size	
			Reaction	
		Left	Size	
			Reaction	
	EOMS	Conjugate	
		Disconjugate	
		Tracking Right	
		Left	
	Blink reflex		
	Gag reflex		
	Facial symmetry		

KEY
MOTOR
5+ Normal power
4+ Weakness
3+ Anti-gravity
2+ Not anti-gravity
1+ Trace
0 No movement

Pupil   B = Brisk
Size   S = Sluggish
           A = Absent

2 mm 3 mm 4 mm 5 mm

6 mm   7 mm   8 mm

↙ = Present
O = Absent
S = Symmetrical
A = Asymmetrical

	TIME
	0700 0800 0900 1000 1100 1200 1300 1400 1500 1600 1700 1800 1900 2000 2100 2200 2300 2400 0100 0200 0300 0400 0500 0600

Date

Speech patterns: _____

Comments: _____

GLASGOW COMA SCALE	Eyes Open	4 Spontaneously
		3 To verbal command
		2 To pain
		1 No response
	Best Motor Response	6 Obeys command
		5 Localize pain
		4 Flexion to pain withdraw
		3 Flexion decorticate
		2 Extension to pain (decerebrate)
		1 No response to pain
	Best Verbal Response	5 Oriented
		4 Confused
		3 Inappropriate words
		2 Incomprehensible sounds
		1 No response

Unit _____

R.N. signature _____ Shift: _____

R.N. signature _____ Shift: _____

R.N. signature _____ Shift: _____

ADDRESSOGRAPH

Form: 408 5/92   **Adult Neuro Flow Sheet**

FIGURE **27-5** A neuro flow sheet is used to record the assessment of neurologic function.

the head and neck, but the vagus nerve also affects cardiac, respiratory, gastric, and gallbladder function. Each nerve may be assessed individually by the examiner with advanced assessment skills (Table 27-2).

Coordination and Balance. Both the cerebellum and the cerebral cortex influence coordination and balance. Cerebellar dysfunction creates loss of steady, balanced posture and gait on the ipsilateral side (same side) as the brain lesion. Lesions of the cortex, however, cause

Table 27-2 | *Cranial Nerves*

NO.	NAME	FUNCTION	TEST
I	Olfactory	Smell	Common odors to one nostril at a time
II	Optic	Vision	Visual acuity Visual fields Optic disc
III	Oculomotor	Movement of eye (medially, upward and inward, downward and outward, upward and outward), accommodation, pupillary constriction, raises upper eyelid	EOMs Doll's eyes (when head is moved, eyes move in opposite direction) Light examination direct and consensual; accommodation
IV	Trochlear	Movement of eye (down and inward)	EOMs Doll's eyes
V	Trigeminal	Facial sensation to hot/cold; light touch Chewing Branches: ophthalmic, maxillary, mandibular	Respective testing of 3 divisions. Clinch jaw and check masseter and temporalis muscles; jaw and corneal reflex
VI	Abducens	Movement of eye (laterally)	EOMs Doll's eyes
VII	Facial	Facial expression; salivation; lacrimation, taste	Smile, frown, show teeth, puff out checks. Taste (anterior $\frac{2}{3}$ of tongue), close eyes
VIII	Acoustic	Hearing (cochlear) Equilibrium (vestibular)	Gross acuity, Rinne and Weber tests. Vestibular usually not tested
IX	Glossopharyngeal	Motor response limited; sensory on posterior tongue Innervates carotid body and sinus	Swallow on command, gag reflex Taste (posterior $\frac{1}{3}$ of tongue)
X	Vagus	Movements of pharynx and larynx (raises the palate) Innervates organs of thorax abdomen	Gag reflex, midline elevation of uvula
XI	Spinal Accessory	Movements of shoulders and neck	Shrug shoulders and turn head against resistance
XII	Hypoglossal	Movement of tongue for speech and swallowing	Protrude tongue (deviates to effected side)

EOMs, Extraocular movements.

motor dysfunction on the contralateral side (opposite side) of the lesion.

Observation of routine activity, such as ambulation, feeding, or performing activities of daily living, can provide valuable information about coordination and balance. In the assessment of balance, ask the patient to walk 10 to 20 feet away from you, turn, and walk back toward you. Observe gait and arm swing. Then ask the patient to walk a straight line in a heel-to-toe fashion.

To perform the Romberg test, have the patient stand, with feet together and arms at sides. Instruct the patient to close the eyes and maintain that position. Stay close by in case the patient starts to fall. Normally, there will be only slight swaying. To evaluate coordination of movements:

1. Ask the patient to pat his or her knees with the palms of the hands and then with the backs of the hands in a rapid, alternating pattern.
2. Hold up one of your fingers and instruct the patient to touch it with his or her index finger.
3. Ask the patient to touch his or her nose with the index finger, first with the eyes open and then with the eyes closed.
4. Ask the patient to run the heel of one foot down the shin of the other leg and then repeat with the opposite heel.

5. Alternate tapping with the heel and then the toes of one foot and then the other foot.

Normally these responses are done smoothly and rapidly.

Neuromuscular Function. Evaluate individual muscle groups by assessing their size, tone, and strength. Upper arm strength is evaluated by having the patient squeeze your fingers. Put one finger on top of another so that a firm squeeze will not painfully press your knuckles together. You can also instruct the patient to lift each hand or to raise a finger on each hand. Another means of assessing upper arm strength is to have the patient extend both arms forward with the palms up. Ask the patient to close his or her eyes and maintain the position for 10 to 20 seconds. With normal strength, the arms remain steady. In the presence of a slight weakness, the weak arm will internally rotate and drift slightly downward. This is referred to as *ulnar* or *motor drift*.

To evaluate strength of the legs, position the patient supine and ask him or her to raise one leg at a time. The patient with normal strength can lift the leg 90 degrees. Test the strength of other muscles as indicated.

Sensory Function. There are many tests of sensory function, including evaluation of the patient's percep-

FIGURE 27-6 Reflexes are elicited by stimulating a sensory nerve, which conveys an impulse to the spinal cord. An impulse is then conveyed by a motor nerve to cause the muscle to contract.

tion of pain, touch, temperature, vibration, position, and tactile discrimination. All sensory testing is done with the eyes closed. Apply various stimuli to the skin and ask the patient to identify the type of stimulus perceived.

Pain. Pain can be evaluated by using a wooden applicator that is broken to create a sharp point. This broken applicator is used as the "sharp" stimulus, whereas the cotton end is used as a "dull" control stimulus. Ask the patient to state whether sharp or dull sensations are felt. Recognition of sharp pricks indicates ability to perceive painful stimuli.

Temperature. Temperature perception can be tested by touching test tubes containing hot or cold water to the patient's skin and asking the patient to distinguish hot from cold.

Light Touch. A wisp of cotton brushed against the skin is used to assess perception of light touch. Ask the patient to state when the sensation is felt.

Vibration. Strike a tuning fork and touch the base to a joint in the great toe or a finger. Ask the patient to report when the vibration is felt and when it stops. The examiner actually stops the tuning fork from vibrating. If the sensation is not perceived, repeat the test on a more proximal joint until the patient perceives it.

Position. Lightly hold the patient's great toe or a finger on the sides and move it up and down. Ask the patient to identify the direction of the movement.

Tactile Discrimination. Tests for tactile discrimination include stereognosis, graphesthesia, and point localization. In testing stereognosis, place a familiar object (paper clip, cotton ball) in the patient's hand and request identification using only one hand. Graphes-

Table 27-3	*Commonly Tested Reflexes*
REFLEX	**EXPECTED RESPONSE**
Biceps	Flexion of forearm
Triceps	Extension of forearm
Brachioradialis	Flexion and supination of forearm
Quadriceps	Extension of lower leg
Achilles (ankle jerk)	Plantar flexion of foot
Clonus	Repetitive movement after brisk dorsiflexion of foot

thesia tests the patient's ability to recognize a number or letter "written" on the palm with a dull object. To test point localization, briefly touch the skin and ask the patient to touch the place where the sensation was felt.

Reflexes. A reflex is an unconscious, involuntary response that is entirely mediated at the level of the spinal cord, without input from higher brain centers. The knee jerk represents a simple reflex. When a stimulus is applied to the patella, the sensory root of the spinal nerve transmits the impulse to the spinal cord. At the cord, the impulse is relayed to the motor nerve root, which then elicits the knee jerk (Fig. 27-6). Other commonly tested reflexes are listed in Table 27-3.

Although these common reflexes are normal, others appear only with pathologic states. The Babinski reflex accompanies abnormalities in the motor pathways originating in the cerebral cortex. Assess for it by stroking the lateral side of the bottom of the foot and across the ball of the foot with a blunt object and observing the resulting movement of the toes.

Normally, the toes curl downward. However, in the presence of cortical dysfunction, the big toe bends upward and the other toes fan out. Figure 27-7 illustrates the response.

Lumbar Puncture

A lumbar puncture is an invasive procedure that is used most often to detect infections and other disorders of the CNS, tumors, and hydrocephalus. A local anesthetic agent is used to anesthetize the puncture site. Then a cannula is inserted into the subarachnoid space at the level of the third lumbar vertebra (Fig. 27-8). Entering at this level allows the physician to avoid traumatizing the spinal cord, which ends at the level of the second lumbar vertebra. Once the needle is in place, a sample of CSF is collected for laboratory analysis. CSF specimens are placed in test tubes and labeled, with the first specimen usually being discarded because it may contain blood from the puncture. Normal CSF has the following characteristics: pressure, 50 to 175 mm H_2O; pH, 7.30 to 7.40; clear, colorless appearance; fasting glucose, 40 to 80 mg/dL; WBC, 0 to 5 small lymphocytes/mm^3.

Injuries resulting from lumbar puncture are rare. However, some patients experience severe headaches resulting from a CSF leak. Leaks are sometimes treated with a blood patch, which is created by injecting a small amount of the patient's blood into the lumbar puncture site. The blood clots, sealing the puncture site and preventing further loss of CSF.

Electroencephalography

The electroencephalogram (EEG) is a graphic representation of electrical activity in brain cells. Small electrodes are placed at various positions on the head to detect electrical signals generated from neurons located near the surface of the cerebral cortex. It is an excellent tool in the diagnosis of seizure activity (Fig. 27-9).

Some people have misconceptions about EEG. Assure the patient that no electrical shock will be experi-

FIGURE **27-7** Babinski reflex. **A,** The examiner scrapes the foot as shown, using a blunt point. **B,** The normal response (absence of Babinski response) is plantar flexion of the toes. **C,** An abnormal response (presence of Babinski response) is characterized by dorsiflexion of the big toe and often fanning of the other toes.

FIGURE **27-8** Lumbar puncture. With the patient in a flexed position to maximize the space between vertebrae, the lumbar puncture needle is inserted between L-4 and L-5 to gain entry to the subarachnoid space. During the actual procedure, the patient would be gowned and draped to protect privacy.

enced, that the examiner is not able to "read the patient's mind," and that the test is not done to detect mental illness. Fatigue stresses the brain and may evoke abnormal activity not usually seen on the EEG. Therefore patients may be evaluated with a sleep-deprived EEG, in which they are awakened after a short sleep period in an effort to elicit such activity during the test.

Electromyography

Electromyography studies the response of peripheral motor and sensory nerves to electrical stimuli. Needle electrodes are placed on several points over a nerve and over the muscles supplied by the nerve. Stimuli are administered, and the effects are recorded on an oscilloscope.

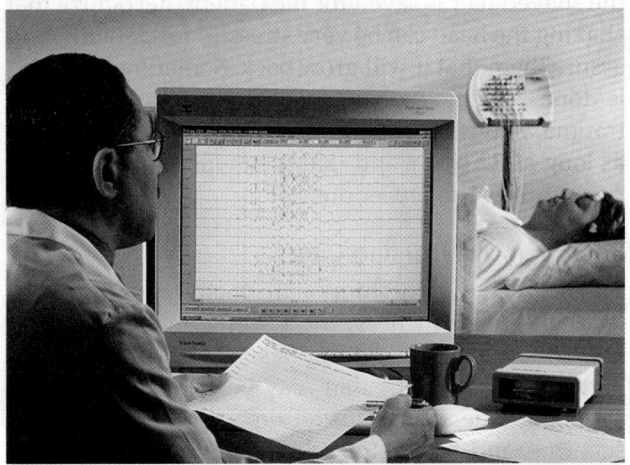

FIGURE **27-9** Client undergoing an electroencephalogram.

Radiologic Studies

Brain Scan. The brain scan shows the pattern of distribution of a radioactive isotope injected intravenously. It is useful in detecting brain abscesses, tumors, contusions, vascular occlusion or hemorrhage, and hematomas. The patient is given potassium chloride 2 hours before the isotope is injected to prevent excessive isotope uptake. The isotope is given immediately before the scan is done. While the patient lies still on a stretcher, the scanner, which is somewhat like an x-ray machine, moves back and forth over the head. There is no sensation associated with the scanning process. The scan is repeated 1 hour later.

Cerebral Angiography and Digital Subtraction Angiography. Cerebral angiography provides images of the cerebral, carotid, and vertebral blood vessels. A catheter is inserted into an artery (usually femoral) and advanced to the carotid or vertebral arteries. A contrast dye is injected, and a series of radiographs are taken. Angiography is the most definitive diagnostic test in the diagnosis of cerebral aneurysm or congenital vascular disorders, such as arteriovenous malformation. Risks include severe allergy to contrast media, embolus, hematoma, hemorrhage, renal toxicity, transient ischemic attack, infection, and loss of consciousness. Digital subtraction angiography (DSA) is a complementary, computer-assisted radiographic procedure for visualization of cerebral vessels.

Computed Tomography. The evolution of computed tomography (CT) represents one of the most significant developments in neurologic diagnostic procedures. CT is an excellent tool in the evaluation of trauma, tumors, and hemorrhage (Fig. 27-10). Enhancement of an area

FIGURE **27-10** Computed tomography scans are taken at various cross sections of the brain. The image in **A** illustrates the cross section used for the scan shown in **B**.

may be achieved by injecting contrast medium; therefore any allergy to such media must be reported to the radiologist in advance. The entire scanning procedure lasts 15 to 20 minutes and generally requires no advance preparation or postprocedure care.

Magnetic Resonance Imaging. One of the latest tools in neuroradiology is magnetic resonance imaging (MRI). Unlike CT, MRI does not expose the patient to radiation. It is a noninvasive examination that involves placing the patient in a strong magnetic field and then applying bursts of radiofrequency waves. Sophisticated technology converts information about the movement of molecules in the tissue into precise, clear images (Fig. 27-11). Magnetic resonance angiography (MRA) is a special technique that allows the measurement of flow through blood vessels. Depending on the type of equipment available, metal prostheses, pacemakers, and various implants may contraindicate MRI. This noninvasive diagnostic procedure is painless, has no known risks, and requires no preparation.

COMMON THERAPEUTIC MEASURES

DRUG THERAPY

A number of drugs are used to treat neurologic disorders. They include antimicrobials, analgesics, anti-inflammatories, corticosteroids, anticonvulsants, diuretics, chemotherapeutic agents, dopaminergics, anticholinergics, cholinergics, and antihistamines. Examples of specific drugs are presented in the Drug Therapy table on pp. 431 and 432.

FIGURE **27-11** Magnetic resonance imaging uses magnetic fields to create cross-sectional views of the brain. This sagittal section shows the cerebrum, ventricles, cerebellum, and medulla.

SURGERY

A craniotomy (surgical opening of the skull) may be done to treat tumors, correct defects, evacuate hematomas, and relieve pressure associated with trauma. A craniectomy is the excision of a segment of the skull, and a cranioplasty is any procedure done to repair a skull defect. General care of the surgical patient is covered in Chapter 17, but interventions specific to neurologic surgery are emphasized here.

Preoperative Nursing Care

Preoperatively, document neurologic status to provide a baseline for evaluating postoperative progress. Encourage the patient to ask questions and to express fears. If the patient has cerebral edema, parenteral corticosteroids may be ordered to help reduce cerebral swelling. All or part of the scalp is usually shaved, and the shaved hair is saved for the patient. Recognize that shaving the head can be very stressful for patients, and assure them that it will grow back. Sometimes shaving is done after the patient is anesthetized to reduce the trauma. Advise the family that a craniotomy can take as long as 12 hours and that they will get progress reports during the procedure.

Postoperative Nursing Care

Postoperative craniotomy care includes monitoring level of consciousness, vital signs, movement and strength, pupil size and response to light, and speech. Signs and symptoms that may be related to complications are headache, visual disturbances, vomiting, seizures, and respiratory depression. Vital signs are recorded and neurologic checks are done hourly until the patient is stable. Maintain intake and output records. Inspect the dressing for bleeding or CSF drainage. Note drainage from the ears or nose. A dressing may be placed loosely to absorb the drainage. Replace it when it becomes wet because the moisture can harbor bacteria. On dressings, CSF appears as a pink stain surrounded by a lighter ring described as a "halo." It is no longer recommended to check CSF with a dipstick for glucose because dipsticks are calibrated only for the specific fluids they were designed to test. Report signs of deteriorating neurologic status to the physician immediately. The physician prescribes the patient's position. The physician usually specifies that the head of the bed be elevated about 30 degrees.

If the patient has an external ventricular drainage system, use strict aseptic technique when changing the insertion-site dressing and the drainage bag. Keep the zero reference point of the drip chamber of the drainage bag at the level of the external auditory canal or at the level prescribed by the physician to prevent drainage of excessive CSF. When the patient is being repositioned, clamp and then restore the drainage tube to the correct level and unclamp.

In addition to the usual surgical complications, the patient having a craniotomy is at risk for increased

DRUG THERAPY *Neurologic Disorders*

DRUG	USE/ACTION	SIDE EFFECTS	NURSING INTERVENTIONS
ANTICONVULSANTS			
Phenytoin (Dilantin)	Reduces neuron hyperexcitability; inhibits seizure activity. Reduces pain of trigeminal neuralgia.	Sluggishness, ataxia, slurred speech, nystagmus, constipation, nausea, vomiting, overgrowth of gingiva, skin rashes. Hypotension with IV route. Unusual: aplastic anemia, agranulocytosis.	With IV doses, monitor BP and pulse and report bradycardia. Do not exceed recommended rate of IV administration per minute. Safety precautions if ataxic, drowsy. Give with food to reduce GI irritation. Provide meticulous mouth care to prevent gingival overgrowth. Identify concurrent drugs to detect possible interactions that enhance or inhibit drug effect.
Fosphenytoin (Cerebyx)	Precursor of phenytoin. Used for acute seizures.	Side effects the same as phenytoin.	IV route. Less irritation at site of IV administration. Do not exceed recommended rate of IV administration.
Gabapentin (Neurontin)	Unique gabapentin-specific binding site in brain; no effect on GABA system.	Somnolence, dizziness, ataxia particularly after initiation of therapy or dosage increase. Weight gain, edema. Dyspepsia, nausea, vomiting, constipation. Rhinitis, pharyngitis.	Safety precautions if drowsy. Give with food to prevent GI distress. Notify physician of side effects. Encourage periodic rest periods to help with fatigue.
Lamotrigine (Lamictal)	Inhibits release of excitatory amino acid glutamate. Blocks Na channels.	Dizziness, headache, insomnia, somnolence, ataxia, diplopia. Nausea, vomiting. Potentially life-threatening rash.	Safety precautions if drowsy. Notify physician of rash. Identify current drugs to detect possible interactions that enhance or inhibit drug effect. Monitor renal and hepatic function. Take drug with food or milk. Medicate for headache.
Topiramate (Topamax)	Blocks voltage-dependent sodium and calcium channels; enhances GABA activity at some GABA receptors; blocks excitatory receptors (kainite/glutamate).	Somnolence, abnormal thinking, dizziness, agitation, confusion, ataxia, nystagmus, nephrolithiasis, nausea, dyspepsia, anorexia, weight loss, dysmenorrhea, upper respiratory tract infection.	Safety precautions if drowsy. Inform physician of agitation, confusion, abnormal thinking. Administer with food if GI upset occurs. Caution not to chew or break tablet because of bitter taste. Maintain adequate hydration to prevent renal stones. Suggest use of barrier contraceptives due to decreased effectiveness of oral contraceptives. Encourage avoidance of alcohol due to increased CNS depression.
Vigabatrin (Sabril)	Inhibits GABA metabolism.	Drowsiness, dizziness, fatigue.	Safety precautions if drowsy. Monitor for possible drug interactions. Encourage rest periods for fatigue.
Tiagabine (Gabitril)	Increases level of GABA by inhibiting reuptake systems.	Tiredness, dizziness, headache, nervousness, asthenia, somnolence, difficulty concentrating. GI upset, pain, serious skin rash.	Safety precautions if drowsy. Note other drugs for possible drug interactions. Give with food. Monitor weight, liver function studies, neurologic status. Avoid alcohol and sleep-inducing drugs.
Zonisamide (Zonegran)	Sulfonamide; mechanism of action is unclear. May decrease seizure activity by inhibiting sodium and calcium channels.	Skin rash; somnolence, anorexia, dizziness, headache, nausea, agitation/irritability. Renal calculi, bone marrow depression. Nausea, vomiting, dry mouth, unusual taste.	Safety precautions if drowsy. Adequate hydration to prevent renal calculi. Monitor hepatic, renal, and cardiac function. Monitor closely at beginning of therapy and with dosage changes.

IV, Intravenous; *BP,* blood pressure; *GI,* gastrointestinal; *GABA,* inhibitory amino acid that increases seizure threshold; *CNS,* central nervous system.

Continued

DRUG THERAPY *Neurologic Disorders—cont'd*

DRUG	USE/ACTION	SIDE EFFECTS	NURSING INTERVENTIONS
Oxcarbazepine (Trileptal)	Inhibits seizure activity by preventing sodium shift that causes neuron hyperexcitability.	Dizziness, drowsiness, double vision, fatigue, ataxia, nausea, vomiting, abdominal pain, tremor, dyspepsia, gait abnormalities.	May be taken with or without food. Implement safety precautions if CNS effects occur. Encourage rest periods for fatigue.
Levetiracetam (Keppra)	Unknown mechanism of action.	Somnolence, dizziness, impaired coordination, abnormal behavior, fatigue, infection.	Safety precautions if drowsy. Give with food to prevent GI side effects. Be aware of interactions with other drugs. Advise to use barrier contraceptives. Implement safety precautions if CNS side effects occur.
BARBITURATES			
Phenobarbital (Luminal) Primidone (Myidone)	Depresses CNS and raises seizure threshold.	Drowsiness, respiratory depression, nausea, vomiting, diarrhea, constipation, rash, photosensitivity, muscle aches. With IV route: laryngospasm, bronchospasm, hypotension.	Safety precautions if drowsy. Monitor respiratory rate and BP, especially with IV route. Note other drugs for possible drug interactions. Tell patient not to stop drug without consulting physician and to avoid alcohol and excessive sunlight.
Carbamazepine (Tegretol)	Slows transmission of impulses in CNS; prevents seizures. Reduces pain of trigeminal neuralgia.	Drowsiness, ataxia, blurred vision, BP increase or decrease, heart failure, urinary retention, rash, hepatitis, aplastic anemia, agranulocytosis.	Safety precautions if drowsy. Monitor BP. Teach patient: avoid alcohol and excessive sunlight, do not change dosage or stop drug without physician's guidance, immediately report fever, sore throat, excessive bruising or bleeding, jaundice.
Diazepam (Valium)	Depresses CNS; inhibits impulse conduction.	Drowsiness, rash, nausea, vomiting, diarrhea, constipation, respiratory depression, psychological and physical dependence. IV route: hypotension, phlebitis.	Safety precautions if drowsy. Monitor infusion site for extravasation. Monitor BP. Give with food to decrease GI distress. Tell patient not to stop or change drug dose without physician's guidance.
Clonazepam (Klonopin)	Raises seizure threshold.	Drowsiness, ataxia, agitation, rash, edema, nocturia, blurred vision, dry mouth, excitement in older adults. Toxicity causes lethargy, confusion, coma.	Safety measures if drowsy. Advise patient that abrupt withdrawal may cause restlessness, insomnia, status epilepticus.

IV, Intravenous; *BP,* blood pressure; *GI,* gastrointestinal; *GABA,* inhibitory amino acid that increases seizure threshold; *CNS,* central nervous system.

ICP, CSF leak, meningitis, and seizures. Other complications depend on the area of the brain affected and could include paralysis, memory loss, confusion, and impaired speech, vision, or hearing. Because increased ICP is a concern with cranial surgery as well as with many neurologic disorders, it is described here.

INCREASED INTRACRANIAL PRESSURE

Increased intracranial pressure (ICP) poses an extremely serious threat to the neurologic patient. Understanding the physiology as well as the signs and symptoms can enable you to recognize the problem and respond appropriately to prevent life-threatening consequences.

Pathophysiology

Anatomically, the skull is an empty cavity with rigid sides and an opening at the bottom. This cavity contains the brain, blood, and CSF, which are the components that exert pressure in the cranium. This pressure, or ICP, is normally 0 to 15 mm Hg.

In the course of a day, ICP fluctuates minimally because alterations are usually corrected rapidly. The Monro-Kellie hypothesis describes the adaptations that must occur in the three components (brain, blood, or CSF) for ICP to remain normal. If the volume of one component increases, ICP will rise unless there is a subsequent decrease in the other two components. For example, if a brain tumor increases the volume of brain tissue, ICP will rise unless the volume of both blood and CSF decreases.

As ICP increases, the perfusion (delivery of blood and oxygen) to brain tissue decreases. This can be measured by calculating cerebral perfusion pressure (CPP), which is obtained by subtracting the ICP from the mean arterial pressure (MAP):

$$CPP = MAP - ICP$$

A minimum perfusion pressure of 70 mm Hg is necessary to ensure adequate cerebral functioning. If perfusion pressure falls to 40 mm Hg, ischemia occurs. A perfusion pressure of 30 mm Hg or less is incompatible with life. Perfusion pressure can be increased by decreasing ICP.

Signs and Symptoms

You can detect increases in ICP and assess the adequacy of perfusion based on the presence of specific signs and symptoms. Assess level of consciousness, pupillary characteristics, motor function, sensory function, and vital signs to detect signs of increasing ICP so that treatment can be initiated promptly.

Level of consciousness is the most reliable indicator of mental status because of its extreme sensitivity to oxygen levels in the cerebral blood. As ICP increases and perfusion is reduced, oxygen delivery to cerebral tissue also is reduced. Changes in level of consciousness are the earliest changes seen in ICP. These changes may be very subtle, with minimal agitation or drowsiness, or may be quite extreme, with profound unresponsiveness.

Classic pupillary changes are seen with increasing ICP. As pressure rises, the pupil progresses from its normal size to a dilated state described as a "blown pupil." The pupil becomes dilated and fixed, and no longer reacts to light. These changes occur because of pressure on the oculomotor nerve (third cranial nerve). This is a late sign of increased ICP.

Another major indicator of increased ICP is altered motor function. As the motor areas of the frontal lobe are compressed by rising pressure, deficits develop on the side opposite the expanding mass. When deficits are on the opposite side from brain injury, they are said to be contralateral to the injury. For example, if there is a tumor in the right side of the brain, motor deficits will appear in the left side of the body. The deficits may involve a single extremity or an entire side. Hemiparesis (weakness on one side) or hemiplegia (paralysis on one side) may be seen.

As increased pressure becomes more extensive, abnormal posturing may be evident. As increasing pressure is exerted on the cerebral tissue above the midbrain, a pattern known as *abnormal flexion* (decorticate)

posturing can be observed. The patient exhibits abnormal flexion in the upper extremities, with extension of the lower extremities. Increasing pressure affecting the midbrain or upper pons causes *extension* (decerebrate) *posturing*. The lower extremities remain extended, and the upper extremities are abnormally extended as well. These motor changes may occur spontaneously or may be seen only with painful stimuli (Fig. 27-12).

Hypothalamic impairment results in the loss of temperature control. As ICP compresses the tissue around the hypothalamus, it becomes ischemic and unable to regulate body temperature.

ICP elevations evoke an increase in systolic blood pressure with little or no associated increase in diastolic pressure. This results in a widening pulse pressure, defined as an increasing difference between systolic and diastolic blood pressure values. Initially, the heart rate may be slightly accelerated. However, as ICP compresses the center for cardiac control in the brainstem, the heart rate becomes slow and irregular. Alterations in respiratory pattern are directly related to the extent of tissue compression. Figure 27-13 illustrates areas of tissue compression (types of "herniation" syndromes).

Although it is extremely important to monitor vital signs in the neurologic patient, remember that changes in pulse, respiratory pattern, and blood pressure are late signs of increasing ICP. The combination of hyper-

A

B

FIGURE 27-12 Abnormal postures may be seen in the patient with neurologic impairment. **A,** Abnormal flexion posturing (decorticate rigidity). **B,** Abnormal extension posturing (decerebrate rigidity).

FIGURE **27-13** Types of intracranial herniation. In *transcalvarial* herniation, edematous brain tissue is extruded through a fracture in the skull. In *central* transtentorial herniation, the lesion is located centrally or superior in the cranium and compression of central and midbrain structures may result. In *lateral,* or *uncal,* herniation, the lesion is located laterally within the cranium and can cause pressure on the midbrain. *Cingulate* herniation occurs between the two frontal lobes; the brain is pressed under the falx cerebri. In *tonsillar* herniation, the cerebellar tonsils are driven between the posterior arch of the atlas and the medulla and may be compressed.

tension, bradycardia, and a widening pulse pressure is known as *Cushing's triad.* Cushing's triad is generally associated with increased ICP, but it is unreliable in determining the severity of neurologic compromise.

Medical Treatment

Prompt treatment of increased ICP is vital for survival. Measures to lower ICP include positioning, hyperventilation, fluid management, mechanical drainage, and drug therapy.

The jugular vein is the primary route for venous outflow from the brain. It has long been thought that raising the head of the bed 30 to 45 degrees improves the flow of venous blood from the brain, thereby decreasing cerebral blood volume and ICP. However, recent research indicates that perfusion pressure may be better preserved if the head of the bed is elevated no more than 30 degrees. Further investigations may lead to some changes in current practice.

As oxygen delivery to cerebral tissue becomes more impaired, the level of carbon dioxide in the tissue increases. Increased carbon dioxide leads to dilation of cerebral blood vessels, thereby increasing the cerebral blood volume and ICP. With controlled hyperventilation, the excess carbon dioxide is eliminated, causing blood vessels to constrict and ICP to fall. Controlled hyperventilation is best achieved by mechanical ventilation. It effectively decreases ICP within 1 to 2 minutes, but its effectiveness is dimin-

ished after 36 to 48 hours. Hyperventilation does have risks. Excessive vasoconstriction reduces cerebral oxygenation and worsens ischemia. Hyperventilation may be reserved for situations in which other treatments fail to reduce ICP.

The patient must have adequate fluids to maintain CPP. Fluid volumes are often increased in an effort to boost perfusion. Patients with questionable cardiac function must be monitored closely for fluid volume excess. A specialized catheter, called a *ventriculostomy catheter,* can be placed in the brain to drain excess CSF. After placement, the catheter is connected to tubing and a collection bag for gravity drainage. Drainage of CSF lowers ICP. Absolute sterility must be maintained in managing this system, because it presents an open avenue for contamination.

Intravenous mannitol administration is one of the mainstays in the treatment of increased ICP. Mannitol is a hyperosmolar diuretic that draws edema fluid from the tissue spaces into the bloodstream. The mannitol and excess fluid are then eliminated through the kidneys. Other diuretic agents, such as furosemide, also may be used in an effort to reduce edema.

Pharmacology Capsule

Diuretics used to treat increased intracranial pressure can cause fluid and electrolyte imbalances.

Corticosteroids, although controversial, may be used to help decrease cerebral edema and ICP. They decrease the edema, thereby lowering the elevated ICP associated with CNS tumors. Dexamethasone (Decadron) is a major agent used for patients with neurologic disorders. Additional information about drugs is presented in the Drug Therapy table pp. 431 and 432.

DISORDERS OF THE NERVOUS SYSTEM

HEADACHE

Headache is the most common type of pain. It is a symptom, rather than a disease, that has many causes. Four common types of headaches are migraine headache, cluster headache, tension headache, and headache related to disorders of the eyes, teeth, or sinuses. For headaches associated with these and other conditions, treatment depends on the underlying cause.

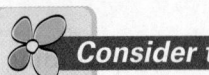
Consider the Alternative

Complementary and alternative therapies are excellent adjuncts in the management of headache. Progressive muscle relaxation techniques, imagery, acupuncture, and electromyography (EMG) biofeedback may reduce the frequency and intensity.

Migraine Headache

Migraine headache is thought to be due to intracranial vasoconstriction followed by vasodilation. Although no single cause is known, it may be triggered by menstruation, ovulation, alcohol, some foods, and stress.

Patients may experience depression, irritability, vision disturbances, nausea, and paresthesias before the onset of pain. The pain is usually unilateral, often begins in the temple or eye area, and is often very intense. Tearing and nausea and vomiting may occur. The patient is hypersensitive to light and sound and prefers a dark, quiet environment.

Mild migraines may be treated with acetaminophen or aspirin, but more severe ones may be treated with ergotamine (Cafergot) or sumatriptan (Imitrex) administered as a tablet or by autoinjector for self-injection. Prevention, however, should be emphasized. Medications such as beta-blockers or calcium channel blockers may help control the vascular influences. Identification and avoidance of triggering agents, such as particular foods (chocolate, yogurt, aged meats, cheeses), beverages (alcohol, red wine), or emotional stress, may also prove helpful.

Cluster Headache

Cluster headaches occur in a series of episodes followed by a long period with no symptoms. They are intensely painful and seem to be related to stress or anxiety. Unlike migraines, cluster headaches usually have no warning symptoms. They are also shorter in duration than migraines. Treatment may include cold application, indomethacin (Indocin), and tricyclic antidepressants.

Tension Headache

Tension headaches result from prolonged muscle contraction associated with anxiety, stress, or stimuli from other sources such as a brain tumor or an abscessed tooth. The location of the pain may vary, and the patient may have nausea and vomiting, dizziness, tinnitus, or tearing. Tension headaches may persist for days or even years. Treatment measures include correction of known causes, psychotherapy, massage, heat application, and relaxation techniques. Analgesics, usually nonopioid, may be prescribed along with other drugs to reduce anxiety.

SEIZURE DISORDER

The electrical impulses generated in the brain normally spread in a very organized fashion. However, in the patient with a seizure disorder, electrical impulses are conducted in a highly chaotic pattern that yields abnormal activity and behavior. Seizure activity involves a large number of hyperactive neurons that use excessive oxygen and glucose. Therefore oxygen and glucose stores may be depleted, leading to permanent neurologic damage.

Seizure activity may be related to trauma, reduced cerebral perfusion, infection, electrolyte disturbances, poisoning, or tumors. There may also be a genetic tendency for such activity.

Medical Diagnosis

Diagnostic testing for seizure activity is often directed toward ruling out specific problems. An accurate history of the seizure disorder can provide clues to the type of seizure disorder, possible triggering events, and the origin of activity. Because unexpected seizure activity is often very frightening to the family, the nurse or other health care provider may be the first reliable eyewitness. If you observe a seizure, note the patient's behavior before, during, and after the seizure as well as the duration of the seizure.

The patient's electroencephalogram (EEG) tracing, which records the electrical activity of the brain, is used to detect abnormal brain activity.

Seizure Classification

The two broad classifications of seizures, based on the patterns of activity, are partial seizures and generalized seizures. Abnormal electrical activity may be generated in a specific area of the brain, remain localized, and stop; or the activity may spread to adjacent neurons but remain fairly localized. These patterns of activity are termed *partial* (or focal) *seizures* because they involve only a part of the brain. The observed activity corresponds to the area of the brain affected.

In addition, partial seizures may recruit a sufficient number of adjacent cells and the activity can spread throughout the cerebral hemispheres. This is known as a *partial seizure with secondary generalization. Generalized seizures* involve the entire brain from the onset and are associated with loss of consciousness.

Some sources use the term *unclassified seizures* for those that are not readily classified as partial or generalized.

Partial Seizures. Partial seizures are described as simple or complex. Simple seizures affect part of one cerebral hemisphere and consciousness is not impaired. A simple partial seizure may include motor, somatosensory, autonomic, or psychic symptoms. Focal motor seizures are a subtype of simple seizures in which the abnormal brain activity remains localized to a specific motor area. This may occur with or without *Jacksonian march,* the term used when the abnormal activity begins in one area and then "marches" (spreads) to adjacent motor areas. For example, the simple focal motor seizure may begin with the eyelid, then spread to the same side of the face, and continue on to involve the arm and leg on that side.

In a complex partial seizure (previously called a *psychomotor* or *temporal lobe seizure*), the patient's consciousness is impaired and the patient may exhibit bizarre, repetitive behavior. Simple partial and complex partial seizures can progress to involve the entire brain. These are referred to as *partial seizures with secondary generalization.*

Generalized Seizures. Generalized seizures involve the entire brain from the onset. Consciousness is lost during the *ictal* (seizure) period. One type of generalized seizure is the tonic-clonic seizure, previously referred to as a *grand mal seizure.* The *tonic phase* of the seizure is characterized by stiffening of the muscles or extremities with loss of consciousness. After the tonic phase, there is a rhythmic movement of the extremities called the *clonic phase* of the seizure. These phases are illustrated in Figure 27-14. The patient may be incontinent of urine during a generalized seizure.

Other types of generalized seizures are absence, myoclonic, and atonic seizures. Absence seizures (previously called *petit mal*) are brief periods of loss of consciousness in which the person may appear to be daydreaming. Absence seizures may be associated with automations such as eye blinking and lip smacking. These seizures are generally identified during childhood. During a myoclonic seizure, the person has only brief jerking or stiffening of the extremities. Atonic seizures were formerly called "drop attacks" because a sudden loss of muscle tone causes the patient to collapse.

Status Epilepticus. Status epilepticus is a medical emergency in which the patient has continuous seizures or repeated seizures in rapid succession for 30 minutes or more. The prolonged seizure activity depletes the brain of oxygen and glucose, which can lead to permanent brain damage.

Tonic phase

Clonic phase

FIGURE **27-14** Phases of a grand mal seizure. **A,** Tonic phase is marked by loss of consciousness, falling, crying, and generalized stiffness. There may be incontinence. **B,** During the clonic phase, there is jerking of the limbs and salivary frothing.

Aura. Some people experience an aura preceding a seizure. The aura is a sensation such as dizziness, numbness, visual or hearing disturbance, perception of an offensive odor, or pain.

Medical Treatment

The most desirable treatment of a seizure disorder is the resolution of the underlying condition. For example, if a tumor is causing seizure activity, surgical excision of the tumor would be the most desirable therapy. However, if a cause is not readily identifiable or correctable, medical management is implemented.

Anticonvulsant drug therapy provides satisfactory chemical control of seizure activity in about 75% of patients. A variety of drugs are available, some being more effective in particular seizure disorders than others. The selected drug is introduced and the dosage is gradually increased until a therapeutic level is achieved. If good seizure control is not accomplished with one drug, combinations of drugs may be prescribed.

Status epilepticus is treated with intravenous anticonvulsant drugs. If the patient does not respond to anticonvulsants, general anesthetic agents and neuromuscular blocking agents may be used. See the Health Promotion Considerations box on p. 437.

Surgical Treatment

Patients whose seizures are poorly controlled with medication may be candidates for surgical procedures to decrease or control seizures. Procedures include re-

Pharmacology Capsule

Sudden discontinuance of anticonvulsant drugs can trigger seizure activity.

Health Promotion Considerations

Seizures

Patients with seizure disorders should receive the following interventions as necessary:

Prevention of Seizure Disorder

- Promote general safety behaviors such as use of helmets and seatbelts
- Obtain perinatal care (for pregnant women and those planning to become pregnant)

Patients with Seizure Disorder

- Avoid alcohol use
- Get adequate rest
- Engage in stress-reducing activities such as meditation and visualization
- Maintain general health through proper diet and exercise

---

moval of seizure foci in the temporal lobe and pallidotomy or vagal nerve stimulator.

NURSING CARE of the Patient with a Seizure Disorder

Assessment

Assessment of the neurologic patient is summarized in Box 27-2. With a seizure disorder, it is especially important to describe the seizure episode including the postictal period (following the seizure) and to document drug therapy.

Nursing Diagnoses, Goals, and Outcome Criteria: Seizure Disorder	
NURSING DIAGNOSES	GOALS AND OUTCOME CRITERIA
Risk for Injury related to seizure activity	Absence of injury: no bruises, breaks in skin, or fractures
Ineffective Coping related to social stigma of seizure disorder or chronicity	Effective coping: patient makes positive statements about life with seizure disorder, patient adheres to prescribed therapy
Deficient Knowledge of seizure disorders, treatment, and self-care	Patient understands self-care: patient and family accurately describe condition, drug therapy, and care; demonstrate appropriate care

Interventions

Risk for Injury

You must protect the patient from injury during and after a seizure. Most agencies require that the side rails of the bed be up and padded, a suction machine be readily available, and the bed be maintained in the low position. Some experts believe that padding the side rails is unnecessary, is cumbersome, and may have a negative emotional impact on the patient and visitors.

Box 27-3 | *Management of Seizures*

"DO'S"	"DON'T'S"
DO remove any objects that could cause harm.	DO NOT restrain unless in grave danger of severe injury.
DO turn the person to one side if possible.	DO NOT attempt to force anything between teeth.
DO note the time the seizure began and how it progressed.	
DO assess and document postictal (postseizure) status.	
DO allow person to rest quietly.	
DO call a medical emergency if a generalized tonic-clonic seizure lasts more than 4 min or if seizures occur in rapid succession.	

It is, however, a common practice used in an effort to protect the patient in case the patient strikes the rails during a seizure.

If the patient has a seizure, quickly move objects away from the patient. If the patient falls to the floor, the head may be cradled in your lap to prevent injury. Do not attempt to restrain the patient. In the past it was common practice to attempt to insert a tongue blade or oral airway between the teeth to prevent biting the tongue. This is no longer recommended. Attempts to force an object between clenched teeth may result in injury to the mouth and do not help if the tongue has already been bitten. The patient will not "swallow his tongue," but it may fall back and occlude the airway. Turning the patient to one side can help maintain a patent airway.

When seizure activity ceases, the patient is typically drowsy and needs to rest. Provide for quiet and privacy. Measures to prevent injury are described in Box 27-3. Afterward, document the conditions and any unusual behaviors that preceded the seizure, the length of the seizure, associated patient activity, deviation of the eyes, and any incontinence. Also, document any lingering effects and the time before recovery.

Ineffective Coping and Deficient Knowledge

Ineffective coping can be related to lack of information or misconceptions and may be reflected in noncompliance with prescribed therapy, in anxiety, or in social isolation. Important aspects of nursing management include not only the care of the patient during hospitalization but also teaching the family and patient about the seizure disorder and the therapy. For guidelines on teaching, see the Patient Teaching Plan on p. 438.

Because a seizure disorder is often a lifelong problem, patient teaching must be directed toward helping the patient and family adjust to a chronic condition.

Seizures

- Factors that may trigger a seizure are fatigue, stress, fever, visual disturbances, alcohol, failure to take medication, and large caffeine intake.
- When you perceive an impending seizure, immediately seek a safe place.
- Know your prescribed drug names, dosages, schedules, and side effects to be reported to the physician.
- Consult your physician regarding the use of generic substitutions for your drugs.
- Never stop taking your seizure medication without direction from your physician.
- Psychological counseling may help you deal with stress associated with this disorder.
- Always wear a medical alert tag, which states that you have a seizure disorder, and carry a card that specifies drug therapy, physician, and individuals to be contacted in an emergency.
- The local chapter of the Epilepsy Foundation is an excellent resource. The telephone number for the Epilepsy Foundation national office is 1-800-332-1000. The Internet address is www.EFA.org.
- A sensation that warns of an impending seizure is called an *aura;* common sensations include dizziness, numbness, visual or hearing disturbance, pain, and perception of an offensive odor.

Patients must adjust physically, psychologically, and vocationally to the changes brought on by the disorder itself as well as to the side effects of the medications. Encourage the patient to ask questions and to express concerns.

HEAD INJURY

Traumatic brain injury is a leading cause of death due to trauma in the United States. The most common causes of head injury are motor vehicle accidents, assaults, and falls, with drug and alcohol abuse being major contributing factors. Several different types of injuries can be identified.

Types of Head Injuries

Scalp Injuries. Scalp injuries include lacerations, contusions, abrasions, and hematomas. They may bleed profusely and may or may not be associated with skull or brain injuries.

Concussion. A concussion is head trauma in which there is no visible injury to the skull or brain. The patient has a loss of consciousness lasting less than 5 minutes and may have a headache, amnesia about the event, nausea, and vomiting.

Contusion. A contusion is more serious than a concussion because there is actual bruising and bleeding in the brain tissue. Contusions can be very serious, especially if the brainstem is affected.

FIGURE **27-15** Epidural hematoma, subdural hematoma, and intracerebral hematoma.

Hematomas. A hematoma is a collection of blood, usually clotted, that may be classified as subdural or epidural.

Subdural Hematoma. A subdural hematoma is usually the result of tearing of the veins that drain the brain, allowing blood to accumulate in the space beneath the dura (Fig. 27-15). The three types of subdural hematomas are acute, subacute, and chronic. Acute subdural hematomas develop within 24 hours of the injury. Subacute subdural hematomas are seen more than 24 hours and less than 1 week after the initial injury. Chronic subdural hematomas occur within weeks or even months of the original injury and are associated with low-impact injuries that cause very slow, diffuse bleeding. Because the bleeding associated with any hematoma can cause potentially serious consequences, astute assessment is needed to determine patient status. Surgical intervention is usually indicated for these types of injuries.

Epidural Hematoma. An epidural hematoma forms in the space between the inner surface of the skull and the outermost meningeal covering of the brain, known as the *dura* (see Fig. 27-15). Generally, epidural hematomas result from arterial bleeding secondary to a laceration and tearing of the middle meningeal artery. The patient typically has a momentary lapse of consciousness, then a period of alertness, followed by rapid deterioration. Therefore you must be alert for any indication of increasing ICP, especially drowsiness progressing to coma. Surgical intervention may be necessary to relieve pressure, remove the clot, and stop the bleeding.

Intracerebral Hemorrhage. Intracerebral hemorrhages result from lesions within the tissue of the brain itself (see Fig. 27-15). These injuries may be small or large and may be accompanied by massive neurologic deficits.

Penetrating Injuries. Penetrating injuries result from sharp objects that penetrate the skull and brain tissue. In addition to the obvious brain injury, there is also a scalp laceration along with the skull fracture. All penetrating injuries require prompt surgical intervention and pose an extremely high risk of infection for the patient because of the wound contamination that occurs.

Surgical Treatment

Surgical intervention for each of these types of trauma is directed at evacuating (removing) hematomas and débriding damaged tissue.

NURSING CARE *of the Patient with a Head Injury*
Assessment

Nursing assessment of the patient with a neurologic disorder is outlined in Box 27-2. See also Nursing Care Plan: The Patient with a Head Injury on p. 440 and the Health Promotion Considerations box on p. 441.

Nursing Diagnoses, Goals, and Outcome Criteria: Head Injury	
NURSING DIAGNOSES	GOALS AND OUTCOME CRITERIA
Ineffective Tissue Perfusion related to increased ICP	Adequate cerebral tissue perfusion: patient alert and oriented
Ineffective Breathing Pattern related to increased ICP	Normal oxygenation: respiratory rate of 12 to 20/min with normal arterial blood gas values
Risk for Injury related to seizures, decreased level of consciousness, disorientation, vision disturbances	Absence of injury: no abrasions, fractures, or severe bruising incurred during seizures or falls
Risk for Infection related to traumatic wounds or invasive procedures	Absence of infection: normal body temperature without signs of wound infection (redness, edema, purulent drainage), urinary infection (cloudiness, foul odor), or phlebitis (redness, tenderness)
Impaired Physical Mobility related to neuromuscular impairment, decreased mental alertness	Absence of complications of immobility (contractures, pressure ulcers, pneumonia, atelectasis, constipation, urinary retention): intact skin, mobile joints, regular bowel movements, no bladder distention, breath sounds clear on auscultation

Disturbed Body Image related to loss of function	Adaptation to altered body function: patient verbalizes way to compensate for changes in body function
Ineffective Role Performance related to neurologic impairment	Adjustment of roles and responsibilities consistent with abilities: patient assumes new roles within abilities

Interventions
Ineffective Tissue Perfusion

Monitor the patient closely for signs of increased ICP and impaired cerebral blood flow: decreasing level of consciousness, pupillary dilation with no response to light, motor deficits, abnormal posture, fever, increased blood pressure, bradycardia, and respiratory depression. Particularly note early signs of deterioration including restlessness, agitation, or lethargy. Promptly report changes to the physician or the registered nurse. Nursing care that can decrease ICP includes positioning to prevent neck and hip flexion, limiting suctioning, spacing nursing care, and preventing isometric muscle contraction. Elevate the head of the bed as ordered. Carefully regulate the rate of administration of intravenous fluids to prevent fluid volume excess. Monitor urine output to assess fluid balance. If a ventriculostomy catheter is in place, inspect and measure the drainage fluid as ordered using strict aseptic technique. Administer diuretics and anti-inflammatory drugs as ordered.

Ineffective Breathing Pattern

Closely monitor the patient's respiratory status using pulse oximetry or measurement of arterial blood gases. Immediately advise the physician of signs of respiratory depression or changes in the respiratory pattern.

Risk for Injury

Nursing measures to prevent injuries associated with seizures and decreased level of consciousness were discussed earlier in this chapter and are summarized in Box 27-3.

Risk for Infection

The patient who has suffered a head injury may have serious lacerations or abrasions that can admit pathogenic organisms. Intravenous lines and urinary catheters also place the patient at risk for infection. Use Standard Precautions when handling all invasive lines and when dressing wounds. Monitor the patient's temperature and inspect wounds for increasing redness, swelling, or foul drainage. Administer antibiotics as ordered.

Impaired Physical Mobility

After a head injury, the patient may have temporary or permanent motor impairment. While confined to bed,

NURSING CARE PLAN

The Patient with a Head Injury

ASSESSMENT

Health History: Austin Mandrel is a 17-year-old boy who was injured in a motorcycle accident 2 days ago. He reportedly struck his head on the pavement and was unconscious on admission. He is now alert and oriented to person and place but not to time. He asks if he has any permanent injuries. He had a seizure the evening of admission but is now being given anticonvulsants and has had no seizures since. His mother reports that he has had no serious illnesses, hospitalizations, or operations and that he has no known allergies. He is a high school junior and football player. He has two close friends who visit frequently. He is receiving intravenous fluids and antibiotics.

Physical Examination: Vital signs: temperature, 98° F orally; pulse, 62; respiration, 12; blood pressure, 150/84 mm Hg. Sutured laceration on the forehead, abrasions on the forehead and right cheek. Edematous, serosanguineous drainage. Pupils equal and react to light. No drainage from the ears. No stiffness of the neck. Reflexes normal in right extremities but decreased in left extremities. Patient moves left extremities on command, but they are weaker ($\frac{4}{5}$) than the right.

Nursing Diagnosis	Goals and Outcome Criteria	Interventions
Ineffective Tissue Perfusion related to increased intracranial pressure (ICP)	Patient will have adequate cerebral tissue perfusion, as evidenced by alertness and orientation to person, place, and time.	Monitor for signs of increased ICP: decreasing level of consciousness, pupil inequality or dilation without response to light, increasing motor deficits, abnormal posture, fever, increasing blood pressure, bradycardia, respiratory depression. If increased ICP is suspected, notify physician, elevate head of bed as ordered. Monitor rate of fluid administration to ensure adequate cerebral perfusion. Administer diuretics and anti-inflammatory drugs as ordered.
Ineffective Breathing pattern related to increased ICP	Patient will have adequate oxygenation, as evidenced by respiratory rate of 12-20 min with normal arterial blood gas values.	Monitor for changes in level of consciousness (LOC); decreasing respiratory rate and depth; and tachycardia. Check results of arterial blood gas studies.
Risk for Injury related to lethargy, possible seizures	Patient will remain free of injury during hospitalization.	Employ seizure precautions per agency policy. Place bed in low position. Have call bell available and within reach of patient's right hand. Provide assistance with transferring.
Risk for Infection related to traumatic wounds	Patient will remain free of infection, as evidenced by normal temperature and white blood cell count.	Assess temperature for elevation. Assess wounds for increasing redness, edema, and foul drainage. Use Standard Precautions for wound care and when handling invasive equipment. Administer antibiotics as ordered.
Impaired Physical Mobility related to neuromuscular impairment, lethargy	Patient will retain normal range of motion in all extremities and will participate in activities to restore strength to left extremities.	Explain importance of frequent position changes (at least q 2 hr) and assist patient to do so. Position affected extremities in functional alignment. Assist in active range-of-motion exercises at least three times a day. Apply antiembolism stockings as ordered. Assess skin, especially bony prominences, for signs of pressure or breakdown. Monitor elimination to detect urinary retention or constipation. Encourage fluids and high-fiber diet as needed.
Disturbed Body Image related to loss of function	Patient will adapt to altered body function, as reflected in positive statements about self.	Encourage patient to ask questions and to express thoughts and feelings about injuries. Include him in planning sessions. Show acceptance through touch and genuine interest. Encourage friends to continue visits. Explain helping process and how rehabilitation measures can help. Emphasize abilities rather than disabilities. Promote independence in light of abilities. Refer to support group.
Ineffective Role Performance related to neurologic impairment	Patient will participate in rehabilitation efforts and explore potential new roles and activities.	Explain healing process and how rehabilitation measures can help. As patient improves, help him learn to perform activities of daily living with limitations.

? CRITICAL THINKING QUESTIONS

- How does increased intracranial pressure affect respirations?

- Why would the patient lose consciousness when the ICP is elevated?

Health Promotion Considerations

Preventing Head Injury

Everyone should practice general safety by using:

- Helmets for sports activities such as football, baseball, skydiving, snowboarding and skateboarding
- Helmets for riding bikes and motorcycles
- Seatbelts while in automobiles
- Helmets on job sites for high-risk jobs such as construction and mining

---

the patient should be turned and positioned and encouraged to deep breathe at least every 2 hours. Routinely inspect the skin for signs of pressure or breakdown. Use antiembolism stockings if ordered. Perform range-of-motion exercises, and position joints in functional alignment. Frequently assess urine and bowel elimination to detect retention or constipation. As soon as permitted, assist the patient out of bed and encourage as much activity as possible. Unfortunately, some head-injured patients have permanent impairments that necessitate lifelong care. Care of the immobile patient is covered in detail in Chapter 21.

Disturbed Body Image and Ineffective Role Performance

The losses associated with a serious head injury can render the patient unable to resume usual activities. The injury also may leave disfiguring scars or distorted features. Demonstrate acceptance of the patient through touch and genuine interest. Encourage the patient to ask questions, express concerns, and anticipate problems and solutions. Be realistic about the patient's disabilities while emphasizing abilities.

Patients with serious deficits are usually treated by a team that includes rehabilitation specialists. These experts help the patient regain physical mobility, learn to carry out activities of daily living, learn new job skills, and deal with the emotional trauma of the injury and its effects.

Include the family in the rehabilitation process. In many cases, family members serve as the caregivers after head injury. Carson (1993) described behaviors of family members of patients who had sustained head injuries. Behaviors included providing personal care, obtaining rehabilitation services, providing a safe en-

Put on Your Thinking Cap!

You are caring for a patient with a head injury. The patient has been lethargic most of the day but now seems more difficult to arouse. His vital signs and pupils are the same as they have been. What do you think is your best course of action in this situation?

---

vironment, seeking reminders of the preinjury person, exploring what abilities might be regained, encouraging return to preinjury activities, encouraging active decision making, becoming active members of the rehabilitation team, and staying open to potential gains.

BRAIN TUMORS

Brain tumors account for a relatively small percentage of cancer deaths annually. Brain tumors develop in some cancer patients as a result of metastasis from other primary sites. Tumor cells can spread to the CNS through the blood and CSF.

Not all brain tumors are malignant. Some tumor types, such as the meningioma, a tumorous growth of the meningeal tissue, are often benign. One might assume that benign tumor cells would suggest an excellent chance of complete recovery. However, the invasion of any kind of tumor into normal brain tissue is never insignificant. This invasion can cause significant damage that may prove fatal because of increasing ICP or surgical inaccessibility of the tumor.

Etiology and Risk Factors

The causes of brain tumors are generally unknown, but some appear to be congenital in origin, whereas others may be related to heredity. In addition, drug influences and environmental factors may play a role in the development of some brain tumors.

Signs and Symptoms

The signs and symptoms of brain tumors are directly related to the area of the brain that is invaded by the tumor. Motor and sensory symptoms, visual disturbances, and headache all may be early manifestations of tumor growth. New-onset seizure activity in an adult patient often indicates the presence of a tumor. Cerebellar tumors may cause difficulties with balance and coordination. Other tumors, depending on their location, may involve cranial nerves.

Medical Treatment

Management of the patient with a brain tumor depends on the type of cells present in the tumor. Surgery can be done to remove as much of the tumor tissue as possible. If the tumor is malignant, surgery is often followed by radiation therapy with or without chemotherapy.

NURSING CARE *of the Patient with a Brain Tumor*

Nursing care of the patient with a brain tumor depends on the specific deficits, treatment, and prognosis and may be similar to the care of the patient with a head injury. Care of the patient with cancer is discussed in Chapter 25.

Assessment

The complete neurologic assessment is summarized in Box 27-2. The assessment is especially important before brain surgery to provide a baseline for comparing postoperative findings.

Nursing Diagnoses, Goals, and Outcome Criteria: Brain Tumor

Nursing diagnoses vary with the patient's specific symptoms and disabilities and the type of treatment employed. Common nursing diagnoses and goals include the following:

NURSING DIAGNOSES	GOALS AND OUTCOME CRITERIA
Acute Pain related to pressure of expanding tumor mass	Pain relief: patient states pain relieved, has relaxed manner
Disturbed Thought Processes related to effects of tumor on brain tissue	Adaptation to altered thinking: improved mental orientation
Disturbed Sensory Perception related to impaired conduction of sensory information	Recognition of disturbed perceptions: absence of injury associated with sensory or perceptual impairment
Impaired Physical Mobility and **Self-Care Deficit** related to motor disturbances, impaired cognition	Accomplishment of activities of daily living: maximum possible patient mobility level and absence of complications of immobility (contractures, pneumonia, constipation, urinary retention)
Ineffective Coping related to life-threatening disease, changes in behavior function	Effective coping: patient and family make positive statements about ability to deal with the illness

Interventions

Acute Pain

Document pain, and administer analgesics as ordered. Codeine or acetaminophen is often used. Small doses of morphine also may be used for pain relief. If pain relief is not achieved, inform the physician and assess for signs of increased ICP.

Disturbed Thought Processes

Monitor for changes in cognitive function by assessing orientation and response to instructions. Patients may demonstrate cognitive dysfunction, including impaired short-term memory, poor judgment, poor decision making, and impaired problem solving. Investigate *sudden* changes in mental status that may be caused by the tumor or by correctable factors such as drugs, hypoxia, and fluid and electrolyte imbalances. Listen carefully to the patient and present reality in a straightforward manner. Devices to help the patient maintain orientation include clocks, calendars, and seasonal decorations.

Disturbed Sensory Perception

Explain that the effects of the brain tumor may cause unusual sensations and perceptual disturbances. Implement safety measures as needed to prevent injury due to impaired vision, spatial perceptual problems, or sensation.

Impaired Physical Mobility and Self-Care Deficits

Patients with brain tumors may have varying degrees of physical impairment. Assess the patient's ability to perform activities of daily living, and provide assistance as needed. Encourage the patient to remain as active as possible. If the patient's mobility is severely impaired, there is a high risk for disuse syndrome and the associated complications. Care of the immobilized patient is described in Chapter 21.

Ineffective Coping

You must assist the patient and family in dealing with a difficult diagnosis in addition to the obvious residual physical effects. A diagnosis of a malignant brain tumor is devastating for the family, and emotional support is vital to help them understand the nature of the disease and the anticipated problems and outcomes. Nursing care depends on the specific deficits, treatment, and prognosis and may be similar to the care of the patient with a head injury. Care of the patient with cancer is discussed in Chapter 25.

INFECTIOUS AND INFLAMMATORY CONDITIONS

Meningitis

Meningitis is inflammation of the meningeal coverings of the brain and spinal cord caused by either viruses or bacteria. Organisms may reach the meninges through the blood, through head wounds, or from other cranial structures such as the sinuses or inner ear. A number of organisms may be responsible for bacterial infection, including *Neisseria meningitidis, Streptococcus pneumoniae,* and *Haemophilus influenzae.*

Complications of meningitis include seizures, septicemia, vasomotor collapse, and increased ICP. *Neisseria meningitidis* is particularly problematic because septicemia develops in approximately 10% of patients.

Signs and Symptoms

The common signs and symptoms of meningitis are generally related to meningeal irritation. These include headache, nuchal rigidity (stiffness of the back of the neck), irritability, diminished level of consciousness, photophobia (sensitivity to light), hypersensitivity, and seizure activity. The presence of Kernig's sign and Brudzinski's sign also is indicative of meningeal irritation. To assess for Kernig's sign (Fig. 27-16, *A*), flex the patient's hip to a 90-degree angle and then extend the knee. In the presence of a meningeal infection, this movement produces pain in the hamstring area. Brudzinski's sign (Fig. 27-16, *B*) is flexion of both hips when the examiner flexes the patient's neck.

FIGURE **27-16 A,** Positive Kernig's sign: When the patient's leg is flexed as shown, the patient is unable to completely extend the leg. **B,** Brudzinski's sign: When the nurse flexes the patient's neck, hip flexion occurs.

Medical Diagnosis

A lumbar puncture is done to obtain a CSF sample for laboratory analysis. The sample is examined to detect the presence of microorganisms in the CSF and to identify the infecting organism. With bacterial meningitis, the CSF appears milky and purulent because of white blood cells suspended in the fluid.

Medical Treatment

Management of bacterial meningitis requires prompt recognition and treatment with antimicrobials. In severe infections, broad-spectrum antimicrobials such as penicillin G are initiated immediately. Changes in therapy may be made when the results of culture and sensitivity tests are reported. Bacterial infections usually respond to antimicrobial therapy, but there are no specific drugs effective against most viral infections of the CNS. Anticonvulsants are used to control seizure activity if necessary.

If needed, Isolation Precautions should be initiated. Organisms responsible for meningococcal meningitis are spread by the respiratory route, and appropriate safeguards must be employed to protect other patients, family, and staff (see Chapter 13).

NURSING CARE *of the Patient with Meningitis*

Assessment

The routine neurologic assessment is summarized in Box 27-2. When a patient has meningitis, assess vital signs and neurologic status frequently to determine further deterioration or the onset of complications. See the Health Promotion Considerations box on p. 444.

Nursing Diagnoses, Goals, and Outcome Criteria: Meningitis	
NURSING DIAGNOSES	GOALS AND OUTCOME CRITERIA
Altered Tissue Perfusion related to increased ICP	Adequate cerebral tissue perfusion: vital signs and level of consciousness consistent with patient norms
Ineffective Breathing Pattern related to depression of the respiratory center	Adequate oxygenation: respiratory rate of 12 to 20/min
Acute Pain related to irritation of meninges and increased ICP	Pain relief: patient states pain has been relieved, relaxed manner
Risk for Injury related to confusion, seizures, restlessness	Absence of injury: no falls or other trauma
Deficient Fluid Volume related to vomiting and fever	Normal fluid balance without vomiting or fever: fluid intake and output approximately equal, moist mucous membranes, blood pressure within patient norms
Risk for Disuse Syndrome related to bed rest	Absence of complications of immobility: clear breath sounds, intact skin, normal muscle strength and joint mobility, regular bowel movements without straining

Interventions

Ineffective Tissue Perfusion

Elevate the head of the patient's bed as ordered. Instruct the patient to avoid coughing and not to hold his or her breath during turning, because these behaviors increase ICP. Do not use restraints unless they are absolutely necessary. Monitor for signs of increasing ICP: decreased level of consciousness, headache, nausea, vomiting, abnormal pupillary responses, and respiratory depression. If ICP does increase, administer prescribed treatments (e.g., diuretics, barbiturates, opioids). Measures to lower the body temperature may be ordered to reduce the metabolic rate.

Ineffective Breathing Pattern

Monitor the respiratory status and gag and swallowing reflexes. Position the patient to maintain a patent airway, and suction if necessary. Arterial blood samples are drawn and analyzed for gas values as ordered. Report a decreasing respiratory rate to the physician.

Acute Pain

Assess the location and severity of any discomfort. Nursing measures to decrease pain include position changes, massage, and a quiet environment. Give analgesics as ordered, and document their effect. Chapter 15 provides additional information about the nursing management of pain.

Risk for Injury

Because of the prevailing risk of seizures, take appropriate precautions to ensure patient safety. A subdued environment should be maintained to reduce irritability and contribute to patient comfort. Keep the bed in a low position, with the side rails padded and raised. Reorient the patient to the setting as needed, and keep the call bell within easy reach. Remind patients who are dizzy not to get up without assistance.

Deficient Fluid Volume

Monitor the patient's vital signs, tissue turgor and moisture, and fluid intake and output. Weight may be measured daily to assess fluid status. Encourage oral fluid intake if it is permitted and if the patient is alert. Provide intravenous fluid therapy as ordered, and monitor to ensure the correct flow rate. Antipyretics may be ordered for fever and antiemetics for vomiting.

Risk for Disuse Syndrome

The patient who is confined to bed is at risk for all the complications of immobility, especially stasis of pulmonary secretions, pressure sores, muscle weakness, joint stiffness, and constipation. Measures to prevent these complications are discussed in detail in Chapter 21.

Encephalitis

Encephalitis is inflammation of brain tissue that is usually caused by one of several viruses. These viruses may be prevalent during certain times of the year or in a specific geographic area. For example,

certain types of mosquitoes found in the United States are carriers of a virus commonly associated with encephalitis. In addition, toxic substances or other types of viral infections, such as herpes simplex, may precipitate encephalitis.

Signs and Symptoms

The patient with encephalitis presents with symptoms directly related to the area of the brain that is involved. Fever, nuchal rigidity (stiff neck), headache, confusion, delirium, agitation, and restlessness are commonly seen. However, the patient also may become comatose or exhibit aphasia, hemiparesis, facial weakness, and other alterations in motor activity.

Medical Treatment

Care for the patient with encephalitis is focused on enhancing patient comfort and increasing strength. Because seizure activity is a potential problem, you must take appropriate safety precautions.

NURSING CARE *of the Patient with Encephalitis*

The nursing plan of care parallels that of the patient with meningitis.

GUILLAIN-BARRÉ SYNDROME

Although its specific cause is unknown, Guillain-Barré syndrome is believed to be an autoimmune response to a viral infection. It is a rapidly progressing disease that affects the motor component of the peripheral nervous system. Although the spinal nerves are usually affected, the cranial nerves also may be involved.

Patients with Guillain-Barré syndrome often report some recent viral infection or vaccination. This apparently triggers an autoimmune response that destroys the myelin sheath around the peripheral nerves, slowing the conduction of impulses across the involved nerves.

Signs and Symptoms

Guillain-Barré syndrome has three phases: initial, plateau, and recovery, as described in Table 27-4. The initial phase is characterized by symmetric muscle weakness that typically begins in the lower extremities and ascends to the trunk and upper extremities. The disease process may affect cranial nerves, resulting in visual and hearing disturbances, difficulty chewing, and lack of facial expression. The muscles of respiration also may be affected, resulting in the need for mechanical ventilation.

Mild paresthesias (abnormal sensations) or anesthesia (numbness) in the feet and hands may be present in a glove or stocking distribution pattern. In addition, some patients experience pain associated with the sensory changes. Despite all the motor and sensory changes, level of consciousness and intellectual functioning remain unchanged.

Table 27-4 | *Phases of Guillain-Barré Syndrome*

PHASE	CHARACTERISTICS	DURATION
Initial	Begins with onset of symptoms Ends when disease ceases to progress	Usually 1-3 wk
Plateau	No further changes; neither deterioration nor improvement	Several days to 2 wk
Recovery	Gradual improvement	May be as long as 2 yr; some residual effects may be permanent

Effects on the autonomic nervous system may include hypertension, orthostatic hypotension, cardiac dysrhythmias, profuse sweating, paralytic ileus, and urinary retention. Dysautonomia, characterized by the effects just mentioned, occurs most frequently in patients with respiratory involvement and is potentially life-threatening.

In the plateau phase, the patient with Guillain-Barré syndrome remains essentially unchanged. There is no further neurologic deterioration, but there is no improvement either.

As recovery begins and progresses, remyelinization occurs and muscle strength returns in a proximal to distal pattern (head to toes). Because the underlying axon generally remains undamaged, approximately 95% of patients with Guillain-Barré syndrome have a nearly complete recovery. Others have residual numbness, stiffness, or paresis.

Medical Diagnosis

The characteristic onset and pattern of ascending motor involvement provide the basis for the diagnosis of Guillain-Barré syndrome. An elevated protein level in the CSF obtained by lumbar puncture provides additional evidence for the diagnosis. Nerve conduction velocity studies reveal slowed conduction speed in the involved nerves.

Medical Treatment

Management during the acute phase of the illness is directed at preserving vital function, particularly respiration. Respiratory status is closely monitored and mechanical ventilation initiated if the vital capacity falls to 15 mL/kg of body weight. Massive doses of corticosteroids may be prescribed to suppress the inflammatory process.

Because Guillain-Barré syndrome is believed to be an autoimmune disease, plasmapheresis has emerged as a major treatment intervention. Plasmapheresis is a process in which blood is removed, centrifuged, and returned to the patient. In the process, antibodies that trigger the autoimmune disease are removed from the blood by a machine equipped with a special filtration system. The patient with Guillain-Barré syndrome generally undergoes a series of treatments, ideally delivered within 7 to 14 days after the onset of the disease. Those patients benefiting from plasmapheresis often recover faster.

NURSING CARE *of the Patient with Guillain-Barré Syndrome*

Assessment

Assessment of the patient with a neurologic disorder is summarized in Box 27-2. When Guillain-Barré syndrome is suspected, the health history describes the progression of symptoms. Note the patient's fears, coping strategies, and sources of support. Record information about important social data such as occupation and family roles and responsibilities. The physical examination focuses on cranial nerve, motor, respiratory, and cardiovascular function.

Nursing Diagnoses, Goals, and Outcome Criteria: Guillain-Barré Syndrome

NURSING DIAGNOSES	GOALS AND OUTCOME CRITERIA
Ineffective Breathing Pattern related to neurologic impairment	Adequate oxygenation: normal arterial blood gases and skin color
Decreased Cardiac Output related to labile blood pressure, cardiac dysrhythmias	Normal cardiac output: regular pulse with rate of 60 to 100 beats/min and blood pressure consistent with patient norms
Risk for Disuse Syndrome related to motor impairment	Absence of complications of immobility: intact skin, no contractures, clear breath sounds, regular bowel movements
Imbalanced Nutrition: Less Than Body Requirements related to dysphagia, endotracheal tube	Adequate nutrition: stable body weight
Risk for Injury related to loss of sensation in hands and feet, motor impairment, inability to speak	Absence of injury in affected body areas: no falls, bruises, corneal damage, or other injuries
Anxiety related to paralysis, doubts about recovery, loss of verbal communication	Decreased anxiety: patient states anxiety is reduced, calm manner
Deficient Knowledge of Guillain-Barré syndrome and its treatment	Knowledge of Guillain-Barré syndrome and its treatment: patient confirms understanding and (if possible) demonstrates self-care

Interventions

Ineffective Breathing Pattern

About 25% of patients with Guillain-Barré syndrome need mechanical ventilation because of neuromuscular failure. Assess the patient's oxygenation status frequently. A respiratory rate greater than 30, abnormal chest and abdominal movements, and decreasing vital capacity signal increasingly ineffective breathing. Turn the patient at least every 2 hours, and suction when indicated by increased pulse or adventitious breath sounds.

Decreased Cardiac Output

Be alert to rapid or slow cardiac dysrhythmias and administer antidysrhythmic drugs as ordered.

Risk for Disuse Syndrome

Immobility is a major issue to address in the patient with Guillain-Barré syndrome. If mobility is severely impaired, the patient is at high risk for disuse syndrome. These patients generally benefit from the use of rotational bed therapy to help promote pulmonary hygiene, peristalsis, and urinary bladder emptying. Careful positioning is crucial, with emphasis on maintaining joint function, muscle tone, and range of motion. Active and passive exercises, splints, and continuous passive motion machines may be used to prevent contractures.

Risk for Injury

Progressive weakness makes the patient susceptible to falls. When the patient is in bed, raise the side rails, place the call bell within reach, and put the bed in low position. If the eyes do not close completely, apply ophthalmic drops or ointments as ordered. A moisture chamber for the eye is used to prevent eye injury from excessive drying. Carefully inspect the skin, especially areas without sensation, to detect pressure or injury.

Imbalanced Nutrition: Less Than Body Requirements

Impaired swallowing or the presence of an endotracheal tube mandates an alternative means of feeding. Enteral feedings are usually provided by way of a gastrostomy or nasoduodenal tube. Feedings may be given continuously or intermittently. Elevate the head of the bed 30 degrees during feedings to reduce the risk of aspiration. Aspirate and measure the residual (amount of feeding remaining in the stomach) at intervals to assess emptying of the stomach and prevent overfilling. In some cases, total parenteral nutrition may be employed.

Anxiety

Anxiety is understandable with progressive paralysis and increasing dependence on others for basic needs. You must work to develop trust and establish a therapeutic relationship with the patient. If the patient is able to speak, encourage discussion of thoughts, fears, and feelings. Explore previously used coping strategies. To promote some sense of control, give the patient some choices about aspects of care. Explain equipment and procedures to the patient. Other strategies to reduce anxiety include the use of imagery, music, deep breathing (if possible), and controlling anxiety-producing thoughts. Boredom is a problem that must be considered for the patient with Guillain-Barré syndrome. Orienting devices such as clocks, calendars, and daily schedules are helpful. The patient may enjoy television, radio, CDs, and visits from friends and family.

One source of anxiety for many patients is impaired communication. While the patient is able to speak, establish a system of communication such as blinking (one blink means *yes*, two blinks mean *no*) or a communication board. Then, if the condition does affect speech or if mechanical ventilation is required, the patient will have a simple means of expression.

Deficient Knowledge

From admission through rehabilitation, the patient with Guillain-Barré syndrome needs education about the condition and its usual course. Patients can deal with the condition better if they know how the symptoms progress and that reversal and improvement are expected.

Rehabilitation

As function is restored, emphasis is placed on both respiratory and physical rehabilitation. Total recovery of respiratory function determines how quickly physical rehabilitation can begin. Once rehabilitation is initiated, attention must be devoted to maximizing motor function through exercises and occupational therapy. Because complete recovery may take several years, a prolonged rehabilitation period is sometimes necessary. Before the patient is discharged from the hospital, referrals may be made to rehabilitation or home health agencies as appropriate. The patient and family may benefit from a support group for people with long-term or chronic illnesses. The Guillain-Barré Foundation is a source of information (telephone number: 1-610-667-0131; website: www.guillain-barre.com).

PARKINSON'S SYNDROME

Parkinson's syndrome is a progressive degenerative disorder of the basal ganglia that results in an eventual loss of coordination and control over involuntary motor movement. It is generally recognized as a disease

---

🌸 Consider the Alternative

Strategies to reduce anxiety include music therapy and massage. The herb *valerian* is used by some people as a sedative; its safety is under study.

of older adults, first appearing in individuals in their 50s, with men affected more often than women. Idiopathic Parkinson's syndrome has no known cause but is related to decreased levels of dopamine in the basal ganglia. A deficiency of dopamine, a neurotransmitter, contributes to the loss of motor function. Other types of parkinsonism are caused by atherosclerosis, the long-term use of phenothiazines, and some toxins.

Signs and Symptoms

Several symptoms are characteristic of Parkinson's syndrome. The major triad of symptoms is tremor, rigidity, and bradykinesia. Tremor is a trembling or shaking type of movement most often seen in the upper extremities of the patient with Parkinson's syndrome. Tremors are more pronounced during resting postures and often relieved by movement. Typically they disappear during sleep. A movement associated with the tremor is pill rolling, in which the tremor repetitively moves the individual's thumb against the fingertips as if rolling a small object. Rigidity is stiffness, and *bradykinesia* refers to extremely slow movements. Other signs and symptoms are loss of dexterity and power in affected limbs, aching, monotone voice, handwriting changes, drooling, lack of facial expression, rhythmic head nodding, reduced blinking, and slumped posture. Those with advanced disease demonstrate cogwheel rigidity (jerky movements with passive muscle stretching) and gait disturbances. The individual may appear to freeze and may have difficulty initiating the action of walking. Depression is common, and dementia develops in some patients. Figure 27-17 illustrates the typical facial appearance, posture, and gait of individuals with Parkinson's syndrome.

Medical Diagnosis

Parkinson's syndrome is diagnosed from the health history and the physical examination results. MRI may be done to rule out other causes of the symptoms.

Medical Treatment

Management of the patient with Parkinson's syndrome is directed toward controlling the symptoms with physical therapy and drug therapy. The most beneficial physical therapy programs incorporate massage, heat, exercise, and gait retraining. Speech therapy has been used with swallowing issues as well as difficulty with speech with variable results.

Drug therapy relieves many of the symptoms of the disease. Early in the course of the disease, dopamine receptor agonists *pramipexole* (Mirapex) or *ropinirole* (Requip) are used to maximize the intrinsic dopamine. The cornerstone of therapy is the use of L-dopa (L-dihydroxyphenylalanine). L-dopa can cross the blood-brain barrier and is converted to dopamine in the basal ganglia, thereby supplementing levels of the neurotransmitter and reducing the symptoms of the disease. The conversion of L-dopa to dopamine

Tremor

Stooped posture

Masklike facies

Rigidity

Arms flexed at elbows and wrists

Tremor

Hips and knees slightly flexed

Short, shuffling steps

FIGURE 27-17 Clinical manifestations of Parkinson's syndrome.

must occur in the basal ganglia and not in the peripheral tissue. To ensure this, inhibitors are administered to prevent the breakdown of L-dopa by decarboxylase enzymes. The decarboxylase inhibitor most commonly used is carbidopa. It is frequently given in combination as carbidopa/levadopa (Sinemet). When the two drugs are used in combination, therapeutic levels may be achieved with lower dosages. Carbidopa/levadopa also comes in orally-disintegrating tablets (Parcopa; Carbilev). The enzyme catechol *O*-methyltransferase (COMT) also breaks down levodopa in the peripheral circulation. Entacapone (Comtan) blocks this break down and prolongs the effectiveness of carbidopa/levadopa (Sinemet). Carbidopa/levadopa/entacapone (Stalevo) provides maximum blocking in the peripheral circulation and decreases the number of pills taken at one time. Because the benefits of L-dopa tend to decline after about 2 years, various other drug combinations may be used in an effort to control symptoms. Selegiline hydrochloride (Eldepryl), a monoamine oxidase (MAO) inhibitor, is used with Sinemet. MAO is the enzyme that degrades dopamine. Selegiline hydrochloride increases the available dopamine.

Anticholinergic drugs such as trihexyphenidyl (Artane) and benztropine (Cogentin) may be used in patients who have less severe symptoms or who are unresponsive to L-dopa. These are useful in managing tremors. Although the exact mechanism of action is unclear, amantadine (Symmetrel), an antiviral compound, also is used in the management of Parkinson's syndrome. Amantadine is thought to release dopamine from storage sites in the neurons. It is often used in combination with L-dopa.

Treatment for depression may include antidepressant drug therapy, psychotherapy, and electroconvulsive therapy. Additional information about drug therapy is presented in the Drug Therapy table on pp. 431 and 432.

Several surgical procedures, among them thalamotomy, thalamic stimulation, and pallidotomy, may be used to treat parkinsonism, although the benefits are variable. Surgical implantation of fetal dopamine-producing cells continues to be done experimentally. Adrenal medullary transplant entails implantation of the patient's own adrenal cells into the brain. It has produced limited improvement in some patients and is not widely accepted. All of these surgical procedures are considered palliative rather than curative.

 Put on Your Thinking Cap!

Write a short teaching plan for a home health patient who has started taking selegiline (Eldepryl) for Parkinson's syndrome.

NURSING CARE *of the Patient with Parkinson's Syndrome*

Nursing management for the patient with Parkinson's syndrome is primarily related to maintaining mobility and preventing injury.

Assessment

The complete neurologic assessment is summarized in Box 27-2. The health history of a patient with Parkinson's syndrome should specifically include assessment for weakness, fatigue, muscle cramps, sweating, dysphagia, constipation, difficulty voiding, and unusual movements. Describe the effects of the disease on the patient's life. During the physical examination, be alert for lack of facial expression, eyes fixed in one direction, drooling, slurred speech, tearing, tremors, muscle stiffness, and poor balance and coordination.

As the disease progresses, the patient becomes more immobilized, requiring additional nursing diagnoses, as addressed in Chapter 21.

Nursing Diagnoses, Goals, and Outcome Criteria: Parkinson's Syndrome	
NURSING DIAGNOSES	GOALS AND OUTCOME CRITERIA
Impaired Physical Mobility and **Self-Care Deficit** related to neuromuscular disease	Maximum possible self-care: patient participates in prescribed exercise program and performs self-care within abilities
Risk for Injury related to poor balance and coordination	Absence of injury: no bruises, lacerations, or fractures due to trauma
Imbalanced Nutrition: Less Than Body Requirements related to dysphagia, difficulty with self-feeding	Adequate nutritional intake: stable body weight
Ineffective Coping related to physical changes and effects of disease on lifestyle	Effective coping with disease effects: patient makes statements confirming ability to deal with condition, adheres to plan of care
Deficient Knowledge of disease, management, and self-care	Compliance with the prescribed plan of care: patient correctly describes and adheres to drug therapy, demonstrates exercise routine, uses resources, adapts to continue self-care

Interventions

Impaired Physical Mobility

Assess the patient's mobility and ability to perform self-care. Provide assistance as needed, but encourage the patient to remain as independent in self-care as possible. Assistive devices, including walkers and wheelchairs, may enable the patient to be mobile despite some deterioration in coordination and balance. Stress the value of exercise in maintaining strength and mobility. Active and passive range-of-motion exercises may be done. Both the physical therapist and the occupational therapist may participate in designing programs to maintain or improve function.

Suggestions to improve mobility with Parkinson's syndrome include the following:

- Scoot to the edge of a chair before trying to stand.
- Use satin sheets to make it easier to move in and out of bed.
- March in place before starting to walk.
- Practice lifting the foot as if to step over an object on the floor to initiate walking.

Risk for Injury

The patient with Parkinson's syndrome is at special risk for injury related to falls. Place the call bell within easy reach and instruct the patient to call for assistance when getting up. If the patient is ambulatory, remove obstacles on the floor. Recommend firm shoes, which provide better support than soft slippers. Provide assistive devices (canes, walkers, wheelchairs) as needed. Allow the patient to move at his or her own speed to decrease the risk of injury. Because this is a chronic condition, the patient's home setting should be evaluated and adapted for safe ambulation.

Imbalanced Nutrition: Less Than Body Requirements

To promote ease of swallowing, position the patient comfortably for meals, with the head elevated and food conveniently arranged. Provide assistance as needed. It may involve only cutting meat and opening containers or may entail actually feeding the patient. Do not rush patients while they are eating. If the patient chokes on liquids, consult the dietitian about the need for semisolids and thick liquids, which are often easier to swallow. Thickening agents can be added to thin fluids to facilitate swallowing. Small, frequent meals may be better tolerated than three large ones. Monitor the patient's weight to assess the adequacy of nutritional intake. Some researchers believe that Parkinson's patients benefit from a low-protein diet during the day and an evening meal high in protein, but this is still experimental.

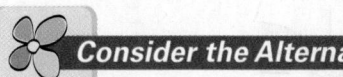

Consider the Alternative

St. John's wort is used widely as an antidepressant. It is an MAO inhibitor and can interact with prescribed drugs. Ask the patient to report use of herbal remedies to the physician. Other measures to treat depression are physical exercise, massage, and light therapy.

Ineffective Coping

Patients with Parkinson's syndrome must deal with loss of mobility that may affect their jobs, home and family responsibilities, social relationships, and leisure activities. Voice changes may severely impair verbal communication. Explore how the patient is dealing with these changes. Nurses and other members of the health care team help the patient identify strategies to adapt to changing abilities. Be alert to expressions of depression and inform the physician of such findings. A referral may be made to a mental health counselor, clinical nurse specialist, or support group. Administer antidepressant drugs as ordered and monitor their effects.

Deficient Knowledge

Management of this progressive condition requires the patient or a caregiver to be knowledgeable about Parkinson's syndrome and how it is treated. Supplement

Patients with Parkinson's Syndrome

Patients with Parkinson's syndrome and those who interact with them should receive the following interventions as necessary:

- Maintain general health and have regular checkups
- Follow a regular routine of stretching and exercise to maintain mobility and balance
- Prevent falls through environmental control

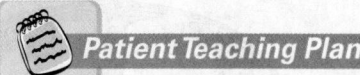

Parkinson's Syndrome

- Drugs relieve symptoms but do not cure Parkinson's syndrome. You must continue therapy as prescribed to control symptoms.
- Know your drug names, dosages, schedule, and adverse effects that should be reported to your physician.
- Exercise is essential to maintain mobility.
- Resources: American Parkinson Disease Association (1-800-223-2732); Parkinson's Disease Foundation (1-222-923-4700, website: www.parkinsons-foundation. org); National Parkinson Foundation, Inc. (1-800-34545), website: http://www.parkinson.org).

Consider the Alternative

Caution patients with Parkinson's syndrome not to use herbal supplements without physician approval. Kava can worsen symptoms of Parkinson's syndrome. Chaste tree fruit interferes with the drug *selegiline*. Indian snakeroot interferes with the actions of levodopa and carbidopa.

information with written material. See the Health Promotion Considerations box below.

MULTIPLE SCLEROSIS

A chronic, progressive degenerative disease, multiple sclerosis (MS) attacks the protective myelin sheath around axons and disrupts the conduction of impulses through the CNS (Fig. 27-18). It may affect motor, sensory, cerebellar, and other pathways. The course of the disease is variable. Several patterns have been identified. The disease may progress steadily (chronic, progressive MS); may be characterized by exacerbations and remissions (exacerbating-remitting MS); may have less stable periods than exacerbating-remitting (relapsing-progressive MS); or may become stable with no active disease for at least a year (stable MS). MS is the second most common neurologic cause of disability. The incidence is highest in persons between 20 and 40 years of age and affects women more often than men.

Etiology

Although the exact cause of MS is unknown, viral infections and autoimmune processes have been implicated. Some studies have implicated a retrovirus in the disease process, but more research is needed to determine whether this is indeed the cause of MS. The myelin sheath surrounding the axons is destroyed, eventually leaving areas of sclerotic tissues (see Fig. 27-18). As the sclerotic tissue develops, the patient may have a period of remission. The involved fibers eventually degenerate, resulting in permanent damage. Nerve impulses, then, are no longer able to travel down the affected axon.

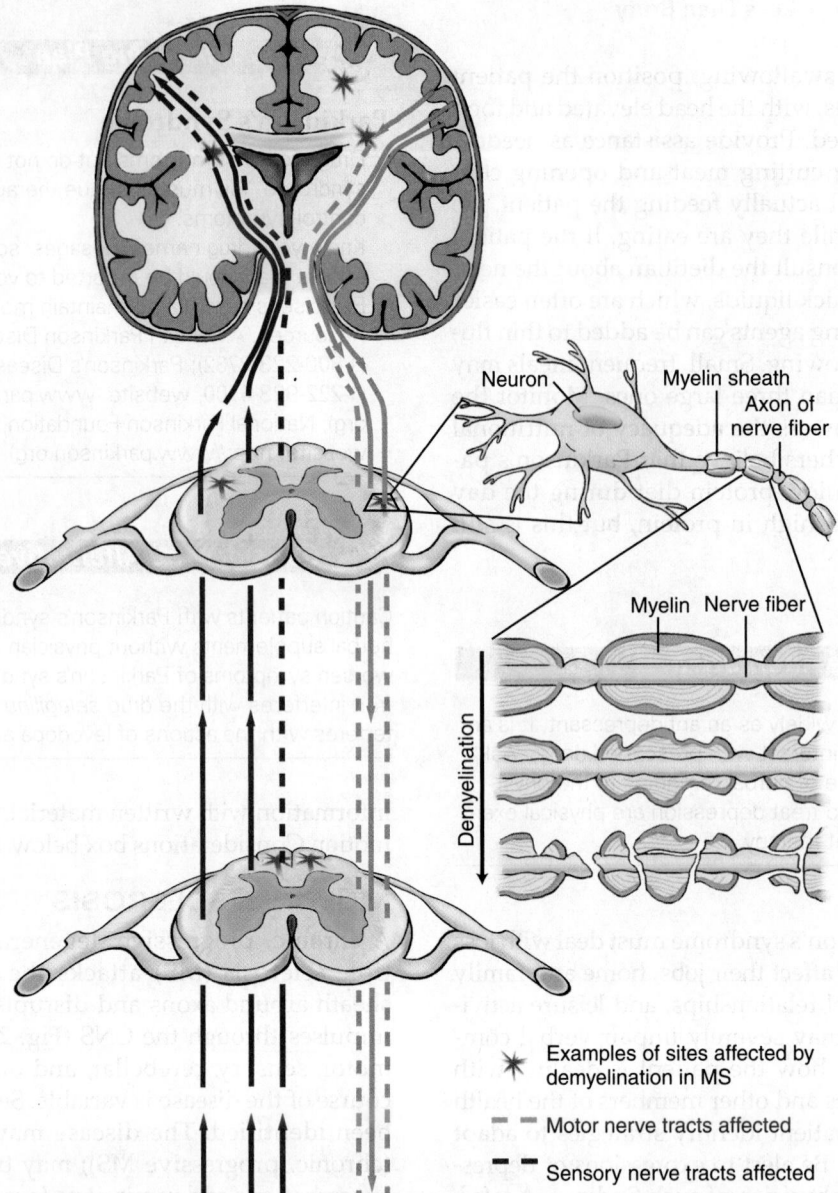

Neuron
Myelin sheath
Axon of
nerve fiber

Myelin   Nerve fiber

Demyelination

✳ Examples of sites affected by demyelination in MS

— — Motor nerve tracts affected

■ ■ ■ Sensory nerve tracts affected

FIGURE **27-18** The lesions in multiple sclerosis: location and effects.

Signs and Symptoms

Because the exact pattern of damage varies from patient to patient, the signs and symptoms are varied as well. The most common symptoms of MS are fatigue, weakness and tingling in one or more extremities, visual disturbances, problems with coordination, bowel and bladder dysfunction, spasticity, and depression.

For patients who have exacerbating-remitting MS, the progression is variable. As the disease progresses, the periods of remission become shorter and the neurologic deficits present during exacerbations become more severe and permanent.

Medical Diagnosis

The diagnosis of MS is based primarily on the physical examination and history of cyclic remission-exacerbation periods. A familial history of the disease is significant, as is worsening of symptoms when the

patient is exposed to warm weather. Magnetic resonance imaging of the brain and spinal cord may reveal plaques characteristic of MS.

Medical Treatment

Because of its chronic, progressive nature, the treatment of MS is symptomatic and supportive. Drug therapy during periods of exacerbation may involve administration of adrenocorticotropic hormone. Corticosteroids (ACTH, Prednisone, Methylprednisolone) may be used to control exacerbations, but they do not slow the progression of the disease. Treatment often includes drugs that modulate the immune response and thus the course of the disease. The specific drug will depend on the type of MS. Drugs in this category include interferon β 1b (Betaseron) and interferon 1a (Avonex). Glatiramer acetate (Copaxone) is an immune modulator that is unrelated to interferon. Immunosuppressants such as mitoxantrone (Novantrone) also are used for exacerbations. When immunosuppressive agents are used, patients must be carefully monitored for bone marrow suppression. The spasticity experienced by MS patients may respond to treatment with baclofen (Lioresal) or tizanidine (Zanaflex). Carbamazepine (Tegretol) and gabapentin (Neurontin) are used to relieve neuropathic pain. Amantadine (Symmetrel) is used to relieve fatigue associated with the disease. Electrical neuromuscular stimulation is being used to decrease spasticity and improve active movement and function, but studies of its effectiveness have not found consistent evidence of improvement. Urinary retention is treated with cholinergics such as bethanechol (Urecholine) or neostigmine (Prostigmine). Urinary frequency and urgency resulting from spasticity of the bladder can be treated with anticholinergics such as propantheline bromide (Pro-Banthine) or oxybutynin (Ditropan). Tolterodine (Detrol) is a competitive muscarinic receptor antagonist and is more specific for bladder than oxybutynin.

NURSING CARE *of the Patient with Multiple Sclerosis*

Assessment

Complete assessment of the patient with a neurologic disorder is summarized in Box 27-2. When a patient has MS, the health history specifically includes the onset and progression of symptoms, especially those that affect mobility, vision, eating, and elimination. Explore the effects of the disease on the person's lifestyle (see the Health Promotion Considerations box below). Identify the patient's usual coping strategies. Important aspects of the physical examination are evaluation of range of motion and strength and observation for gait abnormalities, tremors, and muscle spasms.

Nursing Diagnoses, Goals, and Outcome Criteria: Multiple Sclerosis	
NURSING DIAGNOSES	GOALS AND OUTCOME CRITERIA
Impaired Physical Mobility related to weakness or spasticity	Maximal possible mobility: patient continues physical activity within capabilities
Disturbed Sensory Perception related to neurologic impairment	Absence of injury associated with impaired sensation: intact skin without redness related to pressure, no falls
Self-Care Deficit related to impaired voluntary movements and poor coordination	Achievement of self-care: activities of daily living completed independently or with assistance as needed
Functional Urinary Incontinence related to impaired conduction of bladder nerve impulses	Absence of bladder distention: bladder not palpable, no uncontrolled passage of urine
Risk for Infection related to inadequate resistance	Absence of infection: normal body temperature and white blood cell count

Ineffective Coping related to chronic illness, uncertain course of disease	Adaptation to changes in physical functioning: behavior and statements reflect intent to maximize abilities
Deficient Knowledge of disease, treatment, and self-care	Patient understands disease, treatment, and self-care: patient accurately describes MS, its treatment, and self-care measures to reduce risk of complications

Interventions

Impaired Physical Mobility

Encourage the patient to be as independent as possible. Provide assistance with ambulation as needed. A cane or walker may enable the patient to walk safely. If the patient has muscle spasms, administer muscle relaxants as ordered. Perform range-of-motion exercises to prevent contractures, and teach a caregiver to do the exercises. Physical therapy may be ordered. The patient who is not able to move independently is at risk for disuse syndrome. If the patient becomes disabled to this extent, decisions must be made about home nursing services or care in a long-term facility.

Disturbed Sensory Perceptions

If the patient has impaired sensation, give special attention to the skin. Inspect extremities and pressure points for signs of pressure or trauma. Encourage the patient to wear shoes when out of bed to prevent injury. Other measures instituted to prevent injury include using caution with sources of heat and cold.

Self-Care Deficit

Encourage patients to do as much as they can for themselves. Provide assistance as needed to carry out activities of daily living. Difficulty with feedings, especially if the patient is dysphagic, may result in inadequate food intake. Alternative means of feeding may be necessary. Discuss with the patient and family their needs for assistance with caregiving. Home nursing care can support the patient who wishes to remain in a home setting.

 Health Promotion Considerations

Patients with Multiple Sclerosis

Patients with multiple sclerosis should receive the following interventions as necessary:

- Maintain general health through diet and exercise
- Avoid or minimize effects of triggers for multiple sclerosis such as infections, trauma, climate changes, and immunizations
- Seek regular medical checkups for disease prevention

Functional Urinary Incontinence

Palpate the patient's lower abdomen for bladder distention. Carry out intermittent catheterization as ordered. If urine retention is a problem, assess the patient for signs and symptoms of urinary tract infection: fever, burning on urination, foul odor, sediment. If the patient has urinary incontinence, take steps to reduce the incontinent episodes as described in Chapter 23. Incontinence briefs may be needed, and meticulous skin care is a must. Loss of bladder control is very distressing, and you must be sensitive in helping the patient deal with it.

Risk for Infection

The MS patient who is being treated with immunosuppressive drugs has decreased resistance to infection. Take steps to reduce the risk of infection. Protect the patient from people with infections. Encourage intake of fluids to maintain adequate hydration, and emphasize good hygiene practices. Teach the patient and family the signs of infection that should be reported promptly to the physician.

Ineffective Coping

Multiple sclerosis is a chronic, progressive disease. Patients have increasing disability, requiring considerable adaptation. Because the initial symptoms typically occur in young adults, patients must often learn to balance work, home, and family responsibilities. Provide the patient opportunities to talk about the illness and its effects. Be accepting of the patient's concerns, and guide the patient to identify strengths, abilities, and usual coping strategies. With the patient's permission, a referral may be made to the clinical nurse specialist, mental health counselor, or spiritual counselor. Support groups can be helpful to many patients and their families.

Deficient Knowledge

Assess what the patient knows about MS and what he or she would like to know. The teaching plan is individualized to the patient's needs and may include problems associated with immobility and measures to prevent complications.

Consider the Alternative

Imagery, breathing exercises, and progressive relaxation can help the MS patient reduce stress. Various special diets and nutritional supplements (commonly fatty acids, niacin, zinc, magnesium, selenium, beta carotene, and vitamins C, B$_6$, and B$_{12}$) have been proposed, but research has not consistently shown benefits to the MS patient.

AMYOTROPHIC LATERAL SCLEROSIS

Etiology

Amyotrophic lateral sclerosis (ALS), also known as *Lou Gehrig's disease,* is a degenerative neurologic disease.

It affects males two to four times as often as females and strikes most often those between 40 and 70 years of age. The disease generally progresses rapidly, and death ensues approximately 3 years after the onset of symptoms. Although a viral cause has been suspected, the exact cause is unknown.

Pathophysiology

In ALS, there is degeneration of the anterior horn cells and the corticospinal tracts, so the patient exhibits both upper and lower motor neuron symptoms. Evidence of upper motor neuron disease includes spasticity and hyperreflexia. Lower motor neuron disease is demonstrated by weakness, atrophy, cramps, and muscle twitching. Some patients have difficulty swallowing and slurred speech. Despite involvement of the motor nuclei of the brainstem, intellectual ability, sensory perception, vision, and hearing are all unaffected.

Signs and Symptoms

Initially, the patient exhibits weakness of voluntary muscles of the upper extremities, particularly the hands. In addition, some patients may experience difficulty swallowing and speaking because of progressive weakness of the oropharyngeal muscles. Spasticity of the involved muscle groups may be evident. The disease progresses steadily until the patient is completely incapacitated. Eventually, respirations become shallow and the patient has difficulty clearing the airway of pulmonary secretions. Death results from aspiration, respiratory infection, or respiratory failure.

Medical Diagnosis

The patient's history and physical examination findings lead to the diagnosis of ALS. Electromyography provides supporting evidence of impaired impulse conduction in the muscles. More sophisticated tests are used to rule out other degenerative motor diseases such as MS or myasthenia gravis.

Medical Treatment

Because there is no known cure or treatment for ALS, therapy is supportive, focusing on the prevention of complications and the maintenance of maximum function.

NURSING CARE *of the Patient with Amyotrophic Lateral Sclerosis*

Assessment

The complete neurologic assessment is outlined in Box 27-2. When a patient has ALS, the nurse's history assessment of the patient determines the presence of dyspnea, dysphagia, muscle cramps, weakness, twitching, and joint stiffness. Describe the effects of the disease on the patient's lifestyle. During the physical examination, anticipate finding weakness, muscle atrophy, abnormal reflexes and gait, and paralysis.

Nursing Diagnoses, Goals, and Outcome Criteria: Amyotrophic Lateral Sclerosis

NURSING DIAGNOSES	GOALS AND OUTCOME CRITERIA
Ineffective Airway Clearance related to paralysis of respiratory muscles	Patent airway: respiratory rate of 12 to 20/min without crackles or wheezes
Impaired Physical Mobility related to progressive weakness and atrophy	Maximal possible mobility: patient participates in activities to maintain joint mobility
Imbalanced Nutrition: Less Than Body Requirements related to dysphagia	Adequate nutritional intake: stable body weight
Impaired Verbal Communication related to oropharyngeal muscle weakness	Effective communication: patient conveys needs without excessive frustration
Impaired Skin Integrity related to immobility	Normal skin integrity: intact skin without signs of pressure (redness, blanching)
Anticipatory Grieving related to progressive, fatal disease	Adaptation to losses: patient verbalizes losses, their importance, and acceptance of losses; makes realistic plans
Situational Low Self-Esteem related to loss of independence	Stable or improved self-esteem: patient makes positive statements about self
Interrupted Family Processes related to progressive illness of patient	Family adapts to patient condition: positive family communication and interactions, patient's role shifted

Interventions

Ineffective Airway Clearance

Monitor the patient's respiratory rate and effort, breath sounds, and pulse rate to detect inadequate oxygenation. Instruct or assist the immobile patient in turning, coughing, and deep breathing at least every 2 hours. Chest physiotherapy may be ordered to mobilize secretions to prevent atelectasis and pneumonia. If the patient has difficulty removing secretions, gentle suction may be needed. Oxygen therapy is indicated if there is evidence of hypoxia (restlessness, tachycardia).

Impaired Physical Mobility

Progressive muscle wasting, spasticity, and paralysis cause increasing immobility. Perform active or passive range-of-motion exercises to prevent contractures. Give antispasmodic drugs as ordered. Maintain extremities in functional positions. Encourage use of assistive devices (cane, walker, wheelchair) as needed to maintain mobility as long as possible. Monitor the patient's ability to perform activities of daily living, and provide assistance as needed. The patient who is immobile is at high risk for complications of immobil-

ity. Nursing care of the immobile patient is covered in Chapter 21.

Imbalanced Nutrition: Less Than Body Requirements

Muscle weakness and cranial nerve involvement eventually make it difficult for the patient to consume adequate food for good nutrition. Monitor the patient's weight to assess adequacy of the diet. Meals may be supplemented with high-protein snacks. Recommend high-fiber foods if the patient can eat them, because constipation is a common problem. Adequate fluids are needed but may be difficult to swallow. The patient may be able to increase fluid intake by eating semisolids such as ice cream, milk shakes, or gelatin desserts.

The patient with ALS is at risk for aspiration because of impaired swallowing. While the patient is eating, the head of the bed must be elevated or the patient must be seated in a chair. Consult the dietitian about providing a diet of the appropriate texture for the patient. Arrange dietary instruction for any caregivers who might be involved in preparing foods for the patient. A speech therapist can recommend techniques to facilitate swallowing. Eventually, oral intake becomes inadequate. The decision to insert a feeding tube should be based on the desires of the patient and family. If a feeding tube is in place, administer feedings and monitor for tube placement and residual. Teach the family or other caregivers how to do the feedings.

Impaired Verbal Communication

Speech becomes impaired by muscle weakness and dyspnea. You need to establish alternatives to verbal communication. These might include the use of blinks or gestures or the use of boards with pictures, words, or letters that the patient can select. Use questions that can be answered with "yes" or "no," and allow the patient time to respond.

Impaired Skin Integrity

Muscle wasting, incontinence, and immobility put these patients at risk for skin breakdown. Reposition them at least every 2 hours, and inspect bony prominences for redness. Special beds that alternate or distribute pressure may be used. Promptly change wet or soiled clothing to avoid skin irritation. Meticulous skin care is essential. Once again, if the patient will be cared for at home, be sure caregivers are able to care for the skin.

Anticipatory Grieving

Once the implications of a diagnosis of ALS are understood, patients and their families may begin the grieving process. Encourage patients to talk, listen compassionately, and help them make realistic plans. Remember the stages of grief and be understanding when patients and families show anger, denial, and depression. Referrals to visiting nurse agencies and hospice services can provide needed emotional and physical support at various times in the progress of the disease.

Situational Low Self-Esteem

Explore the patient's thoughts, feelings, and concerns about living with this progressive, terminal disease. Although it is difficult not to offer false reassurance, let the patient ventilate, cry, or express anger. Stress the patient's strengths, abilities, and contributions. Identify and enlist sources of support (family, friends, support groups, spiritual counselors, therapists). Stress-reducing techniques include imagery, breathing exercises, and progressive relaxation. Preserve the patient's dignity by providing privacy during personal care and by helping the patient attend to grooming and appearance.

Interrupted Family Processes

The disease is painful for both the patient and the family as it steadily takes its toll. Patients with ALS are often middle-aged, with family responsibilities, jobs, and places in the community. The family must plan for transfer of responsibilities and care of the patient when he or she becomes disabled. Issues that need to be discussed are patient feelings about advance directives, insurance, and wills. These topics may be difficult for them to address but are best handled while the patient can participate. Care of the dying patient is covered in Chapter 24.

What Does Culture Have to Do with Incurable Illness?

Patients facing progressive, incurable illness may find comfort in religious symbols, charms, incense, candles, and native healers.

HUNTINGTON'S DISEASE

Huntington's disease is an inherited degenerative neurologic disorder. It usually begins in middle adulthood with abnormal movements, emotional disturbance, and intellectual decline. Symptoms progress steadily, with increasing disability and death in 15 to 20 years. Medical and nursing care are supportive only; there is no cure.

MYASTHENIA GRAVIS

Myasthenia gravis is a chronic, progressive disease in which there is a defect at the neuromuscular junction, where electrical impulses are transmitted to muscle tissue.

Pharmacology Capsule

Edrophonium rapidly reverses a myasthenic crisis but has no effect on a cholinergic crisis.

Etiology

There is evidence that myasthenia gravis has an autoimmune basis. Some patients present with an increase in the titer of acetylcholine receptor antibody. The presence of these antibodies interferes with the normal activity at the acetylcholine receptor sites and reduces muscle strength.

Pathophysiology

Normally, as a nerve impulse travels down a peripheral nerve, the neurotransmitter acetylcholine is released at the presynaptic membrane (Fig. 27-19). The impulse is then transmitted across the synaptic junction to postsynaptic receptor sites on the effector muscle. This causes contraction of the involved muscle.

In myasthenia gravis, there are insufficient receptor sites at the junction of the motor nerve with the muscle. With repeated stimulation, the muscle becomes exhausted and is eventually unable to contract at all. If respiratory muscles become involved, death from respiratory insufficiency or arrest is a possibility.

Signs and Symptoms

Myasthenia gravis is characterized by the following features: weakness of voluntary muscles, particularly those of chewing, swallowing, and speaking; partial improvements of strength with rest; and dramatic improvement with the use of anticholinesterase drugs.

The onset of symptoms is gradual, and early weakness may be so subtle that it goes unnoticed. Muscles responsible for fine movements, such as eye, facial, or hand muscles, are often affected early in the disease process. Ptosis and diplopia are commonly seen. The patient becomes unable to perform any activity that demands sustained muscular contractions, such as brushing the hair, walking upstairs, or holding the hands over the head. The fatigue may abate with rest but rapidly returns when the activity is tried again. If the diaphragm or intercostal muscles are involved, breathing is compromised.

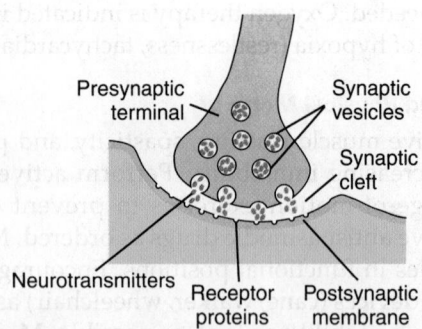

FIGURE **27-19** Neurotransmitters (norepinephrine, acetylcholine, dopamine) are released from the axon, travel across the synaptic cleft, and produce some response in the receptors of target cells.

Medical Diagnosis

The diagnosis is made by administering edrophonium (Tensilon). This is an anticholinesterase agent that increases the relative amount of acetylcholine in the neuromuscular junction by destroying acetylcholinesterase. In the patient with myasthenia gravis, muscle tone is markedly improved within 1 minute of injection, and this improvement persists for 4 to 5 minutes. The serum is tested for antiacetylcholine receptor antibodies. CT and MRI are performed to screen for thymoma.

Medical Treatment

Anticholinesterase Drugs. Therapy is directed primarily toward pharmacologic management with anticholinesterase agents and corticosteroids. Neostigmine and pyridostigmine (Mestinon) are anticholinesterase drugs that increase the availability of acetylcholine at the neuromuscular junction. Both drugs inhibit the action of cholinesterase, the enzyme that destroys acetylcholine. The availability of acetylcholine is improved, thereby enhancing muscle strength. Dosages are individualized for each patient, based on response and needs. Stress or sustained levels of activity can alter the need for these agents.

Neuromuscular blocking agents must be used very cautiously in the patient with myasthenia gravis.

Corticosteroids. Corticosteroids may be useful in those patients who do not respond well to the anticholinesterase agents. Adrenocorticotropic hormone or prednisone is administered concurrently with the anticholinesterase agent in an effort to induce remission. During the first 7 to 10 days of therapy, symptoms may worsen, requiring hospitalization to monitor for respiratory depression. With improvement, corticosteroids may be tapered and maintained at the lowest effective dose.

Cytotoxic Therapies. Cytotoxic therapies are useful in patients who are unable to significantly taper corticosteroids. Azathioprine and cyclosporine have been used in these cases.

Thymectomy. Because a large number of patients with myasthenia gravis have hyperplasia of the thymus gland, thymectomy is performed early after the initial diagnosis. Close monitoring is essential postoperatively because there is a risk of respiratory compromise because of possible pneumothorax. About 40% of patients enjoy some degree of remission after thymectomy.

Plasmapheresis. Plasmapheresis is an adjunctive therapy based on the autoimmune theory of myasthenia. It is a process of plasma exchange in which the acetylcholine receptor antibodies are washed from the plasma. A temporary catheter, similar to a renal dialysis access catheter, is used for venous access. Blood is then routed through a pheresis field, where the antibodies are separated from the plasma. The washed blood is then returned to the patient. The procedure takes 3 to 4 hours and is repeated over several days to ensure adequate treatment. Improvement in muscle strength may be noted within 24 to 48 hours after treatment. As progress is made with plasmapheresis, drug dosages may be decreased.

Myasthenic and Cholinergic Crises

Emergency respiratory support requiring mechanical ventilation may be necessary in the event of myasthenic or cholinergic crises. Myasthenic crisis is marked by a sudden exacerbation of myasthenic symptoms, including difficulty swallowing and breathing, with possible respiratory arrest. Infection often precipitates the event, and symptoms do not decrease even with higher doses of medications.

Cholinergic crisis presents with sudden, extreme weakness and respiratory impairment. It is precipitated by overmedication with anticholinesterase drugs, which literally bombard the receptor sites with excess amounts of acetylcholine. Intubation and mechanical ventilation are required to manage the respiratory compromise.

Because the two crises present similarly, differentiation is critical. Once again, edrophonium is used to distinguish the two entities. Rapid improvement in muscle strength after administration of edrophonium indicates an underlying myasthenic crisis. If no improvement is observed, the patient is experiencing a cholinergic crisis.

Because myasthenia gravis is a chronic neurologic disease, the patient is generally managed at home. However, hospitalization is likely on the initial diagnosis and during periods of crisis and respiratory compromise.

NURSING CARE *of the Patient with Myasthenia Gravis*

Assessment

The complete neurologic assessment is outlined in Box 27-2. When the patient has myasthenia gravis, the health history describes the onset of symptoms, particularly muscle weakness, diplopia, dysphagia, slurred speech, breathing difficulties, and loss of balance. Record the effects of the condition on the patient's lifestyle. In the physical examination, evaluate muscle strength, balance, respiratory effort, and oxygenation status.

Nursing Diagnoses, Goals, and Outcome Criteria: Myasthenia Gravis	
NURSING DIAGNOSES	GOALS AND OUTCOME CRITERIA
Ineffective Breathing Pattern related to impaired conduction of nerve impulses	Adequate oxygenation: respiratory rate of 12 to 20/min without dyspnea
Impaired Physical Mobility and Self-Care Deficit related to muscle weakness, fatigue	Improved mobility and self-care: performance of activities of daily living without excessive fatigue

Continued

Impaired Verbal Communication related to weakness of the muscles involved in speech	Effective communication: patient makes needs known
Impaired Swallowing related to muscle weakness	Adequate intake of fluids and food: stable body weight and absence of respiratory distress associated with aspiration
Deficient Knowledge of disease and treatment	Patient understands disease and treatment: patient accurately describes condition and treatment, follows plan of care

Interventions

Ineffective Breathing Pattern

You must monitor the patient for early signs and symptoms of ineffective breathing and hypoxia (tachycardia, restlessness). Progressive symptoms that do not respond to prescribed drug therapy may require mechanical ventilation. Management of the patient on a ventilator is discussed in Chapter 30.

Impaired Physical Mobility and Self-Care Deficit

Because of weakness, the patient may be relatively inactive and unable to provide self-care. Monitor the patient's capabilities, and assist as needed. Measures to prevent complications, discussed in Chapter 21, include turning and repositioning at least every 2 hours.

Impaired Swallowing

Patients may have difficulty chewing and swallowing. Anticholinesterase drugs may be ordered 30 minutes before meals to improve muscle strength. Seat the patient upright for meals, and allow or assist the patient to eat in an unhurried manner. Teach patients to rest their chins on the chest area when swallowing to help prevent aspiration. Small, frequent meals may be tolerated better than three large ones. A soft diet is usually ordered so that minimal chewing is required. If swallowing is severely impaired, a feeding tube may be inserted and liquid feedings given as ordered. Adequate fluid intake is important to maintain hydration and prevent constipation.

Deficient Knowledge

Patient teaching with myasthenia gravis is essential because this chronic condition requires lifelong treatment. See the Health Promotion Considerations box at right.

TRIGEMINAL NEURALGIA (TIC DOULOUREUX)

Trigeminal neuralgia is characterized by intense pain along the distribution of one of the three branches of the trigeminal nerve (fifth cranial nerve): ophthalmic, mandibular, or maxillary (Fig. 27-20). The pain has an

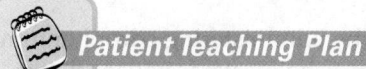

Patient Teaching Plan

Myasthenia Gravis

- Myasthenia gravis is a chronic disease that can be treated but not cured.
- You must know your drug names, dosages, schedule, side effects, and adverse effects that should be reported to the physician. It is very important to take the prescribed drugs on time.
- Myasthenic crisis indicates too little acetylcholine.
- Cholinergic crisis occurs when there is too much acetylcholine.
- Difficulty swallowing and breathing are symptoms of both types of crises, and each requires immediate medical treatment.
- You will need to adjust your routine based on your symptoms.
- A good source of information is the Myasthenia Gravis Foundation (1-800-541-5454; website: www. myasthenia. org), which may have a local chapter where you live.

Health Promotion Considerations

Patients with Myasthenia Gravis

Patients with myasthenia gravis should receive the following interventions as necessary:
- Maintain general health through diet
- Seek regular medical checkups for disease prevention
- Plan rest periods
- Tailor activities to conserve energy

abrupt onset and is usually unilateral in nature, lasting from seconds to a few minutes. Despite the intense pain, there is no associated motor or sensory deficit. The pain may be crippling, restricting the patient's daily routine. Attacks may be triggered by ingestion of hot or cold liquids, chewing, shaving, or washing the face. Between episodes the patient may experience a dull ache or be pain free.

Etiology

Although the exact cause of trigeminal neuralgia is undetermined, various contributing factors can be identified. Trauma or infection may precipitate the characteristic pain, as may compression on the nerve by an aneurysm, artery, or tumor.

Medical Diagnosis

Because there is no specific test, the diagnosis is based on the history. Stimulation of certain trigger points may precipitate the pain.

Medical Treatment

Pharmacologic management is the preferable course of therapy. Phenytoin (Dilantin) and carbamazepine

Ophthalmic division
Ophthalmic nerve
Maxillary nerve
Maxillary division
Mandibular division
Trigeminal nerve
Mandibular nerve

FIGURE 27-20 Distribution of the trigeminal nerve and its three divisions: ophthalmic, maxillary, and mandibular.

(Tegretol) are most commonly used to suppress the pain episodes. During the acute attack, alcohol or phenol may be injected into the affected branch of the trigeminal nerve, with pain relief lasting from 8 to 16 months.

Patients with the most severe, debilitating pain may undergo surgical intervention. Electrocoagulation, a procedure in which heated electrodes are used to destroy the sensory fibers of the nerve, is effective in providing lasting pain relief without compromising motor or tactile function.

NURSING CARE *of the Patient with Trigeminal Neuralgia*

Assessment

Assessment of the patient with trigeminal neuralgia focuses on describing the pain, factors that trigger it, and treatments found to be effective or ineffective. The effects of the condition on the patient's life are recorded.

Nursing Diagnoses, Goals, and Outcome Criteria: Trigeminal Neuralgia

NURSING DIAGNOSES	GOALS AND OUTCOME CRITERIA
Chronic Pain related to disease process	Reduced frequency and severity of attacks: patient reports attacks are less frequent and pain is lessened
Self-Care Deficit related to debilitating pain	Self-care activities accomplished: activities of daily living completed independently
Imbalanced Nutrition: Less Than Body Requirements related to pain associated with chewing	Adequate nutrition: stable body weight
Fear related to anticipated painful episodes	Lessened fear: patient expresses less fear and greater confidence in ability to manage condition
Deficient Knowledge of trigeminal neuralgia and its treatment	Patient understands condition and treatment: patient accurately describes condition, prevention of episodes, and treatment

Interventions

The focus of nursing care for the patient with trigeminal neuralgia is pain assessment and management. It may be beneficial to assist the patient in developing alternative strategies for pain relief, such as guided imagery or relaxation therapy. Because of the debilitating nature of the pain, the patient may need assistance in performing self-care activities. Nutrition may be affected because chewing may trigger pain. Psychological effects are also a consideration in management because the fear of engaging in some activity that may trigger pain can lead to social isolation. Chapter 15 provides additional information about care of the patient in pain. Patient teaching emphasizes the nature of the condition and avoidance of factors that trigger episodes.

NEUROFIBROMATOSIS

Neurofibromatosis, also known as *von Recklinghausen disease,* is characterized by multiple tumors of the peripheral, spinal, and cranial nerves. The tumors are benign but may be removed to relieve compression on the nerves or for cosmetic reasons. The patient also may have bone, muscle, and skin involvement.

BELL'S PALSY

Bell's palsy is acute paralysis of the seventh cranial nerve, which serves the face. The condition usually begins with pain behind the ear or on the face. The patient then has a drawing sensation followed by paralysis of the muscles on the affected side. The affected eyelids do not close, taste is impaired, and eating may be difficult. Most patients recover over a period of weeks or months, but some have residual weakness.

Bell's palsy is treated on an outpatient basis with prednisone and analgesics. Artificial tears are needed if the eyelids do not close, and the affected eye should be closed and an eye shield should be used on the affected eye at night to prevent drying of the cornea. When function begins to return, the patient can do simple exercises to improve muscle tone: grimacing, opening and closing the eye, whistling, and puffing out the cheeks. Be sensitive to the patient's concerns about the condition and his or her appearance.

CEREBRAL PALSY

Cerebral palsy is a paralysis associated with a loss in motor coordination caused by cerebral damage.

Although the etiology is uncertain, the damage is generally believed to occur at birth and to be related to hypoxia, premature birth, or birth trauma.

Individuals with cerebral palsy are often frustrated by people who equate the disorder with mental retardation. Although the staggering gait and unclear speech may resemble a stereotype of a person with mental retardation, the individual with cerebral palsy is fully capable of comprehending his or her situation and is willing to strive for as much independence as possible.

Types of Cerebral Palsy

Three general types of cerebral palsy can be identified, based on symptoms: spastic paralysis, athetoid, and ataxic. Spastic paralysis is characterized by overall exaggerated reflexes and muscle spasms. Random, purposeless movement with extreme muscle tone is indicative of the athetoid type, whereas the ataxic variety is characterized by poor balance, an uncoordinated, staggering gait, and speech or vision defects.

Medical Treatment

Although there is no cure for cerebral palsy, early muscle training and exercises can be beneficial in an effort to prevent complications and promote optimal function. Orthopedic surgery, braces, and casts may be useful in limiting deformities and disabilities.

NURSING CARE of the Patient with Cerebral Palsy

Nursing care of the patient with cerebral palsy is covered in depth in pediatric nursing texts because it is typically a lifelong condition diagnosed in infancy. Therefore, although many adults have cerebral palsy, it is not discussed in detail here.

POSTPOLIO SYNDROME

Before the advent of the polio vaccine, many people suffered varying degrees of motor impairment caused by the polio virus. Many years after having had the initial infection, some patients once again experience progressive muscle weakness, fatigue, pain, and respiratory problems typical of polio infections. The reason for the recurrence of symptoms is not known. Medical and nursing care are primarily supportive, aimed at helping the patient adapt to the symptoms and maintain maximum possible function.

SUMMARY

Management of the patient with a neurologic disorder can be demanding and challenging. Astute observation and assessment are vital to any treatment plan, and other therapies are often based on the nursing assessment. As is apparent from this chapter, many nursing diagnoses and modes of management are common to almost any patient with a neurologic disorder. Because

of the complicated nature of many of these disorders, the management of other body systems also must be considered in a comprehensive care plan.

Key Points

- The functional unit of the nervous system is the neuron (nerve cell), which conducts electrical impulses throughout the nervous system.
- The brain and the spinal cord compose the central nervous system, whereas the nerves in the peripheral parts of the body compose the peripheral nervous system.
- Cerebrospinal fluid circulates through the central nervous system.
- The neurologic assessment includes evaluation of the level of consciousness, pupillary size and response, coordination and balance, sensory function, reflexes, and vital signs.
- Increased intracranial pressure may impair cerebral tissue perfusion, resulting in ischemia and possibly respiratory arrest.
- Signs and symptoms of increased intracranial pressure and impaired cerebral blood flow are decreasing level of consciousness, pupil dilation with no response to light, motor deficits, abnormal posture, fever, increased blood pressure, bradycardia, and respiratory depression.
- Measures to decrease intracranial pressure include positioning, hyperventilation, fluid restriction, mechanical drainage, and drug therapy.
- Seizures are abnormal activity and behavior caused by abnormal electrical impulses in the brain that may be treated with anticonvulsant therapy and, when possible, measures to correct the cause.
- Nursing care of the patient with a seizure disorder addresses Risk for Injury, Ineffective Coping, and Deficient Knowledge.
- Nursing care of the patient with a head injury may focus on Ineffective Tissue Perfusion, Ineffective Breathing Pattern, Risk for Injury, Risk for Infection, Impaired Physical Mobility, Disturbed Body Image, and Ineffective Role Performance.
- Meningitis and encephalitis are infections of the nervous system.
- Guillain-Barré syndrome, thought to be an autoimmune response to a viral infection, is characterized by progressive ascending neurologic deficits that, in most cases, eventually resolve.
- Nursing care of the patient with Guillain-Barré syndrome addresses Ineffective Breathing Pattern, Decreased Cardiac Output, Risk for Disuse Syndrome, Imbalanced Nutrition: Less Than Body Requirements, Risk for Injury, Anxiety, and Deficient Knowledge.
- Parkinson's syndrome, a progressive disorder that results in loss of coordination and control over involuntary movement, is treated with physical therapy and drugs that increase dopamine levels in the brain.
- The focus of nursing care for the patient with Parkinson's syndrome is Impaired Physical Mobility, Risk for Injury, Imbalanced Nutrition: Less Than Body Requirements, Ineffective Coping, and Deficient Knowledge.

- Multiple sclerosis is a progressive degenerative disease that disrupts the motor pathways of the central nervous system and may lead to severe neurologic disabilities.
- Amyotrophic lateral sclerosis is a rapidly progressive degenerative disease that usually results in death from respiratory complications within 3 years.
- The patient with amyotrophic lateral sclerosis has increasing needs for nursing care, eventually becoming completely dependent for all aspects of care.
- Myasthenia gravis is caused by a defect in impulse conduction that is manifested as weakness of voluntary muscles and is treated with anticholinesterase drugs and corticosteroids.

- Trigeminal neuralgia is intense pain along a branch of the trigeminal nerve that may be treated with drug therapy or surgical intervention.
- Cerebral palsy is associated with a loss in motor coordination caused by cerebral damage.

 Go to your Companion CD-ROM for a Pharmacology Tutorial, Audio Glossary, and 3-D animations.

evolve   Be sure to visit the companion Evolve site at http://evolve.elsevier.com/Linton/ for WebLinks and additional online resources.

REVIEW QUESTIONS *Choose the best answer.*

1. The known neurotransmitters include acetylcholine, norepinephrine, epinephrine, and:
   1. Dopamine
   2. Acetylcholinesterase
   3. Dendrites
   4. Interneurons

2. Which statement best describes normal aging of the neurologic system?
   1. The size of neurons increases to make up for the loss in number of neurons.
   2. Decreasing lipofuscin and amyloid slow the transmission of impulses.
   3. Despite loss of neurons, most older people retain normal cognition.
   4. By age 80, only the Achilles tendon jerk reflex remains intact.

3. A patient who is being treated for a closed head injury is lying still and appears to be sleeping even in the noisy emergency room. When you shake his shoulder and call his name, he opens his eyes and says, "huh?" Then he closes his eyes again. A term to describe his level of consciousness is:
   1. Somnolent
   2. Lethargic
   3. Stuporous
   4. Semicomatose

4. To evaluate neuromuscular function, the patient is instructed to raise one leg at a time while lying supine. A patient with normal strength would be able to lift each leg at least:
   1. 25 degrees
   2. 45 degrees
   3. 60 degrees
   4. 90 degrees

5. A postoperative craniotomy patient has an external ventricular drainage system. Proper management of the system includes:
   1. Do not clamp the drainage tube under any circumstances
   2. Use clean technique to cleanse the insertion site every shift
   3. Keep the zero point of the drip chamber at the level of the external auditory canal
   4. Irrigate the tube with sterile normal saline at least every 8 hours

6. A patient with a head injury is being monitored for increased intracranial pressure. The earliest sign of increased intracranial pressure is a change in:
   1. Pupil response to light
   2. Level of consciousness
   3. Blood pressure
   4. Motor and sensory function

7. Factors that may trigger migraine headaches include the following:
   1. Alcohol
   2. Sleep disturbances
   3. Exposure to bright light
   4. Changes in environmental temperature

8. Nursing measures when a patient has a generalized seizure include the following:
   1. Apply soft arm restraints to prevent injury
   2. Insert a tongue blade between the teeth to prevent biting the tongue
   3. Turn the patient to one side to prevent swallowing the tongue
   4. Move objects away from the patient to prevent injury

9. One nursing measure used to decrease intracranial pressure is to:
   1. Suction the patient frequently
   2. Encourage isometric exercises
   3. Avoid flexing the neck and hips
   4. Provide continuous stimulation

Cerebrovascular Accident

JANEAN W. JENKINS

Objectives

After reading and studying this chapter, you should be able to:

1. Discuss the risk factors for cerebrovascular accident (CVA).
2. Identify the two major types of CVA.
3. Describe the pathophysiology, signs and symptoms, and medical treatment for each type of CVA.
4. Describe the neurologic deficits that may result from CVA.
5. Explain the tests and procedures used to diagnose a CVA and nursing responsibilities for patients undergoing those tests and procedures.
6. List data to be included in the nursing assessment of the CVA patient.
7. Assist in developing a nursing care plan for a CVA patient during the acute and rehabilitation phases.
8. Specify criteria used to evaluate the outcomes of nursing care for the CVA patient.
9. Identify resources for the CVA patient and family.
10. Discuss criteria used to identify patients eligible for treatment with rt-PA.

Key Terms

Be sure to check out the bonus material on the Companion CD-ROM, including selected audio pronunciations.

aphasia (ă-FĀ-zhă, p. 468)
diplopia (dĭp-LŌ-pē-ă, p. 477)
dysarthria (dĭs-ĂR-thrē-ă, p. 468)
dysphagia (dĭs-FĀ-jē-ă, p. 468)
dyspraxia (dĭs-PRĂK-sē-ă, p. 468)
expressive aphasia (p. 468)
global aphasia (p. 468)
hemiplegia (hĕm-ē-PLĒ-jă, p. 468)
homonymous hemianopsia
   (hŏ-MŎN-ĭ-mŭs hē-mē-ă-NŎP-sē-ă, p. 469)
intracerebral (ĭn-trăh-sĕ-RĒ-brăl, p. 466)
nonfluent aphasia (p. 468)
ptosis (TŌ-sĭs, p. 477)
receptive aphasia (p. 468)
subarachnoid (sŭb-ăh-RĂK-noid, p. 466)
transient ischemic attack (TIA)
   (TRĂN-zē-ĕnt ĭs-KĒ-mĭk ă-TĂK, p. 462)

The brain is the body's center of thinking, feeling, and physical function. A continuous blood supply is essential to maintain function in the brain. A cerebrovascular accident (CVA) is an interruption of blood flow to part of the brain. Without normal blood flow, the affected area is deprived of oxygen and cell death begins to occur in as little as 4 minutes. The effects of oxygen deprivation vary depending on the area of the brain involved and the length of time the brain is deprived of oxygen. If blood flow is restored to the deprived area in time, recovery of the brain tissue may occur.

ANATOMY AND PHYSIOLOGY

The central structures of the brain include the cerebrum, the brainstem, and the cerebellum. A brief review of the anatomy and physiology of the brain is presented here. Refer to Chapter 27 for a more detailed review.

CEREBRUM

The cerebrum has many complex functions, including initiation of movements, recognition of sensory input, higher-order thinking, regulation of emotional behavior, and regulation of endocrine and autonomic functions.

The cerebrum is divided into two halves, called *hemispheres.* Each hemisphere controls the opposite side of the body; that is, the right hemisphere controls the left side of the body and the left hemisphere controls the right side of the body. For most people, the left hemisphere is dominant. This hemisphere controls the more analytic mental processes such as language acquisition and use, mathematics, and reasoning powers. The right hemisphere encompasses emotional and artistic tendencies.

A folded layer of nerve cells, the *cortex*, covers each hemisphere. The cortex of each hemisphere is divided into the parietal, frontal, temporal, and occipital lobes. Each lobe has a different area of function (Fig. 28-1).

BRAINSTEM

The brainstem includes the midbrain, pons, medulla, and part of the reticular activating system. The brainstem controls vital, basic functions, including respiration, heart rate, and consciousness.

Sensory

- Genitals
- Toes, feet
- Leg, hip, trunk, neck, head
- Shoulder, arm, elbow, forearm
- Wrist, hand
- Fingers, thumb
- Eye, nose
- Face
- Lips
- Teeth, gums, jaw
- Tongue, pharynx
- Intra-abdominal

Motor

- Toes
- Ankle, knee, hip
- Trunk, shoulder
- Elbow, wrist
- Hand
- Fingers, thumb
- Neck, brow
- Eyelid, eyeball
- Face
- Lips
- Jaw, tongue
- Swallowing

Vocalization

FIGURE **28-1** Control zones of the brain. This drawing represents a slice of each side of the brain. The diagram on the left shows the areas of the cerebral cortex that receive sensory information for specific body areas. The diagram on the right shows where motor activity is initiated for various areas of the body.

CEREBELLUM

The cerebellum uses information received from the cerebrum, muscles, joints, and inner ear to coordinate movement, balance, and posture. Unlike the cerebrum, the right side of the cerebellum controls the right side of the body and the left side of the cerebellum controls the left side of the body.

CIRCULATION

The brain is rich with arterial circulation to satisfy its high need for oxygen. Figure 28-2 shows the major cerebral arteries. Although the brain comprises only 2% of the body's weight, it consumes 20% of the oxygen supply and cardiac circulation each minute. The two major arterial systems that supply the brain are the carotid and the vertebral arteries. The carotid system begins as one common artery that later divides into the external and internal carotid arteries. The external carotid arteries divide to supply blood to the face. The internal arteries further divide into the middle cerebral artery and the anterior cerebral artery to supply blood to the brain. The vertebral arteries originate from the subcla-

vian artery and travel up the anterior neck to merge and form the basilar artery at the brainstem. A second division forms the posterior cerebral artery. The internal carotid arteries and vertebral-basilar arteries unite to form the circle of Willis. Some people have anatomic differences in blood vessels that can increase the likelihood that they will sustain a CVA.

CEREBROVASCULAR ACCIDENTS

A cerebrovascular accident is commonly referred to as a *stroke* or "brain attack." Stroke is the third leading cause of death and the leading cause of adult disability in the United States. More than 700,000 Americans experience a new or recurrent stroke each year, resulting in the deaths of approximately 160,000 people annually. (An additional 200,000 to 500,000 individuals experience a transient ischemic attack [TIA]). The economic effect of stroke is estimated to be over $45 billion each year. Despite these statistics, there is reason for hope. Approximately 5,500,000 Americans

FIGURE **28-2** Cerebral circulation.

Box 28-1 *Signs of a Stroke*

- Sudden numbness or weakness of the face, arm, or leg, especially on one side of the body
- Sudden confusion, trouble speaking or understanding
- Sudden trouble seeing in one or both eyes
- Sudden trouble walking, dizziness, loss of balance or coordination
- Sudden, severe headache with no known cause

---

are stroke survivors. Stroke is considered one of the most preventable of catastrophic events in the United States. With risk factor modification and new treatments emerging, the outlook for patients and families continues to improve. Box 28-1 lists the common signs of a stroke.

RISK FACTORS FOR STROKE

Stroke experts believe that the majority of strokes could be prevented. Unfortunately, the public has little knowledge about stroke in relation to signs and symptoms of impending stroke or TIA, prevention of stroke, or medical treatment available. Nurses are becoming more involved in community education through outreach programs directed at assisting the public to learn more about stroke, identify risk factors, and teach individuals methods to adopt a healthy lifestyle to reduce their risk of suffering a stroke.

Risk factors are classified as *modifiable* and *nonmodifiable*. Nonmodifiable factors are risk factors that cannot be changed: age, race, gender, and heredity. Cerebrovascular accidents are more common in men, African

Americans, people ages 51 to 74 years, and those with a family history of CVA. Stroke has been considered mostly a disease of older individuals, but at least 5% of strokes occur in individuals younger than 45 years. Causes of strokes among the young include drug abuse, use of birth control pills in combination with smoking, congenital heart conditions, mitral valve prolapse, atrial fibrillation, infectious endocarditis, sickle cell anemia, rheumatic fever, and leukemia.

Modifiable risk factors are those that can be eliminated or controlled, thereby dramatically reducing the risk for CVA. The modifiable risk factors are listed in Table 28-1 along with the interventions used for each factor. The Health Promotion Considerations box on p. 463 discusses the nation's goals for stroke prevention. A common denominator of many of the risk factors (hypertension, cardiac disease, diabetes mellitus) is atherosclerosis. Therefore many interventions include measures to slow the progression of atherosclerosis (see Chapter 35 for more complete coverage).

TRANSIENT ISCHEMIC ATTACK

A **transient ischemic attack (TIA)** is a temporary neurologic deficit caused by impairment of cerebral blood flow. Blood vessels may be occluded by spasms, fragments of plaque, or blood clots. It is believed that at least 85% of blood flow to an area must be blocked before signs and symptoms of a TIA appear. These episodes of temporary neurologic changes were previously thought to be "benign." It is now known that TIAs are important warning signs for the individual experiencing a full stroke in the future. Although TIA

Table 28-1 | *Modifiable CVA Risk Factors and Related Interventions*

MODIFIABLE RISK FACTOR	INTERVENTIONS TO MODIFY EFFECTS OF RISK FACTOR
PATHOLOGIC DISORDERS	
Hypertension	Antihypertensive drugs. Weight control. Stress management. Smoking cessation. Limited alcohol consumption. Low-fat diet. Reduced sodium intake.
Cardiac disease	Drug therapy to improve blood flow and prevent clots. Treatment of atrial fibrillation.
Diabetes mellitus	Balanced program of drug therapy, diet, weight control, exercise. Blood glucose monitoring.
Hypotension	Maintain good hydration, especially in older adults. Monitor effects of diuretic and antihypertensive therapy.
Migraine headaches	Drug therapy to abort impending migraines or for prophylaxis.
Conditions that increase risk of blood clotting (e.g., sickle cell anemia)	Good hydration. Drug therapy as appropriate.
LIFESTYLE FACTORS	
Excessive alcohol consumption	Limit alcohol to one ounce of pure alcohol or less (not more than 1 ounce of pure alcohol per day: 2 cans beer, 2 small glasses of wine, 2 average cocktails). Avoid binge drinking.
Cigarette smoking	Advise patients of risks of tobacco use. Explain that risk falls with smoking cessation. Recommend self-help programs. Refer to MD for drug therapy.
Obesity	Encourage patient to maintain normal body weight. Instruction in proper diet. Weight control programs that help patients modify eating behaviors and establish healthy nutritional practices. Exercise programs as specified by the physician.
High-fat diet	Instruction in meal planning and preparation. Reduce saturated fats in diet.
Drug abuse	Drug abuse treatment programs.

Health Promotion Considerations

Healthy People 2010: Implications for Nurses

Healthy People 2010 presents a comprehensive set of disease prevention and health promotion objectives developed to improve the health of all people in the United States during the first decade of the twenty-first century. Nurses are in a unique position within the community to promote and participate in this initiative.

Role of the Nurse in Stroke Prevention and Treatment

- Spread the word about risk factors for and warning signs of stroke.
- Participate in community education programs for stroke.
- Get involved in Operation Stroke in your community.
- Participate in stroke and blood pressure screenings.
- Promote evidence-based care and best practices.
- Engage in and promote physical activity.
- Participate in anti-smoking campaigns, and assist patients to locate programs.
- Recognize depression after stroke, and help patients obtain adequate treatment.

has been described as lasting less than 24 hours, most of these temporary changes resolve much more rapidly. Current recommendations suggest that the transient events can cause permanent brain injury and should be evaluated to determine the cause and treated aggressively to prevent a stroke (Albers et al., 2002). It

is recommended that a patient experiencing a TIA receive a full medical evaluation within 24 hours. This may be completed in an inpatient or outpatient setting. Approximately 30% of individuals who experience a TIA continue on to have a stroke within 5 years.

Signs and Symptoms

With a TIA, neurologic signs and symptoms last from a few minutes to 24 hours, often with no permanent effects. Some common signs and symptoms are dizziness, momentary confusion, loss of speech, loss of balance, tinnitus, visual disturbances, ptosis, dysarthria, dysphagia, drooping mouth, weakness, and tingling or numbness on one side of the body. The nature and severity of the symptoms depend on the area of the brain involved and the extent of tissue deprived of oxygen.

Medical Diagnosis

A TIA is generally diagnosed from the health history, physical examination findings, and results of brain imaging studies. In addition, laboratory studies, electrocardiography (ECG), duplex ultrasonography, and cerebral angiography may be ordered to detect risk factors for TIA and stroke. Angiography and radiologic studies can show narrowing of cerebral blood vessels. Doppler studies may also be done to assess cerebral blood flow. Ultrasonic duplex scanning is useful in detecting carotid artery disease. Computed tomography and electroencephalography (EEG) may be employed to rule out intracranial lesions such as tumors, aneurysms, and abscesses. Key features of diagnostic tests are presented in the Diagnostic Tests and Procedures table on pp. 423 and 424.

On auscultation, a swooshing noise may be heard over a carotid artery. Its sound is similar to that of a rush of water through a narrow or dammed-up area. This sound, called a *bruit*, reveals that the artery is partially obstructed as with an atherosclerotic plaque.

Medical Treatment

Treatment of a TIA depends on the cause. The common causes of TIA are thought to be carotid artery disease, large or small artery disease from atherosclerosis, and atrial fibrillation. The treatment of atherosclerotic disease depends on the location of the narrowed vessel and the degree of narrowing. Medical treatment may include drug therapy with acetylsalicylic acid (aspirin), ticlopidine hydrochloride (Ticlid), extended-release dipyridamole (Aggrenox), or clopidogrel bisulfate (Plavix) to decrease platelet clumping. In atrial fibrillation, microscopic emboli are believed to form, which later are released from the heart and travel to the arteries of the brain to cause a TIA or stroke. Warfarin (Coumadin) and heparin are anticoagulants that may be given alone or in combination in patients exhibiting a cardioembolic TIA. The dosage for warfarin therapy is based on the prothrombin time and the international normalized ratio (INR). For therapeutic anticoagulation, the prothrombin time is usually kept in a therapeutic range of 1.5 to 2.0 times normal and the INR at 2.0 to 3.0. The effect of heparin therapy is monitored with the activated partial thromboplastin time (aPTT). Additional information about drug therapy is provided in the Drug Therapy table below.

Because of the operative risks and controversy about the value of surgical intervention in terms of stroke prevention, surgery is often reserved for the

Pharmacology Capsule

When patients are taking antiplatelet or anticoagulant medications, take care to prevent injuries and bleeding.

DRUG THERAPY | Cerebrovascular Accident

DRUG	USE/ACTION	SIDE EFFECTS	NURSING INTERVENTIONS
CORTICOSTEROIDS			
Dexamethasone (Decadron)	Reduces ICP by reducing inflammation in brain after stroke.	Fluid retention, hypertension, hypokalemia, hyperglycemia, suppressed response to infection, fat deposits in cheeks and upper back, gastric ulcers, insomnia, easy bruising, mood swings. Dose usually tapered over 7-10 days to prevent acute withdrawal and adrenal insufficiency.	Monitor I&O, BP, blood glucose in people with diabetes. Protect from infection. Report even minor signs of infection. Protect from bumps and other minor injuries.
HYPEROSMOTIC AGENTS			
Mannitol (Osmitrol) Urea (Ureaphil) Glycerin (Osmoglyn)	Induces diuresis, which reduces ICP. Mannitol is first-choice drug.	Circulatory overload, heart failure, hypertension, renal failure.	15%-25% mannitol solutions should be filtered. Monitor infusion site; stop flow and have restarted if infiltrated to avoid tissue damage. Monitor for signs of fluid volume excess: hypertension, bounding pulse, edema, urine output less than fluid intake.
ANTICOAGULANTS			
Heparin sodium (Liquaemin sodium)	Prevents formation of new blood clots; does not dissolve existing clots.	Bleeding or hemorrhage due to excessive anticoagulation; hyperkalemia; alopecia (hair loss); allergy. Contraindicated with active bleeding.	Effect is monitored by partial thromboplastin time (PTT) or by activated partial thromboplastin time (aPTT). Therapeutic goal is 1.5-2.0 times the control of 30-40 sec. If patient's aPTT is greater, withhold drug and contact physician. Assess for bruises, bleeding from gastrointestinal and urinary tracts, mouth, or nose. Heparin antidote is protamine sulfate. Caution with venipuncture—apply pressure to site.

BP, Blood pressure; *I & O,* intake and output; *ICP,* intracranial pressure; *IV,* intravenous; *MI,* myocardial infarction.

DRUG THERAPY *Cerebrovascular Accident—cont'd*

DRUG	USE/ACTION	SIDE EFFECTS	NURSING INTERVENTIONS
Warfarin sodium (Coumadin, Panwarfin)	Prevents formation of new blood clots; does not dissolve existing clots.	Bleeding or hemorrhage due to excessive anticoagulation. Contraindicated with severe cardiac, renal, or liver disease. Interacts with many other drugs.	Effect is monitored by prothrombin time (PT) and international normalized ratio (INR). Therapeutic goal is a PT of 1.5-2.0 times control and INR of 2.0-3.0. Check PT/INR before initiating medication and daily until maintenance dose is reached. Assess for bruising, bleeding from gastrointestinal and urinary tracts, mouth, or nose. Apply pressure after venipuncture. Antidote for warfarin overdose is vitamin K_1 (AquaMEPHYTON).
THROMBOLYTICS			
Streptokinase	Dissolves fibrin clots and clot components to destroy thrombi.	Increased risk of minor and major bleeding, especially at injection sites. Mild fever, mild allergic reaction. Extensive list of contraindications to be reviewed carefully before administration.	Avoid unnecessary injections; watch puncture sites closely. After arterial puncture, apply pressure at least 30 minutes. For major bleeding, streptokinase infusion must be stopped; whole blood, packed cells, or plasma may be ordered. Antidote for excessive bleeding: aminocaproic acid (Amicar).
Tissue plasminogen activator (tPA) Recombinant tPA (rt-PA)	Initiates dissolution of clots by breaking down fibrin.	Hemorrhage, especially within the first 24 hr after administration.	Minimize venipunctures; protect arterial line sites; assess for bleeding; monitor coagulation sites.
PLATELET AGGREGATION INHIBITORS			
Aspirin	Reduces risk of stroke in male patients with recurrent ischemic attacks.	Excessive bruising, bleeding; bronchoconstriction; nausea, vomiting, gastric bleeding, urticaria, confusion, drowsiness, tinnitus. May be given in combination with other antiplatelet agents.	Tinnitus and confusion suggest overdosage. Teach patients that aspirin can be harmful if not taken properly.
Dipyridamole (Persantine)	Prevents thromboembolism with heart valve prostheses. Used with coumarin anticoagulants.	Hypotension, dizziness. Caution with hypotensive patients. MI, dysrhythmias with IV use. Constipation, dry mouth.	Teach patient to manage orthostatic hypotension. Monitor pulse and blood pressure.
Aspirin/extended-release dipyridamole (Aggrenox)	Prolongs bleeding time, decreasing the risk of stroke.	Rash, diarrhea, itching, bruising. Not associated with neutropenic purpura as with Ticlid.	May be given with or without food; assess for bruising.
Ticlopidine (Ticlid)	Prolongs bleeding time, decreasing the risk of stroke.	Diarrhea, nausea, dyspepsia, rash; occasionally neutropenia, purpura. Overdose: hypotension.	Give with food or after meals; assess for bruising, signs of infection.
Clopidogrel (Plavix)	Reduces risk of stroke by inhibition of clotting.	GI bleeding, epistaxis, neutropenia, intracranial hemorrhage, hypertension, dyspnea.	Give with food. Advise patients of need for periodic lab studies, including liver function tests with long-term therapy.
CALCIUM CHANNEL BLOCKERS			
Nimodipine (Nimotop)	Prevents spasms in cerebral blood vessels after a hemorrhagic stroke.	Headache, fatigue, depression, confusion, dysrhythmias, hypotension, myocardial infarction, renal failure.	Monitor pulse and blood pressure. Assess for edema. Monitor urine output. Count pulse before each dose; withhold if less than 60 beats/min.

most serious stenosis. The most common surgical procedures are carotid endarterectomy (Fig. 28-3) and transluminal angioplasty. Carotid endarterectomy is the surgical removal of plaques in the artery to permit improved blood flow. Patients who are at high risk for surgical intervention due to other health problems may benefit from angioplasty. A stent may be placed in the artery to keep it open. Transluminal angioplasty improves blood flow by dilating the narrowed artery with a balloon that is inserted into the artery. A patent foramen ovale is sometimes identified in the patient with TIA. Closure of this defect can be accomplished through an open surgical approach or a transcatheter closure.

STROKE

As noted earlier, stroke is the third leading cause of death and the leading cause of adult disability in the United States. Approximately 750,000 Americans experience strokes each year, resulting in the deaths of approximately 160,000 people annually. When the occurrence of transient ischemic attacks is added to these numbers, the total may reach 2 million cerebral vascular accidents each year in the United States alone. Acute care and rehabilitation of stroke patients is a long and expensive process. Advances in care have improved the outlook for many individuals who experience a stroke. Over half of stroke victims acquire independence in activities of daily living within 1 year after the stroke. Thirty percent of stroke survivors return to work or productive lives within 1 year. These are important figures to remember when caring for the stroke patient. A stroke is an abrupt impairment of brain function resulting in a set of neurologic signs and symptoms that are caused by impaired blood flow to the brain and that last more than 24 hours. When symptoms progress over hours or days, the condition is described as *stroke in evolution*. When the neurologic deficits do not change for 2 to 3 days, the stroke is said to be completed. Unlike TIA, a completed stroke causes lingering motor, sensory, or cognitive damage with varying disabilities.

Pathophysiology

The two main classifications of stroke are hemorrhagic and ischemic.

Hemorrhagic Stroke. Hemorrhagic stroke accounts for only about 20% of all strokes. In hemorrhagic stroke, a blood vessel in the brain ruptures and bleeding into the brain occurs. As a result, intracranial pressure may increase, disrupting normal cerebral function. Hemorrhagic strokes are further classified by location. An intracerebral (within the cerebrum) hemorrhage is associated with trauma, uncontrolled hypertension, and aneurysms. When a hemorrhage occurs within the spaces of the brain, the terms *subdural, subarachnoid,* or *ventricular* will be used to describe the location. Hemorrhagic strokes are often sudden in onset and require emergent, life-sustaining treatment.

A subarachnoid hemorrhage occurs between the arachnoid and pia mater layers of the brain covering. The pia mater is the thin membrane covering the brain. The arachnoid covers the pia mater. Subarachnoid hemorrhage may be caused by congenital malforma-

Descending branch
of hypoglossal nerve

External carotid artery
Internal carotid artery

Vagus nerve

Common
carotid artery

Incision line

Internal jugular vein

FIGURE **28-3** Carotid endarterectomy. Plaques are removed from the artery to improve blood flow.

tions of blood vessels in the brain or by rupture of an aneurysm.

Ischemic Stroke. An ischemic stroke is caused by the obstruction of a blood vessel by an atherosclerotic plaque, a blood clot, or a combination of the two or by other debris released into the vessel that impedes blood flow to an area of the brain. Brain cells deprived of blood flow become ischemic and die. Ischemic strokes account for 80% of all strokes including embolic and thrombotic strokes. In an embolic stroke, the clot or plaque fragment is "traveling" through a blood vessel from an area outside of the brain until it lodges in a cerebral artery. Mitral valve stenosis, atrial fibrillation, and myocardial infarction are cardiovascular conditions that may lead to the development of clots that become emboli.

A thrombotic stroke develops when an obstruction forms in a blood vessel of the brain. The atherosclerotic process, which often affects large cerebral arteries, produces most of the thrombotic strokes. Patients may experience stroke in evolution, in which symptoms worsen over approximately 48 hours. As the obstruction progresses, neurologic impairment increases. Figure 28-4 illustrates each type of stroke. Patients who have thrombotic strokes may have a history of TIAs.

A lacunar stroke results from occlusion of the small penetrating arteries deep within the brain. The occlusive process in these small arteries is different from that of the larger arteries. The clinical features associated with lacunar strokes are usually less severe and produce less-pronounced neurologic changes.

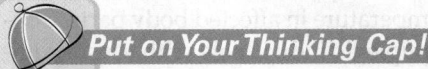

Put on Your Thinking Cap!

Why would patients with atrial fibrillation be treated with anticoagulants?

Signs and Symptoms

A stroke may produce different signs and symptoms, depending on the type, location, and extent of brain injury. Symptoms of a hemorrhagic stroke generally occur suddenly and may include severe headache that the patient describes as "the worst headache of my life." Other symptoms are stiff neck, loss of consciousness, vomiting, and seizures (see Box 28-1).

Symptoms of an embolic stroke also often appear without warning. The specific symptoms depend on the area of the brain affected by the lack of blood supply. One or more of the following signs and symptoms may be present: one-sided (unilateral) weakness, numbness, visual problems, confusion and memory lapses, headache, dysphagia (difficulty swallowing), and language problems. Language problems may be in the form of difficulty understanding, speaking, or both. Reading and writing also may be affected.

The signs and symptoms of a thrombotic stroke may be the same as those of an embolic stroke. Because the obstruction forms gradually through the atherosclerotic process, however, the symptoms may develop more gradually. Sudden onset of symptoms may occur with either embolic or thrombotic stroke.

Regardless of the type of stroke, symptoms can be devastating. Whereas some symptoms improve with time and therapy, others may be permanent. Many signs and symptoms are related to the location of the damage and whether the right or the left side of the brain is affected. Figure 28-5 compares right-sided and left-sided stroke. Long-term effects that merit more discussion are the following: aphasia, dysarthria, dysphagia, dyspraxia, hemiplegia, homonymous hemianopsia, personality change, emotional lability, impaired cognition, and bladder dysfunction.

Aphasia. The speech center is located in the left hemisphere in more than 90% of all people. In left-handed persons, the speech center is sometimes located in the

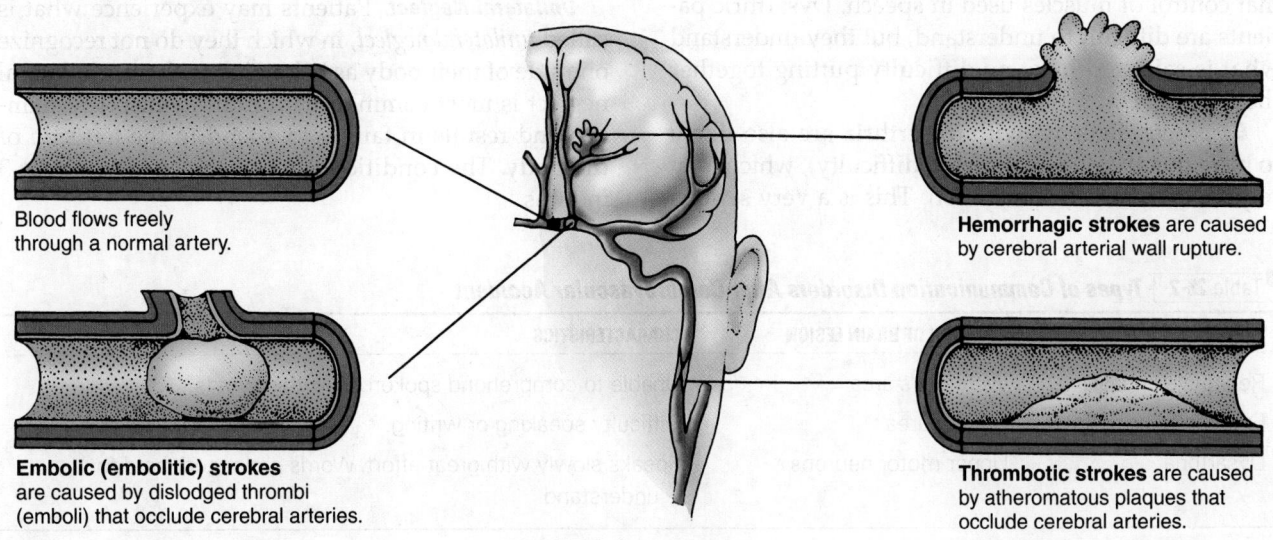

Blood flows freely through a normal artery.

Embolic (embolitic) strokes are caused by dislodged thrombi (emboli) that occlude cerebral arteries.

Hemorrhagic strokes are caused by cerebral arterial wall rupture.

Thrombotic strokes are caused by atheromatous plaques that occlude cerebral arteries.

FIGURE **28-4** Types of stroke.

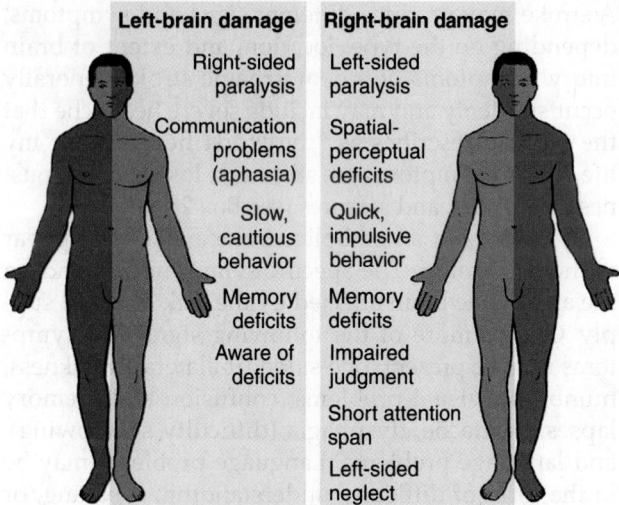

Left-brain damage	Right-brain damage
Right-sided paralysis	Left-sided paralysis
Communication problems (aphasia)	Spatial-perceptual deficits
Slow, cautious behavior	Quick, impulsive behavior
Memory deficits	Memory deficits
Aware of deficits	Impaired judgment
	Short attention span
	Left-sided neglect

FIGURE 28-5 Comparison of right-sided and left-sided stroke.

right hemisphere. If the speech center is damaged, communication is affected. Aphasia is a defect in the use of language: speech, reading, writing, or word comprehension. Aphasia is classified as receptive or expressive. The patient with receptive aphasia has difficulty understanding spoken or written words. The patient with expressive aphasia has difficulty speaking and writing. Aphasia can also be classified as fluent or nonfluent. The patient who has fluent dysphasia sounds normal but makes little sense, whereas the person with nonfluent aphasia has difficulty initiating speech. Although these types of aphasia are distinctly defined, some patients have components of both types. The term global aphasia is sometimes used when speech is impaired to the point that the person has almost no ability to communicate. Terms describing communication problems of the stroke patient are defined in Table 28-2.

Dysarthria. Dysarthria is the inability to speak clearly. It is caused by neurologic damage that prevents normal control of muscles used in speech. Dysarthric patients are difficult to understand, but they understand what is said and have no difficulty putting together their thoughts.

Dysphagia. Patients with dysarthria are also likely to have dysphagia (swallowing difficulty), which may require extensive rehabilitation. This is a very serious

problem because of the risk of aspiration and because it can interfere with adequate nutrition. Dysphagia can be especially discouraging for the patient when attempts to eat result in choking, frustration, and fear. A gastrostomy tube may be inserted for long-term feeding purposes. Speech therapists are trained to help patients with dysphagia.

Dyspraxia. Dyspraxia is the partial inability to initiate coordinated voluntary motor acts. Any part of the body with motor function may be affected. For instance, the patient may not be able to walk or transfer to a chair without assistance even though the patient is not paralyzed. Patients with dyspraxia may be able to spontaneously perform a motor act yet be unable to initiate such an act willfully. This contradictory behavior can lead uninformed family, friends, or caretakers to assume the person is being "difficult." The difficulty initiating motor actions seen in dyspraxia is quite different from the inability to perform motor acts due to hemiplegia. The person who has apraxia can move the affected parts but cannot perform specific purposeful actions such as walking or dressing.

Hemiplegia. Hemiplegia is defined as paralysis of one side of the body. The affected side is opposite from the side of the brain in which the stroke occurred because nerve fibers in the brain cross over as they pass into the spinal cord. Hemiplegia is characterized at first by flaccidity (decreased muscle tone) and then by spasticity (increased muscle tone). Recovery from hemiplegia is a gradual process, and the extent of improvement varies widely.

Sensory Impairment. Impaired sensory function is common after a stroke. The patient may be unable to feel touch, pain, or temperature in affected body parts. Conversely, some hemiplegic individuals with sensory impairment perceive every sensation to the affected area as painful. Patients may feel as if their body were limp or flaccid. Altered sensations put the patient at risk for injury from pressure and excess heat or cold. Injuries may be ignored because the patient is not aware of them.

Unilateral Neglect. Patients may experience what is called *unilateral neglect*, in which they do not recognize one side of their body as belonging to them. Unilateral neglect is most common with right hemisphere damage and results in failure to attend to the left side of the body. The condition often resolves after about 3 months.

Table 28-2 | *Types of Communication Disorders After Cerebrovascular Accident*

TYPE	LOCATION OF BRAIN LESION	CHARACTERISTICS
Receptive aphasia	Wernicke's area	Unable to comprehend spoken or written words.
Expressive aphasia	Broca's area	Difficulty speaking or writing.
Dysarthria	Upper motor neurons	Speaks slowly with great effort. Words prolonged, hard to understand.

Homonymous Hemianopsia. Homonymous hemianopsia is a perceptual problem that involves loss of one side of the field of vision. Homonymous hemianopsia translates to a half-blinded field of vision that occurs on the same side in both eyes. At mealtime, the patient may leave half the plate untouched, the half on the affected side. Or the patient may shave his face completely on one side and leave the whiskers untouched on his affected side.

Intellectual and Emotional Effects. Many patients experience emotional changes after a stroke, sometimes to the point of personality change. Emotional lability is a frequent problem after a stroke. The patient may seem quite happy and then suddenly burst into tears for no apparent reason. Angry outbursts, childlike behavior, and inappropriate sexual behavior may occur. Emotional changes such as these are thought to be caused by neurochemical imbalances in the brain or by loss of the brain's ability to inhibit inappropriate behavior. It has also been found that cognitive processes may be slowed after a stroke even without obvious deficits in thinking and responding.

Elimination Disturbances. In the acute phase of stroke and sometimes into the rehabilitation phase, the patient may experience a neurogenic bladder. A neurogenic bladder is further classified depending on the type of symptoms identified. A flaccid bladder (one without muscle tone) cannot empty completely. In some cases, the coordination to be able to store urine in the bladder or wait once the urge to void is felt is lost (dyssynergia), which also leads to incontinence.

Bowel incontinence may also be a physiologic consequence of stroke. However, confusion, disorientation, and immobility may contribute to incontinent episodes and to chronic constipation.

With both bladder and bowel incontinence, it is important to determine if the cause is physiologic or related to other factors such as infection from a urinary catheter or the inability of the patient to communicate the need to go to the bathroom. Bladder and bowel retraining programs should be implemented as soon as possible.

Medical Diagnosis

When a patient is admitted to a hospital with a tentative diagnosis of a stroke, the following procedures may be ordered: blood studies, electrocardiogram (ECG), computed tomography, magnetic resonance imaging, carotid ultrasound studies, cerebral and carotid angiography, electroencephalography, positron emission tomography, and single-photon emission computed tomography.

Blood studies and the ECG are done to identify the presence of risk factors for stroke such as hyperlipidemia and atrial fibrillation. A lumbar puncture may be performed to obtain cerebrospinal fluid for examination. Grossly bloody cerebrospinal fluid indicates hemorrhagic rather than ischemic stroke. This finding has important implications for treatment, because anticoagulants are contraindicated following hemorrhagic stroke. A lumbar puncture is *not* done if increased intracranial pressure is suspected. The Diagnostic Tests and Procedures table on pp. 423 and 424 summarizes nursing care of patients who have neurologic diagnostic tests and procedures.

Complications

Patients suffering an acute stroke are at risk for many complications related to impaired neuromuscular function. The patient with severe motor impairment is at risk for constipation, dehydration, contractures, urinary tract infections, thrombophlebitis, decubitus ulcers, and pneumonia. Sensory losses put the patient at risk for traumatic and thermal injuries. Swallowing difficulties place the patient at risk for pulmonary complications such as choking and aspiration pneumonia.

Prognosis

The prognosis for patients experiencing a TIA or stroke is becoming increasingly hopeful. The critical variables that affect recovery are the patient's condition before the stroke, the length of time between the occurrence of stroke and the diagnosis, the treatment and support for the patient in the acute phase (usually the first 48 hours), the severity of the patient's symptoms, and access to rehabilitative therapy. Patients with acute stroke who have access to emergent care and are treated with rt-PA within 90 minutes of symptom onset have a better cure rate after 3 months than those treated later or not at all (Bahouth and LaMonte, 2005). To accomplish this requires a structured multidisciplinary approach to stroke care. Current national recommendations include medical systems to offer pre-hospital assessment and transportation, stroke centers, stroke units, and organized stroke teams. Because not all hospitals are equipped to handle the rapid evaluation and treatment of acute stroke, it is important for emergency medical services to work closely with recognized stroke centers to transport patients to appropriate locations for this treatment.

The long-term recovery of the stroke patient may well depend on the care received immediately after the stroke. Most recovery from stroke takes place in the first 3 to 6 months, but progress often continues long after that.

The nurse's role in providing care to stroke patients is a vital one and has a significant impact on patient outcome.

Medical Treatment in the Acute Phase

The acute phase of a stroke begins with the onset of signs and symptoms and continues until the patient's vital signs, particularly blood pressure and neurologic condition, stabilize. This phase usually lasts 24 to 48 hours. The patients are often placed in a monitored setting for close observation and treatment during the acute phase. A challenge for the physician is to provide immediate care for acute problems while considering preexisting conditions as well. Management of chronic conditions such as diabetes mellitus, heart disease, arthritis, and gastrointestinal disturbances must continue during the acute phase of stroke. Many medical management interventions are directed at minimizing complications and deterioration of the patient's condition after a stroke. The four major focus areas are hypertension, oxygenation, hyperglycemia, and hyperthermia. It is very important to monitor patients and report any changes in vital signs, oxygenation, temperature, or glucose levels.

Hypertension. The majority of patients admitted with an acute stroke have high blood pressure during and immediately after a stroke. It is important to be cautious in treating high blood pressure during this phase because sudden reductions in blood pressure have been associated with decreased cerebral perfusion and may lead to worsening of brain tissue damage. Blood pressure naturally decreases within 48 hours, even without treatment. If a patient is to receive thrombolytic therapy, blood pressure control measures will be more aggressive. A small group of patients may present or develop low blood pressure after a stroke. This is often related to dehydration and should be identified and treated right away to avoid a decrease in blood flow to the brain. In patients experiencing a hemorrhagic stroke, blood pressure control will be maintained much tighter and hypertension will be avoided to reduce the risk of more bleeding into the brain.

Oxygenation. Oxygenation is a priority immediately after a stroke, especially if the patient is unconscious, because hypoxemia can extend the area affected and therefore worsen the stroke. Oxygen therapy and monitoring of oxygen saturation may be ordered. For patients who are comatose, intubation and mechanical ventilation may be required to provide adequate ventilation. Respiratory exercises, including incentive spirometry, may be ordered for the alert patient.

Hyperthermia. Fever is common after a stroke. Fever may be related to stress response of the stroke itself. Hyperthermia of any degree has now been shown to extend the area of damage and potentially worsen the outcome after stroke. Recent studies support keeping the patient's temperature as close to normal as possible. Fever can be adequately managed with medications such as Tylenol. Induced hypothermia is not a current recommendation.

Hyperglycemia. Individuals experiencing a stroke will often develop hyperglycemia (elevated blood glucose). This often occurs in the absence of having a history of diabetes. Hyperglycemia during the acute phase of a stroke may represent the body's stress response to stroke. It has been shown to contribute to brain damage and worsen the outcome of a patient.

Current recommendations require treating hyperglycemia aggressively to maintain serum levels of <140.

Drug Therapy. Tissue plasminogen activator (TPA) (alteplase [Activase, Activase rt-PA]) may be given to dissolve clots in patients with acute ischemic strokes. This is the only FDA-approved medication to reverse the effects of an ischemic stroke. To be given intravenously, this medication must be initiated within 3 hours from the onset of stroke symptoms. This narrow window of time has limited the use of t-PA with acute ischemic stroke. Patient selection criteria are also very strict, because this medication is associated with a higher risk of cerebral hemorrhage in patients who have received it. Once it is determined that the stroke is from an ischemic event and hemorrhage has been ruled out, the patient should be evaluated for treatment with t-PA.

Eligibility Criteria for t-PA Administration.
- Age 18 years or older
- Clinical diagnosis of stroke, with an NIH Stroke Scale score under 22
- Time of onset of stroke is known and is 3 hours or less
- Blood pressure: systolic <185; diastolic <110
- Not a minor or rapidly resolving stroke
- No seizure at onset of stroke
- Not taking warfarin (Coumadin)
- Prothrombin time <15 seconds or INR <1.7
- Not receiving heparin during the past 48 hours with elevated partial thromboplastin time
- Platelet count >100,000
- Blood glucose level between 50 and 400 mg/dl
- No acute myocardial infarction
- No prior intracranial hemorrhage, neoplasm, arteriovenous malformation, or aneurysm
- No major surgical procedures within 14 days
- No stroke or serious head injury within 3 months
- No gastrointestinal or urinary bleeding within past 21 days
- Not lactating or postpartum within past 30 days

Thrombolytic agents such as t-PA and streptokinase are being tested for intra-arterial treatment of acute ischemic stroke. None have FDA approval at this time; however, in stroke centers with interventional radiologists, intra-arterial lysis is an option and may be offered for up to 6 hours after the onset of stroke symptoms.

Other Medications. The trauma of a CVA causes edema in the affected tissues and surrounding tissues. Cerebral edema is sometimes treated with osmotic diuretics such as mannitol and with hyperventilation. In severe cases, surgical intervention may be required. Nimodipine (Nimotop), a calcium channel blocker, may be ordered to prevent spasms in cerebral blood vessels after subarachnoid hemorrhage. Phenytoin (Dilantin) and phenobarbital are anticonvulsants that may be ordered if the patient has seizures. The efficacy and safety of heparin and heparinoids have been challenged in recent years and are no longer routinely used as a first-line treatment with a TIA or an acute ischemic stroke unless a cardioembolic stroke is suspected. Small doses of these medications given subcutaneously are recommended in the prevention of deep vein thrombosis associated with acute stroke. When appropriate, heparin is given intravenously followed by oral warfarin. Later the regimen may be changed to aspirin, which decreases the risk of thrombus by preventing platelets from clumping.

Medical management is often directed at preventing a subsequent or future stroke. Examples of drugs given in an effort to prevent strokes caused by thrombi include acetylsalicylic acid (aspirin), ticlopidine hydrochloride (Ticlid), Aggrenox, and clopidogrel (Plavix). Drugs used to prevent or treat CVA are included in the Drug Therapy table on pp. 464 and 465.

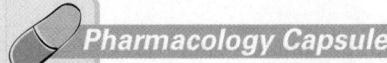

Pharmacology Capsule

Tissue plasminogen activator, which is used to dissolve clots, must be given within 3 hours of the onset of stroke symptoms.

Surgical Intervention. Surgical intervention is an option for some patients with hemorrhagic strokes. Decisions about surgery are based on the patient's age, the intracranial pressure, and the location of the hemorrhage. Clot retrieval methods are under study.

Fluids and Nutrition. An order for intravenous fluids will probably be given for the stroke patient in the acute phase. This route provides fluids, electrolytes, and an access for the intravenous administration of drugs. The dietary order is based on the patient's nutritional requirements and ability to eat. Food may be regular, soft, or pureed, depending on how well the patient can chew and swallow. Vitamins and electrolyte supplementation may also be ordered.

Total parenteral nutrition may be ordered for the malnourished patient. Sometimes a nasogastric tube is inserted for feeding purposes. If long-term enteral feedings are indicated, a gastrostomy tube may be placed.

Urine Elimination. Sometimes an indwelling catheter is ordered to manage urinary incontinence. Intermittent catheterization is a method of controlling incontinence caused by a flaccid bladder that is less likely to lead to infection. Intermittent catheterization is done every 4 to 6 hours as ordered. The frequency of catheterization is based on the amount of urine obtained each time.

NURSING CARE in the Acute Phase of Stroke

Once a stroke has occurred, it is important to rapidly identify the type and extent of the stroke so that appropriate treatment can be initiated. The most important aspects of care during the acute phase of a stroke are assessment and stabilization of the patient to prevent further brain injury This phase is sometimes referred to as the "hyperacute." Management in this phase focuses on identifying the type and extent of the stroke so that appropriate treatment can be initiated, maintenance or improvement of vital physiologic functions, and support of the patient and family (see Nursing Care Plan: The Stroke Patient on pp. 472 and 473).

Assessment

The initial nursing assessment is directed at evaluating the type and extent of the stroke including the time of onset, symptoms experienced, and other details related to the onset of the symptoms (e.g., activity). Several tools are available to use for assessing patients experiencing signs of a stroke. The Cincinnati Pre-hospital Stroke Scale is a quick and easy tool that is often used in the pre-hospital phase by emergency medical technicians. This is a three-step test, shown in Box 28-2, to assess facial muscles, arm movement, and speech function. Abnormality in any one of these strongly suggests the patient may be having a stroke. Nursing assessments should also reveal risk factors for CVA and identify nursing care needs of the patient. Details of the neurologic assessment are covered in Chapter 27 and summarized in Box 27-2. Data specific to the stroke patient are outlined in Box 28-3.

Health History

The health history may be obtained from the patient if he or she is able to communicate. On introduction to the patient, begin to study the patient's ability to understand language and to respond verbally and nonverbally. Responses to simple yes-or-no commands provide a good basis for initial assessment. Evaluate verbal responses, facial expressions, and physical

Box 28-2 | *Cincinnati Pre-Hospital Stroke Scale*

The patient is asked to show teeth or smile.
- **Normal**—both sides of face move equally well.
- **Abnormal**—one side of face does not move as well as the other side.

The patient is asked to close both eyes and hold both arms straight out for 10 seconds.
- **Normal**—both arms move the same, or both arms do not move at all.
- **Abnormal**—one arm does not move, or one arm drifts down.

The patient is asked to repeat a simple phrase, such as "You can't teach an old dog new tricks."
- **Normal**—patient uses correct words with no slurring.
- **Abnormal**—patient slurs words, uses the wrong words, or is unable to speak.

From Kothari R. U., Pancioli A., Liu T., Brott T., & Broderick J. (1999). Cincinnati Prehospital Stroke Scale: Reproducibility and validity. Reprinted from *Ann Emerg Med*, Apr; 33(4): 373-378. Copyright © 1999, with permission from American College of Emergency Physicians.

NURSING CARE PLAN
The Stroke Patient

ASSESSMENT

Health History: An obese 68-year-old male was admitted with weakness on the right side and slurred speech. His daughter assisted with the history because the patient had some difficulty responding verbally. He has had type 2 diabetes mellitus for 10 years, which he treats with an oral hypoglycemic agent, and had a myocardial infarction at age 75. He has no changes in vision but does wear reading glasses. He has good hearing and no headaches. He is right-handed. He was unable to stand when he awoke this morning. He tried to drink some water but had difficulty swallowing. He has had no loss of bowel or bladder control. He is divorced. An adult daughter and her two teenagers live with him. He is a retired construction worker; his hobbies are carpentry and watching television.

Physical Examination: Vital Signs: temperature, 97° F orally; pulse, 96; respirations, 22; blood pressure, 210/104. Patient is alert. Acknowledges he is in the hospital but is uncertain about day or date and time. Uses gestures to respond to some questions when he seems unable to find the right word. Pupils are equal and react to light. Ptosis of right eyelid is noted. Hand grips, voluntary movements, and reflexes of leg, arm, and hand are normal on left side but diminished on right side. Leans toward right side when not supported.

Nursing Diagnosis	Goals and Outcome Criteria	Interventions
Deficient Fluid Volume related to inadequate intake, dysphagia	The patient will maintain adequate hydration, as evidenced by moist mucous membranes, dilute urine, pulse and blood pressure within usual range.	Record fluid intake and output. Administer intravenous fluid as ordered. Monitor oral fluid intake and assess swallowing. Assist patient to sit up while eating and drinking. If thin fluids are difficult to swallow, try semisolids such as ice cream, pudding, and popsicles. Have oral suction device available in case of choking or aspiration. Detect and report signs and symptoms of fluid volume deficit: tachycardia, concentrated urine, dry mucous membranes.
Imbalanced Nutrition: Less Than Body Requirements related to dysphagia, inability to feed self	The patient will maintain adequate nutrition, as evidenced by stable weight.	Assess food intake. Assist with meals as needed. Seat upright for meals. Do not make him feel rushed. Provide alternative means of feeding (nasogastric or gastrostomy tube, total nutrition) as ordered. Weigh weekly to assess adequacy of food intake.
Impaired Verbal Communication related to aphasia	The patient will use nonverbal means to supplement verbal communication and will participate in speech therapy exercises.	Establish a code system of blinks or nods for nonverbal communication, use pictures or cards that patient can select to express his needs. Encourage verbalization but recognize frustration and provide words if patient cannot retrieve them. Discuss referral for speech therapy with physician. Tell the patient that improvement is usually possible with therapy.
Impaired Physical Mobility related to weakness, paralysis, poor balance	The patient will maintain intact skin, joint mobility, regular bowel and bladder elimination, good peripheral circulation, and normal breath sounds.	While on bedrest, assist him to change positions at least every 2 hours. He should not lie on his right side for more than 30 minutes at a time. Use positioning techniques and devices to reduce pressure points. Inspect skin for redness and edema associated with pressure. Position limbs in functional alignment, and perform range-of-motion exercises three times a day. Do not pull on the affected side. Monitor bowel and bladder function. Administer stool softeners and laxatives as ordered. Encourage fluids and fiber when able to take orally. Palpate lower abdomen for bladder distention and catheterize as ordered as necessary. Report tenderness, pain, or swelling in calves. Exercise legs with each position change. Apply elastic stockings or alternating pressure wraps as ordered. Ambulate when able. Encourage coughing and deep breathing with each position change. Assess lung fields for atelectasis, wheezes, or rales. Report temperature elevation.

reactions for appropriateness. If responses are not appropriate, try to identify the source of difficulty. Does the patient have trouble finding words? Do clues help the patient respond? Does the patient speak fluently? If the patient cannot provide the data needed, attempt to obtain them from a family member or friend. Note the informant (person who provides the history). Assess the patient's orientation to person, place, and time.

Chief Complaint and History of Present Illness. In the history of the present illness, identify the events

NURSING CARE PLAN

The Stroke Patient—cont'd

Nursing Diagnosis	Goals and Outcome Criteria	Interventions
Risk for Injury related to paralysis	The patient will have no falls or injuries associated with motor impairment or altered sensory perception.	Keep the bed in low position with the side rails raised according to hospital policy. Put the call bell within reach and instruct patient to call for help to get up. A bed-check device may be implemented when patients have difficulty understanding directions or are in a confused state. Check on him frequently. Monitor position of affected extremities to prevent trauma that might not be detected because of poor sensation. Use sling or brace if ordered to support affected limbs. Assess effects of ptosis on vision. If vision is impaired, approach patient from unaffected side and arrange personal articles on that side. When patient is out of bed, be sure he is seated safely. Use pillows to prevent excessive leaning to one side. When ambulatory, use gait belt if needed and assist as appropriate.
Anxiety related to loss of function or fear of disability	The patient will have a reduction in anxiety, as evidenced by calm manner and patient statement.	Acknowledge signs of anxiety and attempt to identify sources. Provide information about what is happening, what you are doing, and what he can expect. Check on him often. Encourage family to visit.
Interrupted Family Processes related to anticipated need of patient for assistance after discharge	The patient and family will plan for altered roles and responsibilities to support the patient during and after discharge.	Give family members an opportunity to ask questions and share their concerns. Provide information and facilitate communication with physician as needed. Refer to sources of support and resources, including social worker and community agencies. Start planning for discharge. Assess family strengths and resources, willingness to help care for patient after discharge. Identify new responsibilities they might need to assume, and discuss how these can be carried out.

? CRITICAL THINKING QUESTIONS

■ What effect might this patient's stroke have on his daughter and her family?

■ Describe three examples of signs of anxiety that the patient may exhibit.

---

that led the patient to seek medical care. A complete description of the illness includes the initial symptoms and how the symptoms progressed.

Medical History. Record past serious illnesses or conditions, including hypertension, heart disease, diabetes mellitus, liver disease, gout, head trauma, and previous strokes or transient ischemic attacks. Record previous hospitalizations, operations, and injuries.

Family History. The health history includes a family history of neurologic or cardiovascular disease as well as strokes.

Review of Systems. Ask the patient about significant problems in the review of systems. Important items to assess include weakness, impaired movement, pain (especially headache), dysphagia, bowel or bladder incontinence, visual disturbances, mental or emotional changes, and altered sensation.

Functional Assessment. The last component of the health history, the functional assessment, addresses the patient's usual activities and health practices. Inquire about activity level, dietary pattern, occupation, use of alcohol and tobacco, drug use, interpersonal relationships, and current stressors. These are important elements that will be used to identify risk factors for stroke and cardiovascular disease.

Physical Examination

During the physical examination, observe the patient's general appearance, responsiveness, and behavior. Record restlessness or agitation. The level of consciousness is important because subtle changes in level of consciousness such as confusion, irritability, or a decrease in level of consciousness may suggest a stroke in evolution or increasing intracranial pressure. Measure vital signs. The breathing pattern and effort are especially important. Obtain the patient's weight and height if possible.

Inspect the face for symmetry. Assess the mouth for moisture and drooling. Evaluate the alert patient's ability to swallow. Inspect the pupils for size, equality, and reaction to light. Conduct a gross vision assessment by asking the patient to read something. Inspect the skin for color and palpate for moisture and turgor. Assess

Box 28-3 *ASSESSMENT of the Cerebrovascular Accident Patient*

Health History

Source of Data:
Reliability and ability of patient to provide information

Present Illness:
Description of onset and progression

Past Medical History:
Cardiovascular conditions, liver disorder, diabetes mellitus, gout, previous cerebrovascular accidents, head injury, current medications

Family History:
Neurologic or vascular conditions

Review of Systems:
Visual disturbances, motor or sensory impairments, pain, dysphagia, incontinence, mental/emotional changes

Functional Assessment:
Usual activities, diet, occupation, use of alcohol and tobacco, interpersonal relationships, stressors

Physical Assessment

General Appearance:
Level of consciousness, behavior, gait, posture

Height and Weight

Vital Signs:
Blood pressure, temperature, pulse, respiration

Face:
Symmetry

Eyes:
Pupil size, equality, alignment, reaction to light; gross visual acuity, eyelid closure, ptosis

Skin:
Moisture, turgor, color

Abdomen:
Bowel or bladder distention

Genitalia and Anus:
Presence or odor of urine or stool

Extremities:
Muscle tone, strength, voluntary movement, sensation

---

extremities for muscle tone and strength, sensation, and voluntary movement. Instruct the patient to move each extremity individually and observe responses. Impaired movement or inappropriate response may be due to aphasia or dyspraxia as well as to neuromuscular damage. The patient who has aphasia has difficulty interpreting the messages and may not perform the requested movement for that reason. The patient with dyspraxia may comprehend the instruction but be unable to direct the body part to move. Also record any evidence of incontinence or bladder distention.

Frequently repeat neurologic checks consisting of evaluating level of consciousness, pupil appearance and response to light, the patient's ability to follow commands, and the movement and sensation of extremities. For additional neurologic assessment, see Chapter 27.

The National Institutes of Health (NIH) Stroke Assessment Scale (Table 28-3) is a tool often used to assess patients who have experienced a stroke. This tool provides a method to guide systematic assessment of neurologic deficits often associated with an acute stroke. The examination addresses motor function, visual fields, ataxia, speech, language, cognition, and motor and sensory abnormalities. A point system is used to rate function; then points are combined to offer a "score." It was designed by a research neurologist to standardize and document neurologic assessments of stroke patients. Most facilities that use this assessment tool require those administering the examination to go through a certification process to ensure accuracy and consistency among examiners.

Nursing assessment of the stroke patient is summarized in Box 28-3.

Nursing Diagnoses, Goals, and Outcome Criteria:
Acute Phase of Stroke

Depending on location and extent of brain damage, appropriate diagnoses and goals may include the following:

NURSING DIAGNOSES	GOALS AND OUTCOME CRITERIA
Ineffective Airway Clearance related to impaired cough reflex, altered consciousness, impaired swallowing	Patent airway: breath sounds clear to auscultation
Ineffective Breathing Pattern related to impaired cerebral circulation, increased intracranial pressure	Effective breathing pattern: normal respiratory rate and depth, arterial blood gases within normal limits
Risk for Injury related to seizure activity, confusion, motor impairment	Absence of injury: no bruising, skin breaks, falls, or fractures
Risk for Deficient Fluid Volume related to inadequate intake or excessive diuresis	Adequate hydration: balanced fluid intake and output
Risk for Fluid Volume Excess related to overhydration	Normal extracellular fluid volume: pulse and blood pressure consistent with patient norms, no edema, breath sounds clear
Imbalanced Nutrition: Less Than Body Requirements related to dysphagia, inability to feed self, inability to chew	Adequate intake of nutrients: maintenance of body weight

Disturbed Sensory Perception related to neurologic impairment	Adaptation to sensory perceptual alterations
Ineffective Thermoregulation related to effects of neurologic impairment and/or metabolic processes	Effective thermoregulation: temperature within patient's normal range
Disturbed Thought Processes related to impaired cerebral circulation	Improved mental function: patient is oriented to self and environment
Impaired Verbal Communication related to aphasia	Effective communication: patient successfully communicates needs
Impaired Physical Mobility related to weakness, paralysis, spasticity, impaired balance	Absence of complications of immobility: joints have full range of motion, skin intact
Total Urinary Incontinence or Functional Urinary Incontinence related to impaired control, inability to manage toileting process	Improved control of urine elimination: episodes of uncontrolled voiding decrease; patient voids voluntarily
Constipation related to immobility, dehydration, drug side effects	Normal bowel elimination: regular passage of soft, formed stool without straining
Bowel Incontinence related to impaired conduction of impulses	Controlled bowel elimination: no involuntary bowel evacuation
Ineffective Coping related to adapting to neurologic deficits	Effective coping strategies: patient verbalizes acceptance of stroke and strives for maximum recovery
Interrupted Family Processes related to disruption of family roles and functions	Adaptation of the family to the patient's condition: family demonstrates willingness and ability to adapt to patient's condition

Interventions

Ineffective Airway Clearance and Ineffective Breathing Pattern

Closely monitor the patient's respiratory status. Maintaining a patent airway is a priority for patients who have suffered strokes. Neurologic deficits may cause altered breathing patterns and impaired swallowing, gag, and cough reflexes. Increasing intracranial pressure may affect the respiratory center in the brain, causing respiratory depression. If the patient exhibits signs of increased intracranial pressure (rising blood pressure, bradycardia, abnormal pupil response, decreasing level of consciousness), elevate the head of the bed 30 degrees and notify the physician.

After a stroke, the patient is at risk for airway obstruction for a number of reasons. If the patient is unconscious, the tongue may fall back and block the airway. A side-lying position helps prevent such obstruction. An oral or nasal airway is sometimes employed to keep the airway open.

Immobility and dehydration cause thick secretions to be retained in the respiratory tract, possibly leading to pneumonia and atelectasis. Good hydration helps thin respiratory secretions for easier expectoration. Dysphagia may cause the patient to aspirate fluids or food, causing airway obstruction and contributing to the development of pneumonia. Pneumonia is, in fact, the most frequent cause of death after stroke. Feeding the patient with dysphagia is discussed in Chapter 38.

Suctioning and frequent position changes can help prevent aspiration and promote removal of secretions. Respiratory treatments for the patient with regular reminders to do deep-breathing exercises can be helpful. Forceful coughing may be discouraged in the acute phase after a hemorrhagic stroke because it tends to increase intracranial pressure. Ask the physician if and when coughing is permitted. Administer oxygen therapy as ordered.

Risk for Injury

Many factors place the stroke patient at risk for injury. Seizures may occur, causing the patient to lose consciousness and to have abnormal motor activity. Raise side rails and pad them according to agency protocol to reduce trauma if the patient strikes the rails. During a seizure, turn the patient to one side and move hard objects away from the patient. Never force anything between clenched teeth. To do so may injure the teeth and gums. Additional information about seizures is presented in Chapter 27.

Safety precautions are also essential for confused patients and patients with motor impairments. Orient patients to their surroundings, and explain why they should not get up unassisted. The staff must respond promptly to the patient's calls for help. Although restraints are needed at times, they should be used as a last resort because they often agitate the patient and can actually cause injuries. A bed check system may be of more benefit when the patient is having difficulty understanding directions. Get sufficient help or use mechanical devices to assist the patient in and out of the bed.

Deficient Fluid Volume or Fluid Volume Excess

Close monitoring of fluid status is especially important in the acute phase of stroke. Accurate intake and output records are essential. Take vital signs and compare for trends suggesting fluid volume excess or deficit. Assess the mouth for moisture. In a well-hydrated person, the mucous membranes of the mouth are moist. Evaluate tissue turgor, but remember that it is not a very reliable indicator of fluid status in the older person. Age-related changes in the skin and

Table 28-3 | *NIH Stroke Scale*

1a. Level of Consciousness	0 Alert
	1 Not alert, but arousable with minimal stimulation
	2 Not alert, requires repeated stimulation to attend
	3 Coma
1b. Ask patient the month and his or her age	0 Answers both correctly
	1 Answers one correctly
	2 Both incorrect
1c. Ask patient to open and close eyes and grip and release hand	0 Obeys both correctly
	1 Obeys one correctly
	2 Both incorrect
2. Best Gaze (only horizontal eye movement)	0 Normal
	1 Partial gaze palsy
	2 Forced deviation
3. Visual Field Testing	0 No visual field loss
	1 Partial hemianopia
	2 Complete hemianopia
	3 Bilateral hemianopia (blind including cortical blindness)
4. Facial Paresis (ask patient to show teeth or raise eyebrows and close eyes tightly)	0 Normal symmetric movement
	1 Minor paralysis (flattened nasolabial fold, asymmetry on smiling)
	2 Partial paralysis (total or near total paralysis of lower face)
	3 Complete paralysis of one or both sides (absence of facial movement in the upper and lower face)
5. Motor Function—Arm (right and left) **Right arm — —** **Left arm — —**	0 Normal (extends arms 90 (or 45) degrees for 10 seconds without drift)
	1 Drift
	2 Some effort against gravity
	3 No effort against gravity
	4 No movement
6. Motor Function—Leg (right and left) **Right leg — —** **Left leg — —**	0 Normal (holds leg 30 degrees position for 5 seconds)
	1 Drift
	2 Some effort against gravity
	3 No effort against gravity
	4 No movement
	9 Untestable (Joint fused or limb amputated)
7. Limb Ataxia	0 No ataxia
	1 Present in one limb
	2 Present in two limbs
8. Sensory (use pinprick to test arms, legs, trunk, and face—compare side to side)	0 Normal trunk and face
	1 Mild to moderate decrease in sensation
	2 Severe to total sensory loss
9. Best Language (describe picture, read items, read sentences)	0 No aphasia
	1 Mild to moderate aphasia
	2 Severe aphasia
	3 Mute
10. Dysarthria (read several words)	0 Normal articulation
	1 Mild to moderate slurring of words
	2 Near unintelligible or unable to speak
	9 Intubated or other physical barriers
11. Extinction and Inattention	0 Normal
	1 Inattention or extinction to bilateral simultaneous stimulation in one of the sensory modalities
	2 Profound hemi-inattention or extinction to more than one sensory modality (e.g., does not recognize own hand)

subcutaneous structures cause a loss of tissue elasticity that may be mistaken for dehydration. Laboratory studies, including urine specific gravity, serum electrolytes, and hematocrit, are also useful indicators of fluid balance.

The patient is at risk for fluid volume excess if excessive intravenous fluids are administered or if the patient's kidneys are unable to eliminate excess fluid rapidly enough. Fluid volume excess may lead to edema and heart failure. Signs of fluid volume excess are fluid intake greater than output, bounding pulse, venous distention, increased blood pressure, crackles in the lungs, and edema. Report evidence of excess fluid to the registered nurse or the physician. The rate of intravenous fluid may be decreased and diuretics given as ordered. Explain to the patient and family the need to temporarily restrict fluids. If the patient is thirsty, frequently provide small amounts of fluids in small containers and record all intake.

Factors that place the stroke patient at risk for fluid volume deficit include age, dysphagia, drug therapy with diuretics, and immobility. The stroke patient is likely to be older, and older people are less able to conserve water through the kidneys. The patient with dysphagia may be unable to take adequate oral fluids. If diuretics are given for fluid volume excess or increased intracranial pressure, they can precipitate excess loss of water and electrolytes. The patient with motor deficits may not be able to obtain fluids independently.

Fluid volume deficit contributes to constipation, skin dryness, urinary tract infections, and renal calculi (stones). Signs of fluid volume deficit are a thready pulse, tachycardia, low blood pressure, low urine output, concentrated urine, dry mucous membranes, and sometimes confusion. Report evidence of fluid volume deficit to the registered nurse or the physician. If intravenous fluids are being administered, the physician may order an increase in the hourly flow rate. Fluids may also be given through enteral feeding tubes.

To reduce the risk of fluid volume deficit, monitor the fluid intake record to be sure the patient is getting at least eight 8-ounce glasses of fluids each day (unless contraindicated). Be sure all staff and family members know to offer fluids and record the amounts taken. Place fluids within sight and easy reach of the patient, and explain the need for adequate hydration. If the patient has hemiplegia, be sure the fluids are placed on the nonparalyzed side. Spillproof containers that are easily held with one hand can facilitate independent drinking. If the patient is able to take oral fluids but has difficulty swallowing, proceed slowly. Have suction equipment on hand in case of aspiration. Thin liquids are more readily aspirated. Jell-O, ice cream, popsicles, and frozen juice may be substituted to provide adequate fluids. There are also thickening agents that can be added to other liquids as needed.

Imbalanced Nutrition: Less Than Body Requirements

The patient's nutritional status is of concern throughout stroke treatment. Factors that may lead to inadequate nutrition include dysphagia, paralysis, difficulty chewing, and depression. The patient who is malnourished is at risk for skin breakdown and infection. Obesity hampers mobility and can interfere with rehabilitation.

The patient who has dysphagia may not be able to consume adequate nutrients orally. Sometimes a nasogastric tube is inserted for feeding purposes. The physician may order total parenteral nutrition for the malnourished patient. Aggressive treatment of dysphagia is delayed until the rehabilitative phase. Dysphagia often resolves spontaneously during the first few months of recovery. Feeding the dysphagic patient is discussed in Chapter 38.

If the patient has a nasogastric or nasointestinal feeding tube in place, check its placement and residual according to agency policy. Provide the correct formula, and ensure that it flows at the prescribed rate. Bolus feedings may be ordered at intervals, or pumps may be used to dispense continuous feedings. Monitor the rate of administration. Slightly elevate the head of the bed to reduce the risk of fluid flowing back into the esophagus and being aspirated. The nasogastric tube irritates the naris and the nasal passages. Gently cleanse the naris several times a day. Assess tube placement according to agency policy. Concentrated formulas may cause diarrhea. If that happens, the physician should be consulted about diluting the formula or changing to another type of formula.

Total parenteral nutrition is given through an intravenous line inserted into a large vein (a central line). Unlike enteral feedings, the flow of total parenteral nutrition fluids is always controlled with a mechanical infusion pump. The nurse hangs new bottles of prescribed fluids. Take special care to prevent air from entering the tubing. The insertion site also requires special care to prevent infection. Change dressings according to agency protocol, using strict aseptic technique. Patients on total parenteral nutrition may develop hyperglycemia; therefore monitor blood glucose levels at regular intervals. Care of the patient receiving total parenteral nutrition is discussed in detail in Chapter 9.

Disturbed Sensory Perception

Sensory perceptual problems in the stroke patient may include visual disturbances, sensory deprivation or overload, and impaired tactile sensation. Among the visual disturbances are diplopia (double vision), loss of the corneal (blink) reflex, ptosis (drooping of the upper eyelid), homonymous hemianopsia, and inability to close the eyelids on the affected side. All of these pose threats to safety and to self-care. They may also contribute to confusion. The cornea is susceptible to injury when not protected and kept moist by the closed eyelid and the blink reflex. Artificial tears may be used to provide moisture.

Patients who have homonymous hemianopsia see only half the field of vision. Some patients have unilateral neglect, a condition in which visual fields are intact but the patient does not attend to certain parts of the fields. Unilateral neglect is most common in patients with right brain damage. These patients may not attend to one side of the body and may overlook objects on one side of the visual field.

It is helpful to encourage patients to scan the affected side. Differences in the nursing approaches during the acute and rehabilitative phases are well contrasted here. In the acute phase, position patients with homonymous hemianopsia so that their unimpaired side is approached by the staff, to reduce stress to the patient. In rehabilitation, position the patient so that deliberate scanning and use of the affected side are required. This is designed to stimulate return of function. Balanced sensory input is essential to reduce the risk of sensory deprivation or overload. The environment should be pleasant but not overly stimulating.

Another type of sensory disturbance after stroke is diminished sensation in affected body parts. The patient who does not feel pressure or pain is susceptible to injury. A paralyzed foot can easily slip down between the bed frame and side rails. Catheter tubing under the leg may create pressure that the patient cannot feel. Protect susceptible areas, and remind the patient of the need for extra caution. Check positioning of affected extremities to ensure that they are free of pressure, and reposition as needed.

Ineffective Thermoregulation

After a stroke, the body's temperature-regulating mechanism may be impaired, causing the temperature to rise. There are also metabolic processes in play that may increase the body temperature. It is important to monitor the patient's temperature and treat elevations promptly. Fever is treated aggressively, most often with antipyretics. Some studies even suggest a decrease in infarction size in those patients aggressively treated for hyperthermia. Always assess the patient for an underlying infection as a potential cause for any temperature elevation.

Disturbed Thought Processes

After a stroke, patients may suffer functional losses, alterations in sensation and perception, and impaired communication. In addition, they find themselves in the hospital, where they are poked, monitored, and prodded by strangers and where days and nights all seem the same. All these factors combined can cause the patient to become disoriented or confused. Neglect associated with right brain strokes may also be manifested as denial. In extreme cases, patients deny that they have even had a stroke.

To orient patients, introduce yourself, remind patients where they are, and tell them what is being done and why. Be sure that eyeglasses and hearing aids are worn if the patient normally uses them. Place clocks and marked calendars in view. Tell the patient what time it is and what to expect next. Confused patients require frequent reassurance and reinforcement. Instructions and information should be concise and repeated as needed. Sometimes a familiar person is helpful with a confused patient. If the visitor is disturbed by the patient's behavior, provide guidance in how to deal with the patient.

Impaired Verbal Communication

The alert patient who has aphasia is understandably anxious about the inability to speak, to understand words, or both. Use brief, clear statements accompanied by gestures, pictures, and facial expressions. Questions that can be answered *yes* or *no* may allow the patient to respond more easily. Pause attentively when the patient struggles to respond. Excessive chatter can be distressing to the aphasic patient. Explain the communication problem and approaches to the family. Speech therapy may be initiated once the medical condition of the patient is stable. Speech rehabilitation is discussed further in the section Nursing Care in the Rehabilitation Phase on p. 480.

Impaired Physical Mobility

Impaired motor function is common after stroke and places the patient at risk for complications of immobility. Care of the immobilized patient is discussed in detail in Chapter 21 and is summarized here.

Skin Integrity. The potential for skin breakdown in this patient population is great because of motor impairment, altered consciousness or sensation, poor nutritional status, and incontinence. Measures to maintain skin integrity include cleanliness, pressure relief, and good hydration and nutrition. When skin is dry, as it often is in older patients, reduce bathing frequency, use soap sparingly, and apply lotions to retain skin moisture.

It is essential to turn and reposition the acute stroke patient at least every 2 hours. Skin breakdown can occur at vulnerable pressure points after just 30 minutes in one position. If reddened pressure areas remain when it is time to turn the patient, shorten the intervals between turnings. Do not allow the patient to lie on the affected side for more than 30 minutes. Because of impaired sensation, the risk of excessive pressure and trauma is much greater on the affected side. Pressure must be alternated on main pressure points such as hips, knees, heels, and lower back. An air flotation mattress or fluidized bed may be used for the high-risk patient. Some of the newer therapeutic beds automatically turn patients. These beds do not stress the usual pressure points of the patient, but regular skin assessments and breathing exercises are still required. As soon as possible, position the patient comfortably in a chair for brief periods. Remember to monitor for a drop in blood pressure when getting the patient out of bed.

Good nursing care is time-consuming, so take advantage of this time to stimulate the patient with conversation and explanations of care. This is important even if the patient is unresponsive.

Joint Mobility. The immobilized patient is at risk for muscle atrophy and joint contractures. In the stroke patient, the affected side is especially vulnerable when there is loss of voluntary movement. During the acute phase, be concerned with maintaining joint mobility. This can be done with frequent, gentle range-of-motion exercises and proper positioning. Determine whether the patient had any preexisting limitations of joint mobility. Older patients may have arthritic changes that reduce the range of motion. Never force resistant joints. Once the acute phase has passed, the patient is usually referred for vigorous physical therapy.

Support affected extremities. It is important never to grab or pull the extremities on the patient's affected side. Dislocation or further injury can easily occur because the patient may not be able to accurately perceive the pressure or pain that is normally felt.

Circulation. Deep vein thrombosis (DVT) is a major complication of immobility, especially in this patient population. Regular passive and active range-of-motion exercises encourage venous blood return, thereby reducing the risk of thrombus formation. The physician may order elastic stockings or alternating pressure wraps to promote venous return. Low-dose anticoagulation therapy should be initiated to help prevent thrombus formation. Ambulation is generally encouraged (if the patient is able) as soon as possible after the medical condition stabilizes.

Total Urinary Incontinence or Functional Urinary Incontinence

It is not unusual for urinary incontinence to occur after stroke. This may be due to a temporarily flaccid bladder or an inability of the brain to coordinate information to be able to store urine in the bladder or wait once the urge to void is felt. Check the patient hourly for wetness. Promptly remove wet clothing and linens. Wash the skin, rinse, and pat dry. A variety of incontinence products are available to minimize the contact of urine with the skin (see Chapter 23). Sometimes an indwelling catheter is ordered to prevent incontinence. The catheter protects the skin and allows for more accurate measurement of output. The disadvantage is that an indwelling catheter is frequently the cause of urinary tract infections. A regular toileting schedule with intermittent catheterization is a better alternative to indwelling catheterization. External condom catheters are options for male patients. Bladder retraining, discussed in Chapter 23, is actively pursued in the rehabilitative phase.

Many older men have prostatic hypertrophy, which can cause dribbling of urine or urine retention. Scheduled toileting may be helpful, but catheterization may be required. The enlarged prostate makes catheterization more difficult. If the catheter cannot be inserted easily, *never* force it. Notify the registered nurse or physician. Sometimes a special type of catheter is needed for the patient with prostate enlargement.

Constipation and/or Bowel Incontinence

As with urinary incontinence, the ability of the brain to coordinate the information to wait once the urge to move the bowels is felt may be damaged. During the acute phase of stroke, it is especially important to monitor bowel elimination, because the patient may develop constipation or incontinence. It is helpful to know the patient's usual patterns of elimination, although they cannot always be determined.

Constipation may develop as a result of immobility, dehydration, and drug therapy. A bowel program, consisting of a mild laxative or stool softener and a high-fiber diet, can help prompt regular fecal elimination. Explain to patients and family members the importance of sufficient fluids to prevent dry stools. Some older people are laxative dependent. It is unrealistic to try to reverse the effects of years of laxative use during the acute phase of stroke. Inform the registered nurse or physician of the pattern, and document bowel movements. Laxatives and enemas may be needed to maintain bowel elimination in these patients.

Bowel incontinence may be related to the inability to toilet independently or to confusion and can often be prevented in the alert patient by taking the patient to the toilet at the usual time of defecation. A raised toilet seat with arm rests is easier and safer for the patient with hemiplegia. If incontinence occurs, take special care to clean the skin thoroughly. Be careful not to make comments that embarrass the patient. Remember that incontinence, especially with liquid stools, may indicate a fecal impaction. Removal of an impaction usually requires repeated enemas and manual removal of hard stool. Restoration of bowel control receives more attention in the rehabilitative phase and is detailed in Chapter 23.

Ineffective Coping

The effects of stroke may be temporary or permanent. It is difficult to predict how much function will be lost permanently or returned during recovery. Patients typically exhibit responses that reflect the grief process: shock, denial, depression, withdrawal, and bargaining. Determine how the patient is coping and whether the coping strategies are constructive and/or effective.

An example of unhealthy coping is the patient who denies having problems with vision or balance and refuses to call for help when getting out of bed. Another example is the depressed and withdrawn patient who resists doing therapeutic exercises that would minimize complications. You can point out the behavior to the patient, explain its consequences, and encourage the patient to take an active role in rehabilitation activities. Depression is a major problem associated with stroke and can occur in up to 70% of stroke patients. The depression seen after a stroke may be the result of a loss of brain chemicals associated with the injury or a reaction to the loss of one's functional abilities. Antidepressant medications may be ordered for patients experiencing depression after a stroke and have been associated with improved outcomes in those patients treated. Sometimes a mental health counselor or support group is beneficial to help the patient learn to deal with the effects of stroke more constructively.

Interrupted Family Processes

In the acute phase of stroke, family members are often frightened and confused. They may fear the patient's death or severe disability. They may also experience emotional and financial strain during the long rehabilitation process. Family members have to assume roles and responsibilities normally carried by the patient. Recognize that the family, as well as the patient, experiences a sense of loss when a loved one has a stroke. Provide support by telling family members what is happening, what is being done, and how they can help the patient. If necessary, a referral may be made to a social worker, mental health specialist, or spiritual counselor.

NURSING CARE *in the Rehabilitation Phase*

A patient's transition from the acute phase to the rehabilitation phase of stroke is an important one. Early and attentive care for the stroke patient shortens the recovery time and hastens the return of function. The general goals of treatment in the rehabilitation phase are to maximize functional abilities and to teach new ways to compensate for losses. Stabilization of vital signs with no further neurologic deficits indicates that the patient has entered the rehabilitation phase of stroke. At this time, the patient's functional and cognitive problems can vary widely, depending on the location and extent of brain damage. The patient may regain complete independent functioning, partially recover previous abilities, or lose functional abilities completely.

The rehabilitation phase is usually managed by an interdisciplinary team that includes nurses, physicians, physical therapists, occupational therapists, speech therapists, social workers, psychologists, recreational therapists, vocational rehabilitation counselors, and dietitians.

During the rehabilitation phase of a stroke, vast changes can occur in the brain. The extent to which collateral blood circulation and alternative neuronal pathways develop affects the ultimate outcome for the patient. The goals of rehabilitation to enhance the ultimate recovery of functional abilities are reached through a program of stimulation and practice. It has been said that rehabilitation is the respectful challenging of the patient facing a chronic health problem. With this in mind, the next section describes nursing care in

the management of long-term problems that can follow a stroke.

Assessment

Nursing assessment of the stroke patient was described earlier in this chapter and is summarized in Box 28-3. In the rehabilitation phase, reassess the patient's abilities as well as his or her expectations, knowledge, motivation, and resources.

Nursing Diagnoses, Goals, and Outcome Criteria: Rehabilitation Phase of Stroke

NURSING DIAGNOSES	GOALS AND OUTCOME CRITERIA
Self-Care Deficit related to sensory and motor impairments	Self-care needs met: care accomplished with assistance as needed
Risk for Injury related to sensory and motor impairments	Absence of injury: no falls, bruises, skin tears, pressure sores
Ineffective Coping related to cognitive impairments	Effective coping: patient uses adaptive strategies to cope with disability
Impaired Verbal Communication related to aphasia, dysarthria	Effective communication: meaningful verbalizations or effective use of nonverbal communication to make needs known
Imbalanced Nutrition: Less Than Body Requirements related to dysphagia, anorexia	Adequate nutrition: achievement and maintenance of ideal body weight
Impaired Physical Mobility related to residual motor impairment	Improved physical mobility: increasing independent physical activity
Constipation related to inactivity	Normal bowel elimination: regular, formed stools without straining
Total Urinary Incontinence and Functional Urinary Incontinence related to neurologic and motor impairment	Normal urine elimination: voluntary urination, decreasing incontinent episodes

Interventions
Self-Care Deficit

The main focus of the rehabilitation phase is to return the stroke patient to the highest level of functioning possible. One of the most frustrating problems after a stroke for many patients and caregivers is the patient's inability to complete activities of daily living. To improve, patients need to use affected parts as much as they are able. It is important for the nurse to demonstrate patience and a supportive attitude. Allow time for patients to try to do things for themselves. Discouragement is a major factor in unsuccessful rehabilitation and demands prompt attention by the rehabilitation team.

A variety of personal devices and environmental adaptations can foster a return to independence. Prosthetic devices that assist patients with dressing, bathing, and eating are available. Simple measures such as replacing buttons with Velcro fasteners and replacing complicated trousers with elastic-waist pants can make a big difference.

A referral for follow-up at home should be initiated so that the safety and accessibility of the home environment can be assessed before discharge. The trend toward shorter hospital stays means this must be addressed very early. Many patients are discharged to rehabilitation or skilled nursing facilities until they are ready to return home. A home visit by the patient, home health nurse, and occupational therapist can be made to identify problems and make plans for adaptations. Adaptations should promote access in and out of the home and enable patients to be as independent as possible. The addition of a raised commode seat, bathtub handrails, shower seat, or other devices can facilitate toileting and bathing. Cooking may be assisted by adjusting the height of counters, creating shelves that roll out, and rearranging cabinet contents to improve access. Patients need to practice daily tasks under conditions similar to those at home. Rehabilitation centers usually have activity centers that allow patients to practice self-care skills with their disabilities (Fig. 28-6).

FIGURE **28-6** Assistive devices enable the patient to be active at home.

Risk for Injury

Alterations in motor function, sensation, and vision are distressing changes that affect the patient's ability to carry out self-care and pose a threat to safety.

Motor. Alterations in motor functioning may leave the patient at risk for injury. Safety precautions are a vital part of nursing care of the patient. Teaching should include calling for assistance as needed, using assistive devices for mobilization, and adaptation of the environment to promote safety. Physical and occupational therapists are invaluable in assisting with providing a safe environment.

Sensation. As noted previously, patients may have altered sensation in the affected body parts after a stroke. This may appear as loss of sensation or as exaggerated response in which every sensation is perceived as painful. The patient may be injured without even knowing it because of impaired sensation. Teach the patient and family to assess the affected area frequently for signs of pressure and to protect it from injury. In addition to teaching the patient how to avoid pressure, advise the patient not to apply heat or cold to that area because of the risk of injury. Remind the patient and family not to pull on the affected side or use that side to move or support the patient in ambulation.

Patients with abnormal pain perception may benefit from regular physical therapy, using a kind of desensitization. During therapy, the patient is reminded and encouraged that the pain is not real and is only misinterpreted by the brain.

Vision. Homonymous hemianopsia, in which half of the field of vision is lost, also presents problems with self-care and safety. In the acute phase, the patient's environment is arranged so that people approach and important items are available on the unaffected side. In rehabilitation, the patient is challenged more to promote adaptation to the disability. Place objects in the field of the visual deficit. Remind and encourage the patient to scan the affected visual field, especially when walking, wheeling, and eating. The patient forms new habits of observation through constant practice.

Ineffective Coping

Intellectual and emotional changes after stroke are distressing to patients and their families. Explain these changes, and demonstrate how to help patients adapt. Cognitive processes may continue to be slow for quite some time after the stroke. It is important to avoid rushing the patient. The patient may become frustrated and give up trying. Emotional ability is manifested as sudden laughing, crying, or outbursts of anger without apparent reason. Caregivers and families may attribute this emotional unpredictability to depression. It is generally believed that depression is frequently associated with brain trauma of any kind. The patient can often be easily distracted from crying or from anger with simple redirection to the task at hand. This is an indication that the depression, if it exists, may be of a different type than the usual emotional state and require specific interventions. Treatment of depression, whatever the cause, is an important part of the rehabilitation process. Research clearly demonstrates a positive relationship to outcomes when patients are identified and treated aggressively for depression after a stroke.

Impaired Verbal Communication

Helping the patient improve or regain effective communication is an extremely important goal of the rehabilitation phase. Aphasia may affect the ability to understand spoken words or to use words to express oneself. Types of aphasia were explained with signs and symptoms of stroke (see Table 28-2).

Patients with aphasia need encouragement as they struggle to communicate. Be patient, because the aphasic person requires more time to plan and deliver a response. Take time to allow this to happen, but provide verbal cues or picture boards before patients become overly frustrated trying to respond. The physician often refers patients with severe communication impairments to speech therapists.

Imbalanced Nutrition: Less Than Body Requirements

The patient with dysphagia must be reevaluated at intervals for ability to swallow. If the patient is able to swallow saliva, the physician may allow liquids to be introduced. Initially, ¼ teaspoon of ice chips might be given with a spoon. The amount is increased and water may be added until the patient is able to swallow a teaspoon of water. If problems with this simple assessment occur, a video fluoroscopic test of swallowing may be ordered. This test traces the route of swallowed fluid to detect swallowing abnormalities. Because water is thin, some patients find it difficult to swallow. It may be helpful to add a thicker substance to liquids to facilitate swallowing.

The patient who has some difficulty swallowing may be placed on a supervised feeding program. Speech therapists are trained to help patients relearn swallowing, but everyday feeding falls to the nursing staff. The best position for eating is sitting with the head tilted forward and toward the unaffected side. Fluid intake must still be encouraged for the dysphagic person, despite the increased work for patient and staff. Special

FIGURE **28-7** Assistive devices for eating. **A,** Utensils adapted to special needs. A plate that keeps food from being pushed off. **B,** Plate guards keep food on the plate. **C,** The round-blade knife allows a person to cut with only one hand. **D,** Special handle is easier to grasp and hold.

utensils can greatly facilitate self-feeding (Fig 28-7). Acknowledge even small improvements as the patient struggles in rehabilitation.

Impaired Physical Mobility

Mobility can continue to be a problem for patients in the rehabilitation phase. Hemiplegia, dyspraxia, and visual field disturbances all create unique problems. Hemiplegia is rarely a motor problem alone. It is often accompanied by disturbances in balance and spatial perception (Fig. 28-8).

Regular physical therapy and occupational therapy promote optimal return of motor function. Regular exercise can facilitate a dramatic return of function for some patients. Therefore affected arms and legs need to be used to maintain muscular function and circulation if and until neurologic ability is recovered. In the meantime, assistance is needed with motor activities. When the patient is moving, assess gait (if applicable), strength in arms and legs, and balance. Correct body mechanics and transfer techniques are essential when working with the patient. A gait belt helps the patient in transfers and in ambulation and may protect staff members from injury. This is a fabric belt with a toothed buckle that is applied between the nipple line and the waist and is used to support and assist the patient. Assistive devices such as the quad cane and walkers may improve safety with ambulation (Fig. 28-9).

Patients who have dyspraxia are unable to initiate voluntary motor acts. It is interesting to note that they sometimes exhibit those actions spontaneously. To help the patient remember to initiate voluntary responses, provide verbal cues. Teach family members about dys-praxia, and advise them to be patient and employ cues to induce the desired motor performance. Remind the patient who has unilateral neglect to use and support the affected side.

Constipation

Bowel elimination problems may continue into the rehabilitation phase. Incontinence is not usually a problem for the alert patient except when it is caused by inability to access toileting devices or manage clothing. Document the timing of incidents of bowel incontinence so a toileting schedule can be developed. Often simply taking the patient to the toilet at the usual time of defecation eliminates bowel incontinence. There is additional discussion of bowel incontinence in Chapter 23.

Constipation is a more common challenge in the rehabilitation phase. A regular bowel program with toileting, orientation, and reminders is needed. Provide sufficient fluids to promote bowel regularity. Many stroke patients do not receive adequate fluid intake because of dysphagia or fear of incontinence. Also, caregivers may not take the extra time needed to provide fluids for the patient who responds slowly. Stool softeners, laxatives, and suppositories may be used to reestablish regular bowel elimination and then gradually discontinued. Some patients continue to need stool softeners. As noted earlier, some patients with long-standing

Put on Your Thinking Cap!

Use a towel or other material to make an arm sling. Place your dominant arm in the sling while you prepare a meal, eat, and clean up. Immediately after this exercise, write down: (1) what adaptations you had to make, (2) what things you were unable to do unassisted, (3) how you felt during the exercise, and (4) how you behaved during the exercise. Compare responses with your classmates. Discuss implications for patient care.

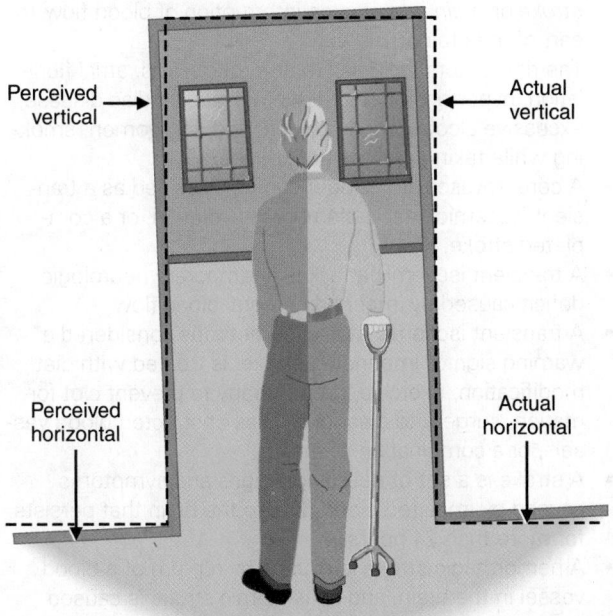

FIGURE **28-8** Perceptual disturbances in hemiplegia may affect the patient's ability to maneuver safely in the environment.

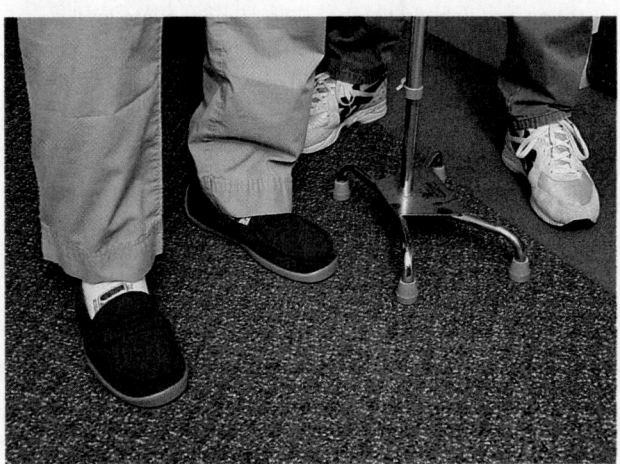

FIGURE **28-9** A quad cane provides good support for a patient with hemiplegia.

laxative dependency may not respond to more conservative measures to promote bowel elimination.

Total Urinary Incontinence and Functional Urinary Incontinence

If an indwelling catheter was inserted in the acute phase of stroke treatment, it will probably be removed and efforts made to restore bladder control. Immediately after the catheter is removed, the patient may have poor sphincter control or may retain urine. Therefore monitor urine output and check for bladder distention until normal voiding is established. Perineal muscle exercises (see Chapter 23) may be prescribed to improve sphincter control.

Intermittent catheterization may continue to be necessary in the rehabilitation phase. The urine volume obtained is measured, and intermittent catheterization is done every 4 to 6 hours, depending on the volume obtained.

Incontinence of urine is more difficult to correct than bowel incontinence. A bladder program should be initiated promptly. Document the patient's fluid intake and frequency of voiding. Scheduled toileting based on the patient's usual pattern often helps control incontinence. Advice for helping patients with dysphagia swallow liquids is given in the Nutrition Concepts box below.

Discharge

Patients may be discharged to their homes or may go to specialized rehabilitation centers for continued therapy. Outpatient therapy is an option for some patients. The rehabilitation phase is defined in various ways. In acute rehabilitation settings, patients will be evaluated by all disciplines and goals will be set. Continuous assessments and goal setting occur throughout the rehabilitation process. When able, patients are transitioned back into the home setting when possible. It is essential to include family, friends, and significant others in this process. Medicare defines the rehabilitation phase as 3 months after the stroke. Rehabilitation specialists say rehabilitation continues indefinitely but progress slows down. There is a great deal of evidence that rehabilitation helps patients recovering from a stroke to achieve a high level of functioning and improve safety after returning home.

During and after the rehabilitation phase, patients and families need to be made aware of resources to help them deal with continuing disabilities. Patients and families should be referred to the American Heart Association/American Stroke Association, National Stroke Association, and other local agencies within the community. There are support groups available in many communities to offer assistance and generally have a positive impact on the stroke survivor.

Although stroke remains a major health problem, the risk can be reduced. The acute phase of stroke, from diagnosis to stabilization of blood pressure, requires support and careful evaluation of the patient's remaining abilities. In rehabilitation, the patient is respectfully challenged to return to the highest level of function possible.

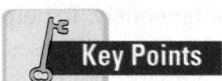 **Key Points**

- A cerebrovascular accident (CVA), commonly called a *stroke* or *brain attack*, is an interruption of blood flow to part of the brain.
- The risk factors for CVA are atherosclerosis, atrial fibrillation, hypertension, diabetes mellitus, cardiac disease, excessive alcohol consumption, and, for women, smoking while taking oral contraceptives.
- A cerebrovascular accident can be classified as a transient ischemic attack, a stroke in evolution, or a completed stroke.
- A transient ischemic attack is a temporary neurologic deficit caused by impaired cerebral blood flow.
- A transient ischemic attack, sometimes considered a warning sign of impending stroke, is treated with diet modification, exercise, drug therapy to prevent clot formation, surgery to clear or bypass obstructed blood vessels, or a combination of these.
- A stroke is a set of neurologic signs and symptoms caused by impaired blood flow to the brain that persists for more than 24 hours.
- A hemorrhagic stroke is caused by rupture of a blood vessel in the brain, and an ischemic stroke is caused by obstruction of a blood vessel by an embolus or a thrombus.
- Signs and symptoms of stroke depend on the type, location, and extent of brain injury but may include one-sided weakness, numbness, visual problems, confusion

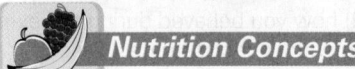 **Nutrition Concepts**

1. A major nutritional concern for the stroke patient is dysphagia (difficulty swallowing), which may lead to malnutrition and dehydration because of inadequate intake.
2. Swallowing thin liquids is frequently a problem. Thin liquids can be thickened with dry milk powder, cornstarch, fruit and vegetable flakes, or commercial thickening agents.
3. Very warm or chilled foods stimulate the swallowing reflex better than bland, lukewarm foods.
4. In addition to thickened liquids, foods that are better for chewing and swallowing are soft bread, cooked cereal, ice cream, yogurt, cooked eggs, moist ground beef, canned fruits and vegetables, thick soups, and puddings.

 Put on Your Thinking Cap!

List all the factors you can think of that might cause a patient recovering from a stroke to be incontinent of urine *besides* the physiologic effects of the stroke.

and memory lapses, headache, dysphagia, and speech problems.

- Some symptoms of stroke improve, but patients may be left with impairments in speech, language comprehension, motor function, vision, cognition, and bladder control, as well as with personality changes and emotional lability.
- Aphasia is the inability to understand words or respond with appropriate messages.
- Dysarthria is the inability to speak clearly because of neurologic damage that affects the muscles of speech.
- Dysphagia is difficulty swallowing.
- Dyspraxia is the partial inability to initiate coordinated voluntary motor acts in an unparalyzed extremity.
- Paralysis of one side of the body (the side opposite the brain injury) is called *hemiplegia.*
- Medical treatment of CVA may employ oxygen therapy, diuretics, corticosteroids, anticoagulants, thrombolytics, intravenous fluids, dietary modifications, and catheterization, as well as treatment of risk factors.
- The focus of nursing care after stroke is on Ineffective Airway Clearance, Ineffective Breathing Pattern, Risk for

Injury, Deficient Fluid Volume, Fluid Volume Excess, Imbalanced Nutrition: Less Than Body Requirements, Disturbed Sensory Perception, Ineffective Thermoregulation, Disturbed Thought Processes, Impaired Verbal Communication, Impaired Physical Mobility, Total Urinary Incontinence or Functional Urinary Incontinence, Constipation, Bowel Incontinence, Ineffective Coping, and Interrupted Family Processes.

- After experiencing a stroke, the patient may regain complete independent functioning, partially recover previous abilities, or lose functional abilities completely.
- The goal of rehabilitation after stroke is to enhance the recovery of functional abilities through a program of stimulation and practice.

 Go to your Companion CD-ROM for a Pharmacology Tutorial, Audio Glossary, and 3-D animations.

evolve Be sure to visit the companion Evolve site at http://evolve.elsevier.com/Linton/ for WebLinks and additional online resources.

REVIEW QUESTIONS *Choose the best answer.*

1. The structures of the brain that control respirations and heart rate are located in the:
   1. Cerebrum
   2. Brainstem
   3. Cerebellum
   4. Cortex

2. Recognition of a transient ischemic attack (TIA) is important because a TIA:
   1. Is a symptom of a brain tumor
   2. Can cause permanent disability
   3. Is a warning sign of future stroke
   4. Occurs shortly before a hemorrhage

3. How are TIAs and strokes different?
   1. Weakness and loss of balance are symptoms of TIA but not stroke.
   2. Imaging studies show circulatory changes with stroke but not with TIA.
   3. Anticoagulants are used with some strokes but not with TIA.
   4. TIA symptoms resolve within 24 hours; stroke symptoms persist longer.

4. When anticoagulants are used to reduce the risk of stroke, the INR should not exceed:
   1. 1.5
   2. 2.0
   3. 2.5
   4. 3.0

5. The most common type of stroke is:
   1. Ischemic
   2. Incomplete
   3. Hemorrhagic
   4. Subarachnoid

6. Ms. Y. is recovering from a stroke. She is able to follow directions and communicate nonverbally. However, she struggles to speak and the words are slurred. When you can understand her, her message is appropriately expressed. This pattern describes:
   1. Amnesia
   2. Dysarthria
   3. Dysphagia
   4. Dyspraxia

7. Modifiable risk factors for stroke include the following:
   1. Age
   2. Race
   3. Gender
   4. Hypertension

8. Successful use of tissue plasminogen activator in the stroke patient requires:
   1. Deep intramuscular administration into a large muscle mass
   2. Administration only to patients who have had hemorrhagic strokes
   3. Intravenous administration within 3 hours of the onset of symptoms
   4. Concurrent use with heparin to prevent additional clots from forming

9. Nursing interventions for patients with aphasia include the following:
   1. Insist that patients try to express needs verbally
   2. Help them find the right word if they become frustrated
   3. Give praise only when patients verbalize successfully
   4. Encourage families to speak for patients rather than forcing patients to speak

Spinal Cord Injury

LESLIE GODDARD

Objectives

After reading and studying this chapter, you should be able to:

1. Explain the impact of spinal cord injury.
2. Describe the diagnostic tests used to evaluate spinal cord injuries and related nursing responsibilities.
3. Explain the physical effects of spinal cord injury.
4. Describe the medical and surgical treatment during the acute phase of spinal cord injury.
5. List the data to be included in the nursing assessment of the patient with a spinal cord injury.
6. Identify nursing diagnoses, goals, interventions, and outcome criteria for the patient with a spinal cord injury.
7. Describe the nursing care for the patient undergoing a laminectomy.
8. State the goals of rehabilitation for the patient with spinal cord injury.

Key Terms

Be sure to check out the bonus material on the Companion CD-ROM, including selected audio pronunciations.

autonomic dysreflexia (ăw-tō-NŌM-ĭk dĭs-rĕ-FLĔKS-ē-ă, p. 493)
dermatome (DĔR-mă-tōm, p. 499)
flaccid (FLĂS-ĭd, p.493)
myelinated (MĬ-ĕ-lĭ-nat-ĕd, p. 487)
paraplegia (păr-ă-PLĒ-jă, p. 491)
quadriplegia (kwŏd-rĭ-PLĒ-jă, p. 491)
spasticity (spăs-TĬS-ĭ-tē, p. 494)

Few injuries are as physically and emotionally devastating to a person as a permanent spinal cord injury. The Spinal Cord Injury Information Network estimates there are 11,000 new cases of spinal cord injury in the United States each year. One third of victims die before reaching a hospital. The remaining injured patients have varying degrees of disabilities, requiring care that costs more than $10 billion annually.

The incidence of spinal cord injury peaks in individuals in their early 20s, with a small increase seen in older adults as a result of falls and degenerative disease. The leading cause of spinal cord injury is trauma sustained in vehicular accidents, falls, assaults, and sports-related mishaps. The cord also can be damaged by degenerative conditions and tumors.

Medical advances and more rapid transport of accident victims to trauma centers have made it possible for an individual with spinal cord injury to achieve a normal life expectancy. The effects of the injury, however, may lead to other health problems that require long-term care and potentially affect quality of life. Quality nursing care during the acute and rehabilitative phases of injury can minimize the impact of lifelong problems that plague the spinal cord–injured person. Consequently, the potential for rehabilitation and full quality of life can be enhanced.

ANATOMY AND PHYSIOLOGY OF THE SPINAL CORD

To understand the effects of spinal cord injury fully, it is important to know the anatomy and physiology of the spinal cord. Normal spinal cord function requires an intact cord with a good blood supply and bony support. Disruption of any one of these components can result in neurologic dysfunction.

VERTEBRAL COLUMN

The bony vertebral column consists of 33 vertebrae: 7 cervical (C1 through C7), 12 thoracic (T1 through T12), 5 lumbar (L1 through L5), 5 sacral (S1 through S5), and 4 coccygeal, which are fused (Fig. 29-1). The individual vertebra consists of a body and an arch, as shown in Figure 29-2. The body is the round structure that forms the anterior portion of the vertebra. The arch is the posterior portion of the vertebra. The spinal cord passes through an opening in the center of each arch. The structures that form the posterior section of the arch are called *laminae*. Each arch has articulating surfaces against which adjacent vertebrae smoothly glide with movement. In addition, each arch has locations for the attachment of ribs and muscles. The bony column is supported by muscles and ligaments, which permit mobility and flexibility.

DISKS

Vertebrae are separated by intervertebral disks, which serve as shock absorbers for the vertebral column (Figure 29-2). Disks are composed of the anulus fibrosus and the nucleus pulposus. The anulus fibrosus is the fibrous ring of tissue that encircles the nucleus pulposus. The nucleus pulposus is the central saclike structure with a gelatinous filling that has a high water content. As a person ages, the nucleus pulposus loses a great deal of its water, so it becomes less effective as a shock absorber. Therefore older people are at greater risk for back injuries and herniated disks.

SPINAL CORD

The spinal cord extends from the brainstem to the level of L2 in the pelvic cavity (Fig. 29-3). It has a central canal, which is continuous with the fourth ventricle of the brain. The cord is surrounded by three protective meningeal layers: the dura mater, the arachnoid, and the pia mater. The dura mater is the outermost layer. The arachnoid, the middle layer, is a network of spaces containing cerebrospinal fluid (CSF). The pia mater is the innermost layer; it directly covers the spinal cord. The cerebrospinal fluid circulates through the brain and spinal column, bathing and protecting the entire central nervous system.

A cross section of the spinal cord reveals an inner area of H-shaped gray matter surrounded by white matter. The gray matter consists of the bodies of nerve cells that control motor and sensory activities. The white matter, which is myelinated (surrounded by a sheath), consists of bundles of fibers. These fibers, known as *columns* or *tracts,* convey information between the brain and the spinal cord. The tracts may be either ascending or descending. Ascending tracts carry sensory information from the spinal cord to the brain. Descending tracts carry motor information from the brain to the spinal cord (Fig. 29-4).

Blood supply to the spinal cord is vital. Any disruption in blood flow can ultimately lead to neurologic damage. The major arterial supply to the spinal cord

FIGURE **29-1** The bony vertebral column consists of 33 vertebrae.

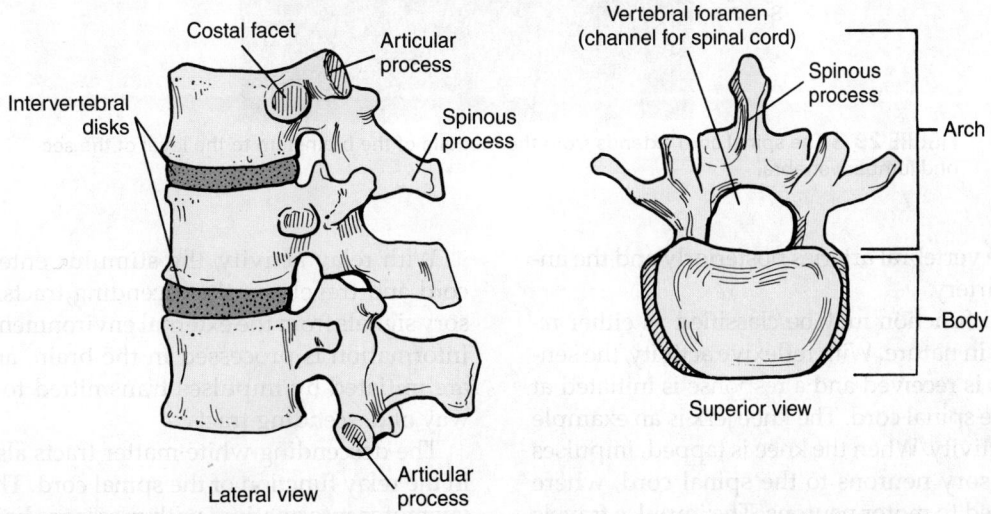

FIGURE **29-2** Intervertebral disks separate the vertebrae, each of which consists of a body and an arch.

Cerebrum

Cerebellum

Mastoid process

Cervical plexus—C–1,2,3,4

Brachial plexus—C–5,6,7,8,T1

Radial n.

Median n.

Ulnar n.

Intercostal nerves

Cauda equina

Lumbar plexus L–2,3,4

Sacral plexus S–3,4,5

Coccygeal plexus S–3,4,5

Pudendal n. S–2,3,4

Posterior cutaneous n. of thigh S–1,2,3

Sciatic n.

FIGURE **29-3** The spinal cord extends from the medulla of the brainstem to the level of the second lumbar vertebra.

consists of the vertebral arteries posteriorly and the anterior spinal artery.

Spinal cord function may be classified as either *reflexive* or *relay* in nature. With reflexive activity, the sensory stimulus is received and a response is initiated at the level of the spinal cord. The knee jerk is an example of reflexive activity. When the knee is tapped, impulses travel by sensory neurons to the spinal cord, where they are relayed to motor neurons. The impulse travels back to the muscles at the front of the thigh, causing muscle contraction and jerking of the leg. This circuit of impulse transmission is called a reflex arc.

With relay activity, the stimulus enters the spinal cord and travels up the ascending tracts to relay sensory signals from the external environment to the brain. Information is processed in the brain, and responses are initiated by impulses transmitted to the body by way of descending tracts.

The descending white matter tracts also participate in the relay function of the spinal cord. These tracts relay motor information, with messages being sent from the brain, down the cord, to muscles, which affect various kinds of responses. Four of the most important spinal cord tracts are summarized in Table 29-1.

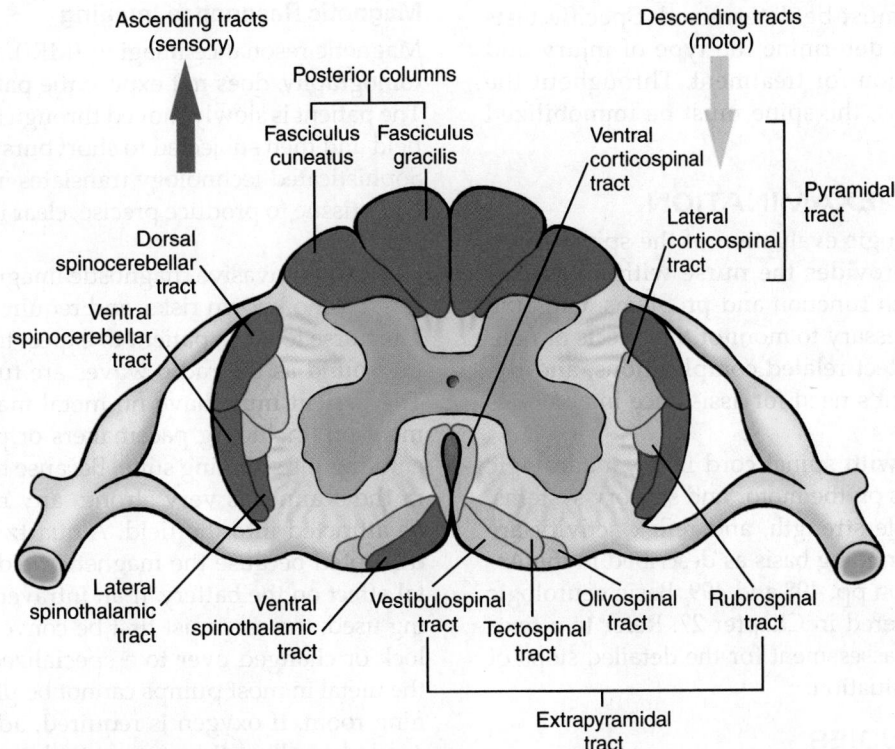

FIGURE 29-4 Cross section of spinal cord. Sensory tracts convey sensory information to the brain. Motor tracts convey information from the brain.

Table 29-1 *Summary of the Four Major Spinal Cord Tracts*

TRACT	TYPE	FEATURES	FUNCTION
Spinothalamic, lateral	Ascending (sensory: pain and temperature)	Originates in spinal cord and ascends to thalamus in brain. On entering cord, impulses cross over to opposite side (contralateral).	Carries pain and temperature sensation from opposite side.
Corticospinal, lateral	Descending (motor)	Initiates in motor tract of brain, crosses over to opposite side at level of medulla, proceeds down to appropriate spinal cord level.	Controls voluntary motor action.
Spinocerebellar	Ascending (sensory)	Initiates in spinal cord and terminates in cerebellum.	Assists in coordination of muscle contraction.
Posterior columns	Ascending (sensory: touch, vibration, position sense)	Made up of several tracts that relay messages from body to brain. Initiates in sensory fibers of spinal nerves, crosses over in medulla, and terminates in sensory cortex of opposite hemisphere.	Carries touch, deep pressure, vibration, and position sense.

Information is conveyed by the senses to the brain and spinal cord via the peripheral nervous system. This system consists of 31 pairs of spinal nerves, (8 cervical, 12 thoracic, and 5 lumbar, 5 sacral, and 1 coccygeal), which branch from the cord and pass between the vertebrae to muscles and visceral organs. Each spinal nerve has a dorsal root, which transmits sensory information, and a ventral root, which transmits motor information. The 12 cranial nerves, arising from the brainstem, also are part of the peripheral nervous system.

DIAGNOSTIC TESTS AND PROCEDURES

Emergency care of the patient with a spinal cord injury is discussed in Chapter 16. When the victim of spinal cord injury arrives at the hospital, the extent of injury must be determined. Specific tests are performed to determine the type of injury and to provide direction for treatment. Throughout the diagnostic process, the spine must be immobilized continuously.

NEUROLOGIC EXAMINATION

The initial neurologic evaluation of the spinal cord–injured patient provides the nurse with a baseline assessment of both function and problems. Ongoing assessment is necessary to monitor the effects of neurologic injury, detect related complications, and determine the patient's need for assistance in activities of daily living.

In the patient with spinal cord injury, neurologic evaluation focuses on the motor and sensory systems. Movement, muscle strength, and reflex activity are evaluated on an ongoing basis as described in the Assessment section on pp. 498 and 499. Basic neurologic assessment is covered in Chapter 27. Refer to a textbook on physical assessment for the detailed steps of the neurologic evaluation.

IMAGING STUDIES

Radiography

Standard radiographs are obtained to detect vertebral compression, fractures, or problems with alignment. The entire spine may be radiographed because patients sometimes have multiple fractures separated by sections of normal spine. The physician also may order special radiographs, called *coned-down views*, which reveal fractures more clearly. Radiography is repeated at intervals to evaluate the achievement of proper alignment with treatment.

Computed Tomography

Computed tomography (CT) provides a noninvasive examination of the specific levels of the spinal cord to be visualized, as well as the bony vertebrae and the spinal nerves. The physician can readily identify bony fractures, floating bone fragments, dislocations, tumors, hemorrhage, and cord and nerve compressions. In some injuries, soft tissue swelling may obscure some structures and make visualization of the cord and vertebrae difficult.

Although no special physical preparation is needed for a patient undergoing computed tomography, this imaging procedure should be explained to the patient. The patient is told that he or she will be asked to lie very still for a period of time while on a small table that slowly moves through the scanner. Enhanced scanning also may be done, in which a radiopaque dye is infused intravenously into the patient. This testing is contraindicated in the patient who is allergic to the dye. The patient receiving the dye must be encouraged to take plenty of fluids after the procedure to promote renal excretion.

Magnetic Resonance Imaging

Magnetic resonance imaging (MRI), unlike computed tomography, does not expose the patient to radiation. The patient is slowly moved through a strong magnetic field and then subjected to short bursts of radio waves. Sophisticated technology translates information about body tissue to produce precise, clear images of internal structures.

This noninvasive diagnostic imaging study is painless, has no known risks, and requires no preparation. The nurse tells the patient to expect to hear a hammering sound as the radio waves are turned on and off. The patient must have no metal materials or equipment on (including pacemakers or prostheses) when entering the scanning suite. Because the magnetic field in the scanner is very strong, any metal object may be attracted into the field. A quartz watch would be disrupted because the magnetic field has a detrimental effect on the battery. If an intravenous pump is being used, the site must first be converted to a heparin lock or changed over to a specialized pump because the metal in most pumps cannot be placed in the scanning room. If oxygen is required, adequate tubing is needed to allow the oxygen tank to be placed a safe distance outside the suite. Patients with pacemakers cannot undergo magnetic resonance imaging because the magnetic field would inactivate the pacer. This is also true of patients with aneurysm clips that are not made of inert metal.

Myelography

A myelogram is obtained to visualize the spinal cord and vertebrae. A puncture is made in the lumbar area between L3 and L4. Radiopaque dye is then injected into the subarachnoid space of the spinal canal. Any obstruction that impedes the flow of the dye can be seen on radiography. Because of the invasive nature of the procedure, informed consent must be obtained. Nursing care before and after myelography is summarized in Box 29-1.

PATHOPHYSIOLOGY OF SPINAL CORD INJURY

Traumatic injury creates abnormal forces on the neck and structural components of the spinal cord. The cervical vertebrae support the head and neck and permit movement in various directions. The thoracic vertebrae, on the other hand, permit little movement because of the restrictions of the ribs. Because the thoracic spine has limited flexibility, the neck and cervical spine are extremely vulnerable to injury.

TYPES OF INJURIES

Spinal cord injuries may be classified (1) by location, (2) as open or closed, and (3) by extent of damage to the cord. Injuries classified by location are described as

Box 29-1 *Nursing Care of the Patient Having Myelography*

Preparation

Ensure that signed consent has been obtained.

Inquire about allergy to dye, iodine, or shellfish; inform radiologist if the patient is allergic.

Allow nothing by mouth for 4-6 hr before the procedure, according to agency protocol.

Administer prescribed premedications.

Have patient empty bladder if able.

Determine whether any medications should be withheld.

Postprocedure Care

Frequently assess vital signs and neurologic status.

Encourage increased fluid intake to promote elimination of dye, if not contraindicated.

Measure and record fluid intake and output.

Position as ordered: flat or head of bed elevated 30-45 degrees, depending on type of contrast medium used.

Administer analgesics as ordered for headache.

Assess for back pain, increased temperature, difficulty voiding, neck stiffness, and nausea and vomiting.

Table 29-2 *Incomplete Injuries and Related Neurologic Deficits*

INJURY	MECHANISM OF INJURY	ACCOMPANYING DEFICIT
Anterior cord syndrome	Herniation of disk occurring with flexion injury or dislocation of vertebrae	Loss of bilateral pain and temperature perception and motor function below level of lesion without loss of position sense
Central cord syndrome	Hyperextension injury	Motor and sensory loss in upper extremities
Brown-Séquard syndrome	Transverse hemisection of cord	Ipsilateral loss of motor function with contralateral loss of pain and temperature perception

cervical, thoracic, or lumbar, depending on the level of the cord affected.

Closed injuries involve trauma in which the skin and meningeal covering that surrounds the spinal cord remain intact. Keep in mind, however, that stretching or twisting the spinal cord can lead to injury as extensive as partial or complete transection. Common causes of closed injuries include compression, flexion, hyperextension, rotation, and blunt trauma (Fig. 29-5). Degeneration of the vertebrae or intervertebral disks, hematomas, or spinal cord tumors also may compress the cord or one of the spinal nerves. Fractures of the vertebral bodies may cause a subluxation (partial dislocation) of bone fragments, which may further damage the cord. Open injuries with damage to protective skin and meninges are most commonly caused by bullets or stabbing.

The injury may be classified as complete or incomplete, depending on the extent to which the cord is transected (cut across). A complete spinal cord injury occurs when the cord has been completely severed, whereas an incomplete injury results from partial cutting of the cord. Open injuries often result in either complete or partial transection (cutting across) of the cord.

EFFECTS OF SPINAL CORD INJURY

Early recognition of the effects of spinal cord injury is vital to maintain maximum possible function. Factors that determine the effects of spinal cord injury include the extent of the cut and the level of the injury. Sometimes the extent of injury cannot be fully determined because the symptoms of spinal cord edema may mimic partial or complete transection. A complete injury cuts all descending and ascending tracts. The result is disruption of all voluntary motor and sensory activity below the level of the injury. However, reflex activity continues below the level of injury because it occurs by completing the reflex arc without the transmission of impulses to and from the brain.

Trauma also may produce a variety of incomplete spinal cord injuries. These are injuries in which some function remains below the level of the injury. Specific tracts may be involved, causing particular patterns of neurologic dysfunction (Fig. 29-6). Table 29-2 describes the major types of incomplete injuries and the resulting neurologic losses.

The higher the level of the injury, the more encompassing is the neurologic dysfunction because increasingly more of the body is affected. High cervical spine injuries may result in the loss of motor and sensory function in all four extremities, known as quadriplegia. Currently the term is more appropriately referred to as *tetraplegia*. Injuries at or below T2 may cause paraplegia, which is paralysis of the lower part of the body. Table 29-3 describes those activities that are possible with spinal cord injury at various levels.

Respiratory Impairment

The diaphragm is innervated by the phrenic nerve, which is formed by the nerve roots of C1 through C4. Therefore injuries at or above the level of C5 (called *high cervical injuries*) may result in instant death because the nerves that control respiration are interrupted. Many

FIGURE **29-5** Mechanisms of spinal cord injury.

patients with high cervical injuries die before reaching the hospital. If these patients receive immediate attention and rapid transport to an acute care facility, mechanical ventilation may be possible. However, they remain dependent on ventilators and face challenges for rehabilitation.

Modern technology affords the ventilator-dependent patient a variety of options for pulmonary rehabilitation. A small portable ventilator can be mounted on the back of a mechanized wheelchair, enabling the patient to be mobile. Phrenic nerve stimulators also may be implanted in the patient to help stimulate diaphragmatic

Complete lesion

Area of cord damage

Total loss of motor, sensory, and reflex activity

Anterior cord syndrome

Pain, temperature

Position, vibration, and touch sense

Motor

Area of cord damage

Loss of motor function with preservation of position, vibration, and touch sense

Brown-Séquard syndrome

Area of cord damage

Loss of pain, temperature, and light touch on opposite side

Loss of motor function and vibration, position, and deep touch sensation on same side as the cord damage

Central cord syndrome

Area of cord damage

Loss of motor function

Incomplete loss of motor function

Conus medullaris and cauda equina syndromes

Loss of motor and/or sensory function in various patterns, with potential for recovery of function with regeneration of peripheral nerves; neurogenic bowel and bladder

Area of cord damage

Conus — T11, T12, L1

Cauda equina — L2, C, S5, S4, S3, S2, S1

T11, T12, T12, L1, L1, L2, L2, L3, L4, L5

FIGURE 29-6 Patterns of injury and neurologic dysfunction.

movement and enhance respiratory function. Even with a ventilator or phrenic nerve stimulator, pulmonary hygiene is an issue because these patients may have difficulty clearing the airway.

Cervical injuries below the level of C4 spare the diaphragm but can involve impairment of intercostal and abdominal muscles. Patients with these injuries can usually breathe independently but often experience some degree of respiratory compromise related to weakened exhalation and cough.

Spinal Shock

Spinal shock is an immediate, transient response to injury in which reflex activity below the level of the injury temporarily ceases. It may appear as early as 30 to 60 minutes after the injury and may persist for days, weeks, or months. During the period of spinal shock, paralysis is described as flaccid, meaning the involved extremity or muscle group has no tone. The involved neurons in the

spinal cord gradually regain their excitability. Resolution of spinal shock is marked by the appearance of spastic, involuntary movements of the extremities.

Autonomic Dysreflexia

One of the most serious and potentially dangerous problems for the spinal cord–injured patient is autonomic dysreflexia, an exaggerated response of the autonomic nervous system to some noxious (painful) stimuli. It occurs in patients whose injury is at or above the level of T6. As spinal shock begins to subside and reflex activity returns, the risk of autonomic dysreflexia increases. It may occur even in patients with long-standing injuries.

Excessive stimulation of sensory receptors below the level of the injury precipitates autonomic dysreflexia. The sympathetic nervous system is stimulated, but an appropriate parasympathetic modulation response cannot be elicited because of the spinal cord injury that

Table 29-3 | *Degree of Loss and Functional Capability with Injury to Each Level of the Spinal Cord*

CORD LEVEL	DEGREE OF LOSS	FUNCTIONAL CAPABILITY
C1 through C4	Motor and sensory function from neck down Respiratory function Bowel and bladder control	Mechanical ventilation with home care
C5	Motor and sensory function below shoulders Intercostal function in ventilation Bowel and bladder control	Has remaining head control, which facilitates use of "joystick" for writing, typing, and control of mechanical wheelchair
C6	Motor and sensory function below shoulders but greater degree of sensation in arm and thumb Intercostal function in ventilation Bowel and bladder control	Requires some assistive devices for upper extremity use but may be able to help feed and dress self Requires mechanical wheelchair but may be capable of utilizing hand control
C7	Motor control of portion of upper extremities Sensation below clavicle Intercostal function Bowel and bladder control	Remaining intact muscles enhance ability to carry out activities of daily living (ADL) Increased ability to manage specially equipped wheelchair and automobile
C8	Motor control of portions of upper extremities Sensation below chest Intercostal function Bowel and bladder control	Improved upper extremity mobility enhances hand grasp, independence in ADL, and use of wheelchair Capable of self-catheterization
T1-T6	Trunk muscles below midchest Sensation from midchest Some intercostal function Bowel and bladder control	Complete control of upper extremities makes independence in wheelchair and ADL possible Employment possible
T6-T12	Motor control below waist Sensation below waist Bowel and bladder control	Capable of unassisted respiratory function Good upper back and abdominal strength, making increased wheelchair activities and athletics possible
L1-L3	Motor and sensory function to lower extremities Sensation to lower abdomen Bowel and bladder function	Full control of upper extremities allows independence in wheelchair and appropriate athletic activity
L3-4	Motor and sensory function to distal portions of lower extremities Bowel and bladder control	Control of hip extensors remains, making ambulation possible with leg braces
L4-S5	Variable motor and sensory function to knee, ankle, and foot Sensation to perineum Variable bowel and bladder control	Ambulation with braces possible Considerable independence in ADL can be expected

separates the two divisions of the autonomic nervous system. Arterioles constrict, causing severe hypertension, which may lead to seizures or a stroke if not corrected. In an attempt to reduce the excessively increased blood pressure, regulatory mechanisms cause the blood vessels to dilate. The vasodilating response is effective only above the level of the injury, where superficial vasodilation, flushing, and profuse sweating occur. The patient experiences nasal congestion, facial flushing, and a pounding headache.

Increased blood pressure also stimulates the vagus nerve, causing bradycardia. Normally, vagal stimulation also would serve to dilate the constricted vessels. But because the cord has been severed, these impulses never reach the affected blood vessels below the level of the lesion.

Autonomic dysreflexia is triggered by a variety of stimuli including a distended bladder, constipation, renal calculi, ejaculation, or uterine contractions, but it also may be caused by pressure sores, a skin rash, enemas, or even sudden position changes. In the event of autonomic dysreflexia, indwelling catheters must be inspected for possible occlusions or kinks. If there is no indwelling catheter and the bladder is distended, intermittent catheterization may be done. If constipation is the triggering event, disimpaction may be necessary. Pressure ulcers need to be treated with a topical anesthetic to decrease the stimuli, and skin rashes can be treated with appropriate topical ointments to decrease itching.

Autonomic dysreflexia is an emergent situation. It is important to obtain a history related to autonomic dysreflexia on any quadriplegic being cared for in a health care setting. This will allow the provider to be on the alert for symptoms and respond in a timely manner.

Spasticity

Most spinal cord–injured patients display some degree of spasticity (increased muscle tone) after their injury. Muscle spasms may prove to be quite incapacitating for these patients, hampering efforts at rehabilitation. Generally, after 1 or 2 years, there is a gradual reduction in spastic episodes.

Muscle tone is evaluated by assessing the amount of resistance to passive movement. The spastic muscle displays a brief period of increased resistance, which is followed by a sudden relaxation. Reflexes also are assessed because hyperactive reflexes accompany spasticity. Spastic activity may be elicited by passive movement, positioning, or even the slight stimulation of a sheet moving over the lower extremities. A number of drugs are available to treat spasticity.

Impaired Sensory and Motor Function

As stated earlier, the higher the level of the lesion, the more extensive is the neurologic dysfunction. Any complete cord injury results in the loss of both motor and sensory function below the level of the lesion. The effects of incomplete lesions on sensation and motor function are variable. Impaired motor function can significantly affect the patient's mobility and self-care and thus result in complications from immobility. Loss of sensation puts the patient at risk for skin breakdown and other injuries because pressure and pain are not perceived.

Impaired Bladder Function

During the period of spinal shock, all bladder and bowel function ceases. An indwelling catheter is inserted to empty the bladder and permit close monitoring of urinary output. As soon as the patient's fluid status is stabilized, the indwelling catheter often is removed and the bladder drained by intermittent catheterization. Once spinal shock resolves, reflex activity returns. The bladder becomes spastic and may spontaneously empty. Bladder retraining protocols can be specifically designed for individual patients.

Medications may be used to aid in the prevention of urinary tract infections. Methenamine mandelate (Mandelamine) is a urinary antiseptic that may be used in the regimen. Because the action of methenamine is enhanced in an acidic environment, vitamin C (ascorbic acid) often is prescribed to lower urine pH.

Impaired Bowel Function

The absence of bowel activity in the first day or two after injury may require insertion of a nasogastric tube for decompression. Peristalsis usually returns by the third postinjury day. Most spinal cord–injured patients can maintain bowel function because the large bowel musculature has its own neural center that responds to distention by the fecal mass. To assist in evacuation of the bowel, the patient must take advantage of the abdominal muscles as well as have an appropriate diet. Bowel retraining programs are initiated to aid in the regular evacuation of the bowel.

Impaired Temperature Regulations

Depending on the level of the injury, the patient may have difficulty maintaining body temperature within a normal range. If a person becomes too cold, the body normally responds with vasoconstriction and shivering to increase the temperature. If a person becomes too hot, sweating helps dissipate heat. The spinal cord–injured patient may lose these regulatory mechanisms and be unable to adapt to temperature extremes. The quadriplegic person is especially vulnerable to environmental temperature changes because such a large part of the body is affected.

Impaired Sexual Function

Spinal levels S2, S3, and S4 control sexual function, so injury at or above these levels results in sexual dysfunction. The ability of the male patient to achieve erection and ejaculation is variable, depending on the level of injury. In females, menses resumes normally after injury. Women with spinal cord injuries can have sexual intercourse but lack vaginal sensation. Some women with spinal cord injuries do experience orgasm, although it is not vaginally triggered. They also can bear children, regardless of the level of the lesion. In the event of pregnancy, vaginal delivery is possible if pelvic proportions are adequate. If the lesion is high, however, the woman will not be aware of labor contractions.

Impaired Skin Integrity

Immobility and loss of sensation put the patient at risk for skin problems. One of the most common complications in the spinal cord–injured patient is pressure ulcers. Because the immobile patient is unable to change positions, skin in the sacral area and across the bony prominences may break down. This presents a portal for infection in the patient. In addition, the presence of a pressure sore in the sacral area impedes early rehabilitation efforts because the patient is unable to begin wheelchair training until the ulcer heals.

Put on Your Thinking Cap!

1. In the community, observe without being noticed a person who is using a wheelchair to determine any difficulties he or she may have with access to public facilities including buildings, transportation, water fountains, and restrooms.
2. Describe any insights this experience provided that could help you take care of a patient with a spinal cord injury who is in a wheelchair.

The complete spinal cord injury also interrupts the vasomotor tone of the vascular system. This loss of tone results in vasodilation and pooling of blood in the periphery, impeding perfusion of the skin and encouraging the development of pressure sores.

Altered Self-Concept and Body Image

The impact of spinal cord injury on the patient's self-concept and body image is tremendous. Depending on the extent of the injury, every aspect of the patient's life (occupation, family roles and responsibilities, socialization, hobbies) may be affected. French and Phillips (1991) have described the effects of spinal cord injury on body image as occurring in four phases: impact, retreat, acknowledgment, and reconstruction. In the impact phase, the patient becomes aware of the devastating changes that have taken place. He or she is in emotional shock and may express a desire to die. The retreat phase is marked by depression and withdrawal as the patient considers the implications of the injury. In the acknowledgment phase, the patient begins to face the injury and deal with it realistically. The patient moves into the reconstruction phase when he or she is ready to tackle the work of rehabilitation and begins to plan for the future. A new body image has been constructed that incorporates the injury.

MEDICAL TREATMENT IN THE ACUTE PHASE

The goals of medical treatment guide the plans for the spinal cord–injured patient through all phases of the injury. The three major medical goals for the patient with spinal injury are to save the patient's life, to prevent further injury to the cord, and to preserve as much cord function as possible. Each medical goal has specific implications for nursing care and is directed at maximizing the patient's potential for recovery and rehabilitation.

SAVING THE PATIENT'S LIFE

The patient with a spinal cord injury may have additional life-threatening injuries. As mentioned earlier, patients with high cervical cord injuries often die from impaired respiratory function before arriving at the hospital.

The first priority is to establish a patent airway. The conventional head-tilt–chin-lift method of opening the airway is inappropriate in spinal injury patients because of the risk of increasing cord damage. The risk of additional damage is especially high with cervical injury. Flexion of the neck, even that caused by a pillow or other support, must be avoided. The jaw-thrust method of opening the airway is preferred for these patients. Once the airway has been opened, 100% oxygen may be administered by mask and manual resuscitator (e.g., an Ambu bag).

An endotracheal or tracheostomy tube may be placed to allow direct access to the airway and to facilitate optimal oxygenation. Any injury that compromises ventilation must be treated immediately.

PREVENTING FURTHER CORD INJURY

Immobilization is essential to prevent further damage to the spinal cord after the initial injury. At the scene of an accident, emergency personnel will apply a hard cervical collar, also known as a *Philadelphia collar*, around the patient's neck to immobilize the spinal column. Various types of devices and traction may be utilized once the patient arrives at an acute care facility.

Traction

Initially, immobilization with skeletal traction often is used to manage cervical spinal cord injuries. A variety of skull traction devices may be used, including Gardner-Wells and Crutchfield tongs. Gardner-Wells tongs are secured just above the ears but do not actually penetrate the skull. Crutchfield tongs, which are less commonly used now than in the past, are applied directly to the skull, just behind the hairline. The tongs allow traction to be applied, which separates and aligns the vertebrae to prevent further cord damage and reduces painful muscle spasms (Fig. 29-7). After the tongs are applied, radiographs are ordered to confirm alignment of the spine. Ongoing neurologic assessment is done to monitor for further deficits.

The halo vest is used to immobilize and align the cervical vertebrae and usually is placed at the time of surgery that is done to internally stabilize fractures and relieve the compression of nerve roots (Fig. 29-8). A ring is applied to the skull using four pins and then attached to a fiberglass vest by adjustable rods. The vest allows the paralyzed patient to be moved out of bed and allows the patient who is not paralyzed to be ambulatory. Because good immobilization of the spine is achieved, attention can be turned to other aspects of treatment and rehabilitation can be initiated.

Special Beds and Cushions

A number of special beds are available to help prevent complications of immobility while maintaining spinal immobilization. A kinetic bed such as the Roto Rest bed slowly but continually rotates the patient from side to side (Fig. 29-9). This rotation is especially helpful in preventing pulmonary complications by mobilizing secretions. Overlay air mattresses are flotation devices that are placed on standard hospital beds. Air-fluidized and flotation beds may be used *after* the spine has been stabilized, but they are *never* used when a patient is in tongs because of the potential damage that could occur if the bed should unexpectedly deflate.

The Wedge-Stryker frame is a canvas and metal frame bed that may be used to help turn the patient. It is not used as often as it was in the past. The patient lies supine on the posterior frame for approximately 2 hours at a time. Then the anterior frame is secured on top of the patient and the device is turned over so

FIGURE **29-7** Gardner-Wells tongs are used to immobilize the cervical spine.

FIGURE **29-8** The halo device immobilizes and aligns the cervical vertebrae.

FIGURE **29-9** The Roto Rest bed slowly turns the patient from side to side.

that the patient is prone on the anterior frame. Two people are needed each time to turn the patient, and the patient must be tightly secured to the frame. Every 2 hours, the patient is turned from the supine to the prone position or vice versa. Many patients have a difficult time adjusting to such a bed because the prone position leaves the patient feeling as though suspended in midair. Because of this, most patients are managed on a conventional or other specialty bed.

Once the patient is able to be up in a chair, cushioning is needed to prevent excessive pressure and pressure ulcers. Types of cushions include those inflated with air, flotation devices, and gel pads. Examples of pressure-reducing cushions are the ROHO cushion, BBD Bye Bye Decubiti cushion, Jay cushion, Akro cushion, and VARILITE cushion. The cushion that best

meets the needs of the individual patient is selected. The physical therapist is a good resource person to consult for this recommendation.

Drug Therapy

Until the early 1990s, management of the spinal cord–injured patient relied almost exclusively on surgical and immobilization techniques. However, the use of methylprednisolone to reduce the damage to the cellular membrane has become standard practice in the acute management of spinal cord injury. The optimal time of administration is within the first 8 hours of injury. Completely paralyzed patients have been found to regain about 20% of function, whereas those partially paralyzed have regained up to 75% of function.

Pharmacology Capsule

The administration of high doses of methylprednisolone sodium succinate during the first 8 hours after spinal cord injury may help limit the neurologic effects of injury.

PRESERVING CORD FUNCTION

Early surgical intervention may be necessary to repair cord damage. Situations in which surgery is required include cord compression by bony fragments, compound vertebral fractures, and gunshot and stab wounds. In these cases, surgery within the first 24 hours is most desirable.

A laminectomy involves removing all or part of the posterior arch of the vertebra. This may be done to alleviate compression on the cord or spinal nerves. If multiple vertebrae are involved, spinal fusion also may be done to stabilize the area. A spinal fusion entails placing a piece of donor bone, commonly taken from the hip, into the area between the involved vertebrae. After healing, the fusion immobilizes the affected section of the spine. Postoperative immobilization of the area is necessary to allow for adequate healing, permanent fusion, and correct alignment. If the cervical area is involved, a halo jacket will be utilized. If the thoracic or lumbar area is involved, other bracelike devices may be fitted to the patient. Neither laminectomy nor spinal fusion can be attempted until the patient has been fully stabilized during the acute phase of the injury.

NURSING CARE *in the Acute Phase*
Assessment

A complete assessment as described here may be delayed until the patient is stabilized. Until then, monitor the patient's level of consciousness, vital signs, respiratory status, motor and sensory function, and intake and output.

Health History

Present Illness. Record the event that brought the patient to the hospital. Note specific injuries incurred in the incident. This may be the initial hospitalization after the injury, or the patient may be admitted at a later time for other reasons. Describe pain and other symptoms in detail.

Past Medical History. It is important not to overlook other medical problems when the patient has a spinal cord injury. Inquire about other accidents or injuries and chronic illnesses such as diabetes, hypertension, heart disease, cancer, or seizure disorder. Record previous hospitalizations and operations. Obtain an obstetric history from the female patient. Identify and record current medications and allergies.

Family History. A routine family history is taken but is not considered specifically relevant to a diagnosis of spinal cord injury resulting from trauma.

Review of Systems. Inquire about signs and symptoms that may be related to neurologic dysfunction or its consequences. Data to be collected include skin condition, headache or dizziness, vision disturbances, hearing impairment or tinnitus, nasal or ear drainage (especially if there was a head injury), dyspnea, nausea and vomiting, constipation or diarrhea, fecal incontinence, bladder dysfunction, sexual dysfunction, and impaired motor and sensory function.

Functional Assessment. Determine the patient's self-care abilities. Explore the patient's roles and responsibilities as a family member. Record occupation, hobbies,

usual activity pattern, habits (including use of tobacco and alcohol), and diet. It is important to know who the patient's significant others are and whether those relationships are supportive. In addition, determine the patient's emotional response to the spinal injury. Ask about usual coping strategies. Determine spiritual beliefs and other sources of support. See the Health Promotion Considerations box below.

Physical Examination

Record the patient's reported height and weight. An actual weight measurement may have to be deferred until the patient can tolerate the procedure. Take vital signs. Be alert for hypotension and bradycardia that may accompany spinal shock (discussed on p. 493). Take the temperature to detect alterations that may reflect failure of regulatory mechanisms or infection. In the general survey, observe the patient's level of responsiveness, posture, and spontaneous movements.

Inspect the skin for lesions (lacerations, bruises) that may have occurred at the same time as the spinal cord injury or for signs of pressure that may have resulted from immobility. Inspect and palpate to evaluate tissue turgor. Inspect the head for lesions, and palpate for masses and swelling. Ask the patient to read available print to assess visual acuity. Examine the pupils of the eyes for size, equality, and reaction to light.

Observe the patient's respiratory effort, and auscultate breath sounds Inspect the abdomen for distention, and auscultate for bowel sounds. Inspect the extremities for open fractures or abnormal positions. Assess range of motion, voluntary and involuntary movement, muscle strength, spasms, and sensory perception in all extremities. If the patient is conscious, ask him or her to move the extremities through the various ranges of motion. This simply indicates whether the patient is capable of such movement and gives some early indication as to the involvement of particular spinal cord levels.

Muscle strength is assessed by using passive range-of-motion exercises and by testing strength against gravity as well as against resistance applied by the ex-

Health Promotion Considerations

Spinal Cord Injury
Prevention
- Identify high-risk populations and provide counseling and education.
- Support safety-focused legislation such as seatbelts, child safety seats, helmet laws, drunk driving.

Following Spinal Cord Injury
- General health screening appropriate to age and gender.
- Promote positive health behaviors (e.g., smoking cessation, healthy diet, exercise programs).
- Spinal cord injury preventive care (e.g., bowel and bladder program, skin care, pressure relief, euthermia).

aminer. Instruct the patient to try to move the extremity against the examiner's hand. Evaluate both upper and lower extremities, and compare one side with the other. Function is graded on a scale of 0 (complete paralysis) to 5 (normal strength) (Table 29-4). If the patient is unconscious, some noxious stimulus, such as pressure on the nail bed, must be applied to determine whether movement is possible. In the event of cranial involvement, such movement in response to noxious stimuli may be described as decorticate or decerebrate posturing. Both of these are described in Chapter 27.

Involuntary movement also may be observed in the injured patient. This type of movement is evidenced by the appearance of muscle spasms. Record the location and severity of such spasms. Techniques for assessing the movement of the major muscle groups in both the upper and the lower extremities are described in Table 29-5.

To evaluate sensory function, determine the patient's ability to perceive sharp and dull sensations and touch with the eyes closed. As with the motor evaluation, compare one side of the body with the other to assess equality. Include the hands, forearms, upper arms, trunk, thighs, lower legs, feet, and perineal area in the assessment. Sensory loss is best described with the aid of a dermatome chart (Fig. 29-10). A dermatome defines an area of the skin that is innervated by a particular subcutaneous nerve root. In the initial postinjury period, frequently reassess sensation because the injury may ascend (rise) and affect vital functions.

To test proprioception (position sense), have the patient close his or her eyes and identify the position of a toe or finger as you move it up or down.

Nursing assessment of the patient with a spinal cord injury is summarized in Box 29-2.

Nursing Diagnoses, Goals, and Outcome Criteria: Acute Phase of Spinal Cord Injury

Nursing Diagnoses	Goals and Outcome Criteria
Ineffective Breathing Pattern related to neurologic impairment	Adequate oxygenation: normal respiratory rate and measures of oxygenation (blood gases, oximeter)
Risk for Injury related to involuntary muscle spasms, lack of motor and sensory function, orthostatic hypotension; and **Disturbed Sensory Perception** (kinesthetic, tactile) related to altered sensory transmission	Reduced risk for injury: protective measures are taken to prevent injury associated with uncontrollable movement or with sensory loss
Absence of injury: patient has no bruises, breaks in skin, signs of pressure, or fractures
Risk for Autonomic Dysreflexia related to bladder or bowel distention, renal calculi, pressure sores	No signs of autonomic dysreflexia: pulse and blood pressure consistent with patient norms
Risk for Disuse Syndrome related to pathologic or prescribed immobility, or both	Absence of complications of immobility: no pressure sores, maximal possible range of motion, clear breath sounds
Bowel Incontinence related to impaired conduction of impulses	Controlled bowel elimination: regular bowel movements under controlled circumstances
Impaired Urinary Elimination related to sensory motor impairment	Absence of urinary retention and urinary infection: no bladder distention, urine clear with normal odor
Risk for Infection related to skeletal traction pins	Pin sites free of infection: minimal redness and swelling around pins, no purulent drainage
Ineffective Thermoregulation related to spinal cord trauma	Maintenance of normal body temperature: temperature within normal range
Self-Care Deficit: Feeding/Dressing/Grooming related to neurologic impairment	Adaptation to self-care deficits: patient participates in self-care as much as possible, accepts help as needed
Sexual Dysfunction related to altered body function	Adaptation to altered sexual function: patient verbalizes sexual capabilities and adaptive techniques
Ineffective Coping related to overwhelming losses and limited potential for recovered function	Effective coping: patient expresses feelings about losses, makes realistic plans for future
Ineffective Therapeutic Regimen Management related to lack of knowledge, denial, depression	Patient effectively manages self-care within capabilities: follows plan of care, plans realistically, uses resources

Interventions

Ineffective Breathing Pattern

Respiratory problems may result from neurologic damage or may be associated with immobility. The patient with an injury at or above C5 has complete loss

Table 29-4 | Grading Scale for Muscle Strength

SCORE	FINDINGS
0	No movement, total paralysis
1	Weak contraction palpated or observed
2	Muscle moves when supported against gravity
3	Active muscle movement against gravity
4	Full active range of motion against gravity but with some weakness when resistance is tested
5	Full active range of motion against gravity and resistance

Table 29-5 *Assessment Techniques for Major Muscle Groups*

NERVE ROOT	MUSCLE ACTION	ASSESSMENT TECHNIQUE
C4-5	Abduction of shoulder	Shrug shoulder against downward pressure
C5-6	Elbow flexion (biceps)	Arm flexed toward body against resistance
C7	Elbow extension (triceps)	Arm extended away from body against resistance
C8	Hand grasp (finger flexors)	Hands grasped around examiner's fingers with attempts to withdraw fingers from grasp
L2-4	Hip flexion	Leg raised against resistance
L2-4	Knee extension	Knee extended away from body against resistance
L5	Foot dorsiflexion	Foot pulled upward against resistance
L5-S1	Knee flexion	Knee flexed toward body against resistance
S1	Plantar flexion	Foot and toes pointed downward against resistance

FIGURE **29-10** A dermatome chart. A dermatome is an area of the skin that is innervated by a particular nerve root.

of spontaneous respirations and requires mechanical ventilation. When a person has an injury to the lower thoracic cord, abdominal and intercostal muscles are affected, resulting in weakened exhalation and cough. Nursing care is individualized for these patients depending on the extent of respiratory impairment. Ventilator-dependent patients may be taught techniques to allow independent breathing for limited periods of time. The ventilator-dependent patient needs special care, as described in Chapter 30.

A variety of techniques may be used to help patients with spontaneous but impaired breathing to clear the airway more effectively. These include breathing exercises, assisted coughing, and vibration and percussion with postural drainage. For assisted coughing, apply firm pressure to the diaphragm just below the rib cage as the patient exhales or coughs. Because timing is important, establish some form of communication with the patient (e.g., a blink) to identify when inspiration is completed. You should be properly trained in this technique before using it.

Turn and reposition the immobile patient as permitted to decrease pooling of secretions in the lungs. If the patient is breathing independently, coach the patient in deep-breathing exercises and use of the incentive spirometer. Adequate hydration helps thin secretions so that they can be more readily removed.

Risk for Injury and Disturbed Sensory Perception

Safety is of prime consideration during the period of spastic paralysis. Involuntary muscle spasms can be so violent that the patient may be thrown from the wheelchair or bedside chair. It is imperative that the patient be adequately secured with a protective strap across the chest. Even while in bed, the patient requires protection. Avoid undue stimulation of the spastic extremity or muscle group. When performing range-of-motion exercises or positioning the patient, avoid grasping the muscle. Rather, support the joints

Box 29-2 | **ASSESSMENT of the Patient with a Spinal Cord Injury**

Health History

Present Illness:
Specific event that caused injury, other apparent injuries, pain location, and severity

Past Medical History:
Past accidents, injuries, hospitalizations, and operations; history of diabetes mellitus, hypertension, heart disease, cancer, seizure disorder; obstetric history; current medications; allergies

Family History:
Routine family history

Review of Systems:
Skin condition, headache, dizziness, vision disturbances, hearing impairment, tinnitus, nasal drainage, dyspnea, nausea, vomiting, constipation, diarrhea, fecal incontinence, bladder dysfunction, sexual dysfunction, impaired motor or sensory function

Functional Assessment:
Self-care abilities, roles and responsibilities, occupation, hobbies, usual activity pattern, use of tobacco and alcohol, diet, interpersonal relationships, emotional response to injury, usual coping strategies, spiritual beliefs, sources of support

Physical Examination

Height and Weight

Vital Signs

Level of Consciousness, Posture, Spontaneous Movements

Skin:
Lesions, bruises, redness, tissue turgor

Head:
Lesions, masses, swelling

Eyes:
Visual acuity; pupil size, equality, reaction to light

Thorax:
Respiratory effort, breath sounds

Abdomen:
Distention, bowel sounds

Extremities:
Range of motion, voluntary and involuntary movements, muscle strength, spasms, sensory perception, abnormal posturing, ability to recognize position of digits without looking

---

above and below the affected muscle groups with the palms of the hands.

For the patient maintained in cervical traction on a conventional bed, position changes must be done by "log-rolling." A minimum of three nurses is needed to correctly log-roll the patient. Some prior planning must be done so that the movement is coordinated. Identify the desired position, and place pillows and equipment in the proper locations before turning the patient. One nurse stands at the head of the bed and stabilizes the traction by placing his or her hands firmly on the patient's head and neck without flexing the neck. The second nurse prepares to move the patient's shoulders while the third prepares to move the patient's hips and legs. After explaining the procedure to the patient, turn the patient as a unit ("log-roll") to the desired position while maintaining proper alignment. Then place pillows to the patient's back and shoulders and between the legs to protect any pressure spots and to promote comfort. The nurse holding the head and neck should not release the patient until all movement has been completed to ensure that traction does not slip out of place.

Venous thromboembolism prevention is essential. Sequential compression devices are important to promote venous return. Use these when the patient is in bed. Pressure stockings can decrease venous stasis and edema.

If injections are necessary, administer them above the level of paralysis. There are two reasons for this. First, circulation is impaired below the level of injury,

causing drug absorption to be poor. Second, the patient is at increased risk for infection when the skin integrity is broken in affected parts of the body.

Sensory loss presents definite implications for nursing care. The spinal cord–injured patient with a complete lesion is unable to detect any temperature or pain sensation below the level of the injury. The individual is not able to determine if a painful stimulus, such as a burn, is present. You must provide meticulous skin care and take all necessary measures to protect the patient from harm.

Risk for Autonomic Dysreflexia

The focus of nursing management for the patient at risk for autonomic dysreflexia is directed primarily toward the prevention of the triggering stimulus. Teach the patient and family members the causes, signs and symptoms, and management of autonomic dysreflexia.

When autonomic dysreflexia occurs, it is a medical emergency. Once it is recognized, immediate action is required. Raise the patient's head to a 45-degree angle or place the patient in a sitting position to help decrease the pressure. If the cause can be identified, make every effort to eliminate it. Check the indwelling catheter for occlusion. If the bladder is distended and no indwelling catheter is present, straight catheterization may be indicated. Fecal impactions, if present, need to be digitally removed after the application of a local anesthetic as ordered. Monitor the patient with severe hypertension for seizures or signs of a stroke. Immediately notify the physician so that appropriate medications or other interventions can be initiated. Administer antihypertensive drugs as ordered. Features of autonomic dysreflexia are summarized in Box 29-3.

Risk for Disuse Syndrome

To avoid the development of pressure ulcers, turn the patient at least every 2 hours. Massage of the bony prominences may be harmful and is not recommended. As the patient is turned, inspect the back and sacral area for skin breakdown or signs of pressure. Provide back care using a gentle lotion or other agent designed specifically to prevent skin breakdown. Relieve pressure on any reddened or broken areas. When the patient is resting in the lateral supine position, place a pillow between the legs to keep the heels free of pressure and to prevent pressure between the knees. Keep bed linens clean, dry, and free of wrinkles. Teach the patient and caregiver how to inspect the skin and recognize signs of pressure.

Specialty beds and cushions also may be used to help alleviate pressure and enhance circulation. Even if special padding is used, patients in wheelchairs should still be instructed or assisted to reposition at least every 15 minutes. Some wheelchairs designed for

quadriplegic patients can be tilted backward to allow shifting of body weight.

Patients with tongs are maintained on strict bed rest. Therefore it is imperative that meticulous skin care be provided. With the vertebral column stabilized, the patient may be turned for position changes and skin assessment.

When the patient has spasticity, nursing management is directed toward preventing contractures and muscle atrophy. Pharmacologic agents, such as diazepam (Valium), baclofen (Lioresal), and dantrolene sodium (Dantrium), may be effective muscle relaxants. Electrical stimulators, used with heat and physiotherapy, also may help relieve spasms. Nursing management of the patient with muscle spasms is summarized in Box 29-4.

During the time of flaccid paralysis, you must diligently perform passive range-of-motion exercises and position and align the patient's extremities to reduce the risk of subluxation or contractures. A more complete discussion of the nursing care of the immobilized person is given in Chapter 21.

Bowel Incontinence

In the early postinjury period, an ileus may develop, meaning that peristalsis ceases. The abdomen becomes distended, and bowel sounds are absent. If this happens, fluids are administered intravenously and nothing is given by mouth. A nasogastric tube may be inserted and connected to suction for decompression. Peristalsis usually returns by the third day after the injury.

Once peristalsis resumes, the patient is given oral fluids and food. Encourage adequate fluids and high-fiber foods to promote soft stools. Administer bulk laxatives, stool softeners, suppositories, and lubricants as ordered. Document bowel movements, and institute measures to prevent constipation and impaction. Work with the patient to determine the best schedule for bowel elimination and to help the patient carry out the program. A bowel retraining program must be a cooperative effort between the caregiver and the patient. The program can succeed only when the patient is prepared physically and

---

Box 29-3 *Autonomic Dysreflexia*

Causes
Distended bladder or plugged catheter
Fecal impaction
Urinary calculi
Pressure ulcer
Ejaculation
Uterine contractions

Signs and Symptoms
Sudden hypertension
Pounding headache
Anxiety
Flushed face
Diaphoresis
Nasal congestion
Bradycardia
Vasoconstriction below lesion with cold skin and "goose flesh"
Vasodilation above lesion with warm, moist skin

Potential Effects
Seizures
Stroke

Management
Assessment to identify cause
Elevation of head of bed
Irrigation or replacement of urinary catheter
Intermittent catheterization
Application of topical anesthetic and digital disimpaction
Removal of pressure from irritated skin
Administration of antihypertensives as ordered

Box 29-4 *Management of Spasticity in the Spinal Cord-Injured Patient*

Perform passive range-of-motion exercises at least four times a day.
Properly position and splint extremities to prevent contractures.
Limit tactile stimuli.
Avoid incidence of noxious stimuli, such as anxiety, pain, bladder or bowel distention, and pressure ulcers.
Turn and reposition at least every 2 hr.
Properly administer medications to reduce spasms.

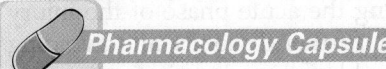

Pharmacology Capsule

Muscle relaxants may be ordered to control muscle spasticity.

---

emotionally. Bowel retraining is discussed in detail in Chapter 23.

Impaired Urinary Elimination

While the patient has an indwelling catheter, meticulous catheter care is essential. Because catheterization increases the risk of urinary tract infections, monitor the patient's temperature and assess the urine for cloudiness and foul odor. Administer prescribed urinary acidifiers, antiseptics, and antimicrobials. Encourage the oral intake of fluids, when permitted, to maintain dilute urine. Discourage the ingestion of dairy products because they contain calcium, which may promote formation of urinary calculi.

In the rehabilitation phase, bladder retraining is addressed. As a bladder retraining program is instituted, work with the patient to carry out the program. To help improve tone and relieve bladder spasms, the catheter may be periodically clamped and then released in an effort to increase bladder capacity. When the bladder can hold 300 to 400 mL of urine, the catheter may be removed for a trial period. Details of bladder retraining are covered in Chapter 23.

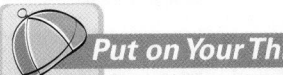

Put on Your Thinking Cap!

D.J. is a 22-year-old who has a spinal cord injury at T5. His physician has indicated that he no longer is experiencing spinal shock. How would you know that spinal shock has resolved? Why is management of the bowel and bladder very important at this time?

Risk for Infection

The risks of pulmonary and urinary infections have already been discussed. If the patient has skeletal traction (Gardner-Wells tongs, halo ring), there also is a risk of infection at the pin insertion sites. Provide specific skin care as ordered or per agency policy. Risk of infection is minimized by cleaning the pin site twice daily with sterile saline and keeping dry. After the initial healing, the area can be cleaned with soap and water. Report increasing redness or purulent drainage at the pin sites to the physician.

Ineffective Thermoregulation

Maintain the environmental temperature at a level that avoids chilling or overheating the patient. A room temperature of 70° F (21° C) will keep the quadriplegic's body temperature stable at 95° F. To prevent hypothermia, provide adequate clothing and blankets. Immediately change wet clothing and linens.

To prevent excessive warming (hyperthermia), the patient should avoid the outdoors during very hot, humid weather. Some patients carry a water spray bottle when outdoors in the heat or during intense activity. The water can be sprayed on the skin, where it evaporates and cools the body. Fans also can help cool the patient. An increase in temperature after exercise is normal.

Self-Care Deficit: Feeding/Dressing/Grooming

Continually reassess the patient's abilities and need for assistance with self-care activities. The patient may need total care initially. As soon as the patient is able, begin preparing him or her for self-care consistent with the patient's expected abilities. During rehabilitation, the patient learns to use specialized equipment and strategies in order to be as independent as possible in self-care.

Sexual Dysfunction

Sexuality and sexual function in the spinal cord–injured patient must be addressed when the patient first brings up the subject. Because sexual gratification is an important aspect of emotional and psychological well-being, it is an issue that requires thoughtful discussion and counseling. Patients must be apprised of their physical abilities to achieve erection or to bear children. Provide information about the possibility of pregnancy and about birth control, if the patient expresses a desire to know.

Advise the patient of resources available in the agency and in the community. The expertise of a trained counselor often is needed, and the counselor is usually a member of the rehabilitation team. Honest discussion must occur between the patient and the counselor. Both parties must be willing to explore the physical and emotional aspects of the injury. Additional information on management of impaired sexual function is presented in Chapters 47 and 48.

Ineffective Coping

Ineffective coping may occur at any phase but is particularly evident during rehabilitation as the patient begins to deal with the realities of the situation. Ineffective coping may present as hopelessness. Hopelessness may be manifested by withdrawal, passive behavior, and decreased affect. A person who feels hopeless sees few or no personal choices available and cannot mobilize the energy needed to move forward. Offer opportunities for the patient to discuss feelings about his or her situation and future. Listen actively, and accept the patient's feelings. When the patient is withdrawn, encourage, but do not force, participation in self-care. As the patient begins to acknowledge the injury and assess its impact, encourage him or her to identify strengths and coping strategies. Refocus attention on things other than the injury and losses. Begin rehabilitation efforts in earnest, and give generous praise for effort.

The health care team also works with the patient's significant others to create a supportive atmosphere that conveys hope, acceptance, and confidence. Patients and families often continue to hope for physical improvement that is unlikely. For example, they may interpret the movement associated with spastic paralysis as a return of voluntary motor function. You can avoid this misconception by explaining this phenomenon in advance and emphasizing that it is expected and does not signify improved function.

Ineffective Therapeutic Regimen Management

During the acute phase of spinal cord injury, explain routines and procedures. The physician or clinical nurse specialist usually informs the patient of the extent of the injury and probable effects. The nurse reinforces that information and helps the patient and family obtain any additional information requested. An important resource is the National Spinal Cord Injury Association (website: http://www.spinalcord.org; telephone: 1-800-962-9629), which has a 24-hour service to provide information about rehabilitation, research, organizations, and local contacts. Many communities have local chapters of the Spinal Cord Society, Paralyzed Veterans of America, and National Spinal Cord Injury Association that can provide information and resources.

The following are the essential components of the teaching plan. The details will vary with the level of the injury:

- Effects of spinal cord injury
- Types of treatments and their purposes
- Breathing exercises and adaptive techniques
- Range-of-motion exercises and positioning
- Management of orthostatic hypotension
- Skin care and assessment (see the Health Promotion Considerations box at right)
- Management of bowel and bladder elimination
- Recognition of signs and symptoms of infection
- Changes in sexual function and resources for information about adaptation
- Protection of body areas that lack sensation
- Adaptive techniques and devices to maximize self-care
- Emotional responses to spinal cord injury and coping strategies
- Community resources

See the Case Study (Box 29-5).

REHABILITATION

The saying "rehabilitation begins at admission" may sound trite, but for the spinal cord–injured patient its truth is astounding. The newly paralyzed person is faced with many sobering physical and psychological challenges. Both the acute care staff and the rehabilitation staff strive to see that the patient is fully equipped to face the challenge.

Nursing care during the acute phase of the injury focuses on preventing further disability and avoiding complications that could prolong hospitalization and hamper rehabilitation. Rehabilitation is best described as those activities that assist the individual to achieve the highest possible level of self-care and independence.

The rehabilitation process involves a well-organized interdisciplinary team that can address all aspects of function. Members of the team include the physician, nurse, physical therapist, occupational therapist, speech

---

Box 29-5 | *Case Study: Spinal Cord Injury*

Todd is a 16-year-old white male who was injured while playing football in the park. His friends called EMS and kept him motionless until their arrival. After his arrival at the hospital, his x-ray films revealed a C5 fracture dislocation. The fracture was immobilized using tongs, and he received methylprednisolone before admission to the ICU. His condition has stabilized, and he now has a halo brace in place for stabilization of the fracture. He is being transferred to your floor before future admission to rehabilitation.

Critical Thinking Questions

1. What strategies would you use to ease his transition to your unit?
2. Identify key components of the nursing care plan to consider based on the level of his injury.
3. Does Todd have a potential risk for autonomic dysreflexia? If it occurs, what assessment data would you gather and what would you do in this crisis?

 Health Promotion Considerations

Skin Care: Key Points for the Patient with a Spinal Cord Injury

- Avoid excessive pressure, shearing force, and trauma.
- Bathe in tepid water with mild soap; dry thoroughly.
- Soak feet for 20 min once a week; keep toenails trimmed and smooth.
- Keep skin dry and free of contact with urine or stool.
- Avoid tight clothing with heavy seams.
- Wear cotton undergarments, and avoid clothing made of fabrics that do not absorb moisture.
- Eat a balanced diet with adequate vitamins A and C and protein.
- Drink 2000 to 3000 mL of fluid (8-12 8-oz glasses) each day unless directed otherwise.
- When in bed, turn at least q 2 hr.
- When in a chair, shift weight at least q 15 min.
- Inspect skin every morning and every evening for redness, bruising, blisters, and dryness, and feel for swelling and hardness.
- If redness is present, try to determine cause. Ask yourself if you are turning or shifting weight often enough, if you are transferring correctly, and if your cushions are in good condition.

therapist, dietitian, social worker, psychologist, and counselor. Each plays a vital role in helping the patient achieve the highest level of independence. What was once regarded by the patient as a normal lifestyle or occupation may no longer be possible. Rather, modifications and adjustments must be made. Both the patient and the family must be emotionally and physically prepared to make those adjustments. The team not only helps the patient accomplish activities of daily living and self-care but also addresses successful adjustment to social integration and gainful employment in the workplace. Although this phase of treatment may take more than a year to accomplish, the patient, family, and rehabilitation team can take pride in the realization that a life can once again be productive and happy.

NURSING CARE OF THE LAMINECTOMY PATIENT

Laminectomy is the removal of part of a vertebra. It usually is done to relieve pressure on spinal nerves. In addition to traumatic cord injury, it may be used to treat herniated disks or spinal tumors. See Chapter 17 for general surgical care.

Preoperatively, assess the patient's vital signs and neurologic status to establish baselines. Determine the patient's understanding of surgical routines. Tell the patient what to expect in the immediate postoperative period.

For the patient who has undergone a laminectomy, postoperative care focuses on ongoing assessment of neurologic status and on promoting healing at the operative site. Specific nursing responsibilities are summarized in Box 29-6.

ASSESSMENT

After a laminectomy, monitor the patient's vital signs, neurologic status, and breath sounds. Frequently assess movement, strength, range of motion, and ability to localize sensory stimulus. Measure fluid intake and output. Auscultate the abdomen for bowel sounds, and palpate for bladder distention. Inspect the surgical dressing for bleeding, clear cerebrospinal fluid drainage, and foul drainage. If the patient has pain, obtain a complete description.

Nursing Diagnoses, Goals, and Outcome Criteria: Post Laminectomy

Nursing Diagnoses	Goals and Outcome Criteria
Risk of Injury related to immobility, neurologic trauma, spinal fluid leakage	Freedom from injury: stable or improving neurologic and vital signs, absence of bleeding or cerebrospinal fluid drainage, absence of fever, normal white blood cell count
Ineffective Tissue Perfusion related to hypovolemia, obstruction to blood flow	Adequate tissue perfusion: normal pulse, blood pressure, respirations, skin color, and tissue turgor
Acute Pain related to tissue trauma, muscle spasms	Pain relief: patient states pain relieved, relaxed expression
Impaired Urinary Elimination related to sensory motor impairment, prescribed position restrictions	Normal urine elimination: spontaneous, controlled voiding; no bladder distention; urine output approximately equal to fluid intake

Continued

Box 29-6   *Nursing Care After Laminectomy*

Neurologic Assessment and Vital Signs

Frequently assess movement, strength, and range of motion.

Assess ability to localize sensory stimulus.

Frequently measure vital signs to determine any postoperative complications, such as hemorrhage or infection.

Circulation and Respiration

Maintain elastic stockings on lower extremities to prevent deep vein thrombosis.

Encourage range-of-motion exercises four times a day.

Encourage deep-breathing exercises every 2 hr.

Auscultate breath sounds every 2-4 hr.

Have patient perform incentive spirometry every 2 hr while awake.

Progressive Ambulation as Appropriate

Help patient progress from sitting at edge of bed to ambulating with assistance.

Encourage increasing distances and independence while ambulating.

Ensure that patient uses back brace or other apparatus as ordered.

Bed or Positioning

Maintain bed flat or only slightly elevated to reduce strain on operative site.

Maintain soft collar for cervical laminectomy.

Encourage position changes every 2 hr.

Bowel and Bladder Function

Measure urinary output.

Assess for urinary distention and complete emptying of bladder after spontaneous void.

Encourage fluid intake.

Perform intermittent catheterization (as needed) if patient is unable to void.

Auscultate bowel sounds.

Initiate bowel program as appropriate.

Surgical Incision

Change dressing aseptically.

Check dressing for blood or cerebrospinal fluid drainage.

Pain or Discomfort

Medicate for pain and spasms as needed.

Encourage ambulation if possible to reduce spasms.

Constipation related to immobility, neurologic trauma, drug therapy	Normal bowel elimination: regular passage of formed stool without discomfort
Impaired Physical Mobility related to neuromuscular impairment, weakness, prescribed restrictions	Improved physical mobility: daily increase in walking distance without fatigue
Deficient Knowledge of course of recovery, self-care activities, and limitations	Patient understands routines, self-care, and limitations: patient describes and demonstrates appropriate self-care

INTERVENTIONS

Risk for Injury

Monitor the patient for complications of surgery. Notify the physician of deviations in vital signs, including increased pulse and respirations, hypotension, and fever. Compare neurologic findings with preoperative assessments. Report decreasing sensory or motor responses to the physician. Assist the patient with measures to prevent complications of immobility (breathing and leg exercises) within the limitations of postoperative restrictions. Inform the physician if clear drainage is observed draining from the incision, because this usually indicates a cerebrospinal fluid leak. When the dressing is changed, use aseptic technique to reduce the risk of wound contamination.

Ineffective Tissue Perfusion

Measures are taken to promote oxygenation and circulation. Apply elastic or pneumatic stockings to the lower extremities as ordered to promote venous return and prevent deep vein thrombosis. Instruct or assist the patient to do range-of-motion exercises at least four times daily or as ordered. Auscultate breath sounds every 2 to 4 hours, and support the patient in deep breathing and coughing to remove pulmonary secretions. The incentive spirometer may be used every 2 hours while the patient is awake. Position the patient in good alignment. Teach the patient to keep the back straight and avoid twisting when turning or getting out of bed.

A soft collar may be ordered after cervical laminectomy. Back braces may be prescribed after lumbar or thoracic spinal fusions. Typically, the braces are worn at all times at first. Use of the device is decreased as muscle strength returns. In some situations, corsets and casts are used to support and stabilize the spine. When supportive devices are worn, inspect the skin carefully to make sure they are not creating pressure that could result in skin breakdown.

Acute Pain

Assess and record the patient's level of discomfort. Keep the bed flat or with the head slightly elevated to reduce strain on the operative site. Administer analgesics and muscle relaxants as ordered. Other pain-control mea-

sures, such as relaxation techniques, cutaneous stimulation, and imagery, are described in detail in Chapter 15. If the prescribed medications and nursing interventions do not provide pain relief, discuss the problem with the physician to see if other measures can be tried.

Impaired Urinary Elimination

Take measures to promote voiding. Intravenous fluids are usually ordered, but fluids also can be given orally as soon as the patient is able to tolerate them. Document voiding, measure urine output, and assess the bladder for emptying. Promote voiding by providing privacy and positioning the patient as comfortably as allowed. Running water may stimulate voiding. If the patient is unable to void, intermittent catheterization may be ordered.

Constipation

Stool softeners may be ordered to prevent constipation. In addition, ingestion of adequate fluids and fiber is helpful. Ambulation, when permitted, also promotes normal bowel elimination.

Impaired Physical Mobility

Patient activity progresses from sitting on the edge of the bed to ambulating with assistance. Encourage the patient to gradually increase distance and independence in ambulating. If the patient is to wear a back brace or other apparatus, ensure that it is properly applied. Physical therapy may be ordered.

Deficient Knowledge

Postoperative teaching is directed toward promoting recovery from the surgery and preventing future injuries. Determine activity restrictions, and discuss these with the patient.

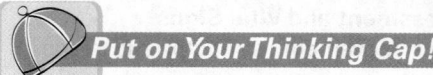

You are assigned to a 19-year-old male who sustained a C8 spinal cord injury 2 weeks ago. His condition is stable at this time, and he is alert and oriented. When the nursing assistant brings his breakfast tray, he closes his eyes, says he isn't hungry, and asks her to turn off the lights and close the drapes.

1. What phase of adjustment do you think the patient's behavior represents?
2. With adequate support, education, and encouragement, the patient will move into the next phase of adjustment. Describe expected behaviors at that time.

- Spinal cord injuries most often result from trauma but also may be caused by degenerative conditions and tumors.

- Spinal cord injuries may be classified by location, as open or closed, and by extent of damage to the cord.
- After spinal cord injury, motor and sensory function is monitored by assessing movement, muscle strength, sensation, and reflex activity.
- Effects of spinal cord injury may include respiratory impairment, spinal shock, autonomic dysreflexia, spasticity, impaired sensory and motor function, impaired bladder function, impaired bowel function, impaired temperature regulation, impaired sexual function, impaired skin integrity, and altered self-concept and body image.
- Injuries at or above the level of the fifth cervical vertebra may result in instant death because of interruption of the nerves that control respirations.
- Autonomic dysreflexia is an exaggerated sympathetic response to stimuli such as bladder distention, constipation, renal calculi, ejaculation, and uterine contractions that produces severe hypertension with the potential for seizures and stroke.
- Muscle tone is usually flaccid immediately after injury, but spasticity develops when spinal shock resolves.
- The goals of medical care after spinal injury are to sustain life, prevent further cord injury, and repair cord damage.

- Immobilization is essential to prevent further damage to the cord after injury.
- Nursing care after spinal cord injury is concerned with Ineffective Breathing Pattern, Risk for Injury and Disturbed Sensory Perception, Risk for Autonomic Dysreflexia, Risk for Disuse Syndrome, Bowel Incontinence, Impaired Urinary Elimination, Risk for Infection, Ineffective Thermoregulation, Hypothermia, Self-Care Deficit: Feeding/Dressing/Grooming, Sexual Dysfunction, Ineffective Coping, and Ineffective Therapeutic Regimen Management.
- Rehabilitation assists the patient to achieve the highest possible level of self-care and independence.
- Laminectomy is a surgical procedure that may be done for several reasons, including spinal cord injury.

 Go to your Companion CD-ROM for a Pharmacology Tutorial, Audio Glossary, and 3-D animations.

evolve   Be sure to visit the companion Evolve site at http://evolve.elsevier.com/Linton/ for WebLinks and additional online resources.

REVIEW QUESTIONS *Choose the best answer.*

1. A patient's chart notes that he has had complete transection of the spinal cord at T8. You would expect the patient to be:
   1. Ventilator dependent
   2. Paraplegic
   3. Comatose
   4. Tetraplegic

2. Which finding would indicate that spinal shock is resolving?
   1. Spastic, involuntary movements of the extremities
   2. Blood pressure returns to normal range
   3. No muscle tone in extremities
   4. Patient responds to light touch and pressure

3. Autonomic dysreflexia in a patient with a spinal cord injury is caused by:
   1. An emotional reaction to pain
   2. Stimulation of the sympathetic nervous system
   3. Dilation of blood vessels below the level of the injury
   4. Constriction of blood vessels above the level of the injury

4. After spinal shock resolved, a patient's bladder began to empty spontaneously. This could be interpreted to mean:
   1. The spinal cord is beginning to heal
   2. The patient is regaining normal bladder control
   3. Intact reflex activity is causing bladder emptying
   4. The patient is not a candidate for bladder retraining

5. Patient teaching for women with spinal cord injuries should include the following:
   1. Pregnancy is unlikely
   2. Sexual intercourse is impossible
   3. If pregnancy occurs, cesarean section will be necessary
   4. Although vaginal sensations are lacking, some women have orgasms

6. Immediate care after a suspected spinal cord injury should include the following:
   1. Gently lift the patient's chin and tilt the head
   2. Prop the patient's head to maintain slight flexion
   3. Administer 100% oxygen by nasal cannula
   4. Use the jaw-thrust method to open the airway

7. The purpose of a skeletal traction device after spinal cord injury is to:
   1. Align and immobilize the vertebrae to prevent further cord damage
   2. Apply tension to the spinal cord to keep it straight
   3. Maintain the neck in the best position to ensure an open airway
   4. Permit healing of the spinal cord injury

8. A patient admitted with a spinal cord injury may be given methylprednisolone to:
   1. Prevent allergic reactions to dyes used in diagnostic procedures
   2. Boost the patient's immune system
   3. Reduce damage to the cellular membrane of the spinal cord
   4. Promote regeneration of neurons

9. Nursing care during the acute phase of spinal cord injury should include the following:

    1. Never use restraints of any kind because the pressure tends to stimulate spastic muscle contractions
    2. Encourage patients in cervical traction to turn themselves every 2 hours to maintain muscle strength
    3. For the best absorption and to avoid injury, administer injections above the level of paralysis
    4. Because the patient will require a permanent indwelling catheter, begin teaching catheter care

10. Postoperative nursing care for the laminectomy patient should include the following:

    1. Inspect the skin under a back brace for signs of pressure or irritation
    2. Adjust the bed to keep the patient in a high-Fowler's position
    3. Discourage use of analgesics that sedate the patient
    4. Observe the bloody drainage, which is usually cerebrospinal fluid

VICTORIA DITTMAR

evolve http://evolve.elsevier.com/Linton/

Objectives

After reading and studying this chapter, you should be able to:

1. Identify data to be collected in the nursing assessment of the patient with a respiratory disorder.
2. Identify the nursing implications of age-related changes in the respiratory system.
3. Describe diagnostic tests or procedures for respiratory disorders and nursing interventions.
4. Explain nursing care of patients receiving therapeutic treatments for respiratory disorders.
5. For selected respiratory disorders, describe the pathophysiology, signs and symptoms, complications, diagnostic measures, and medical treatment.
6. Assist in developing a nursing care plan for the patient who has an acute respiratory disorder.

Key Terms

Be sure to check out the bonus material on the Companion CD-ROM, including selected audio pronunciations.

atelectasis (ă-tĕ-LĔK-tă-sĭs, p. 514)
crackles (KRĂK-ŭlz, p. 514)
dyspnea (DĬSP-nē-ă, p. 511)
hemothorax (hē-mō-THŌ-răks, p. 544)
hypercapnia (hī-pĕr-KĂP-nē-ă, p. 538)
hypoxemia (hī-pŏk-SĒ-mē-ă, p. 524)
hypoxia (hī-PŎK-sē-ă, p. 513)
orthopnea (ŏr-thŏp-NĒ-ă, p. 511)
pneumothorax (nū-mō-THŌ-răks, p. 514)
rhonchus (*pl.* rhonchi) (RŎNG-kăs, RŎNG-kī, p. 514)
tachypnea (tăk-ĭp-NĒ-ă, p. 528)
tissue perfusion (pĕr-FŪ-zhŭn, p. 547)

Respiration is basic to life. The respiratory system provides fuel for bodily activities and energy to sustain life. Respiration is defined as the exchange of oxygen (O_2) and carbon dioxide (CO_2) through the inspiration of air from the atmosphere and the expiration of air from the lungs. The function of the respiratory system is to supply oxygen for the metabolic needs of the cells and to remove carbon dioxide, one of the waste products of cellular metabolism.

ANATOMY AND PHYSIOLOGY OF THE RESPIRATORY SYSTEM

ANATOMY OF THE RESPIRATORY SYSTEM

To reach the lungs, air must travel through several passages, including the nose, mouth, pharynx, larynx, trachea, and bronchi (Fig. 30-1). Each passage has an effect on the quality of the air that reaches the lungs.

Nose

The nose includes the external nose, the part that is seen on the face, and the nasal cavity, which lies over the roof of the mouth. The external nose is made up of bones and cartilage that are covered with skin. The inside lining of the external nose consists of thick mucous membranes and small hairs. The mucous membranes also line the nasal cavity along with the cilia, which are small, hairlike projections.

The mucous membranes warm and moisten the air that enters the nose. If the air is not warmed as it enters the body, the tissue lining the respiratory tract functions poorly. The mucous membranes, the hairs in the external nose, and the cilia filter out dust particles and bacteria from the air. These cilia wave back and forth approximately 12 times per second to help the mucus clean the air. Air that enters via the nose is warmed and filtered, whereas air that enters via the mouth is not.

Pharynx

The pharynx, or throat, is a 5-inch tube extending from the back of the mouth to the esophagus. It is divided into three parts: nasal, oral, and laryngeal. The nasopharynx lies behind the nose, the oropharynx lies behind the mouth, and the laryngopharynx lies behind the larynx. The pharynx serves as a passage for both the respiratory and the digestive systems. It also has an important function in the formation of sounds, especially vowel sounds. The tonsils are located in the pharynx and may interfere with breathing, particularly nasal breathing, if they become enlarged. In addition, speech may have a nasal sound.

Larynx

The larynx, or "voice box," is the air passage between the pharynx and the trachea. It contains vocal cords and several types of cartilage, including the thyroid cartilage and the epiglottis. The epiglottis has a hinged, doorlike action at the entrance to the larynx. During swallowing, it acts like a lid to help prevent aspiration of food into the trachea.

The vocal cords are folds of mucous membranes that are attached to cartilage and extend from the front to the back of the larynx. The space between the folds is known as the *glottis*. Sound is produced when air from the lungs causes a rapid, repeated opening and closing of the glottis. The sounds are transformed into speech through the movements of the lips, jaws, and tongue.

Trachea

The trachea, or windpipe, is a 4- to 5-inch tube descending from the larynx into the bronchi. It is made up of cartilage, smooth muscle, and connective tissue lined by a layer of mucous membrane. The trachea functions as a passageway for air to reach the lungs.

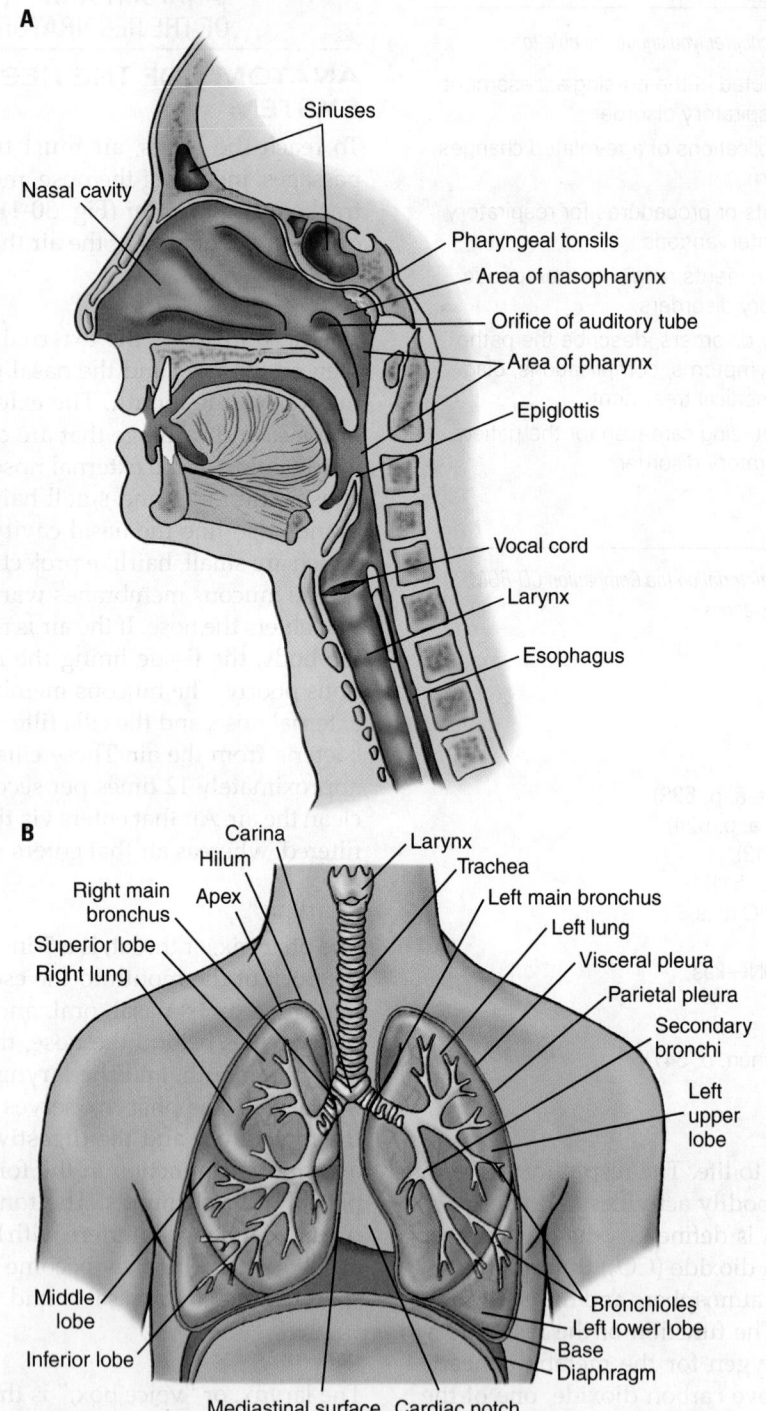

FIGURE 30-1 Structure of the respiratory system. **A,** Upper respiratory tract. **B,** Lower respiratory tract.

Bronchi

The bronchi provide a passageway for air going to and from the lungs. Two primary bronchi split to the right and left from the trachea. The right bronchus is shorter and wider and runs straighter up and down than the left bronchus. Therefore foreign bodies from the trachea usually enter the right bronchus.

The larger bronchi divide into smaller, or secondary, bronchi, which then divide again into even smaller tertiary bronchi. The tertiary bronchi divide into smaller units called *bronchioles*, which eventually lead into tiny air sacs called *alveoli* located in the lungs. It is through the walls of the alveoli that the exchange of oxygen and carbon dioxide takes place (Fig. 30-2).

Lungs

The lungs are located in the right and left sides of the thoracic cavity within the chest wall. The thoracic cavity is separated from the abdominal cavity by the diaphragm, a large sheet of muscle. The lungs are divided into lobes: three lobes on the right and two on the left. Each lung is covered by a membrane called the *pleura*. The pleura is a sac containing a small amount of fluid that acts as a lubricant for the lungs when they expand and contract.

RESPIRATORY PHYSIOLOGY

Mechanism of Breathing

The process of air entering into the lungs is called *inspiration*, and the process of air leaving the lungs is called *expiration*. The terms *inhalation* and *exhalation* are used interchangeably with inspiration and expiration. Both of these processes are accomplished by the movement of the diaphragm and the muscles in the chest. Inspiration involves an active contraction of the muscles and diaphragm and can be noted by an enlargement of the chest cavity. Expiration is a passive process dur-

ing which the muscles relax and the chest returns to its normal size (Fig. 30-3).

During normal, quiet breathing, approximately 500 mL of air is inhaled and exhaled. Most of the air movement occurs because of the contraction and relaxation of the diaphragm. A temporary interruption in the normal breathing pattern in which no air movement occurs is called *apnea*. Difficulty breathing, or shortness of breath, is called **dyspnea**. Difficulty with breathing in a lying position is called **orthopnea**. Different types of breathing patterns are described in Table 30-1.

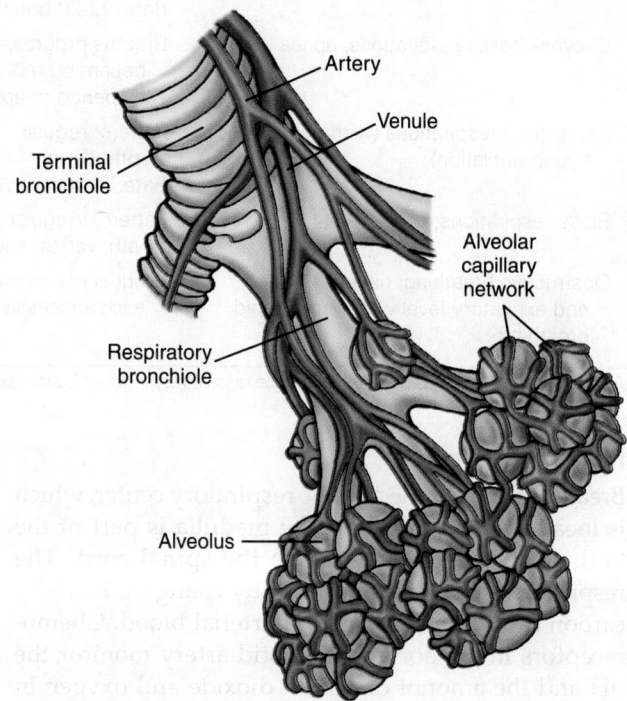

FIGURE **30-2** The terminal bronchioles, alveoli, and capillaries.

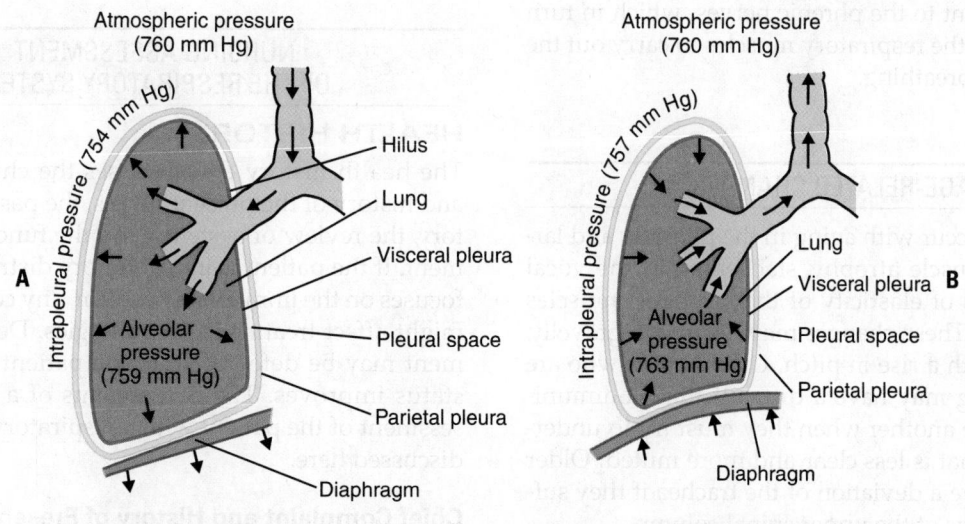

FIGURE **30-3** Normal inspiration (**A**) and expiration (**B**). Note the visceral pleura, pleural space, and parietal pleura and the changes in pressure in the alveoli and pleural space on inspiration and expiration.

Table 30-1 | *Types of Breathing Patterns*

PATTERN	CHARACTERISTICS	CAUSES
Normal	Pattern: regular Depth: even Rate: 12-20 breaths/min	Normal respiratory drive
Tachypnea	Pattern: regular Depth: even Rate: faster than 20 breaths/min	Fever, pain, anxiety
Bradypnea	Pattern: regular Depth: even Rate: slower than 12 breaths/min	Sedatives, opioids, alcohol; brain, metabolic, and respiratory disorders
Sighing respirations	Pattern: regular Depth: uneven: periodic deep breaths (more than 3 sighs/min) Rate: 12-20 breaths/min	Severe anxiety
Cheyne-Stokes respirations, apnea	Breaths progressively deeper, then becoming more shallow, followed by period of apnea	Severe brain pathology
Kussmaul's respirations (with hyperventilation)	Pattern: regular Depth: deep Rate: faster than 20 breaths/min	Metabolic acidosis Diabetic ketoacidosis, renal failure
Biot's respirations; apnea	Pattern: irregular Depth: varies, sudden periods of apnea	Neurologic disorders
Obstructive breathing, rising end-expiratory level with forced rapid breathing	Gradual rise in end-expiratory level with each successive breath	Emphysema

Adapted from Kersten, L.D. (1989). *Comprehensive respiratory nursing* (pp. 279-281). Philadelphia: Saunders.

Respiratory Center

Breathing is controlled by the respiratory center, which is located in the medulla. The medulla is part of the brainstem immediately above the spinal cord. The respiratory center is stimulated by changing levels of carbon dioxide and oxygen in arterial blood. Chemoreceptors in the aorta and carotid artery monitor the pH and the amount of carbon dioxide and oxygen in the bloodstream. Changes in the pH, increased levels of carbon dioxide, or decreased levels of oxygen cause signals to be sent to the phrenic nerves, which in turn send signals to the respiratory muscles to carry out the major work of breathing.

AGE-RELATED CHANGES

Changes that occur with aging in the pharynx and larynx include muscle atrophy, slackening of the vocal cords, and loss of elasticity of the laryngeal muscles and cartilages. These changes may result in a gravelly, softer voice with a rise in pitch. Older adults who are hard of hearing may have a difficult time communicating with one another when they must try to understand speech that is less clear and more muted. Older adults may have a deviation of the trachea if they suffer from scoliosis of the upper spinal column.

Older people may experience difficulty with respiration because they may have loss of lung elasticity, enlargement of the bronchioles, and a decreased number of functioning alveoli. Older adults are also more susceptible to lung infections because of less effective respiratory defense mechanisms. In addition, the respiratory muscles atrophy, the rib cage becomes more rigid, and the diaphragm flattens. The consequences of these changes include reduced chest movement and ability to inhale and exhale, less effective cough, increased work of breathing, and less tolerance for exercise and stress.

NURSING ASSESSMENT OF THE RESPIRATORY SYSTEM

HEALTH HISTORY

The health history encompasses the chief complaint and history of the present illness, the past medical history, the review of systems, and the functional assessment. If the patient is in respiratory distress, the nurse focuses on the immediate problem, any conditions that might affect treatment, and allergies. Detailed assessment may be deferred until the patient's respiratory status improves. The components of a complete assessment of the patient with a respiratory disorder are discussed here.

Chief Complaint and History of Present Illness

Common complaints associated with respiratory disorders are cough, dyspnea, and pain. To describe a cough, include the onset, duration, frequency, type (wet or dry), severity, and related symptoms such as sputum production and pain. Document the frequency of expectoration and the sputum characteristics (color, consistency, odor, amount). Record the patient's effort to treat the cough with measures such as medication, vaporizers, and humidifiers, as well as the response to the treatments.

If the patient complains of dyspnea, determine the onset, duration, severity, and precipitating events. Note whether the dyspnea becomes worse with activity or certain positions and whether it is more frequent during certain seasons. Identify associated symptoms such as fatigue or palpitations. Describe the effectiveness of methods used to manage dyspnea, which might include medications, oxygen, and positioning.

When the patient has chest pain, describe the location, severity, onset, duration, and precipitating events (trauma, coughing, inspiration). Determine whether the pain causes shallow breathing and whether it radiates up to the jaw or down the arms. Record the presence of fever, sweating, or nausea. Document measures that bring relief such as splinting, heat, analgesics, and antitussives.

Past Medical History and Family History

The patient's past medical history determines previous respiratory disorders, allergies, trauma, and surgery. Conditions that are important to document when a patient has a respiratory disorder include allergies, colds, pneumonia, tuberculosis, chronic bronchitis, emphysema, asthma, cancer of the respiratory tract, cystic fibrosis, sinus infections, ear infections, diabetes mellitus, and heart disease. It is especially important to note conditions that suppress the immune response, making the patient more susceptible to infection. Record all recent and current medications, including the use of over-the-counter drugs, and the dates of the most recent chest radiograph and tuberculin skin test. Inquire about immunizations against pneumonia and influenza. Include questions regarding family history. Also describe any major respiratory conditions and the smoking history of members of the household.

Review of Systems

The review of systems assesses signs and symptoms that may be directly or indirectly related to the respiratory disorder. Ask about fatigue, weakness, fever, chills, and night sweats. Other data that may be significant are earaches, nasal obstructions, sinus pain, sore throat, hoarseness, edema, dyspnea, and orthopnea.

Functional Assessment

Describe the patient's occupational history, including any exposure to pathogens or to substances that might irritate or harm the respiratory tract. Document exposure to any fumes, toxins, coal dust, silica, or sawdust. Ask the patient to describe a typical day and to give particular attention to any limitations imposed by

the respiratory disorder. Ask about the usual diet and fluid intake. A smoking history is important and for the cigarette smoker is usually reported in pack years. Pack years are calculated by multiplying the number of years the patient smoked cigarettes times the number of packs smoked each day. To illustrate, a person who smoked two packs a day for 30 years would have a 60-pack-year smoking history. The functional assessment also includes the patient's role in the family, sources of stress, and coping strategies.

 What Does Culture Have to Do with Smoking?

Among adolescents, smoking is most prevalent among whites, followed by Hispanics, and then African Americans. However, programs aimed at smoking prevention and cessation need to target all segments of the population because smoking is a health threat to everyone that typically begins before high school. On a positive note, people who practice Mormonism abstain from using tobacco.

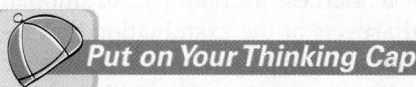 **Put on Your Thinking Cap!**

A patient has smoked one pack of cigarettes each day for 15 years. Calculate the pack years of his smoking history.

PHYSICAL EXAMINATION

Begin the physical examination with observation of the patient's general appearance. Note facial expression, posture, alertness, speech pattern, and any obvious signs of distress. Take the vital signs, and measure height and weight. Be alert to unusually rapid or slow breathing and to tachycardia, which may be a sign of *hypoxia*. The normal respiratory rate is 12 to 20 breaths per minute.

Head and Neck

Examine the head and neck. Inspect the nose for symmetry and for deformity, and gently palpate for tenderness. The patency of each naris can be assessed by closing one at a time and asking the patient to breathe in through the nose. Note flaring of the nares, because it is a common sign of air hunger. Use a nasal speculum to inspect the nasal cavity for swelling, discharge, bleeding, or foreign bodies. The nasal mucosa is normally light red in color. Tilt back the patient's head to inspect for deviation of the nasal septum, the structure that separates the nares. A deviation may be seen as a hump in the nasal cavity. Palpate the sinuses for tenderness by using the thumbs to apply pressure over the frontal and maxillary sinuses (see Chapter 53).

Inspect the lips, the tip of the nose, the top of the auricles, the gums, and the area under the tongue for cyanosis, a bluish color related to inadequate tissue oxygenation. Document the presence of pursed-lip breathing, a common technique for decreasing dyspnea with chronic respiratory disease. Inspect the pharynx for redness and tonsil exudate or enlargement, which are signs of infection.

Inspect the trachea to see if it is midline; if not midline, it is said to be *deviated*. A deviated trachea can be indicative of a large atelectasis, pleural effusion, aortic aneurysm, enlargement of part of the thyroid gland, and/or tension pneumothorax. Place the thumbs on either side of the trachea just above the clavicles, and gently move the trachea from side to side. Compare the spaces between the sternocleidomastoid muscles on either shoulder and the trachea. An experienced examiner palpates for enlargement and tenderness of the lymph glands in the neck.

Thorax

Inspect the chest for deformities and lesions, and observe the breathing pattern and effort. The rise and fall of the chest should be regular and symmetric. Table 30-1 illustrates the different types of breathing patterns. Palpate the thorax for tenderness and lumps. Additional, more sophisticated aspects of the examination that require special training include palpating for symmetric chest expansion and tactile fremitus. The skilled examiner also may percuss (tap) the thorax in a systematic manner to elicit sounds that give clues about the density of underlying tissues.

Using the diaphragm of the stethoscope, auscultate the lungs bilaterally in a systematic manner (Fig. 30-4), usually the posterior, the sides, and then the anterior chest. Listen for the normal movement of air in and out of the lungs and for abnormal breath sounds: wheezes, rhonchi, and crackles. A wheeze is a high-pitched sound caused by air passing through narrowed passageways that may be present with asthma or chronic obstructive pulmonary disease. A rhonchus is a dry, rattling sound caused by partial bronchial obstruction. Crackles, also called *rales*, are abnormal sounds associated with many cardiac and pulmonary disorders. Fine crackles are due to fluid accumulation in the alveoli and do not clear with coughing. To demonstrate the sound of fine crackles, rub a few strands of hair between the thumb and forefinger next to the ear. Coarse crackles are described as sounding like a Velcro fastener being separated. Course crackles are due to secretions accumulating in the larger airways and usually clear with coughing. One other abnormal sound that may be heard on auscultation is a pleural friction rub, which is indicative of pleurisy.

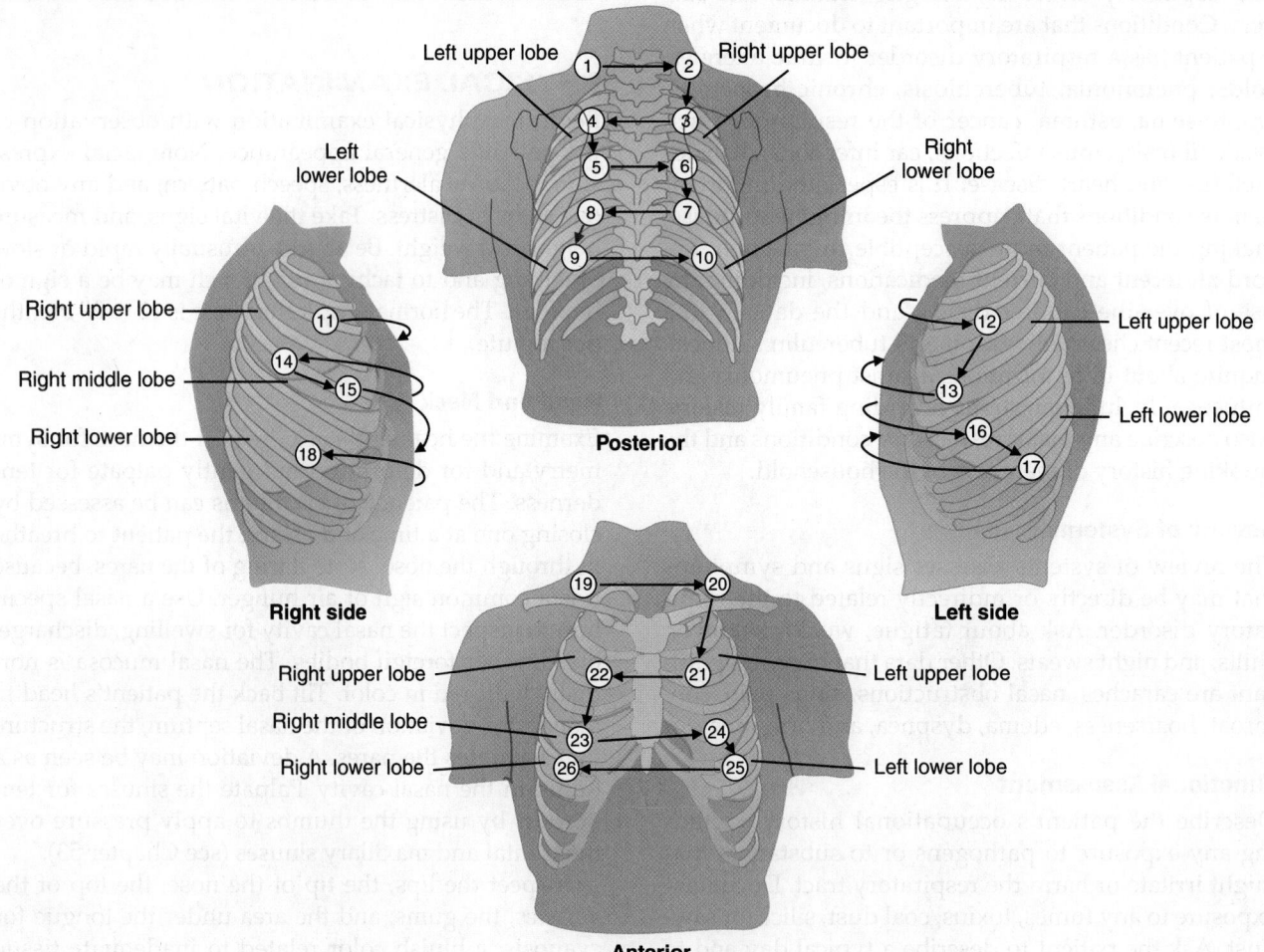

FIGURE 30-4 Sequence for percussion and auscultation of the lungs.

A pleural friction rub is a grating, scratchy noise similar to a creaking shoe.

In addition to the examination of the thorax and the auscultation of lung sounds, assess for signs of circulatory disorders that could affect respirations. Inspect the abdomen for distention that might interfere with full expansion of the lungs. Inspect the extremities for color, and palpate for edema. Examine the fingers for clubbing, which is associated with chronic respiratory problems (Fig. 30-5). Assess Homans' sign by passively dorsiflexing the patient's foot. Suspect thrombophlebitis if this maneuver elicits pain behind the knee or in the calf. This is important because the deep veins in the legs and pelvis are the source of most pulmonary emboli. It is important not to vigorously dosiflex the foot because this could potentially dislodge a clot from the leg. A negative Homans' sign does not completely rule out venous inflammation, nor does a positive sign always indicate inflammation. Nevertheless, it is one piece of data that should be documented.

The nursing assessment of the patient with a respiratory disorder is summarized in Box 30-1.

DIAGNOSTIC TESTS AND PROCEDURES

A variety of tests and procedures may be performed to diagnose disorders of the respiratory system. These tests and procedures are described briefly here. Details of patient preparation and postprocedure care are presented in the Diagnostic Tests and Procedures table on pp. 517 and 518.

Put on Your Thinking Cap!

A patient in respiratory distress usually has tachycardia. Explain why this happens and what purpose the increased heart rate serves.

RADIOLOGIC STUDIES

Chest Radiography

Radiographic examination of the chest is one of the most frequently used methods for respiratory screening and diagnosis. It also is used to assess progression of a disease and response to treatment. The radiograph or roentgenogram produces a picture in which the bony structures (e.g., ribs, sternum, clavicle), heart shadow, trachea, bronchi, and blood vessels are visible. Bone appears white on the film because it is very dense and does not absorb much energy. In contrast, the lungs appear black because they are filled with air and absorb the x-ray energy. Chest films usually are taken posteroanterior (back to front), anteroposterior (front to back), and lateral (side) to view the chest cavity from different angles.

Fluoroscopy

Fluoroscopy is a radiograph of the chest taken to observe deep structures in motion. It is possible to observe both lungs at the same time during inspiration and expiration. Instead of producing a single, still image, the screen registers a constant image of the chest. The fluoroscopic examination can give information about

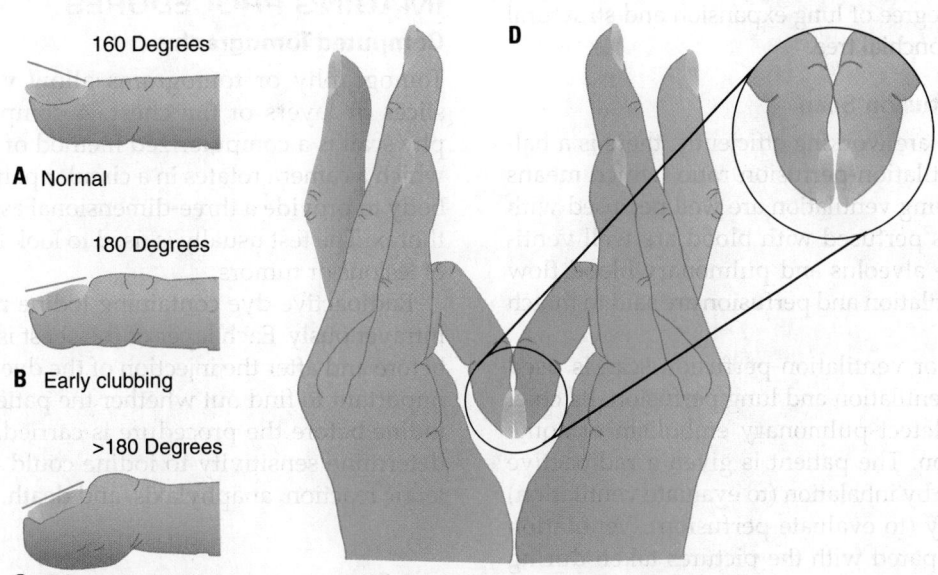

FIGURE **30-5** Clubbing is a flattening of the angle between the nail and the skin. **A,** Normal angle of 160 degrees. **B,** Early clubbing: the angle is flattened to 180 degrees. **C,** Advanced clubbing: the angle is greater than 180 degrees. **D,** The Schamroth technique: the patient puts the nails of the ring fingers of each hand together and holds the other fingers straight up. The examiner looks at the space between the touching nails. If there is no clubbing, the space is diamond shaped.

Box 30-1 | *ASSESSMENT of the Patient with a Respiratory Disorder*

HEALTH HISTORY

Present Illness:
Cough: Onset, duration, frequency, type, severity, sputum production and characteristics, pain

Dyspnea:
Onset, duration, severity, precipitating events, associated symptoms

Pain:
Location, onset, duration, precipitating events, effects on breathing, measures that reduce or relieve, associated symptoms

Past Medical History:
Colds, pneumonia, tuberculosis, chronic bronchitis, emphysema, asthma, cancer of the respiratory tract, cystic fibrosis, sinus infections, ear infections, diabetes mellitus, heart disease, allergies, trauma, surgeries, hospitalizations, conditions that suppress the immune response, immunizations against pneumonia and influenza, last chest radiograph, last tuberculin skin test, recent and current medications

Family History:
Major respiratory conditions, smoking history

Review of Symptoms:
Fatigue, weakness, fever, chills, night sweats, earaches, nasal obstruction, sinus pain, sore throat, hoarseness, edema, dyspnea, orthopnea

Functional Assessment:
Occupation, exposure to pathogens or respiratory irritants, typical day, usual diet and fluid intake, smoking history, role in family, stressors, coping strategies

PHYSICAL EXAMINATION

General Survey:
Appearance, facial expression, posture, alertness, speech pattern, obvious distress

Vital Signs

Height and Weight

Nose:
Nasal shape, tenderness, patency, flaring; swelling, discharge, bleeding, foreign bodies in nasal cavity, septal deviation

Sinuses:
Tenderness

Lips:
Pursed-lip breathing, color

Pharynx:
Redness, tonsil exudate or enlargement

Trachea:
Midline

Lymph Nodes:
Enlargement, tenderness

Thorax:
Breathing pattern and effort, accessory muscles, lung sounds

Abdomen:
Distention

Extremities:
Color, clubbing, edema, Homans' sign

---

the speed and degree of lung expansion and structural defects in the bronchial tree.

Ventilation-Perfusion Scan

When the lungs are working efficiently, there is a balance in the ventilation-perfusion ratio, which means that areas receiving ventilation are well perfused with blood and areas perfused with blood are well ventilated. When the alveolus and pulmonary blood flow are normal, ventilation and perfusion are said to match (Fig. 30-6).

A lung scan or ventilation-perfusion scan is used to assess lung ventilation and lung perfusion. Its chief purpose is to detect pulmonary embolism or some other obstruction. The patient is given a radioactive substance either by inhalation (to evaluate ventilation) or intravenously (to evaluate perfusion). Ventilation images are compared with the pictures taken during the perfusion scan to determine whether there is an equal amount of radioactivity on both the ventilation and the perfusion pictures. Any areas indicating good ventilation but poor perfusion suggest the presence of a pulmonary embolus or obstruction.

IMAGING PROCEDURES

Computed Tomography

Tomography or tomograms allow visualization of slices or layers of the chest. A computed tomography scan is a computerized method of tomography in which a camera rotates in a circular pattern around the body to provide a three-dimensional assessment of the thorax. The test usually is used to look for the presence of lesions or tumors.

Radioactive dye containing iodine may be injected intravenously. Each layer of the chest is photographed before and after the injection of the dye. It is extremely important to find out whether the patient is allergic to iodine before the procedure is carried out. Failure to determine sensitivity to iodine could result in an allergic reaction, anaphylaxis, and death.

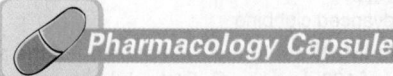
Pharmacology Capsule

Dyes used in computed tomography contain iodine that can produce fatal reactions in people with iodine allergies.

DIAGNOSTIC TESTS and PROCEDURES | *The Respiratory System*

TEST/PURPOSE	PATIENT PREPARATION	POSTPROCEDURE CARE
General nursing implications: Always tell the patient what to expect before, during, and after the procedure. When a venous blood sample is required, tell the patient to expect a venipuncture.		
PULMONARY FUNCTION TESTS (PFTS) Evaluate lung function, gas exchanges, pulmonary blood flow, and acid-base balance.	Advise not to smoke or eat a heavy meal 4-6 hr before test. Patient should be dressed comfortably and should void before the tests. Determine whether any medications or treatments should be withheld.	Resume medications. No special care.
FIBEROPTIC BRONCHOSCOPY Used to visualize abnormalities, take biopsy samples of lesions, or remove foreign bodies.	Obtain signed consent. NPO 6-8 hr or as specified. Have patient remove dentures and provide oral hygiene. Document loose teeth. Ask the patient not to smoke. Administer sedatives and anticholinergics as ordered.	NPO until gag reflex returns. Semi-Fowler's position. Monitor vital signs. Monitor for gross hemoptysis, swelling of face and neck, stridor, decreased or asymmetric chest movement, diminished lung sounds, dyspnea. Report abnormal findings to physician.
THORACENTESIS Pleural fluid is aspirated and examined for pathogens, other abnormal components. Cells studied for malignancy.	Obtain signed consent. Stress the importance of not moving or coughing during the procedure. Support the patient during the thoracentesis, and monitor skin color, respiratory rate, and general response. Label specimens and send to laboratory.	Monitor vital signs, lung sounds, chest movement. Report dyspnea, asymmetric chest movement. Assess for bleeding. Document amount and color of fluid removed. Check dressing for bleeding.
TUBERCULIN SKIN TEST Determine past or present exposure to tuberculosis.	Inform patient the procedure causes pain briefly. Cleanse skin and inject intradermally in lower anterior forearm. Mark and record site. Tell patient skin reaction may persist for a week, do not scratch. Stress need to return in 48-72 hr to read reaction. A reaction (swelling, redness) of 5 mm or more is positive for tuberculosis exposure. A patient who has ever been vaccinated with BCG will test positive regardless of actual exposure.	Follow-up depends on response. If positive, patient will be evaluated for active tuberculosis.
RADIOGRAPHIC AND IMAGING STUDIES **Chest Radiography** Used to screen and diagnose some respiratory disorders.	Patient will be asked to remove jewelry on neck and chest and clothing above waist and to put on hospital gown.	No special care.
Fluoroscopy Motion radiographs of lungs.	Same as chest radiography.	No special care.
Ventilation-Perfusion Scan (Lung Scan) Demonstrates lung ventilation and perfusion. Detects pulmonary embolism and other obstructive conditions.	Assure patient that radiation dose is small and that isotope is quickly eliminated. Procedure is painless except for venipuncture. If sedation is needed for agitated patients or small children, the patient is usually maintained NPO for 4 hr. The procedure takes approximately 2 hr. Monitor patient for 1 hr for anaphylaxis.	Check venipuncture site. Apply small dressing and pressure if needed. Radioactive material is excreted in the urine. Tell patient to wash hands after voiding. Anyone who handles patient's urine should wear rubber gloves. Gloves and hands should be washed after urine is discarded.

BCG, Bacille Calmette-Guérin; *NPO*, nothing by mouth.

Continued

DIAGNOSTIC TESTS and PROCEDURES | *The Respiratory System—cont'd*

TEST/PURPOSE	PATIENT PREPARATION	POSTPROCEDURE CARE
Computed Tomography (CT, CAT, or CAT Scan) Used to visualize lesions and tumors.	Inform the patient that the procedure is painless. Stress the importance of remaining still during the scanning. Assess iodine allergy and report to radiologist in case contrast medium is to be used. NPO status may be required.	Assess for side effects of contrast: headache, nausea, vomiting.
Magnetic Resonance Imaging (MRI) Produces images of multiple body planes without radiation. Used to detect abnormalities, lesions, and tumors.	Obtain signed consent. Inform patient: will lie on a stretcher that slides into a tubelike device. Mechanical clanging noises are heard as the machine operates. Aneurysm clips, intraocular metal, heart valves made before 1964, and middle ear prostheses generally contraindicate MRI. Metal implants such as cardiac pacemakers and orthopedic implants may be affected by MRI but are not absolute contra-indications. Assess for and report claustrophobia. Patients who are anxious or restless may require sedation. Special equipment must be used for oxygen therapy or mechanical ventilation. Have patient remove metal watch and jewelry.	Safety precautions if sedated; otherwise, no special care is needed.
LABORATORY STUDIES **Arterial Blood Gas Analysis** Detects alkalosis or acidosis and alterations in oxygenation status.	Tell the patient a blood sample will be drawn from an artery (usually the radial). An Allen test *must* be done before an arterial puncture to ensure that the arteries to the hand are patent. (Arterial punctures require specialized training.)	Apply pressure to the puncture site for 5-10 min. Note on the laboratory slip the concentration of any oxygen therapy. Transport the blood gas syringe containing the specimen to the laboratory in an ice bath within 15 min.
Sputum Analysis Volume, consistency, odor, color provide clues to clinical disorders. **Sputum Culture and Sensitivity (C&S)** Reveals pathogens and effective antimicrobials. **Sputum for Cytology** Detects malignant cells and inflammatory changes.	Collect the specimen early in the morning before breakfast. Provide a sterile container. Instruct patient to (1) brush teeth and rinse mouth; (2) cough deeply and expectorate directly into the container; (3) immediately cap the container; and (4) inform the nurse that the specimen is ready. *For cytology*, a special container and solution must be used for specimens. Send specimen to the laboratory promptly. Refrigerate if it will be more than an hour before delivery to the laboratory.	No special care.

NPO, Nothing by mouth.

Magnetic Resonance Imaging

A magnetic resonance imaging (MRI) scan is similar to a computed tomography scan but without the harmful radiation. The MRI scanner encloses the patient in a doughnut-shaped magnet and picks up signals from the body to make electronic images. The patient must remain as quiet and as motionless as possible during the procedure. No preparation is necessary, but patients should be warned that no metal may be worn inside the unit (with the exception of dental fillings). Patients with implanted devices such as pacemakers and orthopedic plates, pins, or screws may be ineligible for MRI scanning.

Positron Emission Tomography

Positron emission tomography (PET) scans of the lungs are used most often to distinguish malignant from benign cells and to evaluate the effectiveness of cancer treatment. PET scans use special radionuclides attached to a natural body compound, usually glucose. This substance is administered to the patient as an IV, and the radioactivity localizes in the appropriate areas

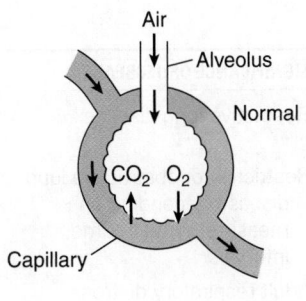

Normal functioning alveolus and pulmonary capillary flow. Ventilation and perfusion match.

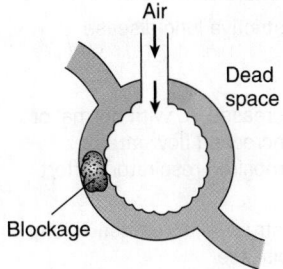

When there is ventilation without perfusion, a dead-space unit exists, e.g., pulmonary embolus preventing blood flow through pulmonary capillary.

When there is no ventilation to an alveolar unit but perfusion continues, a shunt unit exists and unoxygenated blood continues to circulate, e.g., atelectasis, pneumonia. The alveoli collapse.

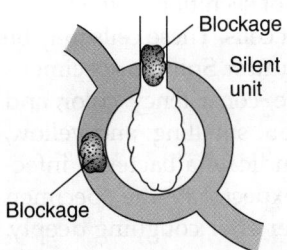

When there is neither ventilation nor perfusion, a silent unit develops, e.g., pulmonary embolus combined with ARDS (adult respiratory distress syndrome). The alveoli collapse.

FIGURE **30-6** Normal functioning alveolus and pulmonary capillary blood flow. When both are normal, the ventilation and perfusion match.

of the body and is detected by the PET scanner. Cancerous tissue, which uses more glucose than normal tissue, will accumulate more of the substance and appear brighter than normal tissue on the PET images. The patient must remain quiet, avoiding movement or talking during the test. Because glucose is the substance most often tagged with the radionuclides, it is important to make sure that the patient has not eaten for at least 4 hours before the test.

PULMONARY FUNCTION TESTS

Pulmonary function tests are used to diagnose pulmonary disease, monitor disease progression, evaluate the extent of disability, and assess the effects of medication. The tests measure lung volumes and capacities including total lung capacity (TLC), forced expiratory volume (FEV), functional residual capacity (FRC), inspiratory capacity (IC), vital capacity (VC), forced vital capacity (FVC), minute volume (MV), and thoracic gas volume (TGV).

A clip is applied to the nose, and the patient breathes through a mouthpiece as directed while various measurements are taken to assess the mechanics of breathing (flow rates of gas in and out of the lungs) and to measure diffusion (the movement of the gas across the alveolar-capillary membrane).

Spirometry

A spirometer is an instrument that measures the ventilatory function of the lung. It measures the volume of air that the lung can hold, the rate of flow of air in and out of the lung, and the compliance (elasticity) of lung tissue. The test enables the physician to detect impaired pulmonary function, classify the pulmonary impairment, estimate the severity of the impairment, monitor the cause of pulmonary disease, evaluate treatment, give information helpful in planning care, and provide preoperative assessment.

The test involves inserting a mouthpiece, taking as deep a breath as possible, and blowing as hard, as fast, and as long as possible. Patients should be encouraged to continue blowing out until exhalation is complete.

Spirometry measures forced vital capacity and forced expiratory volume. These and other lung volumes and capacities are defined in Table 30-2.

People who are to undergo spirometry should be taught what to expect during the test and how to prepare. They may be anxious about taking a breathing test if they have respiratory problems, because they may fear increased dyspnea or exhaustion. They should be advised not to smoke or use bronchodilator medications for 4 to 6 hours before testing.

Pharmacology Capsule

Bronchodilators should not be given before pulmonary function testing because they can alter the results.

Arterial Blood Gas Analysis

Ventilation and diffusion also are measured by testing for concentrations of oxygen and carbon dioxide in the arterial blood to determine whether the exchange is adequate across the alveolar membrane. Blood gas analysis is useful in the care of patients with respiratory disorders, problems of circulation and distribution of blood, body fluid imbalances, and acid-base imbalances. *Drawing an arterial blood sample requires special training.* Samples are often obtained from the radial artery after first performing the Allen test to ensure adequate circulation to the hand from other arteries (Fig. 30-7). After the arterial puncture,

Table 30-2 | *Lung Volumes and Capacities*

VOLUME	DEFINITION	SIGNIFICANCE OF INCREASE	SIGNIFICANCE OF DECREASE
Total lung capacity (TLC)	Total lung volume when fully inflated	Overdistention of lung caused by obstructive lung disease	Restrictive lung disease
Forced expiratory volume (FEV)	Volume of air expired during specified time intervals (0.5, 1, 2, 3 sec)	Not significant	Restrictive or obstructive lung disease depending on measurements at time intervals
Functional residual capacity (FRC)	Volume of air remaining in the lungs after normal exhalation	Chronic obstructive pulmonary disease	Adult respiratory distress syndrome (ARDS)
Inspiratory capacity (IC)	Maximum volume of air that can be inhaled after a normal exhalation	Excessive use of positive end-expiratory pressure	Restrictive lung disease
Vital capacity (VC)	Total volume of air that can be exhaled after maximum inspiration	Not significant Increased or normal VC with normal flow rates: pulmonary edema	Decreased VC with normal or increased flow rates: impaired respiratory effort
Forced vital capacity (FVC)	Total volume of air exhaled rapidly and forcefully after maximum inhalation	Not significant	Obstructive or restrictive lung disease
Minute volume (MV)	Total amount of air breathed in 1 min	Not significant	Restrictive parenchymal lung disease; fatigue
Thoracic gas volume (TGV)	Total volume of air in the lungs, including ventilated and nonventilated areas	Obstructive lung disease with air trapping	Not significant

Data from Chernecky, C.C., & Berger, B.J. (2001). *Laboratory tests and diagnostic procedures.* (3rd ed.). Philadelphia: Saunders; Jaffe, M.S., & McVan, B.F. (1997). *Davis's laboratory and diagnostic test handbook.* Philadelphia: Saunders.

pressure must be applied for 5 to 10 minutes to ensure no bleeding. In the critical care setting, an arterial line, commonly called an *ART line,* may be placed by the physician. This line allows for frequent monitoring of arterial blood gases without repeated arterial punctures.

The arterial blood sample is analyzed for pH, $PaCO_2$, Pao_2, HCO_3^-, and O_2 saturation to detect alkalosis or acidosis and alterations in oxygenation status. Normal values for adults are pH: 7.35 to 7.45; $Paco_2$: 35 to 45 mm Hg; Pao_2: 80 to 100 mm Hg (some references give a lower limit of 75 mm Hg); HCO_3^-: 22 to 26 mEq/L; O_2 saturation: 96% to 100%.

PULSE OXIMETRY

Pulse oximetry permits the noninvasive measurement of arterial oxygen saturation. A sensor is clipped to an earlobe or fingertip. A beam of light passes through the tissue, and the amount of light absorbed by oxygen-saturated hemoglobin is measured. The oxygen saturation is presented as a percentage and registered on a digital readout. Factors that interfere with accurate measurement of the oximeter are hypotension, hypothermia, vasoconstriction, and finger movement. Normal pulse oximetry is ≥95%. Notify your supervisor or the physician of readings <90%.

SPUTUM ANALYSIS

Sputum is material that originates in the bronchi. Sputum analysis may be performed when respiratory dis-

ease is suspected. The mucous membrane lining of the lower respiratory tract responds to acute inflammation by increasing the production of secretions, which may contain bacterial or malignant cells. These cells may be detected by examination of sputum. Sputum specimens are examined also for volume, consistency, color, and odor. Sputum that is thick, foul smelling, and yellow, green, or rust colored may indicate a bacterial infection. Instruct the patient to expectorate the specimen directly into a sterile container after coughing deeply. If the patient is unable to expectorate a specimen, sputum production may be induced with aerosol therapy or obtained by suctioning.

Culture and Sensitivity

Sputum culture and sensitivity tests are ordered to determine the presence of bacteria, identify the specific organisms, and identify appropriate antimicrobials. Collect specimens before antimicrobial therapy is begun to ensure that sufficient bacterial growth is present.

Acid-Fast Test

An acid-fast test on a sputum specimen is performed to determine the presence of acid-fast bacilli, which include the bacteria that cause tuberculosis. Specimens are usually collected on 3 consecutive days. Keep each sputum specimen covered and refrigerated or delivered to the laboratory within 1 hour. Use a new sterile container for each collection.

FIGURE **30-7** The Allen test should be done before each radial arterial puncture to ensure adequate collateral circulation. Because an arterial puncture may injure the radial artery, the adequacy of blood supply to the area by other arteries must be determined. A puncture is not done on an artery if the other blood supply is not adequate. To perform the Allen test, occlude the radial and ulnar arteries and have the patient make a fist (**A**). While maintaining pressure on the arteries, have the patient open the hand. The hand is pale if the arteries are occluded (**B**). Release the pressure on the ulnar artery. If collateral circulation is adequate, color will return to the hand. This is a positive Allen test result; the puncture can proceed on the radial artery. If color does not return, the Allen test result is negative and the radial artery should not be punctured (**C**). A blood sample is drawn from the radial artery after a positive Allen test result (**D**).

Cytologic Specimens

Sputum specimens are obtained for cytologic examination to determine the presence of lung carcinoma or infectious conditions. Because sputum contains cells from the tracheobronchial tree, malignant cells may be detected in the specimen. A special container with fixative solution may be used for this type of specimen collection. Consult the agency laboratory manual for directions.

FIBEROPTIC BRONCHOSCOPY

A bronchoscopic examination is performed by inserting a flexible fiberoptic scope through the nose or mouth into the bronchial tree after local anesthesia of the patient's throat. The scope allows for direct visualization of the bronchial tree structures for assessment, diagnosis, or removal of foreign bodies or mucus plugs. Lesions suggestive of malignancy may be located and a biopsy performed as well. Before the pro-

cedure, signed consent should be obtained. Have the patient remove dentures. Give sedatives as ordered. Afterward, monitor the patient's respiratory status and level of consciousness. The patient should take nothing by mouth until the gag reflex returns. Complications of bronchoscopy include bronchospasm, bacteremia, bronchial perforation, pneumonia, laryngospasm, hemorrhage, and pneumothorax.

Additional details about diagnostic tests and procedures are presented in the Diagnostic Tests and Procedures table on pp. 517 and 518.

COMMON THERAPEUTIC MEASURES

THORACENTESIS

A thoracentesis is the insertion of a large-bore needle through the chest wall into the pleural space. The procedure is usually performed at the bedside by the physician. Thoracentesis is done to remove pleural fluid, blood, or air or to instill medication. Pleural fluid may be removed to reduce respiratory distress caused by fluid accumulation in the pleural space. In addition, fluid obtained in the procedure may be studied to obtain blood cell counts or to measure protein, glucose, lactic dehydrogenase, fibrinogen, or amylase levels. The study of pleural fluids may aid in the diagnosis of infectious diseases and cancer.

The patient sits on the side of the bed and leans the upper torso over the bedside table with the head resting on folded arms or pillows (Fig. 30-8). If the patient is unable to sit up, a side-lying position with the head of the bed elevated 30 degrees may be used. The skin is cleansed thoroughly and a local anesthetic injected. The physician inserts a 20-gauge or larger needle between the ribs and through the parietal membrane. Fluid or air is then aspirated, the thoracentesis needle is removed, and a sterile dressing is applied to the puncture site. The patient is positioned on the unaffected side. A chest radiograph may be ordered after the procedure to detect any pulmonary complications caused by accidental injury to the lung. Complications of thoracentesis include air embolism, hemothorax, pneumothorax, and pulmonary edema. Immediately report uneven chest movements, respiratory distress, or hemorrhage to the supervisor and the physician. Details of nursing responsibilities are included in Box 30-1.

BREATHING EXERCISES

Deep-Breathing and Coughing Exercises

Deep-breathing and coughing exercises are performed to aid in lung expansion and expectoration of respiratory secretions. They are indicated when patients are immobilized or after general anesthesia. Instructions to the patient include the following:

1. Sit in a semi-Fowler's position for maximal lung expansion.
2. Place one hand on the abdomen to feel it rise and fall with breathing.
3. Inhale deeply through the nose, pause 1 to 3 seconds, and exhale slowly through the mouth.
4. After 4 to 6 deep breaths, cough deeply from the lungs to aid in the expectoration of sputum.
5. After thoracic or abdominal surgery, splint the incision with a pillow to minimize discomfort and support the incision.

Pursed-Lip Breathing

Another type of breathing exercise is pursed-lip breathing. It is used to inhibit airway collapse and to decrease dyspnea in patients with chronic lung disease. Instruct patients to pucker the lips as if to whistle, blow out a candle, or blow through a straw. They should then inhale through the nose and slowly exhale through pursed lips. Exhalation should last twice as long as inhalation.

FIGURE 30-8 A, The patient is positioned for a thoracentesis. **B,** The needle is inserted into the pleural space, avoiding lung tissue and the diaphragm. The exact location of the puncture varies.

Sustained Maximal Inspiration

Sustained maximal inspiration is used to ensure deep inspiration for maximal expansion and aeration of the lungs. An incentive spirometer is an instrument that frequently is used to encourage maximal inspiration. Spirometers basically consist of a cylinder that contains balls or disks and a tube through which the patient inhales. As the patient inhales through the tube,

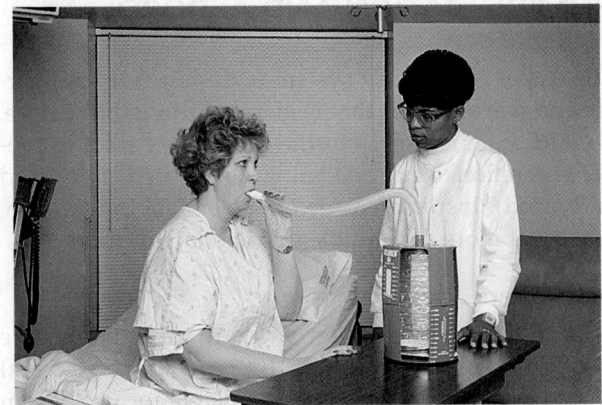

FIGURE **30-9** Incentive spirometry encourages deep breathing by providing a visual cue to the patient about the efficiency of deep breathing.

Chest percussion (with cupped hand)

Chest vibration

FIGURE **30-10** Chest physiotherapy. **A,** Percussion. **B,** Vibration.

the balls or disks rise (Fig. 30-9). Instruct the patient to inhale deeply to move the balls or disks in the cylinder upward. For maximum effect, the spirometer is kept upright because tilting the device reduces respiratory effort. Some spirometers provide a digital readout of the volume of air displaced. If the patient's maximal inspiration can be measured before surgery, that reading can be used as a target after surgery.

CHEST PHYSIOTHERAPY

Chest physiotherapy consists of percussion, vibration, and postural drainage. These mechanical techniques are used to facilitate the mobilization and expectoration of secretions in patients with large mucus-producing or chronic mucus-retaining respiratory disorders such as chronic bronchitis and cystic fibrosis. Although this therapy is usually performed in the acute care setting by a respiratory therapist, the nurse often does this in long-term and home care settings. Therefore you should be familiar with the procedures and be able to evaluate the patient's response. In an outpatient setting, you also may monitor the caregiver's technique in administering the treatment. Chest physiotherapy should be performed before meals to reduce the risk of regurgitation and aspiration of stomach contents.

Chest Percussion and Vibration

Chest percussion and vibration are performed to facilitate the movement of respiratory secretions so sputum can be expectorated. Percussion is clapping of the cupped palms against the chest wall to dislodge and mobilize respiratory secretions (Fig. 30-10, *A*). The procedure is performed with the hands cupped to create a pocket of air when striking the patient's chest—first with one hand and then with the other. Percussion is confined to areas protected by the rib cage and is never done over the sternum, kidney, liver, spleen, stomach, or spine. In general, percussion is done for 20 to 30 seconds, followed by vibration.

Vibration is performed by the therapist placing one hand on the top of the other, keeping the arms

straight, and pressing the hands flat against the patient's chest (see Fig. 30-10, *B*). As the patient exhales, the therapist creates a shaking (vibrating) movement with the palms. The therapist pauses during inhalation. The vibration is repeated over three or four breathing cycles.

Contraindications to percussion and vibration include lung cancer, bronchospasm, pain in the area being treated, hemorrhage, hemoptysis, increased intracranial pressure, chest trauma, pulmonary embolism, pulmonary edema, gastric reflux, pneumonectomy with open pericardium, extreme agitation or anxiety, and high risk for rib fractures.

Postural Drainage

Postural drainage is the technique of positioning the patient to facilitate gravitational movement of respiratory secretions toward the bronchi and trachea for expectoration. Various positions are used to drain all 18 segments of the lungs. If a patient cannot tolerate a specific position, it should be omitted or modified. Instruct the patient to breathe slowly and deeply throughout the procedure. Drain the upper lobes first and the posterior basal segments of the lower lobes last. The patient should not sit up between position changes. Provide tissues and a disposal receptacle. Maintain each position for 5 to 15 minutes. Perform postural drainage before meals or tube feedings. It may be ordered after respiratory treatments with bronchodilators. The frequency is ordered by the physician. Discontinue the procedure and inform the physician if the patient experiences a heart rate over 120 beats per minute, dysrhythmias, hypertension, hypotension, dizziness, or signs of hypoxemia.

SUCTIONING

Suctioning may be required if excessive secretions accumulate in the oral or nasal airway and the patient cannot expectorate. The goal of suctioning is to improve oxygen and carbon dioxide exchange in the lungs by removing excessive mucus secretions with a suction catheter. Consult a procedure manual for details, but key points when suctioning a patient include the following:

1. Use strict aseptic technique (sterile for tracheal, clean for oral).
2. Administer oxygen before inserting the suction catheter because the procedure temporarily interferes with the patient's airflow.
3. Moisten the catheter in sterile water, and insert the catheter through the nose or mouth before applying suction.
4. Apply suction as the catheter is withdrawn from the airway.
5. Maintain the pressure gauge between 80 and 100 mm Hg.
6. Limit each suction pass to 10 seconds.
7. Allow the patient to rest briefly, encourage deep breathing, and rinse the catheter with sterile solution between suction attempts.
8. Monitor the patient's response to suctioning.
9. If tachycardia or increased respiratory distress develops, stop the procedure and give the patient oxygen as ordered.
10. Document the amount, color, odor, and consistency of the patient's secretions as well as the patient's status before and after the procedure.

HUMIDIFICATION AND AEROSOL THERAPY

The upper respiratory system is designed to moisturize and warm the air that is inspired through the nose. Humidity is necessary in the respiratory tract to prevent secretions from becoming inspissated (thickened and dried). Inspissated secretions irritate the mucosa, making it more susceptible to bacterial infection.

Humidifiers

A humidifier creates water vapor to raise the relative humidity of inspired gas to 100%. There are several types of humidifying devices available for use. Room humidifiers deliver water vapor directly into the air. Medical oxygen is humidified as it bubbles through a container of water. Humidifiers that require heat to create water vapor pose a risk of heat injury. The fluid reservoir can become contaminated, making it a source of airborne infection. To prevent the spread of bacteria, sterile water should be used to fill the reservoir and the equipment must be cleaned between each use. Last, the equipment can present an electrical hazard.

Aerosol Therapy

Aerosol therapy is used to liquefy and mobilize respiratory secretions and to deliver medications. Aerosols are suspended liquid particles of bronchodilators or inactive fluids such as water or saline that are delivered by devices called *nebulizers*. Nebulizers deliver a humidified aerosol through large tubing, which may be connected to an oxygen mask or a handheld device. When handheld nebulizers are used, the patient should sit upright and slowly inhale the nebulizer aerosol deeply, hold the breath briefly, and exhale slowly. Once secretions are mobilized, the patient may require deep-breathing and coughing techniques, postural drainage, suctioning, or a combination of these to clear the secretions. Because aerosols can cause bronchospasm, bronchodilators may be ordered before administering some types of aerosol therapy. There is also a risk of fluid retention, infection, and drug toxicity.

OXYGEN THERAPY

Air in the atmosphere contains approximately 21% oxygen. Usually this is sufficient for oxygenation to maintain the tissue's ability to function appropriately. In the presence of cardiopulmonary disease or injury, it may be necessary to provide a patient with supplemental oxygen, that is, to enrich the atmospheric air with higher concentrations than the patient normally

---

Put on Your Thinking Cap!

Why is actual suctioning time limited to 10 seconds for each pass of the catheter?

Pharmacology Capsule

Oxygen should be thought of as a pharmacologic agent with risks of adverse effects.

breathes. Oxygen should be treated as a pharmacologic agent in that there may be serious side effects as well as benefits from its use.

Oxygen therapy requires a medical order that should be carried out like any drug order. If a patient is observed becoming lethargic or bradypneic (abnormally slow breathing), immediately notify a supervisor or physician because these are symptoms of adverse effects of oxygen therapy.

To administer oxygen to the patient, it is necessary to alter the gas from a compressed form such as a bulk oxygen supply or cylinder to a form with a usable, safe flow rate. Modern hospitals have bulk oxygen systems with wall adapters to which flowmeters can be attached. When patients with oxygen must be transported, a cylinder on wheels is necessary. A regulator with a flowmeter must be used. After a flowmeter has been attached to the oxygen source, it may be necessary to humidify the gas before delivering it to the patient. Humidification is usually unnecessary when using a low-flow cannula at a flow setting of 2 or fewer liters per minute or when using an air entrainment (Venturi) oxygen delivery system.

A tube is needed to connect the flowmeter to the specific oxygen delivery device being used. In some of the devices, the tube is incorporated as an integral component, but in others it is not. It is possible to use extension tubes for some devices, but increasing the length of the tube increases the resistance to gas flow, thus causing pressure to back up in the system, so the patient may not receive the desired oxygen flow.

Oxygen therapy is ordered in liters per minute, or FiO_2. FiO_2 means fraction of inspired oxygen. It is written, for example, as 0.30, which means 30% oxygen concentration. Various devices can deliver different amounts of oxygen (Fig. 30-11).

A

Nasal prongs

From oxygen source

B

Metal piece conforms to shape of nose

Exhalation ports

Strap

From oxygen source

C

Exhalation ports

Strap

Inflated reservoir bag

From oxygen source

FIGURE **30-11** Oxygen delivery systems. **A,** Nasal cannula. **B,** Standard oxygen mask. **C,** Partial rebreathing oxygen mask.

Continued

Exhalation ports

Strap

Air entrainment port

Entrained room air

100% Oxygen

Flexible tube

Inhaled mixture of 100% oxygen and room air

Removable adapter

Vocal cords

Tract

Esophagus

Transtracheal catheter

Trachea

Connection to oxygen source

E

FIGURE **30-11** Cont'd **D,** Venturi oxygen mask. **E,** Transtracheal oxygen delivery.

The most commonly used device is the nasal cannula, which fits around the face and directly into the nares by way of two prongs. It is designed to deliver a low flow of oxygen from 1 to 6 L/min with an approximate FiO_2 of 0.24 to 0.40 (24% to 40% oxygen). The nasal catheter is also a low-flow device that is inserted into one naris and then into the pharyngeal space approximately at the uvula. The FiO_2 and flow rates are the same as those for the cannula. This catheter is rarely used, except during short-term procedures.

Four types of masks are available: the simple oxygen mask, the partial rebreathing mask, the nonrebreathing mask, and the air entrainment (Venturi) mask. The simple oxygen mask is designed to deliver an FiO_2 ranging from 0.35 to 0.55 (35% to 55% oxygen). Flow rates from the flowmeter may be adjusted from 6 to 10 L/min. The minimum flow rate of 6 L/min is necessary to prevent any chance of carbon dioxide buildup from occurring. The partial rebreathing mask includes a reservoir bag to elevate the potential FiO_2. It is unique because the patient actually rebreathes part of the exhaled gas in the system. However, it is designed so that the rebreathed gas contains almost no carbon dioxide from the patient's lungs—only enriched oxygen. The expected FiO_2 range is 0.35 to 0.60 (35% to 60%). The flowmeter setting must be from 6 to 10 L/min. The nonrebreathing mask is so named because none of the patient's exhaled gas is rebreathed. Like the previous mask, it also includes a reservoir bag to enhance the FiO_2, but it has a series of valves to direct the flow of oxygen in such a way that the patient receives a fresh supply of gas with each breath. The expected FiO_2 should be near 1.0 (100%). However, research has shown experimentally that the highest FiO_2 is approximately 0.7 (70%). The air entrainment mask is designed to provide a specific FiO_2. This device has been called a *Venti mask* or a *Venturi mask* in the past and still may be referred to by these names. The manufacturers of these devices list a specific flowmeter setting for the desired FiO_2. It is also necessary either to adjust a setting on the device or to place a specific attachment on the mask to obtain the desired results. Read the literature accompanying the mask, and if there is confusion, consult a respiratory therapist.

Transtracheal oxygen therapy delivers oxygen through a small, flexible catheter that is inserted into the trachea through a small incision or with a special needle. This approach is sometimes used when long-term therapy is indicated.

There may be times when an oxygen mask must be removed, as for oral care or for eating or drinking. Ask the physician to write an order for the temporary use of a cannula during these times.

Advances in outpatient oxygen therapy have the potential to improve greatly the quality of life for patients with chronic pulmonary conditions. Whereas patients used to have to rent large cylinders for home use, they can now rent oxygen concentrators that process room air and deliver air with an increased percentage of oxygen. The concentrator is about the size of a canister vacuum cleaner and has a 50-foot tubing connected to a nasal cannula. This allows the patient considerable freedom of mobility in the home setting.

To leave the home, patients can use small tanks of compressed oxygen. The tanks weigh approximately 3 pounds and can deliver 2 L/min for approximately 3 hours. A device that can be used with the canister delivers oxygen only "on demand," when the patient inhales. This conserves the oxygen, making the canister last longer. Portable liquid oxygen canisters that can deliver a very high flow of oxygen are also available. These canisters can be refilled from a larger tank that can be kept in the patient's home. A weekend version of the tank fits in the back seat of a car and lasts several days. These devices allow considerable freedom for the patient.

The nurse must recognize the complications of oxygen therapy, including hypoventilation, toxicity, atel-

ectasis, and ocular damage. Patients at greatest risk for oxygen-induced hypoventilation are those with chronic respiratory disorders. They may have become insensitive to high carbon dioxide levels in the blood, so that low oxygen levels in the blood serve as the stimulus for respirations ("hypoxic drive"). Oxygen administration raises the level of oxygen in the blood, and the patient who has hypoxic drive may hypoventilate or even have apnea. Oxygen toxicity can result from exposure to a high concentration of oxygen for a prolonged period of time. Toxicity progresses from tracheobronchitis to lung fibrosis and atelectasis and may be fatal. Atelectasis can result from the replacement of nitrogen normally in the alveoli with oxygen. Oxygen is readily absorbed, predisposing the alveoli to collapse. Exposure to 100% oxygen can cause retinal injury and visual impairment.

Key points when a patient is receiving oxygen therapy are the following:

1. Monitor the liter flow to be sure it is as prescribed.
2. Assess the patient's response to oxygen therapy; monitor reports of blood gas analyses.
3. Inspect the tubing for kinks, obstructions, loose connections; listen for a hissing sound in the oxygen mask; feel for adequate oxygen flow.
4. Maintain sterile water in the humidifier reservoir.
5. Clean and replace oxygen therapy equipment according to agency policy.
6. Post a "No Smoking" sign and advise the patient and visitors that smoking is not allowed because oxygen supports combustion.

INTERMITTENT POSITIVE-PRESSURE BREATHING TREATMENTS

Intermittent positive-pressure breathing (IPPB) treatments are used to achieve maximal lung expansion. The IPPB equipment delivers humidified gas with positive pressure, which forces air into the lungs with inhalation and allows passive exhalation. This facilitates maximal exchange of oxygen and carbon dioxide gases in the alveoli and promotes a productive cough. Aerosol medications, including mucolytics (agents that liquefy secretions) and bronchodilators, can be administered through IPPB treatments with a nebulizer device. Although most IPPB treatments are administered by respiratory therapists, they are done by nurses in some settings.

In the past, IPPB was used for a wide range of conditions. The American Association for Respiratory Care now recommends it only for specific conditions, including atelectasis, decreased lung compliance with kyphoscoliosis, and cardiogenic pulmonary edema. In addition to its limited usefulness, IPPB is losing favor because it may cause a tension pneumothorax in patients with chronic obstructive pulmonary disease. It also may cause respiratory alkalosis because of hyperventilation. The desired effects of IPPB usually can be achieved by other, less expensive measures such as incentive spirometry and handheld nebulizers.

ARTIFICIAL AIRWAYS

Artificial airways are sometimes required to maintain a patent airway. Artificial airways include the oral airway, nasal airway, endotracheal tube, and tracheostomy tube.

Oral Airway

The oral airway is a curved tube used to maintain an airway temporarily. The oropharyngeal airway is inserted by tilting the head back, opening the mouth, and inserting the airway into the patient's mouth with the tip pointed toward the roof of the mouth. The tube is turned over while being advanced so that the end of the tube rests on the base of the patient's tongue.

Nasal Airway

A nasopharyngeal airway is a soft rubber tube that is inserted through the nose and extended to the base of the tongue. After ruling out a deviated septum, the nasal airway is coated with a water-soluble lubricant and inserted upward into the nose so that the distal end is located in the pharynx at the level of the base of the tongue. A nasal airway should be changed from one naris to the other every 8 hours.

Endotracheal Tube

An endotracheal tube is a long tube inserted through the mouth or nose into the trachea. These tubes have cuffs—inflatable balloons that seal the trachea to prevent aspiration of foreign material and to facilitate mechanical ventilation. Insertion of an endotracheal tube and care of the patient who is intubated require specialized training.

Tracheostomy

A tracheostomy is a surgically created opening through the neck into the trachea. There are a variety of tracheostomy tubes, and they may be used with or without cuffs. Care of the patient with a tracheostomy is covered in Chapter 53.

MECHANICAL VENTILATION

Mechanical ventilation is the process of providing respiratory support by means of a mechanical device called a *ventilator*. Ventilators are required most commonly for patients with acute respiratory failure who are unable to maintain adequate gas exchange in the lungs. This may be evidenced by tachypnea or bradypnea with an elevated or a stable arterial carbon dioxide tension ($Paco_2$), a low arterial oxygen tension (PaO_2), or a low pH. To ventilate a patient mechanically, a cuffed endotracheal or tracheostomy tube must be used to deliver the air. Once the tube is in place, the cuff must be inflated to create a closed system in the patient's airway.

Otherwise, air being forced into the lungs could simply flow back out through the trachea.

A volume-limited ventilator is used most commonly for patients with acute respiratory failure. It inflates the lungs with a preset volume of oxygenated air that is delivered under pressure during the inspiratory cycle. The expiratory cycle may be conducted passively or with pressure as indicated.

There are three types of positive-pressure ventilators: volume cycled, pressure cycled, and time cycled. A volume-cycled ventilator, which delivers a constant preset amount of oxygenated air to the patient, is the most commonly used type. A pressure-cycled ventilator, which pushes air into the lungs until a preset pressure is reached, is not widely used for continuous mechanical ventilation. Time-cycled ventilators deliver oxygenated air over a preset length of time. This type is used most frequently in infants and children.

Depending on the patient's needs, ventilators may be programmed to control or assist the rate of ventilation. The most frequently used modes are intermittent mandatory ventilation and synchronized intermittent mandatory ventilation. These modes provide assistance with ventilation by allowing the patient to breathe spontaneously between a preset number of ventilator breaths. Ventilators deliver oxygen ranging in concentration from 21% oxygen (atmospheric air) to 100% oxygen. The oxygen concentration, or FiO_2, is adjusted for individual patient needs.

Tidal volume is the preset amount of oxygenated air delivered during each ventilator breath. This is usually 10 to 15 mL/kg of the patient's body weight.

The respiratory rate setting is the total number of breaths delivered per minute. The rate may be governed by the ventilator alone or by the ventilator and the patient's spontaneous respirations.

Positive end-expiratory pressure may be prescribed to keep the pressure in the lungs above the atmospheric pressure at the end of expiration. This reduces collapse of small airways and alveoli, thereby increasing the functional residual capacity and improving ventilation.

Other mechanical ventilation modalities include options such as pressure support, flow-by, continuous positive airway pressure, and high-frequency ventilation. These are mentioned only for completeness and not for discussion. If you encounter any of these modalities, specific training is needed that is beyond the scope of this text.

Like much other health care technology, mechanical ventilation can now be managed in the home. With proper training, these devices can be managed by a family member. A device that is used by people with sleep apnea is a continuous positive airway pressure (CPAP) unit. CPAP maintains positive pressure in the airway during sleep, thereby avoiding periods of apnea. CPAP units are small and have a nose mask that is worn during sleep.

Nursing care of patients on mechanical ventilation requires special training, but key aspects of care include the following:

1. Monitor settings to ensure they are set as prescribed.
2. Be sure high and low pressure alarm settings are turned on.
3. Have a manual resuscitator and oxygen source readily available.
4. Do not allow water to accumulate in the tubing.
5. Monitor the patient's vital signs and breath sounds; suction as necessary.
6. Establish an alternate method of communication because the patient cannot speak while intubated.

CHEST TUBES

Chest tubes are inserted to drain air or fluid from the pleural space of the lungs. This permits reexpansion of a collapsed lung in the patient with a hemothorax, pneumothorax, or pleural effusion. Chest tubes are inserted by the physician under sterile conditions in the operating room or at the bedside. Multiple tubes may be inserted. A small incision is made to insert one chest tube in the second to fourth intercostal space to remove air. A tube placed in the eighth or ninth intercostal space is for fluid removal. The tubes are sutured in place, and an airtight sterile dressing is applied. The distal ends of the plastic chest tubes are connected to sterile rubber tubing that leads to a pleural drainage device composed of three compartments: the collection chamber, the water-seal chamber, and the suction chamber (Fig. 30-12). Chest fluid and air drain into the collection chamber. Air is diverted to the water-seal chamber, where it can be seen bubbling up through the water. Suction pressure is controlled in the suction control chamber. The tubing in the suction chamber is partially submerged in water; the depth of the tube in the water regulates the amount of suction. After the tubes have been inserted, a chest radiograph is obtained to confirm placement.

Monitor the patient's vital signs, breath sounds, and oxygen status frequently. Assess the dressing to be sure a tight seal is maintained. Tape tubing connections, and inspect the connections frequently to detect air leaks. Coil extra tubing on the bed to avoid kinks, and keep the drainage system on the floor. Monitor the drainage for blood clots or lung tissue, which may have to be gently kneaded downward to keep the tube patent. Agency and physician preferences dictate whether chest tubes are stripped or milked (Fig. 30-13). Observe the chambers for bubbling. When the system is initially connected to the patient, bubbles are usually seen in the water-seal chamber. After a short time, bubbling in this chamber will stop until the lung has reexpanded or the tubing is occluded. If suction is prescribed, you will also see bubbling in the suction control chamber.

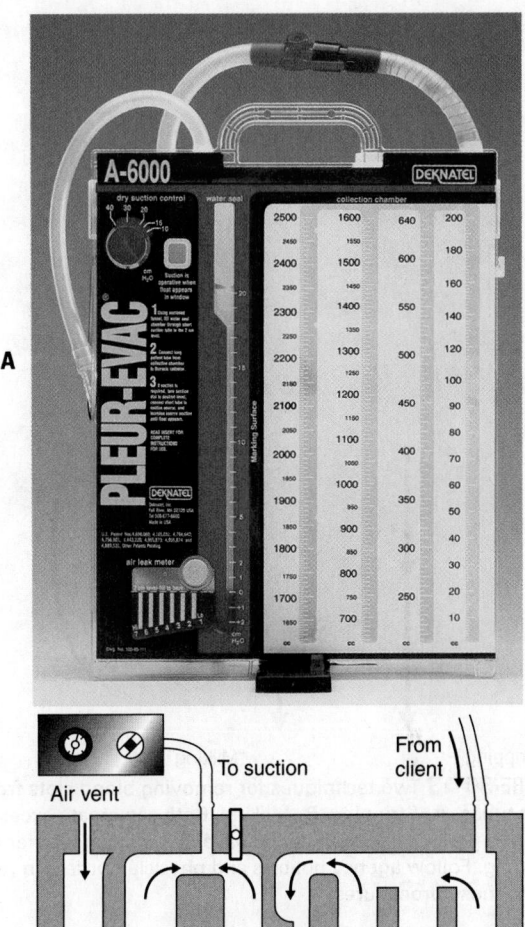

FIGURE 30-12 **A,** A commonly used disposable chest drainage system. **B,** Diagram of chambers of water-seal chest drainage.

The rate of drainage is monitored by marking the drainage level on the drainage receptacle. The middle water-seal chamber is observed for the expected rise in the fluid level with inspiration and the fall with expiration. This is called *tidaling*. Continuous bubbling in the water-seal chamber suggests an air leak. If an air leak is suspected, agency policy may permit the tubing to be clamped for a maximum of 10 seconds while locating the leak. The suction control chamber may be wet or dry. Wet chambers are regulated by maintaining the water level that is ordered by the physician. Gentle bubbling is expected in the wet suction chamber. Dry chambers are regulated by adjusting the dry suction until the float appears. The drainage receptacle is not usually changed unless the drainage chamber is full. Use sterile technique to change the receptacle. Know

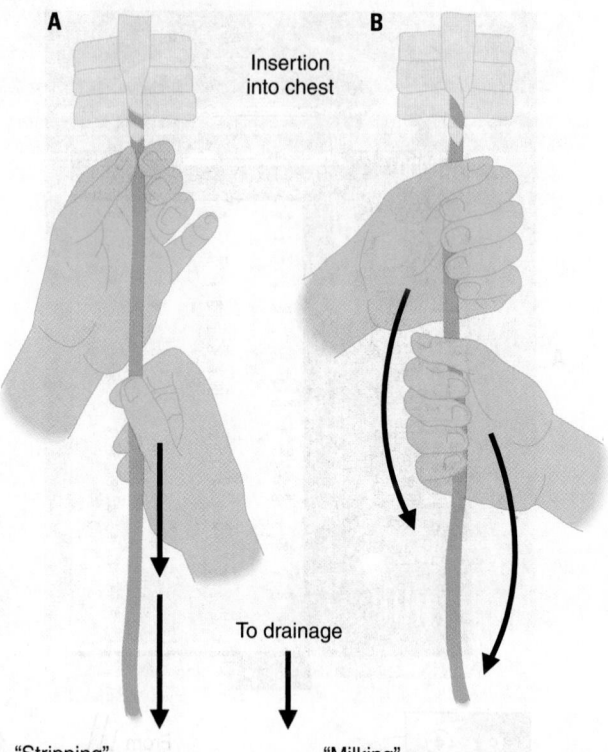

"Stripping"   "Milking"

FIGURE **30-13** Two techniques for removing blood clots from chest tubes. **A,** Stripping. **B,** Milking. Both can create excessive negative pressure in the pleural space, but milking is safer than stripping. Follow agency policies and physician orders in relation to these procedures.

the agency policies and procedures for managing chest tubes.

An alternative to the large chest drainage systems is the Heimlich flutter valve. The valve is a disposable unit that is attached to the chest tube and to a sterile drainage receptacle. Air and fluid can flow into the receptacle but cannot flow backward into the chest. The patient who has a flutter valve can assume any position and can ambulate easily. A system with a flutter valve can be attached to chest suction if necessary.

THORACIC SURGERY

A thoracotomy is the surgical opening of the chest wall. Surgical procedures on the lung include pneumonectomy, lobectomy, segmental resection, and wedge resection. *Pneumonectomy* is the removal of an entire lung, whereas a *lobectomy* is removal of one lobe of a lung. The extensive dissection and removal of a section of the lung is called a *segmental resection*. A *wedge resection* is the removal of a small, triangular section of lung tissue. Other procedures that require a thoracotomy are *decortication* and *thoracoplasty*. Decortication is stripping of the membrane that covers the visceral pleura, and thoracoplasty is the removal of ribs. Among the most common purposes for thoracic surgery are evaluation of chest trauma, removal of tumors and cysts, and treatment of empyema.

PREOPERATIVE NURSING CARE *of the Patient with a Thoracotomy*

Preoperative nursing care is described in Chapter 17. Before thoracotomy, emphasize postoperative breathing exercises. If the insertion of a chest tube is anticipated, explain the procedure to the patient.

POSTOPERATIVE NURSING CARE *of the Patient with a Thoracotomy*

Assessment

After surgery, monitor vital signs, lung sounds, mental status, dressings, and chest tube function and drainage.

Nursing Diagnoses, Goals, and Outcome Criteria: Thoracotomy

General postoperative nursing diagnoses are presented in Chapter 17. Diagnoses and goals specific to the patient who has had a thoracotomy may also include the following:

NURSING DIAGNOSES	GOALS AND OUTCOME CRITERIA
Impaired Gas Exchange related to ventilation-perfusion mismatch	Improved gas exchange: vital signs consistent with patient's norms, arterial blood gases within normal limits
Ineffective Breathing Pattern related to preexisting respiratory disease or pain	Effective breathing pattern: regular respirations without cyanosis or dyspnea
Ineffective Airway Clearance related to dry secretions or ineffective cough	Effective airway clearance: breath sounds clear to auscultation

Interventions

Impaired Gas Exchange

After a thoracotomy, the patient is at risk for pneumonia and atelectasis because of the effects of anesthesia (which impairs ciliary motion), drugs that dry secretions, and immobility. To improve gas exchange, position the patient with the head of the bed elevated 20 to 40 degrees. In the immediate postoperative period, the patient is usually placed on the unaffected side. Thereafter, various positions are permitted depending on the specific surgical procedure. Avoid the operative side after wedge resection or segmentectomy to encourage expansion of remaining lung tissue on the affected side. After pneumonectomy, also avoid the complete side-lying position on the affected side because this may encourage mediastinal shift. Administer oxygen as ordered.

Ineffective Breathing Pattern

Splint the thoracic incision while assisting the patient to breathe deeply and cough. An incentive spirometer may be used to encourage full expansion of the lungs. Adequate pain control enables the patient to breathe more effectively. Chest physiotherapy and bronchodilators are indicated for some patients. When permitted, assist the patient to sit on the edge of the bed with the feet flat on the floor. An overbed table can be placed in front of the patient, who can lean on it with folded arms. This position fosters movement of the diaphragm and chest expansion.

Ineffective Airway Clearance

Good hydration thins secretions; therefore encourage fluids. If the patient cannot tolerate adequate oral fluids, intravenous fluids may be ordered. For management of chronic respiratory conditions, see Chapter 31.

VIDEO THORACOSCOPY

Many procedures that formerly required thoracic surgery now can be done with video thoracoscopy. Thoracoscopy is performed by inserting an endoscope through a small thoracic incision. Procedures that can be done with this instrument include resection of pulmonary and mediastinal lesions, biopsy, drainage of effusions, sympathectomy, vagotomy, and thymectomy. Potential complications of thoracoscopy include atelectasis, pneumonia, air leaks, and injury to thoracic organs. A chest tube is usually needed to promote full reexpansion of the lung on the operative side. Otherwise, patient care is much less complicated than it is after thoracotomy. Monitor the patient's respiratory status, including lung sounds. Immediately report sudden dyspnea or other signs of respiratory distress to the surgeon. Document the amount and appearance of chest tube drainage. Inspect the closed drainage system for proper functioning. Incentive spirometry may be used to encourage lung expansion. Give analgesics as ordered, although pain is usually not as severe as it is after thoracotomy. Patients are usually permitted out of bed 4 to 6 hours after surgery and can return to work in 1 week. Before discharge, instruct the patient to notify the physician of dyspnea or a temperature higher than 38.3° C (101° F).

DRUG THERAPY

Drugs used to treat respiratory disorders include decongestants, antitussives, antihistamines, expectorants, antimicrobials, bronchodilators, corticosteroids, mast cell stabilizers, leukotriene inhibitors, mucolytics, and thrombolytics, as described in the Drug Therapy table on pp. 532 and 533.

Decongestants

Decongestants are adrenergic agents. They mimic the action of epinephrine and norepinephrine, causing constriction of nasal blood vessels and reducing the swelling of mucous membranes. Over-the-counter decongestants such as Sudafed are commonly used to treat the common cold. With oral decongestants, constriction of the blood vessels is not limited to the nasal passages, so that systemic vasoconstriction and elevated blood pressure may result. Systemic effects are less severe with topical drops and sprays. Nevertheless, people with hypertension, heart disease, diabetes mellitus, and hyperthyroidism are usually advised to avoid decongestant drugs except under medical supervision.

Pharmacology Capsule

People with hypertension, heart disease, and hyperthyroidism should not take over-the-counter cold remedies without consulting a pharmacist or a physician. Many cold remedies stimulate the heart and raise the blood pressure.

Antitussives

Antitussives suppress the cough reflex. Antitussive action is not always desirable because coughing removes secretions from the airways. However, when a cough is nonproductive, creates pain, interferes with sleep, or impairs wound healing, temporary cough suppression may be indicated. Codeine is an effective antitussive, but it is an opioid with many side effects and abuse potential. Therefore dextromethorphan, which is not an opioid, is more commonly used.

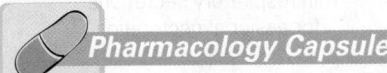

Pharmacology Capsule

Use antitussives cautiously. Cough is a protective mechanism that clears the airway.

Antihistamines

Antihistamines are also called *histamine-1 blockers* because they block the effects of histamine—one of the chemicals that causes allergic symptoms. Antihistamines include a variety of prescription and over-the-counter medications that are frequently used because of their action in drying nasal secretions. First-generation antihistamines such as diphenhydramine (Benadryl) provide short-term relief. However, they also can cause dizziness, dry mouth, constipation, blurred vision, urinary retention, tachycardia, drowsiness, and impaired judgment. Second-generation antihistamines such as loratadine (Claritin) are less likely to cause drowsiness. Antihistamines may worsen a cough by drying up bronchial secretions. These drugs are not usually recommended for people with asthma because dry secretions contribute to difficulty clearing the airway.

Expectorants

Expectorants thin respiratory secretions so they are more readily mobilized and cleared from the airways. Their value is in question, but they are commonly prescribed.

| DRUG THERAPY | Drugs Used to Treat Respiratory Disorders |

DRUG	USE/ACTION	SIDE EFFECTS	NURSING INTERVENTIONS
DECONGESTANTS			
Pseudoephedrine (Sudafed)	Vasoconstriction. Reduce swelling of mucous membranes. Used to treat nasal discharge, common cold.	Occasional mild CNS stimulation, especially in older adults. Toxicity: lightheadedness, tachycardia, palpitations, nausea, vomiting, hallucinations, seizures.	Monitor pulse and blood pressure, mental and emotional state. Contraindicated with severe hypertension, coronary artery disease, lactation. Tell patient to swallow extended-release tablets whole.
ANTITUSSIVES			
Codeine Hydrocodone bitartrate (Hycodan) Dextromethorphan	Suppression of cough reflex. Appropriate uses: control nonproductive cough or cough that interferes with rest or wound healing.	Codeine is an opioid; has abuse potential. Can cause sedation. Dextromethorphan does not have these effects.	Encourage fluids unless contraindicated to facilitate expectoration of secretions. Safety measures with codeine.
ANTIHISTAMINES			
Diphenhydramine (Benadryl)	Block allergic response. Dry respiratory secretions. Also antiemetic and sedative effects.	Drowsiness, dry mouth, blurred vision, photophobia, thickening of mucus secretions, decreased sweating, constipation, urinary retention, increased heart rate.	Safety precautions if drowsy. Monitor respiratory status. Not recommended for patients with asthma. Encourage fluids if not contraindicated. Monitor elimination. Oral hygiene.
EXPECTORANTS			
Guaifenesin (Robitussin)	Thin respiratory secretions for easier expectoration.	Nausea and vomiting with large doses.	Assess cough productivity. Do not crush sustained-release capsules.
ANTIMICROBIALS	Kill or inhibit the growth of bacteria, viruses, or fungi.	Side and adverse effects specific to each antimicrobial classification. Common side effects are nausea, vomiting, and diarrhea. Risk of superinfections such as yeast infections of mouth, genitourinary tract. Risk of severe allergic response.	Assess allergies before administration. Be alert for allergic response: rash, dyspnea, loss of consciousness. Withhold drug if allergy suspected. Instruct patient to complete entire course of therapy. Monitor for improvement and for superinfections. Report continued symptoms.
BRONCHODILATORS	Relax smooth muscle in the bronchial tree to relieve bronchial constriction.		
1. Methylxanthines Theophylline Aminophylline	Methylxanthines also cause increased heart rate and force of cardiac contraction, central nervous system stimulation, and increased gastric acid secretion.	Anxiety, restlessness, tachypnea, tachycardia, dysrhythmias, GI distress. Rapid intravenous administration can cause hypotension, fatal dysrhythmias.	Monitor vital signs, mental state, serum drug levels. Measure intake and output. Give with milk or food to decrease GI distress. Do not administer before bedtime (may keep awake).
2. Adrenergics (sympathomimetics) Epinephrine Isoproterenol hydrochloride (Isuprel) Ephedrine	Adrenergics also decrease mucus secretion, increase mucociliary clearance, and stabilize mast cells.	Restlessness, anxiety, tachycardia, headache, hypertension, disorientation, nausea, vomiting, diarrhea.	Do not exceed prescribed dosage. Teach patient to use inhaler. Rinse mouth after inhalation to decrease dryness and irritation. Avoid excessive caffeine. Monitor respiratory and cardiovascular status.

CNS, Central nervous system; *GI,* gastrointestinal system; *IV,* intravenous.

DRUG THERAPY | *Drugs Used to Treat Respiratory Disorders—cont'd*

DRUG	USE/ACTION	SIDE EFFECTS	NURSING INTERVENTIONS
BRONCHODILATORS— con'td Selective beta₂ agonists: Albuterol sulfate (Proventil) Terbutaline sulfate (Brethine) Isoetharine hydrochloride (Bronkosol)		Less cardiac stimulation with beta₂ agonists than with nonselective adrenergics.	
3. Inhaled muscarinics Ipratropium bromide (Atrovent)	Inhaled muscarinics act directly on the respiratory passages to cause bronchodilation. Not effective for acute asthma attacks.	Increased intraocular pressure with narrow-angle glaucoma. Rare: hypotension.	Monitor respiratory status. Evaluate for improvement. Tell patient not to use more than two inhalations at a time. Rinse mouth after inhaling to reduce dry mouth and throat. Avoid excessive caffeine intake.
CORTICOSTERIODS Systemic (prednisone) Inhalation, oral: beclomethasone (Vanceril, Beclovent) Inhalation, nasal: beclomethasone (Beconase)	Stabilize mast cells to reduce release of mediators that cause inflammation and edema. Restore bronchodilator response to sympathomimetics in treating acute bronchial constriction. Routes: oral, parenteral, inhalation.	Systemic therapy: water and sodium retention, potassium loss, abnormal fat distribution, hypertension, gastrointestinal distress. Masks signs of infection. Abrupt withdrawal can trigger adrenal insufficiency. Inhaled steroids: hoarseness, oral yeast infections, systemic effects possible with long-term use.	Monitor vital signs, weight, and electrolytes. Assess for subtle signs of infection. Rinse mouth after inhalation.
MAST CELL STABILIZER Cromolyn sodium (Intal) Nedocromil (Tilade)	Reduce the production of chemicals by the mast cells that cause bronchial constriction, edema, inflammation. Help reduce frequency/severity of asthma attacks. Do not *stop* asthma attack. Routes: inhalation, nasal.	Wheezing, sneezing, coughing. Occasional bronchoconstriction. Rare: allergies, headache, nausea, urinary frequency.	Instruct patient in self-medication. Advise that excessive use can actually cause bronchoconstriction. Rinsing mouth after use of inhaler reduces dry mouth effects. Monitor effects.
LEUKOTRIENE INHIBITORS Zafirlukast (Accolate) Zileuton (Zyflo)	Inhibit synthesis or receptors of substances that mediate allergic responses. Prevent acute asthma attacks.	Zafirlukast: headache, nausea, diarrhea, infection. Zileuton: elevated liver enzymes, pain, nausea, headache.	Zafirlukast: take on empty stomach. Zileuton: can take with or without food. Monitor liver function.
Montelukast (Singulair)		Montelukast well tolerated; does *not* seem to cause liver damage.	Montelukast: phenytoin can lower blood levels.
THROMBOLYTICS Streptokinase (Streptase) Urokinase (Abbokinase) Alteplase (Activase)	Dissolve clots; used to treat pulmonary emboli. An IV bolus dose is given, followed by an infusion.	Streptokinase: cerebral hemorrhage, hypotension, allergic reaction, bleeding. Alteplase: bleeding, dysrhythmias, rash, itching.	Assess for bleeding. Monitor fibrinogen levels, blood pressure, pulse. Watch for allergic reactions.

Antimicrobials

Antimicrobials kill or inhibit the growth of bacteria, viruses, or fungi. Antibacterials are used to treat only bacterial infections because they are not effective against viruses or fungi. A limited number of antiviral and antifungal drugs are available. Specific antimicrobials are best selected after culture and sensitivity tests are performed on a specimen of respiratory secretions. Antimicrobials can cause allergic responses and have many side effects. Instruct the patient in self-medication and stress the importance of completing the prescribed course of therapy to prevent reinfection and the development of resistant strains of pathogens.

Bronchodilators

Bronchodilators relax smooth muscle in the bronchial airways and blood vessels. They are used to treat airway obstruction from respiratory disorders such as asthma and chronic obstructive pulmonary disease. The primary drawback to many bronchodilators is their tendency to cause cardiac and central nervous system stimulation. Some bronchodilators act primarily to prevent bronchial constriction, whereas others relieve it.

Corticosteroids

Corticosteroids are anti-inflammatory drugs that may be administered parenterally, orally, and by inhalation. The drugs may be inhaled orally or nasally. They are important drugs in the treatment of asthma because they reduce inflammation and edema in the respiratory tract. These drugs are less commonly used to treat chronic obstructive pulmonary disease. Among the many systemic effects of steroids are fluid and electrolyte imbalances, hyperglycemia, hypertension, osteoporosis, reduced resistance to infection, and muscle wasting. Oral and parenteral steroids have more side effects than inhaled forms of the drug. Therefore parenteral use is generally confined to short-term, acute situations and oral use is usually limited to 2 weeks. Advise patients not to discontinue steroid therapy abruptly because that may lead to acute adrenal insufficiency.

Pharmacology Capsule

Inhaled corticosteroids can have systemic effects if used over a long period of time.

Mast Cell Stabilizers

Cromolyn sodium (Intal) and nedocromil (Tilade) reduce the production of chemicals by the mast cells that cause bronchoconstriction, edema, and inflammation. These drugs, *called mast cell stabilizers,* are used to pre-

vent acute asthma attacks. They are not useful in stopping an attack after it starts.

Leukotriene Inhibitors

Leukotrienes are substances that mediate allergic responses, including bronchospasm. Drugs that inhibit leukotrienes are useful in the treatment of asthma because they inhibit the allergic response, thereby helping prevent, but not interrupt, acute asthmatic attacks. Examples are zafirlukast (Accolate), zileuton (Zyflo), and montelukast sodium (Singulair).

Mucolytics

Mucolytics reduce the viscosity (thickness) and elasticity of mucus. Acetylcysteine (Mucomyst) is used as an inhalant to thin the secretions in conditions such as acute and chronic bronchitis, asthma, and acute respiratory distress syndrome. It is important for the patient on mucolytics to be adequately hydrated.

Thrombolytics

Thrombolytics such as streptokinase (Streptase), urokinase (Abbokinase), and alteplase or tissue plasminogen activator (Activase) may be used to dissolve blood clots in the lungs (pulmonary emboli).

DISORDERS OF THE RESPIRATORY SYSTEM

ACUTE VIRAL RHINITIS (THE COMMON COLD)
Etiology and Risk Factors

Acute viral rhinitis, also called *coryza* or the *common cold,* is the most prevalent infectious disease. It is caused by viruses that invade the upper respiratory tract through airborne droplets. The droplets are spread by an infected person through breathing, sneezing, or coughing or by direct hand contact. Touching contaminated surfaces and then carrying the virus to the nasal membranes and eyes is the most important means of spreading a cold. Therefore careful attention to hand washing is one of the best preventive measures for avoiding a common cold.

Signs and Symptoms

Colds occur most frequently during the winter months when people tend to stay indoors and can more easily contaminate one another. A cold lasts 2 to 14 days, and people are most contagious during the first 3 days. Symptoms include a feeling of nasal dryness and stuffiness, sneezing, runny nose, headache, sore throat, lethargy, and fatigue. In severe cases, chills, fever, and marked prostration may be present.

Complications

Although most people with colds recover without incident, viral or bacterial pneumonitis develops in some patients.

Medical Diagnosis

The common cold is diagnosed on the basis of the patient history and physical examination.

Medical Treatment

The most common treatment for a cold is a combination of rest, fluids, proper diet, antipyretics, and analgesics. Antibiotics and currently available antiviral agents are usually not indicated because they are not effective against cold viruses (see the Health Promotion Considerations box below). Studies have been inconclusive about the value of using large doses of vitamin C for treating and preventing a cold. Other drugs that may be used to relieve the symptoms of the common cold by drying secretions are antihistamines and decongestants. Although many people believe that the herb *Echinacea* can prevent or reduce the duration of colds, research to date has not supported its value. Thorough hand washing can help prevent colds (see the Health Promotion Considerations box below).

NURSING CARE *of the Patient with Acute Viral Rhinitis*

Assessment

The complete assessment of the patient with a respiratory disorder is summarized in Box 30-1. The health history may be limited in focus and include a complete description of symptoms, past medical history, and drug history. The physical examination focuses on the nose, throat, ears, neck, and chest.

Nursing Diagnosis, Goal, and Outcome Criteria: Common Cold

The primary diagnosis for the patient with a common cold is Ineffective Therapeutic Regimen Manage-

ment related to lack of understanding of treatment, prevention, and signs and symptoms of complications. The goal of nursing care is effective patient management of the cold with full recovery and no complications. If the patient is at risk for secondary infection, the goal is absence of signs of worsening infection.

Criteria for assessing the effective patient management of the plan of care are the patient's verbalization of content presented and statement of intent to follow plan of care. Absence of infection is evidenced by normal vital signs, clear breath sounds, and clear sputum.

Interventions

The common cold is unlikely to require inpatient care unless a patient is immunocompromised. Therefore the primary nursing intervention is usually patient teaching. Advise the patient to rest and to maintain a daily fluid intake of 2 to 3 L, if not contraindicated. Good hydration is essential for keeping secretions thin for easier expectoration. A room humidifier may provide some comfort by keeping mucous membranes moist. Fever can be treated with antipyretics. If the physician has prescribed or recommended drugs, inform the patient of the proper use, dosages, and side effects. Many drugs used to treat symptoms of the common cold cause drowsiness, so advise the patient to avoid activities requiring mental alertness.

Pharmacology Capsule

Explain to patients that antibacterials are not usually prescribed for the common cold, because the common cold is caused by a virus and antibacterials are effective only against bacteria.

Infection control measures are needed to prevent spread of the cold and to protect the patient who has a cold from secondary bacterial infections. During the first 3 days, the patient is most contagious. The patient should avoid contact with others, especially those who are at increased risk for infection (young children, older adults, people who are immunosuppressed), to prevent the spread of the cold.

ACUTE BRONCHITIS
Etiology and Risk Factors

Acute bronchitis is a common condition that may follow a viral infection such as a cold or influenza. Bronchitis is usually viral in origin, but bacterial causes (*Streptococcus pneumoniae* or *Haemophilus influenzae*) also are common. Irritation and inflammation may

Health Promotion Considerations

Meeting *Healthy People 2010* Objectives for Reducing Antibiotic Use

Immunizations and Infectious Diseases *Healthy People 2010* objective: To reduce the number of courses of antibiotics prescribed for the sole diagnosis of the common cold:
- Teach patients the difference between bacterial and viral infections.
- Teach patients that the common cold from a viral cause does not require antimicrobial therapy.
- Reinforce health promotion considerations such as frequent hand washing using soap and warm water for at least 20 seconds. Instruct to cover mouth and nose when coughing or sneezing.
- Teach patients the importance of adequate nutrition to reduce their susceptibility to infectious organisms.

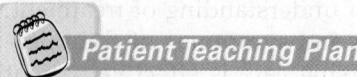

Common Cold

To reduce the risk of spreading the cold or of acquiring secondary bacterial infection:

- Avoid close contact with other people who have bacterial infections.
- Avoid crowded places.
- Avoid sharing drinking glasses or eating utensils.
- Practice good hand washing with antibacterial soap.
- Cover the mouth when coughing or sneezing.
- Use disposable tissues for expectorated secretions; dispose of them promptly.
- If you develop purulent (greenish) sputum; chest pain; a temperature higher than 37.8° C (100° F); a red, sore throat; or lung congestion, contact the physician, because these signs and symptoms suggest a more severe respiratory condition that may require additional treatment.

occur throughout the upper respiratory tract, resulting in an increased production of mucus. Excess production of mucus leads to coughing and sputum production.

Signs and Symptoms

Symptoms of acute bronchitis include fever, cough, yellow or green sputum, rapid breathing, and occasionally chest pain.

Medical Diagnosis

Acute bronchitis is usually diagnosed on the basis of the health history and the physical findings.

Medical Treatment

Treatment consists of a broad-spectrum antibiotic (e.g., ampicillin, tetracycline, erythromycin) for 7 to 10 days; hospitalization is usually unnecessary.

NURSING CARE *of the Patient with Acute Bronchitis*

Nursing care with acute bronchitis is similar to that for the common cold. In addition, encourage patients who are taking antibiotics to take the full course of the medication.

INFLUENZA

The term *flu* is commonly used to describe a number of ailments involving various body systems. However, influenza is actually an acute viral respiratory infection that is accompanied by a fever. There are several strains of the influenza virus (A, B, C). A strain is further subtyped according to the place and year it was isolated. Influenza usually occurs in epidemics during the winter months. Those most susceptible to the influenza virus are very young children, older adults, people living in institutional situations, people with chronic diseases, and health care personnel.

Complications

The most common complications of influenza are bronchitis and viral or bacterial pneumonia. Other, less common complications are myocarditis, pericarditis, Reye's syndrome, confusion, seizures, Guillain-Barré syndrome, toxic shock syndrome, myositis, and renal failure.

Signs and Symptoms

Influenza is similar to the common cold in the way that it is spread, that is, through droplet infection; however, its symptoms differ from those of the common cold. People with colds experience nasal symptoms and malaise and usually are afebrile (without fever), whereas those with influenza typically have chills, fever, sore throat, muscular pain, headache, and dry, hacking cough.

Medical Diagnosis

A diagnosis of influenza is usually based on the patient's history and physical findings. Laboratory tests for confirming infections caused by the influenza virus are improving dramatically and can provide results in less than 48 hours. However, viral tests in general are expensive and may not be available in all facilities.

Medical Treatment

Treatment of influenza is similar to the treatment of the common cold: rest, fluids, proper diet, antipyretics, and analgesics. First-generation antiviral agents such as amantadine hydrochloride (Symmetrel) or rimantadine (Flumadine) can be used to treat type A influenza. Second-generation antivirals such as oseltamivir (Tamiflu) and zanamivir (Relenza) treat influenza types A and B. With either generation, therapy must be started within 24 to 48 hours after the onset of symptoms and continued for 10 days.

The best treatment is prevention through immunization, especially for older adults, people with chronic illnesses, health care personnel, and people living in crowded environments. The Department of Health and Human Services Centers for Disease Control and Prevention National Immunization Guidelines recommends an annual influenza vaccine. Two types of vaccine are available—an inactivated vaccine and a live vaccine. The live vaccine, known as FluMist™ is given intranasally. This vaccine is used only for healthy children, adolescents, and adults, ages 5 to 49 years. The inactivated influenza vaccine is recommended for all others, including health care workers. The immunizations are usually given in the fall of the year. The protection rate for influenza vaccines is approximately 70% in the general population but may be lower among older adults. Although the incidence of adverse reactions to influenza immunizations is small, some people report sore arm, headache, fever, muscle aches, nausea, and diarrhea. Reported intranasal vaccine reactions include runny nose, nasal congestion, or cough. Acetaminophen 325 mg taken every 4 hours for the first 12 hours may reduce these symptoms. Other measures to reduce the risk of influenza are good nutrition and hygiene. An antiviral agent also may be prescribed for people who are at increased risk of acquiring viral infections.

Consider the Alternative

Echinacea is an herb taken orally to stimulate immune function, suppress inflammation, and treat viral infections such as the common cold and influenza. There is little evidence that it prevents colds, but it may decrease the duration and severity of a cold.

Pharmacology Capsule

Antiviral drugs must be administered soon after the onset of influenza symptoms to be effective.

NURSING CARE *of the Patient with Influenza*

Nursing care of the patient with influenza is similar to care of the patient with the common cold. Ongoing monitoring is particularly important with influenza because of the risk of serious complications, especially in older adults. In addition, encourage immunization against influenza for people at high risk: those with serious chronic cardiopulmonary disorders, residents of long-term care facilities, health care providers who have contact with high-risk patients, people older than 65 years, and those who have chronic metabolic disorders such as diabetes mellitus.

PNEUMONIA

Etiology and Risk Factors

The term *pneumonia* describes inflammation of certain parts of the lung such as the alveoli and bronchioles. Pneumonia may be caused by either infectious or noninfectious agents. Examples of infectious agents are bacteria, fungi, and nonspecific viruses. Noninfectious agents may include irritating fumes, dust, or chemicals that are inhaled or foreign matter that is aspirated. Nosocomial pneumonia is a health care–associated infection that may be attributed to inadequate hand washing, poor sterile technique with suctioning, contaminated equipment, and exposure to others who have infectious respiratory conditions.

People who are most likely to contract pneumonia are smokers; those with altered consciousness from alcohol, seizures, anesthesia, or drug overdose; those who are immunosuppressed; chronically ill people who are malnourished or debilitated; and people on bed rest with prolonged immobility.

Patients at increased risk for aspiration pneumonia are those with impaired swallowing or cough reflexes, decreased gastrointestinal motility, esophageal abnormalities, tube feedings, tracheostomies, and endotracheal tubes.

Pathophysiology

Pneumonia may be classified according to the causative organism—usually bacteria or viruses. Gram-positive bacteria cause pneumococcal, staphylococcal, and streptococcal pneumonias, and gram-negative bacteria cause pseudomonal and influenza pneumonias and legionnaires' disease. Pneumococcal pneumonia *(S. pneumoniae)* is the most common cause of bacterial pneumonia. Viral pneumonias are caused by several different viruses, including the influenza virus.

The pathophysiology of pneumonia follows a predictable course. When pathogens invade the lungs, the inflammatory process causes fluid to accumulate in the affected alveoli. In a process called *hepatization,* capillaries dilate and neutrophils, red blood cells, and fibrin fill the alveoli, causing the lung to appear red and granular. Next, blood flow decreases and leukocytes (white blood cells) and fibrin infiltrate the area and consolidate (solidify). As the infection resolves, the consolidated material dissolves and is ingested and removed by macrophages.

Complications

Although most people recover from pneumonia, it remains among one of the leading causes of death, especially in older adults (Minino et al., 2005). Relatively common pulmonary complications of pneumonia include pleurisy, pleural effusion, and atelectasis. Pleurisy is inflammation of the pleura that causes pain with breathing. Pleural effusion is the accumulation of fluid between the pleura that encases the lungs and the pleura that lines the thoracic cavity. A large amount of fluid can lead to collapse of the lung. Atelectasis refers to collapsed alveoli. Other, less common pulmonary complications of pneumonia are lung abscesses, delayed resolution, and empyema. Empyema is the presence of purulent exudate in the pleural cavity. Potential systemic complications include pericarditis, arthritis, meningitis, and endocarditis.

Signs and Symptoms

Usual symptoms of pneumonia are fever, chills, sweats, chest pain, cough, sputum production, hemoptysis (coughing up blood), dyspnea (difficulty breathing), headache, and fatigue. Older adults, however, may present with confusion, anorexia, and weakness but no fever or cough. People with bacterial pneumonia may experience an abrupt, almost explosive onset: severe, shaking chills; sharp, stabbing lateral chest pain, especially with coughing and breathing; and intermittent cough with rusty sputum. Viral pneumonia is characterized by burning or searing chest pain in the sternal area; a continuous, hacking, barking cough producing small amounts of sputum; and headache.

Medical Diagnosis

Diagnosis of pneumonia is based on the findings of the history and physical examination, sputum culture and Gram stain, chest radiograph, complete blood count, and blood culture.

Medical Treatment

Treatment usually consists of increased fluid intake (at least 3 L every 24 hours), limited activity or bed rest, antipyretics, analgesics, and, in some cases, oxygen and aerosol intermittent positive-pressure breathing therapy. Bacterial pneumonias are treated with appropriate antibacterials; however, antibacterials are not used with viral pneumonias because they do not kill viruses.

Vaccination with the pneumococcal conjugate vaccine is recommended for all children under 24 months of age; children ages 24 to 59 months who have sickle cell disease, HIV infection, chronic disease, or immunosuppression; and children ages 24 to 59 months who are African American, Alaskan native, or American Indian.

Vaccination with an unconjugated pneumococcal vaccine (e.g., Pneumovax 23) may be recommended for adults with chronic illnesses, particularly cardiovascular and respiratory diseases and diabetes mellitus; people recovering from a severe illness; people age 65 years and older; and older adults living in nursing homes or other long-term care facilities. Vaccination with the unconjugated vaccine is not recommended for children younger than 2 years. A booster may be given to selected patients after 6 years.

NURSING CARE *of the Patient with Pneumonia*

Assessment

Assessment of the patient with a respiratory disorder is summarized in Box 30-1 (see also Nursing Care Plan: The Patient with Pneumonia on p. 539).

Nursing Diagnoses, Goals, and Outcome Criteria: Pneumonia

Nursing Diagnoses	Goals and Outcome Criteria
Ineffective Airway Clearance related to increased sputum production, thick secretions, ineffective cough	Effective airway clearance: clear breath sounds without wheezes or crackles
Impaired Gas Exchange related to obstruction of airways by edema and secretions or atelectasis	Adequate oxygenation: normal arterial blood gases, heart rate, and respiratory rate
Activity Intolerance related to obstruction of airways by edema and secretions or atelectasis	Improved activity tolerance: performance of daily activities without fatigue or dyspnea
Imbalanced Nutrition: Less Than Body Requirements related to anorexia, dyspnea, fatigue	Optimal nutritional status: stable body weight
Risk for Deficient Fluid Volume related to inadequate fluid intake, fever, mouth breathing	Normal hydration: fluid intake approximately equal to fluid output, moist mucous membranes, blood pressure consistent with patient norms
Acute Pain related to inflammation, cough, muscle aches	Pain relief: patient statement of pain relief, relaxed appearance

Interventions

Ineffective Airway Clearance

Accumulated secretions in the respiratory tract impair gas exchange and may result in alveolar collapse. Therapeutic measures are taken to decrease the production and promote the expectoration of secretions. Administer antimicrobials, decongestants, and expectorants as ordered. A good cough is essential for removal of secretions, but antitussives may be given as ordered if the patient becomes exhausted because of constant coughing. Encourage or assist the patient to change positions at least every 2 hours to help mobilize secretions. Other measures used to mobilize secretions are deep-breathing and coughing exercises, chest physiotherapy, and aerosol therapy. The patient who has a very weak cough may require suctioning. Provide tissues and a receptacle for disposal of secretions. Note the amount, color, and consistency of secretions. Auscultate lung sounds frequently to assess the effects of interventions to clear the airways.

Impaired Gas Exchange

The edema and secretions present with pneumonia interfere with the exchange of gases in the lungs. The patient may have hypoxemia, meaning that the level of oxygen in the blood is low. At the same time, excess carbon dioxide may accumulate in the blood, a condition called hypercapnia. Because normal oxygenation is essential for all body tissues, efforts must be made to improve the patient's gas exchange.

To assess gas exchange, monitor vital signs, lung sounds, and skin color. Be alert for signs of hypoxemia: restlessness, tachycardia, and tachypnea. If arterial blood gases are being measured, report abnormal results to the physician. Hemoglobin may also be measured. A low hemoglobin is significant because it indicates the reduced oxygen-carrying capacity of red blood cells.

Measures that mobilize secretions, discussed earlier, are important in improving gas exchange. In addition, elevate the head of the bed. Some patients are more comfortable in a reclining chair that permits alterations in position. A semi-Fowler's position decreases the pressure of the abdominal organs on the diaphragm

NURSING CARE PLAN

The Patient with Pneumonia

ASSESSMENT

Health History: A 77-year-old retired schoolteacher comes to the clinic complaining of chills and fever, cough, sore throat, and chest pain. The physician diagnosed viral pneumonia and recommended hospitalization. She states she had a cold for about a week and seemed to get progressively worse. She states she has "a little" shortness of breath and tires very easily. Her chest pain is aggravated by coughing. She has been taking over-the-counter cold remedies. She has a history of hypertension and congestive heart failure for which she takes an ACE inhibitor and a diuretic. She lives alone in a one-story apartment. She has a close friend next door who visits frequently.

Physical Examination: Vital signs: temperature, 100.6° F orally; pulse, 92; respiration, 24; blood pressure, 160/94. Alert, slightly dyspneic. Skin color pale. Nail beds slightly dusky. Lung sounds clear to auscultation over right lung fields. Wheezes and crackles auscultated in left lung. Frequent cough producing greenish sputum. No retractions or use of accessory muscles of respiration. Abdomen soft.

Nursing Diagnosis	Goals and Outcome Criteria	Interventions
Ineffective Airway Clearance related to increased sputum production and thick secretions	The patient will have a patent airway, as evidenced by clear breath sounds without wheezes or crackles.	Administer decongestants and expectorants as ordered. Administer antitussives as ordered if cough interferes with rest. Suction only if necessary. Turn, deep breathe, and cough at least every 2 hours. Perform chest physiotherapy and provide aerosol therapy as ordered. Assess response. Monitor lung sounds, respiratory rate, and characteristics of secretions. Dispose of tissues in a sanitary manner.
Impaired Gas Exchange related to obstruction of airways by edema and secretions or atelectasis	The patient will have adequate oxygenation, as evidenced by normal arterial blood gases and vital signs.	Monitor vital signs, lung sounds, skin color, blood gas reports, and level of consciousness. Be alert for signs of hypoxemia: restlessness, tachycardia, tachypnea. Report abnormal findings to physician. Elevate head of bed. Administer oxygen therapy as ordered.
Activity Intolerance related to fatigue or hypoxia	The patient will perform activities of daily living as ordered without excessive fatigue or dyspnea.	Instruct in activity restrictions. Plan care to allow periods of uninterrupted rest. Assist with activities of daily living as needed. Gradually encourage increased activity while monitoring for dyspnea and fatigue. Keep interactions short, and limit visitors.
Imbalanced Nutrition: Less Than Body Requirements related to anorexia, dyspnea, or fatigue	The patient will maintain optimal nutritional status, as evidenced by stable body weight.	Monitor food intake and weight. If intake is poor, consult with dietitian about patient preferences. Suggest small, frequent meals. Provide pleasant environment for meals. Position for comfort. Use oxygen cannula during meals if permitted. Weigh daily.
Risk for Deficient Fluid Volume related to inadequate fluid intake, fever, or mouth breathing	The patient's hydration will remain normal, as evidenced by fluid intake equal to output, moist mucous membranes, and blood pressure consistent with patient's norms.	Monitor fluid status for signs of fluid volume deficit: decreased skin turgor, concentrated urine, decreased urine output, dry mucous membranes, elevated hemoglobin and hematocrit levels. Administer intravenous fluids as ordered. Encourage fluids by mouth up to 3 L/day as permitted. Record intake and output. Monitor temperature and treat fever as ordered. Keep dry and lightly covered. Administer tepid sponge baths as ordered for fever, but do not induce shivering. Use hypothermia blanket as ordered.
Acute Pain related to inflammation, cough, or muscle aches	The patient will report pain relief, as measured with a pain scale.	Use a pain scale to assess pain. Administer analgesics as ordered. Reposition for comfort. Splint painful areas during coughing and deep breathing. Use massage and relaxation techniques. Document effects of interventions.

? CRITICAL THINKING QUESTIONS

■ Identify the factors that make fluid balance a challenge for this patient.

■ What are the risks that occur when patients self-medicate?

so the patient breathes more easily. Maintain oxygen therapy as ordered.

Activity Intolerance

Activity is usually restricted for the patient with pneumonia and may range from complete bed rest to limited activities. Schedule nursing care to prevent overtiring and to allow for periods of uninterrupted rest. Provide assistance as needed until the patient is able to resume self-care. Keep conversations short, and encourage visitors not to tire the patient with long visits. When the patient begins to resume activities of daily living, evaluate the ability to tolerate daily activities.

Imbalanced Nutrition: Less Than Body Requirements

Good nutrition is essential to combat the infection and to promote healing (see the Nutrition Concepts box below). Assess the patient's usual dietary habits to provide baseline information so that the diet may be individualized. Monitor weight to determine the adequacy of nutrition. Weigh the patient before breakfast using the same scale each time. Monitor albumin and lymphocyte blood counts to detect low levels that are common with inadequate protein.

A typical diet for the patient with pneumonia is a high-protein, soft diet. Unfortunately, fatigue, dyspnea, and anorexia may interfere with adequate food intake. Provide the diet as ordered, assist the patient with the meal if needed, and document intake. To enhance the appetite, provide oral care before meals, elevate the head of the bed, and arrange the tray in an attractive and convenient manner. The diet should conform to the patient's preferences as much as possible. If oxygen is needed, a nasal cannula is recommended during meals. If the patient tires quickly, more frequent meals with smaller servings may be better received.

Risk for Deficient Fluid Volume

The patient with pneumonia may lose excess fluid because of fever and mouth breathing, and fluid intake may be inadequate because of fatigue and dyspnea. Dehydration causes respiratory secretions to be thicker and more difficult to mobilize. Signs and symptoms of deficient fluid volume include decreased skin turgor, concentrated urine, dry mucous membranes, and elevated hemoglobin and hematocrit levels. Therefore the patient should consume 3 L of fluid a day unless contraindicated. If the patient's oral intake is low, intravenous fluids may be ordered. Hard candy, if permitted, stimulates thirst and fluid intake. Intake and output records may be kept.

Monitor the patient's temperature every 2 to 4 hours to detect fever. Administer antipyretics as ordered. Keep the patient dry and lightly covered. Keep the room at a comfortable temperature that avoids chilling. Tepid sponge baths may be given for high fevers as ordered, but do not induce shivering. A hypothermia blanket may be needed to reduce body temperature.

Acute Pain

Treat pain with ordered analgesics. Also use positioning, splinting painful areas during deep breathing and coughing, and massage to promote comfort. Other measures to manage pain are detailed in Chapter 15. Document the effects of comfort measures, and notify the physician if pain is unrelieved or worsens.

Prevention of Aspiration Pneumonia

Aspiration pneumonia may be prevented by measures to avoid aspiration or to treat it promptly. If a patient is at risk for aspiration, keep suction equipment on hand. Position patients with dysphagia (difficulty swallowing) upright with the neck in a neutral position or slightly bent forward during meals. Because semisol-

Nutrition Concepts

1. Adequate fluids may help to mobilize pulmonary secretions for expectoration.
2. Approximately 40% of patients admitted to intensive care units with acute respiratory failure are malnourished.
3. Nutritional support for patients with respiratory failure should begin within the first 3 to 4 days of hospitalization.
4. Patients who receive nutritional support are more easily weaned from ventilators than those who receive only intravenous glucose support.
5. A diet for patients who have been in acute respiratory failure should be high in nutrients.
6. Lung disease can substantially increase energy needs.
7. The patient who is malnourished is at increased risk for respiratory infections because of impaired immunity and possible impairment of defense mechanisms.
8. When a patient has a fever, each degree Celsius of elevation increases the metabolic rate 10% to 13%. For each degree Fahrenheit, the metabolic rate rises 7.2%.
9. Excessive intake of vitamin K–rich foods (cabbage, broccoli, cauliflower, asparagus, onions, spinach, fish, liver) can interfere with anticoagulation therapy.

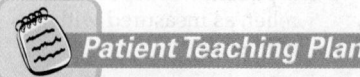

Patient Teaching Plan

Pneumonia

The teaching plan for the patient with pneumonia should include the following points:

- Gradually increase your activities as you recover because fatigue may persist for several weeks.
- Avoid people with colds or other infections.
- You need plenty of rest, good nutrition, and 3 L of fluids each day (unless contraindicated!).
- Complete any prescribed drugs after discharge.

ids are swallowed more easily than thin liquids, thickening agents may be added to liquids.

If a patient is receiving enteral feedings, elevate the head of the bed while the feeding is being delivered and for 30 minutes afterward. Check tube position per agency policy before each bolus feeding or at specified intervals. The aspirated fluid can be tested for acidity to ensure tube placement. Measure residual before each bolus feeding. If it is greater than 100 mL, withhold the feeding and notify the physician.

Stop continuous feedings for 20 to 30 minutes before lowering the patient's head. If a patient must be kept flat, the best position is on the right side. Check residual every 4 hours. If the residual is 20% more than the hourly rate, consult the physician about reducing the rate of feeding.

To reduce the risk of aspiration, position the unconscious patient on alternating sides with the head of the bed elevated unless contraindicated. Do not put fluids in the patient's mouth until the presence of a gag reflex has been established.

If aspiration is suspected, use suction to try to remove the foreign material. A side-lying or slight Trendelenburg position, if not contraindicated, may promote drainage from the airway. Stop the enteral feeding until it is ruled out as the source of the aspirated material. Monitor the patient closely and notify the physician. Administer oxygen as ordered.

PLEURISY (PLEURITIS)

Pleurisy is inflammation of the pleura. The most common causes are pneumonia, tuberculosis, injury to the chest wall, pulmonary infarction, and tumors. The most characteristic symptom of pleurisy is abrupt and severe pain. The pain almost always occurs on one side of the chest, and patients can usually point to the exact spot where the pain is occurring. Breathing and coughing aggravate the pain.

Treatment of pleurisy is aimed at the underlying disease and at pain relief. Analgesics, anti-inflammatory drugs, antitussives, antimicrobials, and local heat therapy may be ordered.

NURSING CARE *of the Patient with Pleurisy*

Assessment

Assessment of the patient with a respiratory disorder is summarized in Box 30-1.

Nursing Diagnoses, Goals, and Outcome Criteria: Pleurisy

The primary nursing diagnoses when a patient has pleurisy are listed here. There may be other diagnoses related to the underlying cause of pleurisy.

NURSING DIAGNOSES	GOALS AND OUTCOME CRITERIA
Acute Pain related to inflammation	Pain relief: patient statement of pain relief, relaxed expression
Ineffective Breathing Pattern related to splinting, pleural effusion	Effective breathing pattern: vital signs within patient norms, normal breath sounds

---

Interventions

Acute Pain

When the patient reports pain, obtain a complete description including location, severity, precipitating factors, and alleviating factors. Use analgesics and splinting of the affected side to relieve pain. It is helpful also to splint the rib cage when coughing. If ordered, apply heat to the painful area and give antitussives to decrease painful coughing. If bed rest is prescribed, assist the patient with regular position changes. Administer nonsteroidal anti-inflammatory drugs (NSAIDs) as ordered to reduce pain and inflammation. Monitor patients on NSAIDs for gastrointestinal distress and bleeding.

Ineffective Breathing Pattern

Monitor the patient's breathing pattern with attention to the symmetry of chest movement. Encourage the patient to turn, take deep breaths and cough, and ambulate if permitted to mobilize secretions and maximize ventilation. Elevate the head of the bed to improve lung expansion. If pleural effusion develops, the patient experiences progressive dyspnea, decreased or absent breath sounds in the affected area, and decreased chest wall movement on the affected side. A thoracentesis may be done to remove the accumulated fluid. If the procedure is done at the bedside, the nurse assists as described in the Common Therapeutic Measures section on pp. 521 and 522.

CHEST TRAUMA

Traumatic chest injuries fall into two major categories: (1) nonpenetrating injuries and (2) penetrating injuries. Nonpenetrating or blunt injuries most commonly result from automobile accidents, falls, or blast injuries. In automobile accidents, 40% of the people killed have sustained blunt injuries from the steering wheel. The extent of the injury depends on the force and impact of the trauma. Common nonpenetrating injuries include rib fractures, pneumothorax, pulmonary contusion, and cardiac contusion. Penetrating injuries most commonly

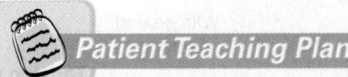

Patient Teaching Plan

Pleurisy

- Take deep breaths every 1 to 2 hours while awake.
- Sitting upright will make breathing more comfortable.
- If being discharged on NSAIDs:
  - Avoid aspirin because it increases the risk of bleeding.
  - Take NSAIDs with food, milk, or antacids if gastrointestinal distress occurs.

result from gunshot or stab wounds to the chest. Common penetrating injuries include pneumothorax and life-threatening tears of the aorta, vena cava, or other major vessels.

Chest trauma can result in changes in normal pressure relationships between air inside and outside the body, interference with normal breathing patterns and protective mechanisms such as cough, disturbances in blood flow to the lungs, swelling, and pain. Patients are therefore at risk for air entering the pleural space, infection and increased secretions in the tracheobronchial tree, hemorrhage, and abnormal fluid collection in the lung.

Signs and Symptoms

Signs and symptoms of chest injury may include obvious trauma to the chest wall (e.g., bruising); chest pain; dyspnea; cough; asymmetric movement of the chest wall; marked cyanosis of the mouth, face, nail beds, and mucous membranes; rapid, weak pulse; decreased blood pressure; deviation of the trachea; distended neck veins; and bloodshot or bulging eyes.

Medical Treatment

Immediate care of a person with a chest injury is directed at stabilization and prevention of further injury. Remove clothing to assess injury sites and to observe

Open pneumothorax

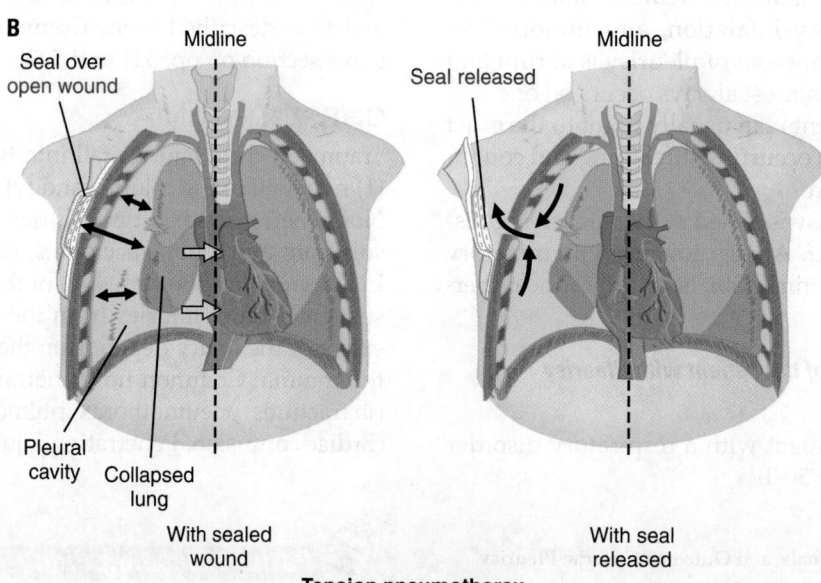

Tension pneumothorax

FIGURE 30-14 **A,** Open pneumothorax. *Solid and dashed arrows* = air movement; *open arrows* = structural movement. On inspiration, air is sucked into the pleural space through the open chest wound and the lung on the affected side collapses. The mediastinal contents shift toward the unaffected side. On expiration, air exits through the open wound and the mediastinal contents swing back toward the affected side (mediastinal flutter). **B,** An airtight dressing can cause a tension pneumothorax when air accumulates in the pleural space through a tear in the lung tissue. The air cannot exit if there is no open chest wound, and pressure builds, shifting the contents of the mediastinum toward the unaffected side and impairing circulatory and respiratory function (mediastinal shift).

for other injuries such as bleeding. Immediately treat bleeding. Cover any open chest wound with an airtight dressing taped on three sides. This is called a *vented dressing*; it permits air to escape through the chest wound but prevents additional air from entering the chest through the wound. If you were to completely seal an open chest wound, air could continue to leak from the lung into the pleural space. With no exit, the leaking air could accumulate in the pleural space and create a tension pneumothorax (discussed in the Pneumothorax section below).

If an airtight dressing has been applied, be alert for worsening respiratory status (increasing dyspnea, cyanosis, distended neck veins, trachea deviated from midline, decreased breath sounds on the affected side), which requires removal of the airtight dressing. Do not remove impaled objects but stabilize them with bulky dressings. Monitor vital signs and level of consciousness, keeping in mind the potential for shock. Oxygen may be administered by nasal cannula. To facilitate breathing, put the client in a semi-Fowler's position or on the injured side (see Fig. 30-14).

PNEUMOTHORAX

Chest injuries often cause pneumothorax, which is an accumulation of air in the pleural cavity that results in complete or partial collapse of a lung. Pneumothorax occurs in nearly half of the people who have chest injuries. Air enters the space between the chest wall and the lung either through a hole in the chest wall or through a tear in the bronchus, bronchioles, or alveoli (Fig. 30-14).

There are two types of pneumothorax: tension and open. With a tension pneumothorax, air repeatedly enters the pleural space with inspiration, causing the pressure to rise. Because air is not escaping from the wound, the accumulating pressure causes the affected lung to collapse. The heart, trachea, esophagus, and great blood vessels shift toward the unaffected side. This is called a *mediastinal shift*, a condition that interferes with blood return to the heart. This is a medical emergency because both the respiratory and circulatory systems are affected. If not corrected, cardiac output falls and the patient dies.

An open pneumothorax results from a chest wound that allows air to move in and out freely with inspiration and expiration. The lung on the affected side collapses. The heart, trachea, esophagus, and great blood vessels may shift back and forth toward the unaffected side with inspiration, then toward the affected side with expiration. This condition is called *mediastinal flutter*. Like mediastinal shift, it is potentially fatal.

Signs and Symptoms

Symptoms of pneumothorax are dyspnea, tachypnea, tachycardia, restlessness, pain, anxiety, decreased movement of the involved chest wall, asymmetric chest wall movement, diminished breath sounds on the injured side, and progressive cyanosis. In trauma cases, there may be a chest wound. If air can be heard or felt moving in and out of the wound, it is called a "sucking" chest wound.

Medical Treatment

The physician may insert an 18-gauge needle through the chest wall into the pleural space and aspirate accumulated air or fluid and then insert a chest tube. An alternative is to omit the needle aspiration and immediately insert the chest tube. If air is entering the pleural space from a tear in the lung or bronchus, surgery may be needed to repair the tear. A variety of materials are being studied for use in sealing persistent air leaks, including intrapleural tetracycline, autologous "blood patches," and fibrin glue.

NURSING CARE *of the Patient with Pneumothorax*

Assessment

The complete assessment of the patient with a respiratory disorder is outlined in Box 30-1. In addition, if the patient has a chest tube, monitor the insertion site as well as the amount and characteristics of any drainage from the tube. Care of patients with chest tubes is covered in the Chest Tubes section on p. 529.

Nursing Diagnoses, Goals, and Outcome Criteria: Pneumothorax

NURSING DIAGNOSES	GOALS AND OUTCOME CRITERIA
Ineffective Breathing Pattern related to decreased lung expansion	Effective breathing pattern: regular respirations, rate of 12 to 20/min, normal arterial blood gases, no dyspnea, normal skin color
Fear related to difficulty breathing	Decreased fear: calm demeanor, patient statement that fear is reduced
Decreased Cardiac Output related to mediastinal shift	Adequate cardiac output: pulse and blood pressure consistent with patient norms
Acute Pain related to trauma, altered pressure in chest cavity, chest tube	Pain relief: patient statement that pain is reduced/relieved, relaxed manner
Risk for Infection related to traumatic injury, chest tube insertion	Absence of infection: normal body temperature, normal white blood cell count

Interventions

Ineffective Breathing Pattern

Monitor the patient closely for increasing respiratory distress as indicated by tachycardia, dyspnea, cyanosis, restlessness, and anxiety. Inspect the trachea for deviation that may be caused by mediastinal shift. Check arterial blood gas results for hypoxemia (low blood oxygen) and hypercapnia (high blood carbon dioxide). Immediately report signs and symptoms of deteriorating respiratory status to the physician. After the chest tube has been inserted, protect the tube and monitor its function as described on p. 529.

Position the patient for comfort in a Fowler's or semi-Fowler's position. Avoid the side-lying position until the affected lung has reexpanded, because this position could foster mediastinal shift. Support and encourage the patient to do deep-breathing and coughing exercises at least every 2 hours while awake. Administer oxygen as ordered.

Fear

A pneumothorax is frightening. Patients feel like they are suffocating and may fear they are dying. Speak to the patient calmly and explain what is happening. Tell the patient that the chest tube will allow the lung to reexpand and relieve the dyspnea. Also, tell the patient how to prevent dislodging the tube. Give the patient the opportunity to ask questions and express fears.

Decreased Cardiac Output

Monitor the patient's pulse and blood pressure. If cardiac output decreases because of mediastinal shift, the blood pressure falls and the pulse rate increases. Immediately notify the physician of signs of this potentially life-threatening change.

Acute Pain

Be alert for signs of pain, and document the characteristics of the patient's pain. Administer analgesics as ordered, and document the effects. In addition to drug therapy, use positioning, massage, distraction, and other measures described in Chapter 15. Notify the physician if pain is not relieved.

Risk for Infection

Monitor the patient for signs and symptoms of infection: fever, increased pulse and respirations, foul drainage from the tube insertion site, and elevated white blood cell count. Various possible sites of infection must be considered: traumatic wounds, chest tube insertion site, intravenous infusion sites, indwelling catheter, and lungs. Use sterile technique for invasive procedures and dressing changes, and administer prescribed antimicrobials. Encourage increased activity when permitted. Monitor hydration status and promote fluid intake of 2 to 3 L/day unless contraindicated. Before discharge, instruct the patient to keep the chest tube insertion site clean and dry and to notify the physician of signs of infection: fever or increasing redness, swelling, or drainage from the insertion site.

HEMOTHORAX

Hemothorax is an accumulation of blood between the chest wall and the lung that is often associated with pneumothorax. Hemothorax results from lacerated or torn blood vessels or lung tissues, lung malignancy, or pulmonary embolus. It may also be a complication of anticoagulant therapy. When air or blood collects in the pleural space, pressure around the lung increases, causing partial or complete collapse. Hemothorax is essentially treated like a pneumothorax, and the nursing care is similar. Surgical intervention may be needed to control the source of bleeding. In addition, the patient is at risk for decreased cardiac output due to hemorrhage.

RIB FRACTURES

Rib fractures are the most common chest injuries. The most common cause is a blunt injury, especially the impact of the steering wheel against the chest in an automobile accident. Ribs 5 through 10 are most frequently fractured because they are least protected by chest muscles. It takes approximately 6 weeks for rib fractures to heal.

Signs and Symptoms

Signs and symptoms of fractured ribs include pain at the site of injury (especially on inspiration), occasional bruising or surface markings, swelling, visible bone fragments at the site of the injury, and shallow breathing or holding the chest protectively to minimize painful chest movements.

Medical Treatment

Treatment is aimed at relief of pain so that the patient can have good chest expansion for adequate breathing. Intercostal nerve blocks with local anesthesia are most frequently used. Analgesics along with mild sedatives also may be given for pain relief. Strapping the chest with tape or binders was once common but is now avoided because this procedure constricts the expansion of the chest and restricts deep breathing, leading to complications such as pneumonia or atelectasis.

NURSING CARE *of the Patient with Rib Fractures*
Assessment

The nursing assessment of the patient with a respiratory disorder is outlined in Box 30-1. After rib fractures, the nurse is especially alert for signs of increasing respiratory distress that may indicate a pneumothorax caused by a bone fragment.

Nursing Diagnosis, Goal, and Outcome Criteria: Rib Fractures

The primary nursing diagnosis for the patient who has fractured ribs is Ineffective Breathing Pattern related to pain that occurs with ventilation. The goal of nursing care when a patient has fractured ribs is for the patient to have an effective breathing pattern. Outcome criteria include vital signs within normal range, absence of dyspnea, and breath sounds clear to auscultation.

Interventions

Breathing exercises are necessary to prevent pulmonary complications after rib fractures. Instruct the patient in supporting the fractured ribs while deep breathing and coughing. The patient will perform these exercises better with adequate pain control. Assess the patient's pain every 2 hours, asking the patient to rank the pain from 0 (no pain) to 10 (worst pain imaginable). Encourage the patient to report pain, and offer reassurance that measures will be taken to provide relief. Because pain typically persists for 5 to 7 days, administer prescribed analgesics. After medications are given, provide a calm environment and encourage the patient to rest. Other nursing measures described in Chapter 15 (guided imagery, distraction, rhythmic breathing) may be used to manage pain as well. Evaluate the effects of pain management measures, and inform the physician if the patient's pain cannot be controlled.

FLAIL CHEST

The term *flail chest* refers to an injury in which two adjacent ribs on the same side of the chest are each broken into two or more segments. The affected section of the rib cage is, in a sense, detached from the rest of the rib cage. This permits it to move independently, so that the segment moves in with inspiration and moves out with expiration. The pattern of movement is exactly the opposite of the movement of an intact chest wall. Therefore it is called *paradoxical movement*. Ventilation is impaired, and the patient becomes hypoxemic. Also, contusion (bruising) of underlying lung tissue may cause fluid to accumulate in the alveoli. Fractured ribs may tear the pleura or the lung itself, resulting in a pneumothorax or a hemothorax. The loss of chest wall stability and collapse of a lung may permit the mediastinum to flutter, swinging back and forth with respirations. Progressive hypoxemia and hypercapnia may be fatal.

Signs and Symptoms

Signs and symptoms of flail chest include severe dyspnea, cyanosis, tachypnea, tachycardia, and paradoxical movement of the chest.

Medical Diagnosis

Diagnosis is based on the history, physical examination, and chest radiographs. Arterial blood gases may be measured to assess the adequacy of ventilation.

Medical Treatment

The treatment of flail chest varies depending on the severity of the condition. If the patient is able to maintain adequate oxygenation, treatment may consist of deep breathing and coughing, IPPB treatment, and pain management. The patient in respiratory distress usually requires intubation and mechanical ventilation. Radiographs and arterial blood gas tests are often repeated at intervals to monitor oxygenation and detect additional pulmonary complications such as pneumonia.

NURSING CARE *of the Patient with Flail Chest*
Assessment

The nursing assessment of the patient with a respiratory disorder is outlined in Box 30-1. When the patient has flail chest, defer the complete assessment until the patient's condition stabilizes. The initial assessment focuses on respiratory status, vital signs, other medical diagnoses, and a drug history.

Nursing Diagnoses, Goals, and Outcome Criteria: Flail Chest

NURSING DIAGNOSES	GOALS AND OUTCOME CRITERIA
Ineffective Breathing Pattern related to loss of rib cage integrity	Effective breathing pattern: normal pulse and respiratory rates, normal arterial blood gases, no dyspnea
Acute Pain related to fractures	Pain relief: patient statement of pain relief, relaxed manner
Anxiety related to lack of understanding of injury and treatment	Reduced anxiety: patient statement of reduced anxiety, calm manner

Interventions

Nursing interventions for patients with flail chest are similar to those for the patient with fractured ribs. Because flail chest is more serious and the patient may be acutely ill, anxiety may be very high. To reduce anxiety, respond promptly to the patient's needs, provide simple explanations, and acknowledge the patient's concerns. Anxiety may be especially high if mechanical ventilation is needed. The detailed care of patients who require mechanical ventilation is beyond the scope of this book. A general discussion of mechanical ventilation is included in the Common Therapeutic Measures section on pp. 528 and 529.

PULMONARY EMBOLUS

An *embolus* is a foreign substance that is carried through the bloodstream. Emboli are usually blood clots but may be fat, air, tumors, bone marrow, amniotic fluid, or clumps of bacteria.

Etiology and Risk Factors

Risk factors for development of emboli include surgery of the pelvis or lower legs, immobility, obesity, estrogen therapy, and clotting abnormalities. Most pulmonary emboli originate in the deep veins of the thigh or pelvis. A thrombus that develops in the veins can break away and become an embolus. The embolus flows with the blood until it reaches a vessel too narrow to pass through. The embolus lodges and obstructs blood flow so that perfusion to the area is diminished. When a portion of a pulmonary blood vessel is occluded by an embolus, the patient is said to have a *pulmonary embolism* (PE). The effects depend on the extent of the lung tissue that is deprived of blood. Small emboli usually do not cause dramatic symptoms but disrupt perfusion nevertheless. The alveoli in the affected area are ventilated, but without blood flow, gas exchange cannot occur. The result is a ventilation-perfusion mismatch that results in hypoxemia. If a large pulmonary vessel is obstructed, alveoli collapse, cardiac output falls, there is constriction of the bronchi and the pulmonary artery, and sudden death may ensue.

Signs and Symptoms

Classic signs and symptoms of PE include sudden chest pain that worsens with breathing, tachypnea, and dyspnea. A spontaneous onset of chest wall tenderness without a history of trauma should raise a red flag. The patient may be apprehensive and diaphoretic with a cough and hemoptysis. Crackles may be heard on auscultation of the lungs, and the patient may have fever and tachycardia.

Medical Diagnosis

A diagnosis of PE is suggested by the history and physical findings and is confirmed by arterial blood gas analysis, electrocardiogram, lung scan, and pulmonary angiogram.

Medical and Surgical Treatment

Anticoagulation therapy is the cornerstone of treatment for PE. Intravenous heparin is usually given to establish and maintain a partial thromboplastin time of 2.0 to 2.5 times the normal rate. Heparin prevents the development of new thrombi; it also prevents the extension of existing thrombi but does not dissolve them. The heparin is eventually discontinued, and the patient is maintained on an oral anticoagulant (warfarin sodium) for up to 6 months. Tissue plasminogen activator, a fibrinolytic, may be given intravenously to dissolve the clots.

Hypoxemia may be managed with oxygen therapy, endotracheal intubation, and mechanical ventilation.

Intravenous fluids and drugs to improve cardiac function are indicated to treat hypotension. Intravenous morphine sulfate is commonly used to relieve chest pain and apprehension.

A number of surgical interventions have been used for PE, including embolectomy, vena cava interruption, and venous thrombectomy. Embolectomy, surgical removal of the embolus from the obstructed pulmonary arteries, is a risky procedure and is reserved for patients who are not candidates for fibrinolytic therapy. Vena cava interruption is most often done by placing a filter in the inferior vena cava to strain clots before they reach the pulmonary circulation (Fig. 30-15). Venous thrombectomy, removal of thrombi from veins, is not often done.

NURSING CARE *of the Patient with a Pulmonary Embolus*

Assessment

Assessment of the patient with a respiratory disorder is outlined in Box 30-1. When a patient has a PE, the nurse must monitor cardiopulmonary function but also must assess risk factors that may have led to the embolism. Homans' sign may be assessed. However, the false-negative and false-positive effects are common. Therefore it is not especially useful to detect thrombophlebitis.

Nursing Diagnoses, Goals, and Outcome Criteria: Pulmonary Embolism	
NURSING DIAGNOSES	GOALS AND OUTCOME CRITERIA
Ineffective Tissue Perfusion related to interruption of blood flow to the alveoli	Normal tissue perfusion: vital signs consistent with patient norms, no dyspnea, normal arterial blood gases

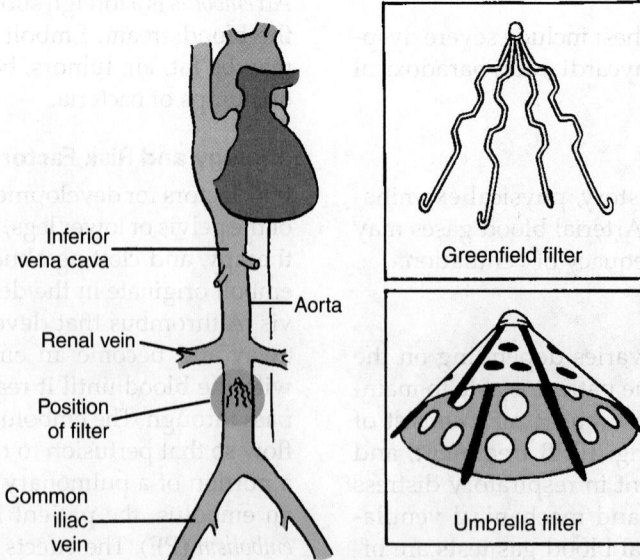

FIGURE 30-15 Greenfield and umbrella filters are examples of filters that may be placed in the inferior vena cava to prevent emboli traveling to the lung.

| Anxiety related to dyspnea, fear of dying | Reduced anxiety: patient statement of less or no anxiety, calm manner |
| Risk for Injury related to anticoagulant therapy | Decreased risk of excessive bleeding: prothrombin time within therapeutic range, absence of excessive bruising or bleeding |

Interventions

Ineffective Tissue Perfusion

Monitor the patient's respiratory rate and effort, breath sounds, skin color, pulse, and blood pressure. Note arterial blood gas results as a measure of tissue perfusion, and notify the physician if they are abnormal. Elevate the head of the patient's bed. Administer oxygen as ordered, usually by nasal cannula. Enforce strict bed rest or other prescribed activity limitations to decrease oxygen demands. Administer prescribed intravenous fluids and inotropic drugs. Measure and record fluid intake and output.

Interventions to decrease the risk of further emboli include active and passive range-of-motion exercises for immobilized patients, early ambulation after surgery, and antiembolism and pneumatic compression stockings. Do not place cushions and pillows under the legs where circulation might be impaired.

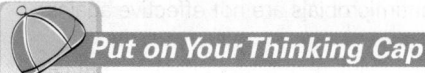

Put on Your Thinking Cap!

To prevent emboli, we recommend compression stockings and avoidance of pressure under the legs. This sounds like a contradiction! How can you explain the value of each intervention?

Anxiety

The patient in respiratory distress and pain is understandably anxious. Remain calm, and tell the patient what is being done. Explain equipment and procedures in terms the patient can understand. Encourage the patient to express concerns and ask questions. Permit a reassuring family member to remain with the patient.

Risk for Injury

Anticoagulant therapy poses a risk of uncontrolled bleeding. While the patient is hospitalized, assess for excessive bruising or bleeding. Symptoms that may be caused by internal bleeding include severe headache and abdominal or back pain. Inspect the urine for hematuria. Apply pressure to venipuncture sites to control bleeding.

To reduce the risk of bleeding, the patient's activated partial thromboplastin time is monitored every

1 to 2 days until stabilized at 1.5 to 2.5 times the normal rate. Anticoagulant therapy for patients with a PE is usually changed to warfarin sodium (Coumadin), an oral anticoagulant, after receiving heparin for a week or so. The effect of warfarin sodium is monitored by assessing the prothrombin time (PT), which should be 1.5 to 2.0 times the normal (control) rate, and the INR, which should be 2.0 to 3.0. The dosage is adjusted daily based on PT and INR.

Pharmacology Capsule

Monitor the patient's activated partial thromboplastin time when on heparin and monitor the prothrombin time and INR when on warfarin sodium to determine the extent of anticoagulation. Watch for bleeding.

RESPIRATORY ARREST

Respiratory arrest, the cessation of breathing, is addressed in Chapter 16.

ACUTE RESPIRATORY DISTRESS SYNDROME

Etiology and Risk Factors

Acute respiratory distress syndrome (ARDS) is a progressive pulmonary disorder that follows some trauma to the lung. From 1 to 96 hours after the trauma, pulmonary infiltrates develop and lung compliance decreases. Fluid shifts into the interstitial spaces in the lungs and into the alveoli, causing pulmonary edema. Production of pulmonary surfactant decreases,

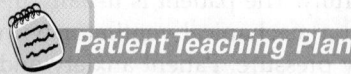

Patient Teaching Plan

Pulmonary Embolism

Patients who have had a PE must be taught how to manage their anticoagulant therapy because they usually remain on these drugs for at least several months. The following are important points:

• Use soft toothbrush and electric razor to avoid trauma and bleeding.

• Report red or dark urine, which suggests urinary bleeding.

• Report vomited blood, nosebleed, and red or black stools, which suggest intestinal bleeding.

• Do not take any over-the-counter medications without consulting with the physician or pharmacist. Some drugs, especially aspirin, prolong the bleeding time, which could cause excessive bleeding.

• To reduce the risk of a future PE, avoid constricting clothing such as garters or tight girdles and avoid prolonged pressure on the back of the knee.

leading to atelectasis. Lung compliance decreases, and the patient rapidly becomes hypoxemic.

Some patients recover and heal completely, whereas lung fibrosis develops in others. The fibrosis may be mild or severe and sometimes occurs after the patient appears to be recovering. Progressive fibrosis may lead to death. Systemic complications of ARDS include cardiac dysrhythmias, renal failure, stress ulcers, thrombocytopenia, and disseminated intravascular coagulation. In addition, these patients are at risk for oxygen toxicity and sepsis.

Signs and Symptoms

The first sign of ARDS is usually increased respiratory rate. Auscultation of the lungs may reveal fine crackles. The patient may be restless, agitated, and confused. The pulse rate increases, and a cough may be present. These early signs are followed by progressively worsening dyspnea with retractions, cyanosis, and diaphoresis. Diffuse crackles and rhonchi may be heard on auscultation.

Medical Diagnosis

Acute respiratory distress syndrome is suspected on the basis of the patient's history and physical findings. Diagnostic studies include arterial blood gas analysis and chest radiographs. The blood pH rises and the $Paco_2$ falls at first because of hyperventilation. The PaO_2 falls below 70 mm Hg despite oxygen concentrations greater than 40% (FiO_2 0.4). Hypoxemia in spite of supplemental oxygen administration is a cardinal sign of ARDS. This hypoxemia causes respiratory acidosis, as evidenced by pH below 7.35.

Medical Treatment

Early detection and treatment are critical factors in treating ARDS successfully. The patient is usually intubated and placed on a mechanical ventilator with positive end-expiratory pressure. Patient anxiety and restlessness may require sedation or even pharmacologic paralysis. Specific drug therapy depends on the underlying cause of ARDS. For example, the patient with sepsis is treated with antimicrobials Corticosteroids are commonly used to reduce inflammation with ARDS, but there is some question about the value of this treatment.

NURSING CARE of the Patient with Acute Respiratory Distress Syndrome

The patient with ARDS is critically ill and should be treated in an intensive care setting. Critical care nursing is beyond the scope of this text. However, all nurses must be aware of the risk of ARDS and respond promptly when a patient exhibits progressive respiratory distress. The rapid progression of the condition is frightening to the patient and the family. Recognize their anxiety and fear and offer emotional support and simple explanations.

Key Points

- The function of the respiratory system is to supply oxygen for the metabolic needs of the cells and to eliminate carbon dioxide, one of the waste materials of cell metabolism.
- Age-related changes in the respiratory system include loss of lung elasticity, enlargement of bronchioles, decreased number of alveoli, thoracic rigidity, atrophy of chest muscles, and flattening of the diaphragm.
- A thoracentesis is the insertion of a needle through the chest wall into the pleural space to remove fluid, blood, or air or to instill medication.
- Chest physiotherapy, which consists of percussion, vibration, and postural drainage, mobilizes respiratory secretions for expectoration.
- Oxygen therapy is widely used and generally safe but must be used cautiously in chronic respiratory patients to avoid respiratory depression.
- Chest tubes drain fluid and air from the pleural space, permitting a collapsed lung to reexpand.
- Nursing diagnoses after thoracotomy may include Impaired Gas Exchange, Ineffective Breathing Pattern, and Ineffective Airway Clearance.
- Drugs commonly used for treatment of respiratory disorders include decongestants, antitussives, antihistamines, expectorants, antimicrobials, bronchodilators, corticosteroids, mast cell stabilizers, and leukotriene inhibitors.
- Acute viral rhinitis (the common cold), the most prevalent infectious disease, is treated symptomatically because available antimicrobials are not effective against the cold virus.
- Influenza is an acute viral respiratory infection that can lead to pneumonia, especially in debilitated people.
- Influenza immunizations do not protect everyone from influenza but do reduce the incidence of the infection and are recommended for people who have poor resistance to infection.
- Pneumonia may be caused by pathogenic organisms or by noninfectious agents such as inhaled irritants, including aspirated gastric contents.
- Nursing diagnoses for the patient with pneumonia may include Ineffective Airway Clearance, Impaired Gas Exchange, Activity Intolerance, Imbalanced Nutrition: Less Than Body Requirements, Risk For Deficient Fluid Volume, and Acute Pain.
- Pleurisy (pleuritis) is inflammation of the pleura that is treated with analgesics, anti-inflammatory drugs, antitussives, antimicrobials, and local heat therapy.
- Nursing diagnoses for the patient with pleurisy may include Acute Pain and Ineffective Breathing Pattern.
- Pneumothorax is the accumulation of air in the pleural space, which may cause the lung to collapse.
- The immediate treatment of an open chest wound is coverage with a vented dressing followed by careful monitoring to detect signs of a tension pneumothorax.
- With a tension pneumothorax, air accumulates in the affected side, collapsing the affected lung and causing the heart, trachea, esophagus, and great blood vessels to shift toward the unaffected side (mediastinal shift, a life-threatening condition).

- Nursing diagnoses when a patient has pneumothorax may include Ineffective Breathing Pattern, Fear, Decreased Cardiac Output, Acute Pain, and Risk For Infection.
- Flail chest is the loss of thoracic integrity caused by fractures of two adjacent ribs into two or more segments on the same side of the chest.
- A pulmonary embolus is a foreign substance carried through the bloodstream into the lung, where it lodges and blocks blood flow.
- Nursing diagnoses for the patient who has a pulmonary embolism may include Ineffective Tissue Perfusion, Anxiety, and Risk for Injury.

- Adult respiratory distress syndrome, a progressive pulmonary disorder that may lead to fibrosis of lung tissue and death, is treated with mechanical ventilation and treatment of the underlying cause.

 Go to your Companion CD-ROM for a Pharmacology Tutorial, Audio Glossary, and 3-D animations.

evolve Be sure to visit the companion Evolve site at http://evolve.elsevier.com/Linton/ for WebLinks and additional online resources.

REVIEW QUESTIONS *Choose the best answer.*

1. Where is the respiratory center located?
   1. Lungs
   2. Alveoli
   3. Brain
   4. Aorta

2. Age-related changes in the respiratory system include the following:
   1. Elevated diaphragm
   2. Atrophy of bronchioles
   3. Respiratory muscle hypertrophy
   4. Rib cage rigidity

3. Which of the following is the best example of documentation of the respiratory assessment?
   1. Patient expectorated moderate amount of tenacious, green sputum.
   2. Patient reports coughing up lots of mucus this shift.
   3. Physical activity seems to cause patient to have severe coughing spells.
   4. Patient is coughing up less sputum today than yesterday.

4. Your patient has a pulse oximeter. The current oxygen saturation is 96%. You should:
   1. Notify the registered nurse or physician immediately
   2. Document the reading and continue routine monitoring
   3. Increase the patient's oxygen to at least 5 L/min
   4. Request arterial blood gases to confirm the oximetry reading

5. Several days after thoracic surgery, your patient's respiratory status is normal. When checking the chest tube drainage system, you observe that there is no bubbling in the water-seal chamber. This could mean that:
   1. There is a leak in the drainage system
   2. The patient's affected lung has reexpanded
   3. It is time to change the drainage receptacle
   4. The patient's affected lung has collapsed

6. A community education project is designed to encourage older adults to have influenza immunizations. A participant asks about the difference between influenza and the common cold. What is the most appropriate reply?
   1. Influenza is actually just a very severe cold.
   2. Colds are caused by bacteria; influenza is caused by a virus.
   3. Influenza is more likely to cause fever and chills.
   4. They are equally likely to have serious complications.

7. A patient who has pneumonia has become restless; vital signs are: T = 100° F, P = 110, R = 28, BP = 130/72. You should suspect:
   1. Fluid volume excess
   2. Dehydration
   3. Excess potassium
   4. Hypoxemia

8. In the emergency care of a patient who has a sucking chest wound, why is a vented dressing preferred over a dressing that completely seals the wound?
   1. The vented dressing permits the drainage of blood from the pleural sac.
   2. Sealing the wound increases the risk of bacterial contamination.
   3. The vented dressing prevents air from escaping from the injured lung.
   4. Sealing the wound could lead to a tension pneumothorax.

9. A patient who comes into the ER after a traffic accident is in respiratory distress. You observe that a part of the rib cage moves inward with inspiration and outward with expiration. This pattern is described as:
   1. Paradoxical movement
   2. Tension pneumothorax
   3. Compensatory breathing
   4. Cheyne-Stokes respirations

10. Measures to prevent pulmonary embolism in postoperative patients include the following:
    1. Splinting extremities to limit movement
    2. Assisting with range-of-motion exercises
    3. Enforcing bed rest until wound healing is complete
    4. Supporting the legs with pillows to promote circulation

CHAPTER 31

Chronic Respiratory Disorders

LOUIS K. LINTON AND ADRIANNE DILL LINTON

evolve http://evolve.elsevier.com/Linton/

Objectives

After reading and studying this chapter, you should be able to:

1. Identify examples of chronic inflammatory, obstructive, and restrictive pulmonary diseases.
2. Explain the relationship between cigarette smoking and chronic respiratory disorders.
3. For selected chronic respiratory disorders, describe the pathophysiology, signs and symptoms, complications, diagnostic measures, and medical treatment.
4. Assist in developing a nursing care plan for the patient who has a chronic respiratory disorder.

Key Terms

 Be sure to check out the bonus material on the Companion CD-ROM, including selected audio pronunciations.

asbestosis (ăs-bĕs-TŌ-sĭs, p. 566)
asthma (ĂZ-mă, p. 550)
brachytherapy (brăk-ē-THĔR-ă-pē, p. 567)
bronchiectasis (brŏng-kē-ĔK-tă-sĭs, p. 561)
bronchitis (brŏng-KĪ-tĭs, p. 553)
cor pulmonale (kŏr pŭl-mō-NĂ-lē, p. 554)
emphysema (ĕm-fĭ-SĒ-mă, p. 554)
granuloma (grăn-ŭ-LŌ-mă, p. 566)
pneumoconiosis (nū-mō-kō-nē-Ō-sĭs, p. 566)
pneumonitis (nū-mō-NĪ-tĭs, p. 566)

CHRONIC OBSTRUCTIVE PULMONARY DISORDERS

Chronic obstructive pulmonary disease (COPD) is the fifth leading cause of death in the United States. It is characterized as varying combinations of asthma, chronic bronchitis, and emphysema. There are people who have only one or two of these conditions, but the three are usually found together. Other terms used to describe COPD are *chronic obstructive lung disease (COLD)* and *chronic airflow limitation (CAL)*.

A common diagnostic procedure for COPD is the pulmonary function test. Pulmonary function tests provide information about airway dynamics, lung volumes, and diffusing capacity. *Airway dynamics* refers to the patient's ability to inhale or exhale by force. Some of the lung volumes measured include vital capacity, inspiratory capacity, expiratory reserve volume, residual volume, and total lung capacity. The diffusing

capacity is a measurement of the ability of gases to diffuse across the alveolar capillary membrane. "Norms" are based on average measurements for healthy people who are the same age, gender, and weight as the patient. Pulmonary function tests should be performed under laboratory conditions by trained personnel to ensure a maximum degree of accuracy. These tests are effort dependent, meaning that the patient must be mentally alert, cooperative, and able to follow directions. Additional information about pulmonary function tests is presented in Chapter 30.

ASTHMA

Asthma is a potentially reversible obstructive airway disorder characterized by airway inflammation and hyperresponsiveness. The incidence of asthma has been increasing. It occurs across the life span, from the very young to the very old. It is a highly complex condition that can be a mild nuisance or a very serious, life-threatening condition. It traditionally has been classified as an obstructive disorder because of the narrowing of the airways and presence of mucus plugs.

 What Does Culture Have to Do with Asthma?

African Americans have a higher incidence of asthma than white Americans.

Pathophysiology

Asthma was once thought to be simply a condition in which allergies induced episodes of bronchoconstriction. We now know that it is much more complicated than that and that it has long-term consequences. Patients with asthma periodically have acute episodes, or attacks, of varying intensity. Attacks have two distinct phases. The early phase of an acute episode begins when "triggers" (e.g., allergens, irritants, infections, exercise, gastroesophageal reflux) activate the inflammatory process. The airways constrict (*bronchoconstriction or bronchospasm*) and become edematous. Mucus secretion increases, forming plugs in the airways, and tenacious sputum is produced. Obstruction causes air to be trapped in the alveoli, creating a ventilation-perfusion mismatch. That is, the alveoli are perfused with blood but not ventilated with fresh air. The effect is hypoxemia with compensatory hyperventilation. Acute episodes usually occur within 30 to 60 minutes after exposure to the trigger and resolve some 30 to 90 minutes later. These events characterize the early phase response to the triggers (Fig. 31-1).

The late phase begins 5 to 6 hours after the early phase response when airway inflammation is pronounced. Red and white blood cells infiltrate the swollen tissues of the airways. During this phase, which lasts several hours or days, the airways are hyperreactive (very sensitive). The patient is at risk for another acute episode until the phase subsides.

When no specific trigger can be identified, the patient may be said to have "intrinsic" asthma. In contrast, asthma associated with known triggers is referred to as "extrinsic" asthma. It is important to note that asthma is not an emotional disorder! Stress does not cause asthma, though there is an understandable emotional response to episodes of difficult breathing. It is

possible that the patient's emotional state plays some role in acute episodes, but this is not fully understood.

Complications

Severe, persistent bronchospasm is called *status asthmaticus*. If not corrected, status asthmaticus can lead to right-sided heart failure, pneumothorax, worsening hypoxemia, acidosis, and respiratory or cardiac arrest. Over time, repeated episodes can cause hypertrophy of bronchial smooth muscle, thickening of the tissues in the airways, hypertrophy of mucus glands, air trapping in the alveoli, and hyperinflation of the lungs.

Signs and Symptoms

During an asthma attack, the patient may exhibit dyspnea, productive cough, use of accessory muscles of respiration (scalenes and sternocleidomastoids), audible expiratory wheezing, tachycardia, and tachypnea. The wheezing is caused by air moving through the narrowed airways. Findings that suggest that respiratory arrest is imminent include drowsiness, confusion, absence of wheezing, bradycardia, and retractions above the sternum.

Medical Diagnosis

A diagnosis of bronchial asthma is based on the health history, the physical examination, and the pulmonary function test results. The pulmonary function tests typically reveal that the airflow coming from the patient's lungs is significantly less than expected. Arterial blood gas measurements may be done if the patient has moderate to severe symptoms.

Medical Treatment

The primary goal of medical therapy is to prevent acute asthma attacks by using bronchodilators and antiinflammatory drugs. Bronchodilators include beta$_2$-receptor agonists, anticholinergics, and the less commonly used methylxanthines. Anticholinergics enhance the bronchodilating action of beta$_2$-receptor agonists. Corticosteroids, mast cell stabilizers, leukotriene inhibitors, and the immunosuppressant monoclonal antibody omalizumab (Xolair) are types of anti-inflammatory drugs. The exact drug therapy varies with the severity of the condition. People with mild asthma may have to use inhaled bronchodilators only when they have symptoms, whereas those with moderate asthma may be advised to use the inhalers daily. Patients with severe asthma may require daily use of inhalers in addition to other agents, such as aerosol corticosteroids (Fig. 31-2). Some combination preparations are available. Advair contains both a corticosteroid and a bronchodilator; Combivent contains an anticholinergic and a bronchodilator.

Drugs used to treat asthma can be classified as those that relieve acute symptoms ("relievers") and those that provide long-term control ("controllers").

A   Normal lungs

Terminal bronchiole

Respiratory bronchiole

Alveoli

B

Swollen mucous membranes

Mucus accumulation

Constriction of muscles

FIGURE 31-1 Comparison of terminal bronchioles, respiratory bronchioles, and alveoli in a normal lung (**A**) and in the lung of a person with bronchial asthma (**B**).

FIGURE **31-2** Use of metered-dose inhaler for administration of inhalant medication.

Beta₂-receptor agonists are the most often used relievers; however, some anticholinergics are effective for this purpose. Controllers include inhaled glucocorticoids, leukotriene modifiers, long-acting beta₂-receptor agonists, mast cell stabilizers, an immunosuppressant monoclonal antibody, and methylxanthines (theophylline, aminophylline). Systemic corticosteroids may be used for asthma that does not respond to other controllers. The course of systemic therapy is usually limited to 2 weeks, although especially severe cases may require them for a longer time. Because older persons may not recognize mild bronchial constriction, some experts recommend that they use inhaled corticosteroids on a regular basis instead of bronchodilators as needed.

Status asthmaticus is treated with inhaled and intravenous bronchodilators and oxygen therapy. Endotracheal intubation and mechanical ventilation are sometimes necessary. Drugs used to treat respiratory disorders are presented in the Drug Therapy table on pp. 532 and 533 in Chapter 30.

Put on Your Thinking Cap!

Write a teaching plan (including at least three facts) for an asthma patient who is prescribed zafirlukast (Accolate).

NURSING CARE *of the Patient with Asthma*

Assessment

The complete assessment of the patient with a respiratory disorder is summarized in Box 30-1 on p. 516 in Chapter 30. When the patient has asthma, obtain essential information (medications, allergies, known cardiac disease, sleep disruption) and immediately take steps to relieve symptoms. Then collect more complete data.

Health History

Determine the frequency and severity of attacks, the factors known to trigger attacks, the impact of the condition on the patient's life, the strategies used to manage the condition, the sources of stress and support, and the patient's knowledge about asthma and its treatment. Explore the patient's ability to afford medical care and drug therapy.

Consider the Alternative

Ma huang is an herbal product that has the same effects as ephedrine: relief of bronchospasm and central nervous system (CNS) stimulation. Because ma huang is available as an herbal supplement, patients may exceed the therapeutic dose. Educate patients that excessive use of ma huang or combining it with other similar drugs could result in toxicity.

Physical Examination

Important aspects of the physical examination include measurement of vital signs and auscultation of lung sounds. In addition, assess the patient's skin color and respiratory effort.

Nursing Diagnoses, Goals, and Outcome Criteria: Asthma	
NURSING DIAGNOSES	GOALS AND OUTCOME CRITERIA
Ineffective Breathing Pattern related to air trapping	Effective breathing pattern: regular respirations, 12 to 20/min, without dyspnea or wheezing
Impaired Gas Exchange related to bronchospasm, air trapping, increased secretions	Improved gas exchange: normal skin color, normal pulse and respiratory rates, arterial blood gases within normal limits
Anxiety related to perceived threat of suffocation, hypoxemia	Reduced anxiety: patient statement of lessened anxiety, calm manner

Interventions

Ineffective Breathing Pattern

Monitor the patient's respiratory rate, pattern, and effort. Support the patient in Fowler's position, and give oxygen as ordered. Administer prescribed bronchodilators, and assess for adverse effects of drug therapy. Remain with the patient during an acute attack. If the patient does not respond to these interventions, immediate medical care is essential because the condition may be life-threatening.

Because asthma is a chronic condition, patient teaching is critical. Patients must understand their drugs, how they should be used, and adverse effects that should be reported to the physician. If the patient is unable to afford these drugs, consult a social worker or case manager for assistance. Many patients are now taught to use peak expiratory flow rate (PEFR) meters routinely. The patient uses the meter twice daily to establish a baseline PEFR and then daily to monitor level of control. If the PEFR drops 20% or more below the patient's usual level, the physician should be notified so that adjustments can be made in the treatment plan.

Impaired Gas Exchange

Monitor for signs and symptoms of impending respiratory failure: tachypnea, shallow respirations, diaphoresis, reddening skin, tachycardia, cardiac dysrhythmias, initial hypertension, later hypotension, restlessness, drowsiness, or loss of consciousness. Check arterial blood gas values, and contact the registered nurse or the physician if the PaO_2 decreases, the $Paco_2$ increases, and the pH falls. Administer oxygen as ordered, usually 4 to 6 L/min unless the patient has chronic bronchitis and emphysema, in which case oxygen therapy is limited to 3 L/min. A nasal cannula is preferred over a face mask because the mask may increase the patient's feeling of suffocation.

If the patient has tenacious secretions that cannot be expectorated, chest physiotherapy and suctioning may be necessary. Because good hydration helps thin

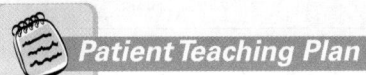

Patient Teaching Plan

Asthma

Because asthma is a chronic condition, the patient must learn to manage it. After the acute attack has subsided, initiate patient teaching. The teaching plan should include the following:

* Acute asthma attacks can be triggered by allergic reactions to substances in the environment, exercise, or infection and can be aggravated by stress.
* To reduce the occurrence of attacks, avoid irritating substances including tobacco smoke, have infections treated promptly, and learn to manage stressful situations.
* If you have symptoms during exercise, use your prescribed inhaler as directed 30 minutes before you exercise.
* Drugs for asthma must be taken as prescribed; report adverse effects to the physician (see the Drug Therapy Table on pp. 532 and 533).
* Seek emergency medical care if your symptoms worsen and do not respond to your medications.
* Drink ten to fourteen 8-ounce glasses of fluids daily if approved by your physician.
* The Asthma and Allergy Foundation of America is a resource for information about treatment and management of asthma.
* To deliver drugs effectively, metered-dose inhalers must be used correctly. (Teach correct use and have patients practice, using the manufacturer's directions.)

secretions, a daily fluid intake of 2500 to 3000 mL is recommended unless contraindicated. Intravenous fluids may be ordered to improve hydration and provide venous access for administration of emergency drugs.

Anxiety

The feeling of not being able to breathe is very frightening. In addition, with moderate to severe asthma, the arterial oxygen decreases, which causes a feeling of restlessness and anxiety. Anxiety may serve to aggravate the physical symptoms. While taking steps to improve the patient's oxygenation, try to reduce anxiety by remaining calm yourself, responding to the patient's needs promptly, providing quiet reassurance, and explaining what is being done. The family also may need information and reassurance to calm their fears so they can be more supportive to the patient.

CHRONIC BRONCHITIS AND EMPHYSEMA

Chronic bronchitis and emphysema can occur independently. Because they most often accompany each other, however, the two conditions are discussed together.

Pathophysiology

Chronic Bronchitis. Chronic bronchitis is bronchial inflammation characterized by increased production of mucus and chronic cough that persist for at least 3 months of the year for 2 consecutive years and by impaired ciliary action (Fig. 31-3). The inflammation is caused by inhaled irritants, including cigarette smoke. At first, only large airways are affected, but smaller

Impaired ciliary action

Increased production of mucus

FIGURE 31-3 Chronic bronchitis.

Centrilobular emphysema

Terminal bronchiole

Distended respiratory bronchiole

Alveoli

Panlobular emphysema

Terminal bronchiole

Respiratory bronchiole

Alveoli

FIGURE 31-4 Types of emphysema.

Put on Your Thinking Cap!

Refer to Chapter 14, Fluids and Electrolytes, to figure out why a patient with COPD might develop respiratory acidosis.

airways are eventually involved. Mucus obstructs the airway, causing air to be trapped in distal portions of the lungs. Alveolar ventilation is impaired, and hypoxemia may develop, leading to heart failure. Cor pulmonale is the term used to describe right-sided heart failure secondary to pulmonary disease. The patient with chronic bronchitis is susceptible to respiratory infections that aggravate the condition.

Emphysema. Pulmonary emphysema is a degenerative, nonreversible disease characterized by the enlargement of the airways beyond the terminal bronchioles. The two types of emphysema are centrilobular and panlobular (Fig. 31-4). Centrilobular emphysema is associated primarily with cigarette smoking, and affects mainly the respiratory bronchioles. The walls of respiratory bronchioles enlarge and break down, whereas the alveoli remain intact. Elastic recoil dimin-

FIGURE 31-5 Patient with chronic bronchitis and all the classic findings of the "blue bloater." Note the elevation of the shoulders and the tense muscles.

Put on Your Thinking Cap!

Why is a patient with emphysema likely to develop failure of the right side of the heart before developing left-sided heart failure?

ishes, and the airways partially collapse. Pockets of air called *bullae* and *blebs* form. Bullae are located between the alveolar spaces, whereas blebs are in the lung parenchyma. Ruptured blebs can cause the lung to collapse. As the functional units of the lung are destroyed, the patient's ability to exchange oxygen and carbon dioxide declines. The lungs become hyperinflated, causing the diaphragm to flatten and increasing the reliance on accessory muscles for breathing. Eventually, as with chronic bronchitis, right-sided heart failure develops. The progression of panlobular emphysema is similar despite differences in the initial pathology. Panlobular emphysema, which affects the respiratory bronchioles *and* the alveoli, is caused more often by a hereditary deficiency of the enzyme inhibitor alpha₁-antitrypsin. The walls of both the alveoli and the respiratory bronchioles break down, causing air to be trapped and decreasing the surface area for gas exchange. A patient may have both types of emphysema at the same time.

Complications

The most serious complications of COPD are respiratory failure and heart failure. Respiratory failure is marked by hypoventilation and ventilation-perfusion mismatch with rising arterial carbon dioxide pressure ($Paco_2$), declining arterial oxygen pressure (Pao_2), and

FIGURE 31-6 Signs and symptoms of chronic obstructive pulmonary disease (COPD).

Speech pattern: a few words between noticeable breaths

Pursed-lip breathing

Cyanosis

Distended neck veins

Overly developed neck and thorax muscles

Barrel chest: increased AP diameter of thorax

Pulsus paradoxus

Clubbing of digits

Nicotine stains

Pitting peripheral edema

Gait and walking pace correspond to breathing; frequent rests to breathe

Prolonged expiration, diminished breath sounds, adventitious breath sounds or hyperventilation; diminished excursions of chest with respiration; hyperresonant to percussion

Enlarged, pulsating liver

Cough nonproductive to productive with mucoid to purulent sputum, which may contain blood

Enlarged heart

Flat or scalloped diaphragm, bullae, abnormal retrosternal space

Exertional dyspnea, or dyspnea at rest; easy fatigability and weakness

Characteristic sitting position with shoulders raised

respiratory acidosis. Factors that may lead to complications include infection, air pollution, continued smoking, left ventricular failure, myocardial infarction, pulmonary embolism, spontaneous pneumothorax, and adverse effects of drugs.

Signs and Symptoms

Chronic bronchitis and emphysema each have specific signs and symptoms because of the differences in pathologic origin. The signs and symptoms of each are presented separately here, but remember that the two conditions are often found together.

Chronic Bronchitis. Signs and symptoms of chronic bronchitis include productive cough, exertional dyspnea, and wheezing. With chronic hypoxemia, the red blood cell count is typically elevated to compensate for the inadequate oxygen in the blood. The patient with cor pulmonale demonstrates signs and symptoms of heart failure, including increasing dyspnea, cyanosis, and peripheral edema. These signs have given rise to the term *blue bloater* to describe the patient with advanced chronic bronchitis (Fig. 31-5).

Emphysema. The main symptom of emphysema is dyspnea on exertion (Fig. 31-6). As the disease progresses, the patient also may have dyspnea when at rest. Patients often are thin and may be observed using accessory muscles of respiration. Increased anteroposterior diameter of the chest creates what is called a *barrel chest*. Despite dyspnea, patients who have emphysema without chronic bronchitis often have normal arterial blood gases until the disease is very advanced. Therefore skin color may be normal. This explains the term *pink puffer* used to describe the patient with em-

FIGURE 31-7 Patient with emphysema and all the classic findings of the "pink puffer." Note the use of accessory muscles in the neck and chest.

physema (Fig. 31-7). Depression and irritability are common in the patient with COPD.

Medical Diagnosis

Chronic obstructive pulmonary disease is suspected on the basis of the patient's health history and physical examination. The most reliable diagnostic tests for COPD are the pulmonary function tests, which reveal a decreased forced expiratory volume and forced vital capacity accompanied by increases in functional residual capacity and residual volume. Total lung capacity can be increased or normal. A computed tomography scan may be done to help differentiate the type of emphysema.

Medical Treatment

Drug Therapy. The goals of medical treatment are improved ventilation and removal of secretions. Drug therapy plays an important part in treating COPD. Bronchodilators, including beta-adrenergics and anticholinergics, are ordered to decrease airway resistance and the work of breathing. The preferred route of administration is by inhalation using a metered-dose inhaler. There is some evidence that anticholinergics such as ipratropium bromide (Atrovent) or tiotropium (Spiriva) are more effective than beta-adrenergics for treating COPD and have fewer side effects.

Oral theophylline is not used as commonly for bronchodilation as it once was because of the risk of drug toxicity, particularly cardiac stimulation. If theophylline is used, the sustained-release form is recommended and periodic blood levels must be determined. Corticosteroids are useful in the treatment of the inflammatory response in asthma, but whether they are effective with bronchitis and emphysema is controversial. Some sources recommend corticosteroids in older persons only if improvement is demonstrated. Antidepressants may be indicated and can improve the quality of life.

Theophylline blood levels must be monitored because toxicity can cause fatal cardiac dysrhythmias. The therapeutic blood level is 5 to 15 micrograms per milliliter (mcg/mL).

Oxygen Therapy. Oxygen therapy may be prescribed but must be used cautiously. The goal of oxygen therapy is to maintain the PaO_2 between 50 and 60 mm Hg. The initial liter flow is usually 1 to 3 L/min. A pulse oximeter may be used while titrating the liter flow to maintain the SaO_2 (saturation of oxygen in the arterial blood) at 90%. Periodically, the pulse oximeter should be correlated with actual blood gas laboratory values. High levels of oxygen are not administered because patients with COPD may rely on *hypoxic drive* to breathe. A comparison of respiratory stimuli in healthy people and people with COPD helps explain the concept of hypoxic drive. A healthy person's respirations are stimulated by rising carbon dioxide levels in the blood. The patient with COPD who retains carbon dioxide, however, has adapted to high blood carbon dioxide and relies on low blood oxygen to stimulate breathing. A high concentration of oxygen may raise the blood oxygen level so that the patient's stimulus to breathe is lost and respiratory depression may result. Not all people with COPD rely on hypoxic drive; retention of carbon dioxide must be confirmed by blood gas analysis.

For outpatient use, patients can rent oxygen tanks or cylinders, oxygen concentrators, and portable oxygen therapy equipment. Oxygen concentrators compress and filter room air and deliver oxygen to the patient through a nasal cannula. Using long tubing, the patient can be mobile in the home setting. Suitcase models can be used for travel. Portable equipment includes liquid oxygen reservoirs that are easily carried on a shoulder strap and compressed gas units that deliver oxygen only "on demand," so that a small quantity lasts longer than standard cylinders.

Patients who meet specific criteria may be prescribed long-term oxygen therapy (LTOT), defined as the use of oxygen therapy for a minimum of 15 hours per day. LTOT has been shown to prolong survival in people with COPD.

Chest Physiotherapy. Chest physiotherapy, described in Chapter 30, may be ordered to mobilize secretions in the patient with COPD.

Exercise. The patient may be referred to a rehabilitation program that includes exercise reconditioning. Programs are individualized but usually use progressive exercise—either walking or pedaling a stationary cycle. A typical program might have the patient walk 10 to 15 minutes every day or every other day. Every week or two, the exercise time is increased by 5 to10 minutes. The goal is to enable the patient to exercise comfortably for 45 minutes to 1 hour daily or every other day. Of course, some patients may not improve this much, but improvement in walking performance and general well-being has been found in patients who consistently walked as little as 12 minutes every day for 2 months. Sometimes bronchodilators are prescribed before exercise.

Nutrition. Nutrition is important for the patient with COPD because malnutrition causes decreased energy and decreased resistance to infection and because obesity increases the work of breathing. No special diet is indicated; however, supplementary feedings may be needed for some patients. Good hydration helps thin pulmonary secretions. See the Nutrition Concepts box on p. 557.

Treatment of Respiratory Failure. Respiratory failure is treated with oxygen therapy, aerosol bronchodilators, chest physiotherapy (possibly), and mechanical ventilation (if the patient is becoming exhausted).

Surgical Treatment

If medical interventions fail, a surgical procedure, lung volume reduction surgery (LVRS), may be used in selected patients. Up to 30% of the hyperinflated lung tissue is excised to improve the mechanics of breathing, enabling the patient to breathe more deeply. The short-term and long-term benefits of such surgery are still being debated. In early studies, about 70% of patients experienced some improvement. However, the recovery period is long, and the mortality rate has been 5% to 10%. One question under study is how to determine which patients are the best candidates for surgical intervention. Other surgical procedures that may benefit selected patients are bullectomy (removal of bullae) and lung transplantation.

Nutrition Concepts

1. Malnutrition and pulmonary disease are strongly related.
2. Starvation and malnutrition often cause impaired pulmonary function, and pulmonary disease may result in malnutrition.
3. Pulmonary disease causes an increase in energy expenditure because of increased work of breathing and chronic infection.
4. Reduced dietary intake in lung disease results from fluid restriction, shortness of breath, anorexia, gastrointestinal distress, and vomiting.
5. Food allergies can be one trigger for asthma attacks.
6. Approximately 70% of patients with chronic obstructive pulmonary disease exhibit weight loss.
7. Strategies for increasing intake and weight gain include eating high-calorie and high-fat foods; small, frequent meals; and resting before meals.

NURSING CARE *of the Patient with Chronic Obstructive Pulmonary Disease*

Assessment

Assessment of the patient with a respiratory disorder is summarized in Box 30-1 on p. 516 in Chapter 30. When a patient has COPD, describe the presenting symptoms—often dyspnea, cough, chest pain, or a combination of these. Obtain a complete medical history unless the patient's symptoms make it difficult to participate in a long interview. Sometimes it is necessary to break the interview into smaller sections so as not to exhaust the patient who is dyspneic. A list of current medications and drug allergies is essential. Obtain a functional assessment to explore the impact of the condition on the patient's activities of daily living. Inquire about exposure to smoke or other respiratory irritants. (See the Nursing Care Plan on pp. 558 and 559.)

During the physical examination, observe the patient's posture, color, respiratory effort, and use of accessory muscles of respiration. Measure vital signs. Observe the patient for signs of hypoxemia, including restlessness, confusion, and lethargy. Note pursed-lip breathing. Inspect the neck for distention of veins. Inspect the shape of the thorax for the classic barrel chest. Auscultate the lung fields for diminished breath sounds. Inspect the nails for clubbing, pallor, or cyanosis. Inspect and palpate the feet and ankles for edema. Note muscle wasting.

Nursing Diagnoses, Goals, and Outcome Criteria: COPD

Nursing Diagnoses	Goals and Outcome Criteria
Impaired Gas Exchange related to damaged alveoli and/or terminal bronchioles, bronchospasm, air trapping	Improved air exchange: vital signs and arterial blood gases consistent with patient norms
Ineffective Airway Clearance related to increased secretions, weak cough	Effective airway clearance: breath sounds clear to auscultation
Anxiety related to hypoxemia	Decreased anxiety: calm manner, patient statement of decreased anxiety
Imbalanced Nutrition: Less Than Body Requirements related to anorexia, dyspnea	Adequate nutrition: stable body weight
Risk for Infection related to decreased ciliary action, increased secretions, weak cough	Absence of infection: normal body temperature, white or clear sputum
Activity Intolerance related to inability to meet oxygen demands	Improved activity tolerance: completion of activities of daily living without excess fatigue
Decreased Cardiac Output related to right-sided heart failure	Improved cardiac output: absence of dependent edema and distended neck veins

Interventions

Impaired Gas Exchange

Monitor the patient's vital signs and arterial blood gases for signs of inadequate oxygenation: tachycardia, tachypnea, increasing $Paco_2$ level, and decreasing pH level. Administer oxygen at 1 to 3 L/min as ordered. Teach the patient and family not to increase the liter flow, because a sudden increase in oxygen in the blood may actually depress respirations in people with emphysema. Place the patient in a high-Fowler's position or seated on the bedside with the arms folded on the overbed table to promote full expansion of the lungs (Fig. 31-8). Teach pursed-lip breathing by instructing the patient to breathe in through the nose and exhale slowly through the mouth with the lips almost closed. Pursed-lip breathing reduces the collapse of airways with exhalation and reduces dyspnea. Administer prescribed bronchodilators, and monitor the patient for therapeutic and adverse effects.

Smoking cessation is an important aspect of the management of chronic bronchitis and emphysema as well as of other cardiovascular and respiratory conditions. One fifth of all deaths in the United States are related to smoking. Health care providers should discourage smoking but must be careful not to be judgmental of the patient. Most patients are aware of the relationship between smoking and respiratory disease, but many find they are unable to overcome the addiction to nicotine. Ask patients if they have considered quitting smoking and if they would like information about programs that might be helpful.

The physician may order nicotine patches, gum, or nasal spray for the patient who wants to try to withdraw from smoking. Some studies have found the success rate for these products is only approximately 25%, but other types of smoking cessation programs typically have less

NURSING CARE PLAN
The Patient with Chronic Obstructive Pulmonary Disease

ASSESSMENT

Health History: A 73-year-old woman is being admitted for increasing dyspnea. She has had chronic bronchitis and emphysema for 3 years. Her past medical history includes frequent upper respiratory infections with two hospitalizations for pneumonia in 2006. She had a myocardial infarction in 2000 and is being treated for hypertension, for which she takes verapamil. She also uses an ipratropium (Atrovent) inhaler four times a day. She is allergic to penicillin. The review of systems notes fatigue, increasing dyspnea both with exertion and at rest, orthopnea, and productive cough with yellow sputum. Patient states she is depressed. She is a retired nurse who volunteers at a local homeless shelter 1 day a week. She lives alone and has no family in the area. She reports that her appetite is poor and that she has lost "a little" weight over the past few weeks. She has smoked one pack of cigarettes daily for 45 years. She states she knows she should quit and has tried many programs but has never lasted more than a week.

Physical Examination: Vital signs: temperature, 100.6° F orally; pulse, 100; respirations, 28; blood pressure, 140/94. Height, 5'6". Weight, 102 lb. The patient is seated with her hands on her knees to elevate her shoulders. She appears to be in mild distress. Skin color is normal. Pulsed-lip breathing noted. Accessory muscles of respiration are tense. The thorax is barrel-shaped. Abdomen soft. Abdominal muscles used in respirations. No peripheral edema.

Nursing Diagnosis	Goals and Outcome Criteria	Interventions
Impaired Gas Exchange related to alveolar destruction, bronchospasm, air trapping	The patient will have improved gas exchange, as evidenced by pulse, respirations, and arterial blood gases with normal pH, Pao_2 minimum 60 mm Hg, and $Paco_2$ at baseline.	Monitor vital signs and arterial blood gases for tachycardia, tachypnea, increasing $Paco_2$, decreasing pH. Administer oxygen at 1-3 L/min per nasal cannula as ordered. Assist to comfortable position: high-Fowler's position in bed or supported at bedside. Reinforce pursed-lip and abdominal breathing techniques. Provide bronchodilator per inhaler as ordered. Assess technique. Assess respiratory status before and after use of bronchodilator. Monitor for adverse drug effects: dry mouth, headache, nausea, blurred vision, palpitations.
Ineffective Airway Clearance related to increased secretions, weak cough	The patient will maintain a patent airway, as evidenced by absence of crackles on auscultation, expectoration of secretions.	Auscultate breath sounds at least q 4 hr. Support patient during coughing and deep breathing. Document sputum amount and color. Encourage 2500-3000 mL of fluid daily. Request chest physiotherapy per order. Have suction equipment available if patient cannot expectorate secretions.
Anxiety related to hypoxemia	The patient will verbalize decreased anxiety and will appear calm.	Respond to the patient's needs promptly. Provide comfort measures. Be accepting of irritability. Acknowledge anxiety and try to identify stressors in addition to hypoxemia. Include patient in planning care.
Imbalanced Nutrition: Less Than Body Requirements related to anorexia, dyspnea	The patient will maintain or increase body weight during hospitalization.	Provide pleasant environment for meals. Schedule respiratory treatments at least an hour before meals. Assist with oral hygiene. Offer to arrange smaller, more frequent meals. Consult with dietitian to consider patient preferences.
Activity Intolerance related to inability to meet oxygen needs	The patient will accomplish activities of daily living without dyspnea or excessive fatigue.	Allow periods of uninterrupted rest during the day. Use comfort measures such as backrub and massage to promote rest. Allow patient to do what she can for herself, but assist when needed to avoid excessive tiring. Include occupational therapist and social worker to discuss plans for discharge and ways to reduce effort of activities at home. Discuss pulmonary rehabilitation program with physician. Encourage ambulation as permitted.

success, with rates of approximately 10% to 20%. Success is defined as abstinence from smoking for at least 1 year. The American Cancer Society and the American Lung Association sponsor programs to support people who are trying to quit smoking.

In addition to nicotine, drugs that have been tried to help people quit smoking include bupropion (Wellbutrin), cimetidine hydrochloride (Tagamet), clonidine (Catapres), doxepin hydrochloride (Sinequan), fluoxetine hydrochloride (Prozac), and calcium channel blockers. Although 70% of smokers indicate they would like to quit, the addictive quality of nicotine makes it very difficult. See Box 31-1 for facts about smoking and Box 31-2 for aids to smoking cessation.

NURSING CARE PLAN

The Patient with Chronic Obstructive Pulmonary Disease—cont'd

Nursing Diagnosis	Goals and Outcome Criteria	Interventions
Risk for Infection related to respiratory infection, effects of continued smoking	The patient will have a normal body temperature, clear or white sputum, no peripheral edema.	Monitor sputum color and body temperature. Administer antimicrobials as ordered. Encourage fluid intake. Protect from people with respiratory infections. Monitor for signs of heart failure, especially peripheral edema.
	The patient will express intent to attempt smoking cessation.	Explore smoking cessation programs that patient has tried. Be nonjudgmental and avoid scolding. Inform her of newer options such as nicotine patches, gum, and nasal spray. Tell her that drug therapy has been helpful for some people and that she may want to ask the physician about this. Provide literature from American Cancer Society and American Lung Association with suggestions to facilitate smoking cessation.
Decreased Cardiac Output related to right-sided heart failure	The patient will have improved cardiac output, as evidenced by no dependent edema or distended neck veins.	Monitor for signs of right-sided heart failure, especially peripheral edema.

? CRITICAL THINKING QUESTIONS

- Explain the basis for this patient's symptoms: fatigue, dyspnea, and productive cough.

- How would you determine whether a patient will be able to use an inhaler properly after discharge?

FIGURE **31-8** Sitting on the edge of the bed with the arms folded and elevated allows the accessory muscles of respiration to function more effectively.

Box 31-1 | **Facts About Smoking**

- Smoking is *the* major preventable cause of death in the United States, where over 400,000 smoking-related deaths occur each year.
- Smoking increases the risk of lung cancer, chronic bronchitis, emphysema, cardiovascular disease, duodenal and gastric ulcers, esophageal reflux, osteoporosis, reproductive complications, premature skin wrinkling, cataracts, and fire-related injuries.
- Environmental tobacco smoke is classified as a carcinogen.
- Smokeless tobacco is not recommended as an alternative to smoking because it has other adverse effects including oral cancers.

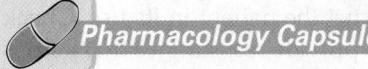
Pharmacology Capsule

Two drugs that have been approved for smoking cessation are nicotine and bupropion (Wellbutrin).

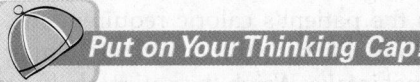
Put on Your Thinking Cap!

Think of some ways to discourage smoking by deglamorizing it. Make a poster to illustrate your strategy.

| Box 31-2 | *Aids to Smoking Cessation* |

MEDICATION	PATIENT TEACHING
Nicotine Replacement	
Gum	Slowly chew 8-10 pieces a day, each for 20-30 minutes, over a period of at least 3 months.
Transdermal patch	Apply patch in the morning and remove at bedtime or the next morning, depending on product instructions. Use the full-dose patch for 1-3 months; then lower-dose patches for 2-4 weeks each to taper off.
Nasal spray (Nicotrol NS)	Deliver one spray to each nostril every 30-60 minutes. Initial irritation (nasal burning, sneezing, watery eyes) resolves after 24-48 hours of use.
Inhaler (Nicotrol Inhaler)	The inhaler resembles a plastic cigarette that delivers nicotine flavored with menthol. Most patients use it 6-16 times a day for 3 months and then taper off over 2-3 months.
Bupropion (Wellbutrin)	Usually prescribed for 7 days before patient attempts to quit smoking and continued for 6-12 weeks. Can be used with nicotine patch.
	Do not exceed prescribed dosage. Overdosage can cause seizures.
	Advise your physician if you have a history of seizures or an eating disorder, both of which are contraindications for bupropion.

Ineffective Airway Clearance

Monitor for signs and symptoms of airway obstruction, including tachycardia, increasing dyspnea, and abnormal breath sounds. Demonstrate effective coughing techniques, and assess the patient's efforts. Encourage the patient to drink at least 2500 to 3000 mL of fluid each day unless contraindicated to help liquefy secretions for easier expectoration. Use a humidifier to decrease the drying of secretions. Perform chest physiotherapy as ordered, and evaluate the effects. If the patient is unable to expectorate, suctioning may be needed to remove secretions.

Anxiety

The most important intervention for relieving anxiety is helping the patient breathe more easily. Positioning and oxygen therapy are two simple measures that can be instituted promptly. Also, explain procedures and equipment to the patient. Remain calm and reassuring until the patient is more comfortable and relaxed. It is important to remember that irritability and anxiety are related to hypoxemia and that the patient is not just being difficult. Encourage a family member who has a calming influence on the patient to remain at the bedside. When leaving the patient, place the call bell within reach and instruct the patient in its use. Check on the patient often to provide reassurance that help is nearby if needed.

Imbalanced Nutrition: Less Than Body Requirements

The work of breathing is increased with COPD, which in turn increases the patient's caloric requirements. Some patients with COPD have difficulty maintaining adequate nutritional intake. Weigh the patient daily or weekly, depending on the situation, to monitor fluid and nutritional status. A patient with heart failure may gain weight because of fluid retention. Weight loss may indicate elimination of excess fluid or loss of body weight as a result of inadequate nutrition. Inadequate nutrition may be associated with dyspnea, anorexia, depression, or inability to obtain and prepare food.

The patient who is dyspneic may be given a soft diet with frequent small meals rather than three large meals daily. High-calorie, high-protein supplements may be provided as well. Try to plan nursing care so that the patient is not excessively tired or coughing during meals. To combat anorexia, consult with the dietitian to provide foods that are appealing to the patient. Assist the patient with oral hygiene before meals. Create a pleasant environment by removing soiled tissues and emesis basins. If the agency permits, encourage a family member to eat with the patient to provide a more social atmosphere. If the patient is unable to consume adequate nutrients, tube feeding or total parenteral nutrition may be instituted. If the patient is obese, discuss the benefits of weight loss.

Risk for Infection

Because of pooled secretions and poor nutritional status, the patient with chronic bronchitis and emphysema is at risk for respiratory infections. Monitor for fever and for green or yellow sputum. Promote good hydration and nutrition. Administer prophylactic antimicrobials as ordered. Advise patients to take annual influenza immunizations and to avoid people who are ill with infectious respiratory diseases. The physician may prescribe a Pneumovax vaccine for pneumococcal pneumonia.

Activity Intolerance

During hospitalization, attempt to schedule treatments, meals, and exercise so that the patient has time to rest. If the patient becomes excessively dyspneic or experiences tachycardia during activity, stop that activity until the patient recovers. When preparing for discharge,

Management and Supervision

Working with the Certified Nursing Assistant

- Demonstrate proper positioning of the patient with dyspnea to the certified nursing assistant (CNA).
- Although the CNA can count the patient's respiratory rate, the nurse should collect additional data including breath sounds.

Chronic Bronchitis and Emphysema

Patients with chronic bronchitis and emphysema need to know how they can manage the condition. However, patient instruction is best done in small units to prevent overtiring and overwhelming the patient. Supplement instruction with written material. Include the following:

- Take your prescribed drugs as instructed; report adverse effects to the physician.
- Avoid substances that irritate the airway.
- Cover the nose and mouth when outside in cold weather.
- To reduce risk of infection, avoid infected people.
- Report fever or increased symptoms to your physician promptly.
- Schedule your activities to allow adequate rest.
- If oxygen therapy is ordered, do not exceed the prescribed liter flow; to do so may depress your breathing.
- Smoking cessation can improve your symptoms. Programs and assistance are provided by the local chapter of the American Lung Association and the American Cancer Society.

help the patient plan a daily schedule that spaces more demanding activities and allows scheduled rest periods. Portable oxygen therapy may be ordered to permit greater mobility while receiving supplemental oxygen. At home, environmental adaptations may be needed, such as rearrangement of furniture to permit easy access to bathrooms and ramps to replace steps.

If the patient is participating in a rehabilitation program to improve exercise tolerance, monitor progress and provide encouragement and feedback.

Decreased Cardiac Output

Patients with chronic bronchitis and emphysema are at risk for right-sided heart failure that eventually affects the left side of the heart as well. Therefore monitor for signs of failure: increasing dyspnea, decreasing urine output, tachycardia, and dependent edema. Management of congestive heart failure is covered in Chapter 35. See the Management and Supervision box above.

BRONCHIECTASIS

Bronchiectasis is an abnormal dilation and distortion of the bronchi and bronchioles that is usually confined to one lung lobe or segment. It typically follows recurrent inflammatory conditions, infections, or obstructions but is sometimes congenital. The most prominent signs of bronchiectasis are coughing and the production of large amounts of purulent sputum. The patient also may have fever, hemoptysis, nasal stuffiness, sinus drainage, fatigue, and weakness.

The goals of medical treatment are to control symptoms and to prevent the spread to other areas of the lungs. Treatment consists of antibiotic therapy, bronchodilators, chest physiotherapy, and oxygen therapy. Severe bronchiectasis may be treated with surgical excision of the affected portion of the lung if the condition is confined to a limited area. Nursing care includes administration of prescribed drugs and treatments and documentation of the patient's response.

CYSTIC FIBROSIS

Cystic fibrosis is a hereditary disorder that is characterized by dysfunction of the exocrine glands and the production of thick, tenacious mucus. Cough is the first pulmonary symptom. It eventually becomes productive of thick, purulent sputum that obstructs the airways. Cystic fibrosis also results in obstruction of

the pancreatic ducts so that pancreatic enzymes cannot be delivered to the gastrointestinal (GI) tract. Without pancreatic enzymes, patients cannot effectively absorb proteins, fats, and fat-soluble vitamins. Their stools become bulky and foul smelling. Most patients do not develop diabetes because the endocrine function of the pancreas is still adequate. In most males, the vas deferens is absent, rendering them infertile. Women have reduced fertility as well. Patients lose more salt in sweat than normal, putting them at risk for salt depletion, especially in hot environments. Over a period of years, symptoms progress, with increasing dyspnea, decreasing exercise tolerance, and weight loss. Airway obstruction and decreased resistance to infections lead to chronic bacterial infections, emphysema, atelectasis, and respiratory failure.

Treatment

At one time, people with cystic fibrosis were unlikely to survive the early childhood years. Improved treatment, however, has resulted in more people with cystic fibrosis surviving to adulthood, so they are now more commonly seen in adult care settings. Treatment consists of pancreatic enzyme replacement, chest physiotherapy, and aerosol and nebulizer treatments to reduce mucus viscosity. Alternatives to manual chest physiotherapy include the flutter mucus clearance device, a handheld tool that vibrates to loosen secretions and promotes movement of secretions out of the lungs. An inflatable vest is also available that achieves similar results. Infections are treated with antibiotic therapy, usually administered parenterally, although some can be given by inhalation. Treatment of infections is complicated by the emergence of bacterial strains that are resistant to commonly used antibiotics. Other treatments that are used less often or in specific circumstances include bronchodilators, anti-inflammatory agents, inhaled deoxyribonuclease, and lung transplantation. It is hoped that gene therapy eventually will provide effective treatment of cystic fibrosis.

NURSING CARE *of the Patient with Cystic Fibrosis*

The goals of nursing care are effective airway clearance, prevention/treatment of infection, adequate nutrition, and effective therapeutic regimen management by patients and their families. Measures to clear the airway include administering prescribed medications, maintaining hydration, and performing chest physiotherapy. Infection prevention focuses on medical asepsis and protecting the patient from others with infections. To maintain adequate nutrition, administer pancreatic enzymes as ordered, allow for rest around mealtimes, and encourage the patient to consume adequate nutrients. Monitor stools to assess the adequacy of replacement enzymes. Frothy, bulky stools indicate inadequate enzymes. For adult cystic fibrosis patients, the therapeutic regimen has been a way of life. Allow the patient to maintain as much control as possible and try to maintain the patient's usual routines during hospitalization. Nevertheless, identify any teaching needs *with* the patient and family and design a teaching plan as appropriate.

CHRONIC RESTRICTIVE PULMONARY DISORDERS

In general, restrictive pulmonary disorders are those that result in reduced lung volumes with a normal to elevated ratio of forced expiratory volume in 1 second to forced vital capacity. Examples of restrictive disorders presented here are tuberculosis, sarcoidosis, pneumoconiosis, interstitial fibrosis, and lung cancer.

TUBERCULOSIS

Etiology and Risk Factors

Tuberculosis is an infection caused by *Mycobacterium tuberculosis*, an acid-fast aerobic bacterium. It is spread by droplets emitted by infected people during coughing, laughing, sneezing, and singing. Tuberculosis was a leading cause of death in the United States until effective drugs became available in the 1940s and 1950s. The incidence declined dramatically until 1986 when the numbers of reported cases began to rise. The rise

What Does Culture Have to Do with Tuberculosis?

In the United States, the incidence of tuberculosis is higher among non-white Americans and immigrants from Asia, Mexico, Africa, the Caribbean, and Latin America. The incidence is greatest in those ages 25 to 44 years among non-whites; among whites, the peak age is 70 years. These populations should be targeted for education and screening.

was variously attributed to the development of drug-resistant strains (multidrug-resistant TB or MDR-TB), the increasing population of immunosuppressed people with human immunodeficiency virus infection, and the influx of immigrants from developing nations. Even though the national incidence has fallen significantly beginning in 1992, the number of new cases continues to rise in many areas. Anyone may become infected with tuberculosis, but most healthy people are not infected through brief contact. Those at increased risk for tuberculosis include older adults; the economically disadvantaged and homeless; people who are substance abusers; children younger than 5 years; people who are immunosuppressed; and some racial and ethnic groups.

Pathophysiology

A patient's initial tuberculosis infection is called the *primary infection.* Most people in whom primary infections develop do not acquire active (symptomatic, progressive) tuberculosis. When the tuberculosis bacterium invades the lung, a small area becomes inflamed. The body's immune response attempts to destroy the infecting organisms, but some may escape and be carried into the lymph nodes or throughout the body. The site of the primary infection may undergo necrotic degeneration. Cavities develop that are filled with infectious material, which eventually liquefies. This material can drain into the tracheobronchial tree and be coughed up as sputum. The infected site usually heals, creating scar tissue (the lesion is called a *tubercle*), and sometimes shelters inactive bacteria. In some patients, however, the infectious process progresses and active tuberculosis develops. Also, it is possible for inactive bacteria to be reactivated, causing illness at a later time.

Tuberculosis is primarily an infection of the lungs, but the organisms may spread and cause infection in the bones, meninges, genitourinary tract, lymph nodes, pleurae, pericardium, abdomen, and endocrine glands. *M. tuberculosis* infection outside the lungs is called *extrapulmonary tuberculosis.*

Signs and Symptoms

Signs and symptoms of pulmonary tuberculosis may include cough, night sweats, chest pain and tightness, fatigue, anorexia, weight loss, and low-grade fever. The cough is often persistent and productive and may produce bloody sputum (hemoptysis). Older adults may have only vague symptoms and fever of undetermined origin. Tuberculosis should be considered in patients who have pneumonia that does not respond to usual therapy.

Medical Diagnosis

The patient's history and physical examination may lead the physician to suspect tuberculosis, especially if there is known exposure to high-risk people. Tests to confirm the diagnosis include sputum cultures, acid-fast smears of potentially infected body fluids, tuberculin skin tests, and chest radiographs. Tuberculin skin tests are commonly used for screening. People who have been infected mount an immune response that causes a local reaction when tuberculin, a protein fraction of the tubercle bacillus, is injected intradermally. The patient is said to have a positive reaction if a hard area (induration) of 5 mm or more develops at the site within 48 to 72 hours. A positive reaction may indicate active or inactive infection (see the Diagnostics Tests and Procedures table on pp. 517 and 518 in Chapter 30).

A number of factors including a history of BCG vaccination may cause false-negative reactions; that is, an induration does not develop even though the patient does have the infection. To determine if a person has the ability to respond to any antigen, additional antigens may be used with the tuberculin. If the patient has no response to any of the antigens, additional testing is needed to rule out tuberculosis.

The Tuberculosis Stat Test detects *M. tuberculosis* in respiratory secretions within 48 hours. The test does not distinguish between active and past infections and is very expensive, so it is used less often than the tuberculin skin test. When tuberculosis is suspected, a chest radiograph is useful in detecting the disease. The use of the CT scan as a diagnostic tool is increasing.

Medical Treatment

Patients who have positive results for tuberculosis on skin tests and negative results on chest radiographs but are at increased risk for the disease are usually treated prophylactically to prevent development of active tuberculosis. The most common preventive treatment is isoniazid (INH) therapy for 9 to 12 months. Individuals with inactive tuberculosis may be treated with INH alone, INH with rifampin, or rifampin with pyrazinamide.

For patients with active tuberculosis, the Centers for Disease Control and Prevention recommends combination drug therapy selected from the first-line drugs that include isoniazid, ethambutol, rifampin or rifabutin, and pyrazinamide. An example of an initial regimen for a person with culture-positive pulmonary tuberculosis caused by drug-sensitive organisms is as follows: INH, rifampin, pyrazinamide, and ethambutol given every day for 56 doses. The patient would then continue therapy with only INH and rifampin daily for 126 doses. Numerous second-line drugs are available for patients who cannot tolerate or do not respond to first-line drugs. These include cycloserine, ethionamide, levofloxacin, moxifloxacin, gatifloxacin, para-aminosalicylic acid, streptomycin, amikacin/kanamycin, and capreomycin.

Pharmacology Capsule

Pyridoxine (vitamin B$_6$) may be ordered with isoniazid to prevent peripheral neuritis.

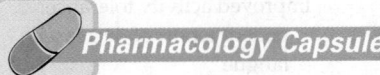

Pharmacology Capsule

A common treatment plan for tuberculosis begins with a 2-month course of isoniazid, rifampin, pyrazinamide, and ethambutol that is followed by 4 months of isoniazid and rifampin alone.

The course of therapy may range from 6 to 24 months. Most drugs can be given in daily doses or twice-weekly doses. Drug therapy for MDR-TB may use various combinations of the drugs just listed with the addition of others as indicated. The risk of adverse effects with long-term drug therapy is significant, so patient monitoring is essential. Adverse effects are especially common in older adults. Hospitalization is sometimes indicated when drug therapy is initiated. Because the organism that causes tuberculosis readily develops resistance to drugs, it is extremely important that patients take the correct drug dosages for the prescribed period of time. Incomplete courses of therapy foster resistant organisms and relapses of the infection. Therefore directly observed therapy (DOT) is recommended to ensure that patients are taking the drugs as prescribed. DOT is recommended in the case of pulmonary tuberculosis with positive sputum smears, treatment failure, disease relapse, drug resistance, HIV infection, psychiatric illness, substance abuse , memory impairment, and history of nonadherence to therapy.

NURSING CARE *of the Patient with Tuberculosis*

Assessment

Assessment of the patient with a respiratory disorder is outlined in Box 30-1 on p. 516 in Chapter 30. When tuberculosis is suspected or confirmed, a complete health history and a physical examination are essential because the infection may not be confined to the lung. The nurse may be responsible for reading the reaction to the skin test.

Nursing Diagnoses, Goals, and Outcome Criteria: Tuberculosis	
NURSING DIAGNOSES	GOALS AND OUTCOME CRITERIA
Impaired Gas Exchange related to respiratory secretions, effects of the infectious process	Improved gas exchange: no dyspnea
Social Isolation related to medically imposed isolation, fear of contagious disease	Reduced social isolation: less feeling of loneliness or rejection
Risk for Injury related to spread of the infection, reactivation of the infection secondary to lowered resistance	Knowledge of measures to decrease disease progression and reactivation of infection: patient demonstrates precautions

Continued

Fatigue related to infection, weight loss, coughing	Improved activity tolerance: patient report of decreased fatigue
Imbalanced Nutrition: Less Than Body Requirements related to anorexia, fatigue, inadequate financial resources, lack of knowledge	Improved nutritional status: stable body weight; normalization of weight if malnourished
Ineffective Therapeutic Regimen Management related to lack of understanding of treatment and risk of reactivation, lack of financial resources	Effective management of prescribed therapy: patient states intention to comply, obtains and takes drugs as prescribed

Interventions

Impaired Gas Exchange

Routinely monitor the patient's respiratory status. Instruct the patient in effective coughing to expectorate secretions. Encourage ambulation as tolerated and within medically prescribed limits. Assist the patient who has limited mobility to change position at least every 2 hours. Although dyspnea is not common except with pleural effusion, elevate the head of the bed for the patient who is dyspneic.

Social Isolation

The patient who is thought to have active tuberculosis is isolated at first. Practice good hand washing and wear masks (disposable particulate respirators) during contacts. Gowns are unnecessary unless there is gross contamination of clothing. The patient may feel rejected and be fearful that others will avoid contact. Encourage expression of feelings about the diagnosis and the isolation. Instruct visitors in measures to reduce the risk of infection.

Risk for Injury

Once antibiotic therapy has been initiated and the patient's sputum cultures demonstrate low counts of acid-fast bacilli, the patient usually can be discharged. Explain to the patient how the infection is transmitted and how to protect others. The patient should always cover the nose and mouth when sneezing or coughing. Disposable tissues should be used and discarded in a sanitary way. Members of the patient's household are tested for active disease. Those who have positive skin tests but are asymptomatic are usually given prophylactic therapy to prevent development of active tuberculosis. One problem with the homeless population is that it may be impossible to locate contacts. Emphasize the importance of the patient completing the full course of therapy. Otherwise, the infection may be reactivated.

Fatigue

Fatigue is fairly common with tuberculosis. Adjust the patient's schedule to allow for periods of rest. Assure the patient that fatigue diminishes as treatment progresses.

Imbalanced Nutrition: Less Than Body Requirements

Anorexia and nausea are common adverse effects of antitubercular drugs. Monitor the patient's weight at regular intervals. Some measures that may reduce the drug's side effects include taking it at bedtime and taking antinausea drugs. Explain the role of nutrition in recovering from an infectious disease, and encourage the patient to eat a balanced diet. Five or six small meals may be more acceptable than three large ones to the patient who has a poor appetite. Respect food preferences as much as possible. For patients who are homeless or have a low income, ask the social worker to locate services that provide food or prepared meals. Some foods can cause serious reactions if consumed with antitubercular medications. Be sure to provide the patient a written list of any foods that should be avoided.

Ineffective Therapeutic Regimen Management

A major problem with treating tuberculosis is failure to complete the lengthy prescribed drug therapy. Nurses must realize that there are many reasons that patients do not take drugs as ordered, including denial of the illness, lack of understanding, adverse drug effects, and inadequate money. Intervention should be based on the reason for the patient's noncompliance. Explain

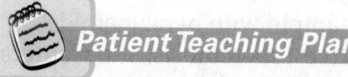

Patient Teaching Plan

Tuberculosis

People with tuberculosis are usually hospitalized for just a short time, so you must implement efficient patient teaching. Supplement verbal instructions with written material. Subjects to include in the teaching plan are the following:

- Tuberculosis is spread by airborne droplets. Protect others by covering your mouth when coughing, laughing, or sneezing. Wash your hands often.
- Effective treatment requires taking drugs exactly as prescribed for the full course of therapy to prevent reinfection. Notify your physician of adverse effects of your drugs, but do not stop taking them unless advised by the physician.
- If you are taking isoniazid, you must avoid foods containing tyramine (e.g., aged cheeses, smoked fish) and histamine (tuna, sauerkraut). These foods combined with isoniazid can make you very ill.
- Good hygiene, nutrition, and hydration can help you recover.
- Rifampin causes body fluids to become red-orange and may stain soft contact lenses.

What Does Culture Have to Do with Patient Teaching?

To be effective, the teaching plan for the patient with tuberculosis must consider the patient's native language, vocabulary, lifestyle, and financial resources.

---

the infectious process and its treatment. Reinforce the physician's instructions for the drugs, and emphasize that failure to complete the course of therapy results in reactivation of the infection that may be more difficult to treat. Encourage the patient to report adverse drug effects, and seek solutions to make them more tolerable. If the patient cannot afford the drugs, consult a social worker to help the patient obtain financial assistance. Patients who are unable to manage daily self-medication can be given doses twice or three times weekly in a health care setting or the patient's worksite or place of residence. This approach is called *directly observed therapy (DOT).*

INTERSTITIAL LUNG DISEASE

Interstitial lung diseases include several conditions in which there is inflammation of the lower respiratory tract and thickening and fibrosis of the alveolar walls, which render the alveoli nonfunctional. The condition may be caused by inhaled substances or connective tissue disorders, but sometimes no specific cause is identified. Some examples of interstitial lung diseases are idiopathic pulmonary fibrosis, including occupational lung diseases, and sarcoidosis.

Idiopathic Pulmonary Fibrosis

Pathophysiology

Idiopathic pulmonary fibrosis is the formation of scar tissue in the lung tissue after inflammation or irritation. It may be related to cigarette smoking, frequent aspiration, or exposure to environmental or occupations substances. Discussion of some specific occupational lung diseases follow.

Complications

Severe fibrosis may lead to pulmonary hypertension (increased pressure in the pulmonary artery caused by obstruction to blood flow in pulmonary vessels), cor pulmonale, and ventilatory failure, in which case the patient is said to have end-stage disease.

Signs and Symptoms

The primary symptoms of diffuse interstitial fibrosis are nonproductive cough and progressive dyspnea. Inspirational crackles are heard in the lungs on auscultation. The patient may have clubbing of the fingertips.

Medical Treatment

The condition is treated with corticosteroids to reduce inflammation, bronchodilators, and oxygen therapy.

Corticosteroid treatment may prevent additional damage but does not correct existing fibrosis. Cytotoxic drugs such as Imuran and antifibrotic agents such as colchicines also may be used. None of these treatments significantly improve survival or quality of life. The patient should avoid additional exposure to the offending substance. Lung transplantation may be recommended for end-stage disease.

NURSING CARE *of the Patient with Idiopathic Pulmonary Fibrosis*

Assessment

The complete assessment of the patient with a respiratory disorder is summarized in Box 30-1 on p. 516 in Chapter 30.

Nursing Diagnoses, Goals, and Outcome Criteria: Idiopathic Pulmonary Fibrosis	
Nursing Diagnoses	Goals and Outcome Criteria
Impaired Gas Exchange related to alveolar damage	Improved gas exchange: normal pulse and respirations, no cyanosis, normal blood gases
Activity Intolerance related to inadequate oxygenation	Improved activity tolerance: lack of dyspnea on exertion, gradual improvement in tolerance of daily activities
Risk for Infection related to immune suppression by corticosteroids	Reduced risk of infection: patient practices infection control measures
Ineffective Airway Clearance related to increased secretions	Effective airway clearance: clear breath sounds, normal pulse, expectoration of secretions
Anxiety related to dyspnea or possible disabling illness	Decreased anxiety: calm manner, patient statement of lessened anxiety

Interventions

Nursing interventions are similar to those described for the patient with COPD.

Occupational Lung Diseases

The inhalation of various particles in the work setting can lead to lung conditions classified as occupational lung diseases. Examples of offending substances are dust, ammonia, chlorine, plant and animal proteins, silica, asbestos, and coal dust. The Occupational Safety and Health Administration provides regulations that are intended to protect workers from exposure that could lead to occupational lung diseases.

Categories of occupational lung diseases are described here briefly. The nursing care of patients with occupational lung diseases varies with the severity of symptoms but is similar to that provided to the patient with COPD.

Acute Respiratory Irritation

The inhalation of gases such as ammonia or chlorine causes acute respiratory irritation. The effects are usually temporary, but if the lower airways are affected, the patient may have pulmonary edema or alveolar damage and airway obstruction. The patient may have coughing, wheezing, and dyspnea. Symptoms resolve within a few days to several weeks, and there is usually no permanent lung damage. The treatment focuses on management of the symptoms and avoidance of future exposure.

Occupational Asthma

Inhalation of plant or animal proteins may cause an allergic reaction referred to as *occupational asthma.* Treatment is the same as that for bronchial asthma. Although the initial acute symptoms usually last only a few hours, the patient may continue to have a hyper-reactive airway for years. This means that future exposure to irritants may trigger acute asthmatic symptoms. The patient should avoid continued exposure to the offending substance.

Hypersensitivity Pneumonitis

Hypersensitivity pneumonitis is an allergic inflammatory response of the alveoli to inhaled organic particles. The reaction may resolve within a few days, or the patient may contract pulmonary edema or interstitial fibrosis with permanent restrictive or restrictive-obstructive disease. The condition may be treated with corticosteroids and avoidance of the irritants. Respiratory support may be needed if symptoms are severe.

Pneumoconiosis

Lung disease caused by inhalation of various dusts is called pneumoconiosis. Pneumoconiosis develops in response to repeated exposure to silica, asbestos, or coal dust and is characterized by diffuse pulmonary fibrosis and restrictive lung disease. The effects are usually aggravated by cigarette smoking, so patients are advised to avoid both the offending dust and the cigarette smoke. Otherwise, treatment is symptomatic.

Asbestosis is a pneumoconiosis caused by occupational exposure to asbestos, an insulating material. Asbestos exposure has been linked to pleural effusions, pleural fibrosis, and malignant mesotheliomas (a specific type of lung cancer). Fear of asbestosis has led to the removal of asbestos insulation from public buildings in many cities, but there is disagreement as to whether the insulation actually poses any public health threat.

Sarcoidosis
Pathophysiology

Sarcoidosis is an inflammatory condition that may affect the skin, eyes, lungs, liver, spleen, bones, salivary glands, joints, and heart. An unknown factor triggers a series of immune processes leading to the formation of clusters of cells and debris in affected tissues called

What Does Culture Have to Do with Sarcoidosis?

In the United States, sarcoidosis more commonly affects African-Americans than white Americans and is twice as common in African-American women as in African-American men.

granulomas. Granulomas in the lungs may resolve or may progress to fibrosis, in which case a restrictive pulmonary condition exists. The course of sarcoidosis is variable. In some patients, it is acute and resolves even without treatment. Others have periods of remission and exacerbations, which may progress to disabling restrictive lung disease.

Signs and Symptoms

Although many patients with sarcoidosis have no symptoms, others experience dry cough, dyspnea, chest pain, hemoptysis, fatigue, weakness, weight loss, and fever.

Medical Diagnosis

A diagnosis of sarcoidosis is based on results of chest radiography, pulmonary function tests, and flexible bronchoscopy with transbronchial lung biopsy.

Medical Treatment

If the patient is asymptomatic, no treatment is indicated. Symptoms usually respond well to a 6- to 12-month course of systemic corticosteroids. Methotrexate has been used as an alternative to corticosteroids in some situations. Lung transplantation is the only option for patients with end-stage pulmonary disease who do not respond to drug therapy. However, the disease may recur in the transplanted lung.

NURSING CARE *of the Patient with Sarcoidosis*

Nursing care of the patient with sarcoidosis focuses on monitoring the patient for progressive dysfunction and teaching about corticosteroid therapy, if prescribed. Care of the patient with severe pulmonary symptoms is similar to that for patients with COPD.

LUNG CANCER
Etiology and Risk Factors

Lung cancer is the leading cause of cancer death in the United States. The incidence is decreasing among men but has been rising steadily among women. Since 1987, the death rate from lung cancer has exceeded that from breast cancer in women.

Cigarette smoking is the leading cause of lung cancer. The risk is increased even more for smokers who are exposed to other carcinogenic substances, such as arsenic, asbestos, and radioactive materials. Evidence is increasing that "secondhand" smoke poses a threat to nonsmokers as well. Air pollution may be an additional risk factor.

Pathophysiology

There are two major categories of lung cancer: small cell ("oat cell") lung carcinoma (SCLC); and non–small cell lung carcinoma (NSCLC). NSCLC includes squamous cell carcinomas, adenocarcinomas, large cell carcinomas, and bronchial carcinoids. Small cell and large cell undifferentiated carcinomas grow rapidly; other lung cancers grow slowly. They all can metastasize to other body organs. Enlarging tumors or metastatic lesions may compress the laryngeal and phrenic nerves, the esophagus, and the major blood vessels. SCLCs, which grow rapidly, tend to metastasize early. They can invade the pericardium, causing pericardial effusion (fluid accumulation in the pericardial sac) and possibly triggering dysrhythmias.

Signs and Symptoms

The warning signs of lung cancer are persistent cough, hemoptysis, chest pain, and recurring pneumonia or bronchitis. Patients also may have dyspnea, weight loss, and pain in the shoulder, arm, or hand. There is some variation with the type of cancer as well as the location. Other signs and symptoms may be related to metastatic lesions. For example, invasion of the tumor into the ribs produces bone pain and invasion of the pericardium may produce cardiac dysrhythmias.

Medical Diagnosis

Diagnostic tests and procedures for lung cancer include radiographic procedures (chest radiography, computed tomography scan, MRI), fiberoptic bronchoscopy, sputum cytology studies, and biopsy of tissue obtained through bronchoscopy, percutaneous transthoracic fine-needle biopsy, thoracotomy, or other methods. Information about specific procedures appears in the Diagnostic Tests and Procedures table on pp. 517 and 518 in Chapter 30. Unfortunately, lesions often are not detectable until they are no longer localized. Radionuclide scans of the bones, liver, or brain may be ordered to detect metastatic lesions.

Medical Treatment

Early detection is the key to survival of lung cancer, but this is difficult because metastasis often occurs before the lesion can be seen on radiographs. Treatment decisions are made on the basis of tumor type, lymph node involvement, evidence of metastasis, and the patient's general state of health. Options include radiotherapy, surgery, chemotherapy, and targeted biologic therapies.

Radiotherapy. Radiotherapy may be used alone or in combination with other treatment methods. It may be curative in some situations but also may be used to temporarily relieve symptoms by reducing the size of the lesion. Radiotherapy for lung cancer may include external beam irradiation and brachytherapy. Brachytherapy is direct irradiation by placement of the radiation source at the site of the tumor. Complications of endobronchial irradiation are pulmonary hemorrhage and radiation bronchitis and stenosis. Other general complications of radiotherapy are discussed in Chapter 25.

Chemotherapy. Chemotherapy may be used alone or with radiation in the treatment of SCLC. There is debate about the value of chemotherapy in other types of lung cancers, but research continues to explore various treatment combinations of agents such as carboplatin, vinblastine, mitomycin C, ifosfamide, and etoposide. Cisplatin and paclitaxel often are used in combination. These and other chemotherapeutic agents are discussed in Chapter 25.

Targeted Biologic Therapies. Targeted biologic therapies that block the activity of growth factor receptors are being studied for their value in cancer treatment. Examples of these agents are gefitinib (Iressa) and erlotinib (Tarceva). Gefitinib has been used to treat advanced NSCLC but is no longer recommended by the FDA except for patients who have been taking it and seem to have benefited.

Surgical Treatment. Surgical intervention is the treatment of choice for early NSCLC. The goal of surgery is to remove the entire tumor while removing as little healthy surrounding tissue as possible. Removal of

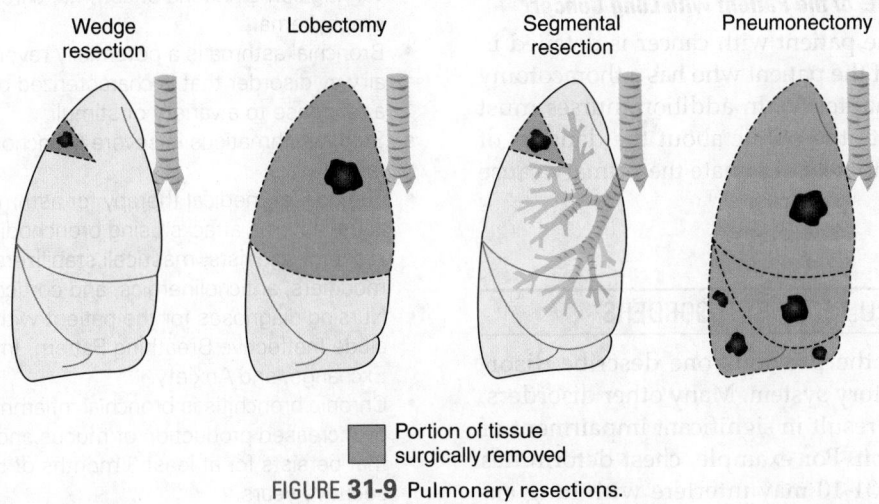

Wedge resection   Lobectomy   Segmental resection   Pneumonectomy

Portion of tissue surgically removed

FIGURE **31-9** Pulmonary resections.

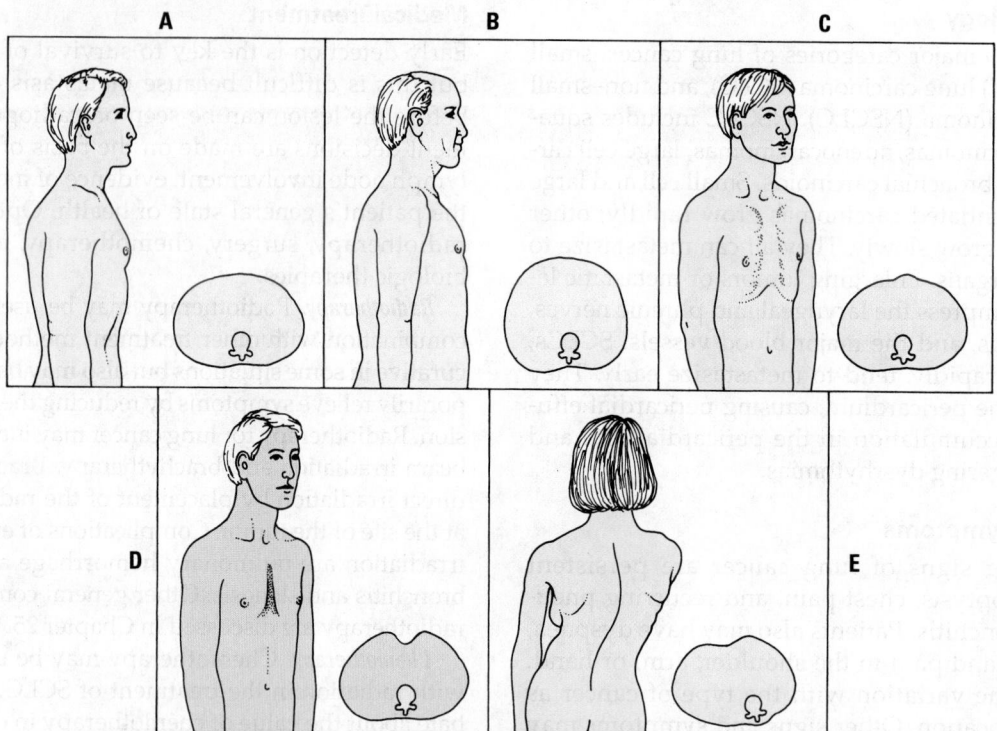

FIGURE 31-10 Normal adult chest (**A**) and chest deformities that may affect respiratory function (**B-E**). **B,** Increased anteroposterior diameter ("barrel chest"). **C,** Pectus excavatum ("funnel chest"). **D,** Pectus carinatum ("pigeon chest"). **E,** Thoracic kyphoscoliosis.

a section of tissue is called a *resection*. With lung surgery, the procedure may be a wedge resection, sleeve lobectomy, segmental resection, lobectomy, or pneumonectomy. These procedures are illustrated in Figure 31-9. Tumors that are accessible with a bronchoscope are sometimes treated with laser therapy. Radiotherapy, chemotherapy, or both may be used before or after surgery.

Despite advances in treatment, the 5-year survival rate for lung cancer remains 15%. Survival improves with early treatment, but American Cancer Society data indicate that only 16% of all lung cancers are detected while still localized. The outlook is best for stages I and II NSCLC treated surgically.

NURSING CARE *of the Patient with Lung Cancer*

Nursing care of the patient with cancer is detailed in Chapter 25. Care of the patient who has a thoracotomy is discussed in Chapter 30. In addition, nurses must continue to educate the public about the dangers of cigarette smoking to help eliminate the primary cause of lung cancer.

EXTRAPULMONARY DISORDERS

This chapter and the previous one describe disorders of the respiratory system. Many other disorders, however, also can result in significant impairment of respiratory function. For example, chest deformities as seen in Figure 31-10 may interfere with lung ex-

pansion. Neuromuscular diseases such as myasthenia gravis and amyotrophic lateral sclerosis affect the muscles of respiration. Head or spinal cord injuries can disrupt the breathing center in the brain or the neural control of the diaphragm. Heart failure with pulmonary edema fills the lungs with fluid, interfering with the exchange of gases. The specific interventions are covered with each of these conditions in other chapters.

Key Points

- Chronic obstructive pulmonary disease (COPD) includes varying combinations of asthma, chronic bronchitis, and emphysema.
- Bronchial asthma is a potentially reversible obstructive airway disorder that is characterized by bronchospasm as a response to a variety of stimuli.
- Status asthmaticus is severe bronchospasm that can be fatal.
- The goal of medical therapy for asthma is to prevent acute asthma attacks using bronchodilators, beta$_2$-receptor agonists, mast cell stabilizers, leukotriene modifiers, anticholinergics, and corticosteroids.
- Nursing diagnoses for the patient with asthma may include Ineffective Breathing Pattern, Impaired Gas Exchange, and Anxiety.
- Chronic bronchitis is bronchial inflammation characterized by increased production of mucus and chronic cough that persists for at least 3 months of the year for 2 consecutive years.

- Pulmonary emphysema, which often coexists with chronic bronchitis, is a degenerative, nonreversible disease characterized by the breakdown of the alveolar septa distal to the terminal bronchioles.
- Centrilobular pulmonary emphysema is characterized by breakdown of respiratory bronchioles; panlobular pulmonary emphysema by breakdown of alveolar walls and respiratory bronchioles.
- Nursing diagnoses for the patient with chronic bronchitis and emphysema may include Impaired Gas Exchange, Ineffective Airway Clearance, Anxiety, Imbalanced Nutrition: Less Than Body Requirements, Risk for Infection, Activity Intolerance, and Decreased Cardiac Output.
- Smoking cessation is an important aspect of management of COPD and other cardiovascular and respiratory conditions, but success rates for stop-smoking programs are low.
- Bronchiectasis is an abnormal dilation and distortion of the bronchi and bronchioles that causes coughing and the production of large amounts of sputum and is often associated with infection.
- Restrictive pulmonary disorders result in reduced lung volumes.
- Tuberculosis is an infectious disease of the lungs and other body tissues that requires long-term drug therapy.
- Nursing diagnoses for the patient with tuberculosis may include Impaired Gas Exchange, Social Isolation, Risk for Injury, Fatigue, Imbalanced Nutrition: Less Than Body

Requirements, and Ineffective Therapeutic Regimen Management.
- Sarcoidosis is an inflammatory condition that may resolve with corticosteroid treatment or may lead to fibrosis.
- Idiopathic pulmonary fibrosis is an inflammatory condition in which there is thickening and fibrosis of the alveolar walls that render the alveoli nonfunctional
- Occupational lung diseases are caused by the inhalation of various substances and include acute respiratory irritation, occupational asthma, hypersensitivity pneumonitis, and pneumoconiosis.
- Nursing diagnoses for the patient with interstitial fibrosis may include Impaired Gas Exchange, Ineffective Airway Clearance, Activity Intolerance, and Anxiety.
- Lung cancer, the leading cause of cancer death in the United States, is usually caused by cigarette smoking and is most treatable if detected while still localized.
- Extrapulmonary causes of respiratory problems may be skeletal, neuromuscular, neurologic, or cardiac.

 Go to your Companion CD-ROM for a Pharmacology Tutorial, Audio Glossary, and 3-D animations.

evolve Be sure to visit the companion Evolve site at http://evolve.elsevier.com/Linton/ for WebLinks and additional online resources.

REVIEW QUESTIONS *Choose the best answer.*

1. The late phase of an acute asthma attack is characterized by:
   1. Bronchospasm
   2. Increased mucus secretion
   3. Hypoxemia
   4. Hyperresponsive airway

2. Drugs that are effective in *relieving* acute symptoms of asthma include the following:
   1. Beta$_2$-receptor agonists
   2. Corticosteroids
   3. Mast cell stabilizers
   4. Leukotriene modifiers

3. Asthma patients use peak expiratory flow rate meters to:
   1. Improve ventilation
   2. Monitor level of control
   3. Prevent hypostatic pneumonia
   4. Measure permanent lung damage

4. A patient's health history includes "reports persistent productive cough for 3 to 4 months each winter for the past 5 years." You recognize these symptoms as typical of:
   1. Centrilobular emphysema
   2. Asthma
   3. Chronic bronchitis
   4. Tuberculosis

5. What is the nursing implication when a COPD patient has hypoxic drive?
   1. The patient needs deep-breathing exercises to improve oxygenation.
   2. The patient's oxygen therapy should not exceed 3 L/min.
   3. The patient is unable to tolerate any activity and should remain in bed.
   4. The patient is in respiratory acidosis and requires emergency care.

6. During a routine visit with a COPD patient, a home health nurse finds the patient to have increased dyspnea since the last visit, heart rate of 92 bpm, and edematous ankles. The nurse should:
   1. Increase the patient's oxygen flow rate to 5 L/min
   2. Encourage the patient to walk more to promote circulation
   3. Document the findings and have the patient return in 1 week for follow-up
   4. Contact the physician to report signs of congestive heart failure

7. The priority nursing diagnosis for the patient with cystic fibrosis is:
   1. Ineffective Airway Clearance
   2. Risk for Infection
   3. Imbalanced Nutrition: Less Than Body Requirements
   4. Risk for Deficient Fluid Volume

8. Patient teaching for the person with active tuberculosis should include the following:
    1. You can stop taking your medications when your symptoms go away
    2. Cover your mouth when coughing to prevent spreading the infection
    3. Antitubercular drugs have no serious side effects
    4. Tuberculosis affects only people who do not have good hygiene

9. The primary drug used for the prevention and treatment of tuberculosis is:
    1. Rifampin
    2. Streptomycin
    3. Ethambutol
    4. Isoniazid

10. The leading cause of lung cancer is:
    1. Asbestos
    2. Smoking
    3. Coal dust
    4. Silica

CHAPTER 32 Hematologic Disorders

STACEY YOUNG-McCAUGHAN*

evolve http://evolve.elsevier.com/Linton/

Objectives

After reading and studying this chapter, you should be able to:

1. List the components of the hematologic system and describe their role in oxygenation and hemostasis.
2. Identify data to be collected when assessing a patient with a disorder of the hematologic system.
3. Describe tests and procedures used to diagnose disorders of the hematologic system and nursing considerations for each.
4. Describe nursing care for patients undergoing common therapeutic measures for disorders of the hematologic system.
5. Describe the pathophysiology, signs and symptoms, medical diagnosis, and medical treatment for selected disorders of the hematologic system,.
6. Assist in planning nursing care for a patient with a disorder of the hematologic system.

Key Terms

Be sure to check out the bonus material on the Companion CD-ROM, including selected audio pronunciations.

anemia (ă-NĒ-mē-ă, p. 581)
ecchymosis (ĕk-ĭ-MŌ-sĭs, p. 576)
hemostasis (hē-mŏ-STĀ-sĭs, p. 571)
orthostatic vital sign changes (ŏr-thō-STĂT-ĭk, p. 575)
oxygenation (ŏk-sĭ-jĕ-NĀ-shŭn, p. 571)
petechiae (pĕ-TĒ-kē-ă, p. 575)
purpura (PŬR-pū-ră, p. 576)
universal donor (p. 578)
universal recipient (p. 578)

The primary functions of the hematologic system are oxygenation and hemostasis (control of bleeding). Disorders of the hematologic system can be either a primary disease or a complication of another disease. The diagnosis and treatment of these disorders can be very complex. The nurse plays an important role in helping assess, plan, and manage the care of these patients.

*The views of this author are her own and do not purport to reflect the position of the Army Medical Department, the Department of the Army, or the Department of Defense.

ANATOMY AND PHYSIOLOGY OF THE HEMATOLOGIC SYSTEM

ANATOMIC STRUCTURES AND COMPONENTS OF THE HEMATOLOGIC SYSTEM

Important structures and components of the hematologic system are the bone marrow, the liver, the spleen, and the blood.

Bone Marrow

The bone marrow is the spongy center of the bones where the red blood cells and platelets are made. The marrow of all bones produces these cells; however, the majority of red blood cells and platelets are produced in the vertebrae, ribs, sternum, skull, pelvis, and long bones of the legs.

Liver

The liver is located in the upper right quadrant of the abdomen, under the rib cage and below the diaphragm. The liver performs many functions for different body systems. As part of the hematologic system, the liver manufactures clotting factors. In addition, the liver clears old and damaged red blood cells from circulation.

Spleen

The spleen is located in the upper left quadrant of the abdomen. Like the liver, the spleen performs many functions for different body systems. As part of the hematologic system, the spleen removes old red blood cells from circulation.

Blood

Blood is a generic term referring to a mixture of red blood cells, platelets, clotting factors, and plasma as well as white blood cells, proteins, electrolytes, hormones, and enzymes that travel through vessels in the body (Fig. 32-1). Blood serves many functions, but as part of the hematologic system, it transports oxygen from the lungs to tissues and maintains hemostasis. A healthy adult has about 6 liters of blood circulating through the body pumped by the heart.

Red Blood Cells (RBCs or Erythrocytes). Red blood cells are made in the bone marrow. Once released from the

FIGURE **32-1 A,** Blood is composed of plasma (about 55%) and cellular elements (about 45%). **B,** Cellular elements include leukocytes (WBCs); thrombocytes (platelets) *(1)*; and erythrocytes (RBCs) *(2).* There are 600 times as many erythrocytes as leukocytes.

marrow, they circulate in the body, transporting oxygen from the lungs to the tissues and carbon dioxide from the tissues back to the lungs. Hemoglobin in the red blood cells makes the transport of oxygen and carbon dioxide possible. The tough, flexible membrane of the red blood cells allows these disk-shaped cells to maneuver through the smallest capillaries. After about 120 days, the old red blood cells are filtered out of circulation by the liver and spleen. The iron and heme in the old red blood cells are recycled to make new red blood cells.

Red blood cells normally have various proteins, called *antigens,* as part of their cell membranes. The two major antigens are named *A* and *B.* Based on the presence or absence of the A and B antigens, a person's blood type is determined. People with type A blood have the A antigen, those with type B blood have the B antigen, those with type AB blood have both the A and B antigens, and those with type O blood have neither the A nor the B antigen. Rhesus (Rh) is another type of red blood cell antigen that is either present or absent. People with the Rh antigen are designated *Rh positive* (Rh), whereas those without the Rh antigen are designated *Rh negative* (Rh̄).

Platelets (Thrombocytes). Platelets also are produced in the bone marrow. Platelets activate the blood clotting system by going to a break in a blood vessel and forming a platelet plug. At the same time, other clotting mechanisms are activated and the body begins repairing itself. Once released into circulation from the bone marrow, the normal life span of a platelet is 10 days.

Clotting Factors. Once platelets activate the blood clotting system, several clotting factors are activated. The clotting factors are numbered I through XIII and include fibrinogen (factor I) and thrombin (factor II). The clotting factors form a stable fibrin matrix over the wounded area, protecting the injured site while the healing process is completed.

Plasma. Plasma is the clear, straw-colored fluid that carries the red blood cells, platelets, and clotting factors through the circulatory system. Plasma is primarily water. The other major components of plasma are the plasma proteins, albumin, and globulins.

PHYSIOLOGIC FUNCTIONS OF THE HEMATOLOGIC SYSTEM
Oxygenation
Red blood cells transport oxygen from the lungs to the tissues and carry carbon dioxide from the tissues back to the lungs for excretion. The hemoglobin in the red blood cells combines easily with both oxygen and carbon dioxide to accomplish oxygenation.

Hemostasis
Hemostasis means control of bleeding. It is how the body maintains the integrity of the circulatory system. If a blood vessel is injured, three things occur: (1) the blood vessel constricts, reducing the amount of bleeding; (2) platelets adhere to the injured blood vessel, forming an unstable platelet plug; and (3) the coagulation cascade is initiated, forming a stable fibrin matrix, which is commonly recognized as a scab. The *coagulation cascade* is a term used to describe the series of events that occur in the process of blood clotting (Fig. 32-2).

AGE-RELATED CHANGES

With advancing age, the bone marrow becomes less productive. Hematologic function is generally not affected unless a person is unusually stressed with trauma, a chronic illness, or treatment for cancer. Yet even with conditions necessitating a higher production of blood cells, the bone marrow can usually respond to the increased demand, given time.

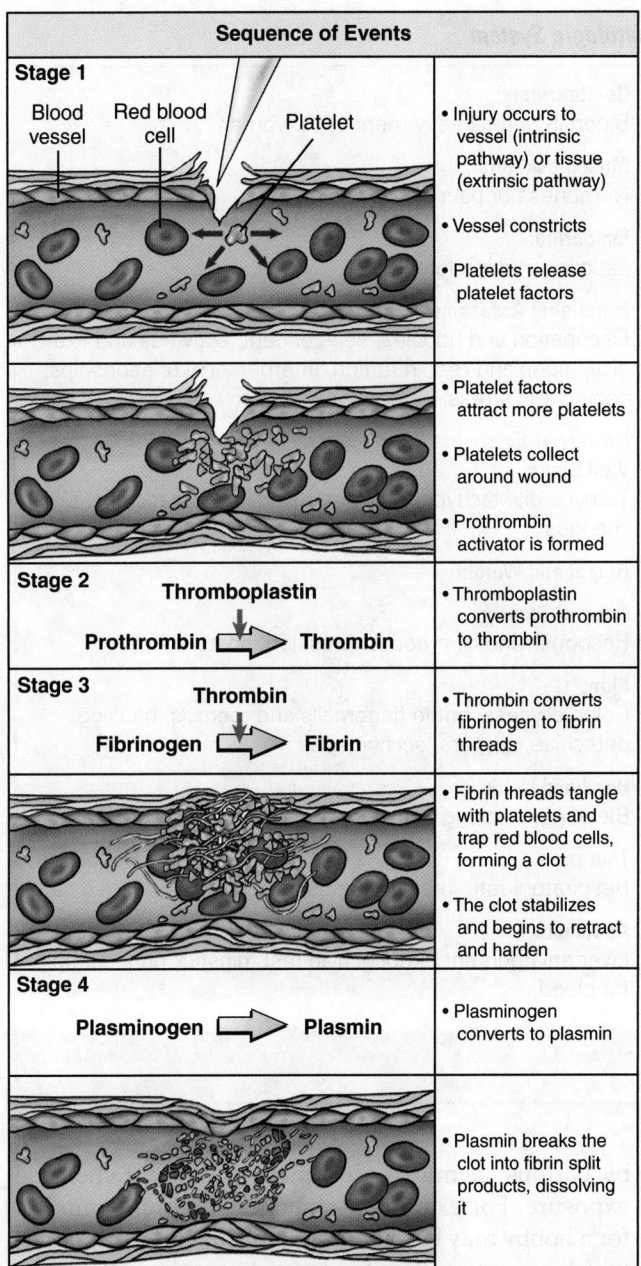

Sequence of Events	
Stage 1 Blood vessel Red blood cell Platelet	• Injury occurs to vessel (intrinsic pathway) or tissue (extrinsic pathway) • Vessel constricts • Platelets release platelet factors
	• Platelet factors attract more platelets • Platelets collect around wound • Prothrombin activator is formed
Stage 2 Thromboplastin Prothrombin ⟹ Thrombin	• Thromboplastin converts prothrombin to thrombin
Stage 3 Thrombin Fibrinogen ⟹ Fibrin	• Thrombin converts fibrinogen to fibrin threads
	• Fibrin threads tangle with platelets and trap red blood cells, forming a clot • The clot stabilizes and begins to retract and harden
Stage 4 Plasminogen ⟹ Plasmin	• Plasminogen converts to plasmin
	• Plasmin breaks the clot into fibrin split products, dissolving it

FIGURE 32-2 Formation of a blood clot.

NURSING ASSESSMENT OF THE HEMATOLOGIC SYSTEM

Many subtle findings on the physical examination can suggest changes in the patient's hematologic system that should be reported to a nurse or physician for evaluation. Box 32-1 outlines the nursing assessment of patients with a disorder of the hematologic system.

HEALTH HISTORY
Chief Complaint and History of Present Illness

Pay special attention to the patient who remarks that he or she bruises easily, bleeds for an unusually long time, or is chronically fatigued. These may be the symptoms of an underlying hematologic disorder.

Past Medical History

A patient could have an underlying hematologic problem if he or she reports any of the following: cancer or prior treatment for cancer, human immunodeficiency virus (HIV) infection, liver disease, kidney disease, malabsorption disease, prolonged bleeding or delayed healing with surgery or dental extractions, a history of blood transfusion, placement of prosthetic heart valves, or placement of an indwelling venous access device, indicating that the patient needed long-term venous access. Note any history of blood transfusions.

Medications the patient is currently using or a recent change in medication may suggest an underlying hematologic problem. It is important to find out what over-the-counter medications the patient uses, because many of these contain aspirin or nonsteroidal anti-inflammatory drugs (NSAIDs) that may prolong bleeding.

Family History

Note any family history of blood disorders such as sickle cell disease or hemophilia. Death of a family member at a young age for reasons other than trauma may indicate a genetic hematologic disorder.

Review of Systems

The review of systems is aimed at finding out what symptoms the patient has been experiencing over the past weeks or months that might provide clues as to what specific medical disorder the patient may now have.

In relation to the integumentary system, ask the patient about changes in skin color, skin dryness, pruritus (itching), and brittle fingernails or toenails. Data relevant to the assessment of the neurologic system include dizziness, vertigo, confusion, and pain. Patients with low red blood cell counts may have headaches. If the patient has had headaches, record the location, duration, and intensity of the pain as well as what, if anything, relieves the pain. Patients with intracranial bleeding from low platelet counts may report sudden mental status changes or severe headaches. Note changes in vision, which may indicate bleeding behind the eye. While collecting data about the respiratory and cardiovascular systems, ask the patient about epistaxis (nosebleeds), hemoptysis (coughing up blood), dyspnea (shortness of breath), heart palpitations, or chest pain, which may be symptoms of a low red blood cell count. Heart palpitations accompanied by dizziness may occur with position changes as the heart beats faster in an attempt to move what little blood there is quickly from the lungs to the body tissues to deliver oxygen. Significant data for assessment of the gastrointestinal system include any changes in eating habits, including changes in appetite or episodes of nausea or vomiting. Inquire about bleeding or pain in the mouth, gums, or tongue. Describe the patient's normal bowel

Box 32-1 | ***ASSESSMENT of Patients with Disorders of the Hematologic System***

Health History

History of Present Illness:
Easy bruising, prolonged bleeding, chronic fatigue

Past Medical History:
Cancer or prior treatment for cancer, HIV infection, liver disease, kidney disease, malabsorption disorder; prolonged bleeding or delayed healing with surgery or dental extractions; history of having blood transfused; placement of prosthetic heart valves, or placement of an indwelling venous access device, indicating that the patient needed long-term venous access; current medications, including over-the-counter medications and any recent changes in medication

Family History:
Blood disorders, death of a family member at a young age for reasons other than trauma

Review of Systems

Integumentary:
Change in skin color, dryness, pruritus, brittle fingernails or toenails

Neurologic:
Dizziness, vertigo, confusion, pain, headache, mental status changes, change in vision

Respiratory:
Epistaxis, hemoptysis, dyspnea

Cardiovascular:
Palpitations, chest pain, dizziness or fainting with position changes

Gastrointestinal:
Change in eating habits, nausea, vomiting, bleeding, pain, change in bowel habits, blood in stool

Genitourinary:
Blood in urine, heavy menses in women

Musculoskeletal:
Numbness or pain in bones or joints

Endocrine:
Fatigue, cold intolerance

Functional Assessment:
Occupation and hobbies, self-concept, activities and exercise, sleep and rest, nutrition, interpersonal relationships, coping and stress, perception of health

Physical Examination

Vital Signs:
Tachycardia, tachypnea, hypotension, orthostatic vital sign changes

Height and Weight

General Survey:
Responsiveness, mood, expression, posture

Skin:
Color, dryness, brittle fingernails and toenails, bruising, petechiae, purpura, ecchymoses

Head and Neck:
Bleeding, cracking at the corners of the mouth

Thorax:
Respiratory rate, breath sounds, heart rate

Abdomen:
Liver enlargement, stool guaiac test, dipstick urine sample for blood

---

function and any recent changes in frequency of bowel movements or consistency of the stool. Record any report of blood in the stool. Likewise, note any report of blood in the urine as an abnormality of the genitourinary system. Ask women about unusually heavy menses, which may indicate a bleeding disorder. Describe any musculoskeletal numbness or pain. Joint pain can occur if bleeding has occurred in the joint. Finally, to collect data about the endocrine system, ask the patient about fatigue or cold intolerance, which may be a symptom of a low red blood cell count.

Functional Assessment

Patients newly diagnosed with blood disorders may not experience dramatic changes in their functional abilities. However, many blood disorders are chronic conditions that the patient has lived with for many years. The functional abilities of these patients may be adversely affected.

Occupation and Hobbies. Knowing a patient's job and hobbies can alert you to unusual chemical exposures. Because the bone marrow and blood can be affected by various chemicals, document any recent chemical exposure. For example, someone who builds models for a hobby may be exposed to unusual glues or paints, which may affect the blood count.

Self-Concept. Assess the patient's self-concept by exploring the patient's feelings about himself or herself. For many people, their self-concept is related to their job. If the patient is unable to work, his or her self-concept can be adversely affected. In addition, medical insurance is often contingent on employment. Loss of medical insurance and the need to receive state or federal assistance can further erode a patient's self-concept. Another factor that can adversely affect the patient's self-concept is a change in appearance because of the disease.

Activity and Exercise. Assess the patient's current activity level and the effects of the disease and treatment on the patient's usual pattern of activity and exercise. Ask about the layout of the patient's home, specifically the location of bathrooms in relation to living areas and bedrooms. Ask if the patient must climb stairs to enter the home or get to a second floor. Having to climb

Health Promotion Considerations

Balanced Diet

A balanced diet should include foods rich in iron, which is required for hemoglobin production. Foods rich in iron include red meats, fish, dried fruits, beans, and dark green vegetables.

stairs can quickly tire a patient with a hematologic disorder. Inquire what the patient does for recreation and whether these activities can still be done during times of decreased energy.

Sleep and Rest. Assess the number of continuous hours the patient sleeps every night, whether any sleeping aids are used, what interrupts the patient's sleep, and whether the patient naps during the day.

Nutrition. Ask the patient to describe his or her usual diet and any recent changes in appetite or weight. Identify factors that might be interfering with eating, such as nausea, vomiting, and taste changes. Depression and loneliness can adversely affect a patient's nutritional status. Limited financial resources can also limit a patient's ability to maintain a nutritious diet.

Interpersonal Relationships. Explore the patient's view of himself or herself as a husband or wife, father or mother, son or daughter, friend, and co-worker. Discuss the effects of the disease on these relationships. Consider the patient's roles in the home. Ask what household chores the patient is responsible for and who does the shopping, cooking, and cleaning. If there are children to care for, ask whether the patient is able to perform the usual child care.

Coping and Stress. Ask what worries the patient and how the patient usually deals with stress. Explore sources of support, which might include family, support groups, and spiritual beliefs and practices.

Perception of Health. Discuss the patient's view of his or her own health and health practices. This might include measures taken to prevent complications from the disease and keeping regular medical appointments.

PHYSICAL EXAMINATION

Begin the physical examination by measuring vital signs, height, and weight. Be alert for tachycardia (pulse greater than 100/min), tachypnea (respiratory rate greater than 20/min), and hypotension (systolic blood pressure less than 90 mm Hg).

Patients with low red blood cell counts may experience orthostatic vital sign changes in pulse and blood pressure when they stand up. The body tries to maintain a normal blood pressure when the patient changes position from lying to standing. If the patient's blood volume is inadequate, the heart rate increases and the blood pressure decreases as the patient stands. This can be why patients complain of feeling dizzy or light-

---

Box 32-2   ***Assessing for Orthostatic Changes in Vital Signs***

1. Have the patient lie down on a bed or in a reclining chair for at least 1 minute.
2. Record the patient's heart rate and blood pressure.
3. Have the patient sit up.
4. After the patient has been sitting 1 minute, record the heart rate and blood pressure again.
5. Have the patient stand up.
6. After the patient has been standing 1 minute, record the heart rate and blood pressure again.
7. If the blood pressure decreases 15-20 points with change from the lying to the standing position and the heart rate increases 15-20 points from lying to standing, the patient is described as having *orthostatic* or *tilt-positive* changes.

---

headed when they stand up quickly. Box 32-2 describes how to assess for orthostatic changes in vital signs. Patients who have orthostatic changes in their vital signs usually need some type of hydration. Often the patient is simply dehydrated and needs extra fluids. However, a patient with a low red blood cell count needing a blood transfusion can also be orthostatic.

Consider the Alternative

Be sure to note any herbal products that the patient uses. Herbs that can affect blood clotting include black cohosh, feverfew, garlic, ginkgo, and ginseng.

General Survey

Note the patient's responsiveness, mood, expression, and posture. Throughout the examination, carefully inspect and describe any reddened, swollen, or painful areas the patient identifies.

Skin

Note the general color of the skin. A patient with a low red blood cell count may appear pale. In dark-skinned people, this may be difficult to assess. Look at the conjunctiva of the eyes, the nail beds, and around the mouth to detect any paleness. Patients also may appear jaundiced, or yellow, if many red blood cells have been destroyed or if the body is having trouble clearing the blood of old red blood cells. Indications of a vitamin deficiency that might cause a blood disorder include dry, itchy skin and scalp or brittle fingernails and toenails.

Describe any bruising. **Petechiae** are small (1 to 3 mm), red or reddish purple spots on the skin resulting from blood capillaries breaking and leaking small amounts of blood into the tissues. Petechiae are often confused with a skin rash. Petechiae almost always signal that the patient has a very low platelet count. Severe coughing can cause petechiae on the chest, neck, and face of a patient. A blood pressure cuff pumped up to greater than 250 mm Hg on a patient with a low platelet count can cause petechiae on the arm below the blood pressure cuff as the small capillaries break with the high cuff pressure. This is not dangerous to the patient but can be frightening to both the patient and the nurse if it happens. Red or reddish purple spots denote pur-pura and are the result of larger blood vessels break-ing. Purpura are larger than petechiae, usually 3 mm or more. Purpura can suggest a low platelet count or a problem with clotting factors in the blood. Ecchymoses are larger purplish areas of skin resulting from a larger amount of blood leaking outside the blood vessels. The common name for ecchymosis is a *bruise*. Ecchymoses do not necessarily indicate a bleeding disorder, but if the patient has a number of these areas or notes that he or she bruises easily, it may be a symptom of a blood disorder.

Head and Neck

When evaluating the eyes, ears, nose, mouth, and throat, note any signs of bleeding. Look for cracking at the corners of the mouth, which may be a symptom of a vitamin deficiency.

Thorax

Lungs. Assess respiratory rate and effort. Auscultate breath sounds, which are usually normal without wheezing, crackles, or rhonchi. Patients with low red blood cell counts often are dyspneic, or short of breath, because they do not have enough red blood cells to carry oxygen to all their tissues. As a result, they are tachypneic, with a respiratory rate greater than 20 per minute, in an attempt to oxygenate what little blood they have. Any strenuous activity may exacerbate the shortness of breath.

Heart and Vascular System. Assess heart rate, rest-ing blood pressure, and adaptation of blood pressure to position changes. Patients with low red blood cell counts can be tachycardic, with a heart rate greater than 100 beats per minute. Again, because there are not enough red blood cells to carry oxygen to all the tis-sues, the heart beats faster in an attempt to move what little blood there is quickly from the lungs to the body tissues to deliver oxygen.

Abdomen

Inspect and palpate the abdomen for distention and tenderness. The examiner with advanced skills may also palpate for organ enlargement. The liver and

---

DIAGNOSTIC TESTS and PROCEDURES *Laboratory Tests*

TEST/STUDY	PURPOSE/PROCEDURE	PATIENT PREPARATION	POSTPROCEDURE NURSING CARE
Blood tests (CBC, RBC count, Hb, Hct, serum iron, TIBC, ferritin, platelet count, PT, PTT, fibrinogen, TT, FSP, D dimers, INR, HbS, serum bilirubin, Coombs' tests)	Blood tests measure various blood components. Different blood tests are collected in different laboratory tubes contain-ing specific reagents or no reagents at all. Usually the tubes have color-coded tops. Be sure and collect the blood in the blood tube specific for the blood test ordered. Usually each institution's laboratory publishes a manual identifying what colored tube to use for each blood test.	Choose the correct blood tubes to collect the blood in. Tell the patient he or she will feel a sharp pain as the needle goes through the skin.	Apply bandage. Have the patient hold pressure to the site for 1 minute. The bandage may be re-moved in 1 hour.
Bleeding time	The bleeding time measures the time it takes for the platelet plug to form.	Tell the patient a blood pres-sure cuff is placed above the elbow and inflated to 40 mm Hg. The forearm is cleaned and a puncture is made. A stop watch is started. The wound is blotted with filter paper every 30 seconds until all the bleeding has stopped. The time is noted.	Apply bandage.

Data from Fischbach, F. (2000). *A manual of laboratory and diagnostic tests* (6th ed.). Philadelphia: Lippincott.
CBC, Complete blood count; *RBC,* red blood cell; *Hb,* hemoglobin; *Hct,* hematocrit; *TIBC,* total iron-binding capacity; *PT,* prothrombin time; *PTT,* partial thromboplastin time; *TT,* thrombin time; *FSP,* fibrin split products; *INR,* International Normalized Ratio; *HbS,* sickle cell hemoglobin.

spleen can become enlarged with blood cell disorders, causing abdominal fullness and tenderness. If a stool specimen is available, a guaiac test may be done to detect microscopic blood. If the patient can provide a urine sample, it also can be tested for blood.

DIAGNOSTIC TESTS AND PROCEDURES

Primarily, blood studies determine the function of the patient's hematologic system. Diagnostic tests and procedures done to diagnose disorders of the hematologic system are described in the Diagnostic Tests and Procedures tables below and on p. 576. The laboratory performing the test should provide normal values for the various blood tests. Ranges of normal values can be found in various textbooks of laboratory and diagnostic tests.

BLOOD TESTS

The red blood cell count, the hemoglobin (Hb or Hgb), and the hematocrit (Hct) are the three main blood tests used to monitor red blood cells. The red blood cell count is the total number of red blood cells found in a cubic millimeter (mm^3) of blood. The hemoglobin indicates the oxygen-carrying capacity in the blood. The hematocrit is the percentage of red blood cells in whole blood. Normally, the hematocrit is approximately three times the hemoglobin value. Iron is an essential part of red blood cells; therefore serum iron, total iron-binding capacity (TIBC), and ferritin are measured to assess the patient's resources for producing red blood cells.

Normal platelet counts range from 140,000 to 440,000 platelets/mm^3 of blood. Many times the platelet count is abbreviated as a multiple of 1000. For example, a platelet count of 200,000 is abbreviated 200K.

DIAGNOSTIC TESTS and PROCEDURES | *Bone Marrow Biopsy*

TEST/STUDY	PURPOSE/PROCEDURE	PATIENT PREPARATION	POSTPROCEDURE NURSING CARE
Bone marrow biopsy	A bone marrow biopsy is used to evaluate how well the bone marrow is making white blood cells, red blood cells, and platelets. The patient is positioned on an examining table according to the location of where the bone marrow biopsy will be collected. The most common site is the posterior iliac crest, although the anterior crest, sternum, and tibia can also be biopsy sites. The selected site is prepared and draped as for a minor surgical procedure. A local anesthetic is injected. A Jamshidi needle is forced into the bone marrow. Bone marrow fluid is aspirated and a core biopsy taken through and with the Jamshidi needle. The needle is removed and a pressure dressing applied to the site. A laboratory technician must be present during the procedure to immediately fix and stain the specimens. Sometimes a short-acting benzodiazepine, such as midazolam (Versed) is used to sedate the patient during the procedure.	Explain the purpose and procedure to the patient. A permit must be signed. No fasting is necessary. Some local discomfort may be experienced as the local anesthetic is injected. The patient usually feels pressure as the Jamshidi needle is inserted into the bone and a momentary sharp pain down the leg as the bone marrow fluid is aspirated. The procedure takes approximately 30 minutes.	If intravenous sedation is used, monitor the patient's pulse, blood pressure, respirations, and pulse oximetry until the patient is fully recovered. The pressure dressing can be removed in 2 hours.

Data from Fischbach, F. (2000). *A manual of laboratory and diagnostic tests* (6th ed.). Philadelphia: Lippincott.

The function of the clotting factors is measured with the prothrombin time (PT), the partial thromboplastin time (PTT), and the bleeding time. If the results of these tests are abnormal, other blood tests that may be done to determine the specific abnormality include measurements of fibrinogen, thrombin time (TT), fibrin split products (FSP), and D dimers. If the patient is taking heparin to anticoagulate the blood, the partial prothrombin time is used to monitor therapy. If the patient is taking warfarin (Coumadin) to anticoagulate the blood, the prothrombin time and/or the International Normalized Ratio (INR) is used to monitor therapy.

BONE MARROW BIOPSY

If blood tests show abnormalities, the physician may perform a bone marrow biopsy to see how well the blood cells are being made in the bone marrow (Fig. 32-3). The Diagnostic Tests and Procedures table on p. 577 describes the bone marrow biopsy procedure.

COMMON THERAPEUTIC MEASURES

Treatment of disorders of the hematologic system is aimed at correcting the underlying problem. Blood product transfusions and colony-stimulating factors are used to symptomatically manage the patient.

NURSING ACTIONS FOR THE PATIENT AT RISK FOR INJURY FROM LOW RED BLOOD CELL COUNTS

Box 32-3 outlines typical nursing actions for the patient at risk for injury from low red blood cell counts.

NURSING ACTIONS FOR THE PATIENT AT RISK FOR INJURY FROM BLEEDING

Box 32-4 outlines typical nursing actions for the patient at risk for injury from bleeding.

BLOOD PRODUCT TRANSFUSIONS

Because of the risk for infections, such as with hepatitis or HIV, blood product transfusions are no longer automatically given when the patient's laboratory values fall below a certain value. Instead, the patient is evaluated clinically and a decision is made with the patient whether to administer a blood transfusion. Symptoms

FIGURE **32-3** Most common site of bone marrow biopsy.

Box 32-3 | *Nursing Actions for the Patient at Risk for Injury From Low Red Blood Cell Counts*

1. Administer oxygen as prescribed.
2. Administer blood products as prescribed (see Table 32-1, Commonly Transfused Blood Products; Box 32-5, Administration of a Red Blood Cell Transfusion; and Table 32-2, Blood Transfusion Reactions).
3. Administer the hematopoietic growth factor *erythropoietin* as prescribed (see Drug Therapy table, Drugs Used to Treat Disorders of the Hematologic System).
4. Allow for rest between periods of activity because the anemic patient can tire easily.
5. Elevate the patient's head on pillows for shortness of breath.
6. Provide extra blankets if the patient feels too cool.
7. Teach the patient and family about the underlying pathophysiology and how to manage the symptoms of anemia.

From Young-McCaughan, S., & Jennings, B. M. (1998). Hematologic and immunologic systems. In J. G. Alspach (Ed.). *Core curriculum for critical care nursing* (5th ed.). Philadelphia: Saunders.

of a low red blood cell count that would prompt a red blood cell transfusion include shortness of breath, tachycardia, decreased blood pressure, chest pain, lightheadedness, or extreme fatigue. For each unit of packed red blood cells transfused, the patient's hemoglobin should increase approximately 1 gm/dL and the hematocrit approximately 3%. Table 32-1 provides an overview of commonly transfused blood components.

Typing for Transfusions

Before a blood transfusion, a sample of the patient's blood is sent to the blood bank for typing and crossmatching. As discussed previously, depending on which antigens are present in the red blood cell membrane, a person has either type A, B, AB, or O blood. Also, depending on the presence or absence of the Rh antigen, a person is either Rh+ or Rh−. People with any of these antigens cannot be given blood containing a different antigen. Therefore persons with type O− blood are considered universal donors because their blood does not contain any of the A, B, or Rh antigens and can safely be given to anyone. Those with AB+ blood are considered universal recipients because their blood contains the A, B, and Rh antigens. They can safely receive any type of blood. However, usually blood banks exactly match the blood to be transfused with the blood of a patient needing a transfusion.

Transfusions of Packed Red Blood Cells

The patient should be counseled by the physician and a consent signed before any blood transfusion. A blood sample is drawn from the patient and sent to the blood bank for type and crossmatch. One procedure for administering a packed red blood cell transfusion is outlined in Box 32-5. The policies for administering blood products vary from hospital to hospital, so be sure

Box 32-4   *Nursing Actions for the Patient at Risk for Injury From Bleeding*

1. Administer blood product transfusions as prescribed. If a platelet transfusion is to be given in preparation for a procedure, it is best to give the transfusion immediately before the procedure so the greatest number of platelets will be available to stop bleeding caused by the procedure (see Table 32-1, Commonly Transfused Blood Products; Box 32-6, Administration of a Platelet Transfusion; and Table 32-2, Blood Transfusion Reactions).
2. Minimize the number of invasive procedures done to the patient that might result in prolonged bleeding by taking the following measures:
   a. Draw blood for as much laboratory work as possible with one venipuncture.
   b. Avoid prolonged tourniquet use.
   c. Apply direct pressure for 5-10 minutes after all invasive procedures such as venipuncture or bone marrow biopsies.
   d. Avoid intramuscular injections.
3. Avoid damage to the rectal mucosa that might cause bleeding by taking the following measures:
   a. Avoid rectal temperatures.
   b. Avoid suppositories.
   c. Avoid enemas.
   d. Prevent constipation by increasing fiber in the diet or administering stool softeners as ordered.
4. When measuring blood pressure, inflate the cuff only until the pulse is obliterated to prevent petechiae along the arm. Set automated sphygmomanometers to the lowest appropriate pressure.
5. Instruct the patient to use a soft-bristled toothbrush. If oral bleeding occurs, toothettes or mouth rinses can be used to maintain oral hygiene.
6. Instruct the patient to use an electric razor to shave, not a straight-edged razor.
7. As much as possible and as prescribed by the physician, avoid the use of drugs that interfere with platelet function such as aspirin, aspirin-containing drugs (e.g., Pepto-Bismol, Percodan), and the nonsteroidal anti-inflammatory drugs (NSAIDs).
8. Teach the patient and family about the underlying pathophysiology that puts the patient at risk for hemorrhage and precautions to minimize the risk of bleeding.

From Young-McCaughan, S., & Jennings, B. M. (1998). Hematologic and immunologic systems. In J. G. Alspach (Ed.). *Core curriculum for critical care nursing* (5th ed.). Philadelphia: Saunders.

Table 32-1   *Commonly Transfused Blood Products*

BLOOD COMPONENT	INDICATIONS	USUAL AMOUNT IN ONE UNIT	RECOMMENDED INFUSION RATE	SPECIAL CONSIDERATIONS
Packed red blood cells (PRBC)	Symptoms due to a low hematocrit or hemoglobin such as shortness of breath, tachycardia, decreased blood pressure, chest pain, light-headedness, or fatigue	250-300 mL/unit	2-4 hr/unit	
Platelets	Bleeding from thrombocytopenia	60 mL/ pack; usually four to six packs are pooled for a platelet transfusion	As quickly as the patient can tolerate	
Fresh frozen plasma (FFP)	Clotting deficiencies, hemophilia, rapid reversal of warfarin (Coumadin), massive red blood cell transfusions	200-280 mL/unit	10 mL/min	FFP contains all clotting factors except platelets
Cryoprecipitate	Hemophilia A, disseminated intravascular coagulation	10 mL/bag; usually 10 bags are pooled for a transfusion	10 mL/min	Cryoprecipitate contains factors I (fibrinogen) and VIII

Data from American Association of Blood Banks, America's Blood Centers, & American Red Cross. (2000). *Circular of information for the use of human blood and blood components.* Stock number 003011OL01. Available on the American Association of Blood Banks website, www.aabb.org; DeVita, Jr. V.T., Hellman, S., & Rosenberg, S.A. (2001). *Cancer: Principles and practice of oncology* (6th ed.). Philadelphia: Lippincott-Raven.

to be familiar with and follow your own institution's policies.

One way to prevent the risks of infection and reactions with blood transfusions is to collect the patient's own blood before a planned procedure and then transfuse the patient's own blood back into the patient if needed as an autologous red blood cell transfusion. The patient donates his or her own blood several times before the planned procedure. The blood is stored by the blood bank and reinfused into the patient if needed intraoperatively or postoperatively. Autologous transfusion—using the patient's own blood—is recommended if significant blood loss is expected during the procedure, especially if the patient has a rare blood type or religious beliefs against receiving donated blood.

Platelet Transfusions

Like red blood cell transfusions, platelet transfusions are not automatically administered when the patient's platelet count falls below a certain value. However, the lower a patient's platelet count goes, the greater is the chance of bleeding. Generally, when the platelet count falls below 20,000 cells/mm^3, platelets are administered. If the platelet count is greater than 20,000

cells/mm^3, platelets usually are not given unless the patient is actively bleeding. For each multidonor (from multiple donors) pack of platelets, the patient's platelet count should increase by 5,000-10,000 cells/mm^3.

The patient should be counseled by the physician and give signed consent for the platelet transfusion. A blood sample is drawn from the patient and sent to the blood bank for typing. If the patient has been previously typed and crossmatched for either a red blood cell transfusion or a platelet transfusion, the blood bank can usually use this information to provide platelets. Platelets are commonly ordered in four-packs or six-packs. Each pack contains approximately 60 mL. One procedure for administering a platelet transfusion is outlined in Box 32-6. The policies for administering blood products vary from hospital to hospital, so be sure to be familiar with and follow your institution's policies.

If platelets are ordered before an invasive procedure that might cause bleeding, such as a lumbar puncture or endoscopy, the platelets should be administered just before the procedure is started. There is no indication to "get the platelets in early" for a procedure scheduled for later in the day. Instead, plan with the physician doing the procedure to administer the platelets just before the procedure begins.

Fresh Frozen Plasma Transfusions

Plasma is separated from whole blood by centrifugation and quickly frozen. So, when plasma is to be transfused,

---

Box 32-5 | *Administration of a Red Blood Cell Transfusion*

1. After the patient has been counseled and has given signed consent for the transfusion, draw a sample of blood and send it to the blood bank with a request for a type and crossmatch. Start an IV of normal saline using an 18- or 20-gauge needle. Blood should not be infused through a cannula smaller than 20 gauge because of the chance of lysing (destroying) the individual blood cells as they go through the cannula.
2. When the blood arrives, it should be checked by two licensed people at the patient's bedside. Be certain to check the expiration date of the blood. Once the blood has arrived from the blood bank, the transfusion should be started within 30 minutes.
3. Take and record the patient's vital signs.
4. To administer blood, use a special blood transfusion tubing that has a filter built in to the system to screen for clots. Piggyback the blood into the normal saline line. Each unit of blood is usually between 250 and 300 mL. Generally blood is infused over 2-4 hours.
5. Stay with the patient for 5-10 minutes after the blood is started to observe for any immediate untoward reactions that might signal a reaction to the transfusion, such as back pain, fever, chills, or a decreased blood pressure.
6. Continue to monitor vital signs during the transfusion per your institution's policy.
7. When the transfusion is complete, document the procedure, the patient's vital signs, and how the patient tolerated the procedure.
8. Subsequent units of blood can be immediately hung as just described. Sometimes the same blood tubing can be used for administering several units of blood.

Box 32-6 | *Administration of a Platelet Transfusion*

1. After the patient has been counseled and has given signed consent for the transfusion, draw a sample of blood and send it to the blood bank with a request for typing and crossmatch. Start an IV of normal saline using at least a 24-gauge needle. Platelets are smaller than red blood cells, and so a smaller IV needle can be used to administer the platelets without risk of lysing the cells.
2. When the platelets arrive, they should be checked by two licensed people at the patient's bedside. Once the platelets have arrived from the blood bank, the transfusion should be started immediately.
3. Take and record the patient's vital signs.
4. Run the platelets through blood transfusion tubing that has a filter built into the system. Piggyback the platelets into the normal saline line. Platelets can be infused as fast as the patient can tolerate.
5. Stay with the patient for 5-10 minutes after the platelets are started to observe for any immediate untoward reactions that might signal a reaction to the transfusion, such as back pain, fever, chills, or decreased blood pressure.
6. Continue to monitor the patient's vital signs during the infusion per your institution's policy.
7. When the transfusion is complete, document the procedure, the patient's vital signs, and how the patient tolerated the procedure.

usually fresh frozen plasma is ordered. Fresh frozen plasma contains all the clotting factors as well as the plasma proteins. Cryoprecipitate, which contains only fibrinogen and factor VIII, can be further separated out from plasma and administered alone if indicated.

Reactions to Blood Transfusions

Four main types of transfusion reactions can occur with transfusions of blood or any of the blood components: hemolytic, anaphylactic, febrile, and circulatory overload. If the patient experiences back or chest pain, fever, chills, a decreased blood pressure, urticaria, wheezing, dyspnea, or coughing during the transfusion, stop the transfusion immediately and keep the intravenous line open with normal saline. Immediately notify the physician, nursing supervisor, and blood bank. Be prepared to administer oxygen, epinephrine, Solu-Cortef, furosemide (Lasix), and antipyretics as prescribed by the physician. Save the unused portion of the blood bag for the blood bank. Be prepared to collect blood and urine samples from the patient for evaluation. Documentation of the event is important. Usually each institution has a blood transfusion reaction form that needs to be completed. Table 32-2 outlines the types, symptoms, and treatments for the different blood transfusion reactions.

COLONY-STIMULATING FACTORS

Colony-stimulating factors are naturally occurring hormones that stimulate the bone marrow to produce more blood cells. Certain of the colony-stimulating factors have been isolated and are available for therapeutic use. Erythropoietin (Epogen) stimulates the bone marrow to produce more red blood cells. The effects of erythropoietin on the hematocrit are not apparent for several days; therefore it is not an option for patients immediately needing to elevate their red blood cell counts. These patients need a red blood cell transfusion. Erythropoietin is predominantly used by hemodialysis patients who are chronically anemic as a result of dialysis, and it has also been used to prevent the complications and relieve the symptoms of anemia in patients with cancer or HIV infection. The Drug Therapy table on p. 582 describes the nursing care of patients receiving these drugs.

DISORDERS OF THE HEMATOLOGIC SYSTEM

RED BLOOD CELL DISORDERS

Patients with red blood cell disorders may have either too many red blood cells (i.e., polycythemia vera) or too few red blood cells (i.e., anemia). Having too few red blood cells is more common. Because the main function of red blood cells is oxygenation, anemia results in tissue hypoxia. Anemia can result from a major blood loss over a short period of time, too few red blood cells being made, or increased red blood cell destruction. Acute blood loss, such as with an arterial rupture, dramatically changes the patient's hemodynamic status, requiring emergency intervention. Chronic blood loss, such as with sickle cell disease, allows the body

---

Table 32-2   *Blood Transfusion Reactions*

REACTION	MECHANISM	SYMPTOMS	OCCURRENCE	TREATMENT
Hemolytic	Antigen-antibody reaction to transfusion of ABO-incompatible blood	Fever, chills, nausea, dyspnea, chest pain, back pain, hypotension	Shortly after starting the transfusion	Stop the transfusion. Notify the physician immediately. Be prepared to provide supportive therapy to maintain heart rate and blood pressure.
Anaphylactic	Type I hypersensitivity reaction to plasma proteins	Urticaria, wheezing, dyspnea, hypotension	Within 30 minutes of starting the transfusion	Stop the transfusion. Notify the physician immediately. Be prepared to administer epinephrine and steroids.
Febrile	Recipient's antibodies react to donor leukocytes	Fever, chills	Within 30-90 minutes of starting the transfusion	Stop the transfusion. Notify the physician immediately.
Circulatory overload	Patient's cardiovascular system is unable to manage the additional fluid load	Cough, frothy sputum, cyanosis, decreased blood pressure	Any time during the transfusion and up to several hours afterward	Stop the transfusion. Call for help. Be prepared to administer oxygen and/or furosemide (Lasix).

| **DRUG THERAPY** | *Drugs Used to Treat Disorders of the Hematologic System* |

DRUG	USE/ACTION	SIDE EFFECTS	NURSING INTERVENTIONS
Epoetin alfa (Epogen)	Stimulates the bone marrow to produce red blood cells	Hypertension, headache, arthralgias	May be given by intravenous or subcutaneous injection. Patient is usually treated three times per week until the hematocrit is 30-33.
Oprelvekin (Neumega)	Stimulates the bone marrow to produce platelets	Fluid and electrolyte abnormalities, dysrhythmias, visual disturbances, dizziness, insomnia, dyspnea, oral candidiasis	Given by subcutaneous injection once a day for up to 21 days. Side effects are experienced by most patients receiving this drug.
Ferrous sulfate (Feosol, Fer-In-Sol)	Iron replacement	Constipation, black stools, mild nausea	Have the patient take the drug with food but not with milk, eggs, or caffeinated drinks because milk, eggs, and caffeine inhibit drug absorption. If the patient is taking liquid iron, dilute the drug and administer through a straw to prevent the drug from staining the teeth.
Iron dextran	Iron replacement	Hypersensitivity reactions, brown skin discoloration at the injection site	Test dose the patient before starting treatment. Give intramuscular injections only in the upper, outer quadrant of the buttock using the Z-track technique. To give an injection using the Z-track technique, firmly pull the skin over the upper, outer quadrant of the buttock laterally. Insert the needle. Withdraw the plunger to check that no blood enters the syringe. Slowly inject the medication. Remove the needle and let go of the skin. Massage the area.
Vitamin B_{12} (cyanocobalamin)	Vitamin B_{12} replacement		Intramuscular injection. For patients with pernicious anemia, vitamin B_{12} injections must be given every month the rest of the person's life.
Hydroxyurea	Prevention of sickle cell crisis	Nausea, vomiting	Reinforce to the patient that this drug must be taken regularly to prevent sickle cell crises and that it is of no use once a crisis occurs.

to compensate. Depending on whether the anemia is acute or chronic, the body compensates in three ways: (1) by increasing heart rate and respiratory rate to circulate the existing red blood cells as quickly as possible with as much oxygen as possible, (2) by redistributing the blood away from the skin, gastrointestinal tract, and kidneys to the brain and heart, and (3) by increasing the production of erythropoietin, the hormone that stimulates the bone marrow to produce more red blood cells. Anemia can be a primary disease or a symptom of another disease. Descriptions of the different types of red blood cell disorders follow.

Polycythemia Vera

Polycythemia vera is a condition in which too many red blood cells are produced. The increased number of red blood cells makes the blood more viscous, or thicker, so that it does not circulate freely through the body. Symptoms of polycythemia vera include headache, dizziness, ringing in the ears, and blurred vision.

Patients with this disorder may have a ruddy (reddish) complexion.

Treatment for polycythemia vera is to have a unit of blood phlebotomized, or taken off, to keep the patient's hematocrit normal. This procedure is usually done in the blood bank. A large-bore intravenous needle is inserted into the patient's antecubital vein, and 1 unit of blood is taken off. This is the same procedure used when a person goes to the blood bank to donate blood; however, the blood taken from the patient with polycythemia vera cannot be used as donor blood.

Aplastic Anemia

Aplastic anemia results from the complete failure of the bone marrow. The term *aplastic anemia* is misleading because patients with this condition have more than an extremely low red blood cell count; they also have extremely low white blood cell counts and low platelet counts because their bone marrow is not making any of these cells. Certain drugs such as streptomycin and chloramphenicol as well as exposure to toxic chemicals or radiation can cause bone marrow failure. Yet in many cases, the cause of a patient's bone marrow failure is never identified.

Signs and symptoms of aplastic anemia can include pallor, extreme fatigue, tachycardia, shortness of breath, hypotension, unusually prolonged or spontaneous bleeding, and frequent infections that do not resolve. In addition to abnormally low red blood cell, white blood cell, and platelet counts on blood tests, patients with aplastic anemia have abnormally low numbers of blood-making cells in their bone marrow.

Medical treatment for aplastic anemia focuses on identifying and treating the cause. Transfusions are given to replace red blood cells and platelets. Antibiotics are given to prevent or treat infections. Corticosteroids also may be given. If the patient's bone marrow does not recover on its own, a bone marrow transplant may be considered if a donor can be found. The patient with aplastic anemia is critically ill and requires intensive nursing support similar to the care provided to a patient who is undergoing a bone marrow transplant, as described in Chapter 33.

Autoimmune Hemolytic Anemia

With aplastic anemia, the bone marrow does not make adequate amounts of the blood cells; with autoimmune hemolytic anemia, the bone marrow makes adequate amounts of the blood cells, but they are destroyed once they are released into the circulation. Causes of autoimmune hemolytic anemia can include certain infections, drug reactions, and certain cancers. Hemolytic anemia of the newborn can occur after delivery if the mother has Rh− blood and the baby has Rh+ blood. Blood transfusions can cause a hemolytic anemia if lymphocytes in the transfused blood make antibodies against the person receiving the blood. As with aplastic anemia, many times the cause of the hemolytic anemia is never identified.

Signs and symptoms of hemolytic anemia include pallor, extreme fatigue, tachycardia, shortness of breath, and hypotension. Patients may appear jaundiced. Patients with hemolytic anemia usually have high bilirubin levels in their blood from all the red blood cells being lysed (broken down). Patients with hemolytic anemia have a positive result on a direct Coombs antiglobulin blood test.

Medical treatment of this type of anemia focuses on identifying and treating the cause. Blood transfusions may be needed to replace red blood cells. Corticosteroids may be administered to the patient. The patient usually recovers in a few days to weeks.

Iron-Deficiency Anemia

Iron-deficiency anemia results from a diet too low in iron or from the body not absorbing enough iron from the gastrointestinal tract. As a result, the body does not have enough iron to make adequate amounts of hemoglobin. Older adults with poor eating habits frequently suffer from anemia. Symptoms of this anemia include fatigue and pallor. In severe cases, patients may have orthostatic changes in their heart rate and blood pressure. In addition to a low red blood cell count, a low hemoglobin value, and a low hematocrit, patients with iron-deficiency anemia have a low serum iron level, a low ferritin level, and a high total iron-binding capacity.

Physicians treat iron-deficiency anemia by prescribing iron supplements such as ferrous sulfate and iron dextran. The Drug Therapy table on p. 582 describes the nursing care of the patient taking iron supplements. Nurses caring for patients with iron-deficiency anemia can suggest incorporating foods high in iron into the diet. Foods that are rich in iron include liver, oysters, red meats, fish, dried fruits, legumes (e.g., dried beans and peas), dark green vegetables, and iron-enriched whole grain breads and cereals. See the Management and Supervision box below.

Pharmacology Capsule

Large doses of supplemental iron can be toxic. Caution patients not to exceed recommended dosage and to keep the drug out of the reach of children.

Pernicious Anemia (Vitamin B₁₂ Anemia)

Pernicious anemia occurs when a person does not absorb vitamin B_{12} from the stomach. The person may lack intrinsic factor, a substance made in the stomach that is essential for B_{12} absorption. The individual may have had a gastrectomy, in which part or all of the stomach was surgically removed, and so cannot make intrinsic factor and therefore cannot absorb vitamin B_{12}. In addition to the fatigue and pallor commonly seen with all anemias, symptoms of pernicious anemia characteristically include weakness, a sore tongue, and numbness of the hands or feet. Physicians treat pernicious anemia by prescribing a monthly intramuscular injection of vitamin B_{12} (cyanocobalamin). The Drug Therapy table on p. 582 describes the nursing care of patients receiving vitamin B_{12}.

Management and Supervision

Helping Certified Nurse Assistants Care for Patients with Blood Disorders

- Instruct the certified nurse assistant (CNA) to allow periods of rest for patients with anemia.
- Show the CNA how to gently handle patients with thrombocytopenia to prevent trauma and bleeding.
- Stress the importance of maintaining accurate records of oral fluid intake of the patient in sickle cell crisis.

FIGURE **32-4** Comparison of normal red blood cells (**A**) and sickled cells (**B**). (Magnification ×875.)

Sickle Cell Anemia

Sickle cell anemia is a disease in which the normally disk-shaped red blood cells become sickle-shaped (Fig. 32-4). These misshapen blood cells are much more fragile than normal red blood cells, and as a result, the sickled cells easily rupture as they pass through small capillaries, resulting in a chronic anemia. In addition, these abnormally shaped, sickled cells become stuck in the small capillaries of the body, obstructing blood flow.

Sickle cell anemia is a genetic disease occurring almost exclusively in African Americans. Eight percent of blacks carry the genetic trait for sickle cell anemia. Because sickle cell anemia is carried on a recessive gene, a person must inherit the gene from both the mother and the father to actually have the disease. Newborn screening for hemoglobin S can be done to identify infants with sickle cell disease and to educate parents about the disease and prevention of crises. Unfortunately, this screening is not required in every state.

Symptoms of sickle cell anemia include persistently low red blood cell counts, fatigue, and jaundice. The chronically low red blood cell counts can cause the heart to enlarge (cardiomegaly) and beat faster in an attempt to oxygenate the body's tissues. A sickle cell crisis occurs when the sickled cells become stuck in larger blood vessels of the body, obstructing blood flow and causing severe pain.

Signs and Symptoms of Sickle Cell Crisis. Various stressors can trigger a sickle cell crisis. They include dehydration, infection, overexertion, cold weather changes, excessive alcohol consumption, and smoking. Symptoms

What Does Culture Have to Do with Recruitment for Clinical Trials?

Diseases like sickle cell occur predominantly in African Americans. This population may be reluctant to join research studies because of unethical studies such as the Tuskegee Syphilis Study started in the 1930s. In the Tuskegee study, African-American men enrolled but were not treated when effective treatment, penicillin, became available in the 1940s.

vary depending upon where circulation is blocked by the sickled red blood cells. Commonly during a sickle cell crisis, circulation to the chest, abdomen, bones, joints, bone marrow, brain, or penis may be compromised. With circulation obstructed, tissue hypoxia occurs, causing severe pain. Patients in a sickle cell crisis often have a fever, either because infection precipitated the crisis or as part of the inflammatory response to tissue hypoxia.

Medical Diagnosis of Sickle Cell Disease. Patients with known sickle cell disease complaining of severe pain are suspected of being in crisis. There is no test to determine that a patient is in sickle cell crisis. Rather, physicians use clinical judgment to make the diagnosis. Crises can last anywhere from 1 to 10 days. Some patients experience crises every few weeks, whereas other patients can go months without experiencing painful episodes. Radiographs and scans of the painful area are usually taken to evaluate for bleeding.

Medical Treatment of the Patient in Sickle Cell Crisis. There is no cure for sickle cell disease. Medical treatment for patients experiencing a sickle cell crisis is symptomatic. The physician usually prescribes intravenous fluids and pain medication. Aggressive intravenous hydration helps the kidneys clear the metabolic wastes from ruptured red blood cells. The pain can be very severe, and the patient needs adequate pain relief during these episodes even if they last for several days. Intravenous morphine commonly is prescribed for pain relief. Patients with sickle cell disease can become addicted to opioids. Therefore physicians try quickly to transition the patient from intravenous opioids to oral opioids to nonopioid pain relievers as the crisis resolves. Red blood cell transfusions may be prescribed to correct the anemia and help the body oxygenate tissues. Although oxygen therapy is often prescribed, it is of little benefit in reversing the crisis.

For patients who experience frequent crises, the drug *hydroxyurea* can be prescribed. Hydroxyurea has been used for many years as a treatment for leukemia. The drug also stimulates the production of a certain type of hemoglobin that is resistant to sickling. Patients with sickle cell disease who regularly take hydroxyurea experience fewer crises. However, once a patient is in crisis, hydroxyurea does not work quickly enough to reduce either the severity or the duration of the crisis. The Drug Therapy table on p. 582 describes the nursing care of patients receiving hydroxyurea.

NURSING CARE PLAN
The Patient in Sickle Cell Crisis

ASSESSMENT

Health History: A 19-year-old African-American woman was diagnosed with sickle cell anemia at age 12. She has been in stable health until 3 days ago, when she complained of nausea and began to have diarrhea and vomiting. She has taken only soup and cola beverages since that time. When she began to complain of severe pain in her abdomen, she was brought to the emergency room by her mother, who suspected sickle cell crisis.

Physical Examination: T, 102° F; P, 106, regular; R, 24; BP, 110/56. Oral mucosa dry. Skin dry and warm to touch. Breath sounds clear to auscultation. Abdomen soft, but tender to light palpation. Bowel sounds hyperactive in all four quadrants. No bladder distention. Mild joint enlargement noted in both knees.

Nursing Diagnosis	Goals and Outcome Criteria	Interventions
Acute Pain related to sickle cell crisis	Pain relief: patient states pain has been relieved, appears relaxed.	Administer analgesics as prescribed. Assess effects and notify physician if pain is not relieved. Have Tabitha rate pain (1 = least, 10 = most) before and after medication. Use distraction technique. Respond to calls quickly. Reassure.
Anxiety related to pain and hospitalization	Reduced anxiety: patient states anxiety is reduced, appears calm.	Respond quickly to her needs. Check on her often. Assign consistent caregiver. Listen. Use attention and touch to convey concern.
Risk for Injury related to orthostatic hypotension	Absence of injury: no falls caused by dizziness.	Assist out of bed when permitted. Have her sit on bedside and exercise legs before rising. Check BP in lying, sitting, and standing positions to detect orthostatic hypotension. Advise her to sit and lower her head if dizzy.
Risk for Deficient Fluid Volume related to inadequate intake and excess loss of fluids	Adequate hydration: consistent intake of 4-6 liters of fluid daily, moist oral tissues, normal urine specific gravity.	Administer intravenous fluids as ordered. Teach importance of fluid intake. Weigh daily to assess change in fluid status. Monitor fluid intake and output. Note urine characteristics.
Ineffective Therapeutic Regimen Management related to lack of knowledge of disease process and self-care	Effective management of condition: patient accurately describes disease process and implications of self-care measures.	Assess what she knows about sickle cell disease. Initiate teaching when crisis has resolved. She should know to avoid smoking, alcohol, and high altitudes. Emphasize need to maintain good hydration (4-6 liters of fluids each day) and to keep regular medical appointments.

? **CRITICAL THINKING** QUESTIONS

- Why would genetic counseling be recommended for a young woman with sickle cell disease?

- Describe the order in which you should implement the listed interventions for this patient.

NURSING CARE *of the Patient in Sickle Cell Crisis*

Patients in sickle cell crisis have specialized needs beyond treatment of the simple anemia. (See Nursing Care Plan: The Patient in Sickle Cell Crisis above.)

Assessment

Obtain a complete description of the pain that the patient in sickle cell crisis is experiencing. Document the location, intensity, duration, and precipitating events. Measure vital signs every 4 hours. Be especially alert for a fever, which may indicate an infection that precipitated the crisis. Investigate any symptoms of an infection, such as sore throat, cough, abnormal breath sounds, dysuria, or diarrhea. Also monitor the patient for signs and symptoms of dehydration, such as concentrated urine, low blood pressure, or poor skin turgor, which may have precipitated the crisis.

Nursing Diagnoses, Goals, and Outcome Criteria: Sickle Cell Crisis	
NURSING DIAGNOSES	GOALS AND OUTCOME CRITERIA
Acute Pain related to sickle cell crisis	Pain relief: patient states pain has been relieved, relaxed manner
Anxiety related to pain and hospitalization	Reduced anxiety: patient states anxiety is reduced, calm manner
Risk for Injury related to orthostatic hypotension	Absence of injury: no falls caused by dizziness

Continued

| Risk for Deficient Fluid Volume related to inadequate intake or excess loss of fluids | Adequate hydration: consistent intake of 4 to 6 liters of fluid daily |
| Ineffective Therapeutic Regimen Management related to lack of knowledge of the disease process and self-care | Effective management of condition: patient accurately describes disease process and implications for self-care measures |

Interventions

Acute Pain

Give pain medications as prescribed. Usually intravenous morphine is prescribed. Initially it is not unusual for patients to need large amounts of medication to control the pain. One option for medication delivery is patient-controlled analgesia. Closely monitor the patient's pain level and medication usage. Good documentation can contribute to effective pain management. Keeping a flow sheet of patient reports of pain on a 10-point scale can be helpful, especially as different nurses care for the patient throughout the day. A "0" represents no pain, and a "10" represents the worst pain a patient ever experienced. The patient report of pain, coupled with the amount of pain medication he or she is receiving, can guide you and the physician as to the appropriate type and amount of pain medication. A detailed discussion of pain management strategies is presented in Chapter 15.

Anxiety

Sickle cell crises can be extremely frightening to a patient, especially because of the severe pain that accompanies these crises. Patients fear not obtaining adequate pain relief. The unpredictability of both the timing and the severity of the crises can be especially frustrating to patients. Provide consistent care to the patient in sickle cell crisis to establish a trusting relationship. Listening closely to the patient helps establish this trust, thereby reducing patient anxiety. Once the patient is discharged from the hospital, he or she

Patient Teaching Plan

Sickle Cell Anemia

- To prevent crises, maintain good hydration and avoid smoking, alcoholic beverages, and high altitudes.
- Drink 4 to 6 liters of fluid each day to maintain adequate hydration.
- Genetic counseling can help you with decisions about having children by exploring the risk of passing on sickle cell trait or disease.
- You can get additional information from the Sickle Cell Disease Association of America or the Sickle Cell Information Center.

can contact one of the many support groups available for patients with sickle cell disease and their families. Patients should be encouraged to attend meetings of these groups so that they can better cope with this chronic disease.

Risk for Injury

The primary treatment for anemia is red blood cell transfusions. Nursing considerations in administering blood transfusions were outlined earlier in this chapter. Nursing actions that should be taken when patients are anemic are outlined in Box 32-3. Procedures for administering a red blood cell transfusion are outlined in Box 32-5.

Risk for Deficient Fluid Volume

Administer intravenous fluids as prescribed, and keep records of fluid intake and output. Measure daily weights to assess gross fluid status. Encourage the patient to drink 4 to 6 liters of fluids each day to maintain adequate hydration.

Ineffective Therapeutic Regimen Management

When patients are not in crisis, they should be taught about their disease. Help patients identify stressors that bring on a crisis, and help them take actions to avoid these stressors. Encourage these patients not to smoke or drink large amounts of alcoholic beverages, because these are two common stressors that can bring on a crisis. Traveling to high altitudes where there is less oxygen can bring on an attack, so patients should be warned about vacationing at high altitudes. Drinking 4 to 6 liters of nonalcoholic fluids a day helps maintain adequate hydration. Regular medical follow-up is extremely important in keeping the patient with sickle cell disease out of a crisis.

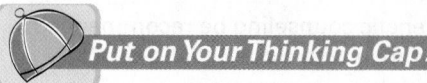

Put on Your Thinking Cap!

How would a high fluid intake decrease the risk of sickle cell crisis?

Genetic counseling can be done with people who have the sickle cell gene to inform them of the risk of passing on the trait or disease to their children. With this information, some people choose not to have their own children and risk passing on this painful, life-threatening disease. There are several resources available for patients, families, and health care providers including (1) the Sickle Cell Disease Association of America (16 South Calvert Street, Suite 600, Baltimore, MD 21202; www.sicklecelldisease.org; telephone: 1-800-421-8453 or 1-415-528-1555; email: scdaa@sicklecelldisease.org) and (2) the Sickle Cell Information Center (PO Box 109, Grady Memorial

Put on Your Thinking Cap!

Why would immunizations be particularly important for people with sickle cell disease?

Hospital, 80 Jesse Hill Jr Drive SE, Atlanta, GA 30303; www.scinfo.org; telephone: 1-404-616-3572; email: aplatt@emory.edu). These organizations provide excellent free literature on sickle cell disease and can help locate groups in specific regions of the country.

COAGULATION DISORDERS

Coagulation disorders can result from a platelet abnormality or from a clotting factor deficiency.

Thrombocytopenia

Thrombocytopenia is a condition in which a person has too few platelets circulating in the blood. This may be because not enough platelets are being made in the bone marrow or because too many platelets are being destroyed in circulation.

The major cause of thrombocytopenia related to inadequate production of platelets is treatment of cancer with chemotherapy or radiation therapy. Both chemotherapy and radiation therapy kill rapidly dividing cells. Unfortunately, the therapy cannot tell the difference between rapidly dividing cancer cells and rapidly dividing normal cells like those that produce platelets. In patients treated with chemotherapy or radiation therapy, thrombocytopenia can be expected 10 to 14 days after treatment and lasts until the bone marrow is able to make more platelets, which is usually a week.

Two examples of thrombocytopenia resulting from too many platelets being either destroyed or consumed are idiopathic thrombocytopenic purpura (ITP) and thrombotic thrombocytopenic purpura (TTP). Both of these disorders are abnormal immunologic processes that result in thrombocytopenia. ITP and TTP are discussed in more detail in Chapter 33.

Symptoms of thrombocytopenia include petechiae and purpura, gingival bleeding, epistaxis (nose bleeds), or any other unusual or prolonged bleeding. The diagnosis is made with blood tests and a bone marrow biopsy. Treatment for thrombocytopenia is to treat or stop the causative factor. If the cause is cancer chemotherapy or radiation therapy, platelet transfusions may be prescribed. Nursing actions for the patient who is at risk for injury from bleeding are outlined in Box 32-4. Procedures for administration of a platelet transfusion are outlined in Box 32-6.

Disseminated Intravascular Coagulation

Disseminated intravascular coagulation (DIC) is a hypercoagulable state, meaning that blood clotting is abnormally increased. DIC occurs when overstimulation of the normal coagulation cascade results in simultaneous thrombosis and hemorrhage. DIC is always secondary to another pathologic process, such as overwhelming sepsis, shock, major trauma, crush injuries, burns, cancer, acute tumor lysis syndrome, or obstetric complications such as abruptio placentae or fetal demise (death). Coagulation occurs at so many sites in the body that eventually all available platelets and clotting factors are depleted and uncontrolled hemorrhage results.

Blood tests that help diagnose DIC include the prothrombin time, partial thromboplastin time, fibrinogen, thrombin time, fibrin split products level, and D dimers.

Blood component replacement therapy may be prescribed. However, some physicians believe additional platelets and clotting factors perpetuate the abnormal DIC feedback loop and so do not prescribe blood component replacement. Heparin may be prescribed to interrupt the DIC cycle and allow the body to replenish platelets and clotting factors. However, heparin therapy is also controversial, because some physicians believe it only makes the bleeding worse. Nursing actions for the patient who is at risk for injury from bleeding are outlined in Box 32-4.

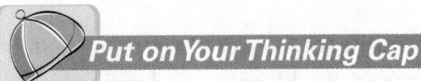

Put on Your Thinking Cap!

Explain how heparin could be helpful for a patient with DIC.

Hemophilia

Hemophilia is a genetic disease in which the affected person lacks some of the blood clotting factors normally found in plasma. The incidence of hemophilia is one case per 5,000 to 30,000 persons, depending on the type of hemophilia. In hemophilia A, factor VIII is missing, whereas in hemophilia B, factor IX is missing. Hemophilia A has a much higher incidence than hemophilia B. Because the trait is carried on the X chromosome, women carry the trait and can pass it on to their sons, who manifest the disease. However, approximately 30% of cases arise from a spontaneous mutation in patients without any family history of hemophilia. Regardless if the trait is inherited or spontaneous, it is rare for women to have this disease.

Signs and Symptoms. Uncontrollable bleeding is the hallmark of hemophilia. Bleeding generally occurs after some sort of trauma; however, bleeding can also occur spontaneously for no clear reason. Most commonly, bleeding occurs into the joints, causing swelling and severe pain. Bleeding also can occur into the skin; from the mouth, gums, and lips; and from the gastrointestinal tract. Because any surgical procedure puts the patient at great risk for bleeding, a complete preoperative evaluation must be done. Also, the availability of replacement factors for transfusion must be confirmed.

Medical Diagnosis. The diagnosis of hemophilia is made by measuring factors VIII and IX in the blood. Also, the partial thromboplastin time is prolonged in people with hemophilia.

Medical Treatment. There is no cure for hemophilia. Medical treatment for patients experiencing a bleeding episode is symptomatic. The physician usually prescribes transfusions of fresh frozen plasma or cryoprecipitate, or both. Patients with hemophilia A need factor VIII, which is found in both fresh frozen plasma and cryoprecipitate. Patients with hemophilia B need factor IX, which is found in fresh frozen plasma. Red blood cell transfusions are frequently used to replace blood lost from the profuse bleeding to which hemophiliacs are prone. The pain can be very severe. The patient needs adequate pain relief during these episodes even if they last several days. Intravenous morphine is commonly prescribed for pain relief. Because patients with hemophilia can become addicted to opioids, pain must be carefully assessed. Usually physicians try quickly to transition the patient from intravenous opioids to oral opioids to nonopioid pain relievers as the crisis resolves.

NURSING CARE *of the Patient with Hemophilia*

Assessment

Assess the patient for bleeding and pain, noting what measures have stopped the bleeding and relieved the pain in the past. Monitor vital signs and urine output.

Nursing Diagnoses, Goals, and Outcome Criteria: Hemophilia

NURSING DIAGNOSES	GOALS AND OUTCOME CRITERIA
Risk for Injury related to bleeding	Cessation of bleeding: no visible bleeding, stable vital signs
Acute Pain related to bleeding into closed spaces, creating pressure on nerves	Pain relief: patient states pain is relieved, relaxed manner
Ineffective Therapeutic Regimen Management related to lack of knowledge about the disease process and self-care	Effective management of condition: patient accurately describes condition and demonstrates self-care measures

Interventions

Risk for Injury

The primary treatment to control bleeding in hemophilia is to transfuse fresh frozen plasma, cryoprecipitate, or both. Nursing considerations in administering these products are outlined in Table 32-1. Bleeding precautions that should be taken when patients have hemophilia are similar to bleeding precautions taken when patients are thrombocytopenic. Refer to Box 32-4 for these bleeding precautions.

Nutrition Concepts

1. Iron-deficiency anemia is caused by inadequate dietary intake of iron or inadequate absorption of dietary iron.
2. The lack of intrinsic factor, which is normally manufactured in the stomach, prevents the absorption of vitamin B$_{12}$ and leads to pernicious anemia.

Acute Pain

Give pain medications as prescribed. If the patient is experiencing a great deal of pain, patient-controlled analgesia may be appropriate. Closely monitor the patient's pain level on a scale of 0 to 10. Keeping a flow sheet of patient reports of pain on a 10-point scale can be helpful, especially as different nurses care for the patient throughout the day. The patient's report of pain, coupled with the amount of pain medication he or she is receiving, can guide the nurse and physician as to the appropriate type and amount of pain medication. A detailed discussion of pain management is presented in Chapter 15.

Ineffective Therapeutic Regimen Management

Hemophiliacs bleed with even the smallest bruise or abrasion. Patients and their families should be taught to prevent injury and to safeguard their environment against accidents as much as possible. Some patients and families are taught to administer the replacement concentrate at home so that if an injury does occur, prompt treatment can be initiated and blood loss minimized. Genetic counseling can be done with people with the hemophilia gene to inform them of the risk of passing

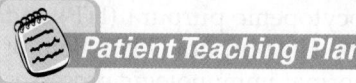

Patient Teaching Plan

Hemophilia

- Protect yourself from injuries by avoiding activities that could result in trauma.
- Know the emergency treatment of bleeding episodes: first aid measures (apply pressure, immobilize and elevate affected part if possible), seek medical attention, administer replacement concentrate (if prescribed).
- A resource for additional information is the National Hemophilia Foundation.

What Does Culture Have to Do with Blood Transfusions?

Members of some religious groups do not accept blood transfusions from other people. Autotransfusion may be an acceptable alternative.

on the disease to their children. With this information, some people choose not to have their own children and risk passing on this painful, life-threatening disease. The National Hemophilia Foundation (116 West 32nd Street, 11th Floor, New York, NY 10001; www.hemophilia.org; telephone: 1-800-42-HANDI or 1-212-328-3700; email: info@hemophilia.org) provides information and support to patients with hemophilia and their families.

Key Points

- The hematologic system includes the bone marrow, liver, spleen, and blood.
- A healthy adult has about 6 liters of blood circulating through the body.
- Components of the blood are red blood cells, platelets, clotting factors, and plasma, as well as white blood cells, proteins, electrolytes, hormones, and enzymes.
- Signs of hematologic abnormalities can include petechiae, purpura, and ecchymoses.
- The four major blood groups are A, B, AB, and O; each group may be Rh negative or Rh positive.
- People with type O-negative blood are universal blood donors, and people with type AB-positive blood are universal blood recipients.
- Types of reaction that can occur when blood or blood components are transfused include hemolytic, anaphylactic, febrile, and circulatory overload.

- Anemia is a deficiency of red blood cells or hemoglobin that may be due to blood loss, an iron-deficient diet, vitamin B_{12} deficiency, bone marrow failure, or genetic abnormalities.
- Sickle cell anemia is an incurable genetic condition in which red blood cells can become abnormally sickle-shaped so that they rupture easily and can obstruct capillaries.
- Sickle cell crisis occurs when blood flow is obstructed. Patients in crisis can experience severe pain.
- Nursing diagnoses during sickle cell crisis focus on the patient's Acute Pain, Anxiety, Risk for Injury, Risk for Deficient Fluid Volume, and Ineffective Therapeutic Regimen Management.
- Thrombocytopenia is a deficiency of platelets that can lead to excessive or prolonged bleeding.
- Hemophilia is an incurable genetic disease in which some of the factors needed for blood clotting are absent.
- Nursing diagnoses for the patient with hemophilia include the patient's Risk for Injury, Acute Pain, and Ineffective Therapeutic Regimen Management.

 Go to your Companion CD-ROM for a Pharmacology Tutorial, Audio Glossary, and 3-D animations.

evolve Be sure to visit the companion Evolve site at http://evolve.elsevier.com/Linton/ for WebLinks and additional online resources.

REVIEW QUESTIONS *Choose the best answer.*

1. If a person has no A or B antigens, what is his blood type?
   1. AB
   2. A
   3. B
   4. O

2. When assessing a patient, you notice multiple ecchymoses and petechiae. This should lead you to suspect a deficiency of:
   1. Red blood cells
   2. White blood cells
   3. Platelets
   4. Protein

3. A patient says he is a universal donor. This means his blood type is:
   1. AB positive
   2. O positive
   3. O negative
   4. AB negative

4. While receiving a blood transfusion, a patient complains of chest and back pain and chills. Your initial action should be to:
   1. Notify the blood bank
   2. Take vital signs
   3. Administer acetaminophen
   4. Stop the transfusion

5. Which nursing intervention is appropriate for a patient with a low red blood cell count?
   1. Avoid rectal temperatures and suppositories.
   2. Allow for rest between periods of activity.
   3. Encourage increased fluids and dietary fiber.
   4. Do not allow fresh flowers in the room.

6. A deficiency of red blood cells, white blood cells, and platelets is characteristic of:
   1. Aplastic anemia
   2. Hemolytic anemia
   3. Sickle cell anemia
   4. Iron-deficiency anemia

7. Sickle cell crisis occurs when:
   1. Cells lack sufficient hemoglobin to transport oxygen
   2. Sickled cells are unable to transport adequate oxygen
   3. Sickled cells form clumps that obstruct blood flow
   4. The bone marrow stops producing red blood cells

8. Factors that can trigger a sickle cell crisis include the following:
   1. Dehydration
   2. Inactivity
   3. Low iron intake
   4. Caffeine consumption

9. Overstimulation of the normal blood clotting process can result in:
   1. Disseminated intravascular coagulation
   2. Idiopathic thrombocytopenic purpura
   3. Thrombotic thrombocytopenic purpura
   4. Hemophilia

10. Hemophilia A is treated with:
    1. Factor VI
    2. Factor VII
    3. Factor VIII
    4. Factor IX

33 Immunologic Disorders

STACEY YOUNG-McCAUGHAN*

evolve http://evolve.elsevier.com/Linton/

Objectives

After reading and studying this chapter, you should be able to:

1. List the components of the immune system and describe their role in innate immunity, acquired immunity, and tolerance.
2. List the data to be collected when assessing a patient with a disorder of the immune system.
3. Describe the tests and procedures used to diagnose disorders of the immune system and nursing considerations for each.
4. Describe the nursing care for patients undergoing common therapeutic measures for disorders of the immune system.
5. Describe the pathophysiology, signs and symptoms, medical diagnosis, and medical treatment for selected disorders of the immune system.
6. Assist in developing a nursing care plan for a patient with a disorder of the immune system.

Key Terms

Be sure to check out the bonus material on the Companion CD-ROM, including selected audio pronunciations.

acquired immunity (p. 594)
antibody (ĂN-tĭ-bŏ-dē, p. 593)
antibody-mediated immunity (p. 594)
antigen (ĂN-tĭ-gĕn, p. 592)
cell-mediated immunity (p. 594)
Compromised Host Precautions (p. 603)
eicosanoid (ī-KŎ-săh-noid, p. 594)
immunity (ĭ-MŪ-nō-tē, p. 594)
immunoglobulin (ĭ-MŪ-nō-GLŎB-ū-lĭn, p. 593)
innate immunity (p. 594)
pathogen (PĂTH-ō-gĕn, p. 591)
phagocytes (FĂG-ō-sīts, p. 594)

The immune system is the body's defense network against infection. It is an inherently complex system that recognizes, isolates, and destroys pathogens as quickly as possible. Disorders of the immune system leave the patient susceptible to overwhelming,

---

* The views of this author are her own and do not purport to reflect the position of the Army Medical Department, Department of the Army, or the Department of Defense.

life-threatening infections. The nurse plays an important role in helping assess, plan, and manage the care of patients with these disorders.

ANATOMY AND PHYSIOLOGY OF THE IMMUNE SYSTEM

ANATOMIC STRUCTURES AND COMPONENTS OF THE IMMUNE SYSTEM

Bone Marrow

The bone marrow is the spongy center of the bones where the white blood cells are made. The marrow of all bones produces these cells; however, in adults the majority of white blood cells are produced in the vertebrae, ribs, sternum, skull, pelvis, and long bones of the legs.

Lymph, Lymphatics, and Lymph Nodes

When blood flows through the capillary beds to deliver oxygen and pick up carbon dioxide, not all the plasma returns to the veins to be recirculated. The lymphatic system is a network of open-ended tubes—separate from the blood circulation system—that collects the plasma left behind in the tissues and returns it to the venous system. In addition, various white blood cells that travel through tissues and organs monitoring for infection reenter the blood circulation via the lymphatic system. This mixture of plasma and cells is known as *lymph fluid*. Lymph fluid is propelled along the lymphatic system by the normal contraction of skeletal muscles. One-way valves located in the lymphatic vessels prevent the lymph fluid from pooling in the periphery. The lymphatic vessels empty into the venous system through the right lymphatic duct of the right subclavian vein and the thoracic duct of the left subclavian vein. Figure 33-1 shows the flow of lymph fluid and where it empties into these ducts.

Lymph nodes are small patches of lymphatic tissue located along the lymphatic system that filter microorganisms from the lymph fluid before it is returned to the bloodstream. Lymph nodes are located throughout the body, as shown in Figure 33-1. The lymph nodes can become swollen with infection and also with some cancers. The nodes closer to the surface of the body in the

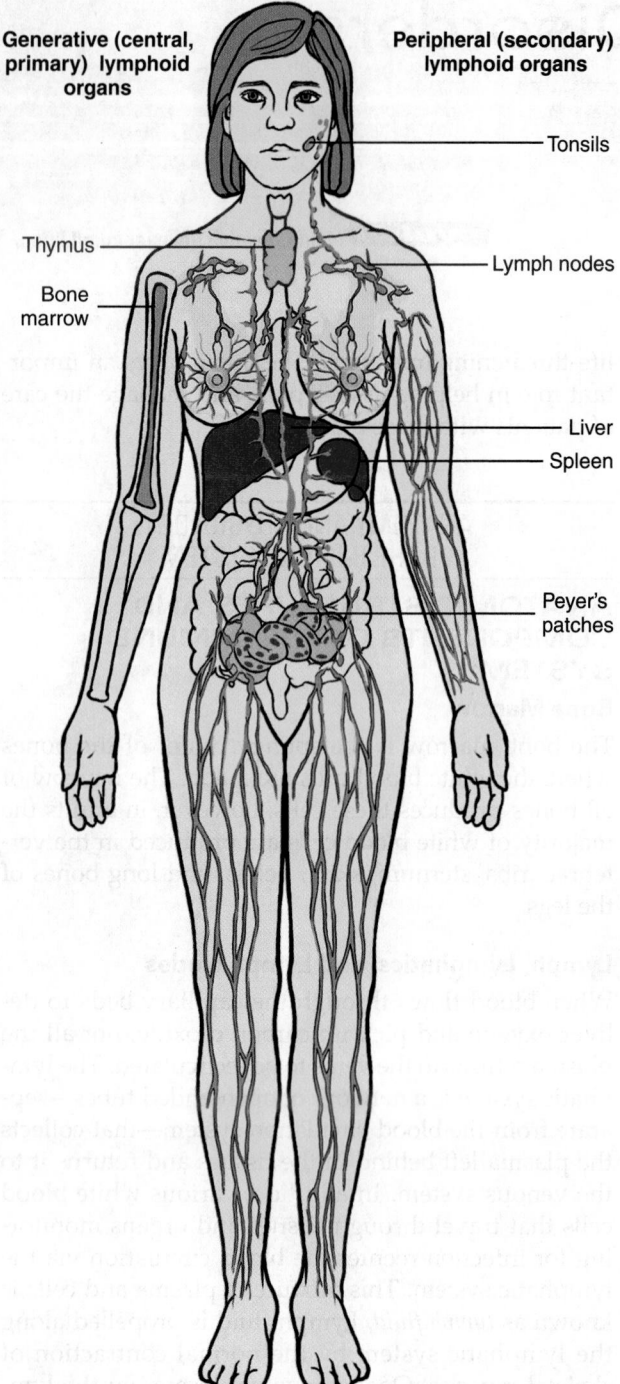

Generative (central, primary) lymphoid organs

Peripheral (secondary) lymphoid organs

Tonsils

Thymus

Bone marrow

Lymph nodes

Liver

Spleen

Peyer's patches

FIGURE **33-1** Diagram of the lymphatic system.

neck, under the arm, and in the groin can be palpated when they are swollen. Usually lymph nodes deeper in the body cannot be palpated but can be visualized on computed tomography if they are larger than 2 cm. During surgery for cancer, the surgeon will usually biopsy nearby lymph nodes and have the pathologist check the specimens to see if the cancer might have spread.

Spleen

The spleen is located in the upper left quadrant of the abdomen. Like the lymph nodes, the spleen filters microorganisms from the blood. Once trapped in the spleen, microorganisms are destroyed by the white blood cells that reside in the spleen.

Under some circumstances the spleen is surgically removed. Trauma from a motor vehicle accident can rupture the victim's spleen, necessitating removal. Patients newly diagnosed with Hodgkin's disease, a form of cancer of the lymph nodes, may have their spleens removed and pathologically examined to help determine the best treatment. Anyone without a spleen is at greater risk for certain kinds of infections such as pneumococcal infections. If possible, patients should receive a Pneumovax vaccine before undergoing splenectomy so that the body can form its own antibodies against pneumococcal bacteria. Vaccinations are not always possible for the individual undergoing an emergency splenectomy.

Thymus

The thymus is a lymphoid organ located in the upper chest below the thyroid. Early in life, certain white blood cells, called *lymphocytes,* migrate from the bone marrow where they are produced to the thymus where they mature into T lymphocytes, or T cells. Mature T lymphocytes are then released into circulation. After puberty, the T cell population has been maximized. The thymus stops growing and eventually shrinks because it is no longer needed to mature T cells.

Stem Cells

Stem cells are called *progenitor cells,* or *precursor cells,* because they are capable of developing into the various white blood cells, red blood cells, or platelets (Fig. 33-2). Although the majority of stem cells are located in the bone marrow, some stem cells circulate in the blood.

White Blood Cells (Leukocytes)

White blood cells are produced by the bone marrow. There are five major types of white blood cells: neutrophils, lymphocytes, eosinophils, basophils, and monocytes. Each type of white blood cell combats certain types of microorganisms. Normally, white blood cells identify and destroy foreign antigens or proteins by ingesting them. Because this process destroys the white blood cells themselves, the normal life span for a white blood cell is only about 12 hours. Other cells called *macrophages* clean up the white blood cell debris. If the dead white blood cells build up faster than the macrophages can clean them up, pus is formed. This is why pus is a classic sign of infection and should immediately be reported to a nurse or a physician and carefully monitored.

Neutrophils. Neutrophils fight bacterial infections. They are the most numerous of the white blood cells, comprising approximately 60% of all the white blood cells. These cells are known by many names, including *polymorphonuclear neutrophils (PMNs, polys), neuts, granulocytes (grans),* or *segmented neutrophils (segs).* The

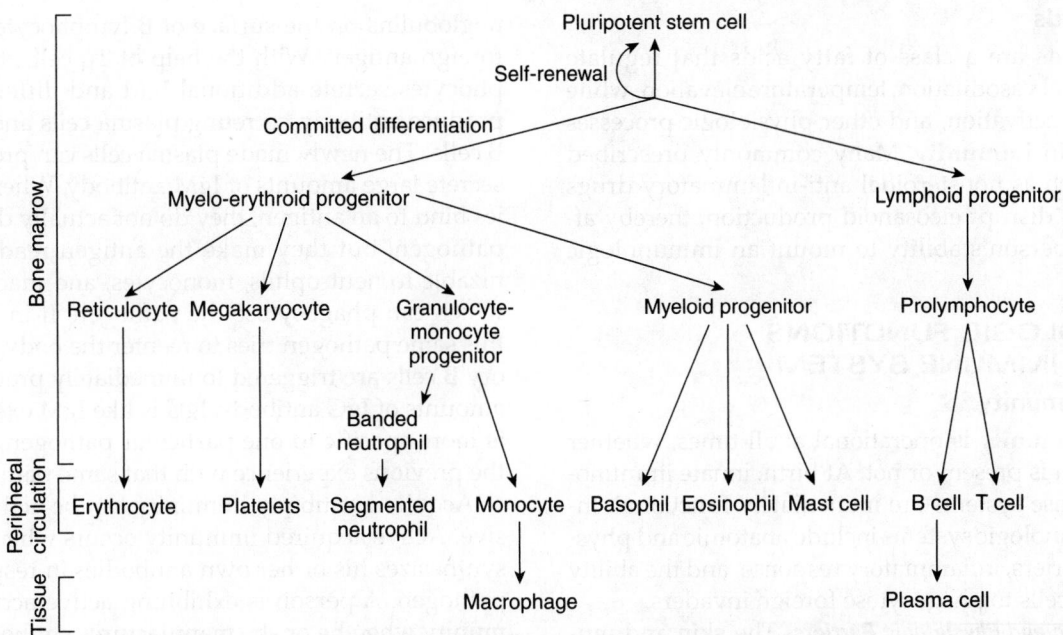

FIGURE 33-2 Maturation of cells constituting the hematologic and immune systems.

bone marrow is capable of producing huge numbers of neutrophils to fight infection.

Monocytes and Macrophages. Once released from the bone marrow, monocytes circulate in the bloodstream for approximately 1 day before leaving the peripheral circulation and entering tissue. When monocytes enter tissue, they are called *macrophages*. Some macrophages move throughout the body, whereas others stay in one particular tissue monitoring for microorganisms. Unlike neutrophils, which are destroyed during phagocytosis, macrophages can ingest many foreign antigens and survive months to years.

Eosinophils. Eosinophils combat parasitic infections. They are also associated with allergic reactions and other inflammatory processes.

Basophils. Basophils can initiate a massive inflammatory response that quickly brings other white blood cells to the site of infection. Basophils work in conjunction with **immunoglobulin** E (IgE). When IgE identifies a foreign antigen, the IgE triggers basophils to release histamine from cell vesicles located in the basophils. Histamine is a potent vasodilator that increases blood circulation to the site, quickly bringing other white blood cells to the site of infection.

Mast Cells. Like basophils, mast cells also store histamine in cell vesicles that can be released by IgE. Whereas basophils normally circulate in the blood, mast cells are located in the tissue.

B Lymphocytes (B Cells). B cells manufacture antigen-binding proteins, called *immunoglobulins*, on their cell membrane. When the B cell immunoglobulin binds with a particular antigen, the B cell is stimulated to produce plasma cells and memory B cells. Plasma cells are **antibody** factories that immediately produce large amounts of immunoglobulin. Memory B cells go into a resting state but can be quickly reactivated to produce plasma cells and antibodies if exposed to the same antigen in the future.

Once the immunoglobulin is released from the membrane of either the B cell or the plasma cell, it is called an *antibody*. There are four major types of antibodies. IgM is the first immunoglobulin to be secreted during the primary immune response to an antigen.

IgG is secreted during the secondary immune response and is more specific to a particular antigen.

IgA is present in secretions such as mucus and mother's milk. IgE attaches to the cell membranes of basophils and mast cells, where it triggers the cell to release histamine.

T Lymphocytes (T Cells). There are two major types of T lymphocytes: T helper (T_H) cells and T cytotoxic (T_C) cells. T_H cells are also called *CD4 cells* because of the protein complex CD4 found on their cell membranes. When T_H cells come in contact with foreign antigens, they secrete cytokines that activate other components of the immune system to facilitate the body's immune response. These are the cells that can become infected with the human immunodeficiency virus (HIV). T_C cells are also called *CD8 cells* because of the protein complex CD8 found on their cell membrane. When T_C cells come in contact with foreign antigens, they can directly destroy the invader.

Cytokines

Cytokines are hormones secreted by cells to signal other cells. Examples of cytokines include interferon, interleukin, tumor necrosis factor (TNF), granulocyte-macrophage colony-stimulating factor (GM-CSF), granulocyte colony-stimulating factor (G-CSF), and erythropoietin (EPO).

Eicosanoids

Eicosanoids are a class of fatty acids that regulate blood vessel vasodilation, temperature elevation, white blood cell activation, and other physiologic processes involved in immunity. Many commonly prescribed drugs, such as nonsteroidal anti-inflammatory drugs (NSAIDs), disrupt eicosanoid production, thereby affecting a person's ability to mount an immunologic response.

PHYSIOLOGIC FUNCTIONS OF THE IMMUNE SYSTEM

Innate Immunity

Innate immunity is operational at all times, whether a pathogen is present or not. At birth, innate immunologic defense systems are immediately functional. Innate immunologic systems include anatomic and physiologic barriers, inflammatory response, and the ability of certain cells to phagocytose foreign invaders.

Anatomic and Physiologic Barriers. The skin and mucous membranes are the body's first line of defense, acting as a protective covering and secreting substances that inhibit the growth of pathogens. Sweat glands secrete a lysozyme, an antimicrobial enzyme. The skin and the mucosa of the gastrointestinal and genitourinary systems are acidic, which inhibits the growth of many pathogenic organisms. Secretions from the respiratory and gastrointestinal tracts contain the antibody IgA, as well as phagocytes. Skin and mucous membrane surfaces are colonized by normal bacterial flora, which prevents pathogens from attaching and gaining access to the body. Also, coughing and sneezing, peristalsis in the gastrointestinal tract, emptying the bladder, and sloughing of dead skin cells all serve to remove microorganisms from the body, thus preventing their invasion and overgrowth.

Inflammation. The body initially responds to an injury or infection by dilating the capillary bed and increasing the capillary permeability of the affected area. This brings white blood cells to the site and allows them to enter the tissue to attack microorganisms. This multistep process is called *inflammation* and is recognized by rubor (redness), tumor (swelling), calor (heat), and dolor (pain) at the site of injury or infection.

Phagocytosis. Phagocytosis is the process of ingesting and digesting invading pathogens, dead cells, and cellular debris. Neutrophils, monocytes, and macrophages are capable of phagocytosis and are sometimes called *phagocytes.*

Acquired Immunity

Whereas innate immunity fights any type of invader and is operational at all times, acquired immunity is specific to a particular pathogen and is activated only when needed. The two types of acquired immunity are antibody-mediated and cell-mediated.

Antibody-Mediated Immunity. An antibody-mediated immune response is initiated when the IgM immunoglobulins on the surface of B lymphocytes detect a foreign antigen. With the help of T_H cells, the B lymphocytes secrete additional IgM and differentiate to produce antibody-secreting plasma cells and memory B cells. The newly made plasma cells can produce and secrete large amounts of IgM antibody. When antibodies bind to an antigen, they do not actually destroy the pathogen, but they make the antigen readily recognizable to neutrophils, monocytes, and macrophages, which can phagocytose the pathogen. If in the future this same pathogen tries to reenter the body, the memory B cells are triggered to immediately produce large amounts of IgG antibody. IgG is like IgM except that it is more specific to one particular pathogen, based on the previous experience with that same pathogen.

Acquired antibody immunity can be active or passive. Active acquired immunity occurs when a person synthesizes his or her own antibodies in response to a pathogen. A person is exhibiting active acquired immunity when he or she manufactures antibodies in response to an infection or a vaccination. Active acquired immunity is permanent. Passive acquired immunity occurs when an antibody produced by one person or an animal is transferred to another person. For example, IgA antibodies in mother's milk confer passive immunity to breast-fed babies. Another example of passive acquired immunity is the gamma globulin that may be given to a person exposed to hepatitis. Gamma globulin contains IgG antibodies that help destroy the hepatitis virus. Passive acquired immunity lasts only 1 to 2 months after the antibodies have been received.

Cell-Mediated Immunity. Antibody-mediated immune responses are aimed primarily at invading microorganisms such as bacteria. In contrast, cell-mediated immunity is aimed primarily at intracellular defects caused by viruses and cancer. Cell-mediated immunity is also responsible for delayed hypersensitivity reactions and rejection of transplanted tissue. T_C cells are the primary component of cell-mediated immunity. When T_C cells recognize foreign antigens in cells, they secrete cytotoxic substances that destroy the defective cells. Unfortunately, a transplanted tissue graft, such as a kidney transplant or a heart transplant, may be recognized by the organ recipient's immune system as foreign and is attacked by T_C cells in this same way.

Tolerance

As part of initiating an immunologic response, the immune system must be able to recognize its own proteins and not mount an immune response against itself. This process of self-recognition occurs as part of normal neonatal growth and development. Autoimmune diseases occur when there is a breakdown of tolerance. The immune system inappropriately identifies its own proteins as foreign and mounts a response to destroy these self-proteins. Examples of autoimmune diseases include idiopathic thrombocytopenic purpura (ITP), thrombotic thrombocytopenic purpura (TTP), acute rheumatic fever, type 1 diabetes mellitus, systemic lupus erythematosus, rheumatoid arthritis, Graves' disease, and Hashimoto's thyroiditis.

AGE-RELATED CHANGES

With advancing age, the bone marrow becomes less productive. Immunologic function is generally not affected unless a person is unusually stressed by trauma, a chronic infection, or treatment for cancer. Yet even with conditions necessitating a higher production of blood cells, the bone marrow usually can respond to the increased demand, given more time. The lymphatic tissue grows very quickly between the ages of 6 and 20 years. With advancing age, lymphatic tissue shrinks, resulting in fewer and smaller lymph nodes. However, as with the bone marrow, this does not generally affect the overall health of an individual.

NURSING ASSESSMENT OF THE IMMUNE SYSTEM

Many subtle findings in the assessment can suggest changes in the patient's immune system that should be reported to the registered nurse or the physician

to evaluate the patient. Box 33-1 outlines the nursing assessment of patients with disorders of the immune system.

HEALTH HISTORY

Chief Complaint and History of Present Illness

Pay special attention to the patient who remarks that he or she has frequent or persistent infections, bleeds for a long time when cut, bruises easily, or has chronic fatigue, because these symptoms may reflect an underlying immunologic disorder.

Past Medical History

A patient could have an underlying immunologic problem if he or she reports any of the following: cancer or prior treatment for cancer, HIV infection, history of splenectomy, or placement of an indwelling venous access device, indicating that the patient needed long-term venous access. Medications the patient is currently using or a recent change in medication may suggest an underlying immunologic problem. It is important to find out what over-the-counter medications (including herbal products) the patient uses, because many of these products contain aspirin or NSAIDs, which may disrupt immunologic function. Ask the patient about any recent changes in medications and any recent immunizations.

Box 33-1   ASSESSMENT of a Patient with Disorders of the Immune System

Health History

History of Present Illness:
Frequent or persistent infections, prolonged bleeding, easy bruising, chronic fatigue

Past Medical History:
Cancer or prior treatment for cancer, HIV infection, history of splenectomy, placement of an indwelling venous access device indicating that the patient needed long-term venous access, recent infections, current medications (including over-the-counter medications, recent changes in medication, herbal products), recent immunizations

Family History:
Cancer, death of a family member at a young age for reasons other than trauma

Review of Systems

Integumentary:
Rash, breaks in the skin, ulcers, lesions, or enlarged lymph nodes; red, swollen, or painful areas

Neurologic:
Weakness, lethargy, malaise, restlessness, apprehension, headache

Respiratory:
Sinus pain, dyspnea, cough

Gastrointestinal:
Sore throat, pain with swallowing, pain with defecation, unplanned weight loss or weight gain, diarrhea

Genitourinary:
Pain or burning with urination

Musculoskeletal:
Pain in bones or joints

Endocrine:
Fatigue

Functional Assessment
Occupation and hobbies, changes in ability to do activities of daily living, roles at home and work, self-concept, activities and exercise, sleep and rest, nutrition, interpersonal relationships, stressors, coping style

Physical Examination

Vital Signs:
Fever, tachycardia, tachypnea, hypotension

Height and Weight

General Survey:
Responsiveness, mood, expression, posture

Skin:
Color

Head and Neck:
Enlarged, swollen, or draining areas; enlarged lymph nodes

Thorax:
Enlarged lymph nodes, respiratory rate, breath sounds, heart rate

Abdomen:
Organ enlargement, enlarged lymph nodes

Family History

Note any family history of immunologic disorders such as cancer. Death of a family member at a young age for reasons other than trauma may indicate a genetic immunologic disorder.

Review of Systems

The review of systems is aimed at finding out what symptoms the patient has been experiencing over the past weeks or months. These symptoms might provide clues as to what specific medical disorder the patient may now have. The primary symptom of an immunologic disorder is infection. The patient should be carefully questioned about any reddened, swollen, painful, or unusually warm areas that might indicate an infectious process. Ask the patient about fever, chills, or night sweats. Night sweats can occur when the patient's temperature rises at night but the patient does not awaken until the temperature falls, causing sweating. Night sweats can occur normally in women undergoing menopause. However, night sweats can also be a symptom of infection (e.g., tuberculosis, malaria), leukemia (cancer of the white blood cells), or lymphoma (cancer of the lymph nodes).

Begin the review of systems with the integument. Ask about any red, swollen, or painful areas, which could be sites of infection. Document any breaks in the skin, ulcers, lesions, or enlarged lymph nodes, which could indicate a site of infection. Relevant data about the neurologic system include weakness, lethargy, malaise, restlessness, apprehension, or headache, which could indicate a central nervous system infection. In relation to the respiratory system, ask about sinus pain, dyspnea, or cough, which could indicate an infection. If the cough is productive, ask the patient to describe the sputum. When assessing the gastrointestinal system, ask about sore throat, any pain with swallowing, and any pain with defecation, which could indicate an infection. Ask if the patient has had any unplanned weight loss or weight gain. When reviewing the genitourinary system, ask about any pain or burning with urination, which could indicate an infection. Describe any musculoskeletal pain. Finally, when assessing the endocrine system, ask about any unusual fatigue.

Functional Assessment

Patients newly diagnosed with an immunologic disorder may not experience dramatic changes in their functional abilities. However, many immunologic disorders are chronic conditions that the patient has lived with—and been treated for—for many years. The functional abilities of these patients may be adversely affected.

Occupation and Hobbies. Knowing a patient's job and hobbies can alert the nurse to unusual chemical exposures. Because the bone marrow and blood can be affected by various chemicals, any recent chemical exposure should be noted. For example, someone who builds models for a hobby may be exposed to unusual glues or paints that may affect the blood count.

Self-Concept. The patient's self-concept can be assessed by exploring the patient's feeling about himself or herself. For many people, one's self-concept depends on one's job. If the patient is unable to work because of an immunologic disorder, his or her self-concept can be adversely affected. In addition, medical insurance is often contingent on employment. Loss of medical insurance and the need to go on state or federal assistance can further erode a patient's self-concept. Another factor that can adversely affect the patient's self-concept is a change in appearance because of the disease or the treatment.

Activity and Exercise. Document the patient's current activity level and the effects of the disease and treatment on the patient's usual pattern of activity and exercise. Ask about the layout of the patient's home, specifically the location of bathrooms in relation to living areas and bedrooms. Ask whether the patient must climb stairs to enter the home or get to a second floor. Stair climbing can quickly tire a patient with an immunologic disorder. Inquire what the patient does for recreation and whether these activities can still be done during times of decreased energy.

Sleep and Rest. Note the number of continuous hours the patient sleeps every night, whether any sleeping aids are used, what interrupts the patient's sleep, and whether the patient naps during the day.

Nutrition. Ask the patient to describe his or her usual diet and any recent changes in appetite or weight. Identify factors that might be interfering with eating, such as nausea, vomiting, and taste changes (see the Nutrition Concepts box below). Depression and loneliness can adversely affect a patient's nutritional status. Limited financial resources can also limit a patient's ability to maintain a nutritious diet.

Interpersonal Relationships. Explore the patient's view of himself or herself as a husband or wife, father or mother, son or daughter, friend, and co-worker. Discuss the effects of the disease on these relationships. The patient's roles in the home must be considered. Ask for what household chores the patient is responsible and who does the shopping, cooking, and cleaning. If there are children for whom to care, ask whether the patient is able to perform the usual child care.

Coping and Stress. Ask what worries the patient and how the patient usually deals with stress. Explore

 Nutrition Concepts

1. Because food contains microorganisms, patients with low white blood cell counts are discouraged from eating raw fruits and vegetables and from drinking milk.
2. Patients with HIV require high calorie and nutrient intake to combat wasting.

sources of support, which might include family, support groups, and spiritual beliefs and practices.

Perception of Health. Discuss the patient's view of his or her own health and health practices. This might include measures taken to prevent complications from disease and keeping regular medical appointments.

PHYSICAL EXAMINATION

The physical examination begins with measurement of vital signs and height and weight. Be alert for fever, tachycardia, tachypnea, and hypotension.

General Survey

Note the patient's responsiveness, mood, expression, and posture. Throughout the examination, carefully inspect and describe any reddened, swollen, or painful areas the patient identifies.

Skin

Inspect the skin from head to toe. Note the general color, texture, turgor, temperature, and integrity of the skin. Palpate for any swollen or painful areas.

Head and Neck

When examining the eyes, ears, nose, mouth, and throat, note any enlarged, swollen, or draining areas that might indicate an infection. Examples might be swollen, draining sinuses; a canker sore in the mouth; or enlarged tonsils with exudate. The examiner with advanced skills may palpate the neck for enlarged lymph nodes.

Thorax

The examiner with advanced skills may palpate the axilla for enlarged lymph nodes.

Lungs. Document respiratory rate and effort. Auscultate for wheezing, crackles, or rhonchi. Patients with a respiratory tract infection may have abnormal breath sounds or a cough.

Heart and Vascular System. Record heart rate and blood pressure. Patients with a severe infection may be tachycardic or hypotensive.

Abdomen

The examiner with advanced skills may palpate the abdomen for tenderness. The liver and spleen can become enlarged with blood cell disorders, causing abdominal fullness and tenderness. Palpate the groin for enlarged lymph nodes.

DIAGNOSTIC TESTS AND PROCEDURES

Various blood studies are used to screen the function of the patient's immunologic system. Blood studies as well as other tests and procedures done to diagnose disorders of the immune system are described in the Diagnostic Tests and Procedures tables on pp. 598 and

600 and 601. The laboratory performing the test should provide normal values for the various blood tests. Ranges of normal values can be found in various textbooks of laboratory and diagnostic tests.

BLOOD TESTS

The complete blood cell (CBC) count is a common blood test done in most laboratories that reports the total number of white blood cells as well as what percentage of the total number of white blood cells are neutrophils, monocytes, eosinophils, basophils, and lymphocytes. Both the total number of white blood cells in the body and the differential, or percentage of each of the specific types of white blood cells in the body, are evaluated. Normal white blood cell counts range between 5,000 and 10,000 white blood cells per cubic millimeter (mm^3) of blood. The majority of the white blood cells, 60%, are neutrophils. Physicians and nurses are interested primarily in the number of neutrophils because these are the cells that fight bacterial infections.

A *shift to the left* on a CBC indicates that the percentage of the white blood cells that are neutrophils is greater than 60%. This usually indicates that the bone marrow has been stimulated to produce more neutrophils to fight a severe infection. In contrast, a *shift to the right* on a CBC indicates that only a small percentage of the white blood cells are neutrophils. This can occur either when the body has been completely overwhelmed with an infection, exhausting the supply of neutrophils, or when the bone marrow is not producing neutrophils. To calculate the absolute neutrophil count, multiply the percent neutrophils indicated on the differential of the CBC by the total number of white blood cells. See Box 33-2 for a sample calculation.

Other blood tests are specific to the diagnosis of a particular disease. The antinuclear antibody test detects antibodies in the blood that may be indicative of systemic lupus erythematosus or other autoimmune disorders. An enzyme-linked immunosorbent assay and Western blot tests are used to diagnose HIV infection. T cell counts and viral load are tests used to determine the severity of the infection. The Diagnostic Tests and Procedures table on p. 598 describes the procedures for collecting blood specimens for these tests.

CULTURES OF BLOOD, URINE, SPUTUM, AND STOOL

Cultures are done to detect infections in the blood, sputum, urine, or stool. When a patient has a fever without an obvious source of infection, all of these specimens are obtained to look for the source of the infection. The table on p. 598 describes the procedures for collecting these specimens for culture.

SKIN TESTS

Skin tests can serve as a barometer of immune system functioning, pointing out either hyposensitivities or

DIAGNOSTIC TESTS and PROCEDURES   Laboratory Studies to Evaluate the Immune System

TEST/STUDY	PURPOSE/PROCEDURE	PATIENT PREPARATION	POSTPROCEDURE NURSING CARE
Blood tests (CBC, ANA, HIV ELISA, HIV Western blot, T cell counts, viral load)	Measure various blood components. Different blood tests are collected in different laboratory tubes containing specific reagents or no reagents at all. Usually the tubes have color-coded tops. Be sure and collect the blood in the blood tube specific for the blood test ordered. Usually each institution's laboratory publishes a manual identifying what colored tube to use for each blood test.	Choose the correct blood tube to collect the blood in. Tell the patient he or she will feel a needlestick as the needle goes through the skin.	Apply bandage. Have the patient hold pressure to the site for 1 minute. The bandage may be removed in 1 hour.
Blood cultures	Detect and identify microorganisms in the blood.	Choose the correct blood culture bottles according to whether aerobic and anaerobic cultures are to be drawn. The vein is prepared with Betadine and allowed to dry. The tops of the blood culture bottles are prepared with Betadine and allowed to dry. Do not touch the draw site except with sterile gloves. Tell the patient he or she will feel a needlestick as the needle goes through the skin. Draw enough blood so that 5 mL of blood can be placed in each culture bottle. Send the specimens to the laboratory immediately. Blood culture results are evaluated at 48 and 72 hours. Tell the patient not to expect any final results for 3-4 days.	Apply bandage. Have the patient hold pressure to the site for 1 minute. The bandage may be removed in 1 hour.
Sputum cultures	Detect and identify microorganisms in the sputum.	Give the patient a sterile cup. Have the patient collect sputum next time he or she coughs. Caution the patient not to collect saliva. Sputum comes from the lungs with coughing. Send the specimen to the laboratory immediately.	No special care after the procedure is required.
Urine cultures	Detect and identify microorganisms in the urine.	Give the patient wipes and a sterile container. Have the patient clean around the meatus of the urethra. Tell the patient to urinate a small amount into the toilet and stop. Then tell the patient to collect a urine specimen. If the patient is unable to collect the specimen, the physician may request a straight catheterization to collect the specimen. Follow the procedures for catheterizing a patient as described in Chapter 40. If the patient has an indwelling catheter, clamp the catheter. In approximately 15 minutes, prepare the withdrawal port on the catheter with Betadine and allow the Betadine to dry. Withdraw a sample of urine through the port with a sterile needle and syringe, and transfer the specimen into a sterile collection cup. Send the specimen to the laboratory immediately.	No special care after the procedure is required.
Stool cultures	Detect and identify microorganisms in the stool.	Have the patient defecate into a clean bedpan or other container. Using a sterile tongue blade, collect a specimen in a sterile container. Send the specimen to the laboratory immediately. Some tests must be done while the specimen is still warm.	No special care after the procedure is required.

Data from Fischbach, F. (2000). A manual of laboratory and diagnostic tests (6th ed.). Philadelphia: Lippincott.
CBC, Complete blood count; ANA, antinuclear antibody; HIV, human immunodeficiency virus; ELISA, enzyme-linked immunosorbent assay.

Box 33-2 | Calculating Absolute Neutrophil Count (ANC) from Complete Blood Count

CBC report

WBC × 10³	6.5
RBC × 10⁶	4.51
HGB g/dL	14.0
HCT %	40.8
MCV fl	90.5
MCH pg	30.9
MCHC g/dL	34.2
PLT × 10³	333

Automated Differential

LYMPH %	35.0
MONO %	10.3
NEUT %	46.3
EOS %	7.3
BASO %	1.0

Manual Differential

SEGMENTED NEUTROPHILS %	49
BANDED NEUTROPHILS %	1
LYMPHOCYTES %	32
MONOCYTES %	8
EOSINOPHILS %	9
BASOPHILS %	1

To calculate the ANC, use the *manual differential* because it is more accurate. Multiply the percent of segmented neutrophils (49% in this example) and the percent of banded neutrophils (1% in this example) by the total number of white blood cells (WBCs) (6500 in this example). Banded neutrophils are included in the calculations of the ANC because they are developmentally nearly mature neutrophils and can function as mature neutrophils (see Fig. 33-2). If a manual differential has not been done, the automated differential can be used; however if the total WBC count is >10,000 µL or <3,000/µL, a manual differential should be requested.

Generic Calculation

(% neutrophils + % bands) (WBC) = ANC

Calculations for this Example

(.49 + .01) (6500) = 3250

---

hypersensitivities to a particular antigen. Examples of allergens used in skin testing include dust, pollen, animal dander, purified protein derivative, tuberculin bacillus, and *Candida albicans*. The Diagnostic Tests and Procedures table on p. 601 describes the procedure for skin tests.

COMMON THERAPEUTIC MEASURES

NURSING ACTIONS FOR THE PATIENT AT RISK FOR INJURY FROM INFECTION

The lower a patient's white blood cell count, in particular the lower the neutrophil count, the greater is the patient's risk of infection. Box 33-3 outlines typical nursing actions for the patient at risk for injury from infection.

BONE MARROW TRANSPLANT AND PERIPHERAL BLOOD STEM CELL TRANSPLANT

Bone marrow transplantation and peripheral blood stem cell transplantation are done to restore the hematologic and immunologic systems in patients with malignancies who have received extremely high doses of chemotherapy and radiation therapy. Bone marrow transplantation is also used in patients with genetic bone marrow defects and aplastic anemia in an attempt to repopulate the bone marrow with blood-producing cells. The donated bone marrow is administered to the patient just like a blood transfusion through an intravenous line. The infused bone marrow finds its way to the patient's bone marrow, where it starts growing and producing healthy white blood cells, red blood cells, and platelets.

There are three main types of transplants: allogeneic bone marrow transplant, autologous bone marrow transplant, and peripheral blood stem cell transplant. *Allogeneic bone marrow transplants* have been done the longest. They originally were used to treat people with leukemia, or cancer of the white blood cells. High doses of chemotherapy and radiation therapy are given to destroy all of the cancerous bone marrow. Then bone marrow from a human leukocyte antigen (HLA)–matched donor is reinfused into the patient to restore bone marrow function. HLA typing is similar to blood typing but is much more specific. Because these HLAs are genetically determined, brothers and sisters of the patient are initially tested to determine whether they can be bone marrow donors for their sibling. There is a 25% chance that a sibling will be an HLA match to a patient needing a bone marrow transplant. There is a possibility that someone in the general population might be HLA matched to the patient, but the chances of finding a matched, unrelated donor are very small. For many patients, an allogeneic bone marrow transplant is not possible because a matched donor cannot be found.

Another type of bone marrow transplant harvests the patient's own bone marrow before chemotherapy and radiation therapy. After therapy, the patient's own bone marrow is returned to the patient. This type of bone marrow transplant, called an *autologous bone marrow transplant*, is the best option for patients with a solid tumor that has not metastasized to the bone marrow—for example, patients with breast cancer or lymphoma. An autologous bone marrow transplant is

DIAGNOSTIC TESTS and PROCEDURES | *Special Procedures to Evaluate the Immune System*

TEST/STUDY	PURPOSE/PROCEDURE	PATIENT PREPARATION	POSTPROCEDURE NURSING CARE
Lymphangiography (LAG)	Lymphangiography demonstrates the anatomy of the lymphatic vessels and nodes. The patient is taken to diagnostic radiology, where a 1- to 2-inch incision is made on the dorsum of each foot or hand. The lymphatic vessels are cannulated and dye is injected. Several radiographs are taken as the dye moves up the extremities. The patient returns to diagnostic radiology 12 to 24 hours later for more radiographs of the lymph nodes and higher lymphatic channels.	Explain the purpose and procedure to the patient and obtain signed consent. Ask the patient about any allergies to contrast media. No fasting is necessary. Some local discomfort may be experienced as the local anesthetic agent is injected to numb the top of the feet or hands. Incisions may stain blue from the dye. The procedure takes approximately 3 hours. The patient returns to diagnostic radiology 12 to 24 hours later for more radiographs.	Check the patient's vital signs q 4 hr for 48 hours. Keep the incisions clean and dry after the procedure. The doctor may order the legs or arms to be elevated. Stitches may be in place that should be removed in 5 to 7 days.
Liver-spleen scan	A spleen scan is used to evaluate the size and function of the spleen. In the nuclear medicine department, a radioactive dye is injected into a vein. The amount of dye taken up by the spleen is measured by a machine 20 to 60 minutes after the dye is injected.	Explain the purpose and procedure to the patient. Ask the patient about any allergies to contrast media. No fasting is necessary. An intravenous line must be in place to inject the dye but may be discontinued after the injection. The procedure takes approximately 60 minutes.	No special care after the procedure is required.
Gallium scan	A gallium scan is used to detect the presence, location, and size of chronic infections, abscesses, and malignant tumors primarily of lymphoid origin. In the nuclear medicine department, a radioactive dye is injected into a vein. The amount of dye taken up by malignant lymphoid tissues is measured by a machine 24 to 72 hours after the dye is injected.	Explain the purpose and procedure to the patient. Ask the patient about any allergies to contrast media. An intravenous line must be in place to inject the dye but may be discontinued after the injection. Scanning is usually done 24 to 72 hours after dye injection. If the abdomen is to be scanned, a laxative is usually given the evening before the scanning. However, the patient may eat breakfast the morning of the scan. During imaging the patient must lie quietly for 45 to 90 minutes while scanning is done.	

Adapted from Fischbach, F. (2000). *A manual of laboratory and diagnostic tests* (6th ed.). Philadelphia: Lippincott.

generally not an option for patients with leukemia or who have a cancer that has metastasized to the bone marrow, because healthy bone marrow must be reinfused into the patient after chemotherapy and radiation therapy to prevent cancer recurrence.

A third type of bone marrow transplant is a *peripheral blood stem cell transplant*. For this type of transplant, colony-stimulating factors are administered to the patient to stimulate the bone marrow to produce large numbers of white blood cells. Then apheresis is performed to collect the patient's peripheral stem cells.

Apheresis is a procedure similar to hemodialysis. A large-bore apheresis catheter is placed into the subclavian vein that allows simultaneous blood withdrawal and blood reinfusion. The patient's blood is first drawn off into the apheresis machine. The apheresis machine centrifuges, or spins, the blood, separating it into white cells, red cells, and plasma. The stem cells in the white blood cell layer are removed and stored, and the rest of the white blood cells, red blood cells, and plasma are returned to the patient. When enough of these peripheral blood stem cells are harvested and stored, the

DIAGNOSTIC TESTS and PROCEDURES | *Special Procedures to Evaluate the Immune System—cont'd*

TEST/STUDY	PURPOSE/PROCEDURE	PATIENT PREPARATION	POSTPROCEDURE NURSING CARE
Skin tests	Skin testing is done for several reasons—to detect sensitivity to allergens such as pollen, to determine sensitivity to microorganisms that cause disease (e.g., tuberculin), and to determine whether cell-mediated immune functions are normal. As part of the evaluation of a patient with HIV infection, skin testing is done to determine whether the cell-mediated immune system is functioning. The inner side of the patient's forearm is cleaned. Generally, 0.1 mL of the test material is injected intradermally using a 26- or 27-gauge needle and tuberculin syringe. A common battery of five skin tests used to test immune function in patients with HIV infection includes mumps, *Candida*, *Trichophyton*, tetanus, and purified protein derivative of tuberculin bacillus.	Explain the purpose and procedure to the patient. Tell the patient he or she will feel a needle prick as the needle goes through the skin.	No special care after the procedure is required. Tell the patient that he or she must be reexamined in 2 to 3 days to determine the results of the testing. Swelling at the site of injection indicates that the body's cell-mediated immune system is functioning.

patient is treated with chemotherapy and radiation therapy. After treatment, the peripheral blood stem cells are returned to the patient. Stem cells re-engraft more quickly than bone marrow, reducing the duration of neutropenia and therefore the risk of infection. Often peripheral blood stem cell transplants are administered concurrently with autologous bone marrow transplants. Peripheral blood stem cell transplants have been so successful that they are quickly becoming the most common type of transplant.

Major complications of bone marrow transplantation and peripheral blood stem cell transplantation include infection, thrombocytopenia, renal insufficiency, hepatic veno-occlusive disease, and graft-versus-host disease. Infection is a constant concern in the care of patients undergoing bone marrow transplantation. For approximately 2 weeks after transplantation, when the new bone marrow is engrafting, patients are severely neutropenic and at very high risk for infection. Even when white blood cells and neutrophil counts approach normal levels, the patient's cell-mediated immune function can be compromised for more than a year.

Thrombocytopenia can be profound and prolonged in the patient undergoing bone marrow transplantation or peripheral blood stem cell transplantation because of the high doses of chemotherapy and radiation therapy.

Renal insufficiency can occur if the kidneys are damaged with high doses of nephrotoxic drugs such as cisplatin chemotherapy or the antibiotic *gentamicin*. Kidney function can be further compromised if blood flow to and through the kidneys is not maintained.

Hepatic veno-occlusive disease can occur if the liver is damaged with high doses of chemotherapy and radiation therapy. Blood flow into and out of the liver can be obstructed, resulting in ischemia, ascites, and increasing serum bilirubin.

Graft-versus-host disease is a complication of allogeneic bone marrow transplants in which T lymphocytes in the transplanted bone marrow identify the patient's tissue as foreign and try to destroy the patient's tissues. The transplanted T lymphocytes attack primarily epithelial cells of the skin, gastrointestinal tract, biliary ducts, and lymphoid system, resulting in a skin rash; large amounts of green, watery, heme-negative diarrhea; and elevated liver enzyme levels.

 Put on Your Thinking Cap!

Compare and contrast the three types of bone marrow transplants in relation to the following: patient preparation, source of cells, advantages, disadvantages, and complications.

Box 33-3 | *Nursing Actions for the Patient at Risk for Injury From Infection: Compromised Host Precautions*

1. The patient should have a private room. It does not have to be an isolation room. The door may be left open. A "Compromised Host Precaution" sign should be posted on the door.

2. All persons entering the patient's room must wash hands before touching the patient for any reason. This is the most important way to prevent infection. The patient and family should be encouraged to remind all staff and visitors to wash their hands before touching the patient.

3. Monitor vital signs every 2-4 hours. Notify physician immediately of temperature >101° F to consider the need for an infectious fever workup and initiating or changing antibiotics. An infectious fever workup usually includes two sets of blood cultures, a chest radiograph, sputum culture, urine culture, wound culture, and cultures of other sites suggestive of infection. Patients with a central line or permanent, indwelling venous access device usually have one set of specimens for culture drawn from the line and one set drawn from a peripheral site. Mark the culture bottles clearly regarding where the specimen was obtained to assist with localization of the infection. Blood cultures are more likely to yield the offending organism if the blood is drawn as the patient's temperature is rising instead of after the patient's temperature has peaked.

4. Invasive procedures should be kept to a minimum. Invasive devices such as catheters and tubes should be removed as soon as the patient's medical condition permits.

5. Careful attention to aseptic technique must be observed, especially when performing phlebotomy, handling intravenous lines, or performing other invasive procedures.

6. Designate a particular stethoscope and thermometer to be used exclusively in caring for the patient.

7. Masks are not required; they are actually discouraged. Staff with upper respiratory tract or other infections should not care for the patient.

8. Clean table tops, equipment, and the floor frequently with hospital-approved disinfectant, clean cloths, and clean mops.

9. The patient should be taught to wash his or her hands before and after eating, using the toilet, and doing any self-care procedure. If possible, the patient should shower every day. Liquid soap instead of bar soap should be used.

10. Encourage the patient to cough and deep breathe every 4 hours. Mobility should be encouraged. Smoking should be discouraged.

11. Only canned or cooked foods should be served. Raw fruits, raw vegetables, and milk products are not served because of the risk of *Escherichia coli*, *Pseudomonas aeruginosa*, and *Klebsiella* species bacteria on or in these food items. The patient should be encouraged to choose appropriate foods from the menu. The diet roster should be annotated "Compromised Host Precautions" so that the nutrition care staff can verify that appropriate choices are being made.

12. Tests, scans, and appointments away from the patient's room should be coordinated in advance to eliminate or minimize waiting time in common waiting areas.

13. The patient should wear a clean mask when outside the room, especially in heavily traveled public areas such as corridors, elevators, and waiting rooms. The mask may be removed when the patient is in less public areas. A new mask should be used for each trip out of the room.

14. Some hospitals allow flowers and plants in the patient's room; however, they should not be handled by the patient because of the possibility of *Escherichia coli* contamination of the water and soil.

15. No humidifiers with standing water should be used in the patient's room. If a wall humidifier is needed, the water should be changed every day.

16. Teach the patient and family about the underlying pathophysiology that puts the patient at risk for infection and about precautions to minimize the risk for infection.

Patients undergoing bone marrow transplantation or peripheral blood stem cell transplantation as treatment for a hematologic or immune system disorder need intensive nursing care and long-term follow-up to be sure their new immune system is functioning and that the underlying disease does not recur.

DISORDERS OF THE IMMUNE SYSTEM

WHITE BLOOD CELL DISORDERS

The main function of the white blood cells is to protect the body against pathogens. Patients are at great risk for infection when the white blood cells are not functioning properly.

Neutropenia

Neutropenia occurs when the total number of neutrophils is abnormally low, putting the patient at increased risk of infection. Neutropenia can be caused by decreased bone marrow production (e.g., because of infiltration with malignant cells), chemotherapy, radiation therapy, certain drugs (e.g., zidovudine, clozapine), or an autoimmune reaction (e.g., systemic lupus erythematosus, rheumatoid arthritis). Neutropenia also can be caused by increased neutrophil utilization because of overwhelming infection. The longer the patient is neutropenic, the greater is the chance of infection. Because these patients do not have adequate numbers of white blood cells to mount an immunologic response, classic signs of infection (redness, swelling, pain) may be absent. Fever may be the only sign of infection.

The most common sites of infection in neutropenic patients are the lung (pneumonia), blood (septicemia), skin, urinary tract, and gastrointestinal tract (mucositis, esophagitis, perirectal lesions). Usually bacteria cause infections in neutropenic patients; however, fungi and viruses can also infect these patients. The goal of antibiotic therapy is to support the patient until the patient's own white blood cells are available to fight the infection. In addition to administering prescribed antibiotics, it is important to minimize the patient's exposure to infectious agents by instituting Compromised Host Precautions, described in Box 33-3.

Leukemia

Leukemia is a cancer of the white blood cells in which the bone marrow produces too many immature white blood cells. These nonfunctioning, immature white blood cells leave the patient unprotected against microorganisms and at a great risk for life-threatening infections. The American Cancer Society statistics estimated that 35,070 cases of leukemia would be diagnosed in 2006, accounting for 2% of all new cases of cancer diagnosed in that year. Although for most cases no cause is identified, factors that may be associated with the development of leukemia are exposure to large doses of ionizing radiation or exposure to certain chemicals such as benzene, a compound found in gasoline. Persons with Down syndrome and certain other genetic abnormalities are at increased risk for developing leukemia.

There are two main types of leukemia—myelogenous and lymphocytic. Each type of leukemia can be either chronic or acute. The chronic leukemias—chronic myelogenous leukemia and chronic lymphocytic leukemia—occur most often in adults. In both types of chronic leukemias, the white blood cell count slowly increases over months or years. The disease usually can be controlled with oral chemotherapy agents for many years. Patients being treated for chronic leukemia generally feel healthy. They do not lose their hair and usually do not experience nausea. Most of these patients can continue to work. A new drug now available for patients with chronic myelogenous leukemia, imatinib mesylate (Gleevec), has revolutionized the treatment of this particular leukemia. Gleevec is a protein tyrosine kinase inhibitor that targets the leukemic cells while sparing normal cells. It is an oral medication taken once a day. Only minimal side effects have been reported. Research continues to determine the optimal length of treatment and follow-up needed for these patients. The average life expectancy after diagnosis for a patient with chronic myelogenous leukemia ranges from 3 to 8 years, depending on the stage of the disease. It is anticipated that life expectancy will increase with Gleevec treatment, but by how much is currently unknown. The average life expectancy for a patient with chronic lymphocytic leukemia ranges from 2 to 10 years, again depending on the stage of the disease when diagnosed. After this time, the chronic leukemias often transform into an acute leukemia that is very difficult to treat. Patients generally die shortly after they enter this accelerated phase.

Each of the chronic forms of leukemia—lymphocytic and myelogenous—also has an acute form. Acute lymphocytic leukemia occurs most often in children between the ages of 2 and 6 years. Acute nonlymphocytic leukemia, also called *acute myelogenous leukemia,* occurs more often in adults. The acute leukemias appear very suddenly. The patient's white blood cell count can skyrocket in days, crowding out the normal red blood cells and platelets and leaving the patient at severe risk for infection and bleeding. Treatment with chemotherapy must be started as soon as possible. Between 70% and 80% of children diagnosed with acute lymphocytic leukemia will be alive in 5 years. Only 20% of patients diagnosed with acute nonlymphocytic leukemia will be alive in 5 years.

Signs and Symptoms of Acute Leukemia

Patients with leukemia commonly have infections because their bone marrow is producing huge numbers of immature white blood cells that cannot effectively fight infection. Usually patients with acute leukemia have fevers and night sweats in response to the infection. Because the leukemic white blood cells crowd out the normal cells in the bone marrow, patients may have symptoms related to low red blood cell counts, such as fatigue, paleness, tachycardia, and tachypnea. Concurrently, patients may have symptoms related to low platelet counts, such as petechiae or purpura, epistaxis (nose bleeds), gingival bleeding (from the gums), melena (blood in the stool), or menorrhagia (heavy menstrual bleeding). Some patients may have bone pain because of the crowding created by rapidly dividing leukemic cells in the bone marrow. Patients may report weight loss and swollen lymph nodes.

Medical Diagnosis of Acute Leukemia

A CBC with an extremely high white blood cell count indicates that leukemia might be present. A bone marrow biopsy enables diagnosis of the specific type of leukemia. The Diagnostic Tests and Procedures tables on pp. 577 and 598 describe the procedure for drawing specimens for a CBC as well as for a bone marrow biopsy.

Medical Treatment of the Patient with Acute Leukemia

The acute leukemias are initially treated using high doses of chemotherapy to destroy the diseased bone marrow and allow the body to regrow healthy bone marrow. Patients are at great risk for infection and bleeding while their healthy bone marrow is growing back, but this is the only way the acute leukemias can be treated. Patients stay in the hospital during the chemotherapy treatments and afterward to receive antibiotics and blood transfusions until their own bone marrow grows back. After the initial high doses of chemotherapy, called *induction therapy,* patients with acute lymphocytic leukemia take lower doses of chemotherapy, called *maintenance therapy,* for 1 to 3 years. Patients with acute nonlymphocytic leukemia immediately receive the same high doses of chemotherapy two to four more times over the next 2 to 4 months but are then finished with treatment. Subsequent chemotherapy for acute nonlymphocytic leukemia is called *intensification* and *consolidation therapy*. Bone marrow transplantation is one form of intensification therapy.

NURSING CARE *of the Patient with Acute Leukemia*

Patients with acute leukemia require intensive nursing care. Patients are normally hospitalized only 2 to 3 weeks and are critically ill most of that time. Once a patient's vital signs stabilize and the patient has no signs or symptoms of infection, he or she can be discharged from the hospital and followed as an outpatient until normal bone marrow function returns and adequate numbers of white blood cells, red blood cells, and platelets are being made. The physical and psychological nursing care of these patients is intensive.

Assessment

Infection is the leading cause of death in patients with leukemia. Therefore patients are frequently assessed for any signs or symptoms of infection. The most common sites of infection are the lungs, blood, skin, urinary tract, and gastrointestinal tract. Take complete vital signs every 4 hours. Fever is the hallmark of infection. Other vital sign changes due to sepsis or to widespread infection include tachycardia, tachypnea, and hypotension. Assess breath sounds every shift and note changes. A cough, especially a productive cough, may indicate an early pulmonary infection. If sputum is produced, note the amount and color. The physician may want the sputum cultured. Each day carefully inspect the skin for any reddened, swollen, painful, or draining areas. This is most easily done when helping the patient bathe. Because patients with leukemia do not have normal white blood cells, pus may not be seen even though an infection may be present. Redness, swelling, pain, or a combination of these may be the only symptoms of a serious infection. Inspect the mouth and pharynx, looking for any reddened, swollen, painful, or draining areas. Ask the patient about any pain or burning on urination, indicating a possible bladder infection.

While assessing for infection, also assess for any evidence of bleeding. The lower the platelet count, the greater is the patient's risk for bleeding. A platelet count below 50,000 cells/mm^3 is cause for concern. Note any petechiae, purpura, or ecchymoses. Patients may have or report epistaxis, gingival bleeding, melena, or menorrhagia. Perform a guaiac test to assess for blood on all bowel movements as directed.

Also note any side effects from the chemotherapy itself, such as nausea and vomiting or stomatitis, so the appropriate interventions can be taken. Most patients lose their hair from chemotherapy for acute leukemia beginning 1 to 2 weeks after treatment. This is to be expected.

While doing a physical examination, also assess how much the patient knows about the disease and

treatment as well as how the patient is coping with this life-threatening disease.

Nursing Diagnoses, Goals, and Outcome Criteria: Acute Leukemia

NURSING DIAGNOSES	GOALS AND OUTCOME CRITERIA
Risk for Injury related to infection, thrombocytopenia, and anemia	Absence of injury from infection, bleeding, and inadequate oxygenation: normal body temperature, no bruising or frank bleeding, pulse and respiratory rates within patient's norms
Fatigue related to the disease process and treatment	Reduction in fatigue: patient reports tolerance of activity has improved
Impaired Oral Mucous Membrane related to stomatitis	Intact mucous membranes: oral tissues normal in color without lesions
Imbalanced Nutrition: Less Than Body Requirements related to nausea and vomiting	Adequate intake of nutrients: stable body weight
Anxiety related to the disease, treatment, and uncertain outcome	Reduced anxiety: patient reports anxiety is reduced, calm manner
Ineffective Therapeutic Regimen Management related to lack of knowledge about the disease process and treatment	Patient manages side effects of treatment effectively: patient resumes self-care; verbalizes disease process, treatment, and implications

Interventions

Risk for Injury

Infection. Infection presents the greatest risk to patients with leukemia. Most hospitals institute Compromised Host Precautions when a patient's absolute neutrophil count falls below 1000 cells/mm^3. Thorough hand washing is of extreme importance in caring for these patients. Microorganisms are transmitted by hospital personnel who do not diligently wash their hands. Encourage patients to shower every day to remove bacteria from the skin and perianal area. Because patients with low white blood cell counts often become infected with their own microorganisms through their gastrointestinal tract, discourage patients from eating fresh fruits or vegetables and from drinking milk products. Any uncooked foods naturally contain the bacteria *Escherichia coli, Pseudomonas aeruginosa,* and *Klebsiella* species. A normal immune system can destroy the bacteria in uncooked foods. However, patients undergoing treatment for leukemia are at high risk for infection after being exposed to even small amounts of these bacteria. Box 33-3 outlines typical Compromised Host Precautions for patients with low white blood cell counts. Once the patient's absolute neutrophil count climbs above 1000 cells/mm³, Compromised Host Precautions can be discontinued and a regular diet resumed without restrictions.

Thrombocytopenia. In addition to infection, patients with leukemia are at great risk for bleeding related to thrombocytopenia (a low platelet count). The primary treatment for thrombocytopenia is a platelet transfusion. However, physicians try not to prescribe platelet transfusions for patients unless they are actively bleeding or their platelet count is below 20,000 cells/mm³ because of the risks associated with blood product administration. Nursing considerations in administering platelet transfusions are outlined in Box 32-6 in Chapter 32. When patients are thrombocytopenic, take bleeding precautions as outlined in Box 32-4 in Chapter 32.

Anemia. Anemia, or hematocrit below 30 and hemoglobin below 10 gm/dL, is a common finding in patients with leukemia. Expect anemia along with neutropenia and thrombocytopenia. As with neutropenia and thrombocytopenia, anemia may be caused by the leukemic cells crowding out the healthy red cells in the bone marrow, or it may be the result of chemotherapy. The primary treatment for anemia is a red blood cell transfusion. Nursing considerations in administering blood transfusions are outlined in Box 32-5 in Chapter 32. Other precautions for patients with anemia are outlined in Box 32-3 in Chapter 32.

Fatigue

Almost all patients with acute leukemia experience fatigue, which has been described as an overwhelming tiredness or exhaustion. Causes of fatigue in these patients can include a low red blood cell count from both the disease and the treatment, the buildup of metabolic wastes as the leukemic cells are being destroyed and cleared from the body, disrupted sleep, and the psychological stress of the disease and treatment. A detailed discussion of the nursing management of fatigue is presented in Chapter 25.

Impaired Oral Mucous Membrane

Stomatitis, or an inflammation of the mucous membranes, is also a common side effect of chemotherapy. A detailed discussion of the nursing management of stomatitis is presented in Chapter 25.

Imbalanced Nutrition: Less Than Body Requirements

Nausea, with or without vomiting, is a common side effect of chemotherapy. Persistent nausea and vomiting can adversely affect a patient's nutritional status and psychological state. You can play an important role in managing this most distressing side effect. A detailed discussion of the nursing management of nausea and vomiting related to chemotherapy is presented in Chapter 25.

Anxiety

A diagnosis of leukemia is always a shock to patients and their families. Patients must deal not only with the disease and treatment but also with the feelings and emotions of facing a life-threatening illness. Encourage patients to ask questions and talk about their feelings. Often a patient's fears are due to a lack of knowledge about the disease and treatment. The oncology clinical nurse specialist or other specially trained oncology nurse can answer many of the patient's and family's questions. Often, information is what the patient and family need to deal with their anxieties. However, a referral to a social worker, chaplain, or mental health counselor may be indicated if the patient and family are having continued anxiety and difficulty in coping. It is important for you to know what the patient understands about the disease, the treatment, and the prognosis so that correct information can be reinforced.

Ineffective Therapeutic Regimen Management

It is very important that the patient receive accurate, consistent information from all members of the health care team. An oncology clinical nurse specialist or other specially trained oncology nurse can usually provide comprehensive information about the disease and its treatment to the patient and family and answer questions as they arise during hospitalization. All nurses reinforce this teaching. The Leukemia and Lymphoma Society (1311 Mamaroneck Avenue, White Plains, NY 10605; website: www.leukemia-lymphoma.org; telephone: 1-800-955-4LSA or 1-914-949-5213) provides excellent, free literature on the different types of leukemia. The National Cancer Institute, through the Cancer Information Service, provides excellent, free literature on chemotherapy for people receiving treatment. They can be reached by calling 1-800-4CANCER or on the Internet at www.nci.nih.gov. The American Cancer Society (1599 Clifton Road, Atlanta, GA 30320; website: www.cancer.org; telephone: 1-800-ACS-2345) has many support services available for people with all forms of cancer, including leukemia.

OTHER IMMUNE SYSTEM DISORDERS
Hypersensitivity Reactions

Hypersensitivity reactions, or allergies, are exaggerated immune responses that can be uncomfortable and potentially harmful to the patient. The four types of hypersensitivity reactions are classified according to the time between exposure and reaction, immune mechanism involved, and site of reaction.

Type I immediate hypersensitivity reactions are mediated by IgE reacting to common allergens such as dust, pollen, animal dander, insect stings, or various drugs. Type I reactions can be either local, resulting in local swelling and discomfort, or systemic, resulting in anaphylaxis and possible death if not recognized and treated promptly. Type I anaphylactic hypersensitivity reactions occur in the following way. After a first, sensitizing exposure to a specific allergen, subsequent exposures to the same allergen trigger an exaggerated antibody reaction. For example, in a person with a hypersensitivity reaction to insect stings, one insect sting results in the production of abnormally large amounts of IgE antibodies. When this person is stung again by the same type of insect, the circulating IgE immediately triggers the release of histamine and other cytokines from mast cells, causing bronchiole constriction, peripheral vasodilation, and increased capillary permeability. These individuals can experience airway obstruction, pulmonary congestion, peripheral edema, hypotension, shock, and circulatory collapse. Prompt diagnosis and treatment of anaphylaxis with epinephrine, antihistamines, steroids, and hemodynamic support are of paramount importance.

Type II immediate hypersensitivity reactions are mediated by antibody reactions. Type II hypersensitivity reactions can occur with a mismatched blood transfusion or as a response to various drugs.

Type III immediate hypersensitivity reactions result in tissue damage resulting from precipitation of antigen-antibody immune complexes. Type III hypersensitivity reactions can occur with autoimmune reactions, some occupational diseases, or as a response to various drugs.

Type IV delayed hypersensitivity reactions result from immune cells migrating to the site of exposure days after the exposure to the antigen. Type IV hypersensitivity reactions can occur with contact dermatitis, measles rash, tuberculin skin testing, or various drugs. Transplanted graft rejection occurs because of a type IV hypersensitivity reaction. Hypersensitivity reactions to drugs, or drug allergies, are one of many possible adverse drug reactions. Drug-induced hypersensitivity reactions can be any of the four types of hypersensitivity.

Idiopathic Thrombocytopenic Purpura

Idiopathic thrombocytopenic purpura (ITP) is an antibody-mediated autoimmune disorder in which IgG mistakenly helps destroy the patient's own platelets. Drugs known to induce ITP include sulfonamides, thiazide diuretics, chlorpropamide, quinidine, and gold. Patients with HIV infection are at increased risk for developing ITP.

Treatment for ITP can include steroids and intravenous immune globulin (IVIG). Approximately 75% of adult patients with ITP will sequester (store) platelets in the spleen, and so splenectomy is done in some patients to remove this storehouse, thereby increasing the

Pharmacology Capsule

Advise patients taking steroids to take them early in the day because these drugs can disrupt sleep.

circulating blood levels of platelets. Immunosuppressive therapy with cytotoxic drugs (e.g., vincristine or cyclophosphamide) can be used in patients who do not respond to splenectomy. Platelet transfusions are *not* indicated because the underlying problem is platelet consumption, not platelet production. If platelets are transfused, they are immediately destroyed. Nursing actions for the patient who is at risk for injury from bleeding are outlined in Box 32-4 in Chapter 32.

Thrombotic Thrombocytopenic Purpura

Thrombotic thrombocytopenic purpura (TTP) is an exaggerated immunologic response to vessel injury that results in extensive clot formation and decreased blood flow to the site. These patients become critically ill, developing fever, thrombocytopenia, hemolytic anemia, renal impairment, and neurologic symptoms.

The main treatment for TTP is plasmapheresis, which presumably removes the immunologic agent that triggered the TTP from the plasma. The patient's blood is centrifuged in an apheresis machine that separates the blood components so that the plasma can be selectively removed. The patient's own white blood cells, red blood cells, and platelets are reinfused during the treatment. Critically ill patients can become hemodynamically unstable during this procedure and need close monitoring and timely interventions to maintain cardiac output and blood pressure. Plasmapheresis usually is done daily or every other day for several weeks until the patient's hematologic parameters stabilize. Other treatments include steroids, antiplatelet agents (e.g., aspirin or dipyridamole [Persantine]), splenectomy, or all three. Platelet transfusions are usually contraindicated because they may contribute to the abnormal clotting process. Nursing actions for the patient who is at risk for injury from bleeding are outlined in Box 32-4 in Chapter 32.

Systemic Lupus Erythematosus

Systemic lupus erythematosus (SLE) is an autoimmune disease in which the person's immune system loses its ability to recognize itself and mounts an immune response against its own proteins. Damage results from antibodies and immune complexes directed against one or many organ systems. The cause of SLE is unknown. Ninety percent of cases occur in women, usually of childbearing age. The disease is much more common in African Americans, Latinos, and Asian Americans as compared with white individuals. Organ damage is progressive in this disease. The most common cause of death in these patients is infection and disease of the cardiovascular, renal, pulmonary, and central nervous systems. Factors associated with a poor outcome include increased creatinine, hypertension, large amounts of protein excreted in the urine, anemia, and low socioeconomic status.

What Does Culture Have to Do with Lupus?

Although the cause of SLE is unknown, there may be a genetic predisposition. The disease is more common in women and is three times more common in African-American women than in Caucasian women.

Signs and Symptoms

Patients with SLE can experience long periods of remission alternating with periods of symptom exacerbation. Almost every organ system can be affected. The most common symptoms, experienced by 95% of patients at some time during the course of their disease, include fatigue, malaise, fever, anorexia, nausea, and weight loss. Musculoskeletal symptoms, also experienced by 95% of patients at some time during the course of their disease, include arthralgias (joint pain) and myalgias (muscle pain). Joints are often swollen, tender, stiff, and painful with movement. Cutaneous symptoms can include a rash and photosensitivity. The classic skin lesion is a butterfly-shaped rash across the bridge of the nose and the cheeks. This rash can extend to the neck, upper trunk, and arms. Life- and organ-threatening symptoms can include inflammation of the kidneys, heart, and/or lungs resulting in organ failure. Inflammation of the retina of the eye can result in sudden-onset blindness, which can be very frightening to patients.

Medical Diagnosis

There is no one test that confirms the diagnosis of SLE. Blood work may detect antinuclear antibody (ANA), but a positive ANA is not specific for SLE. A negative ANA assay makes the diagnosis of SLE unlikely but not impossible. Rather than a blood test, the diagnosis of SLE is based on the constellation of symptoms the patient is experiencing. Because symptoms come and go, the diagnosis of SLE can be very difficult to make and can take a long time. The American Rheumatism Association has established criteria for the diagnosis of SLE. If a patient experiences any four of the following symptoms, a diagnosis of SLE can be made:

- Characteristic rash
- Photosensitivity with exposure to sunlight
- Oral ulcers
- Arthritis
- Pleuritis or pericarditis (i.e., inflammation of the lungs or heart)
- Renal disorder (e.g., proteinuria)
- Neurologic disorder (e.g., seizures, psychosis)
- Hematologic disorder (e.g., anemia, leukopenia, thrombocytopenia)
- Immunologic disorder (as evidenced by detection of abnormal antibodies in the blood)
- Positive ANA

Medical Treatment

There is no cure for SLE. The medical treatment of SLE is symptomatic and aimed at minimizing symptoms, preventing organ damage, and maintaining quality of life. Fever, arthralgias, myalgias, and rash are managed with analgesics, nonsteroidal anti-inflammatory drugs (NSAIDs), antimalarials, and corticosteroids. If symptoms are not controlled with these drugs or if organ function is threatened, cytotoxic agents (e.g., azathioprine, chlorambucil, cyclophosphamide, methotrexate) can be used to suppress the abnormal immune response.

NURSING CARE *of the Patient with SLE*

The nursing care of the patient with SLE varies depending on the severity of the symptoms the patient may be experiencing. Patients are treated primarily as outpatients. Because patients with SLE are frequent consumers of medical care, they often become very knowledgeable about their disease and want to be fully informed of all treatments they are receiving as well as the possible side effects of the treatments. The goal of care is quality of life.

Assessment

The complexity of SLE requires a thorough health history and physical examination. It is critical to do a complete functional assessment to determine the effects of the symptoms on the patient's activities of daily living.

Nursing Diagnoses, Goals, and Outcome Criteria: Systemic Lupus Erythematosus

Nursing goals and diagnoses for the patient with SLE are extremely individualized but may include the following:

NURSING DIAGNOSES	GOALS AND OUTCOME CRITERIA
Fatigue related to the disease process and treatment	Decreased fatigue: patient manages daily routines without excessive tiring
Acute Pain related to inflammation of joints and muscles	Pain relief: patient states pain is relieved, appears relaxed
Disturbed Body Image related to skin rash	Improved body image: patient makes positive statements about self, employs measures to improve appearance
Ineffective Coping related to stress of chronic illness	Effective coping: patient employs positive coping skills to reduce stress
Ineffective Therapeutic Regimen Management related to lack of knowledge about disease process and treatment	Patient resumes self care: patient accurately describes disease process, treatments, and side effects of treatment

Interventions

Fatigue

Almost all patients with SLE report experiencing fatigue. Causes of fatigue in these patients can include a low red blood cell count from both the disease and treatment, chronic pain, disrupted sleep, and the psychological stress of the disease and treatment. A detailed discussion of the nursing management of fatigue is presented in Chapter 25.

Acute Pain

Pain can be caused by inflammation of muscles and joints as well as inflammation of various organs. Closely monitor the patient's pain level and medication usage. Keeping a flow sheet of patient reports of pain on a 10-point scale can be helpful, especially as different nurses care for the patient throughout the day. A "0" represents no pain, whereas a "10" represents the worst pain a patient has ever experienced. The patient report of pain coupled with the amount of pain medication he or she is receiving can guide the nurse and physician as to the appropriate type and amount of pain medication. Pharmacologic and nonpharmacologic pain management strategies are presented in Chapter 15.

Disturbed Body Image

Encourage the patient to avoid prolonged exposure to the sun and to use sunscreen with an SPF rating of >15 to prevent the skin rash and exacerbation of symptoms.

Ineffective Coping

A diagnosis of SLE is always a shock to patients and their families. Patients must deal not only with the disease and treatment but also with the emotions of facing a chronic illness. Encourage patients to ask questions and to talk about their feelings. A referral to a social worker, chaplain, or mental health counselor may be indicated if the patient and family are having difficulty coping.

Ineffective Therapeutic Regimen Management

It is very important that the patient receive accurate, consistent information from all members of the health care team. A clinical nurse specialist or other specially trained nurse can usually provide comprehensive information about the disease and its treatment to the patient and family and answer questions as they arise during hospitalization. It is important for you to know what the patient has been told about the disease, the treatment, and the prognosis so that correct information can be reinforced. Most important, the patient's interpretation and understanding of the information is essential. There are several resources available about SLE for patients, families, and health care providers, including the Lupus Foundation of America (2000 L Street, N.W., Suite 710,

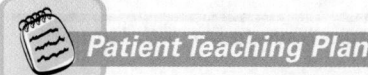

Patient Teaching Plan

Systemic Lupus Erythematosus

- Know the names, dosages, schedule, and side effects of your drugs.
- Avoid prolonged exposure to the sun and use sunscreen with an SPF rating of >15.
- You can get additional information from the Lupus Foundation of America and the American Lupus Society.

Washington, DC 20036; www.lupus.org; telephone 202-349-1155) and the American Lupus Society (260 Maple Court, Suite 123, Ventura, CA 93003-3511; telephone: 1-805-339-0443 and 1-800-331-1802). These organizations provide excellent free literature on SLE and can help locate support groups in specific regions of the country.

HUMAN IMMUNODEFICIENCY VIRUS INFECTION

Human immunodeficiency virus (HIV) is a retrovirus that infects cells expressing CD4 on their cell membranes, primarily T_H cells. HIV/AIDS is covered in detail in Chapter 34.

TRANSPLANT REJECTION

Patients who undergo kidney, heart, liver, or other organ transplantation risk that their own healthy immune system will recognize the transplanted organ (or allograft) as foreign and try to destroy it. Rejections occur through various mechanisms. T_C lymphocytes can directly attack the allograft, resulting in acute transplant rejection within hours of the transplant. B lymphocytes can make antibodies against the allograft. Fibrin accumulates on the transplanted tissue, causing ischemia. In this way, the allograft is slowly rejected over months to years. Tissue matching of donor to recipient minimizes the chance of the recipient's immune system attacking the allograft after transplantation.

Various combinations of drugs are also given to suppress the recipient's immune system and minimize the immune response to the allograft. However, these drugs also suppress the patient's ability to fight bacteria, viruses, fungi, and parasites, putting the patient at increased risk for infection. Combinations of steroids (which inhibit the inflammatory response by inhibiting the production of prostaglandins), cyclosporine (which inhibits T lymphocytes), and azathioprine (which inhibits B cell and T cell proliferation) are commonly used to chronically suppress the immune system after an organ transplant. The Drug Therapy

DRUG THERAPY *Drugs Used to Prevent Rejection of a Transplanted Organ*

DRUG	USE/ACTION	SIDE EFFECTS	NURSING INTERVENTIONS
Steroids, e.g., dexamethasone (Decadron), methylprednisolone (Solu-Medrol), prednisone, prednisolone, hydrocortisone (Solu-Cortef)	Used to prevent rejection of a transplanted organ because glucocorticoids interfere with eicosanoid production. Also used to treat acute hypersensitivity reaction type I (anaphylaxis).	Glucose intolerance, muscle wasting, obesity, hyperlipidemia, redistribution of body fat, growth inhibition in children, increased capillary fragility, osteoporosis, stomach irritation and peptic ulcer disease, hypertension, sodium and water retention, mood changes.	Give these drugs with meals. An H$_2$-receptor antagonist such as ranitidine (Zantac) may be prescribed to decrease gastric acid production. If the patient takes these drugs for an extended period of time, the drug should not be stopped abruptly. Instead, the drug dose should be gradually decreased over time under a physician's direction.
Purine and pyrimidine analogs, e.g., azathioprine, mycophenolic acid, brequinar	Used to prevent rejection of a transplanted organ by interfering with DNA synthesis in rapidly dividing cells such as T cells.	Bone marrow suppression, increased susceptibility to infection, stomach irritation, diarrhea, hepatotoxicity.	Closely monitor the patient's complete blood cell count (CBC) and liver function studies.

table above describes the nursing care of patients taking these drugs. There are also several newer drugs that target the T cells while preserving B cell function and thus more of the patient's immune function. Examples of these drugs are tacrolimus (Prograf), antilymphocyte globulin, antithymocyte globulin, and murine monoclonal antibody to CD3 (OKT3). Patients who have undergone organ transplantation must take immunosuppressive therapy the rest of their lives to preserve the allograft. These immunosuppressive drugs, which are needed to preserve the allograft, paradoxically put patients at an increased risk of infection from environmental bacteria, viruses, fungi, and parasites.

 Put on Your Thinking Cap!

Explain what would happen physiologically if transplant recipients did not take immunosuppressant drugs to prevent organ rejection.

 Consider the Alternative

Herbs that are used to boost the immune system include Echinacea, ginseng, and goldenseal. Patients should consult with their physicians about taking them, because they have adverse effects and can interact with some medications. The actual value of these herbs is under study.

 Key Points

- The immune system is the body's defense network against infection; it provides the body with resistance to invading organisms and enables it to fight off invaders once they have gained access.
- Body organs that are part of a functioning immune system include the bone marrow, lymph nodes, spleen, and thymus.
- Antigens are foreign substances that stimulate a response from the immune system, whereas antibodies are proteins that are produced by the immune system to help eradicate antigens.
- Innate immunity is present in the body at birth, whereas acquired immunity develops after birth as a result of the body's immune response to specific antigens.
- Many types of leukocytes act as nature's cleanup mechanism by migrating to infected or inflamed areas and engulfing and destroying antigens through a process known as *phagocytosis.*
- The two types of acquired immunity are antibody-mediated and cell-mediated.
- Acquired immunity depends on the proper development and functioning of specific white blood cells called *B* and *T lymphocytes.*
- Immunodeficiency occurs when the body is unable to launch an adequate immune response, resulting in an increased risk for infection.
- Because the bone marrow becomes less responsive with age, the older person's immune response may be inadequate under stressful situations.
- The patient with a low white blood cell count is at risk for infection.
- Bone marrow transplantation and peripheral blood stem cell transplantation are procedures that reconstitute the

- hematologic and immunologic systems after certain cancer therapies.
- The two main types of leukemia are myelogenous and lymphocytic.
- Infection is the leading cause of death in patients with leukemia.
- Drugs used to suppress the immune response after organ or tissue transplants also put the patient at risk for infection.
- Allergy or hypersensitivity occurs when a normally inoffensive foreign substance stimulates an atypical or exaggerated immune response.

- Systemic lupus erythematosus is considered an autoimmune disorder.
- Systemic lupus erythematosus can affect multiple body systems.

 Go to your Companion CD-ROM for a Pharmacology Tutorial, Audio Glossary, and 3-D animations.

evolve Be sure to visit the companion Evolve site at http://evolve.elsevier.com/Linton/ for WebLinks and additional online resources.

REVIEW QUESTIONS *Choose the best answer.*

1. A patient has a neutrophil count that is 70% of his total WBC count. You should suspect:
   1. Bacterial infection
   2. Viral infection
   3. Parasitic infestation
   4. Allergic reaction

2. Mr. B. had chickenpox as a child. When he was exposed to chickenpox years later, he did not become infected. His resistance was most likely due to:
   1. Passive acquired immunity
   2. Innate immunity
   3. Active acquired immunity
   4. Idiopathic immunity

3. Which statement best describes the effects of age-related changes in the immune system?
   1. The older person has little resistance to infection.
   2. The immune system functions well under normal circumstances.
   3. Lymphatic tissue enlarges to compensate for decreased activity.
   4. Older people have better immune function than most young adults.

4. Which of the following is an autoimmune disorder?
   1. Type 2 diabetes mellitus
   2. Hypothyroidism
   3. Leukemia
   4. Systemic lupus erythematosus

5. A priority when collecting data about the patient with an immune disorder is:
   1. Signs and symptoms of infection
   2. Unexplained changes in weight
   3. Increased blood pressure
   4. Characteristics of urine

6. During report, it is noted that there is a shift to the right on your patient's CBC. You know that this could mean that:
   1. Your patient has a mild infection
   2. Your patient's infection is resolving
   3. Your patient has an overwhelming infection
   4. Your patient is producing excess neutrophils

7. A patient with leukemia is on Compromised Host Precautions, which include the following:
   1. Visitors and staff should wash their hands before patient contact
   2. The patient can have only fresh, raw fruits and vegetables
   3. Staff should always wear masks when in the patient's room
   4. Vital signs should be monitored at least every 8 hours

8. Shortly after receiving an antibiotic, a patient experienced a type 1 immediate hypersensitivity reaction. Signs and symptoms would include the following:
   1. Mental confusion
   2. Difficulty breathing
   3. Hypertension
   4. Nausea and vomiting

9. Pain management during the acute phase of a sickle cell crisis usually requires:
   1. Nonsteroidal anti-inflammatory drugs
   2. Physical therapy
   3. Nerve blocks
   4. Opioid analgesics

Extrinsic Clotting
and Destruction
Function
...
North American
Coalition...

34 HIV/AIDS

CHAPTER

MARK A. MEYER

evolve   http://evolve.elsevier.com/Linton/

Objectives

After reading and studying this chapter, you should be able to:

1. Describe the history of HIV/AIDS.
2. Explain the pathophysiology and etiology of HIV infection.
3. List risk factors associated with HIV infection.
4. Identify complications associated with HIV infection.
5. Identify criteria for diagnosis of AIDS.
6. Name the major HIV drugs, indications, side effects, and nursing considerations.
7. Describe appropriate nursing care of the HIV/AIDS patient.

Key Terms

Be sure to check out the bonus material on the Companion CD-ROM, including selected audio pronunciations.

AIDS (acquired immunodeficiency syndrome)
(ĬM-mu-nō-dē-FĪ-shĕn-cē, p. 611)
HAART (highly active antiretroviral therapy)
(ĂN-tē-rētrō-VĪ-rŭl, p. 620)
HIV (human immunodeficiency virus, p. 611)
protease inhibitor (PRŌ-tē-āce ĭn-HĬB-ĭ-tĕr, p. 620)

Few diseases have descended on human beings as swiftly and wreaked as much devastation as human immunodeficiency virus/acquired immunodeficiency syndrome (HIV/AIDS). The disease has swept through every country on the globe, claiming victims without regard to age, race, class, or gender. Rich and poor, older adult and newborn, male and female, black and white—all have been vulnerable to HIV infection.

Research and education in the prevention and treatment of HIV infection must continue unabated. Despite advances, there is still no cure, but there is reason for hope. In the developed world, the disease has come to be viewed less as a fatal illness than as a manageable chronic condition. In the developing world, where access to health care and medications is often difficult, the picture is less optimistic. Worldwide, only about one in five people at risk of becoming infected with HIV has access to prevention services.

HISTORY

The origins of **HIV (human immunodeficiency virus)** and the disease it causes—**AIDS (acquired immunodeficiency syndrome)**—are difficult to pinpoint. The virus might have sprung up as early as the 1940s, yet it was not recognized as a new pathogen until the early 1980s. Young men generally have normally functioning immune systems. Epidemiologists (physicians who study patterns of illness) began to take note when immune-deficiency conditions such as oral candida (thrush), herpes, *Pneumocystis jiroveci* pneumonia, and Kaposi's sarcoma (KS), a rare type of cancer, began to show up in the United States, primarily among urban populations of men who have sex with men (MSM). In 1986, HIV-1 and HIV-2 were isolated as the viruses that cause AIDS.

Men who have sex with men were just the first to be affected. Infection was soon seen in other populations, including the following:

- Hemophiliacs (individuals who must use blood products to treat their blood clotting disorder)
- Patients who received a transfusion with HIV-infected blood or blood products
- Newborns and breast-fed infants of HIV-infected mothers (perinatal transmission)
- Injection drug users
- Partners, including heterosexuals, having unprotected sex with those infected with the virus

In some developing countries, such as Sub-Saharan Africa, HIV infects more heterosexuals than homosexuals. It is transmitted by exposure to bodily fluids (blood, semen, breast milk, vaginal secretions) that contain the virus, not by lifestyle or sexual preference.

According to the U.S. Centers for Disease Control and Prevention (CDC, 2004a), more than 42,000 newly diagnosed HIV infections occur annually in the United States. Since the disease was recognized in 1981, nearly 530,000 deaths have been attributed to AIDS in the

What Does Culture Have to do with HIV and AIDS?

HIV is disproportionately represented in some cultural groups. Therefore prevention programs need to be culturally sensitive to reach target audiences.

Eastern Europe
and Central Asia
1.6 million

North America
1.2 million

Western and
Central Europe
720,000

East Asia
870,000

North Africa and
Middle East
510,000

South and
Southeast Asia
7.4 million

Latin America and
the Caribbean
2.1 million

Australia and
the Pacific
74,000

Sub-Saharan
Africa
25.8 million

FIGURE **34-1** Estimated distribution of adults and children infected with HIV and AIDS at the end of 2005. (Data from the World Health Organization Joint United Nations Program on AIDS, December 2005.)

Table 34-1 | *U.S. AIDS Cases by Age*

AGE (IN YEARS)	ESTIMATED NUMBER OF AIDS CASES IN 2004	CUMULATIVE ESTIMATED NUMBER OF AIDS CASES, THROUGH 2004*
Under 13	48	9443
Ages 13 to 14	60	959
Ages 15 to 19	326	4936
Ages 20 to 24	1788	34,164
Ages 25 to 29	3576	114,642
Ages 30 to 34	5786	195,404
Ages 35 to 39	8031	208,199
Ages 40 to 44	8747	161,964
Ages 45 to 49	6245	99,644
Ages 50 to 54	3932	54,869
Ages 55 to 59	2079	29,553
Ages 60 to 64	996	16,119
Ages 65 or older	901	14,410

*Includes persons with a diagnosis of AIDS from the beginning of the epidemic through 2004.

United States (CDC, 2004a), with 25 million deaths worldwide (Fig. 34-1).

DEMOGRAPHICS

Although HIV can infect anyone, infection rates are often reported by demographics, such as race, age, and gender. More than half of all new infections occur among young adults ages 15 to 24 years, at least 27% of whom are women. Infections in teenagers are more frequent among women (61%) than among men (39%). Many older American adults believe they are not at risk for HIV infection. However, since 1981, HIV/AIDS has affected 123,711 adults over age 65, and in 2004, 901 HIV cases were documented in Americans over age 65 (CDC, 2004a). Table 34-1 lists HIV/AIDS cases in the United States by age.

Table 34-2 | *U.S. AIDS Cases by Race/Ethnicity**

RACE OR ETHNICITY	ESTIMATED NUMBER OF AIDS CASES IN 2004	CUMULATIVE ESTIMATED NUMBER OF AIDS CASES, THROUGH 2004†
White, not Hispanic	12,013	375,155
Black, not Hispanic	20,965	379,278
Hispanic	8672	177,164
Asian/Pacific Islander	488	7317
American Indian/ Alaska Native	193	3084

*CDC tracks HIV/AIDS information on five racial and ethnic groups: white, black, Hispanic, Asian/Pacific Islander, and American Indian/ Alaska Native.
†Includes persons with a diagnosis of AIDS from the beginning of the epidemic through 2004.

Table 34-3 | *U.S. AIDS Cases by Exposure Category*

EXPOSURE CATEGORY	ESTIMATED NUMBER OF AIDS CASES IN 2004*		
	MALE	FEMALE	TOTAL
Male-to-male sexual contact	17,691	—	17,691
Injection drug use	5968	3184	9152
Male-to-male sexual contact and injection drug use	1920	—	1920
Heterosexual contact	5149	7979	13,128
Other†	298	279	577

*Includes persons with a diagnosis of AIDS from the beginning of the epidemic through 2004.
†Includes hemophilia, blood transfusion, perinatal, and risk not reported or not identified.

According to the CDC (2004), the racial face of AIDS has changed since 1984, when whites accounted for 49% of AIDS cases, Black Americans 27%, and Hispanics 12%. In 2004, Black Americans accounted for 40%, whites 37%, and Hispanics 22%. Blacks and Hispanics share a disproportionate burden of HIV disease in the United States. In the upper Midwest, a disproportionately large number of American Indians are infected. Table 34-2 presents a summary of the number of AIDS cases in the United States by race and ethnicity.

Another way of reporting HIV rates and AIDS diagnoses is by mode of transmission. The CDC has established five primary transmission categories:

- Male-to-male sexual contact
- Injection drug use
- Heterosexual (male-female) contact
- Mother-to-child (perinatal) transmission
- Other (includes blood transfusions and unknown cause)

Table 34-4 | *Cumulative U.S. AIDS Cases by Exposure Category*

EXPOSURE CATEGORY	ESTIMATED NUMBER OF AIDS CASES THROUGH 2004*		
	MALE	FEMALE	TOTAL
Male-to-male sexual contact	441,380	—	441,380
Injection drug use	176,162	72,651	248,813
Male-to-male sexual contact and injection drug use	64,833	—	64,833
Heterosexual contact	59,939	99,175	159,114
Other†	14,085	6,636	20,721

*Includes persons with a diagnosis of AIDS from the beginning of the epidemic through 2004.
†Includes hemophilia, blood transfusion, perinatal, and risk not reported or not identified.

Table 34-5 | *U.S. AIDS Cases Among Children**

EXPOSURE CATEGORY	ESTIMATED NUMBER OF AIDS CASES IN 2004	CUMULATIVE ESTIMATED NUMBER OF AIDS CASES THROUGH 2004†
Perinatal	47	8779
Other‡	0	664

*The term "children" refers to persons younger than 13 years at the time of diagnosis.
†Includes persons with a diagnosis of AIDS from the beginning of the epidemic through 2004.
‡Includes hemophilia, blood transfusion, perinatal, and risk not reported or not identified.

Tables 34-3, 34-4, and 34-5 list the specific number of AIDS cases diagnosed within each of these exposure categories in the United States in 2004.

HIV is transmitted by blood and body fluids (breast milk, semen, and vaginal fluids). The risk of HIV transmission by various behaviors can be seen on a continuum from low risk to high risk. Table 34-6 identifies the levels of risk of HIV transmission for various behaviors.

PATHOPHYSIOLOGY

HIV falls into a category of viruses called *retroviruses*. In these viruses, transcription of genetic material is reversed. Ribonucleic acid (RNA) is made into deoxyribonucleic acid (DNA) rather than the normal pattern of DNA to RNA. Reverse transcriptase is an enzyme that is responsible for transcribing RNA into DNA (Kirton, 2003).

THE LIFE CYCLE OF HIV

HIV first penetrates the body through blood and body fluids. HIV is spherical in shape and has two protein markers that protrude from the virus. These markers are like keys that attach themselves to protein markers found on macrophages and T4 helper cells or CD4 cells. Macrophages and T4 helper cells are distributed throughout the body, especially in mucous membranes and body orifices. Once the HIV virus attaches to the macrophages and T4 helper cells, it infuses its genetic material into the host cell. The reverse transcriptase enzyme then transcribes HIV RNA into HIV DNA and inserts the HIV DNA into the host's DNA. Once the HIV DNA is incorporated into the host cell's DNA, billions of copies of HIV are made (Colagreco, 2003). Roughly 21 billion new HIV virions (complete viral particles) are produced daily compared with 1 to 2 billion new T4 cells. A person who is HIV positive may have an entire supply of T4 cells depleted every 15 days. Eventually, the body is unable to maintain a healthy immune response and the body will begin to show symptoms of HIV/AIDS (Colagreco, 2003).

THE BODY'S RESPONSE TO HIV INFECTION

Once infected with HIV, the body mounts a defense with antibodies and T cells. *Viral load* is a term used to describe how much virus is found in the blood. Especially high levels of viral load have been documented in the early phases of HIV infection. Approximately 12 weeks after infection, the body produces enough antibodies to be detected by standard HIV testing. Once a sufficient amount of antibodies is produced, the HIV viral load begins to drop, indicating partial effectiveness of the body to rid itself of HIV. Throughout the course of HIV infection, the body maintains high levels of HIV antibodies. However, CD8 cells and CD4 cells continue to decline throughout the course of the illness. Table 34-7 lists normal lymphocyte counts.

STAGES OF HIV INFECTION

The initial stage of HIV infection lasts 4 to 8 weeks from the time of exposure. High levels of virus are in the blood. The patient experiences generalized flu-like symptoms. The virus then enters a latent stage in which it is inactive in the infected, resting CD4 host cells. When the resting CD4 host cell is activated for an immune response, the virus begins to replicate. Levels of virus are high in the lymph nodes where CD4 cells reside, but the levels are low in the blood. The latent stage can last 2 to 12 years, during which time the patient is asymptomatic. During this time, the number of CD4 cells declines. During the third stage of HIV infection, the patient begins to experience opportunistic infections. Levels of CD4 cells are usually below 500 cells/mm^3 and declining, while levels of virus in the blood are increasing. This stage can last 2 to 3 years. Once the CD4 cell levels drop below 200 cells/mm^3, the patient is considered to have AIDS. Virus levels in the blood are high. This stage eventually ends in death, which may occur within a year. According to the Centers for Disease Control and Prevention (2004b), 70% of those diagnosed with AIDS have now survived 8 to 9 years after being diagnosed.

Table 34-6 | *Levels of HIV Transmission Risk for Various Behaviors*

No Risk Behavior	Casual contact Shaking hands Hugging and kissing Eating in restaurants Using restrooms Swimming Insect bites/mosquitoes Donating blood
Little Risk Behavior	Mutual masturbation, rubbing, cuddling, kissing, oral sex with condom, sex toys not shared with a partner, oral sex without contact with glans penis
Moderate Risk Behavior	Oral sex with contact with glans penis Anal or vaginal sex with a condom and a water-based lubricant
Very High Risk Behavior	Use of injection drugs, including steroids (needle sharing) Partners of injecting drug users Unprotected, penetrative sex (anal, vaginal)

Data from Kirton, C. (2001). Risk assessment, identification, and HIV counseling. In Kirton, C., Talotta, D., & Zwolski, K. (2001). *Handbook of HIV/AIDS nursing*. St. Louis: Mosby.

Table 34-7 | *Normal Lymphocyte Counts*

AGE	CD4 ABSOLUTE COUNT (cells/mm^3)	CD8 ABSOLUTE COUNT (cells/mm^3)	CD4:CD8 RATIO
18 years–70 years	600–980	420–660	1.2–1.9

Data from Kirton, C. (2001). Clinical application of immunological and virological markers. In Kirton, C., Talotta, D., & Zwolski, K. (Eds.). *Handbook of HIV/AIDS nursing*. St. Louis: Mosby.

SIGNS AND SYMPTOMS OF HIV INFECTION

Patients in the initial stage of HIV infection may experience only generalized flu-like symptoms such as malaise, nausea and vomiting, decreased appetite, rash, and diarrhea. Because the symptoms are vague, HIV infection often is not diagnosed in the early stage. During the second, latent stage of the disease, patients may not experience any symptoms. Eventually, they begin to experience frequent and persistent infections. Patients may present for medical care complaining of fever, night sweats, swollen lymph nodes, or other symptoms specific to the site of infection such as headache, skin lesions that do not heal, sore throat, dyspnea, burning with urination, or diarrhea. Patients also may report extreme fatigue and weight loss. Any of these symptoms coupled with a history of unprotected sexual contact with persons possibly infected with HIV, a history of intravenous drug abuse using shared needles, or a history of a blood transfusion before 1989 warrants consideration of a diagnosis of HIV infection.

COMPLICATIONS

The major complications of HIV infection are opportunistic infections, wasting, secondary cancers, and dementia. Patients with AIDS are at very high risk for opportunistic fungal, parasitic, and viral infections. Infections these patients commonly experience include oral candidiasis, *P. jiroveci* pneumonia, herpes simplex, cytomegalovirus retinitis, *Cryptosporidium* enteritis, *Cryptococcus neoformans* meningitis, and toxoplasmosis (Fig. 34-2). Almost all patients with HIV infection experience a wasting syndrome characterized by weight loss and malnutrition. Reduced food intake, malabsorption of nutrients, and altered metabolic pathways

FIGURE **34-2** Clinical symptoms of acquired immunodeficiency syndrome (AIDS). **A,** Severe weight loss and anorexia. **B,** Biopsyproven Kaposi sarcoma lesions. **C,** Perianal vesicular and ulcerative lesions of herpes simplex infection. (A from Taylor PK: *Diagnostic picture tests in sexually transmitted disease,* London, 1995, Mosby; B and C from Morse SA, Ballard BC, Holmes KK, et al editors: *Atlas of sexually transmitted diseases and AIDS,* ed 3, London, 2003, Mosby.)

all contribute to this wasting syndrome. Cancers such as Kaposi's sarcoma, non-Hodgkin's lymphoma, anal cancer, and cervical cancer occur in 40% of patients with HIV infection. Presumably this increased incidence of cancer is due to the inability of the patient's crippled immune system to identify and destroy cells that undergo malignant changes. The virus can affect the central nervous system, causing encephalopathy, cognitive impairment, and dementia.

OPPORTUNISTIC INFECTIONS

Once the body's CD4 cells, CD8 cells, and/or HIV antibodies fall below normal, infections and cancers that the body could normally resist take advantage of this opportunity and cause infection or cancer in the body. That is why these infections are called *opportunistic infections.* The leading cause of death in persons with AIDS is pneumonia caused by unspecified organisms. Opportunistic infections can be caused by parasites, fungi, bacteria, and viruses. Figure 34-3 shows tissues that may be affected by HIV.

PARASITIC INFECTIONS

Opportunistic parasitic infections include cryptosporidiosis, isosporiasis, and toxoplasmosis.

Cryptosporidiosis and Isosporiasis

Cryptosporidium and *Isospora,* the causative agents for cryptosporidiosis and isosporiasis, respectively, are fairly common in the environment, particularly in developing countries. They pose a special threat when the HIV patient's CD4 count falls below 200 cells/mm^3. The main symptom of infection with these parasites is watery diarrhea that may be severe and persistent, resulting in severe dehydration and electrolyte imbalances. Diagnosis is based on laboratory examination of a stool specimen (Ownby, 2003).

Nursing care is directed toward preventing dehydration and maintaining fluid and electrolyte balance. Antidiarrheal drugs and intravenous fluids may be ordered. Antimicrobial agents are effective for some parasitic infections, but others can be treated only symptomatically. To reduce the risk of transmission and reinfection, teach the patient to practice good handwashing and personal hygiene and to avoid ingestion of potentially contaminated water (Ownby, 2003).

Toxoplasmosis

Toxoplasma gondii, a protozoon that causes toxoplasmosis, has a worldwide distribution. Cats, mammals, and birds serve as hosts to the causative agent. Humans become infected by ingesting contaminated, undercooked meats or vegetables or by contact with cat feces. Toxoplasmosis can affect any tissue in the body but affects mostly the brain, lungs, and eyes. In immunosuppressed patients, toxoplasmosis encephalitis is the most common form. Unless detected and treated early, toxoplasmosis can be fatal. Symptoms include dull, constant headache, weakness, seizures, altered level of consciousness, hemiparesis, cerebellar tremor, and visual field defects. Pulmonary infections result in a feverish illness that mimics *P. jiroveci* pneumonia with shortness of breath and a nonproductive cough. When it affects the eyes, there is a loss of visual acuity as well as photophobia. Bactrim is used to treat toxoplasmosis. Teach patients to wash hands, avoid undercooked and raw meats, and avoid cat litter boxes (Stanley, Marsco, & McNicholl, 2003).

FUNGAL INFECTIONS

Opportunistic fungal infections include microsporidiosis, *P. jiroveci* pneumonia, aspergillosis, candidiasis, coccidioidomycosis, cryptococcosis, and histoplasmosis. These infections may be treated with various antifungal drugs including amphotericin B, itraconazole, Amphotec, nystatin, clotrimazole, fluconazole, ketoconazole, fluconazole, and flucytosine.

Pharmacology Capsule

Amphotericin B, which is administered intravenously, causes fever, rigors, and headache. Pretreatment with Benadryl, Demerol, and Tylenol as ordered will minimize this reaction. Amphotericin B can also cause electrolyte disturbances and is toxic to the kidneys. Other antifungal drugs are hepatotoxic.

Microsporidiosis

The source of human infection with microsporidiosis is unknown, although some believe it is caused by the ingestion of *Microsporum* spores. Symptoms are watery diarrhea with weight loss, malabsorption, abdominal cramps, and flatulence. Management focuses on treating the symptoms because there is no curative therapy available. Patients are encouraged to drink three liters of fluid each day; milk products should be avoided. A diet low in fat and residue and high in protein and calories is recommended. The best way to avoid being infected with *Microsporum* is to practice good hand washing and good hygiene and to avoid ingestion of food or water contaminated with fecal matter (Kirton, 2003).

Pneumocystis Jiroveci Pneumonia

P. jiroveci is a fungal organism that, when acquired by inhalation, can cause *P. jiroveci* pneumonia. *P. jiroveci* pneumonia is the second leading cause of death among AIDS patients. By lodging in interstitial spaces of the lung tissue, *P. jiroveci* pneumonia cysts prevent the exchange of gases. This causes shortness of breath upon exertion, fever, and a nonproductive cough. Treatment employs Bactrim, Dapsone, Clindamycin, and Pentamidine. Patients considered at high risk for *P. jiroveci* pneumonia are treated prophylactically with Bactrim (Fugate, 2003).

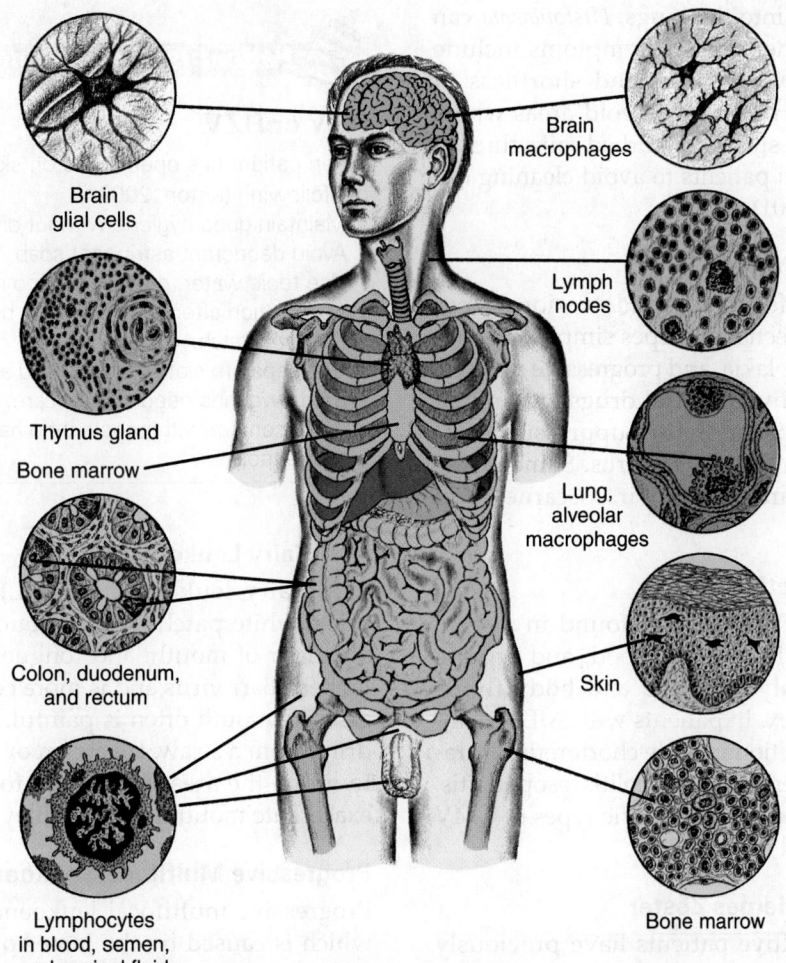

Brain glial cells

Brain macrophages

Lymph nodes

Thymus gland

Bone marrow

Lung, alveolar macrophages

Colon, duodenum, and rectum

Skin

Lymphocytes in blood, semen, and vaginal fluid

Bone marrow

FIGURE 34-3 Distribution of tissues that can be infected by HIV. Infection is closely linked to the presence of CD4 receptors on host tissue, with the possible exceptions of glial cells in the brain and chromaffin cells in the colon, duodenum, and rectum.

Aspergillosis

Aspergillosis is caused by *Aspergillus,* which lives in soil, water, and air. Pulmonary infection can develop when *Aspergillus* spores are inhaled, especially by patients whose CD4 count has dropped below 50 cells/mm^3. Symptoms include fever, cough, dyspnea, chest pain, and hemoptysis. Despite antifungal treatment, aspergillosis is usually fatal within 8 weeks. To decrease the risk of aspergillosis, advise the patient to avoid wet, cool places. Potted plants, marijuana, wicker, and household dust are common sources of *Aspergillus* (Zwolski, 2003).

Candidiasis

Candida albicans is a fungal yeast organism that is found in most foods, soil, and inanimate objects. Approximately 80% of HIV patients will develop candidiasis, which usually affects the mouth, vagina, and/or anus. Symptoms include thrush, which is an oral form of candidiasis. Unlike oral hairy leukoplakia, candida plaques can be scraped off. Any patient with oral or vaginal candidiasis who is not on antibiotic therapy should be tested for HIV. Inform the patient that candidiasis often reappears and to monitor for reinfection (Moran, 2003).

Coccidioidomycosis

The causative agent for coccidioidomycosis is *Coccidioides immitis,* which is endemic in the southwestern United States and northern Mexico. Particles are inhaled into the lungs. Symptoms include fever, weight loss, fatigue, dry cough, or pleuritic chest pain. Dissemination to other organs may occur after infection of the lungs. Persons with HIV should avoid exposure to disturbed soils in endemic areas.

Cryptococcosis

Cryptococcosis is caused by a yeast (*Cryptococcus neoformans*) and is the most common systemic fungal infection in AIDS patients. Symptoms appear approximately 30 days after exposure. Symptoms include fever, headache, malaise, nausea, vomiting, altered mental status, and a stiff neck (Zwolski, 2001).

Histoplasmosis

Histoplasma is a fungus that is endemic in the central and southern parts of the United States. It is found in soil and bird droppings. Infection (histoplasmosis) usually involves the lungs after *Histoplasma* spores are inhaled. Once inhaled into the lungs, *Histoplasma* can be disseminated to other organs. Symptoms include fever, night sweats, weight loss, and shortness of breath. Patients with HIV should avoid areas where *Histoplasma* is common, such as disturbed soils, chicken coops, and caves. Teach patients to avoid cleaning out bird cages (Zwolski, 2001).

VIRAL INFECTIONS

Opportunistic viral infections include various types of cytomegalovirus infections, herpes simplex, herpes zoster, oral hairy leukoplakia, and progressive multifocal leukoencephalopathy. Antiviral drugs are limited in number and work primarily by suppressing viral replication rather than killing the virus. Some of the antiviral drugs used are ganciclovir, foscarnet, and acyclovir.

Cytomegalovirus Infections

Cytomegalovirus (CMV) is a virus found in semen, cervical secretions, saliva, urine, blood, and organs. It is transmitted mainly by blood and body fluids through unprotected sex. In patients with AIDS, complications of CMV infection include chorioretinitis, radiculopathy, subacute encephalitis, colitis, esophagitis, and pneumonia (Porche, 2003). Specific types of CMV infections are described in Table 34-8.

Herpes Simplex and Herpes Zoster

Over 70% of HIV-positive patients have previously been infected with herpes simplex virus-1 (HSV-1), HSV-2, or both. When HSV is reactivated in HIV patients, it can cause serious disease and tissue destruction. HSV infection follows a predictable pattern: primary outbreak, latency, and possible reactivation at some later point in life. Most adults carry herpes zoster virus (HZV) because of exposure to the chickenpox virus as a child. Reactivation of HZV usually occurs as *shingles* and can be very painful and serious in the immunocompromised patient (Robinson, 2003). Refer to the Patient Teaching Plan above.

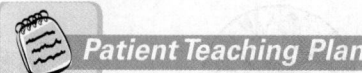

Patient Teaching Plan

HSV or HZV

When patient has open sores on skin, instruct patient to do the following (Kirton, 2003):
- Maintain good hygiene without drying out the skin.
- Avoid deodorant astringent soap.
- Use tepid water; pat skin dry, no rubbing.
- Apply lotion after bathing and at bedtime.
- Do not scratch.
- Use separate cloths for affected areas.
- Some wounds need special care.
- Avoid contact with people who have never had chickenpox.

Oral Hairy Leukoplakia

Oral hairy leukoplakia (OHL) is characterized by thick, white patches on the buccal mucosa, soft palate, floor of mouth, and tongue. It is associated with Epstein-Barr virus and is more common among smokers. The mouth often is painful. Advise the patient to drink from a straw. Ice cream or popsicles can be used to numb the area. Hot/spicy foods and alcohol may exacerbate mouth pain (Keithley, 2003).

Progressive Multifocal Leukoencephalopathy

Progressive multifocal leukoencephalopathy (PML), which is caused by the Jamestown Canyon virus (JC virus), develops in 2% to 4% of AIDS patients and is recognized as an AIDS indicator illness. The JC virus causes progressive degeneration of the white matter of the brain; death ensues within 4 to 6 months after the onset of symptoms. Symptoms include weakness and progressively impaired speech, vision, and motor function. There is no proven effective therapy for treatment of PML. Intrathecal cytosine arabinoside (Ara-C) may be tried, but it causes bone marrow suppression. Maintaining low viral loads through antiretroviral therapy seems to be the best strategy for preventing

Table 34-8 | *Cytomegalovirus*

CMV TYPE	SYMPTOMS	DIAGNOSIS
CMV Retinitis	Decreased visual acuity, presence of floaters, progression to visual field loss leading to blindness	Funduscopic examination
CMV Radiculopathy	Spinal cord syndrome—lower extremity weakness, spasticity, areflexia, urinary retention	Cerebrospinal fluid culture
CMV Subacute Encephalitis	Mental changes, somnolence, headache	Brain biopsy
CMV Esophagitis	Painful swallowing	Endoscopic examination
CMV Pneumonia	Dyspnea on exertion; dry, nonproductive cough	X-ray examination and histological findings
Colitis	Diarrhea, weight loss, fever	Endoscopic examination, ulcerated colon

Data from Zwolski, K. (2001). Viral infections. In Kirton, C. A., Talotta, D., & Zwolski, K. (Eds.). *Handbook of HIV/AIDS nursing*. St. Louis: Mosby.

PML (Kirton, 2003). Both the family and the patient need support to accept and plan for the patient's approaching decline and death. Anticipate grief over loss, and help the family arrange nursing home care and advanced directives (Sellers, 2003).

BACTERIAL INFECTIONS

Opportunistic bacterial infections include bacillary angiomatosis, *Mycobacterium avium* complex (MAC), and tuberculosis. Treatments employ various antibacterial drugs depending on the infecting organism. Patients need to understand the importance of taking antibacterials exactly as prescribed and completing the prescribed course of therapy. In persons with HIV, anti-infective drugs sometimes are ordered prophylactically when the CD4 counts fall below specific levels.

Bacillary Angiomatosis

Bacillary angiomatosis (BA) is a disease caused by bacteria (*Bartonella henselae* and *B. quintana*) that usually cause skin lesions. However, any organ may be affected. BA is usually transmitted by cats and their fleas. Most patients with BA have been bitten or scratched by a cat. Symptoms include papules and plaques that may occur anywhere on the skin. Patients with HIV should be warned about the risk of being around cats. Advise the patient to avoid rough play with cats and to make sure cats are treated for fleas (Stanley, Marsco, & Mc-Nicholl, 2003).

Mycobacterium avium Complex

M. avium, the causative agent for *M. avium* complex (MAC), is found everywhere, including in most food, animal, and soil sources. MAC may affect any organ of the body causing fever, fatigue, weight loss, night sweats, abdominal pain, and diarrhea. It is not contagious. Prophylactic treatment should be considered when CD4 cell counts drop below 50 cells/mm^3 (Kirton, 2003).

Tuberculosis

HIV patients are much more likely than healthy persons to develop tuberculosis (TB) if exposed to the causative agent *Mycobacterium tuberculosis*. This is particularly true if CD4 counts drop below 200 cells/mm^3 (Porche, 2003). TB is covered in Chapter 31.

ONCOLOGIC CONDITIONS

Oncologic conditions that occur most often in persons with HIV include Kaposi's sarcoma and lymphoma. Other cancer sites are the rectum and the vagina.

Kaposi's Sarcoma

Kaposi's sarcoma (KS) is a common type of neoplasm that develops in people with AIDS. It is thought to be caused by the sexual transmission of the human herpes virus 8 (HHV8) (Moran, 2003). KS affects the skin first, appearing as a macular, painless, nonpruritic lesion.

Patient Teaching Plan

The Patient with Kaposi's Sarcoma

* Tumor growth varies from patient to patient.
* Regardless of therapy, KS tends to reoccur.
* Various therapies are available; each has risks and benefits.
* For patients with cutaneous KS: report blood in stool or abdominal pain.

Data from Kirton, C. (Ed.). (2003). *ANAC's core curriculum for HIV/AIDS nursing* (2nd ed.). Thousand Oaks, CA: Sage Publications.

KS can vary in color—pink, red, purple, and brown. When KS is confined to the skin, there are no symptoms. However, symptoms develop when tumors spread to the gastrointestinal system (GI) and lungs. Sometimes when KS shows on the skin, it has already affected the body internally. When KS affects the GI system, bleeding may result, causing anemia. When KS affects the respiratory system, hypoxia may occur (Moran, 2003).

Diagnosis. KS is diagnosed by clinical appearance, but the most definitive method is a biopsy. There is no cure for KS, and treatment is considered palliative.

Treatment. Treatment includes simple observation, HARRT (highly active antiretroviral therapy), surgical removal, cryotherapy, radiotherapy, and chemotherapy. To help patients with self-care, refer to the Patient Teaching Plan above.

Lymphomas

Lymphoma is a type of cancer that originates in lymphoid tissue—bone marrow, spleen, thymus gland. Immunodeficient patients have a 14-times greater risk of getting lymphomas than the general population. The two types of lymphoma are Hodgkin's and non-Hodgkin's. Non-Hodgkin's lymphoma (NHL) is the second most common malignancy found in patients with AIDS.

The prognosis with NHL is poor because the disease has spread widely by the time it is discovered. With chemotherapy, survival rates areas are as follows:

* 24 months with CD4 counts higher than 100 cells/mm^3
* 4½ months with CD4 counts less than 100 cells/mm^3
* 2 months if the central nervous system (CNS) is affected

Symptoms that typically are vague and vary according to the site involved include chills, fever, night sweats, and weight loss. Having a fever for more than 2 weeks strongly suggests lymphoma. Diagnosis is based on results of biopsy of lymphoid tissue. Other diagnostic testing includes x-ray, computed tomography (CT) scan, bone marrow smear, and lumbar puncture. Treatment is chemotherapy (Moran, 2003).

MEDICAL DIAGNOSIS OF HIV

To be diagnosed as HIV positive, one must test positive to an HIV *antibody* test (ELISA or Western blot). The enzyme-linked immunoassay (ELISA) test is usually done first, and it has been shown to have 99% reliability. The Western blot test is used as a confirmation test, which has been shown to have 99.99% reliability (Kirton, Talotta, & Zwolski, 2001). Persons who test negative initially should be retested in 3 to 6 months because of the lag time between exposure and a positive test. It is important to remember that some individuals never test positive for HIV because they never produce enough antibodies to the HIV virus to be detected.

The CDC (2004) criteria for a diagnosis of AIDS include the following:

- CD4 count of less than 200 cells/mm^3, asymptomatic
- CD4 count of less than 200 cells/mm^3, with category B symptoms. Category B symptoms include bacillary angiomatosis; candidiasis; oropharyngeal, vaginal, cervical dysplasias; herpes zoster (shingles); idiopathic thrombocytopenic purpura; listeriosis; oral hairy leukoplakia; pelvic inflammatory disease (PID); peripheral neuropathy
- Category C symptoms regardless of CD4 count. Category C symptoms include candidiasis of bronchi, trachea, or lungs; esophageal, cervical cancer; coccidioidomycosis; cryptococcosis; cryptosporidiosis; CMV; encephalopathy; HSV; chronic ulcers of longer than 1 month's duration or bronchitis, pneumonitis, or esophagitis; histoplasmosis; isosporiasis; KS; lymphoma; *M. avium, M. tuberculosis, P. jiroveci* pneumonia; pneumonia-recurrent; progressive multifocal leukoencephalopathy; salmonella; septicemia, recurrent; toxoplasmosis; wasting due to HIV

In 1996, the Home Access HIV-1 Test System was introduced; it allowed individuals to collect a specimen at home and receive prompt results after submitting it by mail for analysis. At this time, the FDA is considering approval of a true home-testing kit—the OraQuick ADVANCE, which detects HIV-1 and HIV-2 in 20 minutes using a cheek swab. Home testing is controversial because of the risks of false-negative and false-positive results as well as the lack of professional counseling about the results. For example, a person in the early stage of infection who tests negative because there are not yet enough antibodies to be detected might assume he or she is free of infection and fail to protect a partner.

MEDICAL TREATMENT

There is no cure for HIV infection. The medical treatment of HIV infection is symptomatic and is aimed at reducing the viral load, preventing and treating infections, and treating malignancies. Patients also are en-

Health Promotion Considerations

Women with HIV

Women with HIV should be treated with antiretroviral drugs during pregnancy and delivery, and the newborn should be treated the first 6 weeks of life to decrease the risk of transmission of the virus to the baby.

couraged to maintain a balanced diet, exercise regularly, maintain good dental hygiene, avoid smoking and using illicit drugs, limit alcohol intake, minimize stress, and practice safe sexual habits. The Health Promotion Considerations box above addresses reducing the risk of perinatal transmission of HIV infection. The Drug Therapy table on p. 621 outlines drugs used to treat HIV infection.

PHARMACOLOGY

HIV patients commonly are started on a medication regimen titled HAART (highly active antiretroviral therapy), which is recommended when the HIV viral load reaches certain levels. The usual combination of drugs is one protease inhibitor and two nucleoside reverse transcriptase inhibitors (NRTIs). Some protocols use NRTIs with one NNRTI (non-nucleoside reverse transcriptase inhibitor), or three NRTIs. A protease inhibitor interferes with the maturation of viral particles. Zidovudine (AZT) is a common NRTI that works by blocking an enzyme needed for viral replication. Efavirenz (Sustiva) is an example of a NNRTI, which also prevents viral replication. Enfuvirtide (Fuzeon) is a newer type of antiretroviral drug that is called a *fusion inhibitor.* A fusion inhibitor inhibits the binding of the HIV with the human cell.

Before the HIV patient is started on a medication regimen, it is important to assess the patient's ability and willingness to comply with the therapy. Once a medication regimen is started, the HIV patient should not miss doses. When a dose is missed, the serum drug level falls, which allows the HIV virus to mutate and build resistance toward the HIV medications. Resistance is a very serious problem with HARRT therapy. If resistance is built up to enough of the HIV medications, the patient will have no medication options, which will ultimately end in his or her death. Therefore if the patient will not be compliant with the HIV medication regimen, it would be better to not even start the HIV medication regimen. Some of the common side effects of HARRT therapy are as follows:

- Lipodystrophy
- Hepatitis
- Diabetes
- Increase in cholesterol
- Increased low-density lipoproteins
- Increased triglycerides
- Pancreatitis

DRUG THERAPY *Classes of Drugs Used to Treat Patients with HIV Infection*

DRUG	USE/ACTION	SIDE EFFECTS	NURSING INTERVENTIONS
NUCLEOSIDE REVERSE TRANSCRIPTASE INHIBITORS (NRTIs)			
Abacavir, lamivudine, and zidovudine (Trizivir)	Used to slow the progression of HIV by interfering with replication inside the T helper CD4 cell.	Headache	Some of these drugs should be taken on an empty stomach, whereas others can be taken with or without food. Administration recommendations for specific drugs should be reviewed with the patient.
Didanosine or ddI (Videx and Videx EC)		Nausea and vomiting Fatigue Muscle aches	A complete blood cell count will be ordered periodically to monitor the patient's white blood cell and red blood cell counts.
Emtricitabine or FTC (Emtriva)		Neutropenia Anemia Peripheral neuropathy	Liver function tests will also be monitored. Multiple drug interactions are possible between NRTIs and other drugs; therefore the patient's complete medication record must be reviewed before beginning these drugs and before adding other drugs to the patient's regimen after he or she is started on an NRTI.
Lamivudine and zidovudine (Combivir)		Skin rash Elevated liver enzymes Pancreatitis	
Lamivudine or 3TC (Epivir)		Diarrhea	
Stavudine or d4T (Zerit)			
Tenofovir (Viread)			
Zalcitabine or ddC (Hivid)			
Zidovudine or AZT (Retrovir)			
PROTEASE INHIBITORS (PIs)			
Amprenavir (Agenerase)	Used to slow the replication and progression of HIV by blocking protease enzymes so that infected cells cannot produce HIV proteins.	Diarrhea	Some of these drugs should be taken on an empty stomach, whereas others should be taken with food. Administration recommendations for specific drugs should be reviewed with the patient.
Atazanavir (REYATAZ)		Nausea and vomiting Kidney stones Jaundice	
Fosamprenavir (Lexiva)		Abdominal pain Headache	Multiple drug interactions are possible between PIs and other drugs; therefore the patient's complete medication record must be reviewed before beginning these drugs and before adding other drugs to the patient's regimen after he or she is started on a PI.
Indinavir (Crixivan)		Skin rash	
Lopinavir and ritonavir (Kaletra)		Numbness and tingling around the mouth	
Nelfinavir (Viracept)		Drooling	
Ritonavir (Norvir)		Dizziness	
Saquinavir (Fortovase)		Sleepiness Sore throat	
Saquinavir mesylate (Invirase)		Sweating Altered taste	
NON-NUCLEOSIDE REVERSE TRANSCRIPTASE INHIBITORS (NNRTIs)			
Delavirdine (Rescriptor)	Used to slow the progression of HIV by interfering with replication inside the T helper CD4 cell.	Skin rash Headache	Can be taken with or without food. Multiple drug interactions are possible between NNRTIs and other drugs; therefore the patient's complete medication record must be reviewed before beginning these drugs and before adding other drugs to the patient's regimen after he or she is started on an NNRTI.
Efavirenz (Sustiva)		Nausea Diarrhea	
Nevirapine (Viramune)		Fatigue	
FUSION INHIBITORS (FIs)			
Enfuvirtide (Fuzeon)	Fusion inhibitors are a new class of antiretroviral agents called *fusion inhibitors*. Fuzeon is used in combination with other antiretroviral drugs in treatment-experienced patients. This drug prevents the HIV from fusing with the cell membrane.	Irritation at injection site Fatigue Nausea Insomnia Peripheral neuropathy	Reconstitute and store as directed. Inject subcutaneously as ordered, and rotate sites.

- Hemolytic anemia
- Peripheral neuropathy
- Nephrolithiasis/nephrotoxicity
- Stevens-Johnson syndrome
- Myopathy
- Hypersensitivity reaction
- Hepatotoxicity
- Nightmares
- Nausea/vomiting/diarrhea

Gastrointestinal upset is a very common side effect of HARRT and is one of the major reasons for noncompliance. The nurse should make the HIV patient aware that many of the side effects of HAART are transitory and will subside within a few weeks. The Drug Therapy table on p. 621 summarizes drugs used to treat HIV.

NURSING CARE *of the Patient with HIV Infection*

As shown in the Nursing Care Plan on p. 623, care of the patient with HIV infection varies depending on the stage of infection the patient is experiencing. During the early stages of the disease, patients are treated primarily as outpatients. Because patients with HIV infection are frequent consumers of medical care, they often become very knowledgeable about their disease and treatment options and want to be actively involved in all treatment decisions. In the later stages of HIV infection, nursing care is much more intensive as the patient becomes more debilitated. Throughout the course of this disease, the goal of all treatments is quality of life.

Assessment

Infection is the leading cause of death in patients with HIV infection. Therefore it is important to frequently assess the patient for any signs or symptoms of infection. The most common sites of infection are the lungs, mouth, gastrointestinal tract, skin, blood, and central nervous system. Any change in the physical examination findings or any change in function should be reported to a registered nurse or physician. While collecting data about the patient's physical status, determine how much the patient knows about the disease and treatment and how the patient is coping with this life-threatening disease. The complete assessment, as done by the registered nurse, is outlined here. The LPN/LVN may collect some of the data.

Health History

A complete past health and social history should be obtained from each patient with HIV. The history should include the following:

- Sexually transmitted infection (STI) history
- Surgical history
- Medication history: all current drugs, compliance, allergies, response to HIV drugs
- Immunization history
- Family history
- Sexual history—number of partners the patient has had in the past year
- Needle and blood exposure history—exposure to hepatitis B and C
- History of screening for hepatitis B and C
- Tobacco/alcohol use
- Illegal drug use history—use of intravenous drugs or unsafe behavior while on drugs
- Travel history—travel outside the United States where possible exposure to pathogens may have occurred
- Pet history—exposure to cats, birds, or exotic pets
- Occupational history—exposure to pathogens in the workplace
- Nutritional history—usual food and fluid intake
- Gynecological history—number of pregnancies; knowledge of contraceptives

Physical Examination

A complete physical examination should be performed (review the Nursing Care Plan on p. 623). The examination should include the following (Kirton, 2003):

- General examination—measure height, weight, vital signs
- Skin examination—signs of infections, lesions
- Head, ears, eyes, nose, and throat examination
- Lymphatic system—enlarged lymph glands
- Respiratory system—auscultate for quality of breath sounds
- Cardiovascular examination
- Abdominal examination
- Musculoskeletal examination
- Neurologic examination—orientation, alertness, sensory and cognitive functioning
- Genitourinary examination
- Laboratory profile
- CD4 count
- CD8 count
- HIV viral load
- CBC
- Chemistry profile
- Rapid plasma reagin (RPR) (syphilis)
- Lipid profile
- STI screening
- Purified protein derivative (PPD) tuberculosis screening
- Chest x-ray
- Hepatitis A, B, C antibody titers
- Toxoplasmosis antibody titers
- Titers for all immunizations received

Nursing Diagnoses, Goals, and Outcome Criteria: HIV Infection

NURSING DIAGNOSES	GOALS AND OUTCOME CRITERIA
Ineffective Therapeutic Regimen Management related to lack of knowledge about disease process and treatment, denial, fear	Effective self-care management: patient correctly describes and demonstrates self-care measures

NURSING CARE PLAN
The Patient with HIV Infection

ASSESSMENT

Health History: A 25-year-old divorced mother of two children works as a freelance accountant and lives with her parents, who provide financial and emotional support. She was diagnosed with HIV infection during the pregnancy with her daughter, Lindsay. Lindsay, now 3, has shown no signs of HIV infection. The patient and her husband have been divorced since her infection was diagnosed. His HIV status is not known. She reports tiring easily but most days is able to work about 6 hours and care for her children. She is seen monthly by a nurse practitioner at a neighborhood clinic. Her medications are indinavir (Crixivan), stavudine (Zerit), and didanosine (Videx). She reports bouts of depression and anxiety about her own and her children's future. Her most recent blood studies show a decline in the number of T helper (CD4) cells. The CD4 cell level today is 480 cells/mm^3. She has been treated twice this fall for upper respiratory tract infections. She does not sleep well. She has experienced a 10-pound weight loss in the past 3 months and reports poor appetite and frequent diarrhea.

Physical Examination: Healthy-looking young woman. Alert. Converses easily. Vital signs WNL. No fever. Lungs clear on auscultation. No lymphadenopathy. Abdomen soft. Bowel sounds present in all 4 quadrants. Normal reflexes. Full range of motion all joints.

Nursing Diagnosis	Goals and Outcome Criteria	Interventions
Ineffective Therapeutic Regimen Management related to lack of knowledge about disease process and treatment, denial, and fear	Patient will effectively manage self-care, as evidenced by correctly taking prescribed medications, following medical advice for rest and protection from infection.	Provide written and verbal instructions for prescribed drug(s). Advise her of the kinds of side and adverse effects that she might experience. Explain the importance of continuing the drugs under medical supervision. Discuss ways to conserve energy and to promote restful sleep at night. Explore options to obtain assistance with child care.
Anxiety related to disease and treatments	Patient will verbalize decreased anxiety and will appear more relaxed.	Encourage her to ask questions and talk about her feelings. Be accepting of feelings she may express (fear, anger, depression are common). Provide information, or refer to a social worker, chaplain, or mental health counselor if needed.
Risk for Infection related to impaired resistance	Patient will remain free of infection, as evidenced by absence of fever, lesions, or signs of inflammation.	Encourage her to immediately report any signs of infection. If antibiotics are ordered, encourage her to take them as prescribed. Explain the need to avoid people with infections and crowded public places during seasons when upper respiratory tract infections are common.
Impaired Oral Mucous Membrane related to HIV infection and oral opportunistic infections	Patient will have intact oral mucous membranes with normal color and no lesions.	Teach importance of regular dental care. Advise her to use a soft toothbrush and to avoid traumatizing oral tissues. Explain how maintaining good fluid intake keeps mucous membranes moist and reduces oral complications.
Imbalanced Nutrition: Less Than Body Requirements and Deficient Fluid Volume related to HIV infection, diarrhea, and gastrointestinal infections	Patient's intake of food and fluids will be adequate, as evidenced by stable body weight, moist mucous membranes, and normal blood pressure and pulse.	Suggest addition of Carnation Instant Breakfast to daily diet to increase calorie intake. Weigh weekly. Talk to nurse practitioner about prescribing antinausea medication, appetite stimulant, and antidiarrheal agent.

? CRITICAL THINKING QUESTIONS

■ How would you explain to the patient the importance of taking the prescribed drugs as prescribed?

■ What other suggestions could you give this patient to help her increase her intake of food and liquids throughout the day?

Anxiety related to the disease and treatment	Reduced anxiety: patient reports anxiety is lessened, more relaxed manner
Risk for Infection (lung, mouth, gastrointestinal tract, skin, blood, central nervous system, eye) related to decreased immunity	Patient remains free of infection: no fever, signs of inflammation, lesions
Impaired Oral Mucous Membrane related to the disease and oral infections	Intact oral mucous membranes: normal color of mouth tissues, no lesions
Imbalanced Nutrition: Less Than Body Requirements and **Deficient Fluid Volume** related to the disease, diarrhea, and gastrointestinal infections	Adequate intake of nutrients and fluids: stable weight, intake and output approximately equal, moist mucous membranes
Disturbed Thought Processes related to disease-induced dementia	Improved thought processes: patient remains oriented Patient safety: absence of injuries associated with confusion
Acute Pain or **Chronic Pain** related to the disease and treatment	Pain relief: patient states pain in relieved, appears relaxed

Interventions

Ineffective Therapeutic Regimen Management

It is very important that the patient receive accurate, consistent information from all members of the health care team. A clinical nurse specialist or other specially trained nurse can usually provide comprehensive information about the disease and its treatment to the patient and family and answer questions as they arise during hospitalization. You can reinforce this teaching. Excellent sources of current information about HIV and AIDS for patients, families, and health care providers are on the Internet (e.g., www.thebody.com and www.hivinsite.ucsf.edu).

Anxiety

A diagnosis of HIV infection is always a shock to patients and their families. Patients must deal not only with the disease and treatment but also with the emotions of facing a life-threatening illness. Encourage patients to ask questions and to talk about their feelings. Often a patient's fears are due to a lack of knowledge about the disease and treatment. The clinical nurse specialist or other specially trained nurse can answer many of the patient's and family's questions. Often information will help the patient and family deal with their anxiety. A referral to a social worker, chaplain, or mental health counselor may be indicated if the patient and family are having continued anxiety and difficulty in coping. It is important for you to know what the

patient has been told about the disease, the treatment, and the prognosis so that correct information can be reinforced. Most important, the patient's interpretation and understanding of the information are essential.

Risk for Infection

As emphasized earlier, patients with HIV are at high risk for opportunistic infections. Early detection and prompt treatment of infection are vital. Many patients take anti-infective drugs (e.g., trimethoprim-sulfamethoxazole, pentamidine) prophylactically to prevent infection. Educate the patient about the importance of taking drugs exactly as prescribed. If a patient does develop an infection, stress the importance of taking the antibiotics exactly as prescribed. Stopping antibiotic therapy early can result in incomplete treatment and the development of resistant organisms. Many of the antibiotics must be administered intravenously and require nursing coordination for intravenous access and either clinic or home administration.

Impaired Oral Mucous Membrane

Patients with HIV can experience altered oral mucous membrane integrity due to both the disease and oral infections. Encourage patients to regularly clean their teeth and mouth with dental floss and a soft toothbrush. Debilitated patients may need assistance with

 Nutrition Concepts

AIDS wasting is common among AIDS patients. Wasting is caused by lack of nutritional intake or the inability of the body to absorb and use nutrition. Every HIV patient should be seen by a nutritionist. Helpful nutrition teaching for the patient with HIV includes the following:
- Do not buy expired foods.
- Do not buy cracked eggs.
- Thoroughly cook meats and poultry.
- Wash hands thoroughly before preparing foods.
- Wash all fruits and vegetables before eating.
- Thaw frozen foods in the refrigerator and not at room temperature.
- Use wooden cutting boards rather than plastic boards because plastic is more likely to harbor pathogens.
- Avoid leftovers.
- If CD4 cell counts drop below 100 cells/mm^3, boil water for 1 minute or use sterile water products.

Many HIV drugs cause hyperlipidemia. Encourage patients to eat small, frequent meals, low in fat and lactose and high in caloric intake.

Encourage patient to abstain from alcohol and caffeine.

Encourage patient to eat healthy with five to six servings of fruits and vegetables/day.

Teach patient to weigh daily and to report to provider any patterns of weight loss or gain.

Data from Winson, G. (2001). HIV/AIDS nutritional management. In Kirton, C., Talotta, D., & Zwolski, K. (2001). *Handbook of HIV/AIDS nursing*. St. Louis: Mosby.

mouth care. Encourage non-caffeinated fluids to maintain hydration and to keep oral mucous membranes moist. Topical anesthetics to control pain can be applied before eating. Prescribed topical antibiotics should be reapplied after eating and routine mouth care. Regular dental evaluations can help prevent and manage oral disease and infections in these patients.

Imbalanced Nutrition: Less Than Body Requirements

A referral to a dietitian for nutrition education and counseling should be made as soon as the patient is diagnosed with HIV. Strategies to maximize calorie and nutrient intake can be discussed. Oral supplements with Carnation Instant Breakfast, Ensure, Sustacal, or Resource can be added as indicated. Administer medications to improve appetite (e.g., megestrol, dronabinol), relieve nausea (e.g., prochlorperazine, metoclopramide), and control diarrhea (e.g., diphenoxylate hydrochloride with atropine sulfate) as prescribed.

In general, the diet should be high in calories and proteins with supplemental vitamins. Advise the patient to avoid caffeine and food that might contain pathogens (e.g., undercooked meat, raw eggs, unpasteurized milk). (See the Nutrition Concepts box on p. 624.)

Disturbed Thought Processes

Patients with HIV encephalopathy may experience both cognitive and motor impairment. Patients may withdraw from social activities because of embarrassment. Patients may become angry and hostile with the onset of yet another disability. Many patients with HIV-induced encephalopathy improve with zidovudine therapy. Both in the hospital and at home, patient safety needs to be constantly reevaluated based on the patient's mental and physical capabilities.

Acute Pain or Chronic Pain

Pain has been an under-recognized problem for patients with HIV infection. Pain can be caused by opportunistic infections, viral invasion into the nerves and muscles, malignant tumors, and diagnostic procedures. Closely monitor the patient's pain level and medication usage. Keeping a flow sheet of patient reports of pain on a 10-point scale can be helpful, especially as different nurses care for the patient throughout the day. A "0" represents no pain, whereas a "10" represents the worst pain a patient has ever experienced. The patient's report of pain coupled with the amount of pain medication he or she is receiving can guide the nurse and physician as to the appropriate type and amount of pain medication. Pharmacologic and nonpharmacologic pain management strategies are presented in Chapter 15.

Ineffective Coping

A diagnosis of HIV/AIDS, with its life-threatening consequences, can overwhelm the patient's ability to cope. Patients and their significant others may experience many emotions such as fear, anxiety, anger, shame, grief, depression, and a loss of self-esteem. Fearing social stigma, patients may be reluctant to share the diagnosis with others. Other than sexual partners and health care providers, the patient is not obligated to inform other persons.

Nurses must be aware of their own feelings, and even fears, about caring for people with HIV. Education about self-protection and measures to take in the event of body fluid exposure can relieve some of your concerns. Your sensitivity and touch can be very comforting to patients. When changes in a patient's emotional state are noted, encourage the patient to talk about his feelings. Provide information about support groups and mental health care as needed.

 Key Points

- HIV is transmitted by risk behavior and body fluid exposure, including intrauterine exposure. It occurs in both heterosexual and homosexual people of all races.
- Behaviors by which HIV may be shared include needle sharing, unprotected sex, and blood transfusions.
- HIV is a retrovirus that enters the body through blood, semen, vaginal fluids, or breast milk.
- HIV infection eventually exhausts the immune response to pathogens.
- CD8 cells drop drastically in the late stage of HIV infection; CD4 cells slowly decline throughout the course of the infection.
- A patient is considered to have AIDS when the CD4 cell level drops below 200 cells/mm³.
- Initial symptoms of HIV infection are usually flu-like symptoms.
- During the latent stage, which can last 2 to 12 years, patients may have no symptoms.
- During the later stages of HIV, patients may have fever, night sweats, swollen lymph glands, skin lesions, dyspnea, burning with urination, diarrhea, and other symptoms.
- The major complications of HIV infection are opportunistic infections, wasting, secondary cancers, and dementia.
- Opportunistic infections can be caused by parasites, viruses, bacteria, or fungi.
- The most common types of cancer associated with HIV infection are Kaposi's sarcoma and lymphoma.
- Blood tests used to diagnose HIV infection are the ELISA and Western blot; both detect antibodies.
- Infection is the leading cause of death in patients with HIV infection.
- The most commonly used types of drugs for HIV infection are nucleoside reverse transcriptase inhibitors, protease inhibitors, non-nucleoside reverse transcriptase inhibitors, and fusion inhibitors.
- Failure to take HIV drugs as scheduled can encourage resistant strains of the HIV.

- Nursing diagnoses for the patient with HIV infection may include Anxiety, Risk for Infection, Impaired Oral Mucous Membrane, Imbalanced Nutrition: Less Than Body Requirements, Disturbed Thought Processes, Chronic Pain, Deficient Fluid Volume, and Ineffective Therapeutic Regimen Management.
- Wasting is caused by inadequate nutritional intake or the inability of the body to absorb and use nutrition.

 Go to your Companion CD-ROM for a Pharmacology Tutorial, Audio Glossary, and 3-D animations.

evolve Be sure to visit the companion Evolve site at http://evolve.elsevier.com/Linton/ for WebLinks and additional online resources.

REVIEW QUESTIONS *Choose the best answer.*

1. HIV can best be described as a:
   1. DNA virus
   2. mRNA virus
   3. tRNA virus
   4. Retrovirus

2. During the latent stage of HIV infection, which cells host the HIV?
   1. CD4 cell
   2. Neutrophil cell
   3. Macrophage cell
   4. Natural killer cell

3. HIV enters the body through:
   1. The respiratory tract
   2. Blood and body fluids
   3. Contaminated food
   4. Skin contact

4. The usual cause of death in persons with AIDS is:
   1. Infection
   2. Cancer
   3. Dementia
   4. Starvation

5. It is possible for a person with HIV infection to have negative HIV blood tests.
   1. True
   2. False

6. Which of the following is the most reliable test for the HIV antibodies?
   1. ELISA
   2. CD4/CD8 ratio
   3. Western blot
   4. Complete blood count

7. Anal or vaginal sex with a condom can be classified as:
   1. Very high risk behavior
   2. Little risk behavior
   3. Moderate risk behavior
   4. No risk behavior

8. AZT is classified as which of the following drug categories?
   1. Non-nucleoside reverse transcriptase inhibitors (NNRTs)
   2. Nucleotide reverse transcriptase inhibitors
   3. Protease inhibitors (PIs)
   4. Nucleoside reverse transcriptase inhibitors (NRTIs)

9. A serious side effect of AZT is which of the following?
   1. A rash
   2. Elevated liver enzymes
   3. GI upset
   4. Hyperlipidemia

10. HIV diagnosis in an adult is confirmed by:
    1. ELISA
    2. P24 antigen test
    3. Western blot assay
    4. CD4 count

11. A patient with HIV infection has recently become confused. You should explain to the patient's partner that:
    1. Confusion with HIV is rare and irreversible
    2. The patient's confusion is probably related to something other than HIV
    3. The patient's mental status may improve with drug therapy
    4. Confusion usually occurs shortly before death

35 Cardiac Disorders

JUDY L. MALTAS

Objectives

After reading and studying this chapter, you should be able to:

1. Label the major parts of the heart.
2. Describe the flow of blood through the heart and coronary vessels.
3. Name the elements of the heart's conduction system.
4. State the order in which normal impulses are conducted through the heart.
5. Explain the nursing considerations for patients having procedures to detect or evaluate cardiac disorders.
6. Identify nursing implications for common therapeutic measures, including drug, diet, or oxygen therapy; pacemakers and cardioverters; cardiac surgery; and cardiopulmonary resuscitation.
7. Explain the pathophysiology, risk factors, signs and symptoms, complications, and treatment for selected cardiac disorders.
8. List the data to be obtained in assessing the patient with a cardiac disorder.
9. Assist in developing nursing care plans for patients with cardiac disorders.

Key Terms

Be sure to check out the bonus material on the Companion CD-ROM, including selected audio pronunciations.

afterload (p. 631)
arteriosclerosis (ăr-tē-rē-ō-sklĕ-RŌ-sĭs, p. 652)
atherosclerosis (ăth-ĕr-ō-sklĕ-RŌ-sĭs, p. 653)
bradycardia (brăd-ē-KĂR-dē-ă, p. 633)
contractility (p. 631)
diastole (p. 631)
dysrhythmia (dĭs-RĬTH-mē-ă, p. 655)
hemodynamics (hē-mō-dī-NĂM-ĭks, p. 661)
murmur (MŬR-měr, p. 633)
myocardial infarction (ĭn-FĂRK-shŭn, p. 654)
palpitation (păl-pĭ-TĀ-shŭn, p. 632)
perfusion (pěr-FŪ-zhŭn, p. 648)
preload (p. 631)
regurgitation (rē-gŭr-jĭ-TĀ-shŭn, p. 670)
syncope (SĬN-kō-pē, p. 632)
systole (p. 627)
tachycardia (tăk-ē-KĂR-dē-ă, p. 633)
thromboembolism (thrŏm-bō-ĔM-bō-lĭsm, p. 655)

The cardiovascular system carries oxygenated blood and nutrients to the cells and transports carbon dioxide and wastes from the cells. It requires a reservoir for blood coming from the tissues, pumping action to send blood to the lungs and the body, and an intact vascular system to transport the blood. A malfunction in any of these components may affect other body systems and may threaten the life and health of the person.

The heart is a hollow muscular pump located in the mediastinum (Fig. 35-1). The right and left sides of the heart receive blood from and send blood to different parts of the body. The heart is covered and protected by the sternum and the ribs anteriorly and flanked by the lungs laterally. The esophagus, the descending aorta, and the fifth through the eighth thoracic vertebrae are directly behind the heart. The heart rests on the diaphragm, with two thirds of it to the left of the sternum. The right side of the heart is located under the sternum. The heart is approximately the size of the person's fist, weighs 10 to 14 ounces in the adult, and is covered by membranes called the *visceral* and *parietal pericardium*. The space between the pericardial membranes contains fluid that lubricates the membranes and decreases friction.

ANATOMY AND PHYSIOLOGY OF THE HEART

CHAMBERS

The heart is divided into four chambers: two upper atria (right and left) and two lower ventricles (right and left). The four chambers are separated by septa (walls) with two chambers on the right (right atrium and ventricle) and two chambers on the left (left atrium and ventricle). Valves separate the atria from the ventricles.

The right atrium (RA) is a thin-walled reservoir and conduit for systemic blood. It receives blood from the inferior and the superior venae cavae and from the coronary sinuses. The right ventricle (RV) has thicker walls than the RA and receives blood from the RA through the tricuspid valve. Blood moves rather passively from the RA to the RV. When the RV contracts (**systole**), blood is ejected through the pulmonic valve into the pulmonary artery. The pulmonary artery

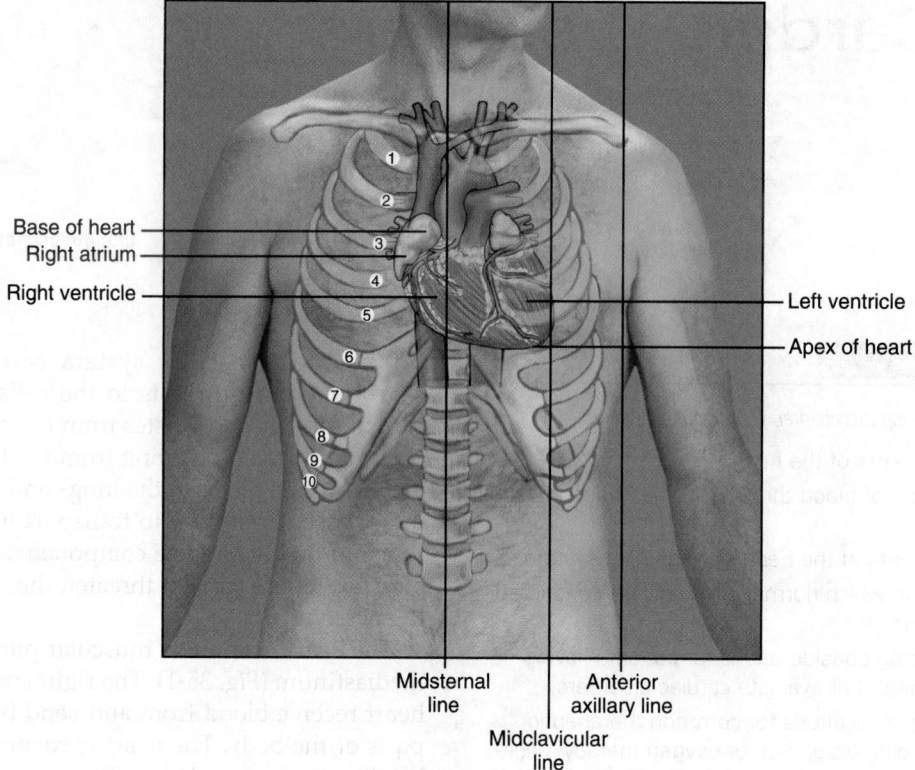

Base of heart
Right atrium
Right ventricle

Left ventricle
Apex of heart

Midsternal line
Anterior axillary line
Midclavicular line

FIGURE **35-1** Anatomic location of the heart.

carries the blood to the lungs, where it releases carbon dioxide as waste and picks up oxygen to be taken to the tissues. Pulmonary veins carry the blood from the lungs to the left atrium (LA).

The blood passes from the LA through the mitral valve into the left ventricle (LV), the chamber with the thickest, strongest muscle. The LV is cone-shaped and contains the apex of the heart located at the midclavicular line at the fourth or fifth intercostal space. An apical pulse is taken by auscultating the heartbeat at this location.

When the LV contracts (systole), blood is ejected through the aortic valve into the aorta and the systemic circulation. The systemic circulation carries oxygen and nutrients to all active cells and transports wastes to the kidneys, liver, and skin for excretion (Fig. 35-2).

The pressures in the RA and RV are very low compared with the pressures in the LA and LV. This is because the LV pumps blood out into the systemic circulation. The pressure in the LV is the highest of all the chambers.

MUSCLE LAYERS

There are three layers of cardiac muscle tissue: the endocardium, the myocardium, and the epicardium. The endocardium is the inner layer that lines the heart chambers. The middle layer, the myocardium, is made of muscle fibers. It is responsible for the pumping action of the heart. The thickness of the myocardium varies with each chamber. The outer layer, the epicardium,

is also the *visceral pericardium*. The coronary arteries are embedded in the epicardium.

VALVES

There are four valves in the heart: the mitral, the tricuspid, the aortic, and the pulmonic. Their purpose is to retain blood in one chamber until the next chamber is ready to receive it. The valves keep blood flowing in one direction. The valves open and close passively in response to changes in pressure and volume. A valve opens when the pressure behind it is greater than the pressure ahead of it. A valve closes when the pressure ahead of it is greater than the pressure behind it.

Atrioventricular Valves

The mitral and tricuspid valves are called *atrioventricular (AV) valves* because they separate the atria from the ventricles. The mitral valve is between the LA and the LV. The tricuspid valve separates the RA from the RV. The cusps, or leaflets, are attached by chordae tendineae to the papillary muscles that line the floor of the ventricles. These valves are closed during systole and open in diastole.

Semilunar Valves

The semilunar valves, called *aortic* and *pulmonic*, separate the ventricles from the aorta and the pulmonary artery, respectively. These valves are open during systole and are closed during diastole. The semilunar valves have three cusps (cup-shaped structures) each.

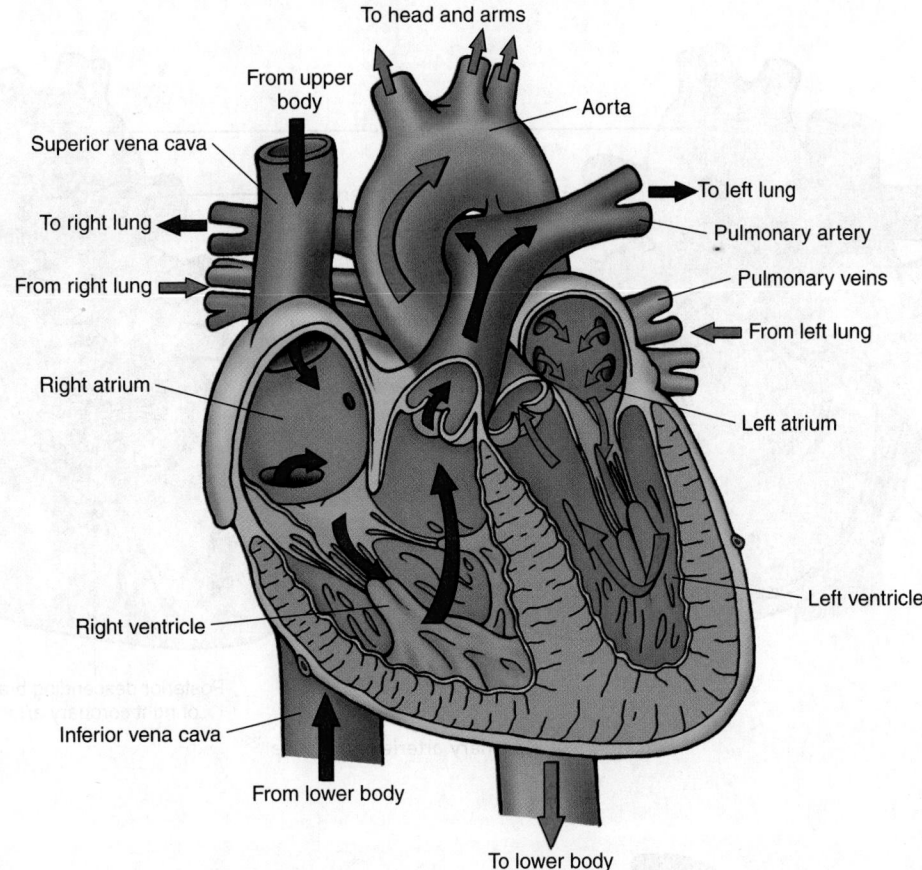

To head and arms

From upper
body

Superior vena cava

To right lung

From right lung

Right atrium

Right ventricle

Inferior vena cava

From lower body

Aorta

To left lung

Pulmonary artery

Pulmonary veins

From left lung

Left atrium

Left ventricle

To lower body

FIGURE 35-2 Normal circulation through the heart.

Heart Sounds

Closure of the valves produces the heart sounds auscultated over the heart. The first heart sound (S_1), referred to as "lub," occurs when the ventricles contract during systole and when the mitral and tricuspid valves close. The second heart sound (S_2), called "dub," occurs during ventricular relaxation or diastole and is caused by the closing of the aortic and pulmonic valves.

CORONARY BLOOD FLOW

The coronary arteries are the first branches of the systemic circulation. These arteries supply blood to the myocardium and the conductive tissue of the heart. The two major coronary arteries, the left coronary artery and the right coronary artery, arise from the aorta just beyond the aortic valve. Blood flow through the coronary arteries occurs during diastole. The left coronary artery, which branches into the left anterior descending and circumflex arteries, supplies blood to the LA, most of the LV, and most of the septum between the two ventricles (interventricular septum). The right coronary artery branches to supply the sinoatrial (SA) and the atrioventricular (AV) nodes, the RA and RV, and the inferior part of the LV. Variations in the pattern of arterial branching are common.

Collateral arteries are connections between two branches of arteries. They are more common in certain areas of the heart. It is thought that collateral cir-

culation protects the heart and that coronary collaterals develop over time as a result of gradual coronary occlusion.

In general, the venous system parallels the arterial system: the great cardiac vein follows the left anterior descending artery; and the small cardiac vein follows the right coronary artery. The veins meet to form the coronary sinus (the largest coronary vein), which returns deoxygenated blood from the myocardium to the right atrium (Fig. 35-3).

CONDUCTION SYSTEM

For the heart to pump blood through the chambers, nerves must stimulate muscle contractions in an orderly fashion. The conduction pattern follows a particular route. The SA node, also called the *pacemaker*, initiates the impulse. The impulse is carried throughout the atria to the AV node, located on the floor of the RA. The impulse is delayed in the AV node and then transmitted to the ventricles through the bundle of His. The bundle is made up of Purkinje cells and is located where the atrial and ventricular septa meet. The bundle of His divides into the left and right bundle branches. The left bundle branch divides into anterior and posterior branches called *fascicles.* The terminal ends of the right and left branches are called the *Purkinje fibers.* When the impulse reaches the Purkinje fibers, the ventricles contract (Fig. 35-4).

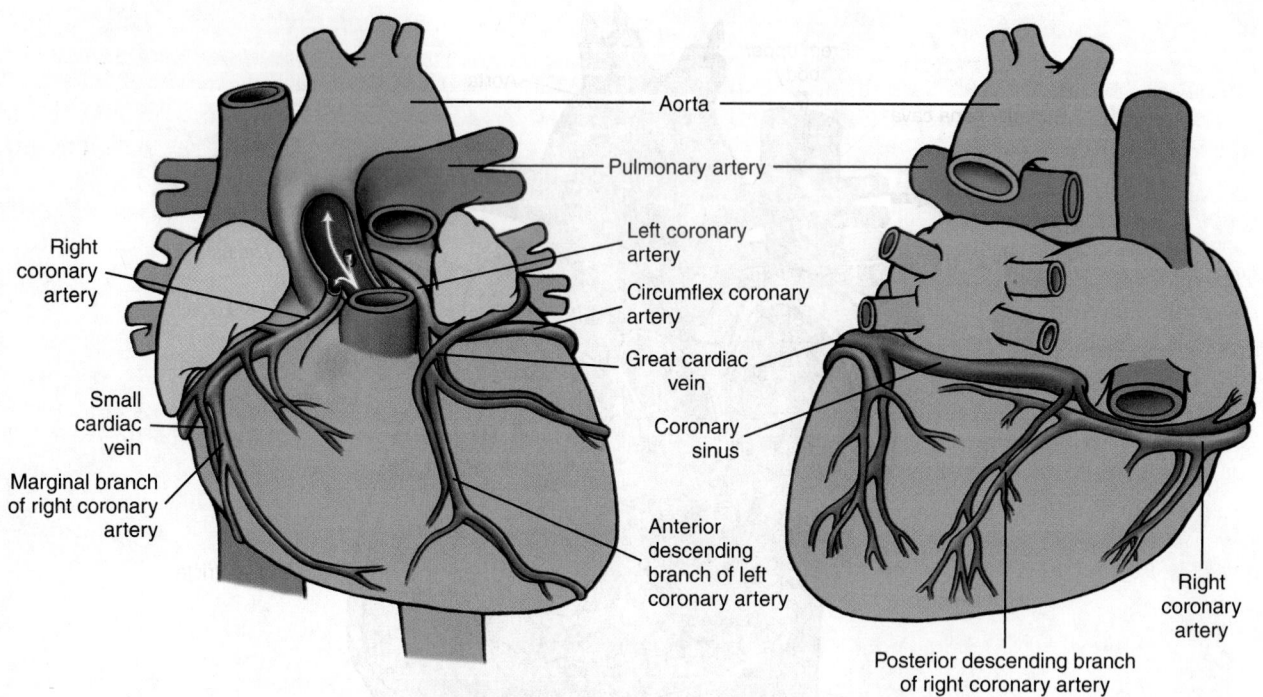

FIGURE **35-3** Coronary arteries and veins.

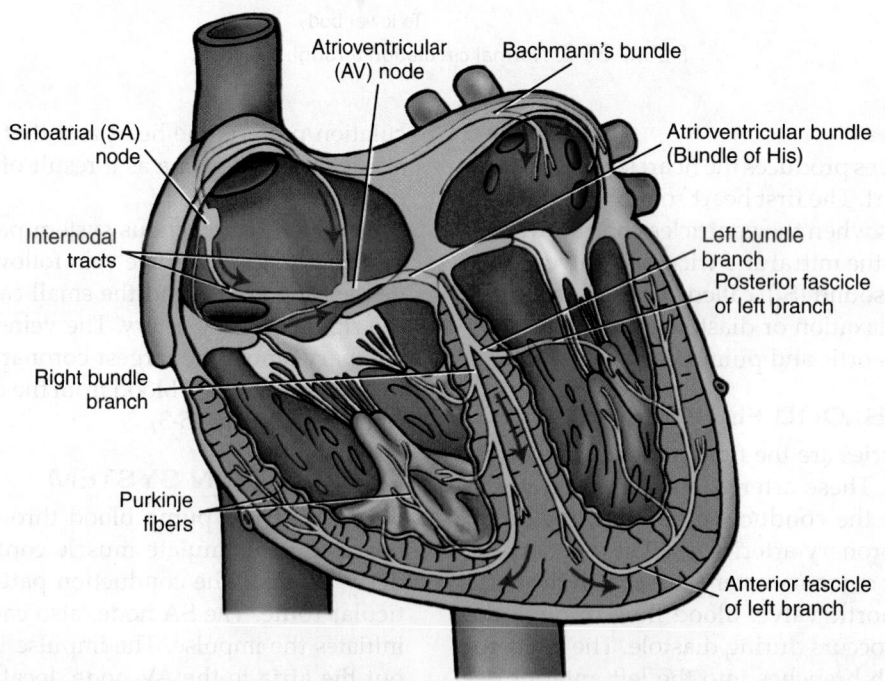

FIGURE **35-4** The conduction system of the heart.

The impulse produces a change in the movement of electrically charged ions across the membrane of cardiac cells. Cardiac cells at rest are electrically polarized, with the inside of the cell negatively charged and the outside of the cell positively charged. When stimulated, cardiac cells lose their internal negativity by a process called *depolarization*. Depolarization moves from cell to cell, producing a wave of electrical activity that is transmitted throughout the heart. Once depolarization is complete, the resting state (i.e., inside of the cell more negative than the outside) is restored through a process called *repolarization*.

The SA node normally generates these impulses at a rate between 60 and 100 beats per minute (bpm). The

SA node is called the *pacemaker of the heart*. The AV node is also capable of generating an impulse if the SA node should fail. The AV node rate is 40 to 60 bpm. The Purkinje network also can generate an impulse, but at less than 40 bpm, which could prevent cessation of heart function for a short time (Table 35-1).

Cardiac Innervation

The heart is innervated by sympathetic and parasympathetic fibers of the autonomic nervous system. Sympathetic fibers are distributed throughout the heart. Sympathetic stimulation results in increased heart rate, increased speed of conduction through the AV node, and more forceful contractions. Parasympathetic fibers, which are part of the vagus nerve, are found primarily in the SA and AV nodes and the atrial tissue. Parasympathetic stimulation results in slowing of the heart rate, slowing of conduction through the AV node, and decreased strength of contraction.

CARDIAC FUNCTION

The primary function of the heart is to pump blood through the pulmonary and systemic circulations. This is accomplished by a continually repeating pattern of contraction and relaxation.

Cardiac Cycle

Contraction and relaxation of the heart make up one heartbeat and are called the *cardiac cycle*. When the ventricles are at rest (relaxation phase), they are filling up with blood coming from the atria. This is called diastole. At the end of diastole, the atria contract to eject more blood into the ventricles (called the *atrial kick*). Once the ventricles have filled with blood and the electrical impulse has reached the terminal fibers of the conduction system, the ventricles contract and eject blood into the pulmonary artery from the RV and into the aorta from the LV. This is called *systole*. In a person with a heart rate of 60 bpm, there would be 60 cardiac cycles per minute.

Cardiac Output

The volume of blood ejected by the heart each minute is determined by the stroke volume and the heart rate. Stroke volume is the amount of blood ejected with each ventricular contraction. The normal stroke volume is 60 to 100 mL. Cardiac output is the amount of blood (in liters) ejected by the heart per minute. It is calculated by multiplying the heart rate by the stroke volume ($CO = HR \times SV$). The normal cardiac output is 4 to 8 L/min. In the normal heart, cardiac output responds to the increased demands for oxygen and nutrients that occur with exercise, infection, or stress.

Three factors affect stroke volume: preload, contractility, and afterload.

Preload. Preload is the amount of blood remaining in a ventricle at the end of diastole or the pressure generated at the end of diastole. Increased preload results in increased stroke volume and, therefore, increased cardiac output. Factors that increase preload include increased venous return to the heart and overhydration. Factors that decrease preload include dehydration, hemorrhage, and venous vasodilation.

Contractility. Contractility is the ability of cardiac muscle fibers to shorten and produce a muscle contraction. *Inotropy* is a term used to refer to the contractile state of the cell. Factors that increase contractility are said to have a positive inotropic effect, and factors that decrease contractility create a negative inotropic effect.

Afterload. Afterload is the amount of pressure the ventricles must overcome to eject the blood volume. It is determined primarily by the pressure in the arterial system. Afterload is decreased by vasodilation and increased by vasoconstriction.

Myocardial Oxygen Consumption

Myocardial tissue routinely needs 70% to 75% of the oxygen delivered to it by the coronary arteries. Skeletal muscles, by contrast, need 35% at rest and up to 75% during exercise. The only ways to increase oxygen supply to the myocardium are to (1) increase the coronary blood flow by coronary artery vasodilation or to (2) increase the oxygen in the blood by administering supplemental oxygen.

AGE-RELATED CHANGES

It is difficult to separate the normal age-related changes in the heart and blood vessels from the changes caused by disease. In general, age-related changes progress slowly, whereas pathogenic changes are more likely to be sudden.

HEART

Changes in the heart muscle include increased density of connective tissue and decreased elasticity. Cardiac contractility may decline, making the heart less able to adapt to changes in circulating blood volume. The valves may thicken and stiffen. If they do not close properly, the patient may have a murmur. The valves may also partially block the path of blood flow, causing incomplete emptying of the chambers.

The number of pacemaker cells in the SA node decreases, as does the number of nerve fibers in the

Table 35-1	*Intrinsic Heart Rates*
INITIATION OF IMPULSE	**RATE**
Sinoatrial node	60-100 bpm
Atrioventricular node	40-60 bpm
Ventricle	15-40 bpm

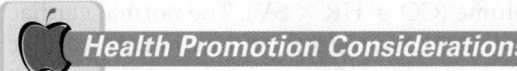
Health Promotion Considerations

Long-Term Conditioning
Long-term conditioning with an exercise program may help decrease arterial stiffening and improve the function of the left ventricle in older individuals. Physical exercise does not have to be strenuous to be helpful. Activity should become a part of an individual's regular routine.

ventricles. The aging heart takes longer to respond to stress and then responds less dramatically. It also takes longer to return to normal after exercise or stress. Cardiac dysrhythmias are more common in older people but should still be evaluated because they can be dangerous.

BLOOD VESSELS

Changes in connective tissue and elastic fibers in arteries cause them to become stiffer. Physical activity can help reverse or delay this process (see the Health Promotion Considerations box above). Pulse pressure (the difference between the systolic and diastolic pressures) and systolic blood pressure generally increase. Experts disagree about what exactly constitutes hypertension in older adults. The veins stretch and dilate, leading to venous stasis and sometimes impaired venous return. Thrombophlebitis and varicosities are more common in older people.

The cardiovascular system adapts more slowly to changes in position; therefore postural hypotension may occur.

NURSING ASSESSMENT OF CARDIAC FUNCTION

HEALTH HISTORY

A complete assessment is important for the cardiac patient. If the patient is having acute symptoms, however, a detailed assessment must be deferred until the patient is stable.

Chief Complaint and History of Present Illness
Determine the patient's reason for seeking medical care. Common symptoms that may be related to cardiac disorders include fatigue, edema, palpitations, dyspnea, and pain. Note when symptoms occur, what aggravates them, and what relieves them.

Medical History
Ask whether the patient has had specific conditions that may be related to cardiac disease. These include hypertension, kidney disease, pulmonary disease, stroke, rheumatic fever, streptococcal sore throat, and scarlet fever. Document previous cardiac disorders and hospitalizations. List recent and current medications and note allergies in appropriate records. It is also important to ask whether the patient is taking any

vitamins, herbs, or homeopathic remedies. It may be easier to ask something such as "What are you doing to stay healthy or to help you feel better?"

Family History
Because cardiovascular problems are often familial or hereditary, ask whether immediate relatives have had hypertension, coronary artery disease (CAD), other cardiac disorders, or diabetes mellitus.

Review of Systems
Inquire whether the patient has experienced the following specific symptoms: weight gain, fatigue, dyspnea (shortness of breath), cough, orthopnea (difficulty breathing in a supine position), paroxysmal nocturnal dyspnea (sudden dyspnea during sleep), palpitations, chest pain, syncope (fainting), concentrated urine, or leg edema.

If the patient has had dyspnea or orthopnea, determine when it occurred and whether the onset was gradual or sudden. Pain also requires detailed descriptions. The pain of heart problems may radiate or be referred to other areas. The pain may radiate down either arm, to the jaw, or to just below the sternum. The severity may range from mild, intermittent discomfort to severe, crushing chest pain. Ask the patient to rate the severity of the pain on a scale of 1 (mildest) to 10 (worst possible). Chest pain may be different in women and may be described as indigestion, as a feeling of anxiety, as nausea, or as a feeling of fatigue. Document the exact description, location, and severity, whether there is radiation, events causing the pain, and what relieves the pain.

Functional Assessment
Determine how this illness has affected the patient's ability to carry out usual activities. Describe activity and rest patterns and usual diet. It is especially important to record salt and fat intake. Ask the patient about sources of stress and coping strategies.

PHYSICAL EXAMINATION

Begin the physical examination with measurement of height and weight and recording of vital signs.

Vital Signs
Blood Pressure. The correct-size blood pressure cuff must be used. Position the arm at the heart level, and check the blood pressure in both arms. Note the pulse pressure (difference between the systolic and diastolic pressures) because it is a noninvasive measure of cardiac output. Next, measure blood pressures and pulse rates in the lying, sitting, and standing positions. A blood pressure decrease of 20 mm Hg or more with a position change indicates decreased blood volume or an autonomic response. As blood pressure decreases, the pulse should increase as a compensatory mechanism.

Pulses. Palpate the radial pulses for rate, rhythm, quality, and equality. Auscultate the apical pulse for rate and rhythm. Apical and radial pulses may be taken simultaneously to detect a pulse deficit. The normal heart rate is 60 to 100 bpm. A rate of less than 60 bpm is considered to be bradycardia; tachycardia is characterized by a heart rate in excess of 100 bpm. The rhythm is described as *regular, irregular,* or *regularly irregular.* The quality of the pulse is graded on a four-point scale: 0, absent pulse (not palpable); 1, weak or thready pulse (pulse easily obliterated by slight finger pressure, returning as pressure is released); 2, normal pulse (easily palpable); and 3, bounding pulse (forceful, not easily obliterated by finger pressure). With a stethoscope, listen at the fifth intercostal space at the midclavicular line to assess the apical pulse. In addition to the radial pulse, assess the carotid, brachial, femoral, popliteal, posterior tibial, and dorsalis pedis pulses at appropriate times in the physical examination.

Respirations. Observe the patient's respiratory effort and skin color. Count the respiratory rate, and auscultate the breath sounds for crackles and wheezes. If the patient produces sputum, describe the color, amount, and appearance.

Skin

Inspect the skin for color, hair distribution, and capillary refill, and palpate the temperature. Skin color and temperature should be relatively the same over the entire body.

Heart Sounds

The heart sounds are systole (lub) and diastole (dub). To auscultate heart sounds, place the diaphragm of the stethoscope firmly on the anterior chest. Avoid auscultating heart sounds through clothing. Figure 35-5 shows where the heart sounds, made by closing of the valves, may be heard best. With practice, you can learn to distinguish these. The following pattern of auscultation is recommended:

1. Listen to the aortic area first and then the pulmonic. As the aortic and the pulmonic valves close, the dub should be louder than the lub in the aortic and pulmonic areas.
2. Listen to the tricuspid and mitral valves in the areas indicated. In these areas, the lub should be louder than the dub.
3. After listening to each area with the diaphragm, repeat the pattern with the bell of the stethoscope. Note additional sounds of S₃ and S₄. The S₃ and S₄ sounds are heard best with the bell of the stethoscope placed at the apex when the patient is positioned on the left side. S₃, also called a *ventricular gallop,* occurs early in diastole. S₃ is normal in children and young adults and may be pathologic after age 30. S₄, also called an *atrial gallop,* occurs late in diastole. S₄ is an abnormal heart sound.

FIGURE **35-5** Auscultation of the heart. **A,** Aortic valve at the second intercostal space to the right of the sternum. **B,** Pulmonic valve at the second intercostal space to the left of the sternum. **C,** Tricuspid valve at the fifth intercostal space to the left of the sternum. **D,** Mitral valve at the fifth intercostal space in the midclavicular line.

Table 35-2 | *Grading of Heart Murmurs*

GRADE	DESCRIPTION
I	Very faint
II	Faint, but recognizable
III	Loud, but moderate in intensity
IV	Loud and accompanied by a palpable thrill
V	Very loud, accompanied by a palpable thrill, and audible with the stethoscope partially off the client's chest
VI	Extremely loud, may be heard with the stethoscope slightly above the client's chest

From Ignatavicius, D.D., Workman, M.L., & Mishler, M.A. (1999). *Medical-surgical nursing across the health care continuum* (3rd ed., p. 735). Philadelphia: Saunders.

Heart Murmurs. A heart murmur is the sound produced by turbulent blood flow across the valves. Murmurs are recorded as having high, low, or medium pitch, and they are located using the anatomic landmarks where they are heard best. The timing of a murmur relates to when it is heard in the cardiac cycle: systole or diastole. Murmurs are graded according to intensity or loudness (Table 35-2).

A rub is heard when the pericardium is inflamed. A scratchy or muffled sound may be heard best by having the patient sit upright and lean forward. This position brings the pericardium closer to the chest wall. A pericardial friction rub is best heard along the left

Box 35-1 **ASSESSMENT of Patients with Cardiac Disorders**

Health History
Present Illness:
Fatigue, edema, palpitations, pain; aggravating and relieving factors

Past Medical History:
Hypertension, kidney disease, pulmonary disease, diabetes mellitus, stroke, rheumatic fever, streptococcal sore throat, scarlet fever, previous cardiac diseases or conditions, previous hospitalizations, recent and current medications, allergies

Family History:
Hypertension, coronary artery disease or other cardiac conditions, diabetes mellitus

Review of Systems:
Weight gain, fatigue, dyspnea, cough, orthopnea, palpitations, chest pain, fainting, concentrated urine, leg edema

Functional Assessment:
Effects of illness on usual activities, activity and rest pattern, lifestyle, diet, sodium and fat intake, sources of stress, coping strategies

Physical Examination
General Survey:
Apparent distress

Height and Weight

Vital Signs:
Blood pressure in both arms and while supine, sitting, standing; apical heart rate and rhythm; peripheral pulses: rate, rhythm, quality, equality; respiratory effort and rate

Skin:
Color, hair distribution, capillary refill, temperature

Thorax:
Heart sounds, heart murmurs, rubs; breath sounds, crackles, wheezes; presence and appearance of sputum

Extremities:
Pulses, color, warmth, edema, hair distribution

sternal border throughout the cardiac cycle. It may help to ask patients to hold their breath briefly. If a rub is heard during this brief time, it is a pericardial rub rather than pleural.

Extremities

Inspect and palpate the extremities for color, edema, warmth, temperature, pulse quality, and hair distribution.

Assessment of the cardiac patient is summarized in Box 35-1.

DIAGNOSTIC TESTS AND PROCEDURES

A number of tests or procedures may be employed to assess cardiac structure and function. More common tests are described here. Patient preparation and postprocedure care are detailed in the Diagnostic Tests and Procedures table on pp. 635 and 636.

ELECTROCARDIOGRAM

The electrocardiogram (ECG) allows study of the electrical activity (conduction system) through the heart muscle. An electrical impulse causes contractions as it passes through the heart muscle. Electrodes placed on the surface of the skin pick up the electrical impulses of the heart. Moving electrodes to various positions permits detection of conduction disturbances in specific areas of the heart.

The ECG is graphed on standardized paper or viewed on an oscilloscope. Each cardiac cycle is rep-

resented by a series of P, Q, R, S, and T waves. The activity represented by each wave is explained in the Interpretation of Electrocardiograms section on pp. 673 to 675. The ECG is interpreted to detect abnormalities in rate, rhythm, or impulse conduction. The normal finding is called a *normal sinus rhythm*, which is characterized by the following:

1. A rate of 60 to 100 bpm
2. A regular rhythm
3. A P wave preceding each QRS complex
4. A PR interval that is within 0.12 to 0.20 second
5. A QRS complex that is 0.10 second or less

AMBULATORY ECG (HOLTER MONITOR)

An ambulatory ECG uses a portable ECG machine with a memory to provide continuous cardiac monitoring for 24 to 48 hours. A complete record of the heart rhythm is stored and analyzed later. This type of monitoring is used to detect dysrhythmias that occur infrequently, to determine if symptoms correlate with any underlying cardiac disease, to assess the effects of medications, and for research purposes. The patient records in a diary all activity that occurs during the monitoring, such as walking, stair climbing, sleeping, and engaging in sexual activity. The monitor strip is computer scanned and then interpreted by a physician.

Even more sophisticated monitoring is accomplished by transtelephonic means. An audio signal is sent over telephone lines to a station operated by personnel trained to recognize potentially dangerous dysrhythmias.

DIAGNOSTIC TESTS and PROCEDURES The Heart

TEST	PURPOSE/PROCEDURE	PATIENT PREPARATION	POSTPROCEDURE NURSING CARE
Electrocardiogram (ECG)	Electrodes are placed on the skin to detect electrical activity of the heart. Detects abnormalities in conduction of impulses, including changes caused by heart damage.	Tell the patient what to expect and that the procedure is painless. No special preparation is needed.	Remove gel from skin. No special care needed.
Holter monitor	Provides continuous ECG monitoring for a 24-to-48-hour period. Detects occasional dysrhythmias that may be correlated with specific activities noted in patient's diary.	Tell patient to wear loose clothing, take only sponge bath, avoid magnets and metal detectors, and monitor placement of electrodes. Emphasize keeping accurate diary of activities and to push "event button" if symptoms occur.	Return at scheduled time. ECG recording will be retrieved for inspection.
Implantable loop recorder (ILR)	Provides ECG monitoring for longer time periods and saves on a memory loop for analysis. Detects dysrhythmias causing syncopal episodes.	Tell patient/family member/significant other to activate recorder when symptoms occur and to keep a written record of events.	Return at scheduled time. ECG recording will be retrieved for inspection.
Echocardiogram	Uses ultrasound to create images of the heart. Gel is placed on the patient's skin and a transducer moved over the area. Detects valve abnormalities, left ventricular hypertrophy, hypertrophic cardiomyopathy.	Tell the patient what to expect and that the procedure is painless. No special preparation is needed.	Remove gel from skin. No special care needed.
Transesophageal echocardiogram	Used when conventional echocardiogram not diagnostic. Probe inserted through esophagus into stomach (behind heart). Same purpose as echocardiogram.	Tell patient what to expect: throat will be anesthetized, may have IV. Signed consent required.	Monitor vital signs, gag reflex, and, if sedated, level of consciousness.
Magnetic resonance imaging (MRI)	Creates images of body structures without radiation. The patient lies on a firm pad that rolls into a circular device. "Open MRI" better tolerated by claustrophobic patients because machine does not surround patient. Clanging sounds are heard as the machine works.	All metal must be removed. Sedation may be ordered if patient is very anxious or unable to be still.	No special care needed. Safety precautions if sedative has been given.
Multiple-gated acquisition scanning	Radioactive material is injected intravenously and the heart scanned to evaluate function. May be done at rest or during exercise.	Tell patient what to expect. Nothing by mouth (NPO) for 2 hr before procedure. Start intravenous infusion as ordered. Signed consent required.	No special care needed.
Stress test (exercise tolerance test)	Assess presence and severity of coronary artery disease by having the patient exercise during ECG monitoring. Blood pressure is monitored. The test is stopped if symptoms of coronary artery disease occur.	Tell the patient what to expect. NPO for 2 hr before test. Give beta-blocker if prescribed. Have patient wear loose clothing and comfortable shoes. Signed consent required.	No special care needed.
Thallium imaging	Thallium-201 is given intravenously and the heart scanned to assess blood flow. Scanning may be done at rest or after exercise.	Same as stress test. Tell patient intravenous injection will be given and that radiation dose is small and quickly eliminated.	No special care needed.

IV, Intravenous

Continued

DIAGNOSTIC TESTS and PROCEDURES *The Heart—cont'd*

TEST	PURPOSE/PROCEDURE	PATIENT PREPARATION	POSTPROCEDURE NURSING CARE
Ultrafast Computed tomography (CT)	Imaging technology that provides images used to assess myocardial perfusion, right and left ventricular muscle mass/function, and measure calcium deposits in coronary circulation.	Tell patient what to expect (lie on table, hold very still, may be asked to hold breath for a few seconds at a time). No special preparation is needed.	No special care needed.
Cardiac catheterization	A catheter is passed through a vein or artery and dye is injected. Radiographs are taken to visualize heart structures and blood vessels. The procedure is done in a special room. Blood pressure, pulse, and ECG are monitored throughout test.	Tell patient what to expect. Assess allergies to seafood or iodine and inform radiologist. NPO for specified time before procedure. Tell patient to expect flushing sensation when dye is injected. Give sedative if ordered. Signed consent required.	Check puncture site; maintain pressure per protocol if a vascular sealing device is not used. Monitor vital signs and peripheral pulses on affected extremity. Enforce bed rest as ordered.
Electrophysiology study (EPS)	A catheter with multiple electrodes is passed into the right side of the heart through the femoral vein. The electrodes record electrical activity of the conduction system and may be used to stimulate the patient's dysrhythmia.	Tell the patient what to expect. NPO for 6 hr before procedure. Premedicate with prescribed sedatives. Signed consent required.	Similar to cardiac catheterization (described above).
Arterial blood gases	Assesses acid-base balance by measuring pH, P_{CO_2}, P_{O_2}, HCO_3^-, and base excess.	Tell patient about arterial puncture. Prepare heparinized syringe and obtain blood sample.	Remove air bubbles from sample. Place tube on ice and send for immediate analysis. Apply pressure to puncture site for 5 min. Report results.
Cardiac enzymes	Measures creatine phosphokinase, lactate dehydrogenase, and aspartate aminotransferase to detect elevation associated with heart damage.	Tell patient a blood sample will be drawn. No special preparation. To detect acute myocardial infarction, draw specimen before other invasive procedures.	Check venipuncture site. Apply pressure if oozing.
Troponin	Measures protein released after myocardial injury. Troponin T (cTnT) and Troponin I (cTnI).	Tell patient a blood sample will be drawn. No special preparation.	Check venipuncture site. Apply pressure if oozing.
Myoglobin	Measures myoglobin levels in the blood.	Tell patient a blood sample will be drawn. No special preparation.	Check venipuncture site. Apply pressure if oozing.
Complete blood count (CBC)	Counts white and red blood cells, hemoglobin and hematocrit, red blood cell indices, and sometimes platelets. (See Normal Values in Table 35-5.)	Tell patient a blood sample will be drawn. No special preparation.	Check venipuncture site. Apply pressure if oozing.
Lipid profile	Measures common serum lipids (cholesterol, triglycerides, lipoproteins). Used to evaluate risk of coronary artery disease.	Tell patient to expect venipuncture. NPO for 12 hr before sample drawn. Usual diet for 2 weeks before test.	Check venipuncture site. Apply pressure if oozing.
B-type natriuretic peptide (BNP)	Measures naturally occurring BNP levels. Elevated in HF. CMP: Helps differentiate dyspnea related to cardiac problems from non-cardiac related dyspnea.	Tell patient a blood sample will be drawn. No special preparation.	Check venipuncture site. Apply pressure if oozing.
C-reactive protein (CRP)	Acute phase protein that is elevated in system inflammation. Elevated levels seen with ACS.	Tell patient a blood sample will be drawn. No special preparation.	Check venipuncture site. Apply pressure if oozing.

ACS, Acute coronary syndrome; *CMP,* cardiomyopathy; *HF,* heart failure.

IMPLANTABLE LOOP MONITOR/ RECORDER

For longer monitoring time periods, to record a patient's ECG during syncopal episodes, an implantable loop monitor/recorder (ILR) may be used. This device, implanted just under the patient's skin in the chest area, continually monitors the ECG activity of the patient in a memory loop. The patient and/or family member/significant other is taught to activate the recorder when symptoms are felt. The ECG can then be analyzed and appropriate treatment implemented. The device can be used for up to 14 months, as needed (Morton, Tucker, & Van Roeden, 2005).

ECHOCARDIOGRAM (HEART SONOGRAM)

The echocardiogram visualizes and records the size, shape, position, and behavior of the heart's internal structures, especially the valves. Ultrasonic waves are beamed into the heart, and their echoes are recorded. This painless test may be performed at the bedside or in a laboratory. Gel is applied to the skin, and a special device called a *transducer* is moved over the precordium. The transducer picks up sound waves and converts them to electrical impulses that are recorded as waveforms on an oscilloscope, a videotape, or a strip chart. Common echocardiogram types include motion mode (M-mode) and two-dimensional mode (2-D mode). Echocardiograms can also be enhanced using Doppler technology (Doppler echocardiogram) and color-flow imaging.

TRANSESOPHAGEAL ECHOCARDIOGRAM

At times, the echocardiogram is not diagnostic and a transesophageal echocardiogram (TEE) is used. A flexible endoscopic probe with an ultrasound transducer is passed down the back of the throat into the esophagus. A local anesthetic to the throat decreases the gag reflex. Occasionally, an intravenous sedative is needed to reduce patient anxiety. Images are obtained from behind the heart as the probe moves down into the stomach. The probe is down for approximately 15 to 20 minutes. The TEE provides information useful in the evaluation of ventricular wall motion and function and possible heart valve disorders.

MAGNETIC RESONANCE IMAGING

A magnetic resonance imaging (MRI) scan provides high-resolution, three-dimensional images of body structures. Cardiac tissue is imaged without lung or bone interference. The patient is enclosed in a chamber for approximately 5 minutes for an MRI scan of the heart. No loose metallic objects are permitted in the chamber during the procedure. Patients with intracranial aneurysm clips, intraocular metal foreign bodies, heart valves manufactured before 1964, and some middle-ear prostheses should not have MRI scans because the devices may be affected by the magnetic field or may interfere with the MRI. Other implanted devices that contraindicate MRI include pacemakers, automatic implantable cardioverter-defibrillators (AICDs), and implanted infusion pumps. For patients who are claustrophobic, an open MRI may be available.

MULTIPLE-GATED ACQUISITION SCAN

In a multiple-gated acquisition scan (MUGA), the patient is injected with technetium 99m, which concentrates in acutely necrotic myocardial tissue. The heart is then scanned to assess left ventricular structure and function, to evaluate myocardial wall motion, to detect intracardiac shunting, to assess valvular disease, and to identify location and size of an acute myocardial infarction (AMI). Assessment of ventricular function can be done while the patient is resting or exercising. Sublingual nitroglycerin may be administered to assess its effect on ventricular function.

STRESS TEST (EXERCISE TOLERANCE TEST)

The stress test is a noninvasive method of assessing the presence and severity of CAD by recording a person's cardiovascular response to exercise. It is also used to measure functional capacity for work, sport, or participation in a rehabilitation program. The stress test is not flawless—false-positive and false-negative results are common. A negative test result does not absolutely exclude CAD. It is, however, the best noninvasive screening procedure available. The alternative is the much more invasive cardiac catheterization.

For the stress test, a continuous ECG is monitored while the patient uses a treadmill or a stationary bicycle. Every 2 to 3 minutes the speed and incline angle of the treadmill are increased (or pedal resistance is increased with a bicycle) until (1) the patient cannot continue for whatever reason, (2) the patient's maximum heart rate is achieved (220 − patient's age = maximum heart rate), (3) symptoms intervene, or (4) significant changes are detected on the ECG. The target heart rate is 85% of the predicted maximum heart rate for the patient's age and gender.

Significant CAD limits blood flow to the myocardium. The increased demands of exercise may cause the patient to have symptoms of CAD, which are angina, dizziness, dyspnea, dysrhythmias, a falling blood pressure, and certain ECG findings. If these symptoms occur, the test must be stopped immediately.

Contraindications for the test include acute systemic illness, severe aortic stenosis, uncontrolled congestive heart failure (CHF), severe hypertension, angina at rest, and significant dysrhythmia. Although the mortality rate for test participants is very low, cardiopulmonary resuscitation equipment must be available.

PERFUSION IMAGING

Perfusion studies, performed most commonly in conjunction with exercise tolerance testing, provide information about the presence of coronary artery disease and the location and extent of ischemic and infarcted myocardium. There are several radioactive tracers approved for perfusion scanning. Thallium-201 is the most widely used over the years and will be addressed here.

Thallium Imaging

Thallium-201 may be administered to assess myocardial blood flow during stress testing. Thallium, which is taken up by normal myocardial cells, is used to detect old or new myocardial ischemia and to evaluate patency of coronary artery bypass grafts. After thallium-201 is injected intravenously, the heart is scanned to assess the areas of concentration. The scan takes approximately 1 hour to complete and is repeated in 2 to 4 hours to assess for redistribution.

Thallium does not enter infarcted or scarred areas and, therefore, shows "cold spots" in areas without blood flow. Exercise-induced ischemia resolves with rest. Scar-induced ischemia, such as that caused by AMI, does not resolve with rest.

For patients who are physically not able to exercise, the heart can be stressed with medications such as dipyridamole (Persantine). These medications mimic the effects of exercise by causing vasodilation of the coronary arteries, which increases blood flow to well-perfused areas, thereby stealing blood from ischemic areas. These differences in flow will show up on the scan.

ULTRAFAST COMPUTED TOMOGRAPHY

Ultrafast CT (also known as *electron-beam CT* or *EBCT*) is a fast form of imaging technology that allows for high-quality images not affected by the movement of the heart as it contracts and relaxes. The images obtained are used to assess myocardial perfusion, along with right and left ventricular muscle mass and function. In addition, Ultrafast CT can measure calcium deposits in the coronary arteries, and a coronary calcium score can be derived. The greater the amount of coronary calcium, the higher the score and the higher the risk of coronary occlusive disease. This procedure is not a substitute for cardiac catheterization (Morton, Tucker, & Van Roeden, 2005).

CARDIAC CATHETERIZATION (CARDIAC ANGIOGRAPHY, CORONARY ARTERIOGRAPHY)

Cardiac catheterization is a procedure in which a catheter is inserted into a vein or artery and is threaded into the heart chambers, coronary arteries, or both, under fluoroscopy (Fig. 35-6). A contrast dye is injected through the catheter, and films are made of the visualized heart structures. Vital signs and ECG are monitored during the procedure.

In a catheterization of the right side of the heart, the catheter is inserted into a vein and threaded into the vena cava, RA, RV, and pulmonary artery. Pressures in the RA, RV, and pulmonary artery may be determined. The function of the pulmonic and tricuspid valves may be assessed.

In a catheterization of the left side of the heart, the catheter is inserted into an artery and threaded against the flow of blood into the coronary arteries or the LV. The femoral vein and artery are the preferred insertion sites. The function of the coronary arteries and the aortic and mitral valves may be assessed. Blood samples may be drawn, and pressures in the various structures are measured.

Complications of cardiac catheterization include bleeding, hematoma formation, infection, and embolus or thrombus formation. Nursing care before and after the procedure is very important.

ELECTROPHYSIOLOGY STUDY

The electrophysiology study (EPS) is used to record the heart's electrical activity from within the heart using catheters with multiple electrodes inserted through the femoral vein into the right side of the heart. The electrodes record the electrical activity of the heart's conduction system. In addition, the electrodes can be used to stimulate dysrhythmias that will help locate the source of the patient's dysrhythmia.

LABORATORY TESTS

Arterial Blood Gases

Arterial blood gases are analyzed to determine the body's ability to maintain the acid-base balance. Acidity or alkalinity is determined by pH. If the serum pH is less than 7.35, the blood is acidic; greater than 7.45 indicates alkalinity. Carbonic acid dissociates into carbon dioxide and water. The lungs regulate carbon dioxide. The partial pressure of carbon dioxide in the blood is abbreviated Pco_2. A Pco_2 greater than 45 with an acidic pH is a respiratory acidosis and indicates that the body is unable to excrete the excess carbon dioxide through the lungs. With a pH in excess of 7.45 and a Pco_2 of less than 35, a respiratory alkalosis is present.

The kidneys regulate bicarbonate (HCO_3^-) through excretion and retention. The HCO_3^- (or base excess—a combination of all serum bases) is assessed to determine metabolic causes of imbalance. If the pH is less than 7.35 and the HCO_3^- is less than 22, the body is in metabolic acidosis. With a pH greater than 7.45 and an HCO_3^- greater than 26, the interpretation is metabolic alkalosis (Table 35-3).

Pulse Oximetry

Pulse oximetry, though not a laboratory test, noninvasively measures arterial oxygen saturation. Light is passed through a pulsating artery and interpreted mechanically to determine the oxygen saturation. The transdermal clip or patch may be applied to a digit (finger or toe), the ear, or the nose (Fig. 35-7).

A **B**

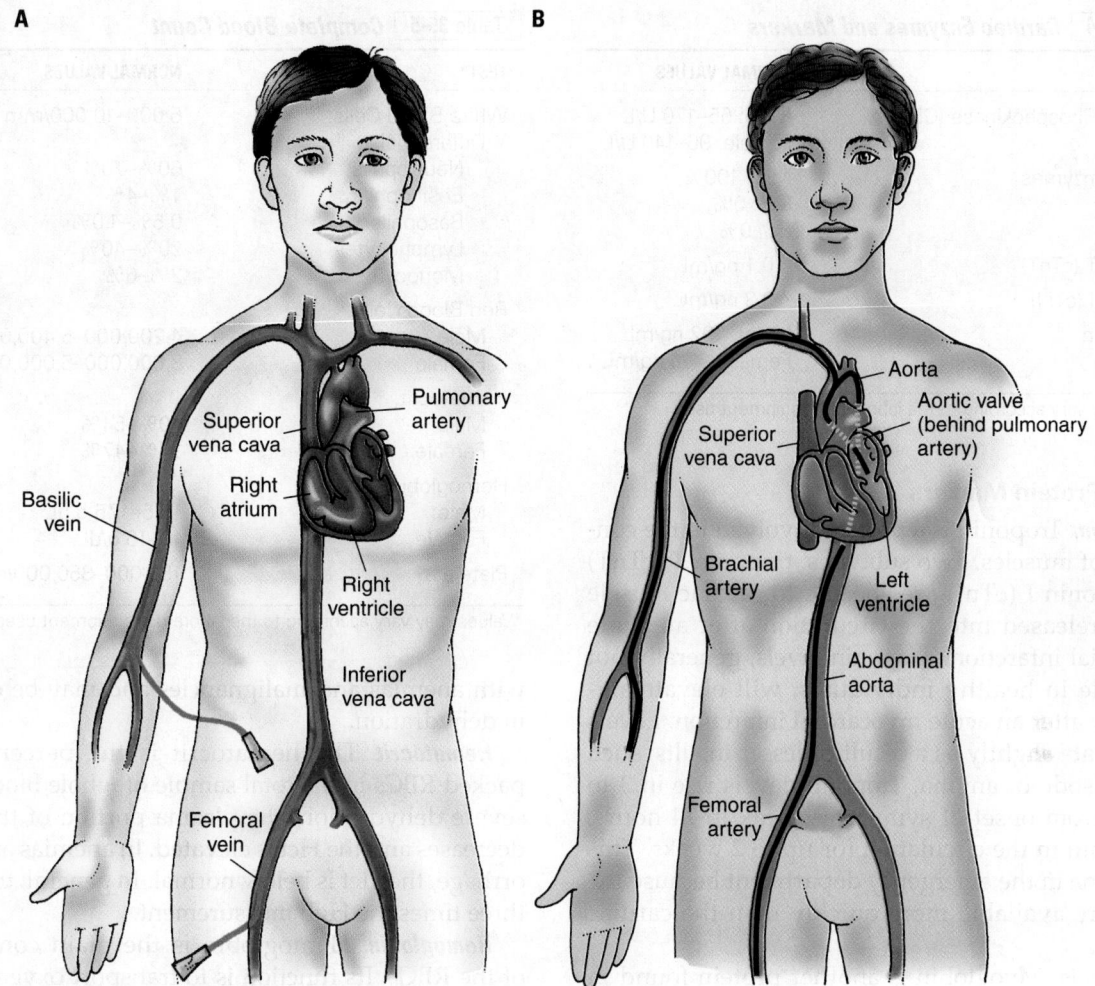

FIGURE **35-6** Right-sided (**A**) and left-sided (**B**) heart catheterization.

Table 35-3 | *Interpreting Arterial Blood Gases*

CONDITION	pH	Pco₂	HCO₃⁻
Normal range	7.35–7.45	35–45	22–26
Respiratory acidosis	↓	↑	Normal
Respiratory alkalosis	↑	↓	Normal
Metabolic acidosis	↓	Normal	↓
Metabolic alkalosis	↑	Normal	↑

↑, Elevated; ↓, decreased. If the arrows are in the same direction, a metabolic problem exists. If arrows are in opposite directions, a respiratory problem exists.

Cardiac Enzymes

Cardiac enzymes are released when heart cells die as a result of damage. These enzymes are measured in the serum, and their values rise as indicators of damage to the heart cells. Table 35-4 lists normal cardiac enzyme levels.

Creatine Phosphokinase. The creatine phosphokinase enzyme is found in high concentration in three tissues: the brain, the heart, and the skeletal muscle. The type of creatine phosphokinase (CPK) specific to heart tissue is CPK-MB. Elevation of the CPK-MB

FIGURE **35-7** Pulse oximeter. **A,** Ear probe. **B,** Clip on finger.

level indicates damage to the myocardial cells. The CPK-MB can be expected to rise 4 to 6 hours after an AMI, peak in 12 to 24 hours at more than 6 times the normal value, and return to normal within 2 to 3 days if no new damage occurs. Serial trends should be observed. The nurse can plot these trends. Musculoskeletal injuries (especially fractures and surgery) and recent excessive athletic activity can also elevate the total CPK level.

Table 35-4	*Cardiac Enzymes and Markers*
TEST*	**NORMAL VALUES**
Creatine Phosphokinase (CPK)	Male: 55–170 U/L Female: 96–140 U/L
CPK Isoenzymes	MM: 100% MB: 0% BB: 0%
Troponin T (cTnT)	<0.1 ng/mL
Troponin I (cTnI)	<0.3 ng/mL
Myoglobin	Male: <92 ng/mL Female: <76 ng/mL

*Values may vary according to the laboratory equipment used.

Cardiac Protein Markers

Troponin. Troponin is a protein involved in the contraction of muscles. Two subtypes, troponin T (cTnT) and troponin I (cTnI) are specific to cardiac muscle and are released into the circulation after an acute myocardial infarction. Troponin levels, generally not detectable in healthy individuals, will elevate significantly after an acute myocardial infarction. Levels may elevate slightly as a result of lesser insults, such as an episode of angina. Troponin levels rise in 3 to 6 hours from onset of symptoms, peak in 24 hours, and remain in the circulation for up to 2 weeks. This test is done in the emergency department because the results are available more quickly than the cardiac enzymes.

Myoglobin. Myoglobin is another protein found in cardiac and skeletal muscle that is released into the circulation very quickly after myocardial infarction. Myoglobin levels increase in 1 to 4 hours after symptoms. Because it is found also in skeletal muscle, myoglobin levels may be elevated by such things as strenuous exercise, renal failure, and neuromuscular diseases. This makes interpreting myoglobin levels difficult in some circumstances.

Complete Blood Count

The complete blood count is a basic screening test. Included in this test are the white blood cell (WBC) count, the red blood cell (RBC) count, the hemoglobin (Hgb) and hematocrit (Hct) measurements, the RBC indices, and, in some laboratories, the platelet count. Components of the complete blood count are presented in Table 35-5.

White Blood Cell Count. The WBC count indicates the body's ability to defend itself against infection and inflammation. The WBC level usually is elevated with inflammatory processes such as AMI and bacterial infections, but it may be below normal with viral infections and bone marrow depression.

Red Blood Cell Count. The RBC count is assessed to determine the ability of the blood to carry oxygen from the lungs to the tissues and carbon dioxide from the tissues to the lungs. The RBC level may be below normal

Table 35-5	*Complete Blood Count*
TEST*	**NORMAL VALUES**
White Blood Cells: Differential:	5,000–10,000/mm^3
Neutrophils	60%–70%
Eosinophils	1%–4%
Basophils	0.5%–1.0%
Lymphocytes	20%–40%
Monocytes	2%–6%
Red Blood Cells: Male Female	 4,200,000–5,400,000/mm^3 3,600,000–5,000,000/mm^3
Hematocrit: Male Female	 40%–54% 37%–47%
Hemoglobin: Male Female	 13.5–17.5 g/dL 12–16 g/dL
Platelets	150,000–350,000/mm^3

*Values may vary according to the laboratory equipment used.

with anemias and malignancies and may be elevated in dehydration.

Hematocrit. The hematocrit is the percentage of packed RBCs in the total sample of whole blood. With severe dehydration, the plasma portion of the blood decreases and the Hct is elevated. In anemias and hemorrhage, the Hct is below normal. In general, the Hct is three times the Hgb measurement.

Hemoglobin. Hemoglobin is the main component of the RBCs. Its function is to transport oxygen to the cells. The Hgb measurement may be below normal in anemias and hemorrhage. It is elevated in dehydration, chronic obstructive pulmonary disease (COPD), and CHF. An Hgb of less than 5 g/dL leads to heart failure and death if not corrected.

Platelet (Thrombocyte) Count. The platelets (thrombocytes) are the smallest of the formed elements in the blood. They are necessary for coagulation. The platelet count is below normal with anemias, bone marrow depression, and bleeding. The count may be increased in acute infections and some heart diseases. A count of less than 20,000 may result in spontaneous bleeding.

Lipid Profile

A lipid profile is a battery of tests that measure the most common serum lipids: cholesterol, triglycerides, and lipoproteins.

Cholesterol is a blood lipid produced by the liver. It is used to form bile salts for the digestion of fat and for the production of adrenal, ovarian, and testicular hormones. The normal adult serum cholesterol level is less than 200 mg/dL. Elevated cholesterol levels (hypercholesterolemia) are associated with increased risk of CAD, hypertension, and AMI. The cholesterol accumulates in the arterial lumen and in time results in decreased blood flow and occlusion.

Low HDL Levels

Low HDL levels can be raised by being physically active at least 30 minutes every day, by not smoking, and by losing weight (or maintaining a healthy weight).

Several forms of cholesterol are identified; however, the high-density lipoproteins (HDLs) and the low-density lipoproteins (LDLs) are the two that most closely correlate with coronary artery disease. The HDLs are desirable because they promote the excretion of cholesterol; therefore higher levels of HDLs are encouraged. On the other hand, elevated LDL levels are associated with a higher risk of CAD; therefore lower LDL levels are encouraged. A good way to remember the difference is that HDLs are healthy and LDLs are lethal. Currently, the recommendations are for HDL levels greater than 40 mg/dL and for LDL levels less than 100 mg/dL (American Heart Association, 2007). See the Health Promotion Considerations box above for advice about increasing HDL levels.

Triglycerides are a major contributor to CAD. They are produced in the liver. Triglyceride levels increase when LDL levels increase. The normal triglyceride level is less than 150 mg/dL.

B-type Natriuretic Peptide

B-type natriuretic peptide (BNP) is a cardiac hormone released when there is ventricular dilation and stretch (such as occurs in heart failure). Less than 100 pg/mL is considered a normal BNP level, and elevated levels relate closely to the severity of heart failure (e.g., the higher the levels, the more severe the failure). In addition, BNP levels can be monitored to assess the effectiveness of treatment.

C-reactive Protein

C-reactive protein (CRP) is an acute-phase protein and a marker for systemic inflammation. Elevated levels of CRP are present in patients with acute coronary syndromes. CRP is being studied to determine its usefulness in predicting recurrent and new cardiovascular events.

COMMON THERAPEUTIC MEASURES

DRUG THERAPY

Commonly used cardiac drugs are cardiac glycosides, antianginals, antidysrhythmics, and miscellaneous and emergency drugs. Examples of these drugs, their actions and adverse effects, and associated nursing considerations are provided in the Drug Therapy table on pp. 642 to 646.

Cardiac Glycosides

The cardiac glycosides are also called *cardiotonics* or *digitalis glycosides*. Examples are digoxin (Lanoxin) and digitoxin. These drugs have several important pharmacologic actions on the heart. They slow the heart rate (negative chronotropic effect) and increase the force of myocardial contraction (positive inotropic effect), causing increased stroke volume and cardiac output. Cardiac glycosides are widely used in the treatment of heart failure (HF). They are also used to treat some cardiac dysrhythmias.

When rapid effects are needed, a patient can be given a loading dose (called a *digitalizing dose*) of cardiac glycosides. Once therapeutic blood levels are obtained, a maintenance dose is prescribed to maintain the therapeutic effects. These drugs have high potential for toxicity and require close monitoring. Common practice is to count the apical pulse before giving each dose. If the rate is below 60 bpm in adults, withhold the dose and contact the physician. Because patients are often on cardiac glycosides for long-term therapy, they must be taught to monitor their own pulse and to report symptoms of toxicity (anorexia, nausea, visual disturbances). Other specific nursing considerations are presented in the Drug Therapy table on p. 642.

Antianginals

Drugs used to treat angina (chest pain related to myocardial ischemia) include nitrates, beta-adrenergic blockers, and calcium channel blockers. Nitrates are used to treat actual anginal episodes and to prevent angina. Beta-adrenergic blockers and calcium channel blockers are used in the long-term management of angina. Examples of each classification and nursing considerations are presented in the Drug Therapy table on pp. 642 and 643.

Antidysrhythmics

Drugs used to treat abnormal cardiac rhythms are called *antidysrhythmics* or *antiarrhythmics*. There are four main classes of antidysrhythmics, each with various actions. In general, they work by slowing the rate of impulse conduction, depressing automaticity, or increasing resistance to premature stimulation. All antidysrhythmics have the potential to cause additional dysrhythmias. Specific drugs and nursing considerations are presented in the Drug Therapy table on pp. 644 and 645.

Angiotensin-Converting Enzyme Inhibitors

Angiotensin-converting enzyme (ACE) inhibitors (ACEI) work against the renin-angiotensin-aldosterone system to dilate arteries and decrease the resistance to blood flow in the arteries (reduced afterload). In addition, less fluid is retained because aldosterone release is blocked. ACE inhibitors are prescribed for patients with heart failure, some cases of hypertension, and in some cases after myocardial infarction Examples of these medications are captopril (Capoten), enalapril (Vasotec), and quinapril (Accupril). Information about

Text continued on p. 647.

| DRUG THERAPY | *Cardiovascular Drugs* |

DRUG	USE/ACTION	NURSING INTERVENTIONS
CARDIAC GLYCOSIDES Digoxin (Lanoxin)	Delays impulse conduction through AV node to slow heart rate (negative chronotropic effect). Increases strength or force of myocardial contraction (positive inotropic effect). Increases stroke volume and CO. Used for HF, atrial fibrillation and flutter, and paroxysmal atrial tachycardia.	Obtain baseline vital signs, ECG, and electrolytes before administering first dose. Assess apical pulse for 1 min; hold and notify physician if <60. Cannot be administered intramuscularly. Monitor K^+ levels; administer K^+ supplements as ordered. Decreased renal function may delay excretion and lead to toxicity. Toxic effects may be indicated by dysrhythmias, pulse <60, anorexia, nausea, syncope, visual disturbances, and abdominal pain. Therapeutic level: 0.8–2.0 ng/mL. Toxic level: >2.0 ng/mL. Teach the patient: • Take radial pulse for 1 min at the same time each day.
ANTIANGINALS Nitroglycerin Available as sublingual tablets, ointment, transdermal patch, buccal tablets, mist, and sustained-release oral tablets	Vasodilator (arteries and veins). Relaxes all smooth muscles, especially vascular smooth muscle. Decreases preload, afterload, BP, CO, and systemic vascular resistance. Used to prevent and treat angina.	Assess BP and pulse before administration. Apply ointment in uniform layer on paper provided; apply to nonhairy skin (chest, back, upper arm); do not touch (causes headache); rotate sites. IV drug is delivered in glass containers with special tubing; use an infusion pump; monitor closely. Teach the patient: • Sit or lie down at onset of chest pain. • Place tablet under tongue; tablet causes tingling sensation if effective (older adults may not detect this). • Repeat q 5 min for total of three doses; if chest pains not relieved, have someone else drive to emergency department. • Keep tablets in containers in which supplied; drug decomposes on exposure to light and air. • Headache decreases with tolerance. • Drug may be taken before activities likely to cause angina (exercise, sex).
Isosorbide dinitrate (Isordil)	Vasodilator that works by relaxing smooth muscles. Decreases preload, afterload, left ventricular end-diastolic pressure, and myocardial oxygen consumption. Used for acute angina and maintenance of chronic angina.	Assess vital signs before administration. Teach the patient: • Take 1-2 hr before meals and at bedtime. • Sit when taking the sublingual or chewable medications. • Change positions slowly to avoid orthostatic hypotension. • Avoid hot showers, tubs, saunas. • Headache decreases over time. • Alcohol potentiates hypotension. • If three sublingual or chewable doses do not relieve angina, go to the emergency department.
Nadolol (Corgard) Dosage increased gradually until optimal response is achieved	Beta-adrenergic blocker. Decreases HR and CO at rest and with exercise. Used in hypertension and prophylactically for chronic stable angina. Decreases conduction velocity through the AV node.	Assess BP and apical pulse before administration. Monitor weight (fluid retention with HF). Teach the patient: • Take radial pulse for 1 min. • Hold medication and notify physician if HR <60. • Weigh daily; report a gain of 3-4 lb. • Do not discontinue this drug abruptly; taper off over 1-2 weeks.

Propranolol (Inderal)	Nonselective beta-adrenergic blocker. Decreases HR, myocardial irritability, and contractility. Decreases BP in hypertension. Decreases CO. Used in dysrhythmia, myocardial infarction, hypertension, migraines, and chronic stable angina.	Monitor vital signs. May be administered with diuretic to decrease Na^+ and water retention. May cause bronchial constriction. Use with caution in all patients with obstructive lung disease. Auscultate lungs for crackles and heart for S_3 and S_4. Monitor weight daily; check for peripheral edema. Monitor blood glucose with diabetes. Teach the patient: • Do not discontinue this drug abruptly; taper over 2 weeks. • Take at the same time(s) each day. • While on this drug, use alcohol only in moderation; no smoking; decrease sodium intake. • There is not the normal increase in heart rate with exercise and stress; increase activity slowly. • Weigh daily; check for edema.
Atenolol (Tenormin) and metoprolol tartrate (Lopressor)	Cardioselective beta-adrenergic blockers used to treat angina and hypertension. Reduce heart rate, BP, cardiac output, and myocardial oxygen consumption.	Monitor vital signs. Continuous ECG monitoring with IV administration. Take apical pulse before each dose. Teach the patient: • Take with or after meals. • Do not discontinue abruptly. • Take pulse and report to physician if below 60 • Avoid alcohol and smoking. • Avoid over-the-counter cold remedies.
Diltiazem hydrochloride (Cardizem)	Calcium channel blocker. Dilates coronary arteries; increases availability of oxygen to the myocardium. Decreases total PVR, afterload, and systolic blood pressure. Slightly decreases myocardial contractility. Prolongs AV node refractory period. Used in chronic stable angina, coronary artery spasm, and hypertension.	Dosage may need to be reduced in older adult patients. Teach the patient: • Take radial pulse for 1 min. • Limit caffeine intake. • Change positions with caution to prevent postural hypotension. • Take before meals and at bedtime.
Nifedipine (Procardia)	Calcium channel blocker. Decreases myocardial oxygen consumption. Dilates coronary arteries. Decreases PVR. Increases CO. Used for angina, mild to moderate hypertension, vascular headaches, coronary artery spasms.	Monitor BP during titration (during dosage adjustment). Teach the patient: • Smoking is contraindicated (nicotine constricts coronary arteries). • Do not discontinue this drug abruptly. • Limit caffeine intake.
Verapamil hydrochloride (Calan, Isoptin)	Calcium channel blocker. Slows AV conduction. Dilates peripheral and coronary arteries. Increases oxygen supply to myocardium. Used to treat supraventricular tachycardias, atrial fibrillation and flutter, angina, hypertension, and vascular headaches.	Assess baseline vital signs, hepatic and renal function. Assess for signs of CHF (pulmonary or peripheral edema). Monitor pulse and BP before each dose. Administer IV bolus more slowly to older adults. Teach the patient: • Take radial pulse for 1 min; report irregular or slow pulse. • No caffeine (opposes calcium channel–blocking effect). • Change position slowly until tolerance develops. • Exercise with caution; drug's effects may give false impression of tolerance.

AV, Atrioventricular; *BP*, blood pressure; *CBC*, complete blood count; *CHF*, congestive heart failure; *CO*, cardiac output; *ECG*, electrocardiogram; *HDL*, high-density lipoprotein; *HF*, heart failure; *HR*, heart rate; *IV*, intravenous; *LDL*, low-density lipoprotein; *MAP*, mean arterial pressure; *NSAID*, nonsteroidal anti-inflammatory drug; *OTC*, over-the-counter; *PVC*, premature ventricular contraction; *PVR*, peripheral vascular resistance; *SVR*, systemic vascular resistance; *VLDL*, very-low-density lipoprotein.

Continued

DRUG THERAPY   *Cardiovascular Drugs—cont'd*

DRUG	USE/ACTION	NURSING INTERVENTIONS
ANTIDYSRHYTHMICS		
Amiodarone hydrochloride (Cordarone)	Antidysrhythmic. Increases action potential duration and effective refractory period. Increases CO. Decreases PVR, coronary artery resistance, and HR. Used for severe tachycardia and supraventricular tachycardias.	Continuously monitor ECG for a decrease in dysrhythmia. Observe for thyroid dysfunction (each 200-mg tablet contains 75 mg of iodine) and neurologic effects (tremors, ataxia, headache, insomnia). Teach the patient: • Take radial pulse daily. • Photosensitivity and photophobia may occur. • Pharmacologic action may have a delayed onset of 5 days to 3 mo. • Skin discolorations fade with time.
Bretylium tosylate (Bretylol)	Adrenergic blocker. Suppresses ventricular fibrillation and ventricular tachycardia. Used for short-time treatment of life-threatening ventricular tachycardias in patients who do not respond to conventional therapy, ventricular fibrillation, and cardioversion.	Monitor vital signs, ECG. Have resuscitation equipment available. If nausea and vomiting occur, decrease the rate of infusion.
Disopyramide phosphate (Norpace)	Reduces the rate of spontaneous diastolic depolarization in pacemaker cells. Increases SVR. Decreases myocardial conductivity. Suppresses ectopic focal activity. Used to suppress and prevent recurrent PVCs and ventricular tachycardia.	Assess apical pulse before administration; hold if <60 or >120 and notify physician. Monitor BP. Monitor intake and output. Urinary retention and constipation may occur. Teach the patient: • Take radial pulse daily. • Weigh daily; observe for edema. • Change position slowly. • No alcohol (severely decreases BP). • Relieve dry mouth with sugarless gum or dry candy. • Avoid sunlight (photosensitivity).
Flecainide acetate (Tambocor)	Antidysrhythmic. Decreases conduction velocity. Increases ventricular refractory period. Used to treat PVCs, atrial tachycardia, and other dysrhythmias not responsive to other antidysrhythmics.	Monitor ECG.
Lidocaine (Xylocaine)	Increases the electrical stimulation threshold of the ventricular conduction system. Used for rapid control of ventricular dysrhythmias during myocardial infarction, cardiac surgery, cardiac catheterization, and digitalis intoxication.	Administer with an infusion pump. Monitor BP and ECG. May precipitate malignant hyperthermia (tachycardia, tachypnea, elevated temperature). Assess breath sounds for crackles.
Mexiletine hydrochloride (Mexitil)	Antidysrhythmic structurally similar to lidocaine. Used to suppress symptomatic ventricular dysrhythmias.	Administer with food or antacids. Monitor ECG. Mix IV solution immediately before administration.
Phenytoin sodium (Dilantin)	Used to treat paroxysmal atrial tachycardia and ventricular dysrhythmias.	May need lower dosage in older adults. Administer only in normal saline (drug crystallizes in dextrose). Do not exceed 50 mg/min IV. Teach the patient: • Alcohol potentiates the action and therefore may precipitate toxicity.
Propranolol (Inderal)	See description under Antianginals.	
Quinidine	Antidysrhythmic. Depresses myocardial excitability, contractility, automaticity, and conduction velocity. Anticholinergic effects increase the ventricular rate. Relaxes muscles. Used for atrial and ventricular dysrhythmias.	If administered with digoxin, may produce toxicity or unpredictable dysrhythmias. Administer with meals to decrease gastric distress. Severe hypotension may occur with large doses. Monitor electrolytes; continuing diarrhea may indicate electrolyte imbalance.

Drug	Action	Nursing Considerations
Tocainide hydrochloride (Tonocard)	Antidysrhythmic. Primary analogue of lidocaine. Used for life-threatening ventricular dysrhythmias associated with prolonged QT interval.	Monitor ECG. Administer with food or antacids to decrease gastrointestinal side effects. Monitor CBC for blood dyscrasias (agranulocytosis, leukocytosis, neutropenia).
Verapamil (Calan, Isoptin)	See description under Antianginals.	

ANTIPLATELET AGENTS

Drug	Action	Nursing Considerations
Clopidogrel (Plavix)	Decreases platelet aggregation. Prolongs bleeding time. Used to prevent thromboembolic disorders such as stroke and MI.	Monitor bleeding time, CBC with differential, platelet count. Avoid OTC medications with aspirin or NSAIDs unless prescribed by physician. Teach the patient: • Report bleeding. • Keep appointments for blood work.
Ticlopidine (Ticlid)	Same as Plavix.	Monitor liver function studies, CBC, prothrombin time. Teach the patient: • Report bleeding. • Take with food. • Keep appointments for blood work.
Abciximab (ReoPro)	Inhibits platelet aggregation. Given IV to reduce ischemic complications with angioplasty or arthrectomy.	Used only in the hospital. Monitor vital signs, ECG, and level of consciousness. Assess hemoglobin, hematocrit, platelet count, and clotting factors frequently. Watch for bleeding. Protect from trauma.

LIPID-LOWERING AGENTS

Drug	Action	Nursing Considerations
Cholestyramine (Questran)	Prescribed when diet, exercise, and weight loss fail to bring cholesterol levels under control. Lowers LDL cholesterol. Increases HDL cholesterol.	Interferes with absorption of some other drugs, so check drug-drug interactions before giving. To get the best effect, teach patients: • Continue diet and exercise. • Increase fluid intake to counter constipating effects.
Gemfibrozil (Lopid)	Decreases synthesis and secretion of VLDL by liver. Decreases triglyceride levels.	For best effect, teach patient: • Continue diet and exercise. • Take with meals.
Nicotinic acid (niacin)	Decreases synthesis/secretion of VLDL and LDL by liver. Increases HDL.	For best effect, teach patient: • Continue diet and exercise. • Take with meals to decrease GI side effects.
Pravastatin (Pravachol) Simvastatin (Zocor) Lovastatin (Mevacor) Atorvastatin (Lipitor)	Increases rate of removal of LDL from plasma. Decreases synthesis of LDL.	Monitor liver function tests. For best effect, teach patient: • Continue diet and exercise. • Report muscle tenderness. • Take as single dose in the evening. • Have routine eye examinations.

AV, Atrioventricular; BP, blood pressure; CBC, complete blood count; CHF, congestive heart failure; CO, cardiac output; ECG, electrocardiogram; HDL, high-density lipoprotein; HF, heart failure; HR, heart rate; IV, intravenous; LDL, low-density lipoprotein; MAP, mean arterial pressure; NSAID, nonsteroidal anti-inflammatory drug; OTC, over-the-counter; PVC, premature ventricular contraction; PVR, peripheral vascular resistance; SVR, systemic vascular resistance; VLDL, very-low-density lipoprotein.

Continued

DRUG THERAPY Cardiovascular Drugs—cont'd

DRUG	USE/ACTION	NURSING INTERVENTIONS
MISCELLANEOUS AND EMERGENCY DRUGS		
Amrinone lactate (Inocor)	Inotropic agent. Vasodilator. Increases myocardial contractions without increasing HR. Increases blood flow through collateral coronary vessels. Increases stroke volume and CO. Decreases preload and afterload. Used to treat HF refractory to other medications.	Administer with an infusion pump. Titrate to target BP. Monitor intake and output. Avoid extravasation. Discard solution 24 hr after preparation.
Atropine sulfate	Vagal blocker. Increases HR and CO in heart blocks and severe bradycardia. Used in symptomatic bradycardia and bradydysrhythmias.	Assess HR and rhythm and BP.
Calcium chloride	Necessary for cardiac rhythm, tone, and contraction. Increases muscle tone and force of contraction. Used in cardiac resuscitation and in cardiac irregularities associated with hyperkalemia.	Monitor ECG, BP, and arterial blood gases. Avoid extravasation; causes necrosis. Alkalosis decreases the absorption of calcium. Acidosis increases the absorption of calcium.
Dobutamine (Dobutrex)	Synthetic catecholamine. Beta-adrenergic agonist. Increases CO with less increase in HR and BP than other catecholamines. Used in CHF and after cardiac surgery to increase myocardial contractility, stroke volume, and CO.	Continuous monitoring of ECG, cardiac parameters, and urinary output; titrate to HR and BP. Urinary output should increase with improved CO and renal function. Often used with nitroprusside or dopamine for additive effects. Causes less increase in HR, PVR, and dysrhythmias than dopamine. At a rate <7 mcg/kg/min, expect increased myocardial contraction, CO, and renal blood flow. At a rate of >7 mcg/kg/min, expect peripheral vasoconstriction and increased MAP.
Dopamine hydrochloride (Intropin)	Neurotransmitter, precursor to norepinephrine. Increases CO and BP. Improves renal blood flow and therefore urine output with lower doses. Used for hemodynamic support in shock.	Avoid extravasation; causes necrosis. Monitor vital signs, ECG, urine output, and extremity color. Titrate to target BP; use an infusion pump. Peripheral vasoconstriction is noted with cold upper and lower extremities.
Epinephrine hydrochloride (Adrenalin chloride)	Catecholamine. Strengthens myocardial contraction; increases BP, HR, and CO. Dilates bronchial tree. Used in anaphylactic shock and to restore cardiac rhythm in cardiac arrest.	Monitor vital signs and ECG continuously. Avoid extravasation; causes sloughing. Titrate to cardiac response. Caution: available in several concentrations (1:100, 1:1000, 1:10,000); be sure to check for prescribed solution. May be administered by endotracheal tube because drug is rapidly absorbed from the lungs.
Isoproterenol hydrochloride (Isuprel)	Cardiac stimulant (positive inotropic and chronotropic effects). Bronchodilator. Peripheral vasodilator. Increases HR and contractility. Decreases PVR and diastolic BP; resulting in increased CO and systolic BP, decreased MAP, and increased myocardial oxygen consumption. Used as a cardiac stimulant in cardiac arrest, cardiogenic shock, ventricular dysrhythmias, and heart block.	Continuously monitor ECG. Monitor vital signs, urine output, and peripheral blood flow. Titrate to desired HR, BP, and urine output. Avoid extravasation.
Sodium nitroprusside (Nipride)	Vasodilator. Decreases preload and afterload. Used in hypertensive crises.	Light-sensitive preparation; wrap in aluminum foil. Administer with an infusion pump. Titrate to maintain CO. Continuously monitor BP. Discard solution 4 hr after preparation. Assess thiocyanate levels daily for patients on long-term therapy.
Norepinephrine (Levophed)	Catecholamine. Vasoconstrictor. Cardiac stimulant: increased BP, myocardial oxygen, and coronary artery blood flow. Used in acute hypertensive states, myocardial infarction, and cardiac arrest.	Mix only with dextrose in water or dextrose in saline. Administer with an infusion pump. Report decreased urine output immediately. Continuously monitor and titrate to desired BP. Monitor peripheral blood flow. Avoid extravasation.
Sodium bicarbonate	Systemic alkalinizer. Used to correct metabolic acidosis in cardiac arrest.	Do not infuse with calcium. Monitor arterial blood gases. Avoid extravasation; causes severe tissue damage.
Milrinone (Primacor)	Inotropic agent. Increases myocardial contractility and cardiac output. Vasodilation decreases preload and afterload. Used to treat CHF that does not respond to usual therapy.	Monitor vital signs, intake and output, and daily weight during therapy. Monitor ECG continuously. Give potassium as ordered for hypokalemia.

AV, Atrioventricular; *BP,* blood pressure; *CBC,* complete blood count; *CHF,* congestive heart failure; *CO,* cardiac output; *ECG,* electrocardiogram; *HDL,* high-density lipoprotein; *HF,* heart failure; *HR,* heart rate; *IV,* intravenous; *LDL,* low-density lipoprotein; *MAP,* mean arterial pressure; *NSAID,* nonsteroidal anti-inflammatory drug; *OTC,* over-the-counter; *PVC,* premature ventricular contraction; *PVR,* peripheral vascular resistance; *SVR,* systemic vascular resistance; *VLDL,* very-low-density lipoprotein.

these medications is presented in the Drug Therapy table on p. 721.

Diuretics

Diuretics are often prescribed for cardiac conditions. Many patients with heart problems have fluid retention that is treated with diuretics. The most frequently used diuretics are the loop diuretics such as furosemide (Lasix), the thiazide diuretics such as hydrochlorothiazide (Esidrix, HCTZ) and the potassium-sparing diuretics such as spironolactone (Aldactone). Information about these and other diuretics is presented in the Drug Therapy table on p. 850.

Anticoagulants

Anticoagulants are used to prevent clot formation. Heparin, low-molecular-weight heparin (LMWH), and warfarin are the most commonly used preventive anticoagulants.

Heparin

Heparin interferes with factor III in the clotting process. It is administered by continuous intravenous drip or subcutaneously. When a patient has a clotting episode, a heparin bolus is administered and a continuous infusion is started. The infusion rate is set to deliver a prescribed number of heparin units per hour. The physician adjusts the heparin dosage based on the activated partial thromboplastin time (aPTT). When the aPTT has stabilized (generally at 1.5 to 2.0 times the control level), the drug can be changed to the subcutaneous route. Because heparin cannot be administered orally, the patient must remain hospitalized during its administration. Heparin is recommended for use with acute coronary syndrome (ACS), during percutaneous coronary interventions (PCI) and surgical revascularization, and in conjunction with fibrinolytic therapy (Ante, 2004; Deglin & Vallerand, 2005).

Low-Molecular-Weight Heparin. Low-molecular-weight heparins (LMWHs), such as enoxaparin (Lovenox), are fragments derived from heparin that work by blocking the formation of thrombin and preventing the development of a clot. The advantages of using LMWHs are that the anticoagulant effect is more predictable, they are administered subcutaneously once or twice a day, and they do not require such close monitoring of aPTT. LMWHs are recommended for patients with deep vein thrombosis, with unstable angina, and in some cases of acute myocardial infarction (before a thrombus occludes the coronary vessel) (Ante, 2004; Deglin & Vallerand, 2005).

Warfarin

The anticoagulant that may be administered orally, warfarin (Coumadin), is started as soon as possible. The warfarin dosage is regulated by the prothrombin time and international normalized ratio (INR). The prothrombin time is kept in a therapeutic range of 1.5 to 2.0 times the normal level. The INR may be kept at 2.0 to 4.5. Patients who have had artificial valve replacements must remain on anticoagulant therapy for life.

All patients on anticoagulants must be monitored closely for any signs of bleeding. Also, patients should be taught how to reduce the risk of bleeding, such as to use an electric razor and a soft-bristle toothbrush.

Pharmacology Capsule

Heparin dosage is adjusted based on the patient's activated partial thromboplastin time (aPTT). Warfarin dosage is adjusted based on the patient's prothrombin time (PT) and international normalized ratio (INR).

Antiplatelet Agents

Antiplatelet therapy is often used after an AMI to prevent additional myocardial infarction and strokes. The dosage of aspirin as an antiplatelet agent in stroke prevention is under investigation. Some studies have shown that one baby aspirin (81 mg) a day is sufficient, and other studies indicate that an even smaller dosage may produce a therapeutic effect. Dipyridamole (Persantine), ticlopidine (Ticlid), and clopidogrel (Plavix) also exhibit antiplatelet effects and may be prescribed for patients who are unable to tolerate aspirin.

Glycoprotein (GP) IIb/IIIa inhibitors block the platelet receptor sites that bind with fibrinogen and lead to platelet aggregation. GP IIb/IIIa inhibitors such as abciximab (ReoPro) and eptifibatide (Integrilin) are used in combination with heparin and aspirin as part of the medical treatment for unstable angina and acute myocardial infarction. They are also being used in conjunction with fibrinolytic therapy and/or percutaneous coronary interventions after acute myocardial infarction.

Pharmacology Capsule

Anticoagulants and antiplatelet agents prevent formation of new clots, but fibrinolytic agents destroy clots that have already formed.

Fibrinolytic Agents

Whereas anticoagulants and antiplatelet agents prevent the continued formation of clots, the fibrinolytic agents (also called *thrombolytics*) act to destroy clots that have already formed. Streptokinase, Reteplase, and tissue plasminogen activator are examples of thrombolytics. They are best used as soon as there is evidence of clot formation. They are administered intravenously when certain criteria have been met. Administration is continued until there is evidence of reperfusion or until the maximum dosage has been given.

Information about anticoagulant, antiplatelet, and fibrinolytic agents is presented in the Drug Therapy tables on pp. 464 and 465 and pp. 697 and 698. Selected antiplatelet agents are also listed in the Drug Therapy table on p. 645.

Lipid-Lowering Agents

Lipid-lowering medications are frequently part of the overall treatment plan, along with diet and exercise, for many patients with heart disease. The goal of therapy is for the patient to have decreased serum triglyceride and LDL levels and an improved HDL level. Patients on this group of medications need to be encouraged to adhere to diet restrictions, exercise, and quit smoking. Serial laboratory tests (lipid profile and liver function) will be closely monitored. Selected lipid-lowering medications are included in the Drug Therapy table on p. 645.

Analgesics

The patient who has an AMI experiences severe chest pain. The first medication administered to a patient with chest pain is nitroglycerin, which is a vasodilator. When this drug does not relieve the pain, morphine is the preferred analgesic. Morphine relieves pain, reduces anxiety, and reduces the workload of the heart by trapping some of the venous blood in the periphery of the body. An alternative to morphine is meperidine hydrochloride (Demerol). Meperidine is less effective in relieving anxiety and cardiac workload than morphine. Morphine and meperidine are most effective when administered intravenously.

DIET THERAPY

Reduction of body weight lessens the workload on the heart. A low-fat, high-fiber diet usually is recommended for cardiac patients. Patients would be encouraged to eat a well-balanced diet that includes an emphasis on fruits, vegetables, grains, and proteins low in fat (fish, legumes, poultry and lean meats). Cholesterol intake should be limited to 200 mg/day for individuals with heart disease or at high risk for heart disease. It is also recommended that foods with *trans* fatty acids be limited (American Heart Association, 2007). An exercise program may help the patient achieve optimal weight.

Sodium

If fluid retention accompanies the cardiac problem, the physician may order sodium restriction. A diet containing sodium 2 g/day is most often prescribed. Restrictions greater than this are difficult to achieve, and studies have shown that patients quickly become noncompliant with the dietary regimen. Salt substitutes are available.

Potassium

Patients taking potassium-wasting diuretics (e.g., furosemide, hydrochlorothiazide) need to include adequate

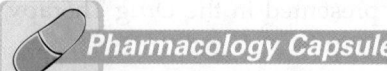

Pharmacology Capsule

Potassium-wasting diuretics such as furosemide and hydrochlorothiazide may cause hypokalemia, which can lead to dangerous dysrhythmias.

Consider the Alternative

Some people use garlic to reduce plasma lipids and lower blood pressure. The best garlic preparation is an enteric-coated dried preparation that contains adequate allicin and allinase—the "active ingredients" in the preparation. Most of the allicin and allinase are destroyed when fresh garlic is cooked or eaten raw. Garlic irritates the GI tract and increases the effects of anticoagulants and insulin.

potassium in the diet to counteract the depletion. Patients taking large doses of potassium-wasting diuretics need to have potassium supplements prescribed.

OXYGEN THERAPY

The myocardium needs an adequate blood supply to function properly. Any patient complaining of chest pain unrelieved by nitroglycerin should have supplemental oxygen administered. A nasal cannula or facemask should be applied and set to deliver the prescribed liter flow, and the patient's response to this therapy should be monitored.

PACEMAKERS

Pacemakers were first introduced in 1958. Their purpose is to restore regular rhythm and to improve cardiac output and tissue perfusion. Pacemakers may be temporary or permanent. Methods for temporary pacing are transcutaneous, transvenous, or epicardial. Transcutaneous pacemakers deliver impulses through the skin from externally placed electrode pads. A transvenous pacemaker has a pacing electrode that is threaded through a vein into the right side of the heart. Epicardial pacing wires are placed into the epicardial wall of the heart during cardiac surgery and the wires are brought through the chest wall. Temporary pacemakers all require an external pulse generator to provide the electrical energy needed to stimulate depolarization. A permanent pacemaker is surgically place subcutaneously in the wall of the chest, with the electrical lead placed into the heart through a vein. Impulses are conducted from the power source (external pulse generator or implanted pacemaker) to the heart to stimulate contraction of the myocardium.

Pacemakers can be used to stimulate the atrium or ventricle (called *single-chamber pacing*), or they can be used to stimulate both chambers (called *dual-chamber pacing*). Dual-chamber pacing produces conduction and contraction that is near normal.

Table 35-6 | Revised NASPE/BPEG Generic Code for Antibradycardia Pacing*

I	II	III	IV	V
Chamber(s) Paced	**Chamber(s) Sensed**	**Response to Sensing**	**Rate Modulation**	**Multisite Pacing**
O = None	O = None	O = None	O = None	O = None
A = Atrium	A = Atrium	T = Triggered	R = Rate modulation	A = Atrium
V = Ventricle	V = Ventricle	I = Inhibited		V = Ventricle
D = Dual (A+V)	D = Dual (A+V)	D = Dual		D = Dual (A+V)
S = Single (A or V)†	S = Single (A or V)†	(T+I)		

From Bernstein, A.D., Daubert, J.C., Fletcher, R.D., Hayes, D.L., Luderitz, B., Reynolds, D.W., Schoenfeld, M.H., & Sutton R. (2002). The revised NASPE/BPEG generic code for antibradycardia, adaptive-rate, and multisite pacing. *Pacing and Clinical Electrophysiology, 25*(2), 261.
*This code differs from the 1987 version that listed programmability and antitachycardia functions. These functions are described in Bernstein, A.D., et al. (1993). NASPE policy statement: The NASPE/BPEG defibrillator code. *Pacing and Clinical Electrophysiology, 16*, 1776-1780.
†Manufacturer's designation only.

Table 35-7 | Pertinent Definitions Related to Pacemakers

Sensing	Ability of the pacemaker to detect intrinsic myocardial electrical activity The pacemaker either is inhibited from delivering a stimulus or initiates an electrical impulse, based on the programmed response
Pulse generation	Occurs when the pacemaker produces a programmed current for a set duration This energy travels through the transvenous lead wires to the myocardium—this is known as pacemaker firing and usually produces a line or spike on the ECG recording
Capture	Refers to the successful stimulation of the myocardium by the pacemaker impulse that results in depolarization Evidenced on the ECG by a pacemaker spike/stimulus followed by either an atrial or ventricular complex, depending on the chambers being paced
Failure of pulse generation	Pacemaker does not discharge a pacing stimulus at its programmed time to the myocardium Evidenced by the absence of a pacemaker spike on the ECG where expected
Sensing failure	Pacemaker has either detected extraneous signals that mimic intrinsic cardiac activity (oversensing) or did not accurately identify intrinsic activity (undersensing) Oversensing is recognized on the ECG by pauses where paced beats were expected and prolongation of the interval between paced beats Undersensing is recognized on the ECG by inappropriate pacemaker spikes relative to the intrinsic electrical activity (pacemaker spikes occurring within the P wave, QRS complex, or T wave) and shortened distances between paced beats
Failure to capture	Pacemaker has delivered a pacing stimulus that was unable to initiate depolarization of the myocardium and subsequent myocardial contraction Evidenced on the ECG by pacemaker spikes that are not followed by a P wave for atrial pacing or spikes not followed by a QRS complex for ventricular pacing

ECG, Electrocardiogram.

Pacemakers have multiple settings related to pacing and sensing. A coding system was developed in the 1970s and has undergone a number of revisions. The most recent revision is found in Table 35-6. A set of pertinent definitions related to pacemakers is found in Table 35-7.

Temporary Pacemakers
Temporary pacemakers can be used electively or for emergency situations. Elective uses include gaining control of very rapid supraventricular tachycardic rhythms, assessing the need for permanent pacing in patients with bradycardias, and following cardiac surgery.

Permanent Pacemakers
Permanent pacemakers are indicated in a number of patient situations in which conduction defects or dysrhythmias compromise the normal function of the heart. Several clinical conditions indicate the need for permanent pacing. A few of these conditions are the following: acquired atrioventricular (AV) block, sinus node dysfunction, chronic bifascicular or trifascicular block, symptomatic tachycardias, and carotid sinus syndrome. A permanent implantable pacemaker is inserted under local anesthesia. The batteries, usually lithium, have an 8- to 10-year expected life. Permanent pacemakers are inserted in the operating room, catheterization laboratory, or special procedures area. The pacing lead is positioned (through the subclavian or cephalic vein) in the right atrium, right ventricle, left ventricle, or a combination of these (depending on the patient's problem). The generator is placed in a subcutaneous pocket, usually under the clavicle or in the abdomen.

NURSING CARE *of the Patient with a Pacemaker*

Patients with inserted pacemakers recover in the post-anesthesia care unit and then go to a unit with telemetry capability. Monitor the patient for proper pacemaker functioning. Examine the ECG for rhythm, pacemaker spike, and dysrhythmias (premature ventricular contractions and ventricular tachycardia are seen most often). The pacemaker spike is a mark observed on the ECG tracing that represents the impulse generated by the pacemaker. Assess vital signs and inspect the incision frequently. Patients rest for 24 hours after the insertion of a permanent pacemaker. Following that, patients are ambulated and are encouraged to resume normal activities.

After insertion of a temporary pacemaker, microshock precautions should be followed. Monitor the ECG and transport the patient with a portable cardiac monitor and a nurse in attendance. Assess the pacemaker for misfiring. Plan a gradual increase in activities.

There are three major problems that can occur with pacing. The first problem, failure to pace, means that the pacemaker did not initiate the electrical stimulus when it was due to fire. Frequently caused by battery failure or lead wire displacement, it is recognized by the lack of a pacer spike on the ECG tracing. The second problem, failure to capture, means that the electrical stimulus from the pacemaker is not followed by electrical activity in the patient's heart. Caused by dislodgement of the lead or the pacemaker output setting set too low, failure to capture is recognized by noting the presence of a pacer spike without ECG activity following the spike. The third problem, failure to sense, means that the pacemaker does not sense the patient's cardiac rhythm and initiates an electrical impulse when it is not needed. Failure to sense is most often caused by displacement of the electrode and can be recognized by pacer spikes that fall too close to the patient's rhythm.

When a permanent pacemaker has been inserted, teach the patient how to count the pulse for 1 full minute daily. Explain wound care and the healing process. Advise the patient to notify the physician of symptoms of decreased cardiac output: dyspnea, dizziness, syncope, weakness, fatigue, and chest pain. Also instruct the patient to carry an identification card describing the type of pacemaker implanted.

CARDIOVERSION

Cardioversion is the delivery of a synchronized shock to terminate atrial or ventricular tachydysrhythmias (rapid abnormal heart rhythms). It may be done as an emergency or elective procedure. The shock is synchronized with the R wave to avoid shocking during the vulnerable period of the T wave. A shock delivered during ventricular relaxation can initiate ventricular fibrillation.

If the patient is receiving digoxin, the drug is withheld for 24 hours before the procedure. Emergency drugs are made available, and the patient has a patent intravenous line in place before the procedure. Explain the procedure, and obtain informed consent. A short-acting sedative is usually given. The cardioverter is set to the synchronized mode, and two electrodes are placed on the chest. One electrode is placed to the right of the sternum just below the clavicle and the other is placed at the apex of the heart. The initial impulse varies from 25 to 100 joules depending on the type of dysrhythmia. If the initial impulse does not convert the dysrhythmia to normal sinus rhythm, the impulse energy is increased and the procedure is repeated.

After cardioversion, the patient usually recovers very quickly from the sedation and does not remember the event. Inspect the skin under the electrodes for irritation. Monitor the patient's heart rate and rhythm, vital signs, and neurologic status. Transient dysrhythmias and a drop in blood pressure are common. Be especially alert for atrial fibrillation, which can contribute to the formation of atrial wall thrombus and emboli.

CARDIOPULMONARY RESUSCITATION

Cardiopulmonary resuscitation is the restoration of heart and lung function after cardiac arrest. The procedure is used in basic cardiac life support and advanced cardiac life support. The reader is referred to materials prepared by the American Heart Association for current, in-depth coverage of the procedure. See Chapter 16 for an overview.

CARDIAC SURGERY

The most common surgical procedures involving the heart are pacemaker insertion, heart surgery to repair or replace valves or septa or remove tumors, and coronary artery bypass surgery. Pacemaker insertion is described earlier in this section. Coronary artery bypass surgery is described as a surgical treatment for AMI on pp. 657 and 658.

With some of the surgical procedures on the heart, the heart muscle must be at rest during the procedure. This requires placing the patient on a machine to direct the blood away from the heart and lungs and to maintain appropriate oxygen and carbon dioxide levels. The heart's rhythm is interrupted by an electrolyte solution and may be restarted after the surgery by electrical stimulation. During this type of surgery, the patient's core temperature usually is reduced to decrease the oxygen needs of the entire body, especially the brain.

PREOPERATIVE NURSING CARE
of the Cardiac Surgery Patient
Assessment

Nursing assessment of the patient with cardiac disorders is summarized in Box 35-1. When a patient is facing cardiac surgery, also assess the patient's fears and anxiety. Patients are usually upset and very concerned when heart surgery is recommended. Determine what patients know about the surgery and what more they would like to know.

Nursing Diagnoses, Goals, and Outcome Criteria:
Preoperative Cardiac Surgery

Nursing Diagnoses	Goals and Outcome Criteria
Fear related to perceived threat of death or unfamiliarity with setting and procedures	Reduced fear: patient states is less fearful, demonstrates relaxed manner
Anxiety related to threat to health status or uncertain outcome	Reduced anxiety: patient states is less anxious, is calmer

Interventions
Fear and Anxiety

Encourage the patient to identify feelings and then explore the basis of those feelings. Do not assume you know how the patient feels. Accept the patient's feelings and do not give trite reassurance ("Don't worry; everything will be fine."). Accurate information about what to expect helps reduce fear of the unknown. Physical comfort measures such as a massage or back rub may also be soothing. If the patient's anxiety level remains high, notify the physician.

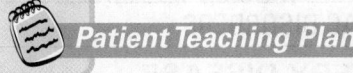
Patient Teaching Plan

Cardiac Surgery, Preoperative

The specifics of the teaching plan depend on the exact procedure and agency/surgeon procedures. General content of the teaching plan incudes the following:

- Preoperative routines: NPO, monitoring, diagnostic tests, any special preparation
- Where the patient will be after surgery: in intensive care unit after extensive procedures; to regular units after pacemaker insertion
- The postoperative care setting: the room and the equipment
- Postoperative routines: how to turn, cough, deep breathe, and exercise the leg muscles; monitoring; procedures
- Postoperative pain: amount of pain to expect, relief measures such as splinting, positioning, medication
- Communication: because most patients are intubated for 4 to 8 hours after surgery, establish a means of communication before surgery

Put on Your Thinking Cap!

A patient is scheduled for extensive cardiac surgery and will be on a ventilator for up to 8 hours postoperatively. What means of communication can you establish in advance? What if the patient is illiterate? What if the patient is deaf?

Good patient teaching is essential to address fear and anxiety. The physician reviews necessary diagnostic tests, the surgical procedure itself, and what to expect after surgery. Nevertheless, the nurse must be able to clarify and further explain what the patient will experience. If the surgery is to be done as an emergency, little time is available to do preoperative teaching. Planned cardiac surgery allows time for the patient to accept the need for surgery and to explore why the procedure is necessary. Include the family in the preoperative teaching to decrease their anxiety and allow them to participate in the patient's recovery. The patient teaching plan must be individualized for the type of surgical procedure.

POSTOPERATIVE NURSING CARE
of the Cardiac Surgery Patient

Nursing care needs vary considerably depending on the type of surgical procedure. Care specific to certain conditions is discussed with those conditions. In addition, see Chapter 17 for thorough coverage of care of the surgical patient. This section addresses needs common to many patients having cardiac surgery.

Assessment

Assessment of the cardiac patient is summarized in Box 35-1. After surgery, be especially alert to changes in vital signs, breath sounds, urine output, mental alertness, and color. In the intensive care unit, monitor cardiac rhythm, arterial blood gases, and hemodynamic pressures. Assess chest tube function. Frequently inspect all dressings for type and amount of drainage. Examine the surgical wound and insertion sites of tubes and cannulas for increasing redness, swelling, and purulent drainage. Assess urine amount, appearance, and odor.

Nursing Diagnoses, Goals, and Outcome Criteria:
Postoperative Cardiac Surgery

Nursing Diagnoses	Goals and Outcome Criteria
Ineffective Breathing Pattern related to mechanical ventilation, general anesthesia, pain, or restrictive surgical dressings	Adequate oxygenation: arterial blood gases within normal limits
Acute Pain related to tissue trauma	Pain relief: patient states pain reduced or relieved, relaxed manner

Continued

Ineffective Thermoregulation related to cooling during surgery	Normal body temperature: temperature of at least 36.7° C (98° F) orally
Decreased Cardiac Output related to fluid loss or decreased fluid intake	Normal cardiac output: fluid intake equal to output
Risk for Infection related to altered skin integrity	Absence of infection: no fever; decreasing drainage, redness, and swelling of wound
Anxiety related to unfamiliar routines and stressful experience	Reduced anxiety: patient states anxiety is reduced

Interventions

Ineffective Breathing Pattern

Patients with open heart or bypass surgery are unresponsive on arrival in the intensive care unit. Ventilatory assistance is of prime importance. Reassess breath sounds and arterial blood gases frequently. Connect chest tubes to underwater seal drainage. (See Chapter 30 for the care of chest tubes.) Reposition the patient often to promote removal of pulmonary secretions and improve respiratory excursion.

When the patient is extubated, provide an oxygen mask or nasal cannula as ordered to provide supplemental oxygen. Assist the patient to cough and deep breathe frequently. A pillow or a blanket in a pillowcase can be used as an incisional splint during coughing. An incentive spirometer is usually ordered. Monitor its use, and remind the patient to use it. Assist with early ambulation, as ordered, to reduce the risk of pulmonary complications.

Acute Pain

Effective pain relief makes it easier for the patient to turn, cough, and deep breathe. Assess the patient's pain: location, severity, aggravating factors, and relieving factors. Administer analgesics as ordered. Intravenous morphine in small doses is most frequently prescribed for analgesia. You may also use independent measures, including position changes, back rubs, relaxation techniques, and imagery. Assess the effectiveness of the interventions in managing pain. Provide for periods of rest and sleep after pain relief efforts.

Ineffective Thermoregulation

Warmed blankets, heating blankets, and warming lights may be used to assist rewarming. Monitor body temperature continuously until the patient is stable.

Decreased Cardiac Output

Monitor cardiac pressures continuously in the intensive care unit until they stabilize. Prescribed medications are adjusted based on vital signs, hemodynamic pressures, and cardiac rhythms. Pacing wires are connected to a temporary pacemaker. Monitor fluid and blood administration, and assess urinary and other drainage outputs. Volume expanders (albumin, dextran, hetastarch) and vasoactive drugs may be necessary to maintain blood pressure. Oral fluids are ordered shortly after extubation.

Risk for Infection

The patient is at risk for incisional, respiratory tract, and urinary tract infections. In addition, the presence of multiple tubes and cannulas provides additional sites for potential nosocomial infection. To reduce the risk of infection, practice good hand-washing technique and use aseptic technique when handling dressings and invasive equipment. Provide wound care as ordered or per agency policy. Administer antibiotics as ordered. Before discharge, begin teaching the patient how to care for the surgical wound. Emphasize signs or symptoms that should be reported to the physician: fever, increasing or purulent wound drainage, increasing redness or swelling, and separation of wound margins.

Anxiety

Inform the patient and the family what is being done and how the patient is responding. Remember to talk to the patient and offer reassurance. When the patient is on a ventilator, use the previously established nonverbal means of communication. It is often necessary to repeat instructions because of the effects of pain, medications, and anxiety. As the patient improves, explain the importance of follow-up care and rehabilitation.

Consider the Alternative

For pain relief, many complementary therapies are used with analgesics. Some examples are massage, relaxation techniques, and imagery.

CARDIAC DISORDERS

CORONARY ARTERY DISEASE

Coronary artery disease (CAD) occurs when the major coronary arteries supplying the myocardium are partially or completely blocked. Blockage of the arteries is caused by coronary artery spasm, arteriosclerosis, or atherosclerosis and may result in ischemia or infarction of myocardial tissue. In 1998, there were 208 deaths per 100,000 population. A *Healthy People 2010* objective is to reduce that number by 20 percent (Centers for Disease Control and Prevention/National Institutes of Health, 2005). See the Health Promotion Considerations box on p. 653 for a review of cardiac risk factor modification.

Arteriosclerosis

Arteriosclerosis is an abnormal thickening, hardening, and loss of elasticity of arterial walls. Smooth muscle cells and collagen migrate into the tunica intima (innermost layer of the artery) and cause the arterial wall to stiffen and thicken and the lumen to decrease in diam-

Health Promotion Considerations

Risk Factor Modification

Risk factor modification will help reduce an individual's risk for developing CAD, angina, and acute coronary syndromes. Controlling HTN, reducing serum cholesterol and LDLs, smoking cessation, participating in regular, moderate exercise, obtaining/maintaining ideal body weight, and learning to handle stress are recommended lifestyle changes that can help decrease risk.

eter. Lipids, cholesterol, calcium, and thrombi adhere to the damaged arterial wall. This process limits the elasticity of the wall and decreases the flow of oxygen-carrying blood to tissues. Some effects of arteriosclerosis are hypertension, impaired tissue perfusion, and aneurysms.

Atherosclerosis

Atherosclerosis, a form of arteriosclerosis, is an inflammatory disease that begins with endothelial injury and progresses to the complicated lesion seen in advanced stages of the disease process. Atherosclerosis begins with injury to the endothelial cells that line the wall of the arteries. Endothelial injury, which leads to inflammation and dysfunction of the endothelial cells, results in the deposit of LDLs along the intima of arteries. These deposits are called *foam cells*. When enough foam cells accumulate, they progress to the lesions associated with atherosclerosis: fatty streaks, fibrous plaque, and complicated (advanced) lesions.

Progression of Lesions.

Fatty Streak. The fatty streak is the earliest lesion to develop in atherosclerosis. Yellow-colored lipids (fat) fill smooth muscle cells, producing streaks of fat that cause no obstruction to the affected vessel. It is commonly found in the aorta by age 10 and in coronary arteries by age 15 regardless of race, gender, or environmental factors. The fatty streak is thought to be reversible. There are no symptoms associated with these lesions.

Fibrous Plaque. The fibrous plaque is the characteristic lesion of progressing atherosclerosis, which develops over time. Smooth muscle cells, chronically stimulated by LDLs and platelet activated growth factors, proliferate, produce collagen, and migrate over the fatty streak. This forms a fibrous plaque that protrudes out from the wall of the artery into the lumen. Other substances (WBCs, platelets, lipids, calcium) adhere to and collect within the plaque. The fibrous plaque is whitish or grayish appearing, may develop in one portion of the artery or circle the entire lumen, and may have smooth or rough edges. Fibrous plaque contributes to the loss of arterial elasticity and impairs the vessel's ability to vasodilate to meet increased oxygen needs.

Complicated Lesions. Complicated lesions develop as ulceration or rupture of the plaque occurs and plate-

lets adhere to the lesion. Platelet adherence can trigger the coagulation cascade with the development of a thrombus that obstructs (occludes) the artery.

Collateral Circulation. If plaque formation occurs slowly, collateral circulation may develop. Collateral blood vessels are new branches that grow from existing arteries to provide increased blood flow.

Risk Factors. Factors that increase the risk of atherosclerosis include increased serum lipids, high blood pressure, cigarette smoking (nicotine), diabetes mellitus with elevated blood glucose, obesity, sedentary lifestyle, age, gender, race, and heredity. These risk factors are divided into two categories: risk factors that can be modified and those that cannot be modified. Risk factors that *cannot* be modified are age, gender, heredity, and race. The focus of patient education is on reducing the risk factors that can be modified. Other factors that may also contribute to the development of coronary heart disease are stress, sex hormones, birth control pills, excessive alcohol intake, and high homocysteine levels.

Healthy People 2010 has set several goals related to serum lipid levels. One of these is to reduce the mean total blood cholesterol in adults from 206 mg/dL to 199 mg/dL. In addition, efforts will be made to reduce the proportion of adults with high blood cholesterol, increase the proportion of adults who have had their blood cholesterol checked within the past 5 years, and increase the proportion of individuals with CAD who have LDL levels treated to the goal of equal to or less than 100 mg/dL (Centers for Disease Control and Prevention/National Institutes of Health, 2005).

Signs and Symptoms

Coronary artery disease usually is asymptomatic until the tissue's blood supply is reduced by at least 50%. Then, the clinical manifestations of CAD include angina pectoris, acute coronary syndrome (unstable angina and acute myocardial infarction), and sudden cardiac death. Acute myocardial infarction has been further categorized into non–ST-segment elevation myocardial infarction (NSTEMI) and ST-segment elevation myocardial infarction (STEMI).

ANGINA PECTORIS

Angina pectoris (shortened to angina), or chest pain, the most common symptom of CAD, results when the demand for oxygen by the myocardial cells exceeds the supply of oxygen delivered. There are different types of angina: stable, unstable, and variant. Stable angina (also called *chronic angina* or *exertional angina*) occurs most often with exercise or activity and usually subsides with rest. Other precipitating factors are smoking, physical exertion, emotional stress, and heavy meals. The pain is usually substernal and described by the patient as viselike, burning, squeezing, or smothering. The pain may radiate to either arm, the shoulder, the jaw, the neck, or the epigastrium. Accompanying symptoms are diaphoresis, dyspnea, nausea, and vomiting. Stable angina occurs intermittently and is often predictable. Usually, stable angina lasts only a few minutes and is relieved by rest or with nitroglycerine (NTG).

Unstable angina (categorized and treated as an acute coronary syndrome) is also called *crescendo angina* or *preinfarction angina.* The pain of unstable angina is more severe, occurs at rest or with minimal exertion, is often not relieved by NTG or requires more frequent NTG administration, and is not predictable. Unstable angina may occur in a patient with a history of stable angina. The patient may describe a change in the pain pattern or in the severity of the pain. Or, unstable angina may be the first clinical manifestation of CAD that a patient experiences. In either case, unstable angina is considered more serious than stable angina and will be treated differently. Patients with unstable angina are at higher risk for acute myocardial infarction (AMI) and are often hospitalized for diagnostic workup and treatment.

Variant angina (also known as *Prinzmetal's angina*) is caused by coronary artery spasm and may not be associated with CAD. This type of angina is unpredictable and often occurs at rest. When the coronary spasm occurs, the patient experiences angina and, if the patient is being monitored, transient ST elevation may be seen. When the spasm subsides, the pain goes away and the ST segment returns to normal. The treatment for variant angina is usually administration of calcium channel blockers to prevent the spasms from occurring.

Medical Treatment

Treatment of CAD includes diet therapy, drug therapy, and reduction of modifiable risk factors (e.g., smoking, obesity, hypertension). Recommendations for medical therapy have been developed for both stable and unstable angina. Initial therapy for patients with angina should follow the mnemonic below (Braunwald, et al., 2002; Gibbons, et al., 2002):

A   Aspirin and antianginal therapy
B   Beta blocker and blood pressure
C   Cigarette smoking and cholesterol
D   Diet and diabetes
E   Education and exercise

Low-dose aspirin is administered to interfere with platelet aggregation and it can reduce the risk of myocardial infarction. If the patient cannot tolerate aspirin, another antiplatelet medication (e.g., Ticlid, Plavix) will be prescribed. Antianginal therapy includes nitrates, beta-adrenergic blockers, and calcium channel blockers. Nitrates such as NTG are used to treat actual episodes of angina and to prevent the occurrence of angina. Various forms of nitroglycerin are prescribed for treatment of acute angina. These are administered sublingually or buccally at the onset of pain. They are quickly absorbed and usually effective. Oral, topical, and transdermal nitrates may be ordered to prevent angina attacks. Beta-adrenergic blockers and calcium channel blockers are prescribed in the long-term management of angina.

After the initial relief and control of the anginal pain, the focus of therapy will turn to risk reduction to include optimizing blood pressure, smoking cessation, lipid control (diet alone or diet plus lipid-lowering medications), healthy diet and tight glucose control for diabetic patients, exercise training, and patient education (i.e., medication therapy, risk reduction, and what to do if symptoms of an AMI occur).

ACE inhibitors may also be prescribed to patients with stable angina to reduce the risk of AMI. In addition, some patients may be recommended for further treatment with percutaneous coronary interventions (PCI), such as angioplasty, stent placement, or atherectomy (Gibbons, et al., 2002).

Additional information about various drug therapies is presented in the Drug Therapy table on p. 646.

Unstable angina may be treated conservatively or more aggressively, depending on the situation. Because unstable angina may be a "warning" of more serious events, it has been classified as an acute coronary syndrome. In current recommendations, unstable angina and NSTEMI are addressed together because they are so closely related. Patients with unstable angina should receive the **A-B-C-D-E's** discussed in the previous section. However, in addition to antiplatelet therapy, anticoagulation therapy with LMWH may be administered. For patients who will be undergoing cardiac catheterization and PCI, a platelet GP IIb/IIIa antagonist will also be administered (Braunwald, et al., 2002).

Surgical Intervention

Surgical procedures to treat CAD are discussed on pp. 656 and 657.

What Does Culture Have to Do with Heart Disease?

American Indians and African Americans develop CAD at an earlier age than other Americans. The incidence of CAD is highest among middle-aged Caucasian males. Latinos have lower death rates from CAD than non-Latinos. Nurses can educate high-risk patients about risk factors that can be modified: obesity, hypertension, and stress. Role models from the target population are especially influential.

ACUTE MYOCARDIAL INFARCTION

An AMI is the death of myocardial tissue as a result of prolonged lack of blood and oxygen supply. Approximately 700,000 Americans have a new myocardial infarction every year and 500,000 Americans have recurrent attacks annually. Approximately 225,000 individuals in the United States will die each year from myocardial infarction. The average age for men having a first heart attack is 65 to 66 years, and the average age in women for a first heart attack is 70 years (American Heart Association, 2007).

Risk Factors

Risk factors for AMI include obesity, smoking, a high-fat diet, hypertension, family history, male gender, diabetes mellitus, sedentary lifestyle, and excessive stress. Smoking, a high-fat diet, hypertension, sedentary lifestyle, and stress are considered modifiable risk factors. This means that risk can be reduced by cessation of smoking, diet modification, management of hypertension, regular exercise, and stress reduction.

Pathophysiology

An AMI begins with the occlusion of a coronary artery. Over a period of 4 to 6 hours, a process of ischemia, injury, and infarction develops. Ischemia results from a lack of blood and oxygen to a portion of the heart muscle. If ischemia is not reversed, injury occurs. Deprived of blood and oxygen, the affected tissue becomes soft and loses its normal color. With continued ischemia, an infarction, or death of myocardial tissue, occurs. Ischemia lasting 20 minutes or more is sufficient to produce irreversible tissue damage.

Within 24 hours after an infarction, the healing process begins. By the third day, necrotic tissue has been broken down by enzymes and removed by macrophages. Collateral circulation develops to supply the injured area, and scar tissue begins to form. About 10 to 14 days after the AMI, the myocardium is especially vulnerable to stress because of the weakness of the healing tissue. Complete healing takes about 6 weeks.

An AMI is considered an acute coronary syndrome, along with unstable angina as mentioned earlier. Health care providers divide AMI into two types: non–ST-elevation MI (NSTEMI) and ST-elevation MI (STEMI) for purposes of diagnosis and treatment. The ST segment of an ECG is usually flat or isoelectric (see the Interpretation of Electrocardiograms section on p. 673). Because the ST segment can be displaced when there is partial or complete lack of oxygen flow to the myocardial cells, the appearance of a patient's ST segment is an important component of the assessment of an AMI. Patients with NSTEMI usually have transient or partial occlusion of a coronary artery, whereas patients with STEMI have total occlusion of a coronary artery from coronary thrombosis.

Complications

The major complications of AMI are dysrhythmias, heart failure, cardiogenic shock, thromboembolism, and ventricular aneurysm/rupture.

Dysrhythmias. Dysrhythmias are disturbances in heart rhythm, including excessively rapid, slow, or irregular heartbeats. They occur in approximately 80% of all patients with AMI. Because some dysrhythmias are life-threatening, continuous cardiac monitoring is usually ordered for patients with AMI. This permits early detection and prompt treatment of dysrhythmias. Recognition and treatment of specific dysrhythmias are addressed on pp. 673 to 682.

Heart Failure. The AMI may cause the heart to fail as a pump if the injured LV is unable to meet the body's circulatory demands. The ventricle fails to empty efficiently. Increased preload leads to systemic and pulmonary edema. Cardiac output and blood pressure fall. Untreated cardiac failure progresses to cardiogenic shock and death. Early symptoms of congestive failure are dyspnea, restlessness, and increasing heart rate.

Cardiogenic Shock. Cardiogenic shock is the most frequent cause of death after an AMI. It is usually related to extensive injury to the LV and is more common when the patient has had a previous infarction. Cardiogenic shock is marked by hypotension; cool, moist skin; oliguria; and decreasing alertness.

Thromboembolism. After an AMI, thrombi may form in the injured heart chambers or in the veins of the legs. The thrombi may break loose, travel through the circulation, and lodge in the lung. Pallor, cyanosis, and heart failure may be caused by pulmonary emboli. Massive pulmonary embolism is characterized by sudden, severe dyspnea. It is usually fatal. Pulmonary emboli are discussed in detail in Chapter 30.

Ventricular Aneurysm/Rupture. Weakened areas of the ventricular wall may bulge during contractions. If scar tissue is inadequate to strengthen the wall, an aneurysm may develop and rupture. Ventricular rupture is fatal.

Signs and Symptoms

Pain is the classic symptom of AMI. It is typically a heavy or constrictive pain located below or behind the sternum, as described with angina. It may radiate to the arms, back, neck, or jaw. The pain may begin with or without exertion. If not relieved by rest and nitroglycerin, it progresses. The patient becomes diaphoretic and lightheaded and may experience nausea, vomiting, and dyspnea. The skin is frequently cold and clammy. The patient experiences great anxiety and often a feeling of impending doom. Not all patients experience the more classic signs and symptoms. Women, older adults, and diabetic patients often have atypical symptoms. Women may complain of fatigue, shortness of breath, and atypical chest pain. Older adults and diabetic patients may not experience chest pain but will complain of other symptoms such as shortness of breath, dizziness, and nausea.

Medical Diagnosis

The diagnosis of an AMI is based primarily on the patient's history and the physical signs and symptoms. The AMI can be confirmed by laboratory evidence and ECG changes.

Cardiac Markers

Troponin. Troponin T (cTnT) and troponin I (cTnI) are proteins released from cardiac muscle when the muscle is damaged. Troponin levels elevate in 3 hours after myocardial injury, peak in 24 hours, and remain in the circulation for up to 2 weeks (cTnI remains elevated for 5 to 7 days; cTnT for 10 to 14 days). Troponin levels may be drawn in the emergency room, helping to establish an early diagnosis.

Myoglobin. Myoglobin is released within 1 hour after an acute myocardial infarction, and levels rise before CK-MB levels; therefore myoglobin levels can be helpful in the early diagnosis of AMI. Myoglobin levels will also be increased after strenuous exercise or renal failure and in the presence of neuromuscular disease.

Cardiac Enzymes. A blood sample is drawn from anyone with prolonged chest pain to measure cardiac enzymes. With sustained ischemia, the cell membrane is impaired and enzymes are released from their intracellular location into the interstitial fluid. These enzymes can be measured in the serum and are assessed at regular intervals to confirm an AMI. CPK and its isoenzyme CPK-MB (myocardial) elevate rapidly with infarction. Beginning 4 to 6 hours after infarction, the CPK rises to 5 or more times the normal level within 12 to 24 hours and returns to normal in 2 to 3 days.

Electrocardiogram. Changes in the normal waveform and dysrhythmias can be seen on an ECG. With ischemia, the ST segment is often depressed and the T wave is inverted. If there has been total occlusion of a coronary artery, the ECG will show ST elevation (STEMI). This is the more common occurrence. If there has been transient or partial occlusion of the artery, the ECG may not show ST elevation (NSTEMI). After infarction, another change often seen on the ECG waveforms is a significant Q wave (Fig. 35-8). A significant Q wave is one that is greater than one-third the height of the R wave. The most frequently observed dysrhythmias are premature ventricular contractions, ventricular tachycardia, and ventricular fibrillation.

Medical Treatment

The goals of medical therapy after an AMI are to limit the amount of cardiac muscle injury, to relieve symptoms, and to prevent or minimize complications.

Drug Therapy. Sublingual or intravenous nitroglycerin is administered to dilate coronary arteries and increase blood flow to the damaged area. If the nitroglycerin relieves the pain, the infarction may not extend. Morphine sulfate is also used for chest pain. It has many effects in addition to analgesia. Morphine causes peripheral pooling of blood, which decreases the blood returning to the heart and lungs. It also diminishes anxiety, decreases tachypnea, and relaxes bronchial smooth muscles, thereby improving gas exchange. If the patient cannot tolerate morphine, meperidine (Demerol) may be ordered, but it does not have all the other beneficial properties of morphine and may increase the heart rate.

Oxygen is administered at 4 to 6 L/min to assist in oxygenating myocardial tissue to support pumping activity and to repair damaged tissue.

Fibrinolytic therapy is recommended for patients with STEMI (patients with total occlusion) (Ante, et al., 2004). Streptokinase and tissue plasminogen activator

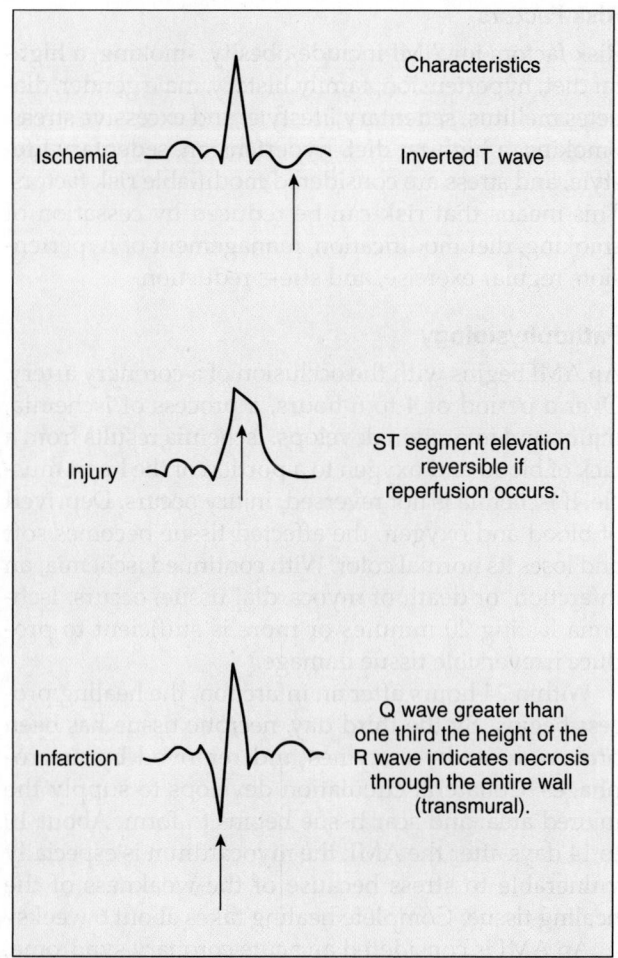

FIGURE 35-8 Electrocardiographic changes with myocardial infarction.

are administered intravenously or into the coronary arteries (during cardiac catheterization) to dissolve the thrombus. This treatment is most effective when initiated early but may be administered up to 12 hours from the onset of chest pain. The patient must meet strict criteria (no recent surgery or active bleeding; no history of a stroke; no bleeding disorders) and provide informed consent before the administration of fibrinolytics. After administration of the fibrinolytics, heparin is administered to prevent further clot formation.

Aspirin and beta-adrenergic blockers should be administered as soon as the patient can tolerate them and if not contraindicated. Beta-adrenergic blockers improve survival rates by decreasing the heart rate, reducing the work of the heart, and lessening the oxygen demand of the myocardium. ACE inhibitors may be prescribed for some patients to minimize the abnormal shaping or remodeling that can occur in the damaged ventricular muscle. Unstable patients may require dopamine or dobutamine, or both, as inotropic agents (Ante, et al., 2004). As the myocardium receives blood and oxygen, reperfusion dysrhythmias that require treatment may be noted.

Percutaneous Coronary Intervention. Emergency percutaneous coronary intervention (PCI) is an option for treatment after AMI, either instead of fibrinolytic therapy or after fibrinolytic therapy (Ante, et al., 2004). There are several PCI procedures that can be performed in the cardiac catheterization laboratory: percutaneous transluminal coronary angioplasty (PTCA), intracoronary stent placement, atherectomy, laser angioplasty, and radiation therapy. PTCA involves passage of a catheter through a peripheral artery (usually the femoral artery) into the occluded coronary artery. The tip of the catheter contains a balloon that is inflated to compress the atherosclerotic plaque and dilate the artery. PTCA is often utilized when there is single-vessel disease, non-calcified lesions, or lesions that are not at bifurcations. PTCA is not recommended for lesions of the left main coronary artery.

When appropriate, this procedure is preferred over coronary artery bypass surgery because it can be done under local anesthetic, it is less invasive, and the recovery time is faster. The procedure is safer than bypass surgery but is not without risks. Complications of PTCA include coronary artery dissection, dysrhythmias, coronary spasm, hematoma at the catheter site, restenosis, and death. In approximately 30% of patients, the vessel narrows again within 6 months.

Intracoronary stents are devices that are positioned within the blockage through a balloon-tipped catheter, expanded into place, and left to support the arterial wall. Over time, endothelial cells will completely line the inner wall of the stent to produce a smooth inner lining (Fig. 35-9). After an intracoronary stent is placed, the patient will be on antiplatelet or anticoagulant agents to decrease the chance of occlusion in the stent. Complications of stents are injury to the vessel wall and bleeding.

The coronary atherectomy is a procedure that widens the coronary artery by removing the atherosclerotic plaque using a device that shaves the plaque off the vessel walls.

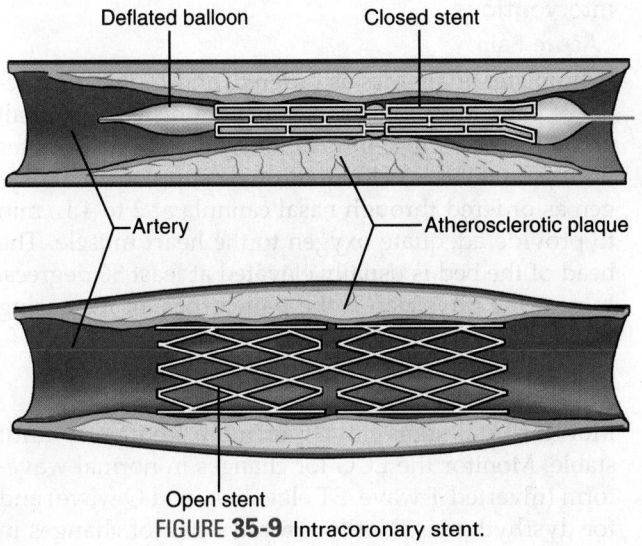

Deflated balloon   Closed stent

Artery   Atherosclerotic plaque

Open stent

FIGURE 35-9 Intracoronary stent.

A newer procedure is laser angioplasty. It uses a catheter with a laser on the tip. The laser is used to widen the lumen of the artery by destroying atherosclerotic plaque.

Radiation therapy is used primarily to treat restenosis of intracoronary stents. Radiation is delivered to the area of stenosis for several minutes. The patient requires no special precautions after the procedure related to the radiation.

Coronary Artery Bypass Graft Surgery. Coronary artery bypass graft surgery may be performed to improve the blood supply to the myocardium. Arterial bypass surgery uses the patient's own vasculature as replacement for occluded coronary arteries. From one to six vessels may be bypassed. The saphenous veins and the internal mammary artery are most commonly used. The saphenous veins are removed from one or both legs, inspected for patency, and reversed so that the valves do not inhibit blood flow. The replacement vessels are attached above and below the occlusions in the coronary arteries and serve as new conduits for oxygenated blood to the myocardium (Fig. 35-10). This is major surgery requiring the heart beat to be stopped and the patient to be placed on a cardiopulmonary bypass (CPB) machine during the surgery. The survival rate is higher in patients who are in stable condition.

Another approach to surgical revascularization is being used on patients requiring surgery on the arteries of the anterior heart. This procedure is called *minimally invasive direct coronary artery bypass grafting* and is performed through a small anterior thoracotomy incision. The patient's internal mammary artery is used to bypass the stenosed vessel, and the bypass is accomplished on a beating heart. The patient does not have to be placed on CPB. Postoperative care is similar to that of other cardiac surgery, although patients do not require as lengthy ventilatory support and total length of hospital stay is shorter.

A third option, off-pump coronary artery bypass (OPCAB), usually uses a full sternotomy incision (as with the traditional CABG) to provide the surgeon access to all coronary vessels (anterior and posterior). The OPCAB surgery is then accomplished on a beating heart without the use of CPB. Specially developed vacuum-assisted stabilizers are used by the surgeon to stabilize the graft site.

A new approach to CABG is done endoscopically. Called *totally endoscopic CAB (TECAB)*, three tiny incisions are made on the patient's chest between ribs, and a small camera and two robotic arms are inserted. The surgeon sits at a console to view the surgical area and manipulates the robotic arms with his or her hands/wrists. The surgery is done on a beating heart, is less traumatic to the patient due to the small incisions, and is easier to recover from.

Another method of revascularization, used for patients with diffuse coronary vessel disease, is transmyocardial laser revascularization. Tiny holes are

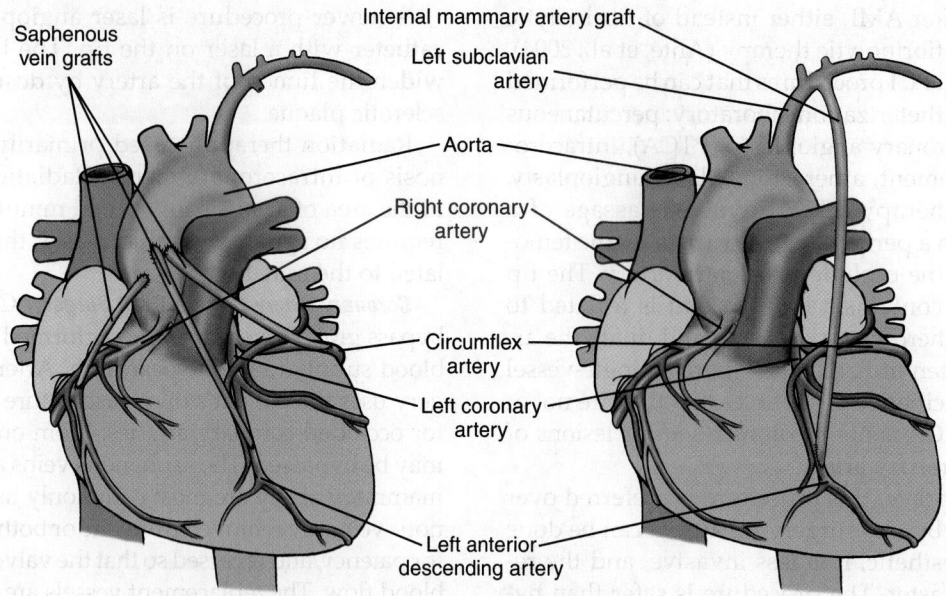

Saphenous vein grafts

Internal mammary artery graft

Left subclavian artery

Aorta

Right coronary artery

Circumflex artery

Left coronary artery

Left anterior descending artery

FIGURE **35-10** Coronary artery bypass graft surgery.

drilled in the myocardium using a laser, which helps provide collateral circulation to the ischemic myocardial muscle (Fig. 35-11).

NURSING CARE *of the Patient with Acute Myocardial Infarction*

Assessment

General assessment of the cardiac patient is summarized in Box 35-1. When a patient has AMI, be especially concerned with assessment of pain. When chest pain is present, early evaluation and treatment are paramount. Ask the patient to describe the pain, including type, location, duration, and severity. It is recommended that chest pain be assessed using the mnemonic PQRST.

P   Precipitating factors, palliative:
    What was the patient doing when the pain began? Did anything make the pain better? Worse?

Q   Quality:
    Have the patient describe what the pain feels like (in his or her own words).

R   Region, radiation:
    Where is the pain located? Does it hurt anywhere else?

S   Severity, symptoms:
    Have the patient rate the pain. Use the pain scale 0-10. Note other symptoms (e.g., nausea, diaphoresis).

T   Time:
    When did the pain start? How long did it last?

Record what the patient was doing when the pain started, what action was taken, and the effects of any actions or treatments. Inspect the patient's skin for color and palpate for temperature and moisture. Frequently assess vital signs. Document the mental status

and level of anxiety. When cardiac monitoring is initiated, evaluate the rate and rhythm.

Nursing Diagnoses, Goals, and Outcome Criteria: Acute Myocardial Infarction

NURSING DIAGNOSES	GOALS AND OUTCOME CRITERIA
Anxiety related to feeling of impending doom, lack of understanding of routines	Reduced anxiety: patient statement of lessened anxiety, calm manner and self-care
Acute Pain related to lack of oxygen to the myocardium	Pain relief: patient statement of relieved pain, relaxed manner
Decreased Cardiac Output related to dysrhythmia and abnormal heart rate	Normal cardiac output: normal pulse, blood pressure, and cardiac rhythm

Interventions

Acute Pain

Administer analgesics as ordered, and monitor for relief of pain. Morphine is usually administered in small amounts (2 to 4 mg) intravenously every few minutes until pain relief is evident. Provide supplemental oxygen as ordered through nasal cannula at 2 to 4 L/min to provide adequate oxygen to the heart muscle. The head of the bed is usually elevated at least 30 degrees. Inform the physician if the patient has an increasing respiratory rate or dyspnea.

Decreased Cardiac Output

Monitor vital signs hourly or more frequently until stable. Monitor the ECG for changes in normal waveform (inverted T wave, ST elevation, and Q wave) and for dysrhythmias. Notify the physician of changes in

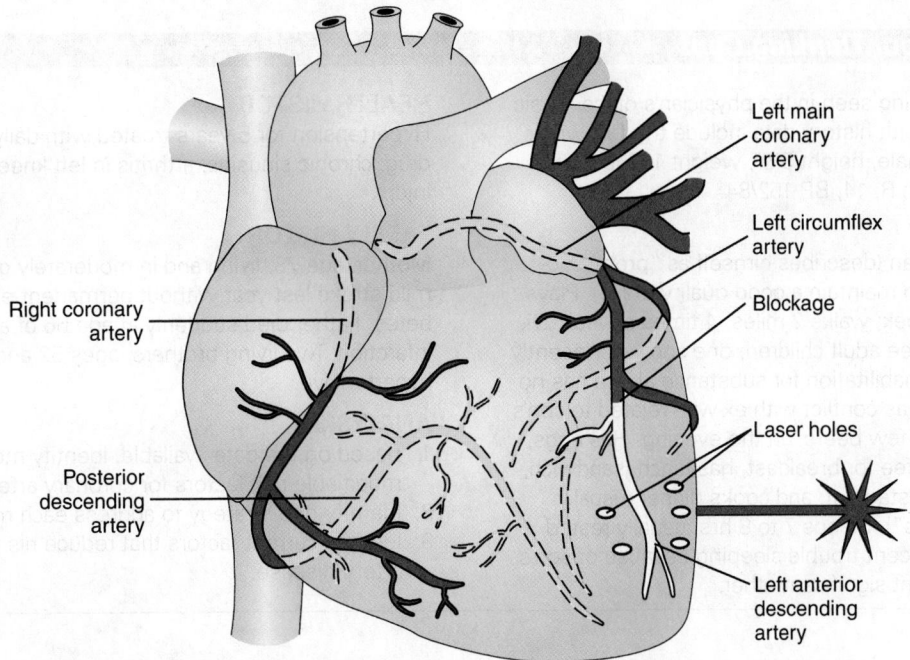

Right coronary artery

Posterior descending artery

Left main coronary artery

Left circumflex artery

Blockage

Laser holes

Left anterior descending artery

FIGURE 35-11 Transmyocardial laser revascularization.

the rhythm. In an intensive care unit, standing orders prescribe drug therapy for specific dysrhythmias. An intravenous line is usually established so that emergency drugs can be administered quickly and directly. Prompt treatment of dysrhythmias may prevent fatal alterations in rhythm. Monitor the patient for fluid volume excess (crackles, cough, jugular vein distention), and report any such evidence to the physician.

Interventions to decrease demands on the heart include assisting the patient to rest, spacing activities and providing rest periods, providing adequate ventilation and oxygenation, relieving pain, and maintaining a calm, quiet environment.

Anxiety

Provide as calm an environment as possible. Explain procedures and equipment to the patient and family, using simple terms. Keep family members informed of the patient's progress. They can be helpful in calming the patient during the acute episode.

During the acute phase of AMI, provide simple explanations of the procedures and routines. Reinforce information given by the physician about the diagnosis and treatment. Patient teaching is especially important in the rehabilitation phase.

Cardiac Rehabilitation

As soon as the patient is stable, begin rehabilitation by teaching the patient and family about exercise, medications, and diet. If surgical intervention has been proposed, you may also teach the patient about that procedure.

The purpose of rehabilitation is to minimize the risk of repetition of adverse cardiac events. The goal of re-

habilitation is to enable patients to attain the highest level of wellness and work ability.

The program is individualized to the patient for maximal success. The four phases of cardiac rehabilitation are (1) inpatient management; (2) immediately after discharge, using telemetry monitoring during exercise; (3) later rehabilitation, which is unmonitored; and (4) maintenance. A team of medical professionals (e.g., nurse, physician, physical therapist, nutritionist,

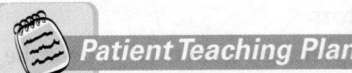
Patient Teaching Plan

Acute Myocardial Infarction

After AMI, the following are some key points in the discharge teaching plan:

- It is very important to take your medications as prescribed and to contact the physician if you have any problems. (Provide written information about drug names, dosages, purpose, interactions with other medications and foods, and adverse effects that should be reported.)
- Your physician may prescribe a low-fat, low-sodium diet to decrease weight and to reduce the workload on your heart.
- Participation in cardiac rehabilitation will help you become active again in a safe manner.
- Stop smoking. Smoking stimulates the heart rate and causes blood vessels to constrict, which makes the heart work harder.
- Maintain normal weight (or lose weight if obese) to decrease the work of the heart.
- The local chapter of the American Heart Association is a helpful resource for information and guidance on diet, smoking cessation, and exercise.

Put on Your Thinking Cap!

A new patient is being seen in the physician's office. Basic information and health history data include the following: 58-year-old white male, height 5'9", weight 190 lbs; vital signs: T, 98° F; P, 82; R, 14; BP, 152/84.

SOCIAL HISTORY

Real estate salesman (describes himself as "pretty successful" and able to maintain a good quality of life). Plays tennis 3 times a week; walks 2 miles, 4 times a week. Divorced father of three adult children; one son who recently was admitted to rehabilitation for substance abuse has no insurance. Patient has conflict with ex-wife related to son's situation. Enjoys a "few beers" in the evening. Has eggs, bacon, biscuits, coffee for breakfast, has lunch (sandwich, fries) at fast-food restaurant, and cooks dinner (usually "meat and potatoes"). Sleeps 7 to 8 hrs; usually rested on arising. Some recent trouble sleeping because of son's problems. No current significant other.

HEALTH HISTORY

Hypertension for 5 years treated with daily antihypertensive drug; chronic sinusitis; arthritis in left knee related to sports injury.

FAMILY HISTORY

Mother, age 78, living and in moderately good health. Had mild stroke last year without permanent effects. Has diabetes. Father died suddenly at age 66 of acute myocardial infarction. Two living brothers, ages 52 and 49. Both are hypertensive.

ANALYSIS

1. Based on the data available, identify modifiable and unmodifiable risk factors for coronary artery disease.
2. Identify one strategy to address each modifiable factor.
3. Identify current factors that reduce his risk of coronary artery disease.

---

social worker) plans the individual program. Education during the rehabilitation process should include normal anatomy and physiology of the heart; pathophysiology of coronary artery disease, angina, and AMI; risk factor modification; activity and exercise; medications; diet; and when to seek medical advice. See the Nutrition Concepts box below for a discussion of dietary considerations for patients with heart disease.

HEART FAILURE

Heart failure is the inability of the heart to meet the metabolic demands of the body. The pumping ability of the heart is ineffective.

Etiology and Risk Factors

Heart failure (HF) is the preferred term used to describe the clinical picture of failure. Congestive heart failure (CHF) is a commonly used term for heart failure; it describes the symptoms seen when the heart fails to pump

effectively and blood "backs up" into the vasculature of the lungs, producing congestion. The two terms (HF and CHF) are often used interchangeably in the clinical setting. Causes of heart failure are primarily of two types: disorders that increase the workload of the heart and disorders that interfere with the pumping ability of the heart. Therefore patients at risk for HF include those with CAD, AMI, cardiomyopathy, hypertension, COPD, pulmonary hypertension, anemia, disease of the heart valves, and fluid volume overload. Other conditions that increase metabolic needs, such as fever and pregnancy, may also precipitate heart failure. Approximately 4.9 million Americans have heart failure and over half a million new cases of heart failure are diagnoses every year. After age 65, 10 of every 1000 individuals have heart failure, and 75% of heart failure patients have a history of hypertension (American Heart Association, 2007).

Pathophysiology

The LV, RV, or both fail as pumps. Usually the left side of the heart fails first. In time, the right side fails as a result of the left-sided failure. Heart failure can be classified as systolic HF resulting from ineffective pumping of the ventricles or as diastolic HF resulting from impaired filling of the ventricles. With either classification, cardiac output is decreased. Heart failure can occur acutely, with onset over several hours or days, or it can be chronic, with onset over months to years.

Compensation. Compensation is a term used to describe the cardiac and circulatory adjustments that maintain or restore cardiac output to normal or near normal. Compensation occurs through three mechanisms: sympathetic nervous system stimulation, regulation of blood volume by the kidneys, and enlargement of the ventricular myocardium.

Sympathetic Compensation. The sympathetic nervous system responds to decreased cardiac output and

Nutrition Concepts

1. A major part of treatment for people with heart disease is reduction of fat and cholesterol in the diet.
2. When fats are used in cooking or eating, unsaturated fats (vegetable oil such as corn oil, canola oil, or olive oil) should be substituted for saturated fats (animal fat such as butter or lard).
3. Fats and oils used in cooking or eating should be limited to five to eight servings daily in normal adults.
4. Saturated fat can be limited by eating only 5 to 7 ounces of meat daily.
5. Foods that contain omega-3 fatty acids (certain fish, walnuts, and soybeans) lower serum triglycerides and decrease the number of deaths resulting from heart disease.

blood pressure. Catecholamines are released that increase heart rate, stroke volume, cardiac output, and venous tone. Increased venous tone increases systemic vascular resistance, venous return, and ventricular filling.

Renal Compensation. The second mechanism that responds to decreased cardiac output is renal compensation. When cardiac output falls, so does renal perfusion. This initiates the renin-angiotensin-aldosterone (RAA) mechanism. Renin, secreted by the kidneys, activates angiotensinogen to convert to angiotensin I. Angiotensin I is converted to angiotensin II, which causes vasoconstriction and triggers release of aldosterone. Vasoconstriction raises the blood pressure by increasing peripheral resistance to blood flow. Aldosterone causes the kidneys to retain sodium and water, which increases blood volume.

Natriuretic Peptides. Natriuretic peptides are neurohormonal substances released with heart failure. Atrial natriuretic peptide (ANP) is released in response to increased volume and stretch in the cardiac atria. B-type natriuretic peptide (BNP) is released when the cardiac ventricles stretch, usually from increased blood volume. The natriuretic peptides are thought to counter the vasoconstrictive and volume-increasing effects of the SNS and RAA systems. BNP levels can be measured in the blood and can be used as a diagnostic tool for HF (Saul & Shatzer, 2003).

Ventricular Hypertrophy. The final mechanism is enlargement of the ventricular myocardium, called *ventricular hypertrophy*, which results from strain. The increased blood volume raises the pressure in the ventricles, which can also cause the ventricles to dilate. The ventricle changes in size and shape, which impairs pumping effectiveness. This process is called *ventricular remodeling*.

After a period, the compensatory mechanisms may no longer be able to meet the increased demands. Contractility decreases; the heart muscle can stretch just so far before becoming inefficient. The force of contraction of the LV decreases. Stroke volume and cardiac output decrease as pumping action fails. Afterload increases with left-sided heart failure. Blood backs up in the LA and then the pulmonary veins. Because of the high pressure in the pulmonary veins (pulmonary hypertension), fluid leaks from the capillaries, causing pulmonary edema. Pulmonary hypertension eventually causes the right side of the heart to fail as well. Then, blood returning to the heart from the body meets resistance, which causes systemic pressure to rise. This results in peripheral edema and enlargement of the liver and spleen. If heart failure is not corrected, death eventually ensues.

With left-sided HF, there is increased left ventricular end-diastolic pressure, increased left atrial pressure, increased pulmonary pressure, and resulting pulmonary edema as the excess fluid leaks into the lung tissues. In right-sided HF, right ventricular pressure increases,

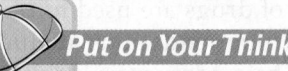
Put on Your Thinking Cap!

1. Explain why a patient with heart failure might (1) feel anxious, and (2) gain weight.
2. A patient with heart failure is advised to try to lose 30 pounds. What nursing strategies would help her achieve this goal?
3. You suspect that a patient with HF and hypertension is not taking her blood pressure medication regularly as prescribed. What strategies might improve her compliance?

right atrial pressure increases, and fluid accumulates in the systemic vasculature.

Signs and Symptoms

The patient with left-sided heart failure is typically very anxious, pale, and tachycardic. Consecutive blood pressure readings may show a downward trend. Auscultation of the lung fields may reveal crackles, wheezes, dyspnea, and cough. When assessing heart sounds, S_3 and S_4 may be heard as a result of the backup of fluid and the heart's inability to handle the excess fluids.

With right-sided heart failure, there is increased central venous pressure, jugular venous distention, abdominal engorgement, and dependent edema. Anorexia, nausea, and vomiting may result from the abdominal engorgement. Fatigue, weight gain, and decreased urinary output are common complaints.

Medical Diagnosis

The diagnosis of HF is made on the basis of the history, physical examination, radiographs, and laboratory test results. A chest radiograph may reveal hazy lung fields, distended vasculature, and cardiomegaly. An echocardiogram may reveal heart enlargement and ineffective ventricular contraction. Laboratory tests indicative of HF are decreased serum sodium and Hct from hemodilution and decreased saturated arterial oxygenation from poor pulmonary perfusion. The blood urea nitrogen (BUN) and creatinine are elevated with decreased renal function. BNP levels are elevated in HF, and the higher the levels, the more severe the failure. Liver function test results are elevated with hepatomegaly (liver enlargement). The patient who is critically ill with HF may require more intensive monitoring of hemodynamics parameters.

Medical Treatment

Medical treatment includes management of the underlying cause, drug therapy to improve cardiac output and eliminate excess fluid, and conservative measures to decrease demands on the heart. Sodium restriction is prescribed for most HF patients.

Treatment of the underlying problem may involve such interventions as correction of dysrhythmias, management of hypertension, and valve replacement or repair.

Drug Therapy. A number of drugs are used to treat heart failure. Current recommendations include ACE inhibitors, diuretics, beta-adrenergic blockers, inotropic agents, cardiac glycosides, and nitrates. In addition, certain patients will benefit from B-type natriuretic peptide. ACE inhibitors decrease preload and afterload by blocking the RAA system, resulting in vasodilation, decreased blood volume, and lower blood pressure. In addition, ACE inhibitors are thought to limit the progression of ventricular remodeling. Diuretics are prescribed to decrease circulating fluid volume and decrease preload. Loop diuretics such as furosemide (Lasix) are usually used in HF. Spironolactone, a weak potassium-sparing diuretic, may be prescribed for some patients because it acts by blocking aldosterone and may slow the process of remodeling. Beta-adrenergic blockers improve survival rates by decreasing the heart rate, reducing the work of the heart, and lessening the oxygen demand of the myocardium. Inotropic agents such as dopamine, dobutamine, and amrinone are prescribed to improve cardiac contractility, improve renal perfusion and decrease fluid retention. Digoxin, a cardiac glycoside with inotropic effects, is prescribed to improve pump function by increasing contractility and decreasing heart rate. Nesiritide (Natrecor) is a recombinant human B-type natriuretic peptide that is often prescribed in patients with decompensated HF. Nesiritide counteracts the vasoconstriction and fluid retention of the RAA system and relieves the severe dyspnea seen in these patients. Nitrates, such as NTG, are venodilators and reduce preload for patients with HF. This helps reduce the workload on the heart. Morphine may be used to decrease anxiety, dilate the vasculature, and reduce myocardial oxygen consumption in the acute stage. The Drug Therapy table on pp. 642 to 646 provides additional information about drugs used to treat HF.

Other Therapy. Other therapies are available for decreasing cardiac workload and increasing myocardial oxygenation. The intra-aortic balloon pump (IABP), ventricular assist devices (VADs), and biventricular pacing may be utilized. The intra-aortic balloon pump is a temporary device used in the intensive care unit to increase cardiac output and coronary artery perfusion. VADs can partially or completely support a patient's failing heart. Currently considered a temporary intervention, VADs are used as a "bridge" to transplantation. Biventricular pacing is useful in approximately 30% of HF patients who have conduction delays in the right or left bundle branch. These conduction delays result in the ventricles being depolarized and contracting out of synchrony. This reduces cardiac output and can contribute to the worsening of HF. In biventricular pacing, leads are placed in both ventricles and they are stimulated at the same time. Cardiac contraction occurs in both ventricles at the same time and cardiac output is improved (Lagrotteria, 2003).

Surgery. Coronary artery bypass grafting is recommended in HF patients who experience angina. Valve repair or replacement is recommended when valve dysfunction contributes to the HF. Partial left ventriculectomy may be useful in some patients. Cardiac transplantation is often the last option for patients with end-stage HF whose symptoms are not responding to conventional therapy.

Complications

Dysrhythmias, pulmonary edema, and cardiogenic shock are possible complications.

NURSING CARE *of the Patient with Heart Failure*
Assessment

Complete assessment of the cardiac patient is outlined in Box 35-1 (see also Nursing Care Plan: The Patient with Heart Failure on p. 663). It is especially important to assess heart sounds, rate, and rhythm. The point of maximum impulse is noted. Assess the apical and radial pulses frequently. Inspect for jugular vein distention. A baseline respiratory assessment of rate, rhythm, and breath sounds is vital. Measure weight and blood pressure accurately. Inspect the skin and palpate for turgor and edema. Intake and output records and daily weights may be done to evaluate fluid retention or loss. If ordered, take central venous pressure and hemodynamic readings as well. If cardiac monitoring is done, observe for dysrhythmias. Nurses who work in intensive care units routinely interpret ECGs. Interpretation is discussed on pp. 673 to 675.

Nursing Diagnoses, Goals, and Outcome Criteria: Heart Failure

Nursing Diagnoses	Goals and Outcome Criteria
Fluid Volume Excess related to ineffective cardiac pumping	Normal fluid volume: no edema or dyspnea, blood pressure consistent with patient norms
Impaired Gas Exchange related to decreased pulmonary perfusion	Adequate oxygenation: clear breath sounds, respiratory rate 12 to 20/min without dyspnea
Anxiety related to edema and difficulty breathing	Reduced anxiety: patient statement of reduced anxiety, calm manner
Decreased Cardiac Output related to mechanical failure	Improved cardiac output: normal heart rate and rhythm, fluid intake and output equal
Activity Intolerance related to inability to meet oxygen demands	Increase activity tolerance: performance of activities of daily living without fatigue

Interventions
Decreased Cardiac Output

Give medications as ordered, and monitor the patient for therapeutic and adverse effects. Older adult patients are more susceptible to adverse drug effects because

NURSING CARE PLAN

The Patient with Heart Failure

ASSESSMENT

Health History: A 73-year-old Chinese-American woman is admitted through the Emergency Department. She is a retired business owner who lives alone and has no immediate family in the area. She began having dyspnea and orthopnea that has become progressively worse over the past 3 days. Her past medical history includes a myocardial infarction 1 year ago and a 10-year history of hypertension treated with diet and verapamil 240 mg daily. In addition to the verapamil, she takes only an occasional laxative. She complains of fatigue, restlessness, nervousness, irritability, insomnia, anorexia, and a productive cough with pink sputum.

Physical Examination: Vital signs: temperature 98° F orally; pulse 104, slightly irregular; respirations 24; blood pressure 168/96. Height 5'2"; weight 152 lbs (a 7-lb increase in 1 week). She is alert but appears anxious. Her skin is pale and diaphoretic. An S_3 is present. Jugular vein distention is noted. Auscultation of the lungs reveals crackles in the lower lobes of both lungs. The abdomen is distended. Bowel sounds are present in all four quadrants. There is 3+ pitting edema in both feet and ankles.

She is being admitted to the telemetry unit for treatment, where she will have continuous electrocardiography and be placed on oxygen.

Nursing Diagnosis	Goals and Outcome Criteria	Interventions
Decreased Cardiac Output related to decreased myocardial contractility	The patient's cardiac output will improve, as evidenced by normal heart rate and rhythm, normal blood pressure, normal hemodynamic measure, and breath sounds clear to auscultation.	Monitor vital signs, heart and lung sounds, level of consciousness, electrocardiography. Enforce bed rest with head of bed elevated. Schedule activities to allow rest. Request small, frequent meals. Administer cardiotonics, vasodilators, and ACE inhibitors as ordered.
Fluid Volume Excess related to decreased glomerular filtration rate, increased aldosterone, sodium and water retention, and increased antidiuretic hormone release	The patient will have normal fluid balance as evidenced by weight of 145 lbs, absence of edema, absence of crackles and wheezes in lungs, and ability to participate in activities of daily living without dyspnea.	Monitor for jugular venous distention and peripheral edema. Auscultate heart and lung sounds q 4 hr. Measure weight daily and intake and output accurately. Maintain intravenous lines and correct fluid infusion rate. Administer diuretics as ordered. Teach about sodium restriction and rationale. Protect edematous extremities from pressure or injury.
Impaired Gas Exchange related to pulmonary congestion	The patient's gas exchange will be evidenced by pulse oximetry >95%, normal skin color, absence of dyspnea, and clear lung sounds.	Assess lung sounds and respiratory status q 4 hr. Monitor O_2 saturation. Elevate head of bed. Administer oxygen as ordered. Assist to cough and deep breathe q 2 hr. Administer diuretics and morphine sulfate as ordered.
Activity Intolerance related to imbalance between oxygen supply and demand	The patient's activity tolerance will improve, as evidenced by performance of activities of daily living without excessive fatigue or dyspnea.	Assess response to activity when permitted. Monitor for dyspnea, changes in vital signs. Limit fatiguing activities. Gradually increase activity as tolerance improves.
Anxiety related to hypoxia, life-threatening situation	The patient's anxiety will be reduced, as evidenced by calm demeanor and statement that she feels less anxious.	Explain procedures and equipment. Tell patient about congestive heart failure and how it is being treated. Point out signs of improvement. Visit often, and respond to call bell promptly. Offer spiritual counselor if desired.
Deficient Knowledge of condition, treatment, self-care, and resources	The patient will verbalize information about her condition, treatment, self-care measures, and resources.	Provide simple explanation of congestive heart failure, its effects, and its treatment. As discharge nears, discuss diet, exercise, and drug therapy. Explain signs and symptoms that should be reported to physician. Advise of services of American Heart Association for information. Explore sources of support and need for visiting nurse or home health services.

? CRITICAL THINKING QUESTIONS

- What is the rationale behind sodium restriction in patients with heart failure?

- Describe three signs of improvement in a patient with heart failure.

they may metabolize and excrete drugs more slowly. This is especially true when the older patient is taking digitalis. Advise the patient to report early signs of digitalis toxicity: anorexia, nausea, and visual disturbances. Bed rest and stress reduction decrease the cardiac workload. When the patient is acutely ill, eliminate unnecessary activity. Give partial baths rather than complete bed baths. Assist the patient to change positions at least every 2 hours so that the skin can be inspected for signs of pressure. Visitors may be permitted, but advise them to sit quietly with the patient for short periods.

Pharmacology Capsule

Before each dose of digitalis, the apical pulse is counted for 1 full minute. If the heart rate is less than 60 bpm, the drug is withheld and the physician is notified.

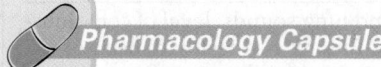

Pharmacology Capsule

The most common adverse effects of diuretic therapy are fluid and electrolyte imbalances.

Impaired Gas Exchange

Hypoxia is a common finding with left-sided heart failure because of pulmonary edema. It is common with right-sided heart failure because of decreased blood flow to the lungs. The patient with HF usually breathes more easily in a semi- or high-Fowler's position. Elevation of the upper body facilitates breathing by reducing pressure of the abdominal organs on the diaphragm. Supplemental oxygen is usually prescribed at 4 to 6 L/min per nasal cannula. The flow rate is reduced to 2 L/min for patients with chronic hypoxia. Assess respiratory status and blood gases frequently.

Prescribed bed rest can lead to other pulmonary complications related to immobility: hypostatic pneumonia and pulmonary emboli. Teach the patient to cough and deep breathe at least every 2 hours to promote respiratory excursion and to mobilize secretions. Other interventions to prevent complications of immobility are detailed in Chapter 21.

On discharge, the physician may order portable oxygen for use at home. The nurse or a respiratory therapist instructs the patient in the use of the equipment and the safety precautions to take when using oxygen (see Chapter 30).

Fluid Volume Excess

Fluid retention is a response to HF, an attempt to maintain normal cardiac output. Unfortunately, it compounds the problem by increasing the workload on the heart. Therefore measures are taken to reduce the fluid volume to normal while improving the function of the heart. Administer diuretics as ordered, and

monitor the patient for adverse effects. The most common adverse effects of diuretic therapy are fluid and electrolyte disturbances. Signs and symptoms that may indicate fluid or electrolyte disturbances include cardiac dysrhythmias, muscle weakness or twitching, cramps, changes in mental status, and abdominal distention. Frequent serum electrolyte measurements are usually ordered. Note the results and notify the physician of abnormal findings. If hourly urine output is being measured, report an output of less than 30 mL/hr to the physician as well. The patient should be weighed daily.

An intravenous catheter is usually placed to provide a line for drug administration. If intravenous fluids are administered, monitor the rate of administration very carefully. If fluid retention is not relieved by other means, fluid restriction may be instituted. All staff should know the exact amount of fluid allowed and must record all intake. Fluid restriction can be very uncomfortable for the patient. Even with fluid volume excess, the patient may feel thirsty because of electrolyte imbalances. Present oral fluids in small containers, and offer them at reasonable intervals. Frequently provide mouth care. The patient and family must understand why fluids are restricted so that the patient does not exceed the prescribed intake.

The most common therapeutic dietary measure for CHF is sodium restriction. The patient may be limited to 2 g of sodium/day. In severe cases, a limitation of 500 to 1000 mg/day may be prescribed. Reduced sodium intake decreases fluid retention, thereby reducing the cardiac workload. For a 2-g sodium diet, advise the patient to avoid foods high in sodium (a list should be provided), not to add salt before or after cooking, and to use no more than 2 cups of milk products daily. Patients often have difficulty changing their use of seasonings. Acknowledge the difficulty, and explain how sodium limitation contributes to improvement of cardiac function.

It is best to identify the type of diet to be prescribed on discharge as early as possible. This allows time for a dietary consultation to be arranged, which should be followed by reinforcement by the nurse. The person who prepares the patient's meals at home must be included in the teaching sessions.

Activity Intolerance

Frequent rest periods, pacing of activities, and relaxation techniques help the patient conserve energy. As the fluid volume is decreased and the cardiac output is increased, the patient can expect to be less fatigued.

The patient may be referred to a rehabilitation facility for exercise training. In general, the patient is advised to plan rest periods before and after tiring activities. Activity should be increased gradually, with rest periods taken when fatigue or dyspnea occurs. The physician may prescribe vasodilators for patients who experience chest pain with some activities. If monitor-

Health Promotion Considerations

Heart Failure: Discharge Instructions

A major goal for heart failure patients is to prevent rehospitalization. A critical factor in reaching this goal is for the patient or family member to recognize early signs and symptoms of worsening failure and to contact their provider. Examples of what to call about are the following: difficulty breathing (especially with activity); dry, hacking cough; weakness, increased fatigue; foot/ankle swelling; dizziness; and weight gain of 3-5 lbs in a week or less.

ing is indicated after discharge, request a referral to a home nursing agency.

Instruct the patient to notify the physician if the following problems develop: increasing dyspnea or edema, excessive fatigue, or pain that is not relieved by rest or prescribed medications. Early recognition of signs and symptoms that the patient's condition is deteriorating is crucial to avoiding rehospitalization (see the Health Promotion Considerations box above). In addition, advise the patient to avoid smoking and smoky environments and to refrain from wearing constricting clothing on the lower extremities.

Anxiety

Factors that may cause the patient to become anxious are dyspnea, unfamiliar setting and routines, and uncertainty about what is happening. Acknowledge the patient's anxiety and attempt to identify the basis. While taking immediate measures to relieve dyspnea, calmly explain what is being done. It may be helpful

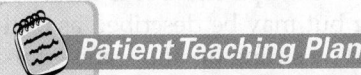

Patient Teaching Plan

Chronic Heart Failure

- Reducing sodium in your diet will help control swelling and reduce the workload on your heart.
- Excess weight makes your heart work harder. Your physician may prescribe a weight-loss diet for you.
- Take your medications as prescribed to improve your heart function. (Provide written information about drug names, actions, dosage, schedule, side and adverse effects, special aspects of administration, and interactions with other medications and food.)
- Gradually increase your activity. Avoid activity that causes shortness of breath or severe fatigue.
- Weigh yourself each morning, before breakfast, on the same scale and with the same amount of clothing.
- Contact your physician if you gain 2 or more pounds in a week, develop a persistent cough, or have shortness of breath or chest pain.
- Resources: The American Heart Association provides information about diet and exercise. The Visiting Nurses Association or a home health agency can monitor your condition and help you in your home.

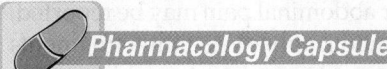

Pharmacology Capsule

Older adults are more susceptible to adverse drug effects because they metabolize and excrete drugs more slowly.

to tell the patient how specific measures help relieve symptoms. The presence of family members may have a calming effect if the relatives understand that they, too, must remain calm.

INFLAMMATORY DISORDERS

Inflammation of the heart most often results from systemic infections. The endocardium, myocardium, and pericardium may be affected.

Infective Endocarditis

Etiology and Risk Factors

Microbial infections of the endocardium affect primarily the valves. Organisms present in the blood easily colonize valves damaged by rheumatic heart disease or congenital defects or a mitral valve that is prolapsed.

Although the incidence of infective endocarditis (IE) has decreased with the use of antibiotics, there has been a resurgence of the problem in intravenous drug abusers. The more frequent use of invasive intravascular catheters for severely compromised patients has also contributed to the frequency with which IE occurs.

Patients with known valvular disease are also at risk for IE. They should be treated with prophylactic antibiotics before dental or invasive procedures. Immunosuppression or any source of bacterial contamination (lacerations, pneumonia, invasive procedures, intravenous drug use with contaminated needles) places patients at risk.

Pathophysiology

Pathogens, usually bacteria, enter the bloodstream by any of the previously mentioned means. The pathogen accumulates on the heart valves and/or the endocardium and forms vegetations. The mitral valve is the most common site for these vegetations. The turbulence of the blood flow through the heart weakens the vegetations and causes pieces to break off. These emboli can then obstruct circulation and impair tissue perfusion in the lungs, brain, kidneys, and heart.

Complications

Complications of IE include HF and embolization. HF is the most frequent cause of death with IE.

Signs and Symptoms

Patients usually present with fever, chills, malaise, fatigue, and weight loss. The fever may be low grade (37.2° to 38.9° C [99° to 102° F]) or higher (38.9° to 40.6° C [102° to 105° F]). The fever is accompanied by chills and night sweats. Chest or abdominal pain may be reported, possibly indicating embolization. Vegetative fragments and microembolizations can produce petechiae inside the mouth and on the ankles, feet, and antecubital areas. Pea-size, tender, red-to-purple lesions known as Osler's nodes may be on the patient's fingertips or toes.

Medical Diagnosis

The diagnosis of IE is based on the history, physical examination, and results of laboratory studies. A history of recent dental or surgical procedures may precede IE. Auscultation may reveal a heart murmur. Echocardiography helps visualize lesions and valvular regurgitation. Right-sided or left-sided heart failure may be evident. Serial blood cultures may give clues to the causative organism or organisms. The WBC count may be elevated.

Medical Treatment

Antimicrobials, rest, and limitation of activities are the primary therapeutic measures for IE. Antimicrobials are given intravenously for 2 to 6 weeks, depending on the organism. The patient is usually hospitalized for at least 1 week and then receives home intravenous therapy if that is available. Prophylactic anticoagulants may be necessary. Surgery may be necessary to replace an infected valve.

NURSING CARE of the Patient with Infective Endocarditis

Assessment

Complete assessment of the cardiac patient is summarized in Box 35-1. With IE, review the patient's history for risk factors, recent invasive procedures, known pathologic cardiac conditions, and onset of symptoms. Assess for temperature elevation, heart murmur, evidence of HF (cough, peripheral edema), and embolization.

Nursing Diagnoses, Goals, and Outcome Criteria: Infective Endocarditis

NURSING DIAGNOSES	GOALS AND OUTCOME CRITERIA
Decreased Cardiac Output related to impaired valve function	Normal cardiac output: normal pulse and blood pressure
Impaired Physical Mobility related to fatigue and prolonged intravenous therapy	Resumption of usual physical activities without symptoms: performance of activities of daily living without fatigue
Ineffective Tissue Perfusion related to embolization	Normal tissue perfusion: absence of dyspnea or signs of circulatory obstruction

Interventions

Administer prescribed antibiotics. Throughout the course of the illness, continue to assess cardiac output and monitor for complications. Teach the patient about the medications prescribed and any restrictions imposed. Encourage adequate rest, which is necessary during the healing process. Range-of-motion exercises may be necessary during the acute stage and until the patient is ambulatory.

Pericarditis

Etiology and Risk Factors

Pericarditis is an inflammation of the pericardium. It may be a primary disease or associated with another inflammatory process. The disease may be acute or chronic. Acute pericarditis is caused by viruses, bacteria, fungi, chemotherapy, or AMI (Dressler's syndrome). Chronic pericarditis is caused by tuberculosis, radiation, or metastases.

Pathophysiology

In acute pericarditis, the inflammatory process causes an increase in the amount of pericardial fluid and inflammation of the pericardial membranes. In chronic pericarditis (also called *constrictive pericarditis*), scarring of the pericardium fuses the visceral and parietal pericardia together. Loss of elasticity results from the scarring. This constrictive process prevents adequate ventricular filling.

Complications

The major complication of pericarditis is pericardial effusion or accumulation of fluid in the pericardial space. This may lead to cardiac tamponade when sufficient fluid accumulation decreases ventricular filling. The resulting drop in cardiac output is an emergency. It is treated with pericardiocentesis to remove the accumulated fluid.

Signs and Symptoms

Chest pain is the hallmark symptom of pericarditis. The pain is most severe on inspiration. It is most often sharp and stabbing but may be described as dull or burning. It is relieved by sitting up and leaning forward. Dyspnea, chills, and fever accompany pericarditis. ST segment elevation may be noted on the ECG. A pericardial rub may be present. Slowly progressing pericardial effusion does not result in hemodynamic compromise until 400 to 500 mL of fluid has accumulated. Rapidly accumulating fluid may precipitate sudden symptoms with only 250 mL of fluid.

Medical Diagnosis

The diagnostic challenge is to differentiate pericarditis from AMI. Serial ECGs show that the ST segment elevation resolves in several weeks. QRS voltage may decrease because of the accumulated fluid in the pericardial space. An echocardiogram may show pericardial thickening and effusion. Atrial fibrillation may occur because of the irritation. The CPK-MB may be elevated. Blood cultures may identify the causative organism or organisms. One differentiating feature to consider is that ischemic chest pain or angina is not relieved by position change and the chest pain that accompanies pericarditis often is relieved by change in position.

Medical Treatment

The patient is treated with analgesics, antipyretics, anti-inflammatory agents, and antibiotics. With constrictive pericarditis, the patient would be treated as for HF. Surgical creation of a pericardial window (removal of a segment of parietal pericardium to allow continuous drainage of pericardial fluid) may be necessary for treating chronic pericarditis with effusion.

NURSING CARE *of the Patient with Pericarditis*

Assessment

General nursing assessment of the cardiac patient is summarized in Box 35-1. With pericarditis, assessment of heart sounds is especially important.

Nursing Diagnoses, Goals, and Outcome Criteria: Pericarditis

NURSING DIAGNOSES	GOALS AND OUTCOME CRITERIA
Acute Pain related to pericardial inflammation	Pain relief: patient statement that pain is reduced, relaxed manner
Decreased Cardiac Output related to pericardial constriction	Improved cardiac output: normal pulse and blood pressure
Anxiety related to illness	Decreased anxiety: patient statement that anxiety is reduced, calm manner

Interventions

Rest and reduction of activity decrease the workload of the heart. Administer medications and teach the patient about the medications. Emotional support from the nursing staff and significant others is vital. The patient can be instructed in relaxation techniques. Moni-

What Does Culture Have to Do with Cardiomyopathy?

African-American males are at increased risk for dilated cardiomyopathy. Be alert to complaints of decreasing exercise tolerance and dyspnea in this population.

tor vital signs and auscultate for a pericardial friction rub. The rub is heard during inspiration with the diaphragm of the stethoscope placed between the second and the fourth intercostal spaces at the left sternal border. It is heard when there is no fluid accumulation. Distant heart sounds may be heard when there is fluid accumulation. Note pain characteristics and response to analgesics and anti-inflammatory agents. Monitor the ECG for dysrhythmias.

CARDIOMYOPATHY

Etiology and Risk Factors

Cardiomyopathy (CMP) is disease of the heart muscle. The cause of CMP is often unknown or CMP may be secondary to another disease process. The disease usually leads to heart failure. Three types of cardiomyopathy are recognized: dilated, hypertrophic, and restrictive (Fig. 35-12). Dilated cardiomyopathy is the most common type, accounting for 87% of cases (American Heart Association, 2007). There are three risk factors associated with dilated CMP: excessive use of alcohol, pregnancy, and infections. A relatively poor prognosis exists for dilated cardiomyopathy, with a 50% mortality in 5 years. Hypertrophic CMP often results from valvular heart disease or HTN. There also appears to be a genetic autosomal dominant link. Hypertrophic CMP is more common in younger individuals; approximately 36% of young athletes who died suddenly were found to have hypertrophic CMP. Restrictive cardiomyopathy is the least common type of CMP. Amyloidosis, sarcoidosis, and other immunosuppressive disorders may predispose individuals to restrictive cardiomyopathy.

Pathophysiology

With dilated cardiomyopathy, there is dilation of the ventricle and severely impaired systolic function. This causes decreased contractility, decreased ejection fraction and stroke volume, and increased left ventricular end-diastolic pressure. Pressure backup results in dilation of all four chambers and is most pronounced in the ventricles. Left ventricular failure and resulting HF

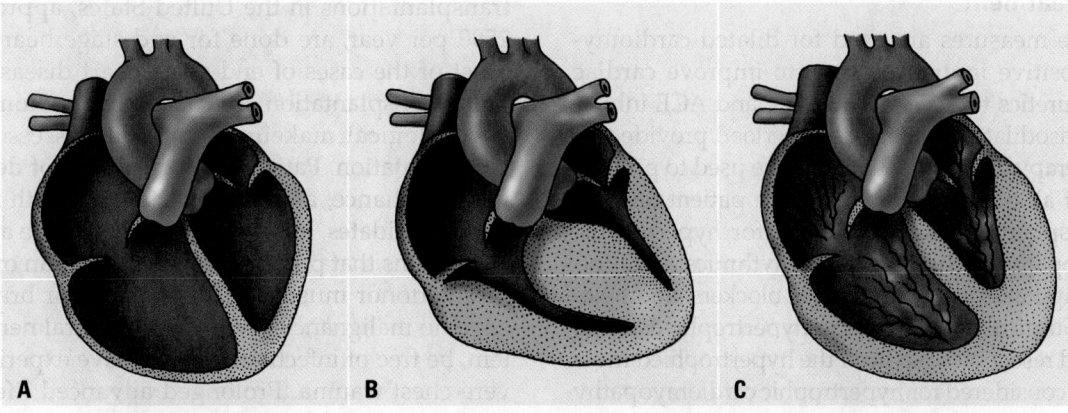

FIGURE **35-12** Cardiomyopathy. **A,** Dilated cardiomyopathy. **B,** Hypertrophic cardiomyopathy. **C,** Restrictive cardiomyopathy.

are seen as the result of excessive back pressure (see Fig. 35-12, *A*).

In hypertrophic cardiomyopathy, the LV hypertrophies and there is thickening of the ventricular septum. The left ventricular capacity decreases, and the outflow track of the left ventricle is decreased in size. The size of the LA increases as a result of the back pressure. The exterior heart size may appear to be normal. Ventricular dysrhythmias are common (see Fig. 35-12, *B*).

In restrictive cardiomyopathy, the myocardium becomes rigid and noncompliant. This reduces ventricular filling and cardiac output. Pulmonary and systemic congestion result (see Fig. 35-12, *C*).

Signs and Symptoms

Dilated cardiomyopathy is a progressive, chronic disease. The onset is gradual, with dyspnea, fatigue, left-sided heart failure, and moderate-to-severe cardiomegaly. Mitral valve regurgitation and S_3 and S_4 sounds are evident.

With hypertrophic cardiomyopathy, the progression of symptoms is slow. Dyspnea, orthopnea, angina, fatigue, syncope, palpitations, ankle edema, and S_4 sounds are found.

With restrictive cardiomyopathy, the primary symptom is exercise intolerance. Dyspnea, fatigue, right-sided HF, S_3 and S_4 sounds, and mitral valve regurgitation are also noted.

Medical Diagnosis

Diagnosis of dilated cardiomyopathy is made primarily on the basis of echocardiography results. Cardiac enlargement may be noted on chest radiography. The echocardiogram and chest radiograph are also used to diagnose hypertrophic cardiomyopathy. Other findings include a systolic murmur and atrial and ventricular dysrhythmias. An enlarged LV may be accompanied by left atrial enlargement. The diagnosis of restrictive cardiomyopathy is demonstrated by decreased cardiac output and HF. It must be differentiated from pericarditis. An echocardiogram may show thickened ventricular walls and small ventricular cavities.

Medical Treatment

Supportive measures are used for dilated cardiomyopathy. Positive inotropic drugs to improve cardiac output, diuretics to decrease preload, and ACE inhibitors and vasodilators to decrease afterload provide this type of therapy. Anticoagulants may be used to prevent thrombi. If all other measures fail, the patient needs a heart transplant. Medical treatment for hypertrophic cardiomyopathy includes antidysrhythmics, antibiotics, anticoagulants, calcium channel blockers, and beta-blockers. Surgical incision of the hypertrophied septal muscle and resection of some of the hypertrophied muscle may be considered for hypertrophic cardiomyopathy An alternative for select patients, nonsurgical reduction of the hypertrophied septum with alcohol ablation, may

be done percutaneously in the cardiac catheterization laboratory. Some patients with hypertrophic CMP may benefit from an implantable cardioverter-defibrillator placed to prevent sudden cardiac death. Treatment of restrictive cardiomyopathy is similar to that of HF therapy. Heart transplantation may be considered. Complications observed with all types of cardiomyopathy are dysrhythmias, HF, and death. There is a poor prognosis with cardiomyopathy. Mortality from CMP is highest in older adults, men, and blacks.

NURSING CARE *of the Patient with Cardiomyopathy*

Assessment

These patients are primarily assessed for heart failure. Be alert for dyspnea, cough, edema, dysrhythmias, and decreased cardiac output.

Nursing Diagnoses, Goals, and Outcome Criteria: Cardiomyopathy	
NURSING DIAGNOSES	GOALS AND OUTCOME CRITERIA
Decreased Cardiac Output related to ventricular failure	Improved cardiac output: normal pulse and blood pressure
Activity Intolerance related to poor tissue perfusion	Increased activity intolerance: performance of daily activities without excessive fatigue
Hopelessness related to poor prognosis	More positive outlook: patient's expression of feelings about condition and hopeful statements

Interventions

The care of these patients is similar to that of patients with HF. In addition, a hopeful atmosphere and a careful explanation of care requirements are necessary. Encourage the family to support the patient. The teaching plan guides the patient to make lifestyle changes. Encourage the patient to make decisions and choices.

CARDIAC TRANSPLANTATION

The first heart transplantation was performed in 1967 in South Africa by Dr. Christiaan Barnard. Today, heart transplantations in the United States, approximately 2500 per year, are done for end-stage heart disease. Most of the cases of end-stage heart disease that require transplantation are caused by cardiomyopathy. Psychological makeup is carefully assessed before transplantation. Patients with a history of depression, noncompliance, and inability to cope with stress are poor candidates. In the United States, there are federal regulations that prohibit the sale of human organs.

The donor must meet the criteria for brain death, have no malignancies outside the central nervous system, be free of infection, and not have experienced severe chest trauma. Prolonged advanced life support measures are avoided. The donor and recipient organs must be carefully matched. The donor heart size must

FIGURE 35-13 Heart transplantation. **A,** After the recipient is placed on cardiopulmonary by-pass, the heart is removed. **B,** The posterior walls of the recipient's left and right atria are left intact. **C,** The left atrium of the donor heart is anastomosed to the recipient's residual posterior atrial walls, and the other atrial walls, the atrial septum, and the great vessels are joined. **D,** Postoperative result.

be sufficient to meet the needs of the recipient. The donor heart may be preserved for 4 to 6 hours before transplantation.

The recipient must be free of infection at the time of transplantation. The patient is prepared for surgery as with any open-heart procedure. Cardiopulmonary bypass is initiated and the recipient's heart is removed except for the posterior portions of the atria (Fig. 35-13). The donor heart is trimmed and anastomosed to the remaining native heart. The patient is removed from bypass, the heart is restarted, and the chest is closed.

Aftercare of the patient with a heart transplant is similar to that of the patient after coronary artery bypass surgery. Hemodynamic monitoring, ventilation, cardiac assessment, care of chest tubes, and accurate intake and output measurements are vital. Immediately after surgery, the patient is placed in a private room in the intensive care unit. Modified protective isolation is used. The use of gowns, masks, and careful hand washing has been found to be superior to strict isolation techniques. Invasive lines/tubes (e.g., endotracheal tube, pulmonary artery catheter, Foley catheter, chest tubes) are removed as rapidly as possible to decrease the chance of infection. The prevention of postoperative infection is a major goal. Pulmonary infections are most frequently found after heart transplantations. Moving the patient from the intensive care unit to a private room and to home as soon as possible decreases the incidence of nosocomial infections. Patients and families are taught the signs and symptoms of infection and to avoid crowds and others with infections.

In addition, the patient with a transplant receives immunosuppressive medications. Lifelong immunosuppression is administered to prevent the body from rejecting the donated heart, which it recognizes as foreign tissue. Initially, large doses of corticosteroids are administered, and the dose is decreased over time. At the first indication of rejection (increased temperature, infection, dyspnea, malaise, fatigue, dysrhythmia), the steroid dose usually is increased. Other drugs used to prevent and treat rejection are azathioprine (Imuran) and cyclosporine (Sandimmune). Protocols using several immunosuppressive agents are considered most effective. Reduced dosages of each drug provide for a lower incidence of toxicity.

Rejection is monitored through endomyocardial biopsies. These are performed frequently in the immediate period after transplantation and less frequently over time. Patients are taught to monitor their own progress and to report problems promptly. Patients are followed closely by the transplant team and are observed for infection, rejection, quality of life, and complications. Common complications noted after heart transplantation are hypertension, elevated cholesterol, obesity, and malignancies.

SUDDEN CARDIAC DEATH

Sudden cardiac death occurs when heart activity and respirations cease abruptly. The most common underlying reason for sudden cardiac death is coronary heart disease.

Pharmacology Capsule

Patients taking immunosuppressive drugs to prevent rejection of transplanted tissue have reduced resistance to infection.

The sudden cardiac death event usually occurs during ordinary activity. It is often preceded by ventricular tachycardia or ventricular fibrillation and occasionally by severe bradydysrhythmias (slow, abnormal cardiac rhythms). An episode of sudden cardiac death may be the first indication of CAD. Other causes include left ventricular dysfunction, cardiomyopathy, hypokalemia, antidysrhythmics, liquid protein diets, and high alcohol consumption.

Those who survive an episode of sudden cardiac death need to have extensive testing done to determine the nature and cause of the sudden cardiac death. Many of these people will need treatment of CAD (medical therapy, PTCA, or coronary artery bypass grafting). Most of these patients have a lethal dysrhythmia that requires intervention. Diagnostic tests include 24-hour Holter monitoring and/or ILR, stress testing, and electrophysiology study. During the electrophysiology study, pacing electrodes are placed in the heart and electrical stimuli are used to elicit the dysrhythmia. This helps the physician determine appropriate medical therapy. In some patients, the dysrhythmia may be treated during the electrophysiology study with catheter ablation. The ablation (removal or "burning") of abnormal conduction pathways or irritable sites in the heart can prevent the dysrhythmia from recurring. Still other patients are treated effectively with antidysrhythmics such as amiodarone (Cordarone). If these therapies are ineffective, the patient may be considered a candidate for an implantable cardioverter/defibrillator (ICD).

Implantable Cardioverter/Defibrillator

The implantable cardioverter/defibrillator (ICD) is used to treat patients with life-threatening recurrent ventricular fibrillation who are unresponsive to medications or pacemakers. Its use has greatly decreased the mortality from sudden cardiac death. The device senses heart rate, diagnoses rhythm changes, and treats ventricular dysrhythmias. The ICD generator is implanted in the subcutaneous tissue over the pectoral muscle. The lead system is placed via a subclavian vein into the endocardium. The cardioverter recognizes ventricular fibrillation and ventricular tachycardia and uses the shocks to convert the dysrhythmia to normal sinus rhythm. When the ICD senses these lethal dysrhythmias, it delivers a shock of up to 35 joules to defibrillate. If the heart rhythm does not return to normal, the device can continue to deliver shocks. The patient is instructed to sit or lie down when experiencing a shock and to keep a record of the number of shocks delivered. Patients report that the shocks feel like a blow to the chest. In addition to defibrillation, the newer generation of ICDs are also able to function as antitachycardia and antibradycardia pacemakers, have event memory/retrieval, and are capable of programmed self-testing.

Complications. Complications associated with the ICD are inappropriate shocks, broken or displaced leads, and failure to deliver shocks as a result of battery failure or failure to recognize a dysrhythmia.

NURSING CARE *of the Patient with an Implantable Cardioverter/Defibrillator*

Nurses can promote psychosocial adaptation in patients with ICDs. The patient may be concerned with body image change and a fear of shocks. It is important to decrease anxiety about being shocked. Some patients become very dependent on the machine. These patients and families need much teaching and support. People who touch the patient during a shock will feel a tingling sensation, which is not harmful. An established support group for the patient and family is very helpful. The family must be instructed in cardiopulmonary resuscitation. An identification bracelet and a card with instructions about the ICD setting are carried at all times. Advise patients to avoid strong magnetic fields (metal detectors, power plants, MRI). The device and batteries should be checked every 2 months. Batteries should last 4 to 7 years.

VALVULAR DISEASE

The purpose of the heart valves is to maintain blood flow in one direction. If the valves are damaged through a congenital defect or acquired disease, their function is compromised. Stenosis and regurgitation are the two major valve problems. Stenosis is narrowing of the valvular opening. A stenotic valve limits the amount of blood ejected from one chamber to the next. Regurgitation, the inability of the valve to close completely, allows the blood to flow backward when a valve does not close efficiently. The left side of the heart is affected most often, and the mitral valve is the most frequently affected of all the valves. The pulmonic valve in the right side of the heart is infrequently affected. Only left-sided valvular disease is discussed here.

Antibiotics have decreased the incidence of valvular disease from rheumatic fever, but the incidence of nonrheumatic valvular disease has increased. Longer life span and intravenous drug abuse are the primary causes of the increasing incidence of nonrheumatic valvular disease.

Mitral Stenosis

Mitral stenosis is a narrowing of the opening in the mitral valve that impedes blood flow from the LA into the LV. The mitral valve leaflets become thickened and fibrotic. Rheumatic heart disease is the leading cause of mitral stenosis. Congenital malformations of the mitral valve occur but are not common. Other causes are calcium accumulation on valve leaflets and atrial myxomas (tumors).

Pathophysiology

The thickening of the valve structures reduces the outflow of blood from the LA to the LV. The LA dilates to accommodate the amount of blood not ejected, and left atrial pressure increases. As left atrial pressure increases, the blood volume backs up into the pulmonary system, increasing pulmonary pressures. This increases the workload on the right side of the heart, leading to right ventricular hypertrophy. Eventually, the RV fails, and cardiac output decreases because less blood is delivered to the LV.

Signs and Symptoms

Symptoms may begin soon after the disease process or may be delayed for many years. Dyspnea, fatigue, cough, chest pain, and activity intolerance are the most frequent symptoms. Exertional dyspnea and pulmonary edema occur as blood backs up in the pulmonary system and serous fluid leaks into the pulmonary tissues. Because stenosis causes turbulent blood flow through the valve, a murmur is present during diastole (best heard at the apex of the heart).

Medical Diagnosis

Diagnosis is made on the basis of the patient history, physical examination, and results of diagnostic procedures. The chest radiograph shows left atrial, right ventricular, and pulmonary vascular enlargement. Echocardiography, often transesophageal echocardiography, is used to visualize the mitral valve. Cardiac catheterization is used to confirm the diagnosis and determine the extent of the disease process.

Medical Treatment

When symptomatic, the patient with mitral stenosis is treated as for CHF with drug therapy, sodium and fluid restrictions, and activity restriction. Digoxin, diuretics, beta-blockers, and antidysrhythmics may be prescribed. If the patient has atrial fibrillation, anticoagulants also may be prescribed. Prophylactic antibiotics are prescribed before any invasive procedure for patients with mitral stenosis because bacteria tend to cluster on the damaged valves.

Surgical Treatment

Surgical treatment includes commissurotomy, mitral valve replacement, and balloon valvuloplasty. Commissurotomy is excision of parts of the leaflets to enlarge the opening. The mitral valve may be replaced with a biologic or synthetic valve (Fig. 35-14). Both commissurotomy and mitral valve replacement require major surgery with cardiopulmonary bypass.

Balloon valvuloplasty, a procedure done in the cardiac catheterization laboratory, has been very successful in dilating stenosed heart valves. It is less invasive than valve replacement or commissurotomy. To dilate the mitral valve, a balloon catheter (like the one used for PTCA) is threaded from the femoral artery to the mitral valve. The balloon is positioned in the valve and inflated until the valve opens sufficiently. After the procedure, the patient is observed closely in an intensive care unit for dysrhythmias and complications.

FIGURE 35-14 Types of prosthetic and tissue valves. **A,** Bileaflet mechanical valve. **B,** Porcine heterograft. **C,** Carpentier-Edwards aortic pericardial valve.

Complications include valve regurgitation, restenosis, perforation of the myocardium, and, rarely, systemic embolization.

NURSING CARE *of the Patient with Mitral Stenosis*
Assessment

It is most important to obtain a complete history as summarized in Box 35-1 and a record of signs and symptoms being experienced. Take the vital signs, and auscultate for heart murmurs. The murmur of mitral stenosis is described as rumbling and low pitched. It is heard best at the apex of the heart. The ECG may show a notched P wave, indicating left atrial enlargement. Atrial fibrillation is frequently seen. Tachycardia and tachypnea are common signs. The pulse pressure may be decreasing, indicating low cardiac output. Jugular venous distention and crackles are found with pulmonary congestion.

Nursing Diagnoses, Goals, and Outcome Criteria:
Mitral Stenosis

The nursing diagnoses and goals for mitral stenosis are the same as those for CHF and for all valvular diseases:

Nursing Diagnoses	Goals and Outcome Criteria
Decreased Cardiac Output related to narrowing or insufficiency of valvular competence	Increased cardiac output: normal pulse and blood pressure
Impaired Gas Exchange related to pulmonary congestion	Improved gas exchange: clear breath sounds, normal arterial blood gases
Activity Intolerance related to imbalance between oxygen supply and demand	Improved activity tolerance: performance of daily activities without excessive fatigue
Fluid Volume Excess related to decreased glomerular filtration rate, increased aldosterone, sodium and water retention, and increased antidiuretic hormone release	Normal fluid balance: no edema, clear breath sounds, fluid output equal to or exceeds fluid intake

Interventions

See the Nursing Care of the Patient with Heart Failure section on pp. 662 to 665 for the remainder of the nursing process.

Mitral Regurgitation

Mitral regurgitation (insufficiency) allows blood to flow back into the LA during diastole. The valve does not close completely because one or both of the valve leaflets becomes rigid and shortens.

The LA and LV hypertrophy as a result of the backflow of blood against the incompetent valve. Left ventricular hypertrophy is compensatory in an attempt to maintain cardiac output. Eventually, the left side of the heart fails, and symptoms are then the same as those with mitral stenosis.

The murmur of mitral regurgitation is high pitched and blowing and occurs during systole. It is best heard at the apex and may radiate to the axilla. With severe disease, S_3 and S_4 sounds may be auscultated. Atrial fibrillation occurs as the LA enlarges.

Mitral regurgitation is treated with vasodilators to decrease the afterload and therefore the regurgitation. Other medical treatment includes activity restriction, dietary sodium limitation, diuretics, and digitalis. Surgical treatment includes annuloplasty and mitral valve replacement. Annuloplasty is reconstruction of the leaflets and the annulus.

Mitral Valve Prolapse

The mitral valve prolapses when one or both leaflets enlarge and protrude into the LA during systole. It has a tendency to run in families and may be caused by heart infections, rheumatic fever, or a wide variety of congenital anomalies. The disease is usually benign but may progress to mitral insufficiency. Mitral valve prolapse occurs in approximately 3% of the population (American Heart Association, 2007). Most victims are women 20 to 55 years of age.

In most patients, symptoms do not occur or may occur with stress. Symptoms include chest pain, palpitations, dizziness, and syncope. Some patients exhibit dysrhythmias. The ECG usually shows normal findings. Evidence of mitral valve prolapse may be found on echocardiography. The problem is often controlled with stress-reduction techniques. Beta-blockers may be prescribed to decrease syncope, palpitations, and severe chest pain. Therapeutic management is matched to the degree of symptoms.

Aortic Stenosis

Etiology and Risk Factors

Stenosis of the aortic valve occurs when the valve cusps become fibrotic and calcify. It may be caused by a congenital malformation or result from rheumatic fever, syphilis, or the aging process (atherosclerosis and calcification). When seen in younger patients, it is most often caused by a congenital malformation. The aortic valve is most commonly diseased in the aging population.

Pathophysiology

The valve opening decreases to one-third normal size before symptoms occur. As flow is impeded through the narrowed valve, the LV hypertrophies to compensate for the extra pressure needed to eject blood. The LA also compensates by delivering a strong atrial kick. These compensatory mechanisms allow normal function until atrial fibrillation disrupts the atrial kick or until the LV hypertrophies to the point of dysfunction, with decreased cardiac output and myocardial ischemia. With left ventricular dysfunction, blood backs up into the LA and the pulmonary system. If uncorrected, eventually the right side of the heart fails.

Signs and Symptoms

The patient complains of dyspnea on exertion, angina, and syncope. Fatigue, orthopnea, and paroxysmal nocturnal dyspnea are late symptoms and indicate heart failure. A systolic murmur may occur.

Medical Diagnosis

The chest radiograph shows atrial and ventricular enlargement, which are late signs. The murmur of aortic stenosis is heard best in the aortic area, the second intercostal space to the right of the sternum. The echocardiogram shows left ventricular wall thickening. An exercise tolerance test may be ordered to evaluate heart function.

Medical Treatment

Prophylactic antibiotics are prescribed to prevent IE with dental and invasive procedures. Heart failure is treated with digoxin, diuretics, a low-sodium diet, and activity restriction. Surgical treatment includes balloon valvuloplasty and aortic valve replacement.

NURSING CARE *of the Patient with Aortic Stenosis*

Monitor for a bounding arterial pulse and widened pulse pressure. The nursing process is the same as for HF (see Nursing Care Plan: The Patient with Heart Failure on p. 663).

Aortic Regurgitation

Fibrosis and thickening of the aortic cusps progress until the valve no longer maintains unidirectional blood flow. Aortic regurgitation (insufficiency) is caused primarily by rheumatic fever. Other causes include IE, blunt chest trauma, calcification of the valve, and chronic hypertension.

Regurgitation of blood into the LV during diastole increases the amount of blood in the LV. The LV dilates and hypertrophies. Myocardial ischemia and left ventricular failure occur. Blood backs up into the pulmonary system and eventually right ventricular failure occurs.

The murmur of aortic regurgitation is high pitched and blowing and occurs in diastole. It is auscultated best at the aortic area. The point of maximal impulse may be shifted to the left and down. Tachycardia and palpitations are compensatory mechanisms. Later signs of HF such as fatigue, dyspnea, and ascites develop. A widened pulse pressure (increased difference between systolic and diastolic pressures) results from a low diastolic pressure. S_3 and S_4 sounds are often auscultated.

Left atrial and ventricular dilation are noted on chest radiography. The echocardiogram shows left ventricular dilation. Cardiac catheterization is used to determine the extent of incompetence.

As with other patients with valve disease, these patients have prophylactic antibiotics prescribed before invasive procedures. Digoxin and diuretics are prescribed for left ventricular hypertrophy. Aortic valve replacement provides long-term correction.

ELECTROCARDIOGRAM MONITORING

Nurses working in critical care areas are responsible for monitoring and interpreting ECGs. Patients usually are monitored continuously at the bedside and have intermittent monitoring through a 12-lead ECG.

12-LEAD ELECTROCARDIOGRAM

A 12-lead ECG looks at the heart from 12 directions or perspectives. This permits more precise evaluation of the heart's electrical activity. Three leads are placed on the limbs (leads I, II, and III), three leads are augmented (aVR, aVL, and aVF), and there are six chest, or precordial, leads (V_1 to V_6). Electricity flows from the negative to the positive lead. If the depolarization wave flows toward the positive pole (electrode), the deflection is upright. If the wave flows away from the positive pole, the deflection is negative.

CONTINUOUS MONITORING

For continuous ECG monitoring, only one or two single leads are used. Most units that perform continuous monitoring use the five-lead system with four limb electrodes and a chest electrode (which is placed at one of the V lead sites). The electrodes are held in place by adhesive pads. Thoroughly clean the electrode sites before applying the pads. Change the pads according to agency policy. Monitor the skin for irritation or breakdown. The lead monitored depends on the purpose of the monitoring (e.g., detect dysrhythmias, detect ischemia).

INTERPRETATION OF ELECTROCARDIOGRAMS

To interpret an ECG strip, the reader is referred to Figure 35-15. The graph paper consists of horizontal and vertical small and large squares. The horizontal axis measures time; the vertical axis measures voltage. Each small square represents 0.04 second on the horizontal axis and 1 mm on the vertical axis. Each large square, bounded by heavy lines, is made up of five small squares and represents 0.20 second and 5 mm. The electrical activity of the heart is represented by deflections, positive and negative, from the baseline. A deflection is an upward or downward movement from the baseline. The baseline is called the *isoelectric line*. The first positive deflection (upward movement) is the small, rounded P wave that represents atrial depolarization. The second positive deflection is the peaked QRS complex that represents ventricular depolarization. The Q is the first negative deflection, meaning the line moves below the isoelectric line. The R wave corresponds to the patient's pulse. Atrial repolarization occurs during ventricular depolarization and is obscured by the QRS complex. The third deflection is the rounded T wave, which represents ventricular repolarization. The fourth deflection, if present, is the U wave. It is small, rounded, and usually indicates electrolyte imbalance (hypokalemia).

The PR interval represents the time it takes the impulse to travel from the atria through the AV node to the ventricles. The PR interval is measured from the beginning of the P wave to the Q wave. The normal PR interval is from 0.12 to 0.20 second. The QRS complex

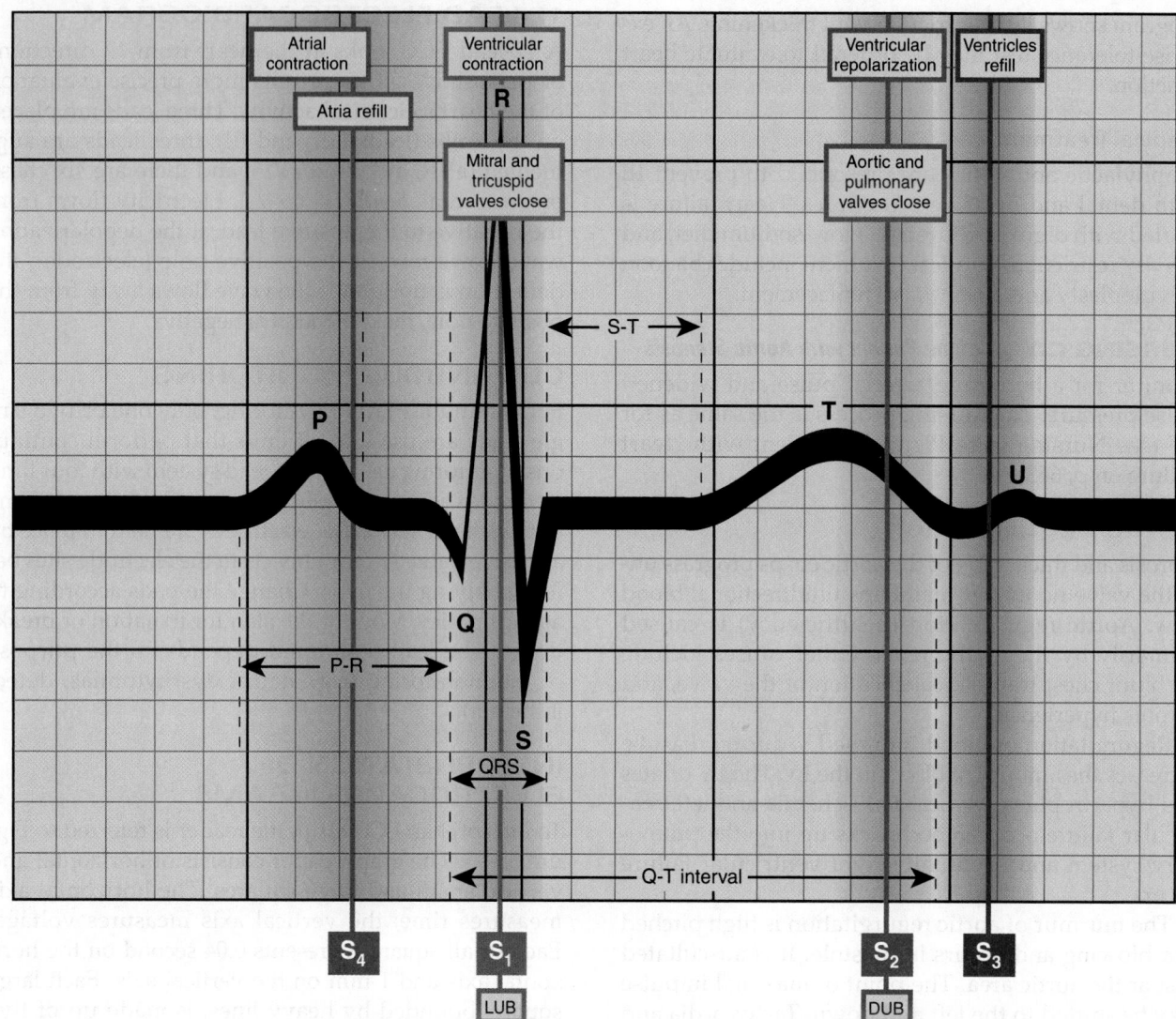

FIGURE **35-15** Relationship between the cardiac cycle and the heart sounds.

is measured from the point at which the Q leaves the isoelectric line to the point at which the S returns to the isoelectric line. The normal QRS complex is 0.06 to 0.10 second. The ST segment represents the time from ventricular depolarization to ventricular repolarization. The ST segment should be along the isoelectric line. The QT segment represents ventricular refractory time. It is measured from the beginning of the QRS complex to the end of the T wave. The normal QT segment time range varies with heart rate; therefore it is necessary to compare the QT obtained with a table (QT tables are available in most textbooks dealing with dysrhythmias). The QT segment is affected by age, gender, and heart rate.

Criteria for Interpreting Electrocardiograms

Criteria have been established for interpreting an ECG strip. The ECG is evaluated for rate, regularity, P waves, PR interval, and QRS complexes (Table 35-8).

Rate Calculation. Most ECG strips have tic marks indicating 3-second time periods. There are several ways to calculate heart rate from the ECG strip. The quickest but least accurate method is to count the number of P waves (for atrial rate) or R waves (for ventricular rate) in a 6-second strip (between 3 tic marks or 30 large squares) and multiply by 10 for the estimate of the number of beats per minute. For example, if there are six R waves in a 6-second strip, the heart rate is 60 bpm.

The more accurate method uses the number of small squares between two P waves (atria) or two R waves (ventricles). Divide 1500 by the number of small squares. For example, if there are 25 small squares between two R waves, the rate is 60 bpm (1500 divided by 25). The atrial rate is determined by the number of P waves and the ventricular rate by the number of QRS complexes. The normal rate is from 60 to 100 bpm.

Rhythm. The consecutive P-P intervals for the atria and the consecutive R-R intervals for ventricles are measured for consistency. Using calipers or a blank piece of paper, note the distance between R waves. If the distances do not vary more than one small square, the rhythm is considered regular. If the distances are greater than one small square, the rhythm is irregular.

Table 35-8 | *Criteria for Electrocardiogram Interpretation*

Rate	Are the atrial and ventricular rates the same as measured by the P-P and R-R intervals?
Rhythm	Is the rate regular or irregular? If irregular, is there a pattern? Are these ectopic beats? Where do they occur?
P waves	Is there a P wave before every QRS complex? Does each P wave have the same size and shape?
PR interval (PRI)	Are all the PRIs the same length? If not, is there a pattern to the irregularity? Are the PRIs within normal range?
QRS complexes	Do all the QRS complexes look alike? Are all the QRS complexes within the normal range (0.06-0.10 sec)?
ST segment	Is the ST segment isoelectric, depressed, or elevated?
T waves	Do all the T waves look alike? Are the T waves upright or inverted?

FIGURE **35-16 Normal sinus rhythm.** Each segment between the dark lines (above the monitor strip) represents 3 seconds, when the monitor is set at a speed of 25 mm/sec. Characteristics: **Rate**—60 to 100 bpm; **Regularity**—essentially regular (P-to-P and R-to-R intervals are regular with only minor variation); **P wave, PR interval**—there is a P before every QRS; each P wave is the same size and shape; PR interval is between 0.12 and 0.20 sec; **QRS**—falls between 0.06 and 0.10 sec; **T wave**—rounded, all the same shape. Interpretation: Normal sinus rhythm.

P Waves. The next evaluation is of P waves. Is there a P wave before each QRS complex? If so, the rhythm originates in the SA node. Do all the P waves appear the same size and shape? If so, the impulse originates in the SA node.

PR Interval. Does the PR interval fall within the normal range of 0.12 to 0.20 second? If so, there is no interference in conduction from the SA to the AV node.

QRS Complex. Does the QRS complex fall within the 0.06- to 0.10-second range? If the QRS is prolonged (0.12 second or greater), there is a delay in conduction through the ventricles.

ST Segment. Examine the ST segment. Is it isoelectric? Or is it depressed or elevated?

T Waves. Are the T waves rounded and the same size and shape? Do the T waves follow the QRS complexes?

QT Interval. Measuring the QT interval is not always part of dysrhythmia interpretation. The QT interval, if measured, should be compared with the QT interval table. The QT interval may be affected by electrolyte imbalances and drugs.

Normal Sinus Rhythm

The most common cardiac rhythm is sinus in origin because the impulse originates in the SA node, is conducted normally, and meets all of the criteria established earlier. Normal sinus rhythm is displayed in Figure 35-16.

Common Dysrhythmias

A dysrhythmia is a disturbance of the rhythm of the heart caused by a problem in the conduction system. Dysrhythmias are categorized according to the site of the origin of the impulse formation. Dysrhythmias originating in the atria are called *atrial dysrhythmias.* Dysrhythmias originating in the AV node are called *junctional* or *escape rhythms.* Dysrhythmias originating below the AV node are called *ventricular.* Blocks are interruptions in impulse conduction. Dysrhythmias and blocks have characteristics that are noted on the ECG. See Figures 35-17 through 35-30 for examples. Antidysrhythmic drugs are used to treat dysrhythmias and restore normal sinus rhythm.

HEMODYNAMIC MONITORING

In addition to noninvasive cardiac assessment and ECG monitoring, more sophisticated measures may be needed to determine what is going on within the heart or vascular system. Nurses who work in intensive care

FIGURE **35-17** **Sinus bradycardia.** Characteristics: **Rate**—less than 60 bpm; **Regularity**—normal; **P wave, PR interval**—normal; **QRS**—normal; **T wave**—normal. Interpretation: All characteristics are within normal ranges except for the rate, which is slow. Causes: Drugs, including digitalis and beta-blockers, vagal stimulation (Valsalva maneuver), severe pain, hyperkalemia, infection, and myocardial infarction. Frequently seen in athletes as a result of conditioning. Symptoms: Dizziness, syncope, chest pain, hypotension, sweating, nausea, dyspnea, and disorientation; sometimes no symptoms. Treatment: Not treated unless the patient is symptomatic. The underlying cause is treated. Atropine may be given to increase the heart rate. Isoproterenol is used with extreme caution. A pacemaker may be needed.

FIGURE **35-18** **Sinus tachycardia.** Characteristics: **Rate**—greater than 100; usually less than 150 bpm; **Regularity**—regular; **P wave, PR interval**—P waves may be buried in T wave of preceding beat with very rapid rates, more than 140 bpm; **QRS**—normal; **T wave**—normal. Interpretation: All characteristics are within normal range except for the rate, which is excessive. Causes: Fever, dehydration, hypovolemia, increased sympathetic nervous system stimulation, stress, exercise, and acute myocardial infarction. Symptoms: Palpitations most common. Angina and decreased cardiac output from the decreased ventricular filling time may also occur. Treatment: Correction of underlying cause. Elimination of caffeine, nicotine, and alcohol. Vagal stimulation may decrease the rate but does not treat the cause. Treatment: Beta-blockers.

areas frequently work with patients who have central venous catheters, pulmonary artery catheters, or arterial lines.

CENTRAL VENOUS CATHETER

The central venous catheter is placed through the skin, into a venous access (brachial, femoral, subclavian, or jugular sites), and threaded into the RA. The catheter may have one to three lumens. With this catheter, the pressure in the RA (called *right atrial pressure* [*RAP*] or *central venous pressure* [*CVP*]) can be measured. This measurement is used as an indication of fluid volume. The normal CVP or RAP is 2 to 6 mm Hg. Measure-

ments below normal indicate hypovolemia, and measurements above normal indicate hypervolemia. This catheter may also be used to infuse fluids, blood and blood products, and medications as well as to withdraw blood for analysis.

PULMONARY ARTERY CATHETER

The pulmonary artery (PA) catheter, frequently called a *Swan-Ganz catheter*, is longer than the central venous catheter. It is inserted like the central venous catheter and is threaded through the RA, the tricuspid valve, the RV, the pulmonic valve, and into the pulmonary artery. The catheter is balloon tipped and flows with

FIGURE **35-19** **Sinus dysrhythmia.** Characteristics: **Rate**—normal; **Regularity**—slightly irregular, varies with respirations; **P wave, PR interval**—P-to-P intervals vary, the difference between the shortest and longest P-to-P interval is greater than 0.12 sec; the PR interval is normal; **QRS**—normal; **T wave**—normal. Interpretation: The rate varies with respirations. Considered normal when the rhythm varies in relation to the respiratory cycle: The R-to-R interval is shorter during inspiration; therefore the rate is increased; the R-to-R interval is longer during expiration; therefore the rate is decreased. Causes: When unrelated to respirations, is often the result of digoxin toxicity, increased intracranial pressure, or inferior wall myocardial infarction. In older adults, marked variation may indicate a condition known as *sick sinus syndrome.* Symptoms: Usually none. Treatment: If treatment is necessary, atropine is used and the underlying problem is treated.

FIGURE **35-20** **First-degree atrioventricular (AV) block.** Characteristics: **Rate**—normal; **Regularity**—regular; **P wave, PR interval**—all P waves are conducted to the ventricles, but AV conduction is prolonged through the AV node; PR interval is greater than 0.20 sec and constant; **QRS**—normal; **T wave**—normal. Interpretation: The PR interval is prolonged. Causes: Increased vagal tone, coronary artery disease, digoxin toxicity, heart infections, and quinidine. Symptoms: Usually none, may be bradycardic. Treatment: Correction of underlying cause.

the blood. Different waveforms are seen on an oscilloscope as the catheter moves through the different areas of the heart. Pulmonary artery catheters have multiple lumens and are approximately 110 cm (44 inches) long. Various lumens are used to measure the pulmonary capillary wedge pressure, inflate the balloon, measure RAP, determine cardiac output, and administer fluids and drugs. Newer catheters incorporate fiberoptics for continuous monitoring of saturated venous oxygenation (SvO_2), a measure of tissue perfusion or continuous cardiac output.

The purpose of a pulmonary artery catheter is to measure right-sided heart pressures and pulmonary artery pressures and to assess left-sided heart func-

tion. The proximal port is used to measure the RAP or CVP (normal value, 2-6 mm Hg). The distal port measures the pulmonary artery pressure (normal value, 20-30/0-10). The lungs are low-pressure organs unless the patient has COPD.

The pulmonary capillary wedge pressure is used to assess the function of the left side of the heart. To determine the pulmonary capillary wedge pressure, the balloon is inflated with up to 1.5 mL of air. This allows the tip of the catheter to float into a pulmonary capillary until it occludes the capillary. This measures the pressure ahead of the catheter, therefore the left ventricular heart function. The normal pulmonary capillary wedge pressure is 4 to 12 mm Hg. Once the pressure is

Mobitz's type I (Wenckebach's)

FIGURE **35-21 Second-degree atrioventricular block: type I (Mobitz I; Wenckebach).** Characteristics: **Rate**—atrial rate is greater than ventricular rate; **Regularity**—atrial rate is regular; ventricular rate is irregular; **P wave, PR interval**—there are more P waves than QRS complexes; the PR interval increases until a P wave is not followed by a QRS; **QRS**—some are absent; **T wave**—absent when the QRS is dropped. Interpretation: Progressively lengthening PR interval and a dropped beat. Causes: Myocardial ischemia with progressive increase in conduction time through the sinoatrial node, inferior wall myocardial infarction, digoxin toxicity, and electrolyte imbalance. Symptoms: Decreased blood pressure and syncope, if any. Treatment: Atropine, pacemaker.

Mobitz's type II

FIGURE **35-22 Second-degree atrioventricular (AV) block: type II (Mobitz II).** Characteristics: **Rate**—atrial rate regular; ventricular rate may be less than atrial; **Regularity**—irregular; **P wave, PR interval**—P-to-P intervals are regular; PR interval is fixed at normal or greater than 0.2 sec; **QRS**—QRS complexes do not always follow P waves; the QRS may be normal or widened; **T wave**—normal after completed conduction. Interpretation: Sudden blocking of a QRS. Causes: Conduction abnormalities in the ventricles, acute myocardial infarction. Symptoms: Hypotension, bradycardia; decreased cardiac output with frequent blocks. Treatment: Pacemaker may be necessary to prevent third-degree AV block or asystole.

recorded, the balloon is deflated. This pressure is lower when fluid is restricted, when diuretics are being administered, and when patients are receiving vasodilators such as nitroglycerin or morphine. The pressure is elevated with excess fluid, when fluid volume expanders such as albumin, dextran, or hetastarch are being administered, or in left heart dysfunction.

Cardiac Output

With a pulmonary artery catheter in place, cardiac output can be measured continuously or by the thermodilution method. The normal cardiac output is 4 to 8 L/min. Stress increases the cardiac output. Cardiac output may decrease with AMI, HF, bradycardia, tachycardia, and some drugs. It is important for the nurse to use consistent technique in measuring cardiac output.

Mixed Venous Oxygen Saturation

PA catheters may have sensors in place that allow for measurement of mixed venous oxygen saturation (SvO_2) or, if the sensor is not part of the catheter, a blood sample can be obtained from the distal port (which opens in the pulmonary artery). Blood in the pulmonary artery is the blood returned from all of the organs and tissues in the body and mixed in the PA. When the oxygen saturation of this mixed venous blood is measured (in

Text continued on p. 682.

FIGURE **35-23** **Third-degree atrioventricular (AV) block.** Characteristics: **Rate**—atrial rate is faster than ventricular rate; ventricular rate is generally less than 45 bpm; **Regularity**—irregular; **P wave, PR interval**—no relationship exists between the P waves and the QRS complexes; **QRS**—atria and ventricles are beating independently; the QRS is ventricular in origin; **T wave**—normal. Interpretation: Impulses originating in the sinoatrial node are blocked at the AV node. The ventricles respond to a secondary pacemaker. Causes: Digoxin toxicity, conduction damage during mitral valve replacement, hypoxia, and rheumatic fever. Symptoms: Hypotension, syncope, decreased cardiac output. The underlying cause is treated. Treatment: Atropine, pacemaker, isoproterenol with extreme caution. Do not administer lidocaine, which could suppress ventricular response.

FIGURE **35-24** **Sinus arrest.** Characteristics: **Rate**—normal or slow before arrest; **Regularity**—regular except when interrupted by a dropped beat; **P wave, PR interval**—normal when present; absent during pause; **QRS**—normal to absent during pause; **T wave**—normal to absent during pause. Interpretation: A pause in the cardiac cycle as the sinoatrial node fails to generate an impulse. Causes: Degenerative heart disease, myocardial infarction, digoxin toxicity. Symptoms: Bradycardia, decreased cardiac output. Treatment: Pacemaker if the patient experiences repeated episodes.

FIGURE **35-25** **Asystole.** Characteristics: **Rate**—none; **Regularity**—none; **P wave, PR interval**—there may be P waves but none is conducted; the PR interval is not measurable; **QRS**—absent; **T wave**—absent. Interpretation: Straight or only slightly wavy baseline. Causes: Severe metabolic deficit, acute respiratory failure, and myocardial damage. Symptoms: Loss of consciousness, no pulse. Treatment: Immediate response with cardiopulmonary resuscitation and advanced cardiac life support; epinephrine, atropine; transcutaneous pacemaker.

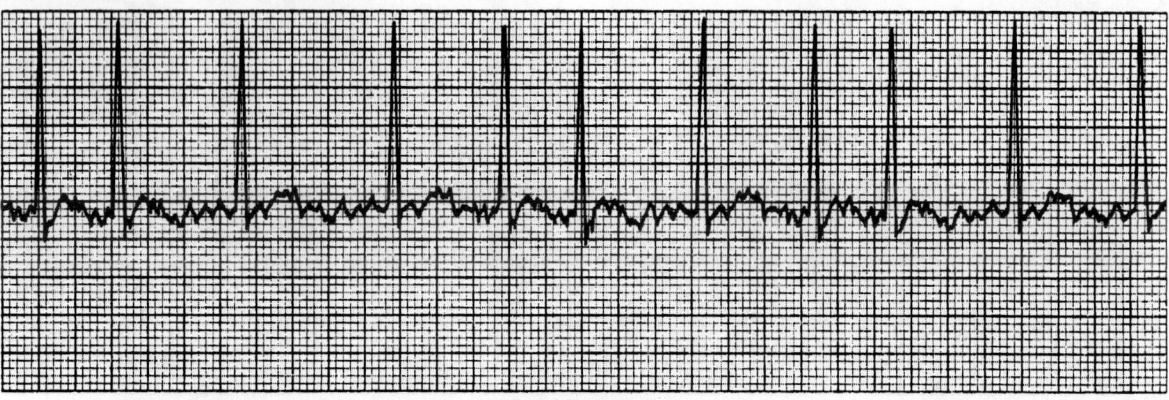

Atrial fibrillation

FIGURE 35-26 Atrial fibrillation. Characteristics: **Rate**—atrial rate is greater than 400 bpm if it can be determined at all; the ventricular rate is 100 to 150 bpm; **Regularity**—very irregular; **P wave, PR interval**—no P waves; PR interval unmeasurable; **QRS**—normal; **T wave**—undeterminable. Interpretation: The baseline between QRS complexes is wavy. Causes: Rheumatic fever, mitral valve stenosis, coronary artery disease, hypertension, cardiomyopathy, myocardial infarction, hyperthyroidism, chronic obstructive pulmonary disease, and heart failure. It is frequently seen in older adults after the administration of anesthetic. Symptoms: May have palpitations, angina, and decreased cardiac output. The concerns with atrial fibrillation are development of an atrial thrombus and loss of atrial kick from ineffective atrial function. Treatment: calcium channel blockers or beta-blockers to reduce a rapid ventricular response; anticoagulants to prevent embolization; synchronized cardioversion or drug therapy (amiodarone or ibutilide) to restore a normal rhythm.

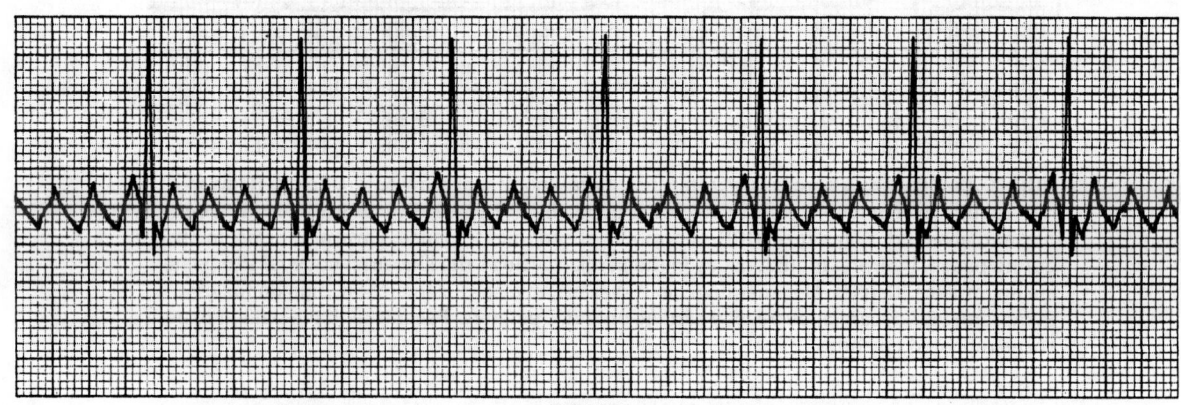

Atrial flutter

FIGURE 35-27 Atrial flutter. Characteristics: **Rate**—atrial rate 250 to 350 bpm; ventricular rate 60 to 100 bpm; **Regularity**—atrial rate regular; ventricular regular or irregular; **P wave, PR interval**—P waves are rounded "F" or flutter waves; PR interval unmeasurable; **QRS**—usually normal; **T wave**—undeterminable. Interpretation: The sawtooth P waves are characteristic; there may be a pattern to the number of flutter waves and ventricular response: 4 to 1, 3 to 1, or 2 to 1. Causes: Coronary artery disease, myocardial damage, valvular disease, heart infections, and digoxin toxicity. Symptoms: Palpitations, decreased cardiac output. Treatment: Harder to treat than atrial fibrillation. Calcium channel blockers or beta-blockers to control the rate. Synchronized cardioversion or drug therapy (amiodarone or ibutilide) to convert the rhythm.

Premature ventricular contraction

FIGURE **35-28 Premature ventricular contractions (PVCs).** Characteristics: **Rate**—normal; **Regularity**—irregular because of PVCs; **P wave, PR interval**—no P wave with the PVC; inverted P wave may follow a PVC; there is no PR interval with the PVC; **QRS**—wide and bizarre in the PVC; **T wave**—opposite deflection to the PVC. Interpretations: Wide QRS. Unifocal PVCs originate from one site. Multifocal PVCs arise from different ventricular sites and have a poorer prognosis. Causes: Digoxin toxicity, hypokalemia, hypercalcemia, sympathetic nervous system stimulation (stress, caffeine, nicotine), and excess catecholamine release. Symptoms: The patient may or may not note a "skipped" beat. The PVCs are not palpable at peripheral pulse sites, but a pause may be observed. Cardiac output diminishes with frequent PVCs. Treatment: No treatment necessary for infrequent PVCs, which probably occur undetected in most people; treat the cause and administer antidysrhythmics for symptomatic or frequent PVCs.

FIGURE **35-29 Ventricular tachycardia.** Characteristics: **Rate**—100 to 250 bpm; there is no relationship between the atrial and the ventricular contractions; **Regularity**—ventricular rhythm usually regular; **P wave, PR interval**—absent; **QRS**—wide, bizarre; greater than 0.12 second; may look like PVCs; **T wave**—opposite deflection to QRS. Interpretation: This is a life-threatening dysrhythmia that often precedes ventricular fibrillation. Causes: Myocardial irritation, myocardial infarction, coronary artery disease, rheumatic heart disease, hypokalemia, and digoxin toxicity. Symptoms: Initially palpitations, dizziness, and chest pain progressing to decreased cardiac output and loss of consciousness. Treatment: Assess for pulse, signs and symptoms. If ventricular tachycardia without pulse, defibrillate and follow advanced cardiac life support algorithm. With pulse but unstable: Synchronized cardioversion. If stable, with pulse: Lidocaine, procainamide, bretylium; then synchronized cardioversion.

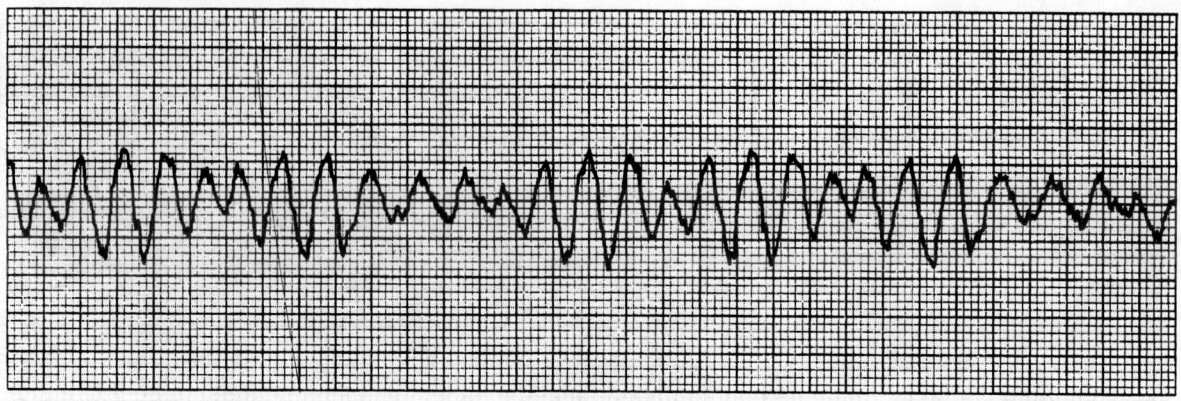

FIGURE **35-30** **Ventricular fibrillation.** Characteristics: **Rate**—undeterminable; **Regularity**—chaotic, wavy baseline; **P wave, PR interval**—undeterminable; **QRS**—undeterminable; **T wave**—undeterminable. Interpretation: This life-threatening dysrhythmia must be terminated quickly if the patient is to resume useful function. Causes: Coronary artery disease, acute myocardial infarction, untreated ventricular tachycardia, electrolyte and acid-base imbalances, electric shock, and hypothermia. Symptoms: Loss of consciousness, cessation of heartbeat and respirations, dilation of pupils. Treatment: Cardiopulmonary resuscitation, defibrillation, and advanced cardiac life support measures are used to treat ventricular fibrillation.

a laboratory or through fiberoptics), the results reflect the degree of oxygen use by the body tissues. SvO_2 can be decreased when oxygen delivery is decreased or the body has increased the use of oxygen (fever, pain, stress). SvO_2 can be increased when oxygen delivery is increased or when oxygen utilization is decreased (hypothermia, general anesthesia). Normal SvO_2 is 60% to 75%.

ARTERIAL LINE

An arterial line may be inserted (most often in the radial artery) to provide a direct measurement of systolic and diastolic blood pressures. Once the line is inserted, it is connected to a pressurized solution to keep the catheter patent and to a transducer to assess pressure. The mean arterial pressure is an indication of tissue perfusion. This pressure is elevated with sympathetic stimulation and increased heart rate.

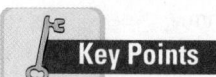
Key Points

- The primary function of the heart is to pump blood through the pulmonary and systemic circulation.
- The heartbeat has two phases: systole (contraction) and diastole (relaxation).
- Cardiac output is the amount of blood ejected per minute by each ventricle; stroke volume is the amount of blood ejected by a ventricle in a single contraction. The factors that affect stroke volume are preload, contractility, and afterload.
- The heart sounds are "lub," heard during systole, and "dub," heard during diastole.
- The most common cardiac surgical procedures are pacemaker insertion, valve repair or replacement, and coronary artery bypass surgery.

- Nursing concerns after cardiac surgery include Ineffective Breathing Pattern, Acute Pain, Ineffective Thermoregulation, Decreased Cardiac Output, Risk for Infection, and Anxiety.
- Pacemakers are electronic devices that deliver impulses to stimulate contraction of the myocardium.
- Coronary artery disease is treated with drug therapy, diet modifications, lifestyle modifications, surgical intervention, or a combination of these.
- Risk factors for atherosclerosis are age, gender, race, heredity, diabetes mellitus with elevated blood glucose, increased serum lipids, nicotine, hypertension, obesity, sedentary lifestyle.
- Angina pectoris is the pain that results from myocardial ischemia. It is treated with vasodilators and rest.
- Procedures used to improve myocardial blood flow include percutaneous coronary balloon angioplasty, laser angioplasty, atherectomy, stent placement, coronary artery bypass grafts, and transmyocardial laser revascularization.
- Acute myocardial infarction, caused by partial or complete occlusion of a coronary artery, can lead to dysrhythmias, heart failure, cardiogenic shock, thromboembolism, and ventricular aneurysm/rupture.
- Nursing care of the patient with myocardial infarction addresses Anxiety, Acute Pain, and Decreased Cardiac Output.
- Patients with acute cardiac conditions often have continuous cardiac monitoring to detect potentially fatal dysrhythmias for prompt treatment.
- Cardiac rehabilitation begins with a cardiac incident, lasts throughout life, and includes the patient and family in teaching about exercise, diet, and medications.
- Heart failure, the inability of the heart to meet the metabolic demands of the body, may be caused by disorders that increase the heart's workload or interfere with its pumping action.
- Treatment of heart failure may include correction of underlying causes, drug therapy to improve cardiac function

and eliminate excess fluid, and measures to decrease demands on the heart.

- Complications of heart failure are dysrhythmias, pulmonary edema, and cardiogenic shock.
- Nursing care of the patient with heart failure focuses on Fluid Volume Excess, Impaired Gas Exchange, Anxiety, Decreased Cardiac Output, and Activity Intolerance.
- Cardiac inflammatory conditions (endocarditis and pericarditis) are treated with drug therapy and rest.
- Cardiomyopathy is a disease of the heart muscle that is treated with supportive measures but may lead to heart failure that eventually requires cardiac transplantation.
- Patients who have received heart transplants require immunosuppressive drugs for the remainder of their lives to prevent rejection of the foreign tissue.
- Signs and symptoms of cardiac transplant rejection are fever, dyspnea, fatigue, and dysrhythmias.
- An implantable cardioverter/defibrillator is an implanted device that monitors cardiac activity, detects life-threatening dysrhythmias, and delivers a shock to convert the rhythm to a normal one.
- The primary disorders of the heart valves are stenosis, which interferes with blood movement from one chamber to the next, and regurgitation, which allows blood to flow backward.
- Valve disease may be treated with drug therapy to improve cardiac function, with balloon valvuloplasty to dilate stenosed valves, with commissurotomy to enlarge the opening, and with valve replacement using a biologic or synthetic valve.
- General measures to maintain perfusion of vital organs are modified Trendelenburg's position, oxygen, intravenous fluids, and drugs to maintain or restore blood pressure.
- A dysrhythmia (also called an *arrhythmia*) is a disturbance of the heart rhythm caused by a problem in the conduction system.

 Go to your Companion CD-ROM for a Pharmacology Tutorial, Audio Glossary, and 3-D animations.

evolve Be sure to visit the companion Evolve site at http://evolve.elsevier.com/Linton/ for WebLinks and additional online resources.

REVIEW QUESTIONS *Choose the best answer.*

1. Normally, the impulse that stimulates a myocardial contraction begins in the:
   1. AV node
   2. Bundle of His
   3. Purkinje cells
   4. SA node

2. Which statement correctly describes one of the three factors that affect stroke volume?
   1. Contractility is the ability of cardiac muscle fibers to shorten and produce a muscle contraction.
   2. Preload is the amount of blood remaining in the atria at the end of diastole.
   3. Cardiac output is the amount of blood ejected by the heart with each ventricular contraction.
   4. Afterload is the amount of blood remaining in the ventricles at the end of systole.

3. Which of the following age-related changes in the circulatory system can cause heart murmurs?
   1. Decreased elasticity of connective tissue in the heart muscle
   2. Arterial stiffening caused by changes in connective tissue and elastic fibers
   3. Heart valves that are stiff and do not close properly
   4. Stretching and dilation of veins resulting in impaired venous return

4. Before administering digoxin, you count a patient's apical heart rate and find that it is 62 bpm. The patient's usual rate ranges from 65 to 75 bpm. What should you do?
   1. Withhold the digoxin and notify the physician.
   2. Administer the digoxin and document the heart rate.
   3. Hold the drug and recheck the heart rate in an hour.
   4. Give half of the prescribed dose of digoxin.

5. An adverse effect common to all antidysrhythmic drugs is:
   1. Fluid and electrolyte imbalance
   2. Drowsiness
   3. Diarrhea
   4. Additional dysrhythmias

6. The usual dietary recommendations for cardiac patients include the following:
   1. No more than 10% saturated fats
   2. Low fiber and carbohydrates
   3. Sodium restricted to 1 g/day
   4. 20% or less of total fat intake

7. Risk factors for atherosclerosis that can be modified include the following:
   1. Gender
   2. Race
   3. Heredity
   4. Sedentary lifestyle

8. Characteristics of angina pectoris include that it:
   1. Most often occurs at rest
   2. Is accompanied by drop in blood pressure
   3. Is usually substernal but may radiate
   4. Is commonly treated with digitalis

9. Which of the following drugs may be administered after acute myocardial infarction to dissolve thrombi?
   1. Heparin
   2. Tissue plasminogen activator
   3. Aspirin
   4. Lidocaine

10. When cardiac output falls, compensatory mechanisms include the following:
    1. Elimination of excess fluid by the kidneys
    2. Dilation of blood vessels in the extremities
    3. Stimulation of the parasympathetic nervous system
    4. Enlargement of the ventricular myocardium

11. Discharge teaching for a patient with heart failure should include instructions to:
    1. Immediately begin a vigorous program of exercise
    2. Inform the physician if you gain more than 2 pounds in a week
    3. Weigh yourself before going to bed each night
    4. Expect to continue having shortness of breath, chest pain, and cough

12. Before invasive procedures including dental work, patients with valvular heart disease usually are prescribed antibiotics to prevent:
    1. Pericarditis
    2. Abscess formation
    3. Infective endocarditis
    4. Cardiomyopathy

13. A patient who has had heart transplantation comes into the physician's office complaining of fever, fatigue, shortness of breath, and an irregular heart beat. You should suspect:
    1. Infection in the surgical wound
    2. Congestive heart failure
    3. Rejection of the transplanted heart
    4. Postoperative anxiety and depression

14. Which of the following findings would you expect in a patient with mitral stenosis?
    1. Increased left atrial pressure
    2. Decreased pulmonary pressure
    3. Increased cardiac output
    4. Decreased right ventricular pressure

CHAPTER 36

Vascular Disorders

evolve http://evolve.elsevier.com/Linton/

Objectives

After reading and studying this chapter, you should be able to:

1. Identify specific anatomic and physiologic factors that affect the vascular system and tissue oxygenation.
2. Indicate appropriate parameters for assessing a patient with peripheral vascular disease, aneurysm, and aortic dissection.
3. Discuss tests and procedures used to diagnose selected vascular disorders and the nursing considerations for each.
4. Describe the pathophysiology, signs and symptoms, complications, and medical or surgical treatments for selected vascular disorders.
5. Assist in developing a plan of care for patients with selected vascular disorders.

Key Terms

Be sure to check out the bonus material on the Companion CD-ROM, including selected audio pronunciations.

aneurysm (ĂN-ū-rĭzm, p. 685)
bruit (BRŪ-ē, p. 691)
embolism (ĔM-bō-lĭzm, p. 696)
hemoconcentration (p. 688)
ischemia (ĭs-KĒ-mē-ă, p. 689)
paresthesia (păr-ĕs-THĒ-zē-ă, p. 688)
phlebitis (flē-BĪ-tĭs, p. 708)
phlebothrombosis (flĕb-ō-thrŏm-BŌ-sĭs, p. 708)
poikilothermy (poi-kĕ-lō-THĔR-mē, p. 688)
thrombophlebitis (thrŏm-bō-flē-BĪ-tĭs, p. 708)
thrombosis (thrŏm-BŌ-sĭs, p. 685)
vasoconstriction (văz-ō-kŏn-STRĬK-shŭn, p. 687)
viscosity (vĭs-KŎS-ĭ-tē, p. 687)

The delivery of oxygen and nutrients to the tissues depends on adequate perfusion (blood flow), which requires a functionally intact cardiovascular system. When the cardiovascular system is compromised by vascular disease, the homeostasis of the body is affected. Risk factors for vascular disease include advanced age, heredity, smoking, obesity, physical inactivity, hypertension, and diabetes mellitus. Vascular diseases can affect both the arterial and the venous components of the circulation. Nearly 1 million people in the United States are affected by atherosclerotic peripheral vascular disease (PVD). Especially among older adults, PVD can lead to functional impairment. Each year, approximately 500,000 people are diagnosed with deep vein thrombosis (DVT), and nearly 140,000 die as a result of complications. Although peripheral aneurysms are less common, abdominal aortic aneurysms are present in 5% to 7% of American males older than 60 years. Of aneurysms larger than 6 cm in diameter, half rupture within 1 year, often with fatal consequences.

Atherosclerosis is covered in Chapter 35. Other peripheral vascular disorders as well as aortic aneurysm and aortic dissection are presented here.

ANATOMY AND PHYSIOLOGY OF THE VASCULAR SYSTEM

The peripheral vascular system comprises arteries, capillaries, veins, and the lymph vessels (Fig. 36-1). The function of this system is to maintain blood flow to supply adequate oxygen and nutrients to all tissues. Any interruption of the blood flow results in tissue hypoxia, which can lead to tissue necrosis (death) if untreated.

ARTERIES

Arteries are the vessels that carry the blood away from the heart toward the tissues. These vessels are normally elastic and have greater tensile strength than the veins. The aorta, which is the largest artery in the body, transports oxygenated blood from the left ventricle of the heart. Arteries that branch from the aortic arch supply the head and arms. The thoracic branch of the descending aorta supplies intercostal muscles, the esophagus, and some respiratory passages. The abdominal branch of the descending aorta supplies the GI organs, the kidneys, the gonads, the lumbar area of the back, and the legs. Arteries branch into progressively smaller vessels as they travel away from the aorta. The smallest branches of the arteries are called *arterioles*.

Arteries and arterioles are thick-walled structures with three layers: the intima, the media, and the adventitia (Fig. 36-2). The *intima* is composed of endothelial cells that form the smooth inner surface of the arteries, allowing the blood to flow with little resistance. The middle layer is the *media*, the primary structure of the artery. The media is composed of smooth muscle, elastic fibers, and connective tissue fibers.

Smooth muscles encircle and control the diameter of arteries and arterioles. Contraction of the muscles constricts the vessels, whereas relaxation of the muscles results in vessel dilation. Smooth muscle contraction and relaxation are governed by the autonomic nervous system and other chemical and hormonal factors.

The outer layer of the arteries and arterioles is the *adventitia*. This layer, which is composed mostly of connective tissue, secures the artery or arteriole to the surrounding structures.

CAPILLARIES

Arterioles branch into progressively smaller and smaller vessels, until they form the capillaries. Capillaries consist of a single layer of endothelial cells that allow the efficient delivery of nutrients and oxygen into the tissues and the removal of metabolic wastes from the tissues. Transfer of oxygen and nutrients between the blood and the tissue cells occurs in the capillaries. Red blood cells have to conform to the size of the capillaries by changing their shape to fit through the small diameter.

The tiny vessels that receive blood from the capillaries are venules, which are the smallest veins. The distribution of capillaries is determined by the metabolic activity occurring in the tissue. Tissues such as skeletal muscles and digestive tract lining have a rich capillary network, whereas tissues such as bone and cartilage have a scanty capillary network.

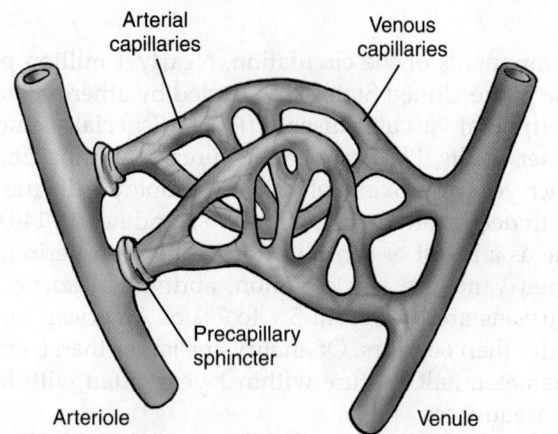

FIGURE **36-1** Capillary bed. Foods, nutrients, and oxygen are delivered to tissues through the capillaries, and wastes are collected from the capillaries for recycling or excretion. Precapillary sphincters help regulate the flow.

FIGURE **36-2** Tissue layers of veins and arteries.

Because capillaries have less smooth muscle than the arteries, the amount of blood in the capillary is controlled by sphincters on the arteriolar side of the capillary. Other factors such as chemical stimulation and hormonal changes also influence blood flow and fluid shifts in the capillaries. For example, histamine causes the capillary permeability to increase, allowing more fluid to shift into the tissues.

VEINS

The blood is returned to the heart by way of the venules and veins These vessels are formed as the capillaries organize into larger and larger vessels. The venous system is less sturdy and more passive than the arterial system. The walls of veins and venules are composed of the same three layers as the walls of the arteries and arterioles, but the layers are less defined (see Fig. 36-2). Because the walls of the veins and venules are thinner and less muscular, they can stretch more than those of the arterial system. Thus the venous system can store a large volume of blood under relatively low pressure. As much as 75% of the body's total blood volume is housed in the venous system.

Valves

The venous system is equipped with valves that are composed of endothelial leaflets (Fig. 36-3). Valves allow the blood to move in only one direction and prevent backflow of the blood in the extremities. Skeletal muscle contractions compress the veins, forcing blood back toward the heart. This action reduces venous pooling and increases the circulating blood volume. As deoxygenated blood moves toward the heart, carbon dioxide and other metabolic wastes are carried to the lungs and kidneys for elimination.

Valve open   Competent valve closed

FIGURE 36-3 Veins contain bicuspid valves that open in the direction of blood flow but prevent regurgitation of flow when pockets become filled and distended.

Innervation

The venous system is innervated by the sympathetic nervous system. The sympathetic nervous system acts on the musculature of the veins to stimulate venoconstriction. Blocking of sympathetic nerve stimulation permits venodilation.

LYMPH VESSELS

The lymph system is an organization of small, thin-walled vessels that resemble the capillaries. These vessels accommodate the collection of lymph fluid from the peripheral tissues and the transportation of the fluid to the venous circulatory system. Because the lymph system interacts with the venous system, it is classified as part of the cardiovascular system. The lymph system comprises two main trunks: the thoracic duct and the right lymphatic duct. Each of these trunks is responsible for collecting and draining fluid from specific areas of the body. (See Chapter 33 for additional information.)

Lymph fluid is composed of plasma-like fluid, large protein molecules, and foreign substances. Because these protein molecules are too large to enter the capillaries or the venules, the lymph fluid carries them to the lymphatic ducts, where they are emptied into the subclavian and the internal jugular veins. The movement of lymph fluid is accomplished by the contraction of muscles that encircle the lymphatic walls and surrounding tissues.

FACTORS THAT AFFECT BLOOD FLOW

The body has multiple homeostatic mechanisms to control the systemic and local blood volume. The mechanisms work by changing resistance within the vessels or by changing the blood viscosity.

Resistance

Resistance within the vascular system is controlled by the diameter of the vessels. When vascular diameter increases, peripheral resistance falls and blood flow increases. When vascular diameter decreases, however, peripheral resistance increases, thereby reducing blood flow. As previously noted, the diameter of blood vessels is controlled by the central nervous system, hormones, some ions, and blood pH.

The sympathetic nervous system plays a major role in adjusting vascular resistance. The diameter of peripheral blood vessels is regulated by the vasomotor center located in the medulla and the pons. Stimulation of the sympathetic nervous system by either physiologic or psychological stressors also triggers the adrenal glands to release norepinephrine and epinephrine, which cause vasoconstriction.

Other factors that cause changes in vascular resistance are angiotensin, serotonin, histamine, the kinins, and the prostaglandins. Angiotensin II is a potent chemical released by the kidneys that causes intense vasoconstriction and retention of salt and water by the kidneys. The kinins, histamine, and prostaglandins cause vasodilation, which decreases peripheral resistance. Serotonin, a chemical that is liberated from platelets when vessel walls are damaged, can cause vasoconstriction or vasodilation, depending on tissue conditions.

Blood Viscosity

In addition to changes in peripheral resistance, modification of blood viscosity also helps regulate blood flow to peripheral tissues. Viscosity describes the thickness of the blood. The blood viscosity is usually constant but can be affected by changes in the proportions of the solid or liquid components. An increase in red blood cells or a decrease in body water produces hemoconcentration, which increases blood viscosity. When blood is concentrated, the kidneys usually begin to retain water and the movement of fluid out of the capillaries is restricted.

An important factor that affects blood viscosity is capillary permeability. Hydrostatic and osmotic pressures normally maintain balanced movement of fluids in and out of the capillaries. Any mechanism that alters capillary permeability changes the amount and direction of fluid movement, resulting in a change in blood viscosity. Factors that increase capillary permeability include histamine, bradykinin, leukotrienes, and prostaglandins. Certain muscle metabolites, hypoxemia, malnutrition, and pH imbalances can also increase capillary permeability. When the proportion of serum to solid components in the blood is higher than normal, blood is less viscous and the kidneys excrete excess fluid.

AGE-RELATED CHANGES

The primary age-related change in peripheral vessels is stiffening of the vessel walls, called *arteriosclerosis*. As arteriosclerosis develops, the delivery of oxygen and nutrients to the tissues is compromised and there is a buildup of waste products in the tissue.

The stiffening of the peripheral vessels associated with aging occurs in both the intima and the media of the vessel wall. The intima is thickened and hardened by the proliferation of cells. It becomes roughened, which increases the risk of thrombus formation and emboli. The connective and elastic tissue fibers in the media become calcified. This process produces a thinner and fragmented layer within the peripheral vessels. Loss of elasticity in the peripheral vessels increases peripheral resistance, which impairs blood flow and results in increased left ventricular workload. As a result, the transportation of oxygen and nutrients to and the removal of wastes from the tissues are affected adversely. The same changes that affect peripheral blood vessels also occur in the aorta of the older adult. The aorta stiffens, thickens, and loses distensibility, which causes increased resistance to blood flow.

The transportation of oxygen also may be compromised by the decrease of hemoglobin seen in some older adults. A reduction of hemoglobin in the blood produces a decline in the oxygen-carrying capacity of the blood. Because the stiffening blood vessels result in decreased blood flow and because a decrease in hemoglobin compromises the oxygen-carrying capacity, peripheral circulation can be substantially affected.

Overall, aging in the vascular system may cause a slowing of the heart rate and a decrease in the stroke volume, which may result in a 30% to 40% decrease in cardiac output. If cardiac output is altered, the older adult may adapt more slowly to changes in the peripheral vascular system.

NURSING ASSESSMENT OF THE VASCULAR SYSTEM

HEALTH HISTORY

Chief Complaint and History of Present Illness

The nursing assessment of a patient who may have a vascular disorder requires a thorough cardiovascular assessment by the registered nurse, as described in Chapter 35. The LPN/LVN may assist in collecting relevant data. Assessment of the peripheral circulation focuses on the six classic "P's" characteristic of peripheral vascular disease: pain, pulselessness, poikilothermy, pallor, paresthesia, and paralysis. Each of these characteristics needs to be evaluated.

Pain. A thorough pain history provides valuable information about vascular disease. Describe the nature of any pain or discomfort in the calf, thigh, hip, or buttock areas. Document the nature of the pain (e.g., sharp, throbbing, continuous, intermittent), the location and duration of the pain, the precipitating factors (e.g., exercise, lying down in bed), and alleviating factors (whatever brings relief). Acute pain is associated with acute arterial obstruction. Intermittent claudication and pain at rest are considered chronic pain.

When pain is caused by a venous disorder, patients typically describe it as tenderness, heaviness, or fullness in the extremity. Note whether the pain was alleviated by elevating the extremity or by wearing support stockings. Pain associated with an aortic aneurysm varies with the location of the aneurysm.

Intermittent Claudication. Intermittent claudication is pain associated with decreased perfusion that is aggravated by exercise and relieved by rest. Intermittent claudication can affect any major muscle group distal to (beyond) the point of arterial occlusion. The pain is described as a feeling of tightness, burning, fatigue, aching, or cramping. Exercise causes the muscle group to become ischemic because blood flow is inadequate to supply nutrients and oxygen and to remove wastes. This results in the development of pain. When the exercise is stopped, the metabolic demands of the muscle tissue decrease, wastes are removed from the tissues, and the pain is relieved.

Rest Pain. Rest pain indicates severe arterial occlusion (obstruction). By impeding blood flow, the occlusion causes tissue ischemia in the extremity. For example, a person with arterial occlusion in the lower extremities may experience severe, burning pain in the legs and feet after lying flat for a period of time. The pain is relieved when the extremity is dangled in a dependent position that promotes blood flow by gravity. Frequently, the patient sleeps best in a chair or with the feet in a dependent position.

Pulselessness. Palpate the peripheral pulses for rate, rhythm, and quality. Compare pulses bilaterally to detect any differences.

Poikilothermy and Pallor. Poikilothermy is decreased temperature at an ischemic site, which is detected by palpating the affected and surrounding areas. The poikilothermic area feels cooler than the rest of the extremity. Pallor, meaning paleness, is apparent over an area of reduced blood supply. Pallor is detected by inspecting the affected site and comparing skin color with other parts of the body.

Paresthesia and Paralysis. Note paresthesia and/or paralysis. Paresthesia is an abnormal sensation such as numbness, tingling, a "pins and needles" sensation, or a crawling sensation. Paralysis is impairment of motor function. These symptoms may be associated with impaired conduction of nerve impulses caused by inadequate oxygen and nutrients to the nerve tissues and the accumulation of waste materials.

Past Medical History

The past medical history includes the cardiovascular assessment, as described in Chapter 35. Document a history of hypertension, coronary artery disease, myocardial infarction, or atherosclerosis. Because atherosclerosis affects the cerebral, renal, and respiratory blood vessels, include each of these areas in the discussion of past medical problems. It is especially significant if the patient has diabetes, because peripheral vascular disease is a common complication of diabetes.

Family History

The family history determines any cardiovascular disorders or other relevant conditions in the immediate family members. Relevant diseases include hypertension, coronary artery disease, myocardial infarction, atherosclerosis, aneurysm, and diabetes.

Review of Systems

Changes in the integument provide important clues to the presence and severity of peripheral vascular disease. Changes that may be associated with PVD are thick and brittle nails; shiny, taut, scaly, and dry skin; skin temperature variations; skin ulcerations; muscle atrophy; localized redness and hardness; and hair loss on the extremities.

Another component of the review of systems is the assessment for chest pain and dyspnea. These symptoms are important because 10% of people with deep vein thrombosis develop a pulmonary embolus.

Aneurysms are often asymptomatic. Depending on the location of the aneurysm, the patient may report hoarseness, dysphagia, dyspnea, abdominal or back pain, or swelling of the head and arms.

Functional Assessment

The functional assessment determines the impact of the disease process on the patient's life. The pain associated with PVD can interfere with work and recreation. Inactivity can reduce the patient's stamina. If the patient has had a limb amputated because of PVD, explore how the limb loss affects the patient's functioning. Other aspects of the functional assessment that are relevant to vascular disease are smoking history and dietary habits. Smoking causes vasoconstriction, and a high fat intake can contribute to arteriosclerosis. Both are associated with peripheral vascular disease.

PHYSICAL EXAMINATION

The physical examination helps determine whether the disease process is arterial or venous in nature. In general, arterial complications involve multiple areas, whereas venous complications remain more localized, usually in the lower extremities. Inspect the skin for color and lesions. Pallor suggests peripheral vasoconstriction or inadequate arterial blood flow. A reddish-brown discoloration called *rubor* in a dependent lower extremity suggests the presence of arterial occlusive disease. In venous disorders, the affected areas of the skin may have a brownish discoloration and be cyanotic when the extremity is dependent. Be alert for open ulcers and for scars around the ankles that may be associated with either arterial or venous disease. Note the presence of stasis dermatitis, a brown pigmentation with flaky skin over the edematous areas of the ankles. It may take on a bluish cast when the leg is in a dependent position. Arterial stasis dermatitis begins as ulcerations in the toes. The ulcers are painful, pale, crusty, and located over bony prominences. Venous stasis dermatitis begins as ulcers in the ankle area. The ulcers develop very slowly, are usually painless, and are difficult to heal.

Determine capillary refill time in the nail beds to determine the adequacy of peripheral perfusion. Press the nail bed until it blanches (turns pale). Then release the pressure and note the number of seconds it takes for the color to return. Capillary refill time greater than 3 seconds denotes a reduction in peripheral perfusion.

Palpate the affected areas to evaluate the temperature, detect edema, and assess peripheral pulses. Palpate skin temperature bilaterally, moving proximally to distally (toward the feet), to detect any ischemic areas. A cool limb suggests an arterial problem, and a warm limb suggests a venous problem. A pulsating mass detected on abdominal palpation may be an aneurysm.

Dependent edema develops as a result of systemic disorders, lymphatic dysfunction, deep vein thrombosis, or chronic venous insufficiency. To determine the severity of edema, press the thumb into the edematous area for approximately 5 seconds. The severity is graded from 1 to 4, depending on the depth of depression: less than ¼ inch = 1; ¼ to ½ inch = 2; ½ to 1 inch = 3; and more than 1 inch = 4. If the depression of the thumb remains in the edematous area, the edema is said to be *pitting.* Compare the same area on both extremities.

Another aspect of the examination is the evaluation of peripheral pulses (Fig. 36-4). Palpate pulses for presence, symmetry, volume, and rhythm. The peripheral pulses to be palpated in the upper extremities include the brachial, ulnar, and radial arteries. The peripheral pulses appraised in the lower extremities are the femoral, popliteal, dorsalis pedis, and posterior tibial arteries. Compare pulses bilaterally. Document absent or asymmetric pulses. The palpation of the arteries provides valuable information concerning the condition of the vessels. A sclerotic vessel feels stiff and cordlike, whereas a normal vessel can be palpated as soft and springy.

When peripheral vascular disease is suspected, Homans' sign traditionally is tested. This test is done by having the patient slightly flex the knee and then sharply dorsiflexing the patient's foot. If dorsiflexion causes pain in the calf area or behind the knee, the patient is said to have a positive Homans' sign. The absence of pain with this action is called a negative Homans' sign. Although a positive Homans' sign is intended to detect DVT, many patients with a positive Homans' sign prove not to have venous thrombosis and individuals with DVT often do not have a positive sign. Therefore this test is not considered reliable for detecting or ruling out thrombosis.

Another test that can be beneficial in the assessment of the peripheral vascular system is the Allen test. The Allen test is used to determine the adequacy of arterial circulation to the hand. The patient is asked to clench the fist tightly while the nurse occludes the radial and ulnar arteries. The patient is then instructed to open the fist, and the nurse releases pressure on the ulnar artery. If the ulnar artery is patent, the palm should promptly return to a normal color. A persistence of pallor in the palm area indicates an occlusion of the ulnar artery. The test can be repeated with the ulnar artery being occluded instead of the radial artery to detect occlusion within the radial artery (see Fig. 30-7).

The nurse with advanced education can further evaluate peripheral vascular function by auscultating

FIGURE **36-4** Palpating distal pulses. **A,** Femoral. **B,** Popliteal. **C,** Dorsalis pedis. **D,** Posterior tibial.

the sounds of blood flow through the arteries. **Bruits** sound like turbulent, fast-moving fluid. The presence of bruits can signal the presence of an aneurysm or the development of chronic arterial occlusive disease long before other signs appear.

Nursing assessment of the patient with peripheral vascular disease is summarized in Box 36-1.

DIAGNOSTIC TESTS AND PROCEDURES

Based on findings of the physical examination, selected diagnostic studies are ordered by the physician to confirm the disease process and to determine the severity of the condition. The procedures and tests that may be used to diagnose peripheral vascular disease are ultrasonography, pressure measurements, stress testing, tomographic angiography, magnetic resonance angiography, and angiography, which includes arteriography and venography, as shown in the Diagnostic Tests and Procedures table on p. 692. Procedures that are useful in the diagnosis of aneurysms include chest radiography, abdominal ultrasound, computed tomography, and transthoracic echocardiography. When pulmonary embolism is suspected, diagnostic tools that might be used include the lung scan, pulmonary angiogram, and spiral CT scan.

ULTRASONOGRAPHY

Doppler ultrasound is used to facilitate the diagnosis of peripheral vascular disease and to monitor the changes in blood flow associated with vascular diseases. It is a noninvasive, inexpensive, highly reliable diagnostic tool. Low-intensity, high-frequency sound waves are directed toward the artery or vein being tested. These sound waves strike the moving blood cells and are reflected back to the receiver. Arteries reflect a high-pitched sound, whereas veins produce sounds that vary with respirations and have a "blowing" tone. In the presence of an occlusion or narrowed vessel, the sounds are diminished. The primary vessels examined are the posterior tibial, popliteal, and common femoral veins. The test takes 10 to 20 minutes. Abdominal ultrasound may be used to screen for abdominal aneurysms. Duplex scanning combines two types of ultrasonography to evaluate blood flow and provide a two-dimension image of the blood vessel and the blood flow.

PRESSURE MEASUREMENTS

Plethysmography is a noninvasive study used to measure blood flow in the extremities. Different procedures are used to assess arterial or venous blood flow. To determine arterial blood flow, three blood pressure cuffs that measure pulse waves are applied to different parts of the extremity. Variations in pressures can indicate arterial occlusion from one area to another. Venous evaluation is done by inflating the proximal cuff and measuring the venous volume in the most distal cuff. If no venous obstruction is present, the distal pressure should rise sharply when the proximal cuff is inflated and quickly return to baseline when the proximal cuff is deflated. Although plethysmography is less accurate than arteriography and venography, it is very safe and can be used to assess patients who are too ill to undergo arteriography.

Pressure measurements can be completed as segmental limb pressures (sometimes called *segmental plethysmography*) and pulse volume measurements. The pulse volumes are recorded as waveforms. These waveforms provide information about the elasticity of blood vessels. Blood pressure is measured at multiple

---

Box 36-1   *ASSESSMENT of the Patient with Peripheral Vascular Disease or Aneurysm*

Health History

Present Illness:
Complaints of pain, pulselessness, poikilothermy, pallor, paresthesia, and paralysis

Past Medical History:
Hypertension, coronary artery disease, myocardial infarction, amputations, atherosclerosis, diabetes mellitus

Family History:
Hypertension, coronary artery disease, myocardial infarction, atherosclerosis, diabetes mellitus, aneurysm

Review of Systems:
Hairlessness on lower extremities; peripheral edema; discoloration of dependent areas; temperature changes in compromised areas; ulcerations on lower extremities; limb pain; thick, brittle toenails; temperature variation over involved area; muscle atrophy; localized redness and induration in affected extremity; chest pain; dyspnea; hoarseness; swelling of head and/or arms; back or abdominal pain

Functional Assessment:
Mobility restricted by pain, decreased stamina

Physical Examination

General Survey:
Posture, gait, presence of pain in affected extremities, edema of face and/or arms

Cardiovascular:
Symmetric peripheral pulses, capillary refill time, Homans' sign

Integument:
Temperature of affected area, edema in dependent area, color of affected extremity, rubor in lower extremities, stasis dermatitis or ulcers

Abdomen:
Palpable pulsatile mass

DIAGNOSTIC TESTS and PROCEDURES | **Peripheral Vascular Disease (PVD)**

TEST	PURPOSE/PROCEDURE	PATIENT PREPARATION	POSTPROCEDURE NURSING CARE
Doppler ultrasound	Uses sound waves to facilitate diagnosis of PVD; monitors changes in blood flow associated with vascular disease.	Tell patient test is painless and has no risks. Patient may be asked to change position of extremity being evaluated and perform breathing exercises.	No special care.
Plethysmography	Used to detect deep vein thrombosis, to screen patients who are at risk for PVD, to investigate the possibility of pulmonary emboli.	Tell patient procedure is safe, painless, and takes about 30-45 min. Leg will be elevated and pressure cuff placed on the thigh. Electrodes record information about blood flow in the veins.	No special care.
Pressure measurement	Types: segmental limb pressures and pulse volume measurements.	Tell patient blood pressures will be measured in multiple sites over the extremities to assess the blood vessels. Pressures are measured during activity and while at rest. The test is noninvasive, painless, and safe.	No special care.
Exercise (treadmill test)	Evaluates the functional abilities of patients with PVD by measuring pulse volumes before, during, and after exercise.	Tell patient test is noninvasive; will be asked to walk for approximately 5 min on a treadmill. The test will be stopped if the patient has pain or dyspnea.	Carefully monitor for any complications that may develop as a result of the test.
Angiography (venography, arteriography, and radiographs)	Taken to identify venous obstruction, confirm PVD, detect clots, or identify suitable vessel for grafting.	Tell patient dye will be injected and radiographs taken. May briefly feel burning sensation when dye is injected. Signed consent required. NPO 4 hr before test. Inform radiologist if allergic to iodine or seafood. Risks: hemorrhage at insertion site, dye-induced allergic reaction, thrombosis/embolism, renal insufficiency, pseudoaneurysm.	Bed rest for several hours; monitor vital signs and pulses hourly for 6 hr. Assess injection site for bleeding, hematoma, and pulsating mass (pseudoaneurysm); neurovascular checks (pulses, sensation, movement, color, warmth).

sites over the extremities to be examined. Pressure readings are reduced at the location of a narrowed or occluded vessel. Measurements are taken while the patient is at rest.

EXERCISE (TREADMILL) TEST

The exercise test is sometimes referred to as a *stress test*. This noninvasive procedure helps evaluate the patient's tolerance for physical activity. Signed consent is required.

The patient is asked to walk for approximately 5 minutes at a rate of 1.5 miles per hour on a treadmill. Continuous ECG and BP monitoring is done. The patient is monitored for any signs of distress such as cardiac dysrhythmias, claudication, or dyspnea. If distress occurs, the test is stopped immediately. After the test, the patient should be monitored until vital signs return to normal.

ANGIOGRAPHY

The purposes of angiography are to confirm the diagnosis of peripheral vascular disease, to distinguish clot formation from venous obstruction, and to locate a suitable vessel for grafting. Angiography is an invasive procedure that requires the injection of dye into the vascular system, which makes the vessels visible on radiographs. The two types of angiography are arteriography, which examines arteries, and venography, which examines veins. Abnormalities can be visualized and assessed during the procedure. The risks that are associated with these tests are hemorrhage at the IV insertion site, dye-induced allergic reactions, thrombosis at the insertion site, and emboli. The patient is exposed to relatively high doses of radiation.

COMMON THERAPEUTIC MEASURES

The primary goals for the patient with peripheral vascular disease are to increase the arterial blood supply to the extremities, reduce venous congestion, dilate blood vessels to increase arterial blood flow, prevent vascular compression, provide relief from pain, attain or maintain tissue integrity, and encourage adherence to the treatment plan.

Exercise programs, stress management, pain management, smoking cessation, elastic stockings, intermittent pneumatic compression units, body positioning, drug therapy, surgical interventions, and patient education are used in the management of the disease process.

EXERCISE

The simple act of walking stimulates the movement of blood from the dependent areas of the extremities toward the heart. Walking contracts the muscles of the lower extremities, pushing venous blood upward toward the heart and promoting the development of col-

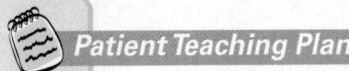

Patient Teaching Plan

Buerger-Allen Exercises

These exercises allow gravity to fill and empty the blood vessels.

- Lie flat on your back and raise your legs above the level of your heart for 2 minutes or until they become very pale.
- Lower the legs to a dependent position, and flex and extend your feet for 3 minutes or until color returns to your legs.
- Keep your legs flat for 5 minutes.
- Go through the entire process six times in each session if you can tolerate it. Three to four sessions a day provide the best results.
- Stop the exercises immediately if you have pain or severe skin color changes.

lateral circulation. For patients with vascular disease, any exercise program must be prescribed by the physician. Patients who have leg ulcers, gangrene, or acute thrombotic occlusion may be restricted to bed rest until the condition improves.

A specific type of exercise program that is effective in the management of peripheral vascular disease is the use of Buerger-Allen exercises or active postural exercises (Fig. 36-5).

STRESS MANAGEMENT

Emotional stress causes peripheral vasoconstriction, which is detrimental to a patient whose circulation is already compromised. Resistance to blood flow is increased, which reduces blood flow to the tissues. Emotional stress cannot be avoided entirely but can be reduced with a stress management plan, which may include lifestyle changes, massage, relaxation, or other stress-reducing activities.

PAIN MANAGEMENT

The patient with peripheral vascular disease often limits ambulation because of pain. However, immobility tends to worsen circulatory problems. Therefore pain management is an important aspect of care. Pain can be managed by promoting circulation to the affected area, by administering prescribed analgesics, or both. When intermittent claudication occurs, the patient should stop the exercise. Rest decreases circulatory demands and alleviates the pain. Once the pain is relieved, the activity may be resumed. Advise the patient to avoid constrictive garments such as girdles, garters, belts, and tight pantyhose that can cause pain by obstructing blood flow.

SMOKING CESSATION

Smoking cessation is critical to effective management of peripheral vascular disease because smoking causes vasoconstriction (constriction of the blood vessels). Vasoconstriction can be documented for up to 1 hour after

FIGURE **36-5** Buerger-Allen exercises for peripheral vascular disease. **A,** Elevate and support the legs at a 45- to 90-degree angle, or until the skin blanches, for 2 to 3 minutes. **B,** Sit with feet in a dependent position so the skin turns red. Support the legs in this position for 5 to 10 minutes. Then flex, extend, pronate, and supinate each foot three times. Finally, lie flat in a supine position for 10 minutes.

a cigarette has been smoked. In addition, the nicotine in tobacco causes vasospasms, which drastically restrict the peripheral circulation. Measures to help the patient include encouragement; reinforcement; teaching about the nature of tobacco addiction, the harm of smoking, and the benefits of stopping; self-help materials or "Quit Kits" that are available from various agencies; and pharmacotherapy. Nicotine (patches, spray, gum, inhalers) and bupropion, individually or together, greatly enhance the chance of success. Even though the best smoking cessation programs have about a 25% to 30% success rate, that rate is significant when you realize that 45 million Americans smoke cigarettes and that smoking is responsible for about 430,700 preventable deaths in the United States annually.

Pharmacology Capsule

Drugs that help some people who are trying to quit smoking are nicotine and bupropion.

ELASTIC STOCKINGS

Another therapy that is useful in the management of peripheral vascular disease is the use of elastic stockings or antiembolism hose. These stockings provide sustained, evenly distributed pressure over the entire surface of the calves and thighs. The correct placement of elastic stockings compresses superficial veins, resulting in improved blood flow to the deeper veins. Take care when applying these stockings because they can become tourniquets if applied incorrectly. The proper size of elastic stockings must be determined for each patient by using the instruction sheet provided by the manufacturer. Elastic stockings are best applied in the morning before rising from bed because swelling is usually at its lowest level at this time of the day. With the stockings inside out, start the placement by pulling the stocking onto the foot with firm, even support (Fig. 36-6). Once the elastic stocking is positioned over the heel, pull from the sides so it distributes evenly over the entire length of the leg. The stockings should be smooth when the application process is completed. If the top is allowed to roll or turn down, circulatory stasis occurs. Remove the stockings for 10 to 20 minutes twice a day. While the stockings are off, it is best for the patient to be resting in bed or with the extremities in a nondependent position. When the elastic stockings are removed, inspect the skin for any signs of irritation, pressure, or tenderness, which could reflect developing complications.

INTERMITTENT PNEUMATIC COMPRESSION

Intermittent pneumatic compression or a pulsatile antiembolism system may be used for patients who are confined to bed after surgery or a traumatic injury. The primary function of these devices is to prevent deep vein thrombosis. With intermittent pneumatic compression, elastic stockings are applied that are sequen-

FIGURE 36-6 Elastic stockings provide sustained, consistently distributed pressure over the entire surface of the calves and thighs to promote venous return.

tially inflated from the ankles, calves, and thighs and then deflated. This expansion and contraction mimics the muscle pumping of the lower extremities, prevents venous pooling, and stimulates the circulation.

POSITIONING

Body positions play an important part in the management of peripheral vascular disease. Frequently, patients are restricted to bed during the acute phases of the disease process. It is important to use different positions to mobilize the blood volume that has become stagnant in the dependent areas. Lowering the extremities below the level of the heart enhances arterial blood supply. Elevating the lower extremities above the level of the heart promotes venous return and reduces venous stasis. For patients who are not restricted to bed, prolonged standing puts strain on the venous system. Instruct the patient to sit down and elevate the extremity to a nondependent position whenever possible.

THERMOTHERAPY

Thermotherapy with either warm or cold can be used for its effects on the circulatory system. Heat, whether dry or moist, works as a vasodilator that promotes arterial flow to the peripheral tissues. Use heat cautiously, however, because patients with peripheral vascular disease may have impaired sensation as a result of tissue ischemia. Blood vessels constrict in response to cold. Clothing can be used effectively to

promote warmth and to prevent vasoconstriction due to chilling.

PROTECTION

Affected extremities must be protected from trauma because the healing process is usually impaired with peripheral vascular disease. To prevent injury to poorly perfused tissues, the patient must avoid scratching and vigorous rubbing. Caution the patient to wear properly fitting shoes and clean socks or hose, to keep fingernails and toenails trimmed and smooth, and not to walk about barefoot. Inform the physician of ingrown toenails, blisters, or skin injuries so prompt treatment can be initiated.

PATIENT TEACHING

Patient education is important in the management of peripheral vascular disease. The patient must understand the disease process and the prescribed therapies. The teaching plan should include cleanliness, warmth, safety, comfort measures, prevention of constricting blood flow, exercise, signs and symptoms that should be reported to the health care provider, drug therapy, and the importance of smoking cessation.

SURGICAL PROCEDURES

As peripheral vascular disease progresses, surgical intervention may become necessary. Embolectomy, percutaneous transluminal angioplasty, endarterectomy, sympathectomy, vein ligation and stripping, and sclerotherapy are procedures that may be used.

Embolectomy

Embolectomy is the removal of a blood clot located in a large vessel. An incision is made into the vessel and the clot is removed under direct visualization of the site or through a catheter. This procedure is used when an arterial embolism is present and the patient has complicating factors that restrict the use of thrombolytic agents. Another method for performing an embolectomy is the use of a Fogarty embolectomy catheter. The catheter, which has a soft, inflatable balloon near the tip, is positioned in the artery. The tip of the catheter is passed through the embolus and inflated. Once the balloon is inflated, a steady tension is placed on the catheter to withdraw the entire embolus and catheter from the vessel.

Percutaneous Transluminal Angioplasty

Percutaneous transluminal angioplasty is used to gain access to the arteries in the lower extremities in people who are poor surgical risks. The primary purpose of this technique is to relieve arterial stenosis in such areas as the superficial femoral and iliac arteries. Under local anesthesia, a balloon catheter is passed into the vessel to the stenotic area. Once the catheter is maneuvered into the optimal position, the balloon is inflated. The inflated balloon presses outwardly against the vessel walls, dilating the lumen of the artery and improving blood flow. Heparin is injected through the catheter at the time of removal to prevent clot formation. Pressure must be applied to the catheter insertion site for approximately 10 to 20 minutes to prevent hemorrhage from the site. Complications of percutaneous transluminal angioplasty are hematoma formation, embolus, arterial dissection, and allergic reactions to the dye used in angiography.

Endarterectomy

An endarterectomy requires an incision into the obstructed vessel. The emboli and atherosclerotic plaque are stripped away from the intima of the vessel, and the vessel is surgically closed.

Sympathectomy

A sympathectomy may be done to improve vascular circulation when the patient has intermittent claudication. The process involves the excision of the sympathetic ganglia, which results in arteriolar dilation and increased blood flow. When poor circulation is related to atherosclerotic vessels, a sympathectomy is not the treatment of choice because the hardened blood vessels have limited ability to dilate. To evaluate the capacity for vascular dilation, a lumbar sympathetic block may be done and the temporary effects monitored.

Vein Ligation and Stripping

Vein ligation and stripping are used primarily to treat varicose veins. The greater or lesser saphenous systems, or both, are the vessels removed in this manner. The surgeon must be certain the deeper veins are patent before the varicosities are removed. Pressure and elevation are used during the procedure to reduce the bleeding. A disadvantage to this procedure is that removal of the saphenous vein means it would not be available if the patient required coronary artery bypass graft surgery in the future.

Sclerotherapy

Sclerotherapy is another method for managing varicose veins, primarily for cosmetic treatment of small, prominent varicosities. Sclerotherapy requires the injection of a chemical that irritates the venous endothelium, causing localized inflammation and fibrosis. The vein becomes thrombosed and eventually closes. Sclerotherapy may be used in conjunction with vein ligation and stripping. The protocol followed after the procedure depends on the physician but usually involves wearing compression stockings or support stockings for a specified period of time. An exercise program of walking is emphasized to encourage and facilitate the blood flow to the extremity. Potential complications include pulmonary embolism, thrombosis, injection site necrosis, vasospasm, hemolysis, and allergic reactions.

NURSING CARE *Related to Surgery*

Preoperative Nursing Care

General preoperative care is covered in Chapter 17. The patient with severe cardiovascular disease may have activity restrictions to reduce the demands on the circulatory system until the surgical procedure is done. The affected extremity should be maintained in a level or slightly dependent position as ordered. To optimize peripheral circulation, keep the extremity warm. Protect the limb from further injury.

Postoperative Nursing Care

The primary goal of the postoperative period is to stimulate circulation by encouraging movement and preventing stasis within the extremity. Closely monitor tissue perfusion in the postoperative period. Evaluate tissue perfusion by assessing the affected extremity for color, temperature, complaints of pain or tenderness, capillary refill time, presence of edema, quality of peripheral pulses, and exercise tolerance. Anticoagulants are usually continued after surgery to prevent the formation of a thrombus at the operative site. If a peripheral pulse disappears, suspect a thrombus. During the recovery period, emphasize that the patient should not cross the legs or place the affected extremity in a dependent position for long periods of time. Elevating the extremity helps prevent edema.

DRUGS

Drugs most often used to treat peripheral vascular disease include anticoagulants, thrombolytics, platelet aggregation inhibitors, vasodilators, nonsteroidal anti-inflammatory drugs, and analgesics. The Drug Therapy table below contains information about these.

Anticoagulants

Anticoagulant therapy is used to prolong the clotting time, hinder the extension of a thrombus, and inhibit the formation of a thrombus during the postoperative period. The primary anticoagulant medications used are heparin, low-molecular-weight heparin (LMWH), and warfarin sodium (Coumadin) derivatives. Heparin is

Consider the Alternative

Many herbal remedies interact with conventional drugs. Feverfew, garlic, ginger root, and ginkgo enhance the effects of antiplatelet drugs. St. John's wort can decrease the effectiveness of warfarin. Caution patients against using herbal remedies while on prescribed anticoagulants.

given intravenously for immediate response and subcutaneously for maintenance or prophylaxis. LMWH is given only subcutaneously, and warfarin is given orally. The clinical indications for anticoagulant treatment are venous thrombosis, pulmonary embolism, and risk for

DRUG THERAPY Peripheral Vascular Diseases

DRUG	USE/ACTION	SIDE EFFECTS	NURSING INTERVENTIONS
ANTICOAGULANTS			
Heparin sodium (Liquaemin Sodium)	Interferes with blood clotting; prevents formation of new clots; does not affect existing clots	Thrombocytopenia, bleeding, hemorrhage, nausea and vomiting, local irritation at injection site	Blood tested regularly to monitor effects on clotting. Check aPTT before each dose. Goal is aPTT 1.5 to 2.5 times normal. Monitor for bleeding. Avoid trauma. Heparin given IV or SC. After SC injection, apply pressure but do not massage. Rotate injection sites.
Low-molecular-weight heparin Enoxaparin (Lovenox) Dalteparin (Fragmin) Ardeparin (Normiflo)	Prevents formation of fibrin and thrombin	Thrombocytopenia, anemia, edema, nausea, fever, confusion, cardiac toxicity, bruising	Given SC only! Do not aspirate. Rotate sites. Leave bubble in syringe when administered. Administer at same time each day. Avoid IM injections. Teach patient to report any bleeding and to use soft toothbrush and electric razor. Do not take aspirin.
Warfarin sodium (Coumadin)	Interferes with blood clotting; may prevent extension of existing clots and formation of new clots	Bruising, hemorrhage, nausea, anorexia	Check prothrombin time/INR before each dose. May be required to notify physician before each dose. Monitor for bleeding. Teach patient not to take aspirin with warfarin.
PLATELET AGGREGATION INHIBITORS/ANTIPLATELETS			
Cilostazol (Pletal)	Inhibits platelet aggregation; used to treat intermittent claudication	Cardiac dysrhythmias, CHF, MI, cerebral infarct Hemorrhage, dizziness, back pain, cough, diarrhea	Monitor for bleeding, signs of heart failure. Blood work must be done during therapy. May take up to 12 weeks for effects.
Aspirin	Inhibits platelet aggregation; decreases inflammation and fever; reduces pain	GI irritation, tinnitus, pruritus, headache, bleeding	Assess for bruising, bleeding. Give with milk or food if GI irritation occurs.
Ticlopidine (Ticlid)	Inhibits platelet aggregation	Rash, diarrhea, hepatitis, cholestatic jaundice, bleeding, blood dyscrasias	Tell patient importance of having regular blood tests done and to report any bleeding. Taking with food decreases GI symptoms.
THROMBOLYTICS			
Streptokinase (Kabikinase) Urokinase (Abbokinase) Alteplase (Activase, t-PA)	Dissolves existing clots	Minor to major bleeding; transient thrombocytopenia and alopecia; hypersensitivity rare; cardiac dysrhythmias	Monitor blood tests of clotting activity. Monitor electrocardiogram and vital signs. Assess for bleeding. Protect from trauma.

aPTT, Activated partial thromboplastin time; CHF, congestive heart failure; GI, gastrointestinal; IM, intramuscular; INR, international normalized ratio; IV, intravenous; MI, myocardial infarction; SC, subcutaneous.

Continued

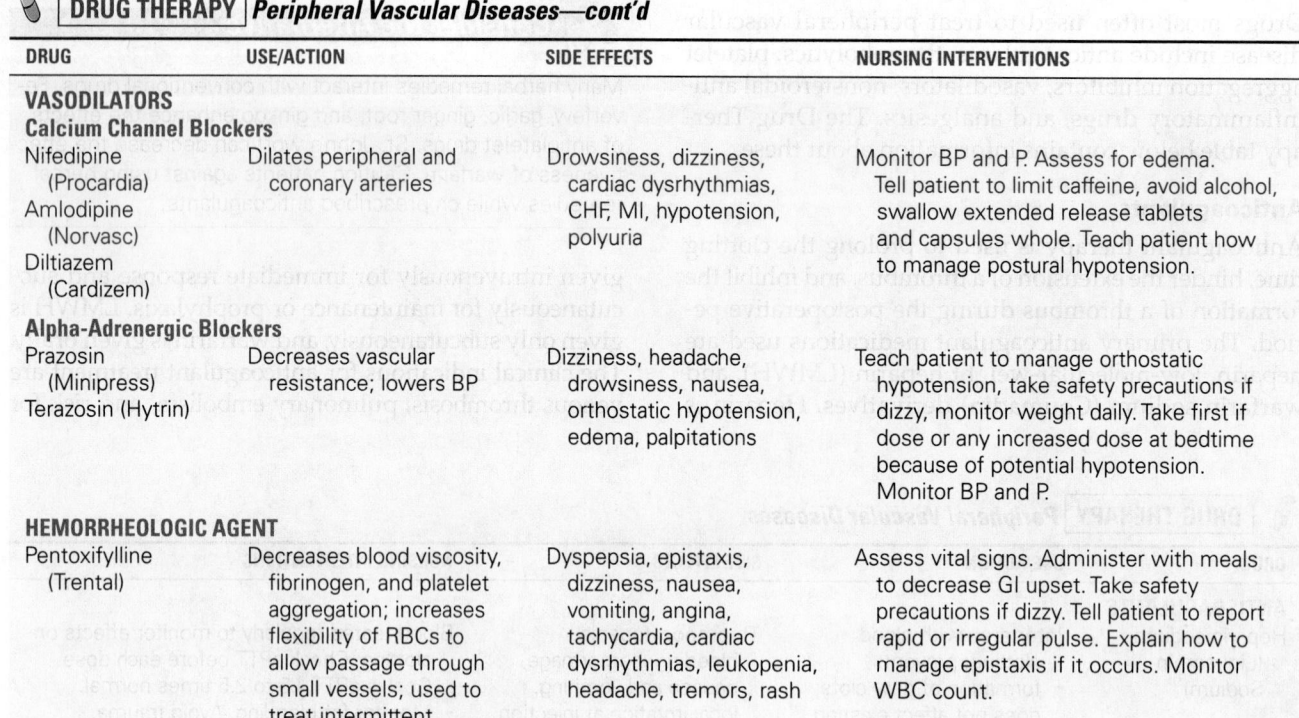

DRUG THERAPY | *Peripheral Vascular Diseases—cont'd*

DRUG	USE/ACTION	SIDE EFFECTS	NURSING INTERVENTIONS
VASODILATORS			
Calcium Channel Blockers			
Nifedipine (Procardia) Amlodipine (Norvasc) Diltiazem (Cardizem)	Dilates peripheral and coronary arteries	Drowsiness, dizziness, cardiac dysrhythmias, CHF, MI, hypotension, polyuria	Monitor BP and P. Assess for edema. Tell patient to limit caffeine, avoid alcohol, swallow extended release tablets and capsules whole. Teach patient how to manage postural hypotension.
Alpha-Adrenergic Blockers			
Prazosin (Minipress) Terazosin (Hytrin)	Decreases vascular resistance; lowers BP	Dizziness, headache, drowsiness, nausea, orthostatic hypotension, edema, palpitations	Teach patient to manage orthostatic hypotension, take safety precautions if dizzy, monitor weight daily. Take first if dose or any increased dose at bedtime because of potential hypotension. Monitor BP and P.
HEMORRHEOLOGIC AGENT			
Pentoxifylline (Trental)	Decreases blood viscosity, fibrinogen, and platelet aggregation; increases flexibility of RBCs to allow passage through small vessels; used to treat intermittent claudication	Dyspepsia, epistaxis, dizziness, nausea, vomiting, angina, tachycardia, cardiac dysrhythmias, leukopenia, headache, tremors, rash	Assess vital signs. Administer with meals to decrease GI upset. Take safety precautions if dizzy. Tell patient to report rapid or irregular pulse. Explain how to manage epistaxis if it occurs. Monitor WBC count.

BP, Blood pressure; *CHF,* congestive heart failure; *GI,* gastrointestinal; *MI,* myocardial infarction; *P,* pulse; *RBC,* red blood cell; *WBC,* white blood cell.

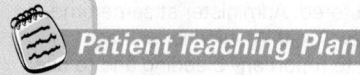

Patient Teaching Plan

Anticoagulant Therapy

- Anticoagulants help prevent blood clots from forming. Take your medications exactly as prescribed.
- Because these drugs can interfere with normal blood clotting, notify your physician of excessive bruising, bleeding gums, or blood in stools or urine.
- Consult your physician before taking any additional medications because some drugs affect the action of your anticoagulant.
- Keep appointments for regular blood tests to monitor the serum level of your drugs. Test results are used to ensure your dosage is safe and effective.
- Wear a medical alert bracelet noting anticoagulant therapy.

embolism. When anticoagulant therapy is used, regular coagulation tests are done to assess the effectiveness of the treatment regimen. The effective range for the activated partial thromboplastin time during heparin treatment is 1.5 to 2.5 times the control. Warfarin dosage is based on the patient's prothrombin time (PT) and international normalized ratio (INR). The target PT and INR depend on the condition being treated. LMWH has advantages over heparin because a fixed dose can be administered, laboratory monitoring is not necessary, and one or two doses daily are sufficient.

The fundamental complication of anticoagulant therapy is spontaneous bleeding that can occur anywhere in the body and may be evident in the urine, stool, emesis, or integument. Because of the risk of bleeding, the antidotes for each type of anticoagulant should be accessible. The antidote for heparin and LMWH is protamine sulfate; for warfarin sodium it is vitamin K.

Medications such as antibiotics, mineral oil, NSAIDs, aspirin, and tolbutamide can intensify the anticoagulant effects of warfarin sodium. Some drugs that decrease the effectiveness of warfarin are antacids, barbiturates, oral contraceptives, and adrenal corticosteroids.

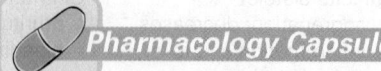

Pharmacology Capsule

Patients taking anticoagulant drugs must be monitored for bleeding.

Thrombolytics

Thrombolytic therapy is given intravenously to dissolve an existing clot. Examples of thrombolytic medications are streptokinase (Kabikinase), urokinase (Abbokinase), tissue plasminogen activator (Activase), reteplase (Retavase), and anistreplase (Eminase). Thrombolytic therapy is used to treat acute myocardial infarction, pulmonary embolism, deep vein thrombosis, and arterial thrombosis or embolism. Uncontrolled bleeding can result from thrombolytics; therefore the patient must be assessed continuously during the treatment regimen.

Pharmacology Capsule

Anticoagulants prevent the formation of blood clots; thrombolytics dissolve existing blood clots.

Other Medications

Many other types of medications are used to treat peripheral vascular diseases. Vasodilators are used to relax the vascular smooth muscle, which reduces resistance in the vessels and results in increased blood flow. Commonly used vasodilators are calcium channel blockers and alpha-adrenergic inhibitors. Analgesics including nonsteroidal anti-inflammatory agents are used to relieve the pain caused by ischemia. With less pain, a patient can participate more in exercises. Platelet aggregation inhibitors (antiplatelets) such as aspirin are used to prevent clot formation by making the platelets less likely to clump together. Pentoxifylline is used to treat peripheral vascular disease by improving the passage of red blood cells through small vessels.

In addition to drugs that prevent clot formation, patients also may be taking medications such as hypoglycemics and antihypertensives to control conditions that contribute to the development of peripheral vascular disease.

Pharmacology Capsule

Monitor patients taking vasodilators for hypotension. Teach them how to manage orthostatic hypotension.

DIETARY INTERVENTIONS

The dietary interventions used with peripheral vascular disease are like those recommended for cardiovascular health. Atherosclerotic plaques create rough vessel walls and contribute to peripheral vascular complications. Low-fat diets reduce serum cholesterol levels, thereby reducing the risk of atherosclerotic plaque formation. A weight-reduction diet may be prescribed if the patient is obese, because obesity causes a strain on the heart, increases venous congestion, and reduces peripheral circulation. Adequate vitamin B, vitamin C, and protein are needed to promote healing and improve tissue integrity. (See the Nutrition Concepts box on p. 712.)

DISORDERS OF THE PERIPHERAL VASCULAR SYSTEM

ARTERIAL EMBOLISM

Pathophysiology

The development of an arterial embolism is a potentially life-threatening event. The arterial embolus usually forms in the heart. However, a roughened atheromatous plaque in any artery can lead to thrombus formation. If a thrombus breaks loose, it becomes an embolus traveling through the circulatory system until it lodges in a vessel, blocking blood flow distal to the occlusion. The effects of arterial occlusion depend on the size of the embolus formed, the organs involved, and the extent to which collateral circulation can maintain sufficient blood supply to affected tissues.

Signs and Symptoms

Whereas some patients with arterial obstruction have no pain, others experience severe pain and other symptoms of tissue ischemia. When the collateral circulation cannot compensate for the compromised blood flow, the patient has distinct symptoms of reduced blood flow to the tissues. Signs and symptoms of inadequate blood supply are the following:

1. Severe, acute pain
2. Gradual loss of sensory and motor function in the affected areas
3. Pain aggravated by movement or pressure
4. Absent distal pulses
5. Pallor and mottling (irregular discoloration)
6. A sharp line of color and temperature demarcation: tissue beyond the obstruction is pale and cool

Medical and Surgical Treatment

Arterial embolism is managed with intravenous anticoagulants and thrombolytic agents. These medications cannot be used with active internal bleeding, cardiovascular accident, recent major surgery, uncontrolled hypertension, and pregnancy. Patients who cannot be treated with medications may be prepared for embolectomy—surgical removal of the embolus.

NURSING CARE *of the Patient with Arterial Embolism*

Assessment

The assessment of the patient with peripheral vascular disease is outlined in Box 36-1.

NURSING DIAGNOSES	GOALS AND OUTCOME CRITERIA
Nursing Diagnoses, Goals, and Outcome Criteria: Arterial Embolism	
Ineffective Tissue Perfusion related to compromised circulation	Improved tissue perfusion: normal skin color, palpable pulses, capillary refill time less than 3 seconds in affected extremity

Continued

Fear related to the treatments, environment, and risk of death	Reduced fear: patient calm, states fear reduced or relieved
Impaired Physical Mobility related to the surgical procedure and compromised circulation	Improved physical mobility: patient increases activity without discomfort
Impaired Skin Integrity related to ischemic changes from the impairment of peripheral circulation	Healthy skin in affected areas: skin intact
Ineffective Therapeutic Regimen Management related to lack of knowledge of self-care	Patient knows and practices prescribed self-care measures: patient correctly describes and demonstrates self-care measures

Interventions

Nursing interventions are designed to improve circulation and prevent further damage to the affected tissue.

Ineffective Tissue Perfusion

To promote circulation, maintain the affected extremities at or slightly below the horizontal, administer prescribed medications, and perform range-of-motion exercises as ordered.

Fear

To decrease fear, orient the patient to the environment and the expected therapies using simple statements to explain the disease process and procedures. Encourage the expression of feelings of helplessness and anxiety, and help the patient identify coping mechanisms that have worked in other situations.

Impaired Physical Mobility

Improved physical mobility requires instruction in range-of-motion exercises and the development of a progressive exercise plan. This exercise plan usually is limited to 15 minutes, three times a day, for the initial days after surgery or treatment. The progression of exercise is determined by the individual patient's response.

Impaired Skin Integrity

With arterial embolism, the affected tissue is highly susceptible to injury. Protect the limb from pressure, trauma, and extreme heat or cold. Edematous tissue is equally susceptible to injury and must be protected.

Ineffective Therapeutic Regimen Management

Patient teaching enables the patient to participate in the plan of care during and after hospitalization. If the patient is on anticoagulant therapy, also see Patient Teaching Plan: Anticoagulant Therapy on p. 698.

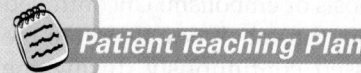

Patient Teaching Plan

Arterial Embolism

Discharge teaching should include the following:
- Protect affected limbs from pressure, trauma, and temperature extremes.
- Exercise improves blood flow; gradually increase your activity as you are able to tolerate it.
- Report pain, numbness, coolness, or pale or bluish skin color to your physician.

Table 36-1 compares features of arterial and venous disease.

PERIPHERAL ARTERIAL OCCLUSIVE DISEASE

Pathophysiology

Peripheral arterial occlusive disease is called *atherosclerosis obliterans, arterial insufficiency,* and *peripheral vascular disease.* It is characterized by pathologic changes in the arteries, typically plaque formations that arise where the arteries branch, veer, arch, or narrow (Fig. 36-7). The most common sites for arterial occlusion are the distal superficial femoral and the popliteal arteries. Occlusions prevent the delivery of oxygen and nutrients to the tissues. Hypoxia affects all tissues distal to

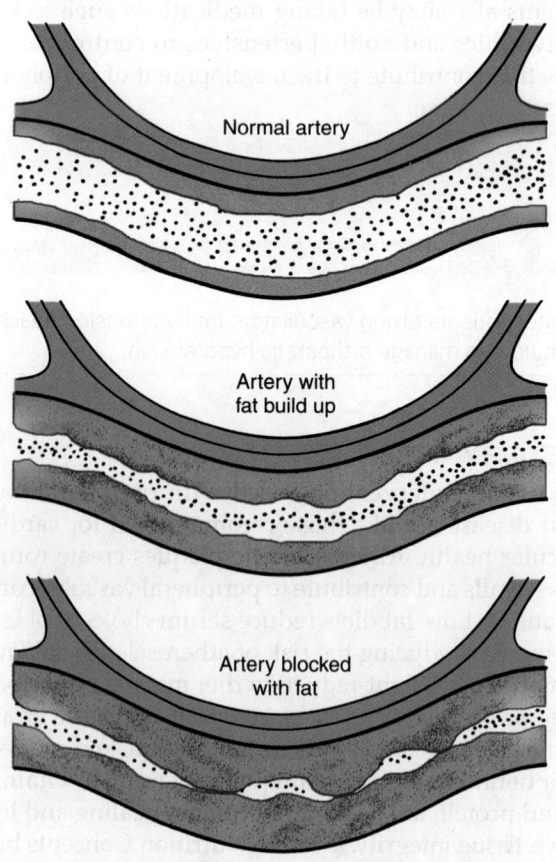

FIGURE **36-7** Development of atherosclerosis.

Table 36-1   *Comparison of Arterial and Venous Insufficiency in the Legs*

CHARACTERISTIC	ARTERIAL	VENOUS
Peripheral pulses	Decreased or absent	Present; may be difficult to palpate because of edema
Capillary refill	>3 seconds	<3 seconds
Edema	None	Lower leg edema
Hair	Loss of hair on legs, feet, toes	Hair may be present or absent
Skin color	Dark reddish color when in dependent position; pale when elevated	Bronze-brown pigmentation; varicose veins may be visible
Skin temperature	Cool	Warm
Pain	Intermittent claudication or rest pain	Dull ache, heaviness in calf or thigh

Modified from Lewis, S.M., Heitkemper, M.M., & Dirksen, S.R. (2004). *Medical-surgical nursing: Assessment and management of clinical problems* (6th ed.). St. Louis: Mosby.

the occlusion. Peripheral nerves and muscles are more susceptible to harm from hypoxia than the skin and subcutaneous tissues. Severe oxygen deprivation may lead to ischemia and then to necrosis (tissue death).

Because peripheral arterial occlusive disease develops gradually, compensatory mechanisms attempt to maintain circulation. These compensatory mechanisms include the development of collateral blood vessels, vasodilation, and anaerobic metabolism. Collateral blood vessels are small, new vessels that branch out to supply blood to poorly perfused tissues. The extent of collateral circulation determines the severity of symptoms.

Peripheral arterial occlusive disease is most common in men older than 50 years. Factors that contribute to the development of this disease include atherosclerosis, embolism, thrombosis, trauma, vasospasm, inflammation, and autoimmune responses. Other risk factors that are more controllable are hyperlipidemia, diabetes mellitus, hypertension, cigarette smoking, and stress.

Signs and Symptoms

The clinical manifestations of peripheral arterial occlusive disease develop gradually. Intermittent claudication is the classic sign. It is experienced as the aching, cramping, tiredness, and weakness in the legs that occur with walking and is relieved by rest. Another manifestation of peripheral arterial occlusive disease is the absence of peripheral pulses below the occlusive area. *Rest pain*, pain that develops during rest, is common. Rest pain is described as persistent and aching. Complaints of tingling or numbness or both in the toes are common. The affected extremity is cold and numb because of the reduction in the flow of blood to the area. Muscle atrophy may be evident. The skin of the affected area is pale because of reduced blood flow. When the extremity is in a dependent position, the color becomes red. Reduced blood supply to toenails can cause the nails to thicken. Other signs of arterial occlusion are shiny, scaly skin; subcutane-

ous tissue loss; hairlessness on the affected extremity; and ulcers with a pale gray or yellowish hue, especially at the ankles. If one extremity is affected more than the other, size differences between the extremities may be apparent.

Medical Diagnosis

The primary diagnostic tests used to confirm a diagnosis of peripheral arterial occlusive disease are duplex imaging and, if surgery is contemplated, angiography.

Medical and Surgical Treatment

The first step in managing peripheral arterial occlusive disease is to make lifestyle changes including smoking cessation, exercise, and weight management. Smoking cessation is a high priority. Success may be enhanced with nicotine replacement therapy and amfebutamone or bupropion. Exercise programs found to be most successful with peripheral arterial disease include at least three sessions of 30 minutes or more each week over at least 6 months, with walking as the preferred type of exercise. Treatment should be initiated for hypertension, hyperlipidemia, or diabetes, if present. Among the drugs used to treat claudication are cilostazol and pentoxifylline. Both prevent platelets from clumping; pentoxifylline also make RBCs more flexible and the blood less thick.

Surgical interventions are percutaneous transluminal angioplasty, atherectomy, and endarterectomy. An endarterectomy with a graft is the surgical replacement of a diseased segment of an artery with a graft of some type—either synthetic or from another blood vessel. Percutaneous transluminal angioplasty (PTA) is used to enlarge the interior diameter of the blood vessel. Possible complications with PTA are hematoma formation, embolus, arterial dissection, and allergic reaction. Low-dose aspirin with or without clopidogrel may be ordered after PTA. If angioplasty fails, a stent may be placed in the vessel to keep the lumen open.

NURSING CARE *of the Patient with Peripheral Arterial Occlusive Disease*

Assessment

Complete assessment of the patient with peripheral vascular disease is summarized in Box 36-1. When the patient has had surgical intervention, it is especially important to assess the pulses distal to the surgical site and compare them with the same pulses in the unaffected extremity. Cessation of a pulse suggests possible arterial occlusion, and the surgeon must be notified immediately. Other important aspects of the postoperative assessment are vital signs, color and temperature of the affected extremity, fluid intake and output, central venous pressure, and mental status. If the patient has pain, document the location, severity, and nature of the pain.

**Nursing Diagnoses, Goals, and Outcome Criteria:
Peripheral Arterial Occlusive Disease**

NURSING DIAGNOSES	GOALS AND OUTCOME CRITERIA
Activity Intolerance related to impaired blood flow to extremities	Improved activity tolerance: patient states is increasingly able to perform activities without pain
Chronic Pain related ischemia	Reduced pain: patient states pain reduced, relaxed manner
Impaired Skin Integrity related to inadequate circulation	Healthy skin: skin intact with normal color and warmth
Disturbed Body Image related to muscle atrophy, stasis ulcers, and skin discoloration	Positive body image: positive patient statements about self, patient makes effort to maintain good physical appearance
Ineffective Tissue Perfusion related to vascular occlusion	Adequate tissue perfusion: palpable peripheral pulses, extremity warm with normal skin color
Ineffective Therapeutic Regimen Management related to lack of knowledge of disease process, treatment, and self-care	Patient carries out proper self-care measures: patient describes and demonstrates self-care

If surgical intervention is performed, additional diagnoses and goals may include the following:

NURSING DIAGNOSES	GOALS AND OUTCOME CRITERIA
Risk for Infection related to surgical incision, graft placement	Absence of infection: normal body temperature, decreasing wound redness and drainage
Decreased Cardiac Output related to hemorrhage, diuresis, fluid shifts	Normal cardiac output: pulse and blood pressure consistent with patient norms
Ineffective Tissue Perfusion related to graft thrombosis	Patent graft: operative extremity warm, with improved color and palpable pulses
Acute Pain related to surgical incision	Pain relief: patient relaxed, states that pain is relieved
Impaired Physical Mobility related to weakness, fear, surgical procedure	Increased physical mobility: increasing activity without pain

Interventions

Activity Intolerance

To monitor the patient's activity tolerance, assess the patient before, during, and after planned activities. Then monitor progress as treatment progresses. When planning an exercise regimen, use the following guidelines:

1. Work with the patient to plan the activity schedule and goals.
2. Gradually increase the exercise time as tolerance increases.
3. Discontinue activity if the patient has chest pain, bradycardia, dyspnea, or intermittent claudication. After rest relieves the pain of intermittent claudication, the patient may resume activity.
4. Reduce the intensity of the activity if the pulse takes longer than 3 to 4 minutes to return to the baseline rate or if the patient has severe dyspnea.
5. For patients confined to bed, start exercises with range-of-motion exercises twice daily.
6. Patients should *not* exercise when they have leg ulcers, cellulitis, deep vein thrombosis, or gangrene.

Chronic Pain

The chronic pain associated with ischemia is exhausting and greatly reduces the patient's quality of life. Therefore pain management must be a priority. The most direct interventions are those that increase circulation or decrease metabolic demands of ischemic tissues. Resting the extremities in a dependent position may help relieve the pain of arterial occlusive disease. Administer analgesics as prescribed, along with other comfort measures. Nonpharmacologic pain relief measures include relaxation techniques, warm baths, breathing exercises, and backrubs. See Chapter 15 for a detailed discussion of pain management.

Impaired Skin Integrity

The nursing interventions for maintaining skin integrity are the same as those for patients with arterial

Consider the Alternative

Relaxation, warm baths, breathing exercises, and backrubs can help the patient with chronic pain.

embolism. To maintain skin integrity, take measures to improve circulation and avoid tissue trauma. If the patient has an ulcerated area, keep it clean and free of pressure. Various wound care products may be prescribed to protect the wound and prevent infection. However, unless circulation is improved, healing is unlikely. The physician will prescribe any activity limitations.

The feet are especially susceptible to injury and require special care. Advise the patient not to go barefoot, to wear only shoes that fit properly, to inspect the feet daily for signs of pressure or lesions, and to keep the toenails neatly trimmed. Because of the risk of ingrown nails, nails should not be trimmed too short. Toenails should always be cut straight across rather than in a curved shape. The patient should see a peripheral vascular specialist promptly if any foot problems develop.

Ineffective Therapeutic Regimen Management

To cope with peripheral arterial occlusive disease, the patient must understand the disease process and treatment. Include the family in patient teaching because their fears and concerns can have an enormous impact on the patient's perception of the situation. The patient teaching plan is the same as for the patient with arterial embolism. Adaptation to lifestyle changes is essential to good management of peripheral arterial disease.

Disturbed Body Image

Encourage the patient to express feelings that result from problems associated with peripheral arterial occlusive disease, such as activity intolerance, stasis ulcers, discoloration of the extremities, and, for some, amputations. Be supportive and help the patient identify coping strategies to deal with the feelings.

Ineffective Tissue Perfusion

Administer vasodilators and other drugs that improve blood flow as ordered. Encourage exercise according to the individualized exercise plan. Maintain adequate warmth, and discourage smoking. Elevation of the extremities usually is *not* recommended with arterial disease.

Additional interventions are indicated for the postoperative patient.

Risk for Infection

After surgery, patients are at risk for infection of the surgical incision and the grafts (especially synthetic grafts) that are used to replace the diseased blood vessel. An infected synthetic graft is very serious because it necessitates removal of the graft and often amputation. Monitor the patient's temperature and report fever to the surgeon. Inspect the incision for increasing redness, edema, and drainage that suggest infection. Antimicrobials are usually ordered before surgery and may be continued after surgery.

Decreased Cardiac Output

Monitor for signs and symptoms of deficient fluid volume: tachycardia, restlessness, decreased urine output, pallor, and hypotension. Provide intravenous and oral fluids as ordered, and keep records of fluid intake and output. Monitor daily weights. Inspect the surgical dressing for bleeding, which must be reported immediately to the surgeon.

Ineffective Tissue Perfusion

Thrombus formation can occur in the graft, causing occlusion and impaired blood flow. Monitor the pulses, warmth, and color of the operative extremity and promptly inform the surgeon of diminishing pulses, coolness, and pallor or cyanosis. Some patients are given anticoagulants or thrombolytics to decrease the risk of graft occlusion. Edema for 4 to 8 weeks is common after bypass surgery. The leg is usually wrapped in a light dressing or vascular boot and kept flat initially. Elastic stockings are not used immediately after a vein graft.

Acute Pain

Acute postoperative pain is treated with analgesics, positioning, and relaxation techniques as described in Chapters 15 and 17.

Impaired Physical Mobility

After surgery, the patient's activities are increased gradually. A specific program of exercises may be prescribed. Assist the patient, and assess muscle strength and tolerance of activity.

THROMBOANGIITIS OBLITERANS

Thromboangiitis obliterans, also called *Buerger's disease*, is an inflammatory thrombotic disorder of arteries and veins in both the lower and upper extremities. It is not an atherosclerotic process. The exact cause is unknown, but it occurs only in smokers. Signs and symptoms may include intermittent claudication, rest pain, skin color and temperature changes in affected areas, cold sensitivity, abnormal sensation, ulceration, and gangrene. Diagnosis is based on physical findings and arteriography.

The most important aspect of treatment is smoking cessation. Palliative treatments include sympathectomy and drugs such as calcium channel blockers, antibiotics, and anticoagulants. If gangrene develops (most commonly below the knee), amputation is the only option. Forty percent of patients who continue tobacco use eventually require amputations. Nursing care is similar to that of patients with peripheral arterial occlusive

What Does Culture Have to Do with Buerger's Disease?

Buerger's disease is very common in India, Korea, and Japan. It is relatively uncommon in the United States. When assessing patients, especially those of Indian, Korean, or Japanese heritage, be alert for related signs and symptoms.

disorders. Emphasis is on smoking cessation measures (see Chapter 30) and protection of the affected extremities.

RAYNAUD'S DISEASE

Pathophysiology

Raynaud's disease and phenomenon are forms of an intermittent constriction of arterioles that affects the hands primarily, although it can affect the toes and tip of the nose. Increased or unusual sensations of coldness, pain, and pallor reflect temporary constriction of the arterioles in the affected areas. Gangrene is not common but can develop in the skin on the tips of the digits. The cause of this condition is unknown, but it may be related to hypersensitivity to cold or release of serotonin. Primarily women from the ages of 16 to 40 years are affected, especially during the winter months or in northern areas where cold weather is more common. Stress seems to aggravate the disease process. Raynaud's phenomenon follows the same general pattern but is typically secondary to connective tissue or collagen vascular disease. The term *primary Raynaud's phenomenon* is synonymous with *Raynaud's disease; secondary Raynaud's phenomenon* is also called simply *Raynaud's phenomenon*.

Consider the Alternative

Biofeedback is sometimes helpful in controlling vasospastic episodes with Raynaud's disease.

Signs and Symptoms

The cardinal signs and symptoms of Raynaud's disease are chronically cold hands, numbness, tingling, and pallor. Finger involvement is not symmetric, and the thumb is not usually affected. During an arterial spasm, the skin color changes from pallor to cyanosis to redness. Pallor is the result of sudden vasoconstriction. Cyanosis reflects inadequate oxygenation. As the spasm resolves, vasodilation allows blood flow to return, which produces a red color.

Medical Diagnosis

The diagnosis of Raynaud's disease is usually based on the signs and symptoms and on the absence of evidence of occlusive vascular disease.

Medical and Surgical Treatment

The goals of the medical treatment plan for Raynaud's disease are to prevent pain and to promote vasodilation in the extremities. Drugs that may be used are calcium channel blockers, transdermal nitroglycerin, an endothelin receptor antagonist (bosentan), phosphodiesterase inhibitors (e.g., sildenafil), and intravenous prostaglandins (e.g., iloprost, alprostadil). In severe cases, the physician may resort to sympathectomy to interrupt the sympathetic nerves. This surgical procedure aids some patients but tends to have temporary effects and is not used routinely.

NURSING CARE *of the Patient with Raynaud's Disease*

Assessment

Assessment of the patient with peripheral vascular disease is summarized in Box 36-1. With Raynaud's disease, assessment of the hands is the priority.

Nursing Diagnoses, Goals, and Outcome Criteria: Raynaud's Disease	
NURSING DIAGNOSES	GOALS AND OUTCOME CRITERIA
Acute Pain related to the ischemia that develops from vasoconstriction	Reduced pain: patient states that pain has decreased, appears relaxed
Ineffective Tissue Perfusion related to vasoconstriction	Improved oxygenation of peripheral tissue: improved warmth and color of affected areas
Fear related to the potential loss of work, difficulty performing activities of daily living	Relief from fear: patient states fear is reduced, appears more relaxed

Interventions

Acute Pain and Ineffective Tissue Perfusion

Nursing interventions to reduce pain and improve tissue perfusion focus on teaching the patient to avoid the stimuli that cause the vasoconstriction: exposure to cold, smoking, and excessive stress. Encourage the patient to take part in a smoking cessation program and to dress warmly when going out in cold weather. Mittens are better than gloves for maintaining warmth. Sometimes the patient can interrupt an acute attack by placing the affected parts in warm water or by using a hair dryer or hand- and foot-warming devices. In addition to alcohol and caffeine, many drugs including over-the-counter cold remedies can aggravate Raynaud's disease. Patients should wear medical alert identification, and inform all new health care providers of their diagnosis so that inappropriate medications will not be prescribed.

Pain can be managed by carefully warming the area when vasoconstriction occurs. However, the affected areas must be protected from trauma. Do not use hot water to warm affected tissue, because the lack of sensation during the period of vasoconstriction could result in serious burns.

Fear

Fear can be addressed in much the same manner as anxiety. Attempt to determine the actual cause of fear, which might be loss of work, loss of limb, or pain. Accept and explore the patient's feelings, provide factual information, encourage problem solving, and help the patient learn to live with the condition and to manage the prescribed therapy.

ANEURYSMS

Pathophysiology

An aneurysm is a dilated segment of an artery caused by weakness and stretching of the arterial wall. Aneurysms can be congenital or acquired. Conditions associated with congenital aneurysms are Marfan syndrome and Ehlers-Danlos syndrome. Acquired aneurysms can be caused by arteriosclerosis, trauma, or infection. The most common cause of aneurysms is atherosclerosis. Hypertension is apparently a contributing factor. The effect of atherosclerosis on the media, the middle layer of the arterial wall, is to weaken elastic fibers, which allows a segment of the vessel to balloon out. Infections, including syphilis, can also damage the media and result in the formation of aneurysms. The abdominal aorta is the most common site of aneurysm formation.

Signs and Symptoms

Signs and symptoms, if any, vary with the location of the aneurysm. People with thoracic aneurysms usually have no symptoms, though some report deep, diffuse chest pain. If the aneurysm puts pressure on the recurrent laryngeal nerve, the patient may complain of hoarseness. Pressure on the esophagus may cause dysphagia (difficulty swallowing). If the superior vena cava is compressed, the patient may have edema of the head and arms. Signs of airway obstruction may be present if the aneurysm presses against pulmonary structures.

Abdominal aneurysms are usually detected during routine physical examinations or radiologic studies. The aneurysm may be palpated as a pulsating mass in the area slightly left of the umbilicus. Although most abdominal aneurysms are asymptomatic, pressure on abdominal organs and nerves may cause back pain, epigastric pain, or constipation.

Complications

Complications of aneurysms include rupture, thrombus formation that obstructs blood flow, emboli, and pressure on surrounding structures.

Medical Diagnosis

Diagnosis is made on the basis of physical findings and radiologic studies. Studies performed to obtain better visualization of the aneurysm include echocardiography, ultrasonography, computed tomography, and aortography.

Medical and Surgical Treatment

Repair of aneurysms may be done by replacing the dilated segment of the artery with a synthetic graft or, in some cases, by suturing or patching the defective area. Repair is usually done as soon as possible but may be delayed until the patient is evaluated for other problems that increase surgical risk.

Decisions to attempt repair of aneurysms are based on the size of the defect and the patient's general status. For example, an abdominal aortic aneurysm smaller than 5 cm is usually monitored with periodic ultrasound studies. If it begins to enlarge, surgical repair may then be recommended.

Complications of aneurysm surgery vary with the location of the defect. Complications of aortic abdominal aneurysm surgery include myocardial infarction, sexual dysfunction, renal failure, emboli, spinal cord ischemia with paralysis, bowel and bladder incontinence, and impaired sensation.

PREOPERATIVE NURSING CARE of the Patient with an Aneurysm

When surgical repair of an aneurysm is planned, prepare the patient physically and emotionally as described in Chapter 17. It is important to document chronic conditions such as emphysema or heart disease that increase the risk of postoperative complications.

POSTOPERATIVE NURSING CARE of the Patient with an Aneurysm

After aortic aneurysm repair, the patient usually is kept in a critical care area for 24 to 48 hours. Mechanical ventilation may be used initially to maintain good oxygenation status.

Assessment

General postoperative assessment is outlined in Box 17-3. After repair of an aortic aneurysm, it is vital to monitor vital signs, hemodynamic status, renal function, and fluid balance. Inspect and palpate the extremities for color, warmth, and peripheral pulses.

Nursing Diagnoses, Goals, and Outcome Criteria: Aortic Aneurysm Repair

In addition to the routine problems of the postoperative patient (see Chapter 17), nursing diagnoses for the patient who has had an aortic aneurysm repair may include the following:

Nursing Diagnoses	Goals and Outcome Criteria
Impaired Urinary Elimination related to interrupted blood flow	Normal urinary function: urine output approximately equal to fluid intake
Risk for Injury related to ileus	Absence of injury related to ileus: wound margins intact, no abdominal distention, bowel sounds present
Ineffective Breathing Pattern related to abdominal incision or splinting	Effective breathing pattern: regular respirations, 12 to 20/min, clear breath sounds
Decreased Cardiac Output related to myocardial infarction, occlusion of blood vessels, graft leakage	Adequate cardiac output: pulse and blood pressure consistent with patient norms
Ineffective Tissue Perfusion related to vascular occlusion	Normal peripheral circulation: warm extremities with palpable pulses

Interventions

Impaired Urinary Elimination

During repair of an abdominal aneurysm, the aorta is clamped for a period of time. This poses a risk of renal damage and subsequent renal failure. Therefore fluid intake and urine output must be measured and recorded hourly. Declining urine output must be promptly reported to the physician. Blood urea nitrogen, creatinine, and electrolyte levels are usually measured daily to detect increases associated with renal failure. Because fluid retention or circulatory obstruction may cause edema, its presence should be noted. Intravenous fluids should be administered as ordered.

Risk for Injury

After abdominal surgery, peristalsis ceases temporarily. A nasogastric tube is usually inserted and attached to suction to prevent gaseous distention of the bowel, which is uncomfortable and places stress on the abdominal incision. Be sure the suction is working properly, and monitor for distention and the return of bowel sounds.

Ineffective Breathing Pattern

Whether the patient has an abdominal or a thoracic incision, there is a risk of poor lung expansion. After thoracic surgery, patients are at especially high risk for atelectasis and pneumonia. Mechanical ventilation in the immediate postoperative period maintains adequate ventilation until the patient is able to breathe effectively. Thereafter, assist the patient to turn, deep breathe, and cough frequently. An incentive spirometer may be used to encourage lung expansion. Support the patient's incision during the breathing exercises. Administer analgesics and use other pain relief measures. The patient can breathe more effectively if good pain relief is achieved. Monitor lung sounds frequently to assess for abnormalities.

Decreased Cardiac Output

Cardiac output may fall as a result of myocardial infarction, cardiac dysrhythmias, heart failure, or hemorrhage. Hemorrhage may occur in the incision or by separation of the graft. Closely monitor the patient's vital signs and hemodynamics. Assess the wound dressing and drains for increasing bleeding. Early signs of circulatory failure are restlessness and tachycardia. Later signs are hypotension, cyanosis, and decreased alertness. Immediately notify the physician if there is evidence of decreasing cardiac output.

Ineffective Tissue Perfusion

There is a risk of impaired blood flow below the level of the aneurysm. Monitor peripheral pulses and the color and warmth of the extremities. This assessment is especially important when a patient has had a femoral or popliteal aneurysm repair. Signs and symptoms of occlusion include pain, pallor or cyanosis, and coldness distal to the repair. If these manifestations occur, they must be reported to the physician at once.

AORTIC DISSECTION

Aortic dissection is different from an aneurysm. A small tear in the intima permits blood to escape into the space between the intima and the media. Blood accumulates between the layers, possibly causing the media to split lengthwise. The split may extend up and down the aorta, where it can occlude major arteries. If no complications occur, the patient may be managed with antihypertensives and drugs to decrease the strength of cardiac contractions. Otherwise, the affected area is replaced with a synthetic graft. A key aspect of postoperative care is keeping the blood pressure at the lowest possible level. In other respects, the care is similar to that of a patient who has had an aneurysm repair.

VARICOSE VEIN DISEASE

Pathophysiology

Varicose veins are referred to as *varicosities*. Varicosities are dilated, tortuous, superficial veins, often the saphenous veins in the lower extremities (Fig. 36-8). The dilation of the vessels results from incompetent valves in the veins—that is, the valves cannot prevent backflow of blood. Vein incompetence is a result of hereditary weakness, aging, pregnancy, obesity, occupations requiring prolonged standing, or a combination of these. Restrictive clothing aggravates the condition. Varicose veins are classified as *primary* (only superficial veins are affected) and *secondary* (characterized by deep vein obstruction). In addition to peripheral veins, varicosities can occur in other areas such as the esophageal and hemorrhoidal veins. Incompetent valves cannot be repaired.

Signs and Symptoms

The onset of varicose vein disease is gradual, but the condition is progressive. When only the superficial veins are involved, the signs and symptoms are minimal except for the cosmetic changes that occur. The dilated veins are seen as oversized, discolored (purplish), and tortuous. Symptoms typically include dull aching sensations when standing or walking; a feeling of heaviness in the affected legs; muscle cramps, especially at night; increased muscular fatigue in the affected area; and ankle edema. Over time, some people develop postphlebitic syndrome, which is evidenced by persistent edema, brownish skin discoloration, and ulcers most commonly on the inner aspect of the ankle.

Medical Diagnosis

Varicose veins typically are diagnosed on the basis of their appearance. Duplex ultrasonography may be used to evaluate obstruction and reflux. Information about other diagnostic tests and procedures is presented in the Diagnostic Tests and Procedures table on p. 692.

FIGURE 36-8 Venous return from the legs. **A,** Normal flow. **B,** Varicosities and retrograde venous flow.

External
iliac
veins

Femoral
veins

Great saphenous
veins

Small saphenous
veins

Perforating veins

A   **B**

Medical and Surgical Treatment

Conservative treatments of varicosities are used whenever possible. Encourage the patient to avoid restrictive garments, prolonged standing or sitting, crossing the legs or knees, and injury to the compromised areas. Inform the obese patient that weight reduction usually reduces pressure on the lower extremities. If the physician recommends support stockings, help the patient learn how to put them on correctly.

Sclerotherapy or laser therapy may be effective in the treatment of superficial varicosities.. Surgery may be recommended for cosmetic reasons or if stasis ulcers develop. The surgical procedure that removes large dilated veins is called *ligation and stripping.*

NURSING CARE *of the Patient with Varicose Vein Disease*

Assessment

When a patient has varicose veins, the health history determines the presence of pain, edema, cramps, and muscle fatigue. Note a family history of varicose veins. Document the patient's occupation and usual activities. When taking a pain and discomfort history, determine what measures the patient has used for pain control.

The physical examination focuses on inspection of the legs for color, edema, turgor, and capillary refill. Palpate the legs for tenderness. Postoperative assessment is especially concerned with monitoring peripheral circulation and tissue perfusion.

Nursing Diagnoses, Goals, and Outcome Criteria: Varicose Veins

Nursing Diagnoses	Goals and Outcome Criteria
Chronic Pain related to engorgement of the veins	Reduced pain: patient states that pain with activity has decreased
Activity Intolerance related to feelings of heaviness and fatigue	Improved activity tolerance: gradual increase in activity with less discomfort
Ineffective Therapeutic Regimen Management related to management of the varicosities	Patient carries out appropriate self-care: patient correctly verbalizes and demonstrates self-care

Interventions

The primary nursing role in the care of the patient with varicose veins is teaching self-care. Interventions to improve activity tolerance and to manage pain are outlined

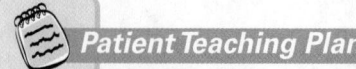
Patient Teaching Plan

Varicose Veins

- Wear antiembolism hose or support hose as recommended by your physician.
- Exercise regularly to promote circulation.
- Avoid prolonged standing, sitting, crossing your legs.
- Avoid restrictive clothing.
- Elevate extremities whenever possible.
- Obesity contributes to the development of varicose veins. People who are overweight usually see improvement with weight loss.
- Nonprescription analgesics and frequent position changes usually control pain.

in the Patient Teaching Plan above. In general, measures that improve venous return also decrease pain.

For the surgical patient, patient teaching also is of paramount importance because the procedure is often done as a same-day surgical procedure. While the patient is still in the surgical suite, pressure bandages are placed on the extremities. The surgeon orders specific aspects of postoperative care such as when the pressure bandages should be removed, what types of stockings are recommended afterwards and how long they should be worn, activity restrictions, and positioning of the legs (usually 15-30 degrees for the first 24 hours). After sclerotherapy or laser therapy, which are outpatient procedures, the patient is advised to wear compression stockings for as long as 6 weeks.

VENOUS THROMBOSIS
Pathophysiology

The terms phlebitis, thrombophlebitis, phlebothrombosis, and *deep vein thrombosis* are often used interchangeably. Each term in reality describes a slightly different process. Phlebitis is an inflammation of the vein wall. With thrombophlebitis, a clot has formed at the site of inflammation within a vein. Phlebothrombosis describes the presence of a thrombus in a vein as a result of stasis, deviation of the intima, or hypercoagulability (an abnormally increased tendency of blood to clot). Deep vein thrombosis (DVT) refers to the presence of a clot in one of the deep veins rather than in the superficial vessels. The deep veins commonly involved with thrombi are the femoral, popliteal, and small calf veins. The superficial vein that is most often the site of thrombus formation is the saphenous vein. A grave complication of deep vein thrombosis is a pulmonary embolism.

Risk Factors

Some of the risk factors that may predispose a person to the development of thrombi are the following:
1. Prescribed bed rest
2. Surgery under general anesthesia for people older than 40 years

3. Leg trauma resulting in immobilization from casts or traction
4. Previous venous insufficiency
5. Obesity
6. Use of oral contraceptives
7. Malignancy

Research has identified three factors (called *Virchow's triad*) that contribute to venous thrombus formation: (1) stasis of the blood, (2) damage to the vessel walls, and (3) hypercoagulability. At least two of the three factors must be present for a thrombus to form.

Signs and Symptoms

The signs and symptoms of each of the disease processes are slightly different, depending on the diagnosis, the size and location of the thrombus, the amount of obstruction, the collateral circulation, and the existence of other medical problems. Phlebothrombosis frequently has no clinical signs because there is no inflammation at the site of thrombosis. As many as 50% of patients with venous thrombosis display no visible signs or symptoms. When obstruction occurs in a deep vein, the affected extremity may be edematous, warm, and tender at the area of compromise; there may be a positive Homans' sign and prominent superficial veins. In comparison, if superficial vessels are obstructed, the symptoms may be limited to pain, redness, warmth, or tenderness in the affected area.

Medical Diagnosis

The primary diagnostic examinations used in the detection of venous thrombi are venography, Doppler ultrasonography, and duplex ultrasonography. These tests are instrumental in the confirmation of the disease process and determination of the treatment plan. A lung scan, pulmonary angiogram, or spiral CT scan may be done if pulmonary embolism is suspected.

Medical and Surgical Treatment

The goals of treatment are to prevent thrombus extension and pulmonary emboli, to reduce the risk of further thrombus formation, and to reduce discomfort. Anticoagulant or thrombolytic therapy or both are begun promptly after diagnosis. The treatment plan typically includes patient teaching about the disease; the ongoing assessment for pulmonary emboli; bed rest; elevation of the extremity; warm, moist soaks to the affected area; and antiembolism hose. Ambulation is initiated after the acute phase. Surgery may be considered when the patient cannot receive anticoagulants or thrombolytic therapy or when the possibility of pulmonary emboli is high.

NURSING CARE *of the Patient with Venous Thrombosis*
Assessment

Assessment of the patient with peripheral vascular disease is summarized in Box 36-1.

Nursing Diagnoses, Goals, and Outcome Criteria: Phlebitis, Thrombophlebitis, Phlebothrombosis, and Deep Vein Thrombosis

Nursing Diagnoses	Goals and Outcome Criteria
Impaired Skin Integrity related to venous stasis	Intact skin: absence of redness, rash, pallor, lesions
Acute Pain related to impaired circulation and tissue ischemia	Pain relief: patient verbalizes pain relief, relaxed manner
Anxiety related to hospitalization and uncertainty of disease process	Reduced anxiety: patient states that anxiety is reduced, calm manner
Activity Intolerance related to leg pain or swelling	Improved activity tolerance: increasing activity without pain
Ineffective Tissue Perfusion related to impaired peripheral circulation	Adequate tissue perfusion: pulses present and symmetric, normal skin color and warmth
Impaired Gas Exchange related to pulmonary emboli	Normal gas exchange: respiratory rate consistent with patient norms, no dyspnea or chest pain
Ineffective Therapeutic Regimen Management related to the developing disease process, treatment, self-care	Patient adheres to prescribed plan of care: correctly describes and demonstrates self-medication, exercises, and precautions

Interventions

Impaired Skin Integrity

Maintaining intact skin is a priority. Carefully inspect the skin to detect early signs of breakdown. Compare the extremities for symmetry in color, warmth, pulses, and circumference. Elevate affected extremities to promote venous return and improve circulation to the area. Because edematous tissue is easily injured and heals poorly, it must be protected from trauma, including pressure.

Acute Pain

The patient's pain must be reduced before activity tolerance can improve. Administer analgesics as prescribed. Implement other prescribed comfort measures such as warm, moist soaks and elevation of the extremity. Massage is contraindicated because it may dislodge a thrombus. A "traveling" blood clot is called an *embolus*. It is very dangerous because it can obstruct blood flow with serious effects including a potentially fatal pulmonary embolism.

Anxiety

Anxiety may be related to lack of knowledge about the disease and its treatment and by concerns about the effects of the condition on employment, activities of daily living, and quality of life. The patient may even restrict activities out of fear of pain. The relief of anxiety can help the patient move toward an acceptable level of activity. Anxiety can be reduced by helping the patient understand the condition and how it best can be managed.

Activity Intolerance

Because inactivity increases the risk of venous thrombosis, make an effort to get the inactive patient mobile again as soon as permitted. Work with the patient to establish a realistic exercise or activity plan. The plan should begin at the patient's current level and slowly add activities over a period of several weeks. Instruct the patient to stop any activity temporarily if pain occurs. Once the pain subsides, the activity may be continued.

Ineffective Tissue Perfusion

Improved peripheral circulation aids in tissue perfusion, which decreases pain, improves skin integrity, reduces anxiety, and increases physical activity. Administer prescribed anticoagulants or platelet aggregation inhibitors to prevent new clots, or administer thrombolytics to dissolve existing clots and reestablish blood flow to the affected area. Check blood test results before giving anticoagulants and take action according to agency policy. Apply warm, moist packs to the affected area as ordered to improve circulation. Assist the patient in the placement of antiembolism hose to prevent stasis and improve circulation. Explain how stress reduction and smoking cessation also improve tissue perfusion by reducing vasoconstriction.

Impaired Gas Exchange

The possibility of a pulmonary embolus developing during the treatment of venous thrombosis is an ever-present threat. When an embolus lodges in the lung, the affected blood vessels can no longer exchange gases. Pressure builds in vessels behind the embolus. Symptoms of pulmonary embolism depend on the amount of tissue affected. Small emboli may produce no symptoms. Larger emboli can cause dyspnea, chest pain, tachycardia, cough, fever, anxiety, and a change in mental status. A massive embolus can cause heart failure and shock. Sixty percent of people do not survive massive emboli.

To improve oxygenation when a patient has a pulmonary embolism, elevate the head of the bed to a 45-degree angle and administer oxygen as ordered. Monitor and document any changes in the patient's respiratory pattern, address anxiety, teach the patient deep-breathing and coughing techniques, and assist with position changes every 2 hours. Administer drugs as ordered to dissolve existing clots and prevent future clots. Surgical removal of the clot, called *pulmonary embolectomy*, is sometimes indicated.

Ineffective Therapeutic Regimen Management

To follow the long-term plan of care, the patient must understand the condition and how it best can be managed. Once the acute process has resolved, discharge planning must include patient teaching as outlined below. If the patient is on anticoagulant therapy, also see Patient Teaching Plan: Anticoagulant Therapy on p. 698.

CHRONIC VENOUS INSUFFICIENCY
Pathophysiology

Chronic venous insufficiency is the culmination of long-standing pressure that stretches the veins and damages the valves. Elevated venous pressure causes edema, primarily around the ankles. Red blood cells seep into the tissues and combine with metabolic wastes to impart a brownish color, called *stasis dermatitis,* around the ankles. Ulcers may form because of the pressure exerted by edema or as a result of trauma. The ulcers develop most often on the medial malleolus (the prominent bone on the inner aspect of the ankle). Because of the poor circulation, the ulcers are very resistant to healing and susceptible to infection. Some ulcers eventually necessitate amputation.

Signs and Symptoms

Signs and symptoms of chronic venous insufficiency include edema around the lower legs, pain, brownish skin discoloration (stasis dermatitis), and stasis ulcerations. Patients often describe pain as "heaviness" or "dull ache" in the calf or thigh. The skin temperature is cool, and nails are normal. Peripheral pulses are present but may be difficult to palpate because of the edema. The feet and ankles often are cyanotic when in a dependent position.

Medical Diagnosis

The physical examination provides evidence of chronic venous insufficiency. Noninvasive screening may be done to confirm the diagnosis of chronic venous insufficiency or assess the severity A culture may be ordered to determine the infectious agent if the stasis ulcer is draining.

Medical and Surgical Treatment

The medical management of stasis ulcerations is constantly changing; however, compression, which promotes venous return, remains the key to healing existing ulcers and preventing new ones. Among the many options, you may see elastic or compression stockings and pneumatic compression devices. High-pressure compression is contraindicated if the patient's arterial blood flow is poor.

If the patient has an ulcer, treatment may include special dressings, systemic antibiotics, topical débriding agents such as Elase, and Unna boots. There is disagreement as to whether oxygen-permeable dressings (e.g., OpSite) or oxygen-impermeable dressings (e.g., DuoDERM) are superior, so you may see either used. Unna boots are medicated dressings used to allow the patient to be ambulatory while protecting the ulcer in a sterile environment. Infected ulcers are treated with systemic antibiotics, which are more effective than topical ointments. Surgery is rarely employed with chronic venous stasis because it is seldom successful. Hyperbaric oxygen therapy may be prescribed in an attempt to promote healing of the ulcer by reducing capillary pressure and hyperoxygenating the blood. The overall goal for medical management of ulcerations is to preserve the extremity by stimulating granulation tissue in the ulcer.

NURSING CARE *of the Patient with Chronic Venous Insufficiency*
Assessment

The complete general assessment of peripheral vascular status is summarized in Box 36-1. When the patient has chronic venous insufficiency, it is especially important to inspect the lower extremities for rubor and stasis dermatitis, palpate skin temperature, and determine the presence of pain in the affected extremity (see Nursing Care Plan: The Patient with a Venous Stasis Ulcer on p. 711).

Nursing Diagnoses, Goals, and Outcome Criteria: Chronic Venous Insufficiency

NURSING DIAGNOSES	GOALS AND OUTCOME CRITERIA
Ineffective Tissue Perfusion related to reduced vascular circulation	Improved peripheral circulation and venous return: absence of edema and lesions, improved skin color
Disturbed Body Image related to chronic, open stasis ulcerations	Patient adapts to changes in appearance: patient expresses concerns about changes, makes effort to maintain/improve appearance
Risk for Infection related to compromised circulation and impaired skin integrity	Absence of infections: normal body temperature, absence of local redness or drainage
Impaired Skin Integrity related to stasis dermatitis and ulcerations	Restored skin integrity: skin intact in affected areas

---

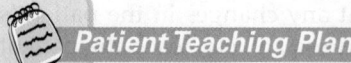

Patient Teaching Plan

Venous Thrombosis

- Protect your legs from pressure and trauma.
- Elevate your legs when sitting to improve circulation.
- Do not massage or rub affected areas.
- Gradually increase your activity; slow down or stop if you have pain during activity.
- Avoid prolonged standing and crossing your legs.
- Notify your physician if you have any chest pain or shortness of breath.

NURSING CARE PLAN

The Patient with a Venous Stasis Ulcer

ASSESSMENT

Health History: A 75-year-old man is being seen in the community clinic for an ulcer on the medial malleolus of the right ankle. The ulcer is shallow and measures 1.5 × 2.5 cm. He describes a "heavy" burning sensation in the lower legs. He worked for many years as a toll booth attendant and has had chronic venous insufficiency for 5 years. He reports having had hypertension in the past but is taking no medication for it. Otherwise he has been in good health and remains active. He is the caregiver for his wife, who has been disabled for 3 years because of a stroke. He has a daughter who helps with her care and who has been dressing the leg ulcer.

Physical Examination: Vital signs: temperature, 97° F orally; pulse, 64; respiration, 16; blood pressure, 194/102. Alert and oriented. Walks with slight limp. 1+ edema both ankles. Varicosities noted in both legs. Stasis dermatitis in ankles and calves. Ulcer is 1.5 × 2.5 cm and shallow. The ulcer is slightly moist, pink, with no drainage or odor. Ankles and feet are cooler than calves. Pedal pulses faint but palpable, slightly stronger in left foot.

Nursing Diagnosis	Goals and Outcome Criteria	Interventions
Ineffective Tissue Perfusion related to compromised circulation	Tissue perfusion will improve, as evidenced by reduced pain, redness, and edema; skin warm to touch.	Instruct the patient in measures to improve circulation: exercise moderately each day, elevate the legs above the level of the heart when resting, avoid smoking, use support stockings as ordered, avoid prolonged periods of walking or standing still. Teach wound care as ordered. At each visit, assess condition of ulcer, peripheral pulses, skin color, and warmth, pain, and edema.
Risk for Infection related to open wound	The patient will remain free of signs and symptoms of infection: fever, increasing redness, purulent drainage.	Teach hygienic techniques of hand washing and wound care. Encourage diet with adequate protein and vitamins. Teach signs and symptoms of infection that should be reported to physician. Instruct in antimicrobial therapy if prescribed.
Chronic Pain related to circulatory impairment	The patient will report pain relief.	Encourage the patient to increase movement and maintain warmth to improve circulation. Teach pain relief measures including relaxation, deep-breathing techniques, cutaneous stimulation, and behavior modification. Explain the use of prescribed analgesics. Assess effectiveness of measures.
Impaired Skin Integrity related to circulatory impairment	The patient's wound will heal completely.	Assess and document the condition of the ulcer during each clinic visit. Advise the patient to use gentle soaps for bathing, to avoid trauma, and not to rub the ulcer. Encourage good nutrition and adequate fluid intake. Discuss wound care with physician or clinical nurse specialist in wound care.
Ineffective Therapeutic Regimen Management related to lack of knowledge of chronic venous insufficiency and treatment of stasis ulcer	The patient will correctly explain chronic venous insufficiency and demonstrate correct care of ulcer.	Assess the patient's understanding of condition and self-care. Advise to avoid restrictive clothing, smoking, and weight gain. Explore sources of stress and coping strategies.
Ineffective Therapeutic Regimen Management related to lack of knowledge of importance of treating hypertension	The patient will verbalize understanding of need to have blood pressure evaluated and will make an appointment for evaluation.	Explain importance of detecting and treating hypertension. Refer to physician or blood pressure clinic for evaluation.

? CRITICAL THINKING QUESTIONS

- What data will contribute to the assessment of the effectiveness of pain and infection control techniques?
- What role does nutrition play in the therapeutic treatment of venous stasis ulcers?
- What data should you collect related to the condition of the ulcer?

Interventions

Ineffective Tissue Perfusion

To improve circulation in areas of compromised vascular function, the patient should elevate the legs when sitting and should wear antiembolism stockings. The patient should avoid standing still, crossing the legs, and wearing restrictive clothing, especially socks or hose with tight, narrow bands.

Disturbed Body Image

Encourage the patient to share feelings about body image changes. Be accepting and supportive. Encourage the patient to pay attention to grooming. The patient may prefer clothing that conceals ulcers and discolored extremities.

Risk for Infection

Carefully monitor for signs of infection such as elevated temperature, chills, general malaise, and localized redness, pain, and purulent drainage. Teach the patient thorough hand washing, good hygiene, and appropriate wound care. The fragile edematous tissue also must be protected from trauma to avoid creating portals for pathogens.

Impaired Skin Integrity

Inspect for dermatitis and ulcerations. Patient education is critical because these ulcerations are frequently treated on an outpatient basis. Instruct the patient and family in the management of the ulcerations while in the home setting. A referral for home health care may be appropriate.

LYMPHANGITIS

Pathophysiology

Lymphangitis is acute inflammation of the lymphatic channels. The inflammation is the result of an infectious process, usually caused by streptococcus.

Signs and Symptoms

The primary characteristic of lymphangitis is enlargement of the lymph nodes along the lymphatic channel. Each node can be palpated along the course of the channel. The patient complains of tenderness as these nodes are assessed. A red streak from the infected wound extends up the extremity along the path of the lymphatics, as each node drains into the lymphatic system and the cardiovascular system. These nodes are located in the groin, the axilla, and the cervical regions. The symptoms of a generalized infection—elevated temperature and chills—are present. The infectious material can localize into an abscess with necrotic, suppurative discharge from the area.

Medical Diagnosis

The classic signs and symptoms, supported by wound culture results, are usually adequate to confirm lymphangitis. Lymphangiography, which uses a contrast medium for the radiologic visualization of the lymphatic system, will also provide evidence of lymphangitis.

Medical and Surgical Treatment

Antimicrobials are used to treat lymphangitis. When an abscess develops, the area is incised to drain the suppurative material. Other supportive measures that may be ordered are rest and elevation of the limb; warm, wet dressings; and elastic support hose.

NURSING CARE *of the Patient with Lymphangitis*

Assessment

Care of the patient with lymphangitis includes inspection of the skin for open wounds, signs of inflammation (redness, warmth, edema), and presence of red streaks along the paths of lymphatic channels. Palpate the lymph nodes in the groin and underarm areas for any enlargements.

Nursing Diagnoses, Goals, and Outcome Criteria: Lymphangitis

Nursing Diagnoses	Goals and Outcome Criteria
Acute Pain related to the inflammatory process in the lymphatic system	Pain relief: patient verbalizes less pain, appears relaxed
Activity Intolerance related to the pain with movement	Improved activity intolerance: patient increases activity without increased pain
Risk for Injury related to infection	Resolution of infection: absence of fever, normal white cell count, decreasing swelling and pain

Interventions

Nursing care of the patient with lymphangitis is essentially the same as that for chronic venous insufficiency.

 Nutrition Concepts

1. Edema frequently is treated with a low-sodium diet, and sodium-restricted diets vary from 4 g (least restrictive) to 250 mg (severe sodium restriction) daily.
2. Foods high in sodium include salt, monosodium glutamate (MSG), smoked or processed meats (ham, bacon, frankfurters, cold cuts), salted foods (potato chips, pretzels, salted nuts, popcorn), prepackaged frozen foods, and canned foods.
3. Older adults taking diuretics generally are not encouraged to restrict sodium intake because they are at risk for the adverse effects of low sodium.
4. Salt substitutes are a source of potassium, which is desirable in patients receiving potassium-wasting diuretics; however, salt substitutes should always be approved by a physician before using.

Interventions to relieve pain include the administration of the prescribed analgesics and antimicrobials and elevation of the extremity to reduce lymphedema. Nonpharmacologic measures should be used, as well as analgesics. The application of warm, moist soaks to the infected areas as prescribed improves the circulation to the area. As the circulation is improved, white blood cells, nutrients, and oxygen are delivered, which aids in the recovery of the healthy tissue. Elastic support hose are used for several months after an acute attack of lymphangitis to prevent the formation of lymphedema.

Key Points

- The peripheral vascular system comprises arteries, capillaries, veins, and lymph vessels, each of which plays a critical role in the oxygenation and nourishment of body tissues.
- Risk factors for peripheral vascular disease include older age, heredity, smoking, obesity, physical inactivity, hypertension, and diabetes mellitus.
- Common age-related changes in the vascular system include arteriosclerosis (stiffening of blood vessel walls), decreased hemoglobin, slower heart rate, and decreased cardiac output.
- The six P's characteristic of peripheral vascular disease are pain, pulselessness, poikilothermy, pallor, paresthesia, and paralysis.
- Intermittent claudication is pain in any major muscle group that is precipitated by exercise and relieved by rest.
- Poikilothermy describes an area of the body that is cooler than the rest of the body because of local ischemia.
- Tests and procedures used to diagnose peripheral vascular disease include Doppler ultrasound, duplex ultrasonography, pressure measurement, exercise testing, and angiography.
- Common therapeutic measures used in the management of peripheral vascular disease are exercise programs, drug therapy, stress management training, pain management, smoking cessation, elastic stockings or intermittent pneumatic compression devices, positioning, thermotherapy, protection, and patient teaching.
- Common surgical interventions for peripheral vascular disease include percutaneous transluminal angioplasty, endarterectomy, embolectomy, sclerotherapy and laser therapy, and vein ligation and stripping.
- Blood flow may be improved with drug therapy using anticoagulants, thrombolytics, platelet aggregation inhibitors, and vasodilators. NSAIDs and other analgesics may be needed for pain and inflammation.
- For persons with vascular disorders, a low-fat diet is usually prescribed and a weight-reduction program may be advised if appropriate.
- The most dangerous complication of venous thrombosis is pulmonary embolism.

- An arterial embolus, an unattached clot or other material in an artery, can lodge in an artery and obstruct blood.
- Nursing care of the patient with an arterial embolus focuses on Ineffective Tissue Perfusion, Fear, Impaired Skin Integrity, Impaired Physical Mobility, and Ineffective Therapeutic Regimen Management.
- Peripheral arterial occlusive diseases impair blood flow and may be treated surgically.
- Nursing care of the patient with peripheral arterial occlusive disease focuses on Activity Intolerance, Chronic Pain, Impaired Skin Integrity, Disturbed Body Image, Ineffective Tissue Perfusion, and Ineffective Therapeutic Regimen Management.
- Thromboangiitis obliterans (Buerger's disease) is an inflammatory thrombotic disorder of arteries and veins in upper and lower extremities of smokers; atherosclerosis is not a factor.
- Raynaud's disease and phenomenon are characterized by intermittent arteriolar vasoconstriction that is usually treated with vasodilators.
- An aneurysm is a dilated segment of an artery, most often the aorta, that can rupture, serve as a site for thrombus formation, and compress surrounding tissues.
- Aortic dissection results from a tear in the intima that allows blood to escape into the space between the intima and the media that causes the media to split lengthwise.
- Varicose veins are dilated, tortuous, superficial veins that result from incompetent venous valves; they may lead to chronic venous insufficiency and are treated with conservative measures to improve venous return and sometimes with surgical intervention.
- Phlebitis is inflammation of a vein wall, whereas thrombophlebitis describes clot formation in an inflamed vein.
- Thrombosis is clot formation, and deep vein thrombosis indicates the clot is located in deep veins—a condition that poses a high risk for pulmonary emboli.
- Risk factors for thrombus formation are bed rest, surgery in people older than 40 years, leg trauma and immobilization, previous venous insufficiency, obesity, oral contraceptives, and malignancy.
- Nursing care of the patient with venous thrombosis addresses Impaired Skin Integrity, Acute Pain, Anxiety, Activity Intolerance, Ineffective Tissue Perfusion, Impaired Gas Exchange, and Ineffective Therapeutic Regimen Management.
- Chronic venous insufficiency causes edema and stasis dermatitis around the ankles.
- Lymphangitis is an inflammation of the lymphatic channels that is treated with antimicrobials, analgesics, heat therapy, and rest.

 Go to your Companion CD-ROM for a Pharmacology Tutorial, Audio Glossary, and 3-D animations.

evolve Be sure to visit the companion Evolve site at http://evolve.elsevier.com/Linton/ for WebLinks and additional online resources.

REVIEW QUESTIONS *Choose the best answer.*

1. The exchange of oxygen and nutrients occurs at the level of the:
   1. Arteriole
   2. Capillary
   3. Venule
   4. Lymphatics

2. Thickening and hardening of the intima put the older adult at risk for:
   1. Anemia
   2. Bradycardia
   3. Emboli
   4. Hypotension

3. A patient complains of pain and cramping in the legs that occurs when walking and is relieved by rest. This complaint is typical of:
   1. Intermittent claudication
   2. Venous thrombosis
   3. Pulmonary embolism
   4. Poikilothermy

4. When inspecting a patient's legs, you press your thumb into an edematous area around the ankles. When you remove your thumb, a depression $\frac{1}{4}$ inch remains on both ankles. You would document:
   1. 1+ edema noted
   2. Pitting edema, both ankles
   3. Mild edema, both ankles
   4. 2+ edema, both ankles

5. Which of the following is an invasive diagnostic procedure used to assess the vascular system?
   1. Ultrasound
   2. Plethysmography
   3. Angiography
   4. Exercise test

6. For the patient with peripheral vascular disease, the common purpose of exercise, elastic stockings, and elevation of extremities is to:
   1. Improve venous return
   2. Stimulate arterial blood flow
   3. Reduce vasoconstriction
   4. Strengthen venous valves

7. The dosage of low-molecular-weight heparin is based on:
   1. Activated partial thromboplastin time
   2. International normalized ratio
   3. Prothrombin time
   4. Fixed recommended dosage

8. Discharge teaching for the patient with peripheral arterial occlusive disease affecting both legs includes:
   1. Advise the patient to elevate the feet when sitting
   2. Tell the patient that exercise is contraindicated
   3. Promptly report any injury to the feet or legs
   4. Explain how to take prescribed vasoconstrictors

9. After repair of an abdominal aneurysm, it is especially important to monitor:
   1. Reflexes in the lower extremities
   2. Intake and output
   3. Mental status
   4. Electrocardiogram

10. The most serious complication of venous thrombosis is:
    1. Pulmonary embolism
    2. Stasis dermatitis
    3. Ankle ulceration
    4. Pitting edema

37 Hypertension

Objectives

After reading and studying this chapter, you should be able to:

1. Define hypertension.
2. Explain the physiology of blood pressure regulation.
3. Discuss the risk factors, signs and symptoms, diagnosis, treatment, and complications of hypertension.
4. Identify the nursing considerations when administering selected antihypertensive drugs.
5. List the data to be collected for the nursing assessment of a person with known or suspected hypertension.
6. Identify the nursing diagnoses, goals, and outcome criteria for the patient with hypertension.
7. Describe the nursing interventions for the patient with hypertension.

Key Terms

 Be sure to check out the bonus material on the Companion CD-ROM, including selected audio pronunciations.

dyslipidemia (dīs-lĭp-ĭ-DĒ-mē-ă, p. 717)
epistaxis (ĕp-ĭ-STĂK-sĭs, p. 717)
hypertension (hī-pĕr-TĔN-shŭn, p. 715)
hypertrophy (hī-PĔR-trŏ-fē, p. 717)
orthostatic hypotension
  (ŏr-thō-STĂT-ĭk hī-pō-TĔN-shŭn, p. 722)
syncope (SĬN-kō-pē, p. 726)
thrombus (*pl.* thrombi) (THRŎM-bŭs) (THRŎM-bī, p. 717)

Hypertension (high blood pressure) is considered the most common cardiovascular problem in the United States today. Approximately 50 million people have hypertension that requires monitoring, treatment, or both. The condition is usually detected in people ages 30 to 50 years; however, it is being found with increasing frequency in children.

What Does Culture Have to Do with Blood Pressure?

Hypertension occurs twice as often in African Americans as in whites and is more common in women than in men. Screening needs to take in all segments of the population, and education should be sensitive to cultural differences.

Hypertension is called "the silent killer" because it often has no symptoms and is not discovered until a serious complication develops. It is estimated that 30% of those with hypertension do not know they have it. Among individuals in the United States with hypertension, 59% are being treated but only 34% are considered to be in control. This is unfortunate because it is believed that hypertension can be controlled in most people.

Complications of hypertension, including damage to the heart, blood vessels, kidneys, brain, and eyes, increase after age 50 years. As blood pressure rises, so does the risk of heart attack, heart failure, stroke, kidney disease, and blindness. Men, especially African Americans, suffer serious complications more often than women. Cardiac disease is the leading cause of death in hypertensive people. Improved management of hypertension has significantly reduced the death rate from stroke in women age 50 and older.

DEFINITIONS

The Seventh Report of the Joint National Committee on Prevention, Detection, Evaluation, and Treatment of High Blood Pressure (JNC 7) defines normal blood pressure as systolic pressure of less than 120 mm Hg and diastolic pressure of less than 80 mm Hg. Patients with systolic pressures between 120 and 139 and with diastolic pressures between 80 and 89 are said to have prehypertension. Readings classified as *stage 1* and *stage 2 hypertension* are specified in Table 37-1. If the systolic and diastolic pressures fall into different stages, the higher measurement is used to classify the stage of hypertension. Complications and death increase directly with the stage of hypertension.

In addition to staging, hypertensive patients are classified as Risk Group A, B, or C. Individuals in Risk Group A have no major risk factors, no target organ damage, and no clinical cardiovascular disease. Individuals in Risk Group B have one or more risk factors, not including diabetes, no target organ damage, and no clinical cardiovascular disease. Individuals in Risk Group C have target organ damage/clinical cardiovascular disease and/or diabetes, with or without other risk factors.

Table 37-1 *Classification of Blood Pressure for Adults 18 Years of Age and Older**

CATEGORY	SYSTOLIC (mm Hg)		DIASTOLIC (mm Hg)
Normal†	<120	and	<80
Prehypertension	120-139	or	80-89
Hypertension‡			
Stage 1	140-159	or	90-99
Stage 2	= or >160	or	= or >100

From Joint National Committee on Prevention, Detection, Evaluation, and Treatment of High Blood Pressure. (2003). *The Seventh Report of the Joint National Committee on Prevention, Detection, Evaluation, and Treatment of High Blood Pressure.* Bethesda, MD: Department of Health and Human Services, National Institutes of Health, National Heart, Lung, and Blood Institute.
*Not taking antihypertensive drugs and not acutely ill.
†Optimal blood pressure with respect to cardiovascular risk is below 120/80 mm Hg. However, unusually low readings should be evaluated for clinical significance.
‡Based on the average of two or more readings taken at each of two or more visits after an initial screening.

Some people have only occasional elevations in blood pressure and normal readings at other times. These findings are called *isolated pressure elevations.* Isolated systolic blood pressure elevations of 160 mm Hg or more frequently occur in older adults. The elevations are usually caused by atherosclerosis.

TYPES OF HYPERTENSION

Hypertension is classified as primary (essential) or secondary. Primary hypertension accounts for 90% to 95% of all cases of hypertension. Its cause is unknown. Secondary hypertension is caused by underlying factors such as kidney disease, certain arterial conditions, some drugs, and occasionally pregnancy.

ANATOMY AND PHYSIOLOGY OF BLOOD PRESSURE REGULATION

Two factors determine blood pressure: cardiac output and peripheral vascular resistance. Blood pressure (BP) equals cardiac output (CO) times peripheral vascular resistance (PVR)—that is, BP = CO × PVR.

CARDIAC OUTPUT

Cardiac output is the volume of blood pumped by the heart in a specific period of time (usually 1 minute). It is determined by the strength, rate, and rhythm of the contraction of the left ventricle and by the blood volume.

PERIPHERAL VASCULAR RESISTANCE

Peripheral vascular resistance is the force in the blood vessels that the left ventricle must overcome to eject blood from the heart. Resistance to blood flow is determined primarily by the diameter of the blood vessels

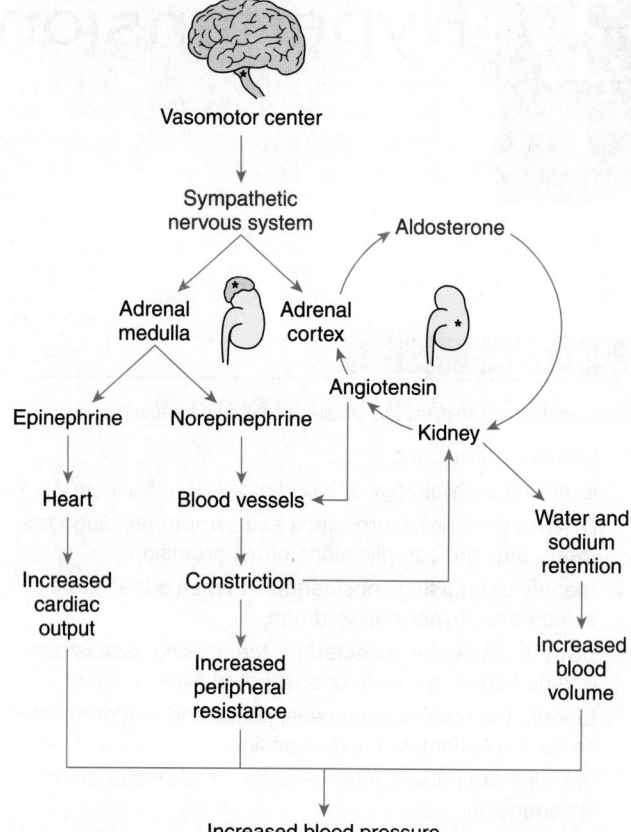

FIGURE **37-1** Factors that increase blood pressure.

and blood viscosity (thickness). Increased peripheral vascular resistance results from a narrowing of the arteries and arterioles or an increased fluid volume in the blood vessels that results from sodium and water retention. Increased peripheral vascular resistance is the most prominent characteristic of hypertension.

The diameter of blood vessels is regulated largely by the vasomotor center. The vasomotor center is located in the medulla of the brain. Sympathetic nervous system tracts from the medulla extend down the spinal cord to the thoracic and abdominal regions. Stimulation of the sympathetic nervous system causes release of the hormones *norepinephrine* and *epinephrine.* These hormones, called *catecholamines,* are vasoconstrictors, meaning that they cause the blood vessels to constrict, making the diameter smaller. By constricting blood vessels, norepinephrine increases peripheral vascular resistance and raises blood pressure. Epinephrine constricts blood vessels and increases the force of cardiac contraction, causing blood pressure to rise.

Vasoconstriction decreases blood flow to the kidneys, which then release renin. Renin leads to the formation of angiotensin, another potent vasoconstrictor. Angiotensin stimulates the adrenal cortex to secrete aldosterone, a hormone that promotes sodium and water retention. This results in an increased blood volume. Vasoconstriction, cardiac stimulation, and retention of fluid all contribute to hypertension. Figure 37-1 illustrates how various factors raise blood pressure.

Some age-related changes affect blood pressure. With aging, atherosclerotic changes reduce the elasticity of the arteries, causing a decrease in cardiac output and an increase in peripheral vascular resistance. After age 60 years, peripheral vascular resistance increases by approximately 1% per year. Systolic pressure rises in response to increased peripheral vascular resistance. In addition, pulse pressure (the difference between the systolic and diastolic pressures) widens in response to a decreased ability of the aorta to distend (stretch).

In the past, elevated blood pressure was considered normal in the older person and was often untreated. Because research has shown that older people do benefit from controlling hypertension, age is no longer considered a barrier to aggressive treatment.

PRIMARY (ESSENTIAL) HYPERTENSION

RISK FACTORS

The most significant risk factors for primary (essential) hypertension are dyslipidemia, atherosclerosis, diabetes mellitus, tobacco use, age over 55 years for men or over 65 for women, family history (father or brother diagnosed with heart disease before age 55; mother or sister diagnosed with heart disease before age 65), and sedentary lifestyle. Obesity, defined as weight 20% over ideal body weight, is also a risk factor. The additional weight and fat cause increases in the number of blood vessels, circulating blood volume, and cardiac workload. Atherosclerosis decreases the elasticity of the arteries and arterioles, causing increased systemic and peripheral vascular resistance. Nicotine in cigarettes constricts blood vessels and causes the release of epinephrine and norepinephrine. These hormones, as already mentioned, also constrict blood vessels and raise heart rate and blood pressure. Lack of physical activity leads to pooling of blood in the extremities and increases the workload of the cardiovascular system.

Other risk factors include stress, overstimulation, and a family history of obesity, hypertension, or dyslipidemia. Dyslipidemia refers to the abnormal amount of specific lipids and lipoproteins in the blood, a factor that contributes to atherosclerosis. Stress caused by such factors as a high-pressure job, financial worries, or family problems increases secretion of catecholamines. Stimulants that may contribute to or aggravate hypertension include caffeine, nicotine, and amphetamines. Caffeine is found in tea, coffee, and chocolate. Nicotine is obtained by smoking or chewing tobacco products.

SIGNS AND SYMPTOMS

Many people who are hypertensive have no symptoms. Symptoms that may accompany hypertension include occipital headaches that are more severe on arising, lightheadedness, and epistaxis (nosebleed). If hypertension has damaged blood vessels in the heart, kidneys, eyes, or brain, the patient may have symptoms of impaired function of those organs.

COMPLICATIONS

The most serious consequences of hypertension are heart attack, heart failure, stroke, kidney disease, and blindness. This occurs because the long-term effect of prolonged hypertension is replacement of elastic arteriolar tissue with stiffer, fibrous collagen tissue. Thickening of the arteriolar wall decreases its ability to distend, resulting in increased peripheral vascular resistance and decreased blood flow to various organs. The organs that are most sensitive to these changes are the heart, kidneys, brain, and eye. Patients with hypertension must be assessed frequently for damage to these sensitive ("target") organs (Fig. 37-2).

Heart

Coronary artery disease develops in patients with hypertension two to three times more frequently than in people with normal blood pressures. Coronary artery disease reduces blood supply to the myocardium, which can result in angina, myocardial infarction, and congestive heart failure. Myocardial infarction, commonly called a *heart attack,* results when the blood supply to the heart muscle is inadequate and the myocardium is deprived of oxygen.

Sustained hypertension requires the left ventricle to work harder to overcome increased peripheral resistance. The increased workload may cause the left ventricle to hypertrophy (enlarge), and it may eventually fail.

Kidneys

Narrowing of the renal arteries may decrease renal function and lead to chronic renal failure. Initial indicators of renal failure are nocturia (need to urinate during the night) and azotemia (accumulation of nitrogen waste products in the blood). In addition, urinalysis may reveal protein (proteinuria) or blood (hematuria) or both in the urine.

Brain

Prolonged hypertension constricts and damages cerebral arteries, putting the patient at risk for transient ischemic attacks and cerebrovascular accidents. A transient ischemic attack, sometimes called a *TIA* or "little stroke," is a temporary neurologic dysfunction caused by cerebral ischemia.

A cerebrovascular accident (CVA, or stroke) results from interrupted blood flow in the brain caused by a thrombus (clot) that occludes the vessel or a rupture of a blood vessel. People with hypertension have a sevenfold greater incidence of cerebrovascular accidents than those with normal blood pressures.

FIGURE **37-2** How hypertension affects major target organs.

Eyes

Damage to the eyes may include narrowing of the retinal arterioles, retinal hemorrhages, and papilledema (edema of the optic nerve). These changes may lead to blindness.

DIAGNOSTIC TESTS AND PROCEDURES

Diagnosis of hypertension is based on direct and indirect data. Hypertension is confirmed by repeated findings of average pressures equal to or greater than 140/90. When elevations are found in clinics or in screenings, the physician might have patients monitor their own blood pressure at home for comparison. Also, ambulatory BP monitors, which are commonly programmed to record readings every 15 to 30 minutes for 24 hours, typically provide readings lower than clinic readings. These readings provide a better foundation for the diagnosis of hypertension than a few isolated readings. The process would not be cost-

effective for all patients but is appropriate in selected situations.

On finding an elevated blood pressure, the physician collects data about the patient's lifestyle, other cardiovascular risk factors, and other medical diagnoses such as diabetes. The patient is examined for effects of hypertension on the heart, eyes, kidneys, and brain. An electrocardiogram should be ordered in addition to blood and urine studies. Blood studies include glucose, hematocrit, potassium, calcium, creatinine, and a lipid profile. If there is kidney damage, the serum creatinine level is elevated. Abnormal serum lipids and lipoproteins may indicate atherosclerosis. A chest radiograph may show enlargement of the heart or pulmonary blood vessels.

Physicians disagree about the need for trying to determine the cause of hypertension. If there is no evidence to suggest an underlying disease process, the consensus is to limit diagnostic tests to those that are most significant. This reduces patient care costs.

Table 37-2 | *Principles of Lifestyle Modification*

- Encourage healthy lifestyles for all individuals.
- Prescribe lifestyle modifications for all patients with prehypertension and hypertension.
- Components of lifestyle modifications include weight reduction, DASH eating plan, dietary sodium reduction, aerobic physical activity, and moderation of alcohol consumption.

LIFESTYLE MODIFICATION RECOMMENDATIONS

MODIFICATION	RECOMMENDATION	AVG. SYSTOLIC REDUCTION RANGE*
Weight reduction	Maintain normal body weight (body mass index 18.5-24.9 kg/m^2).	5-20 mm Hg/10 kg
DASH eating plan	Adopt a diet rich in fruits, vegetables, and low-fat dairy products with reduced content of saturated and total fat.	8-14 mm Hg
Dietary sodium reduction	Reduce dietary sodium intake to ≤100 mmol per day (2.4 g sodium or 6 g sodium chloride).	2-8 mm Hg
Aerobic physical activity	Regular aerobic physical activity (e.g., brisk walking) at least 30 minutes per day, most days of the week.	4-9 mm Hg
Moderation of alcohol consumption	Men: limit to ≤2 drinks† per day. Women and lighter weight persons: limit to ≤1 drink† per day.	2-4 mm Hg

From Joint National Committee on Prevention, Detection, Evaluation, and Treatment of High Blood Pressure. (2003). *The Seventh Report of the Joint National Committee on Prevention, Detection, Evaluation, and Treatment of High Blood Pressure.* Bethesda, MD: Department of Health and Human Services, National Institutes of Health, National Heart, Lung, and Blood Institute.
*Effects are dose and time dependent.
†1 drink = ½ oz or 15 mL ethanol (e.g., 12 oz beer, 5 oz wine, 1.5 oz 80-proof whiskey).

MEDICAL TREATMENT

The goal of therapy for hypertension is to gradually reduce peripheral vascular resistance and blood pressure. Lowering the pressure to less than 140/90 significantly decreases cardiovascular risks. For patients who have diabetes or renal disease, the medical goal is less than 130/80. Optimal blood pressure is usually defined as a diastolic pressure of less than 80 mm Hg and systolic pressure less than 120 mm Hg. Treatment of underlying conditions may lower the blood pressure in people with secondary hypertension.

For treatment of primary hypertension, a conservative, nonpharmacologic method (without drugs) usually is tried first. Drug treatment may be added if needed.

Lifestyle Modifications

A nonpharmacologic approach includes weight reduction, smoking cessation, sodium and alcohol restriction, exercise, and relaxation techniques. Reduction of weight can reduce blood pressure by reducing the cardiac workload. Stopping smoking eliminates vasoconstriction caused by nicotine. Reduction of sodium in the body reduces water retention and decreases the blood volume.

A planned program of exercise improves cardiac efficiency by increasing cardiac output and decreasing

Consider the Alternative

Complementary therapies such as relaxation, biofeedback, and behavior modification may be used along with traditional medical treatment of hypertension.

peripheral vascular resistance. Exercise also decreases the patient's blood glucose and cholesterol levels and promotes a sense of well-being. Isotonic exercises such as walking, bicycling, and swimming help reduce weight and promote relaxation.

Relaxation therapy, biofeedback, and behavior modification techniques also may be used to reduce stress and lower blood pressure. Alcohol intake should not exceed 2 ounces per day because alcohol can increase blood pressure and can alter the effects of some antihypertensive drugs.

Lifestyle modifications are recommended for individuals with high-normal and all stages of hypertension regardless of the risk group (Table 37-2).

Pharmacologic Therapy

Drug therapy is indicated if the blood pressure is very high initially (systolic ≥160, diastolic ≥100) or if conservative therapies for less severe hypertension are not effective within 3 to 6 months. Drug therapy must be individualized for each patient and may be recommended at earlier stages. The goal of drug therapy is to normalize blood pressure using the smallest number of the safest drugs at the lowest effective dosages. A single agent is preferred if good control can be achieved because patients are more likely to take one drug as prescribed than multiple agents. However, most patients require two or more drugs to achieve control. Antihypertensive drugs are listed in the Drug Therapy table on pp. 720 and 721.

JNC 7 Recommendations for Treatment of Hypertension. Figure 37-3 is an algorithm for the treatment of hypertension recommended by the JNC 7. If lifestyle modifications have not achieved the blood pressure goal,

DRUG THERAPY *Antihypertensive Drugs and Nursing Interventions*

GENERAL CONSIDERATIONS

1. Monitor blood pressure (BP) regularly with patient in supine, sitting, and standing positions.
2. Encourage patients to take medications and keep follow-up appointments even when they are feeling well.
3. Teach patients with orthostatic hypotension to rise slowly, avoid prolonged standing, and avoid hot baths and showers.
4. Advise patients to consult physician or pharmacist about safety of over-the-counter drugs.
5. Do not stop drugs abruptly because rebound hypertension may occur.

DRUG CLASSES/EXAMPLE	USE/ACTION	SIDE EFFECTS	NURSING INTERVENTIONS
CENTRALLY ACTING DRUGS (ALPHA₂ AGONISTS)			
Clonidine (Catapres) Methyldopa (Aldomet)	Act on central nervous system to block vasoconstriction, which lowers BP; also reduces anxiety	Drowsiness, dry mouth, weakness, depression, retention of sodium and water. Orthostatic hypotension with some drugs.	Monitor BP. Safety precautions. Oral hygiene. Assess for edema. Teach patient to manage orthostatic hypotension.
GANGLIONIC BLOCKERS			
Mecamylamine (Inversine)	Block transmission of nerve impulses that constrict blood vessels; vessels dilate, reducing BP	Sodium and water retention, bradycardia, impaired ejaculation, nasal stuffiness, gastrointestinal disturbances. Some drugs cause orthostatic hypotension.	Monitor pulse and BP. Assess for edema, sexual dysfunction. Give with meals to reduce gastrointestinal distress. Teach patient to manage orthostatic hypotension.
ALPHA-ADRENERGIC RECEPTOR BLOCKERS			
Phentolamine (Regitine) Prazosin (Minipress) Terazosin (Hytrin)	Block effects of norepinephrine, causing vasodilation	Reflex tachycardia, palpitations, headache, dizziness, drowsiness, nausea. Potentially severe orthostatic hypotension with first or increased dose of prazosin.	Monitor pulse and BP. Advise patient that most side effects diminish over time. Give first or increased dose of prazosin at bedtime. Advise of possible orthostatic hypotension.
BETA-ADRENERGIC RECEPTOR BLOCKERS			
Propranolol (Inderal) Atenolol (Tenormin)	Decrease cardiac stimulation	Bradycardia, fatigue, drowsiness, depression, hypoglycemia, bronchial constriction.	Monitor pulse, BP, and respiration. Assess emotional status. Monitor patients with asthma for dyspnea; patients with diabetes for low blood glucose.

initial drug choices are made on the basis of individual factors. Different recommendations are made depending on whether the patient has stage 1 or stage 2 hypertension. Stage 1 hypertension is defined as a systolic BP of 140 to 159 or a diastolic BP of 90 to 99; stage 2 hypertension is defined as a systolic BP of 160 or more or a diastolic BP of 100 or more. Some patients have "compelling indications for individual drug classes." Specific classes of drugs are recommended for patients with heart failure, diabetes, and chronic kidney disease and for patients who have had a myocardial infarction, are at high risk for cardiovascular disease, or are being treated to prevent a recurrent stroke.

Specific Antihypertensive Drugs. First-line drugs recommended by JNC 7 for antihypertension include diuretics, angiotensin-converting enzyme (ACE) inhibitors, angiotensin II receptor blockers, beta-blockers, and calcium channel blockers. Other categories that may be used are alpha₁ adrenergic blockers, central

alpha₂ agonists and other centrally acting drugs, ganglionic blockers, and direct vasodilators. A number of combination drugs are available that reduce the number of tablets the patient must take.

Diuretics. There are several types of diuretics that may be used to treat hypertension. These include thiazide-type diuretics, loop (high ceiling) diuretics, and potassium-sparing diuretics. The JNC 7 recommends a thiazide-type diuretic such as hydrochlorothiazide (HydroDIURIL) for initial therapy. Thiazide-type diuretics decrease the reabsorption of sodium and water. However, the exact means by which they lower blood pressure is not known. Although they reduce blood volume initially, that effect stabilizes over time but the blood pressure reduction persists. Diuretics are especially effective in treating hypertensive African-American patients.

Patients taking diuretics must be monitored for fluid and electrolyte imbalances, especially hypovo-

DRUG THERAPY | *Antihypertensive Drugs and Nursing Interventions—cont'd*

DRUG CLASSES/EXAMPLE	USE/ACTION	SIDE EFFECTS	NURSING INTERVENTIONS
DIRECT VASODILATORS Hydralazine (Apresoline)	Relax vascular smooth muscle, causing vasodilation	Reflex tachycardia, headache, dizziness, nausea and vomiting, anorexia, hypotension.	Monitor pulse and BP.
CALCIUM CHANNEL BLOCKERS Verapamil (Calan) Nifedipine (Procardia) Diltiazem (Cardizem)	Decrease force of cardiac contraction and dilate peripheral blood vessels	Bradycardia, flushing, dizziness, headache.	Monitor pulse. Elevate legs when sitting to reduce edema.
ANGIOTENSIN-CONVERTING ENZYME INHIBITORS Captopril (Capoten) Enalapril (Vasotec)	Reduce aldosterone secretion and prevent formation of angiotensin II, thus decreasing peripheral resistance and fluid volume	Skin rash, neutropenia. Renal failure in patients with renal artery stenosis. Cough.	Monitor blood cell counts. Report changes in urine output.
DIURETICS Hydrochlorothiazide (HCTZ) Furosemide (Lasix)	Reduce fluid volume; may cause vasodilation; sodium loss may reduce vasoconstriction	Fluid volume deficit, hyponatremia, hypokalemia (except with potassium-sparing diuretics).	Monitor fluid balance: hydration, urine output, mental status, muscle tone. Recommend foods high in potassium (bananas, orange juice) unless on potassium-sparing diuretics.
ANGIOTENSIN II RECEPTOR ANTAGONISTS Losartan (Cozaar) Valsartan (Diovan)	Block action of angiotensin II; vasodilation; reduce blood volume by excretion of water and salt	Dizziness.	Safety precautions.

lemia and potassium imbalances. Intake and output records may be kept on hospitalized patients who are taking diuretics. Hypokalemia is a potentially serious problem except with potassium-sparing diuretics (e.g., amiloride [Midamor]). Older patients are especially susceptible to hypokalemia. Monitor for signs of hypokalemia: confusion, irritability, muscle weakness, cardiac dysrhythmias, and anorexia. Severe hypokalemia can lead to respiratory arrest and disruptions in cardiac rhythm. To prevent hypokalemia, encourage the patient to consume additional dietary potassium. Sources of potassium include bananas and orange juice. Some patients require supplementary potassium.

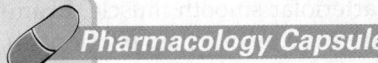
Pharmacology Capsule

When patients are taking diuretics, monitor for signs and symptoms of hypokalemia: cardiac dysrhythmias, muscle weakness, and diminished bowel sounds.

Beta-Adrenergic Receptor Blockers. Beta-adrenergic receptor blockers, commonly called *beta-blockers*, reduce blood pressure by blocking the beta effects of catecholamines. Examples of beta-blockers used to treat hypertension are atenolol (Tenormin), labetalol (Normodyne), metoprolol (Lopressor), and propranolol (Inderal). When beta receptors are stimulated, they stimulate the heart and relax bronchial smooth muscle. Beta-blockers prevent this stimulation, resulting in decreased heart rate, decreased strength of cardiac contraction, and bronchial constriction. There are a number of beta-blockers that have slightly different effects. Some affect cardiac function more; others have a greater effect on the bronchi. Except for labetalol, beta-blockers are less effective for African-American patients than other types of antihypertensive drugs.

Common side effects of beta-blockers include bradycardia and hypotension, hypoglycemia, and increased low-density lipoprotein in the blood. Beta-blockers usually are not recommended in patients with asthma, chronic obstructive pulmonary disease, heart block, or congestive heart failure. When a patient is taking a beta-blocker, the nurse should monitor for bradycardia and hypotension. People with diabetes should be watched carefully for hypoglycemia because beta-blockers lower blood glucose and suppress the usual signs of hypoglycemia. Diaphoresis (excessive perspiration) may be the only sign of hypoglycemia when people with diabetes are taking beta-blockers. Older adult patients are at greater risk than young patients for hypotension and bradycardia associated with beta-blockers. Therefore they should be started on low doses that are cautiously increased if needed.

TREATMENT

Principles of Hypertension Treatment

- Treat to BP <140/90 mm Hg or BP <130/80 mm Hg in patients with diabetes or chronic kidney disease.
- Majority of patients will require two medications to reach goal.

Algorithm for Treatment of Hypertension

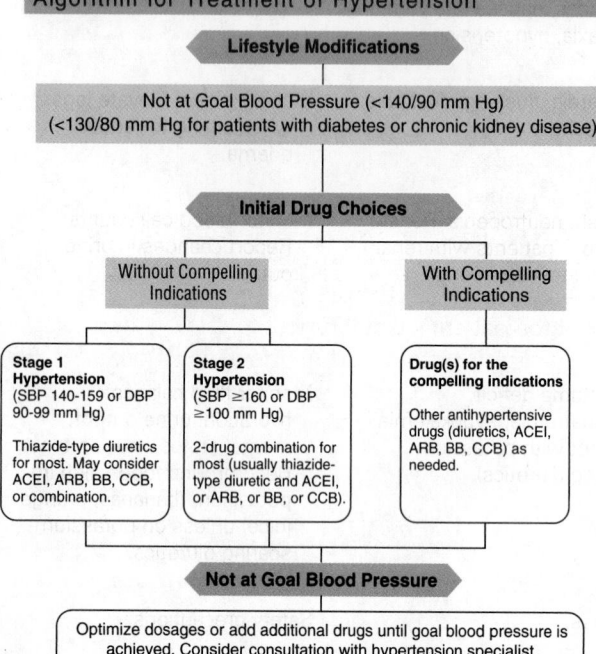

FIGURE **37-3** Algorithm for the treatment of hypertension.

Monitor people with diabetes for low blood glucose if they are taking beta-blockers.

Calcium Antagonists. Calcium antagonists are called *calcium channel blockers* because they block the movement of calcium into cardiac and vascular smooth muscle cells. This action reduces the heart rate, decreases the force of cardiac contraction, and dilates peripheral blood vessels. Because dilated vessels present less resistance to blood flow, blood pressure is reduced. Diltiazem (Cardizem), isradipine (DynaCirc), nicardipine (Cardene), nifedipine (Procardia), and verapamil (Calan) are examples of calcium channel blockers used for hypertension.

Common side effects of calcium channel blockers are flushing, dizziness, and headache. The nurse should also monitor for hypotension, bradycardia, and edema.

Angiotensin-Converting Enzyme Inhibitors. Angiotensin-converting enzyme inhibitors (ACE inhibitors or ACEIs) prevent the conversion of angiotensin I to angiotensin II, a potent vasoconstrictor. Blocking the production of angiotensin II decreases peripheral resis-

What Does Culture Have to Do with Antihypertensive Drugs?

Your genes affect the way you metabolize drugs. Therefore ethnicity and race explain some variations in effects of antihypertensive drugs. For example, Asians respond better to beta-blockers than whites do. Whites respond better than African Americans to beta-blockers and ACE inhibitors.

tance. ACE inhibitors also decrease fluid retention by decreasing the production of aldosterone. Examples of ACE inhibitors are captopril (Capoten) and enalapril (Vasotec). ACE inhibitors with diuretics are often effective for African-American patients. Adverse effects can include a chronic cough, dizziness, headache, fatigue, angioedema, hyperkalemia, and hypotension.

Angiotensin II Receptor Antagonists. Angiotensin II receptor antagonists (ARBs) prevent vasoconstriction in response to angiotensin. They also prevent the release of aldosterone, which increases excretion of salt and water, thereby reducing blood volume. Examples of angiotensin II receptor antagonists are losartan (Cozaar) and valsartan (Diovan). Unlike the ACE inhibitors, the only significant adverse effect of these drugs has been dizziness in some patients.

Central Adrenergic Blockers. Central adrenergic blockers inhibit impulses from the vasomotor center in the brain that maintain the muscle tone in blood vessels. The effect of this type of drug is to reduce peripheral resistance and lower blood pressure. Examples of centrally acting adrenergic blockers are clonidine (Catapres) and methyldopa (Aldomet).

Alpha-Adrenergic Receptor Blockers. Stimulation of alpha receptors produces constriction of arterioles. Drugs such as prazosin (Minipress) and doxazosin (Cardura) block alpha receptor stimulation and lower blood pressure by reducing peripheral resistance. The most important adverse effect is orthostatic hypotension, which is most severe with initial or increased dosages. Patients should lie down for 2 hours after taking a first or increased dose of this drug. For this reason, it is best given at bedtime. Alpha-blockers can also cause dizziness, headache, and drowsiness.

Direct Vasodilators. Direct vasodilators lower blood pressure by relaxing arteriolar smooth muscle. Examples of direct vasodilators are fenoldopam (Corlopam), minoxidil (Loniten), hydralazine (Apresoline), diazoxide (Hyperstat IV), and sodium nitroprusside (Nipride). Fenoldopam, nitroglycerin, sodium nitroprusside, hydralazine, and diazoxide are used to treat hypertensive crisis. Most emergency vasodilators are diluted in intravenous fluids and administered at the rate needed for the desired results. Diazoxide is given by direct intravenous injection (IV push), usually in small, repeated doses until the blood pressure reaches the target reading.

Nursing Implications. You need to be familiar with the drugs commonly prescribed for hypertension. Nursing responsibilities include administering the drugs to inpatients, monitoring for therapeutic and adverse effects, and teaching patients about their drugs. Additional information about antihypertensive drugs and nursing interventions is presented in the Drug Therapy table on pp. 720 and 721.

Older adults respond differently to drug therapy. Older patients are at greater risk for adverse effects of medications because of reduced liver and kidney function. They are especially susceptible to orthostatic hypotension because their blood vessels respond more slowly to position changes. This creates increased risk for falls.

Older people may respond differently to beta-blockers and to diuretics. The effectiveness of beta-blockers may be reduced because beta receptor activity is lessened in older adults. In addition, diuretics may produce a more profound decrease in blood volume in these patients. Also, older patients often are taking medications for other conditions. Drug interactions can alter therapeutic effects or enhance side effects. Dosages for antihypertensive medications may need to be reduced or adjusted depending on what conditions the patient has.

Put on Your Thinking Cap!

You have been asked to give a talk on hypertension to members of a senior center. The members are low income and have minimal education. Some speak limited English.
1. How might you explain the effects of hypertension on the body?
2. Select one lifestyle modification and explain how it reduces the risk of hypertension.

SECONDARY HYPERTENSION

Secondary hypertension, which has a specific known cause, is less common than primary hypertension. Examples of causes are renal disease, excess secretion of adrenal hormones, narrowing of the aorta, and increased intracranial pressure, as well as some drugs such as vasoconstrictors.

NURSING CARE of the Patient with Hypertension

Assessment

Early detection, education, and promotion of adherence are the keys to blood pressure control. Periodic blood pressure checks detect new or unknown hypertensive people and provide data to evaluate the effect of therapy in known hypertensive people.

The nursing assessment of the known or suspected hypertensive person begins with a complete history and physical examination by the registered nurse The LPN/LVN may be involved in initial blood pressure screenings and monitoring and provides important data to evaluate treatment effectiveness.

Health History

The patient's reason for seeking health care should be noted. Because hypertension often has no symptoms, the visit may be related to some other problem. Explore the past medical history to determine whether the patient has ever had hypertension or renal, cardiac, or endocrine disorders. Note the date and readings of the last blood pressure measurement. Ask the female patient about pregnancy and about hormone replacement therapy if appropriate. List current medications, including over-the-counter drugs. In the family health history, inquire about hypertension, myocardial infarction, or cerebrovascular accidents among relatives.

Review the body systems for significant signs and symptoms, particularly headaches, epistaxis, dizziness, visual disturbances, dyspnea, angina, or nocturia. Data about the patient's usual functioning may detect some potential risk factors for hypertension. It includes occupation, exercise and activity, sleep and rest, nutrition, interpersonal relationships, and stressors.

Physical Examination

While taking the health history and beginning the physical examination, observe the patient's general appearance, noting any obvious distress. Measure height and weight and vital signs. The nurse may be the first to detect elevated pressure, so accurate measurement of blood pressure is very important. The patient should be seated comfortably in a chair with his or her feet on the floor and arm resting on a surface at the level of the heart. The proper cuff size is essential. The bladder in the cuff should encircle at least 80% of the circumference of the patient's arm. Too small a cuff may give a false high reading, whereas a cuff that is too large may give a false low reading. For a more accurate reading, determine the systolic pulse first by palpation. Then deflate the cuff and take the pressure by auscultation, being careful to reinflate it above the palpated systolic pressure.

For the initial assessment, multiple readings should be taken. The blood pressure should be assessed in both arms in the supine, sitting, and standing positions. Begin blood pressure assessment with the patient resting supine for at least 10 minutes. After supine blood pressure assessment, take the sitting and then the standing readings after 1 to 3 minutes in each position. When body position is altered from supine to standing, the systolic pressure normally falls approximately 10 mm Hg and the diastolic pressure rises approximately 5 mm Hg. Assess the apical and peripheral pulses for rate, rhythm, and quality or character in each position.

In general, blood pressure readings obtained in the home are more valid measures because patients are more relaxed there than in a clinic or office.

In addition to blood pressure and pulses, assess respiratory rate and effort. Inspect extremities for edema and color. Note any abnormalities in neurologic or muscular function.

Nursing assessment of the patient with known or suspected hypertension is summarized in Box 37-1.

When screening persons for hypertension, if blood pressure is elevated initially, reassess it after 1 to 5 minutes. If the pressure remains elevated, refer the patient for medical evaluation. Remember that a single elevated reading does not mean that the patient has hypertension. If the blood pressure is severely elevated (diastolic pressure of 115 mm Hg or more), the patient is in imminent danger of a stroke and immediate medical care is needed.

Nursing Diagnoses, Goals, and Outcome Criteria: Hypertension

NURSING DIAGNOSES	GOALS AND OUTCOME CRITERIA
Ineffective Therapeutic Regimen Management related to lack of knowledge about management of hypertension, drug side effects, difficulty maintaining lifestyle changes	Effective patient management of prescribed treatment: patient correctly explains hypertension and its treatment. Patient adheres to prescribed treatment plan: lowered blood pressure, evidence of positive lifestyle changes (weight loss, cessation of smoking)
Risk for Injury related to orthostatic hypotension secondary to antihypertensive drug therapy, sedation	Lack of injury: no falls or other incidents associated with orthostatic hypotension or sedation
Ineffective Coping related to depression secondary to drug side effects	Effective coping: patient reports positive emotional state
Sexual Dysfunction related to drug side effects	Satisfactory sexual function: patient's statement of ability to manage effects of drug therapy on sexual function

Interventions

Ineffective Therapeutic Regimen Management

Adherence to therapy requires commitment and active participation on the part of the patient. Lifestyle changes may be required, and pharmacologic side effects may be unpleasant. Failure to follow the prescribed regimen is often referred to as *noncompliance*. Some people prefer the term *nonadherence* as being less judgmental. In counseling the patient, it must be stressed that hypertension is a chronic disease requiring long-term management. Sometimes patients discontinue drug therapy inappropriately because they have no symptoms and current blood pressure readings (on medications!) are normal.

Patient education is critical for effective management of hypertension. Education begins as soon as the condition is diagnosed and continues throughout life. As with any patient teaching, begin by finding out what the person already knows and is most interested in learning. Addressing the patient's immediate concerns first builds trust that should facilitate further

teaching. Present measures to manage hypertension as health practices that are beneficial to everyone rather than a long list of "don'ts." Include members of the patient's household, especially a spouse, in the teaching. Their understanding and cooperation can be very supportive to the patient.

Teaching patients about their medications will, it is hoped, promote adherence. Information in writing and a chart with times for medication administration may be helpful. Patients who do not take their medications as prescribed often cite the adverse side effects as reasons for noncompliance. It is important to teach patients to report unpleasant drug side effects to the physician promptly. A change in dosage or in the medication itself may reduce undesirable effects, but the patient should not make changes unless advised to do so by the physician. Common side effects of antihypertensive drugs that may affect adherence are orthostatic hypotension, sedation, sexual dysfunction, and depression.

Diet Therapy. The goals of diet therapy for the person with hypertension are to maintain ideal body

---

Box 37-1 | **ASSESSMENT of the Patient with Known or Suspected Hypertension**

Health History

Present Illness:
Description of reason for seeking care

Past Medical History:
Hypertension; last blood pressure reading; renal, cardiac, or endocrine disorders; pregnancy; current medications

Family History:
Hypertension, myocardial infarction, cerebrovascular accident

Review of Systems:
Headache, dizziness, epistaxis, visual disturbances, dyspnea, angina, nocturia

Functional Assessment:
Occupation, activity and exercise, sleep and rest, nutrition, interpersonal relationships, current stressors

Physical Examination

General Appearance:
Distress

Height and Weight

Vital Signs

Blood Pressure:
Supine, sitting, standing

Pulse

Respiration

Temperature

Extremities:
Edema

Neuromuscular:
Abnormalities

weight and to prevent fluid retention. Total calorie intake may need to be adjusted to achieve these goals. A diet low in saturated fats with no more than 2 g of sodium is often prescribed. Sodium restriction is more effective for some patients than for others. The National Research Council recommends a maximum daily sodium intake of 2400 mg.

If the patient is taking a potassium-wasting diuretic, dietary potassium intake may need to be increased or potassium supplements may be recommended.

The nurse and the dietitian should cooperate in teaching patients about their prescribed dietary alterations. If someone other than the patient prepares the food at home, that person should be included during the dietary teaching.

What Does Culture Have to Do with Diet?

Cultural dietary practices affect the types of foods eaten and how they are prepared. These practices must be considered and incorporated when teaching patients about healthier dietary practices.

The DASH (Dietary Approaches to Stop Hypertension) eating plan can not only help to lower blood pressure in people with hypertension but can also decrease the risk of a person developing hypertension. Therefore it is a good plan for the whole family (Table 37-3). The DASH plan is high in the following:

- Fruits, vegetables
- Low-fat dairy products
- Whole grains
- Poultry and fish
- Nuts
- Potassium, calcium, magnesium
- Protein and fiber

The DASH plan is low in the following:

- Saturated fat, total fat, and cholesterol
- Red meats
- Sugared beverages
- Salt and sodium

The Nutrition Concepts box on p. 726 also discusses diet and hypertension.

Exercise. Nutrition and exercise go hand in hand. It is very difficult to maintain or lose weight without engaging in some form of exercise. Walking is highly recommended as an exercise that increases cardiovascular

---

Table 37-3 | *The DASH Eating Plan*

The DASH eating plan shown below is based on 2000 calories a day. The number of daily servings in a food group may vary from those listed, depending upon your caloric needs.

FOOD GROUP	DAILY SERVINGS (EXCEPT AS NOTED)	SERVING SIZES
Grains and grain products	7-8	1 slice bread 1 cup ready-to-eat cereal* ½ cup cooked rice, pasta, or cereal
Vegetables	4-5	1 cup raw leafy vegetable ½ cup cooked vegetable 6 ounces vegetable juice
Fruits	4-5	1 medium fruit ¼ cup dried fruit ½ cup fresh, frozen, or canned fruit 6 ounces fruit juice
Low-fat or fat-free dairy foods	2-3	8 ounces milk 1 cup yogurt 1½ ounces cheese
Lean meats, poultry, and fish	2 or fewer	3 ounces cooked lean meat, skinless poultry, or fish
Nuts, seeds, and dry beans	4-5 per week	⅓ cup or 1½ ounces of nuts 1 tablespoon or ½ ounce seeds ½ cup cooked dry beans
Fats and oils†	2-3	1 teaspoon soft margarine 1 tablespoon low-fat mayonnaise 2 tablespoons light salad dressing 1 teaspoon vegetable oil
Sweets	5 per week	1 tablespoon sugar 1 tablespoon jelly or jam ½ ounce jelly beans 8 ounces lemonade

From Department of Health and Human Services, National Institutes of Health, National Heart, Lung, and Blood Institute. (2003). *Your guide to lowering blood pressure.* Bethesda, MD: NIH.
*Serving sizes vary between ½ cup and 1¼ cup. Check the product's nutrition label.
†Fat content changes serving counts for fats and oils: for example, 1 tablespoon of regular salad dressing equals 1 serving, 1 tablespoon of low-fat salad dressing equals ½ serving, and 1 tablespoon of fat-free salad dressing equals 0 servings.

Nutrition Concepts

1. Diet and lifestyle changes, including weight reduction, exercise, and stress management, are important in the treatment of hypertension.
2. Weight loss in obese people lowers blood pressure at a rate of 1 mm Hg per kg (2.2 pounds) of body weight.
3. Sodium-restricted diets help lower blood pressure in many people with hypertension.
4. A high potassium intake may help lower blood pressure as well as replace potassium lost with potassium-wasting diuretics. Foods particularly high in potassium are fresh fruits and vegetables.
5. An adequate calcium intake may help in preventing and treating hypertension. Two to three cups of milk or yogurt per day, 4 ounces of low-sodium cheese, or calcium supplements (calcium carbonate, 1 to 2 g/day) can provide adequate calcium intake.

functioning, burns calories, relieves stress, and promotes a sense of well-being. Thirty minutes of physical exercise most days of the week can make a difference. An exercise program can benefit people of all ages, even older adults. Advise patients to ask their physicians before beginning new exercise programs. Instruct them to increase their activities gradually over a period of time.

A program of good nutrition and exercise may allow a patient to eliminate or reduce medications used to control hypertension. This information may be motivating to some people.

Stress Management. Patients need to understand that stress can raise blood pressure. Help patients identify stressors in their lives and explore ways to reduce them. Referrals to professional counselors may be in order for patients with complicated or multiple stressors. Some agencies or community centers offer classes in stress management or relaxation techniques.

Drug Therapy. Patients need to be well informed about their medications. Review with the patient the name, dosage, purpose, and side effects of any prescribed medications. Advise patients not to discontinue their drugs or change the dosage without consulting with the physician even if they feel well. Blood pressure can be very high with no symptoms. Suddenly stopping antihypertensive drugs may produce adverse effects, including rebound hypertension (sudden return of elevated blood pressure), myocardial infarction, and cerebrovascular accident. Also, explain that many over-the-counter drugs such as cold remedies contain vasoconstrictors that can counteract blood pressure medications.

Box 37-2 summarizes a variety of actions patients may take to help lower their blood pressure.

Risk for Injury

The patient taking antihypertensive medications may be at risk for injury because of drug side effects. The

Box 37-2 *Action Items to Help Lower Your Blood Pressure*

- Maintain a healthy weight:
  - Check with your health care provider to see if you need to lose weight.
  - If you do, lose weight slowly using a healthy eating plan and engaging in physical activity.
- Be physically active:
  - Engage in physical activity for a total of 30 minutes on most days of the week.
  - Combine everyday chores with moderate-level sporting activities, such as walking, to achieve your physical activity goals.
- Follow a healthy eating plan:
  - Set up a healthy eating plan with foods low in saturated fat, total fat, and cholesterol and high in fruits, vegetables, and low-fat dairy foods such as the DASH eating plan.
  - Write down everything that you eat and drink in a food diary. Note areas that are successful or need improvement.
  - If you are trying to lose weight, choose an eating plan that is lower in calories.
- Reduce sodium in your diet:
  - Choose foods that are low in salt and other forms of sodium.
  - Use spices, garlic, and onions to add flavor to your meals without adding more sodium.
- Drink alcohol only in moderation:
  - In addition to raising your blood pressure, too much alcohol can add unneeded calories to your diet.
  - If you drink alcoholic beverages, have only a moderate amount—one drink a day for women, two drinks a day for men.
- Take prescribed drugs as directed:
  - If you need drugs to help lower your blood pressure, you still must follow the lifestyle changes just mentioned.
  - Use notes and other reminders to help you remember to take your drugs. Ask your family to help you with reminder phone calls and messages.

From Department of Health and Human Services, National Institutes of Health, National Heart, Lung, and Blood Institute. (2003). *Your guide to lowering blood pressure.* Bethesda MD: NIH.

effects that pose the greatest potential for injury are orthostatic hypotension and sedation.

Orthostatic Hypotension. Orthostatic or postural hypotension is a sudden drop in systolic blood pressure, usually 20 mm Hg, when going from a lying or sitting position to a standing position. Monitor for lightheadedness, dizziness, and syncope (fainting) in patients who are at risk for orthostatic hypotension. Instruct patients who are prone to orthostatic hypotension to exercise their legs and then to rise slowly from a lying or sitting position. They should avoid activities that cause blood pressure to fall, such as prolonged standing in one place and taking very hot baths or showers.

Sedation. Sedation may be dealt with by taking medications at bedtime to promote sleep. Advise patients if drowsiness is likely so that dangerous activities or those requiring alertness can be avoided during times of peak drug effect.

Ineffective Coping

If depression occurs as a side effect of an antihypertensive drug, consult the physician so that another drug may be substituted. This side effect should be taken very seriously. Refer patients with severe depression to a mental health professional.

Sexual Dysfunction

A common side effect of many antihypertensive medications is sexual dysfunction. Dysfunctions may take the form of decreased libido, inability to achieve an erection, or delayed ejaculation. Many patients consider sexual function to be a very personal subject, so it must be handled in a sensitive manner. Some patients volunteer information about sexual changes. Others may fail to relate the problem to their medications and not report it to the nurse or the physician. You can introduce the subject by saying, "Some people taking this medication have changes in sexual function. Has this been a problem for you?" If it is a problem for the patient, advise the physician so that an alternative medication or other intervention can be considered.

Older Patients

Planning nursing care for older hypertensive patients requires some additional considerations. Response to drug therapy is more difficult to predict, and side effects are more common. Orthostatic hypotension and sedation are especially problematic for the older person, who is prone to fall and suffer serious injuries. Depression also must be taken very seriously because it lowers motivation, impairs quality of life, and can lead to suicide.

Health care providers tend to assume that older adults are not sexually active. Therefore they often fail to assess sexual function or dysfunction in older people. This is a real disservice to the older person whose sexual functioning is impaired as a result of antihypertensive drugs. The older patient should be treated just like a younger patient in the assessment and management of distressing drug effects.

Pharmacology Capsule

Advise patients not to discontinue antihypertensive therapy simply because they feel well. Blood pressure can be very high with no symptoms.

HYPERTENSIVE EMERGENCIES

Hypertensive crisis is a life-threatening medical emergency. The patient presents with severe headache, blurred vision, nausea, restlessness, and confusion. Along with a very elevated diastolic blood pressure (130 mm Hg or more), the heart and respiratory rates are increased. This episode may result from having stopped taking antihypertensive drugs or may be caused by malignant hypertension, hypertensive encephalopathy, eclampsia, pheochromocytoma (adrenal tumor), or a cerebrovascular accident. Malignant hypertension is a specific type of hypertensive emergency in which the diastolic pressure exceeds 140 mm Hg. It has a sudden onset and is seen most often in African-American men ages 30 to 40 years.

Without appropriate treatment, the patient in hypertensive crisis may incur cardiac and renal damage. Death may ensue as a result of a cerebrovascular accident, renal failure, or cardiac failure.

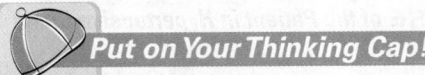

Put on Your Thinking Cap!

Albert Smith, a 34-year-old African-American male, arrives at the emergency department complaining of severe headache and blurred vision. His BP is 220/146. The physician diagnoses malignant hypertension. Mr. Smith is anxious and says his father died of a stroke at age 39. Mr. Smith is a carpenter who reports no history of serious illness except thyroid deficiency. What is Mr. Smith's primary risk factor for malignant hypertension?

MEDICAL DIAGNOSIS

Assessment in the emergency department reveals elevated blood pressure, pulse, and respiratory rate. Retinal hemorrhage or papilledema or both can be

---

Box 37-3 | *Emergency Antihypertensive Drugs*

Vasodilators
Sodium nitroprusside (Nipride)
Nitroglycerin
Fenoldopam (Corlopam)
Diazoxide (Hyperstat)*

Calcium Channel Blocker
Nifedipine (Procardia)

Adrenergic Blocker
Labetalol (Normodyne)

ACE Inhibitor
Captopril (Capoten)

Alpha₂ Agonist
Clonidine (Catapres)

From Lehne, R.A. (2001). *Pharmacology for nursing care* (4th ed.). Philadelphia: Saunders.
*Obsolete when no intensive monitoring is available.

observed in the fundus (back, interior portion) of the eye.

The physician may order blood drawn for arterial blood gases, complete blood count, electrolytes, blood urea nitrogen, creatinine, and cardiac enzymes. A chest radiograph may be requested. Direct blood pressure monitoring through an arterial catheter is preferred.

MEDICAL TREATMENT

The goal of drug therapy is to rapidly reduce the pressure to a non–life-threatening level and then to bring it slowly within normal range. This is done with diuretics and potent vasodilators. Examples of drugs that may be ordered include fenoldopam, nitroglycerin, diazoxide, hydralazine, phentolamine, labetalol, and nitroprusside. An intravenous line is usually established because many drugs are given by that route. Oral options for the management of hypertensive crisis include captopril, clonidine, and nifedipine. Drugs used to treat hypertensive crisis are listed in Box 37-3.

NURSING CARE *of the Patient in Hypertensive Crisis*
Assessment

The patient in hypertensive crisis must be closely monitored. Frequently check the patient's blood pressure, pulse, respiration, and level of consciousness. Some drugs are given in intravenous fluids, requiring continuous monitoring and adjustment. Maintain a careful record of fluid intake and output. Nausea and vomiting may indicate an impending seizure or coma.

Interventions

The nurse's role in caring for the patient in hypertensive crisis includes administering prescribed drugs, monitoring vital signs before and after each drug dose, monitoring cardiac and renal function, starting and

maintaining intravenous therapy and oxygen as ordered, and comforting the patient.

Take appropriate safety measures if the patient shows signs of seizure activity or a decreasing level of consciousness. Bed side rails should be raised and padded if necessary according to agency policy. Elevate the head of the bed to facilitate breathing. Place an oral airway and suction equipment at the bedside. Offer brief explanations or words of encouragement to allay some of the patient's anxiety. Once the patient's condition improves, it is important to explain how to manage hypertension and to prevent future crises from developing.

 Key Points

- Hypertension is called "the silent killer" because it often has no symptoms and is not discovered until a serious complication develops such as damage to the blood vessels in the kidneys, eyes, heart, or brain.
- Hypertension is defined as a persistent elevation of arterial blood pressure of 140/90 mm Hg or greater.
- Primary (essential) hypertension has no known cause, whereas secondary hypertension is caused by an underlying factor such as kidney disease.
- The two factors that determine blood pressure are cardiac output and peripheral vascular resistance.
- The primary risk factors for primary hypertension are dyslipidemia, obesity, atherosclerosis, use of tobacco, diabetes, sedentary lifestyle, age, and family history of early heart disease.
- Blood pressure tends to rise as people age, but age is not a barrier to aggressive treatment of hypertension.
- Hypertension often has no symptoms, but some people experience occipital headaches, lightheadedness, and epistaxis.
- A diagnosis of hypertension is usually based on multiple readings and is accompanied by tests to rule out possible correctable causes.
- Conservative measures to treat hypertension include weight reduction, smoking cessation, sodium restriction, exercise, relaxation techniques, and modified alcohol intake.
- Pharmacologic treatment is based on the stage of hypertension and presence of other factors such as kidney disease and heart failure.
- Types of drugs used to treat hypertension include diuretics, beta-adrenergic receptor blockers, calcium channel blockers, angiotensin-converting enzyme inhibitors, angiotensin II receptor antagonists, central adrenergic blockers, alpha-adrenergic receptor blockers, direct vasodilators, and ganglionic blockers.
- Ethnicity affects response to many antihypertensive drugs.
- Nursing care of the hypertensive person addresses Ineffective Therapeutic Regimen Management, Risk for Injury, Ineffective Coping, and Sexual Dysfunction.

- Hypertensive crisis, defined as a diastolic blood pressure of 130 mm Hg or more, is a life-threatening medical emergency that is usually treated with diuretics and potent vasodilators.
- Complications of hypertensive crisis include stroke, heart failure, and kidney failure.

 Go to your Companion CD-ROM for a Pharmacology Tutorial, Audio Glossary, and 3-D animations.

evolve Be sure to visit the companion Evolve site at http://evolve.elsevier.com/Linton/ for WebLinks and additional online resources.

REVIEW QUESTIONS *Choose the best answer.*

1. A consistent blood pressure of 144/100 is considered:
   1. Normal
   2. High normal
   3. Stage 1 hypertension
   4. Stage 2 hypertension

2. Individuals at greatest risk for severe complications of hypertension are:
   1. White males
   2. White females
   3. African-American males
   4. African-American females

3. The cause of primary (essential) hypertension is:
   1. Kidney disease
   2. Unknown
   3. Arteriosclerosis
   4. Pregnancy

4. Complications associated with prolonged hypertension include the following:
   1. Glaucoma
   2. Damage to heart valves
   3. Chronic renal failure
   4. Alzheimer's disease

5. A patient who is taking hydrochlorothiazide for hypertension complains of weakness, feeling grouchy, and loss of appetite. You should suspect:
   1. Hypotension
   2. Hypokalemia
   3. Hyponatremia
   4. Hypocalcemia

6. Beta-blockers lower blood pressure by:
   1. Eliminating excess body fluid
   2. Inhibiting cardiac stimulation
   3. Blocking the movement of calcium into myocardial cells
   4. Preventing the formation of angiotensin II

7. The initial measurement of blood pressure should include the following:
   1. Determining the diastolic pressure first by palpation and then by auscultation
   2. Taking readings in sequence: supine, sitting, and standing positions
   3. Having the patient rest supine for at least 10 minutes before taking BP
   4. Measuring the pressure only in the patient's dominant arm

8. A patient on antihypertensive drugs complains of feeling dizzy when first getting up. What should you advise the patient to do when this occurs?
   1. Change positions slowly and exercise the legs before standing.
   2. Discontinue all antihypertensive drugs immediately.
   3. Go back to bed and call the physician.
   4. Increase salt intake to bring blood pressure up to normal.

9. An 80-year-old patient who has been diagnosed with hypertension is not taking her prescribed medications. She says, "Wouldn't you expect my blood pressure to be up a bit at my age?" The nurse's most appropriate reply is:
   1. "Blood pressure tends to increase with age, but treatment reduces the risk of complications regardless of your age."
   2. "As long as you are feeling well, it will not hurt for you to skip your medication."
   3. "High blood pressure medications probably offer little benefit to someone your age."
   4. "Your doctor is going to be pretty upset if you don't follow medical orders."

38 Digestive Tract Disorders

evolve http://evolve.elsevier.com/Linton/

Objectives

After reading and studying this chapter, you should be able to:

1. Identify the nursing responsibilities in the care of patients undergoing diagnostic tests and procedures for disorders of the digestive tract.
2. List the data to be included in the nursing assessment of the patient with a digestive disorder.
3. Describe the nursing care of patients with gastrointestinal intubation and decompression, tube feedings, total parenteral nutrition, digestive tract surgery, and drug therapy for digestive disorders.
4. Describe the pathophysiology, signs and symptoms, complications, and medical treatment of selected digestive disorders.
5. Assist in developing nursing care plans for patients receiving treatment for digestive disorders.

Key Terms

Be sure to check out the bonus material on the Companion CD-ROM, including selected audio pronunciations.

anorexia (ăn-ō-RĔK-sē-ă, p. 745)
caries (KĀ-rē-ēz or KĂR-ēz, p. 752)
cathartic (kă-THĂR-tĭk, p. 744)
dyspepsia (dĭs-PĔP-sē-ă, p. 733)
dysphagia (dĭs-FĀ-jē-ă, p. 756)
emesis (ĔM-ĕ-sĭs, p. 750)
eructation (ĕ-rŭk-TĀ-shŭn, p. 761)
flatulence (FLĂT-ū-lĕns, p. 733)
flatus (FLĀ-tŭs, p. 743)
gingivitis (jĭn-jĭ-VĪ-tĭs, p. 752)
laxative (LĂK-să-tĭv, p. 779)
peritoneum (pĕ-rĭ-tō-NĒ-ŭm, p. 730)
peritonitis (pĕ-rĭ-tō-NĪ-tĭs, p. 771)
regurgitation (rē-gŭr-jĭ-TĀ-shŭn, p. 759)
stomatitis (stō-mă-TĪ-tĭs, p. 751)

To remain healthy, the human body must have a steady supply of nutrients and fluids. The primary role of the digestive tract is to extract the molecules essential for cellular function from food and fluids. Disorders of the digestive tract can threaten the patient's nutritional status, leading to disorders in the structure and functioning of other body systems.

ANATOMY AND PHYSIOLOGY OF THE DIGESTIVE TRACT

The functions of the digestive tract are ingestion, digestion, and absorption of nutrients, and elimination of wastes. Digestion is the breakdown of food into simple nutrient molecules that can be used by the cells. The process of digestion requires (1) the adequate intake of food and fluids, (2) the mechanical and chemical breakdown of food, and (3) the movement of food through the digestive tract. Absorption is the transfer of digested food molecules from the digestive tract into the bloodstream. Elimination is the removal of solid food wastes from the body.

The digestive tract is also called the *gastrointestinal tract* (or *GI tract*) and the *alimentary tract* (Fig. 38-1). It is a muscular tube about 30 feet long. The main parts of the digestive tract are the mouth, pharynx, esophagus, stomach, small intestine, large intestine, and anus.

Other organs that are outside the digestive tract but are considered part of the digestive system are called *accessory organs*. Accessory organs include the salivary glands, liver, gallbladder, and pancreas. Each of these secretes fluid, containing specialized enzymes, into the digestive tract. These enzymes play a part in the breakdown or metabolism of foodstuffs (Table 38-1).

A two-layer membrane, the peritoneum, lines the abdominal cavity and covers the surfaces of the abdominal organs. Lubricating fluid between the two layers permits the organs to move without friction during breathing and digestive movements.

MOUTH

Food is taken into the mouth, where the teeth, tongue, and salivary glands begin the process of food digestion. As the teeth cut and grind the food, the salivary glands secrete saliva, a watery solution that contains amylase (ptyalin). Amylase is an enzyme that initiates the breakdown of carbohydrates. The tongue helps by mixing saliva with the food and pressing it against the teeth. When the bolus is to be swallowed, the tongue forces the food into the pharynx.

PHARYNX

The pharynx is a muscular structure that is shared by the digestive and respiratory tracts. It joins the mouth

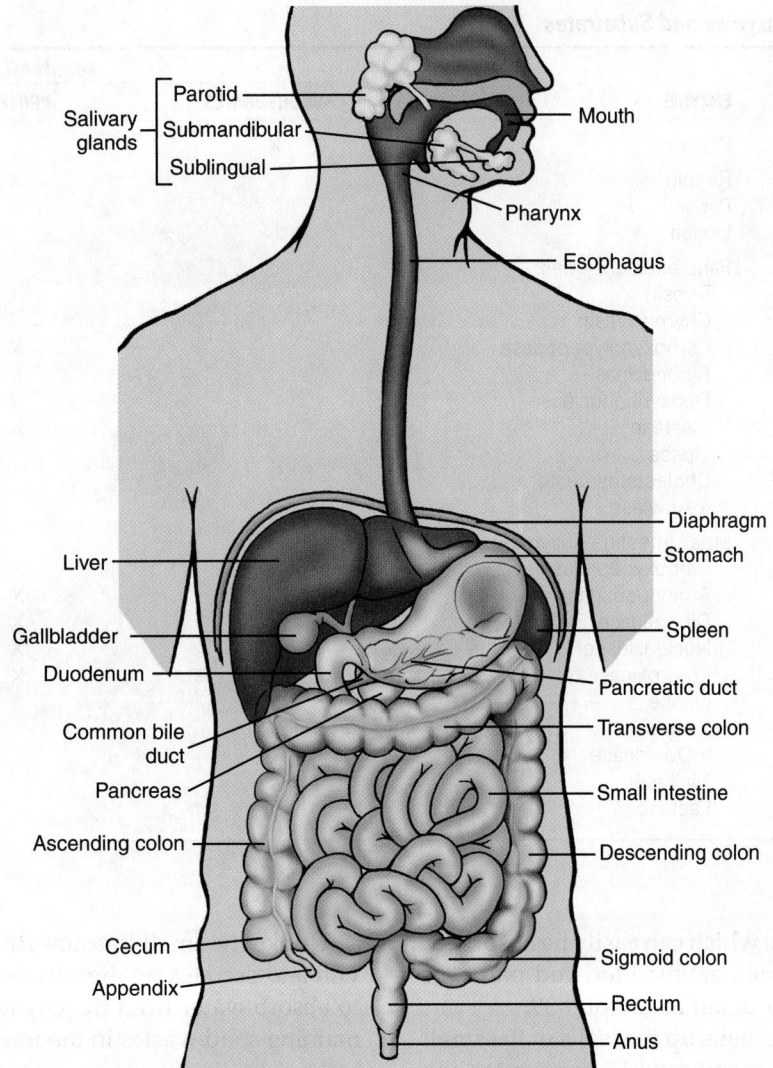

FIGURE **38-1** The digestive tract and associated structures.

and nasal passages to the esophagus. During swallowing, the epiglottis covers the airway like a trapdoor to prevent food from entering the respiratory tract.

ESOPHAGUS

Food moves from the pharynx into the esophagus, a long muscular tube that passes through the diaphragm into the stomach. Gravity helps but is not essential for the movement of food through the esophagus. Circular, wavelike contractions of the muscles of the digestive tract propel food down the tract. This movement is called *peristalsis.*

STOMACH

The stomach is the widest section of the digestive tract. It is separated from the esophagus by the cardiac sphincter. The stomach is not very large when empty, but it expands considerably when food is present. It consists of three sections: the fundus, the body, and the pylorus. A unique arrangement of muscle layers

allows the stomach to churn the food, mixing it with gastric secretions until it becomes a semiliquid mass called *chyme.* Gastric secretions include rennin, pepsin, hydrochloric acid, and lipase. Rennin starts to break down milk proteins, lipase breaks down fats, and pepsin and hydrochloric acid partially digest proteins. The pyloric sphincter between the stomach and the small intestine keeps food in the stomach until it is properly mixed.

SMALL INTESTINE

Chyme leaves the stomach and enters the small intestine, where chemical digestion and absorption of nutrients take place. The small intestine is approximately 20 feet long and consists of three sections: the duodenum, the jejunum, and the ileum.

Liver and pancreatic secretions enter the digestive tract in the duodenum. Bile, produced in the liver and stored in the gallbladder, breaks down large fat globules. Pancreatic enzymes further reduce the fat to

Table 38-1 *Digestive Enzymes and Substrates*

SITE	ENZYME	SUBSTRATE		
		CARBOHYDRATES	PROTEIN	FATS
Mouth	Ptyalin	X		
Stomach	Rennin		X	
	Pepsin		X	
	Lipase			X
Small intestine	Pancreatic enzymes:			
	Trypsin		X	
	Chymotrypsin		X	
	Carboxypolypeptidase		X	
	Ribonuclease		X	
	Deoxyribonuclease		X	
	Elastase		X	
	Lipase			X
	Cholesterase ester			X
	α-Amylase	X		
	Small intestine enzymes:			
	Carboxypeptidase		X	
	Aminopeptidase		X	
	Dipeptidase		X	
	Nucleosidase		X	
	Enterokinase		X	
	Lipase			X
	Sucrase	X		
	α-Dextrinase	X		
	Maltase	X		
	Lactase	X		

glycerol and fatty acids, which can easily be absorbed. The functions of the liver, gallbladder, and pancreas are discussed in greater detail in Chapter 39.

Three layers of tissue make up the walls of the small intestine. The mucous membrane layer secretes the digestive enzymes sucrase, lactase, maltase, carboxypeptidase, aminopeptidase, dipeptidase, nucleosidase, lipase, and enterokinase. Enzymes and their substrates are listed in Table 38-1. The inner layer is lined with thousands of microscopic projections called *villi.* Digested food molecules are absorbed through the villi into the bloodstream. Muscle layers contract to continue mixing the chyme, moving it toward the large intestine.

LARGE INTESTINE AND ANUS

Chyme enters the large intestine through the ileocecal valve. The first section of the large intestine is the cecum, where the appendix is located. The large intestine goes up the right side of the abdomen (the ascending colon), across the abdomen just below the waist (the transverse colon), and down the left side of the abdomen (the descending colon). The part of the descending colon between the iliac crest and the rectum is called the *sigmoid colon.* The last 6 to 8 inches of the large intestine is the rectum, which ends at the anus, where wastes leave the body. The presence of sphincters in the anus allows wastes to be stored until voluntary elimination occurs.

Unlike the small intestine, the large intestine has no villi and secretes no digestive enzymes. Its function is to absorb water from the chyme and eliminate the remaining solid wastes in the form of feces.

AGE-RELATED CHANGES

Normal aging generally does not significantly impair ingestion, digestion, absorption, or elimination. When acute or chronic illnesses occur, however, the older person is at increased risk for problems with digestion and elimination.

The teeth are mechanically worn down with age. They appear darker and somewhat transparent. The gingiva (gum) tends to recede. Although tooth loss is not a normal effect of aging, about 40% of all Americans ages 65 years and older are edentulous. The main reasons for tooth loss are caries and periodontal disease. Many older people have complete or partial dentures. The jaw may be affected by osteoarthritis. There is a significant loss of taste buds with age. The older person may be able to detect sweet better than other tastes. Xerostomia (dry mouth) is common but may be caused more by poor hydration and drug side effects than by aging.

The walls of the esophagus and stomach become thinner with aging, and secretions lessen. The esophageal sphincters that normally prevent the reflux of gastric contents are more relaxed. The production of hydrochloric acid and digestive enzymes decreases. Gastric motor activity slows; thus gastric emptying is delayed and hunger contractions diminish. There are no significant changes in the small intestine with age. The absorption of vitamin A may increase, whereas the absorption of vitamin D, calcium, and zinc may be reduced. In the large intestine, the muscle layer and mucosa atrophy. Smooth muscle tone and blood flow decrease, and connective tissue increases. Movements of contents through the colon are slower. The anal sphincter tone and strength decrease.

Constipation is a frequent complaint among older adults, and they use laxatives more often than young people do. Many experts believe that constipation is not a normal age-related change but rather is caused by such factors as low fluid intake, lack of dietary fiber, inactivity, drugs, depression, and hypothyroidism.

NURSING ASSESSMENT OF THE DIGESTIVE TRACT

HEALTH HISTORY

Chief Complaint and History of Present Illness

Although the registered nurse should perform the complete assessment, the LPN/LVN contributes to the database. Therefore the complete nursing assessment is detailed here. The health history begins with a detailed description of the present illness. Complaints may include weight changes, problems with food ingestion, symptoms of digestive disturbances, or changes in bowel elimination.

Past Medical History

The past medical history may disclose recent surgery, trauma, burns, or infections. Note serious illnesses such as diabetes, hepatitis, anemia, peptic ulcers, gallbladder disease, and cancer. Also identify any alternative methods of feeding or fecal diversion (ileostomy, colostomy). If feedings are given via nasogastric, gastrostomy, enterostomy, or esophagogastrostomy tubes, record the type and amount of feedings as well as the feeding schedule. The past history also includes a list of recent and current medications, both prescription and over the counter. Use of antacids and laxatives is especially important to note. Record any food allergy or intolerance, with a description of the reaction that occurs when the offending food is eaten.

Family History

Inquire whether the patient has a family history of diabetes, cancer of the digestive tract, peptic ulcers, gallbladder disease, hepatitis, alcoholism, intestinal polyps, or obesity.

Review of Systems

The review of systems begins with a description of the patient's general health state. Ask about changes in the skin, including dryness, bruising, and pruritus (itching). Determine whether the patient has any mouth problems, specifically lesions, bleeding, increased or decreased salivation, abnormal tastes or odors, and pain. Document if the patient has dentures, partial plates, or natural teeth, and record the last dental examination. Note any problems with chewing or swallowing. Also inquire about changes in appetite, food intake, and weight. If nausea, vomiting, dyspepsia (indigestion), heartburn, flatus, abdominal distention, or pain is present, identify factors that seem to be related to the symptoms. Describe pain location, along with precipitating factors, relationship to meals, and measures that relieve the pain. Assessment of elimination includes usual bowel habits and recent changes, flatulence (gas), change in stool characteristics (frequency, amount, color, consistency), bleeding, and painful defecation.

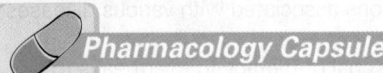

Pharmacology Capsule

Many drugs affect gastrointestinal function, causing anorexia, nausea, vomiting, and diarrhea or constipation.

Functional Assessment

The functional assessment focuses on nutrition, activity, and stressors. Information about general dietary habits should include the daily pattern of food intake (mealtimes, food eaten in a typical day, food likes and dislikes, and use of food supplements), attitudes and beliefs about food, and changes in dietary habits related to health problems. Describe the effects of the chief complaint on usual functioning. Note whether the patient is able to obtain and prepare food and eat independently (See the Nutrition Concepts box on p. 734.)

PHYSICAL EXAMINATION

Begin the physical examination with the measurement of height, weight, and vital signs. Observe the patient's general appearance noting skin color, texture, and turgor; posture; motor activity; and responses to instructions.

Head and Neck

Inspection of the mouth determines the condition of the lips, teeth, gums, tongue, and mucous membranes. Describe caries, moisture, color, and lesions. Note any unpleasant or unusual odors of the mouth. If the patient has dentures, examine the mouth with and without the dentures in place. A tongue blade is needed to depress the tongue and examine the pharynx. Instruct the patient to say *ah* while observing the movement of the uvula rand soft palate. Normally, the uvula and soft palate move upward, with the uvula remaining in the midline.

Abdomen

For the abdominal examination, the patient should be supine, with the head raised slightly and the knees slightly flexed. The areas of the abdomen are commonly described as *quadrants*. An imaginary line is drawn horizontally across the abdomen at the level of the um-

Nutrition Concepts

1. People with gastric ulcers experience increased pain after eating.
2. People with duodenal ulcers experience decreased pain after eating.
3. A peptic ulcer diet is individualized and usually consists of small to moderate-size meals, avoiding foods that cause an increase in gastric acid secretions or consistently cause distress.
4. Diarrhea is caused by pathogenic organisms, diet, intestinal lesions, or irritations associated with various diseases or conditions.
5. The major nutritional goal of therapy for diarrhea is to replace lost fluids.
6. Constipation is caused by insufficient fiber intake, insufficient fluid intake, lack of exercise, some drugs, and the habitual use of laxatives.
7. The dietary treatment of constipation consists of increasing fluid (8-10 glasses of water/day) and fiber intake.
8. A hot drink such as coffee or tea enhances peristalsis and promotes defecation.

bilicus. A second imaginary line extends from the sternum to the pubic bone. This creates the four quadrants: the right upper quadrant, the left upper quadrant, the right lower quadrant, and the left lower quadrant. Findings can then be documented by anatomic location (Fig. 38-2).

Inspection. Inspect the skin of the abdomen for color, texture, scars, striae ("stretch marks"), rashes, lesions, and dilated blood vessels. Describe the general contour of the abdomen. Contour is described as flat, convex (rounded), concave (sunken), protuberant, or distended. Note the location and contour of the umbilicus. Aortic pulsations and peristalsis are sometimes observed, especially in thin people.

Auscultation. After inspecting the abdomen, auscultate the abdomen to assess bowel sounds. Auscultation is done before palpation because palpation can alter normal bowel sounds. The diaphragm of the stethoscope should be warmed and used to listen to each quadrant. Normal bowel sounds include clicks and gurgles that occur 5 to 30 times per minute. Listen for at least 2 minutes in each quadrant. If no sounds are heard, listen for a full 5 minutes before recording bowel sounds as absent. Bowel sounds may be described as present, absent, increased, decreased, high-pitched, gurgling, tinkling, or gushing. Loud gurgling sounds are called *borborygmi*. Record the presence or absence of bowel sounds in each quadrant.

Percussion. Nurses with advanced training in physical examination use percussion and palpation to collect

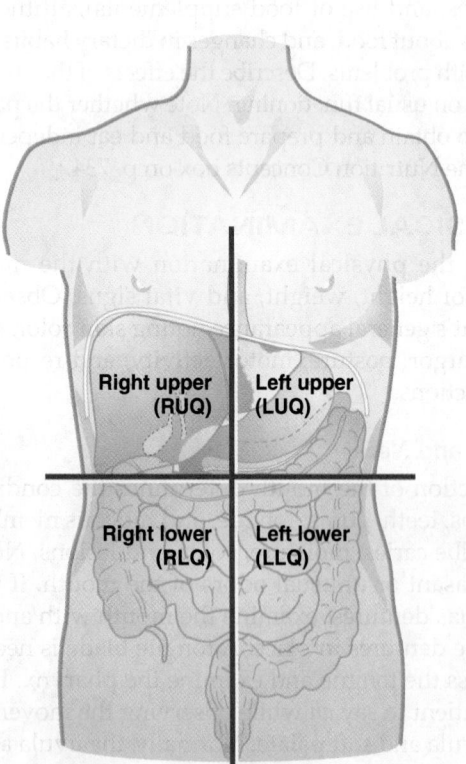

**Quadrants of the abdomen
and their underlying organs***

Right upper quadrant (RUQ)	Left upper quadrant (LUQ)
Adrenal gland (right)	Adrenal gland (left)
Colon (hepatic flexure and portions of ascending and transverse)	Colon (splenic flexure and portions of transverse and descending)
Duodenum	Kidney (portion of left)
Kidney (portion of right)	Liver (left lobe)
Liver (right lobe)	Pancreas (body)
Gallbladder	Spleen
Pancreas (head)	Stomach
Pylorus	
Right lower quadrant (RLQ)	Left lower quadrant (LLQ)
Appendix	Bladder (if distended)
Bladder (if distended)	Colon (sigmoid and portion of descending)
Cecum	
Colon (portion of ascending)	Kidney (lower pole of left)
Kidney (lower pole of right)	Ovary (left)
Ovary (right)	Salpinx (uterine tube; left)
Salpinx (uterine tube; right)	Spermatic cord (left)
Spermatic cord (right)	Ureter (left)
Ureter (right)	Uterus (if enlarged)
Uterus (if enlarged)	

*Small intestine loops in all quadrants.

FIGURE **38-2** The abdomen is divided into four quadrants.

additional data. Percussion is tapping on the skin to detect the presence of air, fluid, or masses in the underlying tissues. It also can be used to locate the margins of internal organs. Percussion over an air-filled organ produces a high-pitched, hollow sound called *tympany*. Tympany is similar to the sound made by a kettle drum. Percussion over a solid or fluid-filled structure sounds dull and flat. Normally, tympany is heard more often than dullness. All four quadrants of the abdomen should be percussed.

Palpation. Palpation is done to detect tenderness, sensitivity, masses, swelling, and muscular resistance. Hold your fingers together and depress the abdomen gently in all four quadrants. Light palpation depresses the abdominal wall only about 1 cm. Deep palpation uses more pressure. To assess for rebound tenderness, the abdomen is depressed and then quickly released. Deep palpation and tests for rebound tenderness should be done only by people who are trained in these techniques.

Rectum and Anus

Wear gloves to examine the anus and perianal area. Inspect the perianal skin for color, rashes, and lesions. Note the presence of any external hemorrhoids. The rectal examination is performed by a trained examiner. You may help position, drape, and comfort the patient. The examiner inserts a gloved, lubricated finger into the rectum and points it toward the umbilicus. The patient is instructed to bear down as if to have a bowel movement. This relaxes the anal sphincter. The examiner palpates for lumps and tenderness in the rectum.

Assessment of the patient with a digestive tract disorder is summarized in Box 38-1.

DIAGNOSTIC TESTS AND PROCEDURES

Diagnostic tests for digestive disorders include radiographic studies, endoscopic examinations, and laboratory studies. Always advise patients about the tests and procedures. Be sure required consent forms are signed.

For radiographs and imaging procedures, follow agency protocol regarding NPO orders and any other preparation. If contrast media will be used, assess for allergy to the "dye," iodine, and shellfish. If the patient is allergic to any of these, notify the radiologist.

For laboratory blood tests, tell the patient a blood sample will be taken and whether NPO is required.

For a urine specimen, instruct the patient in the collection procedure.

Studies are described briefly in the Diagnostic Tests and Procedures table on pp. 736 and 737.

RADIOGRAPHIC STUDIES

Radiographic studies include the upper gastrointestinal (UGI or GI) series (barium swallow), small bowel series, and barium enema examination. Radiographs of the gallbladder are obtained as well and are discussed in Chapter 39. These studies allow the radiologist to study the structure and function of the digestive tract. A contrast medium is used in some studies. This is a substance, such as barium sulfate, that can be given

---

Box 38-1 *ASSESSMENT of the Patient with a Disorder of the Digestive Tract*

Health History

Present Illness:
Weight changes, problems with food ingestion, symptoms of digestive disturbances, alterations in bowel elimination

Past Medical History:
Recent surgery, trauma, infections; history of diabetes mellitus, hepatitis, anemia, peptic ulcers, gallbladder disease, cancer; alternative methods of feeding: type, amount, schedule; fecal diversion: type; allergies: food, drugs

Family History:
Diabetes mellitus, cancer of the digestive tract, peptic ulcers, gallbladder disease, hepatitis, alcoholism, intestinal polyps, obesity

Review of Systems:

Skin Color, Pruritus

Oral Cavity:
Presence and condition of teeth, condition of gums, moisture, pain, abnormal tastes or odors, difficulty chewing

Appetite

Dysphagia

Digestive Disturbances:
Nausea, vomiting, dyspepsia, heartburn, pain

Bowel Elimination:
Changes, pain, flatulence, bleeding, stool characteristics

Functional Assessment:
Dietary pattern, attitudes and beliefs about food, activity, stressors

Physical Examination

Height and Weight

Vital Signs

General Appearance

Head and Neck:
Condition of teeth, gums, tongue, mucous membranes, odors, uvula position

Abdomen:
Skin color, texture, scars, striae, rashes, lesions, dilated blood vessels; abdominal contour, distention; umbilicus location and contour; bowel sounds; abdominal tenderness, masses, swelling, muscular resistance, rebound tenderness

Perianal Skin:
Color, rash, lesions; hemorrhoids

DIAGNOSTIC TESTS and PROCEDURES | The Digestive Tract

TEST/PURPOSE	PATIENT PREPARATION	POSTPROCEDURE NURSING CARE
RADIOGRAPHIC TESTS		
Upper gastrointestinal (UGI or GI) series Barium swallow detects abnormalities of esophagus and stomach	Inform patient he or she will need to drink a solution containing contrast medium. Radiographs will be taken of the esophagus, stomach, and duodenum via fluoroscope. Films will be repeated 6 hr later to see how much barium has passed through the stomach. NPO 6-8 hr before procedure, per agency protocol.	Monitor stools at least 2 days for passage of white stools that show that barium is being eliminated (normal stool color returns in 3 days). Laxatives may be ordered to promote elimination. Provide food, extra fluids, and rest.
Small bowel series detects abnormalities of small intestine	Patient drinks a contrast solution. Films are taken at 20-30 min intervals as solution passes through small intestine. Patient will be asked to assume various positions for x-rays. Procedure may take several hours. Preparation same as UGI series.	Same as for UGI series.
Barium enema detects abnormalities of large intestine	Contrast solution is administered by enema, and radiographs are taken with patient in a variety of positions. May take as long as 1/4 hr. Patient may be restricted to clear liquids day or evening before procedure. Laxative and enemas are given on previous day. Usually NPO after midnight. Enemas are given until intestine is clear on morning of procedure.	Same as for UGI series.
ENDOSCOPIC TESTS **Upper Digestive Tract**		
Esophagoscopy visualizes esophagus Gastroscopy visualizes stomach Gastroduodenoscopy visualizes stomach and duodenum Esophagogastroduodenoscopy visualizes esophagus, stomach, and duodenum Endoscopic retrograde cholangiography visualizes bile ducts and gallbladder	Upper digestive tract examinations: NPO for 6-8 hr. If ordered, give sedative shortly before examination.	NPO until gag reflex returns. Monitor for signs of trauma: bleeding from the throat or rectum. Monitor for signs of perforation: fever, abdominal distention, cramping pain, vague discomfort.
Lower Digestive Tract		
Colonoscopy visualizes colon Proctoscopy visualizes rectum	NPO for 6-8 hr before examination. May be restricted to liquids previous day or evening. Bowel cleansing may be done with cathartics, suppositories, and enemas.	Monitor for signs of perforation: fever, abdominal distention, cramping pain. Assess for rectal bleeding.
Sigmoidoscopy visualizes rectum and sigmoid colon	Cathartics and suppositories are usually given the evening before the test. Enemas until colon is clear may be ordered on morning of test.	
CAPSULE ENDOSCOPY		
Transmits video images of entire digestive tract Especially useful for study of small intestine May detect obscure GI bleeding, inflammatory bowel disease, small bowel tumors, malabsorption disorders, inflammation caused by NSAIDs or radiotherapy	10-hour overnight fast required for small bowel study. Bowel preparation, if any, varies with agency and physician. Study of the esophagus requires 2-hour fast. Simethicone may be given when capsule is swallowed to reduce bubbles and improve visualization.	Capsule normally is eliminated painlessly in the stool. No special care required. If the small intestine is obstructed, the capsule can become lodged at the site, requiring surgical removal.

LABORATORY TESTS

Blood Tests

	Patient Preparation	Aftercare
Serum electrolytes measure electrolytes in the blood to detect imbalances	Medications that affect results may be held until blood is drawn.	Resume medications.
Serum protein electrophoresis measures serum protein, which may be decreased with peptic ulcers, acute cholecystitis, malabsorption	Medications that can alter test results (aspirin, isoniazid, neomycin, bicarbonate, sulfonamides) may be withheld until blood sample is drawn.	Resume medications.
Carcinoembryonic antigen (CEA); presence in the blood may indicate GI malignancy, although test is not specific. Also used to monitor response to cancer therapy	No special preparation. Note whether patient smokes; if smokes, normally will have a positive CEA test.	No special care.

Gastric Analysis

	Patient Preparation	Aftercare
Basal secretion test measures HCl and pepsin secreted in the stomach	NPO for 12 hr. Tell patient an NG tube will be inserted and the stomach contents aspirated and discarded. At 15-min intervals for 1 hr, contents are aspirated again. Collect specimens separately.	Remove tube. Resume meals and medications. Offer comfort measures.
Gastric acid stimulation test; secretions increase with ulcers and decrease with gastric cancer	Same as basal secretion test. Then, a drug will be given to stimulate secretions and additional specimens aspirated at 15-min intervals for another 1-2 hr.	Same as basal secretions test.

Stool Analysis

	Patient Preparation	Aftercare
Stool occult blood detects GI bleeding when blood is not readily seen	Advise patient of need for specimen. See text guidelines for collecting specimen. Instruct patient of need for specimen. If test done at home, explain procedure.	No special care.
Stool ova and parasites detects parasitic infections	Same as stool occult blood.	No special care.
Fecal fat; increased fat in stools occurs with Crohn's disease, malabsorption, and pancreatic disease	Instruct patient in a 60-gm fat diet to be followed for 3-6 days, followed by collection of a stool specimen. No laxatives, enemas, or suppositories may be used for 3 days before the test. See text guidelines for specimen collection.	Resume normal diet.

NPO, Nothing by mouth; HCl, hydrochloric acid; NG, nasogastric.

orally or by enema. Sometimes air is introduced into the bowel for radiographic studies. This is called an *air contrast procedure*. When radiographs are taken, the contrast medium outlines the hollow organs of the digestive tract (Fig. 38-3).

Most hospitals and clinics have a specific protocol to follow before the examination to be sure the GI tract is cleansed. If the patient is not properly prepared for the procedure, it may have to be repeated. Fluid restriction and bowel cleansing can be difficult for older or debilitated patients. If they become exhausted or if their vital signs change, the preparation should be stopped and the physician notified. After the procedure, it is vital that the barium be cleared from the GI tract. Figure 38-4 illustrates the time required for food or other substances to move through the digestive tract.

ENDOSCOPIC EXAMINATION

Traditional endoscopic examinations permit direct inspection of hollow, interior organs through a lighted tube called an *endoscope*. Endoscopes may be rigid tubes or flexible fiberscopes. Endoscopic examinations of the upper gastrointestinal tract include esophagoscopy, gastroscopy, gastroduodenoscopy, esophagogastroduodenoscopy, and endoscopic retrograde cholangiography. Endoscopic examinations of the lower digestive tract include colonoscopy, proctoscopy, and sigmoidoscopy. The names of these examinations sound complicated but can easily be broken down to determine what structures are being studied. Box 38-2 lists prefixes for parts of the digestive system that can be combined with the suffix *-scopy*, meaning *to examine*.

FIGURE **38-3** Contrast medium outlines the hollow organs of the digestive tract.

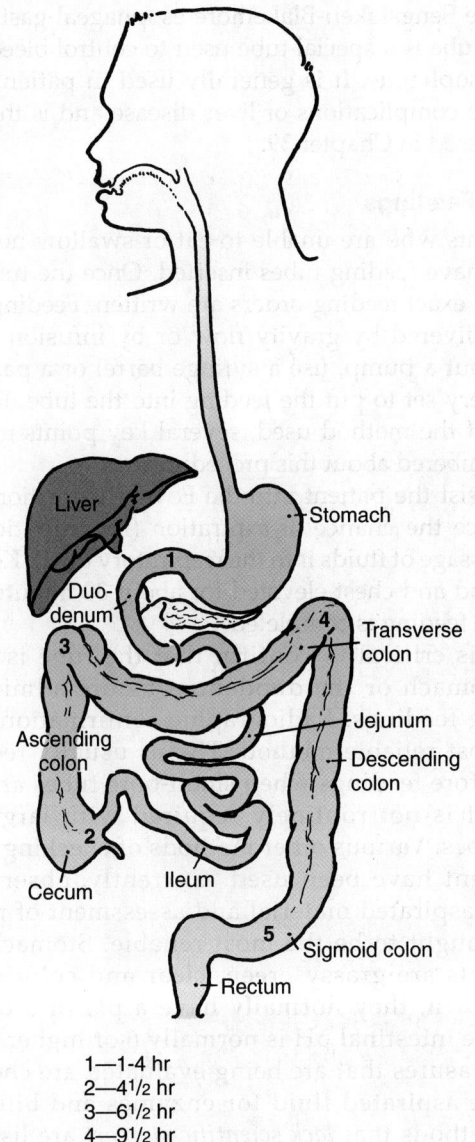

Liver

Stomach

1

Duo-
denum

4

Transverse
colon

3

Jejunum

Ascending
colon

Descending
colon

2

Ileum

Cecum

5

Sigmoid colon

Rectum

1—1-4 hr
2—4½ hr
3—6½ hr
4—9½ hr
5—12-24 hr

FIGURE **38-4** Time required for the passage of substances through the digestive tract.

Box 38-2 | *Terminology for Diagnostic Studies of the Digestive Tract*

ROOT	REFERS TO
Esophag-	Esophagus
Gastro-	Stomach
Duoden-	Duodenum
Sigmoid-	Sigmoid colon
Proct-	Rectum
Cholangi-	Gallbladder
Pancreat-	Pancreas

How to interpret new terms:
scopy = "to examine"
Proctoscopy = *Proct + scopy*
Proctoscopy = to examine the rectum
Esophagogastroduodenoscopy = *esophag + gastr + duoden + scopy*
Esophagogastroduodenoscopy = to examine the esophagus, stomach, and duodenum

the capsule. Bowel preparation may or may not be required depending on institutional practice. A variation on the endoscopic capsule is designed specifically to study the esophagus. With this device, leads are attached to the patient's chest and transmit images to a recorder. For the esophageal study, the patient swallows the pill while lying flat and then is gradually raised to a sitting position.

LABORATORY STUDIES

The most common laboratory studies are performed on gastric secretions and stool specimens.

Gastric Analysis

Gastric analysis is performed to determine the hydrochloric acid content of the gastric fluid. A nasogastric tube is inserted, and gastric secretions are withdrawn every 15 minutes for 1 hour. This enables measurement of basal gastric secretions. If a gastric acid stimulation test is ordered as well, a drug that stimulates acid secretion (e.g., pentagastrin [Peptavlon]) is administered to the patient. Once again, specimens are collected at 15-minute intervals, labeled, and sent for analysis.

Tubeless gastric analysis detects the presence of gastric hydrochloric acid. A gastric stimulant is given, followed an hour later by a resin dye. The dye is given orally. It reacts with gastric hydrochloric acid to release the dye, which is excreted in the urine. If hydrochloric acid is present in the stomach, the dye appears in the urine 2 hours later.

Occult Blood Test

One test that is done often on the nursing unit detects occult blood in body fluids. Occult blood is blood that is not visible with the naked eye. Specimens most often tested for occult blood are vomitus, gastric secretions, and stool. To test for occult blood, a small sample of the body fluid or stool is placed on a special type of paper

Before endoscopic examinations, signed consent may be required. Patients are usually not permitted food or fluids for 6 to 8 hours before the examination. Bowel cleansing may be very thorough or may require just enemas. A sedative may be ordered before the procedure to reduce anxiety. The most serious complication of endoscopy is perforation, or puncture, of the digestive tract.

The newest innovation in endoscopy employs a disposable video camera capsule that is about the size of a large vitamin tablet. The patient swallows the capsule. Leads are applied to the abdomen and connected to a recording device worn on a belt. Images are transmitted as it moves through the digestive tract. The patient can go about usual activities while the capsule is in transit. It is especially usefully for visualizing the small intestine, which is not accessible with traditional endoscopy. Patients fast overnight before swallowing that is then treated with a chemical. If blood is present, specific color changes are observed on the paper.

Stool Examination

Stool specimens are examined most often for blood, bile, pathogenic organisms, and parasite ova (eggs). Fecal fat and the white blood cell count may be determined in certain circumstances. Several important points must be remembered when stool examinations are ordered:

1. Collect the specimen in a clean, dry container. Urine should not be in the container because it destroys parasites. Bathroom tissue should not be discarded in the container because the paper contains bismuth, which interferes with some tests.
2. It is best to deliver stool specimens to the laboratory immediately. If temporary storage is necessary, specimens for ova and parasites must be kept warm. Specimens for pathogens should be refrigerated.
3. When a stool specimen is being tested for occult blood, the patient should not eat red meat for 2 to 3 days before the specimen is collected. Red meat interferes with the test results.
4. Examples of drugs that may interfere with results are salicylates, ascorbic acid, anticoagulants, and steroids.
5. If visible blood or mucus is present in the stool, include it in the specimen sent to the laboratory.

COMMON THERAPEUTIC MEASURES

GASTROINTESTINAL INTUBATION

Tubes are inserted most often into the stomach or intestines to deliver feedings or to keep the digestive tract empty (decompression). Tubes that are passed through the nose are called *nasogastric, nasoduodenal,* or *nasoenteric* tubes, depending on whether the end is located in the stomach or the small intestine.

There are a variety of tubes for special purposes (Fig. 38-5). Levin and gastric sump tubes are nasogastric tubes and may be used for feedings or decompression (Fig. 38-6). Gastrostomy tubes, used for feedings, are placed in the stomach through an opening (stoma) in the abdominal wall. Smaller nasoduodenal tubes, such as the Dobbhoff feeding tube, are weighted so that they pass through the stomach into the duodenum.

Nasoenteric tubes used for decompression of the small intestine include the Miller-Abbott, Cantor, and Harris tubes. Care of the patient with tubes for feeding or decompression is discussed separately.

The Sengstaken-Blakemore esophageal-gastric balloon tube is a special tube used to control bleeding in the esophagus. It is generally used in patients with severe complications of liver disease and is therefore discussed in Chapter 39.

Tube Feedings

Patients who are unable to eat or swallow normally may have feeding tubes inserted. Once the tube is in place, exact feeding orders are written. Feedings may be delivered by gravity flow or by infusion pump. Without a pump, use a syringe barrel or a packaged delivery set to put the feeding into the tube. Regardless of the method used, several key points must be remembered about this procedure:

1. Assist the patient into the Fowler's position to reduce the chance of aspiration (regurgitation and passage of fluids into the respiratory tract). Keep the head and chest elevated for about 30 minutes after the feeding is completed.
2. It is critical to confirm that the tube is in the stomach or the duodenum before administering feedings. Radiographic confirmation is the most reliable method. This is usually required before feedings when small-bore tubes are used but is not routinely required with large-bore tubes. Various other methods of checking placement have been used. Currently, observation of aspirated material and assessment of pH are thought to be the most reliable. Stomach contents are grassy green, clear and colorless, or brown; they normally have a pH of 5 or less. The intestinal pH is normally 6 or higher. Other measures that are being evaluated are checking the aspirated fluid for enzymes and bilirubin. Methods that *lack scientific support* are listening over the stomach area with a stethoscope while injecting air through the tube, placing the end of the tube in water to see if bubbles appear, testing the patient's ability to speak, and observing for respiratory symptoms. When a patient has continuous feedings, placement is usually checked at least once each shift.
3. Residual is monitored to help prevent overfilling of the stomach. Check for residual (formula remaining in the stomach from the previous feeding) before each feeding or according to agency procedure. Use a syringe to withdraw and measure the formula. Agency policies dictate what action should be taken based on the amount of residual formula. The physician may need to be notified. The amount of the residual may be subtracted from the next feeding, or feedings may be discontinued for a specified period of time. The residual formula

FIGURE 38-5 Examples of tubes used in the digestive tract.

Lavacuator tube
An orogastric tube with a large suction lumen and a smaller lavage/vent lumen that provides continuous suction because irrigating solution enters the lavage lumen while stomach contents are removed through the suction lumen. Used to remove toxic substances from the stomach.

Cantor tube
A single-lumen long tube with a small inflatable bag at the distal end. About 5 to 10 mL of mercury is injected with a needle (gauge 21 or smaller or balloon may leak) and syringe into the bag before insertion of the tube.

Levin tube
A plastic or rubber single-lumen tube with a solid tip that may be inserted into the stomach via the nose or mouth. Used to drain fluid and gas from the stomach. Single lumen must be used for irrigation and drainage, so continuous irrigation is not possible.

Sengstaken-Blakemore tube
A three-lumen tube. Two ports inflate an esophageal and a gastric balloon for tamponade, and the third is used for nasogastric suction. This tube does not provide esophageal suction, but a nasogastric tube may be inserted in the opposite naris or the mouth and allowed to rest on top of the esophageal balloon. Esophageal suction is then possible, reducing the risk of aspiration.

Salem sump tube
A short double-lumen tube. The small vent tube within the large suction tube prevents mucosal suction damage by maintaining the pressure in open eyes at the distal end of the tube at less than 25 mm Hg.

Weighted flexible feeding tube with stylet
Access port with irrigation adapter allows maintenance of the tube without disconnecting the feeding set.

should be returned through the tube to prevent loss of electrolytes.

4. Obtain the correct formula. In the hospital setting, feedings are commercially prepared. There are many varieties of formulas. Be sure to give the right formula, in the right amount, at the right dilution, on the right schedule, to the right patient.

5. When tube feedings are first started, they often are diluted to one-half or one-fourth strength. If the patient tolerates the formula well, the concentration is gradually increased.

6. Stop the feeding and notify the physician if the patient has nausea or pain.

7. Rinse the tube by flushing it with at least 30 mL of water after each bolus feeding. Extra water may be ordered.

8. If diarrhea occurs, contact the physician regarding decreasing the concentration or the rate of delivery, or both, of the formula.

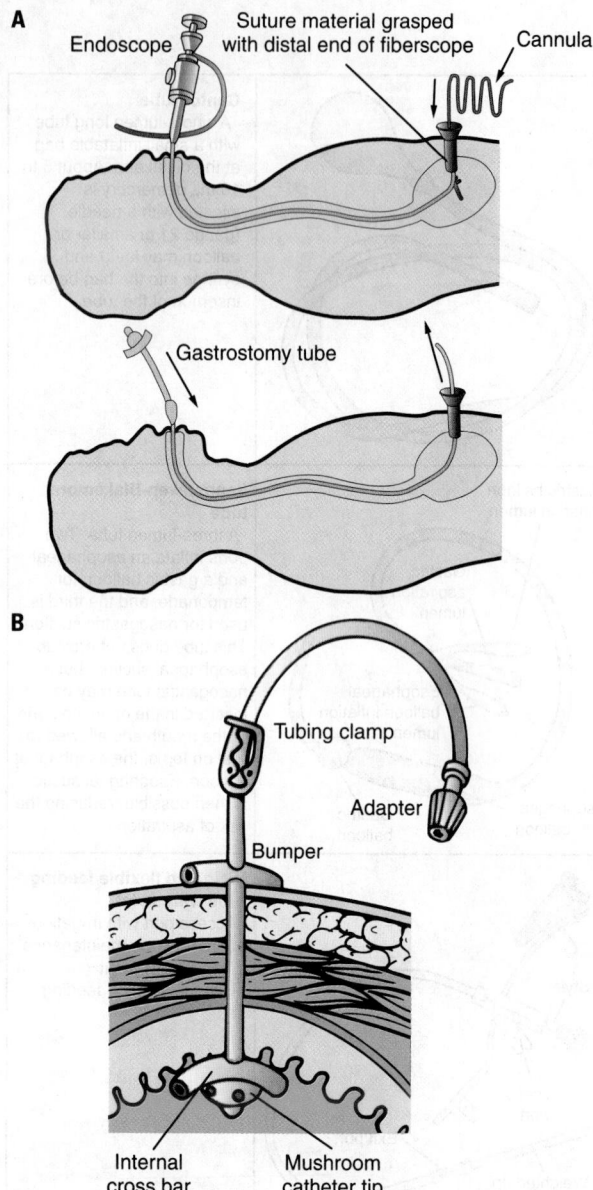

FIGURE **38-6** Percutaneous endoscopic gastrostomy (PEG). **A,** Placement of PEG tube. Using endoscopy, a gastrostomy tube is inserted through the esophagus into the stomach. A cannula is inserted through the abdominal wall into the stomach. The fiberscope grasps the cannula, and the cannula and tube are pulled out through the abdominal wall. **B,** A retention disk and bumper keep the tube in place.

9. Dumping syndrome may occur with rapid feedings of concentrated formula. Signs and symptoms are cold sweat, abdominal distention, dizziness, weakness, rapid pulse rate, nausea, and diarrhea.

10. If using a syringe to give the feeding, do the following:
    - Remove the plunger from the barrel of the syringe.
    - Attach the barrel to the feeding tube.
    - Pinch or kink the tube while the syringe barrel is filled with formula to reduce the amount of air being forced into the stomach.

- Hold the barrel about 12 inches above the level of the stomach, and allow the fluid to flow by gravity.
- Flush tubing with water per agency protocol.

11. If an infusion pump is used to deliver the feeding, fill the tubing with formula before connecting it to the feeding tube to reduce the amount of air forced into the digestive tract. Continuous feedings are usually given at a rate of 80 to 150 mL per hour. No more than 6 hours' worth of formula should be hung because it can become contaminated. Bolus feedings are given at specified intervals. They usually consist of 200 to 300 mL over 30 to 45 minutes for each feeding. Oral drugs can usually be given through a nasogastric tube, but some drugs should not be crushed. Consult a drug reference. The tubing and bag must be changed every 24 hours.

Gastrointestinal Decompression

Gastrointestinal decompression is used for the relief or prevention of distention. A tube is passed through a nostril and into the stomach or intestines (or both) and attached to suction. The suction removes fluid and gases that accumulate when gastrointestinal motility is impaired. Conditions that slow motility include peritonitis, obstruction, and any type of surgery performed while the patient is under general anesthesia. Handling of the bowel in abdominal surgery often causes a temporary loss of peristalsis. Decompression may be ordered until bowel activity returns, usually in 3 to 5 days.

Several types of tubes are used for gastrointestinal decompression. As mentioned earlier, the Levin and gastric sump tubes can be used for gastric decompression (often called *GI suction*). Miller-Abbott, Cantor, and Harris tubes are weighted and are used for intestinal decompression (Fig. 38-7). The patient may return from surgery with the tube in place, or it can be inserted on the nursing unit. The following are key points to remember when caring for the patient with gastrointestinal suction:

1. Attach the tube to a suction apparatus as ordered. Generally, low, intermittent suction pressure is used with single-lumen tubes; low, continuous suction is used with double-lumen tubes.

2. Monitor the patency of the tube. Observe for the movement of fluids through the tubing into the suction container. If the tube does not seem to be draining, change the patient's position. Gently rotate the tube or pull it out very slightly. (*Exception:* Do not reposition tubes after gastric surgery.) Notify the physician if drainage does not resume.

3. Irrigations should not be done routinely, but they may be ordered occasionally as needed. Frequent irrigations cause acid-base disturbances. For adults, irrigations are usually done with 20 to 30 mL of normal saline. Check the physician's order or the agency procedure manual.

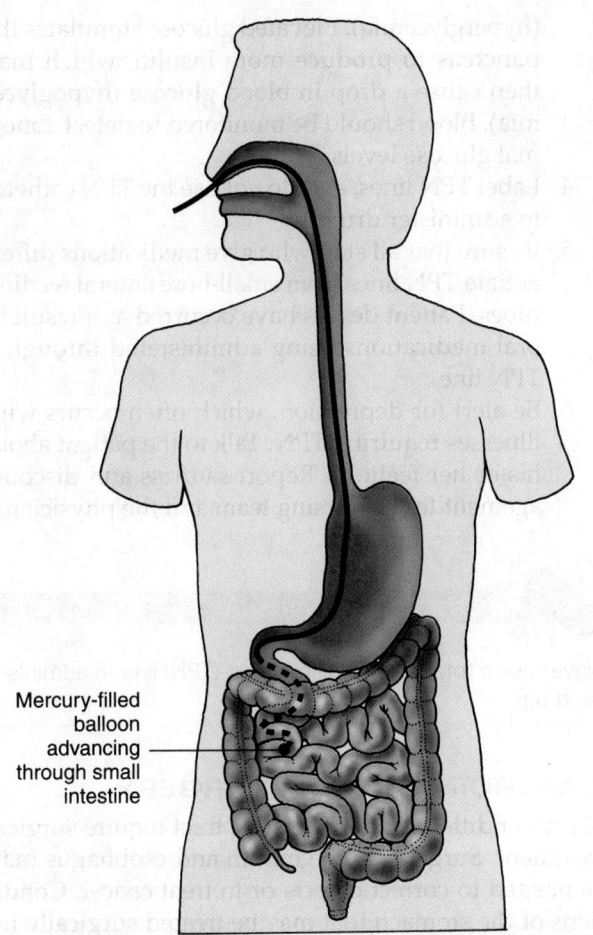

FIGURE **38-7** A nasointestinal tube has a mercury-filled balloon that stimulates peristalsis and advances the tube through the intestines.

Mercury-filled
balloon
advancing
through small
intestine

FIGURE **38-8** This method of taping a nasogastric tube anchors it securely while avoiding trauma to the nose.

4. Monitor the suction output. Record the amount, color, and characteristics every shift. When blood is present, the drainage may be bright red, dark red, brown, or black. Dark brown or green fluid suggests that an obstruction is below the point where bile enters the digestive tract.

5. Monitor the patient for successful decompression. If distention is not being effectively relieved, the patient may have nausea and vomiting, shortness of breath, a feeling of fullness, and enlargement of the abdomen.

6. Assess for the return of peristalsis, indicated by the presence of bowel sounds and passage of **flatus** (gas) through the rectum.

7. Provide comfort measures. The nasopharynx and throat are often very tender. Because the patient is allowed nothing by mouth, mouth dryness is another source of discomfort. Handle the tubing gently. Cleanse the nostrils and apply a water-soluble lubricant to reduce drying and irritation. Provide mouth care frequently. Moisturize the lips. Offer oral spray or lozenges as ordered to provide temporary relief of sore throat.

8. Once the tube is in place, tape it to keep it from being pulled out unless it is the type of tube in-

tended to move through the digestive tract. Tape should secure the tube to the upper lip and cheek or nose (Fig. 38-8). Do not tape the tubing to the forehead because this puts excessive pressure on the nasal tissues. During activity, move the tube carefully to avoid trauma to the nasopharynx. Wrapping the tube with a piece of tape that is pinned to the patient's gown may prevent accidental traction on the tube.

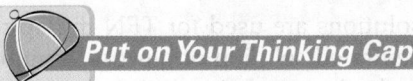

Put on Your Thinking Cap!

What type of acid-base imbalance could result from frequent irrigations of nasogastric tubes? Explain why.

TOTAL PARENTERAL NUTRITION

Sometimes the digestive tract cannot be used for feedings. Total parenteral nutrition (TPN) bypasses the digestive tract by delivering nutrients directly to the bloodstream. A catheter inserted into a large vein such as the subclavian is used for the feedings (Fig. 38-9). The feeding passes directly into the superior vena cava and the right atrium. This placement allows for rapid dilution of the concentrated feeding. If the solution were given in a smaller vein, it would cause thrombophlebitis (inflammation of the vein).

When the catheter is inserted, it is sutured to the skin and the insertion site is covered with a sterile dressing. A radiograph is ordered to check placement before the catheter is used for feedings.

Regular intravenous feedings can provide only water, glucose, electrolytes, minerals, and vitamins. This

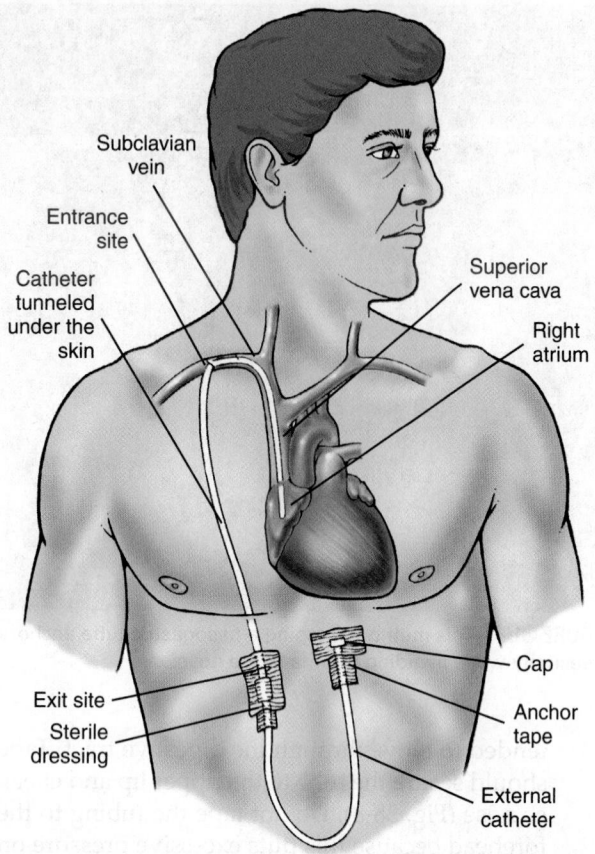

FIGURE 38-9 A catheter inserted into the right subclavian vein for total parenteral nutrition. A transparent waterproof dressing allows vapor to escape while maintaining sterility.

is adequate for short-term problems but does not provide all the nutrients necessary to maintain health or promote healing.

Two types of solutions are used for TPN therapy. The first is a concentrated solution of glucose, amino acids, vitamins, and minerals. It is administered using a special filter. A lipid solution also can be given through a peripheral vein. The lipids are not mixed with the TPN solution.

Important points to remember when caring for the patient receiving TPN include the following:

1. Take great care to prevent infection at the insertion site. Always use sterile technique for site care. The exact procedure should be ordered or written in the agency procedure manual. With each dressing change, inspect the site for signs of infection (redness, swelling, foul odor, or purulent drainage). Monitor the patient's temperature for an elevation.

2. Monitor the flow rate. If the solution is given too rapidly, the patient may have circulatory overload, changes in blood glucose, or excessive diuresis (urine output). If the feeding falls behind schedule, do not speed up the rate to catch up.

3. Monitor the patient for signs and symptoms of blood glucose changes. The concentrated glucose solution can raise the blood glucose excessively

(hyperglycemia). Elevated glucose stimulates the pancreas to produce more insulin, which may then cause a drop in blood glucose (hypoglycemia). Blood should be monitored to detect abnormal glucose levels.

4. Label TPN lines, and do not use the TPN catheter to administer drugs.

5. Be sure that all staff who give medications differentiate TPN lines from small-bore enteral feeding tubes. Patient deaths have occurred as a result of oral medications being administered through a TPN line.

6. Be alert for depression, which often occurs with illnesses requiring TPN. Talk to the patient about his or her feelings. Report sadness and discouragement to the nursing team and the physician.

Pharmacology Capsule

Never use a total parenteral nutrition (TPN) line to administer drugs.

GASTROINTESTINAL SURGERY

Many conditions of the digestive tract require surgical treatment. Surgery on the mouth and esophagus may be needed to correct defects or to treat cancer. Conditions of the stomach that may be treated surgically include bleeding ulcers, hiatal hernia, and cancer. Less commonly, surgery is done to decrease the capacity of the stomach for the treatment of extreme obesity. Conditions of the large intestine that may require surgery include cancer, diverticulosis, appendicitis, polyps, obstruction, and ulcerative colitis. General care of the surgical patient is covered in Chapter 17.

PREOPERATIVE NURSING CARE *of the Patient Having Gastrointestinal Surgery*

Radiographic examinations of the digestive tract often are done before surgery. These may be done on an outpatient basis or after admission to the hospital.

The digestive tract is usually cleansed before gastrointestinal surgery. The extent of the cleansing depends on the exact site of the surgery. Oral preparations such as magnesium citrate or large-volume cathartic (laxative) solutions may be prescribed. Use of enemas until the returning fluid is clear also may be ordered. This process is tiring and may exhaust the very ill or older patient. The nurse should offer assistance with toileting and hygiene. Changes in vital signs (abnormal heart rate or rhythm, hypotension) or mental state during the bowel cleansing process should be reported to the physician.

Diet is usually limited to liquids for 24 hours before the surgery. The patient should have nothing to eat or drink for a specified period before surgery. Intravenous fluids may be ordered, especially if gastrointestinal suction is being used. Oral antibiotics may be given to reduce the bacterial flora in the bowel, thereby decreasing the risk of contamination of the peritoneal cavity during surgery.

General anesthesia and abdominal surgery cause a temporary loss of peristalsis. Therefore, before or during surgery, a nasogastric tube may be inserted and attached to suction. This prevents the accumulation of fluid and gas in the digestive tract until peristalsis returns.

POSTOPERATIVE NURSING CARE
of the Patient Who Has Had Gastrointestinal Surgery

Usual postoperative care, discussed in Chapter 17, includes measures to relieve pain, detect complications (hemorrhage, infection), and prevent adverse effects of immobility, anesthesia, and drug therapy. Immediately after surgery on the digestive tract, be especially concerned with preventing gastric or abdominal distention, replacing lost fluids, and maintaining urine elimination. The patient usually has a nasogastric tube in place for decompression. The continuous removal of fluids and gas decreases the stimulation of the digestive tract and reduces pressure on the internal incisions. Monitor gastrointestinal suction to be sure it is functioning. Inspect, describe, and measure the drainage. Assess the abdomen for distention and bowel sounds. Follow the physician's orders regarding irrigation. After gastric surgery, do *not* irrigate or reposition the tube because of the possibility of traumatizing healing tissue. Inform the physician if the tube is not draining properly or if the abdomen becomes distended.

Intravenous fluids are given until gastrointestinal suction is discontinued and oral intake is adequate. Keep strict intake and output records. The patient is at risk for fluid and electrolyte imbalances when gastrointestinal suction is used. Because patients often have difficulty voiding after abdominal surgery, an indwelling catheter is usually inserted during the procedure. If there is no catheter, nursing measures may be needed to promote voiding. These measures are discussed in Chapter 40.

DRUG THERAPY

Drugs that are commonly used for their effects on the digestive tract include emetics, antiemetics, laxatives, cathartics, antidiarrheals, antacids, anticholinergics, mucosal barriers, histamine-2 (H_2)-receptor blockers, prostaglandins, and antibiotics. These drugs are discussed with the conditions for which they are prescribed. In addition, the Drug Therapy table on pp. 746 to 749 summarizes these drugs, their actions, and nursing interventions.

DISORDERS OF THE DIGESTIVE TRACT

DISORDERS AFFECTING INGESTION

Anything that interferes with the ability to eat a balanced diet can cause nutritional deficiencies. Problems can be as basic as anorexia, inability to feed oneself, or dysphagia, or they may occur secondary to other problems such as oral infection and inflammation, dental problems, oral cancer, and parotitis.

Anorexia

The intake of food depends largely on having an appetite. Lack of appetite is called anorexia.

Causes

Anorexia can occur with many physical and emotional disturbances. Nausea, a decreased sense of taste or smell, mouth disorders, and medications are some physical factors that may decrease one's appetite. Emotional problems such as anxiety, depression, or disturbing thoughts also may cause anorexia. The environment can influence appetite as well. Unpleasant odors or sights can quickly dampen a patient's enthusiasm for a meal. Therapeutic diets such as pureed, low-salt, and low-fat diets are unappetizing to some people. Older people often report decreased appetite. This may be attributed to diminished senses of taste and smell, drug effects, decreased activity, and social isolation.

Medical Diagnosis

The physician assesses the patient for evidence of malnutrition. Weight may be monitored over several weeks. A complete history and physical examination are done to detect underlying problems and the effects of inadequate intake. Initial diagnostic tests that are likely to be ordered include measurements of serum hemoglobin, iron, total iron-binding capacity, transferrin, calcium, folate, B_{12}, and zinc. Tests of thyroid function may be ordered to detect metabolic disorders, and skin tests may be ordered to evaluate allergic responses. A stool specimen may be tested for occult blood. If indicated, the physician may perform additional procedures to detect possible cancers of the digestive system, lungs, and breasts.

Medical Treatment

Correctable causes of anorexia are treated, but sometimes no physical cause is found. Nutritional supplements may be ordered. The oral route is preferred, but, in extreme cases, enteral feedings or TPN may be indicated.

NURSING CARE of the Patient with Anorexia
Assessment

The general assessment of the patient with digestive disturbances is summarized in Box 38-1. In assessing the patient with anorexia, explore factors that may be affecting appetite. Record chronic and recent illnesses, hospitalizations, medications, and allergies. Obtain the female patient's obstetric history as well. The review of systems may provide clues to anorexia. Significant symptoms include pain, nausea, dyspnea, and extreme fatigue. The functional assessment reveals patterns of

Text continued on p. 750.

DRUG THERAPY · Disorders of the Digestive Tract

DRUG	USE/ACTION	SIDE EFFECTS	NURSING INTERVENTIONS
ANTACIDS Magnesium hydroxide Aluminum hydroxide Calcium carbonate Sodium bicarbonate	Reduce pain of peptic ulcers by neutralizing acid in stomach, decreasing irritation of stomach lining, and inhibiting production of pepsin.	Calcium and aluminum salts tend to cause constipation. Magnesium salts tend to cause diarrhea. Combinations may be used to neutralize these effects.	Teach patients that antacids are nonprescription drugs but that they still have side effects, interact with other drugs, and can be abused. Shake liquids before pouring. Follow dose with water or milk to deliver antacid to stomach. Antacids interfere with absorption of oral drugs if given within 1-2 hr of each other. Tablets should be chewed before swallowing.
H_2 RECEPTOR ANTAGONISTS Cimetidine (Tagamet) Ranitidine (Zantac) Famotidine (Pepcid) Nizatidine (Axid)	Reduce secretion of gastric acid and promote healing of ulcers.	Diarrhea, muscle pain, rash, confusion, drowsiness. Cimetidine can cause impotence and gynecomastia and impairs metabolism of many common drugs. Other drugs have fewer side effects; do not cause impotence or gynecomastia.	Give with or after meals. Do not give ranitidine at same time as antacids.
PROTON PUMP INHIBITORS Omeprazole (Prilosec) Esomeprazole (Nexium) Lansoprazole (Prevacid) Pantoprazole (Protonix) Rabeprazole (Aciphex)	Inhibit gastric acid secretion. Uses: peptic ulcer disease, GERD, Zollinger-Ellison syndrome.	Nausea, diarrhea, headache.	Advise patient to swallow capsule whole. For patients who cannot swallow capsules, Prevacid capsules can be opened and the contents mixed in applesauce. A liquid preparation also is available.
MUCOSAL BARRIER Sucralfate (Carafate)	Interacts with acid to form protective gel that coats ulcer surface to permit healing.	Constipation, dry mouth, drowsiness, rash, itching.	Give on empty stomach: 1 hr before meals and at bedtime. Do not give within 30 min of antacids. Interferes with absorption of some other drugs.
SYNTHETIC PROSTAGLANDINS Misoprostol (Cytotec)	Decreases gastric acid secretion and protects gastric mucosa. Often used to prevent gastric ulcers caused by NSAIDs.	Contraindicated during pregnancy. Side effects: diarrhea, abdominal pain, miscarriage, headache, flatulence, nausea/vomiting.	Usually given with meals and at bedtime.
ANTICHOLINERGICS Atropine Pirenzepine (Gastrozepin)	Block action of acetylcholine. Decrease salivary and gastric secretions. Reduce pain by reducing smooth muscle tone in GI tract.	Dry mouth, constipation, visual disturbance, urine retention. Much milder side effects with pirenzepine than with atropine. Older adults may become confused, agitated, or drowsy.	Contraindicated with narrow-angle glaucoma, renal disease, prostatic hypertrophy, or intestinal obstruction. Best given ½ to 1 hr before meals and at bedtime. Provide oral hygiene. Monitor stools and urine output. Report changes in behavior.

Drug	Action/Use	Side Effects	Nursing Considerations
5-HR RECEPTOR ANTAGONISTS Ondansetron (Zofran) Granisetron (Kytril) Palonosetron (Aloxi)	Prevents nausea and vomiting caused by chemotherapy. Aloxi has a very long half-life (40 hours) so a single dose usually controls initial and delayed chemotherapy side effects.	Usually tolerated well. Most common side effects: headache, constipation, diarrhea, abdominal pain, musculoskeletal pain, shivering, fever, hypoxia, urinary retention.	After diluting according to directions, given IV 30 minutes before chemotherapy dose as ordered. Advise patient that drowsiness may occur.
LAXATIVES **Stimulants** Bisacodyl (Dulcolax) Senna (Senokot) *Cascara sagrada* Castor oil	Facilitate bowel elimination. Stimulate GI tract by irritating mucosa. Tend to produce diarrhea-like stool. Castor oil too harsh for routine use.	Bisacodyl suppositories can irritate the anus. Cascara and senna can make urine pink or brownish. Castor oil rapidly produces watery stool.	Monitor stools. Encourage adequate fluids and fiber to reduce need for laxatives. Laxatives are intended for temporary, occasional relief of constipation and are contraindicated with undiagnosed abdominal pain and inflammatory conditions of GI tract. Chill castor oil and follow with fruit juice.
Bulk-Forming Laxatives Psyllium (Metamucil) Methylcellulose (Citrucel)	Retain water in stool to increase bulk and fluid, which stimulates peristalsis with passage of formed, soft stool.	One of safest laxatives for long-term therapy and during pregnancy. Obstruction can occur if not taken with adequate fluids or if passage through the intestine is arrested.	Patient must take adequate fluids, or mass can harden. May take up to 3 days before effect evident, so used primarily for prevention of constipation.
Saline (Osmotic) Laxatives Magnesium citrate Magnesium hydroxide (Milk of Magnesia) Sodium phosphate (Fleet Phospho-Soda)	Draw water into bowel to distend and stimulate evacuation. Short-term use only.	Risk of dehydration with prolonged use.	Contraindicated with kidney disease, heart failure, hypertension, and edema.
Lubricants Mineral oil	Lubricate feces for easier passage.	Risk of lipid pneumonia if aspirated.	Impair absorption of fat-soluble drugs and nutrients, so should be given on an empty stomach.
Fecal Wetting Agents Docusate calcium (Surfak) Docusate sodium (Colace)	Soften fecal mass. May take up to 3 days before effects evident, so used primarily for prevention of constipation.		Liquid forms can be given in milk or juice to mask taste.
Suppositories Glycerin Bisacodyl (Dulcolax)	Stimulate evacuation by irritating or distending bowel. Usually act within an hour.		
Other Lactulose (Cephulac)	Increases fecal water content to stimulate evacuation. Promotes passage of ammonia through rectum. Used in hepatic encephalopathy.	Cramps, flatulence, diarrhea, hyperglycemia with diabetes.	Can be mixed with full glass of water, milk, or juice to disguise taste. More effective on empty stomach.

GERD, Gastroesophageal reflux disease; *GI*, gastrointestinal; *NSAIDs*, nonsteroidal anti-inflammatory drugs.

Continued

DRUG THERAPY *Disorders of the Digestive Tract—cont'd*

DRUG	USE/ACTION	SIDE EFFECTS	NURSING INTERVENTIONS
Other—cont'd			
Polyethylene glycol–electrolyte solution (GoLYTELY)	Rapidly causes diarrhea by allowing a large volume of water to be retained in colon. Four liters given over approximately 3 hr; cleans bowel in about 4 hr. Most often used to prepare GI tract for diagnostic procedures or surgery.		Rapid, dramatic effect, so be sure toilet is convenient.
ANTIDIARRHEAL AGENTS			
Opiates			
Morphine	Decrease intestinal motility so that liquid portion of feces is reabsorbed.	CNS depression, drowsiness dizziness, constipation, nausea, dry mouth.	Sometimes given after each stool for acute diarrhea, but do not exceed maximum dosage. Use safety precautions. Oral hygiene.
Diphenoxylate HCl (Lomotil)			
Loperamide HCl (Imodium)			
Adsorbents			
Kaolin	Bind to substances that may cause diarrhea.		Shake suspension before pouring. Do not administer with other oral drugs because adsorbents will interfere with absorption.
Aluminum hydroxide			
Lactobacillus Products	Replace normal bacterial flora of bowel.		May require refrigeration.
ANTIBACTERIAL AGENTS			
Ciprofloxacin (Cipro)	Treat diarrhea caused by pathogens. Cipro: *Escherichia coli, Campylobacter jejuni, Shigella.*	Varies with specific drug.	Advise patient to complete entire course of therapy and to report worsening symptoms.
Erythromycin (E-Mycin)	E-Mycin: *Entamoeba histolytica.*		
Metronidazole (Flagyl)	Flagyl: *Clostridium difficile.*		
EMETICS			
Ipecac syrup	Cause vomiting. Used to treat some types of poisoning and oral drug overdose.	CNS depression (use cautiously with other CNS depressants).	Follow ipecac with water according to age: <1 yr: ≤1 glass. Older children: 1-2 glasses Adults: 3-4 glasses Emetic action inactivated by charcoal. Milk interferes with action of ipecac.
ANTIEMETICS			
Antihistamines	Prevent and treat nausea.	Drowsiness and confusion, especially if given with other CNS depressants.	Use cautiously with asthma, glaucoma, prostatic hypertrophy.
Promethazine HCl (Phenergan)	Decrease sensitivity of vestibular apparatus of inner ear. Suppress vomiting center.		
Dimenhydrinate HCl (Dramamine)			
Sedatives			
Hydroxyzine	Decrease sensitivity of vestibular apparatus and suppress vomiting center. Often used to prevent motion sickness.		

Drug	Action/Use	Side Effects	Nursing Considerations
Anticholinergics Scopolamine (Transderm-Scop)			Transderm-Scop is a medicated adhesive disk that is placed behind ear.
PROKINETIC AGENT Metoclopramide (Reglan)	Speeds up gastric emptying into small intestine.	CNS depression, GI upset, Parkinson-like symptoms.	Contraindications: GI perforation, obstruction, or hemorrhage; epilepsy.
ANTI-INFECTIVES Sulfasalazine (Azulfidine)	Treatment of ulcerative colitis.	Orange-yellow color to urine and skin, photosensitivity.	Contraindication: allergy to aspirin. Adequate fluid intake needed to prevent crystalluria and urinary stone formation. Avoid direct sunlight.
Olsalazine (Dipentum)	Treatment of ulcerative colitis.	Abdominal pain, diarrhea, headache, nausea.	Discontinue if hives, rash, wheezing occur. Encourage fluids.
Amoxicillin (Amoxil)	Combined with omeprazole, prostaglandins, and/or bismuth subsalicylate to treat *Helicobacter pylori*.	Rash, diarrhea, anaphylaxis, superinfections (colitis).	Instruct patient to take full course of treatment.
ANTIFUNGALS Nystatin (Mycostatin)	Effective against *Candida albicans* (yeast) infections.	Nausea, vomiting, diarrhea with nystatin.	Instruct patient to dissolve lozenges in mouth. Shake suspensions well. Swish nystatin in mouth before swallowing.
Clotrimazole (Mycelex)		Nausea, vomiting, itching with clotrimazole.	Vaginal preparations are available.

GI, Gastrointestinal; *CNS*, central nervous system.

activity and rest, usual dietary patterns, current stressors, and coping strategies—all factors that can affect appetite. During the physical examination, be especially alert for signs of malnutrition: glossitis (inflammation of the tongue), cheilosis (cracked lips), edema, jaundice, and muscle wasting. The examination also should assess for inflammation or lesions of the mouth and dental problems. If the patient has dentures, evaluate the fit. It is very important to have the patient remove the dentures before the gums are assessed.

Nursing Diagnosis, Goal, and Outcome Criteria: Anorexia

NURSING DIAGNOSES	GOALS AND OUTCOME CRITERIA
Imbalanced Nutrition: Less Than Body Requirements related to anorexia	Improved appetite and adequate food intake: patient states appetite is better, increased intake of food, and stable or increased body weight

Interventions

It is helpful if you can identify factors that contribute to the patient's anorexia. Depending on the reason for the anorexia, a number of interventions may be successful in improving the patient's appetite. If the patient has a dry mouth or bad taste in the mouth, assist with oral hygiene before and after meals. If the teeth or gums are in poor condition, teach proper oral hygiene and refer the patient for dental care. Poorly fitting dentures need to be relined for a tighter fit or need to be replaced.

When a patient is nauseated, institute measures to relieve the nausea before presenting a meal tray. Nausea and anorexia both can be related to unpleasant stimuli in the environment. Before serving a meal tray, remove bedpans and emesis basins from sight, conceal drains and drainage collection devices, and deodorize the room if necessary.

Many people enjoy meals more when they are in the company of others. Socialization during mealtime can greatly improve a person's appetite. Encourage a family member to visit during meals or accompany the patient to a dining facility so that they can eat together. Some facilities provide guest trays for patients' family members. In long-term care facilities, a central dining room is usually available for those who enjoy company during meals. On nursing units, small groups of patients often enjoy having their meals together in a sunroom or lounge.

Even people with good appetites eat some foods more willingly than others. For the patient with anorexia, it is especially important to respect food likes and dislikes. If the food being served is unappealing, ask the dietitian to discuss the diet with the patient. Sometimes food from home is a special treat. Before food is brought in by family or friends, advise them of any dietary restrictions. Small servings are more acceptable than large ones to the anorexic person. Additional nutrients can be provided by between-meals snacks. In the inpatient setting, the nurse has little control over the specific food served, but in the home, the meal preparer can be encouraged to provide foods that vary in color, texture, and taste.

Position the patient comfortably and with easy access to the food. If the patient cannot cut food or open packages, be sure to do this. Do not schedule tiring activities immediately before mealtime.

Fortunately, anorexia is a temporary problem for most people. For others, however, it is a chronic problem. Teach the patient the importance of adequate nutritional intake. When they understand how nutrition is related to their health goals, most patients will make an effort to eat. If the patient seems to be anxious or depressed, ask about concerns that he or she may have. Consult the physician about possible counseling if emotional distress persists.

 What Does Culture Have to Do with Anorexia?

Food preferences, including seasoning and methods of preparation, have a strong cultural basis. When a patient is not accustomed to traditional American food, inquire about whether more familiar foods can be provided or brought in by the family.

Feeding Problems

Patients may require assistance with meals because of temporary impairments or long-term disabilities. Patients with paralysis, arthritis, neuromuscular disorders, confusion, weakness, or visual impairment are likely to need assistance. Thorough assessments and individualized interventions are needed to ensure adequate nutrition despite disability.

Medical Diagnosis and Treatment

The medical diagnosis is directed at identifying the basic problems and prescribing treatment as appropriate. Patients often are referred to physical therapy and occupational therapy to help them regain basic self-care skills.

NURSING CARE *of the Patient with Feeding Problems*

Assessment

Assess each patient's ability to feed himself or herself independently. Determine the nature of the patient's difficulty and identify remaining abilities. Some patients are temporarily impaired because they are immobilized or confined to restricted positions as part of their medical treatment. Important aspects of the physical examination are visual acuity, range of motion and muscle strength in both arms, and range of motion and grip strength in both hands. Evaluate the patient's ability to follow instructions as well.

Nursing Diagnoses, Goals, and Outcome Criteria: Feeding Problems

NURSING DIAGNOSES	GOALS AND OUTCOME CRITERIA
Self-Care Deficit, Feeding related to paralysis, weakness, poor coordination, confusion, visual impairment	Improved self-feeding: patient participates in feeding within his or her capabilities
Imbalanced Nutrition: Less Than Body Requirements related to inability to feed self	Adequate food intake: stable body weight or attainment of ideal body weight

Interventions

Encourage patients to be as independent in feeding as possible. For some, proper positioning and arrangement of the meal tray are all that is needed. Assistive devices designed for paralyzed and arthritic patients are available. These can be obtained through the physical therapy or occupational therapy department. Simple adaptations such as padding the handles of utensils may enable the patient with limited grasping ability to feed himself or herself.

When patients need only partial assistance, open milk cartons, cut meat, butter bread, and season food. Sometimes the patient can hold finger foods while you provide food that requires utensils. Before seasoning food or sweetening drinks, ask about patient preferences. Most people feel very strongly about these preferences. Confused patients often can feed themselves if the task is made simple. They may require occasional reminders to continue eating. Sometimes a group dining situation works well for these patients because they may imitate the behavior of others who are eating.

The term *feeder* is sometimes used to refer to patients who must be fed. This label is demeaning and threatens the patient's self-esteem. The patient should be addressed as an adult. Engage the patient in pleasant conversation while he or she is being fed. Remember the following points when feeding a patient:

1. Check the diet and patient's name for accuracy.
2. Seat the patient upright, with the head tilted slightly forward.
3. Tuck a napkin or towel at the patient's chin to catch spills.
4. If the patient is able to communicate, ask in what order the food should be offered. The practice of mixing all food together to make sure the patient gets a little of everything is unappetizing and not recommended.
5. Some patients do not open their mouths voluntarily. Touch the lips with the spoon or gently press just below the lower lip with a finger to encourage them to do so.
6. Pacing is important, so observe that the patient has swallowed before offering more food.
7. In stroke patients, food may accumulate in the affected side of the mouth. Check the mouth at intervals for accumulated food.
8. Offer fluids periodically.

At the completion of the meal, provide mouth care and record the amount of food taken.

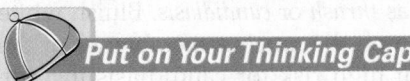 **Put on Your Thinking Cap!**

Practice feeding a classmate a simple meal. Then reverse roles and permit the classmate to feed you. Assume the person being fed is unable to speak clearly but understands what is said. Immediately afterward write down (1) the steps you went through when feeding another person; (2) how you felt while being fed; and (3) what you learned from the experience that you could apply in patient care.

Oral Inflammation and Infections

Stomatitis

Stomatitis is a general term for inflammation of the oral mucosa. It may result from the mechanical trauma of poorly fitting dentures, the irritation of excessive tobacco or alcohol use, poor oral hygiene, inadequate nutrition, pathogenic organisms, radiation therapy, or drug therapy. Disorders of the kidney, liver, or blood also can cause stomatitis. Emotional tension and excessive fatigue seem to make people more susceptible to some types of stomatitis. Medical treatment is directed toward determining the cause and eliminating it. If specific pathogenic organisms are identified, appropriate antibiotics (usually topical) or antiviral agents may be prescribed. A soft, bland diet may be ordered.

Vincent's Infection

Vincent's infection is caused by bacteria. It has been called *trench mouth* because it often developed among soldiers in the field in World War I. It is a bacterial infection that causes a metallic taste and bleeding ulcers in the mouth, foul breath, and increased salivation. The patient also may have signs of a general infection, such as fever, enlarged lymph nodes, and anorexia. Topical antibiotics and mouthwashes are used to treat the infection. Rest, a nutritious diet, and good oral hygiene are helpful.

Herpes Simplex

Herpes simplex is caused by the herpes simplex virus, type 1. Ulcers and vesicles develop in the mouth and on the lips. People commonly refer to these lesions as *cold sores* or *fever blisters*. They tend to occur in people who have upper respiratory tract infections, have had excessive sun exposure, or are under stress. Spirits of camphor, topical steroids, and antiviral agents may be prescribed as treatment.

Aphthous Stomatitis

Aphthous stomatitis ("canker sore") may be caused by a virus. It is characterized by ulcers of the lips and mouth that recur at intervals. Topical or systemic steroids may be used to treat this chronic condition.

Candida Albicans

Candida albicans, a yeast-like fungus, causes the oral condition known as *thrush* or *candidiasis.* Bluish white lesions can be seen on the mucous membranes of the mouth. Patients at high risk for candidiasis include those on steroid or long-term antibiotic therapy. Oral medications are usually prescribed to treat candidiasis. Chronic candidiasis may be treated with topical antifungal agents. Vaginal nystatin tablets can be used like lozenges and allowed to dissolve in the mouth.

NURSING CARE of the Patient with Oral Inflammation or Infection

Patients with only oral inflammation or infections are usually treated as outpatients, so the nurse's role is limited to reinforcing medical instructions. These conditions, however, may develop in patients who are hospitalized for other reasons. The nurse then has a more active role in treating the condition and teaching patients.

Assessment

The nursing history includes a thorough description of the patient's symptoms. Describe pain location, onset, and precipitating factors. Note measures that have helped relieve the pain as well. Record any known illnesses and treatments, including drugs and radiation therapy. Describe habits, including diet, oral care practices, alcohol intake, and use of tobacco. Assess the patient's stress level. Inspect the lips and oral cavity for redness, swelling, and lesions.

Nursing Diagnoses, Goals, and Outcome Criteria: Stomatitis	
NURSING DIAGNOSES	GOALS AND OUTCOME CRITERIA
Acute Pain related to tissue trauma, irritation, infection	Pain relief: relaxed appearance, patient statement that pain is reduced or relieved
Impaired Oral Mucous Membrane related to trauma, ineffective oral hygiene, infection, adverse drug effects	Healthy oral mucous membranes: membranes intact, without redness or lesions
Imbalanced Nutrition: Less Than Body Requirements related to inflamed or infected oral tissue	Adequate nutrition: usual food intake, stable body weight

Interventions

When acute inflammation is present, gentle oral hygiene and the use of prescribed mouthwashes are soothing. The teeth and tongue can be cleansed with a soft-bristle toothbrush, sponge, or cotton-tipped applicator. Medications must be given as ordered. It is important to read the directions for these medications carefully. Instead of just swallowing the medication, the patient may need to swish liquid medication in the mouth or to permit tablets to dissolve in the mouth. If the patient is discharged while taking a medication, emphasize the importance of completing the entire prescription. Teach the patient proper techniques for brushing and flossing the teeth. Emphasize the importance of daily oral hygiene and good nutrition in preventing recurrences.

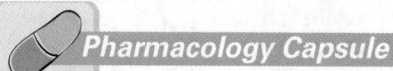 **Pharmacology Capsule**

When drugs are given for stomatitis, the directions may be to "swish and swallow" the medication. Be sure to instruct patients appropriately and evaluate their understanding of directions.

Disorders of the Teeth and Gums

Dental Caries

The term *dental* caries refers to a destructive process of tooth decay. Dental decay starts with the presence of plaque on the teeth. Plaque is a substance made up of bacteria, saliva, and cells that sticks to the surface of the teeth. Bacteria produce acids that destroy the protective tooth enamel, permitting decay. Untreated decay erodes into the canal of the tooth, causing intense pain and death of the pulp. The only treatment for dental caries is removal of the decayed part of the tooth, followed by filling the cavity with a restorative material.

Tooth decay can be prevented largely by good oral hygiene and nutrition. Fluoride is so effective in strengthening tooth enamel that many cities add it to the public water supply. In addition, a dentist may apply fluoride directly to tooth surfaces. Toothpastes containing fluoride are recommended by the American Dental Association to reduce the risk of tooth decay. Patients are encouraged to limit sugar intake as well. Be aware that some mouthwashes contain sugar and others contain alcohol, which are inappropriate for some patients.

Periodontal Disease

Periodontal disease begins with gingivitis (inflammation of the gums) and progresses to involve the other structures that support the teeth. In gingivitis, the gums are typically red, swollen, and painful and bleed easily. Gingivitis results primarily from inadequate oral hygiene. Food particles accumulate between the teeth and the gums, causing irritation. Gingivitis is more common in people who are missing some teeth or whose bite does not close properly. Other contributing factors are poor general health, anemia, vitamin deficiencies, and some blood dyscrasias.

FIGURE 38-10 Acute gingivitis.

Early detection and treatment of gingivitis can stop the progression. Treatment in the early stage consists of professional dental care for teeth cleaning and correction of contributing problems. If the condition is not treated, abscesses develop around the roots, the teeth loosen, and extraction becomes necessary. In more advanced cases, treatment may include not only removing calculus (hardened plaque) but also smoothing root surfaces and surgical removal of the soft, diseased gum tissue. Abnormalities of the teeth and gums are illustrated in Figure 38-10.

NURSING CARE *of the Patient with a Tooth or Gum Disorder*

Assessment

In the health history, determine the presence of oral pain or soreness. Note the patient's usual diet, frequency of dental examinations, and mouth care practices. When examining the mouth, observe the condition of the teeth and gums. Document missing or broken teeth, caries, redness or lesions of the gums, and gum recession. It is especially important for nurses in long-term care to assess patients' mouths at frequent intervals. Oral problems often are overlooked until they are quite advanced.

Nursing Diagnoses, Goals, and Outcome Criteria: Disorders of the Teeth and Gums	
NURSING DIAGNOSES	GOALS AND OUTCOME CRITERIA
Acute Pain related to dental caries, tissue inflammation	Pain relief: relaxed appearance, patient statement that pain is reduced or relieved
Imbalanced Nutrition: Less Than Body Requirements related to oral pain	Adequate nutrition: stable body weight

Interventions

Most patients are treated for dental and gum conditions in dentists' offices. Sometimes, however, dental problems develop when the patient is receiving nursing care for some other reason. In that case, interventions may be directed at minimizing pain until the

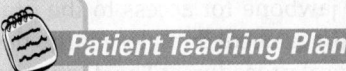

Patient Teaching Plan

Disorders of the Teeth or Gums

You are in a position to teach patients how to prevent dental caries and gingivitis. Include the following in your instructions:

- Seek periodic dental examinations so that problems can be detected early and expert instruction in mouth care may be obtained.
- Brush your teeth at least twice daily and floss every day.
- Eat a balanced diet with limited sugar intake.

problem can be corrected by a dentist. The physician or dentist may order analgesics for acute pain. Gentle mouth care should be performed several times daily.

Provide oral care for patients who cannot do it themselves. Nurse aides and attendants need to understand the importance of regular mouth care and know how to provide it. Clearly include this care in the aide's daily instructions.

Oral Cancer

The most life-threatening disorder affecting the mouth is cancer. Two types of malignant tumors develop in the mouth: squamous cell carcinoma and basal cell carcinoma. Squamous cell carcinomas occur on the lips, buccal mucosa, gums, floor of the mouth, tonsils, and tongue. The most common site for basal cell carcinoma is the lip.

Risk Factors

Cancer of the lip is related to prolonged exposure to irritants, including sun, wind, and pipe smoking. Factors that increase the risk of cancers inside the mouth include tobacco and alcohol use (especially in combination), poor nutritional status, and chronic irritation.

Signs and Symptoms

Symptoms of oral cancer include tongue irritation, loose teeth, and pain in the tongue or ear. Malignant lesions may appear as ulcerations, thickened or rough areas, or sore spots. The presence of hard, white patches in the mouth is called *leukoplakia*. Leukoplakia is considered a premalignant condition.

Medical Diagnosis and Treatment

A biopsy of suspicious lesions is done to make a medical diagnosis. When a malignancy is confirmed, the physician often orders endoscopic examinations and radiographs of the upper digestive and respiratory tracts to see whether there is evidence of metastases. Depending on the extent of the cancer, treatment may include surgery, radiation, or chemotherapy, or a combination of these. Small lesions simply may be excised and sutured. Larger lesions that are more invasive usually require more extensive surgery. An incision can be made along the jawbone for access to the oral cavity. Grafts are sometimes needed to close large defects caused by the surgical procedures. The donor site is usually the patient's anterior thigh. Surgical procedures are illustrated in Figure 38-11.

NURSING CARE of the Patient with Oral Cancer

Assessment

Assessment of the patient with a disorder of the digestive tract is summarized in Box 38-1. When a patient is being evaluated for possible oral cancer, it is especially important to note a history of prolonged sun exposure, tobacco use, or alcohol consumption. Ask whether the patient or immediate family members have a history of cancer. Significant signs and symptoms to record include

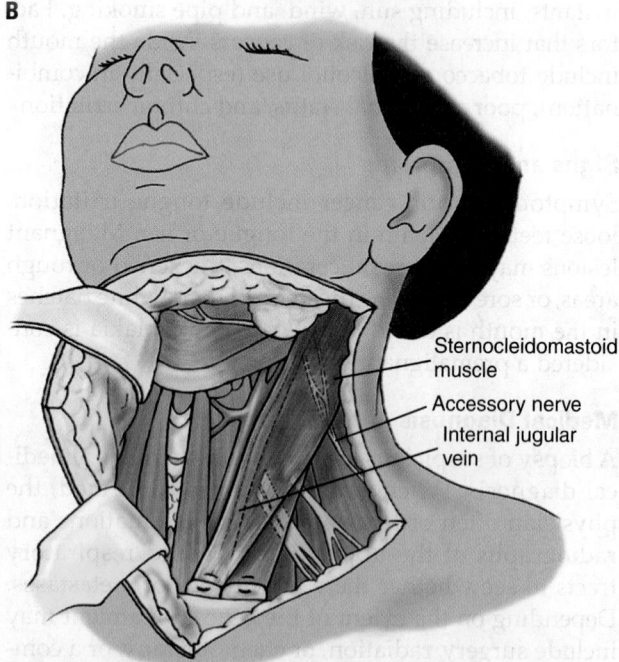

Sternocleidomastoid muscle
Accessory nerve
Internal jugular vein

FIGURE 38-11 Approaches to surgery of the oral cavity for cancer. **A,** Peroral (through the mouth). **B,** Radical neck dissection for advanced oral and pharyngeal cancers.

difficulty swallowing or chewing, decreased appetite, weight loss, change in fit of dentures, and hemoptysis. The physical examination should focus on examination of the mouth for lesions. In addition, assess the neck for limitation of movement and enlarged lymph nodes.

Nursing Diagnoses, Goals, and Outcome Criteria: Oral Cancer

NURSING DIAGNOSES	GOALS AND OUTCOME CRITERIA
Impaired Oral Mucous Membrane related to tumor, edema, secretions	Healthy oral mucosa: membranes intact without lesions, healed surgical incisions
Ineffective Breathing Pattern related to tumor, tissue trauma	Effective breathing patterns: normal respiratory rate and effort

When surgery is performed, additional nursing diagnoses may include the following:

Nursing Diagnoses, Goals, and Outcome Criteria: After Surgery for Oral Cancer

NURSING DIAGNOSES	GOALS AND OUTCOME CRITERIA
Acute Pain related to tissue trauma	Pain relief: relaxed appearance, patient statement that pain is reduced or relieved
Imbalanced Nutrition: Less Than Body Requirements related to pain, edema, medical restrictions on oral intake	Adequate nutrition: caloric intake sufficient to maintain body weight
Impaired Verbal Communication related to edema, tissue trauma	Effective communication: patient communicates needs verbally or nonverbally
Disturbed Body Image related to surgical or radiation treatment	Adjustment to altered appearance or function: patient statement of acceptance of changes, positive statements about self
Risk for Infection related to broken skin, traumatized tissue	Absence of infection: no fever, normal white blood cell count, incision free of excessive swelling and redness, no purulent drainage
Ineffective Tissue Perfusion of graft related to inadequate blood flow	Adequately perfused graft: warm tissue with normal color

Interventions

Impaired Oral Mucous Membrane

Mouth care varies with the type of lesion and the treatment performed. Surgical incisions can be extensive, with considerable tissue trauma. Radiation therapy causes edema. Dry mouth is often a problem after radiation of the mouth. Consult with the physician before doing any mouth care for the patient who has had oral surgery or radiation. Temperatures are usually taken by the tympanic or rectal route after oral surgery. The physician may order specific solutions for rinsing the mouth. One solution that soothes and cleans is half hydrogen peroxide and half normal saline. Another is made by mixing ½ teaspoon of baking soda in 8 ounces of water. Good hydration keeps the oral mucosa moist and thins secretions.

Ineffective Breathing Pattern

Edema, secretions, and an enlarging tumor can cause obstruction of the airway. Monitor respiratory status frequently and report signs of inadequate oxygenation (dyspnea, restlessness, tachycardia). If edema is present, elevate the head of the bed. Steroids may be ordered to decrease inflammation and production of secretions. Oral suction may be ordered to remove secretions that might be aspirated. A tracheotomy may be performed to prevent or treat airway obstruction. Care of the patient with a tracheostomy is covered in Chapter 53.

Acute Pain

Patients with oral cancer may have pain as a result of the lesion, surgical trauma, or the effects of radiation. Patients who have had grafts often report more pain in the donor site than in the grafted site. Administer analgesics as ordered to manage pain. Inform the physician if the medication is not controlling the patient's pain. In addition to drug therapy, use relaxation, imagery, and other strategies, as described in Chapter 15.

Imbalanced Nutrition: Less Than Body Requirements

If the patient is able to swallow, a soft or liquid diet may be prescribed. Mouth care before and after meals may improve appetite and keeps the mouth free of food particles. If the patient cannot or should not take oral nutrition, a feeding tube (nasogastric or gastrostomy) will probably be needed. Another option is TPN. Monitor intake and output records and daily weights to assess adequate intake. With large tumors that cannot be completely removed, or after extensive oral surgery, the feeding tube may be needed indefinitely. See p. 740 in the Common Therapeutic Measures section for care of the patient with a feeding tube. When the patient is able to take oral fluids, assess swallowing and monitor the amount of food taken. Therapy may be needed to help the patient learn to swallow again. Speech therapists are experts in evaluating and managing swallowing disorders.

Impaired Verbal Communication

A large tumor or one that interferes with movement of the tongue is likely to affect speech. In addition, surgical procedures can damage structures involved in normal speech. Assess the patient's ability to read and write. Devise a system to enable the patient to communicate with others. Keep a Magic Slate or pen and pad within the patient's reach. The call bell also must be within reach at all times. Mark the intercom system at the nurse's station so that staff will know to go to the patient's room rather than ask over the intercom what is needed. If the speech organs are intact, the patient may need speech therapy to regain clear oral communication. The nurse and others need to realize how traumatic it is for the patient who is unable to express thoughts verbally. Be patient and do not rush the patient. Compliment successful communication.

Disturbed Body Image

Patients with oral cancer may have body image disturbances as a result of impaired speech, inability to eat, and altered physical appearance. Sometimes external incisions are extensive and disfiguring. Patients need to feel accepted by caregivers and family. Demonstrate acceptance by attentive care, patience, touching, and listening. Assure patients that edema related to surgery will resolve. Some disfigurement, however, may be permanent. Encourage the patient to resume grooming and explore ways to improve appearance. Professional counseling may be needed to help the patient learn to cope with body image changes.

Risk for Infection

Patients with open lesions or surgical incisions are at risk for infection. If a graft has been done, the patient's donor site is also a potential site for infection. Be alert for signs and symptoms of infection (fever, redness, swelling, purulent drainage), and advise the physician if they are present. Prophylactic antibiotics may be ordered. Provide care of external incisions according to physician's orders and agency policy.

Ineffective Tissue Perfusion

Sometimes tissue is grafted to cover a large defect. The primary concern with the graft is maintaining adequate

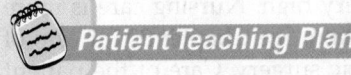
Patient Teaching Plan

Oral Cancer Prevention

- Avoid known risk factors: tobacco and alcohol use, excessive sun exposure.
- Report any dental problem or pain in the mouth to a dentist or physician for early evaluation.
- Good nutrition and mouth care are essential for oral health and wound healing.

If the patient is discharged with a feeding tube or tracheostomy, begin teaching for self-care as soon as the patient is well enough to participate. If the patient and family need assistance, contact the physician about a referral to a home health agency.

blood supply so that the tissue remains alive. Monitor graft color and warmth, and protect the graft from pressure. Report coolness or darkness to the physician.

Parotitis

Parotitis is inflammation of the parotid glands. This condition causes painful swelling of the salivary glands below the ear next to the lower jaw. Pain increases during eating. Parotitis may develop in patients who are unable to take oral liquids for a long time, especially if their oral hygiene is poor. Patients who are very weak and have little resistance to infection also are at risk for parotitis.

The condition is treated with antibiotics, mouthwashes, and warm compresses. If chronic inflammation develops, surgical drainage or removal may be necessary. Otherwise, the infected gland can rupture, spreading infection into surrounding tissues. Parotitis might be prevented in susceptible patients by providing chewing gum or citrus-flavored hard candy (if allowed) to stimulate saliva production. Assess the patient's temperature and comfort level, and monitor swelling of the infected gland. Provide antibiotics and mouth care as ordered.

Achalasia

Achalasia is characterized by progressively worsening dysphagia (difficulty swallowing). It is caused by failure of the lower esophageal muscles and sphincter to relax during swallowing. The cause is unknown but is thought to be a neuromuscular defect affecting the esophageal muscles. Treatment includes drug therapy, dilation, and surgical measures. Isosorbide dinitrate and nifedipine may provide short-term improvement. Botulinum toxin, when injected into the sphincter via endoscopy, may improve achalasia for several months. The procedure, however, is controversial. Esophageal dilation is done on an outpatient basis. The main complication is perforation of the esophagus. Symptoms of perforation are chest and shoulder pain, fever, and subcutaneous emphysema. Esophagomyotomy is a surgical procedure that cuts the esophageal sphincter. Either a thoracic or an abdominal approach may be used. Hospitalization is expected for several days. The success rate for this procedure is very high. Nursing care is more complex than with dilation. See Chapter 30 for care of the patient after thoracic surgery. Care of the patient having abdominal surgery is addressed in this chapter.

Measures to decrease symptoms are usually determined through patient experimentation. The patient can eliminate foods that seem to cause problems, find the eating position that works best, and avoid restrictive clothing. Elevating the head of the bed at night helps control esophageal reflux.

Esophageal Cancer
Pathophysiology

Cancer of the esophagus is not common, but when it does occur, it has a very poor prognosis. Most esophageal cancers are located in the middle or lower portion of the esophagus. There is no known cause, but predisposing factors are cigarette smoking, excessive alcohol intake, chronic trauma, poor oral hygiene, and eating spicy foods.

Cancer of the esophagus often has begun to metastasize by the time it is diagnosed. The liver and lung are common sites of metastasis. The lesion also can extend to the aorta, causing erosion and hemorrhage. Other complications are esophageal obstruction and perforation.

What Does Culture Have to Do with Esophageal Cancer?

In the United States, the incidence of esophageal cancer is higher among African-American males than among white males and is related to tobacco use and dietary factors. The incidence is higher in areas of the world where food and soil contamination and nutritional deficiencies are common.

Signs and Symptoms

Progressive dysphagia (difficulty swallowing) is the primary symptom of esophageal cancer. The patient has difficulty with meat first, then with soft foods, and eventually with liquids. Pain associated with swallowing may be substernal, epigastric, or located in the back and radiating to the neck, jaws, ear, or shoulder. Some patients report sore throats and choking. Obstruction is a late sign of esophageal cancer. Weight loss may be dramatic.

Medical Diagnosis

Radiologic studies used to diagnose cancer of the esophagus include barium swallow and computed tomography. Esophagoscopy may be done to permit the physician to visualize and biopsy the lesion. Endoscopic ultrasonography also may be used to assess the lesion and surrounding tissue. Additional information about common diagnostic tests and procedures is summarized in the Diagnostic Tests and Procedures table on pp. 736 and 737.

Medical and Surgical Treatment

Esophageal cancer may be treated with surgery, radiation, chemotherapy, or various combinations of these. Neither chemotherapy nor radiation alone can cure esophageal cancer. Surgical procedures used to treat this type of cancer include the following (Fig. 38-12):

- Esophagectomy—removal of all or part of the esophagus and replacement of the resected part with a Dacron graft.
- Esophagogastrostomy—resection of the diseased part of the esophagus and attachment of the remaining esophagus to the stomach.
- Esophagogastrectomy—resection of the lower part of the esophagus and the upper part of the

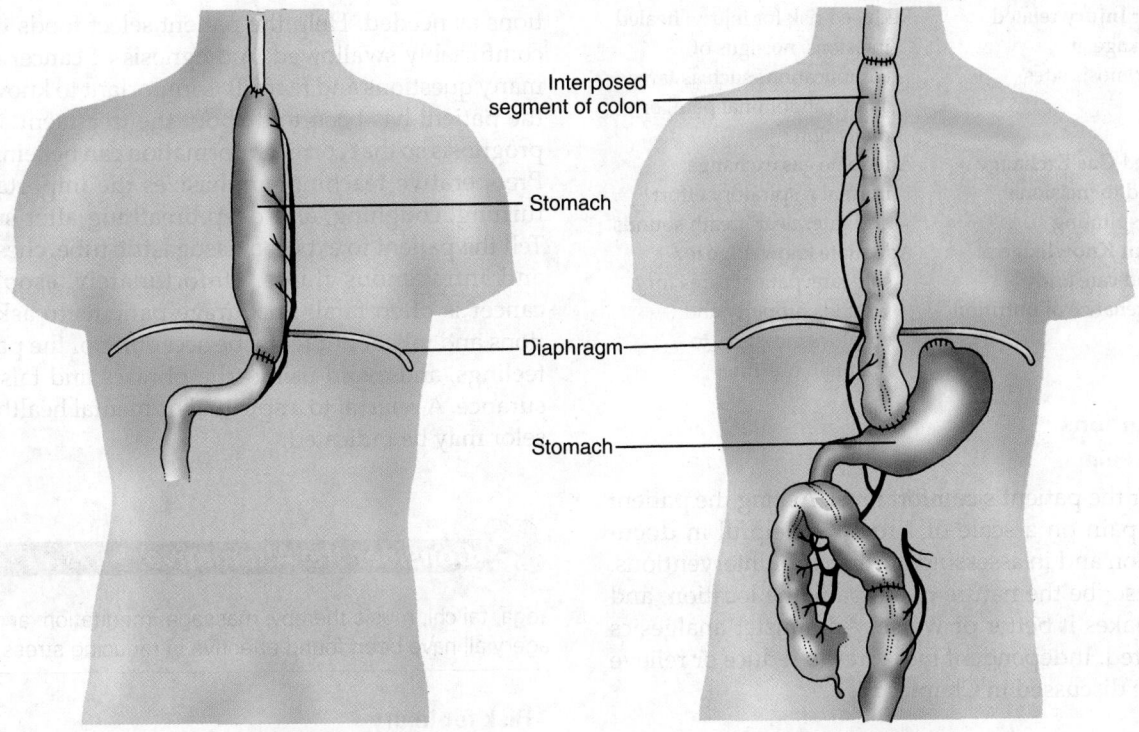

Esophagogastrostomy   **Colon interposition**

FIGURE **38-12** Surgical approaches to the treatment of esophageal cancer.

stomach. The remaining portions of the esophagus and the stomach are reattached.
- Esophagoenterostomy—replacement of the diseased part of the esophagus with a segment of
  colon.

Patients who are considered poor surgical risks may
receive palliative treatment such as the following:
- Dilation of the esophagus to decrease dysphagia.
- Placement of a stent (a rigid tube) in the esophagus to keep it open.
- Laser treatment through an endoscope.
- Radiation therapy, usually a 6- to 8-week course
  of therapy.
- Chemotherapy.
- Photodynamic therapy in which the patient is
  given a light-sensitive drug. Two days later, a
  special fiberoptic probe placed in the esophagus
  activates the drug, which destroys only cancer
  cells.

Because maintaining good nutrition is a major challenge, the physician may insert a feeding tube, often a
gastrostomy tube, to provide adequate nourishment.

NURSING CARE *of the Patient with Esophageal Cancer*

Assessment

Assessment of the patient with a digestive tract disorder is summarized in Box 38-1. When caring for the
patient with cancer of the esophagus, key data in the
health history are dysphagia, pain, and choking. Obtain a thorough description of the patient's pain, in-

cluding location, severity, precipitating factors, and
measures that bring relief. The nursing assessment
of dysphagia includes the patient's description of the
problem and observations of the patient while eating.
Note the conditions under which the patient has dysphagia, as well as the temperature and texture of foods
that cause problems. Assess for the presence of hoarseness, cough, anorexia, weight loss, and regurgitation.
The functional assessment documents the use of alcohol and tobacco and dietary practices.

General physical appearance and height and
weight are important aspects of the physical examination. It is helpful to observe the patient eating.
Note body position, size of bites, chewing efforts, and
speed of eating.

Nursing Diagnoses, Goals, and Outcome Criteria: Esophageal Cancer	
Nursing Diagnoses	**Goals and Outcome Criteria**
Acute Pain related to esophageal lesion, effect of radiation therapy	Pain relief: relaxed manner, patient statement of pain reduction or relief
Imbalanced Nutrition: Less Than Body Requirements related to dysphagia	Adequate nutritional intake: stable or increased body weight
Anxiety related to diagnosis, therapy, uncertain outcome	Decreased anxiety: calm manner, patient statement of lessened anxiety

Continued

Risk for Injury related to leakage at anastomosis sites	Reduced risk for injury: healed incisions; no signs of complications such as tarry stools, abdominal pain, or distention
Impaired Gas Exchange related to incisional pain, splinting	Adequate gas exchange: normal respiratory effort and rate, clear breath sounds
Deficient Knowledge of wound care and maintenance of nutrition	Adequate knowledge for self-care: patient cares for wounds properly and employs measures to maintain nutrition

Interventions

Acute Pain

Monitor the patient's comfort level. Asking the patient to rate pain on a scale of 1 to 10 is helpful in documentation and in assessing the effects of interventions. Also describe the nature of the pain, the location, and what makes it better or worse. Administer analgesics as ordered. Independent measures to reduce or relieve pain are discussed in Chapter 15.

Imbalanced Nutrition: Less Than Body Requirements

Nutrition is a major problem for the patient with esophageal cancer. Daily weights, intake and output measurements, and calorie counts all may be kept to monitor adequacy of intake. A high-calorie, high-protein diet is recommended. The texture of food is adjusted as needed (e.g., soft, semisolid), depending on the patient's ability to swallow.

Some general interventions may be helpful in managing dysphagia. A quiet, relaxed environment helps the patient concentrate on effective swallowing. An erect position is preferred. The head should be tilted slightly forward. Some patients think that they can swallow better with the head thrown back. In reality, that position actually makes swallowing more difficult and increases the risk of aspiration. If dysphagia prevents adequate nutritional intake, an alternative feeding method must be used. Options include nasogastric and gastrostomy feedings and TPN.

Postoperatively, patients usually have nasogastric tubes in place and attached to suction. Do not irrigate or reposition nasogastric tubes in patients who have had esophageal surgery. The physician should be notified if the tube is not draining properly. Drainage is typically bloody for the first 8 to 12 hours and then gradually turns yellowish. After bowel sounds return, the physician orders oral fluids introduced in small amounts. At first, only water is given. Evaluate the patient's ability to swallow. Record intake and output and daily weights to evaluate nutrition.

Anxiety

During the diagnostic period, assess the patient's understanding of tests and procedures and offer explanations as needed. Help the patient select foods that are comfortably swallowed. A diagnosis of cancer evokes many questions and fears. It is important to know what the patient has been told about the treatment and the prognosis so that correct information can be reinforced. Preoperative teaching emphasizes the importance of turning, coughing, and deep breathing after surgery. Tell the patient to expect a nasogastric tube, chest tube, and intravenous fluids. Unfortunately, esophageal cancer is often fatal. Encourage patients to ask questions and talk about fears. Be accepting of the patient's feelings, and avoid using trite phrases and false reassurance. A referral to a spiritual or mental health counselor may be indicated.

Consider the Alternative

Yoga, tai chi, music therapy, massage, meditation, and imagery all have been found effective in reducing stress.

Risk for Injury

Depending on the surgical procedure, the patient may have multiple incisions and wound drains. Assist the patient in supporting the wounds during coughing and position changes. Like any surgical patient, the patient who has undergone surgery for esophageal cancer must be monitored for signs and symptoms of hemorrhage (restlessness, tachycardia, hypotension) and infection (fever, increased white blood cell count, erythema, purulent wound drainage). In addition to the risk of infection, the patient is at risk for leakage at anastomosis sites. If the anastomosis is not secure, digestive fluids leak into the thoracic or abdominal cavity. The risk of leakage is greatest 5 to 7 days after surgery. Signs and symptoms of leakage are fever, tachycardia, tachypnea, and fluid accumulation. The physician should be notified immediately if leakage is suspected.

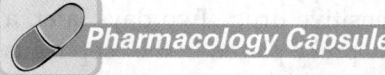

Pharmacology Capsule

The patient with dysphagia may be able to take liquid medications more easily than capsules or tablets.

Impaired Gas Exchange

Immediately after surgery, the patient may be artificially ventilated to maintain adequate oxygenation. Chest tubes are needed to remove fluid from the thoracic cavity. When the ventilator is discontinued, you must encourage and support the patient in turning, coughing, and deep breathing. Chest physiotherapy or incentive spirometry may be ordered. Elevate the patient's head to ease chest expansion and to reduce the risk of reflux of gastric contents into the esophagus.

Patients who have stents placed in the esophagus should be told how to reduce the risk of regurgitation of stomach contents. Instruct them to eat only small meals, to remain upright for several hours after meals, and to avoid lying flat at any time. The head of the bed should be elevated at least 30 degrees at all times.

Deficient Knowledge

Postoperatively, prepare the patient for discharge. Encourage the patient to continue breathing exercises and to gradually increase activity. Discourage bed rest. Point out the characteristics of the healing incisions and teach the patient signs of wound complications that should be reported. Stress the importance of small, high-calorie, high-protein meals. If nasogastric feedings are continued, instruct the patient and family in management of the feedings. Because esophageal cancer often recurs, the patient should know to report increased pain or dysphagia. A referral may be made to a home health agency for assistance after discharge.

DISORDERS AFFECTING DIGESTION AND ABSORPTION

Nausea and Vomiting

Nausea is a feeling of discomfort sometimes referred to as *queasiness*. It may or may not be accompanied by abdominal pain, pallor, perspiration, and cold, clammy skin. Causes of nausea include irritating foods, infectious diseases, radiation, drugs and other chemicals, hormonal changes and imbalances, and distention of the digestive tract. It is common after surgery and in patients with motion sickness and inner ear disorders.

Nausea and vomiting often occur together. Vomiting is the forceful expulsion of stomach contents through the mouth. It occurs when the vomiting reflex in the brain is stimulated. Very forceful ejection of stomach contents is called *projectile vomiting*. **Regurgitation** is the gentle ejection of food or fluid without nausea or retching. Just before vomiting occurs, a person usually senses what is about to happen. Tachycardia and increased salivation are common just before vomiting.

Complications

Prolonged or severe vomiting can lead to significant losses of fluids and electrolytes. In addition to dehydration, metabolic alkalosis may develop due to loss of stomach acids. Patients who are very weak or unable to move are at risk for aspirating the vomited stomach contents. Therefore nausea and vomiting must be treated to relieve patient discomfort and to prevent complications.

Medical Treatment

Drugs that prevent or treat nausea and vomiting are classified as *antiemetics*. Most antiemetic drugs have multiple uses. They may have local effects (adsorbents), they may act on the central nervous system, or they may act in more than one way. Centrally acting antiemetics include anticholinergics, antihistamines, phenothiazines, and marijuana derivatives. Antiemetics classified as 5-HT receptor antagonists affect the small intestine as well as the peripheral and central nervous systems. Examples of these drugs are listed in the Drug Therapy table on pp. 748 and 749. A common side effect of most centrally acting antiemetics is drowsiness. They also may cause tachycardia, hypotension, constipation, urinary retention, and dry mouth. Many antiemetics are contraindicated in patients with glaucoma, myocardial infarction, bowel or urinary obstruction, and pregnancy.

Intravenous fluids may be ordered to prevent dehydration. Oral fluids may be limited to clear liquids or withheld completely until the vomiting stops. At times, a nasogastric tube is inserted and attached to suction to keep the stomach empty. Severe or prolonged vomiting may necessitate TPN to meet the patient's metabolic needs.

Pharmacology Capsule

A common side effect of most antiemetics is drowsiness, so take necessary safety precautions.

NURSING CARE *of the Patient with Nausea and Vomiting*

Assessment

The nursing assessment plays an important part in the management of nausea and vomiting. The health history should elicit a description of the onset, frequency, and duration of the present illness. Note the conditions under which nausea and vomiting occur. For example, is it before or after meals, at a certain time of day, or after taking a certain medication? If vomiting occurs, record the amount, color, odor, and contents of the vomitus. Contents might include undigested food or medications. Vomitus containing bile has a characteristic green color. A bright red color suggests recent bleeding in the esophagus or stomach, although it could be due to recently ingested red food or liquid. When blood has been in the stomach long enough to be acted on by stomach secretions, it turns dark brown and resembles wet coffee grounds.

A complete health history should be obtained when the patient is able to participate. Record surgeries, chronic illnesses, allergies, and medications. Inquire about pregnancy because many drugs are contraindicated in the pregnant woman.

In the physical examination, describe the patient's general appearance and record vital signs and height and weight. Collect data related to hydration status, which would include pulse and blood pressure, tissue turgor, mental status, and muscle tone. Evaluate respiratory rate, effort, and breath sounds. Inspect, auscultate, and palpate the abdomen for distention, bowel sounds, and tenderness.

Nursing Diagnoses, Goals, and Outcome Criteria: Nausea and Vomiting

NURSING DIAGNOSES	GOALS AND OUTCOME CRITERIA
Imbalanced Nutrition: Less Than Body Requirements related to inability to consume or retain food	Adequate nutrition: stable body weight, retention of food and fluids
Deficient Fluid Volume related to loss of fluids by vomiting	Normal hydration: pulse and blood pressure consistent with patient norms, urine output approximately equal to fluid intake, moist mucous membranes
Risk for Aspiration related to decreased level of consciousness, impaired swallowing, wired jaws, depressed gag reflex, vomiting	Absence of aspiration: respiratory rate 12-20 without dyspnea, clear breath sounds

Interventions

Imbalanced Nutrition: Less Than Body Requirements and Deficient Fluid Volume

When a patient complains of nausea, assist him or her in assuming a still, comfortable position. Maintain a cool room temperature, and remove any unpleasant stimuli. Provide an emesis basin. Apply a cool, damp cloth to the face and neck for comfort. Advise the patient that taking deep breaths and swallowing may be effective in suppressing the vomiting reflex. Unless the episode passes promptly, administer an antiemetic drug as ordered. In situations in which nausea can be anticipated, antiemetics are best given before nausea occurs. It is easier to prevent nausea than to treat it.

If the patient does vomit, remain close by and offer reassurance. Empty the emesis basin as promptly as possible and return it to the bedside in case it is needed again. Replace soiled clothing and linen. Offer mouth care to remove unpleasant tastes when the urge to vomit subsides.

Severe or prolonged vomiting puts the patient at risk for deficient fluid volume. Infants and older adults are especially susceptible to deficient fluid volume because their kidneys are less efficient in conserving body fluids. Monitor intake and output, vital signs, and other measures of hydration. Signs of deficient fluid volume include tachycardia, hypotension, oliguria, confusion, and poor tissue turgor.

When the patient is ready to resume oral intake, he or she is usually started on clear liquids. Tea, broth, flat carbonated liquids, and gelatin generally are tolerated best. Other liquids may be added if nausea and vomiting do not recur. If permitted, offer dry toast or crackers to help relieve nausea. Advise the patient to eat slowly.

When regular meals are resumed, encourage the patient to take fluids between meals rather than with meals. As mentioned earlier, alternative methods of feeding will be necessary if nausea and vomiting threaten the patient's fluid or nutritional status.

Risk for Aspiration

The patient who is unconscious or has impaired swallowing or a depressed gag reflex is at risk for aspiration. This risk is much greater when the patient is vomiting. Position the patient on the side so that vomitus can drain from the mouth. Keep the suction apparatus on hand and use it as needed to clear the mouth and upper airway. Monitor the patient's respiratory rate and effort and breath sounds. Notify the physician of increasing respiratory rate, dyspnea, and abnormal breath sounds.

Consider the Alternative

Ginger root is effective in calming upset stomach, reducing flatulence, and preventing motion sickness. Be aware that it enhances anticoagulants and antiplatelet agents.

Hiatal Hernia
Pathophysiology

The esophageal hiatus is the opening in the diaphragm through which the esophagus passes. A hiatal hernia is the protrusion of the lower esophagus and stomach upward through the diaphragm and into the chest. Figure 38-13 illustrates the two types of hiatal hernias, sliding hernia and paraesophageal (rolling) hernia. In a sliding hernia, the gastroesophageal junction is above the hiatus. The stomach slides into the thoracic cavity when the patient reclines. It slides back into place when the patient stands or sits up. Sliding hernias are commonly associated with gastroesophageal reflux disease (GERD). Weakness of the esophageal sphincter permits gastric fluids to flow backward into the esophagus. Acidic gastric fluids can cause inflammation of the esophagus. However, not all patients with hiatal hernias have GERD, and not all patients with GERD have hiatal hernias. GERD is discussed on p. 763.

In a rolling hernia, the gastroesophageal junction remains in place but a portion of the stomach herniates up through the diaphragm through a secondary opening.

Complications of hiatal hernia include ulcerations, bleeding, and aspiration of regurgitated stomach contents. The paraesophageal hernia can also result in strangulation of the hernia, a situation in which the herniated tissue becomes trapped and deprived of blood flow.

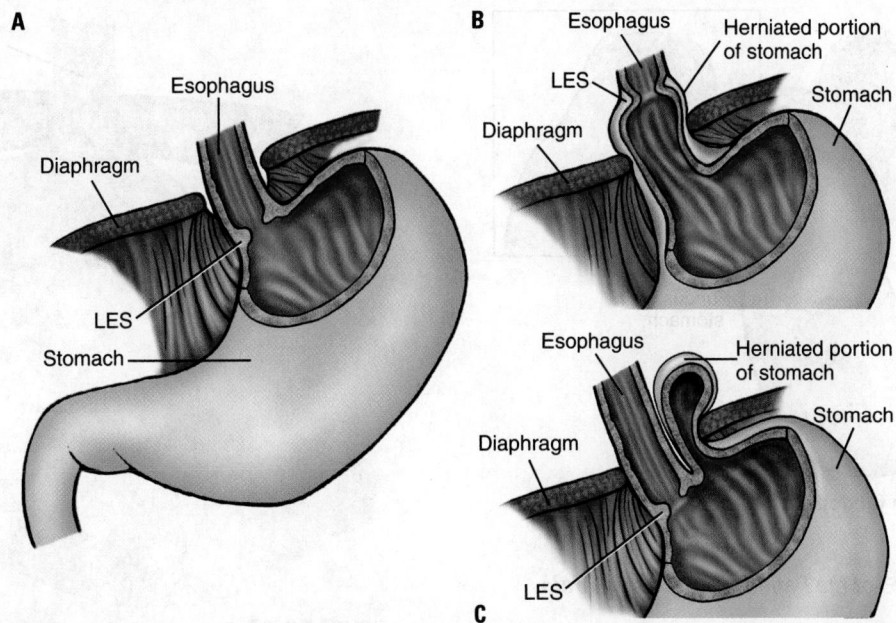

FIGURE **38-13** Hiatal hernia. **A**, Normal anatomy. **B**, Sliding hiatal hernia. **C**, Paraesophageal (rolling) hiatal hernia.

Causes

Hiatal hernia may be caused by weakness of the muscles of the diaphragm in the area where the esophagus and the stomach join (the lower esophageal sphincter [LES]), however, the exact cause is not known. Factors that contribute to development of hiatal hernia include excessive intra-abdominal pressure, trauma, and long-term bed rest in a reclining position. Intra-abdominal pressure is increased by obesity, pregnancy, abdominal tumors, ascites, and repeated heavy lifting or strain. Hiatal hernia develops in about half of all people older than 60 years.

Signs and Symptoms

Many patients with hiatal hernias have no symptoms at all. Others report feelings of fullness, dysphagia, eructation (belching), regurgitation, and heartburn. Heartburn is a feeling of burning and tightness rising from the lower sternum to the throat. It is triggered by foods and drugs that decrease LES pressure and by lying down or bending over.

Medical Diagnosis

When hiatal hernia is suspected, several tests and procedures may be ordered. A barium swallow examination with fluoroscopy outlines the esophagus and demonstrates esophageal peristalsis. A CT scan helps visualize the abnormality. In the patient with hiatal hernia, the reflux of gastric contents is evident. Esophagoscopy is direct examination of the esophagus with an endoscope. Structural abnormalities and tissue inflammation may be detected. Tissue specimens can be taken for biopsy during endoscopy.

Esophageal manometry measures the pressures in the stomach and the esophagus. With the patient sit-ting up, a small tube is inserted through the nose into the stomach. The patient is then placed in a supine position. Small amounts of water or gelatin are given to the patient to swallow. Pressure measurements are taken in the stomach and esophagus. For acid reflux testing, a second probe that is sensitive to acid is inserted through the nose into the esophagus. The detection of acid in the esophagus is consistent with esophageal reflux.

Medical Treatment

In many cases, hiatal hernia can be managed with drug therapy, diet, and measures to avoid increased intra-abdominal pressure. Drug therapy includes antacids and, sometimes, drugs such as H_2-receptor blockers (e.g., ranitidine [Zantac]) or proton pump inhibitors (e.g., omeprazole [Prilosec]) to reduce gastric acid secretion. Bethanechol chloride (Urecholine) may be ordered to increase the tone of the LES.

Surgery may be necessary if severe bleeding or narrowing of the esophagus occurs. Surgical options to treat hiatal hernia include several types of fundoplication and placement of the synthetic Angelchik prosthesis. Fundoplication (Fig. 38-14) strengthens the LES by suturing the fundus of the stomach around the esophagus and anchoring it below the diaphragm. The Angelchik prosthesis, illustrated in Figure 38-15, is a C-shaped silicone device. It is tied around the distal esophagus, anchoring it below the diaphragm. The Nissen and Toupet fundoplication procedures can be done laparoscopically. When laparoscopy is not appropriate, incisions may be made in either the abdomen or the chest. Either way, there is a risk of postoperative respiratory complications.

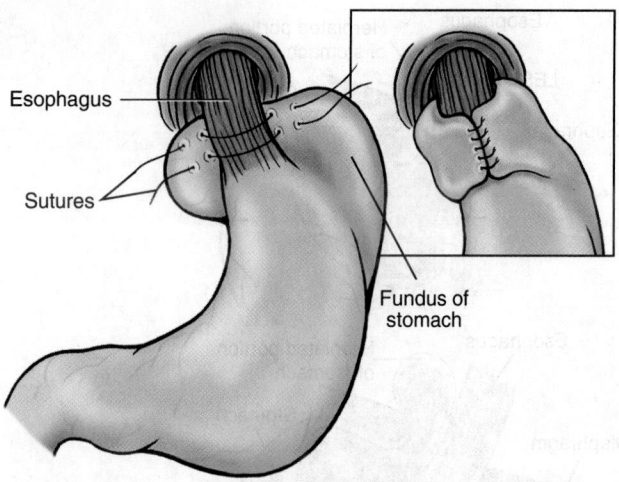

FIGURE **38-14** Nissen fundoplication for hiatal hernia repair.

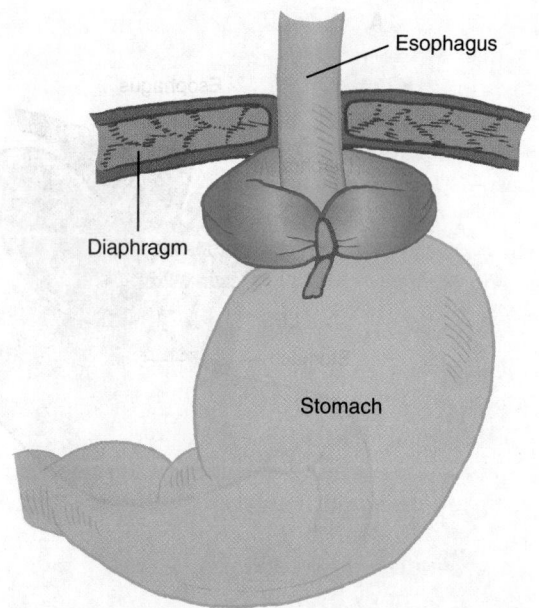

FIGURE **38-15** Placement of the Angelchik prosthesis.

NURSING CARE *of the Patient with Hiatal Hernia*

Assessment

Assessment of the patient with a digestive tract disorder is summarized in Box 38-1. When a patient has hiatal hernia, document the symptoms (pain, dysphagia, eructation). Record factors that trigger the symptoms as well as measures that aggravate or relieve them. Note any abdominal trauma in the past medical history. Describe the patient's dietary habits, use of alcohol and tobacco, and medication history. Inquire about activities requiring lifting or intense physical exertion. In the physical examination, measure the patient's height and weight.

Nursing Diagnoses, Goals, and Outcome Criteria: Hiatal Hernia

NURSING DIAGNOSES	GOALS AND OUTCOME CRITERIA
Chronic Pain related to esophageal inflammation	Pain relief: patient statement of less or no pain, relaxed manner
Risk for Aspiration related to regurgitation of gastric contents	Absence of aspiration: respiratory rate 12-20 without dyspnea, clear breath sounds
Imbalanced Nutrition: Less Than Body Requirements related to dysphagia	Adequate nutrition: stable body weight

Interventions
Chronic Pain

Pain is caused by the reflux of acid into the inflamed esophagus. Therefore pain can be reduced by increasing LES pressure, which keeps gastric contents from passing into the esophagus. Drugs that increase LES pressure, neutralize acid, and reduce acid secretion are administered as ordered. Evaluate the effects of drug therapy. Dietary alterations, discussed on p. 763, are helpful in reducing the symptoms of hiatal hernia.

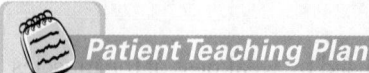

Patient Teaching Plan

Hiatal Hernia

- Drug therapy: know the drugs you take, their dosages, schedule, and adverse effects.
- Eat small, frequent meals. Avoid foods that aggravate the condition (fatty foods, caffeine, alcohol).
- Maintain normal weight to decrease intra-abdominal pressure.
- Elevate the head of your bed to discourage reflux.
- Avoid smoking.
- Learn stress management techniques.
- To prevent increased intra-abdominal pressure, avoid bending forward, lifting, or straining, and avoid clothing that is tight around the waist or abdomen.

Risk for Aspiration

Gastric contents that are regurgitated into the esophagus may be aspirated into the respiratory tract, causing aspiration pneumonia. To reduce the risk of aspiration, food and fluids should not be taken for 2 to 3 hours before bedtime. This reduces reflux of stomach contents during sleep. Patients with hiatal hernia should sleep with their heads elevated 6 to 12 inches. Wooden blocks can be placed under the legs of the head of the bed if a mechanical or electrical bed is not available. This sleeping position requires a period of adjustment but is very important to prevent nighttime reflux.

Imbalanced Nutrition: Less Than Body Requirements

Assess weight changes and note excessive weight loss. Measures to control pain, as discussed earlier, help the patient eat more comfortably. Advise small, frequent meals because large meals increase pressure in the stomach and delay gastric emptying. Encourage the patient to avoid foods that are known to decrease LES pressure: fatty foods, coffee, tea, cola, chocolate, and alcohol. Also, acidic and spicy foods may be irritating when the esophagus is inflamed. Counsel the obese patient about the relationship between obesity and increased intra-abdominal pressure.

POSTOPERATIVE NURSING CARE
of the Patient with Hiatal Hernia Repair

When the patient has had an abdominal or thoracic approach for hiatal hernia repair, care is similar to that after any major surgery. Turning, coughing, and deep breathing are particularly important for these patients. The patient will probably have a nasogastric tube in place and connected to suction for a day or two after surgery. Until bowel function returns, the patient is given only intravenous fluids. Tell the patient to expect mild dysphagia for several weeks.

Gastroesophageal Reflux Disease

Gastroesophageal reflux disease (GERD) is the backward flow of gastric contents from the stomach into the esophagus. A key finding is inappropriate relaxation of the lower esophageal sphincter (LES). GERD is often associated with a sliding hernia, although the two are not always found together.

Pathophysiology

Factors that contribute to the development of GERD include abnormalities around the LES, gastric or duodenal ulcer, gastric or esophageal surgery, prolonged vomiting, and prolonged gastric intubation. The acidic stomach contents flow backwards into the esophagus and eventually cause esophagitis (inflammation of the esophagus).

Signs and Symptoms

The onset of GERD symptoms may be sudden or gradual. Patients typically report a painful burning sensation that moves up and down, commonly occurs after meals, and is relieved by antacids. If severe, the pain may radiate to the back, neck, or jaw. Acid regurgitation, intermittent dysphagia, and belching are common. Symptoms are likely to occur after activities that increase intra-abdominal pressure such as lifting, straining, and lying supine.

Medical Diagnosis

A diagnosis of GERD is suggested by the signs and symptoms. Various diagnostic procedures may be done to confirm the diagnosis, assess the severity, and detect complications. These might include radiographic studies, endoscopy, biopsy, gastric analysis, esophageal manometry, 24-hour monitoring of esophageal pH, and acid perfusion tests.

Medical Treatment and Nursing Care

Medical treatment and nursing care are like those described earlier for hiatal hernia. In brief, drug therapy may include the following:

- H₂-receptor blockers (e.g., ranitidine [Zantac])
- Prokinetic agents (e.g., metoclopramide [Reglan])
- Proton pump inhibitors (omeprazole [Prilosec])

If medical care is unsuccessful, surgical fundoplication may be done.

 Put on Your Thinking Cap!

Draw pictures or create a model to illustrate what a sliding hiatal hernia is and how it causes heartburn.

Gastritis
Pathophysiology

Gastritis is an inflammation of the lining of the stomach. The area of the inflammation and the depth of stomach tissue affected vary with different types of gastritis. Gastritis is commonly classified as acute, chronic type A, and chronic type B. Despite a variety of causes, the pathophysiology is common to all. The mucosal barrier that normally protects the stomach from auto-digestion breaks down. Hydrochloric acid, histamine, and pepsin act to cause tissue edema, increased capillary permeability, and possible hemorrhage.

Among the many causes of gastritis, *Helicobacter pylori* is thought to be the prime culprit. Gastritis induced by *H. pylori* affects primarily the superficial tissues. The type associated with NSAIDs, stress, and alcohol tends to affect deeper tissue and is more prone to hemorrhage. The role of diet in gastritis is not completely understood. Some foods like red and black pepper can cause superficial erosions in the gastric mucosa. It is interesting to note that chili pepper in small amounts stimulates mucus production but in large amounts can damage the mucosa. Other related factors are reflux of bile salts from the duodenum, prolonged vomiting, intense stress, and CNS lesions. Chronic gastritis type A probably is induced by immune mechanisms. The changes in the stomach lining with chronic atrophic gastritis result in decreased production of acid and intrinsic factor. Intrinsic factor is needed for the absorption of vitamin B₁₂, which is essential for the maturation of red blood cells. Without intrinsic factor, a serious condition called *pernicious anemia* develops.

 Pharmacology Capsule

Only the parenteral form of vitamin B₁₂ is effective in pernicious anemia.

The management of pernicious anemia is discussed in Chapter 32.

Signs and Symptoms

Symptoms of acute gastritis usually include nausea, vomiting, anorexia, a feeling of fullness, and pain in the stomach area. In people who abuse alcohol, hemorrhage may be the only symptom. Symptoms of chronic gastritis may be the same as acute gastritis. Some patients, however, have only mild indigestion or no symptoms at all unless they develop pernicious anemia.

Medical Diagnosis

The best means of diagnosing gastritis is gastroscopy. The physician is able to visualize the interior of the stomach and biopsy any suspicious areas. Laboratory studies may be done to detect occult blood in the feces, low blood hemoglobin and hematocrit, and low serum gastrin levels. The presence of *H. pylori* can be confirmed by breath, urine, stool, or serum tests or by gastric tissue biopsy. Because *H. pylori* has been associated with gastric and duodenal ulcers and with gastric cancer, cytologic examination of a tissue specimen commonly is done.

Medical Treatment

The medical management of acute gastritis is concerned with treatment of the symptoms and fluid replacement. If hospitalization is considered necessary, oral fluids and foods usually are withheld until the acute symptoms subside. Intravenous fluids can be ordered to prevent or treat dehydration. Medications to reduce gastric acidity (i.e., antacids, H$_2$-receptor blockers, proton pump inhibitors) and to relieve nausea may be given. Analgesics may be ordered for pain relief and antibiotics for *H. pylori*. When nausea and vomiting stop, oral fluids are gradually increased. Typically, the patient progresses from clear liquids to full liquids and then to a soft, bland diet.

The medical management of chronic gastritis focuses on elimination of the cause (e.g., *H. pylori*, alcohol, drugs) and treatment of pernicious anemia. Treatment of *H. pylori* usually requires a combination of omeprazole (Prilosec), which reduces gastric acid secretion, and one or two antibiotics (amoxicillin and/or clarithromycin). Prepackaged combinations are available. Corticosteroids also may be used to reduce inflammation. Vitamin B$_{12}$ injections must be given regularly to prevent long-term complications. A bland diet given in six small feedings per day is usually prescribed, with antacids ordered after meals when reflux is most common.

Surgical intervention may be needed if conservative measures fail to correct or control gastritis or if the patient is hemorrhaging. Specific procedures and nursing implications are the same as for peptic ulcer disease, which is discussed on pp. 765 to 772.

NURSING CARE *of the Patient with Gastritis*

Assessment

In taking the health history, first describe the patient's present illness. Patients often complain of pain, indigestion, nausea, and vomiting. Determine the onset, duration, and location of pain. Note factors that trigger or relieve the symptoms. Document chronic illnesses, as well as current and recent medications. Ask whether the patient has had any unexplained weight loss and if stools have been bloody or black. The functional assessment provides information about dietary practices, use of alcohol and tobacco, and activity and rest patterns. Ask if there are significant sources of stress at present.

In the physical examination, observe the patient's general appearance for signs of distress. Measure vital signs and height and weight for comparison with previous readings. Note the skin color and check turgor. Inspect the abdomen for distention and palpate for tenderness and guarding. Auscultate the abdomen for increased bowel sounds.

Nursing Diagnoses, Goals, and Outcome Criteria: Gastritis

Nursing Diagnoses	Goals and Outcome Criteria
Acute Pain related to inflammation of the gastric mucosa	Pain relief: patient states less or no pain, relaxed manner
Imbalanced Nutrition: Less Than Body Requirements related to anorexia, pain, nausea and vomiting	Adequate nutrition: stable weight
Deficient Fluid Volume related to vomiting, bleeding	Normal hydration: pulse and blood pressure within patient norms, moist mucous membranes, urine output equal to fluid intake Absence of bleeding: normal stool color, no blood in emesis
Ineffective Coping related to chronic illness	Effective coping strategies: patient employs stress management techniques and resources

Interventions

Acute Pain

Give medications as ordered, including antacids, H$_2$-receptor blockers, proton pump inhibitors, other anti-ulcer agents, analgesics, and antibiotics. Assess drug effectiveness and inform the physician if pain is not relieved. Nonpharmacologic methods of pain control as described in Chapter 15 may be employed as well.

Imbalanced Nutrition: Less Than Body Requirements

The most appropriate diet for the patient with gastritis is controversial. In general, encourage the patient to avoid caffeine and alcohol and any other foods that seem to aggravate the symptoms. Many sources recommend a soft, bland diet taken in small meals; however, this pattern may actually increase the total amount of acid secreted. Most sources agree that the patient should avoid large meals before retiring. Note the patient's dietary intake. Periodic weights may be appropriate to determine whether the patient is receiving adequate nourishment.

Deficient Fluid Volume

Deficit fluid volume may result from dehydration or from hemorrhage. The patient may become dehydrated because of poor oral intake or severe vomiting. Be alert for signs of deficient fluid volume (oliguria, tachycardia, dry skin and mucous membranes, poor tissue turgor, and hypotension). Record intake and output. Inspect

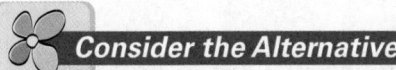

Consider the Alternative

Alternative therapies for stress reduction include acupuncture, therapeutic massage, guided imagery, progressive relaxation, meditation, yoga, and aromatherapy with chamomile, lavender, citronella, and mandarin.

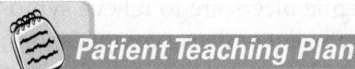

Patient Teaching Plan

Gastritis

- Adjust your diet as recommended, which may include soft, bland, small meals; avoid irritants.
- You need to know the name, dosage, schedule, and adverse effects of your drugs.
- Some stress reduction techniques that you might find helpful are exercise, soft music, and regular leisure activities.
- Notify your physician if you have bloody vomitus or dark, tarry stools.
- It is vital that you avoid using tobacco because it stimulates acid secretion.
- Do not take aspirin or NSAIDs because they aggravate gastritis and increase the risk of hemorrhage.

vomited fluids for bright red blood or dark brown particles that indicate bleeding in the stomach. Inspect the stool for the maroon or tarry black appearance characteristic of bleeding from the stomach. Give intravenous fluids as ordered, monitoring the rate of infusion.

Ineffective Coping

Chronic illness drains the patient physically and emotionally. Explore how the patient is dealing with gastritis and what additional supports are needed. Professional counseling may be needed to help the patient learn relaxation and stress management techniques. When alcohol abuse contributes to gastritis, provide information about community resources such as Alcoholics Anonymous.

Peptic Ulcer

Pathophysiology

A peptic ulcer is a loss of tissue from the lining of the digestive tract. Normally, a mucous barrier protects the lining from the digestive fluids. When that barrier fails, pepsin and hydrochloric acid injure the unprotected tissue.

Peptic ulcers may be acute or chronic, depending on the layers of tissue affected. Acute ulcers affect only the superficial layers of the digestive lining, whereas chronic ulcers extend into the muscle layer. Acute ulcers are sometimes called *acute gastric lesions*.

Peptic ulcers are classified as gastric or duodenal, depending on their location. Gastric and duodenal ulcers differ in depth of injury, amount of gastric secretions, incidence, and signs and symptoms. These differences are presented in Table 38-2.

Gastric ulcers occur most often in men and in older adults. Women who have ulcers are more likely to have gastric ulcers than duodenal ulcers. The incidence rate of gastric ulcers is higher among people with type A blood than among people with other blood types. Although people think of ulcers as a condition of the rich and powerful, gastric ulcers are actually more common among unskilled laborers.

Eighty percent of peptic ulcers occur in the duodenum. Duodenal ulcers are more common in younger men and in people with type O blood. There is an

Table 38-2	*Comparison of Gastric and Duodenal Ulcers*

CHARACTERISTIC	GASTRIC ULCER	DUODENAL ULCER
Incidence	More common in older men, working class, those with blood type A, substance abusers, and people under severe stress.	More common in younger men, all social classes, those with blood type O, people with chronic illnesses.
Ulcer depth	Shallow.	Deep.
Gastric secretions	Unchanged or decreased.	Increased.
Signs and symptoms	Burning and pressure in upper left abdomen below rib cage and in back. Pain 1-2 hr after meals. Relieved by food or fluids.	Burning and pressure in upper middle abdomen and back. Pain 2-4 hr after meals. Relieved by antacids or foods.
Complications	Hemorrhage, perforation, obstruction.	Hemorrhage, perforation, obstruction.

increase in the secretion of gastric acid. Duodenal ulcers are found among people in all occupations and income levels.

Causes

Factors that contribute to the development of ulcers are thought to include drugs, infection, and stress. Drugs that are associated with ulcer disease include aspirin and nonsteroidal anti-inflammatory drugs (NSAIDs) such as ibuprofen. However, most ulcers are caused by the microorganism *Helicobacter pylori.* Also, extremely stressful events such as shock, burns, and trauma are thought to cause a temporary decrease in blood flow to the gastric mucosa. Inadequate blood flow interferes with the mucosal barrier, permitting breakdown of the stomach lining. Ulcers attributed to this process are called *stress ulcers.* Spicy foods often have been blamed for ulcers, but this link has not been proved. With gastric ulcers, gastric acid production is usually normal or decreased.

Conditions that cause excessive gastric acid secretion seem to contribute to the development of duodenal ulcers. Examples of such conditions are chronic obstructive pulmonary disease, cirrhosis of the liver, chronic pancreatitis, and hyperparathyroidism. Heavy alcohol and tobacco use also are associated with duodenal ulcers, as well as with gastric ulcers.

Signs and Symptoms

Gastric ulcers typically produce burning pain in the epigastric area 1 to 2 hours after meals. Nausea, anorexia, and weight loss are sometimes present. Some patients have no pain at all until serious complications develop.

Although some patients with duodenal ulcers have no pain, others experience a burning or cramping pain 2 to 4 hours after meals. The pain is located in the area just beneath the xiphoid process. It is often relieved by antacids or food. The patient commonly reports pain that lasts for several weeks or months, disappears, and returns.

Complications

Peptic ulcers can lead to serious, even life-threatening complications. *Intractability* is the term used to describe symptomatic peptic ulcer disease that does not respond to treatment. Hemorrhage is more common in older adults and in people with gastric ulcers. If the hemorrhage is not brought under control, the patient can bleed to death.

A perforation is a break in the wall of the stomach or the duodenum that permits digestive fluids to leak into the peritoneal cavity, causing inflammation of the peritoneum (peritonitis).

The pylorus is the opening between the stomach and the duodenum. With peptic ulcer disease, pyloric obstruction may develop as a result of edema and scar-ring. Pyloric obstruction causes persistent vomiting that can lead to severe fluid and electrolyte imbalances.

Medical Diagnosis

Tests and procedures used to detect peptic ulcers include barium swallow examination, gastroscopy, and esophagogastroduodenoscopy. These studies, including patient preparation and aftercare, are described in the Diagnostic Tests and Procedures table on pp. 736 and 737. Gastric analysis may be done to determine the acidity of stomach secretions. However, the value of this test is in doubt. The test may be more accurate if pentagastrin is given to stimulate gastric secretions before collection of the specimens. Several laboratory tests are available that can detect *H. pylori* in a specimen obtained from a biopsy of the gastric mucosa. *H. pylori* also can be detected by antibodies in the blood or stool and by a breath test.

Pharmacology Capsule

Antacids are drugs and can have adverse effects if taken excessively!

Medical Treatment

The goals in treating peptic ulcers are to relieve symptoms, promote healing, prevent or detect complications, and prevent recurrence. Interventions include drug therapy, diet, and stress management.

Drug Therapy. Drug therapy is intended to relieve symptoms, heal the ulcer, cure *H. pylori* infections, and/or prevent recurrence. Anti-secretory drugs decrease gastric acid secretion, which relieves symptoms and allows the ulcer to begin healing. H_2-receptor blockers, proton pump inhibitors, and prostaglandins are examples of anti-secretory drugs. H_2-receptor blockers, which are the most commonly used anti-ulcer drugs, include cimetidine (Tagamet), famotidine (Pepcid), ranitidine (Zantac), and nizatidine (Axid). If *H. pylori* infection is confirmed, it is treated with various combinations of antibiotics, bismuth preparations, proton pump inhibitors, and H_2-receptor blockers. Multiple antibiotics are needed to prevent the development of resistant strains.

Antacids were once considered the first-line treatment for peptic ulcer disease. They do neutralize acid and prevent the formation of pepsin. However, they are no more effective than H_2-receptor blockers, which are more convenient and have fewer side effects in most patients. When used, antacids are usually ordered 1 and 3 hours after meals and at bedtime. Because antacids are available without a prescription, patients may think they can do no harm. In fact, they can have serious side effects. They also impair the absorption of many other drugs if they are taken at the same time. The patient should be cautioned to take the exact amount prescribed and not to adjust it on his or her own.

There are some other drugs that you may see prescribed to treat ulcers. Pirenzepine (Gastrozepin) is a unique anticholinergic drug that reduces acid secretion without serious side effects. Metoclopramide (Reglan) is a prokinetic agent that causes the stomach to empty more quickly, removing food and drugs that stimulate acid production. Sucralfate (Carafate) is a mucosal barrier. It clings to the surface of the ulcer and protects it so that healing can take place. It is used less often now than in the past.

In special cases, anti-secretory therapy may be continued as a preventive measure after the ulcer has healed. Misoprostol (Cytotec) and the proton pump inhibitor omeprazole (Prilosec) may be used to prevent ulcers in patients who take NSAIDs. Antacids, sucralfate, and H_2-receptor blockers are not recommended for this purpose.

Diet Therapy. The recommended diet therapy for ulcer patients has changed over the years. The current approach is to permit the patient almost any foods that do not produce discomfort. The patient is usually discouraged from taking in foods that stimulate acid secretion but do not neutralize acids. These foods include coffee, tea, meat broth, and alcohol. The effect of spicy foods is debated, but they should be excluded if they cause pain. Symptoms occur more often when the stomach is empty. Therefore frequent small feedings throughout the day may be recommended. The ulcer patient should be advised not to skip meals.

Managing Complications. Complications may be treated medically or surgically. If hemorrhage is suspected, a nasogastric tube is inserted and attached to suction to remove and measure blood in the stomach. After the stomach has been suctioned, the physician may use saline lavage to control bleeding. The patient is placed on the left side, and 50 to 200 mL of saline (traditionally, iced saline has been used to cause vasoconstriction) is instilled in the stomach through the nasogastric tube. The saline is then suctioned out, and the procedure is repeated until the returning fluid is clear and free of clots. Some experts now recommend that room-temperature saline be used to decrease the risk of damage to the gastric mucosa and to avoid stimulation of the vagus nerve. Vasopressin may be given intravenously to constrict blood vessels and control hemorrhage. Arterial embolization is a procedure that uses the patient's own blood and other substances to seal bleeding arteries. Once bleeding is controlled, antacids and H_2-receptor blockers are usually ordered at frequent intervals.

Perforation is treated initially with gastric decompression and intravenous fluids and antibiotics. A small perforation may close spontaneously. Otherwise, surgical repair is needed.

Obstruction may be due to edema and spasm, which often respond to medical treatment. A nasogastric tube is inserted to decompress the stomach, and intravenous fluids are provided. The nasogastric tube is clamped after 72 hours. If there is no evidence of continued obstruction, oral fluids are introduced. Continued obstruction requires surgical intervention.

Complications of peptic ulcer disease, signs and symptoms, related treatments, and nursing care are summarized in Table 38-3.

Surgical intervention is indicated to reduce acid secretion or for treatment of complications that do not respond to conservative treatment. Procedures that decrease acid secretion include vagotomy, pyloroplasty, gastroenterostomy, antrectomy, and subtotal gastrectomy. In extreme cases, total gastrectomy is necessary. Some of these procedures are described in Table 38-4 and illustrated in Figure 38-16.

Table 38-3	*Complications of Peptic Ulcer Disease*			
COMPLICATION	**SIGNS AND SYMPTOMS**	**TREATMENT**		**NURSING CARE**
Hemorrhage	Thready pulse, restlessness, diaphoresis, chills, oliguria, hematemesis, tarry stools, hypotension.	Saline lavage, vasopressin, arterial embolization.		Assist with procedure. Monitor effects of treatment. Monitor for water intoxication: headache, coma, tremor, sweating, anxiety. Monitor vital signs, intake and output. Maintain patent NG tube. IV fluids as ordered.
Perforation	Sudden, sharp midepigastric pain that spreads over entire abdomen. Rigid abdomen. Absence of bowel sounds. Shock.	NG suction, IV fluids, antibiotics.		Monitor vital signs, intake and output. Enforce NPO order. Give fluids and blood as ordered. Keep NG tube patent.
Obstruction	Feeling of fullness, nausea after eating, persistent vomiting.	NG suction.		Monitor vital signs, intake and output. Keep NG tube patent.

NG, Nasogastric; *IV,* intravenous; *NPO,* nothing by mouth.

Table 38-4 | *Surgical Treatment of Peptic Ulcer Disease*

OPERATION	PROCEDURE	PURPOSE	ADVERSE EFFECTS
Vagotomy			
Truncal	Vagus nerve that supplies stomach is severed.	Decreases stimulation of gastric acid secretion.	May have delayed gastric emptying. Feeling of fullness, dumping syndrome, diarrhea.
Selective or superselective	Severs that part of vagus nerve that stimulates acid production. Spares nerve supply to pyloric sphincter.	Decreases stimulation of gastric acid secretion.	Delayed gastric emptying.
Pyloroplasty	Widens pylorus.	Improves passage of stomach contents into duodenum. Usually done with vagotomy to prevent gastric stasis.	Dumping syndrome due to rapid emptying of stomach into duodenum.
Simple gastroenterostomy	Creates passage between body of stomach and jejunum.	Permits passage of alkaline intestinal secretions into stomach to neutralize gastric acid.	May actually increase gastric acid secretion.
Antrectomy	Removal of antrum of stomach.	Reduces gastric acid by removing source of acid secretion.	Diarrhea, feeling of fullness after eating, dumping syndrome, malabsorption, anemia.
Subtotal gastrectomy			
Gastroduodenoscopy (Billroth I)	Part of distal portion of stomach, including antrum, is removed. Remaining stomach is anastomosed to duodenum.	Reduces acid by removing source of acid secretion.	Dumping syndrome (less often than with other procedures), anemia, malabsorption, weight loss, bile reflux.
Gastrojejunostomy (Billroth II)	Part of distal portion of stomach, including antrum, is removed. Remaining stomach is anastomosed to jejunum.	Removes source of acid secretion.	Dumping syndrome, weight loss, malabsorption, duodenal infection, pernicious anemia, afferent loop syndrome (obstruction of duodenal loop).
Total gastrectomy	Removal of entire stomach. Esophagus anastomosed to duodenum.	Removes source of gastric acid secretion.	Can consume only small, frequent meals of semisolid foods. Pernicious anemia; dumping syndrome.

NURSING CARE *of the Patient with Peptic Ulcer Managed Medically*

Nursing care of the patient with peptic ulcer disease can be quite complicated, depending on the severity of the condition and the medical or surgical treatment. Therefore nursing care of the medical patient and the surgical patient are discussed separately (see also Nursing Care Plan: The Patient with a Peptic Ulcer on p. 770).

Assessment

Complete assessment of the patient with a disorder of the digestive tract is summarized in Box 38-1. Data collected by the LPN/LVN make an important contribution to the patient assessment. When a patient has peptic ulcer disease, describe the symptoms that caused the patient to seek medical care. Document the presence of pain, including location, aggravating factors, and measures that bring relief. Note the relationship between pain and food intake.

Important aspects of the past medical history include recent serious illnesses, previous peptic ulcer disease, and a medication history. Inquire about a family history of ulcers as well. Significant symptoms include nausea, vomiting, and indigestion. Ask if blood has been noted in vomitus and if stools have changed color or consistency. The functional assessment records the patient's usual diet, use of alcohol and tobacco, activities, sleep patterns, and stressors.

Begin the physical examination with general observations of the patient. Take vital signs to detect tachycardia and hypotension, which may indicate complications in the acutely ill patient. Measure height and weight. Assess the skin and mucous membranes for turgor and moisture. Inspect the abdomen for distention and palpate for tenderness. Auscultate for bowel sounds.

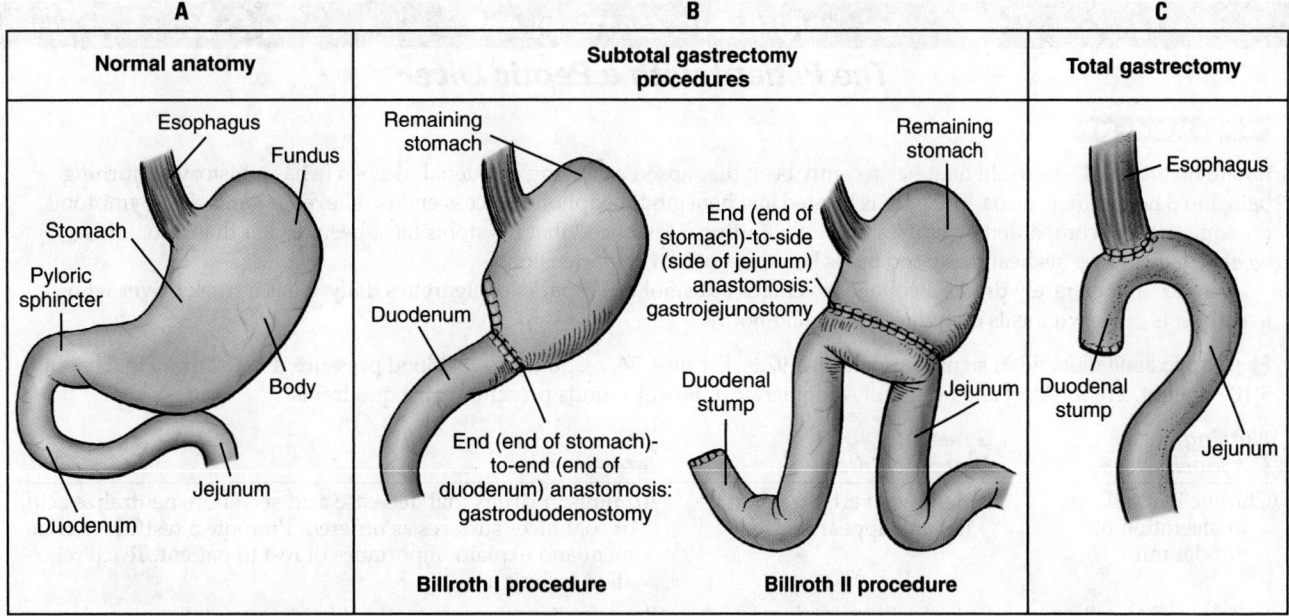

FIGURE 38-16 Gastric surgical procedure. **A,** Normal anatomy. **B,** Subtotal gastrectomy procedures (Billroth I and Billroth II). **C,** Total gastrectomy.

Nursing Diagnoses, Goals, and Outcome Criteria: Peptic Ulcer

NURSING DIAGNOSES	GOALS AND OUTCOME CRITERIA
Chronic Pain related to ulceration of stomach or duodenum	Pain relief: patient states pain reduced or relieved, relaxed manner
Imbalanced Nutrition: Less Than Body Requirements related to nausea, vomiting, anorexia, dietary restrictions, nothing-by-mouth status	Adequate nutrition: stable body weight
Risk for Injury related to hemorrhage, perforation, obstruction	Absence of complications: vital signs within patient norms; no vomiting, hematemesis, or tarry stools
Ineffective Coping related to prescribed alterations in lifestyle	Effective coping: adjustment to prescribed changes in lifestyle, adherence to treatment regimen

Interventions

Chronic Pain

The most important means of reducing pain associated with peptic ulcer disease are drug therapy, rest, and diet. Drugs reduce pain by neutralizing acid, decreasing acid secretion, or coating the ulcer surface. For maximum effect, give the medications at the recommended times. For example, antacids are most effective when given 1 hour after meals and at bedtime. Know the side effects of these drugs and monitor for them. Notify the physician if pain persists or worsens despite drug therapy. Rest reduces symptoms of peptic ulcer disease because physical activity stimulates gastric secretions. The en-

vironment should be as restful as possible. Encourage relaxation techniques and stress management strategies as described in Chapter 15.

Imbalanced Nutrition: Less Than Body Requirements

Dietary restrictions have long been part of the treatment of peptic ulcer disease. Many experts now question the impact of special diets on ulcers. When the patient has acute symptoms, a bland, low-fiber diet often is given in six small feedings. The reason for giving more frequent feedings is because the patient has less pain when there is food in the stomach. However, more frequent feedings also increase the total amount of acid produced. Experts do agree that patients should not consume a large meal shortly before retiring. The patient is advised to avoid any foods that have caused gastric distress in the past. In general, alcohol, tobacco, and beverages that contain caffeine are discouraged because they stimulate release of gastrin. The physician may advise the patient to adhere to a low-fiber diet with limited protein and calcium. Some patients tolerate decaffeinated coffee, but it contains peptides that also can stimulate gastrin release.

When nausea and vomiting are present, oral fluids may be restricted to clear liquids or the patient may be allowed nothing by mouth. Administer antiemetics as ordered. Promptly remove emesis basins and measure vomited fluid. If necessary, help the patient to wash and replace soiled clothing.

Risk for Injury

Monitor the patient for signs and symptoms of complications. Signs of bleeding are hematemesis (vomiting

NURSING CARE PLAN
The Patient with a Peptic Ulcer

ASSESSMENT

Health History: A 47-year-old man has recently been diagnosed as having duodenal ulcers. He has a history of burning pain 2 to 3 hours after meals. The pain is located just beneath the xiphoid process and is relieved by antacids. Symptoms are sometimes accompanied by nausea but not vomiting. He noticed that his stools have been darker than usual this week. He describes his health as good but is being treated for hypertension.

He states that he rarely drinks alcoholic beverages but smokes 1½ packs of cigarettes daily. He is a truck driver who usually eats only two meals each day, at irregular hours.

Physical Examination: Vital signs: temperature, 97.6° F; pulse, 76; respiration, 16; blood pressure, 136/82 mm Hg. Height, 5'10"; weight, 210 lb. Alert and oriented. Abdomen soft. Bowel sounds present in all 4 quadrants.

Nursing Diagnosis	Goals and Outcome Criteria	Interventions
Chronic Pain related to ulceration of duodenum	Patient will verbalize pain relief and appear relaxed.	Administer drugs that decrease acid secretion, neutralize acid, or coat ulcer surfaces as ordered. Promote a restful environment and explain importance of rest to patient. Teach relaxation techniques.
Imbalanced Nutrition: Less Than Body Requirements related to nausea, vomiting, anorexia, dietary restrictions	Patient will maintain adequate nutrition, as evidenced by stable body weight.	Provide diet as ordered: often bland, low-fat diet given in six small feedings. Administer antiemetics for nausea and vomiting. Monitor weight. Consult dietitian if patient is losing weight.
Risk for Injury related to hemorrhage, perforation, and obstruction	Patient will remain free of complications, as evidenced by normal vital signs and no vomiting, hematemesis, or tarry stools.	Monitor for signs and symptoms of bleeding: hematemesis, tarry stools, weakness, tachycardia, pallor, and hypotension. If hemorrhage occurs, notify physician and monitor vital signs. Perform lavage via nasogastric tube as ordered. Keep patient quiet, and enforce nothing-by-mouth order. Maintain intravenous lines to ensure venous access in emergency. Monitor for signs and symptoms of perforation: sudden, sharp pain in midepigastric region that spreads across abdomen, patient drawing knees up toward chest. If perforation occurs, notify physician and monitor vital signs. Withhold oral fluids. Anticipate need for nasogastric suction and intravenous fluids. Monitor for signs and symptoms of pyloric obstruction: persistent vomiting. Carry out orders, including nasogastric suction, intravenous fluids, and antibiotics.
Ineffective Coping related to prescribed alterations in lifestyle	Patient will express intent to implement lifestyle alterations.	Identify behaviors such as use of alcohol and tobacco that aggravate peptic ulcer disease. Explain effects of behaviors on disease. Offer information about resources (American Cancer Society, American Lung Association) that provide services to help patients give up tobacco.
Deficient Knowledge of self-care to manage peptic ulcer disease	Patient will correctly describe self-care measures to promote healing of duodenal ulcers and prevent recurrence.	Advise patient to avoid substances that stimulate release of gastrin: alcohol, tobacco, caffeine. Stress importance of taking drugs as prescribed. Explain side effects and adverse effects and their management. List drugs that are contraindicated: aspirin, nonsteroidal anti-inflammatory drugs, and corticosteroids. Supplement verbal instruction with written information. Encourage follow-up care.

? CRITICAL THINKING QUESTIONS

■ Why might antibiotics be prescribed for the patient with peptic ulcer disease?

■ Describe two relaxation techniques that could help the patient reduce stress.

blood) and the presence of blood in the feces. Blood that has passed through the digestive tract is maroon to black and causes the stool to have a sticky or tarry quality. Stools and vomited fluid may be tested for occult blood. When blood loss is significant, the patient may go into shock. Early signs of shock are weakness, tachycardia, and pallor. Hypotension is a relatively late sign.

If hemorrhage occurs, notify your supervisor or the physician and continue to monitor the patient's vital signs. Anticipate insertion of a nasogastric tube and saline lavage. Assist with the procedures, and reassure the patient. Keep the patient quiet; give nothing by mouth. Maintain intravenous lines, and record fluid intake and output. The patient may have to be prepared for transfer to intensive care or to surgery.

Perforation is characterized by sudden, sharp pain starting in the midepigastric region and spreading across the entire abdomen. Digestive fluids in the abdomen cause peritonitis (inflammation of the peritoneum). With peritonitis, the abdomen is rigid and tender. The patient tends to draw the knees up toward the chest.

When perforation is suspected, the nursing care is much like that provided for hemorrhage. Notify the physician, and monitor the patient's vital signs. Give nothing by mouth. Anticipate the need for nasogastric intubation and decompression and for intravenous fluids. The patient may be prepared for surgery.

The most prominent symptom of pyloric obstruction is persistent vomiting. The patient also may have signs and symptoms of fluid deficit and electrolyte imbalances. Insert a nasogastric tube for decompression as ordered. Administer intravenous fluids and antibiotics. When the nasogastric tube is removed, monitor the patient's tolerance of fluids.

Ineffective Coping

During periods of acute discomfort, patients are often receptive to measures that bring relief. Once acute symptoms resolve, however, many patients return to behaviors such as use of alcohol and tobacco that ag-

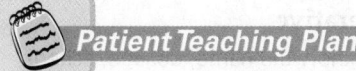

Patient Teaching Plan

Peptic Ulcer

- It is important for you to know the name, dosage, schedule, and adverse effects of each drug you take.
- Avoid aspirin, NSAIDs, alcohol, and smoking because they aggravate peptic ulcer disease.
- Your physician may recommend a specific diet that will decrease irritation to your stomach.
- Follow-up care is important to ensure that your ulcer is healing or has not recurred.
- Resources for stress management techniques and alcohol abuse (if appropriate) are available.

gravate peptic ulcer disease. Explore what the patient thinks about prescribed treatments and how they will affect his or her lifestyle. Resources to help patients who have difficulty giving up alcohol or tobacco are available.

NURSING CARE *of the Patient with Peptic Ulcer Managed Surgically*

Preoperative nursing care is like that outlined in Chapter 17 for any patient having major surgery. This section emphasizes the special postoperative needs of the patient who has undergone gastric surgery for peptic ulcer disease.

Assessment

Postoperatively, the patient should be assessed for pain, nausea, and vomiting. If the patient has pain, describe the severity (using a scale of 1 to 10), location, and related factors. Measure vital signs at frequent intervals until the patient is stable. Note the amount and type of intravenous fluids, and check the infusion site for swelling or redness. If a nasogastric tube is present, document patency of the tube as well as the color and amount of drainage. Inspect the skin around the nostril where the tube is located for irritation. Auscultate breath sounds. Inspect the wound dressing for bleeding. Once the dressing is removed, examine the wound for increased redness, swelling, drainage, and incomplete closure. Describe any drainage from the wound or from drains. Inspect the abdomen for distention and auscultate for bowel sounds. Monitor urine output and palpate for bladder distention.

Nursing Diagnoses, Goals, and Outcome Criteria: Gastric Surgery

NURSING DIAGNOSES	GOALS AND OUTCOME CRITERIA
Risk for Injury related to gastric dilation, obstruction, perforation	Absence of complications: vital signs within patient norms, minimal vomiting
Imbalanced Nutrition: Less Than Body Requirements related to decreased capacity for intake of nutrients	Adequate nutrition: maintains/ attains ideal body weight
Decreased Cardiac Output related to hypovolemia secondary to dumping syndrome	Normal cardiac output: no decrease in blood pressure after meals

Interventions

Risk for Injury

Potential complications of gastric surgery include gastric dilation, obstruction, and perforation. Gastric dilation results from accumulation of fluid in the stomach. The patient complains of feeling full and having epigastric pain. Tachycardia, hypotension, and hiccups may develop. Obstruction can result from edema at the surgical site, causing pain and vomiting.

A nasogastric tube is usually inserted preoperatively and remains in place after surgery. Specific orders for suction will be written. It is very important to maintain suction and drainage as ordered. Excessive fluid and gas in the stomach put pressure on the incision that could cause perforation. Perforation could result in hemorrhage and peritonitis.

After gastric surgery, *do not* irrigate or reposition the tube. To do so may cause the suture line in the stomach to tear. Nasogastric drainage is usually bright red immediately after surgery. The color darkens over the first 24 hours and then turns yellow or green. The tube is removed when peristalsis returns, usually on the third to fifth postoperative day. Document the presence of bowel sounds and the passage of flatus through the rectum.

Imbalanced Nutrition: Less Than Body Requirements

After the tube is removed, the diet is gradually advanced from water or ice chips to clear liquids, full liquids, and then to solid foods. Soft, starchy, low-fat protein foods are tolerated best initially. As the diet is progressed, assess for nausea, vomiting, or abdominal distention. Special dietary needs depend on the type of surgery. After subtotal gastrectomy, small frequent meals are given until the stomach stretches enough to tolerate three regular meals a day. After total gastrectomy, small, frequent meals of semisolid foods often are necessary for the rest of the patient's life.

Gastric surgery can have serious effects on the patient's nutritional status. The absorption of vitamin B_{12}, folic acid, iron, calcium, and vitamin D may be impaired, so supplements will be needed. Without vitamin B_{12}, the patient develops pernicious anemia. Pernicious anemia is more common after a total gastrectomy but can follow a subtotal gastrectomy. As discussed earlier, the parietal cells in the stomach produce intrinsic factor, a substance that is needed to absorb vitamin B_{12}. Vitamin B_{12} is essential for the production of red blood cells. When all or part of the stomach is removed, the patient develops a vitamin B_{12} deficiency and, eventually, severe anemia. The condition is easily treated with regular injections of vitamin B_{12}.

Decreased Cardiac Output

Some patients experience dumping syndrome after gastric surgery. For many years, dumping syndrome was explained as the result of fluid shifting from the bloodstream into the intestine. We now know that this was an oversimplification of the symptoms and that the fluid shift alone is not sufficient to explain the syndrome. The symptoms of dumping syndrome may occur in stages. In the first stage, the patient experiences abdominal fullness and nausea within 10 to 20 minutes of eating. These symptoms are thought to be caused by distention of the small intestine by the consumed food and fluids and the shift of a modest amount of

fluid from the circulation into the intestines. The patient feels flushed and faint, the heart rate races, and the patient breaks into a sweat as a result of pooling of blood in the abdominal organs. In the intermediate stage, the patient has abdominal bloating, flatulence, cramps, and diarrhea that occur 20 to 60 minutes after eating. These symptoms are probably related to the malabsorption of carbohydrates and other foodstuffs because of a deficiency of digestive enzymes. One to 3 hours later, the late stage may occur. The patient may perspire, feel weak, anxious, shaky, or hungry. These symptoms are blamed on hypoglycemia caused by an exaggerated rise in insulin secretion in response to the rapid delivery of carbohydrates into the intestine.

Dumping syndrome usually disappears within a few months. Meanwhile, the following directions for the patient will help:

1. Consume a diet low in carbohydrates and refined sugar, moderate in fat, and moderate to high in protein.
2. Smaller, more frequent meals may be tolerated better than three large meals.
3. Drink fluids between meals, not with them.
4. Lie down for about 30 minutes after meals.

Stomach Cancer

Pathophysiology

Cancer of the stomach is diagnosed in more than 22,000 people in the United States each year. The incidence is highest among males, people older than 70 years, and people of lower socioeconomic status. Asian/Pacific Islanders, African Americans, and Latinos are at greater risk than non-Latino whites.

Stomach carcinoma begins in the mucous membranes, invades the gastric wall, and spreads to the regional lymphatics, liver, pancreas, and colon. Distant metastases are found in the lungs and bones. Unfortunately, there are no specific signs or symptoms in the early stages. Late signs and symptoms are vomiting,

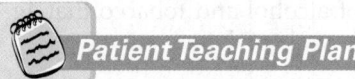
Patient Teaching Plan

Peptic Ulcer, Postoperative

- For each of your drugs, know the name, dosage, schedule, and adverse effects.
- After subtotal gastrectomy, eat small, frequent meals until your stomach capacity expands. After total gastrectomy, you will probably need to eat small, frequent meals for the rest of your life.
- Promptly inform your physician if you have nausea, vomiting, abdominal pain, or dark, tarry stools.
- Reduce the risk of recurrence by avoiding caffeine, alcohol, aspirin, and NSAIDs.
- If you are very stressed, try stress management techniques like relaxation exercises or seek personal counseling.

ascites, liver enlargement, and an abdominal mass. By the time late signs appear, the cancer is advanced and the patient's chance of 5-year survival is very poor.

Risk Factors

No specific cause of gastric cancer is known; however, various factors are known to increase a person's risk for this cancer. Risk factors include *H. pylori* infection, pernicious anemia, chronic atrophic gastritis, achlorhydria (lack of hydrochloric acid), type A blood, and a family history of stomach cancer. Some personal habits that seem to be related to stomach cancer are cigarette smoking, alcohol abuse, and a diet high in starch, salt, pickled foods, salted meats, and nitrates. Patients who have had the Billroth II procedure (gastrojejunostomy) also have increased incidence of stomach cancer. (See the Health Promotion Considerations box on p. 774.)

What Does Culture Have to Do with Stomach Cancer?

The incidence of stomach cancer in African-American males is higher than in whites. Also, culturally based dietary patterns (high intake of starch, salt, pickled foods, salted meats, and nitrates) increase the risk of stomach cancer.

Medical Diagnosis

Gastroscopy is used to examine the interior of the stomach and to take specimens for microscopic study. Other procedures that might be used to establish the diagnosis and extent of the cancer are endoscopic ultrasound, upper GI series, CT scan, PET scan, MRI, and laparoscopy. Laboratory studies include hemoglobin and hematocrit, serum albumin, liver function tests, and carcinoembryonic antigen. Stool specimens may be tested for occult blood.

Medical Treatment

Stomach cancer may be treated with surgery, chemotherapy, and radiation therapy. If the cancer is detected early, surgical options include subtotal gastrectomy with lymph node dissection and total gastrectomy. Sometimes part of the esophagus or duodenum is resected. In more advanced cancer, the surgeon may remove as much of the tumor as possible to relieve or prevent obstruction without removing the entire stomach. Gene therapy and immune-based therapy are in early phases of study and may someday prove useful.

PREOPERATIVE NURSING CARE of the Patient with Stomach Cancer

In the preoperative period, assess the patient's understanding of the condition and what to expect after surgery. It is important to know what the physician has told the patient so that conflicting messages are not sent.

Nursing care focuses on patient teaching. Inform the patient about the nasogastric tube and intravenous fluids, and teach coughing, deep breathing, and leg exercises. Identify and support the patient's usual coping methods. Include sources of support such as family members or a spiritual counselor in the preoperative care.

POSTOPERATIVE NURSING CARE of the Patient with Stomach Cancer

General nursing care for the postoperative patient is covered in Chapter 17. Special needs of patients having surgery for gastric cancer are discussed here. Chapter 25 presents general care of the patient who has cancer.

Assessment

Data related to comfort, appetite, and nausea and vomiting are especially important after surgery for stomach cancer. Monitor weight changes and determine dietary preferences. Identify the patient's support system and coping strategies.

Nursing Diagnoses, Goals, and Outcome Criteria: Stomach Cancer: Postoperative Care	
NURSING DIAGNOSES	GOALS AND OUTCOME CRITERIA
Acute Pain related to tumor or surgical trauma or both	Pain relief: patient states less or no pain, relaxed manner
Imbalanced Nutrition: Less Than Body Requirements related to anorexia, pain, nausea and vomiting	Adequate nutrition: maintains or attains ideal body weight
Ineffective Coping related to diagnosis of cancer, poor prognosis	Effective coping: patient verbalizes concerns, seeks and utilizes resources as needed, makes realistic plans

Interventions

Acute Pain

Give analgesics as ordered, but also employ other nursing measures to manage pain. Massage, relaxation techniques, and mental imagery are examples of measures to treat pain.

Imbalanced Nutrition: Less Than Body Requirements

Nutritional needs are much like those of the patient who has undergone surgery for peptic ulcer disease. When nasogastric suction is discontinued, oral fluids are introduced. If the patient tolerates clear liquids, the diet is gradually advanced. Small servings of bland foods are tolerated best. If dumping syndrome is a problem, it is managed with a diet that is low in carbohydrates and refined sugar, low in fat, and moderate to high in protein. Food is served in six small meals, and fluids should be taken between meals, not with them. Advise the patient to lie down for 30 minutes after eating. Monitor the patient's weight carefully. If weight is not maintained with oral intake, TPN may be instituted.

Ineffective Coping

The patient and family may need help in coping with this life-threatening illness. Encourage the patient to talk. Be accepting of the thoughts and feelings expressed. Guide the patient to think about changes that may be necessary in daily routines after discharge. If chemotherapy or radiation therapy is planned, the patient needs to know what to expect. Share information about community resources such as home health agencies or the American Cancer Society (www.cancer.org).

Health Promotion Considerations

Breaking the Link Between Diet and Digestive Tract Cancers

- People who have a poor diet, do not have enough physical activity, or are overweight may be at increased risk of several types of cancer. Overweight and obese individuals are two times more likely than healthy-weight people to develop a type of esophageal cancer called esophageal adenocarcinoma. A smaller increase in risk has been found for a specific type of stomach cancer that begins in the area of the stomach next to the esophagus.
- Having a healthy diet, being physically active, and maintaining a healthy weight may help reduce cancer risk. For example, the risk of stomach cancer may be reduced by eating whole-grain products and fresh fruits and vegetables that are high in vitamins A and C. The National Institutes of Health recommends the following:
  - **Eat well:** A healthy diet includes plenty of foods that are high in fiber, vitamins, and minerals. This includes whole-grain breads and cereals and 5 to 9 servings of fruits and vegetables every day. In addition, it is important to limit foods high in fat (e.g., butter, whole milk, fried foods, red meat).
  - **Be active and maintain a healthy weight:** Physical activity can help control weight and reduce body fat. Most scientists agree that it is a good idea for an adult to engage in moderate physical activity (e.g., brisk walking) for at least 30 minutes on 5 or more days each week.

Data from www.cancer.gov/cancertopics/factsheet/Risk/obesity and www.cancer.gov/cancertopics/wyntk/ overview/page4.

Patient Teaching Plan

Stomach Cancer: Postoperative Care

- For each of your drugs, know the name, dosage, schedule, and adverse effects.
- Eat six small meals a day, and drink fluids between meals rather than with meals.
- Notify your physician if your wound shows increasing redness, swelling, pain, or drainage.

If the patient is scheduled for chemotherapy or radiation therapy, explain what the patient can expect.

Obesity

Obesity is defined as increased body weight caused by excessive body fat. The term is used when a person's body mass index is 30 kg/m^2 or more. This number is derived by dividing body weight in kilograms by height in meters squared.

Causes

Factors related to obesity include heredity, body build and metabolism, and psychosocial factors. Although many factors may contribute to obesity, the basic problem is that caloric intake exceeds metabolic demands. Excess food energy is converted to fat cells, which are capable of great expansion. When fat cells reach a certain size, they divide to form new fat cells. Fat cells decrease in size, but not in number, when a person loses weight.

Many attempts have been made to explain why some people become obese. There may be a mechanism in the hypothalamus that regulates weight within a certain range. When a person's nutrient intake falls below the level required to maintain the set weight, the body conserves energy to maintain that weight. This may explain why some people always seem to return to a certain weight despite strict dieting and temporary weight loss.

Complications

Complications of obesity include cardiovascular and respiratory problems, polycythemia, diabetes mellitus, cholelithiasis (gallstones), infertility, endometrial cancer, and fatty liver infiltration. Obesity also aggravates degenerative joint disease. In addition, obesity can take its toll on the patient's emotional and social well-being. Very obese people may be ostracized and experience discrimination. Even health care providers sometimes treat obese patients as uncooperative and unmotivated.

Medical Diagnosis

Obesity may be defined based on the formula in Box 38-3 or by comparison with standard weight tables. The amount of body fat can be estimated by measuring skinfold thickness at selected body sites. The physician may order tests of endocrine function to rule out correctable causes of obesity. Additional diagnostic tests and procedures may be done to detect complications associated with obesity.

Box 38-3	*Defining Obesity*

Formula:

$$\frac{\text{Weight (in kilograms)}}{\text{Height (in meters squared)}}$$

Normal: 18.5 to 24.9 kg/m^2
Overweight: 25 to 29.9 kg/m^2
Obese: 30 to 39.9 kg/m^2
Extremely obese: 40 kg/m^2 or more

Medical and Surgical Treatment

The primary treatment of obesity is a weight-reduction diet accompanied by a planned exercise program. The ideal diet consists of foods from the basic four food groups and takes individual preferences into account. The calorie allowance may be as low as 800 calories a day. Amphetamines are effective in suppressing appetite but are not widely prescribed because their effects are temporary and they aggravate cardiac disease and hypertension. Other drugs that are available include benzphetamine (Didrex), phendimetrazine (e.g., Adipost), mazindol (Sanorex), Orlistat (Xenical), and sibutramine (Meridia). To be effective, drugs must be used in combination with diet and exercise. The antidepressant bupropion (Wellbutrin) is being studied for usefulness in weight loss.

When extreme obesity (sometimes called *morbid obesity*) persists over a period of years despite conservative treatment, surgical intervention (bariatric surgery) may be recommended. Bariatric surgical procedures are either restrictive or malabsorptive. Restrictive surgery reduces the size of the stomach so that the patient feels full after eating only a small amount of food. Malabsorptive procedures bypass a portion of the small intestine, which reduces food absorption. Restrictive procedures include the Roux-en-Y gastric bypass (RNYGBP), vertical-banded gastroplasty (VBG), and the lap-band system (LBS). The *Roux-en-Y gastric bypass* decreases the size of the stomach by creating a small pouch that receives food from the esophagus and then connects the pouch directly to the jejunum. This decreases the stomach capacity for food and bypasses much of the absorptive section of the GI tract. The RNYGBP is primarily a restrictive procedure; however, patients absorb less as well. It is one of the best tolerated procedures and has a low rate of complications. In the vertical banded gastroplasty, the stomach is stapled to reduce its capacity, leaving a small opening for food to move from the small pouch into the lower stomach. When the small pouch fills, the patient feels full. Because the pouch empties slowly, the patient feels satisfied and eats less. The LBP is the newest restrictive procedure. It involves the laparoscopic placement of an adjustable band around the fundus of the stomach, which creates a small pouch. The band contains an inflatable balloon connected to a port that is tunneled to the patient's abdominal subcutaneous tissue. The port allows the band to be tightened or relaxed as needed. The *biliopancreatic diversion* is the most common malabsorptive procedure. It involves removal of part of the stomach and anastomosis of the duodenum to the distal ileum. The shortened digestive tract absorbs less food.

Each of these procedures carries the risk of some complications. The Roux-en-Y bypass can cause dumping syndrome because food passes too rapidly into the jejunum. Deficiencies of iron, calcium, and cobalamin may require supplements. The biliopancreatic diversion is more likely to cause metabolic and nutritional complications. Vertical banded gastroplasty can cause persistent vomiting if solids are consumed too rapidly, distention of the walls of the functional pouch, rupture of the staple line, and erosion of the band into the stomach tissue. Simple gastroplasty ("stomach stapling") does not cause dumping syndrome or malabsorption, but weight loss is often less impressive.

Procedures that usually are done for cosmetic reasons include *liposuction*—the removal of adipose tissue through a suction cannula; and *lipectomy*—the surgical excision of flabby folds of adipose tissue.

 Consider the Alternative

Ephedra sinica (ma huang) is an herbal product that some people use as an over-the-counter (OTC) weight loss product. Caution patients that it stimulates the body, especially the heart and central nervous system. The side effects can be most dangerous for people with hypertension, diabetes, prostate enlargement, and seizure disorders.

NURSING CARE *of the Obese Patient*

Assessment

Assessment of the obese patient identifies factors that may contribute to obesity and explores the physical and psychosocial effects. If you are collecting data, record the patient's reason for seeking care. The past medical history documents pertinent chronic illnesses such as cardiac, respiratory, and orthopedic problems and diabetes mellitus. Ask about usual dietary practices. Identify factors that trigger overeating and reactions to overeating. Inquire about interpersonal relationships, stresses, and coping strategies. In addition, collect data about previous efforts to lose weight and current interest in losing weight. Some aspects of the

 Patient Teaching Plan

Obesity

- A balanced, low-calorie diet is more effective over time than a faddish, quick weight loss program.
- Eating habits must be changed or the weight loss will be temporary.
- Goal weight should be determined with the physician and the dietitian. Realistic goals for weight loss should be set at 1 or 2 pounds per week.
- A list of foods to include and those to avoid will be provided.
- Weighing food portions at the beginning of the diet makes you more aware of portion sizes.
- Physical activity is important for weight loss. With your physician's approval, gradually increase your activity as tolerance increases.

physical examination are more difficult when the patient is obese. It may be difficult to auscultate heart, lung, and bowel sounds. Having the patient lean forward or lie on the left side may make it easier to hear heart sounds. Accurate measurement of blood pressure requires a large cuff. Scales must accommodate heavier patients.

When collecting these data, it is essential to convey an attitude of respect and concern. Be aware of your personal feelings about obese people and consider how these feelings affect the nurse-patient relationship.

Nursing Diagnoses, Goals, and Outcome Criteria: Obesity

NURSING DIAGNOSES	GOALS AND OUTCOME CRITERIA
Imbalanced Nutrition: More Than Body Requirements related to excessive calorie intake for metabolic needs	Appropriate nutrient intake: patient attains ideal body weight
Ineffective Tissue Perfusion related to increased workload on heart	Adequate tissue perfusion: pulse and blood pressure within normal ranges
Ineffective Breathing Pattern related to restricted lung expansion	Effective ventilation: respiratory rate 12-20/min without dyspnea
Disturbed Body Image related to excessive weight, perceived unattractiveness	Improved body image: positive patient statements about self, good grooming

Interventions for the Obese Patient Managed Non-Surgically

Imbalanced Nutrition: More Than Body Requirements

Assessment of nutrition, the development of a nutritional plan, and patient teaching should be done by a registered dietitian. However, the nurse can reinforce what the patient has been taught. Before nutrition teaching begins, it is important to determine what the patient already knows and what he or she is motivated to learn.

Ineffective Tissue Perfusion

Monitor the patient's tolerance of physical activity. Tachycardia and dyspnea suggest that the patient's tolerance has been exceeded. When an obese patient is hospitalized for a medical or surgical condition, take extra precautions to maintain circulation and respirations. Position changes, deep breathing, and leg exercises reduce the risk of cardiopulmonary complications.

Ineffective Breathing Pattern

Monitor the patient's respiratory rate, effort, and breath sounds. During hospitalization, position changes and breathing exercises are especially important. The pa-

tient often breathes easier with the head of the bed elevated.

Disturbed Body Image

Demonstrate acceptance of obese patients by spending time with them, avoiding judgmental comments, and touching. Encourage the patient to identify solutions for overcoming perceived limitations imposed by weight. Acknowledge and compliment good grooming and attention to appearance and attributes other than physical size.

Interventions After Bariatric Surgery

After bariatric surgery, patients need the same care as any postoperative patient as discussed in Chapter 17. However, the needs of the obese surgical patient that require special attention are covered here.

Impaired Gas Exchange

Some obese people cannot expand the lungs fully because of the weight of fatty tissue on the chest. This increases the risk of postoperative atelectasis and pneumonia and makes breathing exercises and spirometry especially important. Elevating the head of the bed 30 to 45 degrees decreases pressure on the diaphragm. If the patient normally uses continuous positive airway pressure (CPAP) or bi-level continuous positive airway pressure (BiPAP) equipment for sleep apnea, it will be needed during hospitalization as well. Monitor results of serum electrolytes, blood urea nitrogen, and creatinine studies.

Ineffective Tissue Perfusion

The obese patient is at greater risk for deep vein thrombosis and pulmonary emboli when immobilized. Therefore early ambulation usually is ordered and the patient usually is treated with low-molecular-weight heparin. Be sure to have help when assisting the patient out of bed. Compression devices may be ordered. For the obese patient, the foot device may fit better than the long-leg device.

Impaired Skin Integrity

Skin and wound care are especially important for several reasons. The blood supply to adipose tissue is relatively poor, so healing is slow and pressure ulcers develop more readily. Also, tissue folds tend to stay moist, so the patient may develop candidiasis. Keep the skin clean and dry. Avoid talcum powder and cornstarch; instead, place soft fabric between tissues layers to absorb moisture. Moisture barriers may be needed in the perineal area.

Imbalanced Nutrition: Less Than Body Requirements

Before the patient can be fed, imaging studies are done to ensure that there are no leaks in the surgical sites in the digestive tract. The patient is advanced from water to clear liquids and then to full liquids. Initially the pouch will hold only 15 to 30 mL. Once solid food is permitted, the typical diet is 800 to 1200 calories per day in four to six small meals. The meals are high in protein and low in fat and carbohydrates. Multivitamin, calcium, and vitamin B_{12} supplementation may be needed. Dumping syndrome, which was described earlier, is a common problem. The patient can learn to avoid it by selecting appropriate foods in the proper amounts.

DISORDERS AFFECTING ABSORPTION AND ELIMINATION

Malabsorption

Malabsorption is a term used to describe a condition in which one or more nutrients are not digested or absorbed. Among the many causes of malabsorption are bacteria, deficiencies of bile salts or digestive enzymes, alterations in the intestinal mucosa, and absence of all or part of the stomach or intestines. The specific effects of malabsorption depend on the type of deficiency that is present. Likewise, treatment is directed at replacing deficient enzymes or avoiding substances that cannot be absorbed. Two examples of malabsorption are sprue and lactase deficiency.

There are two types of sprue: celiac (nontropical) and tropical. Celiac sprue is caused by a genetic abnormality. It is characterized by severe changes in the intestinal mucosa and impaired absorption of most nutrients. Tropical sprue is caused by an infectious agent and results in malabsorption of fats, folic acid, and vitamin B_{12}.

People with lactase deficiency do not have adequate lactase to metabolize lactose. These people are said to have lactose intolerance. Lactase deficiency may be inherited or acquired. Causes of acquired lactase deficiency include inflammatory bowel disease, gastroenteritis, and sprue syndrome.

What Does Culture Have to Do with Malabsorption?

Inherited lactase deficiency is most prevalent among African Americans, Asians, and South Americans. The dietitian should be contacted to help the patient design a culturally appropriate diet.

Signs and Symptoms

A common sign of malabsorption is steatorrhea, the presence of excessive fat in the stool. Stools are large, bulky, foamy, and foul smelling. Patients also may have weight loss, fatigue, decreased libido, easy bruising, edema, anemia, and bone pain.

Bloating, cramping, abdominal cramps, and diarrhea are symptoms of lactase deficiency that commonly occur within several hours of consuming milk products.

Medical Diagnosis

The diagnosis of sprue is based on laboratory studies, endoscopy with biopsy, and radiologic imaging studies. Lactase deficiency is diagnosed on the basis of the health history, the lactose tolerance test, a breath test for abnormal hydrogen levels, and if necessary, biopsy of the intestinal mucosa.

Medical Treatment

Sprue is treated with diet and drug therapy. Foods that aggravate the patient's symptoms are eliminated from the diet. Celiac disease is treated by avoiding products that contain gluten (wheat, barley, oats, rye). Severe symptoms may be treated with corticosteroids. Tropical sprue is treated with antibiotics, oral folate, and vitamin B_{12} injections.

Lactase deficiency can be treated by the elimination of milk and milk products from the diet, although many adults can tolerate small amounts of lactose without symptoms. Lactase enzyme can be mixed with milk or taken before drinking milk to avoid symptoms. Some milk and milk products that have been treated with lactase also are available. If milk products are limited, the diet must be assessed for adequacy of calcium, vitamin D, and riboflavin. Supplements may be advised.

NURSING CARE *of the Patient with Malabsorption*

Document the patient's symptoms. Note stool characteristics. In the case of celiac sprue, teach the patient how to eliminate gluten from the diet. Give antibiotics as ordered for tropical sprue. If folic acid therapy is to be continued, instruct the patient in self-medication. The effect of therapy is evaluated by the return of normal stool consistency. Advise the patient with lactase deficiency of dietary restrictions and alternative products.

Diarrhea

Diarrhea is defined as the passage of loose, liquid stools with increased frequency. The patient also may have cramps, abdominal pain, and a feeling of urgency before bowel movements.

Causes

Many factors can cause diarrhea. They include spoiled foods, allergies, infections, diverticulosis, malabsorption, cancer, stress, fecal impactions, and tube feedings. Diarrhea is an adverse effect of some medications.

Complications

Diarrhea is usually temporary and causes no serious problems. It does pose a greater threat, however, to the very old, the very young, and those in poor health. These individuals are more likely to become dehydrated and experience electrolyte imbalances and metabolic acidosis. Chronic diarrhea interferes with absorption of nutrients and can lead to malnutrition and anemia.

Medical Treatment

Acute diarrhea is usually treated by resting the digestive tract and giving antidiarrheal drugs. In the outpatient setting, the patient is advised to consume only clear liquids. A variety of liquids, such as broth, gelatin, and clear fruit juices, provide water, electrolytes, and some calories. Hospitalized patients may be allowed nothing by mouth and be given intravenous fluids. Severe, persistent diarrhea may require TPN. When diarrhea begins to improve, the diet gradually is expanded to include full liquids, bland solids, and then all other foods.

Consider the Alternative!

Natural substances that can help control diarrhea include rice water (made by boiling rice and straining the water), potatoes, and unpeeled apples. An herbal remedy is goldenseal, which is effective for diarrhea caused by some bacteria. High doses of this herb can cause dangerous CNS stimulation and uterine contractions, which contraindicate its use during pregnancy.

NURSING CARE *of the Patient with Diarrhea*

Assessment

Nursing assessment of the patient with diarrhea can help determine possible causes, the severity and progress of the condition, complications, and the effect of treatment. Therefore the data that you collect are very important. The history should record the presence of diarrhea and detail the onset, severity, precipitating factors, and measures that bring relief. Describe pain that accompanies diarrhea. Ask the patient about stool characteristics, including amount, color, odor, and unusual contents such as blood, mucus, or undigested food. The functional assessment focuses on usual diet, dietary changes, recent and current medications, and recent travel to a foreign country. It is also important to assess the patient's ability to get to the toilet independently or to call for assistance with toileting.

Important aspects of the physical examination include vital signs, weight, and tissue turgor. Tissue turgor is often assessed by gently pinching the tissue on the forearm. If the pinched tissue flattens as soon as it is released, tissue turgor is generally considered good. This test is not a good indicator of hydration in older adults because their tissue is less elastic, regardless of hydration. Palpate the abdomen for distention or tenderness, and inspect the perianal area for irritation. A rectal examination should be performed as agency policy permits if the nurse suspects fecal impaction.

Diarrhea is a nursing diagnosis, but other related diagnoses, as included in the following box, also may be appropriate for the patient with diarrhea.

Nursing Diagnoses, Goals, and Outcome Criteria: Diarrhea

Nursing Diagnoses	Goals and Outcome Criteria
Deficient Fluid Volume related to fluid loss from diarrhea	Adequate hydration: pulse and blood pressure within patient norms, moist mucous membranes, urine output equal to fluid intake
Imbalanced Nutrition: Less Than Body Requirements related to failure to absorb nutrients	Adequate nutrition: attain and maintain normal body weight
Acute Pain related to abdominal cramping and rectal irritation	Pain relief: patient states less or no pain, relaxed manner
Impaired Skin Integrity related to irritation of diarrhea stool	Intact skin: no perianal redness, lesions
Self-Care Deficit, Toileting related to weakness or decreased level of consciousness	Improved self-care ability: patient uses toilet independently and without injury

Interventions

Deficient Fluid Volume and Imbalanced Nutrition: Less Than Body Requirements

The prevention of serious fluid and electrolyte imbalances requires careful monitoring and replacement of fluid losses. When patients have severe diarrhea, keep intake and output records. Whenever possible, measure liquid stools. Stool characteristics are also important and should be recorded. Signs and symptoms that suggest possible fluid imbalances include unequal fluid intake and output; decreased blood pressure; changes in pulse rate or rhythm; changes in respiratory rate or depth; confusion; muscle weakness, tingling, or twitching; dry mucous membranes; and poor tissue turgor. These changes may indicate serious imbalances in water and electrolytes. They should be recorded and reported promptly.

If oral fluids are permitted, the patient should take 2000 to 3000 mL of various fluids each day. Carefully monitor the flow rates of intravenous fluids. Excessive or rapid fluid replacement can cause heart failure, especially in older adults.

Impaired Skin Integrity

Liquid stool is very irritating to the anal and perianal areas. With frequent bowel movements, skin breakdown may occur. Assist the patient, if necessary, with perianal care after each stool. Wash the area thoroughly and gently with warm water and mild soap, rinse, then pat dry with a soft towel. Protective creams, sprays, or lotions can be applied.

Acute Pain

Abdominal cramping associated with diarrhea is often relieved by antidiarrheal drugs that reduce intestinal activity. Record the severity, duration, and location of the pain as well as the effects of drug therapy.

Management and Supervision

Helping Certified Nursing Assistants Assist with Toileting

Because certified nursing assistants (CNAs) usually assist patients with personal care, they are most likely to assist with toileting. The CNAs should inform the nurse if the patient has difficulty with defecation or has abnormal stools such as diarrhea or stools containing blood, mucus, or undigested food.

Self-Care Deficit, Toileting

Frail older persons or those who are acutely ill may have difficulty with toileting during diarrhea episodes. If possible, place them in rooms close to the nurses' station. Staff should be aware of the need to respond promptly to call bells. A bedside commode is recommended if the toilet is too far from the bed. Patients who are unable to call for help must be checked frequently for the presence of diarrhea stools. (See the Management and Supervision box above.)

Constipation

The frequency of defecation varies among healthy people. Bowel movements may occur as often as two or three times daily or as seldom as once a week. If the stool is soft and is passed without difficulty, the patient is not constipated. Constipation is a condition in which a person has hard, dry, infrequent stools that are passed with difficulty.

Causes

Many factors can contribute to constipation. When stool is present in the rectum, the urge to defecate occurs. If the urge is ignored, stool remains in the rectum longer than usual and becomes dry. It is then more difficult, and sometimes painful, to have a bowel movement. People who frequently ignore the urge to defecate may become chronically constipated. The frequent use of laxatives or enemas also may contribute to chronic constipation. These agents keep the lower digestive tract empty and eventually interfere with the normal pattern of elimination.

Because physical activity promotes normal bowel elimination, people who are inactive are at risk for constipation. Inadequate water intake can lead to constipation because more water will be reabsorbed from the stool in the large intestine. Diet significantly affects the stool. A diet that is low in fiber and high in foods such as cheese, lean meat, and pasta promotes constipation.

Drugs that slow intestinal motility or increase urine output also contribute to constipation. Examples of these drugs are those used for anesthesia, pain relief, and cold symptoms. Medical conditions that may be related to constipation include diseases of the colon or rectum, as well as brain or spinal cord injury. Abdominal surgery causes a loss of intestinal activity, but it should be temporary.

Many people believe that constipation is normal for older people. Normal age-related changes in the large intestine do not explain the frequent complaints of constipation by older adults. More likely, when constipation does occur, it is related to inactivity, drug therapy, long-term laxative or enema abuse, or some medical condition.

Many older adults grew up believing that a daily bowel movement was necessary for health. If a day passed without a bowel movement, they used laxatives or enemas to produce one. Over time, this practice fosters laxative or enema dependence. Eventually, the person is unable to have a bowel movement without the laxative or enema. This dependence, established over many years, is very difficult to correct.

Complications

When people are constipated, they have to strain to have bowel movements. Straining occurs when a person attempts to exhale with the glottis closed, causing increased pressure in the chest and abdominal cavities. This is called the *Valsalva maneuver*. The pressure slows the flow of circulating blood back into the chest, causing a brief drop in pulse and blood pressure. Relaxation allows a rush of blood back into the chest with a resulting rise in pulse and blood pressure. The rapid changes in blood flow can be fatal to a patient with heart disease. Therefore prevention of constipation and straining is very important in the care of cardiac patients. Chronic constipation contributes to the development of hemorrhoids. Another complication of constipation is fecal impaction, which is discussed on p. 780.

Medical Treatment

Treatment of constipation is directed toward immediate relief of the problem and prevention of future episodes. Laxatives, suppositories, enemas, or a combination is ordered to get prompt results. The physician may prescribe stool softeners as well. Stool softeners, as the name suggests, promote normal elimination by allowing more water to be held in the stool so that it is softer and more easily passed. It takes several days for the effects of stool softeners to be seen, so they are not used for acute constipation. They are relatively safe drugs that are often prescribed over a long period of time. The trade names of some stool softeners are Colace, Surfak, and Metamucil.

Metamucil is an example of a bulk-forming stool softener. In the intestinal tract, it absorbs water to produce a gel-like mass to aid in the passage of a soft stool. If the patient does not take adequate fluids, the mass can harden and cause obstruction in the intestine. The Drug Therapy table on pp. 747 and 748 provides additional information about drugs used to treat constipation.

NURSING CARE *of the Patient with Constipation*

Assessment

The assessment of bowel elimination may detect constipation or risk factors that may cause it. Data that contribute to the assessment include the patient's usual pattern of bowel elimination, including frequency, amount, color, unusual contents (blood, mucus, undigested food), and pain associated with defecation. Note recent changes in any of these factors. Information about diet, exercise, and drug therapy is helpful in revealing potential risk factors for constipation. If any aids to elimination (laxatives, enemas, suppositories) are used, record the type and frequency of use.

Examine the abdomen for distention or visible peristalsis. Auscultate for bowel sounds in all four quadrants of the abdomen. When severe constipation is accompanied by mild diarrhea, a rectal examination should be done to detect a fecal impaction if agency policy permits.

Nursing Diagnoses, Goals, and Outcome Criterion: Constipation	
NURSING DIAGNOSES	GOALS AND OUTCOME CRITERIA
Constipation related to drug therapy, diet, inadequate fluid intake, inactivity, neuromuscular disorders, or laxative abuse	Establishment of normal bowel elimination: regular passage of formed stools without straining

Interventions

Constipation

The first action is directed at relieving the patient's constipation. Sometimes the physician will write an order for a laxative or an enema as needed. An enema or suppository is preferred if the patient is very uncomfortable because it usually acts within an hour. A laxative may take as long as 8 to 10 hours.

When a laxative is truly needed, it should be given. Laxatives are, however, often abused. Frequent use can lead to physical and psychological dependence. Laxatives also can produce diarrhea, which may lead to excessive loss of fluids and electrolytes.

Nurses are often responsible for managing the bowel elimination of severely disabled people. This is especially true in long-term care facilities. It is critical to record and describe all stools so that problems can be found and treated early. Teach nurses' aides the importance of keeping accurate records. If detected early, constipation may be treated easily with a mild laxative or suppository. Severe constipation may require repeated enemas and laxatives for relief.

In many cases, bowel elimination can be maintained with diet, fluids, exercise, and regular toilet habits. Occasional use of elimination aids is not harmful. Some patients, however, require nursing interventions to promote elimination over a long period of time.

Megacolon. Megacolon is a condition in which the large intestine loses the ability to contract effectively enough to propel the fecal mass toward the rectum. These patients usually need regular enemas for bowel cleansing. Other measures are generally not adequate. Patients who have special problems with constipation are those with neurologic conditions such as spinal cord injuries and cerebrovascular accident (stroke). The management of bowel elimination in these patients and the process of bowel retraining are discussed in Chapter 23.

Fecal Impaction. All nursing staff should understand the possibility of fecal impaction in the physically or mentally impaired person. Fecal impaction refers to the retention of a large mass of stool in the rectum that the patient is unable to pass. Some liquid stool trickles around the impaction and may be mistaken for diarrhea.

Suspect impaction when a patient who has not had a bowel movement for several days has repeated episodes of mild diarrhea. If agency policy permits, assess for impaction by inserting a gloved, lubricated finger into the rectum. The fecal mass is usually easily felt. It may be very hard or soft.

Remove the impaction following agency protocol or specific physician's orders. This process usually requires administration of a mineral oil enema to soften hard stool, followed by a soapsuds enema. It may be necessary to break up and remove the mass manually. This procedure is painful and embarrassing for the patient. With good nursing care, manual extraction should rarely be necessary.

Intestinal Obstruction

Causes

Intestinal obstruction can be caused by many factors, including strangulated hernia, tumor, paralytic ileus, stricture, volvulus (twisting of the bowel), intussusception (telescoping of the bowel into itself), and postoperative adhesions. When the bowel is obstructed, digestive contents cannot progress. Volvulus and intussusception are illustrated in Figure 38-17.

Signs and Symptoms

Symptoms are most acute when an obstruction is located in the proximal portion of the small intestine. Early symptoms of obstruction are vomiting (possibly projectile), abdominal pain, and constipation. Gastric contents are vomited first, followed by bile, and then fecal matter. Blood or purulent drainage may be passed rectally. Abdominal distention may develop, especially with colon obstruction.

Complications

Vomiting can lead to fluid and electrolyte imbalances and metabolic alkalosis. If blood supply to the intestine is impaired, gangrene and perforation of the bowel may occur. Untreated obstruction can result in shock and death.

Medical Diagnosis

Intestinal obstruction is suspected on the basis of the history, physical examination, and laboratory studies. It is confirmed by radiologic studies.

Medical Treatment

The initial treatment of obstruction is gastrointestinal decompression. A nasoenteral tube is passed and connected to suction. Intravenous fluids are provided. Depending on the cause of the obstruction, surgical intervention may be necessary.

NURSING CARE of the Patient with Intestinal Obstruction

Assessment

Assess the patient's symptoms, including pain and nausea. Describe the onset and progression of symptoms. The past medical history should include potentially related conditions, such as hernia, cancer of the digestive tract, and abdominal surgeries. Ask when the patient's last bowel movement was and if the characteristics were normal.

Take vital signs to detect signs of infection (fever, tachycardia) and impending shock (tachycardia, hypotension). Assess skin moisture and tissue turgor, along with moisture of the mucous membranes. Inspect the abdomen for distention and visible peristalsis; auscultate for rapid, high-pitched tinkling bowel sounds; and gently palpate for tenderness and guarding. Note rectal bleeding or drainage.

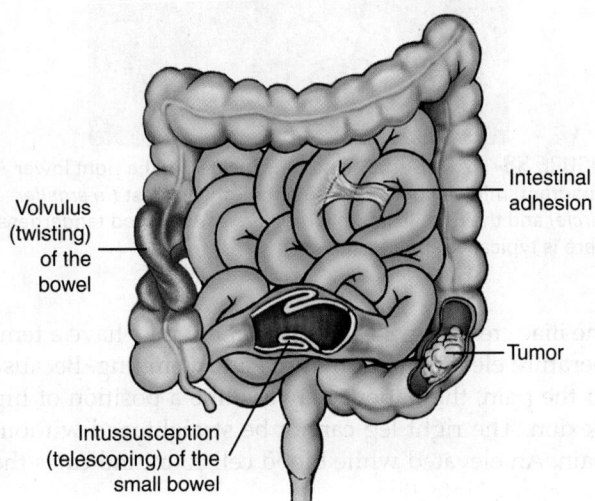

Volvulus (twisting) of the bowel

Intussusception (telescoping) of the small bowel

Intestinal adhesion

Tumor

FIGURE **38-17** Causes of mechanical bowel obstruction.

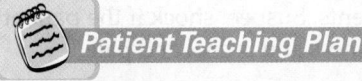

Patient Teaching Plan

Constipation

- Include high-fiber foods such as fruits, raw vegetables, greens, and whole grains in the diet.
- Drink six to eight 8-ounce glasses of water each day unless the physician has restricted fluid intake for some reason.
- Exercise daily. It need not be strenuous; walking is excellent exercise.
- Go to the bathroom promptly in response to the urge to have a bowel movement.
- Contrary to popular opinion, it is not necessary to have a bowel movement every day. A bowel movement every 2 or 3 days without pain or straining is normal for some people.
- Use a toilet that is comfortable. Feet should touch the floor, causing the hips to bend slightly. Use a footstool if necessary. This helps use of the abdominal muscles.
- Laxatives can be used safely for occasional constipation. If they are used frequently, however, they can interfere with normal elimination. Consult your doctor for a recommended laxative.

Preoperative Nursing Diagnoses, Goals, and Outcome Criteria: Intestinal Obstruction	
NURSING DIAGNOSES	GOALS AND OUTCOME CRITERIA
Acute Pain related to distention	Pain relief: patient states less or no pain, relaxed manner
Deficient Fluid Volume related to vomiting, intestinal suction	Normal hydration: pulse and blood pressure within patient norms, moist mucous membranes, equal fluid intake and output
Risk for Infection related to complications of obstruction	Absence of infection: no fever, respiratory rate 12-20/min, normal white blood cell count
Ineffective Breathing Pattern related to abdominal distention	Effective ventilation: respiratory rate 12-20/min without dyspnea
Anxiety related to pain, anticipated surgery	Decreased anxiety: patient states less or no anxiety, calm

Interventions

Acute Pain

Give analgesics as ordered and assess effectiveness. If the physician is withholding analgesics while making a diagnosis, inform the patient of this and use other strategies, such as massage and relaxation.

Deficient Fluid Volume

Promote fluid balance by providing intravenous fluids as ordered. Monitor vital signs and intake and output. If nasoenteral suction is ordered, monitor output and ensure free drainage at all times.

Risk for Infection

Monitor the patient's temperature. Signs of intestinal rupture (increasing tenderness, sudden sharp pain, abdominal rigidity) are reported to the physician immediately.

Ineffective Breathing Pattern

Elevate the patient's head to relieve pressure on the diaphragm. Encourage deep breathing and coughing. Administer oxygen as ordered. When surgery is planned, carry out preoperative orders, which often include giving an enema and intravenous fluids.

Anxiety

Give simple explanations of what is being done and what the patient should expect postoperatively if surgery is scheduled. Stress the importance of deep breathing, turning, coughing, and leg exercises.

POSTOPERATIVE NURSING CARE *of the Patient Treated Surgically for Intestinal Obstruction*

Postoperative care depends on the surgical procedure performed.

Appendicitis

Pathophysiology

The appendix is a blind pouch in the cecum. Appendicitis is an inflammation of the appendix. Inflammation occurs when the opening of the appendix to the large intestine is blocked by feces, tumors, helminths, or indigestible substances such as seeds. The tissue becomes infected by bacteria in the digestive tract. Pus accumulates, the blood supply is impaired, and the appendix may rupture. A ruptured appendix allows digestive contents to enter the abdominal cavity, causing peritonitis—a life-threatening surgical emergency. Early detection of appendicitis may permit treatment before the appendix ruptures.

Signs and Symptoms

The initial symptom of appendicitis is usually pain in the epigastric region or around the umbilicus, which then shifts to the right lower quadrant. The classic symptom of appendicitis is pain at McBurney's point, which is located midway between the umbilicus and

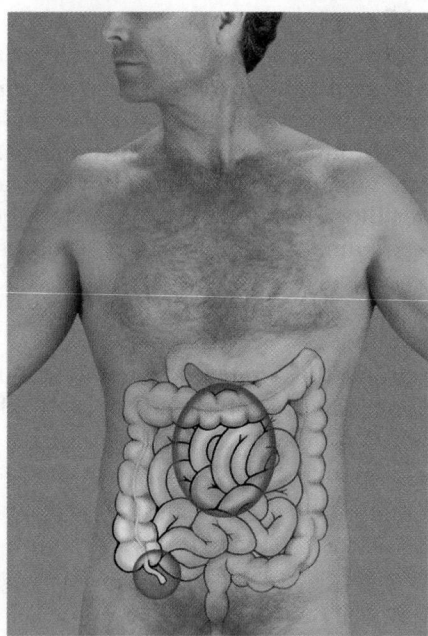

FIGURE **38-18** McBurney's point is located in the right lower quadrant, midway between the anterior iliac crest *(in smaller circle)* and the umbilicus *(in larger circle)*. Localized tenderness here is typical of appendicitis.

the iliac crest (Fig. 38-18). The patient may have a temperature elevation and nausea and vomiting. Because of the pain, the patient may assume a position of hip flexion. The right leg cannot be straightened without pain. An elevated white blood cell count indicates the presence of infection.

Signs and symptoms of peritonitis are absence of bowel sounds, severe abdominal distention, increased pulse and temperature, nausea, and vomiting. The abdomen may be rigid, although this sign is often absent with peritonitis in older patients. Suspect shock if the patient begins to lose consciousness and is cool and pale.

Medical Diagnosis

A diagnosis of appendicitis is based on classic signs and symptoms and a white blood cell count of 10,000 to 15,000/mm^3.

Medical Treatment

When appendicitis is suspected, the patient is allowed nothing by mouth. A cold pack to the abdomen may be ordered. Laxatives and heat applications should *never* be used for undiagnosed abdominal pain. If the appendix is inflamed, heat or laxatives may cause it to rupture.

If rupture has not occurred, immediate surgical treatment is indicated. With a ruptured appendix, surgery may be delayed 6 to 8 hours while antibiotics and intravenous fluids are given.

NURSING CARE *of the Patient with Appendicitis*

Assessment

The patient's chief complaint is usually pain. Describe the location, severity, onset, duration, precipitating factors, and alleviating measures in relation to the pain. In the past medical history, note previous abdominal distress, chronic illnesses, and surgeries. Record allergies and medications as well. The presence of nausea and vomiting is determined in the review of systems. Significant data in the physical examination are temperature; abdominal pain, distention, and tenderness; and the presence and characteristics of bowel sounds.

Nursing Diagnoses, Goals, and Outcome Criteria: Appendicitis

NURSING DIAGNOSES	GOALS AND OUTCOME CRITERIA
Risk for Infection (peritonitis) related to appendix rupture	Absence of infection: normal body temperature and vital signs, bowel sounds present, and abdomen soft
Deficient Fluid Volume related to nausea, vomiting, medical restriction of fluid intake	Normal fluid balance: pulse and blood pressure within patient norms, moist mucous membranes, serum electrolytes within normal limits, fluid intake equal to output
Acute Pain related to inflammation of appendix or surgical tissue trauma	Pain relief: patient states less or no pain, relaxed manner
Ineffective Breathing Pattern related to incisional pain or anesthesia	Effective ventilation: respiratory rate 12-20/min, clear breath sounds
Fear related to sudden emergency status, minimal preoperative teaching	Reduced fear: patient states less or no fear, calm manner

Preoperative Interventions

Before surgery, the patient will probably be most comfortable in a semi-Fowler or side-lying position with the hips flexed. Until the physician determines the diagnosis, analgesics may be withheld. The location and pattern of the pain are needed to make a diagnosis. Explain this to the patient. If rupture is suspected, elevate the patient's head to localize the infection.

Postoperative Interventions

Postoperatively, the patient receives antibiotics, intravenous fluids, and possibly gastrointestinal decompression. Assist the patient in turning, coughing, and deep breathing to promote expansion of the lungs. Incentive spirometry also can be useful. Show the patient how to splint the incision during deep breathing. Early ambulation is usually ordered to reduce the risk of postoperative complications. Assess the abdominal wound for redness, swelling, and foul drainage. Pro-

vide wound care as ordered or according to agency policy.

If there are no complications, the patient is usually discharged in a few days. Normal activities can be resumed in 2 to 3 weeks.

Peritonitis
Pathophysiology

Peritonitis is inflammation of the peritoneum caused by chemical or bacterial contamination of the peritoneal cavity. Chemical contamination may follow rupture of a digestive tract structure, including the appendix. Bacterial contamination may be caused by rupture of a digestive tract structure or fallopian tube or from nonsterile, traumatic wounds.

When a chemical or bacterial contaminant is present, the body's defenses attempt to wall off the area to contain the injury. Fluid shifts out of the bloodstream into the peritoneal cavity. Peristalsis slows or stops. If defenses are adequate, the offending fluid remains localized and is eventually eliminated. Complications of peritonitis include abscesses, adhesions, septicemia, hypovolemic shock, paralytic ileus, and organ failure.

Signs and Symptoms

Signs and symptoms of peritonitis include pain over the affected area, rebound tenderness, abdominal rigidity and distention, fever, tachycardia, tachypnea, nausea, and vomiting. The older patient may have more subtle symptoms with less pain and the absence of abdominal rigidity.

Medical Diagnosis

A diagnosis of peritonitis is suspected on the basis of the patient's history and physical examination. Diagnostic tests and procedures done to confirm the inflammation include a complete blood cell count, serum electrolyte measurements, abdominal radiography, computed tomography, and ultrasound. Paracentesis may be done to obtain a specimen of fluid for culture.

Medical Treatment

A nasogastric tube is inserted for gastrointestinal decompression. Intravenous fluids, antibiotics, and analgesics are ordered. Surgery may be done to close a ruptured structure and to remove foreign material and fluid from the peritoneal cavity.

NURSING CARE *of the Patient with Peritonitis*
Assessment

Begin by assessing the patient's present illness. Pain is the prominent symptom. Record the onset, location, and severity of the pain and any related symptoms. When peritonitis is suspected, record a history of abdominal trauma, including surgery. Take and record vital signs. Inspect the abdomen for distention and auscultate for the presence of bowel sounds. Note measures of fluid status, including tissue turgor, moisture of mucous membranes, and intake and output.

Nursing Diagnoses, Goals, and Outcome Criteria: Peritonitis

NURSING DIAGNOSES	GOALS AND OUTCOME CRITERIA
Acute Pain related to inflammation	Pain relief: patient states pain is reduced or relieved, has relaxed manner
Decreased Cardiac Output related to decreased blood volume	Normal cardiac output: pulse and blood pressure within patient norms, skin warm and dry, fluid output equal to intake
Imbalanced Nutrition: Less Than Body Requirements related to nausea, vomiting, nothing-by-mouth status	Adequate nutrition: stable body weight
Anxiety related to threat of serious illness and invasive treatment	Decreased anxiety: patient states anxiety reduced or relieved, calm manner

Interventions

Acute Pain

Administer opioid analgesics as ordered for pain. Position the patient with the head elevated, and provide comfort measures such as massage and relaxation techniques. Notify the physician if pain relief is not obtained.

Decreased Cardiac Output

The shift of fluid from the blood into the peritoneal cavity may be so great that the patient develops deficient intravascular fluid volume. Cardiac output falls, and perfusion of vital organs is reduced. Administer intravenous fluids as ordered, and monitor fluid intake and output. Monitor vital signs and report increasing pulse, restlessness, pallor, and decreasing blood pressure. In addition to deficient fluid volume, the patient may go into shock because of septicemia (the presence of bacteria in the blood).

Imbalanced Nutrition: Less Than Body Requirements

Gastrointestinal decompression usually eliminates nausea and vomiting, but antiemetics may be ordered as needed. Check to be sure that the nasogastric tube is draining at all times.

Anxiety

The patient is likely to be anxious because of pain and uncertainty about what is happening. Even when there is a sense of urgency in caring for the patient, give simple explanations for procedures and tell the patient what to expect. Encourage the patient to ask questions. If surgery is planned, essential preoperative teaching may have to be done quickly. Explain to the patient

the importance of breathing and leg exercises after abdominal surgery. The physician may order sedatives to calm the patient.

POSTOPERATIVE NURSING CARE
of the Patient Treated Surgically for Peritonitis

Postoperative care is like that for any major surgery and is described in Chapter 17.

Abdominal Hernia

Pathophysiology

Muscles play an important role in keeping the abdominal organs in place. Weakness in those muscles may allow a portion of the large intestine to push through the abdominal wall. The bulging portion of intestine is called a *hernia*. Hernias occur most often in areas where the abdominal wall is already weak. Weak locations include the umbilicus and the lower inguinal areas of the abdomen (Fig. 38-19). Hernias also may develop at the site of a surgical incision.

Hernias are classified as reducible or irreducible. A *reducible* hernia slips back into the abdominal cavity with gentle pressure or when the patient lies on his or her back. When the hernia cannot be manipulated back into place, it is said to be *irreducible*, or *incarcerated*. An irreducible hernia may impair blood flow to the trapped loop of intestine, causing it to become gangrenous. A hernia that is trapped and deprived of blood is said to be *strangulated*.

Signs and Symptoms

Hernias are usually diagnosed when a patient reports a smooth lump on the abdomen. The lump may disappear when the patient is lying down or at rest but returns when standing or straining. Heavy lifting or coughing usually causes the hernia to appear.

Hernias usually are not painful unless they become incarcerated. With incarceration, the patient has severe abdominal pain and distention, vomiting, and cramps.

FIGURE **38-19** Abdominal hernias.

Medical Diagnosis

Hernias are diagnosed on the basis of the health history and physical examination.

Medical Treatment

Surgical repair of hernias is usually recommended even if they are reducible. Repair prevents the possibility of incarceration. Two surgical procedures are used to repair hernias. Herniorrhaphy is the repair of the muscle defect by suturing. If additional measures are needed to strengthen the abdominal wall, a hernioplasty is done. Strong materials are used to cover and reinforce the defect.

Some patients cannot tolerate the stress of surgical hernia repair. For them, a truss may be advised, although trusses are not used as widely as in the past. A truss consists of a pad that is placed over the hernia and a belt that holds it in place. It provides support for the weak muscles.

NURSING CARE *of the Patient with Abdominal Hernia*

Assessment

Begin the assessment with the patient's chief complaint, usually a smooth lump in the abdomen that appears and disappears with various activities and positions. Ask about pain and vomiting, which may be present if the hernia is strangulated. Explore the patient's work and home responsibilities to identify the type of physical exertion required. The most relevant aspect of the physical examination is the assessment of the abdomen. Inspect for abnormalities and listen for bowel sounds in all four quadrants. If the patient wears a truss, inspect the skin underneath it for signs of irritation.

Nursing Diagnoses, Goals, and Outcome Criteria: Abdominal Hernia

NURSING DIAGNOSES	GOALS AND OUTCOME CRITERIA
Risk for Injury related to hernia strangulation or distention	Absence of injury (strangulation): normal pulse and temperature without abdominal pain
Impaired Skin Integrity related to pressure created by the truss	Absence of complications caused by truss: intact skin without redness under truss

Preoperative Interventions

Risk for Injury

Monitor the patient for signs and symptoms of strangulation (nausea, vomiting, pain, abdominal distention, fever, tachycardia). If these symptoms develop, immediately notify the physician. It is important for the nonsurgical patient to know that these symptoms should be reported.

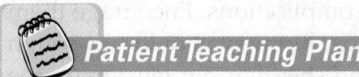

Patient Teaching Plan

Truss

- Put the truss on before rising each morning.
- Check under the pad and the belt several times daily for skin irritation.
- The truss does not cure a hernia, so you still should avoid straining.

Determine what restrictions the patient has in relation to physical exertion, and provide verbal and written instructions to the patient.

Impaired Skin Integrity

Teach patients who use a truss what measures to take to avoid injury to the skin.

Nursing Diagnoses, Goals, and Outcome Criteria: Abdominal Hernia Repair

NURSING DIAGNOSES	GOALS AND OUTCOME CRITERIA
Impaired Urinary Elimination related to abdominal surgery, anesthesia	Normal urinary function: urine output approximately equal to fluid intake, no bladder distention
Constipation related to immobility, effects of anesthesia, and abdominal surgery	Normal bowel elimination: formed stools at regular intervals without pain or straining
Acute Pain related to scrotal swelling	Pain relief: patient states less or no pain, relaxed manner
Risk for Injury related to wound dehiscence	Well-healed wound: margins intact, decreasing redness and swelling

Postoperative Interventions

The general postoperative care of patients who have undergone surgery is discussed in Chapter 17. In addition to the routine postoperative assessments, after hernia repair be especially concerned with assessing bowel and bladder elimination, wound healing, and the patient's knowledge about ways to avoid placing stress on the healing surgical wound.

Impaired Urinary Elimination

Many patients have temporary problems with urination after hernia repair surgery. Keep intake and output records, document voiding, and assess for bladder distention.

Constipation

Bowel activity also may cease temporarily in response to the anesthesia and manipulation of the bowel during surgery. Therefore monitor bowel sounds and note the passage of flatus. Like any other patients having major surgery, hernia repair patients need to keep their lungs clear to prevent complications. Encourage them to turn and deep breathe, but they should not cough or sneeze. Coughing and sneezing put tension on the surgical incision and repaired tissues.

Acute Pain

Scrotal swelling is common after inguinal hernia repair. A scrotal support and an ice pack can greatly reduce the painful swelling.

Risk for Injury

Activities are usually restricted for 2 to 6 weeks. Reinforce the physician's instructions about refraining from exertion and lifting. Advise the patient to report fever or wound drainage to the physician.

Inflammatory Bowel Disease

Pathophysiology

Inflammatory bowel disease (IBD) refers to both ulcerative colitis and Crohn's disease. Crohn's disease is also known as *regional enteritis*. In both conditions, there is inflammation and ulceration of the lining of the intestinal tract. With ulcerative colitis, the inflammation typically begins in the rectum and gradually extends up the bowel toward the cecum. The progression of Crohn's disease is different in that it can affect any area of the gastrointestinal tract. Although the terminal ileum is most often affected, there may be multiple sites interspersed with healthy segments of bowel.

The two conditions have similar symptoms and are treated much the same way medically. Surgical options, however, are different.

A patient with IBD may have a few isolated attacks or may have a chronic condition. With chronic IBD, attacks may last days or even months, followed by periods of remission lasting several weeks to several years.

What Does Culture Have to Do with IBD?

IBD is more common among Caucasians and people of middle-Eastern origin than among African Americans and Asian Americans.

Causes

The exact cause of IBD is unknown. Possible causes that are being studied include infectious agents, autoimmune reactions, allergies, heredity, and foreign substances. In the past, it was thought that IBD might be caused by stress. Current thinking, however, suggests that stress is the result of IBD rather than the cause.

Signs and Symptoms

The symptoms of IBD vary with the extent of the disease. When ulcerative colitis affects only the rectum, the patient may be constipated. More commonly, however, patients have diarrhea with frequent bloody stools and abdominal cramping. In severe cases, the patient also may have fever and weight loss.

Symptoms of Crohn's disease are even more variable, depending on the areas affected. If the stomach and duodenum are involved, symptoms include nausea, vomiting, and epigastric pain. Involvement of the small intestine produces pain and abdominal tenderness and cramping. An inflamed colon typically causes abdominal pain, cramping, rectal bleeding, and diarrhea. Systemic signs and symptoms include fever, night sweats, malaise, and joint pain.

Complications

The local complications of IBD include hemorrhage, obstruction, perforation (rupture), abscesses in the anus or rectum, fistulas, and megacolon. Patients who have had ulcerative colitis for 10 years have a greatly increased risk of cancer of the large intestine. Patients with Crohn's disease also are thought to have an increased risk of colon cancer, although the relationship is less clear.

Systemic complications also may be found with ulcerative colitis. These are conditions outside the intestine but related to the colitis. They include inflammation of the joints and eyes, skin lesions, urinary stones, and liver disease. Of course, severe or prolonged diarrhea can result in malnutrition, anemia, and fluid and electrolyte imbalances.

Medical Diagnosis

Inflammatory bowel disease is suspected on the basis of the history and physical examination. Abdominal radiography may be done to rule out obstruction before additional tests are done. To confirm the diagnosis, the physician may then order a barium enema examination with air contrast and colonoscopy with biopsy, ultrasonography, computed tomography, and cell studies. The video capsule that is swallowed by the patient provides a view of the small intestine that is not accessible by endoscopy.

Medical Treatment

Treatment of IBD addresses both the local and the systemic effects of the disorders. Intestinal inflammation is treated with drug therapy, diet, and rest. The drugs listed here may be used alone or in combination, depending on the specific situation.

- *Corticosteroids* to decrease inflammation in mild to moderately severe episodes
- *Immunosuppressants* to inhibit the immune response
- *Antidiarrheals* to control diarrhea EXCEPT in severe colitis
- *Anticholinergics* to reduce pain and gastrointestinal motility and secretions
- *Antibiotics* to treat mild to moderately severe attacks of Crohn's disease: usually sulfasala-

zine, mesalamine, olsalazine; sometimes metronidazole, ciprofloxacin, cephalexin, or sulfatrimethoprim. Antibiotics are not very useful for ulcerative colitis

- *Aminosalicylates,* specifically 5-ASA (mesalamine oral, suppository, or enema; or sulfasalazine), to reduce symptoms
- *Iron supplements* and *vitamin B₁₂* to treat anemia
- *Infliximab (Remicade)* to block the inflammatory process in Crohn's disease

Patients with ulcerative colitis are usually maintained between acute episodes with aminosalicylates; however, 6-MP is appropriate in some circumstances. Crohn's disease is less responsive to aminosalicylates, so the patient may be maintained on azathioprine or 6-MP.

Research is underway to assess the effects of other drugs including monoclonal antibodies and cytokine interleukin-10. Based on the low incidence of IBD among smokers, therapy with nicotine transdermal patches or gum also is being studied.

A low-roughage diet without milk products is prescribed for mild to moderate IBD. Intravenous fluids or TPN may be needed to provide fluid, electrolytes, and nutrients when symptoms are severe.

Although most patients respond to medical treatment, some require surgery. Removal of the colon (colectomy) is curative for ulcerative colitis. When the colon is removed, an artificial opening from the small intestine through the abdominal wall is needed to allow elimination of digestive wastes. The opening is called an *ileostomy.* Although good health is usually restored after this surgery, an ileostomy is permanent and requires special care. Therefore surgery is not usually done unless all other measures have failed. Care of the patient with an ostomy is covered in Chapter 26.

Surgical treatment of Crohn's disease is more likely to be removal of the diseased portion of the intestine. Recurrence is so common that surgery is not usually done unless necessitated by serious complications. Postoperatively, the disease typically reappears at the site of anastomosis within a year. Newly affected areas also may appear in other sections of the intestine.

Pharmacology Capsule

Corticosteroids suppress the immune and inflammatory responses, so the patient is more susceptible to infection.

NURSING CARE *of the Patient with Inflammatory Bowel Disease*

The nursing care of a patient during an acute attack of IBD is concerned with ongoing assessment, comfort measures, skin care, emotional support, and administering drugs and monitoring the effects. The nursing needs of the IBD patient who undergoes surgery are like those of other patients who have undergone gastrointestinal surgery, as discussed on pp. 744 to 745.

Assessment

Assessment of the patient with IBD should identify the symptoms that caused the patient to seek care—usually pain and diarrhea. Record the onset, location, severity, and duration of pain. Note factors that contribute to the onset of pain, such as specific foods or stressors. Also note the onset and duration of diarrhea as well as the presence of blood. Assess the impact of the illness on the patient's life, and explore how the patient copes.

Important aspects of the physical examination are vital signs, height and weight, and measures of hydration (tissue turgor, mucous membrane moisture). Inspect the perianal area for irritation or ulceration. Maintain accurate intake and output records. Measure diarrhea stools if possible and count as output.

Nursing Diagnoses, Goals, and Outcome Criteria: Inflammatory Bowel Disease	
NURSING DIAGNOSES	**GOALS AND OUTCOME CRITERIA**
Acute Pain related to abdominal cramping, perianal irritation	Pain relief: patient states pain is reduced or relieved, manner is relaxed
Diarrhea related to intestinal inflammation	Cessation of diarrhea: stools formed, less frequent
Deficient Fluid Volume related to diarrhea	Adequate hydration: pulse and blood pressure within patient norms, moist mucous membranes
Imbalanced Nutrition: Less Than Body Requirements related to malabsorption	Adequate nutrition: stable body weight
Ineffective Coping relate to chronic illness	Effective coping: patient reports strategies to deal with IBD; patient sees disease as manageable
Risk for Injury related to adverse drug effects	Absence of adverse drug effects: normal urine output, electrolyte and blood glucose levels within normal limits, no bruising

Interventions

Acute Pain

Perianal pain is treated with gentle cleansing, sitz baths, and skin protectants. Measures to relieve abdominal pain include administration of analgesics and antispasmodics and application of heat to the abdomen as ordered. Positioning, massage, relaxation, imagery, and other strategies described in Chapter 15 also may be used.

Diarrhea

Easy access to a toilet and prompt response to calls for help reduce the chance of episodes of bowel incontinence. After each stool, gently clean and inspect the perianal area. If bedpans or bedside commodes are used, remove and clean them immediately. Use room deodorizers to eliminate odors.

Prescribed drugs for diarrhea usually include antidiarrheals, antispasmodics, anticholinergics, antibiotics, and corticosteroids. The patient may be allowed nothing by mouth or may be given only clear liquids when diarrhea is severe. Bed rest may be prescribed, or the patient may just be encouraged to rest.

Deficient Fluid Volume

Severe diarrhea can quickly deplete the patient's fluid volume. Assess fluid status on an ongoing basis. Signs of fluid volume deficit are dry mucous membranes, hypotension, tachycardia, and decreased urine output. Administer intravenous fluids and TPN as ordered.

Imbalanced Nutrition: Less Than Body Requirements

The patient with ulcerative colitis needs to avoid only foods that worsen symptoms. For the patient with Crohn's disease, total parenteral nutrition and elemental enteral diets (e.g., Ensure) may be prescribed. The patient who is able to take solid food is usually placed on a low-residue diet without caffeine, pepper, or alcohol. Foods that are not allowed include whole grains, nuts, and raw fruits and vegetables. Consult a dietitian to teach the patient about the prescribed diet. Monitor weight on a routine basis.

Ineffective Coping

Inflammatory bowel disease is painful and stressful and can interfere with the patient's everyday life. Try to establish a trusting relationship with the patient. Encourage independence, participation in care and decision making, and realistic goal setting. People who have IBD may benefit from therapy that assists them with stress management. With the patient's approval, initiate a referral to a mental health professional or spiritual counselor. Report sadness and discouragement to the physician.

Risk for Injury

Nursing responsibilities in relation to drug therapy for IBD include administering the drugs, monitoring their effects, and teaching the patient about long-term drug therapy. Sulfasalazine is the antibiotic most often prescribed for patients with ulcerative colitis. It is useful in treating acute attacks and preventing future attacks. After an acute attack has subsided, the drug dosage is gradually reduced. A low-maintenance dose may be given for as long as a year. Teach the patient that discontinuing the drug early may result in another acute attack.

Sulfasalazine can cause crystals to form in the urine (crystalluria), which can damage the kidneys. Therefore patients taking this drug should take enough fluids to maintain a urine output of 1500 mL/day. A high urine output reduces the risk of crystalluria.

Corticosteroids are used in IBD for their ability to reduce inflammation. Unfortunately, this action also decreases the ability of the body to resist infection. Patients on steroids must be monitored for any signs and symptoms of infections. Instruct them to avoid unnecessary exposure to others with infectious conditions.

Long-term steroid therapy can have many other serious side effects as well. These effects include fluid and electrolyte imbalances, ulcers, increased blood glucose, weight gain, elevated blood pressure, acne, capillary fragility, and hirsutism (abnormal growth of hair).

Put on Your Thinking Cap!

Compare and contrast ulcerative colitis and Crohn's disease. How are they similar and how are they different?

Diverticulosis

Pathophysiology

Diverticulosis is a condition characterized by small, saclike pouches in the intestinal wall called *diverticula*. Diverticula occur when weak areas of the intestinal wall allow segments of the mucous membrane to herniate outward (Fig. 38-20). Most diverticula are found in the sigmoid colon, and there is usually more than one.

Risk Factors

Because diverticulosis is most common in developed countries, it is thought that lack of dietary residue is a contributing factor. Other related factors are older age, constipation, obesity, and emotional tension.

Signs and Symptoms

Diverticulosis is often asymptomatic, but many people report changes in bowel habits. The change may be

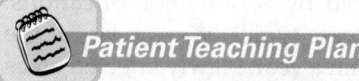

Patient Teaching Plan

Inflammatory Bowel Disease

Topics for patient teaching include the following:
- Stress-reduction measures are recommended to help control your symptoms.
- Because people with IBD have increased risk of cancer, you should have regular colon screening.
- You can facilitate digestion by taking small bites, eating slowly, and chewing well.
- Avoid caffeine and other irritating fluids and foods; consume a high-calorie, low-residue diet.
- You need to know the names, dosages, and schedules of your prescribed drugs and know what effects should be reported to the physician.
- Resources: National Foundation for Ileitis and Colitis (1-212-685-3440); United Ostomy Association, 36 Executive Park, Ste. 120, Irvine, CA 92714.

FIGURE 38-20 Diverticula in the sigmoid colon.

constipation, diarrhea, or periodic bouts of each. Other symptoms might include rectal bleeding, pain in the left lower abdomen, nausea and vomiting, and urinary problems.

Complications

Intestinal contents can lodge in diverticula, causing inflammation or infection. The patient is then said to have *diverticulitis*. Diverticulitis may be related to irritating foods, alcohol, chronic constipation, and persistent coughing. Symptoms of pain and bleeding are more severe with diverticulitis. The patient also may have a fever.

Possible complications of diverticulitis are severe bleeding, obstruction, perforation (rupture), peritonitis, and fistula formation. A fistula is an abnormal opening. In this case, it is most likely to develop between the colon and the bladder or vagina. The fistula permits bowel contents to pass into these other structures.

Medical Diagnosis

Diverticulosis may be suspected on the basis of the patient's symptoms. The stool is tested for occult blood. Abdominal CT and barium enema examination allow the physician to confirm the presence of diverticula. Because these procedures are invasive, they are delayed if there are signs and symptoms of acute inflammation.

Medical Treatment

Diverticulosis is currently being treated with a high-residue diet without spicy foods. Stool softeners or bulk-forming laxatives are used to treat constipation, and antidiarrheals are prescribed for those who have diarrhea. If pain is severe, it may be treated with an-

algesics. Opioids, especially morphine, should not be given because they cause constipation and may increase pressure in the sigmoid colon. Broad-spectrum antibiotics are often prescribed. Anticholinergics may be given to decrease spasms in the colon.

During periods of acute inflammation, the patient is placed on bed rest and given nothing by mouth. Intravenous fluids are ordered. Gastrointestinal decompression also may be instituted.

If symptoms persist and complications occur, surgical intervention may be necessary. The affected portion of the colon is removed. A temporary colostomy may be created to rest the colon while the surgical incisions heal. Sometimes elective surgery is recommended because the risk of surgical complications is much lower than it is with emergency surgery.

NURSING CARE *of the Patient with Diverticulosis*

Assess the patient's comfort and stool characteristics. Note any nausea and vomiting. Monitor the patient's temperature. Assess the abdomen for distention and tenderness.

Nursing Diagnoses, Goals, and Outcome Criteria: Diverticulosis	
Nursing Diagnoses	**Goals and Outcome Criteria**
Deficient Fluid Volume related to diarrhea and vomiting	Adequate hydration: pulse and blood pressure within patient norms, urine output approximately equal to fluid intake, moist mucous membranes
Acute Pain related to inflammation	Pain relief: patient states pain is decreased or relieved, has relaxed manner
Risk for Infection related to perforation	Absence of infection: no fever, normal white blood cell count, abdomen soft and not tender

Interventions

Provide fluids as permitted, and monitor the patient's intake and output. Give antiemetics as ordered for nausea. Analgesics and anticholinergics may be given as ordered for pain. Be alert for signs of perforation (fever, abdominal distention, rigidity). Teach the patient about diverticulosis, including the pathophysiology, treatment, and symptoms of inflammation.

If surgery is performed, the nursing care is similar to that described for any major abdominal surgery. General surgical care is included in Chapter 17, and care of the patient with an ostomy is discussed in Chapter 26.

Colorectal Cancer

Pathophysiology

Colorectal cancer, or cancer of the large intestine, is the third most common cancer in women. People at greater risk for colorectal cancer are those with histories of inflammatory bowel disease or family histories of colorectal cancer or multiple intestinal polyps. There is some evidence that a high-fat, low-fiber diet and inadequate intake of fruits and vegetables also may contribute to the development of this type of cancer.

Colorectal cancer can develop anywhere in the large intestine. Three fourths of all colorectal cancers are located in the rectum or lower sigmoid colon (Fig. 38-21). These portions of the intestine are easy to examine with a sigmoidoscope. Therefore sigmoidoscopy is often included in the routine physical examinations of older adults.

Signs and Symptoms

Signs and symptoms of colorectal cancer depend on the location of the disease. In the early stages, symptoms are usually mild. If the cancer is located on the right side of the abdomen, the patient may have only vague cramping until the disease is advanced. Unexplained anemia, weakness, and fatigue related to blood loss may be the only early symptoms of right-sided colon cancer.

Cancers on the left side or in the rectum cause more obvious changes in bowel function. Patients may develop diarrhea or constipation and may notice blood in the stool. Stools may become very narrow, causing them to be described as pencil-like. This is due to pressure on the bowel from the growing tumor, which causes a narrowed lumen. The patient may report a feeling of fullness or pressure in the abdomen or rectum. If untreated, obstruction of the bowel eventually occurs regardless of the tumor site.

Medical and Surgical Treatment

Colorectal cancers usually are treated surgically. The exact surgical procedure depends on the location and extent of the cancer. For cancers above the rectum, the diseased portion of the intestine often can be removed.

The healthy ends of the remaining intestine are then anastomosed (connected).

Rectal cancers often require more extensive surgery, with incisions in both the abdomen and the perineum (abdominoperineal resection). With removal of the rectum, a permanent colostomy may be created for fecal elimination. However, relatively new procedures may be used to attach the rectal stump to the anus in patients with certain rectal cancers. When this is possible, normal bowel elimination can be maintained and a colostomy can be avoided.

Combination chemotherapy may be recommended postoperatively if the tumor extends through the bowel wall or if lymph nodes are involved. Early-stage rectal cancer is sometimes treated with radiation and surgery.

NURSING CARE *of the Patient with Colorectal Cancer*

Because the primary treatment for colon cancer is surgery, nursing care focuses on the surgical patient. Preoperative care includes bowel preparation, hydration, emotional support, and teaching postoperative routines to prevent surgical complications. Care of the patient with an ostomy is covered in Chapter 26, and care of patients receiving radiation or chemotherapy is covered in Chapter 25.

Assessment

In the postoperative period, assess vital signs, intake and output, breath sounds, bowel sounds, and pain. Describe the appearance of wounds and wound drainage. If there is a colostomy, measure and describe the fecal drainage. Assess the patient's reactions to the surgical procedure and any other anticipated therapies.

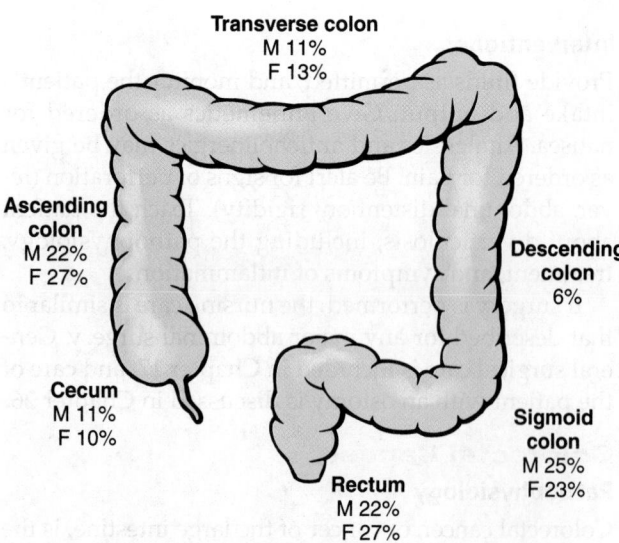

Ascending colon
M 22%
F 27%

Transverse colon
M 11%
F 13%

Descending colon
6%

Cecum
M 11%
F 10%

Sigmoid colon
M 25%
F 23%

Rectum
M 22%
F 27%

FIGURE **38-21** Sites of colorectal cancer.

Nursing Diagnoses, Goals, and Outcome Criteria: Colorectal Cancer	
NURSING DIAGNOSES	GOALS AND OUTCOME CRITERIA
Risk for Injury related to extensive surgical trauma, open wounds	Wound healing without infection: no fever, intact wound margins without excessive redness
Ineffective Tissue Perfusion related to effects of anesthesia, immobility	Adequate tissue perfusion: vital signs consistent with patient baseline norms
Acute Pain related to tissue trauma	Pain relief: patient states less or no pain, relaxed manner
Sexual Dysfunction related to perineal surgery	Patient understanding of potential sexual dysfunction: patient describes possible problems and corrective measures
Ineffective Coping related to life-threatening illness	Effective coping: patient uses strategies that promote adaptation to illness

Interventions

Risk for Injury

The nursing care of a patient after an abdominoperineal resection is very demanding. The patient has three incisions: one on the abdomen, a second for the colostomy, and a third on the perineum. Check all three for bleeding or drainage. The perineal wound normally drains a large amount of serosanguineous fluid. Serosanguineous fluid is made up of serum and blood. It is a pinkish color and thin in consistency. The wound may be open and packed, partly closed with Penrose drains, or closed and drained with a suction device. An example of a suction drainage system is the Jackson-Pratt drain and fluid collection device. Dressings should initially be reinforced when saturated. Disposable waterproof pads under the patient's hips protect bedding and can easily be changed. A T-binder holds the perineal dressing securely in place.

With so many wounds, especially open ones, these patients are at great risk for infection. Any handling of wound dressings should be done wearing sterile gloves. Always assess the wound for signs of infection (unusual odor, excessive redness or swelling around the wound, purulent drainage).

If there is packing in a wound, it will be removed gradually. Once the packing has been completely removed, the physician may order the wound to be irrigated on a regular schedule. Gentle irrigations promote healing by keeping the wound clean. Use strict sterile technique during wound irrigations.

Ineffective Tissue Perfusion

Because the abdominoperineal resection requires several incisions and is a lengthy procedure, the patient is at risk for respiratory and circulatory complications. Coughing, deep breathing, and incentive spirometry help prevent fluid accumulation in the lungs. Encourage and help the patient change positions at least every 2 hours. Leg exercises are important because the pressure on abdominal blood vessels during the long surgery may contribute to the formation of blood clots in the legs.

Acute Pain

Pain is severe for several postoperative days. Give opioid analgesics as ordered. If they do not provide relief, inform the physician. In addition to drug therapy, try comfort measures such as position changes and back rubs. At first, the patient will probably be most comfortable in a side-lying position. Later, he or she will be able to tolerate being supine as well.

When the patient is allowed to be up, sitz baths may be ordered several times a day. The warm water cleans, soothes, and increases circulation to the perineum. Supervise the patient in the sitz bath the first few times in case of dizziness or faintness.

Sexual Dysfunction

Extensive perineal surgery can cause various types of sexual dysfunction. Be open and sensitive to questions that the patient may bring up about sexual function. Refer questions about the specific effects of particular surgical procedures on sexual function to the physician. This is not to say that you should dismiss or ignore patient concerns about sexuality but to stress that the information given must be accurate. Once the correct answers are known, the nurse can reinforce them.

Ineffective Coping

Patients with colorectal cancer and their families often face a difficult period of adjustment. For many people, the thought of having cancer brings up fears of pain, suffering, and a lingering death. These fears may not surface until after the patient recovers from the acute postoperative period. The nurse can help by encouraging the patient to express fears and ask questions and by being a kind listener. Referrals to mental health or spiritual counselors or to support groups can be helpful.

While learning to deal with changes in body image and the threat of a potentially deadly disease, the patient may be faced with receiving chemotherapy as well. Most patients have heard about the side effects of the powerful drugs used in chemotherapy, and they may be justifiably fearful of the treatments. The nursing care of patients receiving chemotherapy is discussed in detail in Chapter 25.

Polyps

Polyps are small growths in the intestine. Most are benign, but they can become malignant. Two inherited syndromes, familial polyposis and Gardner's syndrome, are characterized by multiple colorectal polyps and almost always lead to cancer. Polyps are usually asymptomatic

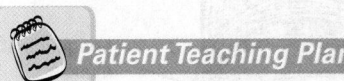

Patient Teaching Plan

Colorectal Cancer

As the patient improves, the nurse needs to consider long-term needs. The teaching plan should include the following:
* Wound care.
* Colostomy care (see Chapter 26).
* Information about resources for treatment of sexual dysfunction (if appropriate).
* Your diet should be high in fiber. Avoid irritating foods and alcohol.
* For each of your medications, know the drug names, dosages, schedule, and adverse effects.
* Symptoms of inflammation are bleeding, fever, and increased pain; promptly notify the physician if these occur.
* Resources: Enterostomal therapist (a nurse who is expert in the care of patients with ostomies); United Ostomy Association, 38 Executive Park, Ste. 120, Irvine, CA 92714.

and are found on routine testing. Potential complications are bleeding and obstruction. Polyps are diagnosed by a barium enema examination or an endoscopic examination. Some of the growths can be removed during the endoscopic examination. Colectomy may be advised for patients with familial polyposis or Gardner's syndrome because of the high risk of malignancy.

Encourage patients who are at risk for cancer to seek medical attention. If the patient has surgery, the postoperative care is similar to that of the patient with cancer of the colon. If a colostomy is created, the patient needs special support and teaching, as described in Chapter 26.

Hemorrhoids

Hemorrhoids are dilated veins in the rectum. They may be above the sphincter muscles of the anus (internal hemorrhoids) or below these muscles (external hemorrhoids) (Fig. 38-22). If blood clots form in external hemorrhoids, they become inflamed and very painful. Hemorrhoids containing clotted blood are said to be *thrombosed*.

Risk Factors

A key factor in the development of hemorrhoids is increased pressure in the rectal blood vessels. Pressure is increased by constipation, pregnancy, and prolonged sitting or standing.

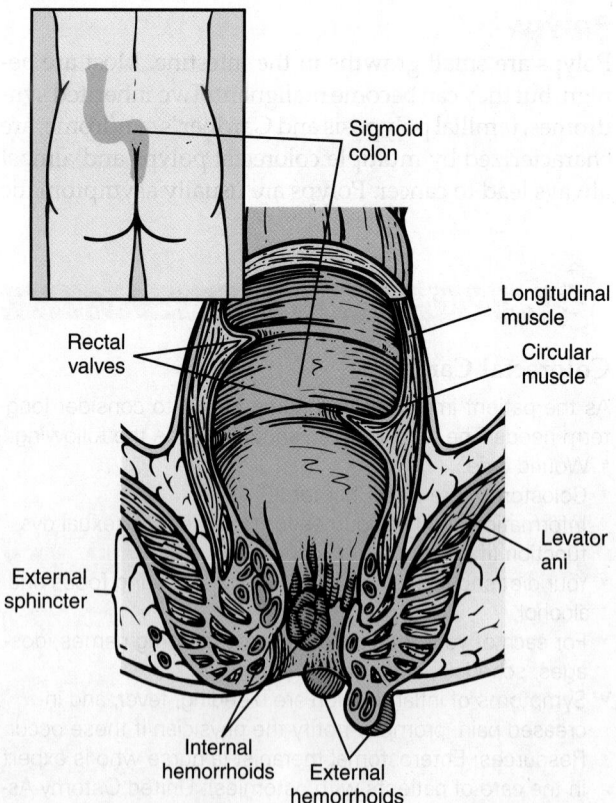

FIGURE **38-22** Internal and external hemorrhoids.

Labels: Sigmoid colon, Longitudinal muscle, Circular muscle, Rectal valves, Levator ani, External sphincter, Internal hemorrhoids, External hemorrhoids

Signs and Symptoms

The most common symptoms of hemorrhoids are rectal pain and itching. Bleeding may occur with defecation, especially if the hemorrhoids are internal. External hemorrhoids are easy to see and appear red or bluish.

Consider the Alternative

Witch hazel compresses applied to the anus after each bowel movement are soothing.

Medical Diagnosis and Treatment

Hemorrhoids are diagnosed upon visual inspection. Nonsurgical treatment of hemorrhoids attempts to relieve pain, swelling, and pressure. Topical medications such as creams, lotions, or suppositories may be ordered to soothe and shrink inflamed tissue. Sitz baths are often comforting. The physician may order heat or cold applications. Sometimes, especially with thrombosed hemorrhoids, ice packs may be applied for a few hours, followed by warm packs.

Outpatient procedures for removing hemorrhoids include the following:

- Ligation—tying off with rubber bands. The bands cut off the blood supply so that the vessels shrink and die. Dead tissue eventually breaks off and is eliminated.
- Sclerotherapy—the injection of an agent into the tissue around the hemorrhoids that causes them to shrink; results often are temporary.
- Thermocoagulation and electrocoagulation—use of different types of devices to remove the hemorrhoid.
- Laser surgery—effective, but more expensive and risky.

A hemorrhoidectomy is the surgical excision (removal) of hemorrhoids. It is necessary when symptoms are very severe. After the hemorrhoids are removed, the wound may be closed with sutures or packed and left open to heal.

NURSING CARE *of the Patient with Hemorrhoids*

Medical management of hemorrhoids usually does not require hospitalization. Therefore this section emphasizes the care of the surgical patient. Preoperative care includes bowel preparation and patient teaching of postoperative measures to prevent complications of immobility and anesthesia.

Assessment

After hemorrhoidectomy, monitor vital signs, intake and output, and breath sounds. Assess the perianal area for bleeding and drainage.

Interventions

Acute Pain

Hemorrhoidectomy patients have severe postoperative pain that requires opioid analgesics for relief. Cold packs over the rectal dressing may be ordered initially. Imagery and relaxation techniques also may help control pain.

Impaired Skin Integrity

The physician removes the wound packing a day or two after surgery. After the packing is removed, assess for rectal bleeding. Sitz baths may then be ordered to soothe and clean the area and to promote circulation. Provide a soft pad or cushion for more comfortable sitting.

Constipation

It is especially important to assess and record any stools passed after rectal surgery. The patient probably will dread the first bowel movement, expecting severe pain. Stool softeners probably will be ordered to reduce the trauma of defecation. Pain medication can be given as ordered before the patient tries to defecate. Someone should stay close by in case the patient feels weak or faint.

Anorectal Abscess

An anorectal abscess is an infection in the tissue around the rectum. Signs and symptoms are rectal pain, swelling, redness, and tenderness. The patient often reports a history of diarrhea. If the abscess becomes chronic, it causes bleeding, itching, and discharge.

Anorectal abscess is treated with antibiotics followed by incision and drainage. The procedure may be done under local or general anesthesia, depending on how extensive the abscess is. Preoperatively, pain is treated with ice packs, sitz baths, and topical agents as ordered. Postoperatively, the nursing care is similar to that after hemorrhoidectomy. Pain is treated with opioid analgesics. Patient teaching emphasizes the importance of thorough cleansing after each bowel movement. Advise the patient to consume adequate fluids and a high-fiber diet to promote soft stools.

Anal Fissure

An anal fissure is a laceration between the anal canal and the perianal skin. Fissures may be related to constipation, diarrhea, Crohn's disease, tuberculosis, leukemia, trauma, or childbirth. Sometimes there is no apparent cause. Signs and symptoms include pain before and after defecation and bleeding on the stool or tissue. If the fissure becomes chronic, the patient may experience pruritus, urinary frequency or retention, and dysuria. Fissures usually heal spontaneously, but they can become chronic. Conservative treatment of anal fissures employs sitz baths, stool softeners, and analgesics. Surgical excision may be necessary. Postoperatively, instruct the patient to cleanse the perianal area after defecation. Pain relief measures and stool softeners are continued.

Anal Fistula

An anal fistula is an abnormal opening between the anal canal and the perianal skin. Fistulas can develop from anorectal abscesses or may be related to inflammatory bowel disease or tuberculosis. The patient typically complains of pruritus and discharge. Sitz baths provide some comfort. The surgical treatment is excision of the fistula and surrounding tissue. Sometimes a temporary colostomy is done to allow the surgical site to heal. Postoperative care includes analgesics and sitz baths for pain.

Pilonidal Cyst

A pilonidal cyst is located in the sacrococcygeal area. It appears to result from an in-folding of skin causing a sinus that is easily infected because of its closeness to the anus. Once infected, it is painful and swollen and may form an abscess. Surgical excision is usually recommended. Care is similar to that for the patient having a hemorrhoidectomy.

Patient Teaching Plan

Hemorrhoids, Postoperative Care

- Notify your surgeon if you have fever or bleeding.
- To prevent recurrence, avoid constipation, prolonged sitting or standing, and straining to have a bowel movement.
- Ingest a high-fiber diet with plenty of fluids to promote regular, soft stools.
- Use stool softeners if prescribed.
- Follow a regular pattern of bowel elimination, and do not delay defecation when the urge occurs.
- Follow the activity limitations prescribed by your physician.

PATIENT EDUCATION TO PROMOTE NORMAL BOWEL FUNCTION

You often have the opportunity to teach patients how to promote normal bowel function and detect problems early. Acute gastrointestinal disorders can be caused by irritants or infectious agents. Identify and avoid foods that create distress.

Good hand washing and proper food handling reduce the ingestion of infectious agents. Food poisoning can be acquired from food that has been improperly stored, poorly cooked, or exposed to contaminated containers or utensils.

Food poisoning is often a problem for frail older adults who live at home. Poor vision and smell can make food management difficult. It is a good idea for the home health nurse to check the patient's refrigerator and food cabinets to identify potential problems.

People who recognize that stress affects their gastrointestinal function may benefit from relaxation techniques and stress management training.

Signs and symptoms of possibly serious digestive problems should be reported for prompt diagnosis and treatment if indicated. Gastrointestinal symptoms that could indicate gastric cancer include persistent gastric distress, anorexia, and weight loss. Rectal bleeding or a change in bowel habits or both often occur with intestinal cancer. As part of the annual physical examination for people older than 40 years, many physicians do a rectal examination and test the stool for occult blood. For both males and females, the American Cancer Society recommends periodic sigmoidoscopy and fecal occult blood tests at intervals beginning at age 50. (See Chapter 25.)

Teaching patients what is normal, how to promote normal function, and how to detect problems can help avoid serious gastrointestinal dysfunction.

Key Points

- Any disorder of the digestive tract can cause nutritional deficiencies by disrupting one or more of its three functions: digestion, absorption, and elimination.
- Anorexia, or lack of appetite, may be caused by illness, drugs, or emotional factors.
- Oral inflammations and infections can be caused by irritants, bacteria, viruses, and fungi and can interfere with food intake and enjoyment.
- Disorders of the teeth and gums require meticulous oral hygiene and professional dental care to prevent tooth loss.
- Cancers inside the oral cavity are usually squamous cell carcinomas related to poor nutrition, chronic irritation, or combined tobacco and alcohol use.
- Cancers of the lip are usually basal cell carcinomas attributed to prolonged exposure to irritants, including sun, wind, and pipe smoking.
- Nursing care of patients being treated for oral cancers focuses on Acute Pain, Impaired Verbal Communication, Imbalanced Nutrition: Less Than Body Requirements, Disturbed Body Image, Risk for Infection, and Ineffective Tissue Perfusion.
- Cancer of the esophagus may be treated with surgery, radiotherapy, chemotherapy, or a combination of these or by palliative measures to maintain a patent esophagus.
- Vomiting, which can result in fluid and electrolyte imbalances, aspiration, and nutritional deficiencies, is treated with antiemetics, fluid and electrolyte replacement, and sometimes gastrointestinal decompression.
- Treatment of hiatal hernia, the protrusion of the lower esophagus and stomach upward through the diaphragm,

may include drug therapy, diet, measures to avoid increased intra-abdominal pressure, or surgery.
- Gastritis is inflammation of the stomach lining usually caused by *Helicobacter pylori* and aggravated by alcohol, caffeine, and other irritants.
- Peptic ulcer is loss of tissue from the lining of the stomach or duodenum that can lead to hemorrhage, perforation, and obstruction.
- Nursing care of patients with peptic ulcer focuses on Acute Pain, Imbalanced Nutrition: Less Than Body Requirements, Risk for Injury, and Ineffective Coping.
- Dumping syndrome may occur after gastric surgery, causing weakness, dizziness, diaphoresis, and palpitations.
- Nursing care of the patient with stomach cancer, which is often advanced when diagnosed, focuses on Acute Pain, Imbalanced Nutrition: Less Than Body Requirements, and Ineffective Coping.
- Persons whose weight is above the ideal are classified as overweight, obese, or extremely obese. Obesity is treated with diet, planned exercise, and, in some cases, drug therapy or surgical intervention.
- There are various types of malabsorption, a condition in which one or more nutrients are not digested or absorbed.
- Diarrhea is the frequent passage of loose or liquid stools. It can lead to fluid and electrolyte imbalances, metabolic acidosis, and malnutrition.
- Constipation is the difficult passage of hard, dry stools. It may be related to inactivity, dehydration, laxative dependence, a low-fiber diet, some drugs, and a variety of medical conditions.
- Fecal impaction is the retention of a large mass of stool in the rectum that the patient cannot pass and that may require removal with enemas and manual extraction.
- Factors that can cause intestinal obstruction include strangulated hernia, tumor, paralytic ileus, stricture, volvulus, intussusception, and postoperative adhesions.
- Appendicitis is inflammation of the appendix that requires surgical treatment to prevent rupture and peritonitis.
- A hernia is a portion of intestine that bulges through a weak area in the muscles of the abdominal wall and can become incarcerated (trapped) and obstructed.
- Inflammatory bowel disease, characterized by inflammation and ulceration of the lining of the intestines, includes ulcerative colitis and Crohn's disease.
- Nursing care of the patient with inflammatory bowel disease focuses on Acute Pain, Diarrhea, Deficient Fluid Volume, Imbalanced Nutrition: Less Than Body Requirements, Ineffective Coping, and Risk for Injury.
- Diverticulosis is characterized by small, saclike pouches in the intestinal wall that can become inflamed, causing obstruction, perforation, peritonitis, and fistula formation.
- Nursing care of the patient with colorectal cancer, which is usually treated surgically, focuses on Risk for Injury, Ineffective Tissue Perfusion, Acute Pain, Sexual Dysfunction, and Ineffective Coping.
- Polyps are small growths in the intestine that are usually benign but may be removed because they may bleed, cause obstructions, or become malignant.

- Hemorrhoids are dilated rectal veins that can become inflamed and thrombosed; they are treated with topical medications, sitz baths, heat or cold, sclerotherapy, or surgical excision.
- Anal disorders include abscesses, fissures, and fistulas, all of which may be treated surgically.

 Go to your Companion CD-ROM for a Pharmacology Tutorial, Audio Glossary, and 3-D animations.

evolve   Be sure to visit the companion Evolve site at http://evolve.elsevier.com/Linton/ for WebLinks and additional online resources.

REVIEW QUESTIONS   *Choose the best answer.*

1. Disease of which part of the digestive tract would most affect absorption of nutrients?
   1. Stomach
   2. Small intestine
   3. Large intestine
   4. Rectum

2. Inspection of the mouth of an older adult reveals all the data listed below. Which is an *abnormal* finding?
   1. Worn chewing surfaces on the teeth
   2. Recession of the gingiva (gums)
   3. Loss of most of the natural teeth
   4. Teeth appear dark and transparent

3. When collecting data about the abdomen, the nurse should perform which technique *last?*
   1. Inspection
   2. Auscultation
   3. Percussion
   4. Palpation

4. Other than a radiograph, the *most reliable* way to assess placement of a nasogastric tube is to:
   1. Auscultate the epigastrium while injecting air into the tube
   2. Examine and check pH of aspirated stomach contents
   3. Place the end of the tube in water and observe for bubbling
   4. Listen for air movement at the end of the tube

5. A patient who has had oral surgery complains of dry mouth. Your most appropriate action is to:
   1. Tell the patient this is normal after oral surgery
   2. Provide a commercial mouthwash for rinsing the mouth
   3. Contact the physician for mouth care instructions
   4. Suction the mouth after giving the patient sips of water

6. You are reviewing the admission papers for a new resident in a long-term care facility. You note a medical diagnosis of achalasia. A relevant part of the nursing care plan should be:
   1. Determine the best position for the patient during meals
   2. Monitor all stools for occult blood
   3. Auscultate bowel sounds in all four quadrants
   4. Maintain strict intake and output records

7. Which of the following types of antiulcer drugs works by inhibiting the secretion of gastric acid?
   1. Antacids
   2. H_2-receptor blockers
   3. Mucosal barriers
   4. Antibiotics

8. A patient who was admitted with severe abdominal pain is being evaluated for possible appendicitis. You should suspect intestinal rupture if:
   1. The patient's WBC count is 15,000/mm³
   2. Palpation at McBurney's point causes pain
   3. The patient keeps both hips flexed
   4. The patient's abdomen is rigid

9. Surgery is used to treat Crohn's disease less often than ulcerative colitis because Crohn's disease:
   1. Usually returns near the site of the anastomosis
   2. Typically involves the entire small and large intestines
   3. Can usually be cured with combination drug therapy
   4. Is associated with a higher risk of surgical complications

10. One method of removing hemorrhoids is to use a rubber band to tie off the hemorrhoid. This is called:
    1. Sclerotherapy
    2. Photocoagulation
    3. Laser excision
    4. Ligation

Objectives

After reading and studying this chapter, you should be able to:

1. Identify nursing assessment data related to the functions of the liver, gallbladder, and pancreas.
2. Identify the nurse's role in tests and procedures performed to diagnose disorders of the liver, gallbladder, and pancreas.
3. Describe the care of the patient who has an esophageal balloon tube in place.
4. Explain the pathology, signs and symptoms, diagnosis, complications, and medical treatment of selected disorders of the liver, gallbladder, and pancreas.
5. Assist in developing a nursing care plan for the patient with liver, gallbladder, or pancreatic dysfunction.

Key Terms

Be sure to check out the bonus material on the Companion CD-ROM, including selected audio pronunciations.

ascites (ă-SĪ-tēz, p. 799)
cholecystectomy (kō-lĕ-sĭs-TĔK-tō-mē, p. 819)
cholecystitis (kō-lĕ-sĭs-TĪ-tĭs, p. 818)
choledocholithiasis (kō-lĕd-ō-kō-lĭ-THĪ-ă-sĭs, p. 819)
cholelithiasis (kō-lĕ-lĭ-THĪ-ă-sĭs, p. 818)
cirrhosis (sĭr-RŌ-sĭs, p. 808)
endocrine gland (ĔN-dō-krĭn, p. 823)
eructation (ĕ-rŭk-TĀ-shŭn, p. 819)
gluconeogenesis (glū-kō-nē-ō-JĔN-ĕ-sĭs, p. 796)
glycogenesis (glī-kō-JĔN-ĕ-sĭs, p. 796)
glycogenolysis (glī-kō-jĕ-NŎL-ĭ-sĭs, p. 796)
hepatic (hĕ-PĂ-tĭc, p. 796)
hepatitis (hĕ-pă-TĪ-tĭs, p. 798)
hepatomegaly (hĕ-pă-tō-MĔG-ă-lē, p. 799)
icterus (ĪK-tĕr-ŭs, p. 799)
jaundice (JĂWN-dĭs, p. 799)

THE LIVER

The liver is the largest internal organ in the body. It is located under the diaphragm in the right upper quadrant of the abdomen, as illustrated in Figure 39-1. The term *hepatic* refers to the liver.

ANATOMY AND PHYSIOLOGY OF THE LIVER

The liver can be divided into four lobes that are made up of many lobules (Fig. 39-2). Blood from the aorta is delivered to the liver via the hepatic artery. The portal vein delivers blood from the intestines to the liver. Portal blood circulates through the liver and is transported to the inferior vena cava by the hepatic veins. Figure 39-3 illustrates hepatic circulation.

Specialized **hepatic** cells allow the liver to carry out many critical functions. Reticuloendothelial cells, called *Kupffer cells,* ingest old red blood cells and bacteria. Parenchymal cells carry out various metabolic functions, including metabolism of carbohydrates, fats, proteins, and steroids and detoxification of potentially harmful substances.

BILE PRODUCTION AND EXCRETION

Bilirubin is a product of the normal breakdown of old red blood cells in the liver. The initial breakdown product is unconjugated or indirect bilirubin. The liver then converts unconjugated bilirubin into conjugated bilirubin and secretes it into the bile. Bile produced in the liver passes through the cystic duct into the gallbladder for storage.

When fats pass into the duodenum, the gallbladder and the liver respond by delivering bile through the common bile duct into the small intestine. Bile emulsifies fat, meaning that it breaks it into small particles that can easily be absorbed. It also neutralizes the acidic chyme as it leaves the stomach. Bile plays a role in the absorption of fat-soluble vitamins and the removal of some toxins.

Bile travels through the intestines with the chyme. In the large intestine, it is converted to urobilinogen and then to stercobilin. This final breakdown product of bilirubin gives stool its characteristic brown color.

METABOLISM

Glucose Metabolism

The liver helps maintain the blood glucose within a certain range. After a meal, excess glucose molecules are taken up by the liver, combined, and then stored as glycogen. This process is called **glycogenesis**. When the glucose level in the blood falls, the process is reversed by **glycogenolysis** and the glucose molecules are returned to the blood. **Gluconeogenesis** is the third process by which the liver maintains blood glucose. Fats and protein are broken down in response to low blood glucose levels, and the molecules are used to make new glucose.

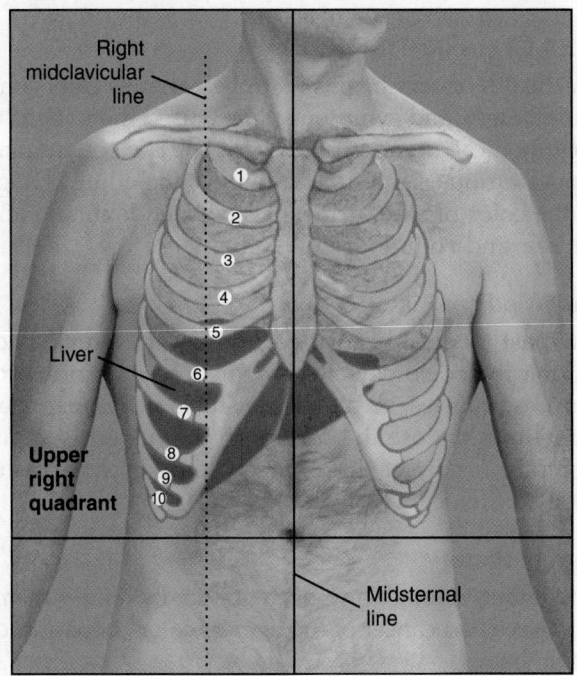

FIGURE **39-1** The liver is located under the diaphragm in the right upper abdomen. Anatomic landmarks are noted.

Protein Metabolism

Some nonessential amino acids, plasma proteins (albumin and globulin), and clotting factors are synthesized in the liver. Another important liver function in relation to protein metabolism is the conversion of ammonia to urea. Ammonia is a byproduct of the metabolism of amino acids. If ammonia accumulates in the blood, it has toxic effects on brain tissue.

Lipid Metabolism

The liver synthesizes lipids from glucose, pyruvic acid, acetic acid, and amino acids. It also synthesizes fatty acids, breaks down triglycerides, and synthesizes and breaks down cholesterol.

Blood Coagulation

Normal blood coagulation (clotting) is a complex process. Two essential elements for coagulation, prothrombin and fibrinogen, are synthesized by the liver.

Detoxification

The liver filters the blood and inactivates many chemicals, including most medications. Therefore medications are prescribed very cautiously for patients with poor liver function. Patients with liver disease are at increased risk for toxic effects of drugs. With age, there is some decrease in liver function, so lower drug dosages may be adequate. Especially with long-term therapy,

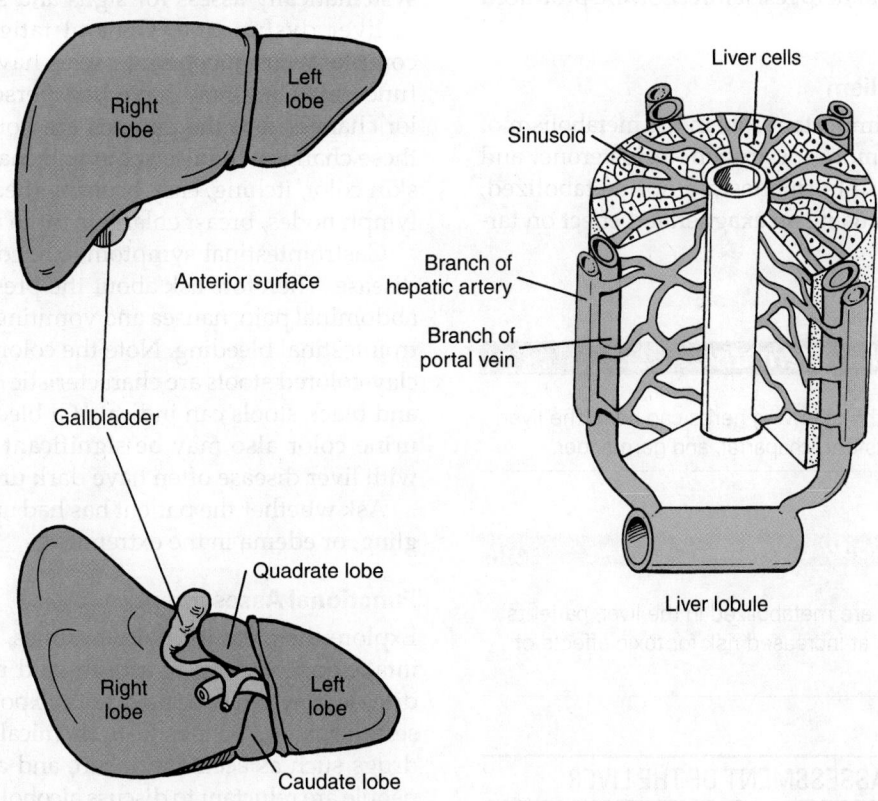

FIGURE **39-2** The liver has four lobes, each made up of many lobules.

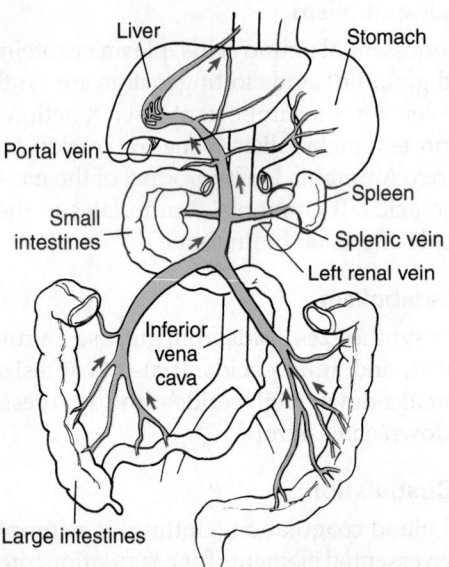

FIGURE **39-3** Hepatic circulation. Venous blood from the spleen, stomach, pancreas, and intestines passes through the liver via the portal vein and is delivered through the hepatic veins to the inferior vena cava.

the older person should be assessed frequently for signs of toxicity.

Immunity

An important protective mechanism is the development of antibodies to resist pathogens. Antibodies and other substances that help resist infection are produced in the liver.

Hormone Metabolism

The liver plays an important role in the metabolism of adrenocortical hormones, estrogen, testosterone, and aldosterone. If these hormones are not metabolized, they accumulate, causing an exaggerated effect on target organs.

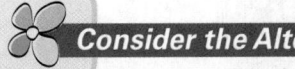

Consider the Alternative

Inform patients that the following herbs can harm the liver: comfrey, borage, coltsfoot, chaparral, and germander.

Pharmacology Capsule

Because many drugs are metabolized in the liver, patients with liver disease are at increased risk for toxic effects of drugs.

NURSING ASSESSMENT OF THE LIVER

The liver has so many important functions that alterations may cause a number of systemic signs and symptoms. The health history and physical examination

may provide clues to liver dysfunction and may be used to assess responses to the treatment of liver disorders. Even though the registered nurse is responsible for the complete patient assessment, the LPN/LVN contributes data.

HEALTH HISTORY

The health history begins with the patient's chief complaint. Signs and symptoms that caused the patient to seek medical attention are described. The patient may report various signs and symptoms, including change in the color of skin, urine, or stools; abdominal pain, nausea, and vomiting; and fatigue.

Past Medical History

The past medical history documents any previous or chronic liver disorders. Record any recent surgical procedures, injuries, or blood transfusions because they sometimes expose the patient to the hepatitis virus. Compile a complete list of medications because many drugs are toxic to the liver.

Family History

Document whether any of the patient's family members have had cancer of the liver or colon, hepatitis, or alcoholism.

Review of Systems

Inquire about the patient's general health status, and systematically assess for signs and symptoms related to liver dysfunction. General fatigue is a common complaint among people who have impaired liver function. They may have had personality or behavior changes, but the patients are not always aware of these changes. Inquire about any changes in weight or skin color, itching, easy bruising, headaches, enlarged lymph nodes, breast enlargement in men, or dyspnea.

Gastrointestinal symptoms are common with liver disease. Therefore ask about the presence of anorexia, abdominal pain, nausea and vomiting, diarrhea, or gastrointestinal bleeding. Note the color of stools because clay-colored stools are characteristic of bile obstruction and black stools can indicate GI bleeding. Changes in urine color also may be significant because patients with liver disease often have dark urine.

Ask whether the patient has had any numbness, tingling, or edema in the extremities.

Functional Assessment

Explore the patient's daily routines, including dietary intake and patterns of activity and rest. Because liver disease may be associated with exposure to toxins, assess the patient's exposure to chemicals, potentially toxic drugs such as acetaminophen, and alcohol use. Some people are reluctant to discuss alcohol use, so the subject must be handled tactfully. People tend to understate the amount of alcohol they typically consume. Note use of street drugs, especially those taken intravenously.

The last part of the functional assessment is the identification of stressors, usual coping strategies, and sources of support.

PHYSICAL EXAMINATION

The physical assessment begins with the measurement of vital signs and height and weight and observation of the patient's general appearance. Skin color is especially important in relation to the liver. Jaundice is a golden yellow skin color associated with liver dysfunction or bile obstruction. It is relatively easy to recognize in fair-skinned people.

Inspect the sclera of the eyes. Like the skin, the sclera may turn yellow, a condition called scleral icterus. This sign is especially useful when jaundice cannot be seen elsewhere in dark-skinned people.

Observe for enlargement of breast tissue in men. Such enlargement is called *gynecomastia*. When inspecting the chest, also look for spider angiomas. Spider angiomas are small, visible vessels shaped like spiders.

The examination of the abdomen is especially important in detecting liver disease. Inspect the shape of the abdomen. Note the presence of prominent veins. If significant ascites (fluid accumulation in the peritoneal cavity) is present, the abdomen appears distended. Measure the abdomen at the largest circumference to permit comparative measurements later (Fig. 39-4).

Palpate the abdomen for distention and tenderness. Experienced examiners may be able to palpate the liver, but unless it is enlarged, it is difficult to locate under the right rib cage. An enlarged, diseased liver may be felt well below the rib margin. Liver enlargement is called hepatomegaly.

Examine the extremities for bruising, edema, muscle wasting, and impaired sensation. Inspect the hands for palmar erythema (redness of the palms).

The assessment of a patient with a liver disorder is summarized in Box 39-1. Findings associated with liver disease are illustrated in Figure 39-5.

DIAGNOSTIC TESTS AND PROCEDURES

The physician uses a number of tools to assess liver function, including endoscopy, laboratory studies, imaging studies, and biopsies. Endoscopy was addressed in Chapter 38. Nursing care of patients having specific tests and procedures is presented in the Diagnostic Tests and Procedures table on pp. 801 to 803.

LABORATORY STUDIES

Laboratory studies of specimens are done to measure bilirubin, urinary and fecal urobilinogen, serum proteins, ammonia, prothrombin time, vitamin K production, international normalized ratio (INR), and serum enzymes. Examples of serum enzymes include alkaline phosphatase (ALP), gamma-glutamyl transpeptidase (GGT), alanine aminotransferase (ALT), also known as

---

Box 39-1   ASSESSMENT of the Patient with Liver Disease

Health History
Present Illness:
Fatigue, weight changes, digestive disturbances, skin changes

Past Medical History:
Previous liver disease, hepatitis B immunization, recent and current medications taken

Review of Systems:
Weakness, fatigue, pruritus, dyspnea, anorexia, abdominal pain, nausea and vomiting, diarrhea, bloody stools, changes in urine or stool color, numbness or tingling of extremities

Functional Assessment:
Diet, alcohol intake, occupation, exposure to toxins, stress, coping strategies, interpersonal relationships

Physical Examination
Vital Signs:
Hypertension, tachypnea

Height and Weight

Skin:
Dryness, scratches, jaundice, bruises

Eye:
Scleral icterus

Thorax:
Spider angiomas

Breasts:
Gynecomastia

Abdomen:
Distention, prominent veins, girth, liver enlargement

FIGURE 39-4 How to measure abdominal girth. Marks are made on the abdominal midline and both sides so that subsequent measurements can always be made at the same place.

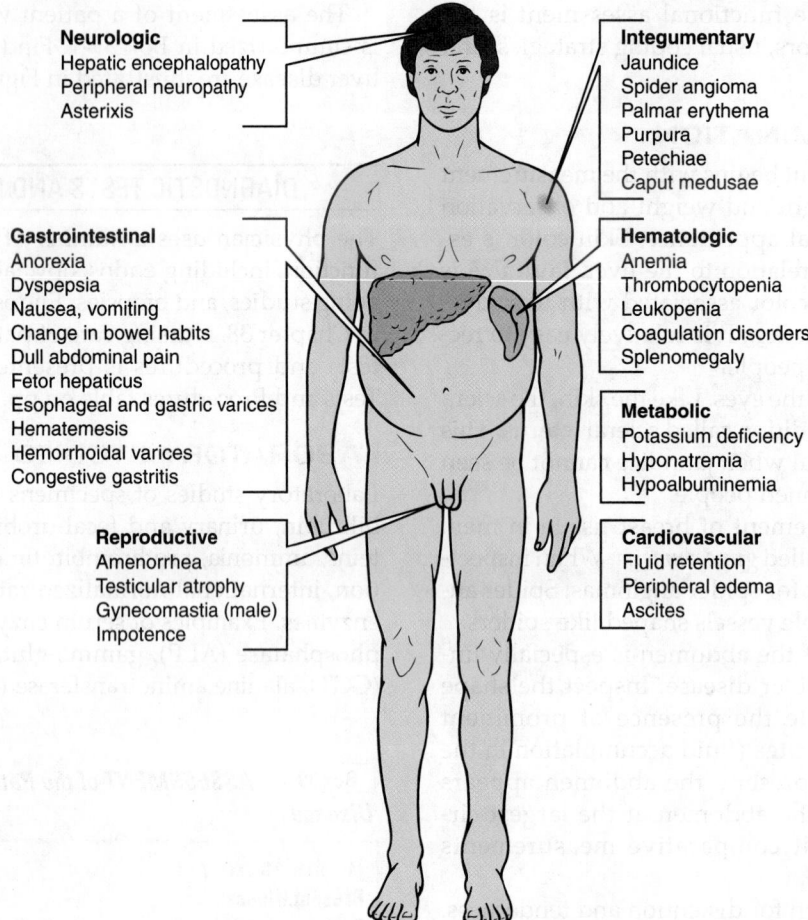

Neurologic
Hepatic encephalopathy
Peripheral neuropathy
Asterixis

Integumentary
Jaundice
Spider angioma
Palmar erythema
Purpura
Petechiae
Caput medusae

Gastrointestinal
Anorexia
Dyspepsia
Nausea, vomiting
Change in bowel habits
Dull abdominal pain
Fetor hepaticus
Esophageal and gastric varices
Hematemesis
Hemorrhoidal varices
Congestive gastritis

Hematologic
Anemia
Thrombocytopenia
Leukopenia
Coagulation disorders
Splenomegaly

Metabolic
Potassium deficiency
Hyponatremia
Hypoalbuminemia

Reproductive
Amenorrhea
Testicular atrophy
Gynecomastia (male)
Impotence

Cardiovascular
Fluid retention
Peripheral edema
Ascites

FIGURE **39-5** Findings associated with liver disease.

serum glutamic-pyruvic transaminase (SGPT); aldolase (ALS); aspartate aminotransferase (AST), also known as serum glutamic-oxaloacetic transaminase (SGOT); and lactate dehydrogenase (LDH). The table on pp. 801 to 803 explains the significance of these laboratory tests.

Because gastrointestinal bleeding is sometimes a problem with liver disease, gastric fluids and stools may be tested for the presence of occult blood. Urine specimens may also be tested for bilirubin and urobilinogen and stool specimens tested for urobilinogen.

IMAGING STUDIES
Radiologic Studies
Radiologic studies are used primarily to visualize the circulatory and biliary systems in the liver. Hepatobiliary scintigraphy (HIDA) is a nuclear imaging scan that employs a radioactive substance. After being injected into a vein, the substance accumulates in the liver. Radiographs are then taken to reveal tumors, cirrhosis, and abscesses.

Computed Tomography and Magnetic Resonance Imaging
Computed tomography (CT) and magnetic resonance imaging (MRI) are used to obtain scans of internal or-

gans, including the liver. They are noninvasive, painless procedures.

Ultrasonography
Ultrasonography uses sound waves to create an image of the liver, spleen, pancreas, gallbladder, and biliary system. It is a noninvasive and painless procedure.

LIVER BIOPSY
A liver biopsy is a procedure that involves removal of a small specimen of liver tissue for examination. The specimen can be obtained through an incision under general anesthesia (open biopsy). Another method (needle biopsy) involves the use of a special type of needle inserted through the abdominal wall to obtain the specimen.

Before either procedure, baseline vital signs should be obtained and blood coagulation studies done. Signed consent is required. When preparing for a needle biopsy, tell the patient what to expect during the procedure. For a needle biopsy, position the patient supine with the right arm behind the head. Place a pad under the right chest. The physician instructs the patient to take a deep breath and hold it during the actual puncture.

DIAGNOSTIC TESTS and PROCEDURES | *Liver and Gallbladder*

General interventions: Check your agency procedure for diagnostic tests and procedures. Always tell the patient what to expect when tests are ordered. Explain if NPO status is necessary. Document the care provided and relevant assessment data. If venipuncture is done, a dressing should be applied and the site checked for oozing. Apply pressure if patient's blood clotting is impaired. Assess allergy to dyes; monitor for reactions.

TEST/STUDY	PURPOSE/PROCEDURE	PATIENT PREPARATION	POSTPROCEDURE NURSING CARE
LABORATORY STUDIES **Blood Studies** Serum bilirubin	Assesses liver function by measuring bilirubin in the blood. Normal values include: Total bilirubin: 0.2-1.0 mg/dL or 3.4-17.1 μmol/L Conjugated bilirubin: 0.0-0.2 mg/dL or 0.0-3.4 μmol/L Unconjugated bilirubin: 0.2-0.8 mg/dL	Tell patient to fast for at least 4 hr before blood sample drawn. Avoid yellow foods for 3-4 days before test. Should not be done within 24 hr after a contrast medium has been given.	No special care.
Alkaline phosphatase	Detects increases associated with liver or bone disease. Normal value: Varies with method.	10-12 hr fast may be required. Some drugs may be withheld for 12 hr.	No special care.
Prothrombin time and INR	Detects prolonged clotting time possibly caused by liver disease or vitamin K deficiency. Normal value: PT: 11.0-12.6 sec INR: 1.0-1.2	No coffee or alcohol for 24 hr before test. Many natural remedies affect result.	No special care.
Serum enzymes AST (SGOT) ALT (SGPT) LDH	Detects elevations in enzymes related to liver diseases. Normal values: AST: Men: 7-21 U/L Women: 6-18 U/L ALT: Men: 6-24 U/L Women: 4-17 U/L LDH: Varies with type of test.	Consult agency guidelines to see if fasting is necessary.	No special care.
Serum protein	Electrophoresis helps diagnose conditions that affect serum proteins.	Avoid high-fat diet for 8 hr before test. Some medications may need to be withheld for several days before blood sample is drawn.	No special care.

AST, Aspartate aminotransferase; *SGOT,* serum glutamic-oxaloacetic transaminase; *ALT,* alanine aminotransferase; *SGPT,* serum glutamic-pyruvic transaminase; *LDH,* lactate dehydrogenase; *PT,* prothrombin time; *INR,* international normalized ratio.

DIAGNOSTIC TESTS and PROCEDURES   *Liver and Gallbladder—cont'd*

TEST/STUDY	PURPOSE/PROCEDURE	PATIENT PREPARATION	POSTPROCEDURE NURSING CARE
RADIOGRAPHIC STUDIES			
Computed tomography (CT)	Creates cross-sectional images of liver and other organs to reveal abnormalities.	Inform radiologist if patient is allergic to contrast media, iodine, or shellfish. Inform patient that the procedure is painless and noninvasive. NPO status may be ordered, but routine drugs can usually be taken. The patient will lie still on a stretcher while a doughnut-shaped machine moves around him or her. Contrast dye is sometimes injected intravenously. It can create a feeling of warmth, a salty taste, and nausea. Sedation can be ordered if the patient has difficulty lying still.	No special care usually needed. Inform the physician of any signs of allergic response to contrast dye. Give antihistamines as ordered for allergy.
T-tube cholangiography	Evaluates whether bile ducts are open after gallbladder surgery.	Contrast agent is injected into T-tube before radiographs are obtained. Takes about 15 min. Same as for intravenous cholangiography.	A fatty meal helps eliminate dye. Report rash, itching, hives, dyspnea that could be allergic reaction to dye.
Intravenous cholangiography	Permits visualization of bile ducts; usually done when gallbladder is not visualized on cholecystography.	Radiographs are taken before and at intervals after intravenous injection of a contrast agent (if done). Withhold food and fluids as ordered. Takes 4-6 hr. Patient is usually NPO after midnight before study. A laxative also may be ordered the night before. Ask about iodine sensitivity, and notify radiologist if patient is sensitive.	Same as for T-tube cholecystography. If solution is given through liver (percutaneous transhepatic cholangiography), watch for signs of bleeding and respiratory distress.
Percutaneous transhepatic cholangiography	Dye is given and radiography is used to visualize the biliary duct system.	Report patient allergies to iodine or seafood before the test. During the procedure, the patient must lie still while a needle is inserted into the liver and dye is injected. Radiography is used to place the needles and observe the outline of the bile ducts or blood vessels.	Bed rest for 8 hr. Check the puncture site for bleeding. Monitor vital signs to detect signs of bleeding. Similar care as for liver biopsy.
Portal venography and hepatic arteriography	Uses intravenous contrast dye followed by radiographs to study blood vessels in liver.		
Liver scan	A radioactive substance is given that collects in liver. A scanner maps uptake of radiation, revealing tumors and abscesses. During procedure, the radioactive substance is given intravenously.	The patient should be assured that a small dose of radiation is harmless. The patient is then helped to assume various positions while radiographs are taken 4-6 hr fast required.	Same as for T-tube cholangiography. Patient must wash hands thoroughly after voiding for 24 hr. Report allergic symptoms.
Gallbladder scan, hepatobiliary scintigraphy, hepatobiliary imaging, biliary tract radionuclide scan, cholescintigraphy, HIDA scan	A radionuclide is injected and images are taken of the biliary tract to assess patency. Detects cholecystitis.	NPO at least 2 hr before procedure. Explain to patient that scan takes about 90 min. Repeat imaging may be needed 24-48 hr later.	Encourage patient to drink fluids to promote elimination of radionuclide, to wash hands after voiding, and to flush immediately. Caregivers should wear gloves to handle urine. Wash gloved hands before removing gloves and wash hands after removing gloves; dispose of gloves as nuclear waste.

	Description	Patient teaching / preparation	Nursing care
OTHER IMAGING PROCEDURES			
Ultrasonography	Uses high-frequency sound waves to create an image of the liver, spleen, pancreas, gallbladder, and biliary system.	May be NPO for 8-12 hr. Patient teaching: The patient will lie on a table. A technician applies gel to the abdomen and moves an instrument called a *transducer* over the abdomen. Images are projected onto a screen. Not painful.	No special care needed after the procedure.
Magnetic resonance imaging (MRI)	Creates cross-sectional images of the liver and other organs without radiation.	Advise the patient that MRI is a painless, noninvasive procedure. All metal must be removed before MRI. The patient must be still on a narrow surface. Older MRI is a circular device that surrounds the body like a tunnel. Closing eyes reduces claustrophobia (open MRI eliminates claustrophobia). Machine is noisy.	No special care needed.
TISSUE EXAMINATION			
Liver biopsy	Removes a small specimen of liver tissue for examination.	Baseline vital signs and blood coagulation studies should be obtained.	With *all* liver biopsies: Monitor vital signs for indications of bleeding (tachycardia, tachypnea, restlessness, hypotension) and pneumothorax (dyspnea, tachycardia).
Needle biopsy	The specimen is obtained by inserting a special needle into the liver through the abdominal wall.	The patient is positioned supine with the right arm behind the head.	Check pressure dressing for bleeding. Position the patient on the right side as ordered.
Open biopsy	An incision is made under general anesthesia.	Done in the operating room and requires standard preoperative procedures. Informed consent must be obtained from the patient.	
ENDOSCOPY			
Cholangiopancreatography, endoscopic retrograde cholangiopancreatography (ERCP)	A flexible endoscope is passed after injection of dye. Study permits visualization of pancreatic, hepatic, and common bile ducts and ampulla of Vater. Used to diagnose pancreatic disease.	NPO for 8-12 hr. Study takes 30-60 min. May feel flushed when dye injected. Rule out iodine allergy.	Advise warm gargles or ice pack to neck for sore throat. Patient may have belching and bloating. Immediately notify physician of severe pain, fever, dyspnea, hematemesis.

HIPA, Heparin-induced platelet activation; *NPO,* nothing by mouth.

A pressure dressing is placed over the puncture site and should be checked for bleeding every 15 minutes for the first hour, every 30 minutes for the next hour, and hourly or according to agency protocol. Monitor for other signs of hemorrhage. The physician usually orders the patient kept on the right side for at least 2 hours to maintain pressure on the site. After a few hours, if nothing has changed, the patient may still be kept flat for up to 14 hours.

The primary complications of liver biopsy are hemorrhage and pneumothorax. Bleeding is a possibility because of the liver's rich blood supply and the potential for impaired coagulation in the patient with liver disease. Pneumothorax occurs if the lung is accidentally punctured during the biopsy. Air escapes into the pleural cavity and the lung on the affected side collapses.

DISORDERS OF THE LIVER

HEPATITIS

Hepatitis is inflammation of the liver. Each year 250,000 cases of viral hepatitis occur in the United States each year. Although many patients have uneventful recoveries, others die of the many conditions that can eventually lead to liver failure and death.

Pathophysiology

Hepatitis has both local and systemic effects. The inflammation process causes the liver to swell. Although swelling is severe, there are no pain receptors inside the liver, its compression can inflame the cells that encapsulate it. This results in the development of a tender, stretched liver capsule. Blood flow through the liver may be impaired, causing pressure to increase in the portal circulation. Systemic effects are related to metabolic functions normally performed by the liver. Other local symptoms depend on the degree of hepatic impairment, and symptoms of hepatitis include jaundice, fever, and malaise.

Types of Hepatitis

Hepatitis can be classified as infectious or noninfectious. Viruses known to cause hepatitis. Hepatitis are classified as types A, B, C, D, and E. Cases that most often cause hepatitis are the cases described for types C and hepatitis D. Noninfectious hepatitis is caused by nonpharmacologic factors, including cancers. Key features of each type of hepatitis are summarized in Table 39-3.

Hepatitis A Hepatitis A is spread by the fecal and enteric transmission. It is caused by hepatitis A virus (HAV), which is transmitted from one person

A pressure dressing is placed over the puncture. It should be checked for bleeding every 15 minutes for the first hour, every 30 minutes for the next hour, and then hourly or according to agency protocol. Monitor vital signs at the same time for signs of blood loss (tachycardia, restlessness, hypotension) or pneumothorax (restlessness, tachypnea). The physician usually orders the patient kept on the right side for at least 2 hours to maintain pressure on the puncture site. After being allowed to change positions, the patient may still be kept flat for up to 14 hours.

The primary complications of liver biopsy are hemorrhage and pneumothorax. Bleeding is a possibility because of the liver's rich blood supply and the potential for impaired coagulation in the patient with liver disease. Pneumothorax occurs if the lung is accidentally punctured during the biopsy. Air escapes into the pleural cavity, and the lung on the affected side collapses.

DISORDERS OF THE LIVER

HEPATITIS

Hepatitis is inflammation of the liver. It is estimated that over 250,000 cases of viral hepatitis are reported in the United States each year. Although many patients have uneventful recoveries, others develop chronic conditions that can eventually lead to liver failure and death.

Pathophysiology

Hepatitis has both local and systemic effects. Locally, the inflammatory process causes the liver to swell. If swelling is severe, there are two important effects. First, the bile channels are compressed, damaging the cells that produce bile. This results in an elevation in serum bilirubin and jaundice. Second, blood flow through the liver is impaired, causing pressure to rise in the portal circulation (see Fig. 39-3).

Systemic effects are related to altered metabolic functions normally performed by the liver and to the infectious response in viral hepatitis. Systemic signs and symptoms of hepatitis include rash, angioedema, arthritis, fever, and malaise.

Types of Hepatitis

Hepatitis can be classified as infectious or noninfectious. Viruses known to cause infectious hepatitis are classified as types A, B, C, D, and E. Other viruses that may cause hepatitis include the recently described hepatitis G and hepatitis GB. Noninfectious hepatitis is caused by exposure to toxic chemicals, including drugs. Key features of each type of hepatitis are summarized in Table 39-1.

Hepatitis A. Hepatitis A has been called *infectious hepatitis* and *epidemic hepatitis*. It is caused by the hepatitis A virus (HAV), which is transmitted from one person to another by way of water, food, or medical equipment that has been contaminated with infected fecal matter. Hepatitis A is the most common type of viral hepatitis. Fortunately, it is rarely fatal and infected persons do not become asymptomatic carriers.

Hepatitis B. Hepatitis B, caused by the hepatitis B virus (HBV), is often called *serum hepatitis.* Because HBV is found in all body fluids of infected persons, modes of transmission include intimate contact with carriers as well as contact with contaminated blood or medical equipment. It also can be transmitted from an infected mother to her baby. Some 6% to 10% of these patients develop chronic hepatitis and become carriers, meaning they can transmit the infection to others. The incidence of hepatitis B has declined dramatically since the 1980s as a result of a comprehensive preventive program that was initiated. This program included screening of pregnant women, treatment of infants born to infected women, and vaccination of children and high-risk groups.

Hepatitis C. Hepatitis C is transmitted by contact with contaminated blood or medical equipment or by contact with infected body fluids. Like hepatitis B, it can be transmitted from an infected mother to her baby. About 40% to 60% of people with hepatitis C develop chronic infections and become carriers. Although the incidence has been falling over the past 25 years, there are still an estimated 2.7 million people with chronic hepatitis C infection.

Hepatitis D. Hepatitis D is caused by a virus known as the *delta agent*, which is a defective RNA virus that can survive only in the company of the hepatitis B virus (HBV). Hepatitis D is transmitted percutaneously (through the skin or mucous membranes) with the B virus. The presence of hepatitis D greatly increases the risk that the patient will progress to chronic hepatitis and possible liver failure.

Hepatitis E. Hepatitis E is similar to hepatitis A and is most commonly transmitted via water or food contaminated with infected fecal matter. Hepatitis E infection is rare in the United States except among people who have traveled in developing countries where the virus is more common. There is no long-term, chronic form of hepatitis E infection.

Hepatitis G. Hepatitis G has been identified in some blood donors and can be transmitted by blood transfusion. Hepatitis G virus (HGV) does not appear to cause chronic hepatitis, but its effects may not be fully known at this time.

Noninfectious Hepatitis. Although the cause is not always identifiable, noninfectious hepatitis can be caused by exposure to toxins such as mercury and arsenic and drugs such as alcohol and acetaminophen.

Signs and Symptoms

Regardless of the cause, the signs and symptoms of hepatitis are similar. Differences occur in the number and severity of the symptoms from one person

| Table 39-1 | **Key Features of Each Type of Viral Hepatitis** |

TYPE	CAUSE	TRANSMISSION ROUTE	INCUBATION PERIOD	PREVENTION
Hepatitis A	Hepatitis A virus (HAV)	Fecal-oral route. Often via contaminated water or food.	3-5 wk	Wash hands after toileting. Use clean water and food supplies. Use gloves to handle stool specimens and soiled articles. Immune globulin is given before or within 48 hr after exposure.
Hepatitis B	Hepatitis B virus (HBV)	Introduction of contaminated blood through skin or mucous membranes. Often via contaminated needles or other medical or dental equipment; also by sexual contact. Newborns may be infected before, during, or after birth.	2-5 mo	Vaccine is given to people at risk for exposure. Use disposable needles. Avoid contaminated articles. Screen blood donors. Use caution with body fluids. Hepatitis B immune globulin is given after exposure.
Hepatitis C (non-A, non-B)	Hepatitis C virus (HCV)	Introduction of contaminated blood through skin or mucous membranes, usually by needles or other medical or dental equipment.	7 wk	Use disposable needles. Avoid contaminated articles. Screen blood donors. Use caution with body fluids. No vaccine is available.
Hepatitis D	"Delta agent" hepatitis D virus (HDV)	Transmitted only with HBV via contaminated blood or equipment, or by sexual contact.	1-6 mo	Hepatitis B vaccine.
Hepatitis E	Hepatitis E virus (HEV)	Fecal-oral route often via contaminated water or food.	3-6 wk	Wash hands after toileting. Use clean water and food supplies. Use gloves to handle stool specimens and soiled articles. Immune globulin is given before or within 48 hr after exposure.

to the next. Many patients have no symptoms at all. For those who are symptomatic, the course of the disease is marked by three phases: preicteric, icteric, and posticteric.

Preicteric Phase. Common findings in the preicteric phase include malaise, severe headache, right upper quadrant abdominal pain, anorexia, nausea, vomiting, fever, arthralgia (joint pain), rash, enlarged lymph nodes, urticaria, and enlargement and tenderness of the liver. The preicteric phase lasts 1 to 21 days and is the period when the patient is most infectious.

Icteric Phase. The icteric phase is characterized by jaundice, light or clay-colored stools, and dark urine typical of impaired bile production and secretion. Pruritus may be present and is caused by the accumulation of bile salts under the skin. Gastrointestinal symptoms from the preicteric phase often persist. The icteric phase lasts 2 to 4 weeks. Hepatitis patients in whom jaundice does not develop are said to have *anicteric hepatitis.*

Posticteric Phase. In the posticteric phase, fatigue, malaise, and liver enlargement persist for several months.

Complications

Most people recover fully from hepatitis A or B, but there can be residual damage and complications. Some patients with hepatitis B or C become carriers. About one fourth of those who become carriers will have chronic active hepatitis, which can lead to cirrhosis. Carriers also are at increased risk for liver cancer. People who have had hepatitis cannot donate blood because of the risk of transmitting the disease to a recipient.

Complications of hepatitis include chronic persistent hepatitis, chronic active hepatitis, and fulminant hepatitis. Chronic persistent hepatitis is characterized by a prolonged recovery with continuing fatigue and liver enlargement that eventually resolves. With chronic active hepatitis, signs and symptoms persist for more than 6 months. Liver damage continues and may lead to cirrhosis. If necrosis of damaged cells occurs without regeneration, fulminant hepatitis results. It is marked by severe liver failure and is often fatal. Hepatitis D virus (HDV), which coexists with HBV, can contribute to the development of fulminant hepatitis.

Medical Diagnosis

A diagnosis of hepatitis is based on the detection of the virus or its antibodies in the blood. The effects of the infection on the liver may cause liver function tests to be abnormal. Typical findings consistent with hepatitis include elevated levels of serum enzymes (AST, ALT, GGT), serum and urinary bilirubin, and urinary urobilinogen. The prothrombin time may be prolonged. Albumin may be normal or low, and gamma globulin may be normal or high. The types of viral hepatitis can be identified by the presence of specific viral antigens and antibodies. A liver biopsy may be done to evaluate harm caused by chronic HBV or HCV.

Medical Treatment

Because there is no cure for hepatitis, treatment is designed to promote healing and to manage symptoms. Research with antiviral drugs is making progress in the treatment of hepatitis. Chronic hepatitis B now is treated with a 4- to 12-month course of interferon, lamivudine (Epivir-HBV), or famciclovir (Famvir). Peginterferon alfa-2a with ribavirin is proving to be far more effective than previous treatments for hepatitis C virus (HCV). The physician's orders usually include antipyretics for fever and antiemetics for nausea. Corticosteroids, although controversial, may be ordered if the patient is very ill or if fulminant hepatitis is suspected. The selection of drugs is important, since hepatotoxic drugs (those that are toxic to the liver) should not be given. Suggested antiemetics are dimenhydrinate (Dramamine) and trimethobenzamide (Tigan). Phenothiazines are contraindicated. If a sedative is needed, chloral hydrate or diphenhydramine (Benadryl) is recommended.

The prescribed diet is usually high-calorie, high-carbohydrate, moderate- to high-protein, and moderate- to low-fat with supplementary vitamins. Recommended activity depends on the patient's signs and symptoms and liver function tests. Bed rest may be ordered during the icteric phase; however, practices vary.

Pharmacology Capsule

Hepatotoxic drugs are contraindicated for the patient with hepatitis because they can cause further damage to liver cells.

Prevention

Vaccines are available to immunize people against hepatitis types A and B. At this time there is no vaccine to prevent other types of hepatitis. Immune globulin (IG) can provide temporary passive immunity and prevent hepatitis A if given within 2 weeks after exposure. Active disease may be averted in patients who have been exposed to HBV by administering the HBV vaccine and hepatitis B immune globulin (HBIG).

NURSING CARE *of the Patient with Hepatitis*

Assessment

Nursing assessment of the patient with liver disease is outlined in Box 39-1. When taking a health history of the person with hepatitis, essential data include information about general health state, drug and alcohol use, chemical exposure, dietary habits, blood transfusions, recent travel, gastrointestinal disturbances, and changes in skin, urine, or stools.

Ongoing physical assessment includes vital signs, inspection of skin, weight changes, and mental status.

Nursing Diagnoses, Goals, and Outcome Criteria: Hepatitis

Nursing Diagnoses	Goals and Outcome Criteria
Activity Intolerance and **Impaired Physical Mobility** related to fatigue, impaired metabolism, prescribed bed rest	Improved activity tolerance: patient report of less fatigue with activity Absence of complications of immobility: skin intact, breath sounds clear, no calf tenderness
Imbalanced Nutrition: Less Than Body Requirements related to anorexia, nausea, and vomiting	Adequate dietary intake: stable body weight
Deficient Fluid Volume related to inadequate intake, vomiting	Normal fluid status: fluid output equal to intake, vital signs consistent with patient norms, moist mucous membranes
Risk for Impaired Skin Integrity related to pruritus and scratching	Intact skin: no abrasions
Disturbed Body Image related to jaundice	Improved body image: patient expresses acceptance of skin discoloration
Anxiety related to hospitalization, unfamiliar procedures, serious illness	Decreased anxiety: patient states that anxiety is decreased or absent, calm manner

Interventions

Activity Intolerance and Impaired Physical Mobility

Most patients with acute viral hepatitis are treated at home, so instructions about activity limitations are needed. The extent of activity limitation depends on the severity of symptoms. While the patient is symptomatic, bed rest may be advised. Explain that rest allows the liver to heal by regenerating new cells to replace those damaged by hepatitis.

Unless the patient has severe complications, complete bed rest is usually not necessary. If complete bed rest is ordered, the patient is at risk for complications of immobility. Inspect the skin for early signs of pressure (redness, especially over bony prominences). If the patient is unable to turn independently, assist with turning at least every 2 hours. Moisturizing lotions protect the skin and can help relieve itching associated with jaundice.

Teach the patient to cough and deep breathe every 2 hours to reduce the risk of pneumonia. Gentle exercise of the legs promotes circulation and discourages the formation of thrombi. Discourage crossing of the legs.

Inactivity tends to lead to constipation and may cause urinary stasis. Therefore record bowel movements and urine output and describe any abnormal characteristics of stool and urine. Promote rest by planning activities to permit times when the patient is not disturbed. Offer diversions such as reading or television to combat boredom. Care of the immobilized patient is discussed in detail in Chapter 21.

Imbalanced Nutrition: Less Than Body Requirements

Good nutrition is essential to decrease demands on the liver (see the Nutrition Concepts box below). Specific dietary orders depend on the extent of liver dysfunction. With uncomplicated hepatitis, protein requirements range from 0.8 to 1.0 gm/kg/day. The recommended daily allowance of protein for healthy adults is 0.75 gm/kg. Fat intake may be restricted. Unfortunately, anorexia is a common symptom of hepatitis. Measures to manage anorexia include small, frequent meals, a pleasant eating environment, frequent oral hygiene, and explanations of the need for a balanced diet. Occasionally, a feeding tube is inserted to increase nutritional intake.

Nausea and vomiting also can contribute to nutritional deficits and fluid and electrolyte imbalances. Best results are usually obtained by administering antiemetics as soon as nausea is reported. A cool, damp cloth applied to the face and neck is sometimes helpful. When the patient vomits, note the amount and contents of vomitus (emesis) as well as any visible or occult blood. Measure emesis, and record the volume as output. Remove soiled clothing, linens, and basins promptly, and handle according to agency infection control guidelines.

Nutrition Concepts

1. People with gallbladder disease should follow a low-fat diet because fat intake usually causes pain.
2. For a person with hepatitis, the diet should be high in calories and vitamins with moderate to high protein and moderate to low fat.
3. When the liver is damaged by cirrhosis, protein may be restricted to lower blood ammonia.
4. In both hepatitis and cirrhosis, carbohydrates should provide most of the calories.
5. A bland, high-carbohydrate, high-protein, low-fat diet is recommended for pancreatitis.
6. Pancreatitis patients must avoid alcohol and spicy foods that stimulate the pancreas.

Deficient Fluid Volume

The patient with hepatitis needs to maintain a fluid intake of 3000 mL/day unless contraindicated. If the patient is hospitalized, maintain intake and output records. Be alert for signs of fluid retention, such as edema, increasing abdominal girth, and rising blood pressure. If the patient's fluid intake is low or if vomiting is present, also monitor for dehydration. Signs of dehydration include dry mucous membranes, tachycardia, concentrated urine, and confusion. Patients who are at risk for dehydration may receive intravenous fluids as prescribed.

Risk for Impaired Skin Integrity

Pruritus, or itching, is an annoying symptom. Patients naturally respond by scratching, which may cause breaks in the skin. Nursing measures are designed to reduce dryness and irritation. Bathe the skin in cool water, and pat dry. Mild soap may be used unless it seems to increase symptoms. Lubricating lotions or topical antipruritics may be applied. Use light strokes in the direction of the heart. Select older, soft sheets. You can suggest that the patient gently pat the skin instead of scratching to reduce the itching sensation. If a patient is confused, trim the fingernails as agency policy permits. Mittens may be needed to prevent excessive scratching. If conservative measures are not effective, consult the physician about ordering an antihistamine.

Disturbed Body Image

The patient may be self-conscious about his or her appearance because of jaundice. Demonstrate acceptance of the patient, and explain that the skin color usually returns to normal in 2 to 4 weeks.

Anxiety

Hospitalization and diagnostic tests and procedures can provoke anxiety in the patient with hepatitis. The patient also may be fearful about the expected course of the disease and the risk of complications. Encourage questions and find out what the patient wants to know. Explanations about what to expect reduce the fear of the unknown. Explore how patients usually deal with stress, and help them identify coping strategies. If the patient has a history of drug or alcohol abuse, provide information about support groups such as Alcoholics Anonymous and Narcotics Anonymous.

Deficient Knowledge

It is particularly important for the patient with chronic hepatitis to learn how to live with the disease. Good nutrition, exercise, adequate sleep, and avoidance of illicit drugs including alcohol can slow the progression of the disease. In addition to the general teaching plan, explain the patient's specific treatment and the importance of taking medications as prescribed. If your patient is a sexually active female who is taking immune globulins or ribavirin, explain that these drugs can cause birth defects. Oral contraceptives may be ineffective, so condoms, spermicidal jelly or foam, or a diaphragm should be used.

Staff Protection

When patients are hospitalized, Standard Precautions are implemented. Nurses are at risk for exposure to hepatitis because they often handle body fluids. The Occupational Safety and Health Administration requires vaccination for hepatitis B for nurses and other health care providers. The vaccine is given in a series of three injections and confers long-term immunity on most people. Follow-up testing may be done to assess the titer level, which is a measure of immunity. If the antibody titer is inadequate, up to three booster doses may be given. Vaccination has significantly decreased hepatitis B among health care providers; however, there is no vaccine for HCV.

Table 39-1 summarizes precautions to be used to prevent the transmission of hepatitis.

CIRRHOSIS

Pathophysiology

Cirrhosis is a chronic, progressive disease of the liver. It is characterized by degeneration and destruction of liver cells. Fibrotic bands of connective tissue impair the flow of blood and lymph and distort the normal liver structure.

As cirrhosis progresses, there is significant disruption of many physiologic processes. The effects of liver disease include metabolic disturbances, blood abnormalities, fluid and electrolyte imbalances, decreased resistance to infection, accumulation of drugs and toxins, and obstruction of blood vessels and bile ducts in the liver.

Incidence

The highest incidence of cirrhosis is in people between the ages of 40 and 60. It is the fifth leading cause of death in people in that age range in the United States. It is more common in men than in women. The pathol-

ogy is most often related to alcoholic liver disease or chronic viral infection.

 What Does Culture Have to Do with Cirrhosis?

Hispanics have the highest rate of deaths from cirrhosis of the liver, followed by African Americans and whites.

Types of Cirrhosis

There are four major types of cirrhosis, classified based on cause: alcoholic cirrhosis, postnecrotic **cirrhosis, biliary cirrhosis,** and cardiac cirrhosis. Several other types occur infrequently.

Alcoholic Cirrhosis. Alcoholic liver disease progresses in three stages: hepatic steatosis, fatty liver, and cirrhosis. This type of cirrhosis was formerly called *Laënnec's cirrhosis* and is caused by exposure to alcohol. The liver enlarges, becomes "knobby," and then shrinks. Fatty liver is reversible if alcohol intake ceases. Alcoholic cirrhosis is not reversible.

Postnecrotic Cirrhosis. Postnecrotic cirrhosis can be a complication of hepatitis in which there is massive liver cell necrosis.

Biliary Cirrhosis. Biliary cirrhosis is also called *obstructive* or *idiopathic cirrhosis.* As the name suggests, it develops as a result of obstruction to bile flow.

Cardiac Cirrhosis. Cardiac cirrhosis follows severe right-sided heart failure. Venous congestion and hypoxia lead to necrosis of liver cells.

Signs and Symptoms

In the early stage, signs and symptoms of cirrhosis are usually subtle. The patient may report slight weight loss, unexplained fever, fatigue, and dull heaviness in the right upper quadrant of the abdomen. These symptoms are probably due to inflammation and enlargement of the liver. The liver may be palpable below the right rib margin.

As the disease progresses, impaired metabolism of carbohydrates, fats, and proteins causes gastrointestinal disturbances such as anorexia, nausea, vomiting, diarrhea or constipation, flatulence, and dyspepsia (heartburn). Resistance to blood flow from the intestines to the liver causes circulation to become congested in the intestines, stomach, and esophagus. Elevated pressure in veins in the gastrointestinal tract causes them to dilate and bulge. Dilated veins in the esophagus are called *esophageal varices,* and those in the rectum are *hemorrhoids.* Prominent veins may be visible on the abdomen.

Anemia, leukocytopenia, thrombocytopenia, and prothrombin deficiency are hematologic disorders associated with cirrhosis. As a result, patients tend to tire quickly and are more susceptible to infections. They bruise easily and may bleed excessively from minor trauma. Epistaxis (nosebleed) is common.

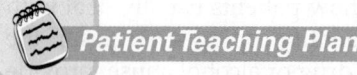 **Patient Teaching Plan**

Hepatitis

Take precautions to avoid exposing others to the virus. Precautions vary with the type of hepatitis, but the following guidelines are helpful:

• People who have had close contact with you should be vaccinated with immune globulin to temporarily boost the body's natural resistance to infection.
• Do not share personal items or utensils with others.
• Wash your hands thoroughly after toileting.
• If you have active hepatitis B, use condoms for sexual intercourse; your partner should be vaccinated against HBV.
• Do not expose others to your blood.

Later signs and symptoms of cirrhosis reflect the liver's inability to perform normal functions. Jaundice develops because of elevated serum bilirubin levels. Two factors contribute to jaundice in the patient with cirrhosis. First, diseased liver cells may be unable to conjugate and excrete bilirubin. Second, structural changes in the liver prevent the normal flow of bile out of the liver. Another effect of impaired bilirubin excretion, as previously mentioned, is the deposition of bile salts under the skin that can cause intense pruritus.

The diseased liver is unable to metabolize estrogen, testosterone, aldosterone, and adrenocortical hormones. The patient, therefore, exhibits signs and symptoms of hormone excesses. Testicular atrophy, impotence, and gynecomastia may be noted in men, and amenorrhea may be noted in women. Palmar erythema and spider angiomas also are attributed to hormone excess. Excess aldosterone contributes to sodium and water retention. The failing liver is also unable to metabolize ammonia, a product of protein metabolism. Excess ammonia affects the central nervous system, leading to confusion and decreasing consciousness.

Cirrhosis impairs the liver's ability to manufacture albumin. Albumin plays a critical role in creating the colloid osmotic pressure that retains water in the vascular compartment. With low serum albumin levels, water leaks from the capillaries, causing decreased blood volume and edema. Ascites is the accumulation of fluid in the peritoneal cavity.

Peripheral neuropathy, characterized by tingling or numbness in the extremities, is common with cirrhosis. This is thought to be caused by dietary deficiencies of vitamin B_{12}, thiamine, and folic acid.

Figure 39-5 illustrates the clinical picture of the patient with liver disease.

Complications

The patient with cirrhosis is at risk for many complications, including portal hypertension, esophageal varices, ascites, hepatic encephalopathy, and hepatorenal syndrome.

Portal Hypertension. The portal vein delivers blood from the intestines to the liver. Changes in the liver with cirrhosis obstruct the flow of incoming blood, causing blood to back up in the portal system. High portal pressure, or portal hypertension, causes collateral vessels to develop. Collateral vessels commonly form in the esophagus, the anterior abdominal wall, and the rectum.

Esophageal Varices. Distended, engorged vessels in the esophagus are called *esophageal varices*. They are fragile and bleed easily, with the potential for fatal hemorrhage. Circumstances that may trigger bleeding include irritation and increased intra-abdominal pressure. Sources of irritation are alcohol, coarse foods, and stomach acid. Intra-abdominal pressure is increased by vomiting, coughing, heavy lifting, and straining at stool.

Ascites. Ascites is an accumulation of fluid in the peritoneal cavity. Factors that contribute to the development of ascites with cirrhosis include portal hypertension, leaking of lymph fluid and albumin-rich fluid from the diseased liver, low serum albumin levels, increased aldosterone levels, and water retention.

Hepatic Encephalopathy. The failing liver is unable to detoxify ammonia, a breakdown product of protein metabolism. Excessive ammonia in the blood causes neurologic symptoms, including cognitive disturbances, declining level of consciousness, and changes in neuromuscular function. If the condition is not reversed, the patient lapses into unconsciousness, referred to as *hepatic coma.*

Factors that may precipitate hepatic encephalopathy are infection, fluid and potassium depletion, gastrointestinal bleeding, constipation, and some drugs.

Hepatorenal Syndrome. Hepatorenal syndrome is renal failure in the cirrhosis patient that often follows diuretic therapy, paracentesis, or gastrointestinal hemorrhage. The kidney structure appears unchanged, so the reason for failure is not known.

Medical Diagnosis

When the patient's history and physical examination suggest cirrhosis, tests and procedures may be ordered to confirm or rule out the disease. These studies include blood tests (liver function tests, CBC, prothrombin time, protein, electrolytes, albumin, bilirubin), urine bilirubin, urobilinogen, liver biopsy, liver scan, ultrasonography, angiography, computed tomography, and magnetic resonance imaging. Results of blood tests that are consistent with cirrhosis include elevated serum and urine bilirubin, elevated serum enzymes, decreased total serum protein, decreased cholesterol, and prolonged prothrombin time. The complete blood cell count may reveal deficiencies of red and white blood cells and platelets.

The liver biopsy is performed to obtain a tissue specimen for microscopic study. Typical cellular changes occur with cirrhosis. Imaging procedures outline the liver features.

The Diagnostic Tests and Procedures table on pp. 801 to 803 summarizes tests and procedures used to diagnose liver disorders.

Medical Treatment

The goals of medical treatment for cirrhosis are to limit deterioration of liver function and to prevent complications, but there is no specific medical treatment. The approach is to promote rest so that the liver can regenerate. The earlier the condition is diagnosed and measures are taken to promote healing, the better is the chance of recovery.

Bed rest is usually ordered if the patient is in liver failure. Malnutrition is common, and the specific diet depends on individual patient factors. A diet high in carbohydrates and vitamins with moderate to high protein intake is typically ordered unless the patient's blood ammonia level is elevated. In that case, protein is restricted until the ammonia level falls. Supplementary iron and vitamins also may be ordered. The amount of fat allowed in the diet varies with the patient's condition. Anorexia is frequently a problem with cirrhosis, so small, semisolid or liquid meals may be better received. Enteral feedings may be needed to provide adequate nutrients.

Other medical treatments may be ordered to correct the complications of cirrhosis. Intravenous fluids may be needed to correct fluid and electrolyte imbalances. Anemia may require blood transfusions. Water and sodium are likely to be restricted in patients with severe fluid retention. Cathartics and antibiotics may be used for hepatic encephalopathy.

Ascites. The medical management of ascites aims to promote reabsorption and elimination of the fluid by means of sodium restriction and diuretics. Combinations of various types of diuretics may yield better results than a single diuretic. Salt-poor albumin may be given intravenously to help maintain blood volume and to increase urinary output. Albumin raises the serum colloid osmotic pressure, causing water to be drawn back into the bloodstream. The Drug Therapy table on pp. 811 to 812 lists drugs used to treat the patient with ascites.

If ascites does not respond to conservative treatment, fluid can be removed with a needle, a procedure called *paracentesis.* An alternative is the placement of a peritoneal-venous shunt.

Paracentesis. Paracentesis is the removal of ascitic fluid from the peritoneal cavity. A special instrument called a *trocar* is inserted through the abdominal wall, and a catheter is placed to allow the fluid to drain. This procedure is indicated only when ascites interferes with the patient's breathing. It is not used frequently because it removes essential protein and electrolytes. In addition, it provides a potential portal of entry for pathogens.

If paracentesis is done to remove ascites, your role is to prepare the patient, assist and support the patient during the procedure, and provide aftercare. The physician should explain what will be done and obtain patient consent. Reinforce explanations and obtain the written consent as agency policy permits. Obtain baseline vital signs, weight, and abdominal girth. Instruct the patient to void.

The procedure is often done at the bedside with the patient in a sitting position. During paracentesis, you should support and encourage the patient. The physician may request monitoring of vital signs during the process. Usually, 2 to 3 L of fluid is removed slowly. Rapid removal of ascitic fluid could result in circulatory collapse. After paracentesis, a sterile dressing is applied to the puncture site. Monitor vital signs every 15 minutes until the patient is stable, and check the dressing for bleeding. Measure the fluid obtained, and send a specimen for laboratory analysis. Document the procedure, including the amount and color of the fluid. Monitor for blood in the urine.

Shunts. Shunts provide a mechanism to collect ascitic fluid and return it to the circulation. Advantages to shunting ascitic fluid rather than removing it are (1) protein-rich serum is retained and returned to the vascular compartment; and (2) urine output increases, which eliminates excess sodium and water. Two types of shunts are the peritoneal-venous shunt and the transjugular intrahepatic portosystemic shunt (TIPS).

Peritoneal-venous shunts may be implanted permanently. Two peritoneal-venous shunts are the LeVeen

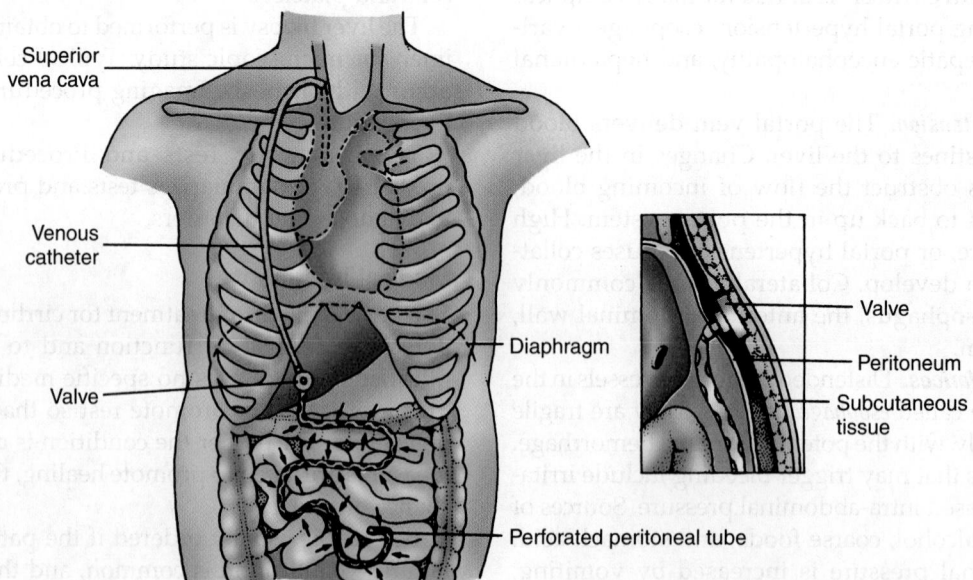

FIGURE 39-6 A peritoneal-venous shunt drains ascitic fluid from the abdominal cavity into the superior vena cava.

and Denver shunts. The LeVeen shunt (Fig. 39-6) is a tube that is placed in the abdomen, running from the peritoneal cavity to the jugular vein or superior vena cava. The tube has a one-way valve that permits excess fluid to drain into the venous circulation when pressure rises in the abdomen. When the patient inspires, intra-abdominal pressure rises, causing the valve to open. The Denver peritoneal-venous shunt involves a manual pump placed under the skin. It can be compressed to cause fluid to flow from the peritoneum to the venous system. Potential complications of peritoneal-venous shunts are peritonitis, tubing obstruction, circulatory overload, disseminated intravascular coagulopathy, variceal hemorrhage, and embolism.

Because of the complications encountered with peritoneal-venous shunts, the TIPS (transjugular intrahepatic portosystemic shunt) is often a preferred treatment. A catheter is threaded through the jugular vein and the inferior vena cava to the hepatic vein. The hepatic vein is punctured and connected to the portal vein with a stent. This procedure reduces pressure in the portal system with fewer complications.

The portacaval shunt and the distal splenorenal shunt are surgically created to reduce portal system pressure while maintaining liver perfusion. The patient with a portacaval shunt is at risk for hepatic encephalopathy because ammonia accumulates in the blood. The incidence of hepatic encephalopathy is lower with distal splenorenal shunts.

Bleeding Esophageal Varices. Several techniques can be used to control bleeding esophageal varices. These include drug therapy, sclerotherapy, and surgical ligation. Although now uncommon, placement of esophageal-gastric balloon tubes may still be useful.

Acute bleeding episodes may be treated with intravenous octreotide, which constricts blood vessels and

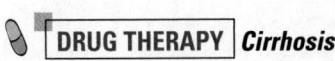

DRUG THERAPY | *Cirrhosis*

GENERAL NURSING IMPLICATIONS
1. No drug can cure cirrhosis.
2. Drug therapy treats symptoms: fluid retention, portal hypertension, encephalopathy, and bleeding.
3. Patients with liver dysfunction may not metabolize drugs normally, so be alert for adverse effects.

DRUG	USE/ACTION	SIDE EFFECTS	NURSING INTERVENTIONS
DIURETICS Spironolactone (Aldactone) Amiloride (Midamor) Furosemide (Lasix) Chlorothiazide (Diuril)	Promote excretion of excess fluid in edema and ascites.	Fluid and electrolyte imbalances, including fluid volume deficit and hyponatremia. Hypokalemia can occur except with potassium-sparing diuretics like spironolactone.	Monitor intake and output, abdominal girth. Check laboratory values for electrolyte imbalances.
HORMONE Sandostatin (Octreotide)	Reduces pressure in portal veins to treat bleeding esophageal varices.	Bradycardia, hyperglycemia, hypoglycemia	Monitor pulse and notify physician if below 60. Monitor glucose levels in patients with diabetes.
BETA-ADRENERGIC BLOCKER Propranolol (Inderal)	Reduces pressure in portal veins to reduce risk of bleeding.	Bradycardia, hypotension, bronchoconstriction. Masks signs of hypoglycemia.	Monitor pulse; if below 60, withhold and notify physician. Monitor blood glucose in people with diabetes.
ANTIBIOTIC Neomycin sulfate	Reduces gastrointestinal bacterial flora, decreasing ammonia production. Used to prevent or treat hepatic encephalopathy.	Toxic to kidney and eighth cranial nerve (hearing and balance). Increases action of neuromuscular blocking agents like anesthetics.	Monitor intake and output. Assess for hearing impairment, tinnitus (ringing in ears), nausea, loss of balance.
LAXATIVE Lactulose (Cephulac)	Promotes elimination of ammonia in feces. Used to prevent or treat hepatic encephalopathy.	Cramps, distention, flatulence, eructation. Hyperglycemia with diabetes.	May be ordered every hour at first. Can be mixed with fruit juice, water, or milk. Monitor diabetics.

Continued

DRUG THERAPY *Cirrhosis—cont'd*

DRUG	USE/ACTION	SIDE EFFECTS	NURSING INTERVENTIONS
DOPAMINERGIC AGENTS			
Levodopa	Replace dopamine lost in process of protein breakdown. Used to prevent or treat hepatic encephalopathy.	Nausea, vomiting, orthostatic hypotension.	Teach patient to manage orthostatic hypotension. Provide comfort measures for nausea. Report vomiting. Give antiemetics as ordered.
VITAMINS			
B complex	Needed for production of red blood cells and for normal growth and development.	Allergic reaction to thiamine (anaphylaxis). Adverse effects rare.	Intradermal test dose may be ordered to detect sensitivity to thiamine. Check site for reaction: redness, swelling. Check reference for incompatibility with other intravenous drugs.
K Menadiol (vitamin K₃) Phytonadione (Aqua-MEPHYTON)	Treats serious bleeding disorders caused by deficiency of prothrombin. Used cautiously with severe liver disease.	Gastric upset (oral route only), rash, urticaria, flushing, hemolytic anemia. Pain and swelling at injection site.	Check laboratory results for prothrombin time. Report abnormalities. Monitor complete blood cell count. Assess for bleeding. Apply pressure to needle puncture sites for 5 min.

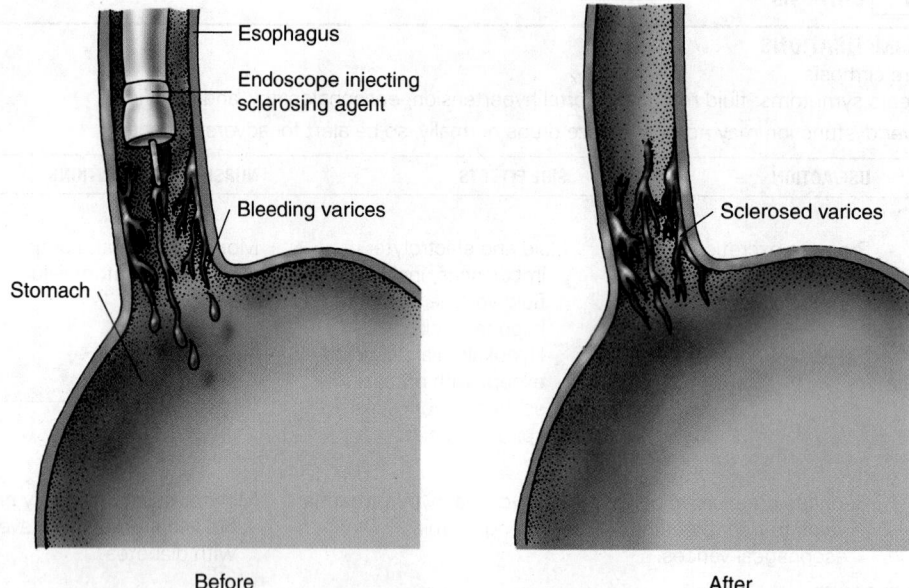

FIGURE **39-7** Injection sclerotherapy.

lowers pressure in the hepatic circulation. In addition to blood transfusions, vitamin K and proton pump inhibitors (PPIs) such as pantoprazole (Protonix) may be ordered. Lactulose may be administered to prevent the breakdown of blood in the intestines that would release ammonia, contributing to hepatic encephalopathy. Beta-adrenergic blockers may be used to reduce blood pressure in the long-term management of patients after acute bleeding episodes.

Surgical Treatment of Bleeding Varices. In an emergency situation, the surgeon may ligate (tie off) bleeding varices directly through an endoscope.

The patient can then be stabilized before a more extensive corrective procedure. Corrective procedures surgically shunt blood from engorged varices to other veins. A portacaval shunt diverts blood to the vena cava, whereas a splenorenal shunt routes the blood to the splenic vein. The incidence of hepatic encephalopathy is lower with the splenorenal shunt than with the portacaval shunt. A third type of shunt that is placed under fluoroscopy is the transjugular intrahepatic portosystemic shunt. A stent is passed into the right internal jugular vein, through the right atrium and into the vena cava and inserted between the hepatic and portal veins. By shunting the blood in this manner, pressure in the portal venous system and the esophageal varices is reduced.

Sclerotherapy. Sclerotherapy is a procedure in which a solution is injected into the varices or into the veins that supply them, causing the varices to harden and close (Fig. 39-7). The procedure can be done through an endoscope or through a small surgical incision. Sclerotherapy can be done to prevent or to treat bleeding.

After sclerotherapy, patients often report chest discomfort for several days. The physician usually orders a mild analgesic. If it does not relieve the pain, the physician should be notified because persistent pain may indicate perforation of the esophagus. Once a patient has had sclerotherapy, extra care must be taken in the insertion of nasogastric tubes.

Esophageal-Gastric Balloon Tube. Although uncommon, esophageal-gastric balloon tubes may be used to apply direct pressure to bleeding veins in the esophagus and stomach if ligation and sclerotherapy fail. Examples of tubes used for this purpose are the Sengstaken-Blakemore esophageal-gastric balloon tube and the Minnesota tube. The Sengstaken-Blakemore tube has three ports. One is used to inflate the esophageal balloon, another to inflate the gastric balloon, and the third to suction the stomach. A second nasogastric tube may be inserted with the Sengstaken-Blakemore tube to collect secretions above the esophageal balloon. The Minnesota tube has four lumina that permit inflation of gastric and esophageal balloons and suctioning of both the esophagus and the stomach (Fig. 39-8).

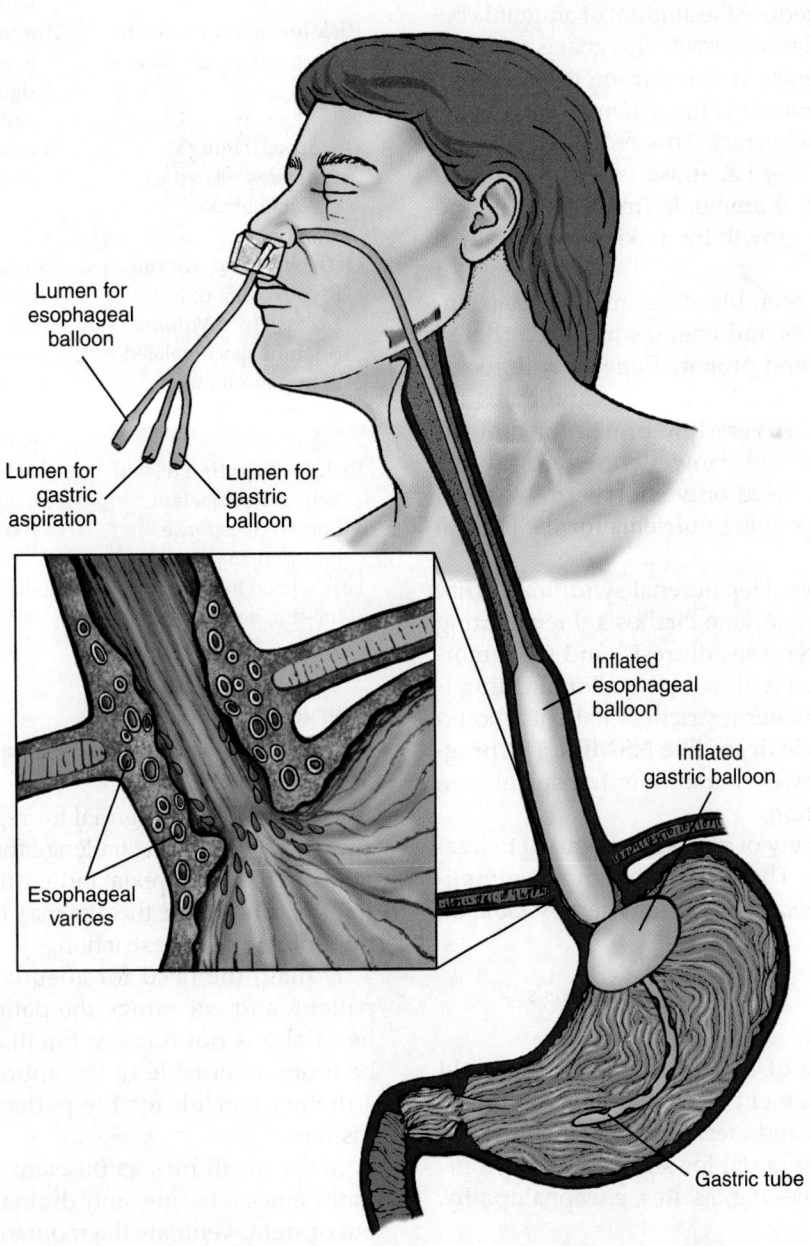

Lumen for esophageal balloon

Lumen for gastric aspiration

Lumen for gastric balloon

Inflated esophageal balloon

Inflated gastric balloon

Esophageal varices

Gastric tube

FIGURE **39-8** Sengstaken-Blakemore tube in place to compress bleeding esophageal varices.

The tube is inserted by a physician. The gastric balloon is inflated first and gently pulled upward to apply pressure to veins in the upper part of the stomach. The esophageal balloon is then inflated. The gastric suction tube is connected to continuous suction. It also may be irrigated to remove clots and maintain patency of the tube. It is important to remove old blood from the stomach so that it will not be digested. Digested blood produces ammonia, which increases the likelihood of hepatic encephalopathy. Gastric suction also reduces the risk of vomiting, which would force the balloons out of place. The tube usually is left inflated for 24 to 48 hours. It then is deflated but left in place so that it can be reinflated if needed.

Hepatic Encephalopathy. Many factors can precipitate hepatic encephalopathy including constipation, GI bleeding, hypokalemia, infection, opioids, dehydration, and renal failure. The goal of drug therapy in hepatic encephalopathy is to reduce the amount of ammonia being produced in the digestive tract. This goal is achieved mainly with drug therapy and reduction of protein intake. A source of ammonia is the action of bacteria on protein in the digestive tract. This reduction may be achieved with lactulose. Lactulose is a cathartic that promotes elimination of ammonia from the colon and discourages bacterial growth by making the intestinal contents more acidic.

If the patient has been bleeding into the gastrointestinal tract, laxatives and enemas may be ordered to remove old blood and protein. Patients with recurring hepatic encephalopathy may be candidates for liver transplantation. A very-low-protein or protein-free diet may be ordered. However, severe protein restriction should be used only short-term to avoid malnutrition and to provide nutrients for the liver to regenerate.

Hepatorenal Syndrome. Hepatorenal syndrome (HRS) is renal failure accompanying cirrhosis. Precipitating factors include paracentesis, diuresis, and GI hemorrhage. It may be treated with salt-poor albumin, diuretics, and sodium and water restriction. Patients should not receive nephrotoxic drugs like NSAIDs. The prognosis is very poor, however, and liver transplantation may be the only solution.

Drug Therapy. A variety of drugs may be used to treat the effects of cirrhosis. These drugs and nursing implications are summarized in the Drug Therapy table on pp. 811 and 812.

NURSING CARE *of the Patient with Cirrhosis*
Assessment

Ongoing assessments of the cirrhosis patient should include daily measurement of weight, measurements of intake and output, and measurement of abdominal girth. Patients are monitored for signs and symptoms of complications—bleeding, ascites, encephalopathy, and renal failure.

Nursing Diagnoses, Goals, and Outcome Criteria: Cirrhosis

Nursing Diagnoses	Goals and Outcome Criteria
Imbalanced Nutrition: Less Than Body Requirements related to anorexia, metabolic imbalances	Adequate nutrition: stable body weight, consumes meals
Activity Intolerance related to fatigue	Improved activity tolerance: performs activities of daily living without excessive fatigue
Risk for Impaired Skin Integrity related to edema, immobility, pruritus, hypoproteinemia	Intact skin: no redness or breaks in skin. No scratching
Ineffective Breathing Pattern related to ascites	Effective breathing: respiratory rate of 12-20 per minute without dyspnea
Risk for Injury related to impaired coagulation	Absence of bleeding: no blood in emesis or stool, vital signs consistent with patient norms
Disturbed Thought Processes related to elevated blood ammonia	Normal cognitive function: mentally alert, oriented
Deficient Fluid Volume (hypovolemia) or **Excess Fluid Volume** (in third space) related to hypoproteinemia, increased aldosterone	Normal fluid distribution in body fluid compartments: balanced fluid intake and output without edema or ascites; pulse and blood pressure consistent with patient norms
Risk for Infection related to liver dysfunction, impaired response to infection, malnutrition	Absence of infection: oral temperature less than 100° F
Fear related to dyspnea, life-threatening illness	Reduced fear: patient states no or less fear, calm manner

Interventions
Imbalanced Nutrition: Less Than Body Requirements

Good nutrition is essential for regeneration of liver tissue. However, it is a challenge for the cirrhosis patient, who often has anorexia, indigestion, nausea, and vomiting. Furthermore, the diet may be made less palatable by protein or salt restriction.

Explain the need for adequate food intake to the patient, and encourage the patient to eat even when he or she is not hungry. Small, frequent meals may be more acceptable to the anorexic patient. Arrange a dietary consult for the patient to report likes and dislikes.

Make mealtimes as pleasant as possible. Put bedpans, emesis basins, and drainage collection devices out of sight. Ventilate the room to reduce odors. Do not schedule tiring activities immediately before meals. Record daily weights as ordered to monitor both nutritional and fluid status.

Activity Intolerance

Some activity limitations are usually imposed, depending on the patient's overall status. Schedule nursing care to allow some periods of undisturbed rest. The patient can generally assume any position that is comfortable. If ascites is present, elevate the head of the bed to facilitate breathing. Some patients are more comfortable sitting in a chair with the feet elevated.

If the patient spends all or most of the day in bed, there is a risk of complications related to immobility. Assist the patient to change positions, deep breathe, and exercise extremities regularly.

Risk for Impaired Skin Integrity

The patient with cirrhosis is at risk for skin breakdown for several reasons. Bile salts that are normally processed by the liver may be deposited under the skin, causing intense pruritus. Loss of muscle and fat tissue with advanced disease reduces the padding that normally protects the skin from pressure. Also, many patients have edema, which makes tissue more fragile and impairs healing.

Nursing measures to relieve the itching of pruritus include gentle bathing with mild soap and warm water, thorough rinsing, and application of moisturizing lotions. The patient's nails should be kept short to reduce trauma from scratching. If scratching persists, put soft cotton mittens or gloves on the patient's hands. If itching is severe, consult the physician about ordering a medication to relieve the discomfort. Cholestyramine (Questran) may be ordered to increase the excretion of bile salts.

Ineffective Breathing Pattern

Ascitic fluid can cause the abdomen to become greatly distended. While in bed, the patient breathes easier with the head of the bed elevated. Sitting in a chair with the feet elevated, if allowed, may be even more comfortable.

Risk for Injury

The patient with cirrhosis is at great risk for injury or hemorrhage due to impaired coagulation and fragile varices. Handle the patient gently to avoid trauma. Use a soft toothbrush or swab for mouth care. Apply firm pressure to injection sites to minimize oozing. Pad side rails if the patient is restless.

An uncommon but effective treatment for bleeding esophageal varices is an esophageal-gastric balloon tube placement. The patient with this type of tube is usually in an intensive care unit, since close monitoring is necessary. The tube is uncomfortable, and the patient is likely to be frightened about both the bleeding

and the treatment. When the tube is in place, monitor the patient for signs of continued or renewed bleeding, including restlessness, increasing pulse and respirations, and falling blood pressure. Note stool characteristics. Bleeding from the esophagus or stomach usually produces a sticky (tarry), maroon to black stool. Examine aspirated stomach and esophageal contents for evidence of fresh bleeding. Old blood in the stomach is usually brownish and may be described as resembling coffee grounds. Fresh blood is bright to dark red.

Because the esophagus and the trachea are adjacent to each other, upward movement of the esophageal balloon can cause airway obstruction. Therefore when the balloon tube is in place, monitor the patient for sudden respiratory distress. If this occurs, both balloon ports must be promptly cut and the tubes removed by a properly trained person.

Disturbed Thought Processes

Cognitive changes in the patient with cirrhosis are usually due to hepatic encephalopathy. Nursing care of the patient with hepatic encephalopathy includes monitoring mental and neurologic status. Inform the registered nurse or physician of changes in status. The patient who is confused or unconscious requires close attention to prevent injury or complications of immobility. Talk to the patient to provide basic information and reassurance. The family also may need an explanation of the patient's behavior. Enforce dietary protein restrictions, and administer prescribed drugs that decrease bacteria in the intestines (e.g., lactulose). Be alert for adverse effects of drug therapy, which may include diarrhea or vitamin K deficiency.

Deficient Fluid Volume or Excess Fluid Volume

Fluid needs vary with the patient's condition. Sodium and water are likely to be restricted if there is marked edema or ascites. Despite the excess in total body water, the patient's blood volume may be dangerously low. Adequate water is present; however, it is not distributed appropriately. Without adequate albumin in the serum, colloid osmotic pressure falls and water shifts out of the capillaries into the tissues. Administer intravenous fluids and salt-poor albumin as ordered. In addition to monitoring vital signs, evaluate fluid intake and output.

Risk for Infection

The patient with cirrhosis is at risk for infection for several reasons. The liver is no longer able to filter bacteria from the blood as it comes from the intestines. The function of the spleen also is impaired, which lowers resistance to infection. In addition, these patients tend to be malnourished, so they lack the building materials for tissue repair. Monitor for fever and malaise, which suggest infection. Protect the patient from others with infections. Practice good hand washing and use aseptic technique for invasive procedures.

Fear

Patients with cirrhosis can experience frightening complications, including confusion, dyspnea, and hemorrhage. With advanced cirrhosis, the prognosis is poor and patients often have repeated emergency admissions. Treatments and diagnostic procedures may be painful and anxiety-producing. The nurse can help by recognizing the patient's fear and acknowledging it.

To provide emotional support to cirrhosis patients, you must be aware of your personal reaction to these patients. There is a stigma attached to cirrhosis because it is often associated with alcohol abuse. Health care providers must treat patients in a nonjudgmental manner. Nurses must realize that alcoholism is a complex chronic disease that is not easily controlled and that cirrhosis can be caused by factors other than alcohol.

Information can help reduce fear. When the patient is acutely ill, give simple explanations and answer questions. When the patient improves, explore what he or she knows about cirrhosis and determine what additional information is needed. General teaching points are noted in the Patient Teaching Plan below.

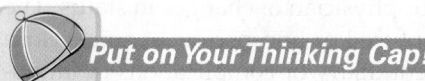

Put on Your Thinking Cap!

Identify three functions of the healthy liver. Describe how cirrhosis affects those functions. State one nursing implication related to the change with cirrhosis in each function.

END-STAGE LIVER DISEASE

End-stage liver disease can result from injury or chronic disease. Hepatic injury may result from acute hepatitis, drug toxicity, or obstruction of the hepatic vein. Liver failure associated with injury is commonly called *fulminant liver failure.*

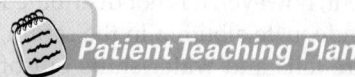

Patient Teaching Plan

Cirrhosis

- A balanced diet will help prevent additional injury to the liver and reduce the risk of complications.
- Avoid specific foods (as advised by the physician and/or dietitian).
- Notify your physician if you have increasing fluid retention, black tarry stools, bloody vomitus, increasing fatigue, or confusion.
- Alcohol is discouraged because of the toxic effects on the liver. Community resources you can use for information and assistance include Alcoholics Anonymous (if appropriate), the American Liver Foundation, and home health nursing services.
- Do not take medications except as approved by your physician. Many drugs, including acetaminophen, can be toxic to the liver.

CANCER OF THE LIVER

Cancer rarely begins in the liver, but the liver is a frequent site of metastasis. Cirrhosis is a predisposing factor for liver cancer. Signs and symptoms of liver cancer include liver enlargement, weight loss, anorexia, nausea, vomiting, and dull pain in the upper right quadrant of the abdomen. As the disease progresses, the signs and symptoms are essentially the same as those of cirrhosis. Because the early signs and symptoms of liver cancer are vague, the condition is often not diagnosed until it is advanced.

Tests and procedures used to diagnose liver cancer are liver scan and biopsy, hepatic arteriography, endoscopy, and measurement of alpha-fetoprotein levels. If the cancer is confined to one area, a lobectomy may be done; otherwise, chemotherapy is the primary treatment. Chemotherapy is generally considered to be palliative, meaning that it may slow the progress of the cancer and increase patient comfort but is unlikely to be curative. In some cases, radiotherapy is prescribed. Transplantation is not generally considered an option with widespread liver cancer.

During the course of the illness, the patient's needs are much like those of the cirrhosis patient, which were covered earlier in this chapter. Additional aspects of nursing care of the patient with cancer are discussed in Chapter 25.

LIVER TRANSPLANTATION

The only possible cure for end-stage liver disease is liver transplantation. Transplantation is also appropriate for patients with cancer that is confined to the liver and for patients with certain congenital disorders.

Patients who are recommended for transplantation are ranked by acuity and need and entered into a national computer network. When a liver becomes available by donation, the best recipient can be identified. Patients awaiting transplantation must be on standby status in case a donor is located. This is a time of alternating hope and fear for patients and families, marked by the recognition that they are waiting for someone else to die.

After liver transplantation, the patient is cared for in a specialized unit. A transplant patient often has a T-tube, wound drainage devices, a nasogastric tube, and a central line for total parenteral nutrition (TPN). Mechanical ventilation also is used initially.

Nursing assessments focus on neurologic status, vital signs, central venous pressure, respiratory status, and indicators of bleeding. If stable, the patient is moved out of the unit after 3 or 4 days. Continue to monitor vital signs, intake and output, and neurologic status. Provide usual postoperative care, including assistance with turning, coughing and deep breathing, and progressive activity.

Lifelong drug therapy is needed to prevent rejection of the donor liver. Some of the current options include cyclosporine, tacrolimus, the monoclonal antibody OKT3, interleukin-2 receptor antagonists, azathioprine, and prednisone. All have significant adverse effects. Prednisone usually is given in combination with another drug and can often be discontinued within a year. OKT3 is a newer agent that may prove to be highly effective and less toxic than other antirejection drugs.

The transplant recipient must be monitored for signs of rejection. These signs include fever, anorexia, depression, vague abdominal pain, muscle aches, and joint pain. Fever is sometimes the *only* sign of rejection. Rejection may be treated with corticosteroids or other immunosuppressants. If this treatment is unsuccessful, retransplantation may be needed.

Before discharge, the patient should know signs and symptoms of transplant rejection and infection, wound care, dietary restrictions (usually sodium restriction), and self-medication.

Pharmacology Capsule

Drugs that suppress rejection of transplanted organs reduce the patient's ability to resist infection.

THE BILIARY TRACT

ANATOMY AND PHYSIOLOGY OF THE BILIARY TRACT

Bile is a yellow-green liquid that has several important functions. It contains bile salts, which are essential for the emulsification and digestion of fats. It also provides a medium for the excretion of bilirubin from the liver.

The biliary tract is made up of the gallbladder and the bile ducts. The function of the biliary tract is to deliver bile from the liver to the duodenum. Bile is produced in the liver and channeled into the common hepatic duct. The common hepatic duct joins the cystic duct to form the common bile duct. The cystic duct leads to the gallbladder, a saclike organ beneath the liver. Bile flows from the liver to the gallbladder, where it is stored and concentrated (Fig. 39-9).

When fats enter the duodenum, the gallbladder contracts and delivers bile to the intestine through the common bile duct.

NURSING ASSESSMENT OF THE BILIARY TRACT

The nursing assessment of the gastrointestinal system was outlined in Chapter 38. Data especially important in a patient with known or suspected gallbladder dysfunction are identified here.

HEALTH HISTORY

Digestive disturbances and pain are common complaints among persons with biliary problems. Obtain a complete description of these symptoms. Note factors that seem to bring on or relieve the symptoms. The relationship between symptoms and meals may be significant. Record the use of estrogen or oral contraceptives. Inquire about factors known to be associated with gallbladder disease: family history, obesity, American Indian ancestry, and inactivity. In the review of systems, ask whether the patient has had dry skin, indigestion, fat intolerance, dyspepsia, nausea, vomiting, light-colored stools, or dark urine.

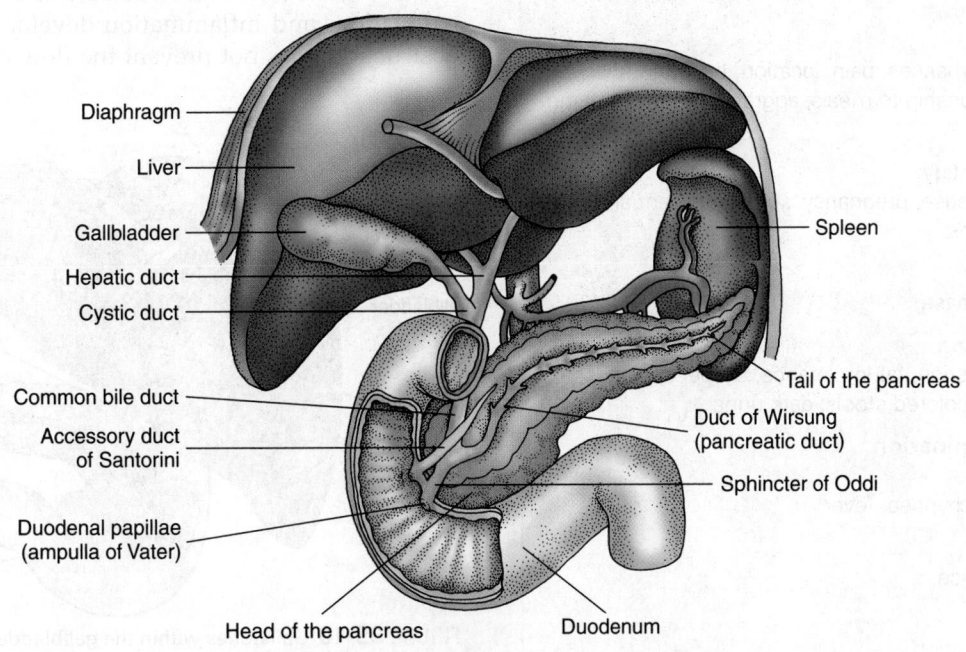

FIGURE **39-9** Anatomy of the liver, gallbladder, and pancreas.

Labels:
Diaphragm
Liver
Gallbladder
Hepatic duct
Cystic duct
Common bile duct
Accessory duct of Santorini
Duodenal papillae (ampulla of Vater)
Head of the pancreas
Spleen
Tail of the pancreas
Duct of Wirsung (pancreatic duct)
Sphincter of Oddi
Duodenum

PHYSICAL EXAMINATION

When a patient has gallbladder disease, significant findings on the physical examination include dry skin, fever, jaundice, tachycardia, tachypnea, and abdominal guarding and distention. Assessment of the patient with a biliary tract disorder is summarized in Box 39-2.

DIAGNOSTIC TESTS AND PROCEDURES

Tests and procedures used to diagnose gallbladder disorders are ultrasonography, oral cholecystography, intravenous cholangiography, T-tube cholangiography, endoscopic retrograde cholangiopancreatography (ERCP), and percutaneous transhepatic cholangiography. Laboratory studies include liver function tests, serum and urine bilirubin measurements, and a complete blood cell count. The Diagnostic Tests and Procedures table on pp. 801 to 803 describes common diagnostic tests and nursing implications.

DISORDERS OF THE GALLBLADDER

Gallbladder disease is one of the most common health problems in the United States. The two most common gallbladder disorders are cholecystitis and cholelithiasis. Carcinoma of the gallbladder occurs but is unusual.

Risk factors for gallbladder disease include obesity, familial tendency, a sedentary lifestyle, and the use of

---

Box 39-2 | **ASSESSMENT of the Patient with Gallbladder Disease**

Health History
Present Illness:
Digestive disturbances; pain: location, onset, intensity, duration, relationship to meals, aggravating and relieving factors

Past Medical History:
Gallbladder disease, pregnancy, surgery, recent and current medications

Family History:
Gallbladder disease

Review of Systems:
Pruritus, indigestion, fat intolerance, dyspepsia, nausea, vomiting, light-colored stools, dark urine

Physical Examination
Vital Signs:
Tachycardia, tachypnea, fever

Skin:
Dryness, jaundice

Abdomen:
Guarding, distention

---

estrogen or oral contraceptives. Women are at greater risk than men, especially women who have had multiple pregnancies. The "5 F's" are sometimes used to describe those at greatest risk for gallbladder disease: female, fat, fair, forty, and fertile.

What Does Culture Have to Do with Gallbladder Disease?
American Indians and whites are at increased risk for gallbladder disease.

CHOLECYSTITIS AND CHOLELITHIASIS

Cholecystitis is inflammation of the gallbladder. It is caused most often by the presence of gallstones but can be due to bacteria, toxic chemicals, tumors, anesthesia, starvation, and opioids. The inflamed gallbladder and cystic duct become swollen and congested with blood. The cystic duct may actually become occluded.

When gallstones are present, the patient is said to have cholelithiasis. Most gallstones are composed of cholesterol mixed with bile salts, bilirubin, calcium, and protein. It is not known exactly why gallstones form, but the process is associated with high concentrations of cholesterol. The concentration of cholesterol rises when there is stasis of bile (as occurs with pregnancy, immobility, and inflammation of the biliary tract).

Gallstones may be found anywhere in the biliary tract: the gallbladder, the cystic duct, or the common bile duct (Fig. 39-10). The stones may move through the biliary tract with bile flow. If a stone cannot pass through the tract, it lodges and causes an obstruction. Ducts respond to obstruction with spasms in an effort to move the stone. This is responsible for an intense, spasmodic pain, called *biliary colic*.

If the cystic duct is obstructed, bile cannot leave the gallbladder and inflammation develops. Cystic duct obstruction does not prevent the flow of bile into the

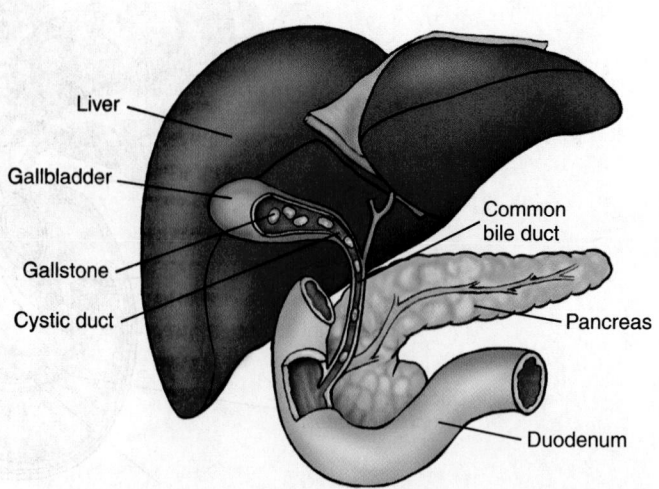

FIGURE **39-10** Gallstones within the gallbladder that could obstruct the common bile duct and the cystic duct.

duodenum from the liver. However, if the common bile duct is obstructed (choledocholithiasis), bile is unable to flow into the duodenum.

Signs and Symptoms

Signs and symptoms of cholecystitis vary from one patient to the next. Some have only mild indigestion, whereas others have severe pain, fever, and jaundice. Other symptoms are nausea, eructation (belching), fever, chills, and right upper quadrant pain that radiates to the shoulder. Symptoms typically occur about 3 hours after a meal, especially if the food had high fat content.

When bile flow is obstructed, bile production in the liver decreases and the serum bilirubin rises, leading to obstructive jaundice. Some excess bilirubin is excreted in the urine, creating a dark amber color. Digestion of fats is impaired, causing intolerance of fatty foods and steatorrhea (excess fat in feces). The absence of urobilinogen in the stool causes it to be a characteristic clay color. The patient is unable to absorb fat-soluble vitamins and may show signs of vitamin deficiencies. Vitamin K deficiency interferes with normal blood clotting, and thus the patient bleeds and bruises easily.

Complications

The most serious complications of cholecystitis and cholelithiasis are pancreatitis, abscesses, cholangitis (inflammation of the biliary ducts), and rupture of the gallbladder.

Medical Diagnosis

A tentative diagnosis of cholelithiasis based on the history and physical examination findings is best confirmed with ultrasonography. Other diagnostic procedures include radiographs and radionuclide imaging.

Blood and urine studies provide additional information. With inflammation or infection, the white blood cell count is elevated. If bile flow is obstructed, levels of serum and urinary bilirubin and serum enzymes may be elevated. Nursing considerations with specific diagnostic tests and procedures are summarized in the Diagnostic Tests and Procedures table on pp. 801 to 803.

Medical Treatment

Acute cholecystitis is managed symptomatically. Analgesics and anticholinergics are ordered to relieve pain and muscle spasms. Antibiotics are given to treat infection. Intravenous fluids are selected to maintain fluid balance, especially if the patient has been vomiting. A nasogastric tube may be inserted and attached to suction. This relieves nausea and vomiting and reduces the stimulation of the gallbladder by intestinal contents.

Among the options available for the treatment of cholelithiasis or choledocholithiasis are drug therapy, shock wave lithotripsy, endoscopic sphincterotomy, and cholecystectomy. Patients with asymptomatic gallstones usually require no treatment except in special circumstances.

Table 39-2	**Drugs Used to Dissolve Gallstones**

GENERAL NURSING IMPLICATIONS
1. Drugs are effective only against small cholesterol stones.
2. Drug therapy is successful in only about one third to one half of patients treated.

DRUG	SIDE EFFECTS	NURSING INTERVENTIONS
ORAL BILE SALTS Chenodeoxycholic acid (Chenix) Ursodeoxycholic acid (UDCA; Actigall)	Diarrhea, cramps, nausea, vomiting, elevated levels of serum enzymes, low-density lipoproteins, and cholesterol. UDCA has milder side effects but is very expensive. Contraindications: biliary tract infection, pancreatitis, pregnancy.	Advise patients not to become pregnant while taking this drug. Stress importance of periodic blood tests to determine liver enzyme and serum cholesterol levels.
DISSOLUTION AGENTS Methyl *tert*-butyl ether (MTBE)	Abdominal pain and nausea during treatment.	Oral contrast dye is given the previous evening. Position patient on right side after the procedure to reduce bleeding. Monitor for hemorrhage, shock, and pneumothorax. Measure vital signs every 15 min until stable; then 3 times at 4-hr intervals. Bed rest for 24 hr.
Monooctanoin (Moctanin)	Anorexia, nausea, vomiting, diarrhea, abdominal pain. Rarely, acute pancreatitis.	Give antiemetics and antidiarrheals PRN, as ordered. With physician's approval, stop infusion for meals. Keep nasal biliary tube securely anchored. Slowing the rate of infusion may control gastrointestinal distress.

PRN, As needed.

Drug Therapy. Two types of drugs are used in a few select patients to dissolve gallstones: oral bile salts and dissolution agents. Ursodeoxycholic acid (UDCA; Actigall) is the oral bile salt in current use. It may be prescribed when the patient has only small cholesterol stones or for those who are poor surgical risks. However, it is very expensive and requires continuous treatment for 6 months to 1 year.

Methyl *tert*-butyl ether (MTBE) and ethyl propionate are dissolution agents. The agent *MTBE* is instilled into the gallbladder through a transhepatic catheter. The physician instills and aspirates the drug repeatedly until fluoroscopy shows that the stones either have dissolved or are not responding to the treatment.

Monooctanoin (Moctanin) is used to treat stones remaining in the common bile duct after cholecystectomy. It is given through a nasobiliary catheter by continuous infusion for 2 to 10 days. The patient is allowed to have a bland diet, and the infusion is stopped during meals. Cholangiograms are obtained periodically to assess the effects of the drug. It is effective about half the time.

Drugs used to treat conditions of the biliary tract are described in Table 39-2.

Extracorporeal Shock Wave Lithotripsy (ESWL). ESWL uses sound waves to break up gallstones. It has been used for patients with few stones and mild to moderate symptoms. With the advent of laparoscopic cholecystectomy, ESWL has been largely abandoned. For general information about lithotripsy, see the Renal Calculi section in Chapter 40.

Endoscopic Sphincterotomy. Endoscopic sphincterotomy involves the use of endoscopic instruments to incise the sphincter of Oddi and extract stones from the common bile duct, as illustrated in Figure 39-11. The patient is given a sedative but remains conscious during the procedure. Lidocaine spray is used to deaden the gag reflex so that the endoscope can be passed through the mouth. A choledochoscope also can be inserted through a T-tube into the common bile duct. A special basket (e.g., Dormia basket) is used to extract the stones.

After endoscopic sphincterotomy, the patient is usually kept on bed rest for 6 to 8 hours. Nothing is given by mouth until the gag reflex returns. The patient is monitored for signs of complications. Bloody stools and tachycardia may indicate hemorrhage secondary to trauma. Fever and abdominal pain may indicate pancreatitis or perforation of the duodenum.

Cholecystectomy. Cholecystectomy is the most frequently used treatment for cholelithiasis. The two procedures that may be used are via laparoscopy or through a right subcostal incision. For laparoscopic cholecystectomy, the surgeon inserts a laparoscope with a camera through a small abdominal incision. Using the camera, the surgeon guides forceps and a laser toward the gallbladder through other small abdominal incisions. The gallbladder is grasped with the forceps,

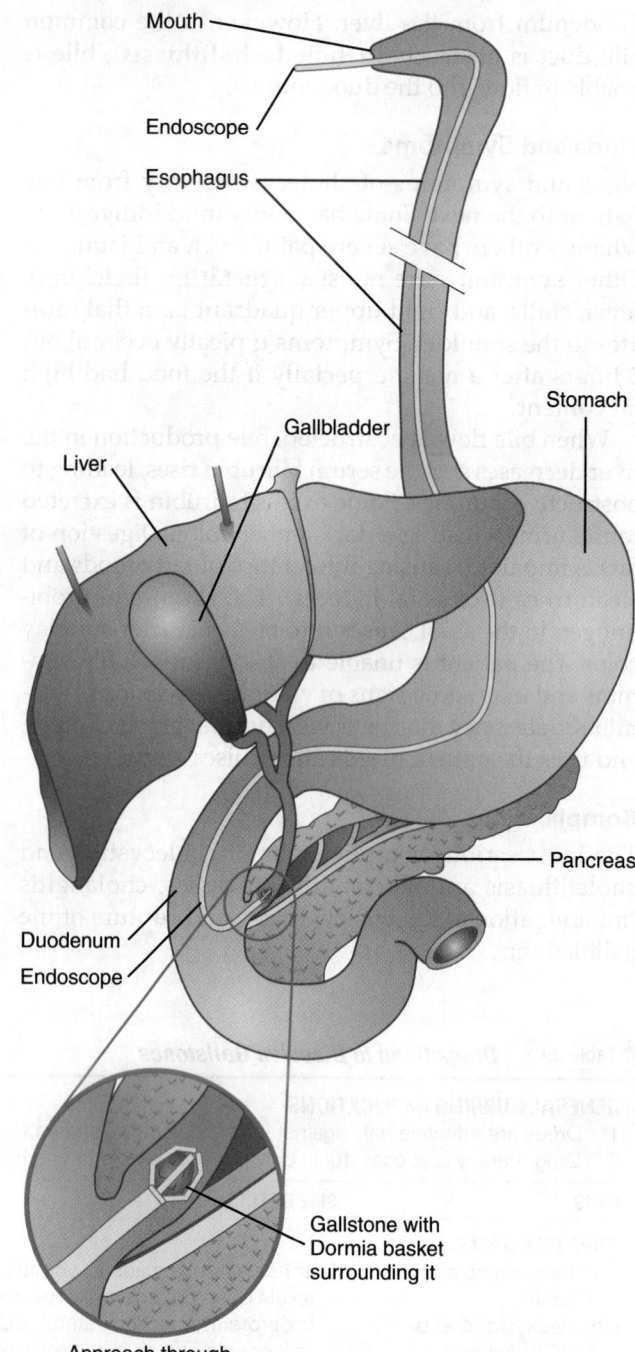

FIGURE 39-11 Choledochoscopic removal of gallstones.

cut free with the laser, and pulled out through one of the small incisions. Stones remaining in the common bile duct can be removed endoscopically. Complications are rare, and patients usually resume regular activities in 3 to 7 days.

In the classic procedure, an incision is made below the right rib margin. The gallbladder is removed, and the common bile duct is explored for stones. Exploration of the bile duct may cause it to swell and obstruct bile flow from the liver. A T-tube may be placed in the common bile duct to maintain bile flow until swelling in the duct subsides (Fig. 39-12). One part of the tubing is brought through the patient's skin and connected

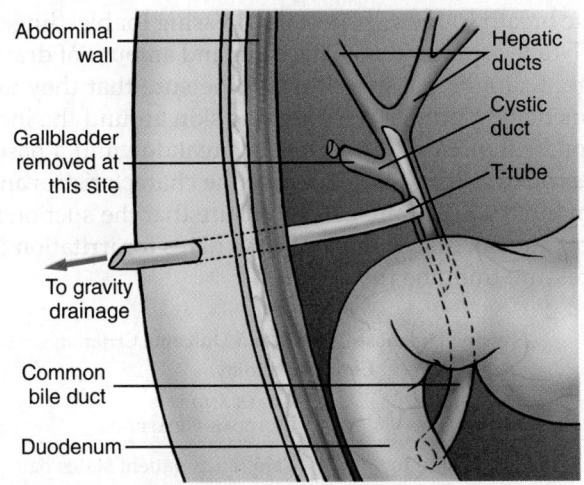

FIGURE 39-12 A T-tube in the common bile duct.

to a closed gravity drainage receptacle. Wound drains also may be present.

When the patient first returns from surgery, the drainage from the T-tube may be bloody, but it should soon become greenish brown. Drainage should gradually decrease as edema subsides in the common bile duct. Measure and record the amount of drainage, and notify the physician if it exceeds 1000 mL in 24 hours.

Place the patient in a low-Fowler's position with the tube arranged to drain freely. Protect the tube during movement to prevent dislodging it. The physician specifies the level of the drainage bag and when it should be clamped. Orders may call for the tube to be clamped for 1 to 2 hours before meals so that bile is available for digestion. The tube is clamped for increasingly longer periods of time. If the patient experiences pain, fever, chills, nausea, or distention, the tube should be unclamped. The physician removes the T-tube when the patient tolerates clamping for a prolonged period of time. Cleanse the area around wound drains using aseptic technique, and dress per agency protocol.

If the patient is discharged with the T-tube in place, you must teach the patient to care for the tube, including emptying the receptacle, caring for the insertion site, and recognizing when to clamp and unclamp it.

NURSING CARE *of the Patient with a Gallbladder Disorder*

Assessment

General assessment of patients with problems of the biliary tract is outlined in Box 39-2.

Nursing Diagnoses, Goals, and Outcome Criteria: Cholelithiasis	
NURSING DIAGNOSES	GOALS AND OUTCOME CRITERIA
Acute Pain related to biliary colic	Reduced pain: patient states pain reduced or relieved
Deficient Fluid Volume related to vomiting, inadequate intake	Adequate hydration: balanced fluid intake and output; vital signs consistent with patient norms

Risk for Impaired Skin Integrity related to pruritus	Decreased itching: no scratching, patient states less or no itching
Anxiety related to disease, anticipation of invasive procedures	Reduced anxiety: patient states anxiety relieved or reduced, relaxed manner
Risk for Injury (bleeding) related to vitamin K deficiency	Absence of bleeding: no abnormal bruising or bleeding

Interventions

Acute Pain

The degree of pain with cholecystitis varies, but many patients experience severe pain. Atropine and opioid analgesics other than morphine are usually ordered. Morphine is not used because it is believed to cause spasms in the common bile duct, which would increase the patient's pain. Evaluate comfort often, and medicate the patient as soon as pain is reported instead of waiting for it to become severe. When opioid analgesics are given, take safety precautions because the drugs cause drowsiness. In addition to medications, use position changes, smooth linens, back rubs, and mouth care to promote comfort.

Attacks of biliary colic are caused by stimulation of the gallbladder, most often by fats in the duodenum. A low-fat diet is recommended to decrease the incidence of acute symptoms.

Deficient Fluid Volume

If nausea and vomiting are present, the patient is at risk for fluid and electrolyte imbalances. Administer antiemetics as ordered. Keep intake and output records. Monitor for signs of deficient fluid volume (hypovolemia): tachycardia, hypotension, dry skin, concentrated urine, decreased urine output.

If vomiting is severe, a nasogastric tube may be inserted and attached to suction. Fluids are provided intravenously. Note the amount and characteristics of aspirated fluid. A problem associated with nasogastric decompression is the continuous removal of gastric secretions. When the fluid is continuously drained, the patient loses significant water, electrolytes, and acid. This puts the patient at risk for deficient fluid volume, potassium deficit, sodium excess, and metabolic alkalosis. Serum electrolytes are monitored, and specific intravenous fluids are ordered to maintain or restore balance.

Risk for Impaired Skin Integrity

Patients who have obstructive jaundice due to blockage of the bile ducts often have pruritus caused by accumulated bile salts under the skin. Measures to promote comfort include tepid baths with baking soda or oily lotions, use of soft linens, and maintaining a comfortable room temperature. Patients should be advised not to scratch, but that can be difficult. Short fingernails or even cotton gloves may be suggested to avoid skin injury from scratching. The physician may order a drug such as cholestyramine (Questran) to reduce the discomfort.

Anxiety

Acute pain and unexpected hospitalization can be anxiety-provoking for patients and their families. Provide clear explanations about what is being done and what they can expect. Acknowledge their anxiety, and take time to answer questions and offer reassurance.

Risk for Injury

A patient who has obstructed bile flow may have a deficiency of vitamin K because absorption of this vitamin in the digestive tract requires bile salts. Vitamin K is needed for the production of prothrombin, an essential element for clotting. Indications of vitamin K deficiency include bleeding gums and oozing of blood at injection sites. Minimize trauma by using a soft toothbrush or swab for mouth care and by applying gentle pressure to injection sites.

Pharmacology Capsule

Caution patients that supplementary bile salts interfere with the effectiveness of oral contraceptives.

NURSING CARE *of the Patient Following Surgery for Cholelithiasis*

Common nursing interventions for the patient who has undergone abdominal surgery for cholelithiasis are presented here. Detailed assessment and care of the surgical patient are presented in Chapter 17. Nursing care after laparoscopic cholecystectomy is much simpler because patients usually recover quickly and are discharged the same day or within 24 hours. They usually do not need postoperative nasogastric intubation or T-tubes.

Assessment

Postoperatively, take the patient's vital signs until the patient is stable. Observe chest expansion, and auscul-

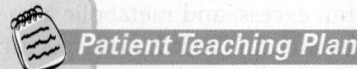

Patient Teaching Plan

Cholelithiasis

- You need to have a low-fat diet with supplementary fat-soluble vitamins (or as ordered by the physician). The dietitian will explain the details of the diet to you.
- Notify your physician of signs of bile duct obstruction: light stools, dark urine, jaundice, and itching.
- If you are taking bile salts, report gastric upset.
- Keep medical appointments to have blood drawn to monitor liver function.
- Do not rely on oral contraceptives; bile salts interfere with their effectiveness.

tate breath sounds. Inspect the dressing for bleeding. If a T-tube is present, note the color and amount of drainage. Examine passive drains to be sure that they are functioning properly. Inspect the skin around the incision or the drain for redness or breakdown. If a nasogastric tube is in place, observe the characteristics and amount of the drainage and ensure that the suction is operational. Inspect the patient's nares for irritation or pressure from the tube.

Nursing Diagnoses, Goals, and Outcome Criteria: Cholecystectomy

NURSING DIAGNOSES	GOALS AND OUTCOME CRITERIA
Acute Pain related to surgical incision, nasogastric tube	Pain relief: patient states pain relieved or reduced, relaxed manner
Ineffective Breathing Pattern related to splinting of the surgical incision	Effective breathing pattern: breath sounds clear on auscultation, respiratory rate of 12-20 per minute
Impaired Skin Integrity related to wound drainage, surgical incision	Wound healing without skin breakdown: clean wound margins without excessive redness
Deficient Fluid Volume related to gastrointestinal suction	Normal fluid and electrolyte status: electrolytes within normal limits, balanced fluid intake and output
Risk for Infection related to surgical incision, invasive procedure	Absence of infection: normal temperature and white blood cell count

Interventions

Acute Pain

When the patient undergoes a procedure that requires a surgical incision, pain is expected. In addition to administering ordered analgesics, reposition the patient for comfort and check to see that any drainage tubes are functioning. Show the patient how to support the incision with the hands or a pillow during coughing and deep breathing. Other pain relief measures are described in Chapter 15. If pain continues despite these measures, notify the physician.

The patient who has a nasogastric tube in place has an additional source of discomfort. The nose and throat may become very sore. Secure the tube to the patient's upper lip or nose so that it is not easily moved or tugged. Gently cleanse the nares, and apply water-soluble lubricant to keep the area moist. Provide frequent mouth care.

Ineffective Breathing Pattern

Potentially ineffective breathing patterns are most likely to be a problem when the patient has a subcostal incision. The incision is located close to the diaphragm, so full lung expansion is painful. The patient tends to guard the surgical area by not breathing deeply. Explain the importance of deep breathing and coughing to prevent atelectasis and pneumonia. Also demonstrate how splinting the area makes breathing and coughing more comfortable. Adequate pain management enables the patient to breathe more effectively. Monitor respiratory rate and breath sounds.

Impaired Skin Integrity

Patients who have subcostal incisions often have wound drains in place. These drains allow for removal of fluids that collect at the surgical site. A Penrose drain diverts fluids directly onto the wound dressings. This requires frequent dressing changes to prevent skin irritation. It is especially important if bile is present in the drainage because bile contains digestive enzymes, which are even more irritating. A pouch collection device like those used for stomas can be applied if needed to protect the skin. A passive drain such as the Jackson-Pratt drain has a fluid collection device that keeps fluid away from the skin.

Deficient Fluid Volume

Postoperatively, measure fluid intake and output. Until oral fluids are permitted, administer intravenous fluids as ordered. Blood studies may be ordered to assess serum electrolytes. If nasogastric suction is ordered, check frequently to be sure it is working properly. Otherwise, the patient may have distention that causes vomiting and further loss of fluids and electrolytes.

Risk for Infection

The patient who has undergone gallbladder surgery is at risk for infection of the surgical wound. Draining wounds provide a moist environment for bacterial growth. Meticulous wound care can reduce that risk.

A complication of endoscopic sphincterotomy is pancreatitis caused by accidental injury to the pancreatic duct. Early signs of pancreatitis are pain and fever.

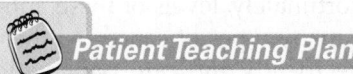

Patient Teaching Plan

Cholecystectomy

- We will teach you how to care for the T-tube before you go home.
- A low-fat diet is usually recommended for 4 to 6 weeks.
- In general, avoid heavy lifting for 4 to 6 weeks or as prescribed. Other activities, including sexual intercourse, can usually be resumed when you feel well enough.
- After laparoscopic cholecystectomy, usual instructions include the following:
  - Avoid fatty foods for several weeks.
  - Remove the dressings and bathe or shower normally the next day.
  - Notify the physician if there is redness, drainage, or pus from the incision.
  - Report any signs of peritonitis: severe abdominal pain, chills and fever, and vomiting.

CANCER OF THE GALLBLADDER

Cancer of the gallbladder is rare and is thought to be related to chronic cholecystitis and cholelithiasis. The diagnosis is often delayed because early signs and symptoms are essentially the same as those of cholecystitis and cholelithiasis.

Treatment options include surgery, chemotherapy, and radiation therapy, but the prognosis is generally poor. Often only supportive, symptomatic care is given. Nursing care is similar to that for other patients with gallbladder disease. You also need to focus on the needs of the cancer patient, as discussed in Chapter 25.

THE PANCREAS

The pancreas is a gland that has both endocrine and exocrine functions. As an endocrine gland, it secretes into the blood hormones that regulate the blood glucose level. The exocrine function is the production of digestive enzymes that are secreted into the duodenum through a duct. This section focuses on disorders of the pancreas, with the exception of diabetes mellitus, which is covered in Chapter 46.

ANATOMY AND PHYSIOLOGY OF THE PANCREAS

The pancreas is a fish-shaped organ located in the upper left quadrant of the abdomen behind the stomach. The head of the pancreas lies against the duodenum, and the tail lies next to the spleen. The pancreatic ducts connect the pancreas to the duodenum. One duct goes directly to the duodenum, and the other merges with the common bile duct, as shown in Figure 39-10.

EXOCRINE FUNCTION

The exocrine function of the pancreas is carried out by acinar tissue. Acinar tissue is composed of tiny grapelike clusters of cells that produce pancreatic fluid. Pancreatic fluid contains enzymes needed for the digestion of proteins, fats, and carbohydrates. It is secreted into the duodenum through the pancreatic duct.

The pancreatic enzymes trypsin, amylase, and lipase act on partially digested foods in the small intestine. Trypsin plays a role in the digestion of protein by breaking proteases and peptones into small polypeptides. Normally, trypsin is not activated until it enters the duodenum. Otherwise, it would digest the protein tissue of the pancreas itself. Amylase acts with intestinal enzymes to reduce starch, sucrose, and fructose to glucose, fructose, and galactose. Lipase acts on emulsified fats to yield fatty acids, glycerides, and glycerol.

ENDOCRINE FUNCTION

The endocrine function of the pancreas is carried out by clusters of specialized cells scattered throughout the pancreas. These cells are called *islets of Langerhans*.

The islets contain alpha, beta, delta, and PP cells. Alpha cells produce and secrete glucagon. Beta cells produce and secrete insulin. Delta cells produce somatostatin, which inhibits the release of glucagon and insulin. PP cells secrete pancreatic polypeptides, a family of peptides known chiefly for their inhibitory functions.

Glucagon is secreted when the blood glucose level falls. It stimulates the liver to convert glycogen into glucose. Insulin is secreted when the blood glucose rises, as after a meal. It stimulates the use of glucose by the cells so that a normal blood glucose level is maintained. The endocrine function of the pancreas is covered more thoroughly in Chapter 46.

NURSING ASSESSMENT of the Patient with a Pancreatic Disorder

Assessment of the patient with a pancreatic disorder is outlined in Box 39-3. The assessment focuses on digestive and metabolic functions.

Health History

Inquire about the patient's general health status because pancreatic disorders are often accompanied by weakness and fatigue. The past medical history may reveal previous disorders of the biliary tract or duodenum, abdominal trauma or surgery, and metabolic

---

Box 39-3 | **ASSESSMENT of the Patient with a Pancreatic Disorder**

Health History
Present Illness:
General well-being, digestive disturbances, pain

Past Medical History:
Disorders of the biliary tract or duodenum, abdominal trauma or surgery, metabolic disorders; medication history, especially thiazides, furosemide, estrogens, corticosteroids, sulfonamides, opiates

Family History:
Pancreatic disorders

Review of Systems:
Pruritus, respiratory distress, nausea and vomiting, abdominal pain

Functional Assessment:
Dietary habits, alcohol intake

Physical Examination
General Survey:
Restlessness, flushing, diaphoresis

Vital Signs:
Low-grade fever, tachycardia, tachypnea, hypotension

Skin:
Jaundice, dryness, scratches

Abdomen:
Distention, tenderness, diminished bowel sounds, discoloration

---

disorders such as diabetes mellitus. The medication history should be detailed and specifically include the use of thiazides, furosemide, estrogens, corticosteroids, sulfonamides, and opiates. Note a family history of pancreatic disorders. In the review of systems, obtain a complete description of any pain in the upper abdomen or epigastric area. Symptoms that may be important in relation to pancreatic disorders are dyspnea, nausea, and vomiting. The functional assessment includes data about the patient's dietary habits and use of alcohol.

Physical Examination

Note any restlessness, flushing, or diaphoresis during the examination. Vital signs may disclose low-grade fever, tachypnea, tachycardia, and hypotension. Inspect the skin for jaundice. Assess the abdomen for distention, tenderness, discoloration, and diminished bowel sounds.

DIAGNOSTIC TESTS AND PROCEDURES

Tests and procedures used to diagnose pancreatic disorders include laboratory analyses of blood, urine, stool, and pancreatic fluid and imaging studies (CT scan, endoscopic ultrasonography, MRI, PET, ERCP).

Specific blood studies used to assess pancreatic function include measurements of serum amylase, lipase, glucose, calcium, and triglycerides. Urine amylase and renal amylase clearance tests also may be ordered. Stool specimens may be analyzed for fat content.

The secretin stimulation test measures the bicarbonate concentration of pancreatic fluid after secretin is given intravenously to stimulate the production of pancreatic fluid.

If cancer is suspected, blood levels of CA 19-9, carcinoembryonic antigen, pancreatic oncofetal antigen, and others that are considered "markers" for cancer may be measured. Unfortunately, levels of these antigens are elevated with many types of cancer, so their presence does not specifically indicate pancreatic cancer.

Additional information about diagnostic tests and procedures for the pancreas is provided in the Diagnostic Tests and Procedures table on pp. 825 and 826.

DISORDERS OF THE PANCREAS

PANCREATITIS

Pancreatitis is inflammation of the pancreas. It may be acute or chronic. Chronic pancreatitis may follow the acute condition but often develops independently.

Pancreatitis is most often caused by biliary tract disorders or alcoholism. Other causes include viral infections; peptic ulcer disease; cysts; metabolic disorders (renal failure, hyperparathyroidism); and trauma from external injury, surgery, or endoscopic procedures. In addition, chronic pancreatitis is sometimes associated with cancer of the duodenum or pancreas.

Normally, pancreatic enzymes are activated in the small intestine. With pancreatitis, digestive enzymes (trypsin, elastase, and phospholipase A) are activated by some unknown mechanism and begin to digest pancreatic tissue (a process called *autodigestion*), fat, and elastic tissue in blood vessels. Pancreatic fluid may leak into the surrounding tissues. The effect of this escaped fluid has been compared to an internal chemical burn, and the effects can be devastating.

Chronic pancreatitis is often related to alcohol abuse. It is usually characterized by obstruction of the pancreatic duct, leading to progressive destruction of the pancreas.

Signs and Symptoms

Abdominal pain is the most prominent symptom of pancreatitis. The pain is typically severe with a sudden onset, is centered in the upper left quadrant or the epigastric region, and radiates to the back. Se-

Put on Your Thinking Cap!

The term *autodigestion* is used to describe the effects of pancreatitis. Explain what this means.

vere vomiting, flushing, cyanosis, and dyspnea often accompany the pain. Other signs and symptoms are low-grade fever, tachypnea, tachycardia, and hypotension.

The abdomen may be tender and distended. Bowel sounds may be absent, suggesting an ileus. Trypsin may damage blood vessels, causing pancreatic hemorrhage and discoloration of the abdomen. You may observe cyanosis or greenish discoloration of the abdominal wall, the flanks, and the area around the umbilicus. Enzymes released into the abdominal cavity increase capillary permeability, permitting protein-rich serum to leak from blood vessels. Bleeding and shifting of fluid reduce blood volume and may lead to shock. Early signs and symptoms of

DIAGNOSTIC TESTS and PROCEDURES *The Pancreas*

TEST	PURPOSE/PROCEDURE	PATIENT PREPARATION	POSTPROCEDURE NURSING CARE
LABORATORY STUDIES			
Amylase	Increases with pancreatitis, parotitis, cholecystitis.	For all laboratory studies, advise patient that a blood sample will be drawn and inform him or her whether fasting is required by agency protocol.	For all laboratory studies, check venipuncture site for bleeding. Apply pressure if necessary.
Serum Enzymes	Lipase increases with pancreatic inflammation, carcinoma. Normal values vary with type of test used.		
Serum Calcium	Decreases with many conditions, including pancreatic disorders.		
Serum Triglycerides	Increase with pancreatitis and many other conditions.		
Tumor Markers			
Carcinoembryonic antigen (CEA); pancreatic oncofetal antigen (POA)	Increase with many types of cancer, including pancreatic; pancreatitis, cirrhosis, hepatitis, and chronic cigarette smoking.		
SECRETIN STIMULATION TEST	Secretin is given intravenously. Gastric and duodenal fluids are aspirated through a double-lumen tube. Fluid is analyzed. Decreased volume of secretions and bicarbonate is consistent with pancreatitis.	Tell patient that a medication will be given in a vein and that a tube will be passed through nose into stomach so that fluid can be removed from stomach for study.	Remove tube unless instructed otherwise. Provide comfort measures.

Continued

TEST	PURPOSE/PROCEDURE	PATIENT PREPARATION	POSTPROCEDURE NURSING CARE
URINE AMYLASE	Increases with acute pancreatitis, peptic ulcer, and choledocholithiasis. Test may be ordered for a 1-, 2-, or 24-hr specimen.	Advise patient of time for collection of specimens. Encourage fluids during test if not contraindicated.	
IMAGING STUDIES			
Abdominal ultrasound	Uses sound waves to visualize pancreas directly. Is noninvasive.	Some laboratories require patient to be NPO before procedure. Study cannot be done if barium or excessive gas is in digestive tract. Tell patient that he or she will lie on back on an examination table. A gel or oil is applied to skin, and an instrument is moved over upper abdomen. Images are seen on a screen and recorded.	No special care.
Computed tomography (CT)	Uses radiographs with a special scanner to provide detailed information about internal organ position and structure. Contrast medium may be given orally or intravenously.	NPO is needed before some CT scans. Tell patient to expect to lie on a narrow stretcher. Scanner is a doughnut-shaped machine that moves back and forth and around stretcher. It makes clicking noises. Contraindicated during pregnancy. Assess allergies to dye, and inform radiologist.	No special care.
Endoscopic retrograde cholangiopancreatography (ERCP)	Uses an endoscope to examine gallbladder and pancreas to evaluate bile obstruction and to confirm pancreatic disease. Contrast medium is injected into bile duct.	A consent form must be signed. Patient will be NPO as long as 12 hr. Physician may order patient to gargle with a topical anesthetic. An intravenous line may be started to administer sedatives.	Monitor vital signs for 4 hr. Check gag reflex before giving fluids or food. Monitor for urinary retention. Report temperature elevation that may indicate inflammation.

NPO, Nothing by mouth.

shock are restlessness and tachycardia. Hypotension is a late sign.

Symptoms of chronic pancreatitis are similar to those of the acute disease but usually appear as periodic attacks that become more and more frequent. In addition, patients with chronic pancreatitis may develop diabetes mellitus and malabsorption with steatorrhea.

Complications

Complications of pancreatitis include pseudocyst; abscess; hypocalcemia; and pulmonary, cardiac, and renal complications.

A pseudocyst is a fluid-filled pouch attached to the pancreas. It contains products of tissue destruction and pancreatic enzymes. The fluid can leak into the digestive tract or the abdominal cavity. Symptoms of pseu-

docyst include abdominal pain, nausea, vomiting, and anorexia. Sometimes a mass can be palpated in the epigastric area. Necrosis within the pancreas can lead to pancreatic abscess, a fluid-filled cavity in the pancreas. Symptoms are similar to those of pseudocyst. Patients usually run a high fever.

Hypocalcemia (low serum calcium) is caused by the action of fatty acids on calcium and increased loss of calcium in the urine. The pulmonary complications of pancreatitis are pneumonia and atelectasis. Pancreatitis can be fatal. In the early stage of acute pancreatitis, causes of death are usually cardiovascular, renal, or pulmonary failure. Later, sepsis and abscesses are the leading causes of death.

A person may recover completely from an attack of acute pancreatitis, have repeated acute episodes, or experience chronic pancreatitis.

Medical Diagnosis

The most important diagnostic findings in acute pancreatitis are elevated serum amylase, serum lipase, and urinary amylase levels. When the kidneys clear amylase more rapidly than they clear creatinine, acute pancreatitis is strongly suspected. Other findings with acute pancreatitis are elevated white blood cell count, elevated serum lipid and glucose levels, and decreased serum calcium level. Ultrasonography and ERCP may reveal the presence of gallstones, cysts, or abscesses and help rule out other disorders that might be causing the patient's symptoms.

Tests for chronic pancreatitis include the secretin stimulation test and fecal studies in addition to the tests used for acute pancreatitis. Findings consistent with chronic pancreatitis are decreased volume and bicarbonate concentration of pancreatic fluid and high fecal fat content.

Medical Treatment

The patient with acute pancreatitis is usually allowed nothing by mouth. This removes the stimulus for secretion of pancreatic fluid. If the patient is vomiting or if an ileus is suspected, a nasogastric tube is inserted and connected to suction. Intravenous fluids are ordered to restore and maintain fluid balance. Blood or plasma expanders are given if the blood volume is low. Urine output is monitored and should be at least 40 mL/hr. A jejunal feeding tube or total parenteral nutrition may be needed to provide adequate nutrients. Once food is permitted, the patient is usually started on a bland, high-carbohydrate, low-fat diet divided into frequent, small meals. Since the inflamed pancreas is susceptible to infection, some physicians order prophylactic antibiotics. Sometimes peritoneal lavage or laparoscopy is used to remove toxic fluid from the peritoneum.

Drug Therapy. Drug therapy for pancreatitis commonly includes analgesics, antispasmodics, anticholinergics, and gastric acid inhibitors. Pain control is a major problem with pancreatitis. Meperidine (Demerol) has traditionally been the analgesic of choice. Opioids (e.g., morphine) traditionally have been avoided because they are thought to cause more spasm in the pancreatic ducts. However, morphine is gaining favor because the pain relief lasts longer and spasms can be managed with the antispasmodic drugs such as nitroglycerin. Anticholinergics decrease secretions, which also can reduce spasms and pain. Reducing the secretion of gastric acid decreases the stimulus for pancreatic secretions. With chronic pancreatitis, addiction to opioid analgesics is a concern.

The patient with chronic pancreatitis is likely to need to take pancreatic enzymes in order to digest food. The enzymes can be taken with meals or snacks. The effect of the enzymes can be determined by examining the stools. Steatorrhea (bulky, frothy stools with a high fat content) results from inadequate enzymes. If diabetes mellitus develops, insulin or oral hypoglycemic drugs are needed, and the patient would require diabetes education.

Other drugs that may be needed are antacids, anticholinergics, and histamine blockers to decrease hydrochloric acid in the stomach. Bile salts also may be needed to enhance absorption of fat-soluble vitamins. Drugs used to treat pancreatitis are described in Table 39-3.

Surgical Intervention. Various surgical procedures may be indicated. For example, if gallstones are present, endoscopic sphincterotomy followed by cholecystectomy may be done. If an abscess, pseudocyst, or severe peritonitis develops, surgical intervention is indicated. Débridement involves resection of necrotic tissue and irrigation of the cavity to remove harmful fluid. The procedure may have to be repeated more than once. After surgical débridement, multiple sumps may be placed in the abdomen for continuous postoperative irrigation. Each sump tube is connected to a separate suction apparatus. Irrigations may be alternated as ordered.

NURSING CARE *of the Patient with Pancreatitis*

Assessment

General nursing assessment of the patient with a pancreatic disorder is outlined in Box 39-3 (see also Nursing Care Plan: The Patient with Pancreatitis on p. 830). When a patient has acute pancreatitis, it is especially important to report signs of hypovolemic shock: restlessness, tachycardia, tachypnea, hypotension, and decreased urinary output. The abdomen should be inspected for discoloration, distention, tenderness, and diminished bowel sounds. The flanks also should be examined for discoloration. In addition, the patient's mental status should be monitored. Altered mental status may be due to metabolic imbalances. The alcoholic patient may develop confusion and agitation due to alcohol withdrawal.

If the patient has surgery, general postoperative assessment should include data covered in Chapter 17.

Nursing Diagnoses, Goals, and Outcome Criteria: Pancreatitis	
NURSING DIAGNOSES	GOALS AND OUTCOME CRITERIA
Acute Pain related to inflammation, infection, biliary obstruction, autodigestion	Pain relief: patient states pain reduced or relieved, relaxed manner
Deficient Fluid Volume related to vomiting, bleeding, fluid shift from the blood to the abdominal cavity	Normal fluid balance: balanced fluid intake and output, pulse and blood pressure consistent with patient norms
Risk for Infection related to tissue necrosis	Absence of infection: normal body temperature and white blood cell count
Impaired Gas Exchange related to pain, pulmonary complications	Adequate gas exchange: breath sounds clear to auscultation, respiratory rate 12-20 per minute

Continued on p. 829

Table 39-3 | *Drugs Used to Treat Pancreatitis*

DRUG	USE/ACTION	SIDE EFFECTS	NURSING INTERVENTIONS
ACUTE PANCREATITIS			
Opioid analgesics Meperidine (Demerol)	Relieve pain.	Sedation, confusion, hypotension, nausea, vomiting, constipation.	Monitor BP, P, R. Assess bowel elimination. Observe safety precautions. Give antiemetics as ordered.
Smooth muscle relaxants Nitroglycerin	Relieve spasm, reduce pain.	Headache, dizziness, flushing, tachycardia, hypotension.	Monitor BP and P. Use special containers and tubing for IV administration.
Antispasmodics Propantheline bromide (Pro-Banthine)	Decrease bicarbonate and pancreatic enzyme secretion.	Tachycardia, dry mouth, constipation, urinary retention and hesitancy, drowsiness.	Administer 30 min before meals. Do not give within 1 hr of antacids or antidiarrheals. Observe safety precautions if patient is drowsy. Provide mouth care. Monitor stools.
Antacids	Neutralize gastric acid; indirectly decrease production of pancreatic secretions.	Constipation with aluminum; diarrhea with magnesium.	Monitor electrolytes. Give 1 hr apart from other oral drugs. Give on empty stomach. Have patient chew tablets and follow with full glass of water. Shake liquids well.
Carbonic anhydrase inhibitors Acetazolamide (Diamox)	Reduce bicarbonate concentration in pancreatic secretions.	Rash, drowsiness, nausea, vomiting, renal calculi, hypercalcemia, aplastic anemia, leukopenia, seizures, hypokalemia.	Encourage 2000-3000 mL fluid/day unless contraindicated. Give with food to decrease GI distress. Observe safety precautions. Monitor electrolytes and blood cell counts.
Somatostatin	Inhibits secretion of pancreatic enzymes.		
Histamine-2 receptor blockers Cimetidine (Tagamet) Ranitidine (Zantac) Famotidine (Pepcid)	Decrease production of HCl so that pancreatic enzymes cannot be activated.	Confusion, nausea, diarrhea, constipation, drowsiness, headache, rash, agranulocytosis.	Administer with or immediately after meals. Discourage smoking, which counteracts these drugs. Observe safety precautions. Report sore throat or fever.
Vitamin and mineral supplements	Supplement poor dietary intake or impaired absorption. Calcium treats hypocalcemia.	Potential for overdose of fat-soluble vitamins and calcium. Calcium potentiates cardiac glycosides.	
Adrenocortical steroids	Decrease inflammation.	Fluid retention, hypokalemia, hyperglycemia, hypocalcemia, decreased resistance to infection, mood swings.	Monitor BP, P, and blood glucose. Assess for edema. Protect from infection. Explain that emotional/personality changes are temporary.
CHRONIC PANCREATITIS			
Pancreatic enzymes Pancreatin Pancrelipase (Cotazym, Viokase, Pancrease)	Supplement normal pancreatic enzyme secretion; aid in digestion of fats, carbohydrates, and proteins. Goal is less frequent stools with lower fat content.	Diarrhea, nausea, stomach cramps, abdominal pain.	Give with meals or snacks. Capsule contents can be sprinkled on food but should not be chewed. Mix powders with fruit juice or applesauce to mask taste. Do not mix with protein foods. Have patient wipe lips with wet cloth to prevent skin irritation. Evaluate drug effect by noting number and consistency of stools.
Hypoglycemic agents Insulin Oral hypoglycemics	Needed when pancreas is unable to produce sufficient insulin.	Hypoglycemia.	See Chapter 46 for details on hypoglycemic drug therapy.

BP, Blood pressure; *P*, pulse; *R*, respiration; *IV*, intravenous; *GI*, gastrointestinal; *HCl*, hydrochloric acid.

Imbalanced Nutrition: Less Than Body Requirements related to anorexia, vomiting, digestive disturbance	Adequate nutrition: stable body weight
Anxiety related to unfamiliar setting and procedures; acute illness	Reduced anxiety: patient states anxiety lessened, calm manner

Interventions

Acute Pain

Describe the patient's pain, and provide ordered analgesics and antispasmodics promptly. Reposition the patient for comfort. Other nursing measures for pain are described in Chapter 15 and include distraction, imagery, and cutaneous stimulation. Evaluate and record the effectiveness of pain control measures. Consult the physician if pain is not relieved.

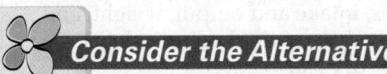

Consider the Alternative

Distraction, imagery, relaxation, and cutaneous stimulation can enhance the effects of analgesics to promote pain relief.

Deficient Fluid Volume

If ordered, insert a nasogastric tube and connect it to suction. Administer prescribed intravenous fluids. Monitor the patient's fluid status by measuring vital signs, intake and output, and weight. Signs of fluid volume deficit include tachycardia, hypotension, dry skin, concentrated urine, and decreased urine output. The physician should be informed if the urine output falls below 40 mL/hr. Depletion of blood volume causes hypovolemic shock and leads to death if not corrected. Other potential fluid imbalances are metabolic alkalosis from severe vomiting, hypokalemia, hyponatremia, hypocalcemia, and hypochloremia.

Risk for Infection

Necrosis of the pancreas and surrounding tissue provides a site for infection. If a surgical procedure is done, there also is risk for wound infection. Inform the physician of fever, purulent drainage, or separation of wound margins—all signs of infection. Take special care to maintain asepsis during wound care. Administer antibiotics as ordered.

Impaired Gas Exchange

Fluid accumulation in the peritoneal cavity puts upward pressure on the diaphragm, thereby limiting lung expansion. Because the acutely ill patient is inactive, secretions may pool in the lungs. Poor lung expansion and inactivity combine to invite pneumonia

and atelectasis. Monitor for tachypnea, dyspnea, and abnormal breath sounds.

Measures to prevent pulmonary complications in the patient with pancreatitis include frequent turning, coughing, and deep breathing. The semi-Fowler's position promotes lung expansion.

Imbalanced Nutrition: Less Than Body Requirements

Initially, the patient will be NPO because food and fluids stimulate pancreatic fluid secretion. When oral intake is resumed, small feedings of a bland, high-carbohydrate, low-fat diet are provided. Spicy foods, caffeine, and alcohol should be avoided. Total parenteral nutrition (see Chapter 9) is usually needed only with severe malnourishment. Daily weights are used to evaluate the adequacy of the nutrition plan.

The patient with chronic pancreatitis commonly requires pancreatic enzyme replacement taken with meals and supplemental vitamins. If the pancreas is severely damaged, insulin secretion will be deficient. The patient will have to be managed like a person with diabetes mellitus (see Chapter 46).

Anxiety

Attempt to determine the reasons for the patient's anxiety. Some concerns can be alleviated by telling the patient what is happening and what to expect. Respond promptly to the patient's needs, and offer comforting reassurance by checking on the patient frequently. Anxiety can be related to pain or hypoxia as well as to emotional distress, so assess comfort and oxygenation status and take appropriate corrective actions. During acute attacks, answer questions and

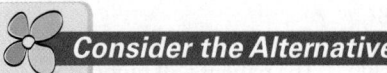

Consider the Alternative

Some patients have found acupuncture helpful for treatment of alcoholism.

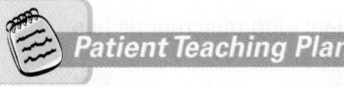

Patient Teaching Plan

Pancreatitis

- Your prescribed diet (usually bland, high-carbohydrate, low-fat) will avoid stimulating your pancreas and will promote healing.
- At first, you may tolerate small, frequent meals better than large meals.
- Abstaining from alcohol decreases your risk of recurrence.
- Community resources such as Alcoholics Anonymous can assist if it is hard for you to abstain from drinking alcohol (website: http://www.alcoholics-anonymous.org; telephone: 1-212-686-1100).

NURSING CARE PLAN

The Patient with Pancreatitis

ASSESSMENT

Health History: Mrs. Sanchez is a 57-year-old Latina admitted with repeated attacks of severe pain in the upper left quadrant that radiates to her back. She reports having vomited repeatedly over the past 24 hours. When the pain is severe, she reports feeling flushed, faint, and short of breath. She has no other related symptoms. Mrs. Sanchez reports having had a gallbladder attack several months ago that resolved without surgery. She is a high school teacher who lives with her husband.

Physical Examination: The patient appears to be in acute distress, but she is alert and oriented. Vital signs: temperature, 100.2° F orally; pulse, 92; respiration, 24; blood pressure, 144/84. Abdomen tender and distended, with hypoactive bowel sounds in all four quadrants.

Nursing Diagnosis	Goals and Outcome Criteria	Interventions
Acute Pain related to inflammation, biliary obstruction, autodigestion	The patient will report decreased pain and will appear more relaxed.	Document painful episodes, and treat promptly with analgesics and antispasmodics as ordered. Use distraction, imagery, and relaxation techniques to enhance drug therapy. Advise physician if pain is unrelieved.
Deficient Fluid Volume related to vomiting, bleeding, fluid shift from bloodstream to abdominal cavity	The patient's fluid status will stabilize, as evidenced by stable blood pressure and pulse, normal skin color, urine output equal to fluid intake.	Insert nasogastric tube and connect to low suction as ordered. Initiate intravenous fluid therapy and administer as ordered. Monitor vital signs, intake and output, weight, and electrolyte studies. Report signs of fluid volume deficit: tachycardia, hypotension, dry skin, concentrated urine.
Risk for Infection related to tissue necrosis	The patient will be free of signs and symptoms of infection: fever, tachycardia, increased white blood cell count.	Monitor vital signs and blood cell counts. Report signs of infection. Administer antimicrobials as ordered. Use Standard Precautions for invasive procedures.
Impaired Gas Exchange related to pain, pulmonary complications	The patient will remain free of pulmonary complications, as evidenced by absence of dyspnea, tachypnea, and abnormal breath sounds.	Assess respirations and breath sounds. Assist to change positions, cough, and deep breathe at least every 2 hours. Use semi-Fowler's position to promote lung expansion.
Imbalanced Nutrition: Less Than Body Requirements related to anorexia, vomiting, digestive disturbances	The patient's body weight will remain stable.	Administer total parenteral nutrition if ordered. Monitor for hyperglycemia, and administer insulin as ordered. Take daily weights. When oral intake is permitted, monitor patient tolerance. Discourage spicy foods, caffeine, and alcohol.
Anxiety related to acute symptoms	The patient will report decreased anxiety and will be calm.	Check on patient often. Respond to her needs promptly. Ask what questions she has, and provide explanations of the condition and the treatment she is receiving.

? CRITICAL THINKING QUESTIONS

- Explain why the patient with pancreatitis has severe pain.

- Explain why it is necessary to monitor respiratory status in the patient with pancreatitis.

---

give simple explanations. As the patient improves, implement your teaching plan.

Deficient Knowledge

The patient with acute pancreatitis is too ill for systematic teaching. Explain simply what you are doing and why. Answer any questions the patient may ask. As the patient improves, the teaching plan should address the

importance of avoiding alcohol to prevent recurrences. Explain the rationale for the prescribed diet.

CANCER OF THE PANCREAS

Cancer of the pancreas is extremely serious. Pancreatic cancer quickly spreads to the duodenum, stomach, spleen, and left adrenal gland. About 32,000 new cases are diagnosed each year in the United States. Only 24%

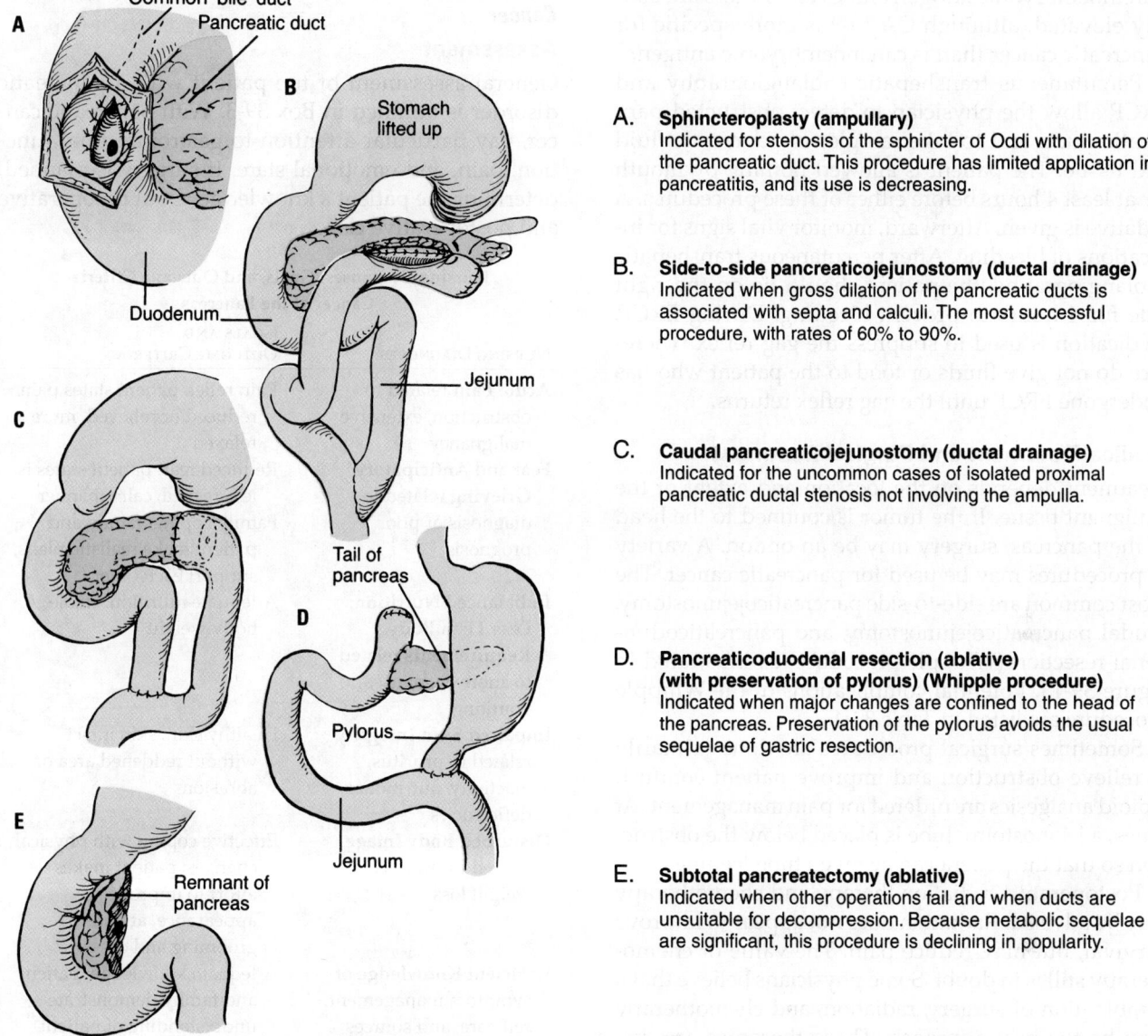

A.   **Sphincteroplasty (ampullary)**
Indicated for stenosis of the sphincter of Oddi with dilation of the pancreatic duct. This procedure has limited application in pancreatitis, and its use is decreasing.

B.   **Side-to-side pancreaticojejunostomy (ductal drainage)**
Indicated when gross dilation of the pancreatic ducts is associated with septa and calculi. The most successful procedure, with rates of 60% to 90%.

C.   **Caudal pancreaticojejunostomy (ductal drainage)**
Indicated for the uncommon cases of isolated proximal pancreatic ductal stenosis not involving the ampulla.

D.   **Pancreaticoduodenal resection (ablative) (with preservation of pylorus) (Whipple procedure)**
Indicated when major changes are confined to the head of the pancreas. Preservation of the pylorus avoids the usual sequelae of gastric resection.

E.   **Subtotal pancreatectomy (ablative)**
Indicated when other operations fail and when ducts are unsuitable for decompression. Because metabolic sequelae are significant, this procedure is declining in popularity.

FIGURE **39-13** Surgical procedures for pancreatic cancer.

of these people will survive for a year; 4% will be alive after 5 years. For persons diagnosed early, about 17% are alive after 5 years. Among the risk factors for pancreatic cancer are chronic pancreatitis and smoking. Other probable risk factors are a high-fat diet and exposure to certain toxic chemicals. Tumors may develop in the head, body, or tail of the pancreas.

Signs and Symptoms

Signs and symptoms of pancreatic cancer vary with the stage and location but often include pain, jaundice with or without liver enlargement, weight loss, and glucose intolerance. When located in the head of the pancreas, tumors typically obstruct the common bile duct, causing jaundice. In the early stage of the disease, jaundice may be the only sign present. If the patient seeks medical care early, the chance of survival is somewhat better. Other signs and symptoms may be weight loss, upper abdominal pain, anorexia, vomiting, weakness, and diarrhea.

When the tumor is in the body or the tail of the pancreas, the patient may not have any symptoms until the disease is advanced. Then the liver, gallbladder, and spleen may be enlarged. Pressure on the portal veins may cause esophageal and gastric varices (dilated veins) that bleed easily into the gastrointestinal tract. Pressure on nerves may cause back pain.

Medical Diagnosis

The most useful diagnostic tests and procedures when pancreatic cancer is suspected are transabdominal ultrasound, computed tomography, ERCP, and endoscopic ultrasonography. Blood studies and other imaging procedures can be helpful as well. Blood values associated with pancreatic cancer include elevated serum amylase, lipase, bilirubin, and enzyme levels.

Carcinoembryonic antigen and CA 19-9 titers are usually elevated, although CA 19-9 is more specific for pancreatic cancer than is carcinoembryonic antigen.

Percutaneous transhepatic cholangiography and ERCP allow the physician to detect obstructed pancreatic ducts and to take samples of pancreatic fluid and tissue. The patient is allowed nothing by mouth for at least 4 hours before either of these procedures. A sedative is given. Afterward, monitor vital signs for indications of bleeding. After percutaneous transhepatic cholangiography, the patient should lie on the right side for 4 hours to prevent bleeding. During ERCP, medication is used to suppress the gag reflex. Therefore do not give fluids or food to the patient who has undergone ERCP until the gag reflex returns.

Medical Treatment and Surgical Treatment

Treatment depends on the location and extent of the malignant tissue. If the tumor is confined to the head of the pancreas, surgery may be an option. A variety of procedures may be used for pancreatic cancer. The most common are side-to-side pancreaticojejunostomy, caudal pancreaticojejunostomy, and pancreaticoduodenal resection (Whipple procedure) as illustrated in Figure 39-13. Potential complications of the Whipple procedure are listed in Table 39-4.

Sometimes surgical procedures are done primarily to relieve obstruction and improve patient comfort. Opioid analgesics are ordered for pain management. At times, a jejunostomy tube is placed below the obstruction so that the patient can be given tube feedings.

Postoperative radiation therapy and chemotherapy may be advised. Radiation does not appear to improve survival, but may reduce pain. The value of chemotherapy still is in doubt. Some physicians believe that a combination of surgery, radiation, and chemotherapy may be the best approach. These therapies are discussed in detail in Chapter 25.

NURSING CARE *of the Patient with Pancreatic Cancer*

Assessment

General assessment of the patient with a pancreatic disorder is outlined in Box 39-3. With pancreatic cancer, pay particular attention to gastrointestinal function, pain, and emotional state. If surgery is planned, determine the patient's knowledge about preoperative and postoperative care.

Nursing Diagnoses, Goals, and Outcome Criteria: Cancer of the Pancreas

NURSING DIAGNOSES	GOALS AND OUTCOME CRITERIA
Acute Pain related to obstruction, extensive malignancy	Pain relief: patient states pain reduced or relieved, more relaxed
Fear and **Anticipatory Grieving** related to diagnosis or poor prognosis	Reduced fear: patient states is less fearful, calm manner Family coping: family and patient make realistic plans, support each other
Imbalanced Nutrition: Less Than Body Requirements related to anorexia, nausea, vomiting	Adequate nutrition: stable body weight
Impaired Skin Integrity related to pruritus, inactivity, nutritional deficiencies	Healthy skin: skin intact without reddened area or abrasions
Disturbed Body Image related to jaundice, weight loss	Effective coping with physical changes: patient makes effort to improve appearance, attends to grooming and dress
Deficient Knowledge of symptom management, self-care, and sources of support	Adequate knowledge: patient and family demonstrate understanding of patient care and resources

Table 39-4 | *Potential Complications of the Whipple Procedure*

COMPLICATION	NURSING INTERVENTIONS
Hemorrhage	Monitor vital signs for tachycardia, falling blood pressure. Assess for restlessness. Check dressings and drains for excess bleeding.
Fluid and electrolyte imbalances	Assess for cardiac dysrhythmias, muscle weakness or twitching, changes in mental status. Monitor intake and output, tissue turgor. Check laboratory reports and notify physician of abnormalities.
Respiratory failure	Monitor respiratory rate and effort, skin color, breath sounds.
Circulatory failure	Monitor for dysrhythmias, tachycardia, falling blood pressure.
Renal failure	Measure intake and urine output. Report output of less than 30 mL/hr. Assess for edema. Maintain prescribed fluid intake.
Hepatic failure	Assess for jaundice, fatigue, confusion, digestive disturbances.
Wound infection, dehiscence, and fistulas	Assess dressing and drains for excess bleeding, foul odor, purulent drainage. Check temperature for fever. Note elevation in white blood cell count.
Hyperglycemia	Monitor blood glucose as ordered. Note drowsiness, thirst, polyphagia, polyuria.

Interventions

In many ways, the care of the patient with pancreatic cancer is like that of the patient with pancreatitis, as discussed on p. 827. Chapter 25 also provides details of caring for the patient with cancer. Areas requiring special attention with pancreatic cancer are discussed here.

Acute Pain

Assess and record pain severity, nature, and location. Opioid analgesics are usually needed for severe pain management; however, nonopioids may be effective for mild to moderate pain. Radiation therapy and chemotherapy can reduce pain by shrinking the tumor. A celiac plexus nerve block can be done during surgery or percutaneously and provides excellent pain control. Other options for intolerable pain are patient-controlled analgesia (PCA) and epidural opioids. The effectiveness of drug therapy may be enhanced by distraction, imagery, and cutaneous stimulation, as discussed in Chapter 15.

Fear and Anticipatory Grieving

You can help the patient by recognizing and acknowledging fear, showing compassion, teaching, and providing attentive care. A referral to a mental health professional or spiritual counselor can be made with the patient's consent.

Imbalanced Nutrition: Less Than Body Requirements

Monitor the patient's dietary intake and weight. If intake is poor, consult the dietitian. Small, frequent meals may be ordered. Pancrelipase tablets are needed if the patient has malabsorption. Sometimes a jejunostomy tube is placed and feeding is delivered by pump. Feedings are usually started with dilute formula given at a slow rate. Both the concentration and the rate are gradually increased. Inform the physician if the patient develops diarrhea. Some patients require total parenteral nutrition for adequate nourishment.

Impaired Skin Integrity

If pruritus is a problem, special skin care and protection are needed. Eliminate bath soaps, and apply emollient lotions. Keep the fingernails short to reduce trauma from scratching. Supply mittens if the patient is unable to avoid scratching. The physician may order diphenhydramine (Benadryl) to reduce pruritus. If a patient has drains or fistulas, irritating digestive fluids may come in contact with the skin. Carefully cleanse the exposed skin. Skin barriers and pouches may be effective in protecting the skin. An enterostomal therapist may be consulted for advice on skin care.

Disturbed Body Image

Weight loss and jaundice alter the patient's appearance and may be distressing. Assist patients with grooming, and encourage them to look their best.

Deficient Knowledge

People under stress retain only part of what they hear, so information often must be repeated and reinforced. Provide written material in addition to verbal instruction. The patient's family also may need information and support when dealing with a diagnosis of pancreatic cancer. Refer questions about medical decisions and prognosis to the physician. The specific teaching plan will depend on the diagnostic and therapeutic measures prescribed. You should advise the patient of community resources, including the American Cancer Society and home health nursing services.

Surgical Complications and Postoperative Nursing Care

In general, the postoperative care of the patient with pancreatic cancer is like that of any patient undergoing major abdominal surgery. If the Whipple procedure is performed, the patient is at risk for many complications. These include hemorrhage; fluid and electrolyte imbalances; respiratory, circulatory, renal, and hepatic failure; wound infection and dehiscence; fistulas; and hyperglycemia. Therefore ongoing nursing assessments are critical. Closely monitor vital signs, intake and output, and blood glucose values. Assess the wound for bleeding, infection, and separation of margins. Evaluate mental status to detect changes associated with electrolyte imbalances, poor circulation, and hepatic or renal failure.

Key Points

- The liver plays an important role in bile production and excretion; glucose, protein, and lipid metabolism; blood coagulation; detoxification; immunity; and hormone metabolism.
- Signs of liver dysfunction include jaundice (a golden yellow skin color) and scleral icterus (yellowing of the sclera of the eyes).
- Hepatitis is liver inflammation caused by a viral infection or exposure to toxic substances; it can lead to hepatic failure.
- Nursing care of the patient with hepatitis addresses Activity Intolerance, Impaired Physical Mobility, Imbalanced Nutrition: Less Than Body Requirements, Acute Pain, Impaired Skin Integrity, Deficient Fluid Volume, Disturbed Body Image, and Anxiety.
- Health care providers should be vaccinated against hepatitis B since it can be spread through contact with body fluids.
- Cirrhosis is chronic, progressive liver failure that disrupts metabolism and causes blood abnormalities, fluid and electrolyte imbalances, decreased resistance to infection, accumulation of drugs and toxins, and obstruction of blood vessels and bile ducts in the liver.

- Cirrhosis may be caused by nutritional deficiencies, toxins (including alcohol), hepatitis, biliary obstruction, and heart failure.
- Complications of cirrhosis include portal hypertension, esophageal varices, ascites, hepatic encephalopathy, and hepatorenal syndrome.
- Nursing care of the patient with cirrhosis addresses Imbalanced Nutrition: Less Than Body Requirements, Activity Intolerance, Risk for Impaired Skin Integrity, Acute Pain, Ineffective Breathing Pattern, Risk for Injury, Disturbed Thought Processes, Deficient Fluid Volume, Excess Fluid Volume, Risk for Infection, and Fear.
- The only cure for end-stage liver disease is liver transplantation, which requires lifelong treatment with antirejection drugs that suppress the immune system and put the patient at risk for infection.
- Signs and symptoms of transplanted organ rejection are fever, anorexia, depression, vague abdominal pain, muscle aches, and joint pain.
- Bile is produced in the liver, stored in the gallbladder, and delivered to the intestine, where it is essential for emulsification and digestion of fats.
- Cholecystitis is inflammation of the gallbladder, usually caused by gallstones; the gallstones may obstruct bile flow, causing symptoms from mild indigestion to nausea, chills and fever, and right upper quadrant pain that radiates to the shoulder.
- Cholelithiasis (stones in the bile) may be treated with cholecystectomy, oral bile salts, dissolution agents, lithotripsy, or endoscopic sphincterotomy.

- Nursing care of the patient with cholecystitis and cholelithiasis focuses on Acute Pain, Deficient Fluid Volume, Risk for Impaired Skin Integrity, Risk for Impaired Skin Integrity, Anxiety, Risk for Injury; *and for surgical patients:* Ineffective Breathing Pattern and Risk for Infection.
- The pancreas has both an endocrine function (insulin secretion) and an exocrine function (secretion of digestive enzymes).
- Pancreatitis is inflammation of the pancreas; it can lead to pseudocyst, abscess, hypocalcemia, and pulmonary, cardiac, and renal complications.
- Nursing care of the patient with pancreatitis addresses Acute Pain, Deficient Fluid Volume, Risk for Infection, Impaired Gas Exchange, Imbalanced Nutrition: Less Than Body Requirements, Anxiety, and Deficient Knowledge.
- Most patients with pancreatic cancer die within a year, especially if the cancer is in the body or the tail of the pancreas.
- Nursing care of the patient with pancreatic cancer usually focuses on Acute Pain, Fear, Anticipatory Grieving, Imbalanced Nutrition: Less Than Body Requirements, Impaired Skin Integrity, and Disturbed Body Image.

 Go to your Companion CD-ROM for a Pharmacology Tutorial, Audio Glossary, and 3-D animations.

evolve Be sure to visit the companion Evolve site at http://evolve.elsevier.com/Linton/ for WebLinks and additional online resources.

REVIEW QUESTIONS *Choose the best answer.*

1. Your focused assessment of a hepatitis patient reveals jaundice, light-colored stools, and dark urine. These findings are typical of which phase of hepatitis?

   1. Preicteric phase
   2. Icteric phase
   3. Posticteric phase
   4. Recovery phase

2. Measures to control pruritus include the following:

   1. Application of lubricating lotions
   2. Assisting with hot baths twice daily
   3. Vigorous massage of affected areas
   4. Administration of prescribed antibiotics

3. Health care providers are routinely vaccinated against which of the following?

   1. Hepatitis A
   2. Hepatitis B
   3. Hepatitis C
   4. Hepatitis D

4. In the cirrhosis patient, esophageal varices and hemorrhoids are caused by which of the following?

   1. Blood vessels weakened by malnutrition
   2. Inability to conjugate and excrete bilirubin
   3. Elevated pressure in gastrointestinal blood vessels
   4. Fluid retention associated with excess aldosterone

5. A patient comes to the clinic for follow-up 1 month after liver transplantation. Which of the following assessment findings would concern you *most?*

   1. Heartburn
   2. Constipation
   3. Pale urine
   4. Fever

6. Which option reflects the correct sequence of bile flow from the liver to the gallbladder?

   1. Common bile duct, common hepatic duct
   2. Cystic duct, common bile duct
   3. Common hepatic duct, common bile duct
   4. Common hepatic duct, cystic duct

7. The purpose of a T-tube after cholecystectomy is to:

   1. Maintain bile flow in the common bile duct
   2. Relieve pressure on the liver
   3. Divert intestinal contents from the surgical site
   4. Prevent bile leakage into the abdomen

8. The exocrine function of the pancreas is which of the following?

   1. Storage and secretion of insulin in response to high blood glucose levels
   2. Conversion of excess blood glucose to glycogen for storage
   3. Breakdown of excessive fats and carbohydrates in the intestine
   4. Production and secretion of digestive enzymes into the duodenum through a duct

9. In a patient with chronic pancreatitis, the effects of pancreatic enzyme tablets can be assessed by:
   1. Monitoring daily weights
   2. Examining the stools for steatorrhea
   3. Recording intake and output
   4. Asking whether pain is relieved

10. The risk of pancreatic cancer can be reduced by which of the following?
    1. Smoking cessation
    2. Increased dietary protein
    3. Regular exercise
    4. Moderate alcohol intake

40 Urologic Disorders

Objectives

After reading and studying this chapter, you should be able to:

1. List the data to be collected when assessing a patient who has a urologic disorder.
2. Describe the diagnostic tests and procedures for patients with urologic disorders.
3. Explain the nursing responsibilities for patients having tests and procedures to diagnose urologic disorders.
4. Describe the nursing responsibilities for common therapeutic measures used to treat urologic disorders.
5. Explain the pathophysiology, signs and symptoms, complications, and treatment of disorders of the kidneys, ureters, bladder, and urethra.
6. Assist in developing a nursing care plan for patients with urologic disorders.

Key Terms

Be sure to check out the bonus material on the Companion CD-ROM, including selected audio pronunciations.

anuria (ă-NŪ-rē-ă, p. 841)
azotemia (ă-zō-TĒ-mē-ă, p. 871)
calculus (*pl.* calculi) (KĂL-kŭ-lŭs) (KĂL-kŭ-lī, p. 841)
cystectomy (sĭs-TĔK-tō-mē, p. 848)
diuresis (dī-ŭ-RĒ-sĭs, p. 868)
diuretic (dī-ŭr-RĔ-tĭc, p. 839)
dysuria (dĭs-Ū-rē-ă, p. 841)
hematuria (hĕm-ă-TŪ-rē-ă, p. 841)
incontinence (ĭn-KŎN-tĭ-nĕns, p. 840)
lithotomy (lĭ-THŎT-ō-mē, p. 859)
lithotripsy (LĬTH-ō-trĭp-sē, p. 859)
nephrotoxic (nĕf-rō-TŎK-sĭk, p. 841)
nocturia (nŏk-TŪ-rē-ă, p. 840)
oliguria (ŏl-ĭ-GŪ-rē-ă, p. 840)
polyuria (pŏl-ē-Ū-rē-ă, p. 840)
uremia (ū-RĒ-mē-ă, p. 871)

The urinary tract plays a vital role in maintaining homeostasis and removing metabolic wastes. Because body systems are interdependent, disease processes in other body systems may have a direct and harmful effect on the urinary system. Similarly, urinary system diseases may affect significantly the respiratory and circulatory systems. Serious alterations in urinary function eventually affect all other systems. A person can live with one functioning kidney, but the body cannot support life with the loss of both kidneys.

ANATOMY AND PHYSIOLOGY OF THE URINARY SYSTEM

ANATOMY

The urinary system consists of two kidneys, two ureters, the bladder, and the urethra (Fig. 40-1).

Kidneys and Ureters

The kidneys are bean-shaped organs located just under and below the twelfth rib near the waist in an area of the body trunk called the *flank* (Fig. 40-2). They each are surrounded by fibrous capsules and layers of fat. They are tightly wedged between the peritoneum, a membrane that separates them from the digestive system, and a layer of muscle in the back.

The hilus, or entry, to the kidney is located on the concave surface of the kidney near the spine (Fig. 40-3). The right and left renal arteries branch off from the abdominal artery and enter the kidneys at the hilus. The entire blood supply circulates through the kidneys every 4 to 5 minutes. Each renal vein returns filtered blood directly to the inferior vena cava. The kidney is divided into an outer layer called the *cortex* and an inner layer called the *medulla*. The cortex receives a large blood supply and is very sensitive to changes in blood pressure and blood volume. The medulla is organized into 8 to 18 pyramid-shaped structures that concentrate and collect urine and drain it into the calices. The calices then drain urine into the renal pelvis. The renal pelvis is at the center of the kidney and forms the funnel-shaped proximal end of the ureter. The ureter carries urine from the renal pelvis to the bladder.

The nephron is the functional unit of the kidney. There are 1 to 1.25 million nephrons in each kidney. The nephron is a vascular tubular system consisting of a glomerulus, a Bowman's capsule, and a tubule. The glomerulus is a mass of blood vessels tucked into the cuplike Bowman's capsule. Each tubule consists of a proximal tubule, the loop of Henle, a distal tubule, and a collecting duct (Fig. 40-4). The nephron is located mostly in the cortex of the kidney, with the loop

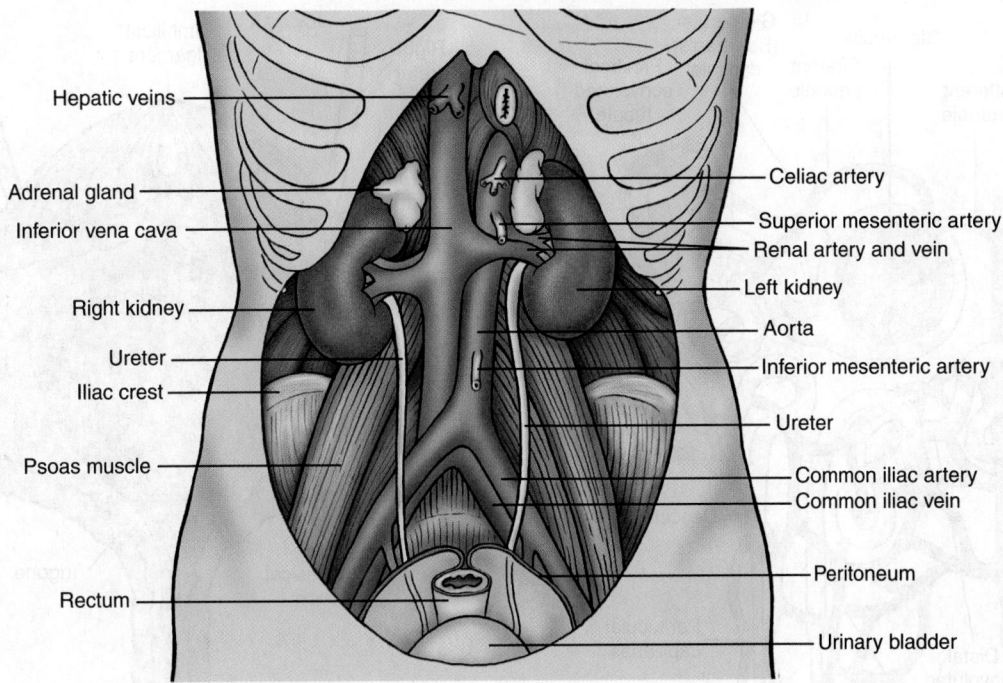

FIGURE **40-1** The kidneys and related structures.

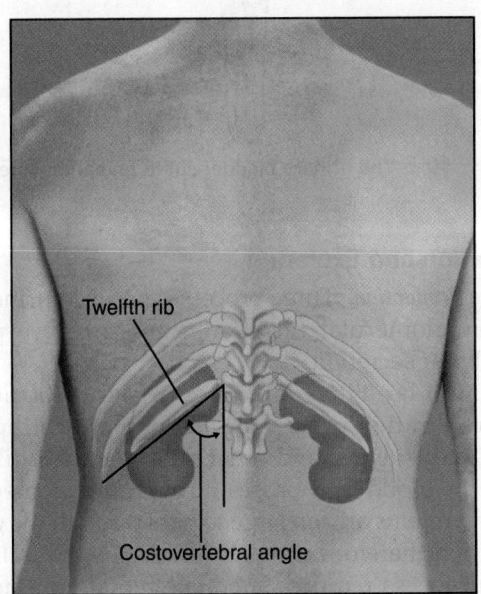

FIGURE **40-2** The kidneys are located just under and below the twelfth rib. The costovertebral angle is illustrated here.

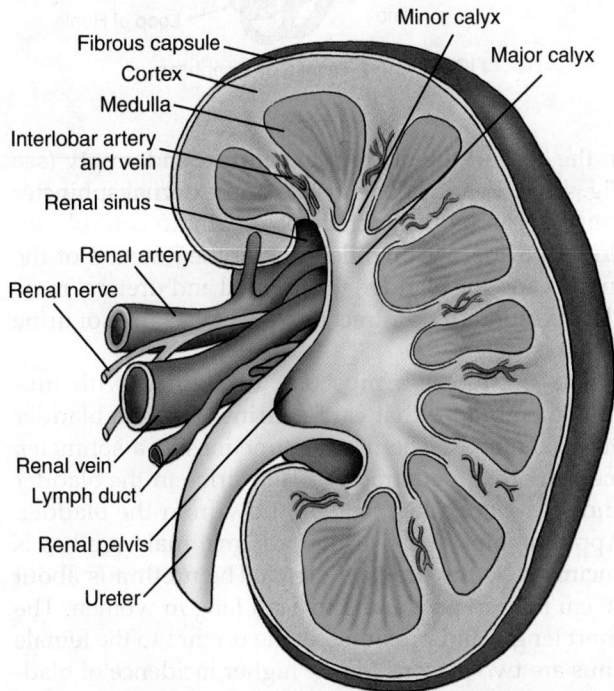

FIGURE **40-3** View of interior kidney structures.

of Henle dipping into the medulla and the collecting ducts traveling through the medulla to the calices.

Bladder and Urethra

The bladder is a muscular sac that readily stretches to store urine. The bladder rests on the floor of the pelvic cavity behind the peritoneum. It is located in front of the rectum in men and in front of the vagina and uterus in women. The upper portion of the bladder is called the *apex,* and the base, or *fundus,* is close to the pelvic floor. The bladder neck, containing the internal

sphincter, is the most inferior portion. The trigone is a triangular-shaped area on the posterior wall as seen in Figure 40-5. The trigone muscles help close the junction of the ureters and the bladder during urination, preventing backflow of urine into the ureters.

Control of the bladder is made possible by both sensory and motor nerves. When 200 to 400 mL of urine collects in the bladder, sensory nerves cause the urge to urinate. Motor nerves stimulate the detrusor muscles

FIGURE **40-4** Details of a nephron.

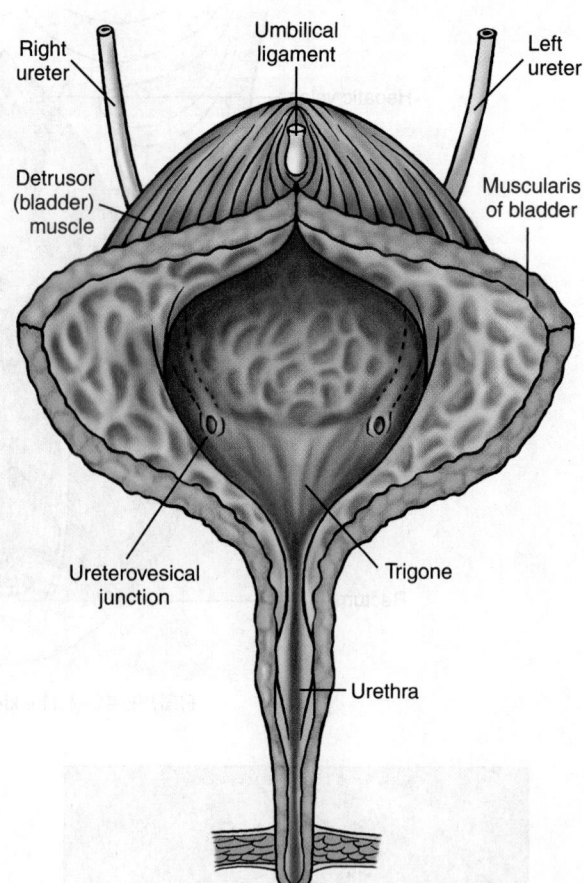

FIGURE **40-5** The urinary bladder cut to reveal the interior.

in the base of the bladder to contract and empty (see Fig. 40-5). Pelvic floor muscles and external sphincter muscles can be contracted voluntarily to control outflow of urine. Meanwhile, back at the junction of the ureters and the bladder, the trigonal and ureteral muscles involuntarily contract to prevent backflow of urine into the ureters.

The urethra is a muscular tube lined with mucous membranes that carries urine from the bladder out of the body. The urethra functions as a sphincter, meaning that it contracts to hold urine in the bladder and relaxes to allow urine to flow from the bladder. Approximately 3 cm of the proximal male urethra is encircled by the prostate gland. The urethra is about 20 cm long in men and 3 to 5 cm long in women. The short length and proximity of the urethra to the female anus are two reasons for the higher incidence of bladder infections in women.

PHYSIOLOGY

The functions of the urinary system are regulatory, excretory, and hormonal. Regulatory functions are performed by the formation of urine and by the secretion of renin, which affects blood pressure. Regulatory processes maintain fluid balance, keep electrolytes in normal range, and maintain acid-base balance. The excretory function of the kidney is the elimination of urine. The hormonal function is to stimulate red blood cell production.

Regulation and Excretion

Urine Production. Three processes occur in urine production: glomerular filtration, tubular reabsorption, and tubular secretion.

Glomerular Filtration. Glomerular filtration is an ultrafiltration process in the glomerular capsule. Fluids, electrolytes, and other substances are filtered out of the blood as it passes through the glomerulus. Plasma proteins are too large to pass through the glomerulus and therefore remain in the blood. The ultrafiltration process requires adequate blood volume and blood pressure. The product of glomerular filtration is called the *glomerular filtrate.* It contains water, electrolytes (sodium, potassium, calcium, magnesium, chloride, bicarbonate, phosphate, other anions), glucose, urea, creatinine, uric acid, and amino acids. Glomerular filtrate and blood plasma are essentially the same except that the filtrate does not have proteins. Most of the filtrate is returned to the blood from the tubules by reabsorption.

Tubular Reabsorption. Water, some electrolytes, and nonelectrolytes are reabsorbed from the tubules of the kidney back into the blood as needed to maintain normal fluid balance. Reabsorption occurs through diffusion, active transport, and osmosis. Some nonelectrolytes (urea, creatinine, uric acid) are not readily reabsorbed and are excreted in the urine. The reabsorption of water reflects the ability of the kidney to concentrate or dilute urine as necessary. The amount of water reabsorbed is influenced by antidiuretic hormone and aldosterone. Antidiuretic hormone, stored in the posterior pituitary, affects the amount of water reabsorbed in the distal tubules and the collecting ducts. If blood volume decreases or blood osmolality (concentration) increases, antidiuretic hormone is secreted from the posterior pituitary. The distal tubules and collecting ducts of the kidney become more permeable to water, so that reabsorption back into the circulating blood increases and urine becomes more concentrated.

Tubular Secretion. Potassium and hydrogen ions are secreted into the tubules from the blood. This secretion process regulates serum potassium levels and is the basis for the kidney's acid-base regulating mechanism. The normal pH of urine is 4.5 to 8.0.

The kidneys and lungs work together to maintain the acid-base balance of the body. The lungs excrete CO_2, a volatile acid, and the kidneys excrete fixed acids produced by normal metabolism. Base levels are maintained by renal conservation of bicarbonate, excretion of sodium for hydrogen, and excretion of ammonia.

The end product of glomerular filtration, tubular reabsorption, and tubular excretion is urine. Urine is composed mostly of water, sodium, potassium, chloride, urea, creatinine, and uric acid. The body normally excretes 1 to 2 L of urine each day, which is approximately 1% of the blood filtered by the glomeruli in the same period of time. Glucose and proteins are substances present in blood but not normally present in the urine. Normally, glucose is completely reabsorbed in the tubules. The presence of proteins in urine indicates glomerular damage. Urine is delivered to the renal pelvis, where it flows into the ureter. The production of urine is illustrated in Figure 40-6.

Urine Elimination. Peristaltic waves move urine from the kidney through the ureter to the bladder. The presence of 200 to 400 mL of urine in the bladder causes the urge to urinate, although the bladder can distend to hold several times that amount. Urination is a complex process that is under a variety of neural controls and is voluntary for the toilet-trained person with intact motor and sensory nerve pathways. Urination generally occurs five to six times a day and may occur once at night. The amount of urine produced is affected by fluid intake, temperature, diaphoresis, vomiting, diarrhea, and medications such as diuretics.

A series of events allow the release of urine from the bladder. The pelvic floor muscles and the urethral sphincter relax. The trigonal muscles contract, closing the ureters to prevent backflow of urine into the ureters. The bladder muscle (detrusor) contracts, and urine is forced through the urethra. After the bladder empties, the bladder muscle relaxes, the bladder neck

FIGURE 40-6 Urine production.

closes, the trigonal muscles relax, and the perineal muscles resume resting tone. Voiding is primarily an involuntary reflex act. Voluntary control of voiding is exhibited in the initiation, restraint, and interruption of urine flow.

Regulation of Serum Calcium and Phosphate. Parathormone is a hormone secreted by the parathyroid glands to maintain serum calcium levels. When serum calcium is low, parathormone is secreted and acts on the tubules to promote reabsorption of calcium ions. At the same time, tubular reabsorption of phosphate is decreased.

This mechanism helps maintain normal serum calcium and phosphate levels.

Regulation of Blood Pressure. Blood pressure is regulated through fluid volume maintenance and release of the hormone *renin* from the kidneys. One way to raise or lower blood pressure is to change blood volume. This can be done by retaining additional fluid or by eliminating excess fluid. For example, suppose a patient has had severe vomiting and diarrhea resulting in dehydration and low blood pressure. Hypertonic plasma caused by dehydration stimulates the release of antidiuretic hormone from the posterior pituitary. Antidiuretic hormone causes reabsorption of water from the renal tubules, decreasing urine volume. The retained fluid expands blood volume, with a subsequent rise in blood pressure.

A second mechanism by which the kidneys affect blood pressure is the secretion of renin. Renin is released in response to inadequate renal blood flow or low arterial pressure. Renin acts on angiotensinogen, a hormone produced by the liver, and converts it to angiotensin I. A lung enzyme converts angiotensin I to angiotensin II. Angiotensin II is a powerful peripheral vasoconstrictor. Also, angiotensin II triggers the release of aldosterone from the adrenal cortex. Aldosterone stimulates tubular reabsorption of sodium and water, and plasma volume is expanded.

With severely decreased cardiac output, as seen in hemorrhage and shock, the renal arteries constrict to prevent fluid loss and to shunt blood to more vital organs (heart, lungs, brain). This vasoconstriction limits renal blood flow. If blood flow is not restored, death of renal tissue may occur.

Hormonal Stimulation of Red Blood Cell Production

Erythropoietin is secreted in the kidneys and stimulates the bone marrow to produce red blood cells. This process is triggered by decreased oxygen in renal blood. Patients in renal failure have a deficiency of erythropoietin, which causes them to become anemic.

AGE-RELATED CHANGES IN THE URINARY SYSTEM

As people age, significant changes occur in the urinary system. Fortunately, the kidneys have enough reserve that normal function is usually maintained. When older people are stressed, however, the kidneys do not adapt as well as they do in younger people.

Structural changes in the kidney include loss of nephrons, thickening of membranes in nephrons, and sclerosis of renal blood vessels. Because of these changes, renal blood flow and glomerular filtration decline. In addition, plasma renin and aldosterone levels fall and tubules are less responsive to antidiuretic hormone. As a result of all these changes, the older person's kidneys are less able to concentrate and dilute urine in response to changes in serum osmolality (concentration).

Creatinine clearance decreases with age. This means that the rate at which the kidneys are able to remove creatinine from the blood is diminished. Creatinine clearance is a better indicator of kidney function than serum creatinine. There also is some decline in erythropoietin, a factor that may contribute to anemia. In an older person, serum glucose may be considerably elevated before it is detected in the urine.

In younger people, urine production peaks during waking hours. This pattern is lost with age such that urine production does not decrease at night. Therefore older people often have nocturia, meaning that they awaken from sleep to void.

The bladder also undergoes changes with age. Bladder muscles weaken, and connective tissue increases. The effect is decreased capacity and incomplete emptying. The mechanism that prevents the reflux of urine from the bladder into the ureters is less effective and can contribute to kidney infections.

Incontinence is not a normal consequence of age, but it is common. Female urinary incontinence is often caused by relaxed pelvic muscles related to childbirth trauma and lack of estrogen after menopause. For detailed information on incontinence, see Chapter 23. In men, urethral obstruction is more often a problem. It is often caused by the enlarged prostate closing in on the urethra. Prostate enlargement is discussed in Chapter 48.

NURSING ASSESSMENT OF THE URINARY SYSTEM

Elimination is considered to be a very personal activity, and people are not accustomed to discussing it with others. Assessment of urinary function and problems, therefore, may be embarrassing to the patient. Privacy and a calm, accepting manner help put the patient at ease.

HEALTH HISTORY
Chief Complaint

Patients with urinary problems most often report changes in urine quality or quantity, pain, or changes in urination.

History of Present Illness

Ask about the patient's normal or usual pattern of urination. Important data include volume of urine, frequency of voiding, and appearance of urine. The patient may have difficulty estimating the amount of urine voided but usually can recognize an increase or decrease from normal. If intake and output records are available, note the recent pattern. Terms used to describe urine volume are *polyuria, oliguria,* and *anuria.* Polyuria refers to a large urine output, oliguria to a low output, and anuria to the absence of output. Urine characteristics to record include color, clarity (clear or cloudy), presence of particles, and odor. Hematuria is the presence of blood in the urine.

Pain may or may not occur, but it is more common with acute conditions. Painful urination is called dysuria. Inquire about the presence of pain or discomfort. Describe the characteristics of the pain: intensity, location, distribution, onset, duration, frequency, relationship to urination, precipitating factors, and measures that provide relief. Urologic conditions also may cause pain in the flank, abdomen, pelvic area, and genitalia. The pain may be so severe that it causes nausea and vomiting.

Include questions about any problem the patient has had initiating or controlling urination. Document circumstances under which these problems occur. For example, involuntary loss of urine with laughing or sneezing is typical of stress incontinence. Urge incontinence is the inability to hold urine when feeling the urge to void.

Past Medical History

After the present illness has been fully described, the patient's past medical history should be explored. Significant findings include a history of streptococcal infections, recurrent urinary tract infections (UTIs), renal calculi ("stones"), gout, or hypercalcemia. Ask if the patient has had urologic surgery, catheterization, examination (e.g., cystoscopy, radiography), or trauma and if the patient uses any type of urinary diversion or collection device. Document recent and current medications, including prescription and over-the-counter drugs and herbal remedies, because some medications are nephrotoxic (harmful to the kidneys). Note exposure to toxic chemicals in the home or the workplace.

Family History

Describe the patient's family medical history. Important conditions to note are congenital kidney problems such as polycystic kidneys or urinary tract malformations, diabetes mellitus, and hypertension.

Review of Systems

Review the body systems to detect other problems that may be related to the urinary tract complaints. Ask if the patient has had changes in skin color, respiratory distress, edema, fatigue, nausea, vomiting, chills, and fever.

Functional Assessment

The functional assessment includes information about habits and practices that might affect or contribute to urinary tract disorders. Ask about daily fluid intake because urine production varies with fluid intake. It is also helpful to determine the patient's usual exercise pattern because excessive exercise or prolonged immobility affects the urinary system. Determine the effects of the chief complaint on daily life as well.

Pharmacology Capsule

Nephrotoxic drugs are harmful to the kidneys.

PHYSICAL EXAMINATION

The physical examination begins with inspection of the skin for color (ashen, yellow) and the presence of crystals on the skin (uremic frost). Evaluate tissue turgor to detect dehydration or edema. Examine the area around the eyes for periorbital edema, which suggests fluid retention. Inspect the mouth for moisture and odor. Patients in renal failure may have an odor of urine on their breath.

Observe respiratory rate, pattern, and effort. Respirations may be rapid with metabolic acidosis, infection, and fluid overload. Kussmaul's respirations, seen with metabolic acidosis, are rapid and deep. Dyspnea may be evident with fluid overload. Auscultate the lungs for crackles or rhonchi that may indicate fluid overload. Heart rhythm irregularities may be noted with potassium imbalances.

Inspect the abdomen for scars and contours, and palpate for tenderness and bladder distention. Auscultate the kidney area over the costovertebral angle (see Fig. 40-2) to detect renal bruits (swishing sounds caused by turbulent blood flow). Renal bruits indicate renal artery stenosis (narrowing). Then percuss the abdomen. A dull sound may be heard over a full bladder. Pain may be elicited over one or both kidneys.

Observe for edema throughout the examination. With renal failure, edema is generalized, not dependent. The skin may be dry, flushed, and shiny over the edematous area.

The last part of the physical examination is inspection of the genitalia. Standard Precautions should be observed. Examine the penis for lesions, scars, or discharge. If there are penile lesions or urethral discharge, smears should be obtained for culture. A nurse with advanced skills or the physician also may perform rectal and pelvic examinations, especially if symptoms suggest problems of the reproductive system. The pelvic examination may reveal gynecologic rather than urologic problems. The male rectal examination helps detect prostate enlargement, which often creates problems with voiding. Nursing assessment of urologic function is outlined in Box 40-1.

DIAGNOSTIC TESTS AND PROCEDURES

Diagnostic tests and procedures for urinary disorders are described here. Related nursing care is presented in the Diagnostic Tests and Procedures table on pp. 843 to 845.

Box 40-1 | *ASSESSMENT of Urologic Function*

Health History

Present Illness:
Changes in urine quality or quantity, voiding pattern, pain

Past Medical History:
Streptococcal infections, urinary tract infections or calculi, gout, hypercalcemia, urologic surgery or instrumentation, urinary diversion, recent and current medications

Family History:
Urinary disorders, diabetes mellitus, hypertension

Review of Systems:
Fatigue, pruritus, dyspnea; urine quantity: polyuria, oliguria, anuria; urine quality: color, odor, components; frequency of voiding; pain: onset, intensity, frequency, location, duration, precipitating and relieving factors

Functional Assessment:
Fluid intake, diet, activity

Physical Examination

General Appearance:
Level of consciousness, orientation

Vital Signs

Height and Weight

Skin:
Color, moisture, turgor, crystals

Respirations:
Rate, pattern, effort, breath sounds

Circulation:
Dysrhythmias, blood pressure alterations

Abdomen:
Scars, contour, tenderness, bruits

Genitalia:
Lesions, scars, discharge

URINE TESTS

Urinalysis

A urine specimen is examined for color, pH, specific gravity, glucose, protein, blood, ketones, and bilirubin. Normal urine is straw colored and slightly acidic. Microscopic examination is used to assess for cells, casts, bacteria, and crystals. Chemical examination to assess electrolytes and osmolality (concentration) of the urine determines the ability of the kidneys to excrete or conserve electrolytes and water. By comparing the osmolality of urine with serum osmolality, it is possible to know if the kidneys are functioning appropriately. If serum osmolality is elevated, the kidneys should reabsorb or conserve water to dilute the serum and excrete more concentrated urine (i.e., urine with high osmolality). If serum osmolality is low (urine is dilute), the kidneys should reduce reabsorption of water to increase serum concentration and produce more dilute urine (i.e., urine with low osmolality). Specific gravity is a measure of osmolality. Data reported from a routine urinalysis are summarized in Table 40-1 on p. 846.

Urine Culture and Sensitivity

Normal urine is sterile. A urine culture permits identification of microorganisms present in the urine. Sensitivity testing determines which antibiotics will be effective against the specific organisms. The specimen can be obtained by the patient, if able, or the nurse. Instructions are given in the Diagnostic Tests and Procedures table on p. 843.

Creatinine Clearance

Creatinine clearance, the rate at which the kidney removes creatinine from the blood, is the best test of overall kidney function. It serves as an estimate of glomerular filtration rate. This test requires collection of all urine for 12 or 24 hours, as ordered. Normal levels vary for men and women. Because values depend on muscle mass, they are usually lower in women. Urine and serum creatinine levels are compared to determine kidney function. If serum creatinine rises and urine creatinine falls, it is an indication of decreased kidney function and glomerular filtration rate.

BLOOD TESTS

Blood Urea Nitrogen

The blood urea nitrogen (BUN) test is a general indicator of the kidneys' ability to excrete urea, an end product of protein metabolism. In addition to renal failure, factors that increase BUN are a high-protein diet (especially with renal disease), gastrointestinal bleeding, dehydration, and some drugs (aspirin, chemotherapeutic agents, diuretics, gentamicin, lithium carbonate, morphine, steroids, sulfonamides, tobramycin).

Serum Creatinine

Creatinine is a waste product of skeletal muscle breakdown. The level of creatinine in the blood is an indication of the kidneys' ability to excrete wastes. Serum creatinine is elevated only in renal disorders and is a better measurement of kidney function than BUN. Unlike BUN, creatinine is not influenced by diet, hydration, nutritional status, or liver function. With normally functioning kidneys, the serum creatinine level is very low and the urine level is high. The normal ratio of BUN to creatinine is 10:1.

Serum Electrolytes

Serum electrolytes must be monitored in the renal patient because imbalances can have very serious consequences. In renal failure, sodium and potassium levels are elevated and calcium levels are decreased.

Text continued on p. 846.

DIAGNOSTIC TESTS and PROCEDURES   *Urinary Disorders*

TEST/PURPOSE	PATIENT PREPARATION	POSTPROCEDURE CARE
LABORATORY STUDIES		
General Considerations: Check agency manual for specific instructions. Tell the patient that a sample (blood, urine, etc.) is needed and why. Determine whether the patient needs to fast before the sample is obtained. Urine specimens should be sent to the laboratory promptly; refrigerate if there is a delay. For blood studies, apply small dressing to venipuncture site. Apply pressure if oozing persists or if patient's blood does not clot normally. For urine samples, instruct patient or assist in sample collection.		
Urine culture and sensitivity: Culture identifies microorganisms in urine. Sensitivity determines which antibiotic will be effective. Normal: no growth. Results in 24-36 hr.	Collect specimen of first voided urine of day. Instruct patient in midstream, clean-catch technique: cleanse penis or vulva thoroughly, void a small amount, stop the urine stream, and then void into a sterile container. If catheterization is necessary, collect the specimen after discarding a small amount of urine. Cap the container and immediately send it to the laboratory. If delivery is delayed, refrigerate the specimen.	Cap specimen and refrigerate or send to laboratory.
Blood urea nitrogen: Indicates kidneys' ability to excrete urea, an end product of protein metabolism. Increases with renal failure, GI bleeding, dehydration, and some drugs. Decreases with alcohol abuse, acromegaly, inadequate protein, hemodialysis, and some drugs.	No special preparation.	
Urine creatinine clearance: Estimates glomerular filtration rate. Decreases with renal disease. Normal value: varies with patient gender and age (usually lower in women).	Provide specimen container. Document first void and save all urine for next 12 or 24 hr as ordered. Keep specimen refrigerated. If patient has a Foley catheter, place drainage bag in basin of ice and empty into refrigerated container hourly.	
Serum creatinine: Measures kidneys' ability to excrete waste based on amount of creatinine in blood. Normal values: varies with method used; should be small. Increased with impaired renal function, urinary obstruction, muscle disease. Decreased with muscular dystrophy.	Patient should avoid strenuous exercise for 8 hours and excessive red meat for 24 hours before the test.	
Serum electrolytes: Detects alterations reflecting inability of kidneys to retain or excrete electrolytes. Sodium and potassium elevated and calcium decreased in renal failure. Normal values: see Chapter 14.	No special preparation.	Check laboratory reports and notify physician of abnormalities. Electrolyte imbalances can be life-threatening. See Chapter 14 for details on specific electrolytes.

Continued

DIAGNOSTIC TESTS and PROCEDURES   *Urinary Disorders—cont'd*

TEST/PURPOSE	PATIENT PREPARATION	POSTPROCEDURE CARE
ULTRASOUND (US)		
Abdominal and renal US: Uses sound waves to detect cysts, tumors, urinary calculi, urinary tract malformations or obstructions. Can be used to guide needle insertion for closed biopsy.	Patient may have to drink a specified amount of water (typically three to four 8-oz glasses of water within 2 hr of the procedure) so that bladder will be full during ultrasound. Tell patient that procedure is painless except for discomfort of full bladder. Takes about 15 min. Enema usually given if transrectal route used. For transabdominal route, gel is applied to skin and an instrument is moved over the lubricated skin surface. Images are recorded for study. Patient instructions will vary if other routes are used.	Wash gel off skin if transabdominal route used.
RADIOGRAPHIC STUDIES		
General Interventions: Explain the test to the patient. Radiation exposure is generally contraindicated during pregnancy. Patients should be questioned about allergies, especially any previous reactions to contrast dye. Special premedication may be ordered for those patients reporting an allergy to iodine. Itching, hives, wheezing, and respiratory distress are symptoms of an allergic reaction. Allergic reactions are treated by discontinuing the administration of the contrast, giving antihistamines, and administering cardiopulmonary resuscitation if necessary. The patient can expect a flushed, warm feeling, a salty taste in the mouth, and maybe nausea when the contrast medium is injected. The procedure takes about 45 minutes.		
Flat plate (KUB [kidneys/ureters/bladder]): Provides radiographic view of kidneys, ureters, and bladder.	No special preparation. Schedule before studies that use contrast media.	No special care.
Intravenous pyelogram (IVP): Uses x-rays and fluoroscope to outline kidneys. Uses contrast medium to show urine flow and obstructions. Detects urinary abnormalities, calculi, ureters, and bladder.	Tell patient that "dye" will be injected and radiographs taken to study urinary tract. Give laxatives and enemas as ordered before test. NPO 8-10 hr before test.	Encourage fluids to flush contrast medium from body. Monitor for signs of iodine allergy: urticaria, rash, nausea, swollen parotid glands. Check injection site for inflammation.
Arteriogram: Uses radiographs and contrast medium to examine blood vessels of kidney.	Tell patient that physician will insert catheter into blood vessel (usually in groin) and inject "dye." Radiographs are then taken as dye circulates through kidneys. Usual preparation: NPO for 8-12 hr, laxatives and enemas. Anticoagulant drugs withheld before test to reduce risk of bleeding. Signed consent required. Premedicate if ordered. Have patient void before sedation.	Assess for signs of bleeding: tachycardia, dyspnea, restlessness, abdominal or flank pain. Check injection site for bleeding. A pressure dressing should be in place. Monitor respiratory status if sedated. ECG monitoring may be ordered. Monitor pulse, color, warmth and sensation of extremity in which catheter was inserted. Maintain bed rest as ordered. Encourage fluids to eliminate dye. Measure intake and output.
Computed tomography (CT): Creates cross-sectional images of kidneys and other organs to reveal abnormalities.	Inform radiologist if patient is allergic to contrast media, iodine, or shellfish. Inform patient that the procedure is painless and noninvasive. NPO status may be ordered, but routine drugs can usually be taken. The patient will lie still on a stretcher while a doughnut-shaped machine moves around him or her. Contrast dye is sometimes injected intravenously. It can create a feeling of warmth, a salty taste, and nausea. Sedation can be ordered if the patient has difficulty lying still.	No special care usually needed. Inform the physician of any signs of allergic response to contrast dye. Give antihistamines as ordered for allergy.

Magnetic resonance imaging (MRI): Creates soft-tissue images using magnets and radio waves.

Tell patient that procedure is painless; must lie still for 30 min or more. Some equipment has videos that patient can view to reduce anxiety. Ask whether patient is claustrophobic. Give sedation if ordered for agitated or anxious patients. Remove any metallic objects such as jewelry. Inquire whether patient has any implanted devices such as cardiac pacemaker or intracranial aneurysm clips, and notify radiologist. Procedure is contraindicated with some implants. Metal may not be a problem with some newer equipment.

No special postprocedure care. Safety precautions if sedated.

Renal scan: Uses radioisotopes and x-rays to study renal blood flow. Detects infarctions, trauma, atherosclerosis, transplant rejection, some renal diseases.

Tell patient that isotope will be injected and radiographs taken. Takes about 1 hr. Radiation dose is small and quickly eliminated.

No special care unless patient is incontinent. Then, wear gloves to handle urine and change linens. Discard per agency protocol. Continent patients can use toilet. Pregnant caregivers should avoid these patients for 24 hr.

INVASIVE PROCEDURES

Renal biopsy: Excision of small amount of kidney tissue for examination. May be obtained through incision (open biopsy) or with special needle (closed biopsy).

Physician explains procedure selected. For closed biopsy, patient is positioned prone with rolled blanket under abdomen for approximately 45 min. Be sure reports of clotting studies (prothrombin time, partial thromboplastin time, platelets) are on chart. Report elevated blood pressure, which increases the risk of bleeding. NPO 6 hr or as ordered. Signed consent required.

Check pressure dressing for hemorrhage. Monitor vital signs for hemorrhage: tachycardia, restlessness, flank pain radiating to abdomen. Position supine with blanket roll or sandbag under flank area. Bed rest for 24 hr. Advise patient to do no heavy lifting, exercise, or sports for 1-2 wk. Hemoglobin and hematocrit are checked at 6 and 24 hr after the biopsy.

Cystoscopy: Uses lighted cystoscope inserted through the urethra to see urethra, bladder, and ureteral openings. Allows diagnosis of problems, removal of bladder calculi, biopsy, some treatments. Local or general anesthesia may be used. Dye may be injected into kidneys through ureters (retrograde pyelography).

Signed consent required. Tell patient that procedure is done in operating room or special room under sterile conditions. For local anesthesia, liquids may be allowed; NPO before general anesthesia. Laxatives or enemas as ordered. Give medications as ordered to reduce anxiety and bladder spasms. Antibiotics may be ordered 2-3 days before procedure and continued several days afterwards.

Safety precautions first time up, because orthostatic hypotension is common. Monitor intake and output, vital signs, urine color: urine may be pink tinged to wine colored; lightens to usual color in 24-48 hr. Report severe pain. Give prescribed analgesics or antispasmodics as ordered, assist with sitz baths for pain or urinary frequency. Encourage 2-3 L of fluids daily. Tell patient that pink-tinged urine is expected for 1-2 days.

URODYNAMIC STUDIES

Cystogram and cystourethrogram: Uses dye injected into bladder through catheter followed by radiographs to outline bladder and demonstrate reflux of urine from bladder to ureters.

For voiding cystourethrogram, bladder and urethra are radiographed during urination. Rate of urine flow is measured. Tell patient that catheter will be inserted and dye instilled into bladder.

Monitor urine output and vital signs. Encourage increased fluids unless contraindicated. Observe for allergic reaction to dye. Assess for urinary retention.

Cystometrogram: Evaluates bladder tone.

Tell patient fluid will be instilled into bladder through urethral catheter. When patient feels urge to void, catheter will be removed. Patient voids, and residual urine is measured. Drugs may be given to test bladder response.

Encourage increased fluids unless contraindicated. Monitor intake and output. Administer drugs as ordered for bladder spasms.

NPO, Nothing by mouth.

Table 40-1 | *Urinalysis Data*

COMPONENTS	NORMAL VALUES	IMPLICATIONS OF ABNORMAL VALUES
Color	Light yellow to amber	Dilute, colorless: overhydration, diabetes insipidus, diabetes mellitus, chronic renal failure Concentrated dark amber: dehydration, some medications or foods Bright red: gross hematuria in acid urine Tea colored: gross hematuria in alkaline urine
Appearance	Clear	Cloudy, hazy: bacteria, pus, small amount of blood
pH	4.5-8.0	<5.0: acidosis, starvation, diarrhea >7.0: alkalosis, bacteriuria, UTI
Specific gravity	1.010-1.025	<1.005: diabetes insipidus, overhydration, renal disease, severe hypokalemia >1.030: dehydration, diabetes mellitus
Protein	Up to 8 mg/dL; reagent strip negative	>8 mg/dL: exercise, severe stress, fever, renal disease, malignancy
Glucose	Negative	Positive: diabetes mellitus, stroke, Cushing's syndrome, anesthesia, severe stress
Ketones	Negative	Positive: diabetes mellitus, starvation, excessive protein ingestion
Bilirubin	Negative	Positive: liver disease (jaundice)
MICROSCOPIC EXAMINATION		
RBCs	0-2.0	>2.0 (hematuria): kidney trauma, renal disease, anticoagulants
WBCs	0-4.0	>4.0: UTI, strenuous exercise
Casts	Negative to occasional hyaline casts	Positive: fever, renal disease, heart failure
Crystals	Negative	Positive: renal stone formation
Bacteria	Negative	Positive: UTI

RBCs, Red blood cells; *UTI*, urinary tract infection; *WBCs*, white blood cells.

RADIOGRAPHIC TESTS AND PROCEDURES

Kidneys, Ureters, Bladder (KUB)

A radiograph of the abdomen, or KUB (for kidneys, ureters, and bladder), provides a general outline of the kidneys, revealing their approximate size and contour. This radiograph is sometimes referred to as a "flat plate." Tumors, malformations, and calculi may be found with this type of radiograph. This procedure requires no special preparation or aftercare. It is not done on pregnant patients, and it should be done before any other studies that require contrast media.

Intravenous Pyelogram

An intravenous pyelogram (IVP) is a diagnostic procedure in which a radiographic contrast medium ("dye") is injected intravenously. Radiographs of the kidneys, ureters, and bladder are taken at 5- to 15-minute intervals. As the contrast is concentrated by the kidneys and excreted through the ureters into the bladder, kidney function and structures, ureter size and patency, bladder size and shape, and presence of calculi (stones) or other obstructions can be assessed. The procedure is contraindicated in older adult patients with known renal insufficiency and in patients with diabetes mellitus or multiple myeloma.

Arteriogram

A renal arteriogram permits study of the renal blood vessels. It is used to diagnose renal artery stenosis, aneurysms, vascular tumors, renal cysts, and renal infarctions. A catheter is inserted through the femoral artery and threaded into the aorta. A contrast medium is injected into each renal artery, and radiographs are taken as the contrast passes through the kidneys.

Cystogram

Contrast media can be instilled into the bladder using a catheter or a cystoscope. Films are then taken to visualize the bladder. This procedure is useful in detecting reflux of urine from the bladder back into the ureters.

Renal Scan

A renal scan indicates the size, shape, and location of the kidneys; detects renal infarction, atherosclerosis, trauma, or rejection of a transplant; and identifies primary renal disease. An intravenous radioisotope is injected, and radiographs are taken to demonstrate blood flow to each kidney. The test is not done on pregnant women but can be used for patients who are allergic to contrast containing iodine.

CT Scan and MRI

A CT scan is useful in detecting kidney size, tumors, abscesses, obstruction, and adrenal masses and tumors. Contrast media may be used to clarify details. MRI also may be used to visualize the kidneys.

ULTRASONOGRAPHY

Ultrasonography (ultrasound) uses high-frequency sound waves to create images of the bladder. It is used to detect urinary tract malformations and obstructions, tumors, renal calculi, perineal fluid accumulation, and cysts. Ultrasound also may be used to guide a needle inserted to aspirate specimens from cysts or tumors. The bladder should be full for visualization of organs and tissues. The procedure may be done through the abdominal wall (transabdominal), the rectum (transrectal), the urethra (transurethral), or the vagina (transvaginal). Preparation and patient instructions are specific for each approach.

INVASIVE PROCEDURES

Renal Biopsy

A renal biopsy is performed to obtain a specimen of renal tissue for direct microscopic examination. It is usually done to evaluate conditions leading to renal failure. The procedure may be done through open or closed methods. The open method is a surgical procedure in which an incision is made in the flank and a specimen of kidney tissue is removed. The closed procedure involves insertion of a needle under fluoroscopy or ultrasonography to aspirate the tissue specimen. For the closed procedure, the patient must be able to lie in the prone position with a blanket roll under the lower abdomen for up to 45 minutes. Patients with breathing problems may not be able to tolerate this position or alter their breathing patterns as needed during the procedure.

The most serious complication of a renal biopsy is hemorrhage. If bleeding is suspected, the patient is given intravenous fluids to restore fluid volume. Persistent bleeding may require surgery.

Cystoscopy

Cystoscopy is the direct visualization of the interior of the urethra, bladder, and ureteral orifices. The procedure may be done in the physician's office for diagnostic reasons or in an outpatient facility for diagnostic or treatment purposes under local or general anesthesia. As a diagnostic procedure, the cystoscopy allows the physician to observe lesions, locate sources of bleeding, and take biopsy samples. Treatments that can be done with this procedure include cauterization of lesions; removal of calculi, tumors, or foreign materials; implantation of radium seeds; insertion of ureteral catheters; and control of bleeding. A lighted tube called a *cystoscope* is inserted through the urethra into the bladder under sterile conditions. Retrograde pyelography, which involves injecting contrast into the ureters, also can be done during cystoscopy.

Back pain, bladder spasms, urinary frequency, and burning on urination are common after cystoscopy. Mild analgesics may bring relief. Belladonna and opium suppositories may be ordered to reduce bladder spasms. Bladder perforation is rare but should be suspected if the patient has severe abdominal pain.

URODYNAMIC STUDIES

Urodynamic studies are performed to determine the physiology of urination. The studies assess innervation of the bladder, incontinence, and other variations in urinary patterns. Urodynamic studies measure the rate and volume of urine flow during voiding. The rate of flow is decreased with obstruction or decreased innervation.

Cystogram and Voiding Cystourethrogram

The cystogram outlines the contour of the bladder and shows reflux or backflow of urine from the bladder into the ureters. Cystograms are useful in diagnosing neurogenic bladders, fistulas, tumors, and ruptured bladders. For a cystogram, a catheter is inserted into the bladder, contrast is injected, and then radiographs are taken.

A voiding cystourethrogram gives the physician additional information on urethral disorders during voiding. The bladder is filled with contrast, and radiographs are taken during and after urination. This procedure may be embarrassing for the patient. Explain the need for the test, and provide as much privacy as possible during the procedure.

Cystometrogram

The cystometrogram is used to evaluate bladder tone in the patient with incontinence or with a neurogenic bladder. A catheter is inserted into the bladder, and fluid is instilled until the patient reports the urge to void. When the patient feels urgency, the catheter is removed, the patient voids, and residual urine is measured. Drugs may be given to see if they effectively enhance or relax bladder tone in the individual patient.

COMMON THERAPEUTIC MEASURES

CATHETERIZATION

Catheterization is the introduction of a catheter through the urethra into the bladder for the purpose of draining urine. Catheters are inserted when patients are unable to void as a result of the effects of anesthesia, paralysis, trauma, unconsciousness, certain surgical procedures, and other factors that inhibit voiding. The major concern with catheterization is the potential for introduction of bacteria into the normally sterile bladder. Catheterization is the primary cause of nosocomial (health care–associated) infections. Therefore it is essential that strict aseptic techniques be followed when catheterization is necessary.

Urinary catheters are available in a variety of sizes for adults (generally from the small 12 French to the larger 20 French) and may be of a retaining or nonretaining design. Examples of retaining catheters are the coudé, Foley, Malecot, and Pezzer. A retaining catheter is one that has a device, like an inflatable balloon, that anchors the catheter in the bladder. Robinson and whistle-tip catheters are nonretaining or straight catheters. Nurses are most familiar with Foley catheters that have either double or triple lumina. Malecot and Pezzer catheters are used most often as suprapubic catheters.

Occasionally, patients are catheterized to measure residual urine. This procedure may be diagnostic, but it is often part of a bladder training program for patients who have lost control over bladder function. To measure residual volume, the patient must be catheterized immediately after voiding. Less than 50 mL of residual urine is considered normal.

The reader should refer to a fundamentals textbook for detailed information on the insertion and care of urethral catheters. Key points to remember when catheterization is necessary are the following:

1. Catheterize only after other noninvasive measures have failed or when absolutely necessary for diagnostic purposes.
2. Use sterile technique and equipment to insert the catheter.
3. With an indwelling catheter, do the following:
   a. Secure the tubing to the female patient's inner thigh or to the male patient's abdomen.
   b. Handle the catheter gently to avoid trauma to the urethra.
   c. Keep the urine collection bag below the level of the patient's bladder and the tubing in a circular fashion *on* the bed.
   d. Keep the drainage system closed as much as possible.
   e. Provide perineal care twice daily. (NOTE: Antibiotic ointments are not recommended.)
   f. Use Standard Precautions before and after handling the catheter.

URETERAL CATHETER

A ureteral catheter is threaded through a ureter into the renal pelvis. It can be inserted through the bladder during cystoscopy or through an abdominal incision. A ureteral catheter permits urine to flow through the swollen ureter after traumatic surgery. The catheter is connected to a drainage system, and output is measured frequently. Record output from this catheter separately from other urine output. Make certain that the catheter is not kinked or clamped because pressure would build up in the kidney, causing tissue damage. The capacity of the renal pelvis is only 3 to 5 mL. If irrigation is ordered, slowly instill no more than 5 mL (or less as ordered) of lukewarm, sterile normal saline. Use strict aseptic technique for the irrigation. Unless both ureters are completely obstructed, urine continues to drain into the bladder. Remember to record urine from each source on the output record.

The patient with a ureterostomy tube is usually kept on bed rest unless a double-J catheter is used. The double-J catheter has one coiled end in the renal pelvis and the other coiled end in the bladder.

NEPHROSTOMY TUBE

When a ureter is completely obstructed, the physician may insert a nephrostomy tube through a flank incision directly into the kidney pelvis. The tube is connected to a drainage system and assessed frequently. You must ensure that the tube is not kinked or clamped at any time because drainage must be continuous. Some urine usually leaks around the tube and flows through the flank incision. Perform sterile dressing changes and skin care as needed. Irrigation with a small amount of sterile normal saline may be ordered. Because of the small capacity of the renal pelvis, no more than 5 mL of irrigating fluid is used. You must use strict aseptic technique.

URINARY STENT

A stent is a hollow tube that is placed in a structure to give it support and allow fluid to flow through. A urinary stent may be placed in the ureter to maintain alignment or to provide a route for urine drainage. The stent is inserted by the physician. It may be completely internal, or it may extend through the urethra or skin. Several types of stents are available.

UROLOGIC SURGERY

Urologic surgery may be done on any part of the urinary tract. *Nephrectomy* is removal of the kidney because of cancer, massive trauma or bleeding, severe chronic failure with infection, polycystic kidney disease, or for donation. Many types of surgery are used to remove calculi, depending on their location. A surgical opening may be made in the renal tissue, renal pelvis, ureter, or bladder. *Lithotripsy* is a noninvasive procedure used to break up calculi, but patient care is similar to that of the surgical patient. Bladder surgery may be necessitated by bleeding, functional problems, or cancer. Removal of the bladder is a cystectomy; an incision in the bladder is a *cystotomy*. Some surgical procedures can be done through a cystoscope, so there is no external incision. Surgical procedures that reroute the flow of urine are called *urinary diversions*. A cystostomy is the formation of an opening or stoma on the abdomen for catheterization or to enable the collection of urine in an external reservoir.

Preoperative Care

Preparation for urologic surgery includes a complete diagnostic workup to rule out other medical problems.

Fluid status is evaluated, and any imbalances are corrected. Usual preoperative care measures are taken as described in Chapter 17. Bowel cleansing may be ordered before some procedures. If the patient will have a stoma for urine drainage, an enterostomal therapist is usually consulted for patient counseling and teaching.

Postoperative Care

After surgery, particular attention is given to urine output, respirations, and bowel function. Output is closely monitored, with drainage from various tubes recorded separately. Urine output of less than 30 mL/hr should be reported to the physician. Flank or abdominal incisions cause pain on deep breathing. Adequate pain management and support of the patient for coughing and deep breathing decrease the risk of atelectasis and pneumonia. Auscultate lungs frequently to assess breath sounds. Urologic surgery often involves manipulation of the bowel, which can lead to paralytic ileus. Therefore food and fluids are usually withheld until bowel sounds are present.

DRUG THERAPY

A number of drugs are available to treat urinary tract disorders. Major classifications of commonly used drugs are diuretics, antihypertensives, phosphate binders, hormones, vitamin and mineral supplements, and immunosuppressants. These classifications, specific drugs, their actions and adverse effects, and nursing interventions are summarized in the Drug Therapy table on pp. 850 to 852. Immunosuppressant drugs are addressed separately in the Drug Therapy table on p. 853.

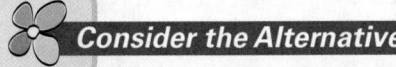

Consider the Alternative

Herbal remedies, like medications, can be harmful to the kidney. For example, aloe can cause nephritis and ephedra (ma huang) can cause kidney stones. Teach patients to always include alternative remedies in their medication histories.

DISORDERS OF THE URINARY TRACT

URINARY TRACT INFLAMMATION AND INFECTIONS

Urinary tract infections (UTIs) are common, especially among women. They can involve any part of the urinary tract and can be acquired through the blood or lymph or may enter through the urethra. Infections are called *ascending* when pathogens move from the urethra to the bladder and *descending* when pathogens travel from the kidney to the bladder. UTIs are the most common nosocomial infections (infections associated with health care). Most UTIs are bacterial, but they can

---

Box 40-2 | *Risk Factors for Urinary Tract Infections*

- Female gender
- Vaginal infections
- Bubble baths and vaginal deodorant sprays
- Dehydration
- Tight-fitting, synthetic undergarments
- Infrequent voiding
- First trimester of pregnancy
- Trauma during delivery

---

be caused by viruses, yeasts, and fungi. It is important to treat UTIs to prevent renal scarring that can lead to failure. Risk factors for UTI are listed in Box 40-2.

Urethritis

Urethritis is inflammation of the urethra. Inflammation may be caused by microorganisms, trauma, or hypersensitivity to chemicals in products such as vaginal deodorants, spermicidal jellies, or bubble bath detergents. The most frequently identified causative microorganisms are *Escherichia coli*, *Chlamydia*, *Trichomonas*, *Neisseria gonorrhoeae*, and herpes simplex virus type 2.

Signs and Symptoms

Signs and symptoms of urethritis include dysuria, frequency, urgency, and bladder spasms. A urethral discharge may be noted.

Medical Diagnosis

Urethritis is diagnosed based on patient signs and symptoms, urinalysis, and urethral smear. Cystitis may be present at the same time.

Medical Treatment

Antimicrobials are used to treat the condition when it is caused by microorganisms. If the patient is sexually active, both the patient and the sexual partner may be treated with antimicrobials to prevent reinfection.

NURSING CARE *of the Patient with Urethritis*
Assessment

Assessment of the urology patient is outlined in Box 40-1. Important aspects of assessment when a patient has urethritis are comfort, possible causative factors, and understanding of treatment and prevention.

Nursing Diagnoses, Goals, and Outcome Criteria: Urethritis

NURSING DIAGNOSES	GOALS AND OUTCOME CRITERIA
Acute Pain related to tissue inflammation	Pain relief: patient states pain relieved, relaxed manner
Ineffective Therapeutic Regimen Management related to lack of knowledge of cause, treatment, and prevention of urethritis	Patient manages treatment plan effectively: patient accurately describes treatment and preventive measures, has no recurrence

Text continued on p. 853.

DRUG THERAPY | *Urinary Disorders*

GENERAL CONSIDERATIONS

1. Drugs are selected carefully because many drugs are nephrotoxic.
2. Drug dosages need to be reduced if renal function is impaired and the drug is excreted in the urine.

DRUG	USE/ACTION	SIDE EFFECTS	NURSING INTERVENTIONS
DIURETICS AND ANTIHYPERTENSIVES			
Diuretics	Cause kidneys to excrete water and sodium. Lower blood pressure.	Dehydration, electrolyte imbalances.	Monitor intake and output, blood pressure, weight. Administer in morning to avoid nocturia. Assess for electrolyte imbalances. Monitor serum potassium level. Potassium supplements may be ordered except with potassium-sparing drugs.
Osmotic diuretics (mannitol, urea)		Dehydration, electrolyte imbalances.	Monitor infusion site for extravasation. Administer only freshly prepared solutions.
Thiazide diuretics (hydrochlorothiazide [HydroDIURIL], metolazone [Zaroxolyn])		Hypokalemia, hypercalcemia.	Monitor patients with diabetes for hyperglycemia. Encourage potassium-rich foods.
Loop diuretics (furosemide [Lasix])		Orthostatic hypotension, hypokalemia, hyponatremia.	Monitor patients with diabetes for hyperglycemia. Encourage potassium-rich foods. Teach patients to cope with orthostatic hypotension.
Potassium-sparing diuretics (spironolactone [Aldactone])		Hyperkalemia, drowsiness. Gynecomastia in men on long-term therapy.	Safety measures. Assess for hyperkalemia: diarrhea, muscle twitching, dysrhythmias.
Antihypertensives	Lower blood pressure.	Orthostatic hypotension. Reflex tachycardia and fluid retention with some types. Rebound hypertension if stopped suddenly.	Monitor blood pressure. Do not discontinue suddenly. For orthostatic hypotension, teach patients to change position slowly and avoid prolonged standing.
Centrally acting antiadrenergics (methyldopa [Aldomet], clonidine [Catapres])		Drowsiness, hemolytic anemia, liver damage.	Administer at bedtime. Safety precautions. Advise patient to discontinue drug only under medical direction.
Peripherally acting antiadrenergics (prazosin [Minipress])		Hypotension (especially with initial dose).	Give first dose or increased dose at bedtime. Teach patient to manage orthostatic hypertension.
Beta-adrenergic blockers (propranolol [Inderal])		Bronchoconstriction, bradycardia, hypoglycemia, heart failure. Masks symptoms of low blood glucose.	Monitor respirations in asthmatics and patients with chronic obstructive pulmonary disease. Assess for edema. Monitor glucose levels.
Vasodilators (hydralazine [Apresoline])		Tachycardia, palpitations, headache, lupus-like syndrome.	Report lupus-like signs: fever, sore throat, skin rash.

PHOSPHATE BINDERS

Aluminum hydroxide gel (Amphojel)	Binds with phosphate in intestines to prevent absorption. Given to prevent renal osteodystrophy. Raises serum calcium.	Hypophosphatemia: muscle weakness, anorexia, bone pain. Constipation.	Monitor for hypophosphatemia. Record bowel movements. Give laxatives and stool softeners as ordered.

VITAMIN AND MINERAL SUPPLEMENTS

Ferrous sulfate	Treats iron-deficiency anemia.	Constipation or diarrhea, dark stools.	Administer on empty stomach with water. Can give liquid with water or fruit juice to disguise taste.
Folic acid	Supplements dietary intake.	Few adverse effects.	Monitor for occasional hypersensitivity.
Calcium gluconate	Treats hypocalcemia.	Hypercalcemia. Constipation.	Monitor blood studies. Administer in divided doses with or after meals. Do not take with other drugs.

HORMONES

Recombinant human erythropoietin (epoetin alfa)	Improves red blood cell formation. Reverses anemia. Requires adequate serum iron and ferritin to be effective.	Headache, tachycardia, hypertension, dyspnea, diarrhea, hyperkalemia, nausea, vomiting, clotted vascular assess, seizures.	Monitor blood pressure. Contraindicated in uncontrolled hypertension. Dosage is adjusted to maintain hematocrit between 30% and 33%.

ANTIBIOTICS

Sulfonamides

Sulfisoxazole (Gantrisin)	Treats UTIs.	Drowsiness, dizziness, agranulocytosis, anemia, thrombocytopenia. Nausea, vomiting, diarrhea. Liver dysfunction. Crystalluria leading to renal tubular damage. Photosensitivity. Allergy. Infertility.	Tell patient urine will be orange. Monitor blood cell counts. Give with full glass of water. Maintain urine output of 1500 mL/day to prevent crystalluria. Have patient avoid excessive sun exposure. Do not give if patient has history of sulfonamide allergy.
Trimethoprim* (Trimpex)	Used to treat acute or chronic UTIs. Especially effective against recurrent UTIs in men.	Nausea, vomiting, glossitis. Skin rash.	Tell patient to report skin rash—may be allergic response.
Aminoglycosides (gentamicin [Garamycin])	Effective against gram-negative bacilli.	Ototoxicity, hepatotoxicity.	Assess hearing. Drug should be stopped if patient has tinnitus or subjective hearing loss. Monitor intake and output. Check BUN and creatinine.
Penicillins (ampicillin)	Effective against most gram-positive and some gram-negative pathogens.	Anaphylaxis, GI distress, rash, blood dyscrasias.	Monitor for allergic reaction: rash, itching, wheezing. Report immediately.

*NOTE: Trimethoprim/sulfamethoxazole is a combination drug. Trade names: Bactrim, Septra, and others. UTIs, Urinary tract infections; BUN, blood urea nitrogen; GI, gastrointestinal.

Continued

DRUG THERAPY Urinary Disorders—cont'd

DRUG	USE/ACTION	SIDE EFFECTS	NURSING INTERVENTIONS
ANTIBIOTICS **Sulfonamides—cont'd**			
Fluoroquinolones (ciprofloxacin)	Broad spectrum. Effective against many gram-positive and gram-negative pathogens.	Drowsiness, headache, agitation, seizures, cardiac dysrhythmias, hepatotoxicity, pseudomembranous colitis. Anaphylaxis, severe skin reactions, crystalluria.	Observe closely for allergic reaction: rash, pruritus, urticaria, wheezing. Notify physician immediately. Monitor liver function tests. Advise patient to drink 1500-2000 mL each day to prevent crystal formation. Do not take within 2 hr of antacids, iron, or zinc. Check for many other drug-drug interactions. Safety measures for drowsiness.
URINARY ANTISEPTICS			
Methenamine (Mandelamine)	Antibacterial. Effective only in acid urine. Used to prevent or suppress recurrent UTIs.	Nausea, vomiting, diarrhea.	Give with meals to reduce gastrointestinal effects. Encourage adequate fluids. Discourage large intake of milk products.
Nalidixic acid (NegGram)	Antibacterial. Used for chronic UTIs.	Headache, malaise, vertigo, syncope, confusion, peripheral neuritis, vision disturbances. Nausea and vomiting. Photosensitivity.	Advise patient to avoid prolonged sun exposure. Administer 1 hr before meals unless gastrointestinal upset occurs. Encourage adequate fluids.
Nitrofurantoin (Furadantin, Macrodantin)	Used to treat acute and chronic UTIs.	Dyspnea. Nausea and vomiting. Numbness and tingling of legs.	Administer with food or milk to reduce gastric distress.
OTHERS			
Pentosan polysulfate sodium (Elmiron)	Increases bladder defense mechanisms or detoxifies irritants that harm the bladder lining.		

UTIs, Urinary tract infections.

DRUG THERAPY | *Immunosuppressants*

GENERAL CONSIDERATIONS

1. Patients on immunosuppressants have reduced resistance to infection, so they must be monitored for subtle signs of infection.
2. Protect patients from infections.
3. Teach patients the importance of taking drugs as prescribed and keeping follow-up appointments.
4. Immunosuppressants increase the risk of malignancies.

DRUG	USE/ACTION	SIDE EFFECTS	NURSING INTERVENTIONS
CORTICOSTEROIDS Prednisone (Deltasone) Methylprednisolone (Medrol) Methylprednisolone sodium succinate (Solu-Medrol)	Anti-inflammatory: prevent movement of leukocytes into transplanted tissue.	Retention of water and sodium; loss of potassium, elevated blood glucose, hypertension, gastrointestinal bleeding, mood swings, psychosis, infections, impaired healing.	Monitor intake and output. Assess for fluid and electrolyte imbalances: edema, increased blood pressure, cardiac dysrhythmias, muscle weakness, confusion. Antacids are often ordered to protect stomach.
CYTOTOXIC DRUGS Azathioprine (Imuran) Cyclophosphamide (Cytoxan) Mycophenolate mofetil (CellCept)	Used with cyclosporine and corticosteroids to inhibit proliferation of B and T lymphocytes.	Diarrhea, bone marrow suppression, vomiting, sepsis, sterility. Azathioprine and mycophenolate are teratogenic.	Be sure pregnancy has been ruled out before starting drugs. Assess for decreased platelets (bruising, bleeding), and decreased white blood cells (frequent infections). Check CBC reports.
MONOCLONAL ANTIBODIES Muromonab-CD3 (Orthoclone OKT3) Basiliximab (Simulect) Daclizumab (Zenapax) Lymphocyte immune globulin (Atgam)	React with T-cell antigens and destroy them. Used to treat acute rejection in renal transplant recipients.	Fever, chills, headache, tremor, dyspnea, flushing, anaphylaxis, nausea, vomiting, diarrhea, chest pain. Potentially fatal anaphylaxis.	Monitor closely for anaphylaxis, especially with first dose. Monitor for fluid overload. Check infusion site. Have site changed if evidence of extravasation.
T-CELL SUPPRESSORS Cyclosporine (Sandimmune and Neoral are NOT interchangeable!)	Interferes with T-lymphocyte activity. Enhances transplant survival with less risk of infection.	Nephrotoxicity (elevated serum creatinine), fluid retention, hypertension, hyperkalemia, hirsutism, venous thrombosis, gingival hyperplasia, tremors, infections, anemia, leukopenia, thrombocytopenia. Anaphylaxis with intravenous administration. Hepatotoxic.	Monitor serum creatinine and electrolytes. Check for edema. Monitor blood pressure. Have epinephrine available during intravenous administration. Monitor liver function studies. Mix oral form with food or chocolate to disguise unpleasant oiliness.

Interventions

Sitz baths are soothing and may reduce the pain of urethritis. Instruct female patients to wipe from front to back after toileting and to void before and after sexual intercourse as a means of preventing urethritis. Discourage bubble baths and vaginal deodorant sprays. Instruct uncircumcised male patients to clean the penis under the foreskin regularly.

Cystitis

Cystitis is inflammation of the urinary bladder. The most common cause is bacterial contamination. Other factors that increase the incidence of cystitis are prolonged immobility, renal calculi, urinary diversion, and indwelling catheters. Women are more susceptible than men to cystitis because the female urethra is shorter and closer to the vagina and rectum. The longer urethra and antibacterial substances in prostatic fluid are thought to decrease the incidence of UTIs in men. Cystitis in the absence of other pathology of the urinary tract is said to be *uncomplicated. Recurring* UTIs are more likely to be associated with urinary tract pathology.

Signs and Symptoms

Symptoms of cystitis include urgency, frequency, dysuria, hematuria, nocturia, bladder spasms, incontinence, and low-grade fever. Urine may be dark, tea-colored, or cloudy. Fever, fatigue, and pelvic or abdominal discomfort are common. Bladder spasms may be manifested by pain behind the symphysis pubis. Spasms may occur during or after urination. Some patients have bacteria in the urine but no symptoms at all.

Medical Diagnosis

A urine specimen is obtained for urinalysis, culture, and sensitivity. The presence of bacteria does not mean the patient has an infection unless the patient also has white blood cells (WBCs) in the urine. The presence of WBCs reflects bacterial tissue invasion—an indicator of infection. Other diagnostic procedures may be indicated to rule out pathology that might be responsible for the infection.

Medical Treatment

Cystitis is treated with antibiotics that concentrate in the urine. The physician may order an antibiotic while awaiting the results of the culture and sensitivity. The order is changed if the results show that another antibiotic would be more effective. For uncomplicated cystitis, treatment may be given in a single dose or in a 1- to 3-day regimen. Patients with recurrent cystitis may be placed on continuous prophylactic antibiotics. A mild analgesic such as acetaminophen is useful for relieving discomfort. Phenazopyridine (Pyridium) may be ordered for 2 to 3 days to decrease discomfort and bladder spasms. Hyoscyamine (Cystospaz) and flavoxate (Urispas) also may be ordered to decrease bladder spasms.

NURSING CARE *of the Patient with Cystitis*
Assessment

The general assessment of the patient with a urinary tract disorder is outlined in Box 40-1. The nursing assessment of the patient with cystitis focuses on patient symptoms, possible causative factors, and understanding of treatment and prevention.

 Put on Your Thinking Cap!

Using the recommended fluid intake for a person with cystitis, calculate how much fluid you would need to take in 24 hours based on your body weight.

Nursing Diagnoses, Goals, and Outcome Criteria: Cystitis

NURSING DIAGNOSES	GOALS AND OUTCOME CRITERIA
Acute Pain related to tissue inflammation	Pain relief: patient states pain relieved, relaxed manner
Ineffective Therapeutic Regimen Management related to lack of knowledge of cause, treatment, and prevention of cystitis	Patient effectively manages treatment plan: patient accurately describes treatment and preventive measures; has no recurrence

Interventions

Cystitis usually is treated on an outpatient basis. Therefore patient teaching is essential. Advise the patient to take analgesics as ordered for pain. Warm sitz baths also are comforting. Patient teaching emphasizes the need for a high fluid intake, instructions about prescribed drugs, and measures to avoid future infections. The patient needs to consume at least 30 mL/kg of fluid per day and void frequently. Fluids should be consumed during the day and at night so that the urinary tract is continually flushed. Instruct the patient

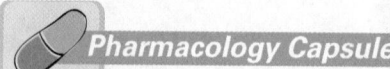 **Pharmacology Capsule**

Instruct patients to complete the entire course of antimicrobial therapy to ensure that the infection is eradicated.

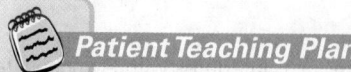 **Patient Teaching Plan**

Cystitis
To reduce the risk of future infections:
- Wear cotton undergarments because they keep the perineum drier than synthetic materials. Moisture encourages bacterial growth.
- Avoid tight-fitting clothing in the perineal area.
- Showers are preferred over tub baths.
- Avoid coffee, tea, carbonated beverages with caffeine, and apple, grapefruit, orange, and tomato juices because these irritate the bladder.
- Maintain a high fluid intake, and empty your bladder often.
- Cranberry juice is sometimes recommended to make the urine more acidic and discourage bacterial growth. Although there is some disagreement about the value of the juice and the amount needed to be effective, it is a safe, simple measure to try.
- Women should wipe from front to back after bowel movements or voiding.
- Drink a glass of water before and after intercourse to "flush" the urethra.
- It is important to keep appointments for follow-up urinalyses to be sure the infection has been eliminated.

to complete the entire course of prescribed antibiotics. Also advise the patient taking phenazopyridine, a drug that relieves burning on urination, that the drug causes an orange-red urine color that may stain clothing.

Interstitial Cystitis
Pathophysiology and Diagnosis

Interstitial cystitis is an inflammatory disease of the bladder that usually is chronic. The cause of the disease, which usually affects females, is unknown. The patient typically reports moderate to severe bladder and pelvic pain and urinary frequency and urgency. Chronic inflammation can cause the bladder to become scarred and stiff, which reduces its capacity. Ulcers may form in the bladder lining, and bleeding may occur. The condition is diagnosed by cystoscopy. Other diagnostic measures may be done to rule out other pathology such as cancer.

Medical Treatment

Treatment is directed toward symptom management and attempts to treat possible causes. Among the drugs that sometimes are helpful are tricyclic antidepressants, antispasmodics, bladder anesthetics, calcium channel blockers, urine alkalinizers, and NSAIDs. A drug that brings symptomatic relief to many is pentosan polysulfate (Elmiron). Other treatments include stretching the bladder under anesthesia, instillation of various medications including dimethyl sulfoxide into the bladder, and electrostimulation. Some sources advise dietary and activity changes and heat application. Cystectomy (surgical removal of the bladder) is an extreme measure that is necessary in some cases.

NURSING CARE *of the Patient with Interstitial Cystitis*

Patients are usually treated as outpatients, so you are more likely to encounter them in clinic or home settings than in hospitals. It is important for you to show acceptance of the patient and empathy for the disruption of lives caused by this disease. It is a physiologic illness, not a psychologic one. Your primary role is teaching and support. The Interstitial Cystitis Association (www.ichelp.com) is a source of general information as well as dietary advice to avoid bladder irritation.

 Consider the Alternative

Biofeedback may help some patients deal with the symptoms of interstitial cystitis.

Pyelonephritis

Pyelonephritis is inflammation of the renal pelvis. It may affect one or both kidneys. Acute pyelonephritis most often is caused by an ascending bacterial infection, but it may be bloodborne. Chronic pyelonephritis

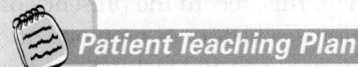 **Patient Teaching Plan**

Interstitial Cystitis

- Avoid acidic foods, coffee, tea, citrus products, aged cheeses, nuts, vinegar, curry, hot peppers, alcohol, and carbonated drinks.
- Prelief is an over-the-counter urinary alkalinizer that your physician may suggest.
- Wear clothing that fits loosely around the waist and lower abdomen.
- A local support group may be available for education and encouragement.

may be persistent or recurrent and results in damage to the renal parenchyma (functional tissue). It most often is the result of reflux of urine from inadequate closure of the ureterovesical junction during voiding. Progressive scarring results in atrophy of the affected kidneys, and hypertension and renal ischemia develop.

Chronic pyelonephritis, usually caused by longstanding UTIs with relapses and reinfections, may lead to chronic renal failure. If the patient progresses to renal atrophy and end-stage renal disease, dialysis or transplantation is the only means of keeping the patient alive.

Signs and Symptoms

Signs and symptoms of acute pyelonephritis include high fever, chills, nausea, vomiting, and dysuria. Severe pain or a constant dull ache occurs in the flank area. The patient with chronic pyelonephritis often complains of bladder irritation, chronic fatigue, and a slight aching over one or both kidneys.

Medical Treatment

The goal of treatment for pyelonephritis is to prevent further damage. Mild symptoms usually can be managed on an outpatient basis. Severe symptoms commonly are treated in the hospital. Antibiotics, urinary tract antiseptics, analgesics, and antispasmodics may be ordered. Long-term antibiotic therapy may be prescribed for patients who have repeated acute infections or chronic infection. Additional medications may be needed to treat hypertension. Adults are advised to drink at least eight 8-ounce glasses of fluids daily. Intravenous fluids may be ordered if the patient has nausea and vomiting. Dietary salt and protein restriction may be imposed on the patient with chronic disease. If an obstruction or congenital anomaly is present, it should be treated. Urine samples must be obtained for follow-up cultures to determine whether the infection has been resolved.

NURSING CARE *of the Patient with Pyelonephritis*
Assessment

The general assessment of the patient with a urinary tract disorder is outlined in Box 40-1. When caring for the patient with pyelonephritis, record the presence of related signs and symptoms, a history of previous urinary tract disorders, any predisposing factors, and the effects of the infection on daily activities.

Nursing Diagnoses, Goals, and Outcome Criteria: Pyelonephritis

NURSING DIAGNOSES	GOALS AND OUTCOME CRITERIA
Acute Pain related to inflammation	Pain relief: patient states pain relieved, relaxed manner
Activity Intolerance related to fatigue	Improved activity tolerance: completes activities of daily living without excessive fatigue
Deficient Fluid Volume related to vomiting, anorexia	Adequate hydration: fluid intake and output equal; pulse and blood pressure consistent with patient norms
Imbalanced Nutrition: Less Than Body Requirements related to anorexia, nausea, vomiting	Adequate nutrition: stable body weight
Ineffective Therapeutic Regimen Management related to lack of knowledge of treatment and future prevention of pyelonephritis	Patient effectively manages treatment plan: patient accurately describes prescribed treatment and preventive measures; has no recurrence

Interventions

Acute Pain

Administer analgesics as ordered when the patient reports pain. Antibiotics and antiseptics do not provide direct pain relief but eventually help by eliminating the cause of the inflammation.

Activity Intolerance

The pain and systemic symptoms of infection contribute to fatigue and activity intolerance. Assist with activities of daily living, and schedule activities to allow for periods of uninterrupted rest. If the patient is being treated at home, advise family members of the patient's need for additional rest. Encourage the family to relieve the patient of some responsibilities until recovered.

Deficient Fluid Volume and Imbalanced Nutrition: Less Than Body Requirements

Adequate food and fluids are very important for the patient with pyelonephritis. If nausea and vomiting occur, inform the physician and administer antiemetics as ordered. Record food and fluid intake and fluid output. If the patient is unable to take the recommended 2 to 3 L of fluid daily, intravenous fluids may be prescribed. Be careful when forcing fluids to avoid circulatory overload. In the older patient, a sudden increase

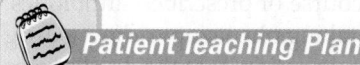

Patient Teaching Plan

Pyelonephritis

- Take your medications exactly as prescribed. Report adverse effects (for specific drugs) to your physician. Be sure to complete the course of therapy.
- Limit your physical activity and exercise as advised by your physician.
- Even after this infection has been treated, drink at least eight 8-ounce glasses of fluids each day to dilute urine and to reduce the risk of recurrence.
- If advised, follow dietary protein and sodium restrictions.

in fluid volume may result in congestive heart failure. Possible signs of this complication are bounding pulse, rising blood pressure, dyspnea, and edema.

Ineffective Therapeutic Regimen Management

If the patient will be taking medications at home, review the drugs and stress the importance of taking them as prescribed. Explain the importance of follow-up evaluation to assess effects of treatment and the need to report suspected recurrence to the physician immediately. Patients with chronic pyelonephritis must be adequately prepared for self-care.

Polycystic Kidney Disease

Polycystic kidney disease is a hereditary disorder. There are two types: childhood and adult. In adults, it usually is manifested by age 40 years. It is characterized by grapelike cysts in place of normal kidney tissue (Fig. 40-7). The cysts enlarge, compress functional renal tissue, and eventually result in renal failure. They also may create pressure on nearby organs. As the kidneys lose the ability to concentrate urine, hypertension and congestive heart failure develop. Often, cystic lesions are found on other organs. Chronic infection contributes to progressive loss of function.

FIGURE 40-7 Polycystic kidney.

Signs and Symptoms

This slowly progressive disorder begins with various types of pain: dull, aching abdominal, lower back, or flank pain; or colicky pain that begins abruptly.

Medical Treatment

Supportive treatment is recommended to preserve kidney function, treat UTI, and control hypertension. Infections should be treated promptly with appropriate antibiotics. As the disease progresses, kidney function decreases and end-stage renal disease develops. Dialysis, nephrectomy, and transplantation are then treatment options. Genetic counseling is advised for these patients because each of their children has a 50% chance of having the condition.

NURSING CARE of the Patient
with Polycystic Kidney Disease

See sections on nursing care of patients with end-stage renal disease and those having renal surgery, dialysis, and transplantation in this chapter.

Acute Glomerulonephritis
Pathophysiology

Glomerulonephritis is an immunologic disease characterized by inflammation of the capillary loops in the glomeruli. There are several immunologic mechanisms that can cause acute glomerulonephritis. For example, the patient may develop antibodies against antigens in the glomeruli. A common type of glomerulonephritis follows an infection of the respiratory tract caused by group A-negative hemolytic streptococcus. An antigen-antibody reaction results in inflammation of the glomeruli, and scar tissue forms. Glomerular permeability increases, allowing proteins to leak into the urine. The glomerular filtration rate decreases, and nitrogenous wastes accumulate in the blood. Both BUN and serum creatinine levels rise. Acute glomerulonephritis usually resolves completely, but some patients develop chronic glomerulonephritis or progress to irreversible renal failure.

Signs and Symptoms

Urine becomes tea colored as output decreases. Peripheral and periorbital (around the eyes) edema is evident. As glomerular filtration decreases, mild to severe hypertension occurs and hypervolemia (increased blood volume) results.

Medical Diagnosis

Diagnosis is based on patient assessment and laboratory tests. A urinalysis is done to detect proteinuria and red blood cell casts. Blood studies measure BUN, creatinine, and albumin. Streptococcal antibody tests indicate whether the patient has had a streptococcal infection. Findings in blood and urine studies tend to vary from one patient to another. Renal ultrasound, renal biopsy, or both also may be ordered.

Medical Treatment

Acute glomerulonephritis is treated with diuretics and, for severe hypertension, antihypertensive medications. Antibiotics are indicated if there is evidence of current streptococcal infection. In the acute phase, bed rest is ordered to prevent or treat heart failure and severe hypertension from fluid overload. Activity restriction usually is continued as long as urine tests show blood or protein, or blood pressure is elevated. Fluids, sodium, potassium, and protein may be restricted until there is sufficient recovery of kidney function. When fluid overload has been corrected, moderate activity is permitted but the patient still needs sufficient rest to allow the kidneys to heal.

Because some patients with acute glomerulonephritis develop renal insufficiency, follow-up is very important. If renal failure develops, dialysis is necessary. Patients who progress to chronic glomerulonephritis acquire end-stage renal disease in 1 to 30 years. (See the Chronic Kidney Disease section on pp. 871 to 878.)

NURSING CARE of the Patient with Acute Glomerulonephritis
Assessment

Assessment of patients with urinary tract disorders is outlined in Box 40-1. For the patient with acute glomerulonephritis, it is especially important to note signs and symptoms, recent infections (especially sore throat or skin lesions), and changes in urine characteristics.

During the physical examination, inspect the area around the eyes, the extremities, and the abdomen for fluid accumulation. Assess tissue turgor. Evaluate respiratory and cardiac function for evidence of excess fluid volume: dyspnea, tachycardia, hypertension. Accurate intake and output records and daily weights help assess the kidneys' ability to excrete excess fluid.

Nursing Diagnoses, Goals, and Outcome Criteria: Acute Glomerulonephritis

Nursing Diagnoses	Goals and Outcome Criteria
Excess Fluid Volume related to renal dysfunction	Restoration of normal fluid balance: balanced fluid intake and output, vital signs consistent with patient norms; no edema
Activity Intolerance related to retention of chemical wastes, fatigue, prescribed bed rest	Improved activity tolerance: patient reports less fatigue with physical activity
Self-Care Deficit related to prescribed bed rest, lack of knowledge of treatment measures	Patient adheres to plan of care: self-care is accomplished within activity restrictions, patient adheres to plan of care
Anxiety related to possibility of chronic illness	Reduced anxiety: patient states anxiety is lessened, appears calm

Interventions

Excess Fluid Volume

Administer diuretics as ordered. Maintain careful records of fluid intake and output. Instruct patients and family members in the importance of accurate records. If fluids are restricted, explain the need for the restriction and help the patient plan the timing and amounts of allowed fluids. Fluid restriction can be very distressing. It helps to present fluids in small containers rather than serving an ounce or two in a large glass. If the patient has edema, special skin care is needed. Handle the patient gently because taut, swollen tissue is easily damaged and heals slowly.

Activity Intolerance

Activity intolerance may be due to infection, accumulated toxins, or anemia. During the acute illness, discourage activity to allow the kidneys to heal. Explain the importance of rest for recovery. Schedule activities to allow for periods of uninterrupted rest. Of course, the patient on bed rest is at risk for complications of immobility: skin breakdown, pneumonia, muscle weakness, joint stiffness, constipation, and thrombus formation. Therefore have the patient change positions, cough and deep breathe, and gently exercise joints periodically. Nursing measures to prevent the complications of immobility are described in Chapter 21.

Self-Care Deficit

Provide assistance with activities of daily living. The patient needs to understand that rest, dietary restrictions, and medications promote recovery. Emphasize the need for follow-up care. When the patient is discharged, reinforce the importance of reporting any signs of recurrence such as changes in urine characteristics or edema. Instruct the patient to increase activities gradually as the edema and fatigue resolve.

Anxiety

The patient with acute glomerulonephritis may be very concerned about the possibility of developing a chronic, life-threatening condition. Give the patient an opportunity to ask questions and share concerns. Helpful interventions may include empathetic listening, providing factual information, or referrals to other professionals.

URINARY TRACT OBSTRUCTIONS

Renal Calculi

Urolithiasis is the formation of calculi (stones) in the urinary tract. It affects 500,000 people in the United States each year, is most common among males, and has a high incidence of recurrence.

Pathophysiology

Most calculi are precipitations of calcium salts (calcium phosphate or calcium oxalate), uric acid, magnesium ammonium phosphate (struvite), or cystine.

All these substances are normally found in the urine. Factors that foster the development of calculi are the following:

- Concentrated urine
- Excessive intake of calcium, vitamin D, protein, oxalates, calcium-based antacids
- Familial tendency
- Hyperparathyroidism
- Immobility, urinary stasis
- Sedentary lifestyle
- Altered urine pH
- Lack of kidney substance that inhibits calculi formation

Urine is normally acidic, with a pH ranging from 4.5 to 8.0. Some substances tend to precipitate in acid urine, causing calculus formation; others precipitate in alkaline urine. UTIs, particularly those caused by *Proteus, Klebsiella,* and *Pseudomonas,* are associated with calculi because these organisms cause the urine to become alkaline. The kidneys excrete substances that are believed to inhibit calculi formation, so a decrease in these substances may contribute to calculus formation.

Most calculi originate in the kidney (nephrolithiasis) and travel through the ureters into the bladder (urolithiasis).

 What Does Culture Have to Do with Urinary Calculi?

The incidence of uric acid stones is high among Jewish males. Caucasians have a greater risk of urinary calculi than do African Americans. Cultural factors such as diet as well as genetic factors probably explain some of these differences.

Signs and Symptoms

The patient's chief complaint is usually pain. The location and characteristics of the pain may provide clues to the site of the calculus. Dull flank pain suggests a calculus in the renal pelvis or stretching of the renal capsule from urine retention (hydronephrosis). If a calculus lodges in a ureter, the patient usually has excruciating pain in the abdomen that radiates to the groin or the perineum. The ureter goes into spasm (colic) in an attempt to move the calculus along and relieve the obstruction. Nausea, vomiting, and hematuria may accompany the pain. The patient also may show signs and symptoms of UTI.

Medical Diagnosis

The presence and location of calculi in the urinary tract may be confirmed by KUB, IVP, retrograde pyelogram, or ultrasound. A CT scan can help rule out other pathology. A routine urinalysis and culture and sensitivity usually are ordered as well. If a calculus can be obtained, its composition can be determined by laboratory analysis.

Medical Treatment

Most calculi are passed spontaneously. Ambulation and adequate hydration facilitate the passage of many calculi. Opioid analgesics and antispasmodics are ordered to relieve the intense, colicky pain. Antibiotics are ordered if infection is present or if internal manipulation of the calculus is necessary. If the calculus does not pass and symptoms continue, several procedures may be used to destroy or remove it.

Lithotripsy. Lithotripsy (shattering of the calculus) may be accomplished by extracorporeal shock wave lithotripsy (ESWL), which uses sound, laser, or dry shock wave energy (electrohydraulic, electromagnetic, piezoelectric) to shatter the stones. ESWL uses a device called a *lithotriptor* to deliver a series of shock waves to disintegrate the calculi. Guided by an ultrasound probe, the energy is directed to the stone through a water-filled cushion. Depending on the type of energy used, conscious sedation, preoperative sedation, or analgesics may be given because the series of 1000 to 1500 shocks is painful. (Fig. 40-8).The shocks are coordinated with the patient's cardiac cycle. The pulverized calculus is excreted in the urine over 1 to 4 weeks. After lithotripsy, the urine is often bright red at first, gradually turning dark red or smoky. A stent may be placed in the ureter before treatment to facilitate passage of the stone fragments. The stent is usually removed in several weeks. Bruising and hemorrhage are possible complications of lithotripsy. However, most patients are able to resume normal activities the next day after the procedure. Antibiotics are generally given for about 2 weeks to prevent urinary tract infection.

Endourologic Procedures. Stones in the bladder often can be crushed and removed using cystoscopic techniques. An instrument called a *ureteroscope* can be passed through the bladder to reach stones located in the renal pelvis and ureters. Along with the ureteroscope, instruments that shatter the stones may be used. For example, with lasertripsy, the calculus is visualized and destroyed with a laser. Like ESWL, fragments are usually passed in the urine. General anesthesia is used, but premedication is commonly omitted because radiographs must be obtained immediately before the procedure.

Surgical Procedures. If calculi are not passed spontaneously or crushed with a lithotriptor, surgery may be necessary. The incision of an organ or a duct to remove a calculus is a lithotomy. A nephrolithotomy is the surgical procedure used if the calculus is in the kidney. The removal of a calculus from the renal pelvis is a pyelolithotomy. A ureterolithotomy is removal of a calculus from a ureter (Fig. 40-9).

Prevention

An important medical goal is to prevent recurrence of renal calculi. Long-term medical management of these patients includes a high fluid intake to keep urine dilute, dietary restrictions for specific elements (i.e., calcium, purines), regular exercise, and occasionally medications to alter the urine pH. Medications are less effective than dietary management.

NURSING CARE *of the Patient with Renal Calculi*

Assessment

Assessment of the patient with a urinary tract disorder is discussed earlier in this chapter (see also Nursing Care Plan: The Patient with Renal Calculi on p. 861). When the patient has known or suspected urinary calculi, pay particular attention to a personal or family history of calculi. Describe the patient's usual fluid intake and diet, including vitamin and mineral supplements. If pain is present, describe the location, severity, and nature of the pain. Also record any changes in

Extracorporeal shock wave
lithotripsy machine

Shock waves
break up stone
in ureter

FIGURE **40-8** Extracorporeal shock wave lithotripsy.

FIGURE **40-9** Surgical procedures for renal calculi. **A,** Nephroscopy. **B,** Pyelolithotomy. **C,** Nephrolithotomy.

urine amount or characteristics. Take the temperature to detect fever. A nurse who is trained in physical examination palpates and percusses the flanks and the abdomen, noting the presence of pain, tenderness, or a distended bladder.

Nursing Diagnoses, Goals, and Outcome Criteria: Urinary Calculi

NURSING DIAGNOSES	GOALS AND OUTCOME CRITERIA
Acute Pain related to obstruction, trauma, and renal colic	Pain relief: patient states pain has been relieved; relaxed manner
Impaired Urinary Elimination related to obstruction	Unobstructed urine elimination: urine output equal to fluid intake
Risk for Deficient Fluid Volume related to anorexia, nausea, and vomiting	Normal fluid balance: fluid intake and output approximately equal, pulse and blood pressure consistent with patient norms
Ineffective Therapeutic Regimen Management related to lack of knowledge of prevention and treatment of calculi	Patient effectively manages treatment plan and takes preventive measures: patient accurately describes prevention and treatment, adheres to preventive measures; has no recurrences

If surgery is performed, additional nursing diagnoses and goals are the following:

NURSING DIAGNOSES	GOALS AND OUTCOME CRITERIA
Risk for Infection related to invasive procedures	Absence of infection: normal body temperature and white blood cell count, clear urine
Decreased Cardiac Output related to blood loss	Adequate cardiac output: pulse and blood pressure consistent with patient norms
Ineffective Breathing Pattern related to splinting of painful incision	Effective breathing patterns: clear breath sounds throughout lung fields, respiratory and depth consistent with patient norms

Interventions
Acute Pain

Because calculi in the urinary tract can cause excruciating pain (renal colic), pain relief is a major nursing concern. Initially, it may be necessary to administer opioid analgesics intravenously to relieve the pain. Antispasmodics are usually ordered to reduce the smooth muscle spasms in the ureters. If pain is intermittent, the patient may be permitted to ambulate when comfortable. Ambulation may actually help the calculus move through the urinary tract. Of course, safety precautions are needed if opioids have been given. The pain may

NURSING CARE PLAN

The Patient with Renal Calculi

ASSESSMENT

Health History: Mr. Frank Scarpino, age 43 years, was admitted with excruciating abdominal pain radiating to the groin. He experienced nausea and vomiting with the pain. Review of systems revealed a history of hypertension controlled with captopril. He also has had repeated urinary tract infections, most recently 1 month ago. At that time, he was treated with antibiotics and the symptoms subsided. Radiologic studies detected a calculus lodged in the right ureter. ESWL was done to shatter the calculus. Mr. Scarpino returned to his hospital room 3 hours ago. He is complaining of soreness in the right lower abdomen.

Physical Examination: Mr. Scarpino is fully oriented but drowsy. Vital signs: temperature, 100° F orally; pulse, 88; respiration, 20: blood pressure, 138/74. His abdomen is soft but tender. There is no bladder distention. He voided 350 mL pink-tinged urine. Intravenous fluids are infusing at 150 mL/hr.

Nursing Diagnosis	Goals and Outcome Criteria	Interventions
Acute Pain related to obstruction, trauma, renal colic	Patient will report pain relief and will appear more relaxed.	Assess pain characteristics. For severe pain, administer morphine as ordered. Administer antispasmodics as ordered. Assist with ambulation when permitted to promote passage of calculus fragments. Milder pain may be treated with nonopioid analgesics. Position changes, back rubs, relaxation, and imagery may be used to enhance analgesia. Document effects of pain relief interventions.
Impaired Urine Elimination related to obstruction	Patient's urine output will be approximately equal to fluid intake.	Measure all fluid intake and output. Report low output to physician. Strain all urine to collect calculi fragments. Send fragments to laboratory for analysis. Maintain intravenous fluids.
Risk for Deficient Fluid Volume related to NPO (nothing by mouth) status, nausea, and vomiting	The patient will be adequately hydrated as evidenced by moist mucous membranes, dilute urine, and vital signs consistent with patient's norms.	Administer intravenous fluids as ordered. Assess for deficient fluid volume: hypotension, tachycardia, sticky mucous membranes, concentrated urine. Encourage oral fluids when permitted. Administer antiemetics as ordered for nausea and vomiting.
Ineffective Breathing Pattern related to abdominal pain, splinting	Patient's breath sounds will be normal throughout the lung fields.	Assess respiratory status: rate, effort, breath sounds. Encourage deep breathing and coughing every 2 hours until fully ambulatory.
Decreased Cardiac Output related to blood loss	Patient's cardiac output will remain normal, as evidenced by vital signs consistent with patient's norms and by absence of tachycardia, hypotension, or restlessness.	Assess the abdomen and groin area for bruising—some is expected. Note red color and increased viscosity of urine associated with bleeding. Report increased redness. Monitor vital signs to detect decreasing cardiac output: tachycardia, restlessness, hypotension.
Ineffective Therapeutic Regimen Management related to lack of knowledge of prevention and treatment of calculi, self-care after lithotripsy	Patient will effectively manage self-care, as evidenced by correct description of self-care after EPL and measures to prevent recurrence of calculi.	Tell the patient that the fragments are usually passed in the urine over a period of several weeks and may cause some pain. Administer antibiotics as ordered, and emphasize importance of treating any new UTIs to reduce the risk of calculi formation. Advise patient to consume 3 to 4 L of fluid daily unless the physician prescribes less. Fluids should be taken around the clock to prevent concentration during the night. If any dietary restrictions are imposed, request a dietary consult to explain them to the patient.

? CRITICAL THINKING QUESTIONS

- Why would the patient continue to have pain after the stones have been shattered with lithotripsy?

- When might a fluid intake such as the recommended 3-4 L/day be contraindicated?

resolve suddenly if the calculus moves into the bladder or is passed through the urethra.

Impaired Urinary Elimination

Depending on its size and location, a calculus may obstruct urine flow. If urine backs up into the kidney, hydronephrosis may develop. Hydronephrosis is distention of the kidney with urine, a condition that can cause permanent damage (Fig. 40-10). Maintain accurate records of fluid intake and output, and report low output to the physician. In addition, urine is usually strained and examined for calculi. If any calculi are recovered, send them to the laboratory for analysis.

Risk for Deficient Fluid Volume

Renal colic is often accompanied by nausea and sometimes vomiting. Give antiemetics promptly as ordered. The physician will probably order intravenous fluids to maintain dilute urine and to flush the urinary tract. A fluid intake of as much as 4 L/day may be recommended. Large volumes of fluids like this must be given carefully to the older patient, in whom fluid volume excess can easily develop. Monitor for signs of circulatory overload (tachycardia, bounding pulse, dyspnea, edema, hypertension).

Postoperative Care

Before surgery, explain the expected procedure to the patient and answer any questions. Goals of postoperative care are maintenance of urine drainage, prevention of UTI, and prevention of pulmonary and circulatory complications.

Risk for Infection

To maintain alignment and urine flow, the patient is apt to have drains, catheters, a ureteral stent, or a combina-

FIGURE **40-10** Hydronephrosis caused by obstruction of the upper portion of the ureter; hydroureter caused by obstruction of the lower portion of the ureter.

tion of these. Each tube is connected to its own closed drainage system. Position tubes for free flow of urine at all times. Keep accurate accounts of drainage from each tube. If the patient has a flank incision, frequently check the area around the dressing for drainage because urine tends to leak from the incision. A large amount of serosanguineous drainage is normal immediately after surgery. In approximately 2 days, the drainage changes to serous. Frequent dressing changes using sterile technique may be required. In some cases, an ostomy appliance is used to collect drainage and to permit accurate measurement of the drainage.

Some patients have nephrostomy tubes placed directly in the kidney. The tube is placed for drainage or for instillation of irrigating fluid. It also diverts urine flow from the ureter until adequate healing has occurred. If irrigations are ordered, use strict aseptic technique and not more than 5 mL of warm, sterile normal saline at a time.

Decreased Cardiac Output

The patient is at risk for the same postoperative complications as any surgical patient. Be especially alert for any signs of excessive bleeding, infection, or pulmonary complications. To detect bleeding, inspect the dressing and drainage hourly for the first 24 hours. Immediately report bright red blood, excessive serosanguineous drainage, increasing pulse, restlessness, or decreasing blood pressure to the physician. Indications of infection such as odor, cloudy drainage, or temperature above 100° F also should be reported. Measures to reduce the risk of infection include maintaining closed drainage systems, changing wet dressings promptly, and using strict aseptic technique when handling tubes or dressings.

Ineffective Breathing Pattern

Monitor the patient's pulmonary status carefully. A flank incision makes taking a deep breath very painful. Assist the patient to turn, cough, and deep breathe at least every 2 hours. An incentive spirometer helps determine how much the patient is able to inflate the lungs. When the patient coughs, the incision needs to be splinted with pillows or folded blankets. For the first 1 or 2 postoperative days, administer analgesics before turning, coughing, and deep breathing to make these activities more comfortable. Adequate fluid intake thins respiratory secretions and makes them easier to expectorate. Early and frequent ambulation promotes improved respiratory function. All of these efforts help prevent atelectasis and pneumonia, a primary treatment goal.

Prevention

When the patient is discharged, reinforce the need to continue to consume 4 L of fluid daily unless contraindicated. The fluid needs to be consumed over the 24-hour period so that urine does not become concentrated at night. Advise the patient to drink two glasses of water before bed and another two glasses when awakening at night to void. This pattern should be followed for life to reduce the risk of calculus formation in the future. If the physician has prescribed a special diet or dietary restriction, provide instructions or have the dietitian do so.

UROLOGIC TRAUMA

The kidneys sustain 50% of all urologic injuries. Trauma may be penetrating or blunt. Penetrating injuries most often result from knives or guns. Blunt trauma occurs when a force is applied to the abdominal wall and the energy is diffused into the abdominal cavity. Examples of blunt force are motor vehicle accidents, contact sports injuries, falls, and intentional injuries. Blunt injuries to the kidneys produce lacerations or contusions. The ureters are rarely injured with blunt trauma. They are disrupted most often by penetration and require surgical anastomosis. The bladder may rupture from blunt trauma if full, but it is rarely harmed when empty. The urethra is most apt to be injured in men because of its unprotected anatomic location.

When blunt trauma is suspected, the patient is observed for bruising on the abdomen or in the flank area. Assess for signs of shock (tachycardia, restlessness, hypotension, pallor), pain, and a palpable abdominal or flank mass. Bruising over the flank and lower back that occur with retroperitoneal bleeding is called *Grey Turner's sign.*

The physician may order a KUB, urography, computed tomography, or ultrasound to determine the extent of injury. Diagnostic peritoneal lavage may be performed to determine whether there is bleeding in the peritoneal cavity. A positive finding necessitates surgery to find and eliminate the source of bleeding.

The most common indication of urologic trauma is hematuria. It is best if the patient can void, but this may not be possible with other injuries. Before catheterizing a patient with suspected trauma, carefully inspect the urethral meatus. If there is blood in or around the meatus, a urologist should perform the catheterization or insert a suprapubic catheter.

If the injury is not severe, if there is little bleeding, and if there are no signs of shock, monitor the patient closely. More severe injuries most likely require surgery to repair damage. Postsurgical care of these patients is similar to the care of the patient with a nephrectomy, urinary calculi, or cystectomy.

CANCERS OF THE URINARY SYSTEM

Care of the patient with cancer is covered in Chapter 25. This section focuses on the specific needs of the patient with cancer of the urinary tract.

Renal Cancer

Malignancies of the kidney account for approximately 35,000 new cases of cancer in the United States each year. Eighty percent of renal malignancies are adenocarcinomas, which affect primarily men 55 to 60 years of age. Less common squamous cell carcinomas of the renal pelvis affect men and women equally.

A renal tumor may reach considerable size before it is detected. Renal malignancies metastasize to the liver, lungs, long bones, and the other kidney. Direct extension of the tumor may be found in the ureter. Early symptoms are anemia, weakness, and weight loss. Painless, gross hematuria is the classic sign, but it usually occurs in the advanced stage. A dull ache in the flank area also is a late symptom.

Medical Diagnosis

The physician may be able to palpate a mass in the flank area. Diagnostic tests and procedures to study the mass may include excretory urography, IVP, retrograde pyelography, ultrasound, arteriography, computed tomography, magnetic resonance imaging, and renal biopsy. Care of the patient undergoing these procedures is detailed in the Diagnostic Tests and Procedures table on pp. 843 to 845.

Medical Treatment

Removal of a kidney is called a *nephrectomy.* Radical nephrectomy is the treatment of choice for renal cancer and involves removal of the kidney and its adjacent tissue, adrenal gland, renal artery and vein, and local lymph glands. Before nephrectomy, the renal artery may be occluded to reduce the blood supply to the tumor. In general, renal tumors are not responsive to radiation or chemotherapy, but radiation is sometimes used as a palliative measure for inoperable cancer. Biotherapy with alfa-interferon and interleukin-2 may be used for the patient with metastatic disease.

NURSING CARE *of the Patient with Renal Cancer*
Assessment

Nursing assessment of the patient with a urologic disorder is outlined in Box 40-1. When a patient has a suspected or confirmed renal malignancy, there may be very few signs and symptoms. Inquire about weakness, fatigue, and any changes observed in the urine. Explore the patient's emotional state, usual coping strategies, and support systems.

Preoperative Care

General preoperative nursing care is discussed in detail in Chapter 17. Before nephrectomy, the patient's primary nursing diagnoses are Ineffective Coping related to potentially fatal disease and Deficient Knowledge of tests, procedures, and effects of nephrectomy. The goals of nursing care are effective patient use of coping mechanisms and understanding of what is being done and what to expect.

Thorough explanations of diagnostic tests and preoperative teaching provide needed information. Assure the patient that one functioning kidney can sustain adequate kidney function. Tests are done to confirm that the unaffected kidney functions adequately before a nephrectomy. Serum and urine laboratory tests are usually ordered to serve as baseline data for postoperative comparison. Older patients are more likely to have renal insufficiency, and they may eventually need renal dialysis after nephrectomy. The teaching plan includes what to expect in the postoperative period and how to turn, cough, and deep breathe. Other preoperative care is the same as that for any other major surgery.

Postoperative Care

Common aspects of postoperative care are covered in Chapter 17. After nephrectomy, monitor vital signs to detect fluid volume alterations related to blood loss or fluid retention. Record intake and output as another measure of fluid balance and renal function. Routinely check drains and tubes to ensure proper function. Monitor dressings for drainage. Once the dressings have been removed, inspect the wound for intactness and signs of infection (excessive redness or swelling, purulent drainage). Determine the patient's comfort level. Auscultate breath sounds and bowel sounds. Anticipate some emotional distress, and encourage the patient to express thoughts and feelings about having cancer.

**Nursing Diagnoses, Goals, and Outcome Criteria:
Renal Cancer, Postoperative**

NURSING DIAGNOSES	GOALS AND OUTCOME CRITERIA
Acute Pain related to incisional tissue trauma	Pain relief: patient states pain is relieved, relaxed manner
Risk for Deficient Fluid Volume related to dehydration, blood loss	Normal hydration and blood volume: pulse and blood pressure consistent with patient norms, normal skin turgor
Ineffective Breathing Pattern related to proximity of incision to diaphragm	Effective breathing patterns: clear breath sounds throughout lung fields
Risk for Injury related to decreased peristalsis caused by bowel manipulation during surgery	Absence of abdominal distention: active bowel sounds, abdomen soft
Risk for Infection related to break in skin	Absence of infection: normal body temperature and white blood cell count
Ineffective Coping related to diagnosis of cancer	Effective coping: patient practices strategies that reduce anxiety but do not interfere with therapeutic plan
Deficient Knowledge of postoperative limitations	Patient understands postoperative restrictions: accurately describes and adheres to activity limitations

Interventions

Acute Pain

Obtain a complete description of the patient's pain. Incisional pain is intense at first and deserves prompt administration of prescribed analgesics. Because of the patient's position in surgery, there may be muscle aches in the opposite side and flank area. Medication can be supplemented with position changes and back rubs. Other comfort measures are described in Chapter 15.

Risk for Deficient Fluid Volume

Intravenous fluids are given initially. The physician normally orders approximately 3 L of fluid daily. Maintain accurate intake and output records. At first, the urine may be measured every 1 to 2 hours. Notify the physician if less than 30 mL is produced in an hour. When the patient is able to be weighed, daily weights are an even better measure of fluid balance than intake and output. BUN, serum creatinine, serum electrolytes, and urine specific gravity are assessed and compared with preoperative values.

Also monitor the nephrectomy patient for bleeding. Frequently check the dressing for drainage. Be careful to check *under* the patient because blood flows to the most dependent area. Sometimes the dressing is dry and intact but the patient is lying in a pool of blood.

Ineffective Breathing Pattern

The location of the flank incision causes pain with expansion of the thorax. Patients tend to protect the area by not breathing deeply. This may lead to pneumonia and atelectasis. It is especially important to have the patient turn, cough, and deep breathe every 1 to 2 hours. You can help by supporting the incision during respiratory exercises. Supervise use of an incentive spirometer to encourage deeper inspiration. As soon as ambulation is permitted, assist the patient out of bed. Be careful not to place tension on tubes and drains. Gradually increase the time and distance walked.

Risk for Injury

Anesthesia and manipulation of abdominal organs cause temporary cessation of peristalsis in the intestines. Until peristalsis returns, the patient is not permitted to take anything by mouth. If peristalsis does not return within 3 to 4 days, the patient is said to have *paralytic ileus*. Because paralytic ileus is fairly common after nephrectomy, a nasogastric tube may be inserted and attached to suction during surgery. Suction keeps the stomach empty, reducing the risk of nausea and abdominal distention. The return of peristalsis is detected by active bowel sounds and the passage of flatus (gas). Auscultate the abdomen for bowel sounds, and observe for abdominal distention. Ambulation promotes the return of peristalsis.

Risk for Infection

During dressing changes, use strict aseptic technique. Montgomery straps may decrease irritation from the adhesive tape if frequent dressing changes are required.

Ineffective Coping

The patient facing cancer fears the possibility of death, mourns the loss of an organ, and may dread additional cancer therapy. You can help by encouraging the patient to talk and clarify concerns, listening empathetically, providing requested information, and referring the patient to expert counselors. Explore usual coping strategies and sources of support. Chapter 25 provides additional detail on nursing care of the cancer patient.

Deficient Knowledge

Before discharge, caution the patient not to lift or participate in strenuous activities for 8 weeks. Contact sports are prohibited for life because trauma to the remaining kidney could eliminate all kidney function.

Bladder Cancer

Cancer of the bladder is the most common malignancy of the urinary tract, with more than 60,000 new cases diagnosed each year in the United States. It occurs most often in men 50 to 70 years of age. The ureteral orifices and the bladder neck are the most common sites of bladder cancer. Over the years, chemical agents have been suspected as carcinogens. The tars found in smoking tobacco, aniline dyes found in industrial compounds, and tryptophan all have been implicated in the development of bladder cancer.

What Does Culture Have to Do with Bladder Cancer?

Risk factors for bladder cancer include cigarette smoking and exposure to chemicals used in the rubber and cable industries. Historically, men have been more likely than women to smoke and to work in industry, which might help explain why this cancer is three times as common among men as among women.

Signs and Symptoms

The most common sign of bladder cancer is painless, intermittent hematuria. Other signs and symptoms include bladder irritability; infection, with dysuria, frequency, and urgency; and decreased stream of urine.

Medical Diagnosis

When the patient's signs and symptoms suggest bladder cancer, the physician may order a urinalysis, IVP, and CT scan. Cystoscopy is done to visualize the bladder and permit biopsy of any observable lesions. Details of these tests and procedures and nursing implications are provided in the Diagnostic Tests and Procedures table on pp. 843 to 845.

Medical Treatment

Bladder malignancies respond more favorably to chemotherapy than do kidney tumors, but surgery is the treatment of choice. The type of surgery depends on whether the cancer is superficial, invasive, or metastatic. Superficial cancers involve only the bladder mucosa or submucosa, or both. Superficial lesions with low recurrence rates may be treated with cystoscopic resection and fulguration or with laser photocoagulation. Cystoscopic resection is the removal of tissue through a cystoscope with a special cutting instrument. Fulguration is the use of electric current to burn and destroy tissue. Laser photocoagulation is the use of an intense beam of light (argon laser) to destroy tissue.

Two other surgical procedures for bladder cancer are segmental bladder resection and radical cystectomy. A segmental bladder resection is done for a single, primary tumor too large to remove by cystoscopic resection. It involves removal of the tumor and adjacent bladder muscle, a procedure that decreases the size of the bladder. A radical cystectomy is removal of the entire bladder and adjacent structures with diversion of the ureters. This procedure is reserved for malignancies that are untreatable with less conservative measures. This is very extensive surgery, and an optimal state of health before surgery is desirable. Radiation and/or chemotherapy may be done before or after surgery depending on the extent of the malignancy. Sometimes chemotherapeutic drugs or immune stimulating agents are instilled directly into the bladder. This procedure is called *intravesical therapy*. Drugs such as thiotepa, doxorubicin (Adriamycin), bacille Calmette-Guérin (BCG), and mitomycin-C are administered into the bladder through a urinary catheter. The patient's position is changed at intervals to ensure the drugs reach the site of the lesion. After about 2 hours, the drugs are drained from the bladder. Treatment may be repeated weekly for 6 to 12 weeks followed by a program of maintenance therapy.

Urinary Diversion. When the bladder and urethra must be removed completely, urine must be allowed to drain through another route, called *urinary diversion*. There are several types of urinary diversions: ileal and sigmoid conduits, ureterostomy, and nephrostomy. These diversions are illustrated in Figure 40-11.

To form an ileal conduit, a portion of the ileum is resected from the small bowel. The ureters are implanted in the ileum, one end of the ileum is closed, and the open end is implanted on the abdominal surface as a stoma. Urine is excreted through the ileal conduit rather than the urethra. A urinary drainage pouch is attached to the skin to collect the urine. A sigmoid conduit is formed by the same procedure except that a section of sigmoid colon instead of ileum is used. A ureterostomy brings the ureter to the abdominal surface, where urine is eliminated through a stoma. A nephrostomy is the placement of a tube in the kidney so that urine may drain through the tube into an

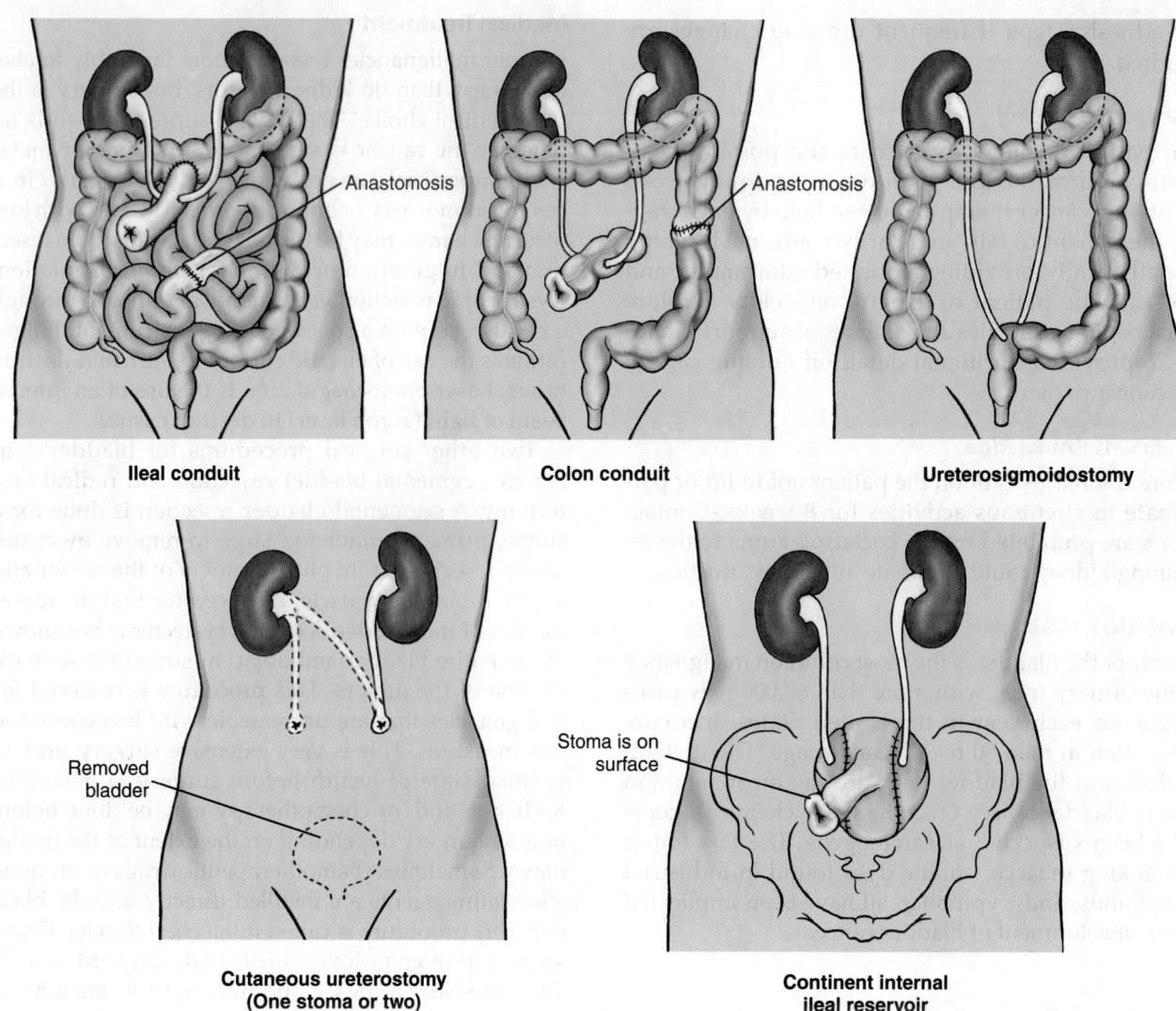

Ileal conduit

Colon conduit

Ureterosigmoidostomy

Anastomosis

Anastomosis

Removed bladder

Stoma is on surface

Cutaneous ureterostomy
(One stoma or two)

Continent internal
ileal reservoir

FIGURE **40-11** Types of urinary diversion procedures.

external collection device. Detailed information about urinary diversion is presented in Chapter 26.

NURSING CARE *of the Patient with Bladder Cancer*

Assessment

Assessment of the patient with possible or confirmed bladder cancer includes a complete description of urinary signs and symptoms. Fatigue and weight loss are significant and should be noted. The health history may reveal use of tobacco or exposure to carcinogenic chemicals. Explore the patient's emotional state, coping strategies, and sources of support.

Preoperative Care

In addition to the common nursing care described in Chapter 17, important preoperative nursing diagnoses for the patient facing segmental resection for cancer may be Fear related to life-threatening diagnosis and In-effective Coping related to lifestyle change. The goals of nursing care are reduced fear and effective coping strategies. To accomplish these goals, explore the patient's fear and provide information and encouragement. The

thought of having cancer is frightening, and nurses must educate the public that it is often curable. Assess coping strategies, and provide resources as needed. The patient needs support to accept the diagnosis and follow through with the treatment.

The patient having radical cystectomy faces a more difficult adjustment—that of permanent urinary diversion. The patient needs to be prepared psychologically as well as physically to deal with a change in body image. The enterostomal therapist is a valuable resource to both you and the patient in preparing for this surgery. The therapist selects the stoma site with the patient. The patient may be advised to wear a water-filled pouch for several days before surgery to help ensure proper stoma placement. If the patient would like to talk to someone who has had a cystectomy, this often can be arranged through a local ostomy club or chapter of the American Cancer Society.

Preoperative care for an ileal or sigmoid conduit includes thorough preparation of the intestinal tract. Bowel preparation requires several days. The patient begins with a low-residue diet and then a clear-fluid diet. Oral neomycin, an antibiotic that is not absorbed from the intestinal tract, is ordered to reduce bacteria in the bowel. Enemas also are ordered before surgery.

The patient who has received effective preoperative nursing interventions demonstrates reduced fear and realistic problem solving.

Postoperative Care

Postoperative assessment includes vital signs, intake and output, patency of tubes, bowel sounds, comfort, and appearance of the drainage, stoma, and wound.

Additional nursing diagnoses such as Disturbed Body Image and Deficient Knowledge of stoma care are appropriate if the patient has ostomy surgery. For the patient with urinary diversion, the outcomes of nursing care are adaptation to disturbed body image, patient demonstration of stoma care, and patient knowledge of significant signs and symptoms that should be reported to the physician.

Nursing Diagnoses, Goals, and Outcome Criteria: Bladder Surgery, Postoperative

Nursing Diagnoses	Goals and Outcome Criteria
Acute Pain related to tissue trauma	Pain relief: patient states pain relieved, relaxed manner
Impaired Urinary Elimination related to urinary diversion	Unobstructed urine drainage: urine clear, flows freely, output equal to fluid intake
Impaired Skin Integrity related to surgical incision	Well-healed incision: wound margins intact, decreasing redness and swelling
Risk for Infection related to tissue trauma	Absence of infection: normal body temperature and white blood cell count
Risk for Injury related to absence of peristalsis secondary to bowel manipulation during surgery	Normal peristalsis: active bowel sounds, soft abdomen
Deficient Knowledge of postoperative self-care	Patient understands self-care after discharge: patient accurately describes and demonstrates care

Interventions

Routine postoperative nursing care aimed at the prevention of complications includes turning, coughing, and deep breathing. Leg exercises and early ambulation are especially important to prevent edema associated with excision of lymph nodes.

Acute Pain

Administer prescribed analgesics and use other comfort measures to control pain.

Impaired Urinary Elimination

Inspect urethral and suprapubic catheters and provide wound care as detailed in Chapter 17. Urine should be free of sediment, blood, or casts. Once the catheters are removed, encourage frequent voiding in the patient who has had a segmental resection. Bladder capacity will increase up to 250 to 300 mL over several months.

If a patient has had a radical cystectomy, inspect the stoma for inflammation and irritation. Details of stoma care are provided in Chapter 26.

Impaired Skin Integrity

Monitor the surgical incision to ensure that it is healing without increasing redness or swelling or purulent drainage. Provide wound care as ordered or per agency protocol. Sites of urine drains and the stoma also must receive care to prevent skin irritation and breakdown.

Risk for Infection

These patients are at risk for infections in the surgical incisions, drain sites, and urinary tract. Monitor the patient's vital signs, blood work, and wounds for evidence of infection (fever, elevated white blood cell count, foul odor). Use strict aseptic technique when providing wound care.

Risk for Injury

Withhold oral fluids as ordered until bowel sounds provide evidence that peristalsis has returned. Administer intravenous fluids as ordered. When oral intake is permitted, encourage an adequate fluid intake (2500 to 3000 mL/day).

Deficient Knowledge

Patient teaching must begin in the early postoperative period because the patient needs to learn self-care before discharge. Allow time for the patient or a caregiver to practice self-care procedures.

RENAL FAILURE

Any condition that decreases blood flow to the kidneys may impair renal function and result in renal failure. Renal failure is classified as *acute* or *chronic* based on onset and reversibility. Acute renal failure has a rapid onset (1 to 7 days) and may be reversible. However, the mortality rate ranges from 35% to 65% depending on

---

Patient Teaching Plan

Urinary Diversion

- Proper stoma care reduces the risk of complications.
- Notify your physician of signs of infection: fever; increasing redness, swelling, and tenderness of incisions.
- Restrict activity as prescribed by your physician to avoid strain on the surgical site.
- Resources include the enterostomal therapist, American Cancer Society, United Ostomy Association (telephone, 1-800-826-0826; or e-mail, info@uoaa.org)

the presence of other diseases or complications. Chronic renal failure has a slow onset (months to years) and is characterized by progressive, irreversible damage.

Acute Renal Failure

Causes

Causes of renal failure can be prerenal, intrarenal, or postrenal. Prerenal failure results from decreased blood flow to the glomeruli. A systolic blood pressure of 70 mm Hg or greater is necessary to sustain glomerular filtration. If the systolic pressure drops below 70 and is not corrected, renal failure may develop.

Intrarenal failure may be caused by nephrotoxic agents, kidney infections, occlusion of intrarenal arteries, hypertension, diabetes mellitus, or direct trauma to the kidney. Antibiotics (particularly the "mycins"), heavy metals (lead and mercury), cleaning compounds, pesticides, and poisonous mushrooms may be toxic to the kidneys. Pyelonephritis, glomerulonephritis, renal tuberculosis, and polycystic kidney disease are examples of kidney conditions that may lead to kidney failure. The arteries in the renal parenchyma may become narrowed as a result of atherosclerosis, hypertension, nephrosclerosis, or blood components (sickled red cells, hemoglobin, or myoglobin). Trauma from motor vehicle accidents, contact sports injuries, and other direct blows also may be intrarenal causes of failure.

Postrenal causes of renal failure are obstructions beyond the kidneys that cause urine to back up. Ureteral calculi and benign prostatic hypertrophy are examples of postrenal causes of failure.

Patients at risk for acute renal failure include those having major surgery, experiencing major trauma, or receiving large doses of nephrotoxic drugs. These patients should have their blood pressure and fluid balance assessed more frequently than usual. Older people also are at risk for acute renal failure because they are less able to adapt to alterations in fluid balance or cardiac output. Renal function should always be assessed with any acute condition in the older patient. Early detection and treatment may significantly decrease the risk of death from acute renal failure.

Pharmacology Capsule

Nephrotoxic antibiotics can lead to acute renal failure.

Stages of Acute Renal Failure

The four stages of acute renal failure are onset, oliguria, diuresis (increased production of urine), and recovery.

Onset Stage. The onset stage is short (1 to 3 days) and characterized by increasing BUN and serum creatinine with normal to decreased urine output. The primary treatment goal during this stage is reversal of failing renal function to prevent further damage.

Oliguric Stage. During the oliguric stage, the urine output decreases to 400 mL/day or less. The serum values for BUN, creatinine, potassium, and phosphorus increase. Serum calcium and bicarbonate decrease. The oliguric stage follows the onset stage and continues for up to 14 days. Urine specific gravity becomes fixed at 1.010 (normal range, 1.010-1.025), indicating the inability of the tubules to concentrate urine. The patient becomes hypervolemic, meaning that the blood volume is greater than normal. Urine osmolality decreases and serum osmolality increases as waste products are retained.

Diuretic Stage. The diuretic stage begins when urine output exceeds 400 mL/day and may rise above 4 L/day. Despite the production of large quantities of urine, few waste products are excreted, and wastes accumulate in the blood. Toward the end of the diuretic stage, the kidneys begin to excrete BUN, creatinine, potassium, and phosphorus and retain calcium and bicarbonate. This is an indication of return of kidney function.

Recovery Stage. As renal tissue recovers, serum electrolytes, BUN, and creatinine return to normal. This recovery stage lasts 1 to 12 months. If complete recovery does not occur, renal insufficiency or chronic renal failure may develop. Renal insufficiency is indicated by loss of approximately 80% of function. It is possible to lead a relatively normal life with renal insufficiency unless other illnesses place an additional burden on kidney function.

Medical Treatment

The primary goal of treatment for acute renal failure (ARF) is to prevent further damage. Supportive measures aim to control symptoms and to prevent complications. Support measures include fluid and dietary restrictions, restoration of electrolyte balance, and dialysis if needed. Nephrotoxic drugs and drugs that reduce renal blood flow must be avoided. Additional treatment depends on the cause of the failure. For prerenal ARF, blood pressure and blood volume must be restored. Treatment of intrinsic ARF is based on efforts to stimulate urine production with IV fluids and with dopamine, furosemide, or both. Postrenal ARF is treated by removal of the cause (typically an obstruction).

Drug Therapy. Oliguria is treated with diuretics, most often an osmotic diuretic like mannitol or a loop diuretic like furosemide (Lasix) or ethacrynic acid (Edecrin). Hyperkalemia, which typically accompanies oliguria, is treated aggressively because it can be life-threatening. Drugs given intravenously to lower

Pharmacology Capsule

Oliguria may be treated with diuretics such as mannitol or furosemide.

serum potassium include hypertonic glucose and insulin, sodium bicarbonate, and calcium gluconate. Sodium polystyrene sulfonate (Kayexalate), given orally or rectally, also lowers serum potassium.

Diet. Dietary modifications for acute renal failure are based on consideration of serum electrolytes and urea. Sodium and potassium allowances are individually determined. Adequate carbohydrates are provided to prevent the breakdown of fat and protein. Essential amino acid supplements may be ordered. If the patient's nutritional needs are not being met by oral intake, enteral nutritional support is instituted. If the GI tract is not functioning, total parenteral nutrition is necessary.

Fluids. Daily fluid needs usually are calculated by adding 500 mL to the previous day's fluid output. The extra 500 mL represents the daily insensible loss (through breathing and perspiration). For example, an oliguric patient who has an output of only 400 mL today would be allowed 400 plus 600 mL, for a total of 1000 mL tomorrow.

Hemodialysis and Peritoneal Dialysis. Conditions that warrant hemodialysis when conservative measures fail include hyperkalemia, severe metabolic acidosis, pulmonary edema, and rising blood urea nitrogen. A temporary cannula can be placed in the jugular, femoral, or subclavian vein. A disadvantage of a femoral

cannula is that the patient must be immobile between dialysis treatments. If the cannula is removed and replaced repeatedly, however, there is a risk of hematoma formation. A subclavian cannula can be left in place between treatments but can cause thrombosis, stenosis, pneumothorax, hemothorax, and brachial nerve damage. The disadvantage of leaving the cannula in place is that the risk of infection increases. Only trained dialysis staff should draw blood or administer medications through the temporary cannula. Peritoneal dialysis is also an option, especially for the patient in congestive heart failure. The Chronic Kidney Disease section on pp. 875 to 878 describes these procedures in more detail.

Continuous Renal Replacement Therapy. Continuous renal replacement therapy (CRRT) offers additional options for treating the patient in acute renal failure. A cannula placed in an artery and a vein (arteriovenous therapy) or two veins (venovenous therapy) is connected to tubing that contains a blood filter and a collection device. The patient's blood flows through the tubing, and excess fluids, electrolytes, and wastes are filtered into the collection device. The blood is then returned to the patient. This procedure does not require dialysate, has little effect on cardiovascular stability, and is continuous. It can be used alone or with hemodialysis (Fig. 40-12).

FIGURE 40-12 Continuous renal replacement therapy.

NURSING CARE *of the Patient in Acute Renal Failure*

Assessment

Complete assessment of the patient with a urinary disorder is summarized in Box 40-1. For the patient in acute renal failure, monitoring fluid status is critical. Intake and output records must be kept carefully. Daily weights are an effective means of assessing changes in fluid status (500 mL of fluid weighs approximately 1 pound). To be useful, daily weights must be done at the same time each day, using the same scale, and with the patient wearing the same amount of clothing. Because hypervolemia (fluid volume excess) is a major problem during the oliguric stage, assess for signs and symptoms of impending heart failure: hypertension, bounding pulse, edema, cough, dysrhythmias.

Electrolyte imbalances can include alterations in serum potassium, sodium, calcium, phosphate, and magnesium. Signs and symptoms of each of these imbalances are discussed in Chapter 14. General assessment of electrolyte balance includes cardiac rate and rhythm, neuromuscular status, edema, and mental status. The acutely ill patient also must be monitored for signs and symptoms related to immobility: pressure sores, impaired circulation, constipation, and atelectasis.

One final area of assessment is the patient's understanding of the condition and its treatment. Identify fears, anxiety, coping strategies, and sources of support.

Nursing Diagnoses, Goals, and Outcome Criteria: Acute Renal Failure

NURSING DIAGNOSES	GOALS AND OUTCOME CRITERIA
Excess Fluid Volume related to impaired kidney function (oliguric stage) OR	Normal fluid and electrolyte balance: normal tissue turgor, absence of dyspnea, normal serum electrolyte values
Deficient Fluid Volume related to high-output renal failure (diuretic stage)	
Decreased Cardiac Output related to fluid and electrolyte imbalances	Normal cardiac output: pulse and blood pressure consistent with patient norms
Anxiety related to life-threatening illness	Decreased anxiety: patient states anxiety reduced, calm manner
Risk for Disuse Syndrome related to immobility	Absence of complications associated with immobility: intact skin, regular bowel movements without difficulty, breath sounds clear to auscultation
Deficient Knowledge of condition, treatment, and self-care	Patient understands condition, treatment, and self-care: patient accurately describes and participates in self-care as allowed

Interventions

Excess Fluid Volume/Deficient Fluid Volume

Assess and document fluid status on an ongoing basis. In the oliguric stage, fluid is likely to be restricted. Explain and reinforce fluid restrictions. The fluid allowance during the oliguric stage may be very limited. Measures to help the patient cope with fluid limitations include considering patient preferences in fluid selection and carefully planning fluid intake throughout waking hours. Remember to plan for fluids needed to take medications. When only a few ounces of fluids is allowed at a time, a small juice cup should be used rather than a large glass that is only one-quarter full. This creates an illusion of volume that may make the patient feel less deprived. To obtain patient cooperation, it is essential for the patient and family to understand the importance of adhering to the fluid restriction.

Give diuretics as ordered, and monitor the patient for adverse effects. A fluid challenge of normal saline may be rapidly infused while diuretics are given to promote improved renal perfusion.

Decreased Cardiac Output

In the diuretic stage, patients produce large volumes of dilute urine. Fluid volume deficit becomes a possibility. The heart rate must increase to make up for the diminished blood volume. Because eventually the heart may fail, it is important to monitor for cardiac dysrhythmias, changes in blood pressure, and shortness of breath. Give oral and intravenous fluids as ordered with careful monitoring of output at the same time.

Anxiety

Anxiety is understandable when a vital organ fails. The patient may fear death or chronic illness, with the potential for financial ruin, loss of vitality, and dependence on medical care. Provide honest responses to questions about renal failure and its treatment. Refer specific questions about the patient's prognosis to the physician.

The patient in acute renal failure may have a complete recovery. This may take up to 1 year. Unfortunately, some patients do not recover but instead progress to chronic renal failure. Those who do not improve need special support to help them learn to accept and deal with this major health deviation.

Risk for Disuse Syndrome

The patient with acute renal failure is very ill and may be immobilized. Therefore you must attend to prevention of complications of immobility as well as to the acute renal problem. This includes skin care, turning, coughing, deep breathing, leg exercises, and measures to promote bowel elimination. Care of the immobilized patient is described in Chapter 21.

Deficient Knowledge

When the patient is acutely ill, provide basic information about the disease, diagnostic tests and procedures, and treatments. Explain the reasons for interventions such as fluid restrictions, turning, deep breathing, and leg exercises. As the patient improves, patient teaching should include management of fluids, diet, drug therapy, activity, and signs and symptoms that should be reported to the physician (dyspnea, edema, fever).

Chronic Kidney Disease

Chronic kidney disease is characterized by progressive destruction of the nephrons of both kidneys. The severity is described in stages with the final stage (5) being end-stage renal disease. The healthy kidneys comprise far more nephrons than needed. Therefore a person can lose about 80% of the nephrons before kidney function becomes impaired. Creatinine clearance is an important measure of renal function. When it falls below 15 mL/min, dialysis or transplantation becomes necessary.

Chronic kidney disease is characterized by **azotemia** (increased nitrogenous waste products in the blood). **Uremia** is the term used when the condition advances to the point that the kidneys are unable to maintain fluid and electrolyte or acid-base balance. Uremia is also called *end-stage renal disease*. All of the causes of acute renal failure listed earlier may lead to chronic kidney disease. In addition, chronic renal infections may predispose the patient to progressive renal failure. The most common causes, however, are hypertension, diabetes mellitus, and atherosclerosis.

Signs and Symptoms

Azotemia. The first function lost in chronic kidney disease is the ability to concentrate urine. This results in an increase of waste products in the blood, despite producing large amounts of dilute urine. As the disease progresses, urine output typically declines until very little to no urine is produced.

Blood urea nitrogen is an approximate estimate of the glomerular filtration rate. It is affected by protein breakdown. Normal BUN ranges from 10 to 20 mg/dL. When BUN reaches or exceeds 70 mg/dL, dialysis is needed to reduce it.

Serum creatinine is a waste product of skeletal muscle breakdown. It is a more reliable measure of kidney function than BUN. It is not affected by diet, hydration, hepatic function, or metabolism. Normal serum creatinine is 0.5 to 1.5 mg/dL. A serum creatinine level that is twice the normal level reflects a 50% loss of function. When the value reaches or exceeds 10 times normal, 90% of function has been lost. The kidneys are able to adapt to a loss of up to 80% of function. The kidneys increase in size in an attempt to maintain function.

Creatinine clearance (a urine test) is the best indicator of renal function. It is ordered less often than serum creatinine, however, because it requires collection of all urine in a 12- or 24-hour period. Normal creatinine clearance exceeds 100 mL/min.

Hyperkalemia. The primary means of potassium excretion is through the kidneys. As kidney function fails,

potassium is retained, which results in hyperkalemia, the most life-threatening effect of renal failure. The normal range for serum potassium is 3.5 to 5.0 mEq/L. Elevated serum potassium interferes with normal cardiac function, causing cardiac dysrhythmias. Dysrhythmias are potentially fatal. The patient becomes apathetic and confused and may have nausea, abdominal cramps, muscle weakness, and numbness of the extremities. Serum potassium greater than 6 mEq/L requires cardiac monitoring. If the serum potassium is not reduced, bradycardia (pulse ≤50 beats/min) or asystole (no heartbeat) may develop.

Hyperkalemia is treated with intravenous glucose and insulin or intravenous 10% calcium gluconate. These drugs drive potassium back into the cells, reducing the serum potassium level. They are used as temporary emergency measures. Kayexalate, given orally or rectally, causes potassium to be drawn into the bowel and eliminated in the feces. The method used most often to reduce elevated serum potassium is dialysis.

Hypocalcemia. Diseased kidney tissue lacks the enzyme that activates vitamin D. Without active vitamin D, calcium absorption from the bowel decreases. The body tries to compensate by shifting calcium from the bones into the blood. Serum phosphate binds with calcium, further depleting calcium levels. The normal serum calcium level is 9 to 11 mg/dL or 4.5 to 5.5 mEq/L. Abnormally low serum calcium is called *hypocalcemia*. Patients with hypocalcemia experience tingling sensations, muscle twitches, irritability, and tetany. Tetany is sustained, painful muscle contraction. Hypocalcemia is treated with calcium supplements, active vitamin D, and phosphate binders. Phosphate binders include calcium carbonate, calcium acetate, or sevelamer (Renagel). Side effects of phosphate binders include hypophosphatemia and constipation. Antacids with aluminum or magnesium, such as milk of magnesia, magnesium carbonate, magnesium oxide, and magnesium trisilicate, should be avoided.

Metabolic Acidosis. Failure of the renal tubules to excrete acid ions and acid waste products causes the body's acid level to rise. Decreased bicarbonate reabsorption renders the body unable to neutralize the excess acid. Excess acid leads to metabolic acidosis. The lungs attempt to compensate by eliminating more carbon dioxide through hyperventilation. Manifestations of metabolic acidosis are headache, lethargy, and delirium.

Fluid Balance. Most patients with chronic kidney disease retain sodium and water, causing hypernatremia and hypervolemia. Elevated blood pressure and edema are signs of hypervolemia. Congestive heart failure may develop in the hypervolemic patient because the patient's heart cannot handle the high fluid volume. Prevention and treatment of hypervolemia include fluid restriction, diuretics, and dialysis if necessary. A few patients are sodium wasters. These patients lose excess sodium and water in the urine and become hyponatremic and hypovolemic.

Insulin Resistance. With renal failure, cells become resistant to the action of insulin. As a result, blood insulin and glucose levels rise. Hyperinsulinemia (high blood insulin) stimulates the liver to produce triglycerides. Patients in chronic kidney disease have high serum levels of very-low-density lipoproteins. Elevated lipids in the blood (hyperlipidemia) contribute to accelerated atherosclerosis.

Anemia. Kidneys of patients with chronic kidney disease produce less erythropoietin, a hormone necessary for red blood cell production. Even the red blood cells that are produced have a shorter life span than usual because of the toxic environment in which they live. Therefore patients with chronic kidney disease have anemia. Iron supplements and folic acid may be ordered. Transfusions may be required if the hematocrit drops below 20% (normal values, 35% to 45% for women and 45% to 55% for men). A genetically engineered erythropoietin (epoetin alfa) can be administered intravenously after hemodialysis or subcutaneously for patients on peritoneal dialysis. This product improves red blood cell formation and has reversed anemia and the need for transfusions in some patients with chronic kidney disease.

Immunologic Function. Because the inflammatory response diminishes with chronic kidney disease, fewer white blood cells gather at the site of an infection or injury. The general immune response is suppressed, and antibody production declines. Therefore the patient has reduced ability to resist infections.

Cardiovascular System. The cardiovascular system is affected by hypervolemia, hyperkalemia, and hypocalcemia. Hypervolemia increases the workload of the heart, possibly leading to congestive heart failure. Manifestations of congestive heart failure are moist breath sounds, bounding pulse, dependent edema, and dyspnea. Dysrhythmias may be caused by hyperkalemia or hypocalcemia.

Neurologic System. Neurologic effects of chronic kidney disease are mental status changes (lethargy, irritability, confusion) and peripheral neuropathy. Peripheral neuropathy may be evident initially as a restless feeling and later as footdrop, loss of feeling in the legs, or paralysis of the legs. Many physicians treat the development of peripheral neuropathy as a signal to begin dialysis.

Disequilibrium syndrome may occur with hemodialysis. The rapid removal of urea from the blood leaves a higher concentration of solutes in the brain and the cerebrospinal fluid (CSF). The solutes increase the osmotic pressure, which draws fluid from the bloodstream into the CSF and brain tissue. Confusion, lethargy, headache, nausea, and vomiting may progress to coma or seizures if not treated. Disequilibrium is corrected with the administration of hypertonic glucose.

Integumentary System. The integumentary system is also affected by the accumulation of waste products.

Calcium phosphate crystals and urea accumulate in the skin, causing itching. Dryness results from decreased oil gland production and decreased perspiration. A pale gray to yellow color may result from anemia and from unexcreted bilirubin and uremic pigments. Hair and nails become dry and brittle. *Uremic frost* is the term used when whitish crystals composed of urea and other salts precipitate on the skin. Uremic frost is most often noted around the mouth. It is a very late sign in chronic kidney disease.

Gastrointestinal System. Ammonia is a breakdown product of urea. When ammonia accumulates in the gastrointestinal tract, it causes irritation, nausea, vomiting, a metallic taste in the mouth, and bleeding. Antacids administered every 2 hours help relieve the irritation. A diet high in carbohydrates and low in protein is prescribed to reduce the accumulation of urea. Other common gastrointestinal disturbances with chronic kidney disease are stomatitis (inflammation of the mouth), anorexia, nausea, vomiting, constipation, and diarrhea.

Musculoskeletal System. *Renal osteodystrophy* refers to the skeletal changes characteristic of chronic kidney disease. The three major changes are metastatic calcification, bone demineralization, and osteitis fibrosa. Metastatic calcification is deposition of calcium phosphate complexes in blood vessels and in joints, lungs, muscles, and eyes. Deposits in blood vessels can impair blood flow so severely that fingers and toes may become gangrenous. Bone demineralization is directly related to hypocalcemia. Low serum calcium triggers increased production of parathormone by the parathyroid glands. Parathormone mobilizes calcium from the bone and shifts it into the blood. Over time, loss of bone mass can be significant. When calcium is lost from bones, it is replaced with fibrous tissue. This condition is called *osteitis fibrosa.*

Reproductive System. Chronic kidney disease affects both the male and female reproductive systems. The production of sex hormones declines, and libido is diminished. Ovulation and menstruation usually cease in women. Men typically have low sperm counts and erectile dysfunction. The general effects of a chronic illness undoubtedly affect sexual desire and function as well.

Endocrine Function. Patients with chronic kidney disease usually appear hypothyroid. Hyperparathyroidism occurs in response to the chronically low serum calcium and high serum phosphates. Patients with diabetes require less exogenous insulin because the enzyme that normally breaks down insulin (renal insulinase) is reduced. Oral hypoglycemics also place the patient at risk for hypoglycemia because the drugs are normally excreted by the kidneys.

Emotional and Psychological Effects. Emotional and psychological effects of chronic kidney disease include emotional lability, depression, anxiety, and slowed intellectual functioning.

Medical Treatment

Treatment of chronic kidney disease aims to promote elimination of wastes, maintenance of fluid balance, and management of the systemic effects of the disease. Conservative treatment of the systemic effects of chronic kidney disease is provided on pp. 875 to 878. To summarize, these treatments include the following:

- Intravenous glucose and insulin, calcium carbonate, calcium acetate, or sodium polystyrene sulfonate to treat hyperkalemia
- Calcium, active vitamin D, and phosphate binders to treat hypocalcemia
- Fluid restriction and diuretics to treat hypervolemia
- Diuretics, beta-blockers, calcium channel blockers, and ACE inhibitors for hypertension
- Iron supplements, folic acid, and synthetic erythropoietin to treat anemia
- Hypertonic glucose to treat disequilibrium syndrome
- High-carbohydrate, low-protein diet to prevent excess urea

Dialysis. When kidney failure can no longer be managed conservatively, dialysis is required to sustain life. Dialysis is the passage of molecules through a semipermeable membrane into a special solution called *dialysate solution.* Dialysis operates like the kidney. Small molecules like urea, creatinine, and electrolytes pass out of the blood, across a membrane, and into a solution.

The goals of dialysis are to:

- Remove the end products of protein metabolism from the blood
- Maintain safe concentrations of serum electrolytes

- Correct acidosis and replenish the body's bicarbonate buffer system
- Remove excess fluid from the blood

Dialysis enables many patients to maintain or regain self-esteem and to be productive members of society. However, initial positive feelings about dialysis sometimes turn to depression as the reality of "being tied to a machine" is recognized. Two primary means of dialysis are hemodialysis and peritoneal dialysis.

Hemodialysis. Hemodialysis is a process by which blood is removed from the body and circulated through an "artificial kidney" for removal of excess fluid, electrolytes, and wastes. The dialyzed blood is then returned to the patient (Fig. 40-13). Hemodialysis requires vascular access (access to the patient's bloodstream). This may be accomplished by catheter, cannula, graft, or fistula. Subclavian or femoral catheters can be used for temporary access for dialysis during acute renal failure while a graft or fistula matures (dilates and toughens) or for patients on peritoneal dialysis who need immediate access for hemodialysis. The catheters may be used for up to 1 week.

Internal connections between veins and arteries do not require dressings. An internal fistula between the patient's artery and vein requires approximately 2 weeks to mature and may be used 3 to 5 years. Connections may be made by using bovine or synthetic grafts that require 1 to 2 weeks to heal before use and last 7 to 9 years.

An arteriovenous shunt or cannula is an external connection between an artery and a vein (Fig. 40-14). By connecting the external ends of the synthetic tubing for dialysis, venipuncture is not necessary. However, because the cannula is external, there is danger of hemorrhage, risk of skin breakdown, restriction of

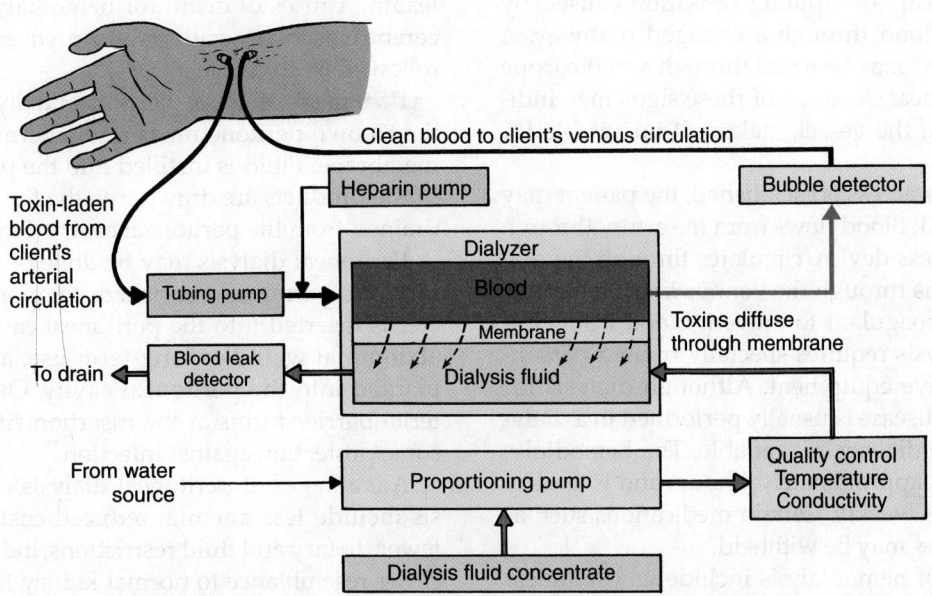

FIGURE **40-13** Schematic diagram of hemodialysis. As the patient's blood passes through the dialyzer, toxins diffuse into the dialysis fluid.

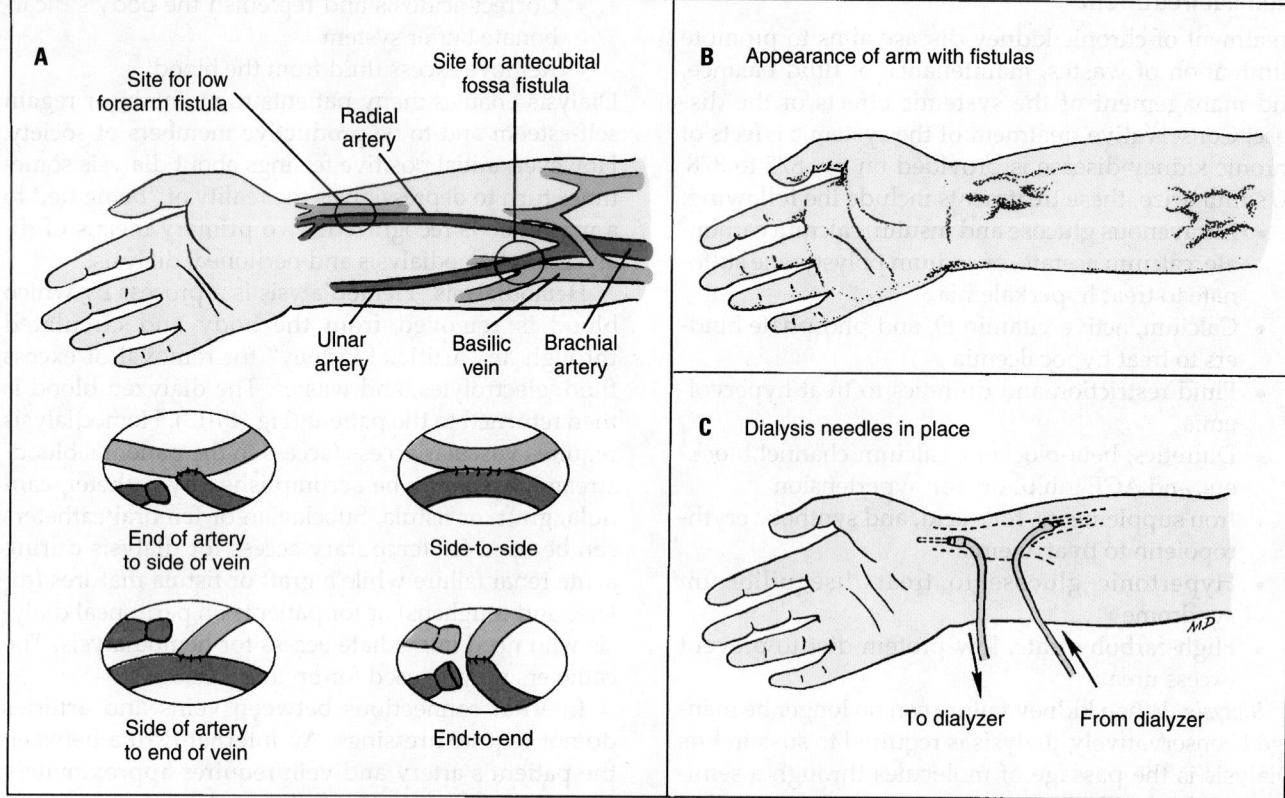

FIGURE **40-14** An internal arteriovenous fistula created by joining an artery and a vein. The fistula will be used for hemodialysis. **A,** Types of fistulas. **B,** The appearance of the arm with fistulas. **C,** Dialysis needles in place in the fistula.

activities, and risk of site infection. The arteriovenous shunt may be used for temporary vascular access but is very rarely used for chronic treatment because of the potential complications.

All vascular access sites must be assessed for patency. Check pulses below the shunt to be sure circulation is adequate. Palpate the venous side of the shunt for a "thrill" or rippling sensation caused by movement of blood through a changed pathway. A bruit or "swoosh" may be heard through a stethoscope with each heartbeat. Absence of these signs may indicate occlusion of the vessel, making it unsuitable for hemodialysis.

Once vascular access is established, the patient may be hemodialyzed. Blood flows from the artery through the vascular access device, circulates through the dialyzer, and returns through the venous line. Heparin is used as an anticoagulant to prevent blood from clotting. Hemodialysis requires specially trained personnel and expensive equipment. Although dialysis for chronic kidney disease is usually performed in a dialysis center, home dialysis is available. The hemodialysis process takes approximately 4 hours and is usually done three times weekly. Certain medications such as antihypertensives may be withheld.

Advantages of hemodialysis include its usefulness in emergencies and the rapid removal of wastes, electrolytes, and fluid. Disadvantages include the need

for vascular access, the use of an anticoagulant, and the potential for hemorrhage, anemia, rapid fluid and electrolyte shifts (dialysis disequilibrium syndrome), muscle cramps, nausea and vomiting, and air emboli.

Complications of hemodialysis include atherosclerotic cardiovascular disease, anemia, gastric ulcers, disturbed calcium metabolism, and hepatitis. The leading causes of death for hemodialysis patients are cerebrovascular accident and myocardial infarction, followed by infection.

Peritoneal Dialysis. Peritoneal dialysis uses the patient's own peritoneum as a semipermeable dialyzing membrane. Fluid is instilled into the peritoneal cavity. Waste products are drawn into the fluid, which is then drained from the peritoneal cavity (Fig. 40-15).

Peritoneal dialysis may be done on either a temporary or a permanent basis. For temporary use, a catheter is inserted into the peritoneal cavity through the abdominal wall. For long-term use, a catheter is implanted into the peritoneal cavity. Over time, a bacterial barrier forms at the insertion site and provides some protection against infection.

Advantages of peritoneal dialysis over hemodialysis include less anemia, reduced cost of equipment, fewer dietary and fluid restrictions, independence, and closer resemblance to normal kidney function. Also, it can be initiated in almost any hospital. Disadvantages include the risk of peritonitis (the major complication)

Tenckhoff catheter
Peritoneal cavity
Dialysis solution
Drainage

FIGURE **40-15** Peritoneal dialysis.

and catheter site infection, hyperglycemia, elevated serum lipids, and body image disturbance. Also, peritoneal dialysis cannot be used for patients with recent abdominal surgery, extensive abdominal trauma, or open abdominal wounds.

Peritoneal dialysis has three phases: inflow, dwell, and drain. The three phases comprise one exchange. During inflow, fluid (commonly 2 liters) is allowed to drain into the peritoneal catheter through an established catheter over about 10 minutes. During the dwell time, fluid remains in the cavity for a specified period of time while ultrafiltration, osmosis, and diffusion occur. The fluid bearing wastes and excess water is then drained from the cavity over 20 to 30 minutes.

Continuous ambulatory peritoneal dialysis (CAPD) allows the patient freedom from a machine and the independence to perform dialysis alone. The exchange process usually is repeated four times each day by outpatients. It may be done more often in acutely ill hospitalized patients. Strict aseptic technique must be used with the initiation of the process and with each exchange. The patient or a reliable caregiver must be taught the process by someone who understands it well.

Automated peritoneal dialysis uses a device called a *cycler* to perform the exchanges during the night. This allows the patient freedom during the day. It also reduces the risk of infection because the system is interrupted less often. There are several variations of this procedure, which may be done from five to seven times a week and may or may not leave the fluid in the abdomen during the waking hours.

Peritonitis, infection of the peritoneum, is the most serious complication of peritoneal dialysis. Infections also may develop at the catheter exit site and tunnel where the catheter is placed under the skin. Cloudiness

and particles in the fluid in the outflow container are evidence of infection. Redness, swelling, and purulent drainage are signs of infection at the exit site. Immediately report any signs of infection to the physician. Peritonitis is usually treated with antibiotics administered through the peritoneal catheter. Other complications include bleeding, abdominal pain, hernias, low back pain, respiratory distress, and decreased serum albumin. Encapsulating sclerosing peritonitis is a condition in which a thick membrane develops around the bowel. The thickened membrane can obstruct the intestines and interferes with ultrafiltration.

NURSING CARE *of the Patient with Chronic Kidney Disease*

Assessment

The general nursing assessment of the patient with a urologic disorder is outlined in Box 40-1. For the patient with chronic kidney disease, frequent monitoring for changes in status is especially important. Fluid balance is evaluated closely. During hospitalization, accurate intake and output records must be kept. Be alert for signs and symptoms of fluid volume excess that can lead to cardiac failure. Warning signs include increasing edema, dyspnea, tachycardia, bounding pulse, and rising blood pressure.

Serum electrolytes are measured frequently, but you must still be alert for signs and symptoms of electrolyte imbalances. With chronic kidney disease, the nurse is most concerned with detecting hyperkalemia, hypocalcemia, and metabolic acidosis. Hyponatremia and hypovolemia are less common. Assessment of fluid and electrolyte imbalances includes characteristics of pulse and respirations, blood pressure, mental status, and neuromuscular activity.

Assessment of nutrition includes appetite, usual daily intake, weight gain or loss pattern, and prescribed diet. Determine how well the patient understands and follows the prescribed diet. See the Nutrition Concepts box below.

Do not overlook mental and emotional status when assessing the patient with kidney disease Increasing confusion or loss of consciousness can be due to accumulated toxins or electrolyte imbalances. Emotional responses to a diagnosis of chronic kidney disease vary. Determine the patient's perceptions of the situation, and identify usual coping strategies. Anxiety, fear, disturbed body image, depression, and lowered self-esteem are common.

The long-term effects of chronic kidney disease and its treatment put the patient at risk for many complications. Monitor bowel elimination for either constipation or diarrhea. Monitor for signs and symptoms of local or systemic infections (redness, swelling, foul drainage, fever, increased white blood cell count). Inspect the skin for bruising, bleeding, or trauma. Evaluate sensation in the extremities. Ask if sexual dysfunction has been a problem and obtain a description of the problem.

Explore patient understanding about chronic kidney disease, its treatment, and self-care measures. Document the patient's ability to perform activities of daily living.

Specific nursing diagnoses and goals vary based on the individual patient data. Many diagnoses and interventions discussed in the Acute Renal Failure section also apply to the patient with chronic kidney disease. The emphasis in this section is on the common problems experienced by the patient in chronic failure.

Nutrition Concepts

1. Renal failure results in an inability of the kidneys to excrete wastes and maintain fluid and electrolyte balance.
2. In renal failure, the nutritional goal is to modify the diet so that the work of the kidneys is reduced.
3. Fluid intake may be restricted to 1000 to 1500 mL/day for patients with renal disease.
4. Sodium and potassium intakes are restricted (including medications) to maintain electrolyte balance in patients who require dialysis.
5. Protein is restricted in patients with renal disease, and any protein ingested should be high in essential amino acids. Examples of these proteins are eggs, meat, poultry, fish, and milk products.
6. People with renal calculi should increase fluid intake to maintain at least 2 L of urine output daily and should avoid foods leading to the formation of calculi.
7. Calcium intake is restricted for those patients having certain types of renal calculi.

Nursing Diagnoses, Goals, and Outcome Criteria: Chronic Kidney Disease

NURSING DIAGNOSES	GOALS AND OUTCOME CRITERIA
Excess Fluid Volume related to fluid retention	Reduced fluid volume and absence of symptoms of heart failure: normal tissue turgor, blood pressure within patient norms, no dyspnea
Imbalanced Nutrition: Less Than Body Requirements related to anorexia, nausea, vomiting, stomatitis, dietary restrictions	Adequate nutrition: consumption of prescribed diet, serum albumin and total protein within acceptable limits
Disturbed Sensory Perception related to effects of uremia on the nervous system	Normal sensory perception: alert and oriented
Ineffective Coping related to multiple life changes	Effective coping: patient uses coping strategies that decrease anxiety without compromising care
Situational Low Self-Esteem related to self-worth, change in appearance, loss of kidney function, venous access devices, inability to fulfill usual roles and responsibilities	Improved self-esteem: positive statements of confidence
Risk for Infection related to impaired immune response, malnutrition, break in skin integrity	Absence of infection: normal body temperature and white blood cell count
Risk for Injury related to coagulation disorder, impaired wound healing, bone demineralization, peripheral neuropathy	Absence of injury: no bruises, bleeding, fractures
Constipation related to inactivity, drug side effects, fluid restriction, electrolyte imbalances	Normal bowel elimination: regular formed stools passed without straining
Diarrhea related to electrolyte imbalances, drug side effects	Normal bowel elimination: formed stools
Sexual Dysfunction related to fatigue, drug side effects, hormone deficiencies, altered self-image	Satisfactory sexual function: patient states intimate relationship is satisfactory
Self-Care Deficit related to lack of knowledge, confusion, anemia, fatigue	Accomplishment of self-care: patient performs activities of daily living within limitations imposed by renal failure and treatments

Interventions

Excess Fluid Volume

As renal failure progresses, the patient's ability to excrete excess fluids continually declines. In the early stages, diuretics may be used to treat fluid retention, but they are not used once dialysis is begun. Fluid intake may be restricted. If intravenous fluids are ordered, closely monitor the rate of infusion. Antihypertensives may be needed to control blood pressure, and digitalis may be given to support cardiac function. Dosage adjustments often are needed because kidney failure affects the ability to excrete these drugs. Administer medications, monitor for side effects, and teach the patient how to take them after discharge and what adverse effects to report.

Patients with fluid volume excess require comfort and safety measures. Edematous legs are easily injured and heal slowly. Protect them from pressure or trauma. If cardiac failure and dyspnea develop, position the patient with the head elevated to ease breathing. Cerebral edema causes confusion and decreasing consciousness. Implement safety measures to protect the confused or semiconscious patient from injury.

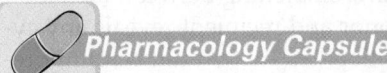

Pharmacology Capsule

Because most drugs are excreted in the urine, people with impaired renal function are at risk for drug toxicity.

Imbalanced Nutrition: Less Than Body Requirements

Adequate nutrition can be a challenge for the patient with chronic kidney disease. Anorexia, nausea, vomiting, and stomatitis interfere with food intake. In addition, sodium, protein, and sometimes fat restrictions make the diet less appealing. Measures to encourage food intake include frequent mouth care and small feedings. Explain the importance of good nutrition to the patient and family. The dietitian can help the patient learn to cope with the diet. The person who prepares the patient's food at home should be included in dietary instructions. Vitamin supplements are routinely ordered because of dietary restrictions. Monitor weight to evaluate both fluid and nutritional status. Teach the patient and the caregivers about medications and status monitors.

Disturbed Sensory Perception

Renal failure affects both the central and the peripheral nervous systems. Cerebral edema and elevated metabolic wastes in the blood can cause confusion, slowed thought processes, lethargy, and loss of consciousness. Protect confused patients, and orient them to person, place, and time. Present information simply, and re-

peat as needed. Avoid sensory overload by reducing environmental stimuli and demands on the patient. For safety reasons, assign the patient to a room close to the nurses' station. Put the bed in low position, and keep the call bell within reach.

The effects of renal disease on the peripheral nerves can lead to loss of sensation in the extremities (peripheral neuropathy). These patients are at risk for injury. Inspect the affected areas daily for any signs of injury. Pressure, ill-fitting shoes, or external heat or cold can cause serious injury before the patient is aware of it. Teach the patient about peripheral neuropathy and how to prevent injuries.

Ineffective Coping

Patients with chronic kidney disease often experience anxiety and fear. They face life-threatening illness, endure invasive treatments and procedures, and undergo radical changes in lifestyle. Explore the patient's coping strategies, and identify factors that interfere with adjustment to renal disease. It helps for the patient to have a regular primary nurse so that a therapeutic relationship can develop. Nurses can help by talking to patients and helping them focus on the sources of their distress. It is important to be accepting of the patient's thoughts and feelings. Do not give false reassurance or tell patients not to worry! Explain routines and procedures, and provide practical advice on the management of everyday problems. Many patients benefit from talking to a mental health professional or attending support groups with people with similar problems. While encouraging patients to accept treatment, respect their rights to be informed and to refuse treatment.

Dialysis patients typically go through stages of adjustment. When dialysis is first started, they usually feel much better. They feel encouraged and view dialysis positively. This might be described as a "honeymoon period." At this stage, the patient is most receptive to teaching. It is wise to take advantage of this opportunity to educate the patient.

After several months of treatment, patients tire of the routine. Depression and disappointment are common. Some cope by denying the need for treatment. They may omit medications or fail to keep appointments for follow-up. Be accepting of the patient but not the behavior at this stage. Confront the patient when ineffective coping behaviors are identified.

Eventually, most dialysis patients accept the need for ongoing treatment. They may try to resume their former levels of activity. At this point, you may need to guide them in realistic goal setting.

Situational Low Self-Esteem

The patient's self-esteem may suffer because of changes in body image and role performance. Encourage patients to talk about the changes they are experiencing and what they mean. Therapeutic communication and touch convey acceptance to patients. Help the patient with grooming to enhance appearance.

Encourage patients to examine their daily routines and look for ways to conserve time and energy. Sources of help and support need to be identified. Family functions may have to be redistributed. It is important for the patient to continue to have roles in the family and to be seen as a contributing family member.

Risk for Infection

Patients with chronic kidney disease must avoid exposure to others with infections. Be sure they know how to take their own temperatures. Instruct them to report fever or other signs of infection to the physician. Practice good hand washing and aseptic technique for invasive procedures.

Risk for Injury

The patient is susceptible to injury because of impaired coagulation and wound healing, bone demineralization, and peripheral neuropathy. Calcium, vitamin D, and phosphate binders are ordered to reduce loss of calcium from the bones. Encourage ambulation, which helps strengthen bones. Assess and protect body parts that lack sensation. Provide an environment with adequate support equipment and few obstacles that might cause bruises or falls.

Constipation

Constipation is a common problem with chronic kidney disease because of inactivity, fluid restriction, electrolyte imbalances, and drug side effects. Encourage activity within the patient's tolerance level. Stool softeners often are ordered to prevent constipation.

Diarrhea

Diarrhea may be caused by drugs or by anxiety. Measure liquid stools and count as fluid output. Give antidiarrheals as ordered. Provide perianal care after each stool.

Sexual Dysfunction

Sexual dysfunction is attributed to both physical and emotional causes. At first you may feel uncomfortable discussing sexual function with patients, but patients need to know that it is acceptable to express concerns. Explain how kidney disease affects sexual function, and explore what this means to the patient. Referral to a counselor who specializes in treatment of sexual dysfunction may be appreciated. Alternative means of sexual expression may enable the patient to continue to feel loved and to be intimate with another person.

Self-Care Deficit

Patients with chronic kidney disease spend more time at home than they do in the hospital. Nurses need to prepare them for self-care.

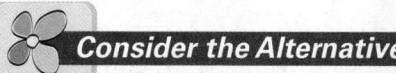
Consider the Alternative

Patients with irreversible chronic diseases are vulnerable to claims of miracle cures. Caution patients to discuss alternative therapies with the physician to prevent potentially harmful outcomes.

RENAL TRANSPLANTATION

KIDNEY DONATION

In 2004, 16,004 kidney transplants were done in the United States with high rates of success. A healthy kidney may be obtained from a live donor (usually a relative) or from a cadaver. When a kidney is obtained from a living related donor, the 1-year recipient survival rate is 97.6%. Of the transplanted kidneys, 94.5% are functioning well 1 year later. Of patients who receive transplants from cadavers, 94% are alive 1 year later, and 88.4% of those transplanted kidneys survive at least 1 year. The tissues of the donor and the recipient must match or the recipient will reject the new kidney. Matching is based on ABO blood groups and human leukocyte antigens. Crossmatching between the blood of the prospective donor and recipient reveals any cytotoxic preformed antibodies that would certainly result in organ rejection. A national network maintains lists of people awaiting donor kidneys. When a cadaver kidney is available, the network tries to locate the best match for the kidney to improve the chances of success.

Kidney donors must be at least 18 years of age, be free of systemic disease or infection, have no history of cancer or renal disease, have normal renal function, and be without major medical problems. People older than 60 years may be considered as candidates for donation on an individual basis. Unfortunately, many older people have advanced cardiac or respiratory disease that makes them ineligible.

Cadavers must meet the same criteria as living donors. Many people carry signed donor cards indicating willingness to have organs used for transplantation in the event of brain death. If brain death does occur, written permission is still sought from the family of the potential donor before organs are removed. The vital organs of the brain-dead person must be kept functioning until the kidney is removed.

PREOPERATIVE NURSING CARE
of the Renal Transplant Recipient

In some respects, preoperative care of the renal transplant recipient is similar to that of any other patient facing major surgery (see Chapter 17). The patient must be prepared mentally and physically for the procedure. The unique aspect of this situation is that the patient awaits an organ from another human being. If a relative is the donor, the surgery can be planned and both people emotionally prepared. Counseling is advised for both the donor and the recipient. The patient may be ambivalent about receiving a relative's organ. The gift of a kidney can restore health, but the recipient may feel guilty about asking a loved one to endure surgery and to give up an organ. The donor also faces the stress of surgery and a future with only one kidney. The donor also has to accept that the kidney could be rejected. Both recipient and donor face the threat of surgical complications.

If awaiting a cadaver kidney, the patient must face the idea that someone must die for a kidney to be available. These potential recipients are on call and must be ready to report to the hospital at any time. In a given year, only about 1 in 4 of the 63,000 patients on waiting lists receives a kidney.

The recipient and the live donor have complete diagnostic workups to rule out other medical problems and to evaluate the function of the urinary tract. Normal function of both of the donor's kidneys must be affirmed. The recipient is given medications to bring blood pressure within normal limits. Immunosuppressant drugs are started to control the body's response to foreign tissue (i.e., the donated kidney; see the Drug Therapy table on p. 853). The recipient also may be given a transfusion of the donor's blood, a measure that has been found to reduce rejection. If the recipient has severe hypertension or a UTI, bilateral nephrectomies may be done before transplantation. The patient is dialyzed shortly before transplantation.

Assessment

In the preoperative period, a complete assessment is done as outlined in Chapter 17. Before renal transplantation, explore the patient's understanding of the surgery. Record baseline vital signs. Identify any specific fears or questions that need to be addressed.

Nursing Diagnoses, Goals, and Outcome Criteria: Renal Transplantation, Preoperative	
NURSING DIAGNOSES	GOALS AND OUTCOME CRITERIA
Fear related to perceived threat of death	Reduced fear: patient states fear is lessened
Deficient Knowledge of surgical routines	Patient understands surgical routines: patient verbalizes accurate information, cooperates in care Nursing Diagnoses, Goals, and Outcome Criteria: Renal Transplantation, Preoperative

Interventions

To achieve these goals, acknowledge and encourage the patient to discuss concerns. Accept fear as understandable and natural. Factual information helps the patient cope by reducing the fear of the unknown. In-

volve the patient in planning and in self-care. When patients are active participants in their care, they feel less helpless and less anxious. Preoperative teaching begins when the patient is identified as a candidate for transplantation. Reinforce information when the actual surgery is imminent. It is somewhat more difficult to teach the patient who is awaiting a cadaver kidney because one never knows when, or if, the transplantation will take place.

Surgical Procedure

The donor kidney is removed from the live donor in an operating room and taken to an adjacent room where the recipient has been prepared to receive it. A cadaver kidney is removed under sterile conditions and transported to the hospital where the recipient is waiting. The donor kidney is placed in the recipient's abdomen and anastomosed (attached) to the bladder via the ureter and also to the blood vessels (Fig. 40-16).

Complications

Complications after renal transplantation include acute tubular necrosis, rejection, renal artery stenosis, hematomas, abscesses, and leakage of ureteral or vascular anastomoses. When the time between organ harvest and implantation is delayed, there is a risk of acute tubular necrosis (ATN). With ATN, urine output may decline or water may be eliminated but not metabolic wastes. This condition requires dialysis until renal function improves (it usually does). Rejection of

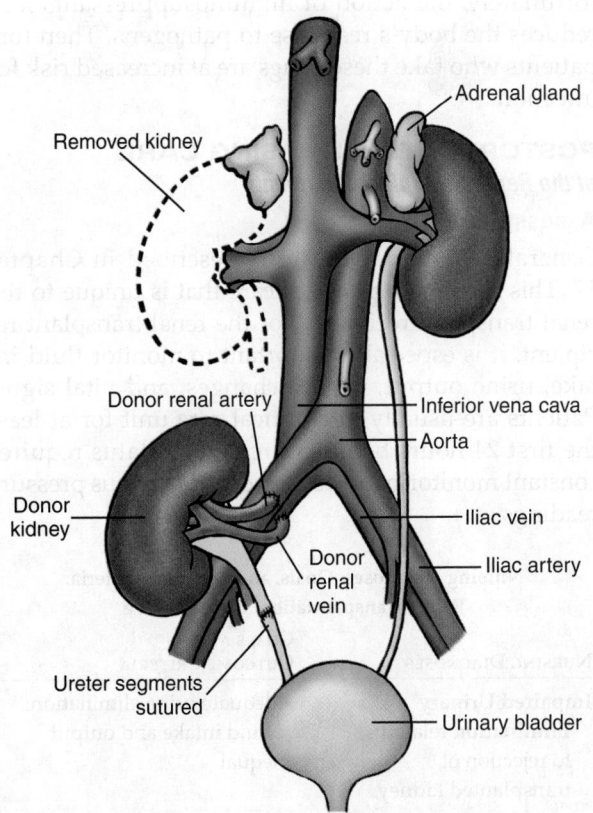

FIGURE **40-16** Placement of a transplanted kidney.

the new organ by the recipient is a major problem with most tissue transplants. Rejection is characterized by fever, elevated blood pressure, and pain over the location of the new kidney. Three types of rejection can occur: hyperacute, acute, and chronic. Hyperacute rejection occurs within 48 hours after transplantation. It is not reversible, and the kidney must be removed. Acute rejection develops between 1 week and 2 years after transplantation and is treated with increased immunosuppressant drugs. Chronic rejection develops and progresses slowly. Eventually, chronic rejection mimics chronic kidney disease, and dialysis may become necessary.

Immunosuppressant drugs, begun before surgery, are continued in the postoperative period to reduce the risk of rejection. These drugs include (1) T-cell suppressors: cyclosporine, tacrolimus, or sirolimus; (2) cytotoxic drugs: mycophenolate mofetil, azathioprine, or cyclophosphamide; and (3) corticosteroids. Antibodies are drugs that are used primarily for short periods to prevent or reverse acute rejection. Those used for transplant patients include polyclonal antibodies (antithymocyte globulin, antilymphocyte globulin) and monoclonal antibodies (muromonab-CD3). Examples of immunosuppressants, their actions and adverse effects, and nursing interventions are provided in the Drug Therapy table on p. 853. They are called *immunosuppressants* because they inhibit the body's immune response to foreign tissue. This action is intended to prevent the donor kidney from being destroyed by the recipient's defenses. Unfortunately, the action of immunosuppressants also reduces the body's response to pathogens. Therefore patients who take these drugs are at increased risk for infection.

POSTOPERATIVE NURSING CARE
of the Renal Transplant Recipient

Assessment

General postoperative care is described in Chapter 17. This section emphasizes care that is unique to the renal transplant recipient. For the renal transplant recipient, it is especially important to monitor fluid intake, urine output, weight changes, and vital signs. Patients are usually in a critical care unit for at least the first 24 hours because circulatory status requires constant monitoring including central venous pressure readings.

Nursing Diagnoses, Goals, and Outcome Criteria: Renal Transplantation, Postoperative	
NURSING DIAGNOSES	GOALS AND OUTCOME CRITERIA
Impaired Urinary Elimination related to rejection of transplanted kidney, renal failure	Adequate urine elimination: fluid intake and output equal
Deficient Fluid Volume related to diuresis, blood loss	Normal fluid volume: pulse and blood pressure consistent with patient norms
Risk for Infection related to suppression of immune response	Absence of infection: normal body temperature and white blood cell count
Ineffective Therapeutic Regimen Management of immediate and long-term postoperative care	Effective management of self-care: patient accurately describes and carries out plan of care
Anxiety related to possibility of organ rejection	Reduced anxiety: patient states anxiety is lessened, calm manner

Interventions

Immediately after surgery, the transplant patient is taken to a special care unit for close monitoring for circulatory and respiratory complications. Assist the patient with turning, coughing, deep breathing, and leg exercises. Institute pain control measures.

Impaired Urinary Elimination

The patient has an indwelling catheter for up to a week to permit constant observation of urine output. Urine is pink to bloody initially and then gradually clears. Maintain catheter patency at all times. You may have an order to gently irrigate the catheter if obstruction by blood clots is suspected. Closely monitor the patient for signs that the transplanted organ is functioning: increasing urine output, normal blood pressure, decreasing BUN and serum creatinine, and stable weight. Commonly, the patient begins to diurese (eliminate excess fluid) as soon as blood flow to the donor kidney is established. The output may be as high as 1 L/hr until BUN and serum creatinine return to normal.

If the patient is oliguric, a fluid challenge and diuretics are prescribed. In addition to the possibilities of renal failure and rejection, be alert for signs and symptoms of cardiac failure related to fluid volume excess: dyspnea, edema, bounding pulse, and cardiac dysrhythmias.

Put on Your Thinking Cap!

What are some measures you can take to maintain catheter patency in the post-transplant patient?

Deficient Fluid Volume

Massive postoperative diuresis causes fluid volume deficit in some patients. With excessive fluid loss, the patient is at risk for electrolyte imbalances and decreased cardiac output. A thready pulse, low blood pressure, and poor tissue turgor suggest dehydration. Serum electrolyte studies are ordered to identify specific imbalances. Intravenous fluid orders must be carefully individualized.

Risk for Infection

Because the immunosuppressant drugs that protect the new kidney also inhibit the body's ability to resist pathogens, you must monitor the transplant recipient carefully for signs and symptoms of infection: fever, elevated white blood cell count, cough, and purulent wound drainage. Signs and symptoms may be very subtle despite a major infection. Use good hand washing and aseptic technique when working with the patient. Separate the patient from others who have infections. Teach the patient and family members the importance of protecting the patient from exposure to infections. Give prophylactic antibiotics as prescribed. The physician prescribes any restrictions on diet, fluids, and activity. Clarify and reinforce these orders. It is critical that the patient knows signs and symptoms of infection, rejection, and renal failure.

Ineffective Therapeutic Regimen Management

Ideally, patient teaching begins before the transplant so it can be reinforced after the procedure.

Anxiety

Anxiety may lessen as renal function improves, but the patient always lives with the possibility of rejection. It is helpful for the patient to talk about feelings and explore ways to deal with them. Some patients find comfort in a support group of people who have had similar experiences or in spiritual resources. Others may need referral to a mental health professional to help them deal constructively with their stress.

THE KIDNEY DONOR

In the excitement over the patient finally receiving a kidney, never forget the role of the donor at this dramatic time. Physical care of the donor is similar to that described earlier for nephrectomy. The nephrectomy may be conventional or laparoscopic. Pain is considerably worse with the conventional approach, so be sure to provide good pain control measures. With the conventional approach, the patient will be hospitalized 4 to 7 days and return to work in 6 to 8 weeks. With the laparoscopic approach, the donor is hospitalized 2 to 4 days and can return to work in 4 to 6 weeks.

Emotionally, the donor usually feels very good about the experience because of the value of the kidney to the recipient. If the kidney fails, however, the donor may be very disappointed. Be sensitive to the emotional needs of the donor.

Key Points

- The urinary system eliminates metabolic wastes in urine, stimulates red blood cell production, and maintains fluid, electrolyte, and acid-base balance.
- Age-related changes in the urinary system include reduced ability to concentrate or dilute urine, nocturia, and decreased bladder capacity.
- Untreated or repeated urinary tract infections can result in renal scarring and lead to renal failure.
- Inflammatory conditions of the urinary tract include cystitis (bladder inflammation), urethritis (urethral inflammation), glomerulonephritis (glomerular inflammation), and pyelonephritis (inflammation of the renal pelvis).
- Risk factors for urinary tract infection include prolonged immobility, renal calculi, urinary diversion, and indwelling urinary catheters.
- Urinary tract infections are treated with antibiotics, urinary tract antiseptics, analgesics, and antispasmodics.
- Acute glomerulonephritis commonly follows a streptococcal respiratory infection and results in an immune response that scars the glomeruli.
- Patients with renal disorders are at risk for excess fluid volume, hypertension, and heart failure.
- Management of renal disorders requires attention to pain management, fluid balance, activity intolerance, and patient education.
- Urinary obstructions anywhere in the urinary tract can lead to hydronephrosis and kidney damage.
- Urinary calculi (stones) form in the urinary tract and may move through the tract with the flow of urine.
- Although most calculi pass spontaneously, some require surgical removal or disintegration by lithotripsy.
- Nursing care of the patient with renal calculi focuses on Acute Pain, Impaired Urinary Elimination, Risk for Deficient Fluid Volume, and Ineffective Therapeutic Regimen Management.
- Complications of urinary tract surgery include urinary tract and wound infection, atelectasis, paralytic ileus, and hemorrhage.
- Renal tumors are often large before they are detected because early symptoms are subtle.
- Cystectomy (bladder removal) requires urine to be diverted to an alternate drainage or collection system. Types of urinary diversion used now are ileal and sigmoid conduits, ureterostomy, and nephrostomy.
- Nursing care after bladder surgery focuses on pain management, unobstructed urine flow, skin integrity, bowel function, and self-care.

Patient Teaching Plan

Kidney Transplant

- Take your medication exactly as prescribed to control rejection and prevent other complications.
- Report adverse effects (specific to your drugs) to the physician.
- Follow the diet prescribed by your physician.
- Avoid people with infections because your resistance is lowered.
- Increase activity as allowed by your physician.
- Immediately notify your physician of signs and symptoms of infection (fever, cough, increasing wound drainage) and rejection (fever, pain in kidney area).

- Renal failure can result from hypotension, toxins, infections, impaired blood flow, trauma, and obstructions.
- The four stages of acute renal failure are onset, oliguria, diuresis, and recovery.
- Management of acute renal failure emphasizes fluid and dietary restrictions, restoration of fluid balance, waste elimination, and maintenance of cardiac output.
- When 90% to 95% of kidney function is lost, the patient is considered to have chronic kidney disease.
- Effects of chronic kidney disease include excess fluid volume, hyperkalemia, hypocalcemia, hyperuricemia, and anemia.
- Dialysis uses a semipermeable membrane to draw excess water, electrolytes, and wastes into a special solution called *dialysate*.

- Renal transplantation is the only alternative to dialysis for the patient with end-stage renal disease.
- Signs and symptoms of rejection of a transplanted kidney are fever, increased blood pressure, and pain over the location of the new kidney.

 Go to your Companion CD-ROM for a Pharmacology Tutorial, Audio Glossary, and 3-D animations.

evolve Be sure to visit the companion Evolve site at http://evolve.elsevier.com/Linton/ for WebLinks and additional online resources.

REVIEW QUESTIONS *Choose the best answer.*

1. An 88-year-old female was seen in the clinic three times last year for kidney infections. Age-related factors that may be contributing to these frequent infections include the following:
   1. Relaxed pelvic muscles related to lack of estrogen
   2. Renal blood flow and glomerular filtration decline
   3. Decreased creatinine clearance by the kidneys
   4. Weak, ineffective contraction of trigonal muscles

2. A patient tells you she has a painful, burning sensation during urination. You should record this symptom as:
   1. Dysuria
   2. Dysphagia
   3. Dysmenorrhea
   4. Dystrophy

3. The first time a patient voids after cystoscopy, you notice the urine is pink-tinged. You should:
   1. Promptly notify the physician
   2. Encourage additional fluids
   3. Recognize that this is normal
   4. Assess the patient's blood pressure

4. The primary cause of health care–associated infections is:
   1. Wound contamination
   2. Catheterization
   3. Tracheal suctioning
   4. Diagnostic procedures

5. Patient teaching to reduce the risk of cystitis in women should include the following:
   1. Tub baths are recommended over showers
   2. Drink a glass of water before and after intercourse
   3. Cleanse the perineum from back to front after elimination
   4. Wear synthetic undergarments that serve as a barrier to moisture

6. Glomerulonephritis is caused by:
   1. Bacteria
   2. Viruses
   3. Urinary obstruction
   4. Immunologic processes

7. A procedure that uses sound, laser, or dry shock wave energy to break up renal calculi is:
   1. Lithotripsy
   2. Lithotomy
   3. Nephrolithotomy
   4. Ureterolithotomy

8. The maximum amount of fluid that can be used to irrigate a nephrostomy tube is:
   1. 1 mL
   2. 5 mL
   3. 30 mL
   4. 100 mL

9. After a nephrectomy, a patient's urine output was 25 mL in the past hour. You should:
   1. Have the patient change positions
   2. Give the patient an 8-ounce glass of water every 2 hours
   3. Increase the flow rate of the patient's intravenous fluids
   4. Notify the physician that the patient's urine output is too low

10. A patient in chronic kidney disease becomes confused. He complains of nausea, abdominal cramps, and lack of sensation in his legs. His heart rhythm is irregular. You should suspect:
    1. Increased blood urea nitrogen
    2. Hyperkalemia
    3. Metabolic acidosis
    4. Hypocalcemia

Connective Tissue Disorders

evolve http://evolve.elsevier.com/Linton/

Objectives

After reading and studying this chapter, you should be able to:

1. Define connective tissue.
2. Describe the function of connective tissue.
3. Describe the characteristics and prevalence of connective tissue diseases.
4. Describe the diagnostic tests and procedures used for assessing connective tissue diseases.
5. Discuss the drugs used to treat connective tissue diseases.
6. Describe the pathophysiology and treatment of osteoarthritis (degenerative joint disease), rheumatoid arthritis, osteoporosis, gout, progressive systemic sclerosis, polymyositis, bursitis, carpal tunnel syndrome, ankylosing spondylitis, polymyalgia rheumatica, Reiter's syndrome, Behçet's syndrome, and Sjögren's syndrome.
7. Identify the data to be collected in the nursing assessment of a patient with a connective tissue disorder.
8. Assist in developing a nursing care plan for a patient whose life has been affected by a connective tissue disease.

Key Terms

Be sure to check out the bonus material on the Companion CD-ROM, including selected audio pronunciations.

ankylosis (ăng-kĭ-LŌ-sĭs, p. 900)
arthroplasty (ĂR-thrō-plăs-tē, p. 894)
Bouchard nodes (boo-SHĂR, [Fig. 41-2, p. 894])
crepitus (KRĔP-ĭ-tŭs, p. 885)
goniometer (gō-nē-ŎM-ĕ-tĕr, p. 885)
Heberden nodes (HĔ-bĕr-dĕnz, [Fig. 41-2, p. 894])
hyperuricemia (hī-pĕr-ŭr-ĭ-SĒ-mē-ă, p. 906)
intra-articular (ĭn-tră-ăr-TĬK-ū-lăr, p. 894)
rheumatoid nodule (ROO-mă-toyd NŎD-ūl, p. 900)
tophi (TŌ-fī, p. 906)
vasculitis (văs-kū-LĪ-tĭs, p. 901)

More than 66 million people in the United States have arthritis or chronic joint symptoms. Often called *rheumatoid disorders*, these conditions affect women more frequently than men but have no particular racial prevalence. Most are chronic and are characterized by alternating exacerbations and remissions, with progressive deterioration. Many have no known cause or cure. Rheumatoid disorders challenge the spirit and body of the patient. They can dramatically alter the patient's lifestyle, self-image, employability, and hope for the future.

A number of the conditions discussed in this chapter are classified as autoimmune disorders. They are included here because their primary effects are on connective tissue. For a thorough explanation of autoimmunity, see Chapter 33.

ANATOMY AND PHYSIOLOGY OF CONNECTIVE TISSUES

Connective tissues bind structures together, providing support for individual organs and a framework for the body as a whole. They also store fat, transport substances, provide protection, and play a role in repair of damaged tissue. The types of connective tissue are loose (areolar, adipose, reticular), dense (tendons, fascia, dermis, gastrointestinal tract submucosa, fibrous joint capsules), elastic (aortic walls, vocal cords, parts of trachea and bronchi, some ligaments), hematopoietic (blood), and strong supportive (cartilage, bone, ligaments).

This chapter is concerned primarily with disorders that affect bone, cartilage, ligaments, and tendons. Although selected autoimmune disorders that significantly affect the musculoskeletal system are included in this chapter, see Chapter 33 for a detailed discussion of autoimmune disorders. Blood disorders are addressed in Chapter 32, and skin disorders other than scleroderma are discussed in Chapter 50.

BONE

Bone is the hard tissue that makes up most of the skeletal system. The functions of the bones are support, protection, movement, storage of calcium and other ions, and manufacture of blood cells.

CARTILAGE

Cartilage is a specialized fibrous connective tissue. It provides firm but flexible support for the embryonic skeleton and part of the adult skeleton. Cartilage differs from bone in that its matrix has the consistency of a firm plastic or gristlelike gel. Cartilage cells are called *chondrocytes* and are located in tiny spaces that are distributed throughout the matrix.

LIGAMENTS

Ligaments are strong and flexible fibrous bands of connective tissue that connect bones and cartilage and support muscles. Yellow ligaments and white ligaments have distinctively different functions. Yellow ligaments, located in the vertebral column, are elastic and allow for stretching. White ligaments, found in the knee, do not stretch but provide stability.

TENDONS

Tendons are composed of very strong and dense fibrous connective tissue. They are in the shape of heavy cords and anchor muscles firmly to bones. One of the most prominent tendons is the Achilles tendon, which can be felt at the back of the ankle just above the heel.

JOINT STRUCTURE AND FUNCTION

Connective tissue disorders are often manifested as joint disorders because joint mobility depends on functional connective tissue. A joint is the site at which two or more bones of the body are joined. Joints permit motion and flexibility of the rigid skeleton. The only bone in the human body that does not articulate with at least one other bone is the hyoid bone, to which the tongue is attached.

Classified on the basis of the extent of movement, joints include synarthroses (fixed joints), amphiarthroses (slightly movable joints), and diarthroses (freely movable joints). Synarthroses, such as those in the skull, allow no movement at all. An example of a slightly movable joint, an amphiarthrosis, is the juncture of the ulna and radius in the forearm. Diarthroses, such as those in the elbows, shoulders, fingers, hips, and knees, allow considerable movement. Diarthroses are sometimes called *synovial joints.* They are encased in a fibrous capsule made of strong cartilage and lined with synovial membrane.

The synovial membrane is very smooth, thus permitting structures to move without friction. Ligaments are tough fibrous cords that bind the capsule. A smooth layer of cartilage also covers the ends of the bones, where it serves as a type of shock absorber. Synovial fluid fills and lubricates the space in the middle of the joint. Bursae are sacs of synovial fluid found in joints that also promote smooth articulation of joint structures. The bursae permit tendons to slide easily with movement of the bones.

AGE-RELATED CHANGES

Age-related changes in connective tissue can significantly impact function. There is a loss of bone mass and bone strength. The progressive loss of bone density during later adult life accounts for the decline in bone strength. Significant bone loss, called *osteoporosis,* is more common in women but affects men as well. These changes put the older patient at risk for fractures.

Age-related joint changes are related primarily to the changes in cartilage. With age, cartilage gradually loses elasticity and then becomes soft and frayed. Water content decreases, and cartilage may ulcerate, leaving bony joint surfaces unprotected and promoting the growth of osteophytes (bony spurs). These joint changes result in pain and limited mobility and can contribute to a loss of independence.

NURSING ASSESSMENT OF CONNECTIVE TISSUE STRUCTURES

HEALTH HISTORY

The nursing assessment requires a detailed health history, because many of the signs and symptoms of connective tissue disorders are insidious. Also, patients with chronic conditions may come to accept their symptoms as a way of life and fail to report them to the nurse. Therefore it may be helpful to have a family member present to assist the patient as historian. The family member may provide a clearer picture of how the changes in health have evolved.

Chief Complaint and History of Present Illness

Determine why the patient is seeking health care. Complaints that suggest possible problems related to connective tissue disorders are aches, pain, joint swelling or stiffness, generalized weakness, a change in ability to work or to enjoy leisure activities, a change in appearance that is significant to the patient, and a change in ability to carry out activities of daily living.

Past Medical History

The past medical history provides information about the patient's prior state of health. Inquire about major childhood and adult illnesses, operations, and current medications and allergies. Ask whether there is a history of tuberculosis, poliomyelitis, diabetes mellitus, gout, arthritis, rickets, infection of bones or joints, autoimmune diseases, and neuromuscular disabilities. Record the dates of immunizations for polio and tetanus, because postpolio syndrome and tetanus are characterized by musculoskeletal symptoms.

Accidents and Injuries. Accidents and injuries, even in the distant past, may be significant because they could be related to the patient's current problem. For example, low back pain in the present may be the result of an injury sustained several years ago. Inquire about participation in sports and the type of work the patient has done. Many types of sports injuries result in osteoarthritis later in life.

Current Medications. Record the use of prescription and over-the-counter drugs. Self-medication is common with musculoskeletal pain, and patients may fail to report it unless specifically asked. Inquire about the use of alternative therapies, including herbal supplements and home remedies. Many herbal supplements interact with traditional medications and have significant side effects. List all medications prescribed previously, and describe their effectiveness. Note any problems associated with current medication and whether the patient thinks the medication is effective. Record any allergies.

Family History

Ask whether the patient or any relative has had osteoporosis, osteoarthritis, rheumatoid arthritis, gout, or scoliosis, because these conditions appear to have some genetic basis. Inquire about any history of other autoimmune diseases such as thyroid disorders.

Review of Systems

Collect data about each body system for significant symptoms. Ask about the patient's general health status to determine the patient's perception of well-being. Specifically, ask whether the patient has had fatigue, malaise, anorexia, weight loss, pain, stiffness, dysphagia, or dyspnea. With joint pain and stiffness, it is especially helpful to determine whether the symptoms are present on arising in the morning and how long they persist. Be aware that many cultures react differently to pain and disability; some may be stoic, whereas others are very expressive. The loss of ability to perform certain daily functions can have a significant impact on the role in the family and therefore cause emotional distress and frustration. For example, a husband crippled with arthritis who can no longer work to support his family will be greatly affected both physically and psychologically.

Functional Assessment

The following questions may be used to determine the patient's functional status and the significance of any changes to the patient:

- How does this problem affect the way you live?
- Have you had to change your everyday activities?
- How do you feel about any changes that you have had to make?
- What have you found helpful in adapting to these changes?
- How do you carry out the treatment program prescribed by your physician?
- Has your treatment plan been effective for you?
- What kind of support systems do you have at home?

PHYSICAL EXAMINATION

The physical examination begins with measurement of the patient's vital signs and height and weight. Be aware that many patients with arthritis have limited physical abilities to stand, step up, or get onto an examination table. A scale-chair is very useful for these patients. Compare findings with the patient's norms, if available. Significant data include fever, tachycardia, tachypnea, weight loss, and loss of height.

Inspect the skin for color, rashes, lesions, scars, or any signs of injuries. Palpate the skin for warmth, edema, and moisture. Palpate lymph nodes for enlargement and tenderness. Inspect joints for swelling and deformity and palpate for warmth, swelling, and tenderness. Assess joint pain and range of motion by asking the patient to move each extremity through the normal range of motion. Be very careful not to extend joints beyond their range/point of comfort. Inflamed joints are extremely sensitive to movement and pressure. During the movement, watch for signs of pain and listen for the crackling sound called **crepitus.** A more precise measurement of joint motion may be done by the physician or other advanced health care provider by using an instrument called a **goniometer,** which measures the range of movement of the joints. Measurement of limb length and muscle strength also may be done. Nursing assessment of the patient with a connective tissue disorder is outlined in Box 41-1.

DIAGNOSTIC TESTS AND PROCEDURES

Procedures used to diagnose connective tissue diseases are mainly laboratory studies of blood and urine and radiologic imaging studies of the bones and joints.

Routine blood studies that are useful in diagnosing connective tissue disorders include a complete blood cell count (CBC), the erythrocyte sedimentation rate (ESR), and C-reactive protein (CRP) determination. These studies help determine whether a disorder is inflammatory or noninflammatory. Other blood studies are the Venereal Disease Research Laboratory (VDRL), rheumatoid factor (RF), creatinine, and antinuclear antibody (ANA) tests. Urine may be tested for creatinine and uric acid levels. Fluids aspirated from joints may be studied to detect uric acid crystals or white blood cells. Most laboratory tests are not diagnostic for a single condition—that is, many factors could cause measures of inflammation to increase. The physician may rely on multiple diagnostic procedures along with the health history and physical examination to reach a diagnosis.

Radiologic imaging studies include radiography, ultrasonography, arthrography, nuclear scintigraphy, magnetic resonance imaging, diskography, tomography, and computed tomography. Other useful measures are biopsy and arthroscopy. The Diagnostic Tests and Procedures table on pp. 887 to 889 summarizes commonly used diagnostic studies and related nursing care. Agency procedure manuals will provide more specific preparation and postprocedure care.

Box 41-1 | ASSESSMENT of the Patient with a Connective Tissue Disorder

Health History

Present Illness:
Changes in movement, activities of daily living; areas of pain, swelling, or tenderness, fatigue

Past Medical History:
Tuberculosis, poliomyelitis, diabetes mellitus, gout, arthritis, rickets, neuromuscular disabilities

Family History:
Rheumatoid arthritis, degenerative arthritis (need for joint replacement surgery), gout, scoliosis, other autoimmune disorders

Review of Systems:
Pain or swelling in joints, limitation of movement, weakness, malaise, change in general appearance of skin

Functional Assessment:
Past or recent injuries due to accidents or falls, use of assistive devices

Physical Examination

General Survey:
Posture, balance, gait, skin condition

Joints:
Warmth, redness, swelling, tenderness, nodules, range of motion, crepitus, function of hands

Skin:
Color, scars, bruising, warmth, swelling, nodules

Upper Extremities:
Symmetry, swelling, tenderness, pain, range of motion, posture

Lower Extremities:
Movement of hips, knees, and ankles; pain; skin condition

COMMON THERAPEUTIC MEASURES

Management of the patient with a connective tissue disorder often requires the services of a team that includes the patient, nurse, physician, social worker, physical therapist, and occupational therapist. The goals of therapy are to reduce inflammation and pain and to promote adaptation to the condition. Therapeutic measures may include physical and occupational therapy, modification of activities of daily living, patient education and support, drug therapy, and surgical intervention. Although none of these measures is curative, they can greatly enhance the patient's function and quality of life.

PHYSICAL AND OCCUPATIONAL THERAPY

Physical therapy employs exercise and positioning to help preserve functional capability and minimize disability. For many patients, braces and splints will be ordered to help support inflamed joints, protect from further injury, and relieve discomfort. Occupational therapy assists the patient in making adaptations in work and personal life that allow maximal possible function.

EDUCATION AND SUPPORT

Education emphasizes the treatment plan and how it will benefit the patient. Team members must be sensitive to the inconvenience and discomfort the disease has caused and must also help the patient identify ways to cope with the condition. Patients and their families need information about community support groups that can offer encouragement, information, and resources. A patient's attitude toward the disease is very important in the successful treatment and management, and psychological support should be provided. Many research studies have shown the connection between a patient's positive attitude and a successful outcome with chronic diseases.

DRUG THERAPY

Drug therapy for connective tissue disorders has traditionally included glucocorticoids and nonsteroidal anti-inflammatory drugs (NSAIDs) to reduce inflammation, detailed in the Drug Therapy table on pp. 890 to 892. When glucocorticoids are indicated, occasional local injections are preferred over systemic therapy. For many patients already on NSAIDs, acetaminophen is often prescribed as a safe analgesic. Other less-safe drugs are gold salts, azathioprine, penicillamine, and cyclosporine.

Recent advances in the treatment of various connective tissue diseases, including rheumatoid arthritis and osteoarthritis, include the development of biologic response modifiers (BRMs), disease-modifying antirheumatic drugs (DMARDs), and cyclooxygenase-2 (Cox-2) inhibitors. BRMs target certain features of the immune system specifically involved in inflammatory disease. Two new BRM drugs are etanercept (Enbrel) and infliximab (Remicade). They work by blocking the action of tumor necrosis factor (TNF), a chemical involved in inflammation.

DMARDs may retard the progression of some diseases. They include leflunomide (Arava), minocycline (Minocin), methotrexate, hydroxychloroquine, and sulfasalazine.

The Cox-2 inhibitors work much like older NSAIDs but are less likely to cause stomach ulcers and bleeding. The first two drugs developed in this new category are celecoxib (Celebrex) and rofecoxib (Vioxx). However, in 2004 Vioxx was voluntarily recalled by its manufacturer, Merck, because of concerns that the drug might increase the risk of heart attack and stroke.

Text continued on p. 893.

DIAGNOSTIC TESTS and PROCEDURES Connective Tissue Disorders

COMMON NURSING IMPLICATIONS:
Always tell the patient what to expect before, during, and after the test/procedure. When blood samples will be needed, inform the patient that blood will be drawn and whether fasting is required.

TEST/PURPOSE	PATIENT PREPARATION	POSTPROCEDURE NURSING CARE
BLOOD STUDIES		
Antinuclear Antibodies (ANA) Positive in SLE, RA, systemic sclerosis, Raynaud's disease, Sjögren's syndrome, necrotizing arteritis.	Fast 8 hr before test.	Apply pressure to venipuncture site. Assess site for bleeding.
C-Reactive Protein Detects active inflammation as in RA, disseminated lupus erythematosus.	Restrict food and fluids for 4 hr.	Apply pressure to venipuncture site. Assess site for bleeding.
Creatinine Assesses renal function. Increased with SLE, PSS, polyarteritis.	Fasting *not* required.	Apply pressure to venipuncture site. Assess site for bleeding.
Erythrocyte Sedimentation Rate (ESR) Determines presence of inflammation. Increased with RA, rheumatic fever. Decreased with osteoarthritis.	Fasting *not* required.	Apply pressure to venipuncture site. Assess site for bleeding.
Red Blood Cell (RBC) Count Detects and differentiates blood dyscrasias. Decreased in RA, SLE.	Fasting *not* required.	Apply pressure to venipuncture site. Assess site for bleeding.
Rheumatoid Factor (RF) Detects antibodies often present with RA.	Fasting *not* required.	Apply pressure to venipuncture site. Assess site for bleeding.
Venereal Disease Research Laboratory (VDRL) Test Measures antibodies to syphilis. Sometimes decreased in SLE.	Fasting *not* required.	Apply pressure to venipuncture site. Assess site for bleeding.
White Blood Cell (WBC) Count Increased in infection, tissue necrosis, inflammation; may decrease in SLE.	Fasting *not* required.	Apply pressure to venipuncture site. Assess site for bleeding.
URINE STUDIES		
24-Hour Urine for Creatinine Measures renal function and status of muscle diseases.	Instruct the patient to collect a 24-hr urine specimen. Discard the first morning specimen. Save rest of urine voided over 24-hr period in a clean, refrigerated 3-L container with or without preservative. Include urine voided at end of 24-hr period. Fasting *not* required.	None.
Urinary Uric Acid (24-Hr Collection) Measures uric acid metabolism; increased in gout, liver disease, chronic myelogenous leukemia, fever.	Requires 24-hr urine specimen (as described above). Fasting *not* required.	None.
RADIOLOGIC STUDIES		
Arthrography Uses contrast medium to show soft-tissue joint structures.	Question patient about allergy to contrast agent, seafood, iodine. If yes, notify radiologist. Tell patient that needle insertion may cause discomfort. May cause swelling that lasts several days.	Assess and document discomfort, swelling. Instruct patient to avoid strenuous activity 12-24 hr after test. Joint may be wrapped.

PSS, Progressive systemic sclerosis; *RA,* rheumatoid arthritis; *SLE,* systemic lupus erythematosus.

Continued

DIAGNOSTIC TESTS and PROCEDURES Connective Tissue Disorders—cont'd

TEST/PURPOSE	PATIENT PREPARATION	POSTPROCEDURE NURSING CARE
Computed Tomography (CT) Detects tumors, some spinal fractures.	Tell patient that procedure may be lengthy (up to 30 min per body part). Patient lies on stretcher while a machine scans area being studied.	None.
Diskography Visualizes vertebral disk after contrast medium injected into disk.	Same as for arthrography.	Same as for arthrography.
Magnetic Resonance Imaging (MRI) Visualizes soft tissue. May detect avascular necrosis, disk disease, tumors, osteomyelitis, torn ligaments.	Tell patient that procedure is painless; must lie still for 30 min or more. Some equipment has videos that patient can view to reduce anxiety. Ask whether patient is claustrophobic. Give sedation if ordered for agitated or anxious patients. Remove any metallic objects such as jewelry. Inquire whether patient has any implanted devices such as cardiac pacemaker or intracranial aneurysm clips, and notify radiologist. Procedure is contraindicated with some implants. Metal may not be a problem with some newer equipment.	No special postprocedure care. Safety precautions if sedated.
Nuclear Scintigraphy (Bone Scan) Detects bone malignancies, osteoporosis, osteomyelitis, some fractures.	Contraindicated during pregnancy. Tell patient that a small amount of radioactive material will be injected intravenously; then a scanner will move slowly back and forth over the body as the patient lies on a stretcher. May take 1 hr. Procedure is painless except for venipuncture. Radioactive isotopes are not harmful except to fetus. Empty bladder immediately before procedure for comfort and to prevent blocked view of pelvis.	No special precaution required for handling urine or stool.
Radiography Shows density, texture, and alignments of bones; reveals soft tissue involvement.	Tell patient to expect to lie on an x-ray table or to stand next to a special device while films are taken. Remove any radiopaque objects (jewelry, etc.) that can interfere with results. Advise radiology of patient's physical limitations r/t moving, turning, climbing.	None.
Tomography Provides details of structures otherwise hidden by bone.	Requires lying in a cylindric scanner; assess for claustrophobia and inform radiologist.	None.
Ultrasonography Reveals masses or fluid in soft tissue.	None.	None.

SPECIAL TESTS

Arthroscopy

A surgical procedure to visualize a joint cavity and structure and to obtain fluid and/or tissue for study.

Inform patient that procedure is performed in operating room under local or general anesthesia.

The patient will have a sterile dressing applied to the wound, which will also be wrapped with compression dressing. Report any drainage of blood or fluid. Instruct patient to limit activity for a few days.

Joint Aspiration

Examination of fluid taken from a joint to diagnose inflammation.

Procedure is usually done at bedside or in examination room. Tell patient that a local anesthetic agent is used to minimize discomfort.

Apply pressure dressing to joint. Instruct patient to rest joint for 8-24 hr. Record on patient's chart and report to physician or nurse supervisor any leakage of blood or fluid. Apply pressure dressing to affected area and keep immobilized for 12-24 hr.

Bone Densitometry (DEXA and DPA Absorptiometry)

Determines bone mineral content and density to detect osteoporosis.

No special advance preparation. Patient will need to remove any metallic objects (zippers, belts, etc.) in the area being examined. Explain that the patient will be positioned on an imaging table and an instrument will pass over the pelvic and hip region. A computer will record density measurements. Radiation exposure is minimal. The procedure is painless.

No special care needed.

Muscle Biopsy

A sample of muscle tissue is taken to detect inflammation reaction, as in polymyositis or myopathic disease.

May be performed under local or general anesthesia.

Apply pressure dressing to affected area and keep immobilized for 12-24 hr.

Skin Biopsy

Studies excised skin to confirm inflammatory connective tissue diseases such as SLE and PSS.

Tell patient a local anesthetic will be injected; there may be slight discomfort when skin sample is obtained.

Keep biopsy site clean and dry with small adhesive bandage until scab develops. Patients who are taking aspirin or NSAIDs are at risk for bleeding and/or bruising at the biopsy site.

NOTE: See agency laboratory manual for specific preparation and norms. Results vary with different types of tests and may be reported in different units of measurement. *NSAID,* Nonsteroidal anti-inflammatory drug; *PSS,* progressive systemic sclerosis; *SLE,* systemic lupus erythematosus.

DRUG THERAPY | *Drugs Used to Treat Connective Tissue Disorders*

DRUG	USE/ACTION	SIDE EFFECTS	NURSING INTERVENTIONS
FIRST-GENERATION NONSTEROIDAL ANTI-INFLAMMATORY DRUGS (NSAIDs)			
Aspirin Diclofenac sodium (Voltaren) Ibuprofen (Motrin, Rufen) Naproxen (Naprosyn) Nabumetone (Relafen)	Analgesic. Antipyretic. Anti-inflammatory (inhibits prostaglandin synthesis). Decreases pain and deformity. Inhibits platelet aggregation (clumping).	Gastrointestinal (GI) upset, GI bleeding may be silent in older adults. Ototoxicity. Bleeding because of anticoagulation. Some may cause drowsiness. Increased blood pressure because of fluid retention.	Instruct patient to take with food or to take enteric-coated aspirin and report ringing in ears (tinitus), abdominal pain, dark stools. Assess for bruising and bleeding. Caution patients not to take aspirin and NSAIDs concurrently and not to drive if drowsy.
SECOND-GENERATION NONSTEROIDAL ANTI-INFLAMMATORY DRUGS: COX-2 INHIBITORS			
Celecoxib (Celebrex)	Analgesic. Antipyretic. Anti-inflammatory (inhibits prostaglandin synthesis).	GI bleeding (less risk than first-generation NSAIDs), fatigue, dependent edema, nausea, increased blood pressure because of fluid retention. Dizziness. FDA is studying for possible increased risk of MI, CVA, and death.	Administer with food or full glass of water. Remain in upright position 15-30 min after taking. Safety precautions if dizzy. Do not confuse with Celexa (antidepressant) or Cerebyx (injectable fosphenytoin to treat seizures). Do not use with aspirin, alcohol, or acetaminophen concurrently.
INDOLE ANALOGUES			
Indomethacin (Indocin) Sulindac (Clinoril)	Analgesic. Anti-inflammatory (inhibits prostaglandin synthesis). Indicated for severe ankylosing spondylitis, painful shoulders.	Gastric bleeding, headaches, dizziness, psychiatric disturbances.	Administer with food. Report any signs of bleeding (tarry stools, hematemesis) to physician.
GLUCOCORTICOIDS			
Hydrocortisone (Cortef, Hydrocortone) Hydrocortisone sodium succinate (Solu-Cortef, cortisol) Cortisone acetate (Cortone) Prednisone (Deltasone) Prednisolone (Delta-Cortef)	Suppress normal immune response and inflammation. Used in inflammatory and allergic conditions.	Muscular weakness, nausea, anorexia, hypotension; sodium retention, hypokalemia; insomnia; nervousness; euphoria; rise in serum glucose. Osteoporosis. Increased susceptibility to infections.	Highest dose usually given in early morning; lowest dose given later in day to mimic normal secretion in body. Stress to patient need to adhere to prescribed schedule. Remember that glucocorticoids mask signs of infection. Observe for any unusual drainage, odors, and elevated temperatures. Must be tapered off rather than stopped abruptly.
DISEASE-MODIFYING ANTIRHEUMATIC DRUGS (DMARDS)			
Methotrexate (Folex)	Treats rheumatoid arthritis.	Anorexia, nausea, vomiting, diarrhea. Toxic effects on oral tissues, liver, lungs, bone marrow, skin, and kidneys. Hemorrhage; hair loss.	Monitor periodic mild immunosuppressant blood and urine studies to detect abnormalities because of toxicity. Encourage fluid intake. Tell patient to avoid trauma because of risk of bleeding; to avoid people with infections; and to report bruising, bleeding, or signs of infection promptly.

Drug	Action/Use	Adverse Effects	Nursing Considerations
Hydroxychloroquine sulfate (Plaquenil)	Basis of antirheumatic effects unknown; may suppress antigens that trigger hypersensitivity reactions.	Headache, nausea, vomiting, anorexia. Ocular toxicity. With prolonged therapy: bone marrow suppression, psychosis.	Ask about known allergy to drug. Tell patient to report visual or hearing disturbances promptly. Monitor complete blood cell count and liver function studies. Instruct patient to see an eye doctor while taking this drug.
Sulfasalazine (Azulfidine)	Antimicrobial, anti-inflammatory. Used to treat rheumatoid arthritis.	Anorexia, nausea, vomiting, headache, oligospermia. Toxic effects on bone marrow, liver, kidneys. Rarely: anaphylaxis.	Monitor liver and kidney function. Ensure urine output of at least 1500 mL/day. Assess for bruising, jaundice, fever, sore throat. Tell patient to avoid direct sunlight.
Leflunomide (Arava)	Treats active rheumatoid arthritis, retards structural damage. Slows disease progression.	Diarrhea, liver toxicity, hair loss. Teratogenic.	Monitor liver studies. Tell patient to report severe diarrhea. Known to cause fetal harm; women of childbearing age should avoid conception. Avoid alcohol consumption while on medication.
ANTIARTHRITIC, BIOLOGIC RESPONSE MODIFIERS			
Etanercept (Enbrel)	Used to treat severe rheumatoid arthritis in adults who do not respond to other DMARDs. Binds tumor necrosis factor, which is involved in immunity and inflammation.	Injection site reaction, abdominal pain, heartburn, headache, dizziness, upper respiratory infections, cough.	Reconstitute supplied diluent, add to powder, swirl to mix (do not shake), and administer immediately. Use only clear, colorless solution. Do not mix with other drugs. Administer SC in upper arm, abdomen, or thigh. Rotate sites. Check injection site for redness, itching. Caution in people with recurring infections or people at risk for infections.
Infliximab (Remicade)	A monoclonal antibody that neutralizes activity of tumor necrosis factor, which decreases inflammation. Used to treat RA, Crohn's disease.	Anaphylaxis, anemia, tachycardia, GI distress, skin rash, headache, dizziness, depression, upper respiratory infections, muscle aches, painful urination, chest pain, hypotension, hypertension.	Given IV q 1-2 months in combination with methotrexate. 2 hr infusion. Reconstitute and use immediately. Monitor for signs of infection, especially upper respiratory tract infections. Cannot be infused in IV line with other agents.
ANTIGOUT AGENTS			
Allopurinol (Zyloprim)	Inhibits synthesis of uric acid.	Drowsiness. Toxicity: maculopapular rash, fever, chills, joint pain. Rarely: bone marrow depression, nausea, diarrhea.	Tell patient to drink 8-10 glasses of fluid daily to maintain output of at least 2000 mL/day. Assess urine for abnormal characteristics. Safety precautions if drowsy. Tell patient it takes several weeks for full effects. Assess and record response.

CVA, Cerebrovascular accident; *FDA,* Food and Drug Administration; *IV,* intravenous; *MI,* myocardial infarction; *NSAIDs,* nonsteroidal anti-inflammatory drugs; *RA,* rheumatoid arthritis; *SC,* subcutaneous.

Continued

DRUG THERAPY *Drugs Used to Treat Connective Tissue Disorders—cont'd*

DRUG	USE/ACTION	SIDE EFFECTS	NURSING INTERVENTIONS
ANTIGOUT AGENTS—cont'd			
Probenecid (Benemid)	Increases urinary excretion of uric acid.	Headache, urinary frequency, GI distress. Rarely: anaphylaxis. Toxicity: maculopapular rash, fever, joint pain, leukopenia, GI distress. Urinary calculi (stones).	Assess allergies. Do not give with penicillin. Use caution with renal impairment. Encourage fluid intake to maintain output of at least 2000 mL/day. Tell patient it takes several weeks for full therapeutic effect.
BONE RESORPTION INHIBITORS			
Ibandronate sodium (Boniva)	Used to prevent and treat osteoporosis in postmenopausal women.	Abdominal pain, hypertension, dyspepsia, arthralgia, nausea, diarrhea.	Main advantage is monthly dosing. Instruct patient to take on empty stomach upon rising. Do not eat or drink anything and remain upright for at least 60 minutes after each dose. Does not replace the need for adequate calcium and vitamin D intake. Contraindicated with uncorrected hypocalcemia.
Alendronate sodium (Fosamax)	Increases bone mineral density by impairing bone resorption.	Abdominal pain, muscle pain, diarrhea, constipation, severe GI disturbances with overdose, hypocalcemia.	Take with 6-8 oz water on arising in AM, nothing else by mouth for 30 min. Patient should not lie down for 30 min after taking.
Calcitonin (Miacalcin)	Impairs bone resorption.	With injections: hypotension, flushing, nausea, vomiting, sweating. With oral form: constipation, edema.	Monitor for hypercalcemia (dry mouth, constipation, headache, depression, weakness). Take tablets with full glass of water ½ to 1 hr after meals. Not to be taken with other oral medications, alcohol, or foods with fiber. Patient must avoid excess tobacco use and caffeine.
Raloxifene (Evista)	Prevents bone loss and lowers cholesterol without stimulating endometrium. Used to prevent osteoporosis in postmenopausal women.	Frequent side effects: infection, flu syndrome, nausea, hot flashes, weight gain, joint pain, sinusitis, thrombosis.	Check for Homans' sign. Seek medical care for chest pain, dyspnea, changes in vision. Should not be taken during pregnancy, before menopause, or during periods of immobility.

SURGICAL TREATMENT

Surgical intervention may be indicated in some musculoskeletal disorders, such as degenerative joint disease and arthritis. Specific surgical interventions are discussed with the particular conditions.

A device used after some types of joint replacement surgery is the continuous passive motion (CPM) machine. This device moves the joints through a set range of motion at a set rate of movements per minute. The movement prevents formation of scar tissue and promotes flexibility of the new joint. The affected extremity may be placed in the CPM machine in the postanesthesia care unit or on the first postoperative day. The CPM machine is used for specific intervals, and the time and degree of flexion and extension are gradually increased. The part of the machine that cradles the limb is padded to prevent pressure or abrasions. Be sure the machine settings are correct as ordered and the limb is properly aligned. Keep the machine clean because it could be a possible source of contamination. Several types of CPM machines are illustrated in the Nursing Care After Total Joint Replacement section on p. 897.

DISORDERS OF CONNECTIVE TISSUE STRUCTURES

OSTEOARTHRITIS

Osteoarthritis is the most common form of arthritis. Although the condition is sometimes called *degenerative joint disease* (*DJD*), not all agree this term is appropriate. Osteoarthritis may be classified as *primary* or *secondary*, depending on the cause. In primary osteoarthritis, some unknown factor triggers the release of chemicals that break down joint cartilage. Osteoarthritis that occurs with aging is generally considered to be primary and may have a genetic basis. Secondary osteoarthritis may be associated with trauma, infection, congenital deformities, or corticosteroid therapy. The incidence of osteoarthritis increases with age, with persons older than 50 years most often affected. It has been estimated that more than 100,000 people in the United States are unable to walk independently to and from the bathroom because of osteoarthritis.

Osteoarthritis generally affects joints under pressure, especially the spine, fingers, knees, hips, and shoulders. People who are obese, who have poor posture, or who experience occupational stress are at greatest risk for the disease. The most common source of major disability is osteoarthritis of the knee.

 What Does Culture Have to Do with Osteoarthritis?

The sites affected most often by osteoarthritis vary with ethnic background. For example, osteoarthritis of the hips is more common among people who live in Japan and Saudi Arabia than among whites in the United States.

Pathophysiology

Osteoarthritis is characterized by the degeneration of articular cartilage with hypertrophy of the underlying and adjacent bone. Normally, the articular cartilage provides a smooth surface for one bone to glide over another (Fig. 41-1). The cartilage transfers the weight of one bone to another so the bones do not shatter. In osteoarthritis, deterioration of the articular cartilage means the shock-absorbing protection is gradually lost. New bone growth is stimulated by exposed bone surfaces, causing bone spurs to develop. Although osteoarthritis is generally classified as a noninflammatory condition, inflammation of the joint is common in advanced conditions due to tissue breakdown.

Signs and Symptoms

Many people with osteoarthritis have no symptoms, but others have pain ranging from mild to severe. The pain is what usually brings the patient to the physician. Pain is commonly associated with activity but relieved by rest. Along with pain in the affected joint, the patient with osteoarthritis may complain of stiffness, limitation of movement, mild tenderness, swelling, and deformity or enlargement of the joint (Fig. 41-2). Sometimes the symptoms subside for long periods of time and then return. The disease usually affects a single joint or only a few joints.

Medical Diagnosis

The diagnosis of osteoarthritis is usually based on the health history and radiographic studies. In the early

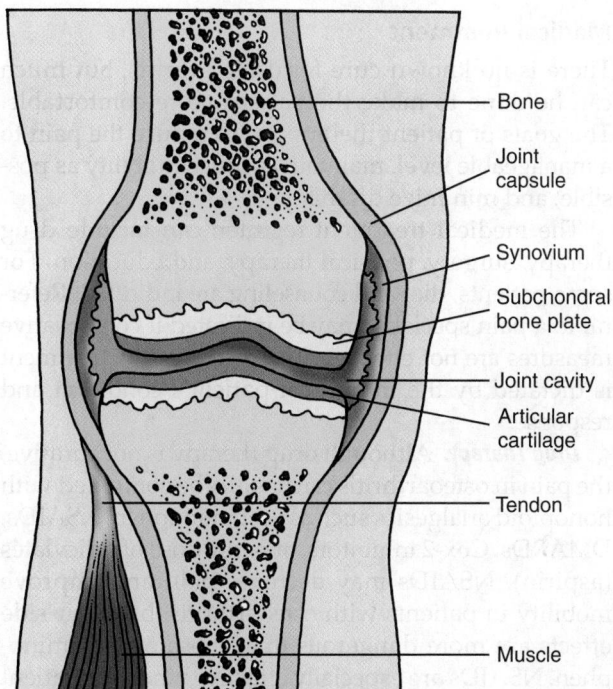

FIGURE **41-1** The structure of a diarthrodial joint. Synovium lines the joint capsule but does not extend into the articular cartilage.

FIGURE **41-2** Osteoarthritis (degenerative joint disease): Heberden nodes at the distal interphalangeal joints and Bouchard nodes at the proximal interphalangeal joints.

stages of the disease, the patient may have no symptoms, even though radiographs reveal classic joint changes. From radiographic evidence, 68% of women older than 65 years have osteoarthritis. The incidence is slightly lower for men of the same age. The extent of the disease process is not necessarily related to the severity of symptoms.

Because plain radiographs do not always reveal cartilage abnormalities, arthroscopy and magnetic resonance imaging may be employed as well. Synovial fluid may be aspirated to assess the presence of leukocytes. A normal ESR, negative RF assay, and synovial fluid with few or no leukocytes are expected. However, it is not unusual for a healthy older person to have a slightly elevated ESR and low titers of RF and ANA.

Medical Treatment

There is no known cure for osteoarthritis, but much can be done to make the patient more comfortable. The goals of patient therapy are to reduce the pain to a manageable level, maintain as much mobility as possible, and minimize disability.

The medical treatment regimen can include drug therapy, surgery, physical therapy, and education. For some patients, diet and counseling are indicated. Referral to a pain specialist may be indicated if conservative measures are not effective. The course of the treatment is dictated by the individual patient's condition and response.

Drug Therapy. Although drug therapy is not curative, the pain in osteoarthritis can usually be controlled with nonopioid analgesics such as acetaminophen, NSAIDs, DMARDs, Cox-2 inhibitors, or a low dose of salicylates (aspirin). NSAIDs may decrease pain and improve mobility in patients with osteoarthritis, but their side effects are more dangerous than those of acetaminophen. NSAIDs are especially effective when the patient shows signs of inflammation, such as warmth, swelling of joints, and erythema (redness). Similar to NSAIDs, indomethacin (Indocin) is effective in reducing inflam-

mation but may cause serious adverse effects (see the Drug Therapy Table on p. 890).

Salicylates are relatively inexpensive, but there is a risk of toxicity. The symptoms of salicylate intoxication in older adults may be atypical. Instead of the common gastrointestinal complaints or ototoxicity, the older person may exhibit confusion, slurring of speech, agitation, or seizures. Although systemic glucocorticoids are not indicated for the treatment of osteoarthritis, intra-articular injections can be beneficial. These injections can be given only three or four times a year, because the drug may cause breakdown of cartilage with frequent use.

A popular dietary supplement widely used for osteoarthritis is glucosamine often combined with chondroitin sulfate. In a recent study funded by the National Center for Complementary and Alternative Medicine (NCCAM), the combination therapy was effective in relieving moderate-to-severe-pain but not mild pain of osteoarthritis. NCCAM recommends additional research to confirm these results and to evaluate whether the supplement can slow the progression of osteoarthritis.

Pharmacology Capsule

Most NSAIDs and indomethacin (Indocin) can cause gastrointestinal irritation and bleeding.

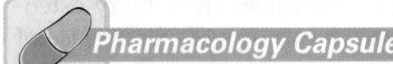

Pharmacology Capsule

Salicylate toxicity may be manifested by tinnitus or, in older adults, by confusion, agitation, slurred speech, or seizures.

Surgical Management. Surgical management is usually reserved for persons with persistent pain and disability despite conservative treatment. Arthroscopic surgery with irrigation and removal of cartilage debris may bring pain relief to some patients. However, this procedure is less common than in the past because there are questions about its value. The surgical treatment of choice for osteoarthritis of the hip or knee is total joint replacement (arthroplasty) (see the Nursing Care Plan: The Patient with a Total Hip Replacement on p. 896). The primary indication for total joint replacement is intractable pain that disrupts sleep and daily activities. Total hip or knee arthroplasty usually relieves pain and restores function to the joint (Fig. 41-3). Joint replacement was once reserved for persons older than 60 years because of concerns that the prosthesis would wear out. This concern is no longer valid, however, because most modern prostheses are predicted to last at least 20 years. A recent development is minimally invasive joint replacement surgery. This type of procedure

FIGURE **41-3** Total joint replacements. **A,** Hip. **B,** Knee. **C,** Shoulder. **D,** Elbow.

Consider the Alternative

Some people use glucosamine and chondroitin to treat osteoarthritis. Both are sold as dietary supplements and are under study to determine safety and effectiveness.

---

requires a much smaller incision than the traditional approach. Some minimally invasive joint replacement procedures are done in outpatient surgical settings.

Physical Therapy. The physical therapy program employs measures to improve range of motion and to maintain muscle mass and strength. Most patients, especially those with mild osteoarthritis, benefit from such a program. Isometric exercises are recommended over isotonic exercises because isotonic movements place greater strain on the joints. Exercise should be followed by periods of rest during the day. When the hips or knees are affected, some activity restriction may be advised. Using a cane to walk can reduce the stress on the affected joints.

Moist heat and occasionally cold can be used to help relieve pain. Heat also prepares the muscles and joints for exercise. Heat may be contraindicated, however, in patients who have had arthroplasty or have metal prostheses, because it may lead to deep thermal burns. Transcutaneous electrical nerve stimulation (TENS) devices are especially effective for treating back pain.

NURSING CARE *of the Patient with Osteoarthritis*

Assessment

The general nursing assessment of the patient with a connective tissue disorder is summarized in Box 41-1. When a patient has osteoarthritis, ask about joint pain or tenderness. Examine the joints for crepitus, enlarge-

ment, deformity, and decreased range of motion. Compare affected and unaffected joints to detect abnormalities. Gently support joints during the examination to minimize the patient's discomfort. Observe the patient's movements and gait, noting abnormalities. Record the location and severity of any problems. Determine how the disease affects the patient's mobility and ability to perform activities of daily living.

Nursing Diagnoses, Goals, and Outcome Criteria: Osteoarthritis

NURSING DIAGNOSES	GOALS AND OUTCOME CRITERIA
Chronic Pain with motion related to loss of smooth joint surfaces	Pain relief: patient states pain reduced or relieved, relaxed manner
Impaired Physical Mobility related to pain, limited range of motion	Improved functional mobility: patient accomplishes activities of daily living with minimal discomfort
Ineffective Coping related to pain, discomfort, disability	Effective coping: patient states is able to make adaptations to cope with condition, makes positive comments about ability to manage
Ineffective Therapeutic Regimen Management related to lack of understanding of osteoarthritis management and self-care	Patient manages disease appropriately: patient demonstrates self-care measures and describes prescribed regimen

Interventions
Chronic Pain

With good pain management, a patient can be more active and have a better quality of life. Administer prescribed analgesics and anti-inflammatory drugs, or instruct the patient in self-medication. Instruct the patient in heat or cold treatments as ordered. Monitor and record the effects of interventions designed to relieve pain. Be sure the physician is aware whether the pain relief measures are ineffective. Measures that protect the joint, discussed in the next section (Impaired Physical Mobility), also help reduce chronic pain. Although it is not unusual for hospitalized patients to have osteoarthritis, most patients manage their own symptoms at home. Therefore everyday management depends on good patient teaching.

Impaired Physical Mobility

Impaired physical mobility can significantly interfere with the patient's ability to carry out usual activities in the home or work setting. Modification of daily activities and joint protection measures can help maintain function. Recommend a regular program of exercise. Stress the importance of balancing rest and activity

---

NURSING CARE PLAN

The Patient with a Total Hip Replacement

ASSESSMENT

Health History: A 74-year-old homemaker has had osteoarthritis for 10 years, with progressive loss of function in both hips. She had a left total hip replacement (arthroplasty) 2 days ago. Her past medical history reveals no other major health problems except poor vision. She lives with her daughter and helps with household chores, which gives her some satisfaction. Postoperatively she is alert and participates in her exercises. The physical therapist assisted her out of bed this morning. She was somewhat weak but was able to walk a short distance.

Physical Examination: Vital signs: temperature, 98° F orally; pulse, 82; respiration, 16; blood pressure, 148/66 mm Hg; height, 5'9"; weight, 162 lb. She is positioned on her right side with an abductor cushion in place. Breath sounds are clear on auscultation. Abdomen is soft, and bowel sounds are present. There is no bladder distention and no redness over bony prominences on back and left side. Warmth, color, and peripheral pulses are symmetric in both legs. She has good sensation in affected leg. The dressing on the surgical incision is dry and intact.

Nursing Diagnosis	Goals and Outcome Criteria	Interventions
Ineffective tissue perfusion related to deep vein thrombosis, decreased mobility, and surgical trauma	The patient will have adequate circulation in the affected extremity, as evidenced by warmth, normal color, and palpable pulses.	Assess neurologic and circulatory status. Check vital signs at least q 4 hr. Report and record any abnormalities. Observe for excess swelling or bleeding at operative site. Assist with exercises as prescribed by physical or occupational therapist. Record and report any change in condition of skin at operative site and pressure areas.
Risk for Injury related to unsteady gait	The patient will experience no falls during hospitalization.	Assist patient in and out of bed. Place call bell within easy reach. Check frequently for patient's need to toilet and need for change of position. Provide assistive devices as ordered.
Risk for Injury related to subluxation (dislocation) of joint prosthesis because of improper position, movement, or activity	The patient will maintain proper body alignment and hip positioning and will not exhibit signs of prosthesis dislocation: sudden, severe pain; abnormal position.	Instruct patient to keep legs slightly abducted. May place pillows between legs to achieve abduction while supine and during turning. Turn only to unaffected side. Tell patient not to cross legs or put on own shoes, socks, or stockings for 2 months. Assess for pain and loss of function. Make home health referral if needed to facilitate transition to home setting.
Risk for Infection related to break in skin integrity from surgical hip replacement procedure	The patient will be free of infection during hospitalization, as evidenced by orientation to person, place, and time; normal body temperature, intact wound with decreasing redness, minimal edema, and no purulent drainage.	Encourage fluids and activity when appropriate. Observe for change in mental status or confusion, which may be first signs of infection in older adults. Keep in mind that previous administration of prednisone may mask symptoms of infection. Turn at least q 2 hr from back to unaffected side only. Use aseptic technique for wound care. Offer fluids at least q 2 hr.

? CRITICAL THINKING QUESTIONS

■ Describe at least two behaviors that could reflect a change in this patient's mental status?

■ What data would suggest the need for a home health referral?

to avoid becoming overly tired. The household may need to be reorganized to reduce demands on the patient. Everyday tasks like dressing and bathing may be affected by the disorder. If the patient's hands are affected, suggest clothing with Velcro closures rather than buttons, pants with an elastic waist, and slip-on shoes. Bathroom grab bars, a shower seat, and a raised toilet seat may promote independence and safety for the patient with poor hip mobility.

Ineffective Coping

Provide an opportunity for the patient to discuss concerns about osteoarthritis and its effects on lifestyle. Help the patient prioritize activities and plan how to

What Does Culture Have to Do with Chronic Illness?

How people react to chronic illness, disability, and dependence is related to their cultural values and beliefs. Consider the older Japanese-American patient who values family interdependence over independence, the Mexican-American patient who accepts illness as God's will, or the person of German heritage who faces pain stoically. Each of these may handle osteoarthritis differently. Nurses must consider these factors when planning patient care.

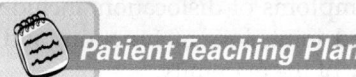

Osteoarthritis

To reduce joint strain and pain:
- Maintain proper posture and body alignment.
- Identify activities that take a long time to do or for which you need assistance.
- Plan activities when help is available or when time is not a major concern, and take periodic rest breaks.
- Wear splints or support devices that rest or relieve painful, unstable joints.
- Push or slide heavy objects rather than pull them.
- Wear shoes with low heels and shock absorbent soles to help decrease stress on the knee joints.
- Avoid stairs whenever possible.
- Sit rather than stand.
- Use high stools when sitting at a counter.
- Use higher chairs rather than low sofas.
- When arising from a chair, inch to the edge of the seat and then use the arm rests to push up from the seat.
- Use large-diameter pencils and pens, and use eating utensils with large, round handles.
- Self-medication:
  - Analgesics are usually more effective if taken routinely as prescribed, rather than only when you have pain.
  - Know the side effects of your medications and notify your physician if they occur (provide specific list).
- Resources: Arthritis Foundation (telephone: 1-800-283-7800; website: http://www.arthritis.org).

continue those activities that are most valued. Practical suggestions for managing the condition help the patient feel a sense of control and confidence in his or her ability to live with the condition.

Ineffective Therapeutic Regimen Management

Determine what the patient already knows about osteoarthritis, and correct any misconceptions. Design and implement an individualized teaching plan.

NURSING CARE *after Total Joint Replacement*

Joints that can be replaced include the elbow, shoulder, phalangeal finger joints, hip, knee, and ankle. Preoperative care prepares the patient for the surgical procedure and the postoperative period. Nurses and physical therapists may instruct the patient in postoperative exercises. Advise the patient and family of postoperative limitations and encourage planning to adapt the home and work environment as needed. General nursing care of the surgical patient is discussed in Chapter 17. This section describes the postoperative nursing care needs of the patient who has had a joint replacement. Surgical orders or protocols are usually very specific for each type of joint surgery and may vary somewhat among surgeons. Common postoperative measures for specific procedures are presented in Box 41-2.

Assessment

Routine postoperative care includes monitoring vital signs, level of consciousness, intake and output, respiratory and neurovascular status, urinary function, bowel elimination, wound condition, and comfort. After total joint replacement, it is especially important to monitor circulation and sensation in the affected extremity. Determine the need for assistance with activities of daily living.

Nursing Diagnoses, Goals, and Outcome Criteria: Total Joint Replacement, Postoperative	
Nursing Diagnoses	**Goals and Outcome Criteria**
Acute Pain related to tissue trauma	Pain relief: patient states pain reduced, relaxed expression
Risk for Injury related to improper alignment, dislocated prosthesis, weakness	Decreased risk for injury: patient maintains proper alignment of operative joint
Impaired Physical Mobility related to immobilization, pain, weakness	Physical mobility without complications of immobility: patient is increasingly mobile without excess fatigue or injury
Ineffective Tissue Perfusion related to trauma, hemorrhage, thrombi, compression of blood vessels	Normal circulation to affected extremity: symmetric color and warmth of extremities, palpable pulse in affected limb, negative Homans' sign

Continued

Box 41-2 | *Guidelines for Nursing Care After Replacement of Specific Joints*

Hip Replacement
1. Do not flex hip more than 90 degrees.
2. Avoid flexion, adduction, and internal rotation.
3. Place a large pillow between patient's legs when turning patient, when patient is supine, and when patient is lying on unaffected side.
4. Advise patient not to cross legs or feet and not to put on own shoes, socks, or stockings for 6 weeks to 2 months, as directed by surgeon.
5. Apply leg abductor splints as ordered.
6. Do not turn onto operative side unless specifically ordered by surgeon.
7. Have patient sit in a chair that has arms to facilitate rising without extreme hip flexion.
8. Arrange for a raised toilet seat to allow toileting without extreme hip flexion.
9. Permit weight bearing as ordered, depending on type of prosthesis used and whether cement was used.
10. Encourage patient to exercise unaffected extremities to maintain strength.

Knee Replacement
1. Encourage quadriceps-setting exercises and straight leg lifts beginning postoperative day 2-5, as ordered.
2. Use continuous passive motion machine as ordered; check alignment and settings.
3. Monitor weight bearing with walker or crutches as ordered.

Finger Joint Replacement
1. Instruct patient to elevate affected hand.
2. Assess sensation and warmth in affected fingers.
3. Instruct patient to use splints during sleep as ordered.
4. Reinforce exercises taught by physical therapist—must be continued for 10-12 weeks.
5. Advise patient not to lift heavy objects with affected hand.

Risk for Infection related to invasive procedure, prosthesis placement

Absence of infection: normal body temperature, decreasing wound redness, normal white blood cell count

Anxiety or **Fear** related to outcome of procedure

Reduced anxiety/fear: patient states anxiety/fear reduced, calm manner

Deficient Knowledge related to postoperative self-care

Patient understands self-care: patient describes and demonstrates self-care

Interventions

Acute Pain

To assist with assessment of the patient's pain, ask about pain location, nature, and severity. Surgical pain is expected, but the patient with osteoarthritis may also have pain in other joints. Administer analgesics as ordered, and document their effects. Reposition the patient as permitted by physician's orders. Use massage, relaxation techniques, imagery, or other strategies described in Chapter 15 to help the patient deal with the pain. Notify the surgeon of sudden, severe pain in the surgical area, which may signal prosthesis dislocation. Uncontrolled pain may make the patient reluctant to participate in rehabilitation measures. Administer analgesics 30 minutes to 1 hour before painful exercises to improve patient participation.

Risk for Injury

Prosthetic joints can become dislocated if they are not maintained in proper alignment. For example, after hip replacement, the affected leg must be kept in a position of abduction to prevent dislocation. Instruct patients not to cross the legs or flex the hip more than

90 degrees. Splints or traction may be used if ordered to maintain the desired position. Progressive exercises are usually prescribed and may be done by the physical therapist. As the patient's activity is increased, teach and reinforce precautions. Teach the patient to recognize signs and symptoms of dislocation, including pain in the affected joint, loss of function, and shortening or deformity of the extremity.

Impaired Physical Mobility

The degree of mobility impairment depends on which joints are affected as well as on the patient's general physical state. In general, early mobility is encouraged. When mobility is severely impaired, the patient is at risk for pulmonary and circulatory complications, urine retention, constipation, and skin breakdown. In addition, unused muscles weaken and unused joints stiffen. Reposition the patient as allowed, carefully inspecting pressure areas for redness caused by circulatory impairment. Coach and support the patient during coughing and deep-breathing exercises and use of the incentive spirometer. Auscultate for breath sounds to detect atelectasis or retained secretions. Inspect and palpate the abdomen for bladder or bowel distention. Administer intravenous fluids as ordered until the patient takes adequate oral fluids. Give stool softeners and laxatives as ordered.

The patient may have self-care deficits related to mobility impairments or restrictions. Identify activities the patient cannot do alone, and provide appropriate assistance. As the patient progresses, encourage increasing independence. Rehabilitation requires patient participation in the prescribed exercise program. The patient may need reassurance that the joint can and should be exercised (Fig. 41-4). A patient generally ex-

Correct positions

Less than 90°

90°

Incorrect position

More than 90°

FIGURE **41-4** Correct and incorrect sitting positions to prevent excessive hip flexion after a total hip replacement.

ercises better if pain control is adequate. A continuous passive motion machine may be used to reduce scar tissue formation and improve range of motion (Fig. 41-5). Some patients are discharged as soon as 3 days after joint replacement surgery. Individuals who may have difficulty at home may go to a rehabilitation facility initially.

Ineffective Tissue Perfusion

Deep vein thrombosis (DVT) is the most serious postoperative complication of hip and knee replacement surgery. Signs and symptoms of deep vein thrombosis include tenderness, swelling, redness, warmth, and firm, palpable blood vessels called *cords.* Although the value of a positive Homans' sign (pain behind the knee or in the calf when the foot is dorsiflexed) is in doubt, some data collection protocols may include it. Monitor body areas distal to the operative joint for circulatory adequacy by collecting data about skin temperature, color, and peripheral pulses. To reduce the risk of DVT

in the legs, antiembolic stockings or pneumatic compression devices may be ordered in addition to anticoagulants Check splints, dressings, and stockings to ensure that they are not restricting circulation. Do not place pillows or pads under the legs. Determine the specific exercises that may be done, based on the physician's orders and protocols. For example, after hip replacement, the patient should flex and extend the toes, feet, and ankles hourly to promote venous return.

The patient is at risk for hemorrhage after joint replacement. Check the dressings and wound drainage for increasing bleeding; monitor vital signs for tachycardia and hypotension; and observe for restlessness and anxiety. Inspect and measure wound drainage in suction devices at least every 8 hours. There is also a risk of fat embolus, which can produce signs of local or cerebral blood vessel occlusion: petechial (pinpoint) hemorrhage of the upper chest and conjunctiva, fat globules in the urine, headache, irritability, confusion, and loss of consciousness.

FIGURE **41-5** A continuous passive motion exerciser in use.

Pressure caused by edema or constrictive dressings can cause nerve damage, which may be manifested by anesthesia (lack of sensation) or paresthesia (abnormal sensation). Therefore monitor sensation distal to the joint and report symptoms of impairment to the surgeon. Check dressings, stockings, and splints to be sure they are not too tight.

Supervise ambulation until the patient is steady and clearly understands the limitations. Keep the environment free of clutter.

Risk for Infection

Monitor the patient's temperature for elevations that may indicate infections. Check the surgical wound for redness, swelling, warmth, and foul-smelling drainage. Use strict sterile technique when handling the wound, drains, or dressings. Keep wound dressings clean and dry. Administer antimicrobials as ordered. Instruct the patient in hand washing and wound care.

Anxiety or Fear

Total joint replacement is usually done after conservative treatments have failed to maintain joint mobility. The patient is typically hopeful but anxious about the outcome of the surgery. Tell the patient what to expect, explain procedures and equipment, and offer to answer questions. Responding promptly to the

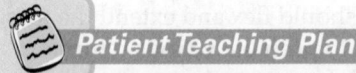
Patient Teaching Plan

Total Joint Replacement

Specifics of the teaching plan depend on which joint was replaced, but all patients need to know the following:
- What activities are permitted
- What activities are contraindicated
- Directions for drug therapy
- Wound care
- Signs and symptoms to be reported to the surgeon
- When to return for follow-up care
- Sources of assistance such as home health care

patient's needs and checking on him or her frequently are reassuring.

Deficient Knowledge

From admission through discharge, teach the patient about self-care, wound care, and signs of possible infection. Ensure understanding by having patients repeat back important information in their own words. Before teaching, assess for pain, fatigue, or communication barriers. Recognize cultural differences in lifestyle, diet, and care issues. Assist patients in planning for care at home, and involve family members in teaching sessions.

RHEUMATOID ARTHRITIS

Rheumatoid arthritis (RA) is a chronic, progressive inflammatory disease. Although it is a systemic disorder, the most notable effect of RA is on diarthroses (synovial joints). The disease has a peak onset in people 30 to 60 years of age and is more common in females than in males. It affects an estimated 1% to 3% of the population in the United States. The course of the disease is variable, ranging from minimal symptoms to severe debilitation.

Pathophysiology

There is no single known cause for RA, but it is considered an autoimmune disorder. Proposed causes include an unknown antigen in the patient's system, one or more viruses, genetic predisposition, and hormonal factors. While research to determine the exact cause continues, many recent discoveries have improved the lives of RA patients.

The onset of the disease is characterized by inflammation of the synovial tissue (the tissues that hold the lubricating fluid of the joints). In RA, the synovium thickens and fluid accumulates in the joint space. Vascular granulation tissue, called *pannus*, forms in the joint capsule and breaks down cartilage and bone. Fibrous tissue invades the pannus, converting it first to rigid scar tissue and finally to bony tissue. These changes result in ankylosis (loss of joint mobility) (Fig. 41-6).

Signs and Symptoms

The most common symptom of RA is pain in the affected joints that is aggravated by movement. Morning stiffness lasting more than 1 hour is almost always a feature of RA, unlike the stiffness of osteoarthritis, which is relieved within minutes. Other symptoms include weakness, easy fatigability, anorexia, weight loss, muscle aches and tenderness, and warmth and swelling of the affected joints. Joint changes are usually symmetric, meaning the same joints in both extremities are affected simultaneously. The distal interphalangeal and metacarpophalangeal joints are affected most often. The wrist, elbow, knee, and ankle are other possible areas affected. Rheumatoid nodules, which are

FIGURE **41-6** Phases in the progression of rheumatoid arthritis. **A,** Early phase: leukocytes increase in inflamed synovium. **B,** Pannus grows over the cartilage; bone edges erode; destruction of articular tissue. **C,** Destruction of bone.

subcutaneous nodules over bony prominences, also may be present (Fig. 41-7).

Any organ of the body may be affected by RA. If blood vessels are affected, they become inflamed, a condition called vasculitis. With vasculitis, the blood supply to body organs is impaired, with possible ischemia or infarction of affected organs. Ischemic lesions of the skin are brownish spots most often seen around the nail beds. Large lesions that tend to ulcerate may appear on the legs. Secondary effects on bone can cause osteoporosis, making the bones susceptible to fractures. The disease may produce inflammatory changes in the tissues of the heart, lungs, kidneys, and eyes. Pleural effusions and pulmonary fibrosis can lead to respiratory impairment or pulmonary hypertension and eventual heart failure.

Some patients with RA develop clusters of symptoms, including Sjögren's syndrome, Felty's syndrome, or Caplan's syndrome. Sjögren's syndrome is characterized by dryness of the mouth, eyes, and vagina. Felty's syndrome, characterized by liver and spleen enlargement and neutropenia, is less common. Caplan's syndrome, marked by rheumatoid nodules in the lungs, occurs most often in coal miners and asbestos workers.

Medical Diagnosis

The diagnosis of RA is based on the health history and physical examination, laboratory findings, and changes detected on radiographic and other imaging studies There is no single test to diagnose RA, but groups of tests and radiographic findings may help confirm the disorder. See the Diagnostic Tests and Procedures table on pp. 887 to 889 for common studies for connective tissue disorders.

Laboratory studies that are likely to be ordered include RF, ESR, and CRP. The presence of RF does not establish the diagnosis of RA; however, its presence may support a diagnosis in persons who have other signs and symptoms. The CRP level and ESR, although not specific, also help support the diagnosis in patients with other suggestive symptoms. Synovial fluid is analyzed for viscosity, white blood cells, and glucose and is subjected to a mucin clot test.

The primary purpose of radiographs is to detect changes brought about by RA and to determine the potential usefulness of disease-modifying drugs or surgery. Magnetic resonance imaging (MRI), bone scans, and dual energy x-ray absorptiometry (DEXA) scans provide more detailed information that may be used to monitor disease progression and response to treatment.

Medical Treatment

The treatment of RA involves combined efforts of medicine, nursing, physical therapy, occupational therapy, and social services. Treatment options include rest, drug therapy, physical and occupational therapy, and surgery.

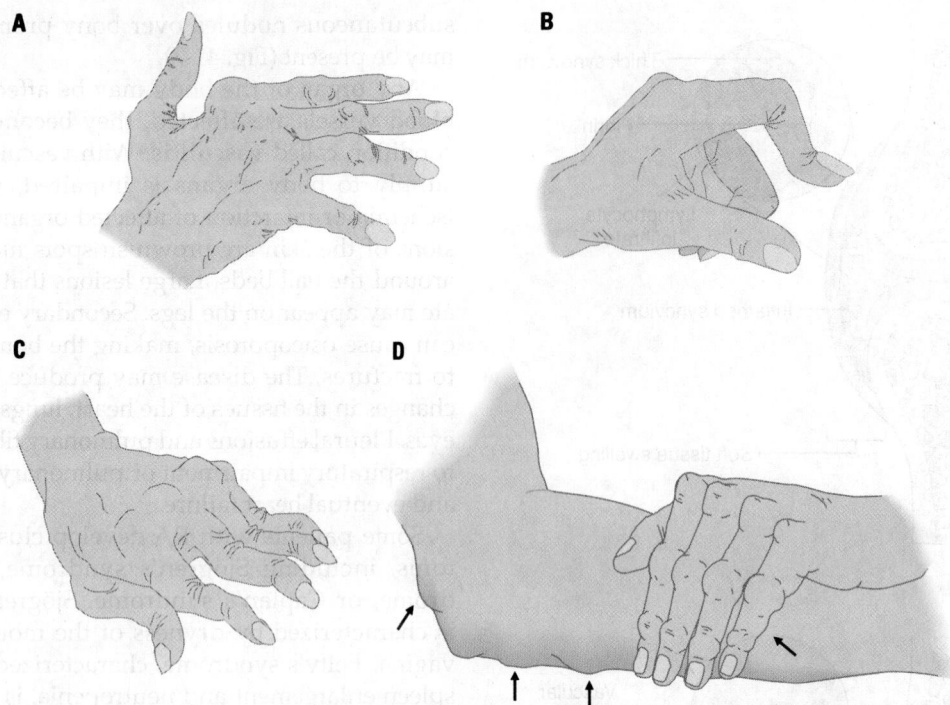

FIGURE **41-7** Four types of hand deformity characteristic of patients with rheumatoid arthritis. **A,** Ulnar drift. **B,** Boutonnière deformity. **C,** Swan-neck deformity. **D,** Rheumatoid nodules.

Drug therapy is aimed at controlling the local inflammatory process and providing symptomatic relief. Traditional agents used for symptomatic relief included aspirin and other NSAIDs for several months, with the addition of gold compounds, *d*-penicillamine, antimalarials, or sulfasalazine if needed. These agents could provide significant clinical improvement for weeks or even months at a time. More aggressive therapies now are used to relieve inflammation within a 3-month period and to prevent deformities. Combinations of NSAIDs, analgesics, COX-2 inhibitors, BRMs, and DMARDs are prescribed to meet the individual patient's therapeutic goal. Leflunomide (Arava) is a newer DMARD that reportedly can slow the progression of the disease. Etanercept (Enbrel) and infliximab (Remicade) are BRMs that have shown great success in rheumatoid patients, with some patients having a remission of the disease. Joint injections of corticosteroids can also be given two or three times a year and may provide significant symptomatic relief. Cytotoxic drugs such as methotrexate sodium (Folex) or cyclophosphamide (Cytoxan) are often very effective in the symptomatic treatment of RA. Systemic glucocorticoids, although effective in reducing the inflammatory process, are the last choice, owing to their adverse side effects (see the Drug Therapy table on p. 890 for details).

In addition to drug therapy, supportive treatments may be employed—including rest, splinting joints to reduce motion that aggravates the inflammation, orthotic devices to support deformed joints, and assistance in modifying activities of daily living. Afternoon rest periods may reduce the fatigue often felt late in the day. Temporary immobilization may be prescribed during acute episodes. However, long-term immobilization contributes to decreased joint flexibility. Types of exercise that may benefit the patient with RA include walking, cycling, aerobics, and aquatics. The physical therapist can recommend the exact exercise program for each patient. Some resources recommend heat treatments before exercise.

Surgical management of RA is reserved for those patients with severe pain and deformities. Among the options are arthroplasty (total joint replacement), synovectomy, tenosynovectomy, and arthrodesis (joint fusion). The most successful procedures are those performed on the knees and hips (see p. 894 in the Osteoarthritis section).

NURSING CARE *of the Patient with Rheumatoid Arthritis*

Assessment

The general assessment of the patient with a connective tissue disorder is summarized in Box 41-1. When a patient has RA, you should collect data related to pain, joint swelling, tenderness, joint deformities and limitation of movement, fatigue, and decreased ability to

Pharmacology Capsule

Aspirin and NSAIDs prolong bleeding time; thus patients must be monitored for bruising and bleeding.

perform activities of daily living (dressing, grooming, eating, toileting).

Nursing Diagnoses, Goals, and Outcome Criteria: Rheumatoid Arthritis	
NURSING DIAGNOSES	GOALS AND OUTCOME CRITERIA
Chronic Pain related to swelling and tenderness	Reduced pain: patient reports decreased pain, relaxed manner
Activity Intolerance related to fatigue	Improved activity tolerance: performance of small tasks without needing a rest period
Ineffective Coping related to frustration, embarrassment, inability to do activities independently	Effective coping: patient identifies ways to deal with physical changes
Social Isolation related to physical impairment and poor body image	Increased social activity: patient resumes as least one social activity that had been abandoned, has realistic view of physical abilities
Ineffective Therapeutic Regimen Management related to lack of understanding of RA, its treatment, and self-care	Patient effectively manages self-care: patient describes and demonstrates correct self-care

Interventions

Chronic Pain

Chronic pain imposes a terrible burden on the patient. Administer prescribed drugs, and teach outpatients about their drug therapy. Teach the patient other measures to control pain including application of heat or cold and administration of medications as ordered. A warm shower on arising may relieve morning pain and stiffness. Maintaining a program of exercise and rest also can help manage joint pain and relieve stress. Care of the patient with pain is discussed in Chapter 15.

Activity Intolerance

With the patient, develop a plan of activities around periods of rest and activity. Provide assistance as needed with getting in and out of bed and going to the bathroom. Patients who are severely disabled may need help with all activities of daily living. If needed, help the patient change positions and provide assistance with meals. Physical and occupational therapy

Consider the Alternative

Nonpharmacologic approaches to pain management include application of heat or cold, balanced exercise and rest, relaxation exercises, meditation, imagery, and music.

may be ordered. Encourage the patient to follow the prescribed therapy program.

Ineffective Coping

A trusting, collaborative relationship is a prerequisite to providing therapeutic care. Spend time with the patient often to explore concerns, answer questions, teach, and plan care. Emphasize the patient's strengths, and explore previously used coping skills. Some patients respond to their physical and functional losses with demanding behavior that others see as manipulative. Patients from other cultures may deal with the pain and disability differently; some may be more stoic and reserved, whereas others may be demanding or helpless. Caregivers must recognize this as an attempt by the patient to maintain some control in his or her life. An important part of coping is learning to maintain maximal possible independence despite the crippling effects of RA. Adaptations in the home and workplace and the use of appropriate assistive devices can promote independence and an improved sense of well-being.

Because a chronic illness affects the family as well as the patient, reach out to the family, offering information, encouragement, problem solving, and resources. Recognize that the family structure differs from one culture to another and the patient's role in the family plays an important part in how they view the effects of the disease. Provide information about community resources such as the local chapter of the Arthritis Foundation. If indicated, consult with the registered nurse or physician about a referral to a home care agency to help the patient learn to manage better at home.

 What Does Culture Have to Do with Pain?

The way people deal with pain is culturally based. For example, people of German, Japanese, and Irish heritage try to be stoic and are reluctant to express pain, whereas people from Italy and the Dominican Republic are more likely to express pain openly. Nurses should not make assumptions about a patient's pain based only on his or her behavior.

Social Isolation

Physical deformities that alter appearance and impair function evoke a great sense of loss in the RA patient. The resulting depression, irritability, and feelings of helplessness can have a devastating effect on the patient's interpersonal relationships. In addition, patients who take corticosteroids often have mood swings, which make their behavior unpredictable. These emotional changes may discourage visits from staff and from family, which increases the patient's isolation. Visit the patient often so he or she does not feel isolated and lonely. Explain the patient's irritability and mood swings to family and friends. Emphasize the importance of their continued support to the patient. Encourage the patient to identify social activities that are appropriate and to remain involved to the extent possible.

Ineffective Therapeutic Regimen Management

The teaching plan should include information about the disease process, drug therapy, and the need for balanced rest and activity.

Put on Your Thinking Cap!

A 30-year-old mother of a 6-month-old infant and a 5-year-old child has just been diagnosed with rheumatoid arthritis. She is married and works full time as a teacher. Identify ways she can modify strain on her joints in the home setting and the work setting.

OSTEOPOROSIS

Pathophysiology

Bone is constantly being formed and absorbed. Until adolescence, bone formation exceeds bone absorption so that bones grow and strengthen. The processes remain equal through the twenties, but beginning around age 30, bone absorption surpasses bone formation. Loss of trabecular bone, the innermost layer, occurs first. The loss of cortical bone, the hard outer shell, begins later in life. The loss of cortical bone begins earlier and progresses faster in women than in men. The net result is loss of bone mass, which leaves the patient susceptible to fractures. Common sites of fractures due to osteoporosis are the wrist, vertebrae, and hip. Age-related loss of bone mass without apparent underlying medical causes is called *primary osteoporosis*. *Secondary osteoporosis* is loss of bone mass due to factors other than age, such as hyperparathy-

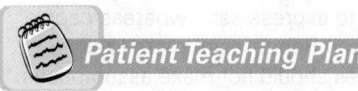

Patient Teaching Plan

Rheumatoid Arthritis

- Take your medications exactly as prescribed, and notify your physician of any adverse effects (provide drug names, dosage, schedule, side and adverse effects).
- Keep follow-up appointments; the effects of many drugs need to be monitored with periodic blood studies.
- You must balance your activity and rest.
- Avoid prolonged bed rest, which can lead to further loss of function.
- Use assistive devices as needed to maintain safe mobility.
- Support your joints in functional positions to reduce the risk of contractures.
- Continue to do as much as you can for yourself, but don't hesitate to ask for help with difficult tasks.
- Avoid straining your joints with heavy lifting.

roidism or long-term therapy with corticosteroids or heparin.

Risk Factors

Many factors appear to increase the risk of osteoporosis. At greatest risk are older women who have small frames, who are white or of northern European heritage, and who have fair skin and blond or red hair. Other risk factors are estrogen deficiency; physical inactivity; low body weight; inadequate calcium, protein, or vitamin D intake; corticosteroid therapy over more than 6 months; and excessive use of cigarettes, caffeine, and alcohol. A number of disorders, such as Cushing's disease and type 2 diabetes mellitus, also seem to be associated with osteoporosis.

Signs and Symptoms

Often the patient has no symptoms of osteoporosis until a fracture occurs. Signs and symptoms of osteoporosis may include back pain, fractures, loss of height due to vertebral compression, and kyphosis. Bone deterioration in the jaw can cause dentures to fit poorly. Collapsed vertebrae can cause chronic pain and decline in function.

Medical Diagnosis

Bone mass can be measured using a technique called *absorptiometry*. Absorptiometry is a quick, painless radiologic procedure that measures the amount of bone tissue in the hip and spine. Blood studies are usually normal with primary osteoporosis, but a battery of tests may be ordered to rule out possible causes of secondary osteoporosis. Radiographs show bone fractures but do not reveal decreased bone density until there is loss of 30% to 50% of the bone mass. A bone specimen may be obtained from the iliac crest for study.

Medical Treatment

It is generally accepted that calcium supplementation and estrogen replacement for postmenopausal women slow bone loss. The recommended elemental calcium intake is 1000 mg/day for premenopausal women and for postmenopausal women who are on estrogen replacement therapy. Postmenopausal women who are not on estrogen replacement therapy need 1500 mg/day of calcium. The only contraindications to supplementary calcium are hypercalcemia, hypophosphatemia, or a history of kidney stones. Estrogen replacement is controversial, but if it is not contraindicated, it may have beneficial effects on the bones for up to 15 years after the onset of menopause. The patient should discuss the issue with her physician. A physical therapist may be consulted to develop an appropriate exercise program for the patient.

Medical treatment has long aimed at preventing fractures and stimulating bone formation, but until recently there were no drugs that actually reversed the progression of osteoporosis. Drugs that may be used to prevent or to treat osteoporosis include the bisphosphonates and selective estrogen receptor modulators (SERMs). Examples of bisphosphonates are alendronate sodium (Fosamax), risedronate (Actonel), and ibandronate (Boniva). Raloxifene (Evista) is a SERM. It is believed that regular exercise promotes bone formation and improves strength, balance, and reaction time, thereby reducing the risk of falls and fractures. Aerobic exercise at least three times a week is encouraged. The incidence or severity of the disorder may be reduced by identifying high-risk people and taking steps to promote healthy bone development.

Patients who have spinal fractures caused by osteoporosis may benefit from percutaneous vertebroplasty, which requires a needle to be inserted into the vertebra so that a special type of cement can be injected directly into the vertebra. This procedure is reported to prevent additional compression of the vertebra and to relieve pain caused by compression. Because percutaneous vertebroplasty is minimally invasive, risks are minimized and the recovery time is short.

What Does Culture Have to Do with Osteoporosis?

Small, fair-skinned women of northern European descent are at greatest risk for osteoporosis. These women should be targeted early for bone-building dietary and exercise programs.

NURSING CARE *of the Patient with Osteoporosis*

Assessment

The nursing assessment of the patient with a connective tissue disorder is summarized in Box 41-1. When a patient has osteoporosis, collect data specifically about the patient's diet, calcium intake, and exercise plan. In the reproductive history, note whether the patient is menopausal or has had an oophorectomy (surgical removal of the ovaries). Measure the patient's height and compare with previous measurements. Describe the patient's posture, clearly noting the presence and degree of deformity. Assist the patient with changes in position during the examination for safety and comfort.

Nursing Diagnoses, Goals, and Outcome Criteria: Osteoporosis

NURSING DIAGNOSES	GOALS AND OUTCOME CRITERIA
Risk for Trauma related to loss of bone strength	Absence of trauma: performance of daily activities without falls or other injuries
Chronic Pain related to fractures, pressure on nerves due to vertebral compression	Pain relief: patient states pain relieved, relaxed manner
Ineffective Therapeutic Regimen Management related to lack of understanding of measures to promote bone formation and prevent bone loss	Effective patient management of condition: patient describes and demonstrates activities to improve bone mass

Interventions

Risk for Trauma

Determine the patient's ability to carry out activities of daily living. Provide assistance if necessary. Advise ambulatory patients to wear good supportive shoes. Provide canes or walkers to improve balance if needed. Keep the environment free of hazards that might cause the patient to fall. Place personal articles within the patient's reach. In the home setting, look for possible hazards and take steps to provide a safer environment. Also evaluate the patient's gross visual acuity. To maneuver safely, the patient must be able to see. If indicated, recommend an eye examination.

Chronic Pain

Obtain a complete description of the patient's pain. Administer analgesics as ordered, but consider nonpharmacologic interventions as well (see Chapter 15). Some patients, especially those with vertebral compression, may have chronic pain that is difficult to manage. You may suggest referral to a clinic that specializes in pain management. Document the effects of pain management strategies.

Ineffective Therapeutic Regimen Management

Patient teaching is key to helping the patient learn to manage osteoporosis.

Put on Your Thinking Cap!

List two different ways a premenopausal woman can obtain her recommended daily calcium intake without supplements.

GOUT

Gout is a systemic disease characterized by the deposition of urate crystals in the joints and other body tissues. There are two forms of gout: primary gout, in which uric acid is elevated because of a metabolic disorder; and secondary gout, in which uric acid is elevated owing to another disease process. Primary gout is more prevalent among men than women, with a peak incidence in men in their 40s and 50s. Women are rarely affected before menopause. Although the cause of most cases of gout is unknown, genetic and environmental factors appear to contribute to the development of this condition. The risk increases with hyperuricemia, obesity, alcohol consumption, and a variety of drugs including thiazide and loop diuretics and low-dose salicylates.

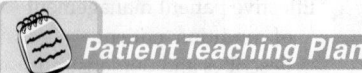

Patient Teaching Plan

Osteoporosis

* Before menopause and while on hormone replacements, you need 1000 mg of calcium daily.
* After menopause, if you do not take hormone replacements, you need 1500 mg of calcium daily.
* There are about 300 mg of calcium in each of the following: 1 cup of milk, 1 cup of yogurt, 1 ounce of Swiss cheese.
* Nonfat and skim milk have as much calcium as whole milk.
* If you take calcium supplements, increase your fluid intake unless advised not to do so by your physician.
* You need 400 IU vitamin D every day (300 IU for men).
* Limit your intake of alcohol and caffeine.
* If Fosamax is prescribed, take it in the morning with a full glass of water on an empty stomach, and sit or stand for 30 minutes after taking it.
* Regular weight-bearing exercise helps maintain bone strength.
* Avoid activities that might lead to falls and fractures.

Pathophysiology

Gout is characterized by hyperuricemia (excess uric acid in the blood) and is related either to an excessive rate of uric acid production or to decreased uric acid excretion by the kidneys. Features of gout may include (1) increased serum urate levels, (2) recurring acute attacks of arthritis, (3) the clumping of urate clusters around the joints of the extremities, causing crippling deformities, (4) renal disease involving blood vessels and interstitial tissues, and (5) uric acid kidney stones.

There are four stages of gout: asymptomatic hyperuricemia, acute gouty arthritis, asymptomatic intercritical period, and chronic tophaceous gout. Infection may develop if the skin breaks open. Kidney stones develop in about 20% of patients with gout.

Signs and Symptoms

In the first stage, the patient's blood uric acid level is elevated but there are no other symptoms. Many people with asymptomatic hyperuricemia never progress to the next stage. The onset of stage 2, acute gouty arthritis, is abrupt, usually occurring at night. The patient is suddenly afflicted with severe, crushing pain and cannot bear even the light touch of bed sheets on the affected joint. The joint commonly affected is that of the great toe. The attack may be precipitated by trauma, diuretics, increased alcohol consumption, or a high-purine diet (food high in proteins). The symptoms usually disappear within a few days, and joint function is completely restored until the next attack. Patients with advanced gout have tophi, which are deposits of sodium urate crystals that are visible as small white nodules under the skin (Fig. 41-8).

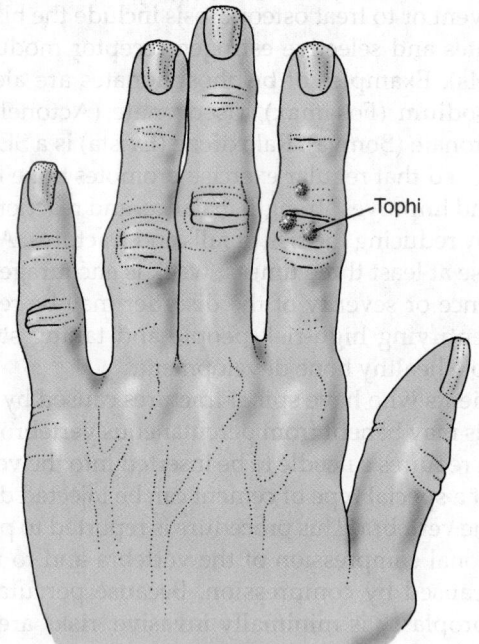

FIGURE **41-8** Typical appearance of tophi, which may occur in chronic gout, on an index finger.

Medical Diagnosis

Gout is usually suspected on the basis of the history and physical examination and confirmed by the finding of urate crystals in synovial fluid. A 24-hour urine specimen may be ordered to measure urinary uric acid, and a fasting blood sample may be drawn to measure the blood uric acid level.

Medical Treatment

Asymptomatic hyperuricemia usually requires no medical treatment. An NSAID alone or with colchicine is used to abort impending attacks of acute gouty arthritis and to treat initial acute episodes. If colchicine is used, it may be given hourly until the acute symptoms ease or until the patient develops nausea and vomiting. For subsequent attacks, other drugs that may relieve symptoms are indomethacin, corticosteroids, and corticotrophin (see the Drug Therapy table on p. 890). Some sources recommend indomethacin and NSAIDs instead of colchicine in older adults. If the patient does not respond to colchicine or NSAIDs, parenteral glucocorticoids or adrenocorticotropin may be prescribed. When a single joint is affected, prednisone may be injected into the joint. Drugs used to inhibit uric acid synthesis during the asymptomatic period include allopurinol (Zyloprim) and probenecid (Benemid). These same agents may be used to treat chronic tophaceous gout.

Pharmacology Capsule

Patients taking antigout drugs need to maintain urine output of at least 2000 mL/day to reduce the risk of urinary calculi formation.

Patients are advised to avoid foods high in purines such as liver, kidney, and sweetbreads. Some sources also recommend a diet that is low in carbohydrates and high in protein and unsaturated fats. If the patient is obese, weight loss will be recommended.

NURSING CARE *of the Patient with Gout*

Assessment

Complete assessment of the patient with a connective tissue disorder is summarized in Box 41-1. When the patient has gout, collect data specifically about pain, joint swelling, tophi, uric acid stones, fever, and a history of trauma, injury, or surgery.

Nursing Diagnoses, Goals, and Outcome Criteria: Gout

NURSING DIAGNOSES	GOALS AND OUTCOME CRITERIA
Acute Pain related to joint inflammation	Pain relief: patient states pain reduction/relief, appears relaxed
Impaired Physical Mobility related to painful joint movement	Improved mobility: patient gradually resumes activities without unbearable pain
Impaired Urinary Elimination related to urate kidney stones	Normal urine output without symptoms of urinary obstruction: fluid intake and output equal; no flank or abdominal pain; no hematuria
Ineffective Therapeutic Regimen Management related to lack of knowledge of gout, its treatment, and self-care measures	Patient effectively manages condition: correctly describes and follows plan of care

Interventions

Acute Pain

Nursing care to decrease discomfort includes elevating the affected extremity, administering prescribed medications, encouraging rest, and avoiding pressure on the area. Because even bed sheets may cause pain, a bed cradle should be used. Hot or cold packs may be ordered. Splints or bandages may be used to immobilize the affected joint. When a patient is taking colchicine, always check laboratory results for abnormalities in blood cell counts. Fatal blood dyscrasias have occurred in patients taking this drug.

Impaired Physical Mobility

Bed rest is usually recommended during the acute period. Provide assistance with activities of daily living as needed. When ambulation is permitted, advise the patient to protect affected joints from trauma by wearing supportive, firm shoes and by keeping walking pathways clearly lighted and free of obstacles that might cause falls.

Impaired Urinary Elimination

When the serum uric acid level is elevated, the excess acid is excreted in the urine, where it may form uric acid stones. Urinary stones can obstruct urine flow from the kidney, causing renal damage. To prevent this complication, advise the patient to drink at least eight 8-ounce glasses of fluid daily unless contraindicated. Drugs may be prescribed to make the urine alkaline because uric acid stones precipitate in acid urine. During hospitalization, intravenous fluids may be given. Monitor intake and urine output. Promptly report signs and symptoms of urinary stones (pain in the flank, lower abdomen, or genitals; fever; hematuria; decreased urine output) to the registered nurse or the physician.

Ineffective Therapeutic Regimen Management

Instruct the patient in measures to prevent or decrease future attacks.

 Put on Your Thinking Cap!

Explain how increased fluid intake will help prevent kidney stones in the patient with gout.

PROGRESSIVE SYSTEMIC SCLEROSIS (PSS OR SCLERODERMA)

Progressive systemic sclerosis is commonly called *scleroderma*. It is a chronic, multisystem autoimmune disease of unknown origin that takes its name from the characteristic hardening of the skin. Other organs affected include the blood vessels, gastrointestinal tract, lungs, heart, and kidneys. The course of the disease varies among individuals, depending on the severity

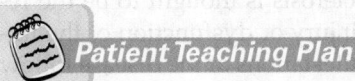 **Patient Teaching Plan**

Gout

Consult a dietitian to help the patient plan a well-balanced diet, and give the patient the following instructions:

- Your diet should be high in carbohydrates, moderate in protein, and low in fat. Limited purine intake is often advised as shown in Box 41-3. Your doctor will advise you of dietary restrictions when you have no symptoms.
- Occasional, moderate alcohol intake may be permitted.
- Maintain a fluid intake of at least eight 8-ounce glasses daily to reduce the risk of uric acid stone formation in the urinary tract.
- Take your drugs as prescribed (provide specific dosage, schedule, list of side effects).
- To prevent severe attacks, report early joint or urinary symptoms to the physician. Severe attacks may be averted if treatment is begun soon after symptoms develop.
- If you are overweight, weight loss may help by reducing stress on joints.

Box 41-3 | *Purine Content of Selected Foods*

High Purine Content
Avoid these foods during both acute and remission stages of gout:

Anchovies	Bouillon	Brains	Broth
Consommé	Goose	Gravy	Heart
Herring	Kidney	Mackerel	Meat extracts
Mincemeat	Mussels	Partridge	Roe
Sardines	Scallops	Sweetbreads	Yeast (baker's and brewer's as supplement)

Moderate Purine Content
One serving (2-3 oz) meat, fish, or fowl or 1 serving (½ cup) of vegetable from these groups is allowed daily (depending on condition) during remissions:

- Fish, poultry, meat, shellfish
- Vegetables: Asparagus, dried beans, lentils, mushrooms, dried peas, spinach

Modified with permission from Mahan, L.K., & Escott-Stump, S. (1996). *Krause's food, nutrition, and diet therapy* (9th ed., p. 895). Philadelphia: Saunders.

---

of involvement of the internal organs. The onset of disease is usually between 30 and 50 years of age, with more women than men affected. Death may occur due to infection or cardiac or renal failure. There are approximately 100,000 to 200,000 individuals with PSS in the United States.

There are two types of PSS: progressively fatal sclerosis and the CREST syndrome. Progressively fatal sclerosis is characterized by thickening of the skin and systemic effects. The CREST syndrome consists of five symptoms: *c*alcinosis (calcium deposits in the tissues), *R*aynaud's phenomenon (vascular spasms), *e*sophageal dysfunction, *s*clerodactyly (scleroderma of the digits), and *t*elangiectasis (dilated superficial blood vessels).

Pathophysiology

Progressive systemic sclerosis is thought to be the result of primary vessel injury or dysfunction of the immune system. The manifestations of the disease follow a chain of events, from inflammation to degeneration of tissues, that results in decreased elasticity, stenosis, and occlusion of vessels.

Signs and Symptoms

The signs and symptoms of PSS reflect problems of the blood vessels, skin, joints, and internal organs. Common manifestations are Raynaud's phenomenon; symmetric, painless swelling or thickening of the skin; taut and shiny skin; morning stiffness; frequent reflux of gastric acid; difficulty swallowing; weight loss; dyspnea; pericarditis; and renal insufficiency.

Medical Diagnosis

A complete history and physical examination may lead the physician to suspect fibrotic changes typical of PSS in the skin, lungs, heart, or esophagus. A positive ANA assay result, elevated ESR, and increased serum muscle enzyme levels support the diagnosis.

Medical Treatment

Even though there is no cure for PSS, treatment with high doses of steroids or other immunosuppressants may bring about remission. Additional aims of treatment are management of symptoms and prevention of complications. Treatment includes physical therapy to maintain joint mobility and preserve muscle strength. Esophageal reflux may be treated with drugs to decrease the acidity of gastric secretions, periodic dilation of the esophagus, and other measures, such as small, frequent feedings and elevation of the head of the bed.

The management of Raynaud's phenomenon is aimed at elimination of anything that causes vasospasm: smoking, cold environmental temperature, and vasoconstricting drugs. Topical nitroglycerin ointment and oral alpha-blockers such as prazosin or calcium channel blockers such as nifedipine are often effective.

Various drugs can be used to treat the symptoms of PSS. *d*-Penicillamine is used to decrease skin thickening and reduce the severity of visceral organ involvement. Antihypertensives are used to control hypertensive crisis, with ACE inhibitors being most effective in averting kidney complications, and anti-inflammatory drugs can be used to control joint pain and stiffness.

NURSING CARE of the Patient with Progressive Systemic Sclerosis

Assessment

The general assessment of the patient with a connective tissue disorder is summarized in Box 41-1. When a patient has PSS, you should seek information in the health history specifically about pain and stiffness in the fingers and intolerance for cold. In the review of systems, identify signs and symptoms suggestive of cardiovascular, respiratory, renal, and gastrointestinal problems.

During the physical examination, inspect for skin rash, loss of wrinkles on the face, limitations of joint range of motion, muscle weakness, and dry mucous membranes. Carefully examine the hands for contractures of the fingers and for color changes or lesions on the fingertips. Palpate the fingers to determine warmth.

Nursing Diagnoses, Goals, and Outcome Criteria: Progressive Systemic Sclerosis

The nursing diagnoses and goals for patients with PSS are similar to those of patients with other connective tissue diseases. The following are the major diagnoses:

NURSING DIAGNOSES	GOALS AND OUTCOME CRITERIA
Impaired Skin Integrity related to thickening of tissues	Optimal skin integrity: warm, intact skin with normal color and texture
Self-Care Deficits related to pain, contractures of fingers, discomfort	Independent self-care: patient performs activities of daily living without excessive discomfort
Chronic Pain related to swelling and stiffness, vasospasm	Pain relief: patient states pain relieved, relaxed manner
Social Isolation related to poor self-concept, changes in physical appearance	Decreased social isolation: patient maintains or increases social interactions
Imbalanced Nutrition: Less Than Body Requirements related to esophageal dysfunction	Adequate nutrition: stable body weight, maintains weight within standards recommended for height
Ineffective Therapeutic Regimen Management related to lack of understanding of PSS, medical management, and self-care	Effective management of condition: patient correctly describes and follows plan of care

Interventions
Impaired Skin Integrity

Keep the skin clean and dry. Encourage the patient to wear protective clothing as needed to maintain warmth and reduce skin discomfort. Cool baths with mild soaps followed by skin lotions may be soothing. Meticulous mouth care is warranted to prevent oral lesions. Administer anti-inflammatory drugs as ordered. Advise the patient to avoid practices that trigger vasospasm, such as exposure to cold and smoking.

Self-Care Deficits

Encourage the patient to participate in self-care as much as possible. Monitor the patient's tolerance for activity, and provide assistance as needed. Schedule rest periods after activities to prevent overtiring. Permit the hospitalized patient to maintain independence in activities within abilities.

FIGURE **41-9** Late-stage skin changes seen in patients with progressive systemic sclerosis. **A,** Edema of the hands and fingers. **B,** Typical facial appearance.

Chronic Pain

The patient with PSS usually has chronic joint pain and episodes of severe pain in the hands and feet associated with Raynaud's phenomenon. Measures to treat joint pain are like those described for rheumatoid arthritis. During acute episodes of Raynaud's phenomenon, the patient may be unable to tolerate anything touching the affected skin. A bed cradle can be used to keep the linens off the body. Adjust the room temperature to prevent chilling, which could provoke vasospasm. Be sure the patient is aware that smoking and severe stress can also trigger vasospasm.

Social Isolation

Swelling of the hands and facial changes can create a birdlike appearance that may cause the patient to withdraw from social interactions (Fig. 41-9). Explore the patient's concerns about the altered appearance, and help the patient anticipate how to deal with various social situations. Demonstrate acceptance of the patient by expressing concern and using touch.

Imbalanced Nutrition: Less Than Body Requirements

If the patient has esophageal involvement, suggest smaller, more frequent meals, which may be better tolerated. A relaxing environment before and after meals is helpful. Spicy foods, alcohol, and caffeine are discouraged because they stimulate gastric secretions. Give antacids and histamine-2 receptor blockers as ordered to neutralize gastric acid and reduce the risk of esophagitis and ulceration caused by esophageal reflux. After meals, the head of the bed should remain elevated for 1 to 2 hours to discourage reflux. Monitor and assess the adequacy of nutritional intake. For more information about diet and connective tissue disease, see the Nutrition Concepts box below.

Ineffective Therapeutic Regimen Management

As with other chronic illnesses, the patient must learn to implement the medical plan and manage the signs and symptoms of the condition. Patient teaching with PSS includes the nature of the disease, measures to prevent episodes of Raynaud's phenomenon, measures to maintain good nutrition and prevent esophageal reflux, signs and symptoms that should be reported

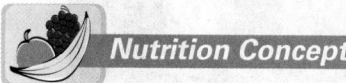

Nutrition Concepts

1. A diet high in calcium (1000 to 1500 mg/day) and vitamin D (400 IU/day) is important for the prevention of osteoporosis.
2. Eight ounces of milk (whole, low-fat, or skim) provides 300 mg of calcium.
3. A well-balanced diet, including foods high in vitamin E and zinc, is recommended for persons with rheumatoid arthritis.
4. A weight-loss program for persons with osteoarthritis helps reduce stress on weight-bearing joints.
5. Patients with gout may be advised to limit purine intake.
6. The patient with esophageal involvement of progressive systemic sclerosis needs small, frequent meals and limited spicy foods, alcohol, and caffeine.

Patient Teaching Plan

Progressive Systemic Sclerosis

- To prevent vasospasm, keep your hands warm and reduce stress and exhaustion.
- Take drugs as prescribed, and report adverse effects to your physician (provide specific information about drug names, dosage, schedule, and adverse effects).
- Esophageal reflux can be managed with drug therapy; relaxing meals; avoiding spicy foods, caffeine, and alcohol; and maintaining an upright position for 1 to 2 hours after eating.

to the physician, and self-medication. Key points are listed in the teaching plan.

DERMATOMYOSITIS/POLYMYOSITIS

Dermatomyositis and polymyositis are relatively rare acute or chronic inflammatory diseases that affect primarily the skeletal muscle. The term *polymyositis* is applied to the condition when there is no skin involvement, and *dermatomyositis* is used when there is a characteristic skin rash. There is no known cause for these conditions, but they are frequently seen in patients with scleroderma, rheumatoid arthritis, vasculitis, systemic lupus erythematosus, or Sjögren's syndrome.

Pathophysiology

The major activity producing pathology in polymyositis is infiltration of inflammatory cells, causing destruction of muscle fibers. Inflammation of tissues surrounding blood vessels is an outstanding pathologic feature of the disease. The condition is sometimes associated with malignancy.

Signs and Symptoms

The primary symptom of polymyositis is muscle weakness, reflected in inability to do normal activities like climbing stairs, raising the arms over the head, and turning over in bed. Other symptoms are Raynaud's phenomenon and joint pain and inflammation. Patients with dermatomyositis typically have periorbital edema (swelling around the eyes) as well. The onset may be abrupt or slow.

Medical Diagnosis

The diagnosis is based on the presence of proximal muscle weakness, a muscle biopsy positive for muscle degeneration, elevated muscle enzymes, and myopathic electromyographic changes.

Medical Treatment

Drug therapy includes high-dose glucocorticoids such as prednisone and chemotherapeutic agents such as methotrexate. Supportive treatment centers on the balancing of rest and exercise to prevent contractures. This goal is difficult to achieve, because range-of-motion exercises may aggravate the condition.

NURSING CARE *of the Patient with Polymyositis*

Because polymyositis is seen in conjunction with other connective tissue diseases, see earlier sections of the chapter for applicable nursing interventions.

OTHER CONNECTIVE TISSUE DISORDERS

Other connective tissue disorders described in Table 41-1 are bursitis, carpal tunnel syndrome, ankylosing spondylitis, polymyalgia rheumatica, Reiter's syndrome, Behçet's syndrome, Sjögren's syndrome, and periarteritis nodosa.

| Table 41-1 | *Other Connective Tissue Disorders* |

DISORDER	PATHOPHYSIOLOGY	MANAGEMENT
Bursitis	*Description:* Acute or chronic inflammation of the bursae caused by trauma, strain, or infection. Calcification of bursae may occur. *Etiology:* Usually excessive use of joint. *Signs and symptoms:* Pain and limited movement in affected joints. Shoulder and hip most often affected.	NSAIDs, rest, splinting. Cold compresses first 24 hr; heat thereafter. Lidocaine injections for temporary pain relief. Once pain resolves, progressive range of motion such as "walking" the fingers of the affected arm up the wall.
Carpal tunnel syndrome	*Description:* Common condition in which the median nerve in the wrist becomes compressed, causing pain and numbness. *Etiology:* Caused by pressure on median nerve as it passes through structures of the wrist. People who do repetitive wrist movements like typing are at risk. *Signs and symptoms:* Pain and numbness in palmar side of fingers, weakness of thumb.	Splinting to prevent flexion and hyperextension. Glucocorticoid injections. Surgical release of transverse carpal ligament. Postoperatively, assess color and temperature of hand. Notify surgeon of pallor, cyanosis, or numbness.
Ankylosing spondylitis	*Description:* Inflammatory disease that affects vertebral column, causing spinal deformities. Chronic but not usually disabling. *Etiology:* Unknown but appears to be linked to HLA-B27 antigen. *Signs and symptoms:* First symptom usually dull, aching pain in buttocks. Also, low-back morning stiffness of several hours' duration that improves with activity. Fatigue. *Complications:* Spinal fractures, iritis (inflammation of the iris of the eye), arthritis.	NSAIDs, physical therapy.
Polymyalgia rheumatica	*Description:* Rheumatic disease. *Etiology:* Unknown but likely has hereditary link. *Signs and symptoms:* Aching and morning stiffness in neck, shoulders and hips, proximal extremities, and torso. Symptoms resolve in 1-2 hr and return after a period of inactivity. Fatigue, weight loss, low-grade fever, anemia.	Prednisone: 30 days or less; NSAIDs.
Reiter's syndrome	*Description:* Connective tissue disease. *Etiology:* Often follows venereal disease or dysentery; incidence higher in people with certain familial tendencies. *Signs and symptoms:* Triad of arthritis, urethritis, conjunctivitis. Fever, malaise, fatigue, anorexia, weight loss, conjunctivitis, heel pain, skin lesions.	NSAIDs, physical therapy.
Behçet's syndrome	*Description, signs and symptoms:* Chronic syndrome characterized by oral and genital ulcers, skin lesions, uveitis, joint pain, phlebitis, GI ulcers. *Etiology:* Not considered hereditary, but there seems to be a familial link.	Treatment varies, based on specific manifestations. May include anticoagulants, glucocorticoids, cyclosporine, chlorambucil, azathioprine, methotrexate, retinal protein S.
Sjögren's syndrome	*Description:* Inflammatory disease that obstructs secretory ducts in the eyes, mouth, and vagina. *Etiology:* Autoimmune disorder; often seen with rheumatoid arthritis, polymyositis, scleroderma, or systemic lupus erythematosus. *Signs and symptoms:* Dry eyes, mouth, and vagina.	Artificial tears and lubricant ointments; artificial saliva, pilocarpine hydrochloride to stimulate salivary flow, dental care; perineal hygiene. Glucocorticoids.
Periarteritis nodosa	*Description:* A form of systemic necrotizing vasculitis; also called *polyarteritis nodosa.* Inflammation of small- and medium-size arteries; can result in thrombosis, infarction, hemorrhage. *Signs and symptoms:* Onset insidious. Fever, weight loss, skin lesions, hypertension, joint swelling, malaise, abdominal pain, change in urinary pattern, anemia, ischemia of fingers, pleuritis. Symptoms of renal, GI, and cardiac involvement.	Glucocorticoids, methotrexate, cyclophosphamide, antihypertensives, diuretics. Other drugs are prescribed for specific manifestations of the disorder.

NSAIDs, Nonsteroidal anti-inflammatory drugs; *GI,* gastrointestinal.

Key Points

- The major connective tissues are bone, blood, cartilage, ligaments, skin, and tendons.
- Age-related changes in connective tissue can have a significant effect on function and quality of life.
- Osteoarthritis is characterized by degeneration of articular cartilage, hypertrophy of underlying and adjacent bone, and inflammation of surrounding synovium that leads to pain with joint movement.
- Osteoarthritis may be treated with drug therapy, education, physical therapy, modification of daily activities, and surgery.
- Nursing care of the patient with osteoarthritis focuses on Chronic Pain, Impaired Physical Mobility, Ineffective Coping, and Ineffective Therapeutic Regimen Management.
- Total joint replacements can be done on the elbow, shoulder, phalangeal finger joints, hip, knee, and ankle.
- Nursing care after total joint replacement addresses Acute Pain, Risk for Injury, Impaired Physical Mobility, Ineffective Tissue Perfusion, Risk for Infection, Anxiety or Fear, and Deficient Knowledge related to postoperative self-care.
- Rheumatoid arthritis, a chronic, progressive inflammatory disease that leads to deformity and loss of joint mobility, is treated with drug therapy, supportive treatments, and modification of activities of daily living.

- Gout, a systemic disease characterized by the deposition of urate crystals in the joints and other body tissues, usually responds to drug therapy that lowers the serum uric acid level.
- Progressive systemic sclerosis, commonly called *scleroderma,* is characterized by thickening of the skin and may affect the blood vessels, gastrointestinal tract, lungs, heart, and kidneys.
- Nursing care for the patient with progressive systemic sclerosis addresses Impaired Skin Integrity, Self-Care Deficits, Chronic Pain, Social Isolation, Imbalanced Nutrition: Less Than Body Requirements, and Ineffective Therapeutic Regimen Management.
- Less common connective tissue disorders are polymyositis, ankylosing spondylitis, polymyalgia rheumatica, Reiter's syndrome, Behçet's syndrome, Sjögren's syndrome, and periarteritis nodosa.
- Most connective tissue disorders are chronic and, although they are not specifically curable, can be improved with symptomatic treatment.

 Go to your Companion CD-ROM for a Pharmacology Tutorial, Audio Glossary, and 3-D animations.

evolve Be sure to visit the companion Evolve site at http://evolve.elsevier.com/Linton/ for WebLinks and additional online resources.

REVIEW QUESTIONS *Choose the best answer.*

1. The joints between the bones of the skull are classified as:
   1. Synarthroses
   2. Amphiarthroses
   3. Diarthroses
   4. Synovial

2. Age-related changes in connective tissue include the following:
   1. Hardening of bone tissue
   2. Increased water content
   3. Loss of cartilage elasticity
   4. Decreased osteophytes

3. A patient who has gout calls the clinic to report having flank pain and blood in her urine. You should:
   1. Recognize signs and symptoms of urinary stones, and notify the physician immediately
   2. Tell her these symptoms are normal with gout and that they will improve soon
   3. Make an appointment for her to see the physician within 1 week
   4. Document her complaints in her record, and ask her to call the next day if symptoms continue

4. A continuous passive motion machine (CPM) has been ordered for a patient after a total joint replacement. The primary purpose of the CPM machine is to:
   1. Prevent postoperative boredom
   2. Prevent scar tissue formation
   3. Restore muscle strength
   4. Test the prosthetic joint

5. One week after total hip replacement surgery, a patient complains of sudden severe pain in the affected hip and inability to bear weight on that leg. You should suspect:
   1. Wound dehiscence
   2. Prosthesis rejection
   3. A new hip fracture
   4. Prosthesis dislocation

6. Common nursing diagnoses for a patient with rheumatoid arthritis (RA) include the following:
   1. Activity Intolerance related to fatigue
   2. Risk for Injury related to sensory losses
   3. Ineffective Tissue Perfusion related to vasoconstriction
   4. Risk for Aspiration related to esophageal dysfunction

7. What is the recommended daily calcium intake for a patient who is postmenopausal and not taking hormone replacement therapy?

   1. 100 mg
   2. 500 mg
   3. 1000 mg
   4. 1500 mg

8. When probenecid (Benemid) is prescribed for a patient with gout, patient teaching should include which of the following pieces of advice?

   1. You must be careful to avoid people who have infections because your immune system is depressed.
   2. Drink at least eight 8-ounce glasses of fluid each day to prevent urinary stones.
   3. You can expect to feel the results of this medication within 72 hours.
   4. Remain in an upright position for at least 30 minutes after taking this medication.

9. Which statement should be included in the teaching plan for a patient with progressive systemic sclerosis (PSS/scleroderma)?

   1. Keep the temperature in your home below 70 degrees.
   2. Remain upright for 1-2 hours after meals.
   3. This is an acute condition that will improve over time.
   4. PSS affects only the skin.

10. A disorder in which the eyes, mouth, and vagina become dry because of obstructed secretory ducts is:

    1. Behçet's syndrome
    2. Periarteritis nodosa
    3. Reiter's syndrome
    4. Sjögren's syndrome

Objectives

After reading and studying this chapter, you should be able to:

1. Identify the types of fractures.
2. Describe the five stages of the healing process.
3. Discuss the major complications of fractures, their signs and symptoms, and their management.
4. Compare the types of medical treatment for fractures, particularly reduction and fixation.
5. Describe common therapeutic measures for fractures, including casts, traction, crutches, walkers, and canes.
6. Discuss the nursing care of a patient with a fracture.
7. Describe specific types of fractures, including hip fractures, Colles' fractures, and pelvic fractures.

Key Terms

Be sure to check out the bonus material on the Companion CD-ROM, including selected audio pronunciations.

bone remodeling (p. 916)
closed reduction or manipulation (p. 919)
comminuted fracture (KŎM-ĭ-nūt-ĕd, p. 919)
compartment syndrome (p. 917)
complete fracture (p. 914)
delayed union (p. 917)
fat embolism (ĔM-bō-lĭzm, p. 916)
fixation (fĭx-SĀ-shŭn, p. 919)
fracture (p. 914)
greenstick fracture (p. 914)
incomplete fracture (p. 914)
malunion (măl-ŪN-yŏn, p. 917)
nonunion (nŏn-ŪN-yŭn, p. 917)
open or compound fracture (p. 914)
open reduction (p. 919)
reduction (p. 919)
stress fracture (p. 914)

A fracture is defined as a break or disruption in the continuity of a bone. With a fracture, injury to surrounding soft tissue also occurs. The severity of soft tissue injury depends on the location and severity of the break.

All fractures are either complete or incomplete. A complete fracture is one in which the break extends across the entire bone, dividing it into two separate pieces. An incomplete fracture is one in which the bone breaks only part way across, leaving some portion of the bone intact. The term greenstick fracture has been used to describe the incomplete fractures most commonly seen in children. In this case, the bone is splintered on one side, but only bent on the other.

CLASSIFICATION OF FRACTURES

Fractures may be classified as open or closed, depending on the type and extent of soft tissue damage. A closed or simple fracture is one in which the broken bone does not break through the skin. In an open or compound fracture, the fragments of the broken bone break through the skin. Open fractures have three grades of severity:

- Grade I: least severe injury, with minimal skin damage
- Grade II: moderately severe injury, with skin and muscle contusions (bruises)
- Grade III: most severe injury (wound larger than 6 to 8 cm), with skin, muscle, blood vessel, and nerve damage

Fractures also may be classified as stress or pathologic fractures, depending on their cause. A stress fracture is caused by either repeated or prolonged stress. Stress fractures are often related to sports such as track or basketball. A pathologic fracture occurs because of a pathologic condition in the bone such as a tumor or disease process that causes a spontaneous break. Figure 42-1 illustrates common types of fractures.

ETIOLOGY AND RISK FACTORS

Fractures are most commonly caused by trauma to the bone, especially as a result of automobile accidents and falls. Bone disease such as bone cancer also can lead to a fracture. Hip fractures in older adults usually are associated with falls. Risk factors for hip fractures include osteoporosis, advanced age, white race, use of psychotropic drugs, and being female.

In adults, the bones most commonly fractured are the ribs. Fractures of the femur are most common in young and middle-aged adults, whereas hip and wrist

Avulsion

Comminuted

Displaced

Greenstick

Impacted

Interarticular

Longitudinal

Oblique

Pathologic

Spiral

Stress

Transverse

FIGURE 42-1 Common types of fractures.

fractures are most common in older adults. The number of hip fractures in the United States has been rising, with 338,000 reported in 1999. Each year, more than $7 billion is spent in direct and indirect cost associated with hip fracture.

FRACTURE HEALING

A bone begins to heal as soon as an injury occurs. New bone tissue is formed to repair the fracture, resulting in a sturdy union between the broken ends of the bone. Healing occurs in the following five stages:

- STAGE 1: *Hematoma formation.* Immediately after a fracture, bleeding and edema occur. In 48 to 72 hours, a clot or hematoma forms between the two broken ends of the bone.
- STAGE 2: *Fibrocartilage formation.* The hematoma that surrounds the fracture does not resorb, as does a hematoma in other parts of the body. Instead, other tissue cells enter the clot and granulation tissue forms, replacing the clot. The granulation tissue then forms a collar around each end

What Does Culture Have to Do with Fractures?

Older white women have a high incidence of osteoporosis and therefore are at greater risk for fractures. This risk can be reduced by targeting these women for preventive measures throughout life. Osteoporosis is easier to prevent than to treat.

of the broken bone, gradually becoming firm and forming a bridge between the two ends.

- STAGE 3: *Callus formation.* Within 1 to 4 weeks after injury, the granulation tissue changes into a callus formation. Callus is made up of cartilage, osteoblasts (bone cells that form new bone), calcium, and phosphorus. The callus is larger than the diameter of the bone and serves as a temporary splint.
- STAGE 4: *Ossification.* Within 3 weeks to 6 months after the break, a permanent bone callus, known as *woven bone,* forms. It is during this stage that the ends of the broken bone begin to knit.

- STAGE 5: *Consolidation and remodeling.* Consolidation occurs when the distance between bone fragments decreases and eventually closes. During **bone remodeling,** the immature bone cells are gradually replaced by mature bone cells. The excess bone is naturally chiseled away by stress to the affected part from motion, exercise, and weight bearing. The bone then takes on its original shape and size (Fig. 42-2).

Healing is affected by many factors, including the location and severity of the fracture, the type of bone, other bone pathology, blood supply to the area, infection, and the adequacy of immobilization. Other factors that affect healing include age, endocrine disorders, and some drugs. The healing time for fractures increases with age, and it may take six times as long for the same type of fracture to heal in an older adult as in an infant. In the absence of bone disease, most older adults eventually heal as well as younger adults. However, many older adults, especially women, have a loss of bone mass.

COMPLICATIONS

Complications of a fracture can delay or impede healing and may even be life-threatening. Short-term complications include infection, fat embolism, deep vein thrombosis, compartment syndrome, and shock. Long-term complications include joint stiffness and contractures, malunion, nonunion, delayed union, post-traumatic arthritis, avascular necrosis, and complex regional pain syndrome.

INFECTION

Infection of the bone, called *osteomyelitis,* can result from contamination of the open wound associated with a fracture or from contamination of the indwelling hardware used to repair the broken bone. When an infection is inadvertently brought by surgery or other treatment, it is known as *iatrogenic.* Any infection can interfere with normal healing. Osteomyelitis occurs most commonly after an open fracture and surgical repair and may become chronic. In deep, grossly contaminated wounds, gas gangrene may develop.

Signs and symptoms of bone infection are local pain, redness, purulent wound drainage, chills, and fever. With gas gangrene, there is a foul-smelling watery drainage with significant redness and swelling of affected tissue.

Osteomyelitis requires aggressive antibiotic therapy. Intravenous antibiotics may be given for 4 to 8 weeks, followed by an additional 4 to 8 weeks of oral drug therapy. Wound care may include irrigation, treatment with antibiotic beads, and surgical removal of dead bone tissue and/or hardware.

FAT EMBOLISM

Fat embolism is a condition in which fat globules are released from the marrow of the broken bone into the bloodstream. Once the fat droplets enter the circulation, they migrate to the lungs. Because they are too large to pass through the pulmonary circulation, they lodge in the capillaries and obstruct blood flow. The fat particles break down into fatty acids, which inflame the pulmonary blood vessels, leading to pulmonary edema.

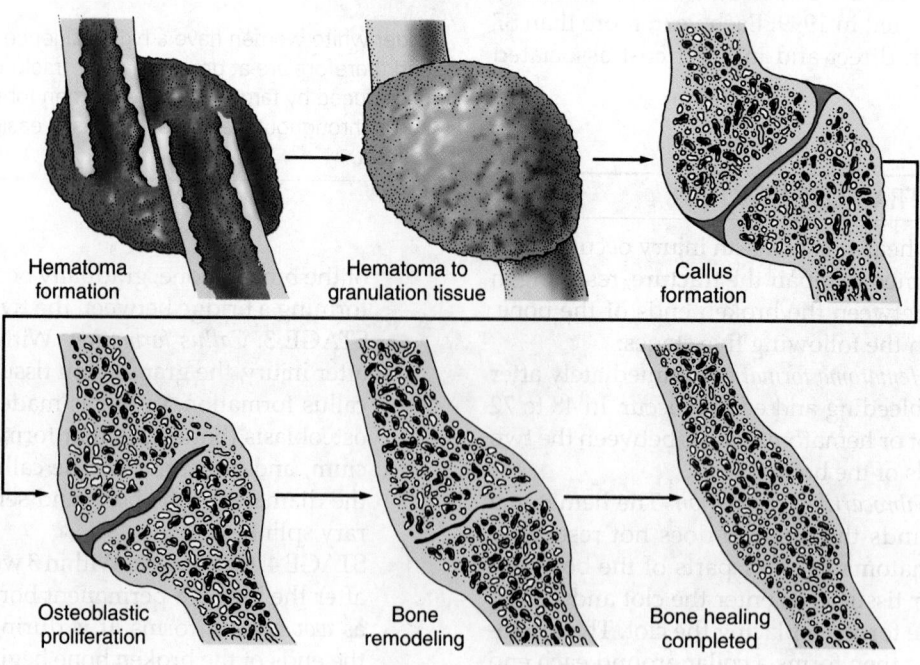

Hematoma formation

Hematoma to granulation tissue

Callus formation

Osteoblastic proliferation

Bone remodeling

Bone healing completed

FIGURE **42-2** Stages of fracture healing.

Fat embolism syndrome is most commonly associated with fractures of the long bones, multiple fractures, and severe trauma. It occurs 24 to 48 hours after injury, most often in young men ages 20 to 40 years and in older adults ages 70 to 80 years. An older patient with a hip fracture is at highest risk.

Respiratory distress is the first sign of a fat embolism, followed by tachycardia (rapid heartbeat), tachypnea (rapid breathing), fever, confusion, and decreased level of consciousness. Another characteristic feature is petechiae, a measles-like rash over the neck, upper arms, chest, or abdomen. Treatment of fat embolism consists of bed rest, gentle handling, oxygen, ventilatory support, and fluid restriction and diuretics for pulmonary edema. Though controversial, corticosteroids sometimes are used. The prognosis is generally good; however, the condition can be fatal.

DEEP VEIN THROMBOSIS

Venous stasis, vessel damage, and altered clotting mechanisms all contribute to the formation of blood clots (thrombi), most commonly in the deep veins of the legs. This complication is increased with immobility often associated with a fracture. Like fat particles, thrombi can break off and travel to the lungs, causing a pulmonary embolism. The prevention and treatment of deep vein thrombosis and pulmonary embolism are covered in Chapter 30.

COMPARTMENT SYNDROME

Compartment syndrome is a serious complication that results from internal or external pressure on the affected area. Compartments are located in the muscles of the extremities. They are enclosed spaces made up of muscle, bone, nerves, and blood vessels wrapped by a fibrous membrane, or fascia. Internal pressure can be caused by bleeding or edema into a compartment; external pressure can be caused by a cast or tight dressing. When there is bleeding or edema into a compartment, there is nowhere for the drainage to go because it is trapped in the space. The increased fluid puts pressure on the tissues, nerves, and blood vessels, so blood flow is decreased, resulting in pain and tissue damage. External pressure also can decrease blood flow to the area.

Although compartment syndrome is relatively rare, it is a serious condition and can create an emergency situation. Within 4 to 6 hours after the onset of compartment syndrome, irreversible muscle damage can occur. Paresis (partial paralysis) can result if the condition is not treated within 24 hours. In 24 to 48 hours, the limb can become useless.

A primary symptom of compartment syndrome is pain, especially with touch or movement, that cannot be relieved with opioid analgesia. Other signs and symptoms are edema, pallor, weak or unequal pulses, cyanosis, tingling, numbness, paresthesia, and, finally, severe pain.

The goal of treatment is to relieve pressure. When there is internal pressure, a surgical fasciotomy, which entails making linear incisions in the fascia, may be done to relieve pressure on the nerves and blood vessels. For external pressure, the cast or dressings are removed and replaced.

SHOCK

After a fracture, there is a risk of excessive blood loss. Tissue trauma may rupture local blood vessels, and vascular internal organs may be punctured, with resultant internal bleeding. Loss of blood leads to shock, which is evidenced by tachycardia, anxiety, pallor, and cool, clammy skin. Careful immobilization of fractures reduces the risk of hemorrhage. If severe external bleeding is evident, external pressure should be applied and medical assistance summoned immediately. Management of hypovolemic shock is discussed in Chapter 19.

 Put on Your Thinking Cap!

A 16-year-old male was admitted after a motorcycle accident. He had a compound fracture of the thigh with severe soft tissue injury. After surgery, he has an external fixation device on the affected leg. A Jackson-Pratt drain is in place. Daily wound care is ordered. List all potential sources of bone infection that you can.

JOINT STIFFNESS AND CONTRACTURES

Joint fractures or dislocations may be followed by stiffness or contractures, especially in older people, due to immobility often associated with a fracture. Prevention requires appropriate positioning and progressive exercise programs as prescribed. Treatment may employ splints, traction, casts, surgical manipulation, and aggressive physiotherapy.

MALUNION, NONUNION, AND DELAYED UNION

Malunion is when expected healing time is appropriate but unsatisfactory alignment of bone results in external deformity and dysfunction. Nonunion occurs when a fracture never heals. Failure of a fracture to heal in the expected time is called delayed union. With delayed union, the bone usually heals eventually—it may just be slower. These complications may be caused by inadequate immobilization or excess movement, poor alignment of the bone fragments, infection, or poor nutrition.

When there is nonunion of a fracture, a variety of methods may be used to stimulate fracture healing. The implantation of bone grafts is an *osteogenic method*. *Osteoconductive methods* employ synthetic materials to provide a matrix for bone growth. The use of substances such as platelet-derived growth factor is called *osteoinduction.* In addition, several types of electric stimulation devices may be used to stimulate bone growth. The stimulation may be internal or external and is done up to 10 hours a day for 3 to 6 months. Although the procedure is time-consuming, it can prevent further surgery and bone grafts.

POST-TRAUMATIC ARTHRITIS

Weight-bearing joints are most vulnerable to post-traumatic arthritis. Excessive stress and strain on the joint or fracture must be avoided to reduce the risk of this complication. Post-traumatic arthritis can be a result of nonunion of a fracture.

AVASCULAR NECROSIS

A variety of factors can interfere with the blood supply after a bone injury. Once bone cells are deprived of oxygen and nutrients, they die and their cell walls collapse. This condition is called *avascular necrosis.* Signs and symptoms include increasing pain, instability, and decreased function in the affected area. Treatment measures include relief of weight bearing and removal of part of the bone to decrease pressure. If conservative measures fail, a variety of surgical procedures may be recommended. Sometimes amputation is necessary.

COMPLEX REGIONAL PAIN SYNDROME

Complex regional pain syndrome type 1 (CRPS–type 1), also called *reflex sympathetic dystrophy,* is usually precipitated by a fracture or other trauma. It is characterized by severe pain at the injury site despite no detectable nerve damage, edema, muscle spasm, stiffness, vasospasms, increased sweating, atrophy, contractures, and loss of bone mass. Symptoms persist longer than expected with the type of injury suffered. The condition is treated with nerve blocks, physical therapy, transcutaneous electrical stimulation, and drugs including analgesics, muscle relaxants, and antidepressants. The effects and treatment of CRPS–type 2, also called *causalgia,* are similar, but nerve damage can be detected.

SIGNS AND SYMPTOMS

The signs and symptoms of a fracture depend on the type and location of the break. Some fractures have so few clinical manifestations that they can be detected only with x-ray. The most common signs and symptoms are swelling, bruising, pain, tenderness, loss of normal function, abnormal position, and decreased mobility. Box 42-1 lists various signs and symptoms of fractures and their causes.

DIAGNOSTIC TESTS AND PROCEDURES

A thorough history and physical are important when fracture is suspected because it may provide valuable information such as mechanism of injury and often helps direct treatment. The most common diagnostic tests used to confirm the presence of a fracture are radiologic studies. Standard radiographs are used first

---

Box 42-1 | *Signs and Symptoms of Fractures and Their Causes*

Pain
There is immediate, severe pain at the time of injury. After injury, pain may result from muscle spasm, overriding of the fractured ends of the bone, or damage to adjacent structures.

Deformity
Strong muscle pull may cause bone fragments to override; therefore alignment and contour changes occur, such as (1) angulation, rotation, and limb shortening; (2) bone depression; or (3) altered curves in the injured site, especially when compared with the opposite site. Swelling (edema) may appear rapidly from localization of serous fluid at the fracture site and extravasation of blood into adjacent tissues. Bruising (ecchymosis) may result from subcutaneous bleeding. Muscle spasms—involuntary muscle contractions near the fracture—may occur.

Tenderness
Tenderness over the fracture site is due to underlying injuries.

Impaired Sensation (Numbness)
Sensation may be impaired as a result of nerve damage or nerve entrapment from edema, bleeding, or bony fragments.

Loss of Normal Function
Normal function may be lost because of instability of the fractured bone, pain, or muscle spasm.

Paralysis
Paralysis may be caused by nerve damage.

Abnormal Mobility
Movement of a part that is normally immobile is due to instability when the long bones are fractured.

Crepitus
Crepitus results from broken bone ends rubbing together. Grating sensations or sounds are felt or heard if the injured part is moved.

Hypovolemic Shock
Hypovolemic shock may result from blood loss or other injuries.

Modified from Black, J.M., Hawks, J.H., & Keene, A.M. (2001). *Medical-surgical nursing: Clinical management for positive outcomes* (6th ed., pp. 588, 590). Philadelphia: Saunders.

to reveal bone disruption, deformity, or malignancy. Computed tomography (CT) may be used to detect fractures of complex structures, such as the hip and pelvis, or compression fractures of the spine. A bone scan may be useful for detecting small bone fractures or fractures caused by stress or disease. Diagnostic tests for fractures are the same as those for connective tissue disorders described in Chapter 41 in the Diagnostic Tests and Procedures table on pp. 887 to 889.

MEDICAL TREATMENT

The goals of medical treatment for a fracture are to realign the bone fragments, establish a sturdy union between the broken ends of the bone, and restore function. The most common therapeutic techniques to accomplish these goals are closed or open reduction and internal or external fixation.

REDUCTION

Reduction is the process of bringing the ends of the broken bone into proper alignment. Closed reduction or manipulation is the nonsurgical realignment of the bones that returns them to their previous anatomic position. No surgical incision is made; however, general or local anesthesia is given. Closed reduction may be done by using traction, manual pressure, or a combination of these (Fig. 42-3). After reduction of a fracture, a radiograph is taken and a cast is usually applied.

Open reduction is a surgical procedure in which an incision is made at the fracture site. It is usually done for open (compound) or comminuted fractures (bone is broken or crushed into small pieces) to clean the area of fragments and debris.

Effective pain management of a fracture is essential for patient mobilization and healing. Once the fracture is aligned, immobilization is necessary for healing to occur. Immobilization of the bones is important be-

cause it prevents movement and increases union. It can be accomplished in many ways such as fixation, casts, splints, and traction.

FIXATION

Fixation is an attempt to attach the fragments of the broken bone together when reduction alone is not feasible because of the type and extent of the break. Internal fixation is done during the open reduction surgical procedure. Internal fixation includes the use of rods, pins, nails, screws, or metal plates to align bone fragments and keep them in place for healing (Fig. 42-4). Figure 42-4, C, illustrates an open reduction and internal fixation of a fractured femur in which a nail was used to maintain alignment. Internal fixation promotes early mobilization and is often preferred for older adults who have brittle bones that may not heal properly or who may suffer the consequences of immobility.

External fixation is similar to internal fixation, but the pins in the bone are inserted directly into the bone, above and below the fracture. The pins are then attached to an external frame and adjusted to align the bone (Figs. 42-5 and 42-6). When there is extensive soft tissue damage or infection, external fixation allows easier access to the site and facilitates wound care. In addition, the device allows for early ambulation and mobility while relieving pain. Pin track infection occurs in approximately 10% of patients with external fixation. Pin care is extremely important to prevent the migration of organisms along the pin from the skin to

FIGURE **42-4** Examples of different types of internal fixation devices. **A,** Tension band wiring technique using Kirschner wires for fracture of a phalanx. **B,** Compression plate applied to the lateral aspect of the femur. **C,** Intramedullary nail fixed to both proximal and distal fragments of the femur.

FIGURE **42-3** Closed (manipulative) reduction to realign a fracture of the arm.

FIGURE **42-5** External fixators. Mini Hoffman system in place on hand.

FIGURE **42-6** The Hex-Fix external fixation system for tibial fractures.

the bone. Patients should be taught to do their own pin care and to recognize signs of infection.

COMMON THERAPEUTIC MEASURES

CASTS, SPLINTS, AND IMMOBILIZERS

Casts, splints, and other immobilizers are used to secure the position of the body parts being treated. They hold the bone in alignment while allowing enough

movement of other parts of the body to carry out activities of daily living. Types of materials used for a cast are plaster of Paris, fiberglass, thermoplastic resins, thermolabile plastic, and polyester-cotton knit impregnated with polyurethane. A variety of materials are used to make splints and immobilizers.

Plaster of Paris consists of anhydrous calcium sulfate embedded in gauze. It is the least expensive type of cast to use. After a well-fitting stockinette has been applied, the gauze is immersed in water and wrapped around the affected part. The stockinette must not be too tight because it may impair circulation. A stockinette that is too loose can wrinkle and result in pressure sores. The strength of the cast is determined by the number of layers of wrapped gauze and the technique of application.

Initially the wet cast is hot, and the heat may cause edema of the underlying tissues from the increased circulation. The cast quickly becomes damp and cool. It dries after about 24 to 72 hours, depending on the size and location. When the cast is dry and strong, it can withstand weight bearing and other stresses. The underlying stockinette covers the edges of the cast to prevent scratching and irritation from the rough plaster. Short pieces of tape are sometimes placed over the edges of the casts to prevent skin irritation by rough edges and to protect the cast from moisture and soiling. This is referred to as "petaling."

Fiberglass is a synthetic material used for casts that is lighter and has a shorter drying time than plaster of Paris. Drying time is 10 to 15 minutes, and the cast can withstand weight bearing 30 minutes after application. Sometimes physicians use plaster of Paris casts on lower extremities for heavier weight bearing and fiberglass casts on upper extremities.

Other types of synthetic materials are thermolabile plastic (Orthoplast) and thermoplastic resins (Hexcelite). They are heated in warm water and molded to fit the torso or extremity. Polyurethane is formed from chemically treated polyester and cotton fabric. The fabric is immersed in cool water to start the chemical process for wrapping.

Sometimes the cast is split down the front to allow the casting material and padding to spread. This is referred to as a *univalved cast*. A *bivalved cast* is cut down both sides so that the front portion can be removed while the back portion maintains immobilization. When an opening is cut into the cast to allow inspection of the body area or to relieve pressure, it is said to be a windowed cast. Always save the cut out "window," because it may be reinserted later.

The four main groups of casts are (1) upper extremity, (2) lower extremity, (3) cast brace, and (4) body or spica cast. Examples of various types of casts are described in Table 42-1. An upper extremity cast is used for breaks in the shoulder, arm, wrist, and hand. A patient who is wearing an arm cast should keep the arm elevated above the heart when lying in bed to prevent swelling. The arm is kept in a sling for support when the patient is up.

Lower extremity casts are used for breaks in the upper and lower leg, ankle, and foot. A leg cast is used to allow mobility and may be used with crutches. A cast shoe or rubber walking pad protects the cast and pre-

vents falls. The affected leg should be elevated on several pillows during the first few days after the break to prevent swelling.

After an adequate amount of healing has taken place and edema has subsided, cast braces may be used for injury to the knee. A cast brace supports the affected

Table 42-1   Cast Types and Common Uses

TYPE	ILLUSTRATION	COMMON USES
Short leg cast		Fracture of foot, ankle, or distal tibia or fibula Severe sprain or strain Postoperative immobilization after open reduction and internal fixation Correction of deformity, such as talipes equinovarus
Long leg cast		Fracture of distal femur, knee, or lower leg Soft tissue injury to knee or knee dislocation Postoperative immobilization after open reduction and internal fixation
Bilateral long leg hip spica cast		Fractures of femur, acetabulum, or pelvis Postoperative immobilization after open reduction and internal fixation
Body jacket cast		Stable spine injuries of the thoracic or lumbar spine

Continued

Table 42-1 *Cast Types and Common Uses—cont'd*

TYPE	ILLUSTRATION	COMMON USES
Short arm cast		Fracture of hand or wrist Postoperative immobilization after open reduction and internal fixation
Long arm cast		Fracture of forearm, elbow, or humerus Postoperative immobilization after open reduction and internal fixation Can be weighted to create traction

Drawings from Maher, A.B., Salmond, S.W., & Pellino, T.A. (1994). *Orthopedic nursing* (pp. 279-280). Philadelphia: Saunders; Body jacket cast drawing from Lewis, S.M., Heitkemper, M.M., & Dirksen, S.R. (2000). *Medical-surgical nursing: Assessment and management of clinical problems* (5th ed., p.1776). Philadelphia: Saunders.

part while allowing the knee to bend. This is accomplished by applying a cast above and below the knee and connecting them with a hinge.

Body or spica casts are used when a fracture is located somewhere in the trunk of the body. A body cast encircles the trunk, whereas a spica cast encases the trunk plus one or two extremities. Body or spica casts severely limit mobility and may cause complications related to lack of movement, such as skin breakdown, respiratory problems, constipation, and joint contractures. In addition, a condition known as *cast syndrome* is caused by compression of a portion of the duodenum between the superior mesenteric artery and the aorta and vertebral column. Signs and symptoms of cast syndrome include nausea and abdominal distention.

The cast is removed only on physician's orders. A special device called a *cast cutter* is used to cut the plaster. Blunt scissors are then used to cut the padding. Tell the patient that the cutter blade is noisy but will not cut

the skin. However, when the cast is removed, the skin that had been under the cast will be tender and dry and may have crusts of dry skin. Gently wash the area, and explain that the skin will regain its normal appearance after a few days. Muscle atrophy may be apparent. Assure the patient that muscle mass will be restored with use of the limb.

TRACTION

Traction exerts a pulling force on a fractured extremity to provide alignment of the broken bone fragments. It also is used to prevent or correct deformity, decrease muscle spasm, promote rest, and maintain the position of the diseased or injured part.

Traction may be applied directly to the skin (skin traction) or attached directly to a bone by means of a metal pin or wire (skeletal traction). Examples of skin traction such as Buck's traction are shown in Figure 42-7. It is used for hip and knee contractures, muscle spasms, and alignment of hip fractures. Weight used during skin traction should not be more than 5 to 10 pounds to prevent injury to the skin.

Skeletal traction provides a strong, steady, continuous pull and can be used for prolonged periods of time. Examples of skeletal traction are Gardner-Wells, Crutchfield, and Vinke tongs and a halo vest, in which pins are inserted into the skull on either side (see Fig. 29-8). Heavier weights can be used with skeletal traction, usually from 15 to 30 pounds. Crutchfield traction and a halo vest are used for reduction and immobilization of fractures of the cervical or high thoracic vertebrae.

Traction may involve complications such as impaired circulation, inadequate fracture alignment, skin breakdown, and soft tissue injury. As noted earlier, pin track infection and osteomyelitis can occur with skel-

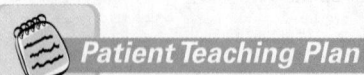

Patient Teaching Plan

Cast Care

- Keep plaster casts dry; follow the physician's instructions regarding wetting synthetic casts.
- Do not remove any padding.
- Do not insert any foreign object inside the cast.
- Do not bear weight on a new plaster cast for 48 hours (with synthetics, may be less than an hour).
- Do not cover the cast with plastic for prolonged periods.
- *Do* report the following to a health care provider: swelling, discoloration of toes or fingers, pain during motion, and burning or tingling under the cast.

Buck's traction

Russell's traction

Head halter traction

Pelvic traction

Balanced suspension traction

FIGURE **42-7** Examples of skin traction.

etal traction. The following are important points to remember when patients are in traction:

- Weights always must hang freely.
- Be sure the amount of weight used is correct as ordered, clamps are tight, and ropes move freely over pulleys.
- Maintain good body alignment so the line of pull is correct.
- Use padding to prevent trauma to skin where traction is applied. Report skin breakdown or irritation to physician.
- Assess affected extremities for temperature, pain, sensation, motion, capillary refill time, and pulses.
- With skeletal traction, assess pin sites for redness, drainage, or odor, which may indicate infection.

ELECTRICAL STIMULATION

Electrical stimulation may be used to promote bone healing by promoting bone growth. An electrical current is delivered through one of three methods: a surgically implanted device, a device with pins that are inserted through the skin to the fracture site, or a pack of electrical coils that is applied to the skin around the fracture site. Electrical bone stimulators are successful

in approximately 80% of cases, with an average healing time of 16 weeks.

ASSISTIVE DEVICES

CRUTCHES

Crutches increase mobility and assist with ambulation after a fracture of the lower extremity. Success in crutch walking depends on many factors, including the patient's motivation, age, interests and activities, and ability to adjust to the crutches. Crutch use requires good upper body strength, so it may not be appropriate for older or frail patients.

In most cases, a physical therapist measures the patient for proper fit and instructs the patient in crutch-walking techniques. The nurse reinforces the instructions and evaluates whether the crutches are being used properly. A properly fitted crutch should reach to 3 fingerbreadths below the axilla to avoid pressure on the axilla and nerves when walking (Fig. 42-8). Axillary pressure could result in temporary or permanent numbness in the hands. When walking, the patient's weight should be put on the hand grips. The hand grips are adjusted so that the elbow is flexed no more than 30 degrees when

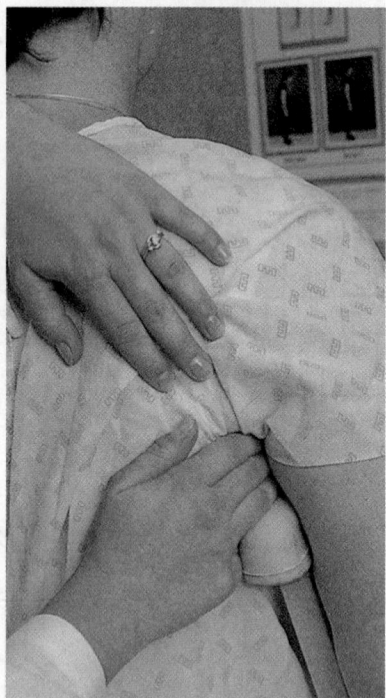

FIGURE **42-8** The distance between the crutch pad and the patient's axilla should be 3 to 4 fingerbreadths.

the patient is standing in the tripod position, which is the basic crutch stance: feet parallel, crutches 6 inches in front of and 6 inches to the side of each foot.

Gait Patterns

Several types of gait patterns are used with crutches. The type of gait used depends on the severity of the patient's disability and the patient's physical condition, trunk strength, upper and lower extremity strength, and balance. All of the gaits begin with the tripod position.

The five types of gait patterns used with crutches are the following:
1. *Two-point gait:* The crutch on one side and the opposite foot are advanced at the same time. This gait is used with partial weight-bearing limitations and with bilateral lower extremity prostheses.
2. *Three-point gait:* Both crutches and the foot of the affected extremity are advanced together, followed by the foot of the unaffected extremity. This gait requires strength and balance. It is used for partial weight bearing or no weight bearing on the affected leg.
3. *Four-point gait:* The right crutch is advanced, then the left foot, then the left crutch, and then the right foot. This gait is used if weight bearing is allowed and one foot can be placed in front of the other.
4. *Swing-to gait:* Both crutches are advanced together and then both legs are lifted and placed down again on a spot behind the crutches. The feet and crutches form a tripod.

5. *Swing-through gait:* Both crutches are advanced together and then both legs are lifted through and beyond the crutches and placed down again at a point in front of the crutches. This gait is used when there is adequate muscle power and balance in the arms and legs.

To sit down after walking with crutches, the patient walks up to a chair, turns using the crutches, and backs up until the unaffected leg touches the seat of the chair. One hand then grips both crutches by the hand grips, and the crutches are placed to the unaffected side. The patient bends at the waist, places the hand on the affected side on the seat, moves the affected leg forward, and lowers onto the seat slowly (Fig. 42-9). To get up from a sitting position, the patient pushes off against the chair with the hand of the affected side and pushes down with the other hand, which is holding both crutches by the hand grips.

Going up and down stairs on crutches is challenging. For stair climbing, the unaffected leg goes up the step first while the body is supported by the crutches. The full body weight is transferred to the unaffected leg, followed by movement of the crutches and the affected leg to the step. To descend stairs, the affected leg and the crutches move down one step first and then the unaffected leg follows. So, when climbing stairs, the good leg goes first, and when descending stairs, the bad leg goes first. ("The good leads up, and bad leads down.")

WALKERS

A walker is used for support and balance, usually by older clients. A modified swing-to gait is used with a walker so that the walker is pushed or lifted forward and then the legs are brought up to it. Rather than lifting both legs forward together, as with crutch walking, one foot is brought forward at a time.

CANES

Canes are used to provide minimal support and balance and to relieve pressure on weight-bearing joints. The cane is placed on the unaffected side with the top of the cane even with the patient's greater trochanter. The elbow should be flexed to approximately 30 degrees. Two-point or four-point gaits are used with a cane. The cane should be held close to the body on the unaffected side and advanced along with the affected leg. When walking, it is better to lift the cane rather than slide it along to prevent catching the cane tip and tripping or falling.

NURSING CARE *of the Patient with a Fracture*

Once the initial emergency treatment and medical management of a patient with a fracture have been provided, nursing care becomes very important. The focus of nursing care is on preventing complications and restoring the patient to independent function. (See Nursing Care Plan: The Patient with a Fracture on p. 927, and see Chapter 16 for a discussion of emergency care.)

FIGURE **42-9** Standing to sitting with crutches.

Assessment

Health History

Even after the initial medical care has been given and the fracture has been set, it is helpful to gather information on the cause, type, and extent of the injury. This information is important because it allows you to observe for complications or other injuries that may have been overlooked during the emergency situation. Ask the patient, family members, or witnesses about the events leading up to the accident and exactly what happened during the accident. In addition, describe symptoms associated with the injury, including the type and extent of pain, the presence of numbness or tingling or both, the loss of motion and sensation, and the complaint of muscle spasms.

Assess the number and types of prescription and over-the-counter medications taken by the patient to determine whether they played any role in the development of the fracture or will affect the recovery and rehabilitation. It is also helpful to find out about other medical problems that either may have been related to the cause of the fracture, such as a pathologic fracture, or that may affect healing. Determine the patient's occupation and usual roles and responsibilities, and discuss with the patient and family the effects of the injury on usual activities.

Physical Examination

Because fractures usually involve some type of accidental injury, be alert for signs of serious complications, such as head, thoracic, or abdominal injuries. In addition, examine the patient for associated tissue trauma, such as bleeding, bruising, and lacerations.

When inspecting the suspected fracture area, observe for deviations in bone alignment. The limb may appear to be deformed. The length of the extremity may change, usually becoming shorter. Inspect the skin over the fracture for lacerations, bruising, or swelling.

Compare the affected extremity with the unaffected extremity. Do neurovascular checks (pulse, skin color, capillary refill time, sensation) in the areas distal to the wound to compare circulation and sensation. Assess pulse rate and volume, as well as capillary refill time in the nails distal to the injury. Observe capillary refill time by applying pressure to the nail and checking the time required for color to return to the area. Skin color is a good indication of circulation to the extremity, and pallor indicates poor circulation. Determine sensation by pinprick, especially in the web space between the first and the second toes or between the thumb and the forefinger.

Nursing Diagnoses, Goals, and Outcome Criteria: Fracture	
NURSING DIAGNOSES	GOALS AND OUTCOME CRITERIA
Acute Pain related to bone fracture, edema, soft tissue damage, or muscle spasm	Pain relief: relaxed manner, patient statement of pain relief
Ineffective Tissue Perfusion related to tissue trauma or pressure caused by edema, bone fragments, hemorrhage, or therapeutic devices	Adequate circulation: affected tissue warm, normal pulses, normal skin color, minimal edema
Risk for Infection related to break in skin, bone trauma, soft tissue damage	Absence of infection: normal body temperature and white blood cell count, clear wound drainage, decreasing edema and redness

Continued

Impaired Physical Mobility related to pain and immobilization	Improved physical mobility: patient performs daily activities as permitted while protecting fracture
Risk for Impaired Skin Integrity related to injury, immobility, and immobilizing devices	Intact or healing skin: absence of open wounds, redness, or pallor due to pressure; skin warm
Activity Intolerance related to prolonged immobilization	Improved activity intolerance: performance of daily activities without fatigue

Additional nursing diagnoses may include Imbalanced Nutrition: Less Than Body Requirements related to additional metabolic needs of healing bone and soft tissues (see the Nutrition Concepts box below); Constipation related to prolonged immobility and pain medication; Self-Care Deficit related to pain and immobility; Ineffective Coping related to prolonged immobility, hospitalization, or altered lifestyle; Disturbed Sleep Pattern related to pain or immobility; and Deficient Diversional Activity related to immobility.

Interventions

Acute Pain

Fractures are painful. The degree of pain experienced depends on the extent and type of injury and the pain tolerance of the patient. The primary method of pain relief is immobilization of the affected part. Elevating the affected area will help manage edema. Analgesic medications and muscle relaxants, as well as cold therapy, also are used. Other methods of pain relief include repositioning, massage, and diversion. General pain management is discussed in more detail in Chapter 15.

Ineffective Tissue Perfusion

Factors that cause ineffective peripheral tissue perfusion are soft tissue injury resulting from trauma, fracture fragments, hemorrhage, edema, compartment syndrome, and positioning. The treatment of the fracture also can interfere with peripheral circulation, including moving or splinting the fracture, manipulation during reduction, and application of a cast, a splint, traction, or a brace.

Frequent neurovascular checks determine whether circulation is adequate and detect signs of pressure on nerves. For patients at risk for circulatory impairment, elevate the affected part above the level of the heart, apply cold packs as ordered to minimize edema, and encourage finger and toe movement. Evidence of impaired circulation includes abnormal coolness or warmth, weak or absent pulses, pale or bluish skin color, and sluggish capillary refill. Pressure on a nerve can cause pain or numbness. Immediately report signs of impaired circulation to the physician. If a cast is too tight, it may have to be cut or replaced.

Risk for Infection

Disruption of skin may occur with a fracture, and when there is open reduction with external fixation, the potential for infection always exists. Infection can delay healing and rehabilitation. Bone infections are especially difficult to treat. Use strict aseptic technique for dressing changes, wound irrigations, and pin care. Observe wounds and pin sites for signs of infection, such as drainage, redness, swelling, and warmth, and monitor the patient's temperature for fever. If an infection develops, employ standard infection control precautions and administer antibiotics as prescribed. The management of infection is discussed more completely in Chapter 13.

Impaired Physical Mobility

Interventions for immobility are aimed at promoting independence and preventing related complications. Patients may experience anxiety and powerlessness when their activity is restricted because of the enforced immobilization related to traction, casts, or other equipment. In addition, they may experience secondary complications of immobility such as deep vein thrombosis, pulmonary embolism, contractures or muscular atrophy, skin breakdown, and gastrointestinal problems, especially constipation. Older individuals are particularly vulnerable to the effects of immobility. Adequate hydration and nutrition are important.

Encourage all patients with fractures to engage in regular movement of some kind. Passive or active range-of-motion exercises are helpful for both bedridden and ambulatory patients. Support the joints above and below the injury in functional positions. Periodic elevation of the affected limb promotes venous return and reduces edema. Gait training with crutches, walkers, and canes promotes mobility and independence. A physical therapist usually works out an activity and exercise program for patients recovering from fractures, and the role of the nurse is to reinforce and encourage

 Nutrition Concepts

1. Calcium in the diet and calcium supplements are recommended to help *prevent* fractures due to osteoporosis in older age.
2. Prolonged immobilization, which often is required after multiple fractures, contributes to the loss of calcium and protein.
3. Essential nutritional elements for optimal bone healing are protein, calcium, and vitamins D, B, and C.
4. Supplemental feedings that are high in calories, protein, and calcium, such as milkshakes, may be served between meals to promote healing.
5. During periods of immobilization, a daily fluid intake of 2000 to 3000 mL is recommended to promote bowel and bladder function.
6. Advise the patient in a hip spica that overeating may cause abdominal pressure and cramping.

NURSING CARE PLAN

The Patient with a Fracture

ASSESSMENT

Health History: Mrs. Jacobson, age 80, was admitted for a Colles' fracture in the left wrist 2 days ago. Before the injury, she lived alone and cared for herself. She was active, alert, and independent. Since the fracture repair, she has complained of pain over the area of the break but has had no signs of infection. Her physician is ready to discharge her to her home.

Physical Examination: Vital signs: temperature, 97.4° F orally; pulse, 98 with slight irregularity; respiration, 20; blood pressure, 165/95 mm Hg. Height 5'3". Weight, 132 lb. Alert and oriented to time, place, and person. Needs assistance with activities of daily living, particularly bathing, dressing, and toileting. Cast on left arm from above her elbow to her fingers.

Nursing Diagnosis	Goals and Outcome Criteria	Interventions
Acute Pain related to bone fracture, edema, soft tissue damage, muscle spasm	The patient's pain will be relieved, as evidenced by absence of verbal complaints, anxiety, and moaning or wincing; patient confirms pain relief.	Provide adequate pain relief using medications and other comfort measures such as positioning and massage.
Ineffective Tissue Perfusion related to decreased blood flow caused by injury	The patient will have adequate tissue perfusion, as evidenced by normal skin color in areas distal to the fracture, adequate capillary refill, and adequate sensation.	Relieve edema by elevating the affected limb above the level of the patient's heart while she is lying in bed and applying cold for brief periods of time; encourage patient to wiggle fingers to increase circulation to the area.
Impaired Physical Mobility related to pain and treatment modalities for fracture	The patient will maintain as much mobility as possible, as evidenced by independence in activities of daily living (ADL) and absence of secondary complications.	Encourage regular movement, including passive or active range-of-motion exercises. Reinforce activity and exercise program for the patient. Seek referral to home health for assistance at home.
Risk for Impaired Skin Integrity related to cast	The patient will maintain skin integrity, as evidenced by intact skin.	Inspect the skin around cast edges for pressure or irritation. Monitor circulation and sensation in fingers.
Deficient Knowledge related to lack of experience with immobilization devices (e.g., casts)	The patient will demonstrate understanding of the immobilization device and will describe its proper care and complications that could arise.	Teach the patient interventions that promote bone and tissue healing; teach patient to recognize signs and symptoms of complications that should be reported to a physician. Instruct patient in cast care.
Self-Care Deficits related to immobilization of wrist	The patient performs activities of daily living independently or with assistance.	Assess ability to do ADL and to perform tasks such as cooking and grocery shopping. Determine whether she has anyone to assist her if needed. If not, request a home health or social work evaluation so that home care or assistance can be provided.

? CRITICAL THINKING QUESTIONS

■ What interventions can the patient perform that will promote bone and tissue healing?

■ What signs and symptoms require physician intervention?

---

patients to carry out the program. More discussion of immobility appears in Chapter 21.

If patients are unable to care for themselves independently at home, assistance from formal agencies such as home health services or social services may be needed. Areas to be assessed for home care needs include ability to carry out activities of daily living, mobility, mental status, and skilled nursing needs. If you

think home care will be needed, consult the case manager or social worker about the appropriate referral.

Risk for Impaired Skin Integrity

Skin integrity may be impaired as a result of the injury itself or the treatment of the injury. A compound fracture causes a break in the skin, and soft tissue injury occurs with almost every kind of fracture. Treatment

Table 42-2 *Tips on Positioning*

FRACTURE	POSITIONING
Cervical	Before treatment: with victim supine, immobilize neck with sandbags or Philadelphia collar If patient *must* be turned, be sure head and neck alignment is maintained
Thoracic spine	Position of comfort
Lumbar spine	Avoid high sitting positions, log-roll
Pelvis	Stable fracture or after fixation: turn to side opposite fracture Unstable: do not turn

Hip	Before surgical treatment: turn toward fracture (avoid dislocation or further displacement of fragments)
	    with pillows between legs
	Postoperatively: turn away from fracture until comfortable enough to turn on operative side, with pillows
	    between legs
	Arthroplasty: maintain abduction at all times with abduction pillow or regular pillows between legs

Shoulder/humerus	Elevate head of bed to comfort Turn to side opposite fracture
Forearm/foreleg	Elevate distal portion of extremity higher than heart

From Maher, A.B., Salmond, S.W., & Pellino, T.A. (1994). *Orthopedic nursing* (p. 281). Philadelphia: Saunders.

Put on Your Thinking Cap!

Assume you are going home with a walker. Assess the barriers in your home and modifications that would be needed for you to get around safely.

measures such as immobilization or devices such as casts or traction may cause pressure on areas of the skin and result in pressure sores. In addition, the improper use of equipment can cause pressure on certain areas of the skin. Individuals who are at highest risk for skin breakdown are older adults, people with preexisting conditions such as diabetes mellitus, and people whose general condition was poor before the injury.

To prevent skin breakdown, patients should begin moving around as soon as possible after the fracture has been treated. Proper positioning and frequent turning are essential for the prevention of skin breakdown. Guidelines for proper positioning are listed in Table 42-2. Good nutrition and fluid intake help maintain healthy tissues.

Activity Intolerance

With prolonged immobility, people become weaker and their ability to participate in activities diminishes. Encourage patients to keep their strength up by carrying out range-of-motion exercises, resistance exercises of the unaffected extremities, and, when possible, ambulation. Participation in activities of daily living and recreational activities also is helpful. Rest periods between activities help preserve strength.

Teaching should take place in the hospital immediately after the fracture is treated to prepare for the patient's discharge home. Assess the patient and family members for their readiness and ability to learn. Patient teaching after fractures should include the types of medical and nursing interventions that will be carried out to promote bone and tissue healing, signs and symptoms of complications that should be reported to a physician, how to use equipment and assistive devices, and techniques for managing activities of daily living.

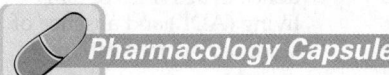

Pharmacology Capsule

Patients who administer their own pain medications are more in control and better able to manage their pain successfully.

MANAGEMENT OF SPECIFIC FRACTURES

FRACTURE OF THE HIP

By age 90, 17% of men and more than 30% of women sustain hip fractures. Most hip fractures are in the femoral neck and intertrochanteric regions (Fig. 42-10). The most common direct cause is a fall on a hard surface; however, it is thought that many fractures in older individuals result from decreased bone mass or brittle bones associated with osteoporosis (see the Health Promotion Considerations box on p. 929). Among older adults, 3% to 5% of all falls result in fractures. Signs and symptoms of a hip fracture are a history of a fall, severe pain and tenderness in the region of the fracture site, evidence of soft tissue trauma, the affected leg shorter than the unaffected leg, and the hip on the affected side rotated externally.

Medical Diagnosis

The diagnosis of hip fracture is confirmed by radiography. Other studies may be done in preparation for sur-

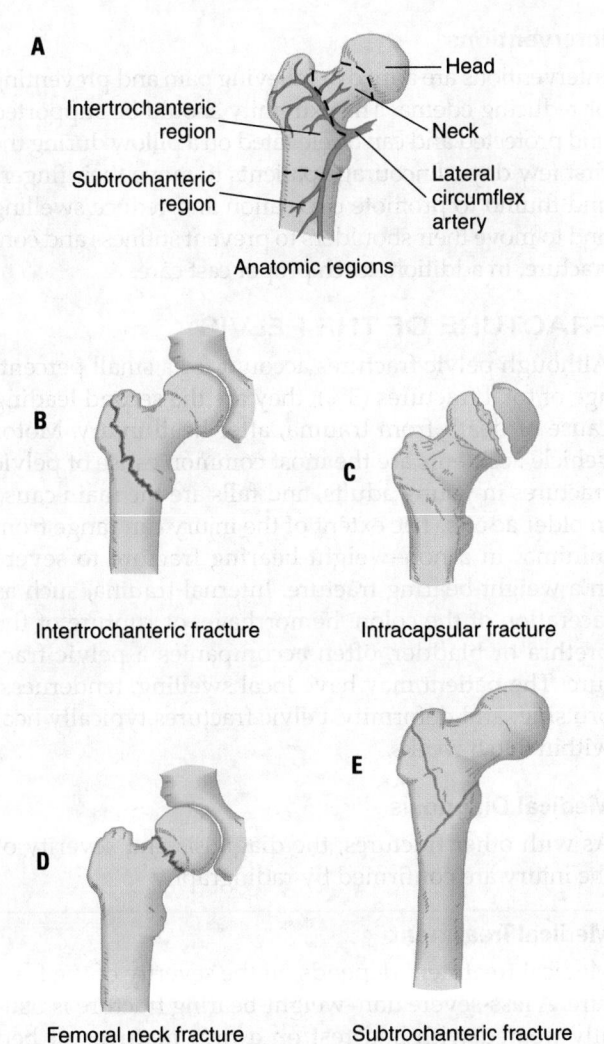

FIGURE 42-10 Femoral fractures. **A,** Anatomic regions of the proximal end of femur. **B,** Intertrochanteric fracture. **C,** Intracapsular fracture. **D,** Femoral neck fracture. **E,** Subtrochanteric fracture.

gery, such as a complete blood cell count, a urinalysis, and electrocardiography.

Medical Treatment

Traction and surgical repair (internal fixation, femoral head replacement, or total hip replacement) are the standard treatments for hip fracture. For older patients, surgical repair of the fracture is often the treatment of choice because it allows them to move around sooner and results in fewer complications related to immobility. Traction may require 12 to 16 weeks of immobilization for healing.

Postoperatively, patients may begin physical therapy as early as 1 day after surgery, depending on the type of repair. They may begin by sitting in a chair and then progress to walking with a walker. After internal fixation, weight bearing on the affected side is limited initially and then gradually increased as tolerated. After total hip replacement, weight bearing can begin almost immediately.

Health Promotion Considerations

Once Is Enough: Preventing Future Fractures in Patients with Osteoporosis

Osteoporosis is a public health threat for an estimated 44 million Americans. The disease makes bones more prone to fractures, especially of the hip, spine, and wrist. In the United States today, about 10 million people already have the disease and almost 34 million more are believed to have low bone mass, which leaves them at increased risk for osteoporosis. Of the 10 million Americans estimated to have osteoporosis, 8 million are women and 2 million are men.

One in two women and one in four men will have an osteoporosis-related fracture in their lifetime. Women near or past menopause who have sustained a fracture in the past are twice as likely to experience another fracture. Yet, unfortunately, only 5% of patients with osteoporotic fractures are referred for an osteoporosis evaluation and medical treatment.

Be sure your patients receive the necessary referrals for bone mineral density testing and other appropriate evaluations. Patients may be reluctant to exercise for fear of breaking another bone. Explain that engaging in weight-bearing exercises and resistance exercises preserves bone density and prevents falls by enhancing balance, flexibility, and strength. As appropriate, you can recommend the following activities to your patients:

• Walking
• Strength training
• Dancing
• Tai chi
• Stair climbing
• Hiking
• Bicycling
• Swimming
• Gardening

Adapted from National Institute of Arthritis and Musculoskeletal and Skin Diseases, *Once is enough: A guide to preventing future fractures*, May 2006, www.niams.nih.gov/bone/ hi/prevent_fracture.htm.

NURSING CARE *of the Patient with a Hip Fracture*

Assessment

Patients with a hip fracture are assessed in the same way as patients with other types of fractures. Monitor for pain, impaired peripheral circulation on the affected side, complications of immobility, skin breakdown, and ability to carry out activities of daily living. Older patients are particularly prone to developing delirium after a broken hip, particularly from the use of anesthesia during surgery; therefore, note mental status and problem behaviors related to confusion.

Nursing Diagnoses, Goals, and Outcome Criteria: Hip Fracture

General nursing diagnoses, goals, and outcome criteria for the patient with a fracture were presented on p. 927. The special needs of the patient with a hip fracture are discussed here.

Interventions

Nursing interventions are geared toward relieving pain, promoting mobility and independence, and preventing complications. Older patients have special nursing care needs because they are vulnerable to complications of immobility and confusion. Pain management is of utmost importance. Confused patients may not be able to tell you the extent or degree of their pain, and many times they may be undermedicated. Problem behaviors such as agitation, trying to climb out of bed, pulling out intravenous tubes or other tubes, and alterations in sleep patterns may be related to pain. Employ comfort measures such as repositioning, body massage, and diversional activities to enhance the effect of medications.

Proper body alignment is extremely important in preventing injury to the fracture area after it has been treated. Turn patients from side to side as ordered. After total hip replacement, the affected hip must not be adducted and must not be flexed more than 90 degrees because excessive flexion or adduction can dislocate the prosthesis. Instruct these patients to use elevated toilet seats, sit in supportive chairs with straight backs and seats, and avoid crossing their legs even at the feet. Care of the patient who has undergone joint replacement surgery is detailed in Chapter 41.

COLLES' FRACTURE

Colles' fracture is a break in the distal radius (wrist area). Colles' fractures often occur in older adults, particularly older women, when an outstretched hand is used to break a fall. The major signs and symptoms are pain and swelling in the area of the injury and a characteristic displacement of the bone in which the wrist has the appearance of a dinner fork. The most common complication is impaired circulation in the area resulting from edema.

Medical Diagnosis

The diagnosis is confirmed by the characteristic bone deformity of the wrist and by radiography.

Medical Treatment

Colles' fractures are managed by closed reduction or manipulation of the bone and immobilization in either a splint or a cast. The elbow is immobilized as well, to prevent misalignment.

NURSING CARE *of the Patient with a Colles' Fracture*
Assessment

Assess patients for pain and swelling following medical treatment of the fracture.

Nursing Diagnoses, Goals, and Outcome Criteria: Colles' Fracture

General nursing diagnoses, goals, and outcome criteria for the patient with a fracture were presented on p. 927. The special needs of the patient with a Colles' fracture are discussed here.

Interventions

Interventions are aimed at relieving pain and preventing or reducing edema. The extremity should be supported and protected and can be elevated on a pillow during the first few days. Encourage patients to move their fingers and thumb to promote circulation and reduce swelling and to move their shoulders to prevent stiffness and contracture. In addition, teach proper cast care.

FRACTURE OF THE PELVIS

Although pelvic fractures account for a small percentage of total fractures (3%), they are the second leading cause of death from trauma, after head injury. Motor vehicle accidents are the most common cause of pelvic fractures in young adults, and falls are the main cause in older adults. The extent of the injury can range from minimal in a non–weight-bearing fracture to severe in a weight-bearing fracture. Internal trauma, such as laceration of the colon, hemorrhage, or rupture of the urethra or bladder, often accompanies a pelvic fracture. The patient may have local swelling, tenderness, bruising, and deformity. Pelvic fractures typically heal within 6 to 8 weeks.

Medical Diagnosis

As with other fractures, the diagnosis and severity of the injury are confirmed by radiography.

Medical Treatment

Medical treatment depends on the severity of the fracture. A less-severe non–weight-bearing fracture is usually treated with bed rest on a firm mattress or bed board for a few days to 6 weeks. A more-severe weight-bearing fracture may require a pelvic sling, skeletal traction, a double hip spica cast, or external fixation. Because of the high risk of internal trauma, monitor the patient so that specific injuries can be treated immediately. Check for the presence of blood in the urine and stool, and watch the abdomen for any signs of rigidity or swelling.

NURSING CARE *of the Patient with a Pelvic Fracture*
Assessment

Observe for signs of bleeding, swelling, infection, thromboembolism, and pain. Assess urine output because the absence of urine may indicate a perforated bladder.

Nursing Diagnoses, Goals, and Outcome Criteria: Pelvic Fracture

General nursing diagnoses, goals, and outcome criteria for the patient with a fracture were presented on p. 927. The special needs of the patient with a pelvic fracture are discussed here.

Interventions

Interventions are designed to alleviate pain, promote mobility, and prevent complications. When handling patients, take extreme care to prevent displacement of the fracture fragments. Turn the patient only on the order of a physician. Provide back care when the patient is raised from the bed using the trapeze or with adequate assistance from others. Because of the potentially severe consequences of immobility, ambulation may be encouraged even though painful. Follow the physician's orders regarding ambulation.

Key Points

- A fracture is a break or disruption in the continuity of a bone, usually causing injury to surrounding soft tissue.
- Open or compound fractures have three grades of severity, ranging from least severe injury with minimal skin damage to most severe injury with skin, muscle, blood vessel, and nerve damage.
- Fractures of the femur are most common in young and middle-aged adults, and hip and wrist fractures are most common in older adults.
- Fractures are usually caused by trauma to the bone, especially as a result of falls and automobile accidents.
- Risk factors for hip fractures include osteoporosis, advanced age, white race, use of psychotropic drugs, and being female.
- The most common signs and symptoms of a fracture are swelling, bruising, pain, tenderness, loss of normal function, and abnormal mobility.
- Bone healing occurs in five stages: (1) hematoma formation, (2) fibrocartilage formation, (3) callus formation, (4) ossification, and (5) consolidation and remodeling.
- Healing time for fractures increases with age, and it may take six times as long for the same type of fracture to heal in an older person as it does in an infant.

- Complications of a fracture include infection, fat embolism, deep vein thrombosis and pulmonary embolism, joint stiffness and contractures, post-traumatic arthritis, compartment syndrome, malunion, nonunion, delayed union, avascular necrosis, and complex regional pain syndrome.
- The goals of medical treatment for a fracture are to realign the bone fragments, establish a sturdy union between the broken ends of the bone, and restore function.
- The most common therapeutic techniques used to treat a fracture are closed and open reduction and internal and external fixation.
- Casts are used for external fixation of extensive fractures and fractures of the extremities.
- Traction provides alignment of the broken bone fragments, prevents or corrects deformity, decreases muscle spasm, promotes rest and exercise, and maintains the position of a diseased or injured part.
- Crutches increase mobility and assist with ambulation after a fracture of the lower extremity.
- A walker is used for support and balance, usually by older patients.
- Canes provide minimal support and balance and relieve pressure on weight-bearing joints.
- The focus of nursing care for a patient with a fracture is on prevention of complications, pain relief, and restoration to independent function.

 Go to your Companion CD-ROM for a Pharmacology Tutorial, Audio Glossary, and 3-D animations.

evolve Be sure to visit the companion Evolve site at http://evolve.elsevier.com/Linton/ for WebLinks and additional online resources.

REVIEW QUESTIONS *Choose the best answer.*

1. A patient is brought to the ER with an injury to his arm that was incurred in a fall. A bone end protrudes from his forearm. The surrounding skin is bruised and swollen. Exposed muscle tissue is also swollen. The patient has normal sensation in his fingers. His injury is best described as:

   1. Closed complete fracture
   2. Grade III incomplete open fracture
   3. Grade I complete closed fracture
   4. Grade II complete open fracture

2. During which stage of bone healing do the ends of the broken bone begin to knit?

   1. Stage II
   2. Stage III
   3. Stage IV
   4. Stage V

3. A patient with a femoral fracture suddenly complains that he cannot catch his breath. His pulse is 106, respirations 30. You notice a measles-like rash on his neck and chest. You should suspect:

   1. Shock
   2. Fat embolism
   3. Avascular necrosis
   4. Compartment syndrome

4. Methods used to stimulate bone growth include the following:

   1. Traction
   2. Thermoplastic resins
   3. Fixation
   4. Electrical stimulation

5. A patient is being discharged with a plaster of Paris cast on her arm. Patient teaching should include the following:
   1. Notify the physician if your fingers become discolored
   2. Use a cotton-tipped applicator to scratch underneath the cast
   3. After the cast dries, you can take a shower without damaging it
   4. Loss of sensation is normal; it will return when the cast is removed

6. Crutches are properly fitted when the:
   1. Patient says they are comfortable
   2. Elbows are bent at 45-degree angles
   3. Crutch is 75% of the patient's height
   4. Crutch pad is 3 to 4 fingerbreadths from the axilla

7. The main advantage of surgery over traction for older patients with hip fractures is:
   1. Traction is more expensive because a longer hospitalization is required
   2. Surgery allows earlier mobilization, which results in fewer complications
   3. After a few days, surgical treatment is generally less painful than traction
   4. Bones of older people heal better with surgery than with traction

8. The most common cause of Colles' fracture is:
   1. Using an outstretched hand to break a fall
   2. Jumping from a high place onto a hard surface
   3. Landing in a sitting position after falling
   4. Falling with the leg in a position of outward rotation

9. The diet for a patient with a serious fracture should include the following:
   1. Reduced fat and calories to prevent weight gain
   2. Increased protein and calcium to build new bone
   3. Large doses of vitamin A and zinc for healing
   4. Decreased fluid intake to prevent bladder distention

10. A grating sound heard when fractured bone ends rub together is called:
    1. Crackling
    2. Bruits
    3. Crepitus
    4. Ecchymosis

43 Amputations

STEPHANIE ELMS

Objectives

After reading and studying this chapter, you should be able to:

1. Identify the clinical indications for amputations.
2. Describe the different types of amputations.
3. Discuss the medical and surgical management of the amputation patient.
4. Identify appropriate nursing interventions during the preoperative and postoperative phases of care.
5. Assist in developing a nursing care plan for the amputation patient.

Key Terms

💿 *Be sure to check out the bonus material on the Companion CD-ROM, including selected audio pronunciations.*

amputation (ăm-pū-TĀ-shŭn, p. 933)
amputee (ăm-pū-TĒ, p. 933)
closed amputation (p. 935)
congenital amputation (kŏn-JĔN-ĭ-tăl ăm-pū-TĀ-shŭn, p. 934)
gangrene (găng-GRĒN, p. 933)
guillotine amputation (GĬL-ō-tēn ăm-pū-TĀ-shŭn, p. 936)
open amputation (p. 935)
phantom limb (p. 942)
replantation (rē-plăn-TĀ-shŭn, p. 933)
residual limb (rē-ZĬ-dū-ăl lĭm, p. 935)
staged amputation (p. 936)
stump (p. 941)

Derived from the Latin word meaning "cutting around," the term amputation refers to the removal of body limbs or parts of limbs. Amputations have been performed since the beginning of mankind, according to findings by archaeologists. Ancient amputations were originally performed to remove gangrenous or damaged limbs; they also were performed for ritual sacrifice, punishment, exorcism of evil spirits, and, in some cases, beautification.

In the past two decades, many advances have been made in surgical amputation and replantation (limb reattachment) techniques, prosthetic devices (artificial limbs), and rehabilitation programs. This has allowed many amputees (people with amputations) to remain active and productive despite their disabilities. In the United States, the vast majority of amputees have had lower extremity amputations.

AMPUTATION

Amputation can occur through a joint (between the bones) or through a bone itself. *Disarticulation* is the term used for an amputation through the joint. The general site of the amputation is described by the joint nearest to it. For example, removal of the lower leg at the middle of the shin or calf is called a *below-knee amputation*. Some of the most common sites of amputation are shown in Figure 43-1.

INDICATIONS AND INCIDENCE

Conditions or situations that lead to the need for an amputation can generally be grouped into four categories: trauma, disease, tumors, and congenital defects.

Trauma

In some serious accidents, part or all of a limb may be removed. This often is referred to as a *traumatic amputation*. In other situations, the limb may be damaged so severely that it must be removed surgically. Common types of accidents and injuries leading to amputation include those involving motorcycles and automobiles, farm machinery, firearms and explosives, electrical equipment, power tools, and frostbite. Trauma tends to be the most common reason for upper extremity amputations. Because these accidents are typically occupational hazards, the victims are usually young men.

Disease

Vascular diseases account for the majority of the estimated 30,000 lower extremity amputations performed in the United States each year. In these cases, blood supply to the tissues is inadequate and the tissues become deprived of oxygen and other important nutrients. Without these nutrients, necrosis or death of the tissue occurs. Some examples of diseases leading to impaired circulation are peripheral vascular disease, diabetes mellitus, and arteriosclerosis. These problems also can be complicated by infection because wounds sustained by limbs without a good blood supply do not heal well and gangrene can set in quickly. Circulation

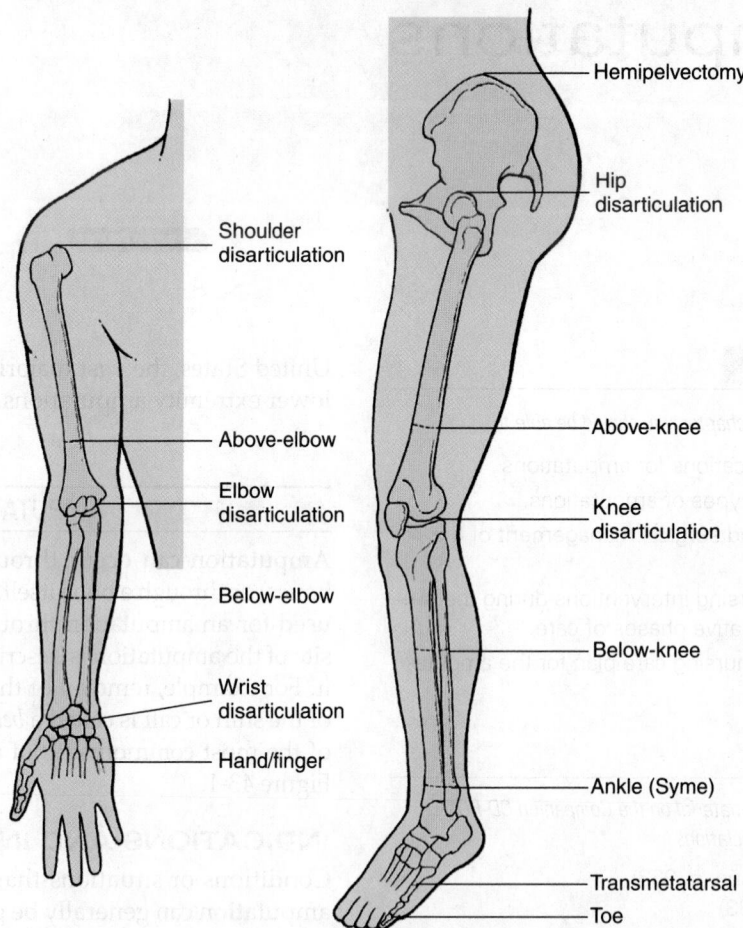

FIGURE **43-1** Common sites of amputation in the upper and lower extremities.

problems are more common among older adults and in the lower extremities. Chronic osteomyelitis, an infection of the bone, bone marrow, or surrounding soft tissue, can also lead to amputation. Sometimes when disease leads to severe necrosis, auto amputation can occur. *Auto amputation* is when the limb, most often a toe, self-amputates itself without surgery.

Tumors

Amputations also may be performed for bone tumors that are very large and invasive. Treatment may require amputation and disarticulation of an entire limb. Primary bone tumors occur most frequently in adolescents but can occur at any age. Approximately one third of these individuals are 11 to 20 years of age.

Congenital Defects

In some situations, a limb or part of a limb may be absent or deformed at birth. These are sometimes called congenital amputations. They result from factors that affect the developing fetus in such a way that the infant is born with a missing, deficient, or abnormal limb. Sometimes surgery is performed to convert a deformed limb into a more functional one that can be fitted with a prosthetic device.

DIAGNOSTIC TESTS AND PROCEDURES

The types of diagnostic studies done for a patient requiring amputation depend on the underlying disease or injury. For example, in a patient with vascular disease, tests to assess circulation are indicated. An elevated white blood cell count is consistent with infection. The Diagnostic Tests and Procedures table on p. 935 lists examples of diagnostic findings associated with some of the contributing factors in amputations.

Vascular Studies

Vascular studies may be done for a patient with compromised circulation, such as in trauma or vascular disease. Angiography is a procedure that involves the injection of a radiopaque dye into blood vessels, which are then viewed radiographically to determine their patency.

Pulse Volume Recording

Pulse volume recording uses a noninvasive device that gives general information about the volume of blood flow to an extremity. Another name for this procedure is *plethysmography.*

DIAGNOSTIC TESTS and PROCEDURES | *Diagnostic Procedures Associated with Indications for Amputation*

TEST/PURPOSE	PATIENT PREPARATION	POSTPROCEDURE CARE
WBC count detects elevation associated with infection.	Tell patient a blood sample will be drawn. Fasting not necessary.	Apply small dressing to site. Assess for bleeding.
Arteriography detects arterial occlusion.	Inquire about allergy to contrast medium, iodine. Inform radiologist if allergic. Mark peripheral pulses. NPO 8 hours before. Signed consent required. Tell patient "dye" will be injected into arm or groin; may briefly feel flushed or nauseated. Then radiographs will be taken to assess blood flow. Should void just before procedure. Remove jewelry and metal objects. Must remain still during test.	Maintain pressure dressing on puncture site as ordered. Assess for bleeding. Frequent neurovascular checks on extremity used to inject dye. Encourage increased fluid intake if permitted.
Pulse volume recording (plethysmography) used to evaluate arterial blood flow to an extremity.	Pressure cuffs are placed on extremities, and arterial pressure is measured during inflation and deflation. Explain procedure to patient. Signed consent not required.	No special care.
Doppler ultrasound used to assess pulses, patency of blood vessels.	Tell patient procedure is noninvasive and painless. Conductive gel is applied and a sensor passed over the extremity to detect pulses.	Cleanse gel from skin.
Bone biopsy usually done after imaging procedures reveal suspicious lesions.	Signed consent required. Sample of bone surgically excised for study.	Inspect site for bleeding. Administer analgesics as ordered.

Thermography

Thermography involves the use of a device that detects and records heat in various parts of the body. Relatively hot or cold spots are revealed, indicating the amount of blood flow to that part of the body. Cool areas generally indicate a decreased blood flow as compared with warm areas.

Doppler Ultrasound

Doppler ultrasound uses sound waves to determine the presence of pulses in the extremities. This technology is much more sensitive than using the fingertips to try to palpate a pulse.

Biopsy

In patients with tumors, a biopsy is often done to determine the nature of the tumor. A biopsy involves removing a small portion of tissue, which is then examined for malignancy.

MEDICAL AND SURGICAL TREATMENT

The management of amputations requires both medical and surgical approaches by the physicians involved in the care of the patient.

Medical Treatment

The medical care of the patient undergoing amputation must include the appropriate treatment and control of any underlying diseases or injuries. For example, diet, medication, and exercise are used to help patients with diabetes and poor peripheral circulation attain good control of their diabetes. Patients with peripheral vascular disease are encouraged to stop smoking because nicotine causes vasoconstriction. The patient who has experienced trauma may have to be stabilized with measures that will maintain his or her heart rate and blood pressure within a normal range.

Surgical Treatment

Amputation is recommended only when other options are not possible or have failed. In an effort to avoid amputation, the physician may perform angioplasty or surgical bypass of obstructed vessels.

Surgical management of the patient aims for amputation at the lowest level that will still preserve healthy tissue and favor wound healing. The surgeon chooses one of two basic types of surgical procedures, depending on the condition of the extremity and the reason for the surgery. These two types are closed amputations and open amputations.

Closed Amputations. Closed amputations are usually performed to create a weight-bearing residual limb, which is especially important for lower extremity amputations. In this procedure, a long skin flap with soft tissue and muscle is positioned over the severed end of the bone and sutured in place. The sutures are usually placed so that they do not bear the full weight of the patient. This technique has many variations.

Open Amputations. In open amputations, the severed bone or joint is left uncovered by a skin flap. This type of amputation is required when an actual or potential infection exists, as may occur with gangrene or trauma.

FIGURE **43-2** Upper extremity prostheses. **A,** Cosmetic. **B,** Cable-activated. **C,** Myoelectrically controlled.

FIGURE **43-3** Lower extremity prostheses.

The wound is left open for 5 to 10 days, sometimes longer, and is closed surgically when infection no longer poses a problem. Another term for this procedure is a staged amputation or guillotine amputation.

Prostheses. Prostheses are artificial substitutes for missing body parts. A prosthetist creates and supervises the use of a prosthesis. He or she explains the type of device to be used as well as the process of fitting the patient and instructing the patient in its use. In some situations, a limb prosthesis may be placed while the patient is still in the operating room. This requires placement of a rigid dressing to accommodate the temporary prosthesis. In other cases, particularly with lower extremity amputations, older or debilitated patients, and infection, fitting of the prosthesis is delayed until the residual limb has healed adequately. Provided there are no problems, a patient can usually bear full weight on a permanent prosthesis approximately 3 months after amputation. Various prostheses are depicted in Figures 43-2 and 43-3.

COMPLICATIONS

Many complications are associated with amputations, including hemorrhage and hematoma, necrosis, wound dehiscence, gangrene, edema, contracture, pain, infection, phantom limb sensation, and phantom limb pain. Factors contributing to each of these complications are listed in Table 43-1.

NURSING CARE *of the Patient Having Amputation Surgery*

PREOPERATIVE NURSING CARE

Nursing care of the amputation patient is based on a preoperative phase and postoperative phase. Routine preoperative and postoperative care are detailed in Chapter 17. This section focuses on the specific needs of the patient having an amputation (see also Nursing Care Plan: The Patient with an Upper Extremity Amputation on p. 939). Preoperative nursing assessment of the patient having an amputation is summarized in Box 43-1. The patient needs to prepare both physically and psychologically for an impending amputation.

Assessment
Health History

Record the conditions that resulted in the need for an amputation (diseases such as diabetes mellitus or peripheral vascular insufficiency, traumatic injuries, neoplasms, birth defects). Take a complete health history, including information on the patient's past medical and surgical conditions. Note preexisting cardiovascular problems because hypertension, coronary artery disease, congestive heart failure, and cardiac murmurs or defects can affect greatly the patient's ability to tolerate surgery and to recover successfully. Also, determine whether the patient has ever had phlebitis, varicosities, thromboses, emboli, or stasis ulcers in either the affected or the unaffected extremities.

Table 43-1　*Complications of Amputation*

COMPLICATION	DESCRIPTION AND CONTRIBUTING FACTORS
Hematoma and hemorrhage	Bleeding into tissue in and around residual limb due to inadequate hemostasis
Necrosis	Tissue destruction and death due to ongoing disease; requires surgical débridement or revision, or both
Wound dehiscence	Opening of suture line due to early removal of sutures or trauma; requires reclosure
Gangrene	Death of tissue associated with inadequate blood supply and bacterial destruction of tissue; requires reamputation
Edema	Swelling and discomfort in residual limb due to dependent position or incorrect wrapping; requires elevation and rewrapping
Contracture	Flexion of joints with loss of range of motion due to prolonged elevation or immobilization of extremities; may be prevented by frequent position changes and range-of-motion exercises
Pain	Extreme, sharp pain at incision site due to scar formation on nerve fibers (neuroma); may require surgical treatment
Infection	Redness, warmth, swelling, and exudate formation at residual limb site due to invasion of tissues by pathogens; may require antibiotics and surgical drainage
Phantom limb sensation	Patient experiences sensations (tingling, numbness, itching, warmth/cold) as if the limb were still present; caused by stimulation along a nerve pathway in which sensory endings were in the amputated part
Phantom limb pain	Patient experiences pain as if the limb were still present; more common when patient had pain in limb before amputation; pain may be enhanced by anxiety and depression; usually diminishes over time but may become chronic

Box 43-1　*ASSESSMENT of the Patient Undergoing an Amputation*

Health History

Chief Complaint and History of Present Illness:
Condition or incident leading to amputation

Past Medical History:
Previous illnesses, operations, hospitalizations, trauma, hypertension, coronary artery disease, congestive heart failure, cardiac murmurs or defects, phlebitis, varicosities, thromboses, emboli, stasis ulcers, diabetes mellitus

Family History:
Diabetes mellitus, hypertension, vascular diseases

Review of Systems
Pain:
Nature, location, severity, precipitating factors, alleviating factors

Sensation:
Loss or change, abnormal perception of heat and cold

Skin:
Color, lesions, ulcers

Leg Ulcers:
Location, size, color, drainage

Sexual:
Dysfunction

Functional Assessment:
Usual diet and fluid intake
Intake of salt and alcohol
Use of tobacco
Exercise, rest, and sleep habits
Occupation, roles, and responsibilities

Coping Strategies

Fears and Concerns

Physical Assessment
Height and Weight

Vital Signs

Skin:
Color, texture, temperature, turgor, lesions

Peripheral Pulses:
Presence, quality, symmetry

Capillary Refill

Sensation

Mental Status:
Level of consciousness, emotional state

Cognition:
Ability to follow directions

Record relevant disorders in the family history, including diabetes, hypertension, and vascular diseases.

Systematically assess signs and symptoms that relate to the vascular condition or other chronic and acute problems. Significant signs and symptoms are pain (location, severity, type, precipitating factors, alleviating factors), loss of sensation or abnormal sensations, intolerance of local heat or cold, color changes in the extremities, leg ulcers, and sexual dysfunction.

Significant data in the functional assessment are usual diet and fluid intake, intake of salt and alcohol, and use of tobacco. Describe exercise and rest and sleep habits as well as the effects of the current symptoms on the patient's usual activities. Identify the patient's occupation and responsibilities to determine how amputation will affect that aspect of his or her life.

A review of the patient's psychosocial background may offer insight into how the patient will tolerate treatments and procedures. Knowledge of how the patient copes with stress may help in planning care to reduce anxiety and fear. The patient about to undergo an amputation will undoubtedly have a number of fears and concerns about the surgical procedure, the loss of a body part, the potential loss of independence, and pain and disfigurement. Open discussion of these concerns may help alleviate those fears.

Physical Examination

Perform a total physical examination, with special attention to the neurologic, cardiovascular, and integumentary systems. Begin with measurement of height and weight and vital signs to uncover factors that may affect circulation, including obesity and hypertension. Throughout the examination, assess neurovascular status. Record the patient's skin color, texture, temperature, and turgor. The overall color, condition, and temperature of the skin are good indicators of blood supply to the extremities. Cool or cold, clammy, mottled skin that is pale or cyanotic may indicate a poor blood supply. Palpating both legs simultaneously makes it easier to detect circulatory differences between the two legs. In addition, there may be open areas on the skin. Describe any skin lesions and drainage from them. Wounds to the extremities are common when blood supply is inadequate.

Palpate the peripheral pulses for presence, quality, and symmetry. If pulses are not palpable, a Doppler ultrasound device can be used to assess them. Assess capillary refill by applying pressure to the nail bed of a finger or toe until it blanches (turns white). When the pressure is released, the nail bed normally regains its normal pink color within 3 seconds. In extremities with a diminished supply of blood, capillary refill may take 5 seconds or longer. Assess sensation by asking the patient to identify touch on the extremities. Experienced examiners may evaluate the patient's ability to sense sharp, dull, warm, and cold stimuli.

Collect data about the patient's mental and emotional status and general cognitive abilities to determine the patient's understanding of the illness and its implications.

Nursing Diagnoses, Goals, and Outcome Criteria: Amputation, Preoperative	
NURSING DIAGNOSES	GOALS AND OUTCOME CRITERIA
Anxiety related to anticipated change in body image and in function	Decreased anxiety: relaxed manner, patient statement that anxiety is reduced
Anticipatory Grieving related to expected loss of body part and function	Progress toward grief resolution: patient expresses feelings about impending losses, demonstrates healthy coping strategies

Interventions

Anxiety

Emotional support is important throughout all phases of care of the patient with an amputation. The patient needs time to prepare psychologically and emotionally for the surgery. Encourage the patient to express thoughts and concerns about the impending amputation. Accept the patient's responses. Allow the patient to express anger or to cry without being judged or given false reassurances. Tell the patient about physical and occupational therapy programs designed to restore maximal independent function.

Anticipatory Grieving

Recognize that the loss of a limb or part of a limb as well as the loss of functional abilities is stressful. Most patients experience a period of grief and mourn over this loss. Grief experienced before the loss actually occurs is called *anticipatory grief*. The patient may be concerned about altered physical appearance as well as loss of function. Explore the patient's expectations and fears about these changes. Gently encourage the patient to focus on what he or she will be able to do despite physical limitations. Allowing patients to grieve is an important part of their recovery and rehabilitation. Nursing care of the grieving patient is discussed in Chapter 24.

POSTOPERATIVE NURSING CARE

The postoperative phase begins immediately after the surgical amputation and includes immediate postoperative care as well as the long-term rehabilitation that is necessary for these patients.

Priorities for the postoperative patient are based on three distinct needs: pain relief, restored mobility, and avoidance of complications. The most common problems in the early postoperative period for patients with amputations are hemorrhage, edema, infection, and pain.

NURSING CARE PLAN

The Patient with an Upper Extremity Amputation

ASSESSMENT

Health History: A 32-year-old man sustained an injury in an industrial accident that required amputation of his right forearm just below the elbow. The patient's right hand was his dominant hand. He has had no other serious physical injuries or illnesses. He is a machinist who is a senior employee in his department. He is married and is the father of three children. His wife is a housewife who has never worked outside the home.

Physical Examination: Lethargic but responds to commands. Vital signs: temperature, 98.2° F orally; pulse, 80; respiration, 16; blood pressure, 126/68 mm Hg. A bulky dressing is in place on the residual limb of the right arm; dressing is dry and intact. A Jackson-Pratt drain is in place, and the receptacle contains approximately 30 mL of sanguineous fluid. Intravenous fluids are infusing into the left arm.

Nursing Diagnosis	Goals and Outcome Criteria	Interventions
Decreased Cardiac Output related to blood loss	The patient's blood volume will remain normal, as evidenced by stable vital signs, urine output equal to fluid intake, and absence of restlessness or frank bleeding.	Reinforce dressing, apply pressure, and elevate residual limb if bleeding is apparent. Monitor for signs of hypovolemia: tachycardia, restlessness, decreased urine output. Check brachial pulse on affected arm if dressing allows.
Acute Pain related to surgical incision, trauma, edema	The patient will state pain is relieved and will appear more relaxed.	Assess pain nature, location, and severity. Administer analgesics as ordered. Provide comfort measures such as back rub, distraction, imagery. Inform surgeon if pain is not relieved.
Risk for Infection related to surgical wound, traumatic injury	The patient will remain free of infection, as evidenced by normal body temperature and absence of foul drainage, excessive redness, warmth, or edema.	Monitor temperature for elevation. Assess dressing for foul drainage. When dressing is removed, inspect residual limb for excessive redness, warmth, or edema. Use Standard Precautions when handling dressing and residual limb. Teach the patient good hygiene to decrease the risk of infection. Administer antimicrobials as ordered.
Impaired Skin Integrity related to incision	The patient's residual limb will heal completely.	Keep the residual limb dressing smooth and snug to mold the residual limb for future prosthesis use. Use caution not to impair blood flow. Check the residual limb for irritation or signs of pressure. Maintain elevation as ordered to minimize edema and pressure on suture line. Apply cold to residual limb dressing as ordered. After the first week, massage the residual limb as ordered to promote circulation.
Disturbed Sensory Perception related to phantom limb sensation or phantom limb pain	The patient will report phantom limb sensations or pain if they occur.	Tell the patient that these sensations sometimes follow amputation. Notify the surgeon. Medicate as ordered. Advise the patient that several therapies are available for the treatment of this problem.
Risk for Injury related to loss of part of limb, weakness	The patient will identify activities requiring adaptation and will avoid dangerous activities.	Help the patient identify usual activities that cannot be safely done without the dominant hand or that require modification. Discuss strategies to adapt activities or to learn to use the left hand. Consult rehabilitation specialist for adaptation in work setting.
Self-Care Deficit related to loss of part of limb, inability to carry out activities of daily living	The patient will accomplish self-care with minimal assistance from others.	Assist the patient with self-care but encourage increasing effort on his part. Praise efforts. Organize environment to facilitate self-care (e.g., place bedside objects on the patient's left).
Anxiety related to perceived threat of disability	The patient will verbalize concerns about injury.	Explore the patient's fears and anxiety. Encourage the patient to talk about the loss. Express concern but not pity. Request services of mental health or spiritual counselor if the patient desires. Include family in care, and explore their needs as well.
Ineffective Coping related to overwhelming injury	The patient will demonstrate realistic goal setting and express intent to participate in rehabilitation program.	Explain the importance of proper residual limb care in preparing for rehabilitation. Consult social worker to assist patient in obtaining rehabilitation services.

Continued

NURSING CARE PLAN

The Patient with an Upper Extremity Amputation—cont'd

Nursing Diagnosis	Goals and Outcome Criteria	Interventions
Disturbed Body Image related to loss of body part	The patient will express feelings about loss of the hand and will consider strategies to improve function and appearance.	Gradually encourage the patient to take more responsibility for care of the residual limb. Counsel family members to demonstrate acceptance of the injury and not to promote excessive dependence. Facilitate meeting with prosthetist to discuss cosmetic and functional options.
Deficient Knowledge of therapy, self-care	The patient will verbalize personal role in recovery and rehabilitation.	Teach the patient to care for the residual limb and any prosthesis: 1. Wash residual limb with soap and water daily, rinse, and dry. 2. Inspect residual limb daily for irritation, redness, edema. 3. Keep prosthetic socket and residual limb sock clean and dry. 4. Do not apply lotions, powders, or creams except as prescribed by the physician. 5. If residual limb is red or irritated, temporarily remove the prosthesis; see physician. 6. Prosthesis will require periodic adjustments.

? CRITICAL THINKING QUESTIONS

- What data should you collect to assess the patient's pain?
- What sensations might this patient feel after the amputation?

- List three activities that are likely to require modification after loss of the dominant hand.
- How would you help this patient explore his fears and anxieties?

 Patient Teaching Plan

Amputation

- A rehabilitation team, including a prosthetist (if applicable), physical therapist, and occupational therapist, will work with you to help you regain the best function possible.
- If a prosthetic device is appropriate for you, the prosthetist will fit the device and teach you about it.
- Many modern prostheses are nearly lifelike in appearance and function.
- Phantom limb sensations are sensations perceived in the limb that has been removed; they are commonly experienced by amputees and may disappear spontaneously or continue for years.
- Medications and other treatments can be used to treat phantom pain.
- For lower extremity amputation (if applicable): upper body training is important to strengthen your arms.
- If you will be using crutches, we will teach you crutch walking and you will need to practice.
- We can arrange for a person who has recovered after an amputation like yours to visit, if you would like that.

Assessment

Monitor vital signs frequently in the first 48 hours postoperatively to detect early signs of problems. Inspect the dressing frequently for any bleeding. Some nurses try to monitor the amount of oozing by marking the stained area on the dressing with a pen, although this is a very rough assessment of bleeding. Sometimes the dressing is dry but blood is draining around the dressing and under the patient. If a drain receptacle is present, note the color and amount of the drainage. The drainage should gradually decrease in amount and lighten in color. Monitor the patient's temperature for elevations that may indicate infection. Also note any foul odor from the dressing. After the dressing is removed, inspect the residual limb for edema. Document the patient's pain, including type, location, severity, and response to treatment. Other aspects of postoperative assessment are detailed in Chapter 17.

Nursing Diagnoses, Goals, and Outcome Criteria: Amputation, Postoperative

Nursing Diagnoses	Goals and Outcome Criteria
Decreased Cardiac Output related to blood loss	Normal cardiac output: pulse and blood pressure consistent with patient norms; skin warm and dry
Acute Pain related to surgical wound	Pain relief: relaxed manner, patient statement that pain is relieved
Risk for Infection related to surgical disruption of skin integrity	Absence of infection: normal body temperature; decreasing redness and edema of wound margins; drainage that decreases in volume and becomes clear
Impaired Skin Integrity related to incision	Healed wound: incision margins intact
Risk for Impaired Skin Integrity related to advanced age and decreased mobility	Absence of new skin lesions: skin intact, no redness due to pressure
Disturbed Sensory Perception related to phantom limb sensations or phantom limb pain	Patient understanding of phantom limb sensation: patient statement of reduced pain
Risk for Injury related to loss of a limb or part of a limb, weakness, debilitation	Absence of injury: no falls or evidence of injury due to weakness or problems with balance
Impaired Physical Mobility related to loss of a limb or part of a limb	Restored mobility: patient performs activities of daily living; gradually returns to preoperative level of functioning
Activity Intolerance related to weakness	Improved activity tolerance: patient carries out daily activities without excessive fatigue, gradual increase in activity level
Self-Care Deficit related to loss of limb or part of a limb, inability to carry out activities of daily living	Resumed self-care: patient performs self-care within limits imposed by limb loss; learns new ways to care for self
Anxiety or **Fear** related to perceived threat of disability, possibility of death	Decreased anxiety/fear: calm manner, patient statement of lessened anxiety and/or fear
Ineffective Coping related to inadequate support system, use of inappropriate coping mechanisms	Effective coping with loss: patient talks about loss, participates in rehabilitation efforts and self-care
Disturbed Body Image related to loss of a body part	Positive body image: patient accepts limb loss, demonstrates proper care of residual limb, makes positive remarks about self and abilities

Interventions

Decreased Cardiac Output

Hemorrhage is the greatest danger in the early postoperative period. Hemorrhage may be detected by observations of excessive bleeding or changes in vital signs. Check vital signs frequently. Restlessness and increasing pulse and respiratory rates may be early signs of hemorrhage. Hypotension and cyanosis are late signs.

A portable wound suction system, such as a Hemovac or a Jackson-Pratt drain, may be placed to collect drainage. Inspect the dressing and the bed linens under the patient. Bright red bleeding, either from the drains or from the dressing itself, is *not* normal. If this is observed, apply a pressure dressing over the existing dressing, elevate the residual limb (also called a **stump**), and notify the surgeon immediately. A large blood pressure cuff may be placed at the bedside for emergency use as a tourniquet.

 Put on Your Thinking Cap!

Sometimes an immediate postoperative prosthesis is applied to the residual limb while the patient is in surgery. The surgical site is heavily covered and makes it difficult to assess the condition of the wound, so you must rely on other assessment data. Explain what data would cause you to suspect excessive blood loss in that situation.

Pain

Postoperatively, the patient has incisional pain that is treated with prescribed pain medications, usually opioid analgesics. Sometimes a sympathectomy is done during the amputation to prevent pain. This involves excising sympathetic nerves supplying the area. A second source of pain may be a neuroma, which may develop when severed nerve endings attempt to regenerate. This can cause a great deal of sharp, severe pain and requires excision by the surgeon. Assess and document the effects of analgesics, and notify the physician if pain

 What Does Culture Have to Do with Amputations?

Values related to body appearance, function, and independence are culturally influenced and will affect the way individuals react to amputation. Also, religious beliefs may dictate the disposal of amputated body parts by burial or cremation. For example, Orthodox Jews require that such body parts be made available for burial.

 Consider the Alternative

Many complementary therapies may be used with analgesics to control pain. Examples are imagery, relaxation, meditation, and acupuncture.

relief is not achieved. Pain management is discussed in detail in Chapter 15.

Risk for Infection

Use aseptic techniques when handling the residual limb, the dressing, and the drains to help reduce the risk of infection. Monitor for signs and symptoms of infection. The incision should be dry, intact, and only slightly red. Suspect infection if a foul or unpleasant odor comes from the dressing, if the patient has a sudden temperature elevation, or if the residual limb is red, excessively warm, or edematous. Laboratory results also may detect an elevated white blood cell count. Treatment for infection may include antibiotics and incision and drainage of the infected residual limb. In severe cases, the infection may cause further tissue damage and require reamputation at a higher level. Therefore it is very important to take measures to prevent infection and to act promptly if there is evidence of infection.

Impaired Skin Integrity and Risk for Impaired Skin Integrity

The care of the residual limb depends on the overall condition of the patient and the type of prosthesis. If the amputation is closed, there is some type of compression dressing with elastic bandages and, in some cases, a cast. The residual limb is bandaged to promote healing and to shrink and shape the residual limb to a tapered, round, smooth end that will fit the prosthesis. Wrap the bandage smoothly with even, moderate tension to all parts of the residual limb. Rewrap the residual limb as needed to maintain pressure. It is very important to avoid a tourniquet-like effect caused by pulling the bandage too tightly or unevenly. Figure 43-4 illustrates the correct bandaging of a residual limb. Commercial "shrinker socks" are available that maintain compression; however, they are expensive and it is difficult to find the right size and length for many patients.

Inspect the residual limb frequently for irritation and edema. Edema in the residual limb is most common during the first 24 hours postoperatively. To minimize this, a heavy cast or pressure dressing is applied in the operating room. Elevate the affected lower extremities by raising the foot of the bed. Pillows can be placed under a below-knee amputation, although the continuous use of pillows is discouraged because it can cause contractures of the hip. For the same reason, position the patient in a low-Fowler's rather than high-Fowler's position. If ordered, apply ice bags to the residual limb. Ice should be used for only brief periods of time because it can cause cold injury. After the fifth to seventh postoperative day, the residual limb can be massaged to promote circulation. If permitted, a patient with a lower extremity amputation should lie prone part of the day.

Disturbed Sensory Perception

As mentioned earlier, phantom limb sensation is common. It tends to lessen with activity, weight bearing, and exercise. It is often described as a burning, stinging, or crushing pain. If the patient reports such pain, notify the surgeon. Treatment for this type of pain may include diversional activities, whirlpool, massage, injection of the residual limb with an anesthetic, or

FIGURE **43-4** Proper techniques for wrapping a lower extremity residual limb.

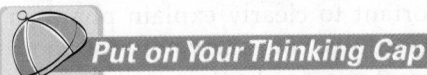
Put on Your Thinking Cap!

The home health nurse is visiting an older woman who had a lower leg amputation 1 month ago. The wound appears to be well healed, but the woman complains of pain that is sometimes severe in the amputated limb. She asks if she is going crazy. What would you tell her?

transcutaneous electrical nerve stimulation (TENS). A properly fitting dressing helps some patients. Drugs that are sometimes helpful include beta-blockers, anticonvulsants, neuroleptics, benzodiazepines, and antidepressants.

Risk for Injury

The patient must learn to function without the amputated limb. He or she must also learn to compensate for the lost extremity in unexpected ways, such as maintaining balance in sitting and standing positions. After lower extremity amputation, safe mobility is a priority. Reinforce the proper use of assistive devices (crutches, walkers) as taught by the physical therapist. Also encourage and assist the patient to do exercises to strengthen remaining limbs. Keep the environment free of clutter to prevent tripping. Patients with upper limb amputations must learn adaptations to perform activities of daily living. Everyday activities such as cooking may result in injury. The occupational therapist helps the patient learn to perform these tasks safely. Rehabilitation centers typically have demonstration homelike settings that allow patients to practice meal preparation and other daily activities. Occupational therapy services also extend to the home, where the therapist helps the patient and family plan for any needed environmental alterations.

Impaired Physical Mobility

An exercise program is usually initiated by a physical therapist. An important goal is the prevention of contractures. These are most common in the knee, hip, and elbow. The patient with a lower extremity amputation may be instructed to lie prone (if tolerable) with the head turned away from the affected side for 30 minutes three or four times a day. Traction, trochanter rolls, and a firm mattress may keep the body in alignment while the patient is in bed. An overbed trapeze may be ordered to facilitate moving back and forth between the bed and the chair. Avoid prolonged flexion of the hip (as when propped on a pillow). Prolonged sitting can lead to hip and knee contractures. Active and passive range-of-motion exercises also are an important part of maintaining mobility and preventing debilitation. Explain the value of exercises to the patient to encourage cooperation and participation.

The patient may have either an immediate or a delayed prosthetic fitting. An immediate fitting allows the patient to become accustomed to weight bearing, ambulation, and balance shortly after surgery. A delayed fitting is usually performed in above-knee amputations, bilateral extremity amputations, or cases of infection in which an open amputation has been performed. The appropriate time frame for fitting a prosthesis in these situations depends on the healing of the residual limb and the overall condition of the patient. A general goal for weight bearing of a lower extremity amputation is about 3 months. When the residual limb has healed satisfactorily, the patient is fitted for a prosthesis. A suitable choice for a prosthesis is based on the site of the amputation and the age, intelligence, health, motivation, occupation, and financial status of the patient.

Activity Intolerance

Surgery and bed rest may adversely affect the patient's tolerance for any type of sustained activity. It is extremely important to plan care to avoid too much patient exertion. Encouraging the patient to resume the preoperative level of activity too soon can impair physical and psychological healing. A typical activity order is for the patient to be assisted out of bed two or three times on the first postoperative day for 1 hour at a time. Over the next few days, the patient with a lower extremity amputation is usually encouraged to remain out of bed for longer periods and to begin to practice ambulation gradually. This may initially involve only a few steps, but these will gradually be increased over time. The patient's level of activity and the rate at which he or she regains endurance depend on many individual factors.

Self-Care Deficit

During the immediate postoperative period, assist the patient in performing activities of daily living as needed. Gradually, guide the patient to adapt to the lost limb and encourage more independence. Patients feel less helpless when they regain the abilities to provide self-care.

Anxiety, Fear, and Ineffective Coping

Provide opportunities for patients to talk about their concerns. It may be helpful to explore how the patient's usual coping strategies can be employed in this situation. Encourage and support effective coping strategies. Identify inappropriate behaviors, and attempt to help the patient find alternatives. Referral to a local amputee support group may be helpful. As mentioned earlier, it is important to expect the patient to experience a grieving process, especially if the amputation is traumatic.

Disturbed Body Image

The patient may have difficulty looking at and caring for the affected extremity. It takes time for the patient to incorporate the change into his or her body image.

Encourage the patient to talk about the change and what effects it will have. Emphasize ways to adapt to the loss and, if the patient wishes, to conceal it. Gradually encourage the patient to participate more in care of the residual limb. Patient instruction for residual limb care is extremely important. Counsel family and friends to support the patient and not to encourage excessive dependence.

THE OLDER ADULT WITH AN AMPUTATION

The older adult with an amputation may have some additional needs that should be considered when planning and providing care. For example, when constructing a teaching plan for the older adult, keep in mind that the healthy older person is completely capable of learning but often requires smaller units of information, more repetition, and more time. Skip unnecessary details, and make sure that during the teaching process patients with glasses or hearing aids have them in place.

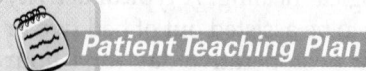

Patient Teaching Plan

Care of Residual Limbs and Prostheses

Residual Limbs

- Wash the residual limb with soap and water every night. Rinse and dry the skin thoroughly.
- Each day use a mirror to inspect the entire residual limb, especially the incision, for irritation, redness, and edema.
- Expose the residual limb to air when possible.
- Residual limb socks should be hand washed, rinsed well, and dried flat. A clean sock should be used every day. Having several socks will allow time for the socks to dry between washings.
- Do not wear mended socks, because a seam is irritating and creates pressure.
- Shoes with uneven heels will change the weight distribution of the residual limb and lead to irritation and possible skin breakdown.
- Do not use lotions, ointments, or powders unless prescribed by the physician.
- If redness or irritation develops on the residual limb, discontinue use of the prosthesis until you have the area checked.

Prostheses

- Keep the prosthetic socket (the opening in which the residual limb is seated) clean.
- The residual limb may shrink in size for up to 2 years after surgery. Annual visits to the prosthetist are recommended for necessary adjustments (more frequently for children as their residual limb grows in size with them).
- Each day, wipe the inside of the prosthesis socket with a damp, soapy cloth, then remove the soap with a clean, damp cloth. Dry thoroughly.
- Consult a prosthetist if there are any problems with the prosthesis. Do not attempt to make adjustments yourself.

It is also important to clearly explain phantom sensations to older adults. Some may not wish to report phantom sensations or phantom pain for fear of seeming foolish. Reminding the older patient that phantom sensations are not uncommon or bizarre can reduce the fear or anxiety that these sensations can cause.

Many older adults have one or more chronic health problems. This factor should be considered when choosing a prosthetic device. A patient with diabetes, for example, is prone to circulation problems and poor wound healing and may need a prosthesis with extra padding or support. Poor vision and decreased sensation may keep the older person from recognizing complications.

Because many older adults have decreased appetites, their nutritional status may be poor. Emphasizing high-calorie and high-protein intake is essential to promote healing and to maintain or build strength. See the Nutrition Concepts box on p. 945.

Remembering that the loss of a limb or part of a limb can be especially difficult for older adults is important in providing psychological support. This is because many older individuals have had to deal with other losses in their lives, such as the loss of loved ones, the loss of independence, and the loss of income associated with retirement. Older people may lack confidence that they can adapt and gain strength.

If the patient is unable to participate fully in his or her care, instruct family members along with the older patient. Home health nursing services may be arranged to facilitate adaptation in the home setting and to monitor for complications. Empathy, patience, and respect are essential in approaching older patients.

REPLANTATION

In some amputation injuries, a type of surgical technique called *replantation* may be performed. This generally involves the use of a microscope and highly specialized instruments to reanastomose (reconnect) blood vessels and nerve fibers in a severed limb. The limb is then sutured into its correct anatomic position. Advances in microsurgical techniques and preservation of severed limbs have made this technique increasingly successful.

INDICATIONS

A number of factors are considered by the surgeon before performing replantation surgery—for example, the type of injury and location. Replantation surgery is most likely to be performed for amputations through the hand or wrist. Amputated thumbs are reattached whenever possible because of the thumb's importance in total hand function. In a severely injured hand in which two or more fingers are detached, an attempt is

Nutrition Concepts

1. A nutritional assessment should be made preoperatively for patients undergoing surgical amputation, especially for older, immobilized, or chronic alcoholic patients.
2. Patients undergoing surgical amputation should be well hydrated; intravenous fluids may be given if oral fluids are not tolerated.
3. Surgical amputation is accompanied by a stress response, resulting in an increased need for calories and protein for healing.
4. Dietary supplements such as Sustacal or Ensure may be needed for patients whose intake of regular foods is inadequate for healing.
5. Patients are encouraged to become mobile as soon as possible after an amputation to prevent loss of calcium and protein.
6. Dietary choices high in protein, zinc, and vitamin C promote wound healing.

---

made by the surgeon to restore as many fingers as possible. Amputations above the wrist do not lend themselves as readily to replantation because of the extensive tissue, muscle, and bone damage accompanying the injury. A large muscle mass injury involves a great amount of tissue damage. Severely traumatized tissue can become ischemic, leading to death of the tissues and loss of the replanted limb. Severe crushing injuries or avulsion injuries in which the limb is mutilated also are not appropriate for replantation. In general, the greater the muscle mass injury, the less likely that replantation will be possible.

Another factor that is considered in deciding whether to attempt replantation is the length of warm or cold ischemia time.

EMERGENCY CARE

Proper handling of amputated parts is extremely important for successful replantation. Current preservation techniques include wrapping the amputated parts in a clean cloth saturated with normal saline or Ringer's lactate solution. These parts are then placed in a sealed plastic bag that is placed in ice water. Direct contact between the amputated part and the ice can lead to further tissue damage and cell death. Partially amputated parts should remain attached to the patient and also should be kept cool if possible. Extra care should be taken to avoid detaching any parts, since even small connections increase the chances for successful repair.

The patient may require treatment for shock due to blood loss. This may include intravenous fluids and blood products. Blood loss from the residual limb may be minimized by using a clean, dry dressing, which can be reinforced as needed. Tourniquets should not be used unless absolutely necessary, because they can cause ischemia of the residual limb.

NURSING CARE *of the Patient Having Replantation Surgery*

PREOPERATIVE NURSING CARE

Assessment

General preoperative care of the replantation patient includes careful assessment of circulatory status, close monitoring of vital signs, and inspection of the residual limb (or dressing) for bleeding. Assess pain at the site of the injury and at other locations. Measure and record fluid intake and output. Note the patient's emotional status, and assess understanding of the preoperative activities and postoperative routines. Identify sources of support.

Nursing Diagnoses, Goals, and Outcome Criteria: Replantation, Preoperative Care	
NURSING DIAGNOSES	GOALS AND OUTCOME CRITERIA
Decreased Cardiac Output related to decreased blood volume	Normal cardiac output: pulse and blood pressure within patient norms, skin warm and dry
Fear related to severe injury or possible failure of replantation	Reduced fear: calm manner, patient statement of less fear
Anxiety related to lack of knowledge of surgical routines	Decreased anxiety: relaxed manner, patient statement of reduced anxiety
Acute Pain related to tissue trauma	Decreased pain: patient statement of less pain, relaxed manner, pulse and blood pressure within patient norms

Interventions

Administer intravenous fluids and blood as ordered. If the dressing becomes saturated with blood, reinforce the dressing. Report continued or excessive bleeding to the physician. Even though preparations for replantation are hurried, be sensitive to the patient's fear and anxiety. Accept the patient's feelings. Provide brief, simple explanations. Administer analgesics as ordered for pain.

POSTOPERATIVE NURSING CARE

Routine postoperative care is discussed in detail in Chapter 17. This section emphasizes the special needs of the replantation patient.

Assessment

Postoperative assessment includes monitoring vital signs, intake and output, and level of consciousness. An essential aspect of care after replantation is hourly neurovascular assessment of the replanted limb. A Doppler device or pulse oximeter may be used to evaluate circulation. When the patient arrives on the nursing unit, immediately assess and document circulatory status to establish a baseline for comparison. Note and record the limb's color, capillary refill, turgor, temperature, and sensation. Signs of arterial occlusion are pale or blue color, slow capillary refill, shriveled appearance, and coolness. Signs of venous congestion are cyanosis, rapid capillary refill, edema, and warmth. Assess the limb for edema because massive edema often accompanies replantation.

Nursing Diagnoses, Goals, and Outcome Criteria: Replantation, Postoperative Care

NURSING DIAGNOSES	GOALS AND OUTCOME CRITERIA
Ineffective Tissue Perfusion related to trauma, edema, compensatory vasoconstriction	Adequate circulation to replanted limb: warmth, normal skin color, arterial pulses
Acute Pain related to tissue trauma	Pain relief: relaxed expression, statement of less pain
Disturbed Body Image related to disfigurement, loss of function	Improved body image: patient touches and looks at affected part, makes positive statements about self

Interventions

Measures to promote circulation to the replanted limb include elevation of the limb and microvascular precautions. Elevation of the limb promotes venous and lymphatic drainage. Take care not to elevate the limb above the level of the heart, because this may impair arterial flow. Several soft pillows or a stockinette connected to an intravenous pole may help achieve this. Microvascular precautions include avoiding any substances or conditions that contribute to blood vessel spasm or constriction. Encourage the patient to abstain from nicotine- and caffeine-containing products for 7 to 10 days postoperatively. Enforce a strict ban on cigarette smoking. In addition, maintain room temperature at 80° F to prevent compensatory vasoconstriction of the peripheral tissues in response to cold. Loosen tight or restrictive gowns or pajamas. Explain the importance of these measures to the patient and family.

The physician may order intravenous low-molecular-weight dextran (Dextran 40), aspirin, or heparin to reduce the risk of thrombosis. Administer the drugs as ordered, and monitor for adverse effects.

Inadequate arterial blood flow to the replanted limb is a medical emergency. If there is evidence of inadequate arterial circulation (no pulse, pallor or cyanosis, cool skin), immediately notify the surgeon and prepare the patient for a return to the operating suite. In some facilities, venous congestion is treated with leeches. Leeches are attached to a selected area of the replanted limb. The saliva of these worms contains an anticoagulant, a local vasodilator, and a local anesthetic. The leech extracts excess blood, reducing venous congestion.

Provide the patient with an opportunity to discuss thoughts and feelings about the replantation, disfigurement, and loss of function. It may take a while before

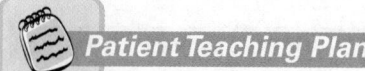

Postoperative Replantation

- Avoid nicotine and caffeine for 7 to 10 days, or as directed by the surgeon.
- Avoid tight clothing that could impair circulation to the replanted limb/digit.
- Keep the limb positioned as instructed.
- A rehabilitation team will teach you proper care to promote improved function.
- Immediately advise your surgeon of changes in the color or warmth of the replanted limb/digit.

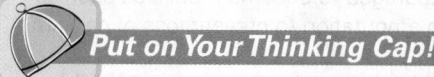

Put on Your Thinking Cap!

What could you do or say to support the patient whose replanted limb must be amputated?

the patient is able to look at and touch the replanted limb. Support the patient, and demonstrate acceptance of him or her. Your comfort with handling the limb can help the patient feel accepted. The rehabilitation team works with the patient to restore maximum possible function.

If the replantation is not successful, the limb is surgically removed. This represents a significant loss to the patient. Recognize this loss, and support the patient.

Other essential aspects of care include routine postoperative measures such as frequent position changes, pulmonary toilet, and pain management.

Key Points

- Amputation is the surgical removal of body limbs or parts of limbs.
- Conditions or situations that can lead to an amputation include trauma, disease, tumors, and congenital problems.
- The medical management of patients who have amputations involves the appropriate treatment and control of underlying diseases such as diabetes mellitus and peripheral vascular disease.
- Complications of amputation include hemorrhage, hematoma, necrosis, wound dehiscence, gangrene, edema, contracture, pain, and infection.
- Preoperatively, the patient needs to prepare physically and psychologically for an impending amputation.
- Postoperative nursing care focuses on Decreased Cardiac Output, Acute Pain, Risk for Infection, Impaired Skin Integrity, Risk for Impaired Skin Integrity, Disturbed Sensory Perception, Risk for Injury, Impaired Physical Mobil-

ity, Activity Intolerance, Self-Care Deficit, Anxiety or Fear, Deficient Knowledge, Ineffective Coping, and Disturbed Body Image.

- Replantation of severed limbs is sometimes possible.
- Before replantation, nursing and medical care focus on preserving the severed part and managing the patient's blood loss.
- Priorities after replantation include assessing for and managing Ineffective Tissue Perfusion, Acute Pain, and Disturbed Body Image.

- If there is evidence of inadequate arterial circulation in a replanted limb, immediately notify the surgeon and prepare the patient for a return to the operating suite.

 Go to your Companion CD-ROM for a Pharmacology Tutorial, Audio Glossary, and 3-D animations.

evolve Be sure to visit the companion Evolve site at http://evolve.elsevier.com/Linton/ for WebLinks and additional online resources.

REVIEW QUESTIONS *Choose the best answer.*

1. The most common cause of lower extremity amputation is:
   1. Trauma
   2. Vascular disease
   3. Tumors
   4. Congenital defects

2. Smoking is contraindicated after replantation because nicotine:
   1. Causes vasoconstriction
   2. Increases the risk of bleeding
   3. Impairs the immune system
   4. Causes arteriosclerosis

3. In which situation would an *open* amputation be most likely?
   1. A teenager with bone cancer
   2. A diabetic patient with vascular disease
   3. A child with a congenital deformity
   4. An accident victim with a crushing injury

4. A patient complains that her amputated foot itches and feels hot. This represents which of the following?
   1. Poor psychological adjustment
   2. Phantom limb sensation
   3. Early symptoms of infection
   4. Denial of the amputation

5. In the early postoperative period, the greatest danger to the patient who has had an amputation is:
   1. Infection
   2. Wound dehiscence
   3. Dehydration
   4. Hemorrhage

6. A compression dressing or a cast is applied after amputation to:
   1. Reduce pain
   2. Shape the residual limb
   3. Prevent wound contamination
   4. Prevent stimulation of nerve endings

7. Measures to prevent contractures in a residual limb after lower extremity amputation include the following:
   1. Keep the patient up in a chair as much as possible
   2. Guide the patient through active range-of-motion exercises
   3. Have the patient lie supine for 30 minutes three or four times a day
   4. Prop the residual limb on a pillow when the patient is supine

8. Patient teaching related to care of a residual limb and prosthesis should include which of the following statements?
   1. Clean, rinse, and dry the prosthetic socket every day.
   2. Always powder the residual limb before putting on the sock.
   3. Redness and irritation of the residual limb are normal.
   4. Wash the residual limb with soap and water once a week.

9. The best way to preserve an amputated body part for possible replantation is to:
   1. Cover the part with ice
   2. Wrap the part in a clean, dry cloth
   3. Wash the part carefully, dry, and wrap in plastic
   4. Seal the part in a plastic bag and put in ice water

10. When you examine a patient's replanted hand, it is slightly bluish, swollen, and warm. These findings indicate:
    1. Arterial occlusion
    2. Rejection of the replanted hand
    3. Venous congestion
    4. That the replantation was successful

44 Pituitary and Adrenal Disorders

Objectives

After reading and studying this chapter, you should be able to:

1. Identify data to be collected for the nursing assessment of adrenal and pituitary function.
2. Describe the tests and procedures used to diagnose disorders of the adrenal and pituitary glands.
3. Describe the pathophysiology and medical treatment of adrenocortical insufficiency, excess adrenocortical hormones, hypopituitarism, diabetes insipidus, and pituitary tumors.
4. Assist in developing nursing care plans for patients with selected disorders of the adrenal and pituitary glands.

Key Terms

Be sure to check out the bonus material on the Companion CD-ROM, including selected audio pronunciations.

acromegaly (ăk-rō-MĔG-ă-lē, p. 952)
Addison's disease (ĂD-ĭ-sŏnz dĭ-ZĔZ, p. 966)
adrenalin (ă-DRĔN-ă-lĭn, p. 965)
androgens (ĂN-drō-jĕnz, p. 966)
catecholamines (kăt-ĕ-KŌL-ă-mēnz, p. 965)
Cushing's disease (KŪSH-ĭng dĭ-ZĔZ, p. 973)
Cushing's syndrome (KŪSH-ĭng SĬN-drōm, p. 973)
diabetes insipidus (DI) (dĭ-ă-BĒ-tēz ĭn-SĬP-ĭ-dŭs, p. 961)
dwarfism (DWORF-ĭ-zm, p. 959)
endocrine gland (ĔN-dō-krĭn, p. 948)
estrogens (ĔS-trō-jĕnz, p. 966)
gigantism (JĬ-găn-tĭzm, p. 952)
glucocorticoid (gloo-kō-KŌR-tĭ-koyd, p. 965)
hypophysectomy (hī-pō-fĭ-SĔK-tŏ-mē, p. 954)
mineralocorticoid (mĭn-ĕr-ăl-ō-KŌR-tĭ-koyd, p. 965)
syndrome of inappropriate antidiuretic hormone (SIADH) (ăn-tĭ-dĭ-ū-RĔT-ĭk HŌR-mōn, p. 963)

Virtually every cell in the human body is affected by the endocrine system. The endocrine system is a complex communication network composed of glands and glandular tissue that make, store, and secrete chemical messengers called *hormones*. Hormones are delivered to target organs and body tissues by the bloodstream. The endocrine glands are depicted in Figure 44-1.

Another class of glands includes the exocrine glands. The exocrine glands pass secretions through ducts or tubes that empty outside the body or into the lumen or opening of other organs. Examples of this type of gland are sweat glands and the portion of the pancreas that secretes digestive enzymes.

HORMONE FUNCTIONS AND REGULATION

The term *hormone* was coined in 1905. It is derived from the Greek word meaning "I arouse to activity." This definition is appropriate because hormones are usually released in response to the body's needs. Hormones are responsible for important functions related to reproduction, fluid and electrolyte balance, host defenses, responses to stress and injury, energy metabolism, and growth and development. The overall mission of the endocrine system is to maintain homeostasis. Homeostasis is the maintenance of physiologic stability despite the constant changes that occur in the environment. A hormone is a substance composed of amines, peptides, or steroids. These substances bind to receptors located inside the cell nucleus or on the cell membranes of target organs or tissues. Receptors are specific for certain kinds of hormones. Once the hormones bind with their receptors, they exert their effects on the organ or tissue.

Regulation of endocrine activity is controlled by mechanisms, called *feedback mechanisms*, that either stimulate or inhibit hormone synthesis and secretion. Feedback mechanisms are triggered by blood levels of specific substances. These substances may be hormones or other chemical compounds regulated by hormones. Feedback may be either positive or negative (Fig. 44-2).

In negative feedback, high levels of a substance inhibit hormone synthesis and secretion, whereas low levels stimulate hormone synthesis and secretion. A simple example of this is the household thermostat. As the environmental temperature rises, the production of heat is decreased or stopped; however, as the temperature drops, heat production increases. In positive feedback, high levels of a substance stimulate hormone synthesis and secretion, whereas low levels inhibit additional hormone synthesis and secretion.

Regulation of hormone production and activity varies with the time of day. Humans and most other animals have a circadian or diurnal rhythm. This rhythm is based on a 24-hour cycle, during which

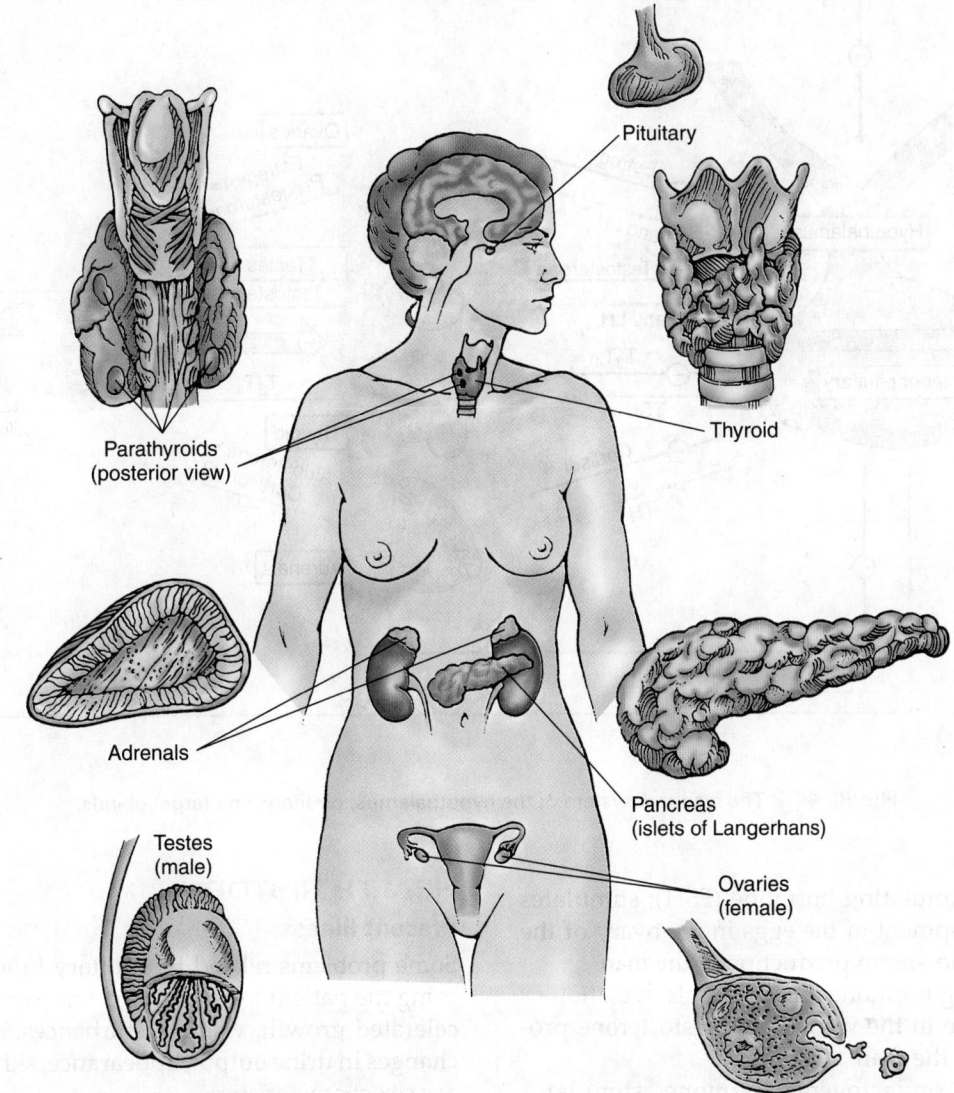

FIGURE **44-1** The endocrine system. The organs of the endocrine system include the pituitary gland, thyroid gland, parathyroid glands, adrenal glands, pancreas, testes (in the man), and ovaries (in the woman).

hormone synthesis and secretion are at their slowest rate during the early morning hours and at their highest rate during the evening hours.

THE PITUITARY GLAND

ANATOMY AND PHYSIOLOGY OF THE PITUITARY GLAND

The pituitary gland, also called the *hypophysis,* is a structure that weighs approximately 0.6 gm and is located in the sella turcica, a small indentation in the sphenoid bone at the base of the brain. It is connected to the hypothalamus by the infundibular (hypophyseal) stalk. The pituitary gland is small and oval and has a diameter of approximately 1 cm. It consists of

two parts, or lobes. The larger of the two lobes, which accounts for 70% to 80% of the gland's weight, is the anterior lobe. The anterior lobe is also called the *adenohypophysis.* The hormones of the anterior pituitary and their actions are as follows:

1. Growth hormone (GH), or somatotropic hormone: stimulates the growth and development of bones, muscles, and organs.
2. Adrenocorticotropic hormone (ACTH): controls the growth, development, and function of the cortex of the adrenal glands; controls release of glucocorticoids and adrenal androgens; necessary for secretion of aldosterone but does not control rate of aldosterone secretion.
3. Thyroid-stimulating hormone (TSH) or thyrotropic hormone: controls the secretory activities of the thyroid gland.

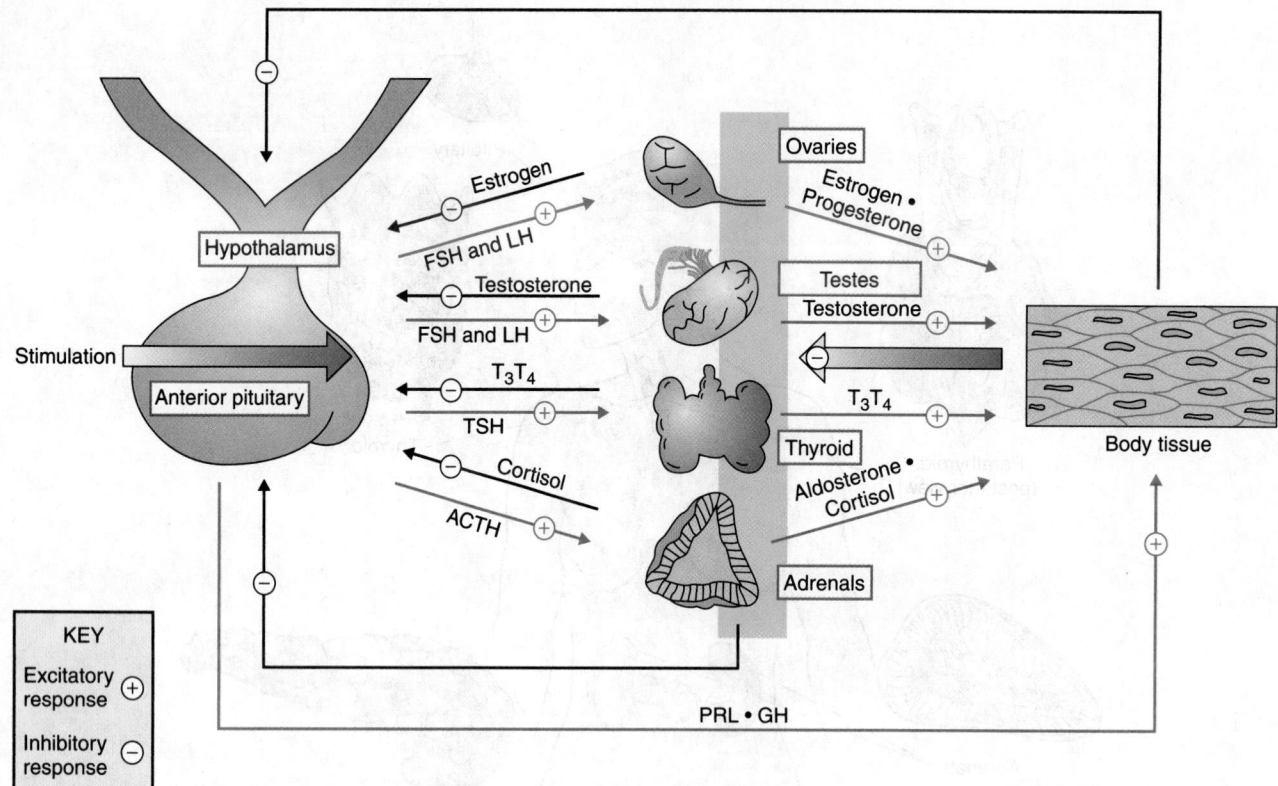

FIGURE **44-2** The feedback system of the hypothalamus, pituitary, and target glands.

4. Follicle-stimulating hormone (FSH): stimulates the development of the eggs in the ovary of the woman and sperm production in the man.
5. Luteinizing hormone (LH): controls ovulation or egg release in the woman and testosterone production in the man.
6. Prolactin, or lactogenic hormone: stimulates breast milk production in the woman.
7. Melanocyte-stimulating hormone (MSH): promotes pigmentation.

The smaller lobe of the pituitary is known also as the *posterior pituitary* because of its location in the sella turcica behind the anterior lobe. It is sometimes referred to as the *neurohypophysis*. The hormones secreted by the posterior pituitary and their actions are as follows:

1. Antidiuretic hormone (ADH), or vasopressin: causes the reabsorption of water from the renal tubules of the kidney. By doing so, water excretion from the body in the form of urine is decreased.
2. Oxytocin: causes contractions of the uterus in labor and the release of breast milk.

NURSING ASSESSMENT OF THE PITUITARY GLAND

The nursing assessment of the patient with a pituitary disorder is outlined in Box 44-1. The LPN/LVN assists with the collection of relevant data.

HEALTH HISTORY

Present Illness

Some problems related to pituitary function that may bring the patient to seek medical care are slowed or accelerated growth, visual disturbances, headache, and changes in urine output, appearance, skin, and secondary sex characteristics.

Past Medical History

A history of brain tumors, pituitary surgery, head trauma, central nervous system infection, vascular disorders, chronic renal failure, hypothyroidism, and disease of the pancreas, liver, or bone should be documented.

Family History

Note a family history of diabetes insipidus (DI).

Review of Systems

Ask about the patient's general health state, and note fatigue, weakness, restlessness, or agitation. Inquire about skin moisture and changes in body hair distribution. Note reports of significant sensory changes such as blurred vision and diplopia (double vision). For both men and women, ask about changes in the breasts. Also inquire whether the patient has experienced chest pain, constipation, polyuria, changes in genitalia, sexual dysfunction, joint pain, abnormal sensations, edema, seizures, and intolerance of heat or cold.

Box 44-1 | *ASSESSMENT of the Patient with a Pituitary Disorder*

Health History

Chief Complaint/Present Illness:
Slowed or accelerated growth; change in appearance, urine output, and/or secondary sex characteristics

Past Medical History:
Brain tumors, pituitary surgery, head trauma, central nervous system infection, vascular disorders, chronic renal failure, hypothyroidism, diseases of the pancreas, liver, or bone

Family History:
Diabetes insipidus or diabetes mellitus

Review of Systems:
Fatigue, restlessness, agitation, skin moisture and hair distribution, vision disturbances, changes in breasts, chest pain, constipation, polyuria, changes in genitalia, sexual dysfunction, joint pain, abnormal sensations, edema, seizures, intolerance of heat or cold

Functional Assessment:
Sleep pattern, usual diet, effects of disease on self-concept and daily life

Physical Examination

General Survey:
Body proportion, behavior, mental emotional state

Vital Signs

Height and Weight

Skin:
Moisture and edema

Head and Face:
Thickened lips, broad nose, prominent forehead and jaw

Neck:
Jugular venous distention

Eyes:
Visual acuity

Breasts:
Enlargement, discharge

Extremities:
Edema, range of motion, crepitus

Neurologic:
Slow reflexes

Genitalia:
Loss of pubic hair, testicular atrophy

Functional Assessment

In the functional assessment, determine whether the patient has had sleep disturbances. Obtain a description of usual diet, and note the effects of symptoms on the person's self-concept and usual activities.

PHYSICAL EXAMINATION

Measure vital signs and height and weight. Palpate the skin for moisture and edema. Inspect the head and face for thickened lips, broad nose, and prominent forehead and jaw. Test visual acuity. Inspect the breasts for enlargement in men, atrophy in women, and nipple discharge. Inspect and palpate the extremities for edema. Perform joint range of motion, noting any limitations or crepitus. Test reflexes for slowness of response. Inspect the male genitalia for loss of hair and palpate for testicular atrophy.

AGE-RELATED CHANGES

In healthy older adults, pituitary function remains adequate. Decreased ADH secretion impairs the ability to concentrate urine, increasing the risk of dehydration.

DIAGNOSTIC TESTS AND PROCEDURES

RADIOGRAPHIC STUDIES

Conventional radiographs, computed tomographic (CT) scans, and magnetic resonance imaging (MRI) may be used to detect a pituitary tumor. Cerebral angi-ography, in which a radiopaque dye is injected into the cerebral arteries, may reveal the presence of aneurysms or arteriovenous malformations. Vascular anomalies can interfere with the supply of blood in the brain and lead to pituitary damage.

LABORATORY STUDIES

Because hormones are circulated in very small quantities, tests to identify normal levels must be sensitive and precise. The radioimmunoassay is a commonly performed test that measures levels of hormones in the blood. A similar type of test is the enzyme-linked immunosorbent assay (or ELISA). This is also thought to be an accurate test for levels of hormones in the blood.

Hormone reserve activity also can be measured using a number of "suppression" or "stimulation" tests. In these tests, hormone levels are measured after administration of an agent that stimulates or suppresses hormonal function. Stimulation will cause a healthy endocrine gland to increase hormone production. Suppression will cause a healthy endocrine gland to decrease hormone production. The response helps the physician determine whether the target gland (e.g., thyroid, adrenal, gonads) or the hypothalamic-pituitary regulatory mechanism is responsible for abnormal hormone levels.

A glucose tolerance test for GH suppression may be done by administering a standard amount of glucose (100 gm or 0.5 gm/kg body weight) intravenously and measuring serial blood glucose levels for 120 minutes.

The rationale is that the glucose will suppress GH levels through a negative feedback process. In normal patients, GH levels fall less than 5 mg/mL. In patients with hyperpituitarism, large decreases in GH occur. This constitutes a positive result. Other studies measure serum levels of GH, insulin-like growth factor 1, gonadotropin, and prolactin. Additional information about diagnostic tests and procedures for pituitary disorders and related nursing care is presented in the table on p. 953.

DISORDERS OF THE PITUITARY GLAND

Dysfunction of the pituitary gland can result from a problem in the gland itself or from a problem in the hypothalamus. The hypothalamus is an organ in the brain that secretes factors that can directly inhibit or stimulate the pituitary (see Fig. 44-2). Pituitary disease is usually manifested by excess or deficient production and secretion of a specific hormone. These hormone imbalances lead to disorders that can be manifested in a variety of ways, including changes in physical appearance, emotional state, mental status, metabolism, and homeostatic mechanisms essential for survival. The pituitary disorders that are discussed in this chapter are hyperpituitarism, hypopituitarism, diabetes insipidus (DI), and syndrome of inappropriate ADH (SIADH).

HYPERPITUITARISM
Etiology

Hyperpituitarism is a pathologic state caused by excess production of one or more of the anterior pituitary hormones. GH and prolactin are the hormones most often produced in excess. GH is responsible for the growth and development of the body's muscles, bones, and other tissue. Overproduction of GH can lead to gigantism or acromegaly. Overproduction of prolactin causes hyperprolactinemia.

The most common factor in hyperpituitarism is the presence of a pituitary adenoma. An adenoma is a benign tumor composed of epithelial tissue. It may vary in size and invasiveness. Those that are larger than 10 mm are called *macroadenomas;* those that are smaller than 10 mm are called *microadenomas.* Adenomas tend to occur most commonly in young women in their teens through early 30s. Pituitary adenomas that secrete hormones may cause amenorrhea, galactorrhea (abnormal milk secretion), hyperthyroidism, and Cushing's syndrome, in addition to gigantism or acromegaly.

Growth hormone, in addition to regulating tissue growth, mobilizes stored fat for energy. As a result of lipolysis of body adipose, excess levels of GH elevate free fatty acids in the bloodstream. This can stimulate the development of atherosclerosis, which causes coronary artery disease and cerebrovascular disease over time. Excess GH also antagonizes insulin and interferes with its effects, thus leading to hyperglycemia and possibly diabetes mellitus.

Prolactinemia. Excess prolactin can cause prolactinemia, characterized by abnormal lactation (galactorrhea), amenorrhea, decreased vaginal lubrication, impotence and decreased libido in men, depression, anxiety, and visual loss.

Gigantism. Gigantism occurs in early childhood or puberty while the long bones of the body are still growing. The long bones consist of epiphyses, which are the end portions of the bone, and a diaphysis, which is the middle or shaft of the bone. Toward the end of puberty or in early adulthood, the line between these structures seals or closes, thus preventing further growth. Before the epiphyseal plates on the ends of these bones close, the diaphysis or long shaft of the bone may continue to grow to great lengths when stimulated by excess GH. The growth in these bones is usually proportional and may cause affected people to reach heights of up to 8 feet and weights of over 300 pounds. These people tend to have multiple health problems and often die in early adulthood. Figure 44-3 illustrates gigantism.

Acromegaly. Acromegaly, although rare, is more common than gigantism. Most patients with acromegaly are found to have pituitary macroadenomas that secrete excess GH. Symptoms usually appear in the fourth or fifth decade of life and affect men and women equally. In these people, excess GH production occurs after epiphyseal closure. The closed epiphyses prevent longitudinal growth of the bones; instead, bones increase in thickness and width. Acromegaly also affects the cardiovascular, digestive, nervous, and genitourinary systems.

FIGURE 44-3 Clinical features of growth hormone excess. Robert Wadlow, nicknamed "The Alton Giant," weighed 9 pounds at birth but grew to 32 pounds by 6 months of age. By his first birthday, he weighed 62 pounds. He died at age 22 because of complications from cellulitis of the feet. At the time of his death, he was 8 feet, 11 inches tall and weighed 475 pounds.

DIAGNOSTIC TESTS and PROCEDURES Pituitary Disorders

TEST/PURPOSE	PATIENT PREPARATION	POSTPROCEDURE NURSING CARE
Cerebral computed tomography scan: Uses radiographs to create images of internal structures; detects tumors, edema, structural abnormalities.	Tell patient he or she will lie still on a stretcher while circular scanner moves around the head. Clicking sounds are heard, but no sensations are felt. Remove jewelry and hairpins. If contrast medium is to be used, assess sensitivity to iodine or previous contrast allergy. Inform radiologist.	If contrast medium is used, assess for side effects: nausea, vomiting, headache, delayed allergic reaction.
Cerebral angiogram: Radiographs are taken to study cerebral blood flow and blood vessels.	Signed consent required. General anesthesia needed for patients who cannot cooperate. Tell patient there may be a burning sensation when contrast medium is injected. Stress importance of lying still. Remove jewelry and hairpins from head. Assess for sensitivity to contrast medium.	Apply pressure to arterial puncture site for 15 min. Assess for bleeding afterward. Record VS per agency protocol. Immobilize extremity as ordered. Bed rest 12-24 hr. Neurologic checks hourly 4 times, then every 4 hr 20 times.
Glucose tolerance test: Evaluates response to glucose dose to detect diabetes mellitus and hyperpituitarism.	Tell patient fasting blood glucose will be measured; then intravenous or oral glucose solution given, and blood samples taken to measure glucose levels at specified intervals. Enforce NPO.	Check venipuncture site. Apply bandage if needed. Provide ordered diet.
Dexamethasone suppression tests: Measure cortisol, which increases with adrenal hyperplasia, Cushing's syndrome, oat cell carcinoma; decreases with histoplasmosis and tuberculosis.	Tell patient that baseline serum and urine cortisol will be measured. For overnight test, a dose of dexamethasone is given, usually around 11 PM, and a blood sample is drawn for cortisol level at 8 AM. Alternative tests are the low-dose test and high-dose test with various schedules for obtaining blood and urine specimens. Explain 24-hr urine collection, if ordered.	Send blood sample to laboratory within 30 min. Apply dressing to venipuncture site. Check for bleeding.
Pituitary hormone levels (luteinizing hormone, follicle-stimulating hormone, growth hormone, adrenocorticotropic hormone, thyroid-stimulating hormone, prolactin) Serum levels are measured to detect elevations or deficiencies of pituitary hormones.	Tell patient a blood sample will be required. Check agency manual for any special preparation.	Check venipuncture site. Apply dressing, and check for bleeding.
Hypertonic saline test: An infusion of hypertonic saline is given to stimulate release of ADH; used to detect DI.	Tell patient IV fluids will be given. Urine output and specific gravity will be measured hourly. Explain urine collection process.	No special care.
Fluid deprivation: Detects changes in specific gravity and osmolality after aqueous vasopressin is given subcutaneously. Specific gravity and osmolality decrease with primary and secondary DI. No response with nephrogenic DI.	NPO for specified time. Tell patient vital signs will be taken; urine specimens collected; body weight measured hourly. A medication will be given and additional measurements done. Administer ordered medication, and collect designated specimens.	No special care.

VS, Vital signs; NPO, nothing by mouth; ADH, antidiuretic hormone; DI, diabetes insipidus.

Signs and Symptoms

Visual deficits and headaches are common in hyperpituitarism and may be the first symptoms of a problem. Visual problems are most often a result of pressure on optic nerves where they are joined near the pituitary gland. Physical features of the disease include enlargement of the hands, feet, and paranasal and frontal sinuses and deformities of the spine and mandible. In addition, soft tissues may become enlarged, especially the tongue, skin, liver, and spleen. This may in turn lead to speech impediments, coarse or distorted facial features, abdominal distention, and sleep apnea. People with acromegaly also may report excessive perspiration (diaphoresis), oily skin, peripheral neuropathies, degeneration of the joints, and proximal muscle weakness. The effects of excess growth hormone impede the activity of insulin, causing patients to have symptoms of diabetes mellitus.

In addition to the features just described, patients with gigantism and acromegaly initially present with increased strength, progressing rapidly to complaints of weakness and fatigue. The examiner also may detect organomegaly (enlargement of internal organs), hypertension, dysphagia, and a deep voice due to hypertrophy of the larynx. Those patients who also have elevated levels of prolactin may present with galactorrhea in women and hypogonadism in men. A dramatic example of acromegaly is presented in Figure 44-4.

Medical Diagnosis

The diagnosis of hyperpituitarism is based on a number of data sources, including physical assessment, radiographic studies, and laboratory findings.

Radiographic Studies. Radiographic films of the skull may show a large sella turcica and increased bone density. Enhanced CT scans using a water-soluble dye or MRI scans may be performed to locate and evaluate potential intracellular or extracellular lesions or tumor formation. Angiography also may be of use to rule out any vascular abnormalities such as aneurysms or arteriovenous malformations.

Laboratory Studies. As mentioned earlier, in hyperpituitarism usually only one pituitary hormone is produced in excess, such as GH or prolactin. Pathologic conditions producing elevated levels of LH or FSH are extremely rare. In suspected cases of hyperpituitarism, levels of anterior pituitary hormones are measured. Elevation of any hormone level requires further evaluation and follow-up. It is normal for LH and FSH to be slightly elevated in postmenopausal women. The glucose tolerance test is the most reliable test for acromegaly. Whereas the GH concentration normally falls during the oral glucose tolerance, it is unchanged in the patient with acromegaly.

Dexamethasone suppression tests are used to rule out problems related to dysfunction of the adrenal glands (see detailed discussion in the Disorders of the Adrenal Glands section on p. 973).

Medical Treatment

Typically, the patient with hyperpituitarism that is manifested as acromegaly or gigantism has skeletal changes and disfigurement that cannot be reversed with treatment. However, soft tissue hypertrophy can improve with treatment. Treatment options include surgery, radiation, and drug therapy.

Drug Therapy. Several types of drugs are effective in the treatment of acromegaly. These include somatostatin analogs, dopamine agonists, and GH receptor antagonists. Octreotide (Sandostatin), a somatostatin analog, is the most commonly prescribed drug for patients with acromegaly. It is given 3 times weekly by subcutaneous injection. Common side effects of octreotide acetate are nausea, vomiting, diarrhea, abdominal pain, and pain at the injection site. Because this drug also suppresses insulin secretion, the patient's blood glucose must be monitored. Blood pressure and weight are monitored to detect fluid retention. Newer drugs in this category are given intramuscularly every 2 to 4 weeks. Dopamine agents such as cabergoline (Dostinex) suppress the secretion of GH. Pegvisomant (Somavert) is a GH receptor antagonist. It is most often used after radiotherapy. Bromocriptine (Parlodel) once was the primary drug, but it has been largely replaced by the newer options that are effective and have fewer side effects. Some of the most common side effects of bromocriptine are headache, dizziness, drowsiness, confusion, nausea, vomiting, dry mouth, and urticaria.

The Drug Therapy table on pp. 956 and 957 provides additional information about drugs used to treat hyperpituitarism.

Pharmacology Capsule

Drugs used to treat gigantism and acromegaly decrease hormone secretion but do not reverse the existing skeletal effects of the condition.

Radiation. Radiation therapy is sometimes used to treat tumors that produce excess GH, but the overall response is slow and numerous complications, such as hypopituitarism, optic nerve damage, and visual defects, can occur. It may be used in combination with surgery or drug therapy. Gamma knife radiotherapy (stereotactic radiosurgery), which uses radiation delivered to the site from multiple angles, may be used to treat acromegaly. Patients usually require hormone replacement after radiotherapy.

Surgical Management

For patients diagnosed with pituitary tumors, the surgical removal of the adenoma or of the pituitary itself (hypophysectomy) is the treatment of choice. A transsphenoidal approach is the most commonly used surgical method. A transsphenoidal hypophysectomy is a

FIGURE 44-4 The progression of acromegaly. A series of photographs of the same person over the course of her lifetime depict the physical changes that occurred. The woman was affected after reaching maturity.

microsurgical procedure performed under general anesthesia with the patient in the semi-Fowler's position. An incision is made at the inner aspect of the upper lip through the maxillary bone, and the sella turcica is entered through the sphenoid sinus (Fig. 44-5). After the gland or a portion of it is removed, a small piece of adipose tissue is harvested from the abdomen and is used to pack the dura mater (one of the meningeal layers) to prevent leakage of cerebrospinal fluid (CSF). An absorbent gauze or similar dressing is used to pack the nasal passages, and an external nasal dressing is applied to keep the packing in place. If the entire pituitary is removed, the patient will require lifelong replacement of glucocorticoids, thyroid hormone, and sex hormones.

An earlier surgical approach, called a *transfrontal craniotomy*, is sometimes used if a tumor is especially large or is invading other structures. This is a more invasive procedure that involves the removal of a portion of the frontal bone of the skull. The cranial vault is then entered, and structures superior to the pituitary gland are displaced to reach it. This involves manipulation of the meningeal layers and the frontal and temporal lobes of the cerebrum, as well as the optic nerve. As a result, the risk of complications and brain damage is great.

NURSING CARE *of the Patient with Hyperpituitarism*

Education and emotional support are vital components in the nursing care of the patient with hyperpituitarism. Patients presenting with hyperpituitarism need to know that many body changes, such as visual disturbances and visceral enlargement, are not reversible. Surgical treatment is aimed primarily at preventing further symptoms and complications.

DRUG THERAPY | *Pituitary*

DRUG	USE/ACTION	SIDE EFFECTS	NURSING INTERVENTIONS
ADH HORMONE PREPARATIONS	All promote conservation of water.	All can cause water intoxication, inadequate tissue perfusion due to vasoconstriction.	Monitor for early signs and symptoms of water intoxication: drowsiness, listlessness, headache. Patient should reduce fluid intake first few days of treatment.
Lypressin (Diapid) nasal spray	Treats diabetes insipidus (DI).	Rhinorrhea, nasal irritation, and congestion. Rarely, dyspnea, hypertension, coronary vasoconstriction.	Teach patient use of intranasal inhaler: hold bottle upright, place nozzle in nostril, spray prescribed number of times, do not inhale. Explain how to monitor intake and output. With DI, stress need for lifelong therapy. Monitor BP, pulse.
Desmopressin (DDAVP) nasal spray, parenteral, oral preparations	Treats DI, hemophilia (increases production of clotting factor VIII), nocturnal diuresis, headache.	Same as lypressin.	Same as lypressin.
Vasopressin (Pitressin) Synthetic for SC and IM	Treats DI, postoperative abdominal distention, used to dispel gas before abdominal radiography. Powerful vasoconstrictor.	May cause angina, MI in patients with coronary artery disease.	Same as lypressin. Also, assess cardiac and peripheral circulation. Extreme caution with cardiac disease.
PITUITARY HORMONE SUPPRESSANTS			
Octreotide acetate (Sandostatin)	Suppresses secretion of growth hormone. Most effective drug for acromegaly.	Nausea, vomiting, diarrhea, headache, flushing, edema, dizziness, altered blood glucose, drowsiness, orthostatic hypotension, visual disturbances, cholelithiasis.	Monitor weight, BP, pulse, respirations, urine output. Assess for edema. Refrigerate ampules. Discard if discolored or contains visible particles. Teach patient to give self-injections; advise to take exactly as prescribed and never take double doses. Assess for changes in blood glucose. Caution about drowsiness and dizziness. Very expensive.

Assessment

Assessment of the patient with a pituitary disorder is summarized in Box 44-1. When a patient has gigantism or acromegaly, areas that merit special attention are energy level, height and weight, vital signs, contours of the face and skull, visual acuity, speech, voice quality, and abdominal distention. If surgical intervention is planned, determine what the patient knows and expects.

Nursing Diagnoses, Goals, and Outcome Criteria: Hyperpituitarism

NURSING DIAGNOSES	GOALS AND OUTCOME CRITERIA
Disturbed Body Image related to changes in physical appearance	Adjustment to physical changes: patient verbalizes feelings about body and indicates acceptance of changes
Activity Intolerance related to fatigue	Improved activity tolerance: accomplishment of daily activities without excessive tiring
Chronic Pain related to musculoskeletal overgrowth, headache	Pain relief: patient verbalizes relief of pain, appears relaxed
Ineffective Therapeutic Regimen Management related to lack of knowledge of condition, treatment, and expected outcomes	Patient manages own treatment with realistic expectations: patient correctly describes self-medication, therapeutic effects and drug adverse effects

Interventions

Disturbed Body Image

Demonstrate acceptance of the patient, and provide opportunities for the patient to share feelings and con-

💊 DRUG THERAPY | Pituitary—cont'd

DRUG	USE/ACTION	SIDE EFFECTS	NURSING INTERVENTIONS
PITUITARY HORMONE SUPPRESSANTS—cont'd			
Bromocriptine (Parlodel)	Inhibits release of prolactin from anterior pituitary. Suppresses lactation. Restores ovulation. Treats acromegaly.	Nausea, vomiting, constipation, hypotension, drowsiness, MI, pulmonary infiltrates, nasal stuffiness, vasoconstriction, anorexia, headache. Rarely, visual disturbances, confusion.	Safety measures if dizzy. Monitor BP. Record bowel movements and stool consistency. Assess effects. Teach patient to report chest pain and/or dyspnea immediately, to rise slowly to standing position, that driving may be dangerous because of drowsiness and dizziness, and that the drug may restore fertility.
Dopamine receptor antagonist: cabergoline (Dostinex)	Prevents/inhibits secretion of prolactin. May lower GH secretion in some patients with acromegaly.	Nausea, constipation, abdominal pain, headache, dizziness, asthenia, fatigue, drowsiness.	Contraindicated with uncontrolled hypertension.
GH receptor antagonist: pegvisomant (Somavert)	Used to treat acromegaly. Prevents growth hormone (GH) from exerting effects on body tissues.	Infection, pain, injection site reaction, chest pain, back pain, flu syndrome, abnormal liver function tests, diarrhea, dizziness, edema, sinusitis.	Contraindicated with latex allergy because vial stopper contains latex. Teach patient or family member to prepare and give SC injections. Do not shake vial when reconstituting drug. Solution should be clear. Discard leftover reconstituted drug.

SC, Subcutaneous; *IM,* intramuscular; *MI,* myocardial infarction; *BP,* blood pressure; *GH,* growth hormone.

FIGURE **44-5** The transsphenoidal surgical approach to the pituitary gland.

cerns. Encourage the patient to pay attention to grooming. If he or she has difficulty adjusting, a referral to a support group or mental health professional may be appropriate.

Activity Intolerance

Because the patient with acromegaly tires quickly, plan activities to allow for adequate rest periods. Help the patient develop a daily schedule that permits achievement of necessary activities balanced with rest requirements.

Chronic Pain

Monitor and document pain. Teach relaxation techniques as discussed in Chapter 15. Administer prescribed analgesics, and evaluate effects.

 Consider the Alternative

Imagery, relaxation exercises, and massage all can be used with analgesics to manage pain.

Ineffective Therapeutic Regimen Management

Advise patients on drug therapy to take prescribed medications exactly as prescribed and not to take double doses if a dose is missed. Other nursing implications are in the Drug Therapy table above and on p. 956.

If the patient has surgery (in this case, hypophysectomy), general preoperative and postoperative care is provided, as described in Chapter 17. This section describes specific nursing care of the patient having pituitary surgery. The patient may be admitted to a critical care unit for the first 24 hours after surgery because of the risk of a number of complications.

POSTOPERATIVE NURSING CARE
of the Patient with Hyperpituitarism
Assessment

Even though the RN is responsible for the complete assessment, the LPN/LVN collects data that are essential to caring for the patient during the postoperative period. Neurologic status and vision must be monitored closely, with particular attention to level of consciousness, pupil size and equality, and vital signs. Data used to assess for meningeal inflammation are obtained by asking the patient to place his or her chin to the chest (severe head or neck pain with this movement is associated with meningeal inflammation). Changes in data that may indicate edema caused by the manipulation of tissues or intracranial bleeding are decreasing alertness, slow pupil response to light, and decreased or asymmetric muscle strength.

Strict documentation of intake and output and measurement of specific gravity are important because these patients are at risk for DI or possibly SIADH. These disorders are discussed in detail in the Diabetes Insipidus section on p. 961 and the Syndrome of Inappropriate Antidiuretic Hormone section on p. 964.

Inspection of nasal packing for drainage is important because CSF leaks may sometimes occur. Document clear, colorless drainage, and notify the surgeon. To confirm whether the drainage is CSF, a specimen of the drainage should be sent to the laboratory for glucose testing. A high level of glucose supports the diagnosis of a CSF leak. A bedside test using a testing strip is no longer recommended. CSF leaks often resolve within 72 hours with rest and head elevation; however, severe, persistent headaches may be treated with a spinal tap to reduce CSF pressure. A return to surgery is rarely indicated.

Monitoring the patient for signs and symptoms of infection also is an important aspect of nursing care. An elevated white blood cell count, sudden rise in temperature, headache, or nuchal rigidity may be indications of meningitis (inflammation of the meninges, the protective layer of membranes that cover the brain and spinal cord).

The patient who has had gamma knife surgery (stereotactic radiosurgery) will return from the procedure with a stereotactic frame in place. Because the frame is secured to the skull with pins, pin care is needed. If the patient has a history of seizures, he or she is at increased risk for seizures for at least 24 hours. In an emergency, the frame may have to be quickly removed by trained personnel. The nursing unit should have a protocol for this procedure.

Nursing Diagnoses, Goals, and Outcome Criteria: Hypophysectomy, Postoperative

NURSING DIAGNOSES	GOALS AND OUTCOME CRITERIA
Anxiety related to lack of knowledge of surgical postoperative care and routines	Reduced anxiety: patient calm, states he or she feels less anxious
Disturbed Sensory Perception (visual) related to tissue trauma and swelling	Absence of visual disturbances: patient reports no change in vision
Acute Pain related to tissue trauma	Pain relief: patient statement of pain relief, relaxed manner
Impaired Oral Mucous Membrane related to surgical incision	Healed surgical incision: incision closed, minimal swelling and redness
Excess Fluid Volume or **Deficient Fluid Volume** related to abnormal ADH production	Normal fluid balance: fluid intake and output approximately equal, normal tissue turgor
Risk for Infection related to impaired tissue integrity	Absence of infection: normal white blood cell count; no neck stiffness, fever, or headache
Risk for Injury related to disruption of packing	Absence of CSF drainage: no clear nasal drainage

Interventions
Anxiety

Orient the patient to the environment, and explain all procedures. Give drugs as ordered to replace pituitary hormones. When the patient is well enough, provide information about drug therapy and self-medication. The patient who has a complete hypophysectomy requires hormone replacements for the rest of his or her life. Replacement therapy typically includes ADH, cortisol, and thyroid medication (see the Disorders of the Adrenal Glands section on p. 965 for a more detailed discussion of glucocorticoids).

Disturbed Sensory Perception

Be aware of existing visual disturbances, and collect data to identify new disturbances that might indicate increased intracranial pressure. Treatment usually does not correct existing disturbances but can prevent further harm.

Acute Pain and Impaired Oral Mucous Membrane

The immediate postoperative period is uncomfortable because the nasal packing remains in place for 2 to 3 days and the patient is forced to breathe through the mouth. Administer analgesics as ordered, and follow up to see if the medication was effective. The presence of a "moustache" dressing also may make the patient feel uncomfortable or embarrassed. Frequent mouth care with moistening of the lips increases comfort. Tooth brushing is not permitted until the incision heals. With gamma radiosurgery, the pin insertion sites may cause discomfort.

Risk for Injury

To prevent dislodgment of the fat pad or adipose graft at the surgical site, instruct the patient to avoid any activities that can cause a Valsalva maneuver. Coughing, straining, vomiting, or sneezing can create enough intracranial pressure to disrupt the surgical site and cause CSF leakage or even bleeding. Stool softeners and laxatives may be ordered to prevent straining. Instead of coughing, incentive spirometry and deep-breathing exercises help maintain pulmonary function without increasing intrathoracic and intracranial pressure. Advise the patient to avoid lifting heavy objects and bending from the waist. Instruct patients to avoid these activities at home as the physician directs (usually 2 to 3 months after surgery).

Excess Fluid Volume or Deficient Fluid Volume

Provide intravenous fluids as ordered, and monitor pulse, BP, and intake and output. Monitor for transient diabetes insipidus (large volume of dilute urine). Notify the physician of excessive fluid retention or diuresis. Changes in vital signs, mental status, and neuromuscular status suggest fluid and electrolyte imbalances.

Risk for Infection

Administer antibiotics as ordered. Monitor body temperature. Be especially alert for stiffness of the neck and headache because these are symptoms of meningitis.

HYPOPITUITARISM
Etiology and Pathophysiology

When inadequate secretion of GH occurs during preadolescence, a syndrome called dwarfism may result.

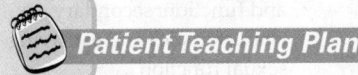

Patient Teaching Plan

Hypophysectomy, Postoperative

- If the anterior pituitary is removed, you will need hormone replacements for the rest of your life.
- For 3 months (or as advised by your physician), avoid any activities that cause straining, heavy lifting, and bending from the waist.
- It is important to prevent constipation because straining increases intracranial pressure.
- Numbness of the incision area and decreased sense of smell are temporary.
- Follow-up care is essential to monitor for any signs of tumor recurrence.

Put on Your Thinking Cap!

Explain why some people with excess growth hormone (GH) develop gigantism and other people with excess GH develop acromegaly.

Dwarfism is defined as attainment of a maximum height that is 40% below normal. In addition, chronic diseases associated with inadequate growth may be present. The causes of dwarfism may be hereditary or may be related to damage to the anterior portion of the pituitary gland. The anterior pituitary may be damaged by necrosis after hemorrhage, trauma, infection, radiation, or autoimmune disorders. Inadequate secretion of GH or an inability of the target organs to respond to GH is usually considered to be the major cause. In rare instances, hypothalamic dysfunction can lead to dwarfism as well. It is important to note that although an actual or relative deficiency of GH may exist, other anterior pituitary hormones also may be deficient.

If growth has been completed and some pathologic process impairs the function of the pituitary, a syndrome known as *panhypopituitarism* can occur. In this situation, all hormones of the anterior pituitary are usually affected. There are a number of causes for panhypopituitarism, which are identified as follows:

1. Sheehan's syndrome: shock and hypotension during the postpartum period leading to infarction of the pituitary gland
2. Tumors of the pituitary gland itself or cranial tumors that impinge on the pituitary
3. Chronic recurrent infections
4. Total or subtotal destruction or removal of the pituitary as a result of trauma, surgery, or radiation therapy
5. Suppression of pituitary tropic hormones by excess target gland hormones (e.g., as is seen in patients on prolonged corticosteroid therapy)

Signs and Symptoms

The manifestations of hypopituitarism depend on the stage of life when the deficiency occurs and which hormones are deficient. In dwarfism, which occurs early in life, the person is remarkably short in stature, sometimes as short as 36 inches, but with proportional physical characteristics. These people often have delayed or absent sexual maturation. There is a greater frequency of mental retardation than in the population at large. Dwarfs also have an accelerated pattern of aging and thus have a shorter life span than the general population, by as much as 20 years.

When a state of panhypopituitarism exists, a syndrome called *Simmonds' cachexia* is present. The patient has muscle and organ wasting and disruptions of both digestion and metabolism. Decreased muscle and organ size is attributed to decreased GH. An absence of ACTH affects the person's ability to cope effectively with stress. (See the Adrenal Hypofunction section on p. 966.) This in turn affects the person's ability to metabolize glucose, and hypoglycemia may result. Because TSH is depleted, the thyroid is unable to produce thyroid hormone. A lack of thyroid hormone produces a state referred to as *hypothyroidism*. In hypothyroidism, insufficient thyroid hormone is available for normal metabolism and thermogenesis, or heat production. Consequently, people who are hypothyroid may be unable to maintain a normal basal metabolic rate or body temperature.

If there is a lack of MSH, decreased pigmentation of the skin occurs. This results in extreme pallor. Finally, with the absence of gonadotropins, gonads may become atrophied. In both men and women, there may be loss of libido, decreased body hair, and sexual dysfunction, and in women, amenorrhea (absence of menstruation).

General signs and symptoms may include fatigue, weakness, malaise, cold intolerance, and lethargy. Again, the type and degree of symptoms depend on specific hormones affected. If the pituitary dysfunction is caused by a tumor, the patient may have headaches, vision disturbances, seizures, and loss of the sense of smell.

Medical Diagnosis

A diagnosis of dwarfism or panhypopituitarism is based on the health history, physical examination, and diagnostic tests. In cases of dwarfism, the physical examination findings are fairly diagnostic. Diagnostic tests and procedures may include conventional radiographs and CT scans to detect pituitary or cranial tumors. Cerebral angiography may be ordered to detect malformed blood vessels. Serum levels of pituitary hormones may be measured as well.

Medical and Surgical Treatment

Deficient hormones are replaced as needed depending on the specific deficiencies of the patient. Deficiency of TSH necessitates thyroid replacement with drugs such as levothyroxine (Synthroid) or liothyronine (Cytomel), usually for the rest of the person's life. Gonadotropin deficiency requires lifelong therapy. To produce or maintain libido, secondary sexual characteristics, and well-being, men also should receive testosterone and women should receive estrogen. In patients for whom childbearing is desirable, FSH and LH are administered to both men and women. However, gonadotropin replacement is contraindicated is some conditions including breast cancer in women and prostate cancer in men. GH replacement is necessary for growth in children. In most instances, GH is administered until the person reaches a height of 5 feet. Replacement of GH in adults produces improved energy, increased lean body mass, and a general feeling of well-being. The use of human GH produced by bacteria through recombinant DNA technology such as somatrem (Protropin) is considerably safer than products used previously. The annual cost of therapy with GH is very expensive. If a tumor is causing hypopituitarism, surgery or radiation is the treatment of choice. (See Surgical Management on pp. 954 and 955 in the Hyperpituitarism section.) The Drug Therapy table on pp. 956 and 957 provides additional information about drug therapy for hypopituitarism.

NURSING CARE *of the Patient with Hypopituitarism*
Assessment

The general assessment of the patient with a pituitary disorder is summarized in Box 44-1. When collecting data for assessment of the patient with hypopituitarism, be especially aware of mental acuity, emotional stability, and affect. Document the patient's general sense of well-being, energy level, and appetite. In reviewing the systems, ask the patient about changes in skin texture, body temperature, hair, and libido. Determine the patient's usual activities and whether there has been any difficulty carrying out those activities.

In the physical examination, measure height and weight and compare with previous measurements. Inspect the hair for distribution, texture, and thickness. Inspect and palpate the skin and nails for color, texture, and moisture. Document the development of secondary sex characteristics, including axillary and pubic hair, genital maturity, breast development, and onset of menarche.

Nursing Diagnoses, Goals, and Outcome Criteria: Hypopituitarism	
NURSING DIAGNOSES	GOALS AND OUTCOME CRITERIA
Disturbed Body Image related to lack (or loss) of secondary sex characteristics	Improved body image: patient makes positive statements about self and takes measures to improve appearance
Sexual Dysfunction related to hormone deficiency	Enhanced sexual development and function: secondary sex characteristics and satisfying sexual function
Imbalanced Nutrition: More or Less Than Body Requirements related to hormone imbalance	Adequate nutrition: body weight normal for height
Deficient Fluid Volume related to hormone deficiency, impaired homeostasis	Normal fluid balance: normal tissue turgor, pulse, and blood pressure
Ineffective Therapeutic Regimen Management related to lack of understanding of condition, treatment, and self-care	Patient follows prescribed treatment regimen: correctly demonstrates self-care, diminishing signs and symptoms of hormone deficiency

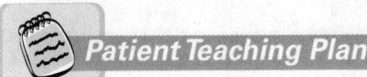

Patient Teaching Plan

Hypopituitarism

* It will be necessary for you to take medications for the rest of your life to replace the pituitary hormones.
* You must become familiar with the signs and symptoms of inadequate or excessive hormone replacement (provide written descriptions) and appropriate actions.
* You must have periodic follow-up care.
* Wear a medical alert bracelet or necklace so that your condition can be quickly recognized in an emergency.
* Carry a card that lists prescribed drugs and dosages and your physician's name and phone number.

Interventions

Patient education is the most important aspect of nursing care because disturbances in body image, sexual function, nutritional status, and fluid balance all can be improved if the patient understands and follows the prescribed therapy. Meanwhile, acknowledge the patient's feelings and encourage expression of concerns. Referral to a mental health counselor is appropriate if the patient has difficulty dealing with the effects of the disease. Good teaching is essential for patients and families to understand hypopituitarism and to participate in the treatment plan.

POSTERIOR PITUITARY DISORDERS

Disorders of the posterior pituitary or neurohypophysis are characterized by deficient or excess ADH production. Another name for ADH is *vasopressin*. ADH helps maintain fluid balance by promoting reabsorption of water in the renal tubules when body water is decreased or very concentrated. The amount of ADH secreted is reflected in the amount of water retained by the kidney. Increased ADH release causes increased water retention. This results in increased intravascular volume and decreased urine output.

Two disorders are associated with dysfunction of the neurohypophysis: DI and SIADH. DI is the more common of the two disorders.

Diabetes Insipidus
Etiology

Diabetes insipidus (DI) is characterized by excessive output of dilute urine. It can be caused by a number of factors. Thus DI is classified as nephrogenic, neurogenic (central or hypothalamic), or dipsogenic DI (primary polydipsia). Nephrogenic DI is an inherited defect in which the renal tubules of the kidney do not respond to ADH, resulting in inadequate water reabsorption by the kidneys. In this case, ADH is produced in sufficient amounts but the kidneys do not respond to it appropriately. Some cases are caused by drugs such as lithium carbonate (Eskalith-CR) or demeclocycline

(Declomycin), which affect the kidney by inhibiting its response to ADH. In neurogenic DI, there is a defect in either the production or secretion of ADH. Neurogenic DI can result from hypothalamic tumors, head trauma, infection, surgical procedures (hypophysectomy), or metastatic tumors originating in the lung or breast. It also can be triggered by a cerebrovascular accident, aneurysm, or intracranial hemorrhage. Dipsogenic DI is a disorder of thirst stimulation. When the patient ingests water, serum osmolality decreases, which causes reduced vasopressin secretion. Other factors that may be associated with dipsogenic DI are habitual excessive water intake and psychiatric conditions. The severity of symptoms in dipsogenic DI varies.

Pathophysiology

Antidiuretic hormone deficiency or an inability of the kidneys to respond to ADH results in the excretion of large volumes of very dilute urine, a symptom referred to as *polyuria*. The distal tubules and collecting ducts do not reabsorb sufficient water. Massive diuresis occurs, resulting in increased plasma osmolarity, which stimulates the osmoreceptors. The osmoreceptors in turn relay information to the cerebral cortex, causing the person to feel thirsty. Increased thirst serves as a compensatory mechanism in that it causes the person to increase water ingestion. Unfortunately, this compensatory mechanism cannot keep up with the demand for water, and diuresis continues. Massive dehydration ensues, which leads to decreased intravascular volume, hypotension, and circulatory collapse. This is accompanied by neurologic changes such as a decreased level of consciousness and severe electrolyte imbalances. Electrolyte imbalances contribute to circulatory collapse by causing dysrhythmias and impaired contractility of the heart. If left untreated, severe cases of DI can lead to cardiac arrest and death.

When DI follows intracranial surgery, a typical pattern occurs. The initial acute phase is marked by the sudden onset of polyuria. In the next phase, urine volume returns to normal. Then, the third phase, which occurs 10 to 14 days postoperatively, results in permanent DI. When DI is associated with head trauma, it is more likely to resolve with treatment.

Signs and Symptoms

Common signs and symptoms of DI are massive diuresis, dehydration, and thirst. Dehydration is characterized by hypotension, tachycardia, dizziness, decreased skin turgor, weakness, and possible fainting episodes. Additional findings include malaise, lethargy, and irritability. An irregular heartbeat may be detected.

Medical Diagnosis

The diagnosis of DI is made primarily on the basis of the health history, physical examination, and laboratory findings. A history of any known etiologic factors, such as surgery, infection, injury, or medication ingestion, should be noted.

The loss of free water is apparent in laboratory studies of blood and urine. An initial diagnosis of DI is made based on a 24-hour urine output of greater than 4 L, without food or fluid restrictions. Patients with DI can excrete up to 30 L/day, depending on the severity of the ADH deficiency or relative deficiency. Because the urine is very dilute, the specific gravity is also extremely low and the osmolarity of the urine is decreased. For the water deprivation test, water is withheld for 8 to 16 hours during which time BP, weight, and urine osmolality are measured each hour. The test is stopped when the osmolalities stabilize, the patient loses 5% of his or her body weight, or the patient develops orthostatic hypotension. A dose of ADH is then given and the urine osmolality measured an hour later. If the patient has neurogenic DI, the urine osmolality should increase (i.e., the urine is more concentrated). Additional details of this and other studies used to diagnose DI are listed in the Diagnostic Tests and Procedures table on p. 953.

Medical Treatment

The management of DI is geared to controlling the signs and symptoms of the disease and possibly reversing the cause of the syndrome. Intravenous fluid volume replacement and vasopressors often are required to maintain adequate blood pressure. Treatment also includes a variety of pharmacologic therapies. A list of these agents can be found in the Drug Therapy table on pp. 956 and 957. Most of these agents act by augmenting existing ADH or replacing it. The most common hormone replacement drug for neurogenic DI is desmopressin acetate (DDAVP), which can be given orally, intravenously, or by nasal inhalation. Short-term therapy is usually managed with subcutaneous injections of aqueous vasopressin. This is usually indicated in situations in which the cause of DI is reversible, such as infection- or medication-related DI. Patients on long-term therapy are placed on nasal spray (lypressin), which may be required for life. This long-term therapy may be necessary after hypophysectomy or other surgical procedures. Patients with primary polyuria related to a psychiatric condition may require ADH supplementation while psychotherapy is used to treat the underlying disorder.

The administration of ADH does not help with nephrogenic DI because the kidneys do not respond to the hormone. Sodium intake may be restricted and thiazide diuretics prescribed for nephrogenic DI. This depletes sodium and decreases the glomerular filtration rate, which increases the reabsorption of water in the proximal tubules.

A variety of other drugs (chlorpropamide [Diabinese], clofibrate [Atromid], carbamazepine [Tegretol], indomethacin [Indocin]) may be used to treat DI depending on the circumstances.

Pharmacology Capsule

Adverse effects of vasopressin administered as a nasal spray are mucous membrane ulcers, chest tightness, and upper respiratory infections.

NURSING CARE *of the Patient with Diabetes Insipidus*

Assessment

A complete history of the patient's symptoms, medical history, and drug history should be obtained by the registered nurse. The LPN/LVN can assist by monitoring for thirst, change in urine appearance or volume, dizziness, weakness, fainting, and palpitations. The physical examination focuses on the symptoms of DI. Monitor hydration, including skin turgor, moisture of mucous membranes, pulse rate and quality, blood pressure, and mental status. Maintain records of intake and output, daily weights, and urine specific gravities.

Nursing Diagnoses, Goals, and Outcome Criteria: Diabetes Insipidus	
NURSING DIAGNOSES	GOALS AND OUTCOME CRITERIA
Anxiety related to physical symptoms and diagnosis	Decreased anxiety: patient states anxiety is reduced, appears calm
Disturbed Body Image related to altered function	Adaptation to physical changes: patient adjusts routines to minimize symptoms
Deficient Fluid Volume related to excessive urine output	Normal fluid balance: fluid intake approximately equal to fluid output
Activity Intolerance related to fatigue and weakness	Improved activity tolerance: patient performs activities of daily living without tiring
Ineffective Therapeutic Regimen Management related to lack of understanding of symptom management and treatment of DI	Appropriate self-care: patient describes and demonstrates self-care and self-medication

Interventions

The patient with a pituitary disorder may be experiencing mild to moderate symptoms or may be critically ill. Specific nursing care depends largely on the type of DI, the severity of the symptoms, and the needs identified in the nursing assessment.

Anxiety and Disturbed Body Image

The patient who is able must be allowed adequate time to ventilate feelings and discuss the disorder. Changes in body function can be very disturbing. Assure the patient that some changes can be controlled with proper treatment. Be alert to the patient's emotional status, and provide support and make referrals as necessary.

Deficient Fluid Volume

Carefully measure intake and output. When the urine output is excessive, as in DI, the physician may order measurement of output at 15- to 30-minute intervals. Because adequate hydration is essential, administer intravenous fluid replacements as ordered. Encourage oral intake, with the prescribed amount based on the volume of urinary output. In addition, weigh the patient at least once daily to identify significant weight loss secondary to water loss.

In situations in which the patient is experiencing an excessive fluid loss, administer exogenous ADH as ordered (see the Drug Therapy table on p. 956). Be familiar with routes of administration, side effects, and contraindications associated with the use of these agents. Be aware that reversal of the fluid volume deficit with ADH can result in water intoxication. Continued monitoring of urine output and osmolality is essential.

Activity Intolerance

Extreme fatigue or muscle weakness can interfere with the patient's ability to participate in activities of daily living, such as hygiene and grooming. Frequently observe the functional ability of these patients, and address the amount of assistance required in the patient's care plan.

Ineffective Therapeutic Regimen Management

Patients who require long-term treatment of DI must learn to manage their symptoms and medications. If the patient has difficulty doing this, a family member or friend may be included in the teaching sessions.

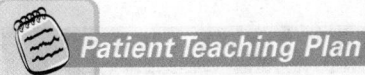
Patient Teaching Plan

Irreversible Diabetes Insipidus

- Continue your prescribed drug therapy, and notify your physician of any side or adverse effects (provide written details).
- Notify your physician if you have increased urine output, thirst, weight loss, and general feelings of malaise or weakness. You may need additional treatment.
- Prolonged use of nasal sprays can cause ulceration of mucous membranes, chest tightness, upper respiratory infections, and respiratory problems.
- Keep office or clinic appointments to identify any changes in pituitary function.
- Schedule activities and regular rest periods to avoid excessive fatigue.
- Wear a medical alert bracelet.
- Drowsiness, listlessness, and headache are signs of water intoxication, which may result from vasopressin therapy.

Some patients are taught to adjust dosages based on urine output, specific gravity (using a hydrometer), and thirst. If the patient's self-care abilities are in doubt, initiate a referral to a home nursing service.

Syndrome of Inappropriate Antidiuretic Hormone

Etiology

The syndrome of inappropriate antidiuretic hormone (SIADH) is characterized by a water imbalance related to an increase in ADH synthesis or secretion, or both. Factors that may cause or contribute to the development of SIADH include brain trauma, surgery, tumors, and infection; some drugs, including vasopressin, general anesthetic agents, oral hypoglycemics, and tricyclic antidepressants; some pulmonary diseases; hypothyroidism; lupus erythematosus; and some types of cancer, including small cell lung cancer, duodenal cancer, and pancreatic cancer.

Pathophysiology

When ADH is elevated despite normal or low serum osmolality, the kidneys retain excessive water. Plasma volume expands, causing the blood pressure to rise. Body sodium is diluted (hyponatremia), and water intoxication develops. There are several types of SIADH with various patterns of abnormal ADH secretion.

Signs and Symptoms

The main symptoms of SIADH initially reflect the effects of dilutional hyponatremia and water retention: weakness, muscle cramps or twitching, anorexia, nausea, diarrhea, irritability, headache, and weight gain without edema. When the central nervous system is affected by water intoxication, the level of consciousness deteriorates. The patient may have seizures or lapse into a coma.

Medical Diagnosis

The diagnosis of SIADH is confirmed by laboratory tests of serum and urine electrolytes and osmolality. Simultaneous measurements of urine and serum osmolality are especially useful. When measured simultaneously, urine osmolality much higher than that of the serum indicates SIADH. In this case, the serum is very dilute and the urine is very concentrated. Major characteristics include hyponatremia, hypochloremia, hypouricemia, reduced blood urea nitrogen and creatinine clearance, increased urine sodium, and fluid volume excess without edema. Urine osmolality may be high considering the level of serum osmolality or it may be extremely dilute. Radiographic studies of the brain and lungs also may be done to detect causative factors.

Medical Treatment

The treatment is intended to correct the cause, if possible, and promote elimination of excess water. Acutely ill patients (those with neurologic symptoms and serum sodium of <120 mEq/ L) are treated with hypertonic saline given very slowly over a 4- to 6-hour period. Once neurologic symptoms resolve, principles of chronic therapy are instituted. One approach is to restrict fluids to 800 to 1000 mL/day with a high intake of dietary sodium. Another approach is administration of normal saline with loop diuretics. A diuretic can be used only if the serum sodium is at least 125 mEq/L because the diuretic will cause further loss of sodium. Patients on diuretic therapy may require sodium and potassium supplements. Patients who cannot adhere to fluid restriction with high sodium intake may be given demeclocycline or lithium carbonate, which blocks the effects of ADH on the renal tubules thereby increasing water excretion. Adverse effects of these drugs can cause complications (see the Drug Therapy table on p. 956).

NURSING CARE of the Patient with Syndrome of Inappropriate Antidiuretic Hormone

Assessment

The health history records the presence of anorexia, nausea, vomiting, diarrhea, headache, irritability, and muscle cramps and weakness. Document a history of cancer, pulmonary disease, nervous system disorders, hypothyroidism, or lupus erythematosus. Note any prescription drugs the patient is taking. Measure the patient's vital signs, weight, intake and output, and urine specific gravity. Palpate the skin for moisture and edema. Test muscle strength by having the patient grip your hands and push and pull against resistance. Document seizures and muscle weakness, twitching, or cramps. Describe mental status (level of consciousness, orientation) at least every 4 hours in the alert, oriented patient and hourly if there is evidence of impairment.

Nursing Diagnoses, Goals, and Outcome Criteria: SIADH

Nursing Diagnoses	Goals and Outcome Criteria
Risk for Injury related to confusion associated with water intoxication, cerebral edema	Absence of injury: no seizures or associated trauma
Excess Fluid Volume related to excess ADH secretion	Normal fluid balance: normal tissue turgor, fluid intake and output approximately equal
Ineffective Therapeutic Regimen Management related to lack of understanding of management of chronic SIADH	Patient effectively manages prescribed therapy: takes drugs correctly, monitors for and reports adverse effects

Interventions

Risk for Injury

If the patient becomes confused, take measures to ensure safety, including putting the bed in low position and checking on the patient frequently. With cerebral

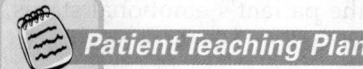

Syndrome of Inappropriate Antidiuretic Hormone

- Weigh daily and notify the physician if you gain 2 lb or more in one day.
- In addition to weight gain, signs and symptoms of excessive water retention (water intoxication) are drowsiness, listlessness, and headache.
- Do not take any nonprescription drugs without consulting your physician or pharmacist.
- See your physician on a regular basis.
- If taking demeclocycline or lithium carbonate, report adverse effects to your physician (provide specifics).

edema, position the patient with the head elevated 30 to 45 degrees or as specified by the physician.

Excess Fluid Volume

Advise the physician of declining neurologic status or weight gain in excess of 2 lb/day. Enforce fluid restrictions, which may be as little as 500 mL/24 hr. Explain the restriction to the patient and family. Remove the large water pitcher. Space fluids over waking hours to reduce thirst and feelings of deprivation. Serve oral fluids in small containers to create the illusion of volume. Encourage frequent mouth care.

Ineffective Therapeutic Regimen Management

Although SIADH is usually temporary, it may not resolve during hospitalization and the patient may need to learn how to manage the condition at home. Provide verbal and written information about prescribed drugs, dosages, and adverse effects. Be sure the patient has a scale at home to monitor weight.

THE ADRENAL GLANDS

ANATOMY AND PHYSIOLOGY OF THE ADRENAL GLANDS

The adrenal glands are a pair of small, highly vascularized, triangular-shaped organs. They are located in the retroperitoneal cavity on the superior poles of each kidney, lateral to the lower thoracic and upper lumbar vertebrae. Each gland weighs approximately 4 gm and measures 3.3 cm in length. The adrenal gland itself is composed of two parts: an outer portion called the *cortex* and an inner portion called the *medulla*. The cortex and medulla have very different, independent functions.

MEDULLA

The medulla constitutes 10% of the gland and contains sympathetic ganglia (groups of nerve cell bodies) with secretory cells. Stimulation of the sympathetic nervous system causes the medulla to secrete two types of catecholamines: norepinephrine (noradrenaline) and epinephrine (adrenalin). Both of these substances act as neurotransmitters. They are released into the circulation and transported to target organs or tissues, where they exert their effects by binding to adrenergic receptors. Catecholamine effects vary depending on the specific receptor in the cell membrane of the target organ. There are multiple adrenergic receptors including alpha$_1$-, alpha$_2$-, beta$_1$-, and beta$_2$-receptors. Norepinephrine binds to alpha-adrenergic receptors, whereas epinephrine affects primarily beta-adrenergic receptors. Table 44-1 lists the specific effects of these catecholamines and the types of receptors with which they bind. The major function of these substances is adaptation to stress, as characterized by the "fight-or-flight response," and maintenance of homeostasis.

CORTEX

The adrenal cortex, which comprises 90% of the adrenal gland, is the outer portion of the gland. This is the portion that is considered to be a part of the endocrine system. The cortex is essential for maintenance of many life-sustaining physiologic activities. The cells of the cortex are organized into three distinct layers or zones. Proceeding from the outermost to innermost layers, they are the zona glomerulosa, zona fasciculata, and zona reticularis. The hormones synthesized and secreted by the cortex are known as *steroids* and consist of mineralocorticoids, glucocorticoids, and androgens or estrogens.

FUNCTION OF THE ADRENAL GLANDS

MINERALOCORTICOIDS

The zona glomerulosa produces mineralocorticoids, the most abundant of which is aldosterone. Mineralocorticoids play a key role in maintaining an adequate extracellular fluid volume. Aldosterone functions at the renal collecting tubule to promote the reabsorption of sodium and the excretion of potassium by the kidney. The secretion of aldosterone is regulated by several factors: serum levels of potassium, the renin-angiotensin mechanism, and ACTH.

RENIN, ANGIOTENSIN, AND ALDOSTERONE

Renin is produced by the juxtaglomerular cells of renal afferent arterioles. Its release is stimulated by a decrease in extracellular fluid volume. Any factor that can cause this decrease (blood or fluid loss, sodium depletion, or changes in body position or posture) can stimulate renin release. Renin acts on plasma proteins to release angiotensin I, which is catalyzed in the lung to angiotensin II. Angiotensin II stimulates the secretion of aldosterone, which results in sodium and water retention. Retention of sodium and water preserves or increases extracellular fluid volume and subsequently increases blood pressure. This compensatory mechanism plays a very important role in maintaining intravascular volume in shock states.

GLUCOCORTICOIDS

The glucocorticoids are produced by the zona reticularis and zona fasciculata. The most abundant and potent of the glucocorticoids is cortisol. Approximately 92% of circulating cortisol is bound to a plasma protein. Free cortisol (8%) binds with receptors in the cytoplasm and nuclei of target cells. Cortisol has a permissive effect on other physiologic processes, meaning that the glucocorticoid must be present for other processes, such as catecholamine activity and excitability of the myocardium, to occur. Glucocorticoid functions include control of carbohydrate, lipid, and fat metabolism, regulation of anti-inflammatory and

Table 44-1 | *Receptors and Effects of Adrenal Medullary Hormones on Selected Organs and Tissues*

ORGAN OR TISSUE	RECEPTOR	EFFECT
Heart	β$_1$	Positive inotropic action (increases myocardial contractility)
		Positive chronotropic action (increases heart rate)
Blood vessels	α	Vasoconstriction (except in cardiac and skeletal muscles)
	β$_2$	Vasodilation
Gastrointestinal tract	α, β	Increased sphincter tone, decreased motility
Kidney	β$_2$	Increased renin release
Bronchioles	β$_2$	Relaxation, dilation
Bladder	α	Sphincter contractions, urinary retention
	β$_2$	Relaxation of detrusor muscle
Skin	α	Increased sweating, piloerection
Adipose tissue	β	Increased lipolysis
Liver	α	Increased gluconeogenesis and glycogenolysis
Pancreas	α	Decreased glucagon and insulin release
	β	Increased glucagon and insulin release
Eyes	α	Dilation of pupils

α, alpha; β, beta.

immune responses, and control of emotional states by the following:

- Increasing hepatic gluconeogenesis and inhibiting peripheral glucose use to maintain glucose levels
- Increasing lipolysis and release of glycerol and free fatty acids
- Increasing protein catabolism
- Degrading collagen and connective tissue
- Increasing polymorphonuclear leukocytes released from bone marrow
- Decreasing capillary permeability, movement of white blood cells into the injured tissue, phagocytosis
- Stabilizing lysosomal membranes
- Suppressing lymphocyte reproduction
- Maintaining behavioral and cognitive functions

SEX HORMONES

Adrenal androgens are another class of steroids produced in the zona fasciculata and zona reticularis of the adrenal cortex. Their primary function is masculinization in men. Other sex hormones include estrogen and progesterone. In men, these substances contribute little to reproductive maturation. In women, however, estrogens are supplied by both the ovaries and the adrenal glands. In postmenopausal women, the adrenal cortex is the primary source of endogenous estrogen.

NURSING ASSESSMENT OF THE PATIENT WITH AN ADRENAL DISORDER

HEALTH HISTORY

Present Illness

Symptoms of adrenal dysfunction that may cause the patient to seek medical attention include decreased energy, mental changes (depression, anxiety, nervousness, confusion), sexual dysfunction, gastrointestinal disturbances, and abnormal skin pigmentation.

Past Medical History

Aspects of the past medical history that may be significant include radiation to the head or abdomen, intracranial surgery, and recent and current medications. Tuberculosis is the most common cause of primary adrenal insufficiency.

Review of Systems

Determine the patient's perception of his or her general state of health. Ask about changes in skin color, especially bronzed or smoky pigmentation, and increased facial hair in women. Note changes in weight and appetite. Symptoms that may be related to adrenal dysfunction are headache, lightheadedness with position changes, muscle weakness, nausea, vomiting, abdominal pain, anorexia, menstrual dysfunction, and erectile dysfunction.

Functional Assessment

Document usual dietary and activity patterns and disruptions in lifestyle.

PHYSICAL EXAMINATION

Measure the patient's height, weight, and vital signs. Take the blood pressure when the patient is reclining and after the patient has moved to an upright position to detect a significant decrease. Note patient responses and ability to follow instructions. Inspect the skin for a bronzed or smoky pigmentation (especially in surgical scars, the skin over the knuckles, in skinfolds, and the areola), bruising, petechiae, vitiligo (loss of pigmentation), and pallor. Inspect the face of the female patient for excess facial hair. Examine the oral mucous membranes for color changes. Inspect the anterior thorax for fat pads under the clavicles, and the posterior thorax for the "buffalo hump." Note obesity of the trunk. Examine the breasts for striae and darkening of the areola. Inspect the abdomen for striae and the extremities for muscle wasting and edema. During examination of the external genitalia, assess for atrophy, hair loss, and appropriateness for age.

Assessment of the patient with an adrenal disorder is summarized in Box 44-2.

AGE-RELATED CHANGES

Under normal circumstances, adrenal function remains adequate in the older person. Some patients have a decline in cortisol secretion, but this is balanced by a decrease in cortisol metabolism such that blood levels remain normal. Secretion of aldosterone and plasma renin activity decline with age, and thus the abilities to conserve sodium and adapt to position changes become less efficient.

DIAGNOSTIC TESTS AND PROCEDURES

Because only two deviations from normal adrenal function are covered here, the appropriate diagnostic tests and procedures are discussed with each condition.

DISORDERS OF THE ADRENAL GLANDS

ADRENAL HYPOFUNCTION (ADDISON'S DISEASE)

Etiology

Adrenal insufficiency may be classified as either *primary* or *secondary*. Primary adrenal insufficiency, which is also called Addison's disease, is frequently due to a destructive disease process affecting the adrenal glands that results in deficiencies of cortisol and aldosterone. The most common cause of Addison's disease is idiopathic atrophy, an autoimmune disease in which

Box 44-2 | ASSESSMENT of the Patient with an Adrenal Disorder

Health History

Present Illness:
Decreased energy, mental changes, sexual dysfunction, gastrointestinal disturbances, abnormal skin pigmentation

Past Medical History:
Radiation to head or abdomen, intracranial surgery, recent and current medications

Review of Systems:
General well-being, bronzed or smoky skin color, increased facial hair in women, headache, lightheadedness with position changes, muscle weakness, nausea, vomiting, abdominal pain, anorexia, menstrual dysfunction, erectile dysfunction

Functional Assessment:
Changes in height and weight, changes in diet, salt craving, disruption of lifestyle by symptoms

Physical Examination

Height and Weight

Vital Signs

Mental Status

Skin:
Smoky or bronzed pigmentation prominent on surgical scars, knuckles, in skin folds, areola; bruising, petechiae, vitiligo, pallor

Head and Face:
Excess facial hair

Mouth:
Color change of oral mucous membranes

Thorax:
Supraclavicular fat pads, "buffalo hump"

Trunk:
Obesity

Breasts:
Striae, darkening of areola

Abdomen:
Striae

Extremities:
Muscle wasting, edema

Genitalia:
Atrophy, loss of hair, appropriate development for age

---

adrenal tissue is destroyed by antibodies formed by the patient's own immune system. Other causes of Addison's disease are tuberculosis, hemorrhage related to anticoagulant therapy, fungal infections (histoplasmosis, coccidioidomycosis), acquired immunodeficiency syndrome, metastatic cancer, gram-negative sepsis (Waterhouse-Friderichsen syndrome), adrenalectomy, adrenal toxins, and abrupt withdrawal of exogenous steroids.

Secondary adrenal insufficiency is a result of dysfunction of the hypothalamus or pituitary (decreased corticotropin, ACTH), which leads to decreased androgen and cortisol production. Unlike primary adrenal insufficiency, in which all steroids are affected, aldosterone may or may not be affected. Causes of secondary adrenal insufficiency include pituitary tumors, postpartum necrosis of the pituitary (Sheehan's syndrome), hypophysectomy, radiation therapy, pituitary or intracranial lesions, or high-dose, long-term glucocorticoid treatment, which suppresses the adrenal glands' intrinsic activity.

Pathophysiology

Insufficiency of adrenocortical steroids causes defects associated with the loss of mineralocorticoids and glucocorticoids. Impaired secretion of cortisol results in decreased gluconeogenesis and decreased liver and muscle glycogen. This in turn decreases supplies of available glucose, causing hypoglycemia. In addition, the glomerular filtration rate of the kidneys and gastric acid production by the parietal cells of the stomach both slow significantly. The cumulative effects of these processes cause decreased urea nitrogen excretion, irritability, anorexia, weight loss, nausea, vomiting, and diarrhea.

Decreased levels of aldosterone alter the clearance of potassium, water, and sodium by the kidney. Potassium excretion is decreased, and hyperkalemia may occur. Because hyperkalemia promotes hydrogen ion retention, metabolic acidosis also can occur. Hypovolemia and hyponatremia may result from accelerated sodium and water excretion.

Other manifestations of adrenal insufficiency are progressive weakness, lethargy, unexplained abdominal pain, and malaise. Skin hyperpigmentation, particularly in sun-exposed areas, pressure points, joints, and creases of the body, is another possible sign. It is most likely due to increased secretion of a beta-lipoprotein or a melanocyte-stimulating hormone, which is released by a part of the pituitary. This is a direct result of hypocortisolism and a lack of negative feedback.

If adrenal androgen levels are lowered, there may be a decrease or loss of body, axillary, and pubic hair. In prepubescent people, facial, pubic, and axillary hair may fail to grow entirely. The severity of these symptoms is linked to the degree of hormone deficiency. This lack of secondary sex characteristics tends to be seen in primary adrenal insufficiency rather than in secondary adrenal insufficiency.

Symptoms of chronic insufficiency are generally less dramatic and life-threatening than symptoms presented during acute adrenal crisis, which is discussed next.

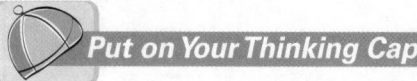

Put on Your Thinking Cap!

Explain how a pituitary disorder could cause adrenal insufficiency.

Acute Adrenal Crisis (Addisonian Crisis). Patients with either primary or secondary adrenal insufficiency are at risk for episodes of acute adrenal crisis, also called *addisonian crisis,* which is a life-threatening emergency. This usually results from a sudden marked decrease in available adrenal hormones. Precipitating factors are adrenal surgery, pituitary destruction, abrupt withdrawal of steroid therapy (often a result of a patient unwittingly stopping medications), and stress. Any factor that causes stress in the person can initiate a crisis. Examples of stressors include infection, illness, trauma, and emotional or psychiatric disturbances.

Manifestations of an addisonian crisis include symptoms of mineralocorticoid and glucocorticoid de-

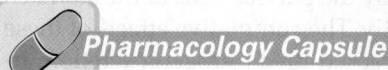

Pharmacology Capsule

When steroid therapy is discontinued, the drug is tapered gradually. An abrupt decline in adrenal hormones could precipitate acute adrenal crisis.

ficiency but are more severe: hypotension, tachycardia, dehydration, confusion, hyponatremia, hyperkalemia, hypercalcemia, and hypoglycemia. If left untreated, fluid and electrolyte imbalances can lead to circulatory collapse, cardiac dysrhythmias, cardiac arrest, coma, and death. The management of an addisonian crisis is outlined in Table 44-2.

Medical Diagnosis

Laboratory Studies. Addison's disease is diagnosed on the basis of clinical manifestations and a variety of laboratory findings, including a low serum and urinary cortisol level, decreased fasting glucose, hyponatremia, hyperkalemia, and increased blood urea nitrogen. In addition, 24-hour urine tests may be performed. This type of testing reflects steroid secretion over a 24-hour period and is the most accurate measurement of steroid secretion, which varies with the diurnal rhythm. Urinary 17-hydroxycorticosteroids also are sometimes measured as an indicator of glucocorticoid metabolites and are specific for this category of steroids. Androgen metabolites can be determined by measurement of 17-ketosteroids. Both of these substances are low or borderline low in adrenal hypofunction. See Box 44-3 for a list of drugs that interfere with urine tests for 17-hydroxycorticosteroids and 17-ketosteroids.

Measurement of plasma ACTH concentration before treatment is begun helps define the basis of the patient's symptoms. If the plasma ACTH level is low, the pituitary is at fault for not producing adequate ACTH. An increased plasma ACTH level suggests that the adrenals are at fault because they are unable to respond to stimulation to produce corticoids. An ACTH stimulation test is necessary for a definitive diagnosis of hypoadrenalism. One common tech-

■ Table 44-2 | *Emergency Medical Care: Acute Adrenal Crisis*

INTERVENTION	RATIONALE
1. Complete blood count, electrolytes, blood urea nitrogen, plasma cortisol levels.	1. To establish a baseline and obtain data for diagnosis and treatment.
2. Initial dose of hydrocortisone (Solu-Cortef) IV push, followed by infusion over 8 hr.	2. To provide a loading dose and maintenance infusion. The half-life of IV hydrocortisone is 60-90 min so blood level must be maintained by continuous infusion. If blood level falls, the patient may have a relapse.
3. Concomitant doses of hydrocortisone IM every 12 hr as ordered by physician.	3. To ensure constant source of glucocorticoids in case of IV failure (infiltration, infusion phlebitis).
4. After resolution of crisis, medications and dosage adjusted to include: a. Oral glucocorticoids started. b. Decreased dosage of oral glucocorticoids over several days as maintenance levels are reached. c. Supplemental mineralocorticoids as glucocorticoid dosage is tapered.	4. To ensure adequacy of mineralocorticoid activity with minimal glucocorticoid dose.
5. Provide emotional support to patient and family.	5. To minimize excess anxiety and fear during a crisis period.

Modified from Ignatavicius, D.D., Workman, M.L., & Mishler, M. (1999). *Medical-surgical nursing across the health care continuum* (3rd ed., p. 1602). Philadelphia: Saunders.
IV, Intravenous; *IM,* intramuscular.

nique used in this test is the administration of a dose of synthetic ACTH (cosyntropin), which is given intramuscularly. Plasma cortisol levels are measured at onset of administration and at 30 and 60 minutes after administration. In primary adrenal insufficiency, the cortisol response is absent or markedly decreased. In secondary insufficiency, there is a decrease in serum cortisol levels; however, it is not as significant a decrease as in cases of primary insufficiency. An eosinophil count may be performed during ACTH stimulation. The eosinophil count drops significantly after ACTH administration in normal people. Patients with Addison's disease show little or no change in the number of circulating eosinophils. If a glucose fasting test is performed, the serum glucose does not rise as high as it would in normal people and returns to a fasting level more rapidly.

Electrocardiogram. Alterations in electrolyte levels often are reflected as deviations in the normal electrocardiogram. For example, hyperkalemia results in peaked T waves, a widened QRS interval, and an increased PR interval.

Radiographic Studies. Skull films, arteriograms, CT scans, and MRI may be performed to rule out causative factors in secondary adrenal insufficiency. They may reveal intracranial lesions that impinge on the pituitary, aneurysms, or other defects. Abdominal imaging may detect atrophy of the adrenal glands and identify a possible cause of primary insufficiency.

Medical Treatment

The mainstay of treatment of patients with Addison's disease is replacement therapy with glucocorticoids and mineralocorticoids. Hydrocortisone commonly is used because it contains both. If glucocorticoids such as cortisone are given, they are typically divided into doses: two thirds of a daily dose is taken in the morning and one third in the evening. This dosage schedule is based on human hormonal variations. Glucocorticoids normally peak in the early morning and are at their lowest level in the evening. A mineralocorticoid (fludrocortisone), if needed, is typically given in the afternoon or evening. See the Drug Therapy table on p. 970 for details. Secondary adrenal insufficiency is treated with glucocorticoids, but mineralocorticoids are usually unnecessary. If the patient has an acute illness, additional glucocorticoids are needed to prevent a life-threatening condition called *Addisonian crisis*. Addisonian crisis is treated with intravenous fluids, electrolytes, and dextrose to restore normal blood pressure.

 Pharmacology Capsule

Addison's disease is treated with glucocorticoids given in divided doses to mimic the body's normal hormonal cycles.

| Box 44-3 | ***Drugs that Interfere with Urine Tests for 17-Hydroxycorticosteroids and 17-Ketosteroids*** |

Acetaminophen	Medroxyprogesterone
Acetazolamide	Meperidine
Acetylsalicylic acid	Metyrapone
Amphetamines	Mitotane
Ascorbic acid	Morphine
Barbiturates	Nalidixic acid
Calcium gluconate	Oral contraceptives
Carbon disulfide	Paraldehyde
Chloral hydrate	Penicillin
Chlordiazepoxide	Pentazocine
Chlorthalidone	Perphenazine
Colchicine	Phenobarbital
Corticotropin	Phenothiazines
Cortisone	Phenylbutazone
Dexamethasone	Phenytoin
Diazepam	Promazine
Digoxin	Propoxyphene
Diphenhydramine	Quinidine
Erythromycin	Quinine
Estrogens	Reserpine
Fructose	Secobarbital
Glutethimide	Spironolactone
Hydralazine	Testosterone
Iodides	Vitamin K

Modified from Ignatavicius, D.D., Workman, M.L., & Mishler, M. (1999). *Medical-surgical nursing: A nursing process approach* (3rd ed., p. 1604). Philadelphia: Saunders.

DRUG THERAPY | *Adrenal Disorders*

DRUG	USE/ACTION	SIDE EFFECTS	NURSING INTERVENTIONS
GLUCOCORTICOIDS Cortisone acetate (Cortone Acetate) Prednisolone (Delta-Cortef, Prelone) Prednisolone acetate (Econopred) Hydrocortisone (Cortef)	All stimulate formation of glucose, promote storage of glucose as glycogen, affect fluid and electrolytes, increase hemoglobin, suppress inflammation. Used to treat adrenal insufficiency. Some have mineralocorticoid effects also.	All: hypokalemia, hypocalcemia, nausea and vomiting, edema, hypertension, increased risk of infection, hyperglycemia, muscle wasting, osteoporosis, ulcer development, acne, pathologic fractures. May cause death if suddenly discontinued.	Monitor weight, intake and output, BP, blood glucose. Assess for edema. Protect from sources of infection. Report signs of infection even if subtle. Assess for hypocalcemia: muscle weakness and twitching. Assess for hypokalemia: muscle weakness and tingling, cardiac dysrhythmias, irritability. Protect from falls and possible fractures. Give oral drugs with food or milk. Many patients with adrenal insufficiency manage with only glucocorticoids.
MINERALOCORTICOIDS Fludrocortisone (Florinef Acetate)	Stimulates reabsorption of sodium and excretion of potassium and hydrogen ions in renal tubules. Used to treat adrenal insufficiency.	Hypokalemia, nausea and vomiting, edema, hypertension, muscle weakness, dizziness, tendon contractures, congestive heart failure.	Monitor weight, intake and output, BP, heart rate and rhythm, serum electrolytes. Assess for hypokalemia-prescribed sodium intake. Do not discontinue suddenly. Tell patient to carry drug identification card.
ADRENOCORTICAL CYTOTOXIC AGENTS Mitotane (Lysodren)	Suppresses adrenocortical function.	Nausea and vomiting, diarrhea, lethargy, dizziness, hypouricemia, hearing and vision disturbances, BP changes, dyspnea.	Monitor BP. Report infections or trauma so drug can be temporarily discontinued. Tell patient not to have immunizations without physician approval and to avoid contact with people who have recently had polio or DPT (diptheria, pertussis, and tetanus) vaccine. Increase fluid intake, and monitor uric acid.
ANTIFUNGAL AGENTS Ketoconazole (Nizoral)	Fungistatic. Suppresses adrenocortical function.	Nausea and vomiting, pruritus, diarrhea or constipation, GI bleeding, lethargy, headache, dizziness, adrenocortical insufficiency. Occasionally, thrombocytopenia, hemolytic anemia, hepatotoxicity.	Monitor stools. Administer antipruritics or apply topical agents as ordered. Safety measures if dizzy or drowsy. Monitor liver function tests, and assess for pale stools, dark urine, fatigue, and anorexia. Avoid alcohol.

BP, Blood pressure; *GI*, gastrointestinal.

Patients with Addison's disease are not at great risk for harmful side effects of corticosteroids because the goal is only to restore the blood level to normal.

NURSING CARE *of the Patient with Addison's Disease*

Assessment

Assessment of the patient with an adrenal disorder is summarized in Box 44-2 (see also Nursing Care Plan: The Patient with Addison's Disease on p. 972). Details of the health history that are especially relevant to Addison's disease are weight loss, salt craving, nausea and vomiting, abdominal cramping and diarrhea, muscle weakness and aches, poor stress response, decreased libido, and amenorrhea. The patient may be irritable or confused. The physical examination may reveal pale skin with bronzed areas, emaciation, sparse body hair, poor skin turgor, hypotension, and muscle wasting. The patient with acute episodes of Addison's disease requires ongoing monitoring of fluid and electrolyte levels and measurement of daily weights.

Nursing Diagnoses, Goals, and Outcome Criteria: Addison's Disease

Nursing Diagnoses	Goals and Outcome Criteria
Ineffective Tissue Perfusion related to electrolyte imbalance, hypovolemia, cardiac dysrhythmias	Improved tissue perfusion: warm, dry skin with strong peripheral pulses
Risk for Injury related to acute adrenal insufficiency, postural hypotension, impaired physiologic response to stress	Decreased risk for injury: blood pressure within patient norms, absence of faintness with position changes
Imbalanced Nutrition: Less Than Body Requirements related to impaired metabolism, inability to ingest sufficient nutrients, lack of interest in eating	Adequate nutrition: weight within 5 pounds of patient's baseline
Fatigue related to fluid, electrolyte, and glucose imbalances	Improved stamina: patient states fatigue is lessened, performs activities of daily living without tiring
Disturbed Body Image related to changes in appearance and function	Adaptation to physical changes: patient makes efforts to improve appearance, makes positive comments about self
Ineffective Therapeutic Regimen Management of long-term glucocorticoid and mineralocorticoid replacement therapy	Patient manages self-care and prescribed treatment: patient explains disease process and treatment with stated intent to adhere to prescribed regimen

Interventions

Ineffective Tissue Perfusion

Monitor for signs and symptoms of inadequate tissue perfusion: confusion, disorientation, tachycardia, apical-radial pulse deficit, general weakness and malaise, and hypotension (including orthostatic changes). Administer prescribed intravenous normal saline, plasma expanders, and vasopressors to maintain blood volume. The patient whose fluid output is greater than intake is at risk for hypovolemia. Because the patient is at risk for hyperkalemia, monitor serum electrolytes and assess for weakness, paresthesia, dizziness, and electrocardiogram changes. Promptly report these signs and symptoms of hyperkalemia to the physician.

Risk for Injury

Be alert for postural hypotension and other signs of hypovolemia. Instruct the patient who has dizziness with position changes to call for help when getting out of bed and to rise slowly to prevent falls. Exercising the legs before standing promotes venous return and may minimize the drop in blood pressure.

Sudden profound weakness with postural hypotension is characteristic of acute addisonian crisis and leads to shock and death if not corrected. Administer fluid replacement and hormones as ordered to treat addisonian crisis.

Imbalanced Nutrition: Less Than Body Requirements

Daily weights provide important data to assess fluid balance. Weight changes also provide information about the adequacy of the patient's diet (see the Nutrition Concepts box below). If nutrition is a problem, consult the dietitian. The prescribed diet is usually high protein, low carbohydrate. Salt may be used liberally because patients with Addison's disease tend to lose sodium. Respect the patient's food preferences as much as possible. The mealtime atmosphere should be conducive to eating.

Nutrition Concepts

1. Early symptoms of Addison's disease may include anorexia, nausea, vomiting, diarrhea, and weight loss, resulting in impaired nutrition.
2. Patients with Cushing's syndrome may experience sodium and water retention.
3. Diet therapy for Cushing's syndrome may include decreased caloric and sodium intake and increased potassium intake.
4. Reducing sodium intake can decrease edema and related weight gain with Cushing's syndrome.
5. Patients with diabetes insipidus usually experience excessive thirst or urination, so they must drink liquids almost continuously to avoid dehydration and hypovolemic shock.

NURSING CARE PLAN

The Patient with Addison's Disease

ASSESSMENT

Health History: A 52-year-old white man is admitted with Addison's disease. He considers himself healthy but has had some joint pain in his knees. He had an appendectomy 20 years ago. The patient complains of weight loss, anorexia, weakness, and darkening of the skin on his face and arms. His usual weight is 170 pounds. He has had bouts of nausea, vomiting, and diarrhea accompanied by vague abdominal pain. The patient is a salesman and reports that his symptoms are making it difficult for him to keep up with his work. He is embarrassed about the change in his skin color.

Physical Examination: Vital signs: blood pressure, 110/80 (sitting) and 88/42 (standing); pulse, 102 with slight irregularity; respiration, 20; temperature, 98° F orally. Height, 5'8". Weight, 155 lb. The patient is oriented but somewhat lethargic. The skin on his face and arms and his abdominal scar are darkly pigmented. His body hair is sparse. The patient's oral mucous membranes are slightly dry.

Nursing Diagnosis	Goals and Outcome Criteria	Interventions
Ineffective Tissue Perfusion related to electrolyte imbalance, fluid volume deficit, and cardiac dysrhythmias	The patient will have improved tissue perfusion, as evidenced by warm, dry skin, strong peripheral pulses, and fluid output equal to fluid intake.	Monitor for signs and symptoms of inadequate tissue perfusion: confusion, disorientation, tachycardia, hypotension, apical-radial pulse deficit, fluid output exceeding intake. Administer intravenous fluids (normal saline, plasma expanders) and vasopressors, as ordered. Monitor for hyperkalemia: weakness, paresthesia, dizziness. Report evidence of inadequate tissue perfusion or hyperkalemia to physician.
Risk for Injury related to acute adrenal insufficiency, impaired stress response, postural hypotension	The patient will remain free of injury due to hypotension, shock, or falls.	Monitor for postural hypotension. If the patient has dizziness with position changes, instruct him to exercise his legs before rising, to rise slowly, and to call for help when getting out of bed. Administer fluids and hormones as ordered.
Imbalanced Nutrition: Less Than Body Requirements related to impaired metabolism, inability to ingest sufficient nutrients, and lack of interest in eating	The patient will be adequately nourished, as evidenced by weight within 5 lb of baseline.	Weigh daily to monitor fluid balance and nutritional status. Request dietary consult for patient education so that food preferences can be respected. Provide high-protein, low-carbohydrate diet as ordered. Tell the patient salt may be used freely. Provide a pleasant atmosphere for meals. Report signs of hypoglycemia: headache, trembling, tachycardia, sweating.
Fatigue related to fluid, electrolyte, and glucose imbalances	The patient will report improved stamina.	Explain medically prescribed activity limitations. Plan care to allow for periods of rest. Discuss energy conservation after discharge.
Disturbed Body Image related to changes in appearance and function	The patient will adapt to altered physical appearance and function, as evidenced by efforts to improve appearance and positive comments about self.	Explore how the patient feels about skin changes. Discuss strategies to deal with changes: long sleeves, avoidance of excess sunlight. Advise to arrange work with rest periods. Encourage attention to grooming. Compliment efforts.
Ineffective Therapeutic Regimen Management related to lack of understanding of long-term glucocorticoid therapy	The patient will manage self-care and prescribed treatment; correctly explain the disease, its treatment, and medication therapy; will state intent to adhere to prescribed regimen.	Implement teaching plan, to include the following: Patient Teaching Plan: Addison's Disease • Wear a medical alert tag and carry emergency kit with dexamethasone. • Take glucocorticoids in divided doses in morning and afternoon with food. • Increase medication dosage as ordered when under stress. • Notify physician or go to emergency room if unable to take oral medications for more than 24 hours. • Lifelong therapy and monitoring are needed. • Report signs and symptoms of inadequate and excessive hormone replacement.

? **CRITICAL THINKING** QUESTIONS

■ Name three strategies for energy conservation.

■ How might you encourage the patient to share his feelings about the skin changes?

Hypoglycemia may develop as a result of decreased cortisol secretion. Encourage frequent rest periods to avoid depletion of glycogen stores. Meals should be taken regularly, and between-meal snacks may be needed to maintain blood glucose. Monitor for and teach the patient symptoms of hypoglycemia: headache, tachycardia, trembling, sweating. Periodic laboratory studies are done to assess nitrogen balance, liver function, and serum albumin, glucose, electrolytes, blood urea nitrogen, and creatinine.

Fatigue

Explain any prescribed activity limitations to the patient. Plan specific rest periods to conserve energy. Provide assistance with activities of daily living as needed. If the patient is on bed rest, intervene to prevent complications of immobility as described in Chapter 21.

Disturbed Body Image

Explore the patient's reaction to the physical changes experienced. Discuss strategies to cope with changes. When the patient's condition has stabilized, encourage attention to grooming and compliment the patient's efforts.

Ineffective Therapeutic Regimen Management

Care of the patient with a chronic disease requires indepth education and information about stress management. It is critical for the patient to understand Addison's disease and to know how to recognize the effects of the disease as well as those of overmedication. The patient must learn to make adjustments in replacement hormones depending on various stressors. Provide written material to supplement the teaching sessions.

ADRENAL HYPERSECRETION (CUSHING'S SYNDROME)

Etiology

Hypersecretion of the adrenal cortex may result in the production of excess amounts of corticosteroids, particularly glucocorticoid. The condition that results

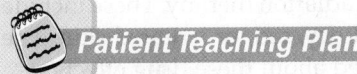

Patient Teaching Plan

Addison's Disease

- Wear a medical alert tag and carry emergency kit with dexamethasone.
- Take glucocorticoid in divided doses in morning and afternoon with food.
- Increase medication dosage as ordered when under stress.
- Notify physician or go to emergency room if unable to take oral medications for more than 24 hours.
- Lifelong therapy and monitoring are needed.
- Report signs and symptoms of inadequate and excessive hormone replacement.

from excessive cortisol is called Cushing's syndrome. The overproduction of adrenocortical hormones may result from endogenous (internal) as well as exogenous (external) causes.

Endogenous causes include corticotropin-secreting pituitary tumors, a cortisol-secreting neoplasm within the adrenal glands, and excess secretion of corticotropin by a carcinoma of the lung or other tissues. Excessive production of ACTH because of a pituitary tumor is called Cushing's disease. The incidence of Cushing's syndrome caused by disease is infrequent, affecting women eight times more often than men. Approximately 25% of cases of Cushing's syndrome are due to adrenal tumors.

The single exogenous cause of Cushing's syndrome is prolonged administration of high doses of corticosteroids. This is also the most common cause of Cushing's syndrome.

Pathophysiology

Clinical manifestations of Cushing's syndrome affect most body systems and are related to excess levels of circulating corticosteroids. In some instances, signs and symptoms of mineralocorticoid and androgen excess may appear; however, signs and symptoms of glucocorticoid excess usually predominate.

Hyperadrenalism produces marked changes in the personal appearance of the affected person, including obesity, facial redness, hirsutism (excess hair), menstrual disorders, hypertension of varying degrees, and muscle wasting of the extremities (Fig. 44-6). Additional findings can be delayed wound healing, insomnia, irrational behavior, and mood disturbances such as irritability and anxiety. The following are hallmark findings that lead to a diagnosis of Cushing's syndrome:

- Truncal obesity (excess adipose in body trunk)
- Protein wasting (slender extremities and very thin and friable skin)
- Facial fullness, often called a "moon face"
- Purple striae on the abdomen, breasts, buttocks, or thighs
- Osteoporosis (a significant finding in premenopausal women)
- Hypokalemia of uncertain etiology

Medical Diagnosis

In addition to physical signs and symptoms, some laboratory, radiographic, and imaging results may be useful in determining a diagnosis.

Laboratory Studies. When Cushing's syndrome is suspected, a 24-hour urine collection for free cortisol usually is ordered. A low-dose dexamethasone suppression test may be done as well. In normal people, the cortisol and 17-hydroxycorticosteroid levels are suppressed. If these levels are not suppressed (compared with the baseline sample), the test is repeated using a higher dose of dexamethasone.

FIGURE **44-6** Clinical manifestations in the patient with Cushing's syndrome.

Abnormal laboratory findings include polycythemia, hypokalemia, hypernatremia, hyperglycemia, leukocytosis, glycosuria, hypocalcemia, and elevated plasma cortisol. ACTH may be high or low, depending on whether the basic problem lies in the adrenals or in the pituitary. In some cases, malignant tumors, especially small cell cancer of the lung, can secrete ACTH, which stimulates excess cortisol secretion.

Radiographic Studies. If a tumor is suspected as a causative factor in Cushing's syndrome, a CT scan and MRI may be done to localize the site of the tumor. Radiographic films also may reveal osteoporosis of the spinal column, especially in women.

Medical Treatment

Depending on the specific patient and the etiology of the disease, various therapies may be used. These include drug therapy, radiation, and surgery. If Cushing's syndrome is caused by administration of synthetic glucocorticoids, the physician may gradually withdraw them. Most patients affected with hyperadrenalism due to a single benign adrenal tumor undergo surgical intervention. Bilateral benign tumors more often are treated with an aldosterone antagonist, that is, a drug that reduces aldosterone secretion or blocks its effects. An example of an aldosterone antagonist is the potassium-sparing diuretic spironolactone (Aldactone). Patients with metastatic adrenal cancer are usu-

ally treated with surgery and chemotherapy. However, a cure for metastatic adrenal cancer is yet to be found. When Cushing's syndrome is caused by a pituitary tumor, removal of part of the pituitary or radiation may reduce ACTH secretion without disturbing other pituitary functions. If this fails, the remaining pituitary tissue may be removed.

Drug Therapy. When surgery is contraindicated, certain agents that interfere with ACTH production or adrenal hormone synthesis may be administered. One example is mitotane (Lysodren), a cytotoxic substance that is used as a palliative treatment for inoperable adrenal tumors. Agents that interfere with cortisol production include ketoconazole (Nizoral), aminoglutethimide (Cytadren), and metyrapone (Metopirone). Metyrapone is also used in combination with mitotane for enhanced effects. There is a risk of acute adrenal crisis when patients are on drugs that suppress adrenal function. In addition, the drugs must be promptly discontinued if trauma or shock occurs, because the patient's ability to adapt is diminished. The Drug Therapy table on p. 970 provides additional information.

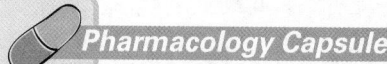

Pharmacology Capsule

Drugs that suppress adrenal function can lead to acute adrenal crisis and must be promptly discontinued if shock or trauma occurs.

Radiation. In cases in which a pituitary adenoma causes excessive secretion of ACTH, the adenoma may be treated with radiation therapy. Radiation can be administered either externally or internally. Internal radiation involves the transsphenoidal implantation of a radioactive material that remains in place for a specified period of time. Radiation therapy is not always effective and can destroy healthy tissue. If radiation therapy is being used to treat a patient with a pituitary adenoma, you must be alert for any significant changes in the patient's neurologic status, such as a complaint of headache or a change in mental status or pupillary responses. In addition, the patient may experience side effects associated with radiation therapy. These include alopecia (hair loss) and dry, red, or irritated skin. The patient must be educated about these drug effects.

Surgical Management

The surgical treatment of hyperadrenalism depends on the specific cause of the disorder. For example, if adrenal hypersecretion is due to a pituitary adenoma that is producing ACTH, a transsphenoidal hypophysectomy is performed (see Surgical Management in the Hyperpituitarism section on p. 954). If adrenal adenoma or carcinoma is the cause of the adrenal hypersecretion, an adrenalectomy (removal of the adrenal gland) is performed. If only one gland is removed, the procedure is referred to as a *unilateral adrenalectomy*; the removal of both of the glands is called a *bilateral adrenalectomy*. An adrenalectomy may be performed in situations in which drug and radiation therapies are unsuccessful. Patients who are undergoing a unilateral adrenalectomy can expect to require replacement therapy for up to 2 years after surgery. A bilateral adrenalectomy necessitates lifelong replacement of both glucocorticoid and mineralocorticoids. Depending on the tumor size, a laparoscopic procedure may be an option. Surgery and chemotherapy are indicated for metastatic adrenal cancer. These treatments may induce remission but are not curative.

NURSING CARE *of the Patient with Cushing's Syndrome*

Assessment

Initial assessment of the patient with Cushing's syndrome includes a detailed history and physical examination done by the registered nurse. The LPN/LVN may collect specific information about the onset of symptoms, prior treatments, drug allergies, and current medications. The complete nursing assessment of the patient with an adrenal disorder is summarized in Box 44-2.

Nursing Diagnoses, Goals, and Outcome Criteria: Cushing's Syndrome	
NURSING DIAGNOSES	GOALS AND OUTCOME CRITERIA
Risk for Infection related to high serum cortisol levels	Absence of infection: normal body temperature and white blood cell count
Disturbed Thought Processes related to fluid and electrolyte imbalance	Normal thought processes: stable mood, patient denial of depression
Risk for Impaired Skin Integrity related to changes in skin and connective tissue and edema	Absence of injury to skin: skin intact with minimal or no bruising
Risk for Injury (fracture) related to osteoporosis	Absence of fractures: no skeletal trauma or fractures
Disturbed Body Image related to changes in physical appearance and function	Adaptation to altered body image: patient attends to appearance, grooming; makes positive comments about self
Ineffective Therapeutic Regimen Management related to lack of understanding of disease, drug therapy, diet, and self-care	Patient follows prescribed treatment: verbalizes and demonstrates self-care; condition stabilizes

Interventions

Risk for Infection

Exposure to people with infections should be avoided because of the patient's decreased resistance to infection. Minor symptoms, such as a low-grade fever (99.5° F or higher), sore throat, or aches, can indicate the onset of a potentially serious infection. Any symptoms indicative of a cold or other problem should be brought to the attention of the physician.

Disturbed Thought Processes

Personality changes often accompany adrenal disorders. When they do occur, discuss them with the patient and the family. Understanding that mood swings are a part of this disorder may help the patient and family cope more effectively. If the emotional changes, particularly depression, become severe, carefully monitor the patient. A psychiatric referral may be necessary.

Risk for Impaired Skin Integrity

The skin of the patient with Cushing's syndrome is extremely fragile. Inspect the skin daily to detect early signs of pressure or injuries. Assist the patient with limited mobility to change positions at least every 2 hours. Keep bed linens clean and dry. Advise the patient to wear shoes when out of bed to reduce the risk of foot injuries. During transfers and position changes, be careful to prevent trauma to the skin.

Risk for Injury

Because fractures occur very easily, protect the patient with Cushing's syndrome from falls or trauma. Keep the bed in low position and the call bell within reach. If the patient is very weak or confused, raise the side rails. Instruct the patient to call for assistance when getting in and out of bed.

Disturbed Body Image

Bruises, abnormal fat distribution, and hirsutism may embarrass the patient. Provide an opportunity for the patient to share thoughts and concerns about these changes. If they are distressing, suggest clothing to conceal them. Encourage and assist patients to be well groomed. Women may choose to shave or to use depilatories to remove unwanted hair. Reassure the patient that physical changes usually improve gradually after medical or surgical treatment.

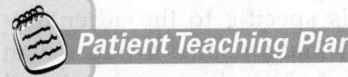 *Patient Teaching Plan*

Cushing's Syndrome

- Avoid people with infections because you have increased risk of infections; report any temperature elevation to your physician.
- Mood swings and changes in appearance are usually corrected with treatment.
- Avoid activities that could result in trauma because you have increased risk of bleeding and fractures.
- It is critical that you continue drug therapy under medical supervision.

Consider the Alternative

Patients with Cushing's syndrome should be cautioned that long-term use of some herbs, including celery, juniper, licorice, and parsley, can cause hypokalemia.

Ineffective Therapeutic Regimen Management

To manage Cushing's syndrome, the patient must understand the condition, complications, treatment, and self-care. Provide written information to supplement verbal teaching about drugs, including drug names and dosages, schedules, and adverse effects. A referral may be made to the dietitian for nutritional counseling. The diet is typically low in calories with sufficient protein and calcium. The following patient teaching plan includes the key patient teaching points.

NURSING CARE *of the Adrenalectomy Patient*

General nursing care of the surgical patient is discussed in Chapter 17. This section addresses the specific needs of the adrenalectomy patient.

PREOPERATIVE NURSING CARE

Preoperative care of the patient undergoing an adrenalectomy involves monitoring for and correcting any existing electrolyte imbalances. Strict hand washing and observance of aseptic technique are key in the prevention of infections in these susceptible patients. Preoperative education involves a discussion of glucocorticoid replacement therapy, including dosage, side effects, and complications.

POSTOPERATIVE NURSING CARE

After adrenalectomy, patients are sent to a critical care unit for at least 1 to 2 days for close observation and assessment. During this period, monitor the vital signs for signs and symptoms of impending shock, which may be evident as hypotension, a weak or thready pulse, decreased urinary output, and changes in level of consciousness. Pulse and blood pressure may be unstable for 24 to 48 hours after surgery, and vasopressors may be needed to maintain blood pressure in the immediate postoperative period.

A nursing diagnosis specific to the adrenalectomy patient is Risk for Injury related to addisonian crisis as a result of the sudden decrease in adrenal hormone secretion. Assess for signs and symptoms of acute adrenal insufficiency: vomiting, weakness, hypotension, joint pain, pruritus, and emotional disturbances. Closely monitor fluid and electrolyte balance. Intravenous fluids may be prescribed to restore or maintain balance. High doses of cortisol are given intravenously during and for several days after surgery to enable the patient to deal with the physical stress of surgery. The dosages are adjusted on the basis of the blood pressure, blood glucose, serum elec-

trolytes, and serum cortisol levels. Later, glucocorticoids are administered orally.

Because the patient's resistance to infection is lowered, be especially careful to protect the patient by using strict aseptic technique for wound care and invasive procedures. Signs of infection may be very subtle.

Assess comfort at frequent intervals, and treat pain with opioid analgesics. Document the effects of treatment. To minimize the risk of pulmonary complications, such as stasis of secretions and pneumonia, instruct the patient to turn, cough, deep breathe, or use an incentive spirometer.

PHEOCHROMOCYTOMA

A pheochromocytoma is a tumor, usually benign, of the adrenal medulla that causes secretion of excessive catecholamines (i.e., epinephrine, norepinephrine). Patients with a pheochromocytoma exhibit episodes of hypertension, hypermetabolism, and hyperglycemia. The classic clinical findings are hypertension with a diastolic pressure of 115 mm Hg or higher; severe, pounding headache; and diaphoresis (profuse sweating). Other signs and symptoms include pallor, dilated pupils, orthostatic hypotension, and blurred vision. Episodes may be triggered by emotional distress, exercise, manipulation of the tumor, postural changes, and major trauma, including surgery.

The condition is treated by surgical removal of the tumor. Before surgery, the surgeon attempts to normalize vital signs with adrenergic antagonists (drugs that block the effects of catecholamines) and stabilize the patient's fluid status. The nurse monitors cardiovascular status and prepares the patient for surgery as detailed in Chapter 17. Postoperative nursing care is generally the same as that described for the patient having an adrenalectomy. However, special postoperative problems in the patient with pheochromocytoma include a greater risk for fluctuations in blood pressure and hypoglycemia. These problems require close monitoring and treatment.

Key Points

- The endocrine system secretes hormones—chemical messengers that affect target organs and body tissues.
- Endocrine activity is regulated by feedback mechanisms that either stimulate or inhibit hormone synthesis and secretion.
- Pituitary hormones affect growth, fluid and electrolyte balance, metabolism, ovulation, milk production, uterine contractions, and skin pigmentation.
- Pituitary and adrenal function usually remain adequate in older people.
- Hyperpituitarism, caused by excess anterior pituitary hormones, leads to gigantism or acromegaly.
- Hyperpituitarism is treated with drugs or surgery to remove the tumor or the entire pituitary (hypophysectomy).

- Treatment of hyperpituitarism can prevent further changes and complications. Soft tissue hypertrophy may be reduced, but skeletal changes are not reversible.
- Dwarfism is the result of inadequate growth hormone.
- Panhypopituitarism is a deficiency of all anterior pituitary hormones and is treated with replacement hormones.
- Diabetes insipidus, caused by a deficit in antidiuretic hormone, results in massive diuresis and is treated with vasopressin.
- Syndrome of inappropriate antidiuretic hormone, caused by excess antidiuretic hormone, results in fluid retention and is treated with diuretics and demeclocycline.
- The adrenal medulla secretes the catecholamines epinephrine and norepinephrine, which promote adaptation to stress.
- The adrenal cortex secretes steroids in the form of mineralocorticoids, glucocorticoids, and androgens or estrogens.
- Primary adrenal insufficiency (Addison's disease) causes hypoglycemia, hyperkalemia, hyponatremia, and hypovolemia and requires lifelong replacement of glucocorticoids and mineralocorticoids.
- Acute adrenal crisis is a life-threatening emergency caused by a sudden marked decrease in adrenal hormones that can lead to circulatory collapse and death.
- Cushing's syndrome results from hypersecretion of cortisol, a glucocorticoid, or from prolonged administration of corticosteroids.
- Cushing's syndrome is characterized by polycythemia, hypokalemia, hyperglycemia, leukocytosis, and glycosuria.
- Cushing's syndrome is treated with drug therapy, radiation, and hypophysectomy or adrenalectomy.
- Nursing care for the patient with Cushing's syndrome is concerned with Risk for Infection, Disturbed Thought Processes, Risk for Impaired Skin Integrity, Risk for Injury, Disturbed Body Image, and Ineffective Therapeutic Regimen Management.
- All chronic pituitary and adrenal conditions require patient teaching to enable the patient to manage the condition by taking medications properly and recognizing the need for medical intervention.
- A pheochromocytoma is an adrenal tumor that increases secretion of catecholamines, causing hypertension, hypermetabolism, and hyperglycemia.

 Go to your Companion CD-ROM for a Pharmacology Tutorial, Audio Glossary, and 3-D animations.

evolve   Be sure to visit the companion Evolve site at http://evolve.elsevier.com/Linton/ for WebLinks and additional online resources.

REVIEW QUESTIONS *Choose the best answer.*

1. The overall mission of the endocrine system is to:
   1. Maintain electrolyte balance
   2. Control metabolic rate
   3. Maintain homeostasis
   4. Resist infection

2. Hormones secreted by the posterior pituitary include the following:
   1. Antidiuretic hormone
   2. Adrenocorticotropic hormone
   3. Growth hormone
   4. Luteinizing hormone

3. A patient who has recently started treatment for acromegaly says, "I will be so glad to look like myself again!" The most appropriate response is:
   1. "I know you are looking forward to that."
   2. "The process of reversing the effects of acromegaly is very slow."
   3. "Treatment will keep your symptoms from getting worse but will not reverse all of them."
   4. "These drugs can slow down the progression of acromegaly, but you will have additional bone enlargement."

4. After surgery to remove a pituitary adenoma, a patient complains of neck stiffness. You should:
   1. Give a gentle neck massage
   2. Administer a prescribed analgesic
   3. Lower the head of the bed
   4. Look for other signs of infection

5. Patients with hypopituitarism who wish to have children must be treated with follicle-stimulating hormone and:
   1. Luteinizing hormone
   2. Thyroid hormone
   3. Corticosteroids
   4. Prolactin

6. The main symptom of SIADH is:
   1. Increased blood glucose
   2. Water retention
   3. Generalized edema
   4. Hypotension

7. The patient with diabetes insipidus must maintain records of:
   1. Daily diet
   2. Sodium intake
   3. Urine specific gravity
   4. Blood pressure and pulse

8. Fluid and electrolyte imbalances associated with Addison's disease include the following:
   1. Hypokalemia
   2. Hyponatremia
   3. Hypervolemia
   4. Metabolic alkalosis

9. A patient who is brought to the emergency room has BP 88/40; pulse 108, thready; and dry skin and mucous membranes. He is confused. A medical alert card in his wallet states that he takes drugs for Addison's disease. You know he has signs and symptoms of:

   1. Acute adrenal crisis
   2. Cushing's syndrome
   3. Diabetic ketoacidosis
   4. Cushing's disease

10. Nursing care of the patient with Cushing's syndrome should include the following:

    1. Apply moisturizers to dark, toughened areas of skin
    2. Protect the patient from visitors and other patients with infections
    3. Tell the patient that mood swings and irritability will not be tolerated
    4. Encourage the patient to use salt liberally to offset excessive loss in the urine

Objectives

After reading and studying this chapter, you should be able to:

1. Identify nursing assessment data related to the functions of the thyroid and parathyroid glands.
2. Describe tests and procedures used to diagnose disorders of the thyroid and parathyroid glands and nursing responsibilities relevant for each.
3. Describe the pathophysiology, signs and symptoms, complications, and treatment of hyperthyroidism, hypothyroidism, hyperparathyroidism, and hypoparathyroidism.
4. Assist in the development of nursing care plans for patients with disorders of the thyroid or parathyroid glands.

Key Terms

Be sure to check out the bonus material on the Companion CD-ROM, including selected audio pronunciations.

Chvostek's sign (KVŎS-tĕks, p. 994)
cretinism (KRĒ-tĭn-ĭzm, p. 988)
exophthalmos (ĕk-sŏf-THĂL-mŏs, p. 980)
goiter (GOI-tĕr, p. 993)
goitrogen (GOI-trō-jĕn, p. 988)
laryngospasm (lă-RĬNG-gō-spăzm, p. 987)
myxedema (mĭk-sĕ-DĒ-mă, p. 988)
nodule (NŎD-ūl, p. 979)
parotiditis (pă-rŏt-ĭ-DĪ-tĭs, p. 983)
tetany (TĔT-ă-nē, p. 987)
thyroiditis (thī-roid-Ī-tĭs, p. 983)
thyrotoxicosis (thī-rō-tŏk-sĭ-KŌ-sĭs, p. 982)
Trousseau's sign (troo-SŌZ, p. 994)

THE THYROID GLAND

ANATOMY AND PHYSIOLOGY OF THE THYROID GLAND

The thyroid gland is located in the lower portion of the anterior neck. It consists of two lobes, one on each side of the trachea. The lobes are connected in front of the trachea by a narrow bridge of tissue called the *isthmus* (Fig. 45-1).

The thyroid gland plays a major role in regulating the body's rate of metabolism and growth and development. When the metabolic rate falls, the hypotha-la-mus stimulates the pituitary gland to secrete thyroid-stimulating hormone (TSH). This hormone in turn stimulates the thyroid gland to secrete hormones that affect the production and use of energy.

The hormones produced by the thyroid gland are thyroid hormone, triiodothyronine, and calcitonin. Each of these is known by several names. Thyroid hormone also is called *thyroxine, tetraiodothyronine,* or T_4. Triiodothyronine is referred to as T_3. Both T_4 and T_3 increase the body's metabolic rate. Calcitonin, or thyrocalcitonin, plays a role in regulating the serum calcium level. It is secreted when serum calcium levels are high, limiting the shift of calcium from the bones into the blood.

AGE-RELATED CHANGES IN THYROID FUNCTION

With age, there is an increased incidence of thyroid nodules. Serum levels of T_4 remain approximately the same in the healthy older person, but levels of T_3 more often decline. The incidence of hypothyroidism increases with age, especially among women. Thyroid conditions are often overlooked in older adults because signs and symptoms may be subtle and attributed to the aging process. Weight changes may not occur in the older person as they do with younger people with thyroid disorders. Treatment of thyroid disorders can have a profound positive effect on the patient's quality of life.

NURSING ASSESSMENT OF THE THYROID GLAND

Thyroid disorders may escape detection until they are rather severe because the symptoms are often vague. Periodic assessment of the patient with a thyroid disorder is necessary for the physician to evaluate the response to treatment and make adjustments if necessary. Data collected by the registered nurse and the LPN/LVN contribute to this assessment and evaluation.

HEALTH HISTORY

To elicit information about common symptoms of thyroid disorders, ask if the patient is aware of any changes in energy level, sleep patterns, personality, mental func-

Box 45-1 *ASSESSMENT of the Patient with a Thyroid Disorder*

Health History

Present Illness:
Fatigue, weight changes, mental-emotional changes

Past Medical History:
Recent surgery or trauma, radiation of the head or neck, recent and current medications, history of thyroid or renal disorders

Review of Systems:
Fatigue, changes in hair or skin, voice changes, palpitations, edema, constipation or diarrhea, polyuria, nervousness, weight loss, temperature intolerance, excessive perspiration, changes in libido or sexual function

Functional Assessment:
Sleep disturbances, usual dietary intake, anorexia, ability to cope with stress

Physical Examination

Vital Signs:
Abnormal heart rate and rhythm, blood pressure changes, tachypnea

Height and Weight

Skin:
Changes in moisture, temperature, and texture

Hair:
Changes in texture

Eyes:
Exophthalmos

Neck:
Enlargement

Hands:
Tremor

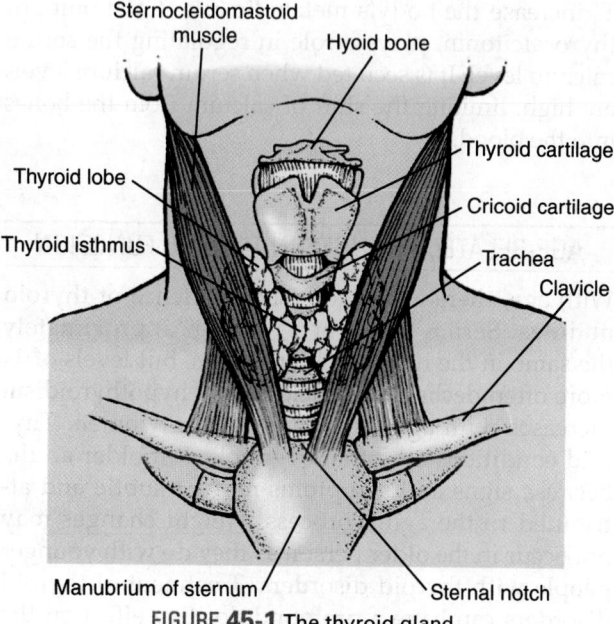

FIGURE **45-1** The thyroid gland.

Labels: Sternocleidomastoid muscle, Hyoid bone, Thyroid cartilage, Cricoid cartilage, Trachea, Clavicle, Thyroid lobe, Thyroid isthmus, Manubrium of sternum, Sternal notch

the facial expression and characteristics as well as the mental alertness. Vital signs are important because they reflect the metabolic rate. Thyroid disorders may cause increased or decreased heart rate, respirations, blood pressure, and temperature as well as irregular heart rhythms. Inspect and palpate the skin for moisture, temperature, and texture. In the head and neck examination, note the hair texture. Examine the eyes for **exophthalmos** (bulging). Inspect the neck for enlargement typical of goiter. Observe the hands for tremor. Nurses with advanced physical examination skills may palpate the neck for thyroid enlargement or nodules.

Key components of the nursing assessment of the patient with a thyroid disorder are outlined in Box 45-1.

DIAGNOSTIC TESTS AND PROCEDURES

Diagnostic studies of the thyroid gland include laboratory blood tests and studies employing radioactive iodine. The Diagnostic Tests and Procedures table on p. 981 summarizes the use of each test and identifies nursing implications.

The most useful tests of thyroid function are measurements of serum T_3, free T_4, T_4, and TSH. These tests have become increasingly more sophisticated; thus more specialized tests are rarely needed. The thyroid-releasing hormone (TRH) stimulation test measures the blood level of TSH after administration of TRH. This test shows whether thyroid hormone abnormalities are caused by a disorder of the thyroid gland itself or by altered production of stimulating hormones by the hypothalamus or the pituitary.

The thyroid gland uses iodine to manufacture hormones. Therefore radioactive iodine isotopes (^{131}I, ^{123}I, ^{99m}Tc) are useful for diagnostic purposes because they concentrate in the thyroid. The amount of iodine taken up by the thyroid is measured to assess the activity

tion, or emotional state. Fatigue may be found with both hypothyroidism and hyperthyroidism. Because thyroid hormones affect the metabolic rate, patients may have unexplained weight changes. Hormone deficiency lowers the metabolic rate, so patients may gain weight. At the other extreme, hormone excess increases the metabolic rate, often causing weight loss.

In the review of systems, pay particular attention to changes in menstrual cycles, sexual function, hydration (thirst, changes in urine output, tissue turgor, moisture of mucous membranes), bowel elimination pattern, and tolerance of heat and cold.

PHYSICAL EXAMINATION

The physical examination begins with measurement of the patient's vital signs and height and weight. Note

DIAGNOSTIC TESTS and PROCEDURES | *Thyroid Disorders*

TEST/PURPOSE	PATIENT PREPARATION	POSTPROCEDURE CARE
LABORATORY STUDIES		
Serum T$_3$ (triiodothyronine) and serum T$_4$ measurements of free and total T$_4$ detect abnormal levels of thyroid hormones. Elevated T$_3$: Graves' disease, toxic adenoma, and toxic nodular goiter. Elevated T$_4$: hyperthyroidism, excessive thyroid hormone replacement. T$_3$ and T$_4$ decrease with hypothyroidism.	Tell patient that blood sample will be drawn. Nonfasting. Some medications may be withheld before blood is drawn.	After blood sample is drawn, assess for oozing. Apply small dressing.
Serum thyroid-stimulating hormone (TSH) increases with hypothyroidism; decreases with hyperthyroidism.	Tell patient a blood sample will be drawn.	After venipuncture, assess for oozing. Apply small dressing.
Thyroid-releasing hormone (TRH) stimulation test assesses response of the pituitary to TRH. Differentiates types of hypothyroidism. TRH normally increases after TRH given intravenously.	Tell patient that a drug will be given intravenously; then several blood samples must be drawn.	Assess venipuncture site for oozing. Apply small bandage.
UPTAKE AND IMAGING PROCEDURES		
Radioactive iodine uptake test. After radioactive iodine is given orally, the amount of ^{131}I taken up by thyroid is measured with a special instrument. High uptake with hyperthyroidism; low with hypothyroidism.	Tell patient the procedure is painless. Ask about pregnancy, in which case radiation is contraindicated. Advise patient that radiation dose is small and will not harm others.	For 24 hours after test, patient should wash hands with soap and water after voiding. If caregiver discards urine, gloves should be worn. Then, gloves should be washed, removed, and bare hands washed. Pregnant women should avoid patient contact for 24 hours.
Thyroid scan ^{131}I, ^{123}I, or ^{99m}Tc is given orally and a scanner used to detect pattern of uptake by the thyroid gland. Can differentiate benign and malignant nodules and detect other abnormalities.	Tell patient about test. If ^{131}I is used, patient will be given isotope in liquid form and will return to radiology 24 hours later for scan. With ^{123}I, scan is done after 3 to 6 hours. Patient will have to lie still on back for 20 minutes during scan. For 1 week before test, patient should not consume iodine. Iodine is in radiographic dyes, some oral contraceptives, weight control drugs, multivitamins, all thyroid drugs, and some food, especially seafood.	Same as for radioactive iodine uptake test.
Thyroid ultrasonography provides high-quality images of thyroid and any nodules.	Advise patient that procedure is painless and noninvasive. An instrument is moved over the neck area and uses sound waves to create an image of the gland.	
Fine-needle aspiration biopsy. Material from thyroid nodules can be aspirated using a needle and guided by ultrasonography.	Same as thyroid ultrasonography. Also, tell patient the physician will use a small needle to remove a tissue sample.	Assess for any signs of bleeding: swelling in the area of the biopsy site, bleeding from the puncture site, increasing pulse.

level of the gland. This test is called a *radioactive iodine (RAI) uptake test*.

For a thyroid scan, the patient ingests radioactive iodine. Then a specialized instrument is used to scan the area of the thyroid gland. It creates a picture of the gland based on the distribution of the iodine. The picture aids in diagnosing cancer because the patterns of iodine concentration in normal and malignant tissue are different. The scan may be repeated at specific intervals. Because a low dose of radiation is used for diagnostic purposes, it poses no danger to the patient or others. However, pregnancy is a contraindication because of possible harm to the fetus.

Thyroid ultrasonography yields very clear images of the thyroid gland and any nodules present. The cytopathologist can use this technology to guide a needle inserted to aspirate material from the nodules. For evaluation of metastatic disease or to image

Put on Your Thinking Cap!

A patient's blood studies show a high level of TSH and a low level of T$_4$. Explain what this finding means.

the portion of the thyroid concealed by the sternum, magnetic resonance imaging (MRI) or computed tomography (CT) is used.

DISORDERS OF THE THYROID GLAND

HYPERTHYROIDISM

Hyperthyroidism is characterized by abnormally increased synthesis and secretion of thyroid hormones. Several forms of hyperthyroidism occur. The most common types are Graves' disease (also called *toxic diffuse goiter*) and multinodular goiter (also called *toxic nodular goiter*).

Graves' disease, which is the most common type of hyperthyroidism, is thought to be an autoimmune disorder. Antibodies activate TSH receptors, which in turn stimulate thyroid enlargement and hormone secretion. Graves' disease develops most often in young women. Regardless of whether the patient has treatment, the condition tends to have periods of remission and exacerbation. Some patients with Graves' disease eventually develop hypothyroidism.

Multinodular goiter occurs most often in women in their sixth and seventh decades. It is most likely to develop in people who have had goiter for a number of years. Hyperthyroidism in this case is caused by small thyroid nodules that secrete excess thyroid hormone. Unlike Graves' disease, the increased hormone production is independent of TSH. The nodules can be benign or malignant. Symptoms of hyperthyroidism are usually less severe with multinodular goiter than with Graves' disease.

Because all types of hyperthyroidism have many common features and because Graves' disease is the most common form, it will be used as the example of hyperthyroidism.

Signs and Symptoms

Many of the signs and symptoms of hyperthyroidism are caused by an increased metabolic rate and can range from mild to severe. Weight loss and nervousness may be the only symptoms in patients with a mild form of the disease. In more severe cases, the patient's history may reveal restlessness, irritable behavior, sleep disturbances, emotional lability, personality changes, hair loss, and fatigue. Weight loss, even when the patient is eating well, is common. Some patients overcompensate for the increased metabolism, overeat, and gain weight. Many patients report poor tolerance of heat and excessive perspiration. Changes in menstrual and

bowel patterns may occur. Examination findings may include warm, moist, velvety skin; fine tremors of the hands; swelling of the neck; and ophthalmopathy including exophthalmos. Exophthalmos is the most apparent effect of hyperthyroidism on the eyes. Tearing, light sensitivity, decreased visual acuity, and swelling occur around the orbit of the eye. Exophthalmos is more common with Graves' disease than with nodular goiter (Fig. 45-2).

Excess thyroid hormones stimulate the heart, causing tachycardia, increased systolic blood pressure, and sometimes atrial fibrillation. The heart rate may be as rapid as 160 beats/min. Even during sleep, the pulse may remain above 80 beats/min.

Complications

If untreated, hyperthyroidism may lead to thyrotoxicosis (thyroid storm/crisis). Thyrotoxicosis is excessive stimulation caused by elevated thyroid hormone levels that produce dangerous tachycardia and hyperthermia. There is a risk of heart failure. The patient is restless and agitated and may lapse into a coma. Thyrotoxicosis is a medical emergency. Fortunately, modern treatment of hyperthyroidism makes this complication rare.

Medical Diagnosis

Laboratory findings consistent with hyperthyroidism are decreased TSH and elevated serum T$_4$. TSH can be so low that it cannot be detected in the blood. Measurement of thyroid-stimulating antibodies and results of a radioactive iodine uptake test are useful in specifically diagnosing Graves' disease.

Medical Treatment

Three methods are used to treat hyperthyroidism: drug therapy, surgery, and radiation therapy. In addition,

FIGURE **45-2** This patient has exophthalmos, bulging eyes, associated with Graves' disease.

beta-adrenergic blockers like propranolol (Inderal) may be given to relieve some of the cardiovascular symptoms associated with hyperthyroidism.

Drug Therapy. Hyperthyroidism may be treated initially with antithyroid drugs. Antithyroid drugs block the synthesis, release, or activity of thyroid hormones. The drugs that may be used as antithyroid agents are thionamides and iodides. These drugs are effective in treating hyperthyroidism; however, they often are used temporarily to lower the level of hormones in the blood before surgery. This process reduces the risk of bleeding and lowers the danger of releasing large amounts of thyroid hormones into the bloodstream during surgery. When a patient is on drugs that interfere with T_4 secretion, monitor for symptoms of hypothyroidism (cold intolerance, edema, weight gain).

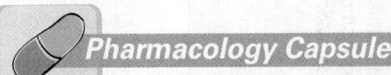

Pharmacology Capsule

Patients on antithyroid drugs must be monitored for hypothyroidism.

Thionamides. Examples of thionamides are propylthiouracil (PTU) and methimazole (Tapazole). It usually takes several weeks before the effects of thionamides are noticeable. The drugs may be given for months or years. The goal is to induce a remission that will allow the drugs to be discontinued. A disadvantage of thionamides is that they can cause agranulocytosis, a condition in which the production of neutrophils is suppressed. Without adequate neutrophils, the patient is unable to resist infection. Any signs of infection, such as sore throat or fever, should be reported to the physician immediately.

Iodides. Iodides are useful because iodine inhibits the synthesis of thyroid hormones. They are used most often after a course of propylthiouracil to suppress hormone secretion before thyroidectomy. The iodides also may be used to treat thyrotoxicosis. Potassium iodide (SSKI) can be given to people who have been exposed to radiation to prevent damage to the thyroid gland.

The iodides most often used to treat hyperthyroidism are Lugol's solution (5% iodine and 10% potassium iodide) and saturated solution of potassium iodide. Iodides may bring some relief within 24 hours, but it takes several weeks for maximum effect. The effect does not last as long as that of thionamides; therefore they are not generally used as the sole treatment for hyperthyroidism.

Iodine solutions can cause discoloration of the teeth and gastric upset. These effects are minimized if the iodine solution is diluted with milk, fruit juice, or some other beverage and sipped through a straw. Signs of iodine toxicity include swelling and irritation of the mucous membranes and increased salivation.

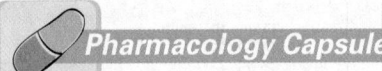

Pharmacology Capsule

Iodine solutions can stain the teeth! They should be mixed with a beverage and sipped through a straw.

Radioactive Iodine. Radioactive iodine (^{131}I) can be used alone or with antithyroid drugs to treat hyperthyroidism. It quickly accumulates in the thyroid gland, where it causes destruction of thyroid tissue. The resulting decrease in thyroid hormone production is not evident for several months. Meanwhile, beta-adrenergic blockers can be given to control cardiac symptoms.

The radiation dose used to treat hyperthyroidism does not pose a threat to others. It should not be used during pregnancy, however, because it affects the thyroid gland of the fetus. Side effects of the treatment are minimal. Inflammation of the thyroid gland (thyroiditis) and the parotid glands (parotiditis) may occur. Parotiditis causes the mouth to be dry and irritated. Hypothyroidism may develop years after treatment. Drugs used to treat thyroid disorders are summarized in the Drug Therapy table on p. 984.

Surgical Treatment

Graves' disease is often treated by removing most of the thyroid gland. This procedure is called a *subtotal thyroidectomy.* The procedure may be done endoscopically or through a larger incision across the top of the clavicles. As mentioned earlier, patients are commonly given antithyroid drug therapy for several weeks before surgery. Before these drugs were commonly used, patients often had dramatic postoperative responses because of the escape of thyroid hormones into the bloodstream during surgery. This severe episode of hyperthyroidism, called *thyroid storm* or *thyroid crisis,* is a medical emergency because it is potentially fatal.

NURSING CARE *of the Nonsurgical Patient with Hyperthyroidism*

Most patients with hyperthyroidism are treated as outpatients. Therefore the nurse in the community or clinic setting may need to help the patient learn to adapt until treatment brings relief.

Assessment

Complete assessment of the patient with a thyroid disorder is summarized in Box 45-1. Data collected by the LPN/LVN help provide a detailed picture of the patient's status. For the patient with hyperthyroidism, significant data would include activity tolerance, heat tolerance, bowel elimination pattern, appetite, weight changes, and food intake. Also consider the patient's mental-emotional state, adaptation to the condition, and understanding of the treatment. Measure vital signs and height and weight. Document skin texture and edema.

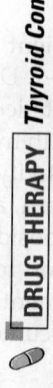

DRUG THERAPY | *Thyroid Conditions*

DRUG	USE/ACTION	SIDE EFFECTS	NURSING INTERVENTIONS
THYROID HORMONE REPLACEMENT DRUGS			
Desiccated thyroid (thyroid USP) Levothyroxine (Synthroid) Liothyronine (Cytomel) Liotrix (Euthroid)	Treat hypothyroidism and thyroiditis. Increase metabolic rate.	Overdose: irritability, insomnia, nervousness, tachycardia, diarrhea, weight loss.	Older patients more susceptible to toxicity. Low doses of one or more preparations given initially. Dosage gradually increased and patient maintained on one preparation. Hypothyroid patients usually require lifelong therapy. Patient teaching needed. Monitor pulse and blood pressure of older patients. Withhold and notify physician if pulse >100. Thyroid preparations interact with many other drugs by affecting metabolic rate.
ANTI-THYROID DRUGS			
Thionamides Methimazole (Tapazole) Propylthiouracil (PTU)	Treat hyperthyroidism by interfering with synthesis of thyroid hormones.	Agranulocytosis, rash, thrombocytopenia, skin discoloration, fever, headache, drowsiness, diarrhea, nausea, vomiting.	Avoid use during pregnancy. Monitor patient for bleeding due to decreased platelets and prothrombin, signs of liver toxicity (jaundice, abdominal pain), agranulocytosis (fever, sore throat, malaise), and hypothyroidism (weight gain, fatigue). Teach patient to report any of these signs and symptoms. Safety precautions if drowsy. Encourage patient to adhere to drug prescription and to keep follow-up appointments.
Iodides Strong iodine solution (Lugol's solution) Saturated solution of potassium iodide (SSKI)	Reduce size and vascularity of thyroid gland in hyperthyroidism. May be used with other drugs to treat hyperthyroidism or alone before surgery for hyperthyroidism.	Excess iodine: fever, rash, oral lesions, metallic taste, diarrhea, parotitis, hypothyroidism.	Dilute liquids in water, fruit juice, or milk. Reduce unpleasant taste and tooth staining by using a straw. Monitor for symptoms of excess iodine. Give SSKI after meals.
Radioactive iodine Sodium iodide ¹³¹I and ¹²³I	Concentrates in thyroid tissue for diagnostic scans. Higher therapeutic dose destroys thyroid tissue in hyperthyroidism and thyroid malignancies.	Diagnostic dose: none. Therapeutic dose: nausea, vomiting.	Diagnostic dose usually requires no radiation precautions except precautions with urine for 24 hours after the test (see Diagnositic Tests and Procedures table on p. 981. Therapeutic dose requires isolation measures. Monitor patient for signs of hypothyroidism (fatigue, weight gain).

Nursing Diagnoses, Goals, and Outcome Criteria: Hyperthyroidism

NURSING DIAGNOSES	GOALS AND OUTCOME CRITERIA
Decreased Cardiac Output related to excessive thyroid hormone stimulation	Normal cardiac output: pulse and blood pressure within patient norms; no signs/symptoms of heart failure: edema, dyspnea
Disturbed Sleep Pattern related to metabolic disturbance	Improved sleep pattern: absence of insomnia, patient describes feeling rested on awakening
Hyperthermia related to increased metabolic energy production	Improved heat tolerance: patient statement of comfort in relation to environmental temperature, no excess perspiration
Imbalanced Nutrition: Less Than Body Requirements related to increased metabolic requirements	Adequate nutrition: stable body weight if no significant recent loss, weight gain if underweight
Risk for Injury related to exophthalmos	Decreased risk of eye injury: lids cover eyeball, eyeball is moist, no pain associated with corneal injury
Disturbed Sensory Perception related to ophthalmopathy	Reduced visual disturbance, eye pain, photosensitivity, periorbital edema
Diarrhea related to excessive thyroid hormone stimulation	Normal bowel elimination: formed stools at regular intervals

Put on Your Thinking Cap!

Explain why people with hyperthyroidism do not tolerate heat well.

Interventions

When a patient is treated as an outpatient, teaching is related to preparing the patient for self-care. If the patient is hospitalized for hyperthyroidism or other conditions, the nurse provides more direct care.

Decreased Cardiac Output

Monitor the patient's pulse and blood pressure at intervals. Give beta-adrenergic blockers as ordered to counteract the stimulant effects of the elevated thyroid hormones. Signs of heart failure include tachycardia, tachypnea, dyspnea, confusion, and edema. Older adults require especially careful monitoring because they are more susceptible to cardiovascular stress with thyroid disease. Immediately report any signs of heart failure to the registered nurse or the physician. Medical treatment of heart failure usually includes oxygen, intravenous fluids, sedatives, and cardiac drugs.

Disturbed Sleep Pattern

Despite fatigue and weakness, the hyperthyroid patient often feels restless and has trouble sleeping. Encourage the patient to arrange the day to allow periods of rest. Caffeine should be avoided because of its stimulating effects. Encourage bedtime rituals, which may be helpful in preparing for sleep. For the hospitalized patient, provide a restful environment and a soothing back rub to promote relaxation. Give sedatives as ordered to promote sleep.

In addition to physical rest, patients need emotional rest. The patient and the family may be able to cope better if they understand the reason for the patient's irritability and nervousness. Patients need to recognize stressful situations and avoid them.

Hyperthermia

Hyperthyroid patients usually have some heat intolerance because of their high metabolic rate. They tend to feel too warm even when others are comfortable. Only light clothing may be needed. Adjust the environmental temperature as much as possible for comfort. A private room allows the patient more freedom to select the room temperature. If the patient perspires heavily, frequent bathing and clothing changes help promote comfort.

Imbalanced Nutrition: Less Than Body Requirements

Despite a normal dietary intake, the patient may not be meeting the increased caloric needs (see the Nutrition Concepts box below). Weigh daily to monitor nutritional adequacy. A diet high in calories, vitamins, and minerals is recommended. Depending on the severity of the condition, the patient may need additional full meals or between-meal snacks. Some patients require as many as 4000 to 5000 calories daily to maintain body weight. The physician may order supplementary vitamins. Additional fluids are recommended to replace fluids lost through increased insensible loss (fluid lost through the skin and the lungs).

Nutrition Concepts

1. Hypothyroid and hyperthyroid patients may require adjustments in calorie intake that are appropriate to metabolic needs.
2. Lack of iodine is associated with the development of a goiter (enlargement of the thyroid gland) in adults and cretinism in infants.
3. Iodized salt is the best way to obtain an adequate amount of iodine in the diet.
4. Another important source of iodine is saltwater seafood.
5. Parathormone, secreted by the parathyroid gland, and thyrocalcitonin, secreted by the thyroid gland, maintain serum calcium levels.

Risk for Injury

Exophthalmos is a condition in which deposits of fat and fluid behind the eyeballs make them bulge outward (see Fig. 45-2). Both eyes are usually affected. If the condition is severe, the eyelids do not cover the eyeballs. The eyeballs are not kept moist and are susceptible to injury. It may be necessary to tape the lids shut. Lubricated eye pads or artificial tears may be used. Raising the head of the bed at night and limiting salt intake may be helpful.

The patient with exophthalmos has a startled appearance. This may make the person self-conscious and embarrassed. Dark glasses help conceal the eyes. For these patients, Disturbed Body Image is an important additional nursing diagnosis. Reassure the patient that the condition usually goes away after treatment of hyperthyroidism.

Disturbed Sensory Perception

In addition to exophthalmos, the hyperthyroid patient has a variety of eye symptoms that may include double vision, periorbital edema, tearing, photosensitivity, and a feeling of "sand" in the eyes. It helps to elevate the head of the bed, reduce bright lighting, and advise use of tinted glasses. Methylcellulose eye drops and diuretics may be ordered to decrease inflammation and swelling. Severe inflammation is treated with a 2- to 4-week course of prednisone. After acute inflammation subsides, surgical procedures on the eyeball muscles and the eyelids may be needed to eliminate double vision and to restore coverage of the eye.

Diarrhea

If the patient has diarrhea, electrolyte imbalances and skin irritation may result. Give antidiarrheal medications as ordered, and monitor the effect. Thorough perianal cleansing after each stool reduces the risk of skin breakdown.

NURSING CARE *of the Patient Having a Thyroidectomy*

General care of the surgical patient is discussed in Chapter 17. This section covers the special needs of the thyroidectomy patient.

Assessment

Preoperative

The preparation of the patient undergoing thyroid surgery is essentially the same as for any major surgery. Ask what the patient knows about surgery and what to expect before and after the procedure. Nursing diagnoses may include those listed earlier for hyperthyroidism, but the condition is usually brought under control before surgery is scheduled. In addition, identify and address learning needs. Teaching is the primary preoperative nursing intervention. The goals of preoperative teaching are patient understanding of the usual preoperative and postoperative procedures and

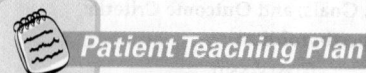

Patient Teaching Plan

Hyperthyroidism

- This is a chronic condition that requires long-term care.
- You must take your medications exactly as prescribed.
- Notify your physician of excessive fatigue and depression, which may indicate hypothyroidism caused by your antithyroid drug.

decreased anxiety. Tell the patient to expect a dressing on the front of the neck. The size of the incision will depend on the surgical approach used. Demonstrate how to avoid straining the neck incision by supporting the head when rising.

To evaluate the effectiveness of preoperative teaching, ask the patient to repeat the information presented. Ask patients to return demonstrations of activities such as deep breathing and supporting the head during position changes.

Postoperative

The patient usually recovers quickly from a thyroidectomy and may be discharged in 1 or 2 days. Rare but serious complications are airway obstruction, recurrent laryngeal nerve damage, hemorrhage, and tetany. One other complication, thyroid crisis, is usually prevented by preoperative treatment with antithyroid drugs.

If part of the thyroid gland is left (subtotal thyroidectomy), it should eventually regenerate and produce adequate hormones. The patient may be somewhat hypothyroid at first, but replacement therapy is not recommended. Giving thyroid hormone would interfere with the regeneration of thyroid tissue.

Immediately after thyroidectomy, it is especially important to *assess* and *document* respiratory status, level of consciousness, wound drainage or bleeding, voice quality, comfort, and neuromuscular irritability (a sign of hypocalcemia associated with damage to the parathyroids).

Nursing Diagnoses, Goals, and Outcome Criteria: Thyroidectomy

Nursing Diagnoses	Goals and Outcome Criteria
Ineffective Airway Clearance related to airway obstruction, laryngeal nerve damage, laryngeal spasm	Effective airway clearance: normal breath sounds, respiratory rate of 12 to 20, no dyspnea
Decreased Cardiac Output related to blood loss, heart failure secondary to thyroid crisis	Normal cardiac output: pulse and blood pressure within normal limits; no edema
Disturbed Body Image related to surgical scar	Adaptation to change in appearance: looks at scar, verbalizes acceptance of scar

Acute Pain related to tissue trauma	Pain relief: patient statement of less or no pain, relaxed manner
Risk for Infection related to impaired skin integrity	Absence of infection: wound margins intact, minimal redness, no purulent drainage, normal body temperature

Interventions

Ineffective Airway Clearance

Turning and deep breathing are recommended to prevent respiratory complications, as with any other surgical patient. The surgeon may not want the patient to cough, however, because of possible stress on the suture line.

It is especially important to monitor and document the rate and ease of respirations after thyroidectomy. Respiratory distress can result from compression of the trachea or from a spasm of the larynx due to nerve damage or hypocalcemia. Before the patient returns from surgery, suction equipment, a laryngoscope, an endotracheal tube, oxygen, and an emergency tracheotomy tray must be available. Your agency may require the tracheotomy tray at the bedside. Elevate the head of the bed to decrease edema. Use pillows to prop and support the head to avoid stress on the suture line.

Because of the location of the thyroidectomy incision, edema or bleeding can cause pressure on the trachea. Signs and symptoms of poor oxygenation due to airway obstruction or blood loss include restlessness, increasing pulse and respiratory rates, and dyspnea. Without prompt intervention, the patient with airway obstruction could die.

The laryngeal nerve innervates the vocal cords. If it is damaged during surgery, vocal cord paralysis can occur. Paralysis of both cords may cause spasms (laryngospasm) that close the airway. An emergency tracheotomy is needed to restore the airway. Signs of laryngeal nerve damage are hoarseness and inability to speak. This is more severe than the usual hoarseness most people have after general anesthesia. Ask the patient to respond verbally to simple questions to determine voice quality.

Before the function of the parathyroid glands was understood, patients having a thyroidectomy often experienced unexplained muscle contractions and respiratory difficulty that sometimes led to death. Eventually, it was determined that the symptoms were caused by hypocalcemia due to a deficiency of parathyroid hormone. Surgeons are now careful to locate and spare the small parathyroid glands. Occasionally, however, the parathyroid glands are injured or accidentally removed during thyroidectomy.

Without parathyroid hormone, the serum calcium level falls, thus causing tetany. Muscle contractions begin as twitches around the mouth and eyes. The face,

fingers, and toes begin to tingle. The patient may have painful "cramps," including the classic signs depicted in Figure 45-3. The most serious effect of hypocalcemia is spasm of the larynx. As the larynx closes, the patient has difficulty breathing and can suffocate. Cardiac dysrhythmias and seizures also can occur.

Tetany is treated with calcium salts given intravenously or orally. The condition usually improves as the injured parathyroid glands recover. Rarely is hypoparathyroidism permanent. If it is, lifetime treatment is required, as described on p. 998.

Decreased Cardiac Output

Frequently inspect the dressing to detect bleeding and take the vital signs. Because the dressing is on the front of the neck, blood might flow under the dressing to the

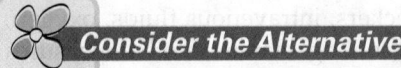
Consider the Alternative

Position changes and back rubs enhance the effects of prescribed analgesics.

A

B

FIGURE **45-3** Signs of hypocalcemia. **A,** Chvostek's sign (facial twitch). **B,** Trousseau's sign (carpopedal spasm).

back of the neck. Therefore be sure to check behind the patient's neck and upper back to detect this.

Thyroid crisis (thyroid storm) can develop when large amounts of thyroid hormone enter the bloodstream during surgery. Approximately 12 hours after surgery, the patient in thyroid crisis shows signs of severe hyperthyroidism (tachycardia, cardiac dysrhythmias, vomiting, fever, and confusion). It can also occur in patients with severe hyperthyroidism who develop a severe illness or infection.

If not treated promptly, the patient will die as a result of heart failure. Early detection of thyroid crisis requires careful monitoring of vital signs during the first postoperative day. The risk of thyroid crisis is reduced if serum hormone levels are reduced before surgery with medications.

Treatment of thyroid crisis consists of antithyroid drugs, intravenous sodium iodide, corticosteroids, beta-adrenergic blockers, intravenous fluids, oxygen, and a hypothermia (cooling) blanket or other measures to reduce body temperature.

Disturbed Body Image

The patient may be worried about the appearance of the surgical scar. Thyroidectomy incisions follow the natural contours of the neck. Once the scar fades, it usually is not noticeable. Meanwhile, it is easy to conceal the fresh scar with clothing. If an endoscopic procedure is used, the incisions will be very small.

Acute Pain

Frequently inquire about the postoperative patient's comfort level. Promptly administer prescribed analgesics, and evaluate and document effects.

Risk for Infection

Any time the skin is broken, the potential for infection exists. Practice good hand washing and use aseptic technique when handling dressings. Tell the patient to avoid touching the fresh incision and to report any signs and symptoms of infection (fever, increasing

Patient Teaching Plan

Thyroidectomy

- If all of your thyroid gland was removed, you will need lifelong replacement of thyroid hormones.
- If only part of your thyroid gland was removed, you may feel tired for a while but this should improve as the remaining gland increases hormone production.
- Thyroidectomy scars usually heal so that they are eventually barely noticeable.
- Take your drugs exactly as prescribed.
- Nervousness and palpitations may be adverse effects of thyroid replacement drugs (hyperthyroidism); notify the physician if they occur.

wound redness and swelling, and foul drainage). Protect the incision from strain and possible dehiscence by supporting the neck when arising and reclining.

HYPOTHYROIDISM

Hypothyroidism is the result of inadequate secretion of thyroid hormones. It is seen in infants, children, and adults. If not treated early, hypothyroidism during infancy causes permanent retardation of physical and mental development (cretinism) (Fig. 45-4). The effects in adults can be quite serious but usually are reversible with treatment. The term myxedema sometimes is used for hypothyroidism. Myxedema actually refers to facial edema that develops with severe, long-term hypothyroidism (Fig. 45-5). Not all hypothyroid patients have myxedema.

Etiology and Risk Factors

Hypothyroidism has many causes—including atrophy of the thyroid gland after years of Graves' disease or thyroiditis, treatment for hyperthyroidism, dietary iodine deficiency, high intake of goitrogens, and defects in thyroid hormone synthesis. These are examples of *primary* hypothyroidism. They account for 90% to 95% of all cases of hypothyroidism. Some foods and drugs act as goitrogens, meaning that they suppress

What Does Culture Have to Do with Hypothyroidism?

The incidence of hypothyroidism is 10 to 20 times higher in iodine-deficient parts of the world (e.g., Zaire, Nepal) than in the United States.

FIGURE **45-4** Cretinism is a condition of permanent physical and mental retardation resulting from untreated hypothyroidism in infancy.

thyroid hormone production. Examples of foods that are goitrogens if taken in large quantities are soybeans, turnips, and rutabagas. Goitrogenic drugs that often are used to treat hyperthyroidism are propylthiouracil, methimazole, and iodine.

Hypothyroidism caused by pituitary or hypothalamic disorders is called *secondary hypothyroidism.* Deficiency of TSH lowers the secretion of thyroid hormones even though the thyroid gland itself remains normal. Of course, patients who have had their entire thyroid or pituitary gland surgically removed also will be hypothyroid. Hypothyroidism also can result from tissue resistance to thyroid hormone—that is, the hormone is present, but the body cells are unable to use it normally.

Signs and Symptoms

The signs and symptoms of hypothyroidism in general are the opposite of those of hyperthyroidism (Table 45-1). The onset is usually gradual. The metabolic rate slows, often causing weight gain even with decreased food intake. Hypothyroid patients commonly report lethargy, forgetfulness, and irritability. They may experience frequent headaches, constipation, menstrual disorders, numbness and tingling in the arms and legs, and intolerance to cold. The pulse tends to be slow, and dyspnea may be present.

Examination may reveal swelling of the lips and eyelids; dry, thick skin; bruising; thin, coarse hair; and hoarseness. Generalized nonpitting edema and facial edema may be present. The patient may seem slow, depressed, or apathetic. Pallor may be present, associated with anemia. Signs and symptoms may be more subtle in the older patient or may be masked by signs and symptoms of other acute or chronic disorders.

FIGURE **45-5** Typical appearance of the patient with myxedema.

Therefore thyroid function in older adults should be assessed as part of routine checkups.

Medical Diagnosis

Hypothyroidism is diagnosed based on the laboratory determination of free T_4 and TSH. A TRH stimulation test also may be ordered. Free T_4 is low with hypothyroidism except when the problem is tissue resistance to the hormone. TSH level enables the physician to determine whether the basic problem is primary or secondary hypothyroidism.

Complications

Severe, untreated hypothyroidism can progress to myxedema coma. Infection, trauma, excessive chilling, and some drugs (opioids, sedatives, tranquilizers) may precipitate myxedema coma in a hypothyroid patient. The main signs of this life-threatening condition are hypothermia, hypotension, and hypoventilation.

Medical Treatment

Hypothyroidism is treated with hormone replacement therapy, most commonly levothyroxine (Synthroid) or liothyronine (Cytomel). Hypothyroid patients usually require lifelong replacement therapy. They should be monitored periodically to evaluate the response to therapy. A patient with heart disease may have difficulty adapting to a sudden increase in metabolic rate. For that reason, replacement therapy for older patients or those with heart disease is usually started with a low dose and gradually increased. If these patients have any chest pain once therapy is started, the physician should be notified immediately.

Pharmacology Capsule

Opioids, sedatives, and tranquilizers can precipitate potentially fatal myxedema coma in a severely hypothyroid person.

NURSING CARE *of the Patient with Hypothyroidism*

Hypothyroidism usually does not require hospitalization, but it may be detected when patients are hospitalized for other reasons. Because the onset of symptoms is often subtle, the nurse in the community or long-term care setting must be alert for signs and symptoms of hypothyroidism (see Nursing Care Plan: The Patient with Hypothyroidism on p. 992).

Assessment

Box 45-1 summarizes the general assessment of the patient with a thyroid disorder. Relevant data include measurement of vital signs, height, and weight. In addition, ask about activity and temperature tolerance, voice quality, bowel elimination pattern, and changes in weight and dietary intake. Inspect and palpate the

Table 45-1 *Comparison of Signs and Symptoms of Hypothyroidism and Hyperthyroidism*

SYSTEM	HYPOTHYROIDISM	HYPERTHYROIDISM
Integumentary	Coarse, dry skin and hair Thick nails	Smooth, moist skin Silky hair Diaphoresis
Musculoskeletal	Muscle aches and pains Weakness Slow movements	Weakness
Cardiovascular	Bradycardia Dysrhythmias Hypotension Anemia Capillary fragility	Tachycardia Dysrhythmias Palpitations Systolic hypertension Angina
Respiratory	Hypoventilation Dyspnea	Increased respiratory rate Dyspnea
Gastrointestinal	Anorexia Nausea and vomiting Constipation Weight gain	Increased appetite Increased bowel sounds Diarrhea Weight loss
Neurologic	Apathy Lethargy Slowed mental function Depression Slow speech Paresthesias Decreased tendon reflexes	Nervousness and irritability Insomnia Personality change Agitation Inability to concentrate Fine tremor of fingers and tongue Hyperreflexia

Reproductive	Women
	  Amenorrhea or prolonged menses
	  Infertility
	  Decreased libido
	Men
	  Decreased libido
	  Erectile dysfunction
		Women
		  Menstrual irregularities
		  Decreased libido
		Men
		  Decreased libido
		  Erectile dysfunction
		  Gynecomastia

Other	Cold intolerance Decreased body temperature Facial puffiness or coarseness Thick tongue Nonpitting edema of hands and feet Sensitivity to central nervous system depressants	Increased body temperature Exophthalmos Goiter Sensitivity to central nervous system stimulants

skin for turgor, texture, and moisture. Note level of consciousness and emotional state. Ask if the patient has noticed a change in mental alertness. Also explore the patient's understanding of hypothyroidism and its treatment.

Nursing Diagnoses, Goals, and Outcome Criteria: Hypothyroidism

NURSING DIAGNOSES	GOALS AND OUTCOME CRITERIA
Activity Intolerance related to decreased metabolic energy production	Improved activity tolerance: patient report of less fatigue with daily activities
Imbalanced Nutrition: More Than Body Requirements related to intake greater than metabolic needs	Balanced nutrition: stable body weight or gradual return to weight before thyroid disorder
Hypothermia related to cold intolerance	Improved cold tolerance: warm hands and feet, no complaints of coldness
Constipation related to decreased peristalsis	Normal bowel function: regular stools without difficulty
Risk for Impaired Skin Integrity related to dryness and edema	Decreased risk of skin breakdown: skin moist, intact
Decreased Cardiac Output related to cardiovascular changes secondary to hypothyroidism	Normal cardiac output: improved stamina, pulse and blood pressure within normal limits; no dyspnea, edema, dysrhythmias
Disturbed Thought Processes related to decreased cerebral oxygenation	Improved thought processes: oriented to person, place, time; patient reports improved mental function

| Disturbed Body Image related to altered physical appearance, disturbed thought processes, lack of energy | Improved body image: patient makes positive statements about appearance, tends to personal appearance |
| Self-Care Deficit related to fatigue | Improved self-care: patient gradually resumes responsibility for personal care, completes care with less fatigue |

Interventions

Activity Intolerance

The hypothyroid patient lacks energy and tires easily. Arrange the schedule to allow for rest periods. Sedatives and barbiturates should be avoided because they may cause excessive sedation. If they are given, lower dosages are recommended. Monitor and document the patient's respirations and level of consciousness. Families and employers need to understand the patient's fatigue and make adjustments until the patient recovers. Improvement is gradual but is usually evident after 2 to 3 weeks.

Imbalanced Nutrition: More Than Body Requirements

Despite having a poor appetite, the patient may have gained weight. Weekly weights are helpful in evaluating the effects of hormone replacement therapy. Calorie reduction may be prescribed for the patient who is overweight. Encourage a balanced diet.

Hypothermia

Cold intolerance is a very uncomfortable effect of hypothyroidism. Provide extra clothing and blankets as needed. Maintain the room temperature at a level comfortable to the patient. This is easier to manage if the patient has a private room. Once thyroid replacement is initiated, the cold intolerance gradually improves.

Constipation

Constipation is a common problem. Until the hypothyroidism is corrected, take measures to promote normal elimination. Adequate fluids, dietary fiber, and physical activity all help reduce constipation. Bulk laxatives or stool softeners may be indicated if other measures do not solve the problem. Remember that adequate fluids are essential to prevent bowel obstruction with bulk laxatives. Older patients should increase activity levels gradually to avoid excessive stress on the heart.

Risk for Impaired Skin Integrity

Dry skin, which is common with hypothyroidism, is prone to breakdown. Liberally apply lotions and creams to help maintain moisture and control itching.

Reduce the frequency of bathing to prevent additional drying of the skin.

Decreased Cardiac Output

Atherosclerosis and heart disease develop in patients whose hypothyroidism is uncorrected for a long time. Monitor these patients for any signs and symptoms of heart failure, such as dyspnea and increasing edema. After hormone replacement therapy is begun, there is some risk of excessive cardiac stimulation. Tell the patient that any chest pain should be reported promptly. Monitor the pulse to detect potentially serious changes in rhythm or rate. Remember that the older adult's circulatory system adapts more slowly to increased thyroid hormone.

Disturbed Thought Processes

Mental dullness and depression can significantly affect the patient's life. Explain that these symptoms are related to hypothyroidism and that correction of hypothyroidism usually results in marked improvement. (An exception is the person who has cretinism caused by untreated hypothyroidism during fetal development or early infancy. The mental retardation of cretinism is not reversible.) Until mental function improves, be careful not to demand too much of the patient. Break teaching into small units, and reinforce at intervals.

 What Does Culture Have to Do with Cretinism?

Neonatal hypothyroidism, which causes cretinism if not corrected early, is much more common among whites than blacks.

Disturbed Body Image

The puffy, apathetic look and weight gain associated with hypothyroidism can be very distressing to the patient. Be accepting of the patient's concerns but encourage good grooming and attention to appearance. Tell the patient that treatment will gradually eliminate these changes.

Self-Care Deficit

The hypothyroid patient can expect to need lifelong hormone replacement therapy. Explain this to the patient, and stress the need for periodic medical evaluation. Describe the name, dosage, and adverse effects of the prescribed drug therapy. Teach the patient the

 Put on Your Thinking Cap!

A patient who was recently diagnosed with hypothyroidism complains that she has no appetite but has gained 20 pounds over the past few months. How would you explain this to her?

NURSING CARE PLAN
The Patient with Hypothyroidism

ASSESSMENT

Health History: A 53-year-old woman comes to the physician's office complaining of fatigue and irritability. Her symptoms have gradually worsened and are now interfering with her work as an executive assistant. She reports that her health has generally been good, with only one hospitalization for an appendectomy 7 years ago. The review of systems reveals frequent headaches, anorexia, constipation, menstrual irregularity, numbness and tingling in the legs, and intolerance to cold. She has noticed a 10-lb weight gain over the past 6 months without a change in diet or exercise.

Physical Examination: Vital signs: temperature, 97° F orally; pulse, 56; respiration, 18; blood pressure, 90/60. (Her record indicates that her previous blood pressure was 128/76 and that pulse was 74.) Height, 5'5". Weight, 155 lb. She is oriented but lethargic. Her hair is coarse, and her skin is dry.

Nursing Diagnosis	Goals and Outcome Criteria	Interventions
Activity Intolerance related to decreased metabolic energy production	The patient will report less fatigue with activities of daily living.	Advise patient to schedule additional rest periods until condition improves. Assure her that these symptoms are temporary.
Imbalanced Nutrition: More Than Body Requirements related to intake greater than metabolic needs	The patient's weight will stabilize within 2 lb of her usual 145 lb.	Weigh during each office visit. Encourage balanced diet. Tell her that weight should normalize when condition is corrected.
Hypothermia related to cold intolerance	The patient will report adequate warmth and increased tolerance of cool temperatures.	Adjust room temperature for patient comfort. Provide adequate covering during physical examination.
Constipation related to decreased peristalsis	The patient will have regular bowel movements passed without straining.	Encourage increased fluid intake, high-fiber diet with fresh fruits and raw vegetables. Instruct in taking stool softeners if advised by physician. Encourage gradual increase in physical activity as tolerance improves.
Risk for Impaired Skin Integrity related to dryness	The patient's skin will remain intact, and usual moisture will be restored.	Advise to decrease bathing frequency and to use moisturizing creams or lotions. Advise to avoid scratching.
Decreased Cardiac Output related to cardiovascular changes secondary to hypothyroidism	The patient's cardiac output will improve, as evidenced by improved stamina, regular pulse between 60 and 100, blood pressure consistent with patient norms, no dyspnea.	Monitor for tachycardia, hypertension, and dysrhythmias after hormone replacement therapy is begun.
Disturbed Thought Processes related to decreased cerebral oxygenation	The patient will report improved mental functioning and will appear less lethargic; is oriented to person, place, and time.	Explain that mental slowness is related to hypothyroidism and that it will improve with treatment. Do not overload patient with information. Teach only critical information initially and supplement with written information. Ask her how her work expectations could be adjusted to accommodate her symptoms temporarily.
Self-Care Deficits related to fatigue	The patient's activities of daily living will be accomplished with only normal fatigue.	Ask patient to consider her daily activities and set priorities. Encourage rest periods. Delay difficult or strenuous tasks until condition improves.

? **CRITICAL THINKING** QUESTIONS

■ What is the most critical information you should teach the patient about hypothyroidism?

■ How can you help the patient set priorities and determine daily activities?

symptoms of hyperthyroidism that might occur with excessive hormone replacement (tachycardia, weight loss, nervousness). Document patient teaching.

GOITER

Goiter is the term used to describe enlargement of the thyroid gland. Enlargement may be due to simple goiter, thyroid nodules, or thyroiditis.

Simple Goiter

Thyroid enlargement with normal thyroid hormone production is called *simple goiter* (Fig. 45-6). Causes include iodine deficiency and long-term exposure to goitrogens. The gland may enlarge to compensate for hypothyroidism. Sometimes the enlarged gland produces excess hormones, making the patient hyperthyroid.

The type of treatment depends on the degree of enlargement and level of thyroid hormone production. If enlargement is mild and hormones are normal, no intervention is required. Some patients need hormone replacement therapy. Surgery is indicated if there is pressure on the trachea or esophagus or if the condition is disfiguring.

Nodules

Multinodular goiter is discussed on p. 982 in the Hyperthyroidism section. As noted, nodules can be benign or malignant. To help determine whether cancer is present, the physician may order a scan that uses radioactive iodine. Nodular goiters are usually surgically removed. In benign conditions, only the nodule may be removed.

THYROID CANCER

Thyroid cancer is not common. It is fatal in less than 1% of all cases. In the early stages, the only sign may be a nodule that can be felt on the thyroid gland. Later, if the cancer spreads, enlarged lymph nodes are felt in the neck. The patient may not show dramatic changes in thyroid hormone levels. Total thyroidectomy is the usual treatment. Nursing care of the thyroidectomy patient is covered on p. 986 in the Hyperthyroidism section. If the malignancy has spread beyond the thyroid gland, more radical surgery may be indicated.

Surgery may be followed with radioactive iodine treatment to destroy any remaining tissue that might harbor malignant cells. This is the same type of iodine used in diagnostic studies, but a larger dose is used. The patient needs to be isolated and on radiation precautions. Body fluids must be handled according to radiation precaution guidelines because they are contaminated. The care of the patient receiving internal radiation therapy is discussed in Chapter 25.

The patient will be alarmed at the diagnosis of cancer. He or she may find some comfort in know-

FIGURE **45-6** Goiter.

ing that the 5-year survival rate for thyroid cancer is among the highest of all types of cancer. Long-term care after thyroid cancer includes management of hypothyroidism and monitoring for recurrence. Scans using radioactive iodine are sometimes ordered at intervals to detect the presence of any remaining cancerous tissue. Periodic TSH and thyroglobulin tests may be ordered. Thyroid replacement therapy is based on the TSH level. Thyroglobulin rises if thyroid cancer recurs.

THE PARATHYROID GLANDS

ANATOMY AND PHYSIOLOGY OF THE PARATHYROID GLANDS

The parathyroid glands are small glands usually located on the back of the thyroid gland (Fig. 45-7). Occasionally, some glands are found in the mediastinum as well. Most people have four parathyroids, but some people have more. Even though they are typically embedded in the thyroid, the parathyroids function independently. They secrete only one hormone, but it is a vital one. Parathyroid hormone, or parathormone (PTH), plays a critical role in regulating the serum calcium level.

Calcium is an essential component of strong bones and plays a vital role in the functions of nerve and muscle cells. When the serum calcium level falls, PTH is secreted. PTH increases the absorption of calcium from the intestines, transfers calcium from the bones to the blood, and signals the kidneys to conserve calcium. In general, calcium retention by the kidney is balanced by phosphate loss.

NURSING ASSESSMENT OF THE PARATHYROID GLANDS

HEALTH HISTORY

Although the registered nurse is responsible for the complete assessment, the LPN/LVN may assist with data collection. Relevant data from the health history include change in mental-emotional status, such as memory problems, irritability, or personality changes. Ask about a history of musculoskeletal problems, including weakness, skeletal pain, backache, and muscle twitching or spasms. Note if the patient has experienced urinary frequency, polyuria, urinary calculi (stones), or constipation. Document a past medical history of head or neck radiation, renal calculi, or chronic renal failure. List medications, including calcium and vitamin D supplements.

PHYSICAL EXAMINATION

Important data in the physical examination include heart rate and rhythm, blood pressure, respiratory effort, muscle strength, muscle twitching, and hair and skin texture. Simple tests are used to elicit Chvostek's sign and Trousseau's sign, which are both indicative of hypocalcemia. Chvostek's sign is a spasm of the facial muscle when the face is tapped over the facial nerve. Trousseau's sign is a carpopedal spasm that occurs when a blood pressure cuff is inflated above the patient's systolic blood pressure and left in place for 2 to 3 minutes (see Fig. 45-3).

Nursing assessment of the patient with a parathyroid disorder is outlined in Box 45-2.

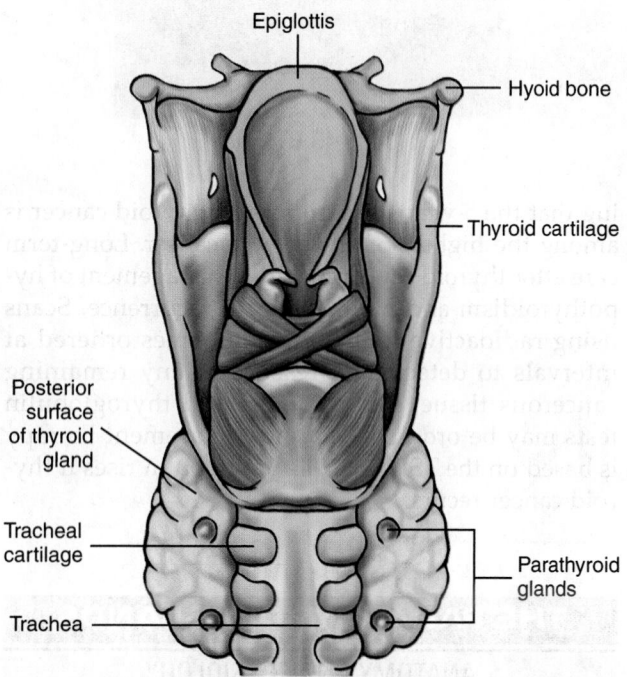

FIGURE **45-7** Posterior view of the neck and thyroid gland, showing the approximate location of the parathyroid glands.

Labels in figure: Epiglottis; Hyoid bone; Thyroid cartilage; Posterior surface of thyroid gland; Tracheal cartilage; Trachea; Parathyroid glands

DIAGNOSTIC TESTS AND PROCEDURES

The diagnosis of parathyroid disorders is based on blood and urine studies and skeletal radiographs. Blood tests include measurements of calcium, phosphate, creatinine, uric acid, magnesium, alkaline phosphatase, and PTH. The presence of parathyroid antibodies also may be identified through blood studies. A 24-hour urine specimen may be collected to determine how much calcium is being excreted in the urine.

If excessive calcium has been drawn from bones, demineralization will be apparent on radiographs. Bone cysts and tumors may be found. A dental examination may be done to detect changes in the teeth consistent with parathyroid dysfunction. An electrocardiogram also may be ordered because calcium imbalances can cause alterations in the electrical activity in the heart.

Box 45-2 **ASSESSMENT of the Patient with a Parathyroid Disorder**

Health History

Present Illness:
Changes in mental-emotional status, neuromuscular symptoms

Past Medical History:
Head or neck radiation, renal calculi, chronic renal failure, recent and current medications, including calcium and vitamin D supplements

Review of Systems:
Fatigue, irritability, muscle tremors or spasms, bone pain, urinary frequency, polyuria, constipation or diarrhea, depression, personality changes

PHYSICAL EXAMINATION

Vital Signs:
Dysrhythmias, hypertension or hypotension

Skin and Hair:
Changes in moisture and texture

Urologic:
Flank pain

Musculoskeletal:
Weakness, tremors

Neurologic:
Abnormally active or depressed reflexes, irritability, headache, confusion, positive Chvostek's sign, positive Trousseau's sign

DISORDERS OF THE PARATHYROID GLANDS

HYPERPARATHYROIDISM

The secretion of excess PTH is called *hyperparathyroidism*. It is caused most often by a tumor called an *adenoma*. The tumors can be benign or malignant. Other factors that may stimulate excess PTH secretion are vitamin D deficiencies, malabsorption, chronic renal failure, and elevated serum phosphate. People who receive a kidney transplant after having been on dialysis for a long time also may have hyperparathyroidism.

The most notable effect of hyperparathyroidism is elevation of serum calcium (hypercalcemia). High levels of PTH cause calcium to shift from the bones into the bloodstream. Excess PTH also promotes retention of calcium and loss of phosphate by the kidneys. If hyperparathyroidism is untreated, severe demineralization of bone tissue occurs. Bones can become brittle, thus resulting in serious fractures. The high level of calcium in the urine can lead to the formation of urinary calculi. Obstruction of the urinary tubules by calculi can lead quickly to severe kidney damage. The effects of hyperparathyroidism on the heart can cause dysrhythmias and hypertension.

Signs and Symptoms

Because hyperparathyroidism usually develops gradually, symptoms are vague at first. The patient may report weakness, lethargy, depression, anorexia, and constipation. Other findings might include mental and personality changes, cardiac dysrhythmias, weight loss, and urinary calculi. Additional signs and symptoms of hyperparathyroidism are outlined in Table 45-2.

Medical Diagnosis

The diagnosis of hyperparathyroidism is based primarily on blood and urine studies. Typical findings include elevated serum calcium and decreased serum phosphate, elevated PTH, and elevated 24-hour urine calcium. Skeletal radiographs and bone density studies reveal bone demineralization if the condition is severe. Sometimes the condition is not recognized until the patient has a spontaneous fracture. Other procedures that may be employed include CT, MRI, ultrasound, fine-needle aspiration, and selective arteriography.

Medical Treatment

Surgical Intervention. If a tumor is causing hyperparathyroidism, it usually is removed surgically. In some cases, more than one gland is removed. The surgeon attempts to leave some parathyroid tissue to prevent hypoparathyroidism. It often is possible for the procedure to be done with an endoscope. However, parathyroidectomy can be a complicated procedure because some parathyroid glands may be located in the mediastinum. Sometimes the patient's normal parathyroid tissue is transplanted to a muscle in the forearm or the neck where it will continue to secrete PTH.

Drug Therapy. If the condition is mild or the patient is not a good candidate for surgery, medical treatment is aimed at lowering the serum calcium level. The patient is instructed to maintain a high fluid intake to dilute the urine. Calcium intake may be restricted. Sodium and phosphorus replacements may

Table 45-2	*Comparison of Signs and Symptoms of Hypoparathyroidism and Hyperparathyroidism*	
SYSTEM	**HYPOPARATHYROIDISM**	**HYPERPARATHYROIDISM**
Musculoskeletal	Fatigue Weakness Cramps Twitching	Poor muscle tone Weakness Bone pain Demineralization Fractures
Urinary	Frequency	Polyuria Renal calculi
Cardiovascular	Decreased cardiac output Dysrhythmias	Hypertension Dysrhythmias
Neurologic	Hyperactive reflexes Memory impairment Depression Anxiety Irritability Personality changes Confusion Numbness and tingling of hands and feet and around mouth Muscle spasms	Depressed reflexes Decreased mental function Depression Mood swings Confusion Coma Poor coordination
Gastrointestinal	Abdominal cramps	Anorexia Nausea and vomiting Constipation
Integumentary	Brittle nails, dry skin	Moist skin

be ordered. When it is necessary to lower the calcium level quickly, an infusion of normal saline is often prescribed. Several drugs can be used to treat hypercalcemia. Calcitonin (Calcimar), gallium nitrate (Ganite), bisphosphonates (etidronate, pamidronate), and plicamycin (Mithracin) inhibit the release of calcium from bones. Oral phosphates inhibit the absorption of calcium from the digestive tract. Furosemide (Lasix) may be given to promote the excretion of calcium in the urine. Propranolol reduces PTH secretion. Because plicamycin has severe toxic effects, it is usually reserved for patients with metastatic parathyroid cancer. If hypercalcemia is caused by vitamin D intoxication, glucocorticoids are highly effective. Drugs used to treat parathyroid disorders are described in the Drug Therapy table on p. 997.

Pharmacology Capsule

Furosemide (Lasix) is a diuretic that promotes the excretion of calcium in the urine.

NURSING CARE of the Patient with Hyperparathyroidism

Assessment

When caring for the hyperparathyroid patient, monitor vital signs, urine output, weight, muscle strength, bowel elimination, and digestive disturbances.

Nursing Diagnoses, Goals, and Outcome Criteria: Hyperparathyroidism

NURSING DIAGNOSES	GOALS AND OUTCOME CRITERIA
Activity Intolerance related to weakness and fatigue	Improved activity tolerance: patient reports performing daily activities with less fatigue
Risk for Injury related to weakness and decreased bone mass	Reduced risk for injury: improved muscle strength, no falls
Impaired Urinary Elimination related to urinary calculi	Normal urinary output: urine output equal to fluid intake
Constipation related to altered intestinal motility	Normal bowel elimination: regular stools without straining
Disturbed Thought Process related to hypercalcemia	Improved mental-emotional state: less irritability, depression
Imbalanced Nutrition: Less Than Body Requirements related to nausea and vomiting	Adequate nutrition: stable body weight, no nausea or vomiting

Interventions

Activity Intolerance and Risk for Injury

Determine the patient's ability to perform self-care safely, and provide help as needed. Move and handle the patient gently. Evaluate the environment for any safety hazards, and take corrective measures. Plan care to allow for periods of rest. If the patient is being treated at home, stress the need to plan for rest periods. Assure the patient that weakness and fatigue are caused by the parathyroid disorder and will improve as the condition is corrected.

Impaired Urinary Elimination

Maintain accurate intake and output records because hypercalcemia can cause urinary calculi and serious kidney damage. Decreasing urine output; sharp pain in the flank (kidney area), lower abdomen, or genitalia; and hematuria are consistent with urinary calculi and should be reported to the physician. A high fluid intake, sometimes as much as 4000 mL/day, may be ordered. Closely monitor urine output and vital signs when large volumes of fluid are administered. Older adults and people with heart disease are at risk for excess fluid volume and congestive heart failure. Patients with cardiac or renal disease may be unable to tolerate this much fluid. Urine may be strained and examined for crystals or calculi. A low-calcium diet and urine acidifiers may be ordered to decrease the risk of calculi formation.

Constipation

Chart bowel movements, including frequency and characteristics of stools. Constipation can often be managed with adequate fluids and fiber in the diet. If these measures are not effective, the physician may order bulk laxatives or stool softeners. It is especially important to monitor bowel elimination in the older patient. Illness, inactivity, and multiple medications combine to increase their risk of constipation and even fecal impaction.

Disturbed Thought Processes

Recognize that irritability, personality changes, and depression are common with hyperparathyroidism. Patients and their families appreciate knowing that these symptoms improve with treatment.

Imbalanced Nutrition: Less Than Body Requirements

Take measures to control nausea and vomiting if present. Monitor weight to detect inadequate nutrition if the patient's intake is poor. Small feedings may be better tolerated. Provide a pleasant mealtime environment.

Postoperative Care

After parathyroidectomy, the patient requires care like that of any surgical patient, as detailed in Chapter 17. Two potential complications specific to parathyroidectomy are airway obstruction and hypocalcemia. When the patient has a neck incision, accumulated fluid and blood in the surgical site can compress the trachea, thus causing airway obstruction. Monitor and document the respiratory rate and effort and the pulse rate. Increasing pulse and respiratory rates, especially accompanied

DRUG THERAPY | *Parathyroid Conditions*

DRUG	USE/ACTION	SIDE EFFECTS	NURSING INTERVENTIONS
CALCIUM SALTS Calcium chloride Calcium gluconate Calcium carbonate	Correct calcium deficiency due to hypoparathyroidism.	Overdosage (hypercalcemia): weakness, hypertension, dysrhythmias, polyuria, bone pain.	Take with food. Serum calcium levels should be monitored. Notify physician of signs of hypercalcemia.
VITAMIN D Calcitriol Dihydrotachysterol Ergocalciferol	Promotes calcium absorption from digestive tract.	Overdosage (hypercalcemia): weakness, hypertension, dysrhythmias, polyuria, bone pain.	Serum calcium levels should be monitored. Notify physician of signs of hypercalcemia.
BISPHOSPHONATES Pamidronate (Aredia)	Inhibits bone resorption, reduces serum calcium. More effective than etidronate.	Local pain, inflammation at infusion site. Potassium, magnesium, and phosphate deficiencies. GI distress. Fluid overload, hypertension.	Assess infusion site. Do not mix with IV solutions that contain calcium. Monitor pulse, blood pressure, fluid intake, and urine output.
Etidronate disodium (Didronel)	Reduces serum level in calcium hyperparathyroidism.	Diarrhea, nausea, metallic taste, bone pain, and tenderness. Hypocalcemia: weakness, muscle spasms.	Dividing dose through the day may control diarrhea. Advise that metallic taste is temporary.
OTHER Furosemide (Lasix)	Promotes excretion of excess calcium in hypoparathyroidism.	Fluid and electrolyte imbalances: metabolic alkalosis, hypovolemia, dehydration, hyponatremia, hypokalemia. Dizziness, headache, tinnitus, hyperglycemia.	Monitor intake and output, serum calcium and potassium levels, pulse, blood pressure, blood glucose.
Parathormone	Short-term treatment of hypoparathyroidism.	Overdosage (hypercalcemia): dysrhythmias, hypertension, weakness, polyuria, bone pain.	Available only for parenteral use.
Calcitonin (Calcimar, Cibacalcin)	Treats hypercalcemia caused by hyperparathyroidism.	Nausea, vomiting, injection site reactions, facial flushing, anaphylaxis.	Monitor for tachycardia due to hypocalcemia. Have epinephrine, antihistamines, and oxygen available. Sensitivity test should be done before giving. Tell patient that flushing is temporary. Teach self-medication. Encourage adequate fluid intake.
Plicamycin (Mithracin)	Treats hypercalcemia by inhibiting release of calcium from bones.	Hypocalcemia: weakness, muscle spasms. Hypokalemia, thrombocytopenia, leukopenia, bleeding, drowsiness, depression, anorexia, nausea, vomiting.	Reserved for patients with metastatic parathyroid cancer because of severity of toxic effects. Monitor for bleeding. Avoid injections. Apply pressure to venipuncture sites for 10 minutes. Assess for signs of infection. Discontinue infusion if extravasation occurs.
Gallium nitrate (Ganite)	Reduces serum calcium level in hypercalcemia.	Hypotension, nausea, and vomiting, decreased serum calcium and bicarbonate, increased blood urea nitrogen and creatinine.	Administer intravenously with normal saline. Monitor serum electrolytes, blood pressure, complete blood count, and urine output.

GI, Gastrointestinal; *IV,* intravenous.

by restlessness, suggest inadequate oxygenation. Notify the physician of any indications of respiratory distress. Keep an emergency tracheotomy tray at the bedside in the event of acute obstruction.

A second possible cause of airway obstruction is related to severe hypocalcemia. Be alert for tetany, a symptom of hypocalcemia, caused by the postoperative decrease in parathyroid hormones. A tingling sensation around the mouth and in the fingers is an early symptom of tetany. It may progress to severe muscle spasms or cramps and even to laryngospasm. To prevent this happening, calcium and other electrolytes are monitored closely in the postoperative period. Promptly inform the registered nurse or the physician of signs of tetany or abnormal electrolyte values. Tetany is treated with oral or intravenous calcium supplements. Treatment of hypocalcemia is discussed in detail in the Hypoparathyroidism section below.

The classic incision is on the front of the neck or upper chest, or both, and usually is covered with a bulky pressure dressing. As with the thyroidectomy patient, this patient's suture line should be protected from stress. Show the patient how to support the head when changing positions. The incisions created by an endoscopic surgical procedure are much smaller. Inspect the dressing and the back of the patient's neck for bleeding. Elevate the patient's head to help reduce swelling.

HYPOPARATHYROIDISM

Hypoparathyroidism is a deficiency of PTH. It is an uncommon condition, usually caused by accidental removal of or damage to parathyroid glands during surgery. Primary hypoparathyroidism can be caused by an autoimmune process and by several conditions, including Wilson's disease (copper overload). Inadequate secretion of PTH leads to hypocalcemia. Severe hypocalcemia can progress to convulsions and respiratory obstruction due to spasms of the larynx. Laryngospasm can be fatal.

Signs and Symptoms

The possibility of parathyroid dysfunction requires close monitoring after thyroid surgery. Trauma or accidental removal of one or more parathyroid glands may lead to symptoms of hypoparathyroidism, as discussed on p. 986 in the Nursing Care of the Patient Having a Thyroidectomy section.

Signs and symptoms of hypocalcemia are painful muscle cramps, fatigue and weakness, tingling and twitching of the face and hands, mental and emotional changes, dry skin, and urinary frequency. With severe hypocalcemia, the patient may have difficulty breathing, convulsions, and cardiac dysrhythmias.

Medical Diagnosis

The diagnosis of hypoparathyroidism is based on patient signs and symptoms and blood studies. Typical findings include low serum calcium, elevated serum phosphate, low urine calcium, and sometimes low serum magnesium. Two classic signs of hypocalcemia that support a diagnosis of hypoparathyroidism are Chvostek's sign and Trousseau's sign.

Medical Treatment

Acute hypoparathyroidism is sometimes treated with parenteral PTH, which is not practical for chronic management. Severe hypocalcemia is treated with intravenous calcium salts. Other electrolyte imbalances must be treated as well.

On a long-term basis, the patient with chronic hypoparathyroidism is treated with oral calcium salts and a form of vitamin D. Chronic hypoparathyroidism that normally is well controlled may be affected when the patient is under severe stress or is very ill. If the patient is unable to take oral calcium, hypocalcemia can develop quickly. Temporary intravenous calcium may be needed.

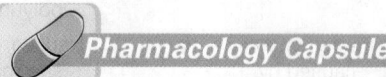
Pharmacology Capsule

Lifelong calcium supplementation is required to treat chronic hypoparathyroidism.

NURSING CARE *of the Patient with Hypoparathyroidism*

Assessment

Assessment of the hypoparathyroid patient is summarized in Box 45-2.

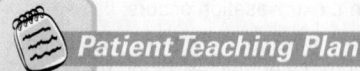
Patient Teaching Plan

Hyperparathyroidism

- Take drugs exactly as ordered, and report adverse effects to the physician.
- Eat a balanced diet.
- Notify the physician of bloody urine or pain in the kidney area or groin.
- Increase fluid intake to the amount recommended by the physician.

Nursing Diagnoses, Goals, and Outcome Criteria: Hypoparathyroidism	
NURSING DIAGNOSES	GOALS AND OUTCOME CRITERIA
Risk for Injury related to hypocalcemia	Decreased risk for injury: serum calcium level within normal limits; no muscle spasms, convulsions, or respiratory distress; negative Chvostek's and Trousseau's signs

| Decreased Cardiac Output related to dysrhythmias and heart failure secondary to hypocalcemia | Normal cardiac output: normal pulse rate and rhythm; normal blood pressure; no dyspnea or edema |

Interventions

Administer drugs as ordered for hypoparathyroidism and hypocalcemia. When administering calcium salts intravenously, monitor the infusion site carefully because the leakage of calcium salts into body tissues causes inflammation. The infusion site should be changed if extravasation occurs. Frequently assess the patient for signs and symptoms of calcium imbalances. Hypocalcemia may appear as a result of inadequate calcium supplementation. Hypercalcemia can result from excessive calcium intake.

If there has been any recent seizure activity or if the patient shows severe neuromuscular irritability, follow seizure precautions. Any signs of respiratory distress may suggest laryngospasm and should be documented and reported to the physician immediately. Monitor the pulse and blood pressure to detect dysrhythmias and heart failure. Report cardiac irregularities, edema, and dyspnea to the physician.

Teach patients with chronic hypoparathyroidism signs and symptoms of calcium imbalances, and provide instructions for self-medication. Advise them to carry medical identification cards to alert health care providers to the disorder in the event of an emergency.

 Key Points

- Thyroxine (T_4), triiodothyronine (T_3), and calcitonin are hormones produced by the thyroid gland that affect metabolic rate, growth and development, and serum calcium regulation.
- Hyperthyroidism is the abnormally increased production of thyroid hormones that may be treated with antithyroid drugs, surgery, or radiation therapy.

- Nursing care of the hyperthyroid patient may address Disturbed Sleep Pattern, Hyperthermia, Imbalanced Nutrition: Less Than Body Requirements, Decreased Cardiac Output, Risk for Injury, and Diarrhea.
- Nursing care after thyroidectomy is concerned with Ineffective Airway Clearance, Decreased Cardiac Output, Disturbed Body Image, Acute Pain, and Risk for Infection.
- Hypothyroidism is inadequate secretion of thyroid hormones that is treated with hormone replacement therapy.
- Nursing care of the hypothyroid patient addresses Activity Intolerance, Imbalanced Nutrition: More Than Body Requirements, Hypothermia, Constipation, Risk for Impaired Skin Integrity, Decreased Cardiac Output, Disturbed Thought Processes, Disturbed Body Image, and Self-Care Deficit.
- Goiter is enlargement of the thyroid gland that may be associated with hypothyroidism or hyperthyroidism.
- The parathyroid glands secrete parathormone, which regulates the serum calcium level.
- Hyperparathyroidism raises the serum calcium level and may cause bone demineralization and obstruction of kidney tubules.
- Nursing care of the patient with hyperparathyroidism focuses on Activity Intolerance, Risk for Injury, Impaired Urinary Elimination, Constipation, Disturbed Thought Processes, and Imbalanced Nutrition: Less Than Body Requirements.
- Hypoparathyroidism, a deficiency of parathormone that sometimes follows thyroidectomy, causes the serum calcium level to fall, producing neuromuscular irritability that can progress to seizures, cardiac dysrhythmias, and laryngospasm.
- Nursing diagnoses for the hypoparathyroid patient are Risk for Injury and Decreased Cardiac Output.

 Go to your Companion CD-ROM for a Pharmacology Tutorial, Audio Glossary, and 3-D animations.

evolve   Be sure to visit the companion Evolve site at http://evolve.elsevier.com/Linton/ for WebLinks and additional online resources.

REVIEW QUESTIONS *Choose the best answer.*

1. The primary function of thyroid hormones is to regulate:

    1. Metabolism
    2. Temperature
    3. Appetite
    4. Thirst

2. You are notified that a patient with severe hypothyroidism is being admitted to your nursing unit. Which action is appropriate?

    1. Obtain an emergency tracheostomy tray.
    2. Close the blinds to dim the room light.
    3. Have extra blankets put in the room.
    4. Pad the side rails on the bed.

3. Which of the following findings is most likely in a patient with severe hyperthyroidism?

   1. Respiratory rate of 12
   2. Heart rate of 120 bpm
   3. Blood pressure of 110/60
   4. Oral temperature of 96° F

4. During shift report, it is stated that a hyperthyroid patient has exophthalmos. You would expect to see:

   1. Enlargement of the patient's neck
   2. Edema of the face and hands
   3. Thin, dry skin that bruises easily
   4. Prominent, bulging eyeballs

5. A 6-week course of treatment with propylthiouracil (PTU) is prescribed for a patient who is scheduled for a thyroidectomy. The patient asks why she has to take this medication. Your best response is:

   1. "PTU will help you eliminate excess thyroid hormone."
   2. "It reduces your thyroid activity, which makes surgery safer for you."
   3. "PTU will provide replacement thyroid hormones after your thyroid gland is removed."
   4. "This drug will cause your thyroid gland to shrink, which will reduce pressure on your airway."

6. In the immediate postoperative period after thyroidectomy, the *first* priority is to:

   1. Maintain a patent airway
   2. Inspect for hemorrhage
   3. Monitor for hypocalcemia
   4. Prevent strain on the suture line

7. The purpose of measuring serum thyroglobulin in a patient who has had thyroid cancer is to:

   1. Determine adequacy of thyroid hormone replacement
   2. Detect any recurrence of the thyroid cancer
   3. See whether all radioactive iodine has been eliminated
   4. Determine whether parathyroid function is normal

8. Which statement accurately describes the relationship between parathyroid hormone (PTH) and serum calcium?

   1. The secretion of PTH decreases when serum calcium is low.
   2. Increased secretion of PTH causes the kidneys to retain calcium.
   3. Chronically decreased PTH can lead to bone demineralization.
   4. Decreased serum PTH causes calcium to shift from the bones to the blood.

9. A patient had a parathyroid adenoma removed 2 days ago. She is now complaining of muscle cramps in her hands and feet. You should suspect:

   1. Poor circulation
   2. Thyroid storm
   3. Hypocalcemia
   4. Metabolic acidosis

10. Nursing implications in administering iodide solutions to a patient include which of the following?

   1. Dilute in milk or juice, and provide a straw.
   2. Take the pulse and blood pressure before each dose.
   3. Tell the patient to report any changes in hearing acuity.
   4. Carefully maintain accurate intake and output records.

CHAPTER 46

Diabetes Mellitus and Hypoglycemia

LISA HOOTER

evolve http://evolve.elsevier.com/Linton/

Objectives

After reading and studying this chapter, you should be able to:

1. Describe the role of insulin in the body.
2. Explain the pathophysiology of diabetes mellitus and hypoglycemia.
3. Describe the signs and symptoms of diabetes mellitus and hypoglycemia.
4. Explain tests and procedures used to diagnose diabetes mellitus and hypoglycemia.
5. Discuss treatment of diabetes mellitus and hypoglycemia.
6. Explain the difference between type 1 and type 2 diabetes mellitus.
7. Differentiate between acute hypoglycemia and diabetic ketoacidosis.
8. Describe the treatment of a patient experiencing acute hypoglycemia or diabetic ketoacidosis.
9. Describe the complications of diabetes mellitus.
10. Identify nursing interventions for a patient diagnosed with diabetes mellitus or hypoglycemia.
11. Identify nursing interventions for a patient diagnosed with ketoacidosis.

Key Terms

Be sure to check out the bonus material on the Companion CD-ROM, including selected audio pronunciations.

endogenous (ĕn-DŎJ-ĕn-ŭs, p. 1001)
euglycemia (Ū-glī-sē-mē-ă, p. 1017)
exogenous (ĕks-ŎJ-ĕn-ŭs, p. 1001)
glycosuria (glī-kō-SŪ-rē-ă, p. 1004)
hypoglycemia (hī-pō-glī-SĒ-mē-ă, p. 1005)
ketoacidosis (kē-tō-ă-sī-DŌ-sĭs, p. 1007)
ketone bodies (KĒ-tōn, p. 1007)
lipoatrophy (lĭp-ō-ĂT-rō-fē, p. 1014)
lipohypertrophy (lĭp-ō-hī-PĔR-trō-fē, p. 1014)
macrovascular (MĂK-rō-văs-cū-lăr, p. 1004)
microvascular (MĬK-rō-văs-cū-lăr, p. 1004)
nephropathy (nĕ-FRŎP-ă-thē, p. 1004)
neuropathy (nū-RŎP-ĕ-thē, p. 1005)
polydipsia (pŏl-ē-DĬP-sē-ă, p. 1002)
polyphagia (pŏl-ē-FĂ-jē-ă, p. 1002)
polyuria (pŏl-ē-Ū-rē-ă, p. 1002)
retinopathy (rĕt-ĭ-NŎP-ă-thē, p. 1004)

DIABETES MELLITUS

Symptoms of diabetes mellitus (DM) have been reported in the literature throughout history, but not until the early twentieth century was the cause identified. In an experiment, the pancreata of several sheep were removed, which caused diabetes to develop in the sheep. Through this experiment, insulin and its role in the body were discovered. The search then began for a way to provide insulin to people whose bodies did not produce enough. Before insulin became available for commercial use in 1921, people with diabetes were placed on high-protein diets until they went into acidosis and died, usually a short time after the onset of the disease.

The National Institutes of Health estimate that 20.8 million people in the United States have DM, which is 7% of the total population. This estimate includes over 6 million people with undiagnosed diabetes. Diabetes is a major health problem and a leading cause of death by disease. People with diabetes are at increased risk for heart disease, renal disease, blindness, amputation, and complications during pregnancy. Fortunately, with early diagnosis and better management, it is possible to reduce the risk of serious complications.

PATHOPHYSIOLOGY

Diabetes mellitus is a chronic disorder characterized by impaired metabolism and by vascular and neurologic complications. A key feature of diabetes is elevated blood glucose, called *hyperglycemia*. The blood glucose level is normally regulated by insulin, a hormone produced by the beta cells in the islets of Langerhans located in the pancreas. In health, small amounts of insulin are secreted continuously into the bloodstream. The ingestion of carbohydrates triggers the secretion of a larger volume of insulin. Insulin that is produced in one's own body is called endogenous, meaning it is internally produced. Insulin that is obtained from other sources and administered to a person is called exogenous, meaning it comes from an external source.

Diabetes mellitus is classified as type 1 (previously called *insulin-dependent DM*, or *IDDM*) or type 2 (previously referred to as *non–insulin-dependent DM*, or *NIDDM*). Both types have a genetic component, but most people with diabetes have no genetic predisposition.

Type 1 DM is characterized by the absence of endogenous insulin. It used to be called *juvenile-onset diabetes* because it occurs most commonly in juveniles and young adults. However, it can also occur in middle-aged and older adults. An autoimmune process, possibly triggered by a viral infection, causes destruction of the beta cells, the development of insulin antibodies, and the production of islet cell antibodies (ICAs). Affected people require exogenous insulin for the rest of their lives.

Type 2 DM is characterized by inadequate endogenous insulin and the body's inability to properly use insulin. Initially, beta cells respond inadequately to hyperglycemia, resulting in chronically elevated blood glucose. The continuous high glucose level in the blood desensitizes the beta cells so that they become progressively less responsive to the elevated glucose. In relation to the use of insulin, specific receptor sites become insensitive to insulin ("insulin resistance") so that glucose is not admitted to cells. Although type 2 DM is more common among adults, it is increasingly found in children as well. One inherited form (maturity-onset diabetes of the young) causes type 2 DM among all age-groups in affected families.

Type 2 DM may be controlled by diet and exercise alone or may require oral hypoglycemic agents or exogenous insulin. Some patients are treated with insulin initially to normalize blood glucose and then are treated with diet, exercise, and perhaps oral agents.

Gestational diabetes mellitus (GDM) is diagnosed when a woman is found to have glucose intolerance for the first time during pregnancy. After delivery, the condition resolves. See a maternity nursing text for information on the management of GDM.

Role of Insulin

We usually think of insulin as a critical hormone for glucose metabolism, and that is correct. However, insulin also is needed for the synthesis of fatty acids and proteins (Box 46-1).

Glucose. Insulin stimulates the active transport of glucose into the cells. When insulin is absent, glucose cannot enter most cells, so it remains in the bloodstream. The blood then becomes thick with glucose, which increases its osmolality. Increased osmolality stimulates the thirst center, causing the patient to experience polydipsia (excessive thirst) and take in additional fluid. The increased fluid does not pass into body tissues, however, because the high serum osmolality retains the fluid in the bloodstream. As the blood passes through the kidneys, some excess glucose is eliminated. The osmotic force created by the glucose draws extra fluid and electrolytes with it, causing abnormally increased urine volume (polyuria).

Because most cells are not able to use glucose without insulin, stored fat is broken down in an effort to provide fuel for heat and energy. Tissue breakdown and loss of lean body mass send hunger signals to the hypothalamus. The patient experiences excessive hunger (polyphagia). The patient may take in more food but, unfortunately, cannot use the extra glucose without insulin. Weight loss occurs despite increased appetite and food ingestion.

Insulin is needed to transport glucose into resting muscle cells. During heavy exercise, however, muscle fibers are highly permeable to glucose even in the absence of insulin. Therefore exercise must be considered in the regulation of serum glucose levels. Other tissues that can use glucose without insulin are the brain, nerves, heart, and the lens of the eye.

Insulin regulates the rate of glucose metabolism. The greater the insulin response to carbohydrate ingestion, the faster the carbohydrates are metabolized.

In a healthy person, when blood glucose falls, insulin production is inhibited and stored glycogen is converted to glucose by a process called *glycogenolysis*. When blood glucose rises, insulin production is stimulated and the conversion of glycogen to glucose is inhibited. This process usually maintains the blood glucose within a normal range. However, when insulin secretion is inadequate, glycogen is converted to glucose in an attempt to nourish glucose-starved tissues but hyperglycemia occurs because cells cannot use the glucose.

Fatty Acids. Insulin promotes fatty acid synthesis and the conversion of fatty acids into fat, which is stored as adipose tissue. Insulin also spares fat by inhibiting the breakdown of adipose tissue and the mobilization of fat and by inhibiting the conversion of fats to glucose.

Without adequate insulin, fat stores break down and increased triglycerides are stored in the liver. The liver can store up to one third of its weight as fat. Increased fatty acids in the liver can triple the production of lipoproteins, which promotes the development of atherosclerosis. This helps explain why people with DM have a high incidence of cardiovascular disease.

Box 46-1 *Insulin: Actions and Effects of Deficiency*

Insulin
- Increases the transport of glucose into the resting muscle cell
- Regulates the rate at which carbohydrates are used
- Promotes the conversion of glucose to glycogen
- Inhibits the conversion of glycogen to glucose
- Promotes fatty acid synthesis
- Spares fat
- Inhibits the breakdown of adipose tissue
- Inhibits the conversion of fats to glucose
- Stimulates protein synthesis in the tissues
- Inhibits the conversion of protein into glucose

Lack of Insulin
- Stimulates the conversion of glycogen to glucose
- Permits fat stores to break down
- Increases triglyceride storage in the liver
- Halts the storage of proteins
- Causes protein to be dumped into the bloodstream

Protein. Insulin enhances protein synthesis in tissues and inhibits the conversion of protein into glucose. Amino acids are admitted into cells, which enhances the rate of protein formation while preventing the degradation of proteins. Without adequate insulin, the storage of proteins halts and large amounts of amino acids are dumped into the bloodstream. High levels of plasma amino acids place people with diabetes at risk for development of gout. Changes in protein metabolism lead to extreme weakness and poor organ functioning.

ETIOLOGY

Type 1 DM has been attributed to genetic, immunologic, and environmental (viruses, toxins) factors. The tendency toward type 1 DM is found in families with a genetic predisposition. There is evidence of a strong genetic component in type 2 DM as well.

It is possible that an autoimmune disorder triggers the sudden onset of diabetes in the young (Fig. 46-1). Our bodies are guarded by an elaborate and extensive immune system. When a microbe and its antigen enter the blood, they encounter white blood cells called *macrophages* that have antigen receptors on their surfaces. These antigen receptors steer the antigens to lymphocytes, which have antigen-specific receptors. When a specific antigen is present, it activates the immune response. The lymphocytes begin producing custom-made antibodies against the antigens, at the same time signaling other types of cells in the immune system to attack the invaders. The lymphocytes and the antibodies are unable to destroy the foreign cells independently without the help of phagocytes and complement cells. This group of cells is selective in identifying and destroying foreign protein. Unfortunately, this part of the immune system can become a renegade faction and turn on its own healthy cells. It is this autoimmune malfunction that may cause complete destruction of the islets of Langerhans in the pancreas, creating type 1 diabetes. In fact, islet cell antibodies are identified in more than 80% of all people with type 1 diabetes at the time of diagnosis.

RISK FACTORS

Risk factors for type 1 DM, other than genetic ones, are not known. According to the American Diabetes Association (ADA), risk factors for type 2 DM include the following:

- Obesity
- Sedentary lifestyle
- Family history of diabetes
- Age 40 years and older
- History of gestational DM
- History of delivering infant weighing more than 10 lbs
- African American (33% higher risk for type 2 DM)
- Latin American/Hispanic (>300% higher risk for type 2 DM)
- American Indians (33% to 50% higher risk for type 2 DM)

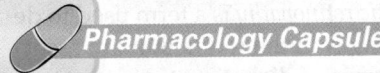

Pharmacology Capsule

Pharmacologic use of glucocorticoids can elevate the blood glucose level. Although unlikely to cause DM in people with normal pancreatic function, glucocorticoid therapy may unmask latent diabetes. It also complicates management of known DM.

What Does Culture Have to Do with Diabetes?

The risk of diabetes mellitus among Latin Americans/Hispanic Americans is 300% that of white Americans. Effective measures to decrease this risk must be sensitive to cultural practices and values.

Metabolic Syndrome

Metabolic syndrome is the common name used to describe a syndrome that is thought by many to be a precursor to diabetes. This syndrome is also referred to as *syndrome X, insulin resistance syndrome* and *cardiovascular dysmetabolic syndrome.* Patients with metabolic syndrome typically have impaired glucose tolerance, high serum insulin, hypertension, elevated triglycerides, low HDL cholesterol, and altered size and density of LDL cholesterol. It is believed that metabolic syndrome represents a chronic low-grade inflammatory

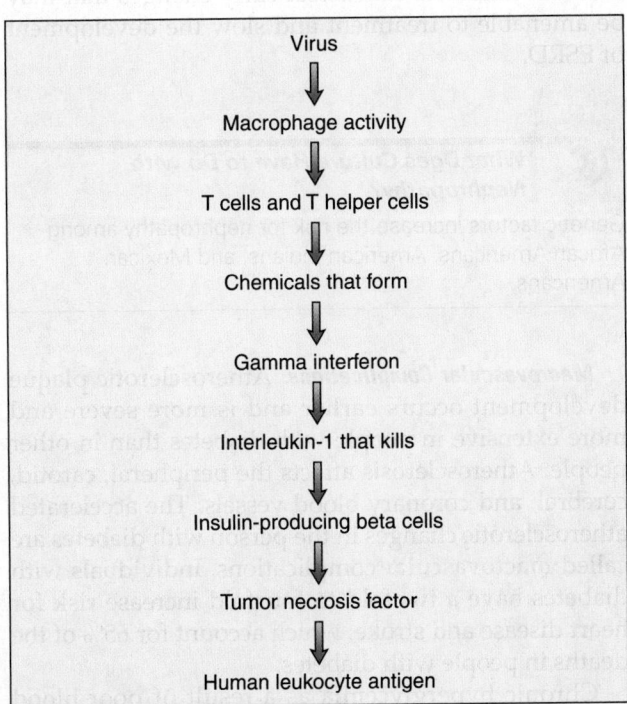

FIGURE 46-1 Possible immunologic cause of diabetes mellitus.

Virus
↓
Macrophage activity
↓
T cells and T helper cells
↓
Chemicals that form
↓
Gamma interferon
↓
Interleukin-1 that kills
↓
Insulin-producing beta cells
↓
Tumor necrosis factor
↓
Human leukocyte antigen

process affecting endothelial tissue (the lining of the heart, blood and lymph vessels). The long-term effects include atherosclerosis, ischemic heart disease, left ventricular hypertrophy, and sometimes type 2 DM. Research is now directed at learning how to detect this syndrome early and what interventions might slow or arrest the progress.

COMPLICATIONS

Long-Term Complications

The duration of diabetes and poor control of blood glucose are the best predictors of the severity of complications. These complications affect almost every organ of the body. They may be classified as microvascular, macrovascular, or neuropathic.

Microvascular Complications. Microvascular complications result from changes in small blood vessels that are unique to diabetes and occur in both type 1 and type 2 disease. The basement membrane of capillaries thickens, which impairs the exchange of nutrients, gases, and wastes. Tissues that are most vulnerable to microvascular complications are the eyes (retinopathy) and the kidneys (nephropathy). Changes in the capillaries appear to be related to persistent hyperglycemia and are aggravated by hypertension and smoking. Neuropathy is sometimes classified with microvascular complications; it is discussed on p. 1005.

Retinopathy. Among people ages 25 to 74 years, DM is the leading cause of blindness. People with diabetes are at increased risk for retinopathy, cataracts, and glaucoma. *Diabetic retinopathy* is a term used to describe pathologic changes in the retina that are associated with DM. Two types of diabetic retinopathy have been identified: nonproliferative and proliferative. Both types may be present at the same time. Manifestations of nonproliferative disease include small hemorrhages and aneurysms in the retina, hard lipid and protein exudates that leak from the blood vessels, infarcted nerve fibers (described as "cotton wool spots"), and changes in retinal veins. Proliferative disease is characterized by the growth of abnormal capillaries on the retina and the optic disc. These fragile vessels can penetrate the vitreous humor and rupture. When there is hemorrhaging into the vitreous, it becomes cloudy and vision is lost. The blood is eventually reabsorbed, but scars may remain, which places traction on the retina and may result in retinal detachment.

Macular edema occurs with both types of diabetic retinopathy. The macula is the center of vision, and edema causes loss of central vision. To illustrate the effect, imagine this page with only the outer margins clearly visible. The center would be clouded.

Signs and symptoms that suggest impending eye problems are the presence of spots ("floaters") in the field of vision, seeing "cobwebs," or sudden visual changes. Often there are no warning signs of retinal changes. Therefore patients with diabetes should have eye examinations at least once a year so that early changes in the eye can be detected and measures taken to try to prevent further deterioration and possible blindness. One strategy that may reduce the risk of injury to the eye is control of hypertension. Early laser treatment of macular edema can halt the progression of retinopathy and may even improve vision.

Nephropathy. Diabetes is the most common cause of end-stage renal disease (ESRD) in the United States. Renal disease develops in about 20% to 30% of people with diabetes, but a higher percentage of those with type 1 diabetes (50%) progress to ESRD than those with type 2 diabetes (20%). Factors that contribute to the development of nephropathy (kidney damage) include poor control of blood glucose, hypertension, long-standing diabetes, and genetic susceptibility. High concentrations of glycosuria (glucose in the urine), along with hypertension, gradually destroy the capillaries that supply the renal glomeruli. Increased permeability of the glomeruli permits serum proteins to be lost in the urine. There are no symptoms in the early stages, but rising microalbuminuria signals the onset of kidney damage. When the level of protein in the urine exceeds 300 mg/day of albumin or 500 mg/day of total protein, the condition will surely progress to ESRD. Signs and symptoms of kidney failure include persistent proteinuria, elevated blood pressure and serum creatinine, hematuria, and oliguria or anuria. Diagnosis is based on laboratory values (see Chapter 40).

Measures to reduce the risk of damage to the kidneys include good glycemic control, control of hypertension, use of angiotensin-converting enzyme inhibitors, maintaining good hydration, and avoiding nephrotoxic chemicals, including drugs. Modest protein restriction may be recommended. Screening for microalbuminuria can detect early changes that may be amenable to treatment and slow the development of ESRD.

 What Does Culture Have to Do with Nephropathy?

Genetic factors increase the risk for nephropathy among African Americans, American Indians, and Mexican Americans.

Macrovascular Complications. Atherosclerotic plaque development occurs earlier and is more severe and more extensive in people with diabetes than in other people. Atherosclerosis affects the peripheral, carotid, cerebral, and coronary blood vessels. The accelerated atherosclerotic changes in the person with diabetes are called macrovascular complications. Individuals with diabetes have a twofold to fourfold increase risk for heart disease and stroke, which account for 65% of the deaths in people with diabetes.

Chronic hyperglycemia as a result of poor blood glucose control may play an important role in the premature development of atherosclerosis in patients with diabetes. However, there is evidence that the elevated insulin level that occurs with insulin resistance also plays a role in the development of atherosclerosis. This is especially apparent in white, middle-aged men. It has been suggested that hyperinsulinemia may affect the endothelium of blood vessels, permitting lipids to be easily deposited on the cell walls of the blood vessels. Other risk factors for macrovascular complications are central obesity, hyperlipidemia, hypertension, genetics, sedentary lifestyle, and smoking.

Macrovascular changes are associated with coronary artery disease (CAD), cerebral vascular accidents (CVA or stroke), and peripheral vascular disease (PVD). Signs and symptoms of PVD may include diminished pedal pulses and claudication (pain in the calf, back, or buttocks while walking). When arteries in the lower extremities can no longer deliver oxygen and nutrients to peripheral tissues, gangrene may develop, necessitating amputation of affected parts of extremities.

Treatment for macrovascular disease is directed toward weight loss and exercise. Patients who smoke are strongly encouraged to quit because of vasoconstriction caused by nicotine. With weight loss, insulin uptake improves and circulating insulin levels decrease. As a result of aerobic exercise, insulin receptor sites increase and serum insulin levels decrease. Exercise, in conjunction with weight loss, reduces the amount of exogenous insulin needed. Because it is thought that exogenous insulin may create immune complexes that damage arterial walls, reduced exogenous insulin needs may reduce the risk for macrovascular disease in DM.

For additional information about CAD, CVA, and PVD, see Chapters 28, 35, and 36.

Neuropathic Complications. Pathologic changes in nerve tissue, called **neuropathy,** are related to poor glucose control, ischemic lesions of nerves, and chemical changes in peripheral nerve cells. Almost 30% of individuals with diabetes over age 40 have impaired sensation in as least one area of the foot. Neuropathy affects approximately 13% of all people with diabetes. Patients who have had diabetes for more than 25 years have a 50% chance of experiencing neuropathies. Neuropathy can be classified as mononeuropathy, polyneuropathy, or autonomic neuropathy.

Mononeuropathy. Mononeuropathy affects a single nerve or group of nerves. It results from inadequate blood supply and is experienced as sharp, stabbing pain. Pain and atrophy occur in muscles enervated by the affected nerve. Sometimes the pain is relieved by walking.

Polyneuropathy. Polyneuropathy involves both sensory and autonomic nerves. Sensory polyneuropathy commonly affects both legs symmetrically. Symptoms range from tingling, numbness, and burning sensations to complete loss of sensation. Pain is often worse during the night. Sometimes polyneuropathy resolves spontaneously.

Autonomic Neuropathy. Autonomic neuropathy affects the sympathetic and parasympathetic nervous systems. It can affect the pupillary response and functions of the cardiovascular, gastrointestinal, and genitourinary systems. Cardiovascular involvement may be manifested as postural hypotension, resting tachycardia, exercise intolerance, and failure of the heart rate to increase with vigorous exercise. Common gastrointestinal symptoms include constipation or, less commonly, diarrhea, as well as anorexia, nausea, vomiting, gastric reflux, and bloating after meals. The stomach may dilate and lose muscle tone so that gastric emptying is delayed, a condition called *gastroparesis.*

The patient may have urinary problems such as an atonic bladder, in which the bladder capacity increases and eventually causes retention with overflow. Sexual problems in men such as erectile dysfunction and retrograde ejaculation are common. Women may have painful intercourse.

Some areas of the body may cease to sweat (anhidrosis), whereas there is excessive sweating (hyperhidrosis) in other areas. Gustatory sweating (facial sweating after eating) may occur after a meal containing cheese or spicy foods.

Diabetic amyotrophy (loss of muscle mass) causes pain in the muscles of the pelvic girdle and thighs. This pain may be so severe that it interferes with activity and sleep. The muscles look wasted, and fasciculation (involuntary twitching of muscle fibers) may be visible under the skin. These contractions do not produce movement.

Hypoglycemic Unawareness. Normally, patients recognize signs and symptoms of **hypoglycemia** (abnormally low level of glucose in the blood) so that they can take corrective action. With hypoglycemic unawareness, the usual symptoms of tachycardia, palpitations, tremor, sweating, and nervousness may be absent. Without this "early warning system," the patient may suddenly have changes in mental status as the first sign of hypoglycemia. This phenomenon has been attributed to autonomic neuropathy, but that relationship has not been consistently demonstrated.

Foot Complications of Diabetes. People with diabetes may have foot problems associated with neuropathy, inadequate blood supply, or a combination of both. When neurologic function is impaired but blood flow is adequate, the foot is warm and pink with good pulses but lacks normal sensation. The patient may have a foot injury but fail to recognize it in the absence of pain.

If the blood supply is impaired but neurologic function is adequate, the foot is cold but sensation is normal. When the foot is raised, it turns pale. When the foot is lowered, it becomes red. Pulses are weak or absent.

Neuropathic ulcers can result from injury to the foot caused by the following:

- *Mechanical irritation,* such as that caused from rough shoe linings or amateur attempts at shaving calluses or cutting toenails

- *Thermal injury,* such as burns caused from heat exposure such as hot-water bottles and sitting too close to a fire or radiator
- *Chemical irritation* caused by substances such as salicylic acid, found in many corn plasters

Patients who cannot see or feel their feet may fail to notice injuries or dangerous situations. A neglected callus may become inflamed and blood and fluid may accumulate beneath the lesion, creating a site for infection. An abscess may form that ruptures to create an ulcer. Treatment is difficult and not always effective, so the best treatment is prevention.

Prevention of Long-Term Complications. The landmark Diabetes Control and Complications Trial (DCCT) found that intensive treatment of type 1 DM delayed the onset or slowed the progress of diabetic retinopathy, nephropathy, and neuropathy. The trial evaluated the effects of tight control of blood glucose levels with multiple daily insulin injections or programmable external insulin pumps. Patients were closely monitored and treated by a team of diabetes experts. The outcomes of the United Kingdom Prospective Diabetes Study (UKPDS) demonstrated similar benefits of tight control with type 2 DM. Tight control means that the blood glucose is maintained in the normal range with carefully balanced drugs, diet, and exercise.

The ADA acknowledges that other factors increase the risk for developing complications. They recommend that individuals with diabetes strive to keep blood pressure readings less than 130 systolic and less than 80 diastolic. Lipid goals should include total cholesterol less than 200 mg/dL, LDL less than 100 mg/dL, HDL more than 45 mg/dL for men (>55 mg/dL for women) and triglycerides less than 150 mg/dL. Individuals with diabetes should be given information regarding smoking cessation. Use of aspirin and ACE inhibitors is recommended for those with increased cardiovascular risk factors.

Acute Emergency Complications

Acute Hypoglycemia. Patients being treated with insulin or other hypoglycemic agents are at risk for acute hypoglycemia. Events that may trigger this dangerous drop in blood glucose include taking too much insulin, not eating enough food or not eating at the right time, and an inconsistent pattern of exercise. Other variables that lower blood glucose are gastroparesis, renal insufficiency, and certain drugs including aspirin and beta-adrenergic blockers. Glucose levels between 50 and 70 mg/dL are considered moderate hypoglycemia. However, some people with diabetes have been known to have serum glucose levels below 50 mg/dL without signs and symptoms of hypoglycemia.

The signs and symptoms of hypoglycemia are classified as adrenergic and neuroglucopenic. Adrenergic symptoms appear first and reflect the response of the

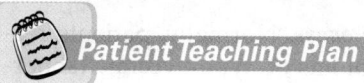
Patient Teaching Plan

"Dos and Don'ts" Regarding Foot Care

Do
- Check your feet every day. Look for red spots, cuts, swelling, and blisters. Use a mirror if you can't see the bottom of your feet.
- Be more active.
- Wash your feet every day. Dry them carefully, especially between the toes.
- Keep your skin soft and smooth. Rub a thin coat of lotion over the tops and bottoms of your feet but not between your toes.
- Trim your toenails across, and file the edges with an emery board.
- Protect your feet from hot and cold.
- Wear shoes at all times.
- Test the water before putting your feet in to make sure the water is not too hot.
- Inspect the insides of your shoes for foreign objects, torn linings, and rough or sharp points.
- Buy shoes that are comfortable at the time of purchase. Wear shoes that are supportive and flexible and do not create pressure on any area of the feet.
- See your physician regularly, and ask him or her to examine your feet at each visit.

Don't
- Smoke.
- Never use hot water bottles, heating pads, or electric blankets. You can burn your feet before you realize it.
- Soak feet in hot water.
- Walk barefoot, even in the house.
- Walk on hot surfaces such as sidewalks or sandy beaches.
- Remove corns or calluses yourself. See a podiatrist for their removal.
- Wear stockings that have been darned or mended.
- Wear shoes without stockings.

Modified from the ADA Position statement: Preventive foot care in diabetes. *Diabetes Care 27* (Suppl 1):S63-S64, 2004; and ADA patient guidelines for foot care (www.diabetes.org).

nervous system to inadequate glucose for cell function. These symptoms are shakiness, nervousness, irritability, tachycardia, anxiety, lightheadedness, hunger, tingling or numbness of the lips or tongue, and diaphoresis.

If treatment is delayed, a second set of symptoms may appear. These symptoms are called *neuroglucopenia* because they are caused by a shortage of glucose to the brain. If the glucose level falls rapidly, however, they may be the first signs of hypoglycemia. These include drowsiness, irritability, impaired judgment, blurred vision, slurred speech, headaches, and mood swings progressing to disorientation, seizures, and unconsciousness. Even more severe hypoglycemia progresses to loss of consciousness, convulsions, coma, and death.

Treatment. To treat hypoglycemia, give the conscious patient 10 to 15 gm of quick-acting carbohydrate such as the following:

- 4-6 ounces of undiluted orange or apple juice, soft drink (not diet)
- 8 ounces skim milk
- 3-4 teaspoons of table sugar
- 4 tablespoons of a light or dark corn syrup, jelly, or jam
- Five or six pieces of hard candy
- Two or three glucose tablets or 15 gm of glucose gel

Repeat every 15 to 30 minutes until the patient's blood glucose is above 70 mg/dL for adults and 80 to 100 mg/dL for older adults and children.

Any patient on insulin always should have injectable glucagon on hand. If the patient is unable to swallow, an intramuscular or subcutaneous injection of 1 mg of glucagon or an intravenous dose of 50 mL of 50% dextrose should be given as ordered or per protocol. On regaining consciousness, the patient should be given an additional treatment of some form of glucose. If it will be an hour or more until the next meal, give the patient some form of complex carbohydrate and protein such as a slice of cheese or meat with crackers.

Consider the Alternative

Among the many herbal supplements that can lower blood glucose are dandelion, onion, garlic, and ginseng. Patients should consult with their physician if they consider using these products.

Diabetic Ketoacidosis. Diabetic **ketoacidosis** (DKA) is a life-threatening emergency caused by a relative or absolute deficiency of insulin. This results in disorders in the metabolism of carbohydrates, fats, and proteins. The sequence of events is as follows:

1. Tissues cannot utilize glucose without insulin, resulting in an increase in serum glucose levels.

2. The high osmotic pressure created by excess glucose leads to osmotic diuresis. As glucose is eliminated in the kidneys, so are large amounts of water and electrolytes.
3. The patient voids large amounts of dilute urine (polyuria).
4. To make matters worse, the sympathetic nervous system responds to the cellular need for fuel by converting glycogen to glucose and manufacturing additional glucose.
5. As glycogen stores are depleted, the body begins to burn fat and protein for energy.
6. Fat metabolism produces acidic substances called **ketone bodies** that accumulate and lead to metabolic acidosis.
7. Protein metabolism results in the loss of lean muscle mass and a negative nitrogen balance.

Early signs and symptoms of DKA are anorexia, headache, and fatigue. As the condition progresses, the classic symptoms of polydipsia, polyuria, and polyphagia develop. If untreated, the patient becomes dehydrated, weak, and lethargic with abdominal pain, nausea, vomiting, fruity breath, increased respiratory rate, tachycardia, blurred vision, and hypothermia. Late signs are air hunger (seen as Kussmaul's respirations: rapid and deep), coma, and shock. Death can result if prompt medical care is not instituted.

The patient with ketoacidosis has hyperglycemia (≥ 300 mg/dL); ketonuria; and acidosis, with a pH of less than 7.3 or a bicarbonate level of less than 15 mEq/L.

The National Diabetes Data Group indicates that 10% of all deaths of people with DM, as recorded on death certificates, result from DKA. It is most likely to occur when diabetes is undiagnosed, when the patient does not take enough insulin, when the patient with uncontrolled type 1 DM exercises too vigorously, or when the patient experiences stress linked to illness, infection, surgery, or emotions. Some drugs such as corticosteroids, sympathomimetics, and thiazide diuretics also can raise serum glucose. In about a quarter of patients with DKA, no cause is identified. Treatment is aimed at correction of the three main problems: dehydration, electrolyte imbalance, and acidosis.

Dehydration. The patient with ketoacidosis may have lost a large volume of fluid as the result of vomiting, polyuria, and hyperventilation. In addition to the risk of shock due to depleted blood volume, the patient is at risk for development of blood clots.

The first need is to replace the fluid, which will aid the kidneys in eliminating excess glucose. The physician usually orders 1000 mL of normal saline to run over the first hour, followed by an additional 2000 to 8000 mL of intravenous fluids for the next 24 hours. If the patient has hypertension or hypernatremia or is at risk for congestive heart failure, the order may be given for 0.45% saline solution instead of normal saline. Also, the rate and total amount of fluid may be decreased in older patients who may not tolerate rapid changes in fluid volume.

Electrolyte Imbalance. The electrolyte of primary concern in ketoacidosis is potassium. Potassium shifts out of the cells, causing transient hyperkalemia. The hyperkalemia associated with hyperglycemia should be treated with fluid replacement and insulin administration. As the patient is rehydrated and normal urine output is reestablished, potassium is lost in the urine. Also, insulin replacement enhances the movement of potassium from the extracellular compartment back into the cells. During this time, the patient is at risk for developing severe hypokalemia that can cause life-threatening cardiac dysrhythmias.

Replacement of potassium is initiated only after adequate urine output is established. During potassium replacement, you must monitor the patient closely. Large doses of potassium may be required even though the serum potassium level is normal at the onset of treatment, because the plasma level will drop during treatment. Because potassium is irritating to the veins and a potassium drip must be carefully regulated, it is better to run the intravenous fluid containing potassium by the piggyback method at a prescribed rate, which is slower than the hydration rate. Remember that potassium must *always* be diluted before intravenous administration.

Sodium deficiency is generally corrected by infusion of normal saline. Phosphate, magnesium, and calcium levels also should be monitored. Once therapy begins, phosphate and magnesium may fall and calcium can rise to dangerous levels.

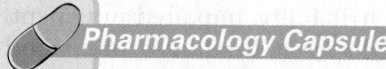

Pharmacology Capsule

When a patient is given insulin to treat diabetic ketoacidosis, monitor for hypokalemia because insulin causes potassium to move from the extracellular fluid into the cells.

Acidosis. Ketoacidosis is a problem primarily with type 1 DM. It occurs when ketone bodies accumulate as the result of the breakdown of fats for energy associated with inadequate insulin. Ketoacidosis can occur also in individuals with type 2 diabetes when severe hyperglycemia is associated with another acute condition, such as sepsis or a myocardial infarction.

Ketoacidosis is treated with the slow intravenous infusion of insulin. When the serum glucose level reaches 250 to 300 mg/dL, dextrose solution is added. The intravenous insulin is given continuously or as a bolus until subcutaneous insulin can be given, or else the patient may become ketoacidotic again. The serum glucose level returns to normal several hours before the serum bicarbonate level. As long as the serum glucose level is normal but the serum bicarbonate level remains abnormal, the insulin drip must be maintained

and glucose level corrected. More glucose is added to the intravenous fluid to cover the insulin. Normal levels of glucose *do not* mean that the acidosis has been corrected. The insulin drip must be maintained until the serum bicarbonate is 15 to 18 mEq/L. When the patient is able to eat and all laboratory values are normal, subcutaneous insulin can be given and the insulin drip discontinued.

Pharmacology Capsule

For continuous IV infusion, insulin is usually diluted in a 100-mL bag of solution. Because insulin binds with plastic, flush plastic tubing with the intravenous solution before adding insulin to the solution.

Hyperglycemic Hyperosmolar Nonketotic Syndrome. Hyperglycemic hyperosmolar nonketotic syndrome (HHNKS) is a condition in which a patient goes into a coma from extremely high glucose levels (>600 mg/dL) but there is no evidence of elevated ketones. Apparently, the patient's pancreas produces just enough insulin to prevent the breakdown of fatty acids and the formation of ketones but not enough insulin to prevent hyperglycemia.

The basic defect is the lack of effective insulin or the inability to use available insulin. The patient's persistent hyperglycemia causes osmotic diuresis, resulting in the loss of fluid and electrolytes. To maintain osmotic equilibrium, fluid shifts from the intracellular fluid space to the extracellular space. Dehydration and hypernatremia develop. Dehydration and neurologic changes may be more pronounced with HHNKS than with DKA. Patients with HHNKS do not experience gastrointestinal symptoms, nor do they experience Kussmaul's respirations because they lack significant lactic acid levels. These patients often tolerate polyuria and polydipsia for weeks before seeking treatment. For some patients, HHNKS is the first sign of diabetes. Others have been previously diagnosed with borderline diabetes.

HHNKS may be caused by the same factors that trigger ketoacidosis. It also can be brought about by total parenteral nutrition or dialysis. In both of these procedures, intravenous solutions that contain large amounts of glucose are administered to the patient. Because the digestive system is bypassed, there is no stimulus to trigger the pancreas to release insulin.

MEDICAL DIAGNOSIS

The diagnosis of DM is based on serum glucose levels. Normal fasting serum glucose levels are between 70 and 100 mg/dL. The official criteria for a diagnosis of DM were published in 1997 by the Expert Committee on the Diagnosis and Classification of Diabetes Mellitus and updated in 2003. A patient who meets one or more of the following criteria on two separate occasions is considered to have DM:

1. Symptoms of diabetes (polyuria, polydipsia, polyphagia, unexplained weight loss) plus random glucose level ≥200 mg/dL. A random reading is based on a blood sample drawn any time of day without regard to mealtimes.
2. Fasting serum glucose level ≥126 mg/dL (after at least an 8-hour fast).
3. Two-hour postprandial glucose level ≥200 mg/dL during an oral glucose tolerance test (OGTT) under specific guidelines. The test must use a glucose load of 75 gm of anhydrous glucose dissolved in water. This test is often unnecessary.

Pre-Diabetes

Individuals with impaired fasting glucose (IFG) and/or impaired glucose tolerance (IGT) are referred to as having *pre-diabetes*. IFG and IGT are risk factors for developing diabetes and cardiovascular disease. The individuals should receive education on weight reduction and increasing physical activity.

- IFG: fasting glucose level from 100 to <126 mg/dL.
- IGT: diagnosis based on (1) a fasting serum glucose level between 100 and 125 mg/dL and (2) a 2-hour OGTT result from 140 to <200 mg/dL.

Oral Glucose Tolerance Test

The OGTT is performed when a patient is suspected of having DM. The patient should consume a diet composed of 150 to 300 gm of carbohydrates for 3 days before the test. However, some physicians tell their patients to eat their normal diets. The night before the test, the patient is instructed to fast after midnight. On the morning of the test, a sample of blood is drawn for a fasting serum glucose test. The patient is then given a drink (Glucola) containing 75 gm of carbohydrates and instructed to remain quiet. This drink is quite sweet and should be served very cold to make it palatable. In certain situations, the glucose can be given by the intravenous route, but this method is not as accurate as the oral route. Blood is then drawn at 30 minutes and 1 hour after the ingestion of glucose. After these two samples, blood is drawn at hourly intervals until the test is completed. Most physicians order either a 3-hour or a 5-hour OGTT. Because blood must be drawn several times, it may be best to insert a heparin lock into the vein at the time blood is obtained for the fasting blood sugar. This eliminates the need for multiple venipunctures.

MEDICAL TREATMENT

The goals of managing diabetes are to normalize the blood glucose, serum lipids, and body weight while meeting energy needs and achieving healthy body weight.

Nutritional Management

Medical nutrition therapy (MNT) is an important part of diabetes management and should be included in diabetes self-management education. (See the Nutrition Concepts box below.) Due to the complexity of nutritional management, a registered dietitian should be part of the diabetes management team and the individual with diabetes should be included in decision making. The goals of MNT are the following:

1. Attain and maintain optimal metabolic outcomes (glucose, lipids, blood pressure).
2. Prevent and treat the chronic complications of diabetes (obesity, dyslipidemia, cardiovascular disease, hypertension, nephropathy).
3. Improve health through healthy food choices and physical activity.
4. Address individual nutritional needs while considering lifestyle, personal, and cultural preferences.

To maintain weight, a caloric intake of 28 calories/kg of body weight is required. To reduce weight, the caloric intake is calculated based on 15 to 20 calories/kg body weight. To arrive at a person's weight in kilograms, divide the weight in pounds by 2.2. If a woman weighs 110 pounds, her weight in kilograms is 55 kg. To maintain her weight, she needs to consume 1540 calories daily. Diets that advocate extreme reductions in carbohydrates (<130 grams/day) are not recommended for individuals with diabetes.

Several nutrition planning approaches are in use. Carbohydrate counting is particularly useful for people who use intensive insulin therapy or pumps. Insulin doses are based on the total grams of carbohydrate to be ingested. For most patients, the emphasis is on a well-balanced diet within the prescribed distribution of proteins, fats, and carbohydrates using the My Pyramid food guide. The Health Promotion Considerations box

 Nutrition Concepts

1. Diet is an essential component in the management of both type 1 and type 2 diabetes mellitus.
2. The goal of the diabetic diet is to maintain plasma glucose as near to the normal physiologic range as possible.
3. A person who requires insulin to control diabetes mellitus should coordinate insulin administration with mealtime patterns.
4. A person with type 2 diabetes can spread food intake throughout the day and eat consistently every day.
5. Diet plans are individualized based on glucose and lipid levels, weight management goals, and what the patient is willing to do.
6. When hypoglycemia is attributed to an overproduction of insulin in response to carbohydrate ingestion, a low-carbohydrate, high-protein diet with smaller meals may control the condition.

below lists the American Diabetes Association's recommendations for optimal calorie distribution.

Patient teaching should include sample menus that include as many favorite foods as possible. People with diabetes require considerable education and support to learn to manage the dietary guidelines. It is vital to consider their personal and ethnic choices. Most nursing care situations do not lend themselves to the in-depth teaching, planning, and reinforcement needed. Outpatient education and visits with a certified diabetes educator (CDE) can help meet this need.

Previously, rigid diabetic diets using exchange lists were recommended for meal planning. Exchange lists are groups of measured foods that represent the same number of calories and the same amount of carbohydrate, fat, and protein. Foods on the same list may be exchanged to add variety to meals. For example, two bread exchanges are equal to a bagel or a plain bun such as a hot dog roll. The patient was taught to select a specific number of foods from each exchange list for the daily meal plan. Exchanges for a variety of foods are published in several books that are available to the public. In addition, food companies often include the exchanges on the packaging of their frozen dinners and other products. Advise patients to read nutrition facts on the labels of prepared foods. Many people—patients and nurses alike—found the original exchange lists difficult to use. You may, however, encounter people who have learned to use them and are reluctant to change their approaches to food selection.

Consider the Alternative

Caution patients who take herbal supplements for diabetes that the supplements should not be used to *replace* conventional therapy. Be sure the physician is aware of supplements being used.

Exercise

Exercise is a very effective treatment adjunct for people with diabetes. It aids in weight loss in obese patients, improves cardiovascular conditioning, improves insulin sensitivity, and promotes a sense of well-being. Exercising muscle uses glucose at 20 times the rate of a muscle at rest and does not require insulin. Much of the morbidity and mortality in patients with type 2 disease occurs because of the atherosclerosis that accompanies long-term uncontrolled diabetes, which places the patient at risk for CVA (stroke) and cardiovascular disease. Exercise is known to improve low-

Health Promotion Considerations

Recommended Calorie Distribution for Patients Who Take Insulin

The American Diabetes Association recommends that the daily calorie intake be distributed as follows:

- Proteins: 15% to 20% (as long as kidney functions are normal)
- Carbohydrates and monosaturated fats (peanut oil, olive oil, canola oil, sesame oil, avocado): 60% to 70%
- Saturated fats (animal fats, egg yolks, coconut oil, palm kernel oil, palm oil, hydrogenated vegetable oils): less than 10%
- Polyunsaturated fats (corn oil, safflower oil, most nuts): less than 10%

Sodium intake should not exceed 2400 mg/day or sodium chloride 6000 mg/day. These levels may be modified for medical reasons and may be restricted further in some clinical situations.

Greater than 20% of the daily intake of calories in protein may be associated with an increase in the glomerular filtration rate. Sustained increases in glomerular filtration rate cause renal and retinal vasodilation, leading to renal damage and retinopathy.

Elevated serum cholesterol and triglyceride levels are often associated with type 2 DM, increasing the risk of cardiovascular disease. Cholesterol should not exceed 300 mg/day. If the patient has elevated low-density lipoprotein levels, saturated fats may be restricted to 7% of the total calories and dietary cholesterol restricted to less than 200 mg/day. Research in the past several years has indicated that replacing some of the allotted fat calories with calories from carbohydrates and fiber has a positive effect on the lipid profile. The exception is the patient who has glucose intolerance.

The addition of water-soluble fibers in the daily diet may lower total cholesterol and low-density lipoprotein levels. In addition, the lower fat intake permits increased insulin binding to receptor sites, resulting in insulin sparing. Foods containing soluble fibers include oatmeal, rice, dried beans, oat bran, lentils, squash, whole-wheat breads, and some fruits. The potential glucose-lowering effect of fiber in the diet received considerable attention in the past. Research, however, has shown that the effect is minimally significant and requires fiber intake far above that usually recommended. In general, people with diabetes need the same amount of fiber as other adults: 20 to 35 gm/day from soluble and insoluble sources. When fiber is added to the diet, it should be done gradually. A sudden addition of large amounts of fiber to the diet may reduce the amount of glucose available for the exogenous insulin or hypoglycemic agent taken by the patient and may result in hypoglycemic episodes.

A simplified method of planning diets for people with diabetes has been designed by the American Diabetes Association and the American Dietetic Association. Foods are divided into three clusters: carbohydrates, proteins, and fats. Meal planning is presented in a booklet entitled *The Exchange Lists for Meal Planning* that can be ordered by calling 1-800-ADA-ORDER.

density lipoproteins, serum glucose, blood pressure, some blood coagulation parameters, and triglycerides. However, exercise must be accompanied by appropriate nutrition to have long-term beneficial results.

The metabolic adjustments that maintain glucose levels during exercise are regulated largely by hormones. A decrease in plasma insulin levels and the presence of glucagons are necessary for hepatic glucose production during physical activity. Increases in plasma glucagon and catecholamine levels are key factors for hepatic glucose release during prolonged exercise. Exercise affects individuals with type 1 diabetes differently from those with type 2 diabetes who do not require insulin. Hyperglycemia may occur with exercise in the patient with type 1 diabetes when insulin levels are inadequate. An excessive release of counterregulatory hormones and mobilization of free fatty acids result in ketone production, which can lead to the development of DKA. In patients with type 2 diabetes, exercise makes insulin receptor sites more sensitive to insulin and lowers plasma glucose levels, which can result in hypoglycemia.

Because of this, it is important for individuals with diabetes to monitor blood glucose levels before and after exercise. Individuals taking insulin may also need to monitor blood glucose levels during prolonged exercise. Caution should be taken when exercising during peak activity of injected insulin to decrease the risk of hypoglycemia. Additional carbohydrate intake may be necessary during prolonged exercise and any time glucose levels are less than 100 mg/dL. Physical activity should be avoided if the fasting glucose levels are more than 250 mg/dL and ketones are present. Caution should be used if glucose levels are more than 300 mg/dL in the absence of ketones.

An appropriate combination of aerobic and anaerobic exercises should be determined. Aerobic exercise produces the most therapeutic effect. The patient should exercise for 30 to 60 minutes three to four times a week. Warm-up exercises such as stretching and walking are recommended before exercise, followed by cool-down exercises afterward. The best aerobic exercises are walking, swimming, bicycle riding, and jogging. Anaerobic exercises are done to build muscle mass. These include activities such as weightlifting, yoga, and sit-ups. Very strenuous exercises can raise blood pressure, which is undesirable with retinopathy and nephropathy. Eventually, the patient with type 2 disease who adheres to a sound nutritional plan and exercise regimen may be able to decrease the amount of exogenous insulin or oral hypoglycemic agents needed. See the Health Promotion Considerations box on p. 1012.

Insulin Therapy

All patients with type 1 disease need insulin injections, and some patients with type 2 disease may eventually need insulin. Insulins are classified by their source and time course of action. For many years, all insulin was obtained from beef and pork. However, beef and pork insulin are not identical to human insulin, and patients could form antibodies against them. The advent of recombinant DNA technology has allowed the manufacture of insulin that is identical to endogenous insulin. This "human" insulin causes fewer problems than that from animal sources. Pork insulin is still available in the United States, but beef insulin is being phased out. Over time, most patients taking insulin from animal sources have been switched to human insulin.

In relation to time course of actions, insulins are classified as rapid acting, short acting, intermediate acting, and long acting. Rapid-acting insulins include insulin lispro (Humalog) and insulin aspart (NovoLog). Regular (Humulin R, Novolin R) insulin is classified as short-acting insulin. Intermediate-acting insulins are NPH (Humulin N) and Lente insulin (Humulin L). Long-acting insulins are Ultralente (Humulin U, Humulin Ultralente) and insulin glargine (Lantus). All rapid-acting and short-acting insulins are clear. Except for insulin glargine (Lantus), which also is clear, the other insulins all are cloudy. Onsets, peaks, and durations are compared in the Drug Therapy table on p. 1013. The effect of insulin on blood glucose levels is shown in Fig. 46-2.

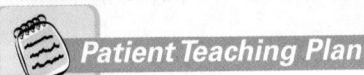

Patient Teaching Plan

Exercise and Diabetes

Have a complete medical examination before initiating a new exercise program:

- Because circulating insulin may be inadequate to ensure glucose uptake, avoid exercise when your serum glucose is greater than 250 mg/dL and ketosis is present.
- Exercise with caution if your serum glucose is greater than 300 mg/dL and no ketosis is present.
- Wear comfortable athletic shoes that provide good support.
- Before every exercise session, warm up with 5 to 10 minutes of slow, continuous aerobic exercise and stretching.
- Discuss with your physician whether to alter food or insulin intake before exercise. A general recommendation is to exercise shortly after eating or to have a small snack before exercising if your serum glucose is less than 100 mg/dL.
- Avoid exercise during the peak action of insulin and oral hypoglycemic agents when hypoglycemia is more likely to occur.
- Carbohydrate snacking may be necessary with prolonged or intense exercise.
- If you take insulin, inject it in the abdomen rather than an extremity before a workout because the drug is absorbed much more quickly from the abdomen.
- Some people experience hypoglycemia several hours after exercise; have food available for these situations.

Health Promotion Considerations

Physical Activity for People with Pre-Diabetes and Diabetes

Research has shown that physical activity has the following benefits for patients with diabetes—and for the rest of us:

- Lower blood glucose and blood pressure.
- Lower LDL cholesterol, and raise HDL cholesterol.
- Improve the body's ability to use insulin.
- Lower the risk of heart disease and stroke.
- Strengthen bones.
- Keep joints flexible.
- Lower the risk of falling.
- Aid in weight loss.
- Reduce body fat.
- Increase energy level, and reduce stress.

Physical activity also plays an important part in preventing type 2 diabetes. A major government study, the Diabetes Prevention Program, showed that a healthy diet and a moderate exercise program resulting in a 5% to 7% weight loss can delay and perhaps prevent the onset of type 2 diabetes.

For those who already have diabetes, physical activity offers all the benefits listed above. However, because some exercises may worsen diabetic complications, care should be taken in starting and maintaining an exercise program. For example, activities that increase the ocular blood pressure, such as lifting heavy weights, can worsen any existing ophthalmologic complications.

To avoid blisters that go unnoticed, leading to a serious infection, patients who walk or engage in other aerobic activities should wear cotton socks and shoes that are designed for the activity. After exercise, the feet should be checked for cuts, sores, bumps, or redness. Patients with numbness in their feet might try swimming instead of walking for aerobic exercise.

Because exercise can cause hypoglycemia, the following precautions are recommended.

Before Exercise
- Patients should be careful about exercising after skipping a recent meal.
- Patients who take insulin should ask their health care team whether they should change their dosage before engaging in physical activity.

During Exercise
- Patients should wear a medical identification bracelet or other ID.
- Patients with type II diabetes should always carry food or glucose tablets so that they are prepared to treat hypoglycemia.

If patients exercise for more than an hour, blood glucose should be checked at regular intervals.

After Exercise
- Patients should check to see how exercise affected their blood glucose level.

Adapted from the National Diabetes Information Clearinghouse, National Institute of Diabetes and Digestive and Kidney Diseases, http://diabetes.niddk.nih.gov/dm/pubs.

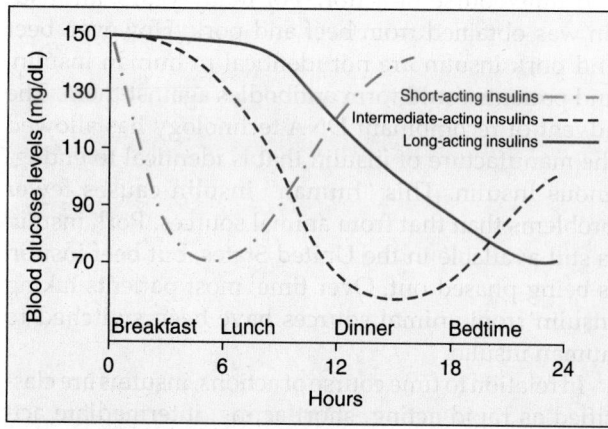

FIGURE **46-2** Effect of insulin on blood glucose levels.

Route. Insulin cannot be given orally because it is rendered useless in the gastrointestinal tract. All insulins can be given subcutaneously, but *only* Regular insulin can be given intravenously. A form of insulin that can be taken by inhalation has recently been approved but is not yet widely used. It is discussed on p. 1015 in the Intranasal Route section..

Concentrations. Insulins are available in varying concentrations. The U-100 insulin has a concentration of 100 units/mL, and U-500 has 500 units/mL. U-100 is

Pharmacology Capsule

Insulin lispro and insulin aspart act rapidly. Regular insulin is short acting, NPH and Lente insulins are intermediate acting, and Ultralente insulin is long acting. Be sure to administer the correct type!

most commonly used. U-500 insulin is used only in emergencies and for patients who are extremely insulin resistant. The insulin with the lowest concentration, U-40, meaning 40 units of insulin per milliliter, is not available in the United States.

Premixed Insulin Products. Premixed insulins that contain both Regular and NPH insulin products are available. There are three mixtures. One contains 70% NPH and 30% Regular insulin; another consists of 50% NPH and 50% Regular insulin, and the third contains 75% NPH and 25% Lispro. Premixed solutions are easier to prepare and decrease the risk of errors associated with drawing up two types of insulin in the same syringe.

Dosing Schedules. The pancreas secretes minute amounts of insulin continuously except after the ingestion of a meal, when it secretes a bolus of insulin into the system. Exogenous insulin is administered in an effort to mimic the action of a normal pancreas. Therefore

💊 | **DRUG THERAPY** *Insulin Preparations: Time Course of Action*

INSULIN TYPE	APPEARANCE	ONSET	PEAK	DURATION
RAPID-ACTING				
Insulin lispro (Humalog)	Clear	<15 minutes	1-2 hours	3-4 hours
Insulin aspart (NovoLog)	Clear	<15 minutes	1-2 hours	3-4 hours
SHORT-ACTING				
Regular insulin (Humulin R, Novolin R)	Clear	30 minutes-1 hour	2-3 hours	3-6 hours
INTERMEDIATE-ACTING				
NPH insulin	Cloudy	2-4 hours	4-10 hours	10-16 hours
LONG-ACTING				
Ultralente insulin	Cloudy	4-8 hours	Does not peak	24-36 hours
Insulin Glargine (Lantus)	Clear	1-2 hours	Does not peak	20-24 hours
INHALED RAPID-ACTING, SHORT-ACTING				
Insulin human rDNA origin (Exubera)	Powder in blister packs		30-90 minutes	

Modified from *Diabetes Forecast*, January 2005.

the person with diabetes requires a bolus of rapid- or short-acting insulin before meals to prevent too rapid a rise in glucose. A long- or intermediate-acting insulin may be prescribed as well in an effort to keep glucose levels even at other times.

Conventional Therapy. Conventional therapy uses one of several dosage schedules and typically uses a combination of a short-acting and an intermediate- or long-acting insulin. One example is the one-fifth rule some physicians use for prescribing insulin. In the morning, the patient takes two fifths of the day's supply in an intermediate-acting insulin such as NPH. In addition, the patient takes one fifth of the daily requirement of insulin as Regular insulin. The latter covers breakfast glucose. Because the NPH peaks at lunchtime, the patient does not need Regular insulin for this meal. At suppertime, the patient takes one fifth of the daily insulin requirement in the form of an intermediate-acting insulin and one fifth as rapid-acting insulin to cover supper carbohydrates. For example, a patient who is prescribed 50 units of insulin a day might take it as follows:

- AM: 20 units of NPH insulin
- AM: 10 units of Regular insulin
- PM: 10 units of NPH insulin
- PM: 10 units of Regular insulin

Another conventional dosage schedule has the patient receive two thirds of the total daily dose in the morning and the remainder late in the day. The doses are fixed so that the patient must maintain a consistent schedule and dietary intake.

Patients on conventional therapy should monitor their blood glucose before meals at least two times each day. A major problem with conventional therapy

is nocturnal hypoglycemia: blood glucose falls between 3 and 4 AM.

Intensive Therapy. Intensive therapy is designed to achieve tight control (i.e., maintain the blood glucose in the normal range). The patient's regimen may require three or four injections each day. The four-injection regimen requires rapid- or short-acting insulin before each meal and intermediate- or long-acting insulin at bedtime.

The preprandial (before meal) doses are adjusted for the caloric content of the meal. The timing of the injection depends on the type of insulin used. Rapid-acting or short-acting insulins should be taken 30 to 60 minutes before a meal, and insulin lispro should be taken within 15 minutes before eating. Dosage adjustments also can be made to accommodate physical activity. Home blood glucose monitoring is essential with this program because testing should be done three to five times daily. The intensified program permits more flexibility in meal composition and timing.

Continuous Subcutaneous Insulin Infusion. The last dosing schedule uses continuous subcutaneous insulin infusion. The patient has an indwelling subcutaneous catheter connected to an external portable infusion pump. The pump delivers Regular insulin continuously. Before meals, the patient triggers the pump to provide the appropriate amount of insulin for the meal to be consumed. Patients who use pumps also must do self-monitoring of blood glucose (SMBG).

Insulin Mixing. If the two types of insulin that the patient takes are consistent with available premixed forms, a single injection is needed for each dose. However, many patients have to mix their own insulins to achieve the exact prescribed proportion of the two insulin types.

In this case, the two types of insulin can be mixed in one syringe to avoid two injections. Suppose you were to give 20 units of Humulin N and 10 units of Humulin R in a single dose. The following are directions for mixing the two types of insulin:

1. Select vials of the prescribed insulins. The Humulin N is cloudy, and the Humulin R is clear.
2. To mix the Humulin N suspension, roll the vial of intermediate-acting insulin between your hands. Do not shake the vial because this would create bubbles.
3. Wipe tops of both vials with alcohol swabs.
4. Draw 20 units of air into a syringe and inject it into the Humulin N vial.
5. Draw 10 units of air into the syringe and inject the air into the Humulin R vial; withdraw 10 units of Humulin R into the syringe.
6. Insert the needle into the Humulin N vial, invert the vial, and withdraw 20 units of Humulin N, being careful not to inject the Humulin R insulin into the Humulin N vial.
7. If you draw up too much Humulin N, you must discard the syringe and start over.

Pharmacology Capsule

Remember "clear to cloudy!" When mixing short-acting (clear) and longer-acting (cloudy) insulins, draw the short-acting insulin into the syringe first. *NOTE:* **Insulin glargine (Lantus) cannot be mixed with other insulins!**

Insulin Injection. The suggested sites for subcutaneous insulin injections are illustrated in Figure 46-3. Site rotation helps prevent lipohypertrophy (swelling or lumps) or lipoatrophy (hollowing or pitting of the subcutaneous tissue). Patients with the latter problem should see a physician about changing the insulin to human insulin (Humulin). In some cases, injecting these sites with their prescribed daily human insulin has resolved the problem. Because lipohypertrophy interferes with the absorption of insulin, affected areas should be avoided as injection sites.

The absorption rate of insulin varies with different body sites. The rate of absorption from the abdomen is approximately 50% faster than from the thighs. For this reason, the American Diabetes Association recommends rotating sites within one anatomic area rather than moving among all areas. Heat and massage increase the absorption rate, as does exercise. As mentioned earlier, if insulin is injected into the thigh before exercise such as jogging, the absorption rate is greatly increased.

Insulin Pump. An external insulin pump looks much like a pager. It consists of a battery-driven syringe with a long piece of tubing (usually made of Teflon) that

FIGURE **46-3** Insulin injection sites.

is attached to a small needle. The needle is inserted subcutaneously in an appropriate part of the anatomy (Fig. 46-4). The syringe usually contains a 2- to 3-day supply of insulin. The pump is programmed to deliver a steady trickle of insulin throughout the day and can provide a bolus of insulin at mealtimes. In this manner, the unit mimics the pancreas. The patient calculates the bolus based on self-monitored blood glucose levels. Every 2 days, the syringe, needle, and tubing are replaced.

One advantage of the external insulin pump is that patients do not have to use intermediate- or long-acting insulins, with their uncertain fluctuations in glucose. Other advantages are that it gives the patient more flexibility regarding mealtimes, travel, and exercise. Potential problems with the pump are occlusion of the tubing or the needle and infection at the site of needle insertion. The pump also is a constant reminder that the patient has diabetes, and because it is worn externally, the patient may feel self-conscious about it. To use the pump, the patient must undergo intensive education and be willing to self-monitor blood glucose levels several times a day while on pump therapy. Some medical insurance companies do not cover the cost of the pump or pump therapy, which makes the cost prohibitive to many. Efforts to develop an "artificial pancreas" are underway. The device would be implanted under the skin and would dispense insulin in response to changing blood glucose levels.

Other less commonly used devices for insulin administration are the jet injector, pen injector, and im-

"FOR INVESTIGATIONAL USE ONLY"

B

FIGURE **46-4** Insulin pumps. **A,** MiniMED 507 external insulin pump with Quick-Release Infusion Set. **B,** MiniMED 2001 implantable insulin pump and handheld programmer.

planted insulin pump. The jet injector delivers insulin through the skin without a needle. The injection does sting and may bruise thin and older people. The high cost of the jet injector is a deterrent to its use. The pen injector looks like a fountain pen and holds preloaded cartridges with the prescribed insulin dose. Implantable pumps work like the portable pump described earlier but are surgically placed under the skin of the abdomen.

Intranasal Route. Intranasal insulin has recently been approved. Only approximately 10% of the drug is absorbed through the nasal mucosa, making it relatively expensive to use. Also, nasal irritation is a frequent side effect. The inhalation form still is being studied to determine whether there are any long-term adverse effects on the lungs. At this time, only Regular insulin is given intranasally, so the patient must still administer longer-acting insulin by injection.

Insulin Catheter. Indwelling subcutaneous catheters may be placed in the abdomen to permit repeated

insulin injections without repeated needlesticks. The catheter can remain in one location for up to 1 week. With each dose of insulin, the site should be assessed for signs of irritation or infection.

Oral Hypoglycemic (Antihyperglycemic or Antidiabetic) Agents

If patients with type 2 DM are unable to control their blood glucose with a nutrition program and exercise, the physician may prescribe one or more oral hypoglycemic agents. If the serum glucose level rises above 300 mg/dL, insulin may be prescribed temporarily until the blood glucose levels are back below 300 mg/dL. Oral hypoglycemic agents include sulfonylureas (three generations), alpha-glucosidase inhibitors, biguanides, thiazolidinediones, D-phenylalanines, and meglitinides.

Sulfonylureas. Sulfonylureas lower blood sugars by stimulating the pancreas to secrete more insulin and increasing the sensitivity of insulin receptors. First- and second-generation sulfonylureas are equally effective in controlling serum glucose but have some important differences, as shown in the Drug Therapy table on p. 1016. Because of the long duration of action, first-generation sulfonylureas are not often used now.

A significant adverse effect of the sulfonylureas is the risk of hypoglycemia. First-generation sulfonylureas also have the potential for interactions with many other drugs, which is problematic in the patient who is taking multiple medications. First-generation drugs are not recommended in patients with liver or renal disease. Because the sulfonylureas are chemically similar to sulfonamide antibacterials, patients who are allergic to one also may be allergic to the other. Be sure to assess for allergy to sulfonamides before a patient starts taking a sulfonylurea.

The second-generation drugs are more potent (so require lower dosage), pose less risk of hypoglycemia, have fewer other side effects, and have fewer drug interactions. Many older people have diminished renal and liver function, which affects metabolism and elimination of drugs, and increases the risk of hypoglycemia. When a sulfonylurea is ordered for the older patient, it is usually glipizide (Glucotrol), which must be taken on an empty stomach; glyburide (DiaBeta, Micronase); or glimepiride (Amaryl). Drugs with long durations of action are more likely to accumulate and cause toxic effects in older patients.

Alpha-Glucosidase Inhibitors. Examples of alpha-glucosidase inhibitors are acarbose (Precose) and miglitol (Glyset). These drugs delay digestion of complex carbohydrates into glucose and other simple sugars. Sometimes they are given in combination with insulin or a sulfonylurea. Side effects include abdominal cramping and distention, flatulence, and diarrhea. Acarbose does not cause hypoglycemia. However, if the patient becomes hypoglycemic because of another hypoglycemic agent taken in combination with the alpha-glucosidase

💊 **DRUG THERAPY** *Oral Hypoglycemics for Type 2 Diabetes*

DRUG CATEGORY	MEDICATION	ACTION	POSSIBLE SIDE EFFECTS
Sulfonylureas	Glipizide (Glucotrol) Glyburide (Diabeta, Micronase) Glimepiride (Amaryl)	Stimulates pancreatic secretion of insulin.	Hypoglycemia, weight gain, sulfa allergy.
Biguanides	Metformin (Glucophage, Fortamet)	Inhibits hepatic glucose production, increases insulin sensitivity.	Lactic acidosis, hypoglycemia when used with sulfonylurea or meglitinide.
Meglitinides/ D-phenylalanines	Repaglinide (Prandin) Nateglinide (Starlix)	Stimulates pancreatic secretion of insulin.	Hypoglycemia, weight gain.
Thiazolidinediones	Pioglitazone (Actos) Rosiglitazone (Avandia)	Increases insulin sensitivity in the tissues.	Hypoglycemia when used with sulfonylurea or meglitinide, weight gain, decreased effectiveness of oral contraceptives, possible liver dysfunction.
Alpha-glucosidase inhibitors	Acarbose (Precose) Miglitol (Glyset)	Delays absorption of carbohydrates in the intestine.	Gastrointestinal side effects.

Modified from Capriotti, T. (2005). Type 2 diabetes epidemic increases use of oral anti-diabetic agents, *Medsurg Nursing 14*(5), pp. 341-347.

inhibitor, oral sucrose will not effectively raise the blood sugar because the acarbose will interfere with absorption of the sucrose. The patient will instead require treatment with oral glucose.

Biguanides. Metformin (Glucophage and Fortamet) is a biguanide that decreases glucose production by the liver and increases the use of glucose by muscle cells. Adverse gastrointestinal effects are fairly common. A rare, but potentially fatal, adverse effect is lactic acidosis, which usually occurs in the presence of impaired renal function. Glucophage XR is an extended-release form of metformin that is taken only once a day instead of two or three times.

Thiazolidinediones. Thiazolidinediones are a newer class of antihyperglycemic agents that includes rosiglitazone maleate (Avandia) and pioglitazone HCl (Actos). Classified as insulin-sensitizing agents, they increase the uptake of glucose by skeletal muscle and fat tissue. These drugs do not cause hypoglycemia when used alone but may when used with a sulfonylurea. Because the first drug in this class (Rezulin) was found to have serious adverse effects on the liver, liver function must be monitored when this class of drugs is used. To date, Avandia and Actos appear to pose low risk to the liver. Side effects include weight gain, edema, and mild transient anemia. Patients should be aware that these drugs decrease the effectiveness of oral contraceptives. They are contraindicated with class 3 or 4 heart failure and during pregnancy.

Meglitinides and D-Phenylalanines. Repaglinide (Prandin) is a meglitinide, and nateglinide (Starlix) is a D-phenylalanine. Because of the similarity of these two types of drugs, called *mealtime insulin secretogogues*, they will be discussed together. Meglitinides and D-phenylalanine stimulate the release of insulin from the pancreas. Taken before each meal, they prevent postprandial blood glucose elevations and prolonged hypoglycemia. Patients should omit the medications if they skip a meal. Hypoglycemia may occur with strenuous exercise or alcohol consumption. Weight gain is a side effect. They are used cautiously with moderate to severe liver failure.

Combination Oral Medications. With increasing use of combination therapy, patients must take more medication doses—a factor that often reduces compliance. Several combination drugs have been released that help simplify dosing schedules. These medications include Actoplus Met (pioglitazone and metformin), Avandamet (rosiglitazone and metformin), Avandaryl (rosiglitazone and glimepiride), Glucovance (glyburide and metformin), and Metaglip (glipizide and metformin). The actions and side and adverse effects are the same as for each individual drug.

In 2005, two new injectable medications to treat diabetes were approved by the FDA. Pramlintide (Symlin) is a synthetic form of the hormone *amylin*, which plays a role in glucose homeostasis. Pramlintide, used to treat type 1 and type 2 diabetes, increases the risk for hypoglycemia and gastrointestinal side effects. Exenatide (Byetta) is classified as an incretin mimetic that has been shown to lower blood glucose levels by increasing insulin secretion. It is used only with type 2 diabetes. Exenatide works only in the presence of elevated glucose levels, so there is no increased risk for hypoglycemia unless the patient is also on sulfonylureas. Most individuals on this medication experience a decreased appetite and weight loss. Both of these new medications have somewhat complex dosing schedules and require injections before each meal. They are also very costly and not covered by many insurance companies.

These drugs and the newly approved inhaled insulin are detailed in the Drug Therapy table on p. 1018.

Approximately 30% to 40% of patients with type 2 diabetes fail to respond to oral agents. Another 10% cease to respond after a period of successful treatment. To maintain optimal glucose control, it is beneficial for these patients to use insulin. Some of them may have to take one dose of insulin, often at night, and then are able to control serum glucose for the rest of the day with oral drugs. A variety of combination regimens (using oral agents and insulin) are being studied.

Newly diagnosed patients with type 2 disease may be placed on insulin to bring their plasma glucose levels within normal limits. They then are placed on a diet and exercise program with or without oral agents to maintain euglycemia (blood glucose within normal range).

Self-Monitoring of Blood Glucose. People with diabetes need to monitor their blood glucose levels so they can regulate their diet, exercise, and medication regimens to remain euglycemic and lead lifestyles as normal as possible. The self-monitoring of blood glucose levels is seen as the greatest breakthrough in managing diabetes since the advent of insulin. It reduces the complications of long-term diabetes by helping the patient normalize blood glucose levels.

The use of portable electronic glucose meters has largely replaced other methods of self-monitoring. The patient puts a drop of blood on a special reagent strip and inserts the strip in the meter. In less than a minute, the glucose level appears on a monitor. Some meters give plasma glucose values, whereas others give whole blood readings. Factors that may affect the use of these meters include cost, comfort with technology, fine motor coordination, intellectual ability, and willingness to use the meter. Self-monitoring of blood glucose is a useful tool in managing diabetes during pregnancy, when glucose levels may change hourly. It also is a must in managing unstable diabetes and for patients who are prone to sudden hypoglycemic episodes or ketoacidosis or who have abnormal renal glucose thresholds.

Goals for glycemic control should be clearly set with consideration to age and co-morbidities (medical conditions in addition to DM). For nonpregnant adults, pre-meal plasma glucose levels should be between 90 and 130 mg/dL (80 and 120 mg/dL for whole blood). Bedtime plasma glucose readings should be between 110 and 150 mg/dL (100 and 140 mg/dL for whole blood). Results falling outside of these recommended parameters warrant alterations in the diabetes regimen.

Glycosylated Glucose Levels

Determination of glycosylated hemoglobin (HbA$_{1c}$) or fructosamine levels every 2 to 3 months is an essential check of glycemic control. The HbA$_{1c}$ reflects glucose levels over the past few months, whereas the fructosamine levels reflect those over several weeks. When the glucose level is elevated, a certain percentage of the glucose molecules bind to the hemoglobin on the red blood cell. The glucose stays on the cell for the life of the cell, which is approximately 3 months. By measuring HbA$_{1c}$ or fructosamine levels, the physician is able to determine how well the blood glucose has been regulated in the recent past. It also allows patients who monitor their own blood glucose levels to evaluate their methods of control. The American Diabetes Association recommends an HbA$_{1c}$ level less than 7% as a treatment goal, or as close to normal as possible without risking hypoglycemia. Less stringent control is advocated for those with episodes of severe hypoglycemia, those who are very young or very old, and those with increased co-morbidities.

Complications of Therapy

Hypoglycemia. The major complication of insulin therapy is hypoglycemia. If a person injects too much insulin, does not eat enough, eats at the wrong time, or exercises inconsistently, serum glucose levels may suddenly drop. Treatment of hypoglycemia is covered on p. 1007 in the Acute Emergency Complications section, but the main thing to remember is that the patient needs some form of glucose immediately.

Somogyi Phenomenon. Too much insulin can actually cause hyperglycemia. The Somogyi phenomenon is characterized by rebound hyperglycemia occurring in response to hypoglycemia. The phenomenon begins with an episode of hypoglycemia, often during the night. Hypoglycemia triggers the body's stress response in an attempt to restore homeostasis. Epinephrine is secreted, which stimulates the liver to convert stored glycogen to glucose, thereby raising the blood glucose level to the point of hyperglycemia.

The Somogyi phenomenon should be suspected when a patient reports awakening with a headache and complains of restless sleep, nightmares, enuresis (involuntary voiding during sleep), and nausea and vomiting. The blood glucose records reflect fluctuation between hypoglycemia and hyperglycemia. The patient may have tried without success to correct the hyperglycemia by increasing the insulin.

To confirm suspected Somogyi phenomenon, the patient's blood glucose needs to be measured between 2 and 4 AM and again at 7 AM. The 2 and 4 AM levels below 60 mg/dL and a 7 AM level above 180 mg/dL support the diagnosis of Somogyi phenomenon.

This vicious cycle can be broken by gradually decreasing the evening dose of exogenous insulin by 2 or 3 units every 3 or 4 days until the rebound hyperglycemia is brought under control. A bedtime snack also may be helpful.

Dawn Phenomenon. Some people with diabetes who are insulin dependent experience an increase in fasting blood glucose levels between 5 and 9 AM that is not related to a period of hypoglycemia. The cause is unknown, but it may reflect release of growth hormone

DRUG THERAPY | *Additional Drugs Used to Treat Diabetes Mellitus*

DRUG	ADMINISTRATION	USE	FEATURES	ACTIONS	MAJOR ADVERSE EFFECTS
INHALED RAPID-ACTING, SHORT-ACTING INSULIN					
Insulin human rDNA origin (Exubera)	Powdered drug doses in blister packs. Inhaled with a special inhaler device. Short-acting insulin; peaks in 30-90 minutes. Does not replace the need for longer-acting insulin in type 1 DM.	For type 1 DM, used with longer-acting insulin. For type 2 DM, used alone or with a longer-acting insulin or oral hypoglycemic drugs.	Should be taken within 10 minutes before a meal. Can cause hypoglycemia. Contraindicated for smokers and people with lung disease. Not yet recommended for children and teenagers.	Promotes insulin secretion by the pancreas; may also increase tissue response to insulin.	Hypoglycemia (more risk with first generation). Weight gain.
Pramlintide (Symlin)	Given by injection at mealtimes at same time as insulin, but the two cannot be mixed in the same syringe. Slows movement of food through digestive tract, which slows rate of glucose absorption. May decrease amount of insulin needed before meals.	Treats types 1 and 2 DM.	Increases risk for hypoglycemia and gastro-intestinal side effects (nausea, vomiting, stomach pain). Complex dosing schedule. Can delay absorption of other drugs. Expensive.	Decreases glucose production by liver, and increases glucose uptake by muscle.	GI symptoms: decreased appetite, nausea, diarrhea. Lactic acidosis (rarely) GI symptoms: flatulence, cramps, abdominal distention, borborygmus Hypoglycemia, but only in the presence of excessive insulin.
INCRETIN MIMETIC					
Exenatide (Byetta)	Given by injection within 1 hour before morning and evening meals. Used in addition to metformin or a sulfonylurea. Increases insulin secretion, but does not replace need for insulin in patients who require it. Works only in the presence of elevated glucose levels, so there is no increased risk for hypoglycemia unless the patient is also on sulfonylureas.	Treats type 2 DM.	Can cause hypoglycemia and gastro-intestinal side effects (decreased appetite and weight loss common, also diarrhea, nausea, vomiting), dizziness, headache. Complex dosing schedule. Comes in a prefilled pen. Expensive.	Inhibits carbo-hydrate digestion and absorption, thereby decreasing the postprandial rise in blood glucose. Decreases insulin resistance, thereby increasing glucose uptake by muscle and decreasing glucose production by the liver.	Weight gain, edema, transient anemia. Monitor liver function, even though risk of liver damage is thought to be small.

Data from U.S. Food and Drug Administration. *Diabetes Information.* www.fda.gov/diabetes/.

and cortisol, which increase blood glucose during early morning rapid eye movement sleep. The blood glucose level is typically normal at 3 AM but elevated at 6 or 7 AM. The condition may be treated with a bedtime snack and delay of the evening intermediate-acting insulin until 10 PM.

NURSING CARE of the Patient with Diabetes Mellitus

Assessment

When a person with diabetes seeks medical care in an emergency situation, a complete assessment must be delayed until the patient is stable. The LPN/LVN collects data that assist in the management of this situation. If the patient is in ketoacidosis, the assessment is likely to show ketonuria, Kussmaul's respirations, orthostatic hypotension, hypertension at times, nausea, vomiting, and lethargy or change in level of consciousness. In the hypoglycemic patient, expect to find tachycardia, anxiety, trembling, and decreasing level of consciousness. Be alert for indications of hyperosmolar nonketotic coma (decreased level of consciousness, polyuria, and polydipsia in the absence of ketosis). In each of these situations, attempt to determine the following:

- Type of diabetes
- Hypoglycemic agents: name, dosage, when last dose was taken
- Food and fluid intake for the past 3 days
- Relevant laboratory values: blood glucose, blood pH, bicarbonate levels, electrolytes, and serum and urine osmolality

Once the patient is stabilized, a complete health history and physical examination should be done by the registered nurse.

Health History

The health history focuses on the signs and symptoms of chronic hyperglycemia and possible complications. Physical and psychosocial factors that may have an impact on the patient's capacity to learn and perform self-care activities should be documented.

Chief Complaint and History of Present Illness. The patient should be asked to describe the signs and symptoms that prompted him or her to seek medical care. The patient might report unexplained weight loss, dryness of skin, vaginal itching, or sores that are slow in healing. Polyphagia, polydipsia, and polyuria, the 3 P's, are classic signs of diabetes mellitus.

Past Medical History. If the patient is known to have DM, the type and duration should be noted. The name and dosage of prescribed medications and when they were last taken should be documented. If the patient monitors blood glucose, the type of equipment used, the testing schedule, and recent test results are recorded.

The history should note diagnoses of circulatory, cardiac, or renal problems. Previous hospitalizations and surgeries are noted. If the patient is female, an ob-

stetric history is recorded, including number of pregnancies if any, outcomes of all pregnancies, and birth weights of full-term infants. For patients who had gestational diabetes, the interviewer should ask whether insulin was required or if diet and exercise maintained adequate control. Other important data to collect are immunization records and allergies.

Family History. A family history of diabetes, heart disease, stroke, hypertension, and hyperlipidemia is significant when a person has or is suspected of having DM.

Review of Systems. The review of symptoms begins with a description of the patient's general health. Changes in skin moisture or turgor are noted. To detect possible changes in the eyes associated with diabetes, the interviewer should inquire whether the patient has had floaters (dark spots that cross the field of vision), diplopia (double vision), or blurred vision or has seen white halos around objects. Significant abdominal symptoms including diarrhea, abdominal bloating, and gas are documented. Problems passing or holding urine should be noted. If the patient has had any pain in the legs, note when the pain occurs. Describe numbness, tingling, or burning sensations in the extremities. Last, the patient should be asked if he or she has experienced changes in mental alertness or seizures.

Functional Assessment. The functional assessment explores factors that can affect the patient's ability to perform self-care, including literacy, financial resources such as health insurance, and family support. The patient is asked to describe the usual pattern of activity and rest. A typical 24-hour dietary history is useful in evaluating how well the patient understands and adheres to the prescribed diet. The impact of diabetes on the patient's life should be explored, including self-concept, social relationships, and employment.

Physical Examination

In the general survey, the patient's level of consciousness, posture and gait, and apparent well-being should be noted. Vital signs, including blood pressure, and height and weight are recorded. Throughout the examination, the skin color, warmth, turgor, and lesions are noted.

The trained examiner inspects the eye grounds for evidence of diabetic retinopathy or cataracts. The vision assessment is important because visual defects may affect the patient's ability to read vital medication instructions or labels. Gross visual acuity may be assessed by having the patient read available print. Snellen's test and other more sophisticated measures also may be used to evaluate the function of the eyes. During the examination of the head and neck, the examiner should be alert for a sweet, fruity odor to the patient's breath that is common with ketoacidosis.

The feet receive special attention. Blisters, lesions, pallor, discoloration, deformities, and edema must be documented. The condition of the nails, particularly thickened or ingrown nails, should be documented. Palpating both ankles and feet simultaneously for warmth and pedal pulses helps identify poor circulation in either or both extremities. Strength in the legs is evaluated by having the patient sit and try to raise and lower each foot while the examiner applies pressure to it. Range of motion in the ankles and feet should be assessed.

Testing gait, balance, and motor coordination provides data about neurologic integrity. This is important because patients who have problems walking or feeding themselves have problems manipulating syringes and glucose monitors. Also, the lower extremities should be tested for the ability to perceive hot and cold, sharp and dull sensations, and painful stimuli.

Assessment of the patient with DM is outlined in Box 46-2.

The diagnoses below are not an exhaustive list because there may be many other nursing diagnoses if a patient has complications associated with DM. The nursing care plan must be individualized based on the assessment. Management of emergencies is discussed in the Acute Emergency Complications section beginning on p. 1006.

Nursing Diagnoses, Goals, and Outcome Criteria: Diabetes

Nursing Diagnoses	Goals and Outcome Criteria
Ineffective Health Maintenance related to lack of knowledge of dietary management of glucose, faulty metabolism, nausea and vomiting, imbalance between food intake and activity expenditure	Effective health maintenance: patient correctly describes self-care measures, maintains blood glucose within limits of 80 and 120 mg/dL, achieves optimal weight
Ineffective Therapeutic Regimen Management related to financial, personal, family pattern disruption	Effective management of self-care using prescribed treatment regimen: patient verbalizes understanding of and intent to adhere to treatment regimen; patient uses resources needed for DM management
Risk for Deficient Fluid Volume related to hyperglycemia, alterations in urine output	Normal extracellular fluid volume: patient correctly describes fluid needs, recognizes the significance of polyuria and oliguria; pulse and blood pressure remain within patient norms
Risk for Injury related to adverse effects of drugs, diminished alertness, increased susceptibility to infection	Decreased risk for injury: blood glucose 80-120 mg/dL, and absence of signs of infection (normal body temperature and white blood cell count)

Activity Intolerance related to impaired tissue perfusion, decreased mobility	Stable or improved activity tolerance: patient performs daily activities without excess fatigue
Chronic Pain related to neuropathy	Pain relief; patient states pain relieved or reduced; appears relaxed
Disturbed Sensory Perception (visual, auditory, tactile) or **Impaired Skin Integrity** related to neurologic and circulatory changes	Absence of injury associated with sensory loss: skin intact, no redness or blisters
Disturbed Thought Processes related to abnormal blood glucose, metabolic imbalances	Normal thought processes: patient is alert and oriented to person, place, and time
Ineffective Coping related to diagnosis, dietary restrictions, disturbed body image, sexual dysfunction, anxiety, fear	Effective coping: patient verbalizes feelings about diabetes and expresses willingness to follow plan of care and to use resources as needed

Interventions

Immediate nursing care of the patient with DM is geared toward urgent needs and complications. After urgent needs are met, nursing care focuses on teaching the patient to manage diabetes.

Ineffective Health Maintenance

Patient education requires that the patient understand the physiology of glucose metabolism and the signs and symptoms of hypoglycemia, ketoacidosis, and hyperglycemic hyperosmolar nonketotic coma. Teach the patient how and when to monitor blood glucose and urine ketone levels, how to interpret the results, and the appropriate actions to take based on the results. If the patient is using a glucose meter, explain and demonstrate calibration and operation of the device, collection of blood samples, and disposal of lancets.

The teaching plan also prepares the patient for self-medication as prescribed. Drug names, dosages, actions, and adverse effects are presented. If insulin is prescribed, demonstrate proper techniques for drawing up and injecting insulin and explain site rotation. Explain how adjustments in insulin or diet and exercise are used to maintain blood glucose levels between 90 and 130 mg/dL before meals and less than 180 mg/dL after meals. Not only provide verbal instruction but also allow the patient to handle equipment and demonstrate skills multiple times. If the patient cannot correctly draw up insulin, a caregiver can prepare the syringes in advance. If refrigerated, the insulin in the prefilled syringes is stable for 1 week. The syringes should be stored in a vertical or tilted

Box 46-2   ASSESSMENT of the Patient with Diabetes Mellitus

Health History

Present Illness:
Polydipsia, polyuria, polyphagia, unexplained weight loss, dry skin, vaginal itching, delayed healing, blood glucose, urine ketones

Past Health:
Established diagnosis of diabetes mellitus, type, onset; cardiovascular or renal disorders; previous hospitalizations; obstetric history: number of pregnancies, outcomes, birth weights, gestational diabetes; immunizations; allergies; and current medications: drug name(s), dosage, schedule, time last dose taken

Family History:
Diabetes, heart disease, stroke

Review of Systems:
Changes in skin moisture or turgor; changes in vision; diarrhea, abdominal bloating, gas; urine retention or incontinence; pain, tingling, or numbness in extremities; changes in mental status; seizures

Functional Assessment:
Literacy, financial resources, usual activity and rest pattern, diet, personal impact of diabetes on life. Self-monitoring of blood glucose: type equipment used, testing schedule, recent test results

Physical Examination

General Survey:
Level of consciousness, posture and gait, well-being

Vital Signs:
Tachycardia, hypertension, hypotension, Kussmaul's respirations

Height and Weight:
Current and usual

Skin:
Color, warmth, turgor, lesions

Eyes:
Changes in eye grounds, acuity

Mouth:
Sweet, fruity breath odor

Lower Extremities:
Blisters, lesions, color, edema, pulses, deformities, strength, range of motion

Neurologic:
Gait and balance; motor coordination; perception of temperature, touch, and pain

---

position (needle up) to reduce clogging of the needle. Before administering, tell the patient to pull back the plunger slightly and gently rock the syringe to remix the solution.

Advise the patient to consult the physician or pharmacist before taking new medications, because many medications interact with drugs given for diabetes.

Consult the dietitian regarding diet, and reinforce nutritional information. During hospitalization, record food intake. Details of medical and dietary management are presented on p. 1009 in the Medical Treatment section.

Ideally, you should present small units of content in each teaching session. Unfortunately, there may be time to provide the patient only with "survival skills" during a brief or busy hospitalization. Therefore verbal instructions should be accompanied by written material and/or videotapes, CDs, or DVDs and information about local resources such as the hospital's certified diabetes educator and the local chapter of the American Diabetes Association. Office nurses, community health nurses, and home health nurses also often participate in teaching the patient with diabetes.

Ineffective Therapeutic Regimen Management

When a patient has had diabetes education but does not follow the prescribed plan, explore possible barriers to carrying out the plan. Some patients may think the program is too hard to follow and not even try. Others may think complications are inevitable and that treatment will not really make a difference. Another reason for noncompliance is lack of financial resources for drugs, supplies, and a balanced diet. Nursing interventions depend on the barriers identified. They are designed to provide practical help, support, and encouragement.

Teach family members how to support and help the family member with diabetes. Treat the family as integral members of the health care team. It is especially important in the nutrition teaching to include the person who does the shopping and cooking. A referral to social services is necessary if the patient cannot afford syringes and insulin. A referral to a diabetes educator, home health nurse, or community health nurse for follow-up teaching and monitoring also is recommended.

Risk for Deficient Fluid Volume

Teach the patient the relationship between blood glucose and urine output. Explain that abnormally increased output may signal hyperglycemia and may eventually lead to dehydration and ketoacidosis.

Pharmacology Capsule

Many drugs can affect blood glucose. For example, beta-adrenergic blockers lower the blood glucose and hydrochlorothiazides raise it.

Risk for Injury

Advise the patient to keep immunizations current because of increased susceptibility to infection and impaired healing. Teach patients to see a physician promptly if they have signs and symptoms of infection such as fever, cough, painful urination, or lesions with purulent drainage.

On sick days, insulin or oral agents should be taken as usual and blood glucose checked every 2 to 4 hours. If the blood glucose exceeds 250 mg/dL, urine should be tested for ketones. Glucose levels greater than 300 mg/dL or ketonuria should be reported to the physician. Patients with type 1 disease may need additional insulin. To prevent dehydration and ketoacidosis, the patient should eat 10 to 15 gm of carbohydrates every 1 to 2 hours and drink small amounts of fluid every 15 to 30 minutes: 4 ounces of orange or apple juice, non-diet soda, or Jell-O provides approximately 15 gm of carbohydrates. If nausea and vomiting occur, suggest soft foods or liquids instead of solid foods. Tell the patient to report nausea, vomiting, and diarrhea to the physician at once because severe fluid loss may occur. The patient who is unable to retain oral fluids may require hospitalization to restore fluid and electrolyte balance.

Activity Intolerance

An exercise regimen can be designed with the hospital rehabilitation department. "All things in moderation" is the best rule of thumb. Lack of exercise or too vigorous activity just before bedtime may contribute to sleeplessness. Details about the effects of exercise on blood glucose and activity recommendations are discussed on pp. 1010 to 1011 in the Exercise section.

Chronic Pain

Leg pain due to long-term complications may require analgesics. Document pain, administer medications as ordered, and evaluate effects of interventions. If the patient is taking analgesics at home, explain how the medication is to be taken and any significant side effects such as drowsiness.

Disturbed Sensory Perception or Impaired Skin Integrity

Instruct the patient on the importance of having yearly eye examinations. The patient should inform the ophthalmologist of the diagnosis of diabetes. If the patient has impaired vision, audiotapes, CDs, special reading materials, and special devices for preparing and administering insulin and for testing blood glucose may be needed.

If the patient has a hearing problem, give directions while facing the patient at eye level and speak clearly. Ask the patient to repeat or demonstrate instructions to make sure that they were heard correctly. Supplement verbal information and demonstrations with written material.

Alterations in tactile sensations may result in burns or frostbite. The patient and the family need to be aware of the danger of impaired sensation. Instruct the patient to avoid injury from heat or cold when outdoors in extreme weather. Caution the patient about the possibility of burns when using heating pads or electric blankets, working around a hot stove, or sitting next to a hot radiator. When taking a bath, measure the temperature of the bath water with a bath thermometer. The temperature should not exceed 43° C (109.4° F). Tissue may be burned before the patient is aware of the excessive heat.

The patient or someone else should examine the patient's feet daily for signs of trauma. Injuries or blisters should be seen promptly by a physician. Foot care for the diabetic is summarized in the Patient Teaching Plan on p. 1023.

Disturbed Thought Processes

Disturbed thought processes may be due to hypoglycemia, ketoacidosis, or HHNKS. Without treatment, the hypoglycemic patient may be irritable at first, then confused, irrational, and lethargic, and eventually comatose. In ketoacidosis, the patient becomes drowsy and the level of consciousness decreases and may progress to coma. HHNKS also is characterized by altered levels of consciousness, progressing from confusion to coma. Emergency and medical treatments are covered on p. 1008 in the Acute Emergency Complications section.

When the patient is confused or disoriented, first initiate actions to determine the cause and seek appropriate medical care. Meanwhile, have someone remain with the patient to ensure safety until the condition improves. Because of the risk of disturbed thought processes, people with diabetes should wear a medical alert tag. The tag identifies the patient as having diabetes so that medical attention will be sought.

Ineffective Coping

Patients may be anxious about the immediate and long-term effects of diabetes and how it will affect their lives. They may be overwhelmed by what they need to learn for self-care. They also may be fearful about lifestyle changes, self-medication, glucose testing, adverse drug effects, and possible complications. Encourage patients to express these concerns so that they can be addressed. Talking with other people who are coping successfully with diabetes can have positive effects.

Encourage patients to express their feelings regarding diabetes and to ask for help or advice when needed. Make every effort to encourage them to resume normal activities and to continue their usual social activities. Help patients identify their strengths and weaknesses and explore coping strategies for managing areas of concern.

One source of stress to some patients is altered sexual function. Listen to the patient's concerns and encourage consultation with the physician on the matter. Altered sexual function may be due to diabetes, but there also may be other causes. Some diagnostic procedures may be done to assess erectile dysfunction. For irreversible erectile dysfunction, the physician can offer the male patient several options (see Chapter 48). Research is ongoing into treatments for female dysfunction. You can explore with the patient the importance of sexual intercourse and his or her willingness to consider alternative means of sexual expression. Patients and their partners may wish to seek counseling from therapists with expertise in sexual dysfunction.

Patient teaching for self-medication cannot be done at the last minute. Supplement teaching with written material and information about outpatient resources.

See the Nursing Care Plans for The Patient with Type 1 Diabetes Mellitus and The Patient with Type 2 Diabetes Mellitus on pp. 1024 to 1027.

HYPOGLYCEMIA

PATHOPHYSIOLOGY

Hypoglycemia may result from causes other than the pharmacologic treatment for diabetes. Regulation of blood glucose depends on insulin levels, available glucagon, and the secretion of catecholamines, growth hormone, and cortisol. Hypoglycemia may occur if there are abnormalities in these regulators. Hypoglycemia is defined as a syndrome that develops when the blood

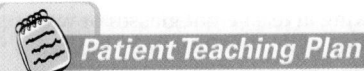

Patient Teaching Plan

Diabetes Mellitus

- Learn the names of your prescribed drugs, dosages and schedule, and (if on insulin) technique for injections.
- Take some form of carbohydrate if you have symptoms of hypoglycemia: nervousness, palpitations, hunger.
- Monitoring your blood glucose helps you see how well your diabetes is being controlled.
- We will teach you how to check your blood glucose and interpret the findings, and what actions, if any, to take.
- Nutrition is an important part of managing your diabetes. The dietitian will discuss dietary guidelines with you.
- Regular exercise helps control your blood glucose and improves circulation.
- Because your feet are susceptible to injury and may not heal well, wear properly fitting shoes, inspect feet daily, and immediately seek medical care for wounds, blisters, and calluses.
- When you are sick, monitor your blood glucose and urine ketones; continue your insulin (if taking), take in carbohydrates that provide 10 to 15 gm of carbohydrates every 1 to 2 hours, and take small amounts of fluids every 15 to 30 minutes.
- Although there is no cure for diabetes at this time, you can reduce your risk of complications with good management.

glucose level falls to less than 45 to 50 mg/dL. Symptoms can occur at different blood levels according to individual tolerances and how rapidly the level falls. The causes of hypoglycemia may be divided into three categories: exogenous, endogenous, and functional.

Summaries of each of these three categories are presented in Table 46-1. *Exogenous hypoglycemia* results from outside factors acting on the body to produce a low blood glucose. These include insulin, oral hypoglycemic agents, alcohol, or exercise. *Endogenous hypoglycemia* occurs when internal factors cause an excessive secretion of insulin or an increase in glucose metabolism. These conditions may be related to tumors or genetics.

Functional hypoglycemia may result from a variety of causes, including gastric surgery, fasting, or malnutrition. Alimentary hypoglycemia occurs in a patient who has undergone gastric surgery. The gastric contents empty rapidly, resulting in increased glucose absorption. In response to the increased glucose, excessive insulin production occurs, causing the hypoglycemia. In impaired glucose tolerance hypoglycemia, there is an excessive response of insulin to glucose. Spontaneous reactive hypoglycemia has received much publicity by the lay and medical communities alike. Symptoms occur as a result of an extreme insulin response to ingestion of foods containing carbohydrates. Low blood glucose levels need to be verified for the diagnosis to be accepted.

SIGNS AND SYMPTOMS

Signs and symptoms of hypoglycemia vary according to how quickly the blood glucose levels are falling. When the levels fall rapidly, epinephrine, cortisol, glucagon, and growth hormone are secreted by the body in an attempt to increase glucose levels. Symptoms that result from these physiologic responses include weakness, hunger, diaphoresis, tremors, anxiety, irritability, headache, pallor, and tachycardia. The symptoms of a blood glucose level that falls over several hours are attributed to lack of essential glucose to brain tissue. These symptoms include confusion, weakness, dizziness, blurred or double vision, seizure, and, in severe cases, coma.

MEDICAL DIAGNOSIS

The diagnosis of hypoglycemia not associated with diabetes can be based on fasting blood glucose, OGTT, intravenous glucose tolerance test, and 72-hour inpatient fasting. The diagnosis should be based on three criteria known as *Whipple's triad:* (1) the presence of symptoms, (2) documentation of low blood glucose when symptoms occur, and (3) improvement of these symptoms when blood glucose rises. These criteria must occur in the absence of sulfonylurea treatment or abnormal plasma insulin and C-peptide.

MEDICAL TREATMENT

Treatment of hypoglycemia depends on the cause of the problem and the patient's condition. In an unconscious patient who has diabetes, hypoglycemia

NURSING CARE PLAN

The Patient with Type 1 Diabetes Mellitus

ASSESSMENT

Health History: A 17-year-old female who has recently been diagnosed with type 1 diabetes mellitus is hospitalized to begin her insulin therapy and stabilize her blood glucose. She sought medical attention because of persistent thirst and increased urination. She has no other health problems but has had frequent upper respiratory infections the past few years. The review of systems reveals periodic blurred vision, itching, increased appetite, weight loss of 7 pounds in 3 months, and fatigue.

Physical Examination: Vital signs: temperature, 98.4° F orally; pulse, 88; respiration, 14; blood pressure, 92/58. Height, 5′2″. Weight, 107 lb. Physical findings are all within normal limits.

Nursing Diagnosis	Goals and Outcome Criteria	Interventions
Ineffective Health Maintenance related to lack of knowledge of diabetes management	The patient will correctly describe type 1 diabetes and its treatment. The patient will demonstrate self-medication, meal planning, and understanding of management of exercise and drug effects.	Explain the physiology of glucose metabolism, signs and symptoms of ketoacidosis, and hypoglycemia. Teach to perform self-monitoring of blood glucose and urine ketone testing and how to interpret results. Explain insulin types, actions, and administration. Have patient practice insulin injection. Explain relationship between diet, exercise, insulin, and blood glucose. Obtain dietary consult regarding diet. Monitor food intake, and replace food not eaten with substitute identified by dietitian.
Ineffective Therapeutic Regimen Management related to financial, personal, or family pattern disruption	The patient will express intent to adhere to prescribed regimen of care.	Request patient education by certified diabetes educator if available. If not, present information in a positive manner and in small units. Identify barriers to self-management. Determine resources and sources of support. Have patient repeat aspects of care and consequences of nonadherence to program. Acknowledge difficulty in making major changes in eating and activity patterns and in administering self-injections. Identify community resources such as the local chapter of the American Diabetes Association. Teach the patient and family members to recognize and respond to hypoglycemia and ketoacidosis.
Deficient Fluid Volume related to altered urine output	The patient will maintain normal blood volume, as evidenced by normal tissue turgor, pulse, and blood pressure.	Stress the importance of drinking at least eight glasses of water daily. Point out that excessive urine output may indicate hyperglycemia. Assess hydration, including tissue turgor, mucous membrane moisture, and vital signs.
Risk for Injury related to adverse effects of drugs, increased susceptibility to infection	The patient's blood glucose will remain within goal range established by physician. The patient will state measures to reduce risk of infection and will identify symptoms that should be reported to the physician.	Teach patient to recognize signs and symptoms of hypoglycemia: shakiness, nervousness, irritability, tachycardia, anxiety, light-headedness, hunger, tingling or numbness of lips and tongue. Instruct to take concentrated sugar if hypoglycemia occurs, followed by a complex carbohydrate (milk, bread) to prevent rebound hypoglycemia. The patient should contact the physician if ill and unable to take food or fluids. Caution the patient that impaired sensation could develop in the extremities and that healing of injuries may be impaired. Encourage to avoid trauma and to inspect the feet daily to detect any injuries.
Activity Intolerance related to metabolic imbalance	The patient will perform usual activities of daily living and carry out planned exercise program without excess fatigue.	An exercise regimen is built into the plan of care. Exercise must be done as part of a regular routine. Tell the patient to avoid injecting insulin into a body area that will be affected by exercise soon after the injection. Patient should not exercise during peak insulin activity and should eat a snack before or during exercise if the blood glucose is <100 mg/dL to avoid hypoglycemia.
Disturbed Sensory Perception (visual) related to abnormal serum glucose	The patient will report correction of blurred vision.	Advise the patient that blurred vision may be due to hyperglycemia. Encourage annual ophthalmologic examination to detect vision changes or problems.

NURSING CARE PLAN
The Patient with Type 1 Diabetes Mellitus—cont'd

Nursing Diagnosis	Goals and Outcome Criteria	Interventions
Disturbed Thought Processes related to abnormal serum glucose	The patient will continue to be alert and fully oriented.	Monitor the patient's mental status. Recognize confusion as a sign of abnormal serum glucose. Tell the patient and family that mental changes are best treated with carbohydrates. If the patient does not improve, the blood glucose should be measured and medical attention must be sought.
Ineffective Coping related to diagnosis, dietary restrictions, disturbed body image, anxiety, and fear	The patient will identify concerns about living with diabetes mellitus and plan strategies for dealing with it.	Encourage the patient to express feelings about diabetes and to ask questions. Assure her that most regular activities can be resumed. Identify the patient's strengths and resources. Explore knowledge about diabetes and any misconceptions. Tell her that pregnancy must be carefully monitored but that it is a future option. Offer support groups if available.

? CRITICAL THINKING QUESTIONS

- How are type 1 and type 2 diabetes alike, and how are they different?

- Diagram the mechanisms by which the body tries to adapt to (1) high blood glucose, and (2) low blood glucose.

- Describe the signs and symptoms of ketoacidosis and hypoglycemia.

---

should be suspected until it is ruled out. Fifty milliliters of 50% glucose solution should be administered IV immediately. The patient with a milder form of hypoglycemia is treated with 15 gm of carbohydrate. If the patient's condition does not improve, another 15 gm of carbohydrate should be given after 10 minutes. Giving more than 15 gm initially may lead to rebound hyperglycemia. In terms of food exchanges, one bread exchange contains 15 gm of carbohydrate, one fruit exchange contains 15 gm of carbohydrate, and one milk exchange contains 12 gm of carbohydrate.

Prevention of hypoglycemia by proper food intake is an important treatment component. The diet is directed by the underlying cause. If the cause is related to an overproduction of insulin after carbohydrate ingestion, a low-carbohydrate, high-protein diet is commonly ordered. Restriction of carbohydrates to no more than 100 gm/day is recommended. Simple sugars are avoided, and complex carbohydrates are encouraged. Because no significant increase in blood glucose is noted with protein ingestion, a high-protein diet is recommended. The remaining calories in the diet are obtained from fat. Because carbohydrates are restricted, the calories required from fat are high. Patients may tolerate smaller, more frequent meals. Alcohol should be avoided. Remember, hypoglycemia associated with treatment of diabetes uses different guidelines for treatment.

NURSING CARE of the Patient with Hypoglycemia
Assessment

The health history is especially important in the diagnosis of hypoglycemia. Describe the present illness, which may include the following symptoms: shakiness, nervousness, irritability, tachycardia, anxiety, lightheadedness, hunger, tingling or numbness of the lips or tongue, nightmares, and crying out during sleep. Note when the episodes occur in relation to meals and particular food intake. The past medical history documents diabetes, previous gastric surgery, abdominal cancer, or adrenal insufficiency. Record medications, paying particular attention to hypoglycemic agents. Note the names of hypoglycemic agents, prescribed dose, and the time that the last dose was taken. The functional assessment elicits information about current diet, exercise, alcohol intake, and the effects of symptoms on daily activities. Important aspects of the physical examination include general behavior, appearance, pulse, and blood pressure.

Nursing Diagnoses, Goals, and Outcome Criteria: Hypoglycemia	
NURSING DIAGNOSES	GOALS AND OUTCOME CRITERIA
Deficient Knowledge of management of hypoglycemia	Patient understands and can manage hypoglycemic episodes: the patient accurately describes and demonstrates self-care measures
Risk for Injury related to episodes of dizziness and weakness	Absence of injury: no falls or injuries as a result of hypoglycemic episodes
Impaired Adjustment related to effects of illness on lifestyles	Adjustment to living with hyperglycemia: patient describes and practices measures to manage hypoglycemia

NURSING CARE PLAN
The Patient with Type 2 Diabetes Mellitus

ASSESSMENT

Health History: An 80-year-old Latino was seen in her physician's office and diagnosed with type 2 diabetes mellitus. A referral has been made to a home health agency. The assessment was done in the patient's home. She is three blocks from a grocery store, which also has a pharmacy. Her physician prescribed glyburide (Micronase), 2.5 mg daily before breakfast. Mrs. Garcia sought medical treatment for fatigue, weight loss (10 lb in 2 months), and symptoms of a urinary tract infection. Mrs. Garcia has a history of hypertension, which is treated with verapamil, and venous insufficiency. When asked, she states she has had some problems with her vision and vaginal pruritus. She reports that her appetite is very good, so she could not understand why she was losing weight. Her usual diet is primarily Mexican-American food, but she reports trying not to eat "too much fat." She expresses concern that a diabetic diet will be too expensive because she has only Social Security income. She said that her father died of a heart attack at age 57, and her mother died at age 73 from kidney failure. One of her brothers has diabetes mellitus, one is deceased from heart disease, and a third is alive and well at age 70. Mrs. Garcia says her symptoms have interfered with performance of usual daily activities and that she is getting up frequently during the night to void, which has affected the quality of her rest. She is a widow who lives alone. She has four adult children, but only one lives in the same city and visits her mother on weekends.

Physical Examination: Vital signs: temperature, 97° F orally; pulse, 86; respiration, 16; blood pressure, 160/95. Patient is alert and oriented. Her skin is dry, and tissue turgor is poor. She has kyphosis and walks slowly. Heart and breath sounds are normal; 2+ edema in both legs. Popliteal pulses are weak; pedal pulses are not palpable. Skin is dark around the ankles. Feet are cool. Capillary return in toenails is 4 seconds. Toenails are unevenly cut. There is a reddened area on one heel, but she says it is not painful.

Nursing Diagnosis	Goals and Outcome Criteria	Interventions
Ineffective Health Maintenance related to lack of knowledge of dietary management of DM, drug therapy, and self-monitoring	The patient will demonstrate the ability to adhere to prescribed diet and drug therapy and to monitor blood glucose.	Assess the patient's understanding of her condition and treatment, and explore her attitude toward managing type 2 diabetes. Assess gross visual acuity, and assist her to get an eye examination and corrective lenses as needed. Contact local Lions Club if she cannot afford prescribed lenses. Design a teaching plan to explain key aspects of care. Emphasize skills needed immediately: how to take medications, what foods to avoid, and how to recognize and treat hypoglycemia. If home blood glucose monitoring is prescribed, practice the process with the patient and evaluate her ability to perform the test and interpret the results. Develop a plan with the patient to cover additional topics. Discuss home health referral with physician.
Ineffective Therapeutic Regimen Management related to financial limitations and difficulties with transportation for food, drugs, and medical care	The patient will manage her prescribed diet and drug therapy.	Assess any barriers the patient perceives to managing her prescribed diet and drug therapy. If there are financial problems, consult a social worker or determine what assistance is available. If transportation and shopping are difficult, explore how daughter can help or provide information about public transportation available for older adults and the disabled. Provide dietary information that incorporates Mexican dishes. Discuss the advantages of using senior nutrition programs or Meals-on-Wheels to provide some meals and ease the burden of food preparation. Monitor weight and blood glucose to assess effects of treatment.
Risk for Injury related to adverse effects of drugs, circulatory impairment, decreased sensation, and increased susceptibility to infection	The patient will take measures to reduce the risk of injury associated with hypoglycemia, inadequate circulation, and diminished sensation; the patient will remain free of fever.	Explain the importance of eating properly while on oral medications that lower the blood glucose. Describe the related signs and symptoms, and advise the patient to consume a glucose source such as sweetened orange juice to reverse hypoglycemia. Stress the importance of contacting the physician if ill and unable to take oral food and fluids. Explain how diabetes affects the blood vessels and nerves, making the extremities especially vulnerable to injury. Emphasize the importance of protecting the feet from injury by wearing properly fitting shoes and keeping the nails trimmed correctly. She should be told to avoid heating pads and to test bath water with a bath thermometer. Advise her to have foot care done by a physician or other specialist (see Patient Teaching Plan on p. 1023).

NURSING CARE PLAN

The Patient with Type 2 Diabetes Mellitus—cont'd

Nursing Diagnosis	Goals and Outcome Criteria	Interventions
Activity Intolerance related to fatigue, venous insufficiency, and circulatory impairment	The patient will resume previous level of activity without excessive fatigue.	Assess energy level. Explore usual day, and discuss ways to conserve energy.
Ineffective Coping related to diagnosis of serious chronic illness that requires alterations in daily life	The patient will demonstrate effective coping with management of diabetes.	Encourage patient to share her thoughts and feelings about having diabetes and her ability to deal with it. Assure her that many older people learn to manage quite well and that resources are available to help her. Communicate with her frequently until her confidence increases. Let her know how she can reach ready sources of information.

? CRITICAL THINKING QUESTIONS

- What effect does nutrition have with regard to blood glucose?

- What barriers might the patient perceive to managing diet and drug therapy?

Table 46-1   Exogenous, Endogenous, and Functional Causes of Hypoglycemia in Adults

CAUSES	PREDISPOSING FACTORS	OCCURRENCE
EXOGENOUS CAUSES		
Insulin	Intentional or accidental overdose; may be combined with inadequate food intake, usually increased exercise, decrease in insulin requirement, or potentiating medications	Most frequent cause of hypoglycemia
Oral hypoglycemic agents	Intentional or accidental overdose; may be combined with inadequate food intake, increased exercise, or potentiating medications	Frequent cause of hypoglycemia with sulfonylureas and meglitinides
Alcohol	Particularly likely in chronically malnourished or acutely food-deprived people	Occurs within 6-36 hr of ingesting moderate to large amounts of alcohol
Exercise	Increased duration and intensity of exercise increases glucose uptake and normally decreases insulin secretion	Occurs with both insulin sulfonylurea administration and intense exercise, but may be unpredictable in onset
ENDOGENOUS CAUSES		
Organic hypoglycemia	Insulinoma (a tumor of the beta cells of the pancreatic islets of Langerhans)	Uncommon neoplasm of beta cells of islets of Langerhans
Extrapancreatic neoplasms	May be mesenchymal tumors, hepatomas, adrenocortical carcinomas, gastrointestinal tumors, lymphomas, or leukemias	Rare; most common in adults 40-70 yrs of age
FUNCTIONAL CAUSES		
Alimentary hypoglycemia	Rapid dumping of carbohydrates into upper small intestine	Postgastrectomy
Drug related (ethanol, haloperidol, pentamidine, salicylates) reactive hypoglycemia	Syndrome with symptoms such as diaphoresis, tachycardia, tremulousness, headache, fatigue, drowsiness, and irritability	Rarely diagnosed throughout the world; widely diagnosed in the United States, prompting American Diabetes Association and Endocrine Society to issue statement that entity is probably overdiagnosed
Abrupt discontinuation of hyperalimentation	Drinking alcohol on an empty stomach	More common with drinks containing both alcohol and glucose or saccharin (e.g., beer; gin and tonic; rum and cola; whiskey and ginger ale)

Modified from Shamoon, H. (2001). Hypoglycemia. In P. Felig, J.D. Baxter, A.E. Broadus, & L. Frohman (Eds.). *Endocrinology and metabolism* (4th ed.). New York. McGraw Hill.

Continued

Table 46-1 *Exogenous, Endogenous, and Functional Causes of Hypoglycemia in Adults —cont'd*

CAUSES	PREDISPOSING FACTORS	OCCURRENCE
FUNCTIONAL CAUSES—cont'd		
Rapid discontinuation of total parenteral alimentation	Endocrine deficiency states (cortisol, growth hormone, glucagons, epinephrine)	Easily prevented
Glucocorticoid deficiency	Critical illness (cardiac, hepatic, and renal disease)	A danger for any person with adrenal insufficiency
Severe liver deficiency	Insufficient glucose output by liver	Fasting hypoglycemia
Lack of body stores for protein, fat, and carbohydrates	Profound malnutrition	Common; also found with relative frequency in kwashiorkor
Prolonged muscular exercise	Metabolism of energy-producing substances	Occurs if exercise is too prolonged or severe or if nutritional intake and carbohydrate stores are insufficient

Modified from Shamoon, H. (2001). Hypoglycemia. In P. Felig, J.D. Baxter, A.E. Broadus, & L. Frohman (Eds.). *Endocrinology and metabolism* (4th ed.). New York. McGraw Hill.

Interventions

Deficient Knowledge

Patient education is a priority after a confirmed diagnosis to prevent future occurrences. Teach patients to recognize the signs and symptoms and to treat them promptly. Advise the patient of factors that may trigger hypoglycemic episodes, such as foods, medications, alcohol, fasting, and exercise. Basic concepts of the diet described earlier need to be stressed and reinforced. A referral for a consultation with a registered dietitian may be helpful for the patient. As a patient educator, you are very influential in promoting self-monitoring and treatment of hypoglycemia.

Risk for Injury

The hypoglycemic patient is at risk for injury as a result of weakness and dizziness. Be alert for signs and symptoms of hypoglycemia. Monitor serum glucose levels. Administer carbohydrates as prescribed by the physician. Until the episode passes, keep the patient in bed with the side rails up and the call bell nearby. Advise the patient not to get up unassisted.

Impaired Adjustment

Emotional support for the patient with hypoglycemia is necessary during both diagnosis and treatment. Prepare the patient for diagnostic tests, and tell the patient what to expect. Once the diagnosis is made, explore the patient's feelings and concerns. Support the patient in learning to incorporate management of hypoglycemia into his or her lifestyle. Guide the patient to anticipate problem situations and possible solutions.

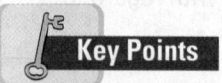

Key Points

- Diabetes mellitus is a condition characterized by impaired metabolism related to tissue resistance to insulin or insulin deficiency.
- Diabetes mellitus is managed with diet, exercise, and insulin and/or oral hypoglycemic agents.
- The major complications of diabetes mellitus are ketoacidosis, hyperosmolar nonketotic coma, vascular changes, and neuropathy.
- Ketoacidosis causes dehydration, electrolyte imbalance, and metabolic acidosis and is treated with fluid and electrolyte replacement and insulin.
- Hyperosmolar nonketotic coma is loss of consciousness due to extremely high serum glucose without ketoacidosis.
- The major complications of insulin therapy are hypoglycemia, insulin shock, and hyperglycemia (Somogyi effect).
- Nursing care of the patient with diabetes mellitus focuses on Ineffective Health Maintenance, Ineffective Therapeutic Regimen Management, Deficient Fluid Volume, Risk for Injury, Activity Intolerance, Chronic Pain, Disturbed Sensory Perception, Disturbed Thought Processes, and Ineffective Coping.
- Hypoglycemia (low serum glucose) in the absence of diabetes mellitus can be caused by pancreatic tumors, adrenal insufficiency, liver disease, and pituitary disorders, but sometimes no specific cause is identified.
- Nursing care of the nondiabetic patient who has hypoglycemia focuses on Deficient Knowledge, Risk for Injury, and Impaired Adjustment.

Go to your Companion CD-ROM for a Pharmacology Tutorial, Audio Glossary, and 3-D animations.

 Be sure to visit the companion Evolve site at http://evolve.elsevier.com/Linton/ for WebLinks and additional online resources.

REVIEW QUESTIONS *Choose the best answer.*

1. A function of insulin is to:
   1. Serve as an energy source
   2. Help transport glucose into cells
   3. Metabolize glucose for energy
   4. Eliminate excess serum glucose

2. The incidence of diabetes mellitus is greatest among people of which ethnicity?
   1. Hispanic
   2. African
   3. European
   4. Asian

3. One type of macrovascular complication of diabetes mellitus is:
   1. Retinopathy
   2. End-stage renal disease
   3. Neuropathy
   4. Coronary artery disease

4. You are collecting data from a patient who has had type 2 diabetes mellitus for 10 years. He complains of dizziness when rising to a standing position and increasing fatigue with his usual exercise program. His vital signs are normal except for a heart rate of 108. You should report these data to the registered nurse because you suspect:
   1. Coronary artery disease
   2. Inadequate control of blood glucose
   3. Autonomic neuropathy
   4. Hyperglycemic episodes

5. A patient who has just been diagnosed with diabetes and started on oral medications says, "I feel strange and my mouth feels numb. Something is wrong!" You note that his hands are trembling and that he is perspiring. What is your best response?
   1. These are common symptoms of diabetes. They will go away soon.
   2. Let's check your blood sugar. It is probably low.
   3. Your doctor will probably need to increase your medication dose.
   4. This is very unusual. I will call your physician.

6. What is the rationale for limiting protein intake in the patient with diabetes mellitus?
   1. Metabolism of excess protein causes ketoacidosis.
   2. Protein needs are decreased because excess glucose meets metabolic needs.
   3. High protein intake interferes with absorption of other nutrients.
   4. High protein intake indirectly contributes to the development of nephropathy.

7. The advantage of human insulin over beef and pork insulin is:
   1. Human insulin is less expensive
   2. People do not form antibodies for human insulin
   3. Human insulin has a longer duration of action
   4. Human insulin does not cause hypoglycemia

8. Which type of oral medication is least likely to cause hypoglycemia?
   1. Alpha-glucosidase inhibitors
   2. Sulfonylureas
   3. Meglitinides
   4. D-phenylalanines

9. The classic signs and symptoms of diabetes mellitus are:
   1. Thirst, tachycardia, tremor
   2. Hyperglycemia, hyponatremia, hyperkalemia
   3. Polyphagia, polydipsia, polyuria
   4. Nephropathy, retinopathy, neuropathy

10. A patient who was newly diagnosed with diabetes says, "Everyone I know with diabetes has had one or both legs amputated." What is the most appropriate reply?
    1. "Try not to think about that."
    2. "Most people with diabetes eventually have to have amputations."
    3. "The ones who had amputations did not follow their doctor's orders."
    4. "There are many things you can do to reduce your risk of future amputations."

47 Female Reproductive Disorders

Objectives

After reading and studying this chapter, you should be able to:

1. List data to be collected when assessing the female reproductive system.
2. Describe the nursing interventions for women who are undergoing diagnostic tests and procedures for reproductive system disorders.
3. Identify the nursing interventions associated with douche, cauterization, heat therapy, and topical medications used to treat disorders of the female reproductive system.
4. Explain the pathophysiology, signs and symptoms, complications, diagnostic procedures, and medical or surgical treatment for selected disorders of the female reproductive system.
5. Assist in developing a nursing care plan for patients with common disorders of the female reproductive system.
6. Describe the nursing interventions for the patient who is menopausal.

Key Terms

Be sure to check out the bonus material on the Companion CD-ROM, including selected audio pronunciations.

cystocele (SĬS-tō-sēl, p. 1058)
dysmenorrhea (dĭs-mĕn-ō-RĒ-ă, p. 1053)
dyspareunia (dĭs-pă-ROO-nē-ă, p. 1050)
dysplasia (dĭs-PLĀ-sē-ă, p. 1035)
endometriosis (ĕn-dō-mē-trē-Ō-sĭs, p. 1052)
hysterectomy (hĭs-tĕr-ĔK-tō-mē, p. 1053)
mastitis (măs-TĪ-tĭs, p. 1048)
menarche (mĕ-NĂR-kē, p. 1032)
menopause (MĔN-ō-păwz, p. 1033)
menorrhagia (mĕn-ō-RĀ-jă, p. 1044)
metrorrhagia (mĕ-trō-RĀ-jă, p. 1044)
rectocele (RĔK-tō-sēl, p. 1058)
retroversion (RĔT-rō-vĕr-zhŭn, p. 1061)
salpingo-oophorectomy (săl-pĭng-gō-ō-ŎF-ō-RĔK-tō-mē, p. 1053)
vaginitis (vă-jĭ-NĪ-tĭs, p. 1045)
vulvitis (vŭl-VĪ-tĭs, p. 1045)

The female reproductive system includes external and internal genitalia and the breasts. The term *vulva* refers to the external genitalia, which comprise the mons pubis, labia majora, labia minora, clitoris, and pudendum (Fig. 47-1). Also included in the vulva are mucus-secreting glands. Bartholin's glands are located on both sides of the posterior edge of the vaginal opening, and Skene's glands are located just inside the urethral opening. The perineum is the area between the posterior junction of the labia minora and the anus. The internal genitalia include two ovaries, two fallopian tubes, the uterus, and the vagina (Fig. 47-2).

ANATOMY AND PHYSIOLOGY OF THE FEMALE REPRODUCTIVE SYSTEM

EXTERNAL GENITALIA

The mons pubis is a pad of fatty tissue that covers and protects the symphysis pubis. The labia majora are extensions of the fatty tissue that cover and protect inner vulvar structures. The labia majora extend from the mons pubis to the perineum. The inner folds of the labia majora are smooth and moist.

The labia minora are thin folds of smooth skin that form a hood, called the *prepuce,* over the clitoris. The clitoris is a small structure that corresponds to the male penis. Like the penis, the clitoris is composed of erectile tissue with sensory nerve endings that are responsive to psychological and physical stimuli. The labia minora are richly endowed with sebaceous glands, nerves, and blood vessels that also respond to psychological and physical stimulation. The labia minora may be entirely covered by the labia majora or may be visible between the outer labia.

The urethral (urinary) meatus is below the clitoris. The openings of Skene's glands are located on both sides of the urinary meatus. The vaginal opening, the introitus, is partially or entirely covered by a thin fold of tissue called the *hymen.* The hymen may be intact, distended, or ruptured. The size of the introitus varies from very small to large and gaping.

INTERNAL GENITALIA

The vagina is a canal that extends from the vulva to the uterus. This structure has the ability to expand and lengthen to accept an erect penis and to provide an exit for a term fetus. The mucous membranes of the vaginal walls secrete lubricating fluid that cleanses the vagina and interacts with bacteria to maintain an acid pH.

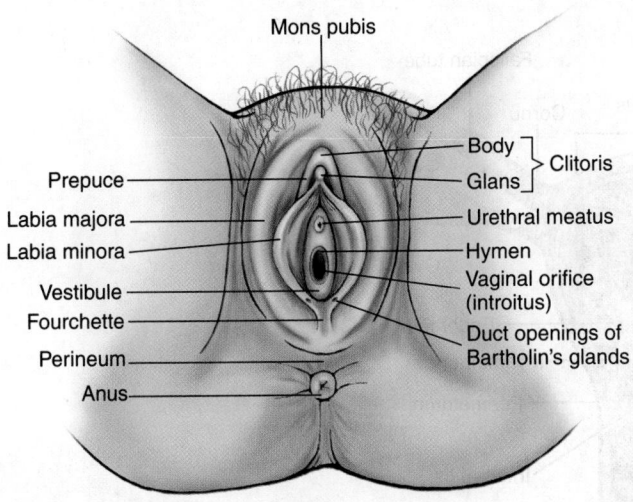

FIGURE **47-1** External female genitalia.

The uterus is a firm, muscular organ that is pear-shaped and hollow. Its lower segment is called the *cervix*. The end of the cervix extends into the upper aspect of the vagina. The os is the opening of the cervix into the vagina. The inner lining of the uterus is called the *endometrium*. The upper segment of the uterine body, or corpus, is called the *fundus*.

The two fallopian tubes are thin, hollow, cilia-lined, tubular structures that extend from the uterine fundus. The fallopian tubes have funnel-shaped ends that partially surround the ovaries and that receive the ovum from the ovary. The fallopian tubes serve as passages for ova from the ovaries and for sperm that travel through the vagina and into the tubes. Fertilization, the union of sperm and ovum, takes place in the fallopian tubes.

The two ovaries are almond-shaped structures located on each side of the uterus. They correspond to the male testes. Ovarian functions include maturation and release of ova (ovulation) and secretion of hormones—estrogens, progesterone, androgens, and relaxin.

It is important to note that the pathway through the female reproductive tract, intended to serve as a route for reproduction, also provides a route for infectious organisms to access the pelvic cavity and its organs.

BREASTS

Although the breasts are not directly involved in the reproductive process, they are addressed as accessories to reproduction because of their function: to nourish the infant after birth. Breast structure is illustrated in Figure 47-3. The inner structure is composed of glandular and ductal tissue, fibrous tissue, and fat. (The fat is responsible for most of the variation in breast size and shape.) The breast is divided into several lobes, each divided into lobules. Lobules contain many hollow, grape-shaped alveoli that produce milk when stimulated by the pituitary hormone *prolactin*. Ducts carry milk from the lobules, through the lobes, to the opening in the nipple.

The nipple with its surrounding areola is a pigmented structure located at the midline of each breast. Breast milk passes through the openings of the lactiferous ducts. Small, round sebaceous glands called *Montgomery's tubercles* are visible under the skin of the areolae. These glands produce a lubricating secretion that protects nipple tissue. Except during normal lactation, there should be no discharge from the nipple.

MENSTRUAL CYCLE

The menstrual cycle, or female reproductive cycle, consists of the ovarian cycle and the uterine cycle. It results from a complex interaction of the hypothalamus, the anterior pituitary, and the ovary (Fig. 47-4). The interaction causes the ovary to release a mature ovum (ovulation) and prepares the uterine lining to receive and nourish the ovum if it is fertilized. If the ovum is not fertilized, the menstrual cycle begins with the onset of menstruation. Menstruation is the passage through the vagina of a mixture of blood and other fluids and tissue formed in the lining of the uterus to receive the fertilized ovum.

The length of the menstrual cycle averages 28 to 30 days, but the range may be 21 to 40 days and may be affected by various factors such as stress, physical activity, and illness. Regardless of the length of the cycle, the progression is the same:

1. Menstruation (day 1 through days 4 to 7).
2. Maturation of an ovarian follicle, with subsequent rupture and release of an ovum in response to follicle-stimulating hormone and luteinizing hormone from the anterior pituitary (days 1 to 14 in a 28-day cycle).
3. Estrogen production (days 6 to 14) by the maturing follicle; progesterone production (days 15 to 26) by the corpus luteum that is formed from the ruptured follicle.
4. Preparation of the uterine lining for implantation of the fertilized ovum, stimulated by estrogen and progesterone from the follicle and corpus luteum (days 6 to 26).
5. The fertilized ovum implants in the uterine lining and secretes human chorionic gonadotropin, which maintains the corpus luteum and estrogen and progesterone levels; menstruation does not occur (day 14).

OR

6. The unfertilized ovum does not implant. Absence of human chorionic gonadotropin causes the corpus luteum to degenerate, which in turn causes a drop in estrogen and progesterone levels and necrosis of the uterine lining (days 27 to 28). The necrotic lining is shed as menstrual flow and begins another cycle at day 1.

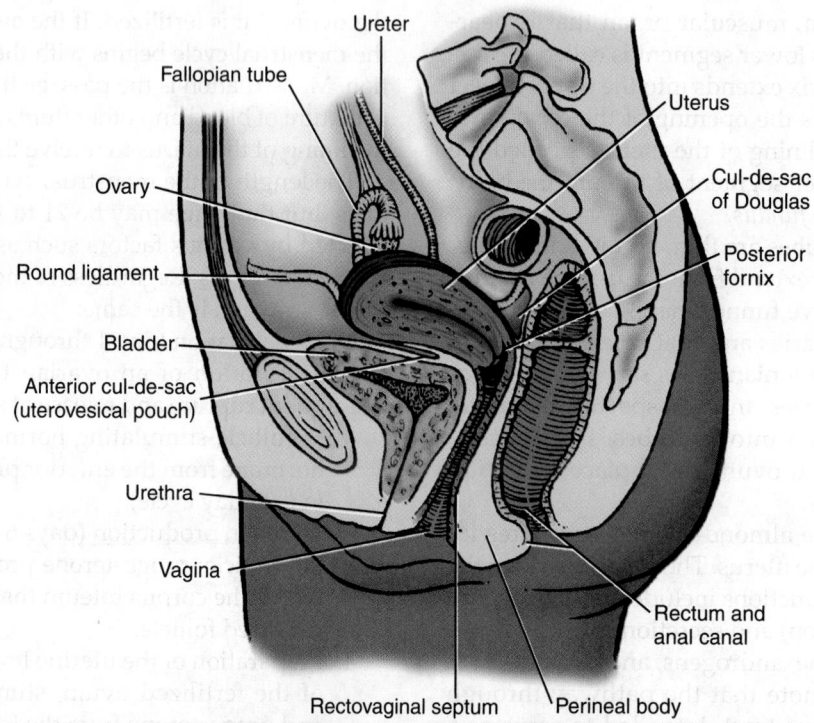

FIGURE **47-2** Internal female genitalia.

NURSING ASSESSMENT OF THE FEMALE REPRODUCTIVE SYSTEM

HEALTH HISTORY

The LPN/LVN collects data that contribute to the professional nurse's complete assessment. The complete assessment is described here even though the LPN/LVN would not be responsible for all of it.

Chief Complaint and History of Present Illness

The basic assessment begins with the patient's reason for seeking medical care. "What is the reason for your visit?" is an opening question that allows the patient to describe in her own terms the reason for the visit and to include related information that may guide subsequent questions. If the reason for the visit is an existing problem, include related signs and symptoms and their onset, frequency, and effect on normal functioning.

Past Medical History

Menstrual History. Record the age at which menstruation began (menarche), the date of the onset of the last menstrual period, the usual number of days between the onset of one period and the onset of the next, the total amount of menstrual flow, the usual number

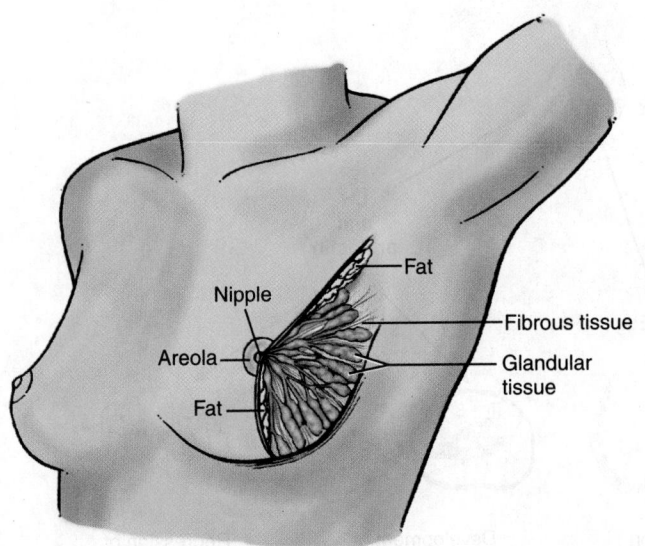

FIGURE **47-3** Structure of the mature female breast.

of days of menstrual flow per period, and the use of tampons.

"Many women experience problems with their periods. What problems have you noticed?" is a questioning technique that implies acceptance of a wide variety of problems and invites the patient to provide additional relevant information. Problems commonly reported include spotting or frank bleeding between periods, abdominal pain at the time of ovulation, abdominal cramping or pain before or during periods (or both), and premenstrual mood changes.

For women who have stopped menstruating owing to menopause, important data include the age at which menstruation ceased as well as related details, such as whether menopause occurred naturally or resulted from surgery, chemotherapy, or radiation therapy. Include information about menopausal symptoms and prescribed or over-the-counter medications taken to relieve menopausal symptoms.

Obstetric-Gynecologic History. "How many times have you been pregnant?" is an appropriate opening question for the obstetric history. If the response indicates that the woman has been pregnant, inquire about the number of term and preterm births, number of living children, number of abortions (spontaneous or induced), and the number of multiple pregnancies (e.g., twins, triplets). Note blood type and Rh factor and a history of rubella or rubella immunization. Terms related to obstetric history are *gravidity* and *parity*. Gravidity refers to the total number of pregnancies. Parity refers to the number of pregnancies that terminated after 20 weeks of gestation, considered the "age of viability." Parity may be recorded according to a number of different codes that use from one- to five-digit numbers. Each institution provides direction on how parity is to be coded for obstetric histories.

The gynecologic history addresses such problems as infections and sexually transmitted diseases, cysts and

tumors, structural and functional abnormalities, infertility, and stress incontinence.

Family History

Record a family history of diabetes mellitus, cancer, complications of pregnancy, multiple pregnancies, genetic disorders, or congenital anomalies.

Review of Systems

Information regarding symptoms and any prescribed or self-selected treatments should be recorded. Commonly reported symptoms are pain, itching, burning, vaginal bleeding between periods or after menopause, heavy or prolonged bleeding with periods, vaginal discharge, and urinary frequency or urgency.

Functional Assessment

The functional assessment includes a diet history, use of dietary supplements including calcium and iron, exercise pattern, sexual history, occupational exposure to potential teratogens, and effects of symptoms on usual activities.

PHYSICAL EXAMINATION

In the general survey, important data include the patient's appearance, facial expression, and any obvious signs of distress. Measure vital signs and height and weight. Skin color, texture, and moisture should be noted. The breasts should be examined for dimpling and abnormal skin texture. The patient is instructed to lean forward so the examiner can observe for asymmetry in the breasts. The examiner asks the patient about changes from usual contours. All breast tissue should be palpated for thickening or lumps (see discussion on p. 1038 in the Breast Self-Examination section). The abdomen is inspected for distention and palpated for tenderness. The legs are inspected for swelling and palpated for tenderness. Nurses with advanced training may do the pelvic examination, but it is more commonly performed by the physician. Therefore it is discussed in detail on p. 1034 in the Diagnostic Tests and Procedures section. Basically, the examiner assesses the external genitalia for lesions, lumps, swelling, and discharge. The vagina and uterine cervix are inspected for lesions, growths, discharge, and redness. The vagina, abdomen, and rectum are palpated for abnormalities. Assessment of the female reproductive system is summarized in Box 47-1.

DIAGNOSTIC TESTS AND PROCEDURES

Most diagnostic tests and procedures are performed by the physician or by the nurse practitioner. The responsibilities of the nurse usually focus on patient instruction regarding the procedure, preparation of the patient, support of the patient throughout the tests and procedures, and assistance to the physician or nurse practitioner. Regardless of the test or procedure to be

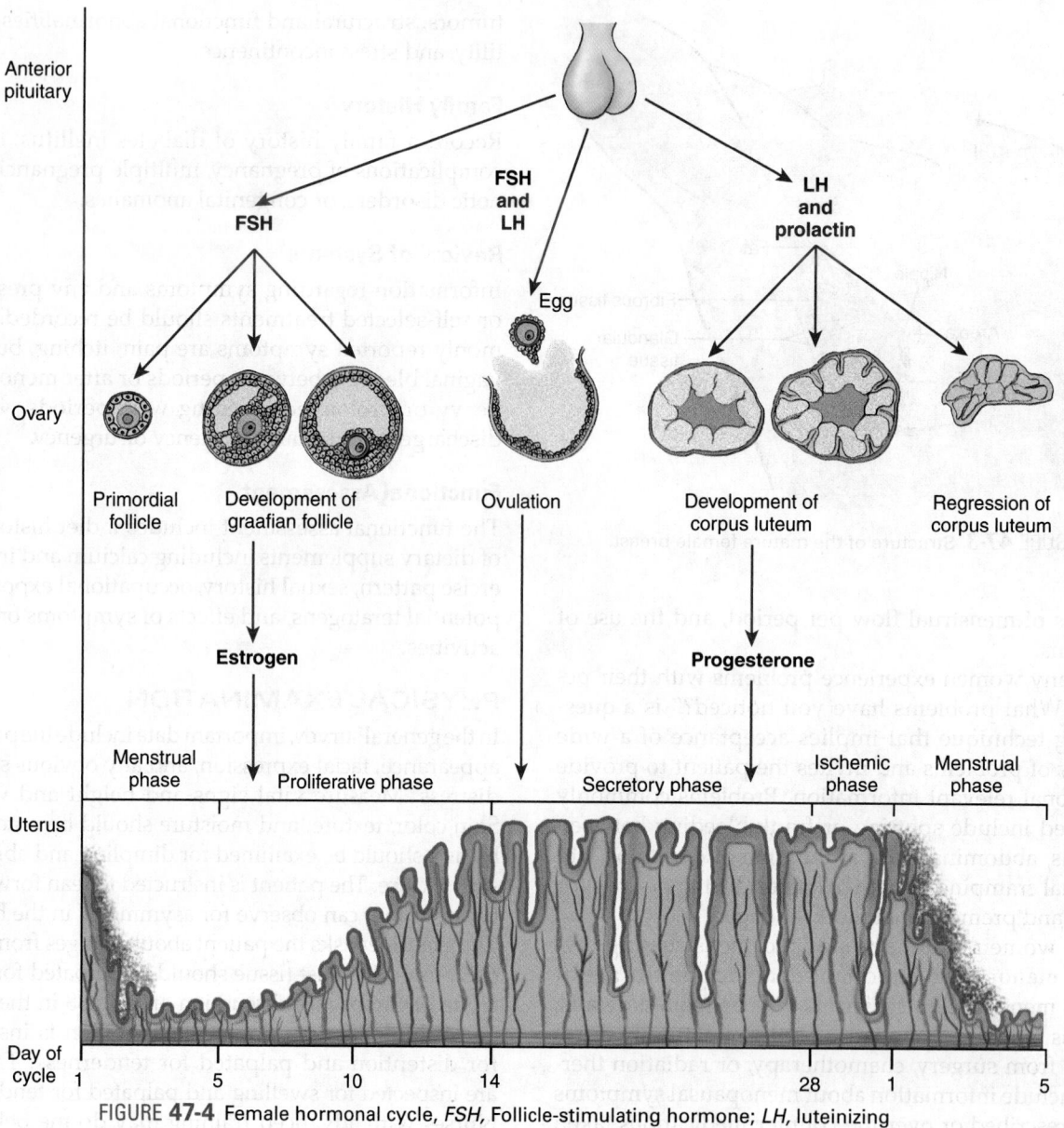

FIGURE **47-4** Female hormonal cycle. *FSH,* Follicle-stimulating hormone; *LH,* luteinizing hormone.

performed, provide anticipatory guidance by telling the patient what to expect. Check the institution's procedure manual for specific preparations and assistants' responsibilities for each test or procedure.

PELVIC EXAMINATION

The pelvic examination allows inspection and palpation of external and internal reproductive structures to identify deviations from normal, to provide information for medical diagnoses, and to collect specimens for laboratory analysis.

The patient assumes the lithotomy position, with her buttocks at the edge of the examination table, her hips and knees flexed, and her feet in stirrups. Many women report that the position is unpleasant because of the sense of vulnerability that they experience. To decrease this effect, delay positioning until just before the examination begins, carefully drape to preserve modesty, and provide verbal and nonverbal support.

To decrease physical discomfort associated with use of the stirrups, cover them with thick footlets or encourage the patient to keep socks or shoes on.

The pelvic examination is divided into three parts: (1) visual inspection and palpation of the external genitalia; (2) visual inspection of the vagina and uterine cervix after introduction of a plastic or metal speculum (Fig. 47-5); and (3) bimanual palpation of the vagina and abdomen. The latter procedure may be performed with two fingers of one gloved hand in the vagina or with one finger in the vagina and one finger in the rectum (Fig. 47-6) and the other hand on the abdomen to allow compression of internal structures between the two hands. The final step is a rectal examination with a gloved finger.

Discomfort varies among women. Some women report no discomfort other than feelings of pressure; other women report pain. One common discomfort is related to a cold speculum. You can prevent this by warming the

Box 47-1   *ASSESSMENT of the Female Reproductive System*

Health History
Present Illness:
Reason for visit, related signs and symptoms, onset and frequency of symptoms, effects on normal functioning

Past Medical History:

Menstrual History:
Age at menarche, date of onset of last menstrual period, duration of menstrual period, amount of menstrual flow, use of tampons, pain, bleeding between periods, premenstrual mood changes. If menopausal: age at which menopause occurred, whether menopause was natural or surgical, related symptoms, medications taken to relieve symptoms

Obstetric and Gynecologic History:
Number of pregnancies, number of term and preterm births, number of living children, number of abortions (spontaneous and induced), number of multiple pregnancies, past problems with reproductive organs, fertility, stress incontinence, history of rubella or rubella immunization, frequency of breast self-examination

Family History:
Diabetes, cancer, complications of pregnancy, genetic disorders, multiple pregnancies, congenital anomalies

Review of Systems:
Pain, itching, burning, vaginal bleeding between periods or after menopause, heavy or prolonged bleeding with periods, vaginal discharge, urinary frequency or urgency

Functional Assessment:
Diet; use of dietary supplements including calcium and iron; exercise pattern; sexual history; occupational exposure to potential teratogens

Physical Examination
General Survey:
Appearance, facial expression, obvious distress

Vital Signs

Height and Weight

Skin:
Texture, moisture, color

Breasts:
Dimpling, texture changes in skin, asymmetry when leaning forward, changes from usual contours, changes in texture, lumps, nipple discharge

Extremities:
Homans' sign, temperature, swelling, tenderness

Abdomen:
Contour, distention, tenderness

Pelvic Examination:

External Genitalia:
Appearance, lesions, lumps, swelling, discharge

Vagina and Uterine Cervix:
Appearance, lesions, growths, discharge, redness
Rectal Examination

---

speculum in water or by wrapping the packaged speculum in the folds of a heating pad. Supportive measures include talking to the patient and directing breathing and relaxation techniques to relieve pain and tension.

After the pelvic examination, assist the patient to sit up and to get off the table. Provide tissues to wipe the perianal area and, if possible, an adhesive panty liner to absorb lubricant as it is expelled from the vagina.

SMEARS AND CULTURES

Collection of specimens for laboratory analysis is one of the purposes of the pelvic examination (Fig. 47-5, D). Institutional policy specifies the necessary equipment and the care of slides for each specimen.

Specimens are routinely collected for a Papanicolaou (Pap) smear for detection of cervical cancer and other abnormal cervical cells (dysplasia). Additional specimens may be collected for identification of suspected infections such as herpes, *Chlamydia*, and gonorrhea.

ENDOMETRIAL AND CERVICAL BIOPSIES

Endometrial biopsies generally are performed for three reasons: (1) to assess the endometrium for readiness to accept and nourish a fertilized ovum; (2) to indirectly assess corpus luteum function in cases of suspected infertility; and (3) to diagnose uterine cancer. The nurse's responsibilities are similar to those for a pelvic examination and collection of specimens for smears and cultures. The physician or nurse practitioner dilates the cervix and scrapes tissue specimens from the endometrium. The procedure may cause cramping so severe that an anesthetic is necessary.

Cervical biopsies are performed to diagnose suspected cervical cancer. There are two types of biopsy: multiple punch and conization. Multiple punch biopsies are done in a physician's office or an outpatient clinic. Because several specimens are obtained by punching out small samples of cervical tissue, the process is usually painful. The nurse's responsibilities are similar to those for endometrial biopsies. You can support the patient by coaching her to use breathing and relaxation techniques to minimize discomfort.

The cone biopsy is invasive surgery and requires admission to an outpatient surgery facility or a hospital. Under general anesthesia, a large amount of cervical tissue is removed. Although the cone biopsy is rarely used for diagnosing cancer, its advantage lies in its potential both to diagnose and to remove cancerous tissue.

COLPOSCOPY

An instrument called a *colposcope* is used to inspect the cervix under magnification and to identify abnormal and potentially cancerous tissue. Colposcopy

A

Vaginal speculum

Urinary bladder

Uterus

Rectum and anal canal

B

Vagina

C

Cervix

External os

D

FIGURE **47-5** Internal examination of the cervix. **A,** Insertion of the speculum. **B,** Open speculum within the vagina. **C,** Examiner's view of the cervix through an open speculum. **D,** An instrument called an Ayre spatula is inserted through the speculum to obtain a cervical specimen for a Papanicolaou test.

is commonly done before cervical biopsies. Patient preparation and nursing care are similar to those for a pelvic examination.

CULDOSCOPY

A culdoscopy is an invasive surgical procedure usually performed with light sedation and local anesthetic on an outpatient basis. When performed by a skillful physician, culdoscopy is the simplest way to directly visu-

alize the female pelvic cavity. With the patient in the knee-chest position, the culdoscope is inserted through a small incision in the posterior vagina. The culdoscope permits examination of the patient's uterus, ovaries, and fallopian tubes. It is performed to obtain tissue specimens and to identify ectopic pregnancy, pelvic masses, and causes of infertility or pain.

The nurse's responsibilities are similar to those for other outpatient procedures, with details specified

FIGURE **47-6** Bimanual palpation. **A,** Bimanual pelvic examination. **B,** Bimanual rectovaginal examination.

by institutional policies. Scrupulous asepsis must be maintained. Many women consider the knee-chest position physically uncomfortable, embarrassing, and humiliating. Assure the patient that she will be draped throughout the procedure, and be conscientious about following through with that assurance. When the procedure is completed, help the patient get out of the knee-chest position without exposure. Advise her that she may experience shoulder pain caused by air entering the pelvic cavity during the procedure. Also reassure her that the incision will close and heal without sutures but that nothing should be inserted in the vagina (e.g., no vaginal intercourse, douching, or tampons) for the period of time specified by the physician.

LAPAROSCOPY

Laparoscopy (Fig. 47-7) is a surgical procedure that may be performed under local anesthesia on an outpatient basis or under general anesthesia in an outpatient surgical facility or a hospital. The physician uses an instrument called a *laparoscope* to visualize abdominal organs and to perform minor surgery such as a tubal ligation. The laparoscope is inserted through a small abdominal incision. Instruments may be inserted through the laparoscope itself or through a small second incision. Before the laparoscope is inserted, a small quantity of gas is injected into the abdomen to create a pocket in which to insert the laparoscope and to allow a clear view of the organs. This gas eventually is absorbed, but in the immediate postoperative period it tends to cause shoulder pain and/or pain below the rib cage. Inform and reassure the patient that the discomfort is expected and is temporary.

DILATION AND CURETTAGE

Dilation and curettage (D&C) is used for diagnostic and treatment purposes. The D&C is used to diagnose uterine cancer and causes of abnormal uterine bleeding. It also may be used to treat some causes of bleeding.

Dilation and curettage is performed in two steps. The first is dilation of the cervix by insertion of a series of progressively larger rods. The second step is endometrial curettage, or scraping of the entire uterine lining. The scraped tissue sample is removed by vacuum aspiration (suction). Tissue samples are prepared for laboratory analysis according to institutional procedures.

Most D&Cs can be performed under local anesthesia in the physician's office or outpatient clinic. Patient preparation and positioning are similar to those used for the pelvic examination. As for all procedures, institutional policy directs the nurse's role and responsibilities.

MAMMOGRAPHY

Mammography is a radiologic test used to detect breast cysts or tumors, especially those not palpated on physical examination. The American Cancer Society recommends that baseline mammograms be obtained in women between the ages of 35 and 39 years. Subsequent tests should be done every 1 to 2 years for women 40 to 49 years of age and annually for women age 50 and older. The test takes only a few minutes and is performed by a trained technician. For the proce-

Put on Your Thinking Cap!

A 47-year-old woman who has never had a mammogram states that her friends have told her it is extremely painful. What approaches might you use in encouraging her to have a mammogram?

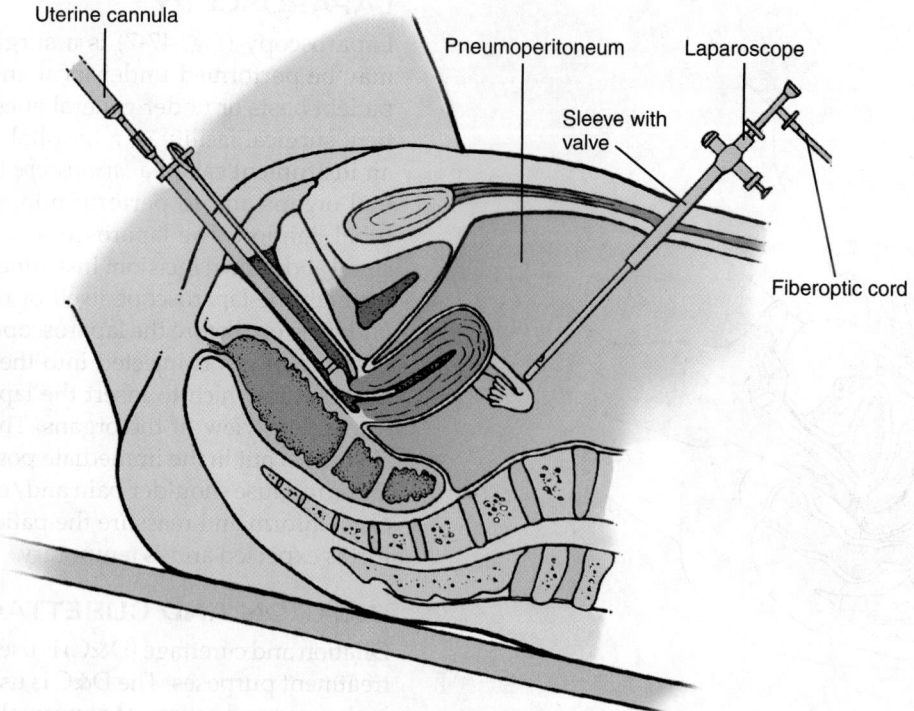

FIGURE **47-7** Laparoscopy.

dure, each breast is compressed in a mammography machine and two views are taken of each breast, one from above and one from the side. The images are usually immediately available, allowing a radiologist to view them before the patient leaves the setting. Most mammograms are obtained in settings that do not routinely employ nurses. However, you need to be familiar with the process so that you can prepare the patient.

BREAST SELF-EXAMINATION

Through regular monthly breast self-examination (BSE), a woman learns to recognize her normal findings, which helps her detect changes if they occur. Every woman who has begun to menstruate should know the correct way to perform breast self-examination.

The BSE should be done at the same time each month: at the end of the menstrual period for menstruating females or on the same date each month for women who have ceased menstruating. The nurse's responsibilities include teaching the importance of BSE, demonstrating the examination, and evaluating the patient's ability to perform a return demonstration on herself.

The BSE begins with inspection of the breasts while the woman is sitting or standing before a mirror. She looks for changes in her breasts as she assumes each of four positions: (1) with her arms relaxed at her sides, (2) with her arms held straight above her head, (3) with her hands pressed against her waist or hips and her elbows brought forward, and (4) leaning forward. She looks for any changes from the previous examination: for dimpling, puckering, or texture changes of the skin; for elevation or enlargement of one breast when she

leans forward or when she brings her elbows forward in the third position; and for other, new differences between the breasts.

The second step of the breast self-examination is palpation of the breasts and the axillary area. The position of choice is for the woman to lie on her back with a folded towel under the shoulder of the breast to be examined. The arm on the same side is raised above her head. Lotion or powder should be applied to the examining hand to help the fingers move smoothly over the skin. The fingers are positioned flat against the skin and moved to cover the entire breast area in one sliding motion. Firm pressure is used, beginning at the nipple and traveling in a circular track around and around the breast until the breast has been covered. Areas to be covered extend from the midaxillary line, to the sternum, and to the top and bottom boundaries. The process is repeated on the opposite side.

Some practitioners prefer to begin at the midaxillary line and palpate the breast tissue in a vertical pattern. The fingers travel up and down in closely spaced strips without leaving the skin surface until the entire breast has been palpated.

Women with small breasts may examine their breasts while showering. This method is less acceptable for women with larger breasts because it does not allow the breasts to flatten for thorough palpation. Any changes in breast texture, particularly any lumps, and any nipple discharge should be reported as soon as possible to the physician or nurse practitioner.

Although many women learn to perform breast self-examination from reading magazine articles or pamphlets, it has been observed that women perform the examination more accurately when they have received direct instruction and demonstration and when they have returned the demonstration for correction of technique.

BREAST BIOPSY

When breast changes are discovered, a breast biopsy may be done to determine the reason for the change. A biopsy is the definitive test for diagnosing breast cancer.

The physician decides which diagnostic procedures are appropriate. Breast biopsies for palpable small lumps can be performed under local anesthesia on an outpatient basis (Fig. 47-8). A needle may be used to aspirate fluid from cysts. Solid masses require a surgical approach to obtain a specimen of the questionable tissue or to remove the mass. Biopsies of large masses are performed under general anesthesia in a hospital setting. All removed tissue and aspirated fluid are sent to the laboratory for analysis. Decisions for further treatment are based on biopsy reports.

The patient admitted to the health care setting for a breast biopsy needs a great deal of supportive care. She needs an opportunity to talk about her fears, and she needs a thorough explanation of what she can expect during the preoperative, operative, and postoperative periods.

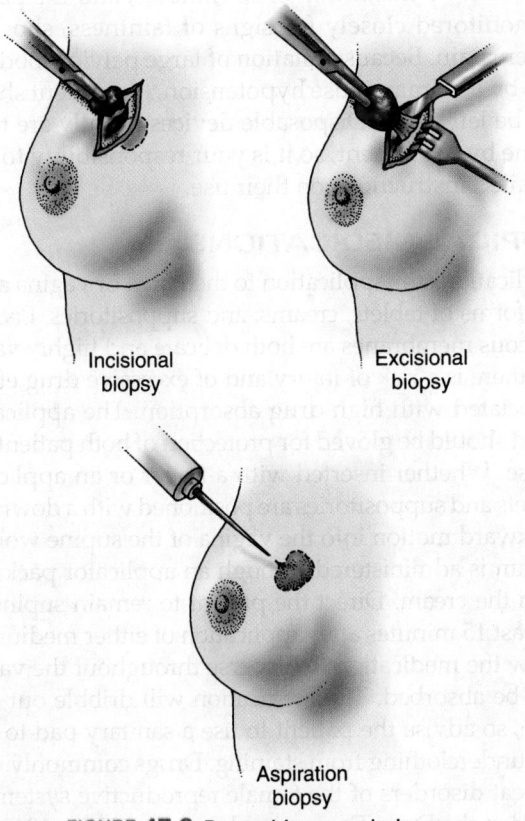

Incisional biopsy

Excisional biopsy

Aspiration biopsy

FIGURE **47-8** Breast biopsy techniques.

Information about diagnostic tests and procedures is summarized in the Diagnostic Tests and Procedures table on p. 1040.

COMMON THERAPEUTIC MEASURES

DOUCHING

Douching is a procedure in which the vagina is flooded with fluid containing various cleansing or perfumed agents. Douching is not recommended for regular hygiene, because it washes away some of the elements that maintain the normal acidic pH. The acidic environment helps the vagina maintain its self-cleansing properties and fight off pathogenic organisms.

Douching is potentially dangerous, because it may force tissue and microorganisms up into the uterus. In addition, cleansing and perfumed agents may cause allergic or irritant reactions. Contrary to common belief, douching is not an effective contraceptive practice.

Douching may be ordered by the physician or nurse practitioner to wash the vagina with a bactericidal solution in preparation for surgery, radiation therapy, or other treatment. If ordered, prepare the douche solution, using exact measures of prescribed ingredients and administer the douche according to your institutional procedure.

Because it is also the nurse's responsibility to teach the patient about appropriate vaginal hygiene, you can teach while the douche is administered. Points to be addressed are in the Patient Teaching Plan below.

CAUTERIZATION

Cauterization is a method of deliberate tissue destruction by means of heat, electricity, or chemicals. The physician or nurse practitioner may cauterize small growths or polyps during the pelvic examination.

APPLICATION OF HEAT

Heat is used as treatment for many reproductive system conditions and disorders. Both dry and moist heat are used to relieve pain, to promote healing by increasing blood flow and tissue metabolism, and to stimulate rupture of abscesses. Because potential damage is associated with excessively high temperature and with conditions such as impaired circulation, edema,

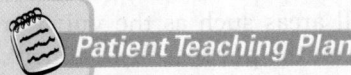
Patient Teaching Plan

Genital Hygiene

- Wash the external genitalia with plain soap and water at least once a day.
- Keep the genital area clean and dry.
- Wear cotton panties.
- Do not douche unless it is ordered by the physician or nurse practitioner.

DIAGNOSTIC TESTS and PROCEDURES *The Female Reproductive System*

TEST/PURPOSE	PATIENT PREPARATION	POSTPROCEDURE NURSING CARE
Pelvic examination includes assessment of external genitalia, vagina, uterine cervix, abdomen, and rectum: to identify abnormalities and to collect fluid or tissue specimens.	Explain the examination; then assist the patient into the lithotomy position immediately before the examination. Drape for privacy. Warm the vaginal speculum. Encourage relaxation.	Assist the patient to assume a sitting position and to get down from the examining table. Offer tissues to wipe the perineal area and a panty liner to absorb lubricant as it drains.
Papanicolaou smear: to detect abnormalities of cervical cells, including cervical cancer. **Cultures:** to detect pathogens that cause herpes, *Chlamydia*, gonorrhea, etc.	Obtain appropriate equipment for specimen collection and preparation.	Same as for pelvic examination. Proper handling of specimens is essential for accurate studies. Prepare specimens, label, and send to the laboratory. Properly dispose of used supplies.
Endometrial biopsy: to study fertility or to detect cancer. **Cervical biopsy:** to detect cancer.	Endometrial and cervical biopsies: assist her to assume the lithotomy position; drape for privacy. Procedure is painful; encourage breathing and relaxation exercises.	Same as for pelvic examination.
Breast biopsy (or fluid aspiration): to diagnose breast cancer. (Done under local or general anesthesia.)	Recognize patient anxiety about outcome and possible implications. Explain procedure.	Check incision for bleeding. Safety precautions if sedated. Provide opportunity to express fears.
Colposcopy: a colposcope is used to inspect the cervix under magnification to identify abnormal tissue. Usually done before cervical biopsy.	Same as for pelvic examination.	Same as for pelvic examination.

and bleeding disorders, any form of heat must be used judiciously.

Dry heat in the form of a hot water bottle, a disposable chemical pack, an electric heating pad, or an aquathermia pad (K-pad) may be applied to the breasts or abdomen to relieve pain and to enhance circulation. The commonly recommended temperature range for most of these devices is 40° to 56° C (104° to 133° F). Institutional policy and physician's orders dictate the exact temperature and the duration of application time. Although the exact procedure for each method varies among institutions, key points when applying dry heat are the following:

1. A physician's order is required.
2. Protect the skin by using a barrier between the heating device and the skin.
3. Monitor the patient's response.
4. Maintain the dry heat source temperature in the appropriate range.

Moist heat in the form of hot compresses and sitz baths is employed for the same general purposes as dry heat. Hot compresses are particularly useful for applying heat to small areas such as the vulva or perineum. Depending on the purpose of treatment, the acceptable temperature range for hot compresses is 40.5° to 46.0° C (105° to 115° F).

Sitz baths provide heat to the perianal area to relieve pain, to cleanse the area, to promote healing or drainage, or to stimulate urination. The patient sits in warm water that may be in a special tub or in a disposable plastic device that fits on the rim of a regular toilet bowl. A continuous flow of fresh, temperature-

controlled warm water is provided by the plumbing apparatus of the sitz bathtub or by a suspended plastic water bag with tubing extended to the disposable device. Water temperature is maintained within the 38° to 46° C (100° to 115° F) range; the treatment is employed for a maximum of 25 minutes; and the patient is monitored closely for signs of faintness, shock, or severe pain. Because dilation of large pelvic blood vessels by heat may cause hypotension, the patient should not be left alone. Disposable devices usually are taken home by the patient, so it is your responsibility to give detailed instructions on their use.

TOPICAL MEDICATIONS

Medications for application to the vulva or vagina are in the forms of tablets, creams, and suppositories. Because mucous membranes are both delicate and highly vascular, there is a risk of injury and of excessive drug effects associated with high drug absorption. The application hand should be gloved for protection of both patient and nurse. Whether inserted with a finger or an applicator, tablets and suppositories are positioned with a down and backward motion into the vagina of the supine woman. Cream is administered through an applicator packaged with the cream. Direct the patient to remain supine for at least 15 minutes after application of either medium, to allow the medication to disperse throughout the vagina and be absorbed. The medication will dribble out over time, so advise the patient to use a sanitary pad to protect underclothing from staining. Drugs commonly used to treat disorders of the female reproductive system are listed in the Drug Therapy table on pp. 1041 to 1043.

DRUG THERAPY Drugs Used to Treat Disorders of the Female Reproductive System

DRUG	USE/ACTION	SIDE EFFECTS	NURSING INTERVENTIONS
OVARIAN HORMONES Conjugated estrogens (Premarin, Cenestin), estradiol (Estrace, Depogen, Dioval, Estinyl)	Replacement of natural hormones after menopause, palliative treatment of advanced breast cancer, treatment of osteoporosis caused by estrogen deficiency. Stimulates endometrial growth and thickening. Enhances bone formation. Depresses beta lipoprotein and cholesterol plasma levels.	Breast tenderness, breakthrough bleeding, vaginal candidiasis, headache, dizziness, depression, elevated blood pressure, thromboembolism, stroke, myocardial infarction (MI), nausea, skin hyperpigmentation, and decreased glucose tolerance. Increased risk of endometrial cancer, especially in postmenopausal women who take estrogens continuously for a year or more.	Advise patients to report signs/symptoms of the following: 1. Thromboembolism: calf pain or swelling, chest pain, numbness, visual disturbances. 2. Cardiovascular problems: weight gain, edema. 3. Liver disorders: abdominal pain, jaundice. 4. Breast lumps. 5. Vaginal bleeding. Discourage smoking, which increases risk of adverse effects. Take with evening meal to reduce nausea. Reinforce physician's instructions.
Oral progestins: Medroxyprogesterone acetate (e.g., Provera), norethindrone (Micronor), norethindrone acetate (Aygestin), micronized progesterone (Prometrium)	Promote secretory function in endometrium. Influence contractile activity of the uterus. Used to treat uterine bleeding, some types of amenorrhea, and premenstrual syndrome (PMS). Palliative treatment of endometriosis and some cancers. Used with estrogens as oral contraceptives.	Breakthrough bleeding, amenorrhea, breast tenderness, edema, pruritus, increased blood pressure, thromboembolism, depression, photosensitivity.	Monitor weight and blood pressure. Assess for pruritus. Tell patient to report signs of circulatory impairment: swelling, numbness, pain in calf or thigh. Advise patient to avoid excessive sun exposure. Assess mental state. Contraindicated with history of thromboembolism, undiagnosed vaginal bleeding, liver dysfunction, cerebral hemorrhage.
Intramuscular progestins: medroxyprogesterone acetate (Depo-Provera), hydroxyprogesterone caproate (Hylutin)			

NOTE: Recent research evidence has revealed increased risks of coronary heart disease and invasive breast cancer when combination estrogen and progestin therapy is used in women with intact uteruses.

Continued

DRUG THERAPY | Drugs Used to Treat Disorders of the Female Reproductive System—cont'd

DRUG	USE/ACTION	SIDE EFFECTS	NURSING INTERVENTIONS
OVARIAN HORMONES—cont'd			
Intravaginal progestin: progesterone (Crinone)			Intravaginal: Use applicator to apply cream or tablet high into vagina.
Transdermal progestin: norethindrone with estradiol (CombiPatch)			Transdermal instructions: Apply to clean, dry skin (not on breast or waistline), press for 10 seconds. Replace once or twice weekly as ordered or if patch falls off. Rotate sites.
SELECTIVE ESTROGEN RECEPTOR MODULATORS (SERMS)			
Tamoxifen (Nolvadex) Toremifene (Fareston) Raloxifene (Evista)	Stimulate estrogen receptors in some tissues and block them in other tissues. Intended to provide benefits of estrogen with fewer risks. Tamoxifen and toremifene used to treat breast cancer and to protect against osteoporosis. Raloxifene is approved only to prevent osteoporosis.	Hot flashes, fluid retention, vaginal discharge, nausea, vomiting, blurred vision, bone pain, menstrual irregularities, confusion. Increases risks of endometrial cancer, stroke, thromboembolism. Teratogenic.	Do not double up if a dose is missed. Tell patient to report severe bone pain to physician so analgesics can be prescribed. Pain is evidence of drug effectiveness; resolves over time. Also, report weight gain, edema, or dyspnea. Patient should use non-hormonal barrier method of contraception during and for 1 month after therapy.
ANDROGENS			
Danazol (Danocrine)	Inhibits production of pituitary gonadotropins. Used to treat endometriosis and fibrocystic breast disease.	Acne, oily skin and hair, hirsutism, edema, weight gain, nervousness, deepening of the voice, decreased breast size, muscle cramps, sleep disorders.	Monitor weight and blood pressure. Assess for signs of liver dysfunction: jaundice, abdominal pain, light-colored stools. Explain side effects to patient. Contraindications: undiagnosed vaginal bleeding; severe cardiovascular, renal, or hepatic disorders.
GONADOTROPIN-RELEASING HORMONE (GNRH) AGONISTS			
Leuprolide acetate (Lupron) Goserelin acetate (Zoladex) Nafarelin acetate (Synarel)	Initially increases, then decreases testosterone levels. Used to treat endometriosis and advanced prostate cancer (see Chapter 48).	Hot flashes, decreased libido, dizziness, headache, nausea, constipation, or diarrhea.	Lupron should be discarded if discolored or if precipitate forms. Use only diluent provided to reconstitute. Administer immediately after reconstituting. Zoladex is gradually dispersed from an implant placed under the skin. Synarel is inhaled nasally. Tell patient to expect hot flashes that usually decrease after time. Pregnancy should be ruled out before giving any of these drugs, because they may cause abortion.

ORAL CONTRACEPTIVES

Estrogen-progestin combinations
(Ortho-Novum, Norinyl, Loestrin, Oval)

Progestin only
(Norplant system)

Estrogen only
(diethylstilbestrol)

Suppress ovulation to prevent pregnancy. Prevent implantation of fertilized ovum. Oral used as emergency postcoital contraceptive ("morning-after pill"); must be given within 24 hours after intercourse.

Nausea, vomiting, headache, edema, weight gain, breast tenderness. Increased risk of thromboembolism (especially among smokers). Severe nausea and vomiting.

Reinforce instructions for self-medication. Monitor weight. Tell patient to report signs of circulatory impairment: swelling, pain, numbness in an extremity. Contraindicated during pregnancy and in patient with a history of thromboembolism, myocardial infarction, cerebral vascular disease. Follow manufacturer's instructions if a dose is missed.

OVULATORY STIMULANT AND FERTILITY DRUGS

Clomiphene citrate (Clomid)

All stimulate or mimic actions of natural pituitary gonadotropins. All can result in multiple births.

Hot flashes, breast tenderness, nausea, vomiting, visual disturbances, headache, depression, fatigue, reversible hair loss, weight gain, dizziness, ovarian enlargement.

Contraindicated with liver dysfunction, pregnancy, abnormal bleeding. Safety precautions if patient is dizzy or has visual disturbances. Stop drug and contact physician if visual disturbances occur. Tell patient to report vaginal bleeding or weight gain, signifying ovarian hyperstimulation, in which case monitor fluid status, weight, and possible signs of internal bleeding. Tell patient to avoid sexual intercourse with ovarian enlargement because of possible rupture.

Menotropins (Pergonal)

Pain and irritation at injection site. Ovarian enlargement and abdominal distention. Rarely, flu-like symptoms: nausea, vomiting, fever.

Reconstitute with sterile saline and administer immediately.

Urofollitropin (Metrodin)

Stimulates ovarian follicular growth. Used to treat selected patients who have not responded to clomiphene citrate.

Same as with menotropins.

Note: Recent research evidence has revealed increased risks of coronary heart disease and invasive breast cancer when combination estrogen and progestin therapy is used in women with intact uteruses.

SURGICAL PROCEDURES

Many disorders of the female reproductive system are treated surgically. Specific examples are given throughout this chapter. Abdominal procedures may be performed through an abdominal incision, vaginally, or endoscopically. The surgeon selects the specific approach according to the diagnosis and the patient's condition. Nursing care varies with each approach. An abdominal approach results in an external excision that requires assessment and care. You must also assess vaginal discharge in these patients since the vagina provides an exit route for blood and other fluids. Vaginal procedures leave no visible incisions, so the patient must be assessed for excessive bleeding through the vagina or for indications of infection such as purulent or foul-smelling vaginal discharge. Laparoscopic procedures require care similar to that for abdominal incisions, but the incisions are much smaller. Again, the patient may have vaginal discharge that should be assessed after laparoscopic pelvic procedures.

DISORDERS OF THE FEMALE REPRODUCTIVE SYSTEM

UTERINE BLEEDING DISORDERS

Pathophysiology

Normal menstrual patterns vary widely in length of cycles (21 to 40 days), duration of menstruation (2 to 8 days), and amount of blood lost (40 to 100 mL). Bleeding patterns that are irregular in both spacing and amount are common in the first 2 years after the onset of menarche and in the 5-year period before menopause. Deviations from the normal cycles are viewed as uterine bleeding disorders. Two of the most common abnormal bleeding patterns, metrorrhagia (bleeding or spotting between menstrual periods) and menorrhagia (menstrual periods characterized by profuse or prolonged bleeding), are addressed in Table 47-1. *Amenorrhea* is the absence of menses.

Etiology and Risk Factors

Both metrorrhagia and menorrhagia are symptoms of underlying factors, rather than being specific definable conditions in themselves. Underlying causes for each vary widely. Common causes include hormonal dysfunction, both benign and malignant tumors, coagulation disorders, systemic diseases, use of some contraceptives, endometrial hyperplasia, inflammatory processes, and systemic diseases. The amount of blood loss varies with the type of disorder. Causes of amenorrhea include pregnancy; excessive weight loss, physical activity, or stress; pituitary, hypothalamic, thyroid, or adrenal disorders; ovarian failure; and uterine abnormalities.

Medical Diagnosis and Treatment

The diagnosis of uterine bleeding is based on the health history and physical examination as well as on the results of various diagnostic tests and procedures. Colposcopy, biopsy, and cauterization as well as laboratory analyses of blood components, hormone levels, and tissue specimens or smears provide diagnostic information. Because anemia may result from excessive bleeding, hemoglobin and hematocrit levels are usually measured as well. The treatment of amenorrhea depends on the cause and whether pregnancy is desired by the patient.

NURSING CARE *of the Patient with Uterine Bleeding*
Assessment

Complete assessment of the female patient with a disorder affecting the reproductive system is summarized in Box 47-1. When a patient has metrorrhagia or menorrhagia, the menstrual history is especially important.

Nursing Diagnoses, Goals, and Outcome Criteria: Metrorrhagia or Menorrhagia	
NURSING DIAGNOSES	GOALS AND OUTCOME CRITERIA
Deficient Knowledge of condition and treatment	Patient understands condition and treatment: patient accurately describes the condition and treatment
Anxiety related to unknown cause of menorrhagia, metrorrhagia	Reduced anxiety: patient states she feels less anxious, calm manner

Interventions
Deficient Knowledge

When the course of treatment has been selected, it may be your responsibility to teach the patient her role in the treatment process and to make sure that she is able to follow through appropriately.

Anxiety

You can be a source of emotional support for the patient, who often is fearful or anxious about the unidentified cause of abnormal bleeding. The underlying causes of abnormal uterine bleeding may be relatively simple and easily treatable or complex and life-threatening. Therefore you must be prepared to help patients cope with all eventualities. Supportive measures such as encouraging the patient to express her feelings, use of touch, and listening convey concern to the patient. Generally it is your responsibility to provide information regarding procedures to be done. Give explanations in terms the patient can understand.

INFECTIONS

Infections of the female reproductive tract affect patients both physiologically and psychologically. The physiologic effects range from short-term reversible changes to long-term changes that result in infertility. The potential psychological effects are numerous. Changes in relationships, feelings of distrust toward

Table 47-1 | *Uterine Bleeding Disorders*

DISORDER	ETIOLOGY	SIGNS AND SYMPTOMS	MEDICAL TREATMENT
Metrorrhagia	Ovulation.	Spotting occurs with regularity 14 days before menses.	None—this is regarded as a normal deviation.
	Intrauterine contraceptive device.	Intermittent spotting between menses.	None if bleeding is not severe and if other causes are ruled out. Monitor serum hemoglobin; if low, iron supplements are prescribed. Remove intrauterine device if bleeding is severe.
	Oral contraceptive use.	Irregular spotting. Early cycle spotting. Late cycle spotting.	Patient is directed to take pill at same time each day. Estrogenic potency of oral contraceptive is increased. Progestational potency of oral contraceptive is increased.
	Trauma; introduction of foreign objects.	Sudden onset of frank bleeding or spotting.	Foreign object is removed. Tissue damage is repaired.
	Vaginitis, cervicitis.	Spotting, combined with vaginal discharge characteristic of infectious organism.	Vaginal examination; culture and Papanicolaou smear to identify underlying cause; cause treated as warranted.
	Ectopic or molar pregnancy.	Spotting or frank bleeding, in addition to symptoms specific to molar pregnancy, ectopic pregnancy.	Ultrasonography and laboratory tests (serum human chorionic gonadotropins level) done. Surgical removal of products of conception.
	Reproductive tract pathology: Endocervical polyps Cervical eversion Cervical dysplasia Endometriosis Salpingitis Ovarian cyst Benign neoplasm Malignant neoplasm	Spotting or frank bleeding, in addition to other symptoms characteristic of specific pathology.	Diagnostic procedures and treatment specific to identified pathologic condition: hormone therapy, antimicrobial or other drug therapy, surgery.

Continued

sexual partners, shame, embarrassment, and diminished self-esteem are but a few.

The majority of infections covered in this chapter often are transmitted through sexual intercourse. In addition, the causative organisms often are those associated with sexually transmitted diseases (STDs), as covered in Chapter 49. However, this chapter focuses primarily on the effects of the microorganisms on the female reproductive tract and on subsequent medical and nursing interventions rather than on the specific disease processes.

Because of their association with sexuality and sexual function, many women view reproductive tract infections as threats or insults to their self-image. They may react with guilt, embarrassment, denial, defensiveness, or a combination of these that cause them to delay seeking diagnosis and treatment. Others are coping with infertility problems that result from infectious processes. When interacting with women who have reproductive tract infections or their effects, you must be sensitive, tactful, and absolutely nonjudgmental.

Vulvitis and Vaginitis

Pathophysiology

Inflammation of the vulva is called **vulvitis**. Depending on the causative agent, vulvitis may be viewed as an infection, as a local manifestation of a general skin disease, as a reaction to a chemical irritant or allergen, or as a common consequence of the aging process. Regardless of its cause, the most common characteristics of vulvitis are inflammation usually with intense pruritus of the vulva and perianal region.

Like vulvitis, **vaginitis** is characterized by a local inflammatory response to various factors. Vaginitis and vulvitis differ in that a significant vaginal discharge is usually present with vaginitis.

Etiology and Risk Factors

Vulvitis and vaginitis are caused by a number of factors that precipitate an inflammatory response. The two most common causes of infection are *Candida albicans* (fungus, or yeast infection) and *Trichomonas vaginalis* (protozoal infection). Both most commonly

Table 47-1 | *Uterine Bleeding Disorders—cont'd*

DISORDER	ETIOLOGY	SIGNS AND SYMPTOMS	MEDICAL TREATMENT
Menorrhagia	Intrauterine contraceptive device.	For all: By definition, profuse or prolonged bleeding during menstruation, in addition to other symptoms characteristic of specific cause.	Substitution of intrauterine device with structural incorporation of progesterone (Progestasert-T) or discontinuation or removal of intrauterine device, with substitution of alternative contraceptive method. Use of PGSIs may be effective in reducing menstrual blood loss. Treatment for remaining causes is specific for each cause.
	Hormonal disturbances.		Determination of hormone status is critically important before hormone therapy or other drug therapy is initiated.
	Endometrial hyperplasia.		Endometrial hyperplasia may be diagnosed and treated by dilation and curettage. For women past childbearing age, hysterectomy may be performed.
	Benign neoplasm.		Benign tumors may be left alone and monitored.
	Malignant neoplasm.		Malignant tumors require a combination of surgical and medical interventions.
	Inflammatory process.		Specific cause is treated.
	Systemic diseases.		Specific cause is treated.

PGSI, Prostaglandin synthesis inhibitor.

infect the vagina and produce characteristic vaginal discharges that are irritating to the vulva and vagina. The discharge associated with *C. albicans* has a distinctive odor and a cottage cheese–like appearance; the discharge associated with *T. vaginalis* is profuse, frothy, and yellow-gray in color and has a fishy odor. Both can be transmitted sexually, although yeast infections often are associated with disruption of the normal vaginal flora by antibiotic therapy or with diabetes mellitus. Other common infective microorganisms are streptococci, staphylococci, and intestinal tract organisms.

Generalized skin diseases that may involve the vulva include psoriasis and inflammation of sweat glands. When these conditions affect the vulva, the constant moist state intensifies the inflammation and subsequent itching.

Vulvar reactions to chemical irritants are common. The vulva is exposed to a wide variety of chemicals that may act as irritants and thus elicit an inflammatory response; the response often extends into the vagina. Perfumed soaps, scented toilet tissue and perineal pads, feminine hygiene sprays, laundry detergent residues, and spermicides are a few examples of common irritants.

Estrogen deficiency associated with the aging process frequently results in nonpathogenic vulvitis and vaginitis due to a combination of tissue atrophy and a decrease in the acid vaginal secretions that normally maintain healthy mucous membranes.

Signs and Symptoms

Regardless of the cause, signs and symptoms include local swelling, redness, and itching. Some infectious agents cause characteristic signs and symptoms that aid in their identification.

Complications

Ascending infection (an infection that moves through the vagina to internal structures) is a potential complication of vulvitis and vaginitis. Infection confined to the lower reproductive tract seldom poses a threat to life or fertility.

Medical Diagnosis

The diagnosis is based on the patient's symptoms and on inspection of the vulva and vagina. Discharge specimens may be collected to aid in identification of specific microbes if microbial infection is suspected.

Medical Treatment

Treatment specific to the causative agent may include topical antifungal creams, oral antiprotozoal agents or antibiotics, vaginal suppositories to reestablish normal vaginal flora, topical or systemic estrogen replacement therapy, improved diabetes control, and avoidance of offending chemical agents. Symptoms are managed with frequent cleansing with neutral agents; wearing cotton panties, cotton-crotched pantyhose, and nonconstricting clothing; and heat in the form of sitz baths and perineal irrigations. Advise the patient not to scratch the itching tissues, which can cause further mechanical trauma and infection. During the course of treatment, she should avoid sexual intercourse or use condoms. The woman's sexual partner or partners may be treated for some infections to avoid reinfection.

NURSING CARE of the Patient with Vulvitis or Vaginitis

Vulvitis and vaginitis usually are diagnosed and treated on an outpatient basis. Because patients usually manage their own treatment, you may be responsible for making sure that the patient understands all self-care instructions and for reinforcing other instructions given by the physician or nurse practitioner. General nursing care of patients with reproductive tract infections is addressed in Table 47-2.

Bartholin's Gland Abscess (Bartholinitis)

Pathophysiology

Because of their location on either side of the vaginal opening, Bartholin's glands are vulnerable to a wide variety of infectious microorganisms. The resultant edema and pus formation occlude the duct of the affected gland and form an abscess.

Etiology and Risk Factors

Various microorganisms can be transmitted from the anus, vulva, or vagina to the Bartholin's gland duct. Commonly cultured organisms include normal intestinal bacterial flora, *Staphylococcus aureus*, *Streptococcus*, *T. vaginalis*, *Neisseria gonorrhoeae*, and *Mycoplasma hominis*. The organisms are often introduced through improper perineal hygiene (i.e., wiping from the anus toward the vagina).

Signs and Symptoms

Perineal pain is the symptom that most commonly motivates the woman to seek medical assistance. Additional signs and symptoms include fever, labial edema, chills, malaise, and purulent discharge.

Complications

Without proper treatment, bartholinitis may progress from a local infection to a systemic infection.

Table 47-2	*Care of Patients with Reproductive Tract Infections*

PATIENT PROBLEM	NURSING INTERVENTIONS

Denial, embarrassment related to questions about infection	Convey acceptance of patient. Use tact in eliciting information about hygiene and sexual practices. Relevant data might include the following:
	    All products applied on or near the vulva or in the vagina: feminine hygiene products, "love potions" (i.e., flavored or scented lubricants, massage oils)
	    Anal contact with penis, fingers, or other objects before contact with vulva or vagina
	    Number of sexual partners; accessibility to partners if their treatment is indicated

Deficient knowledge regarding treatment and self-care	Explanation of teaching about use of creams, jellies, suppositories:
	    Purpose
	    Position for application or insertion
	    Application or insertion method
	    Position after insertion
	    Care of equipment (i.e., applicator)
	    Use of tampon or perineal pad to hold medication in place
	Instructions about perineal hygiene:
	    Frequent washing with neutral soap
	    Thorough rinsing
	    No douching unless specifically ordered
	    No commercial perineal deodorants
	    Frequent change of underpants (preferably cotton)
	    Sitz baths to relieve pain, itching
	    Wiping perineal-anal area from front to back; one stroke per tissue
	    Complete full course of prescribed drug therapy

Medical Diagnosis

Visual inspection reveals a swollen, often reddened mass on the affected side of the vaginal introitus. Gentle palpation causes pain, tenderness, or both. If there is drainage, a specimen may be obtained for culture and sensitivity testing. Because causative microorganisms include those responsible for transmission of STDs, the patient is usually screened for these diseases (see Chapter 49).

Medical Treatment

Conservative treatment consists of oral analgesics and moist heat in the form of frequent sitz baths or hot wet packs. The moist heat relieves pain and facilitates spontaneous rupture and drainage of the abscess. Surgical incision and drainage of the abscess may be done by the physician. More aggressive treatment with broad-spectrum antibiotics is indicated if symptoms of systemic infection are present.

NURSING CARE *of the Patient with Bartholinitis*

Basic nursing interventions are outlined in Table 47-2. Provide the appropriate instruction to help the patient comply with the prescribed treatment. Tactful instruction in basic perineal hygiene principles is in order if the evidence indicates that inappropriate or inadequate practices are being followed. Basic practices include soap-and-water cleansing at least once daily and wiping the perineal area with a clean tissue from front to back after urination or defecation.

Cervicitis

Pathophysiology

Cervicitis is inflammation of the cervix. It may be acute or chronic. Although cervicitis is usually due to an infectious process associated with STDs, the inflammation may be associated with physical or chemical trauma.

Etiology and Risk Factors

Cervicitis is caused by a variety of agents: infectious organisms, scraping of cells for diagnostic tests, cryosurgery, use of vaginal tampons or medications, childbirth, decreased estrogen levels after menopause, and use of oral contraceptives.

Signs and Symptoms

Cervicitis is usually asymptomatic, although it may cause pain, visible vaginal discharge, bleeding, or dysuria. Unsuspected cervicitis may be detected on pelvic examination or on routine Pap smears. When viewed via a speculum, the cervix appears swollen and reddened; gentle touch may precipitate bleeding. Mucopurulent discharge and vesicular or ulcerated lesions most often are associated with STDs.

Complications

Cervicitis itself is considered to be a relatively benign condition. However, if the causative agent is an infec-tion, the infection may ascend through the reproductive tract and cause pelvic inflammatory disease. Certain microorganisms that cause cervicitis also alter the vaginal pH and exert a spermicidal effect that results in infertility.

Medical Diagnosis and Treatment

Cervicitis may be diagnosed on the basis of the pelvic examination or results of the Pap smear. Treatment depends on the causative agent(s). Infections are treated with systemic or topical antimicrobial agents. Cervicitis related to menopause is treated with topical or oral estrogen. Additional treatment options include topical application of acidic preparations in the form of douches or jellies, cauterization with silver nitrate, and cryosurgery or laser surgery. Cryosurgery is the use of a cold probe to destroy selected tissue.

NURSING CARE *of the Patient with Cervicitis*

Cervicitis usually is diagnosed and treated in outpatient settings. Treatment is administered by a physician or nurse practitioner or by the patient herself. Nursing care is limited to assisting with assessment procedures, patient support, and teaching the patient to carry out the prescribed treatment and posttreatment procedures.

Pharmacology Capsule

Instruct patients to complete the full course of antimicrobial therapy to treat infections.

Mastitis

Pathophysiology

Mastitis is an infection-induced inflammation of breast tissue most commonly occurring in the lactating woman. Historically, early postpartum mastitis epidemics were common among women who delivered in hospitals and who were hospitalized for the then-usual 10 or more days. With today's short hospital stays, mastitis is associated not with hospitalization but rather with a combination of ineffective breast-feeding techniques that result in poor drainage of mammary ducts and alveoli, lowered resistance to infection due to stress and fatigue, and exposure of breast tissue to infection-causing organisms.

Etiology and Risk Factors

S. aureus is the microorganism most commonly associated with mastitis; *Escherichia coli* and streptococci also may be the agents of infection. The nipple serves as the portal of entry for the organism. Cracked nipples are especially susceptible. A common mechanism of organism transmission is touching the nipples with unclean hands.

Signs and Symptoms

Mastitis is usually confined to one breast and may be asymptomatic except for breast tenderness and low-grade (and often unsuspected) fever. The infection therefore may be undetected if frequent breast-feeding empties breast ducts and alveoli and if the woman's natural immune response prevents spread of the infection. In symptomatic mastitis, the causative organism invades the breast connective tissue or the lobes and ducts and stimulates an inflammatory response that results in localized pain, fever, tachycardia, general malaise, and headache. The affected breast tissue feels hard and warm on palpation; the skin over the infected area is reddened.

Complications

Untreated symptomatic mastitis may result in abscess formation as the sepsis becomes localized. Enlargement of axillary lymph nodes also may result.

Medical Diagnosis and Treatment

The diagnosis is based on presenting symptoms. Symptomatic mastitis is unmistakable. If there is a purulent discharge from the nipple, a specimen can be collected for culture and sensitivity testing. However, treatment is initiated based on the symptoms alone and consists primarily of immediate and aggressive antibiotic therapy.

Symptoms are managed by frequent emptying of the breast, heat application, rest, and administration of an analgesic. The question of whether to empty the breast by breast-feeding or by artificial pumping is a controversial one. The physician will determine whether breast-feeding should continue. Many broad-spectrum antibiotics are tolerated well by both mother and infant. This is significant because antibiotics taken by the mother will be present in her breast milk.

If an abscess forms, surgical excision and drainage of the abscess may be necessary and a longer period of antibiotic therapy will be required.

NURSING CARE *of the Patient with Mastitis*

The most effective nursing intervention is teaching patients how to prevent mastitis.

Assessment

Explore the breast-feeding woman's knowledge of measures to prevent mastitis. Take the patient's temperature. Palpate the breasts for pain, tenderness, warmth, and hardness, and inspect for purulent discharge from the nipple.

Nursing Diagnoses, Goals, and Outcome Criteria: Mastitis

NURSING DIAGNOSES	GOALS AND OUTCOME CRITERIA
Risk for Injury related to possible abscess formation	Recovery without complications: absence of fever, pain, redness, and purulent drainage
Deficient Knowledge of mastitis prevention and treatment	Patient understands how to treat mastitis and prevent recurrence: patient accurately describes and demonstrates self-care measures

Interventions

Risk for Injury

If mastitis or breast abscess occurs, reinforce the prescribed treatment. If heat treatments or drug therapy are prescribed, be sure the patient understands the instructions.

Deficient Knowledge

The points commonly addressed in breast-feeding education are those that also prevent the infectious process from occurring.

FIBROCYSTIC CHANGES

Pathophysiology

Fibrocystic breast changes represent an exaggerated response to hormonal influences. Excess fibrous tissue develops accompanied by overgrowth of the lining of the mammary ducts, proliferation of mammary ducts, and the formation of cysts. Fibrocystic nodules do not "become cancerous," but their presence may make it more difficult to detect malignant tumors by palpation.

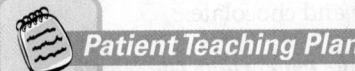

Patient Teaching Plan

Mastitis

- Be sure to complete your course of antibiotics as prescribed.
- Report continued or additional symptoms.
- Pain usually can be managed with analgesics as prescribed.
- Allow for extra rest periods.
- To prevent recurrence during breast-feeding:
  - Breast-feed frequently, and completely empty the breasts.
  - Wash hands thoroughly before handling breasts.
  - Avoid cracked nipples:
    - Make certain that the infant's lips and gums are around the areola and not on the nipple itself.
    - Break suction before removing the nipple from the infant's mouth.
    - Cleanse with plain water to prevent chemical trauma from soap, alcohol, and other drying agents.
    - Leave milk on nipples and expose them to the air or a heat lamp after breast-feeding.
- Wear a supportive but nonconstrictive bra.
- Get adequate rest, nutrition, and fluids.
- Promptly report early symptoms of breast infection to health care provider.

Etiology and Risk Factors

Fibrocystic changes are more common among women who have never given birth, have had a spontaneous abortion, and who had an early menarche and late menopause. The risk also is greater for women who have premenstrual abnormalities and do not use oral contraceptives.

Signs and Symptoms

This painful condition usually affects both breasts. Smooth round lumps that are freely movable may be felt. Sometimes there is milky yellow or green discharge from the nipple. Symptoms commonly are most apparent during the premenstrual phase of the menstrual cycle and typically improve after the menstrual period.

Medical Diagnosis and Treatment

Diagnosis is based on the physical examination and health history. A mammogram or ultrasound can help distinguish lumps as fibrocystic changes rather than cancer. If indicated, fluid for study may be aspirated from a mass or the mass may be surgically removed for examination. Women with fibrocystic changes should learn to perform breast self-examination and should have periodic professional breast examinations.

There is no specific cure for fibrocystic changes. Danazol reduces symptoms by decreasing estrogen production. However, the side effects (acne, edema, excess hair growth) make it unacceptable to many women. Other therapies that lack scientific support but seem to help some women include vitamin E, diuretics, low-salt diet, wearing a good support bra, stress reduction, and restriction of coffee and chocolate.

NURSING CARE of the Patient with Fibrocystic Changes

Fibrocystic breast changes are treated on an outpatient basis. Therefore the primary role of the nurse is to instruct the patient in self-examination and to encourage scheduled professional examinations.

PELVIC INFLAMMATORY DISEASE

Pathophysiology

Pelvic inflammatory disease (PID) is an infectious process that may affect any or all structures in the pelvic portion of the reproductive tract and peritoneal cavity. It is called an *ascending infection* because causative organisms migrate upward from the portal of entry, the vulva or vagina.

PID is a major female reproductive health problem and a major cause of infertility in the United States. The infectious process results in scarring and adhesions in the fallopian tubes that can cause total or partial obstruction. Total obstruction results in infertility. Partial obstruction often results in ectopic pregnancy, in which the fertilized ovum implants in a site other than the uterus, usually in the fallopian tube or the pelvic

cavity. Unfortunately, the incidence of PID is particularly high in adolescent girls.

Etiology and Risk Factors

Because the majority of PID cases are caused by sexually transmitted organisms, PID is generally classified as an STD syndrome. *N. gonorrhoeae, Chlamydia trachomatis,* and *M. hominis* are recognized as the organisms most associated with PID. *Chlamydia* infection is thought to be the most commonly occurring STD and the one most often responsible for PID. As such, it is often implicated in infection of the fallopian tubes (salpingitis) and is considered to be the primary cause of ectopic pregnancy and infertility associated with tubal obstruction.

However, non-STD organisms also have been identified as causative agents. Staphylococcal, streptococcal, and other organisms have been cultured from women with PID. Sources of non–STD-associated PID include contaminated hands or instruments during gynecologic surgery, childbirth, abortion, and pelvic examinations. Women with compromised resistance to infection and women who are poorly nourished are particularly prone to developing non–STD-associated PID.

The risk of PID increases as the number of sexual partners increases. This factor is most applicable to PID caused by organisms implicated in STDs.

Vaginal douching also is considered to be a possible risk factor for PID. It is thought that the force of the fluid used in douching may propel microorganisms from the vagina through the cervical os (opening) and into the uterus, fallopian tubes, and pelvic cavity.

Signs and Symptoms

Pelvic inflammatory disease may be a silent infection with no symptoms. As a result, it may remain untreated while causing damage to pelvic structures. Symptomatic PID may appear with either the gradual onset of dull, steady, low abdominal pain or the sudden onset of severe abdominal pain, chills, and fever. Other symptoms may include dysuria, irregular bleeding, a foul-smelling vaginal discharge that may cause inflammation and skin breakdown of the vulva, and dyspareunia (pain during sexual intercourse).

Symptomatic PID is much more likely to be diagnosed and treated than asymptomatic PID. In many instances, evidence of PID is first discovered during surgery for ectopic pregnancy, blocked fallopian tubes, ovarian abscess, or other pelvic disorders.

Complications

The risk of complications of PID increases with each repeated infection. Common effects of PID include ectopic pregnancy, infertility, and chronic abdominal discomfort. Without prompt diagnosis and aggressive treatment, infection of the entire peritoneal cavity (peritonitis) and systemic septic shock also are potential complications.

Medical Diagnosis

The diagnosis is based on the presenting symptoms (if any) and the pelvic examination. The definitive diagnosis is based on culture of the causative organism or organisms. Sonography, laparoscopy, and culdocentesis are additional diagnostic procedures that may be employed.

Medical Treatment

PID usually can be treated at home. However, very acute symptoms and severe pain may require inpatient care. Treatment includes rest; application of heat via warm compresses, a heating pad, or sitz baths; and a regimen of analgesics and broad-spectrum antibiotics. Depending on the severity and extent of the infection, oral and/or parenteral antibiotics are prescribed. The woman should avoid sexual intercourse for at least 3 weeks. If the causative organism is thought to have been transmitted sexually, the woman's sexual partner or partners should be treated to avoid repeated infection.

NURSING CARE of the Patient with Pelvic Inflammatory Disease

Assessment

Nursing assessment of the woman with a disorder of the reproductive system is summarized in Box 47-1. Preparation of the patient for physical examination includes anticipatory guidance, positioning and draping, and emotional support (see Table 47-2). You need to simultaneously assist the examiner and provide support for the patient. Precautions to avoid transmission of infection to yourself and others are summarized in the Patient Teaching Plan above.

Nursing Diagnoses, Goals, and Outcome Criteria: PID

Nursing Diagnoses	Goals and Outcome Criteria
Acute Pain related to inflammation	Pain relief: patient states pain relieved
Impaired Skin Integrity related to infectious drainage	Restored skin integrity: intact skin without excessive redness or edema
Deficient Knowledge of treatment and prevention of reinfection	Patient understands and carries out treatment and preventive measures: patient verbalizes instructions and states intent to follow prescribed measures

Interventions

Care of the patient with PID includes rest with limited activity, application of heat as ordered, administration of prescribed antibiotics, patient education, and recognizing and reporting signs and symptoms of the side effects of antibiotics.

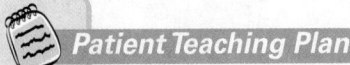

Patient Teaching Plan

Precautions to Avoid Reproductive Tract Infection

- Maintain optimum general health: adequate nutrition and sleep, good stress management.
- Cleanse perianal area daily with neutral soap followed by thorough rinsing; apply no other products unless ordered by health care provider.
- Wipe perianal area with one front-to-back swipe per tissue.
- Avoid sharing of any equipment (including washcloths) used for perineal or vaginal hygiene.
- Change perineal pads or tampons frequently during menses even when flow is slight. Increase soap-and-water cleansing to at least twice per day.
- Inspect genitalia of partner before intercourse or other contact with perianal area. Avoid contact if any lesions or discharge is noted. The same precautions should be followed for any part of the partner's anatomy (e.g., mouth, hands, fingers) that will contact perianal area during sexual encounter.
- Wash with soap and water the penis, hands, or other objects that contact anus before contact with vulva or vagina.
- Use condoms with spermicidal cream or jelly for penis-vulva-vaginal contact when monogamous relationship is not well established.
- Avoid intercourse during treatment for reproductive tract infection. Use condom if intercourse cannot be avoided.

Acute Pain

Prescribed analgesics are administered for pain control. Additional pain relief measures are discussed in Chapter 15. Monitor and record the efficacy of analgesics.

Impaired Skin Integrity

If perineal pads are needed for collection of vaginal discharge, change them frequently. Note the character, amount, color, and odor of vaginal discharge. Frequent perineal cleansing is done with mild soap and water, followed by rinsing and patting dry. Inspect the vulva for signs of inflammation or excoriation, and monitor and record the temperature.

Deficient Knowledge

Nurses play a significant role in the primary prevention of PID and in fostering early diagnosis and treatment of reproductive tract infections so that they do not result in PID. Primary prevention includes measures to reduce risk factors. All women should practice good reproductive tract hygiene habits. The patient with PID needs to understand the importance of taking antibiotics as prescribed. Failure to complete the course of therapy encourages the development of resistant strains of bacteria. Other teaching points include

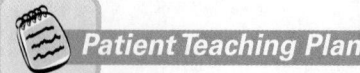

Patient Teaching Plan

Prevention of Pelvic Inflammatory Disease

When teaching prevention of PID to the sexually active woman with multiple partners or with a single partner with an unknown sexual history, include the following:

- During sexual intercourse, always use protective mechanical or chemical barriers such as a condom, diaphragm, vaginal sponge, and spermicidal vaginal jelly or cream.
- Recognize signs and symptoms of common STDs.
- Seek prompt medical diagnosis and treatment of STDs or other suspected reproductive tract infections.
- Have routine yearly pelvic examination by a physician or nurse practitioner, with cultures done to detect *N. gonorrhoeae*, *C. trachomatis*, and other organisms.
- Routinely inspect the sexual partners' genitalia for signs of infection before each contact for sexual intercourse.

the need to abstain from intercourse for the prescribed period and the need for the sexual partner to be treated if advised.

BENIGN GROWTHS

Endometriosis

Pathophysiology

Endometrial tissue that lines the uterus responds to hormonal influences during the menstrual cycle. During menstruation, small amounts of menstrual fluid are ejected through the fallopian tubes into the pelvic cavity (retrograde menstruation) rather than through the cervical os into the vagina. In some women, the endometrial cells deposited in the pelvic cavity implant on structures within the cavity. There, they continue to respond to menstrual cycle hormonal stimulation. The result is the periodically painful and potentially destructive condition called endometriosis. In women with endometriosis, the ectopic (out-of-place) endometrial tissue behaves in the pelvic cavity as it does in the uterus: it proliferates and then bleeds if fertilization of the ovum does not occur. As a result, more and more endometrial cells attach to pelvic structures. These cell clusters, called *implants*, are sometimes referred to as *chocolate cysts* because of their color. The implants can migrate to other areas of the body, possibly transported by blood or lymph. Bleeding by endometrial tissue causes local inflammation and pain wherever the site of implantation may be. The number of implants gradually increases, creating multiple sites of inflammation and pain. In response to the inflammation, fibrous tissue forms that results in scarring and adhesions (Fig. 47-9).

Etiology and Risk Factors

Although it is known that almost all women experience retrograde menstruation to some degree, it is not known why some women develop endometriosis and others do not. Several theories have been explored; one is that endometriosis may be linked to a defect in the immune system of its victims. The disease is believed to occur in 10% of all women of reproductive age. The incidence and severity are greatest in women with relatives who have endometriosis.

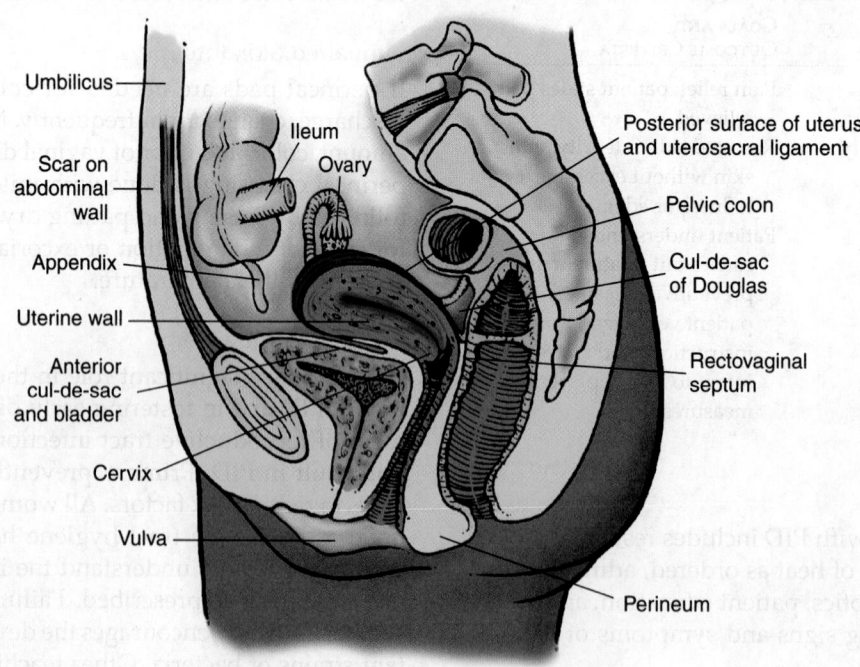

FIGURE **47-9** Common sites of endometriosis.

Signs and Symptoms

As noted previously, the major symptom is pain, although some women are asymptomatic. Because the uterine endometrial tissue is bleeding simultaneously, pain appears as dysmenorrhea and may extend to a feeling of general pelvic heaviness. Additional symptoms include pain with defecation, dyspareunia, and abnormal bleeding. Emotional symptoms, including anger and depression, also are common. Infertility may be a sign of endometriosis when adhesions affect uterine position or fallopian tube patency, movement, or both.

Complications

The most common complication of endometriosis is constriction of pelvic structures by endometriosis-related adhesions. Constriction of the bowel, ureters, or both may cause partial or complete obstruction within the affected structure, creating a medical emergency.

Medical Diagnosis

Visualization and excision of endometrial implants via laparoscopy provide specimens for laboratory analysis and are the primary diagnostic procedures for endometriosis. Ultrasonography may be employed as a preliminary diagnostic tool to determine the presence of pelvic masses.

Medical Treatment

Medical management includes the use of nonsteroidal anti-inflammatory agents to relieve pain. The most commonly used drugs for pharmacologic treatment of endometriosis are gonadotropin-releasing hormone (GnRH) agonists or a synthetic androgenic steroid. GnRH agonists suppress the secretion of gonadotropin-releasing hormone, causing the estrogen level to fall, which permits endometriosis implants to shrink. There are several such drugs, including leuprolide acetate (Lupron) or goserelin acetate (Zoladex) and nafarelin acetate (Synarel). Leuprolide therapy requires monthly intramuscular injection. Goserelin is released slowly from a subdermal implant, and nafarelin is taken by nasal inhalation. Side effects are similar to those seen with danazol. Danazol (Danocrine), a synthetic androgenic steroid, inhibits gonadotropin excretion, resulting in amenorrhea and atrophy of intrauterine and ectopic endometrial tissue. Many women find the common side effects of danazol to be unacceptable: masculinizing characteristics such as voice deepening, hirsutism (excess hair growth), clitoral enlargement, and skin changes; and menopausal symptoms such as hot flashes, vaginal atrophy, and dryness. Both classes of drugs are contraindicated during pregnancy, so the patient should know to use a barrier contraceptive during and for 1 to 3 months after the first normal menstrual period following therapy. Oral contraceptives may be prescribed on a long-term basis to inhibit endometrial proliferation, thereby relieving symptoms.

Androgens have masculinizing effects on females. The effects usually resolve when the drugs are discontinued.

Oral contraceptives are contraindicated in a woman with a history of cardiovascular disease, cerebrovascular disease, or thrombophlebitis.

Surgical management is commonly employed and includes laparoscopy for both diagnosis and removal of endometrial implants via resection, electrocauterization, or laser excision. Because it is difficult to visualize and remove all implants and because the underlying cause continues to exist, such surgery does not constitute a permanent cure and may need to be repeated at intervals. When fertility is no longer desired or complications develop, total abdominal hysterectomy with bilateral salpingo-oophorectomy (excision of the uterus, fallopian tubes, and ovaries) may be performed. Removal of the ovaries prevents the production of estrogen that would stimulate endometrial tissue. However, estrogen replacement therapy is not an option to relieve menopausal effects for these women as long as endometrial implants remain, because the implants continue to respond to the estrogen and symptoms return.

NURSING CARE *of the Patient with Endometriosis*

Endometriosis is usually treated on an outpatient basis, so nursing care is limited unless the patient is admitted for surgery. Perhaps the most significant nursing interventions are validating that the pain is real and providing information about pain relief measures (see Chapter 15). The office or clinic nurse may be involved in patient teaching. Patient teaching is based on the treatment method selected and includes anticipatory guidance and treatment-specific instructions. Because periodic bleeding of all endometrial sites may cause anemia, teaching should include symptoms of anemia and the need for dietary or supplemental vitamin and mineral therapy. Preoperative and postoperative nursing care of the patient who has had a hysterectomy is addressed in the nursing care plan (see Nursing Care Plan: The Patient with a Hysterectomy on pp. 1056 and 1057).

Cysts

A cyst is a closed, saclike structure that is lined with epithelium and that contains fluid, semisolid, or solid material. Cysts are classified as neoplasms and may be benign or malignant; the majority are benign. The most common ovarian and breast cysts are covered individually in Table 47-3.

Table 47-3 | *Common Ovarian and Breast Cysts*

TYPE OF CYST	PATHOPHYSIOLOGY	SIGNS AND SYMPTOMS	DIAGNOSIS AND MANAGEMENT
Follicular ovarian cyst	Forms when a dominant follicle fails to rupture and release its ovum and thus continues to grow. Occasionally formed in response to ovarian hyperstimulation by fertility drugs. May rupture and bleed into the pelvic cavity, causing sudden, severe abdominal pain.	Usually asymptomatic unless very large, then: pelvic heaviness or congestion and an aching feeling.	Usually detected during a pelvic examination. Most disappear spontaneously in 2-3 months without treatment. If it remains on reexamination after 6-10 weeks, the cyst may be examined and removed via laparoscope or drained by needle aspiration.
Corpus luteum ovarian cyst	Forms after ovulation; characterized by excessive bleeding into the luteal cavity and by increased progesterone secretion. Use of fertility drugs is associated with ovarian hyperstimulation and formation of multiple cysts. Associated with more complications than follicular cysts. May rupture and hemorrhage into the pelvic cavity, causing a degree of pain related to the amount of bleeding.	Initial symptom: delayed onset of the menstrual period, followed by irregularities in menstrual amount and duration of flow. Patient may have dull, aching pelvic pain or cramping.	Is palpable as a small, tender mass on the affected ovary. If severe abdominal pain exists, ectopic pregnancy should be ruled out. May be visualized via laparoscopic or culdoscopic examination if diagnosis is questionable. Usually no treatment is indicated. Normally disappears spontaneously.
Dermoid ovarian cyst	Composed of tissue from the three embryonic germ cell layers. May contain remnants of fat, hair, teeth, cartilage, and nerve tissue. Usually arises from the ovary on a pedicle (stalk). A small number (3%-5%) of dermoid cysts become malignant.	Asymptomatic when small. Pelvic aching or heaviness with large cyst. Moderate pain if pedicle gradually becomes twisted; extremely severe pain with sudden twisting.	Palpated as a dense, firm mass during pelvic examination. With long pedicle, the mass may be found some distance from the ovary to which it is attached. A pregnancy test is needed to rule out ectopic pregnancy. If radiographs show teeth in the mass, the diagnosis of dermoid cyst is confirmed. Any dermoid cyst should be removed surgically because of the potential for malignancy.

For women with ovarian or breast cysts, nursing intervention focuses on teaching. Instruct the patient to keep a diary of symptoms, detailing when they occur and any factors that may be associated with the symptoms. Teaching is specific to the prescribed therapy.

Fibroid Tumors (Myomas, Leiomyomas)

Pathophysiology

Uterine fibroid tumors are both benign and common. It is predicted that at least 25% of all women will develop fibroid tumors during their reproductive periods. Fibroid tumors grow slowly during the reproductive years but tend to atrophy after the onset of menopause.

Etiology and Risk Factors

Although the exact cause is unknown, it is widely thought that fibroid tumors form and grow in re-

 What Does Culture Have to Do with Uterine Fibroid Tumors?

The incidence of fibroid tumors is increased among African-American women. These women should be advised to report menstrual irregularities and pain so that the condition can be diagnosed early and treatment can be initiated.

sponse to stimulation by estrogen, primarily estradiol. Human growth hormone and human placental lactogen may also promote the tumors' development and growth.

Signs and Symptoms

Fibroid tumors may be asymptomatic, but the most common symptoms are menstrual irregularities—menorrhagia and dysmenorrhea. Discomfort from pressure on pelvic structures and dyspareunia may be associated with a large tumor. For some women,

Table 47-3	*Common Ovarian and Breast Cysts—cont'd*		
TYPE OF CYST	**PATHOPHYSIOLOGY**	**SIGNS AND SYMPTOMS**	**DIAGNOSIS AND MANAGEMENT**
Breast cyst	Most commonly identified cause is ovarian estrogen secretion. Additional contributing factors may be stress and caffeine. Is an exaggerated response to hormonal influence. May enlarge during the premenstrual period and shrink from the onset of menstruation until the next ovulation. Commonly called *fibrocystic disease*. Controversial: Some fibrocystic subtypes are considered precancerous.	Most are round, freely movable, benign cysts. May be soft or firm, depending on contents. Small cysts are numerous; breasts have lumpy "cottage cheese" consistency. Varying degrees of pain between ovulation and menstruation.	Methods of preliminary diagnosis: Palpation, mammography, and ultrasonography useful for initial study. Contents of fluid-filled cysts may be aspirated for laboratory study or just observed over time. Accurate diagnosis of solid cysts requires surgical biopsy. Treatment: Oral analgesics, heat application, and caffeine restriction. Other possible dietary measures include decreased salt intake and supplementary vitamins and fatty acids. Most aggressive surgical treatment is mastectomy, which occasionally is an option selected by women who undergo repeated surgical biopsies. Hormone therapy: 1. Danazol (Danocrine): Decreases secretion of estrogen. Dosage is generally low enough to avoid serious side effects. 2. Low-dose estrogen with progesterone or progestins.

the initial hint that something is wrong is the gradual enlargement of the lower abdomen, which may be mistaken for pregnancy.

Complications

A very large fibroid tumor may compress the urethra, obstructing urine flow and causing secondary hydronephrosis. More common complications include infertility, crowding and malpositioning of the fetus during pregnancy, and degenerative changes related to interruption of blood supply.

Medical Diagnosis

On pelvic examination, the uterus is found to be enlarged and distorted. A pregnancy test, Pap smear analysis, and complete blood cell count should be done to rule out other conditions.

Medical Treatment

Many women need no treatment, and their tumors atrophy after menopause. Methods of contraception are limited by fibroid tumors: intrauterine devices are contraindicated, the estrogen in oral contraceptives may stimulate growth of the tumors, and diaphragms may be uncomfortable. For women who desire to be-

come pregnant, some gynecologic surgeons perform myomectomy (removal of the tumor alone), usually by laser surgery. Some small tumors can be removed endoscopically or destroyed with cryosurgery. A procedure to block blood flow to the tumor has also been employed to destroy the tissue. For tumors that are very large or that are associated with complications, hysterectomy is the usual surgery of choice. Pregnancy should be delayed for 4 to 6 months after myomectomy. Leuprolide (Lupron), a GnRH agonist, may be ordered to shrink large tumors before surgery. However, there are concerns that this drug causes bone demineralization.

NURSING CARE *of the Patient with Fibroid Tumors*

Assist the physician or nurse practitioner with diagnostic procedures, and provide support to the patient. Women tend to equate the word *tumor* with malignancy. Therefore you may need to give repeated reassurance that the fibroid tumor is benign. If the practitioner elects a conservative approach of monitoring tumor growth, the patient may need reassurance that this approach is commonly used (see Nursing Care Plan: The Patient with a Hysterectomy on pp. 1056 and 1057.) If the patient with fibroid tumors has heavy

NURSING CARE PLAN
The Patient with a Hysterectomy

ASSESSMENT

Health History: A 42-year-old married woman has a diagnosis of uterine fibroid tumors. She has been pregnant three times and has three living children, two boys and one girl, all of whom are teenagers still living at home. Her menstrual periods have been regular, with onset every 30 days and lasting for 6 days. She describes her menstrual flow as heavy. She states that she saturates six to eight heavy-day pads and six to eight super tampons per 24 hours for the first 3 days of each period, after which flow tapers off and she can manage the remainder of each period with four to six tampons per 24 hours. Her last period ended 6 days ago. She describes her health as excellent, with the exception of the uterine fibroids that were diagnosed when she was 33 years old. She is admitted for a total abdominal hysterectomy with bilateral salpingo-oophorectomy. This will be her first experience with surgery.

Physical Examination: Vital signs: temperature 97.8° F orally; pulse 72; respiration 18; blood pressure 116/74. Lungs clear on auscultation. Weight: 116 lbs. Height: 5'3". Alert. Skin color medium tan; nail beds pink with rapid capillary refill. Appears to be in good physical condition: body is firm with little evidence of adipose tissue and with excellent muscle tone; abdomen firm but protruding, appears about 5 months pregnant.

Laboratory: Urinalysis, complete blood count: All reports indicate no deviation from normal ranges except for hemoglobin (Hgb) concentration 10.4 g/dL (normal, 11 to 16 g/dL) and hematocrit 30% (normal, 31% to 44%). She has been typed and cross-matched for two units of whole blood "on hold" for surgery.

Nursing Diagnosis	Goals and Outcome Criteria	Interventions
Preoperative Nursing Diagnoses		
Risk for Situational Low Self-Esteem related to perceived potential changes in femininity, effect on sexual relationship	The patient will verbalize understanding of expected changes in anatomy and physiology and of ability to resume a satisfying sexual relationship with husband after recovery from surgery.	Explain the following: 1. The only expected noticeable effects of loss of uterus and ovaries will be cessation of menstrual periods and ability to become pregnant, in addition to cessation of symptoms for which she is seeking surgery. 2. She may experience vaginal numbness for a short period of time. 3. Many women experience improved libido and sexual satisfaction after hysterectomy; sexual spontaneity may increase with lack of need for contraception. 4. Although penile or vaginal intercourse should not be resumed until at least 6 weeks after surgery, oral sex and masturbation to orgasm are safe. 5. Positions for sexual intercourse should avoid pressure on the abdominal incision for as long as incisional tenderness persists. 6. Orgasmic contractions of the uterus will no longer be present; this change of uterine sensation is noted by some but not by most women. 7. Estrogen replacement therapy (ERT) will prevent atrophy of vagina and decreased lubrication associated with removal of ovaries.
Deficient Knowledge related to information or misinterpretation of effects of hormone replacement therapy (HRT)	The patient will verbalize understanding of potential side effects of HRT and strategies to minimize side effects.	Explain the following: 1. The dosage of estrogen replacement may be adjusted for optimum therapeutic effect; she should report any concerns to her gynecologist. 2. Estrogen may increase fluid retention, which may make one "feel fat." Dietary control of sodium intake will reduce tendency for fluid retention. 3. Gradual resumption of presurgical physical activity and a well-balanced diet should maintain weight and fitness at presurgical levels.
Postoperative Nursing Diagnoses (see Chapter 17 for general postsurgical diagnoses and care)		
Ineffective Tissue Perfusion related to anemia, surgical trauma, effects of anesthesia	The patient will have adequate oxygenation of tissues, as evidenced by a pulse rate of 66 to 80, respiratory rate of 12 to 20, stable skin color, alert mental status, negative Homans' sign.	Monitor pulse, respiration, and blood pressure rates and auscultate respirations on schedule according to institutional policy. Assist patient to turn, deep breathe, cough on schedule; assist with incentive spirometer if ordered. Monitor skin color, temperature, and capillary refill, including lower extremities. Instruct and assist with foot and leg exercises while patient is confined to bed; encourage and assist with am-

NURSING CARE PLAN

The Patient with a Hysterectomy—cont'd

Nursing Diagnosis	Goals and Outcome Criteria	Interventions
		bulation when allowed. Assess ability to answer questions appropriately. Check for Homans' sign by dorsiflexing foot; report positive sign (calf pain) to physician. If elastic hose are ordered, make sure they are applied and removed according to schedule when patient is in bed and at all times when out of bed; instruct patient about self-application. Monitor laboratory reports. Report to appropriate person any deviations from normal ranges. Medicate with analgesics to maximize comfort status.
Risk for Deficient Fluid Volume related to postoperative bleeding	The patient will maintain adequate fluid volume, balanced fluid intake and output, moist mucous membranes, stable pulse and blood pressure.	Check abdominal dressing and perineal pad at least every hour for the first 12 hours; report any drainage observed on dressing, excessive vaginal bleeding. Should saturate less than one perineal pad per hour. Compare fluid intake (intravenous, oral) with urinary output (indwelling catheter collection bag or voided); report discrepancies. Monitor intravenous infusion; carry out related responsibilities according to institutional policy. Encourage fluid intake when allowed. Check mucous membranes for moisture; offer frequent mouthwashes during nothing-by-mouth status. Monitor pulse and blood pressure; compare with baseline levels; report deviations from acceptable ranges.
Urinary Retention related to surgical manipulation, local tissue edema, temporary sensory or motor impairment	The patient will empty bladder at regular intervals without catheterization.	Assist patient to bathroom or commode; use bedpan only if absolutely necessary. Assist patient to assume comfortable position. Provide privacy but remain within calling distance. If patient is unable to void without assistance, employ assistive measures: run water in sink or shower; pour warm water over perineum. Teach or assist patient to perform perineal hygiene at least every 8 hours: wash vulva with warm, soapy water; rinse with warm water from irrigating apparatus; rinse perineum after every voiding. Measure and record urine output; note color, clarity, and odor of urine. Palpate for bladder fullness above symphysis pubis to assess for urinary retention. If patient is unable to void or is retaining urine, allow her to rest for 30 minutes and repeat attempt for spontaneous voiding. Follow order for intermittent catheterization or repeat insertion of indwelling catheter if patient is unable to void a sufficient quantity. Continue to monitor and to assist with voiding until patient consistently empties her bladder without assistance.
Constipation related to weakening of abdominal musculature, abdominal pain, decreased physical activity, dietary changes, drug side effects	The patient will have bowel movement on or before the fourth day after surgery.	Auscultate abdomen for bowel sounds, palpate for distention. Insert rectal tube as ordered, if appropriate. When oral intake is allowed, administer antiflatulent if ordered; teach patient self-administration if allowed. Encourage early and frequent ambulation. Encourage oral intake of fluids, especially of fruit juices. Assess for nausea and vomiting; administer antiemetic if nausea and vomiting are present. Follow protocol for diet; encourage selection of high-fiber foods when patient is allowed options. Administer stool softener or laxative if ordered. Assist patient to splint abdomen while attempting to pass feces. Report inability to have a bowel movement within the allotted time period.

? CRITICAL THINKING QUESTIONS

■ How would you explain the effects of HRT to a patient who has deficient knowledge related to this intervention?

■ Outline your strategy for helping this patient deal with the emotional trauma of a hysterectomy.

bleeding, she should be advised to avoid aspirin and other drugs that enhance bleeding.

UTERINE DISPLACEMENT
Cystocele and Rectocele
Pathophysiology

Cystocele and rectocele are vaginal disorders caused by weakness of supportive structures between the vagina and bladder (cystocele) or the vagina and rectum (rectocele). They typically occur together. Bulging of the bladder and rectum through the vaginal wall is visible and palpable on vaginal examination. Although small cystoceles and rectoceles may cause no problems, larger herniations may cause problems with emptying of both bladder and bowel. Stress incontinence, incomplete bladder emptying, difficulty with expulsion of fecal matter collected in the area of herniation, and incontinence of gas or liquid feces are problems typically reported.

Etiology and Risk Factors

During pregnancy and childbirth, the muscles that support the pelvic floor may be weakened. Repeat pregnancies result in further weakening that may eventually allow the bladder and the bowel to press through the vaginal wall.

Signs and Symptoms

Symptoms other than the already described common bladder and bowel problems include dyspareunia, lower back and pelvic discomfort, and recurrent bladder infections.

Medical Diagnosis and Treatment

The diagnosis is made on the basis of inspection and palpation. Treatment of small cystoceles and rectoceles may be limited to pelvic floor (Kegel) exercises, which improve muscle tone. Estrogen replacement therapy may be prescribed to improve tone and vascularity of supportive tissues. A pessary may be helpful with cystocele. A pessary is a device that is inserted into the vagina to provide support. Surgical intervention via anterior colporrhaphy and posterior colporrhaphy (A&P repair) to tighten the vaginal wall has long been the treatment of choice for larger or symptomatic cystoceles and rectoceles. An anterior colporrhaphy reduces the size of the anterior vaginal wall and is used to treat a cystocele. Posterior colporrhaphy reduces the size of the posterior vaginal wall and is used to treat a rectocele. There is a risk of vaginal stenosis, which results in painful intercourse after posterior repair. These procedures usually are not done during the childbearing years because vaginal delivery would disrupt the repair.

It is interesting to note that nurse researchers who utilize noninvasive methods based on pelvic floor exercises report long-term success rates comparable to those found with colporrhaphy.

NURSING CARE *of the Patient with Cystocele and Rectocele*
Assessment

Assessment of the patient with a disorder of the reproductive system is outlined in Box 47-1. When a patient has uterine displacement, also record problems related to urinary and bowel function. If surgery is planned, assess the patient's understanding of the procedure, the preoperative and postoperative care, and the patient's concerns.

Nursing Diagnoses, Goals, and Outcome Criteria: Cystocele and Rectocele

Nursing Diagnoses	Goals and Outcome Criteria
Urinary Stress Incontinence related to pelvic muscle weakness	Control of urine elimination: patient reports improved bladder control
Constipation related to collection of feces in herniated bowel	Normal bowel elimination: regular bowel movements without straining
Sexual Dysfunction related to painful intercourse	Satisfying sexual practices without pain: patient's statement of lack of pain during intercourse
Risk for Infection related to incomplete bladder emptying	Absence of urinary tract infections: normal body temperature; no pain on urination

After surgical intervention, additional nursing diagnoses and goals are the following:

Nursing Diagnoses	Goals and Outcome Criteria
Acute Pain related to tissue trauma	Reduced pain: patient states pain relieved, relaxed manner
Risk for Injury related to infection and stress on surgical incisions	Wound healing without disruption or infection: intact surgical incisions without increasing redness or purulent drainage
Deficient Knowledge of postoperative self-care	Patient understands surgical routines and self-care: patient accurately describes postoperative self-care

Interventions

Nursing interventions vary depending on the medical treatment.

Urinary Stress Incontinence

For conservative treatment, you can teach Kegel exercises. (See Chapter 23.) The exercise is viewed as a preventive measure that can be adopted in early adulthood to maintain optimum pelvic floor muscle support throughout life.

Constipation

For the patient who reports problems with expelling feces, teaching includes directions to maintain soft stool consistency and regular bowel elimination. Dietary support focuses on frequent ingestion of fluids and a wide variety of high-fiber foods such as fruits, vegetables, and grains. Regular use of bulk stool softeners may be necessary.

Sexual Dysfunction

For the patient who is treated with colporrhaphy, preoperative nursing care includes anticipatory guidance regarding the impending surgery and postsurgical period and carrying out the physician's orders. The patient may fear painful intercourse postoperatively or may be concerned about the effects of surgery on sexual function. Explain that intercourse should be delayed for a prescribed period of time for healing to occur. No permanent impairment of sexual function is expected.

Risk for Infection

Preoperative orders commonly include a vaginal douching with an antibacterial solution, a cleansing enema, and hair removal according to agency procedure. Postsurgical nursing care is directed at prevention of infection and protection of the suture line. Perineal care is provided at regular intervals. In addition to incisional infections, the patient is at risk for urinary tract infections. An indwelling urethral or suprapubic catheter commonly is left in place for several days to keep the bladder empty and thus to prevent strain on sutures and to let local edema subside. Instruct the patient to report urinary frequency, burning, or foul odor, which suggests infection of the urinary tract.

Acute Pain

Postoperative perineal care includes cleansing of the perineum at regular intervals, initial application of cold to reduce pain and swelling, and subsequent application of heat via sitz baths and heat lamps. Because postoperative pain may be severe, administer analgesics as ordered. Assess the effects of comfort measures, and inform the physician if pain is not relieved.

Risk for Injury

A low-residue diet reduces fecal bulk, and stool softeners are recommended to prevent straining during defecation after surgery. Encourage adequate fluids and ambulation.

Deficient Knowledge

Discharge teaching focuses on the patient's responsibility for continued self-care as ordered by the physician. Reinforce instructions regarding diet, medications, activity restrictions, and avoidance of sexual intercourse for the time specified by the physician. Reassure the patient that loss of vaginal sensation is expected and will resolve after a few months. To minimize vaginal stenosis after posterior repair, the surgeon may instruct the patient to use dilators and vaginal lubricants and to resume intercourse 6 weeks after surgery.

Uterine Prolapse

Uterine prolapse is a condition in which the uterus descends into the vagina from its usual position in the pelvis (Fig. 47-10). Descent is rated as *first degree* if the cervix is above the vaginal introitus, *second degree* if the cervix protrudes from the introitus, and *third degree* if the vagina is inverted and both the cervix and the body of the uterus protrude from the introitus. If the vagina inverts, it carries with it the adjacent bladder and rectum. Although uterine prolapse can occur in women who have never been pregnant, it is most common in postmenopausal women who have had multiple pregnancies.

Etiology and Risk Factors

Cardinal ligaments support the uterus in its anatomic position. The ligaments may be congenitally weak or may become stretched during pregnancy or injured during childbirth, resulting in weakening of support. As the woman ages, other supportive structures and uterine walls tend to relax, resulting in some degree of uterine prolapse.

Signs and Symptoms

Dyspareunia, backache, and a feeling of pelvic heaviness and pressure are commonly reported symptoms. Cystocele and rectocele usually accompany uterine prolapse.

Complications

In second-degree and third-degree prolapse, the protruding uterine portion is subject to trauma and may become eroded and necrotic.

Medical Diagnosis

Second-degree and third-degree prolapse are readily detected by visual inspection. First-degree prolapse is diagnosed through pelvic examination, although early first-degree prolapse may escape detection as the uterine descent is not evident when the patient is supine.

Medical Treatment

Vaginal hysterectomy with anterior and posterior colporrhaphy is the most common surgical treatment for uterine prolapse. For the woman who desires to preserve childbearing capability, it is possible to shorten the supportive ligaments surgically and return the uterus to the correct anatomic position.

For women who are poor surgical risks or who refuse surgical treatment, pessaries may be used. Pessaries are instruments that are inserted into the vagina to apply pressure on the vaginal wall, thereby supporting the uterus in the pelvis. There are several types of pessaries, including ring ("doughnut") pessary and lever pessary. After placement of a pessary, advise the patient to return within 24 hours for the physician to assess placement, effectiveness, and problems related to pressure on surrounding structures. Pessaries must be removed, cleaned, and replaced periodically. If they are not maintained or are fitted improperly, they may act as irritants and cause tissue erosion, malignant tissue changes, or both. Be sure to document that the patient has a pessary so that it will not be forgotten and neglected. Topical estrogen creams or vaginal tablets may improve the tone of the muscles in the pelvic floor.

NURSING CARE *of the Patient with Uterine Prolapse*

Assessment

Nursing assessment of the patient with a disorder of the reproductive system is outlined in Box 47-1. When the patient has uterine prolapse, record related symptoms. If the prolapsed uterus is visible, note any signs of trauma or tissue breakdown.

Interventions

You can serve as a source of emotional support and information for the patient. Nursing care depends on the treatment selected. Proper use of a pessary can reduce the risk of uterine trauma. When a pessary is the treatment of choice, explain the importance of frequent

examinations by a physician or nurse practitioner, the need to report pessary-related discomfort to the health care provider, and the need for pessary care. Although some primary health care providers prefer to remove, clean, and replace pessaries, capable patients can be taught to do this themselves.

Nursing Diagnoses, Goals, and Outcome Criteria: Second- or Third-Degree Uterine Prolapse	
NURSING DIAGNOSES	**GOALS AND OUTCOME CRITERIA**
Disturbed Body Image related to interference with daily activities	Improved body image: positive patient remarks about self and ability to manage uterine prolapse
Sexual Dysfunction related to abnormal uterine position	Satisfying sexual function: patient states sexual activity is satisfying and without pain
Risk for Injury related to trauma of the exposed uterus	Absence of uterine trauma: no breaks in tissue integrity of uterus
Deficient Knowledge of self-care	Patient understands and practices self-care: patient accurately describes self-care, keeps follow-up appointments

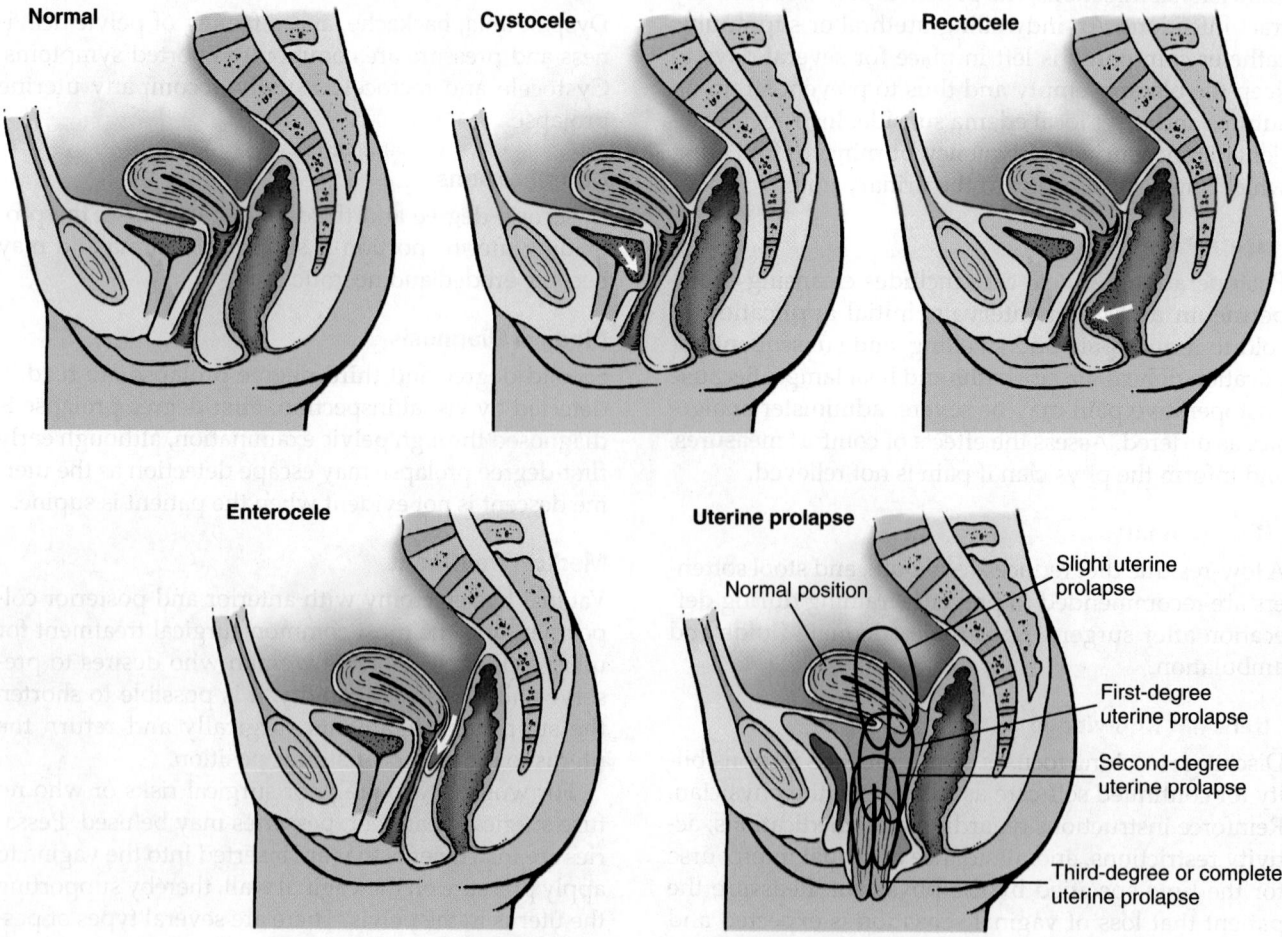

FIGURE **47-10** Types of genital prolapse.

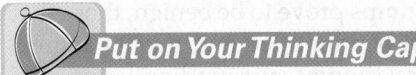

Put on Your Thinking Cap!

A newly hired nurse in a long-term care facility is surprised to learn that some patients have pessaries. The nurse says, "Nobody uses those things any more!" How would you explain the use of pessaries in this population?

Retroversion and Retroflexion, Anteversion and Anteflexion

The uterus is normally positioned at a 45-degree angle anterior to the vagina, with the cervix pointed downward toward the posterior vaginal wall (Fig. 47-11). Displacement from the normal position may be a normal congenital variation or may be related to a number of other factors (Fig. 47-12). Posterior displacement may be retroversion or retroflexion. Retroversion is a backward tilt of the uterus with the cervix pointed downward toward the anterior vaginal wall. With retroflexion, the body of the uterus bends backward on itself. Anterior displacement may be anteversion or anteflexion. With anteversion, the entire uterus tilts forward at a sharper angle to the vagina. With anteflexion, the uterus bends forward as if folding on itself.

FIGURE **47-11** Normal position of the uterus.

Etiology and Risk Factors

Weakening and stretching of the round, broad, and uterosacral ligaments and weakened pelvic floor musculature related to childbearing are the most common causes of uterine displacement. Other causes include surgical trauma, pelvic tumors, pelvic inflammatory disease, and endometriosis.

Signs and Symptoms

Most uterine displacement is asymptomatic, although dyspareunia and low back pain may occur with retroversion.

Complications

Difficulty with conception has been associated with uterine displacement, particularly with retroversion. However, most complications are now thought to be associated with an underlying pathology (e.g., endometriosis, pelvic inflammatory disease) rather than with displacement itself.

Medical Diagnosis and Treatment

The pelvic examination reveals uterine displacement. Treatment is seldom employed, although some women find relief from backache by assuming a knee-chest position. Kegel exercises may be employed to strengthen the pelvic floor muscular support system. For patients who are not candidates for surgery, a pessary may be used (see pp. 1059 and 1060 in the Uterine Prolapse section).

NURSING CARE *of the Patient with Retroversion and Retroflexion, Anteversion and Anteflexion*

The nurse's role is usually limited to history taking and providing information. If a pessary is inserted, provide instructions similar to those described on pp. 1059 and 1060 in the Uterine Prolapse section.

VAGINAL FISTULAS

Vaginal fistulas are abnormal passageways between the vagina and other pelvic organs. A fistula between the vagina and the urinary bladder is called a *vesicovaginal fistula;* a *urethrovaginal fistula* is located between

In **retroversion**, the uterus *tilts posteriorly*, and the cervix rotates anteriorly.

In **retroflexion**, the uterus *bends posteriorly.*

In **anteversion**, the uterus *tilts anteriorly.*

In **anteflexion**, the uterus *bends anteriorly.*

FIGURE **47-12** Types of uterine displacement.

the urethra and the vagina. Both of these fistulas permit urine to flow into the vagina. A *rectovaginal fistula* is located between the vagina and the rectum and permits flatus and feces to pass into the vagina. Urine or fecal matter in the vagina can lead to severe vaginal and vulvar irritation and infection. Vaginal fistulas often can be diagnosed on the basis of the health history and physical examination findings. Dye may be injected into the vagina and radiographs may be made to locate the fistula.

Surgical correction is often needed, although some small fistulas close spontaneously. Surgery may be delayed until the infection and inflammation have subsided. Preoperatively, instruct the patient in perineal hygiene and measures to control odor. Encourage fluid intake to reduce the risk of infection. The physician may prescribe sitz baths and deodorizing douches. Remember that excessive pressure during douching may force fluid through the fistula. Perineal pads are needed but must be changed frequently, and perineal care should be done every 4 hours.

After repair of a urinary fistula, the patient will have a urinary catheter that must be kept patent. Encourage fluids to promote urine output and to maintain catheter patency. After repair of a rectovaginal fistula, a liquid, low-residue diet is ordered initially to delay the need for a bowel movement so the surgical site can heal. After several days, stool softeners and laxatives may be ordered to promote bowel elimination. Enemas are contraindicated because they may disrupt the sutured area. Unfortunately, surgical correction is not always successful.

CANCER

A diagnosis of cancer of the female reproductive system can have profound psychological impact. For example, cancer implies threats to personal survival, sexual relationships, family integrity, and a woman's concept of herself as a female. You can play a potentially significant role in helping the patient cope with decision making, treatment methods and their effects, the inevitable grieving process, and the reactions of family members and friends.

Breast Cancer

Breast cancer is the most prevalent form of cancer in American women; the current prediction is that one of every eight or nine women will develop breast cancer at some point in her life. It is the second leading cause of cancer deaths in women. Men can have breast cancer also, although it accounts for only 0.22% of all cancer deaths among men. It once was thought that survival rates were poorer for men, but that is not true.

For early detection of breast cancer, the American Cancer Society recommends periodic mammography and clinical breast examinations. Regular monthly breast self-examination is described as an option for women beginning in their 20s. Although it is estimated that 80% of breast lumps prove to be benign, those that are malignant must be identified and treated aggressively to prevent invasion of surrounding tissue, metastasis to distant structures, and death.

The three major types of breast cancer, according to the type of cells undergoing malignant changes, are ductal, lobular, and nipple. Malignant growths usually are singular and unilateral (affecting only one breast), and they can be found in any part of the breast. However, nearly one half of all malignant breast tumors are located in the upper outer quadrant, and nearly one fourth are located in the nipple-areolar complex. Most malignant lumps are painless and are palpated as firm, irregularly shaped, and fixed to underlying structures or skin. However, they sometimes resemble benign lumps: soft or semifirm, symmetric in shape with discrete borders, and freely movable. Therefore no lump should be ignored because it "feels" benign. Prompt evaluation is vital and may include tissue examination of cells obtained by needle aspiration or surgical biopsy.

Etiology and Risk Factors

White non-Latino women have the highest incidence of breast cancer. African-American women are most likely to die from it.

Although no cause has been identified for breast cancer, statistical evidence indicates the existence of several risk factors (Box 47-2). Women who have a mutation of the BRCA genes have a 50% to 85% lifetime risk of developing breast cancer. However, these women account for only 5% to 10% of all breast cancers.

Family history is important. The risk rises if one or more first-degree family members (mother, sister, daughter) have had breast cancer and if that cancer was premenopausal and bilateral. Additional risk factors reported in some studies are radiation exposure, late menopause, obesity, excessive alcohol intake, hormone replacement therapy, sedentary lifestyle, nulliparity, high-fat diet, and oral contraceptives. The risk of developing breast cancer rises as the number of factors rise. However, it is important to remember that most women diagnosed with breast cancer have none of these known risk factors. See the Nutrition Concepts box on p. 1063.

Box 47-2 | *Established Risk Factors for Breast Cancer*

- Sex: female
- Family history: mother, sister, or daughter diagnosed with breast cancer
- Age: 50 years and older
- Age at menarche: 11 years or younger
- Age at first childbirth: 30 years or older (or nulliparous)
- Personal medical history: benign breast biopsy, atypical hyperplasia in the breast, breast cancer
- BRCA1 or BRCA2 gene mutation

What Does Culture Have to Do with Breast Cancer?

Some genetic factors increase the risk of breast cancer. Other suspected risk factors—including high-fat diet, obesity, and sedentary lifestyle—may be culturally based. No race or culture is free of breast cancer.

Nutrition Concepts

1. Long-term dieting is associated with amenorrhea and reduced fertility.
2. Factors that may interfere with optimal nutrition for women of childbearing age include lack of resources, lack of nutrition knowledge, self-imposed dietary restrictions, and genetic idiosyncrasies.
3. High dietary fat intake has been linked to breast cancer.

Prognosis

Relative survival rates are determined by comparing survival rates among cancer patients with overall survival rates in similar groups of people who do not have cancer. When cancer is confined to the breast, the 5-year relative survival rate is 96.8%. When cancer has spread to surrounding tissue, the 5-year survival rate is 75.9%; when the disease has metastasized, the rate is 20.6%.

What Does Culture Have to Do with Breast Cancer Survival?

Low-income African-American women more often have advanced disease when diagnosed and are more likely than white women to die from breast cancer. This population should be targeted for instruction in breast self-examination. Resources for evaluation and treatment that are available to these women must be identified.

Signs and Symptoms

Painless breast tissue thickening or lump is the initial sign, palpated during breast self-examination or visualized on a mammogram. Most late symptoms are associated with the tumor's invasion of surrounding tissues—dimpling of the skin, nipple discharge, nipple or skin retraction, edema, dilated blood vessels, ulceration, and hemorrhage. Dry, patchy nipple skin is suggestive of Paget's disease, an uncommon cancer of the nipple and areola. Chest pain may be associated with metastasis to the lung.

Complications

Infiltration of adjacent breast and axillary tissue and metastasis to distant sites are the major complications of advanced breast cancer.

Medical Diagnosis

Routine screening methods for breast cancer follow specific guidelines:
- Clinical breast examination every 3 years until age 40, and every year after age 40
- Baseline mammogram by age 40, followed by repeat mammogram every 1 to 2 years from ages 40 to 49, and every year beginning at age 50
- Breast ultrasound, digital mammography, or magnetic resonance imaging for questionable mammogram readings
- Biopsy of suspicious tissue for histologic analysis: fine-needle aspiration, core-needle aspiration, incisional biopsy, or excisional biopsy

Medical Treatment

If tissue examination confirms the malignancy, the patient and her physician consider surgical options based on the type, size, and extent of the cancerous growth. Women are playing increasingly active roles in the decision-making process and may "shop" for surgeons with whom they can agree on the selected surgical method. An oncologist may serve as a consultant in the decision-making process. Surgical options include lumpectomy, simple mastectomy, and radical mastectomy. Lumpectomy is removal of the tumor with a margin of surrounding healthy tissue but with preservation of most of the breast. A simple mastectomy is removal of the entire breast. Radical mastectomy is removal of all breast tissue, overlying skin, axillary lymph nodes, and underlying pectoral muscles. A variation of radical mastectomy adds removal of the internal mammary lymphatic chain. Four commonly employed options are depicted in Figure 47-13. Lymphatic mapping and sentinel node biopsy uses dye or radioactive material to locate the lymph node that drains first from the site of the tumor. Study of this node enables the surgeon to determine whether and how far the cancer has spread. This procedure may avoid more extensive and unnecessary node dissection. For treatment of early-stage cancer, there is evidence that lumpectomy plus radiotherapy offers the same long-term survival rate as more extensive surgery with radiotherapy. Additional treatment options depend on staging, which is outlined in Figure 47-14.

Breast cancer is staged according to the tumor-node-metastasis classification explained in Chapter 25. The stages are summarized in Figure 47-14. Another critical factor is determined—whether the cancer cells are estrogen receptors (ER+) or nonreceptors (ER−). If cells are ER+, indicating that the tumor needs estrogen for growth, the drug *tamoxifen citrate* may be prescribed. Tamoxifen is a selective estrogen receptor modulator (SERM). SERMs block circulating estrogen from reaching the receptor cells. The use of SERMs *tamoxifen* and *raloxifene* to prevent initial malignancy in selected women who are at high risk for the development of breast cancer is under study.

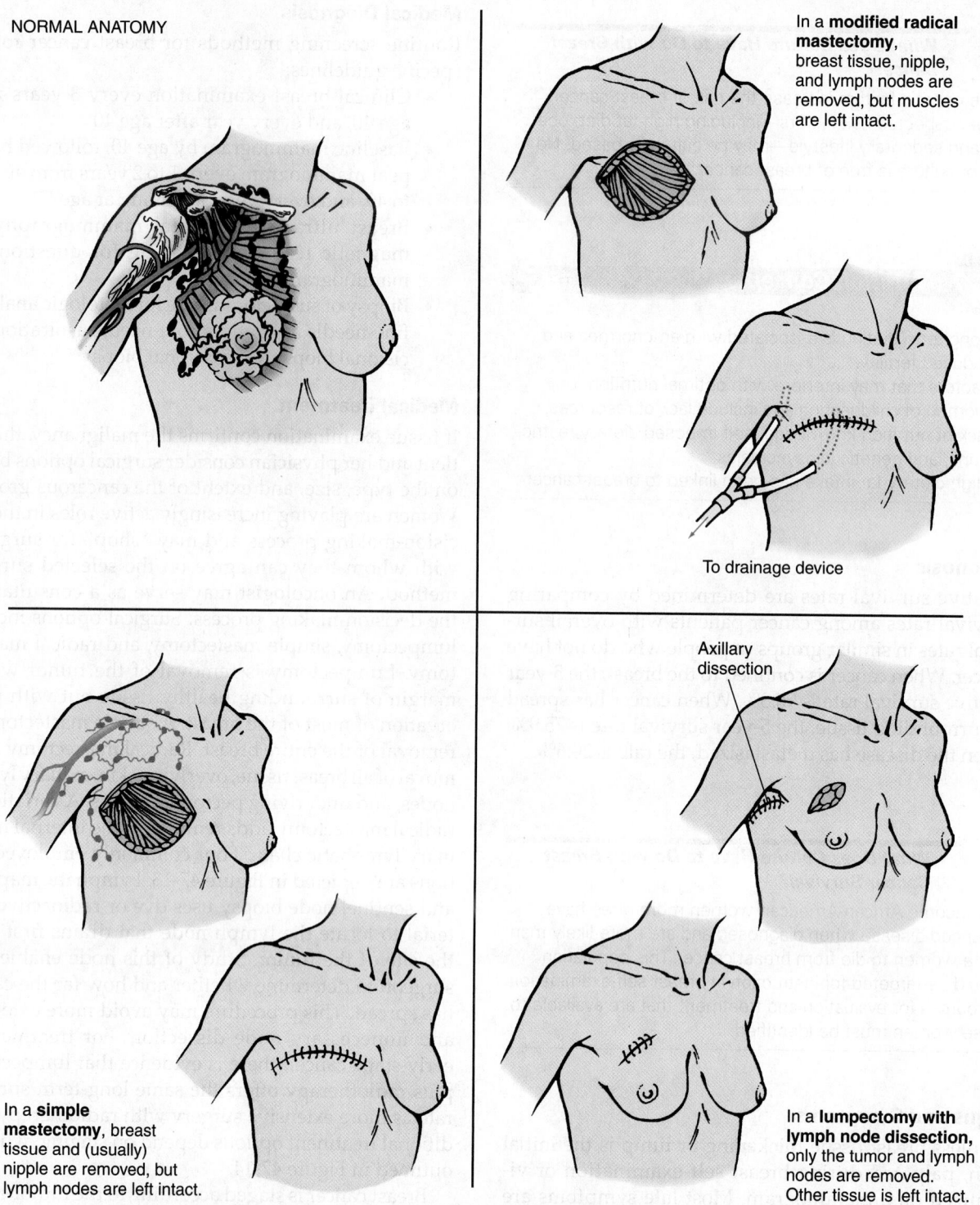

NORMAL ANATOMY

In a **modified radical mastectomy,** breast tissue, nipple, and lymph nodes are removed, but muscles are left intact.

To drainage device

Axillary dissection

In a **simple mastectomy,** breast tissue and (usually) nipple are removed, but lymph nodes are left intact.

In a **lumpectomy with lymph node dissection,** only the tumor and lymph nodes are removed. Other tissue is left intact.

FIGURE **47-13** Options in the surgical management of breast cancer.

The oncologist plays a critical role in continued management of care. Chemotherapy, hormone therapy, radiation therapy, biologic therapy, or a combination of these may be employed before, during, or after surgery. Most physicians routinely follow lumpectomy with radiation therapy, even though evidence indicates that all malignant cells were removed. Radiation therapy is used because studies indicate that there may be small

metastases without nodal involvement. See Chapter 25 for a discussion of treatment modalities.

Many women elect breast reconstruction after modified radical mastectomy or radical mastectomy. Reconstruction is performed by a plastic surgeon and may be initiated immediately after the mastectomy and before closure of the wound, or it may be delayed. Reconstruction usually begins with implantation of a

Stage I
Tumor smaller than 2 cm, with 0 lymph nodes positive for cancer and no metastases evident

Stage II
Tumor 2-5 cm, with 0-1 lymph nodes positive for cancer and no metastases evident

Stage III
Tumor larger than 5 cm, with 0 lymph nodes positive for cancer and no metastases evident

Tumor smaller than 2 cm, with axillary lymph nodes positive for cancer cells and no metastases evident

Tumor 2-5 cm, with axillary lymph nodes positive for cancer cells and no metastases evident

Lateral axillary nodes
Supraclavicular node
Suprascapular nodes
Apical nodes
Anterior pectoral nodes
Ulcer
Peau d'orange

Stage IV
Tumor of any size, with or without lymph nodes positive for cancer cells and distant metastases present

Brain
Lungs
Bone
Breast (other)
Liver

FIGURE **47-14** Stages of breast cancer.

| Table 47-4 | *Examples of Breast Reconstruction Procedures* |

PROCEDURE	DESCRIPTION
Implantation	An implant matching the size of the other breast is placed under the muscle of the operative side to create a breast mound.
Tissue expansion	A tissue expander is placed under the muscle and gradually expanded with saline to stretch the overlying skin and create a pocket. After several weeks, the tissue expander is exchanged for an implant.
Myocutaneous flaps	A flap of skin, fat, and muscle is transferred from the donor site to the operative area. The flap contains an appropriate amount of fat to match the other breast and is similar in appearance to breast tissue. A blood supply is established by reanastomosis of vessels from the operative area to those with the flap when possible. A new nipple may be created with tissue from the other nipple, labia, or thigh. Nipples can also be created by tattooing.

---

tissue expander placed under the pectoralis muscle. Small amounts of normal saline are periodically injected into the expander until the expander creates a space the size of the prosthesis that will replace the expander in a future surgical procedure. Other reconstruction methods employ transfer of tissue from other areas of the patient's own body, including the abdomen and back (Table 47-4). The last stage of breast reconstruction is creation of a natural appearing nipple. The new nipple is constructed from tissue taken from the other breast or the upper, inner thigh. Permanent pigment may be used to create the appearance of the nipple and areola.

NURSING CARE *of the Patient with Breast Cancer*

Assessment

Nursing assessments are focused on physical manifestations of disease, physical and psychological responses to treatments, review of all body systems, presence of pain, psychosocial factors, and level of knowledge. In the immediate postoperative period, the LPN/LVN may monitor the patient's vital signs, the wound dressings and drainage, and the arm on the affected side for edema.

Care of the surgical patient is covered in Chapter 17, and care of the patient who has cancer is covered in Chapter 25. Additional specific nursing diagnoses and goals for the mastectomy patient are listed in the following box.

Nursing Diagnoses, Goals, and Outcome Criteria: Postoperative Mastectomy

NURSING DIAGNOSES	GOALS AND OUTCOME CRITERIA
Disturbed Body Image related to altered appearance, loss of breast, perceived loss of attractiveness	Improved body image: patient demonstrates comfort with the new body image
Risk for Injury related to lymphedema secondary to excision of lymph nodes	Absent or minimal lymphedema: arm circumference unchanged
Impaired Physical Mobility of affected arm related to axillary lymph node dissection	Normal mobility of affected arm: patient has full range of motion in affected arm within 6 weeks
Deficient Knowledge of self-care and resources	Patient understands self-care: patient demonstrates self-care and identifies resources

Interventions

Disturbed Body Image

The breasts are an important part of a woman's self-image. To many women, loss of a breast represents loss of femininity. Even with immediate reconstruction, the breasts do not look completely normal. The patient may see herself as sexually unattractive and fear rejection by her sexual partner. These feelings are superimposed on the fear created by a diagnosis of cancer.

Be accepting of the patient, whose feelings may surface in a variety of ways, including anger, denial, and depression. From the early postoperative period, encourage the patient to attend to her appearance. Provide information about breast prostheses and clothing designed for women who have had mastectomies. If the patient has had chemotherapy, hair loss also may contribute to her body image disturbance. Strategies and resources for the cancer patient with a body image disturbance are discussed in Chapter 25.

Risk for Injury

A radical mastectomy includes the removal of lymph nodes in the axilla on the affected side. Because lymph nodes normally help return tissue fluid to the blood-stream, their removal can result in lymphedema (the accumulation of fluid in the affected area). An important aspect of postoperative care after mastectomy is directed toward preventing and minimizing lymph-edema in the arm on the affected side. Interventions to manage lymphedema include the following:

- Elevate the arm to a height above the level of the heart.
- Measure blood pressures on the arm on the unaffected side, *never on the affected side.*

- Do not use the affected arm for venipuncture, injections, or parenteral fluid administration.
- Do not apply deodorant to or shave the axilla on the affected side.
- Frequently measure the circumference of the affected arm; immediately report an increase.
- Encourage frequent and progressive exercise of the arm on the affected side.
- Encourage the patient to use the arm for as many activities of daily living as possible.

Position the patient alternately on her unaffected side and her back, observing regular postoperative care as described in Chapter 17.

Impaired Physical Mobility

Dissection of the lymph nodes in the axilla may or may not be done with a mastectomy. If the axilla is dissected, the patient is at risk for contractures unless proper positioning is maintained and exercises are begun as soon as permitted by the surgeon. Postoperatively, place the patient in semi-Fowler's position with the affected arm elevated on a pillow. Encourage her to flex and extend her fingers. Offer analgesics 30 minutes ahead of time so the exercises can be done more comfortably. The exercises should be done 3 to 5 times each day until full arm and shoulder range of motion is restored (Fig. 47-15).

Deficient Knowledge

With the patient's permission, arrangements can be made for visits from a representative of the American Cancer Society's Reach for Recovery program. The representatives are volunteers who have experienced breast cancer themselves and who have learned to cope successfully with the diagnosis, treatment, and related stressors. They assist patients by providing information, anticipatory guidance, and emotional support.

Patient teaching should have begun preoperatively but must be reinforced postoperatively. Content to cover includes signs and symptoms of infection, wound care, arm exercises, prevention of lymphedema, resources, and (if appropriate) management of the effects of chemotherapy or radiotherapy. With the patient's permission, include her significant other in the teaching process. This provides an opportunity for the partner to understand the patient's experience, to demonstrate support, and to participate in her recovery. With simple mastectomies, patients are sometimes discharged in less than 24 hours. This makes patient teaching especially challenging. Be sure to provide written information and resources along with verbal instructions.

Cervical Cancer

Cervical cancer generally grows slowly. For patients who have regular pelvic examinations and Pap smears, cervical cancer is usually diagnosed and treated in its early stage. Advanced cervical cancer may invade such surrounding structures as pelvic walls, bowel, and bladder.

FIGURE **47-15** Arm exercises for mastectomy patients.

Etiology and Risk Factors

Research indicates that the risk for cervical cancer is increased in women who have been infected with the human papillomavirus (HPV) or human immunodeficiency virus (HIV). Additional factors associated with cervical cancer are cigarette smoking, initial sexual intercourse in early adolescence, multiple sexual partners, and dietary deficiencies in folic acid and in vitamins A and C. A new vaccine, Gardasil, is available to protect against HPV infection and therefore to prevent cervical cancer. In the past, a drug called *diethylstilbestrol* was used to prevent spontaneous abortion. It has since become apparent that this therapy increased the risk of reproductive system cancers in offspring that were exposed to the drug. Diethylstilbestrol is no longer used for this purpose, but you may encounter women who have had cancer related to the drugs given to their mothers during pregnancy. There is no evidence that family history or the patient's menstrual history increases the risk of cervical cancer. Although cervical cancer formerly was thought to be linked to sexual intercourse with uncircumcised males, current research does not support this speculation.

What Does Culture Have to Do with Cervical Cancer?

Cervical cancer is more common among Latino, African-American, and American Indian women than among Caucasians. Cultural practices including diet may explain the difference.

Signs and Symptoms

Early cervical cancer is asymptomatic. Advanced cancer also may be asymptomatic or may be associated with blood-tinged or frank bloody vaginal discharge, menstrual irregularities, or bleeding after intercourse.

Complications

Invasion of cervical cancer into adjacent structures causes site-related symptoms such as pain, backache, and bleeding. Anemia due to chronic bleeding may develop.

Medical Diagnosis

Cervical cancer often is first suspected when a positive Pap smear result reveals atypical cells. Tissue specimens obtained by multiple punch biopsy, endocervical curettage, or conization are studied for microscopic evidence of malignancy. Cervical cancer is preceded by changes in cells called *dysplasia*.

Cervical cancer is staged according to the extent of invasion, with stage 0 signifying limitation to the cervical epithelium and with stage IVb indicating metastasis to distant organs.

Medical Treatment

Treatment depends on the stage of the tumor and on various general health factors. Mild dysplasia may be treated with loop electrosurgical excision. This procedure, which can be done in an outpatient setting, uses electricity to destroy abnormal tissue. Localized carcinoma (in situ) may be treated with laser destruction, cryosurgery, or conization alone; total hysterectomy may be performed if childbearing is not desired.

Invasive cancer is treated with radiation, surgery, or both. Radiotherapy may be external or internal. If the therapy is internal, a sealed source is placed in the vagina for a specified period of time. Because effective treatment requires proper placement, the patient is immobilized as much as possible for the duration of the treatment. Radiotherapy and related nursing care are discussed in detail in Chapter 25.

If surgery is elected, the extent of the surgery depends on the extent of invasion. It ranges from radical hysterectomy (removal of the uterus, fallopian tubes, upper third of the vagina, and usually the ovaries) to total pelvic exenteration (removal of the uterus, ovaries, fallopian tubes, vagina, bladder, urethra, descending colon, rectum, anal canal, and pelvic lymph nodes). Nursing care of the patient with cervical cancer is discussed on p. 1070 in the Nursing Care of the Patient with Cancer of the Cervix, Ovaries, Vulva, or Vagina section.

Ovarian Cancer

Ovarian cancer occurs most often in women between the ages of 55 and 65. Although the incidence is relatively low compared with that of other cancers, the mortality rate from ovarian cancer is the highest of all female reproductive system cancers. The high mortality is because ovarian cancer is asymptomatic until it is advanced, so it usually grows for an extended period of time before it is diagnosed. In most cases, abnormal cell growth occurs in both ovaries.

Etiology and Risk Factors

No specific causes have been found for ovarian cancer. However, risk factors include a family or personal history of ovarian cancer; a personal history of ovarian dysfunction or of breast, endometrial, or colorectal cancer; high-fat diet; nulliparity (has not produced a viable offspring); and early menarche and late menopause. Ovarian cancer rarely is found in women who have had children or who have used oral contraceptives. Therefore birth control pills or prophylactic bilateral oophorectomy (surgical removal of the ovaries) may be suggested for women at high risk for ovarian cancer.

Signs and Symptoms

Ovarian cancer is asymptomatic in its early stage. Because symptoms of even advanced ovarian cancer tend to be vague and nonspecific, they usually are attributed to various other conditions before ovarian cancer is considered. Abdominal pain and bloating, gastrointestinal tract symptoms such as flatulence, and urinary tract complaints may be reported. Abnormal uterine bleeding is not common. In extremely advanced cancer, ascites may be noted.

Complications

Ovarian cancer can spread to the peritoneum, omentum, and bowel surface via direct invasion, peritoneal fluid, and the lymphatic and venous systems.

Medical Diagnosis

Palpable tumors may be discovered on pelvic and rectal examinations. Abdominal and vaginal ultrasound with color Doppler imaging may be used as diagnostic tools. Blood may be drawn for a CA-125 serum marker test, which, if elevated, may indicate ovarian epithelial cancer. If evidence supports a diagnosis of ovarian cancer, an exploratory laparotomy or laparoscopy is done to directly visualize the tumor or tumors and to obtain tissue for definitive diagnosis and for staging and grading of the malignancy.

Some practitioners advocate routine screening of blood serum for CA-125 for early detection of ovarian cancer. However, elevated CA-125 levels can be caused by other factors in addition to ovarian cancer.

Medical Treatment

Treatment depends on the staging of the tumor or tumors. Options include surgery (usually total abdominal hysterectomy and bilateral salpingo-oophorectomy), systemic or intraperitoneal chemotherapy, intraperitoneal radioisotope instillation, and external radiation therapy. Even with advanced disease, treatment can improve comfort. Regardless of the stage and prognosis for survival, CA-125 levels may be monitored to assess tumor progression or regression. Nursing care of the patient with ovarian cancer is discussed on p. 1069 in the Nursing Care of the Patient with Cancer of the Cervix, Ovaries, Vulva, or Vagina section.

Vulvar Cancer

Cancer of the vulva is the rarest but also the most visible of the cancers of the female reproductive system. It may appear as a visible and palpable lump on the vulva or as a deviation from the normally pink, moist mucosa. The lesion may be scaly; red, white, or irregularly pigmented; and edematous. Drainage from the lesion may be pink (serosanguineous) or bloody. The most common site is the labia majora.

Although it is rare, malignant melanoma may occur in the vulva. Its incidence is highest in postmenopausal women. The symptoms are similar to those of the more common vulvar cancers.

Etiology and Risk Factors

The cause of vulvar cancer is unknown, but it may be related to STDs, particularly HPV. Other risk factors are diabetes mellitus and hypertension.

Signs and Symptoms

The most commonly reported symptom is pruritus (itching). Pain and bleeding are additional symptoms.

Complications

Although cancer of the vulva generally remains localized, it may become invasive if not discovered and treated. It can invade adjacent structures or metastasize via the lymphatic system.

Medical Diagnosis

A preliminary diagnosis is made through palpation of a mass or by visualization of tissue that appears suspicious. Biopsy is necessary for definitive diagnosis.

Medical Treatment

Treatment depends on the extent to which the malignant cells have spread. For localized lesions, conservative removal of the malignant tissue by laser surgery or topical chemotherapy may be employed. For wider, deeper, or invasive lesions, radical surgical removal through hemivulvectomy or vulvectomy and bilateral dissection of groin lymph nodes or through pelvic exenteration may be necessary. Radical hemivulvectomy is generally preferred because radical vulvectomy results in greater scarring and loss of function and is more prone to wound breakdown. Pelvic exenteration is the removal of all pelvic organs including the bladder; the descending colon and anal canal may or may not be removed. Chemotherapy, radiation therapy, or both may follow surgery. Nursing care of the patient with vulvar cancer is discussed on p. 1070 in the Nursing Care of the Patient with Cancer of the Cervix, Ovaries, Vulva, or Vagina section.

Vaginal Cancer

The vagina seldom is the primary site for cancer; rather, it is the site for the extension of cancer that originates in the vulva, cervix, or endometrium. Except for young women whose vaginal cancers are associated with intrauterine exposure to diethylstilbestrol, vaginal cancer is found most commonly in postmenopausal women.

Etiology and Risk Factors

No definite cause has been identified for vaginal cancer. However, researchers have identified the following risk factors: STDs (syphilis, herpes virus type 2, HPV), a previous diagnosis of cervical or vulvar cancer, previous radiation therapy, and intrauterine exposure to diethylstilbestrol.

Signs and Symptoms

In its early and most easily treated form, vaginal cancer usually is asymptomatic. Later symptoms include a burning sensation, vaginal discharge that may have a foul odor, dyspareunia, spotting after intercourse, and vaginal bleeding. Pelvic pain usually is associated with invasion of adjacent structures.

Complications

Invasion of adjacent structures and metastasis are the most common complications of epithelial vaginal cancer. The prognosis is poor for vaginal malignant melanoma, with an extremely low 5-year survival rate.

Medical Diagnosis and Treatment

Most cases are detected during inspection of the vagina and from routine Pap smears. A definitive diagnosis is made via colposcopy and biopsy of suspicious areas followed by tissue studies. Treatment of vaginal cancer depends on the extent of invasion. In situ (localized) cancer may be treated relatively simply with local laser surgery or cryosurgery. More radical treatment is indicated if the cancer is more invasive. Possible treatments employed either alone or in combination include topical chemotherapy, internal or external radiotherapy, partial or total vaginectomy, and pelvic exenteration.

 What Does Culture Have to Do with Body Image After Mastectomy?

The importance of reproductive capacity as a measure of a woman's value depends on cultural values. In cultures that associate the breasts with sexuality, the loss of a breast can cause a woman to feel undesirable.

NURSING CARE *of the Patient with Cancer of the Cervix, Ovaries, Vulva, or Vagina*

The patient with cancer of the cervix, ovaries, vulva, or vagina presents many challenges. She has a life-threatening condition whose treatment very often threatens not only her self-concept but also her sexual function. Treatments beyond local excision of affected tissue may result in disfigurement or in anatomic changes that hinder penile-vaginal intercourse, or both. The patient's psychosocial needs are as critical as her physical needs.

Assessment

Complete assessment of the patient with a disorder of the female reproductive system is summarized in

Box 47-1. When the patient has or may have cancer, the health history documents signs and symptoms and possible risk factors. When reviewing the systems, changes or problems that may be related such as fatigue, pain, and bowel or bladder dysfunction should be described. The effects of the symptoms on normal functioning should be explored. The patient may react to the diagnosis with anxiety, fear, depression, anger, or withdrawal. A complete physical examination should be done. The physician or nurse practitioner performs a pelvic examination that may reveal lesions, masses, and lymph node enlargement.

Nursing Diagnoses, Goals, and Outcome Criteria: Cancer of the Cervix, Ovaries, Vulva, or Vagina

Nursing Diagnoses	Goals and Outcome Criteria
Anxiety and **Fear** related to threat to health and lack of knowledge about the cancer and prescribed treatment	Reduced anxiety and fear: patient's statement of reduced anxiety and fear, with calm manner
Disturbed Body Image related to change in body appearance or function	Improved body image: positive patient statements about self and efforts to maintain or improve appearance
Ineffective Sexuality Pattern related to physical and emotional effects of cancer of the reproductive system	Satisfactory sexual patterns: patient's discussion of effects of disease or treatment on sexuality and coping strategies
Compromised Family Coping related to lack of knowledge, situational crisis, role changes, or patient preoccupation with self	Appropriate family-patient interactions: family demonstration of support and positive coping
Risk for Injury (to patient and others) related to effects of radiotherapy, chemotherapy	Decreased risk of injury from treatment: maintenance of applicator position and adherence of patient and others to radiation precautions

Interventions

Anxiety and Fear

The woman needs to be able to express her feelings about her diagnosis and prescribed treatment without being judged. Listen carefully to determine any knowledge deficits or misconceptions. Provide information or sources of information as appropriate. Many women of all ages are computer-literate and therefore have access to endless sources. However, patients should be cautioned that not all Internet information is accurate or appropriate for her situation. National organizations like the American Cancer Society have excellent patient education materials. Community agencies may have a lending library of books and videotapes. Support groups are often helpful because patients learn from others who have had similar experiences. Many patients appreciate follow-up phone calls or the ability to call a resource person when needed.

Disturbed Body Image

The patient may be distressed if there is a change in appearance or function caused by the cancer or the treatment. Loss of reproductive capacity can be especially painful for women who still wish to bear children. You can listen kindly when the patient wishes to express her thoughts. Patients who are severely disturbed should be offered the benefit of a mental health professional or spiritual counselor. Encourage measures to improve the appearance, and praise the patient's positive efforts. Management of alopecia (hair loss) associated with cancer therapy is discussed in Chapter 25.

Ineffective Sexuality Pattern

The physician should present realistic expectations for future sexual functioning. The patient may be advised to abstain from sexual intercourse during the treatment and healing. Permanent effects of the disease and treatment may require alternative sexual practices. The patient may wish to discuss this topic with you. It is critical that you show an accepting attitude toward sexuality in general and toward any specific sexual practices acceptable to the patient and her partner. A counselor or therapist may be consulted to help the patient adapt.

Compromised Family Coping

Include the family or identified support system in care. The family needs to understand the effects of the cancer and the treatments. They also need to understand the patient's need for support and for assistance during therapy and recovery. Encourage members of the household to consider ways to reduce demands on the patient. In addition, be sensitive to the needs of family members who may fear losing a loved one. Inclusion of the woman's sexual partner is particularly critical if altered sexual expression is expected after treatment.

Risk for Injury

Physical care of the patient varies with the prescribed treatment and is based on physician's orders, institutional policies and procedures, and nursing diagnoses. General guidelines for the care of the patient who is having radiotherapy are covered in Chapter 25.

Internal radiation poses a nursing challenge. If a sealed radiation source is to be implanted in the vagina, an indwelling urinary catheter is inserted first. An applicator that will contain the radiation source is inserted into the vagina while the patient is in the operating room. The placement is checked on radiographs and is maintained by vaginal packing. The radiation source may be placed in the applicator before the applicator is inserted, or it may be placed in the applicator after the patient is transferred to her room and positioned in bed. The radiation dosage is determined and ordered by a radiologist; the duration of implantation is based on the total dosage but generally ranges from 24 to 72 hours.

The patient poses a source of radiation exposure to anyone within a radius of several feet, so usual radiation precautions are in force. For each nurse who is allowed to care for the patient, exposure should not exceed a total of 30 minutes per 24 hours. Visitors are screened according to protocol; those cleared to visit should be instructed to remain outside a 6-foot radius of the patient and to limit the duration of visits according to policy.

The patient is assigned a private room for the duration of internal radiotherapy. Enforce strict bed rest to prevent dislodgment of the applicator. Movement is restricted to cautious turning from side to side. The facts that radiation therapy may precipitate nausea, vomiting, and diarrhea; that movement must be restricted; and that total time for nursing care is restricted make care particularly challenging. You need to be exceptionally well organized and able to anticipate and to act efficiently. Administration of antiemetics, sedatives, and antidiarrheal medications may control radiation side effects and thus facilitate patient comfort, maintenance of applicator position, and efficiency of nursing care time.

Effects of radiation on local tissue produce a profuse, foul-smelling vaginal discharge that is largely absorbed by the packing and thus cannot be controlled with cleansing. A room deodorizer may be partially effective in making the odor tolerable. After removal of the packing and applicator at the conclusion of therapy, a cleansing vaginal douche may be ordered. The patient then is no longer a source of radiation and can resume her normal activities. Consider transfer of the patient to another room to remove her from a noxious environment and to allow housekeeping personnel to clean and air the room. External radiation therapy sometimes is used instead of internal treatment. See Chapter 25 for care of the patient having external radiation.

Care of the patient admitted for a pelvic exenteration is exceptionally complex and is beyond the scope of this textbook. An expert nursing staff is essential to provide the emotional support and physical care demanded for this patient.

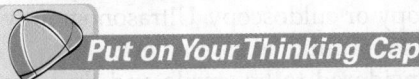
Put on Your Thinking Cap!

A patient with pelvic cancer has had a surgical procedure that includes removal of the vagina. She tearfully says, "I will never be able to make love to my husband again." What are some things you could say or do to show acceptance of her feelings at this time?

INFERTILITY

Infertility generally is defined as the inability to conceive within 1 year of regular unprotected sexual intercourse. Infertility is categorized as *primary infertility* if the woman has never conceived or if the man has never impregnated a woman. *Secondary infertility* refers to the woman who has conceived at least one time but is not able to conceive again. An estimated 15% of American couples are infertile. Treatment enables approximately 60% of those couples to conceive and carry pregnancies to term.

In recent years, the entertainment and news media have provided mechanisms for the frank discussion of components of infertility: causes, psychosocial effects, and treatments. Associated problems and treatments have been described by professional health care providers and scientists, and personal accounts have been given by affected individuals. For many, the acceptance of infertility as a topic for public discussion has removed the stigma of infertility as a source of shame and embarrassment; myths have been debunked; and lay and professional people are becoming more knowledgeable about the subject. As a result, infertility has become a major subspecialty of gynecology and infertility researchers have developed highly sophisticated and effective diagnostic techniques and treatments.

Etiology and Risk Factors

Causes of infertility may be related to the female, the male, or both. Sometimes the cause cannot be determined. Conception depends on a number of factors, broadly categorized as follows:

1. Timing and techniques used for sexual intercourse:
   A. Impregnation of the ovum by the sperm must occur within 24 hours after ovulation. Intercourse should be scheduled for every other day around ovulation time to optimize the potential for fertilization of the ovum.
   B. Semen should be deposited deeply in the vagina, in proximity to the cervical os.
2. Production and release of a healthy ovum by the female and of numerous (approximately 200,000,000 per ejaculate) healthy sperm by the male.
3. Anatomically and physiologically correct female and male reproductive systems:
   A. Female: patent fallopian tubes with active fimbriated ends, uterine endometrium prepared for reception and implantation of a fertilized ovum.
   B. Male: epididymis temperature that maintains sperm viability during storage, patent seminiferous tubules, and vas deferens with enervated musculature.
4. Biochemical compatibility between female vaginal-cervical-fallopian environment and male ejaculate.

Faulty timing or technique for sexual intercourse is easily corrected through patient education. Many other causes for infertility exist. As mentioned previously, untreated or inadequately treated STDs can impair fertility by altering anatomy, physiology, and patency of the reproductive tracts of either or both partners. Additional identified influences on conception include dysfunction of any part of the hypothalamic-pituitary-endocrine system, malnutrition or obesity, smoking, drug and alcohol use, exposure to toxic chemicals or radiation, nervous system disorders that affect reproductive structures that transfer ova and sperm, and male practices that maintain above-normal epididymal temperature (i.e., wearing tight underwear and pants, frequent and prolonged immersion in hot water or sauna). Causes of infertility are summarized in Box 47-3.

Medical Diagnosis

The diagnosis is based on data obtained from exhaustive psychosocial and physical health and sexual health histories of both partners. If the histories provide clues that may explain possible detriments to fertility, such as poor timing or techniques of sexual intercourse or habitual epididymal exposure to high temperatures, further diagnostic attempts may be delayed until the couple has had time to remediate the potential problem or problems. If such simple factors

are not identified, history taking is followed by systematic, comprehensive physical examinations and laboratory tests.

The male partner usually is the initial focus of diagnostic procedures because tests for diagnosis of male-associated infertility problems are generally easier, less invasive, less expensive, and (unlike a complete female fertility workup) not cycle-dependent. A semen specimen for analysis is collected by masturbation after a period of sexual abstinence that approximates the male's average frequency interval for intercourse. The specimen is then assessed for volume and for sperm count, morphology (shape), duration of viability, motility, and liquefaction. A second specimen is examined if variations from normal are found. He may be referred to a urologist or endocrinologist for further diagnosis and possible treatment.

Evaluation of the female partner includes a battery of tests. The woman may be instructed to maintain a record of her basal body temperature, which is taken each morning upon awakening. The basal body temperature rises when ovulation occurs, which suggests the timing of intercourse. Another tool is the ovulation prediction kit that measures luteinizing hormone (LH) in the urine. Daily measurements detect a rise in LH, which usually is followed by ovulation in 28 to 36 hours. Other diagnostic data are obtained with cervical and vaginal smears, endometrial biopsy, and measurement of plasma progesterone.

If the diagnostic tests indicate normal hormonal functions, a postcoital test may be done. The couple has intercourse around the expected time of ovulation and 2 to 12 hours before the scheduled test. A specimen of cervical and vaginal secretions is aspirated from the cervix by the physician or nurse practitioner. The characteristics of the mucus are assessed by gross inspection and by microscopic examination. The examiner also inspects the specimen for number and motility of sperm. If a previous test of the male's semen indicated normal motility and viability of sperm but the postcoital test indicates nonviable sperm, this suggests that the cervical mucus is not conducive to sperm survival, perhaps because of an antigen-antibody response to the semen.

Determination of fallopian tube patency usually is accomplished with hysterosalpingography. A radiopaque dye is injected through the cervix. Radiographs then are taken to visualize the uterus and tubes. Physical assessment of the peritoneal cavity, if required, employs laparoscopy or culdoscopy. Ultrasonography may be employed for additional assessment.

Women are considered to be sterile and thus are not candidates for infertility diagnosis and treatment if they have congenital reproductive tract anomalies that cannot be corrected by surgery. Absence of one or more reproductive tract structures is also untreatable.

Box 47-3 | *Causes of Infertility*

Female
- Developmental: uterine abnormalities
- Endocrine: pituitary, thyroid, and adrenal dysfunctions; ovarian dysfunctions (inhibit maturation and release of ova)
- Diseases: pelvic inflammatory disease (especially from gonococcus); fallopian tube obstructions; diseases of cervix and uterus that inhibit passage of active sperm
- Other: malnutrition, severe anemia, anxiety

Male
- Developmental: undescended testes, other congenital anomalies (inhibit development of sperm)
- Endocrine: hormonal deficiencies (pituitary, thyroid, adrenal) (inhibit development of sperm)
- Diseases: testicular destruction from disease, orchitis from mumps, prostatitis
- Other: excessive smoking, fatigue, alcohol, excessive heat (hot baths), marijuana use

Both Male and Female
- Diseases: sexually transmitted diseases (STDs), cancer with obstructions (inhibit transport of ovum or sperm)
- Other: immunologic incompatibility (inhibit sperm penetration of ovum), marital problems
- Diethylstilbestrol exposure in utero (suggested but not proved as a cause of male infertility)

From Phipps, W.J., Monahan, F.D., Sands, J.K., Marek, J.F., & Neighbors, M. (2003). *Medical-surgical nursing: Health and illness perspectives* (7th ed., p. 1784). St. Louis: Mosby.

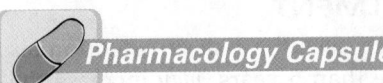
Pharmacology Capsule

Ovulatory stimulants can cause ovarian hyperstimulation with possible rupture of the enlarged ovary.

Medical Treatment

Treatment for infertility depends on specific diagnostic findings. A brief overview of specific problems and related treatments is presented in Table 47-5.

NURSING CARE of the Patient with an Infertility Disorder

Assessment

Assessment of the female reproductive system is summarized in Box 47-1. The LPN/LVN assists with data collection for the assessment.

Nursing Diagnoses, Goals, and Outcome Criteria: Infertility

NURSING DIAGNOSES	GOALS AND OUTCOME CRITERIA
Situational Low Self-Esteem related to inability to conceive or feeling of failure	Improved self-esteem: positive expressions about self
Ineffective Sexuality Pattern related to structured efforts to conceive or loss of spontaneity	Acknowledgment of the effects of the situation on one's sexual relationship: patient identifies ways to maintain a satisfying sexual relationship
Ineffective Coping related to unmet expectations or feelings of loss	Effective coping: patient uses healthy coping strategies

Deficient Knowledge of diagnostic and treatment procedures	Patient understands diagnostic and treatment procedures: patient verbalizes diagnostic and treatment procedures

Interventions

Fertility tests and treatments are generally done on an outpatient basis. The woman who undergoes the process usually has a prolonged relationship and frequent contacts with the nurse in the outpatient setting.

Situational Low Self-Esteem

Invasion of personal privacy is necessarily greater in fertility diagnosis and treatment than in any other condition. Gently explore the feelings of the patient and her partner about their difficulty conceiving. An open, empathetic attitude is vital if the patient is to be open. Support groups or professional counselors may help the couple maintain self-esteem.

Ineffective Sexuality Pattern

The most intimate details of her sexual relationship with her partner are elicited, and diagnostic and treatment procedures repeatedly violate the desire for modesty. Lovemaking becomes scheduled rather than spontaneous.

Ineffective Coping

You may be the only person with whom the woman shares her psychological reactions to the diagnosis of infertility and her subsequent emotional highs and lows throughout diagnosis and treatment. You therefore play a critical role in assisting the patient to cope with infertility. Give the patient the opportunity to

---

Table 47-5 | Common Causes of Female Infertility and Related Medical Treatment

ETIOLOGY	MEDICAL TREATMENT
Failure to ovulate, associated with the following:	
Delayed follicular maturation	Clomiphene citrate (Clomid)
Hypogonadotropin secretion	Menotropins (Pergonal)
Hypothalamic-pituitary dysfunction	Gonadotropin-releasing hormone
Elevated prolactin level	Bromocriptine mesylate (Parlodel)
Hypothyroidism	Thyroid-stimulating hormone
Ovarian tumors	Surgical excision
Poor-quality midcycle cervical mucus	Conjugated estrogens (Premarin) therapy
Inadequate endometrial development	Progesterone therapy
Endometriosis	Lupron therapy
	Gamete intrafallopian transfer
Reproductive tract infections	Antimicrobial therapy
Tubal construction	Hysterosalpingogram
Sperm-inhospitable cervical mucus	Therapeutic intrauterine insemination
	In vitro fertilization
Immunologic reaction to sperm	Use of condoms to reduce antibody titer, followed by unprotected intercourse at time of ovulation only
	In vitro fertilization

discuss her thoughts and feelings about infertility and to explore coping strategies.

Deficient Knowledge

The needs of her sexual partner must be considered as well, and he should be included in patient teaching. Patient teaching includes information about diagnostic procedures, treatments, causes of infertility, and resources.

MENOPAUSE

Menopause is the cessation of menstruation that marks the end of a woman's reproductive capacity. Natural menopause is part of normal aging, but surgical menopause results from removal of the ovaries. Natural menopause occurs gradually and may permit better adaptation than surgical menopause, which suddenly eliminates the source of natural estrogen. Diminished ovarian function associated with aging causes ovulation to cease and estrogen production to decline. The onset of menopause may begin as early as age 35 but more commonly occurs between ages 40 and 55. With natural menopause, the woman's first sign may be menstrual irregularity. Menstrual periods tend to be spaced farther apart, and the amount of bleeding gradually diminishes. The entire process from earliest signs to complete cessation of menstruation usually is 2 years or less. A woman is said to be menopausal when she has not had a menstrual period for 1 year. Some women experience a surgical menopause brought on by the surgical removal of the ovaries. Unless estrogen replacement is begun promptly, the patient develops the signs and symptoms of menopause rapidly.

SIGNS AND SYMPTOMS

The signs and symptoms of menopause may include hot flashes—a warm feeling caused by vasodilation that affects the face, neck, and upper body. Hot flashes are typically accompanied by perspiration and sometimes by a feeling of faintness. Other common symptoms are vaginal dryness, insomnia, joint pain, headache, and nausea. Without estrogen, the uterus becomes smaller, the vagina shortens, and vaginal tissues become drier. Breast tissue may lose its firmness, and pubic and axillary hair become sparse. Supporting pelvic structures relax, causing some women to have stress incontinence. There may be significant loss of bone mass, thus leading to fragile bones, a condition called *osteoporosis*. Some women report emotional instability, irritability, and depression, but the impact of menopause on a woman is very individualized. Some grieve for the loss of reproductive capacity, and some feel a loss of femininity and sexual attractiveness. Others welcome the end of menstrual periods and no longer having to worry about the risk of pregnancy.

MEDICAL TREATMENT

Estrogen therapy decreases the risk of osteoporosis but, if taken for more than 5 years, *may* increase the risk of breast cancer. Therefore each woman's health history must be considered so that she and her physician can decide whether hormone replacement therapy will be used. Estrogens are contraindicated with estrogen-dependent cancer, undiagnosed abnormal vaginal bleeding, and current or past thromboembolic disorders.

There are many drug regimens. The patient who still has her uterus and ovaries has typically been treated with estrogen and progestins (compounds that have actions like progesterone). Because progestin decreases the risk of endometrial cancer related to estrogen therapy, it is not needed in women who no longer have a uterus. Findings from the Women's Health Initiative indicate the combination therapy in women with intact uteruses increases the risk of invasive breast cancer and coronary heart disease.

Oral drug therapy is most commonly used, but a transdermal form of estrogen is also available. The transdermal drug is delivered by an adhesive bandage–like patch. Estrogen creams, vaginal tablets, and suppositories may be used to relieve vaginal dryness. Drugs used to control "hot flashes" include clonidine patches, Bellergal-S, venlafaxine, and paroxetine.

 Consider the Alternative

Black cohosh is sometimes used to treat menstrual cramps and as an alternative to estrogen for treatment of menopausal symptoms. Black cohosh can potentiate antihypertensive and hypoglycemic drugs. Patients are advised to limit its use to 6 months because of lack of information about long-term effects.

Consider the Alternative

Over-the-counter options for treating hot flashes include vitamin E 400-800 IU PO daily, vitamin B complex 200 mg PO daily, and selenium per manufacturer's instructions.

NURSING CARE *of the Menopausal Patient*
Assessment

Assessment of the woman with a disorder of the reproductive system is summarized in Box 47-1. When a woman has menopausal symptoms, record them and explore how the patient is coping with this significant life change.

Nursing Diagnoses, Goals, and Outcome Criteria: Menopause

The primary nursing diagnosis for the menopausal patient is usually Ineffective Therapeutic Regimen

Management related to lack of understanding of the effects and treatment of menopause. The goals of nursing care are effective management of prescribed therapy and decreased signs and symptoms of menopause. The outcome criterion is the patient's report of reduced symptoms.

Interventions

Assess the patient's understanding of menopause and how she feels about it. The patient may need reassurance that her symptoms and responses are normal and common. If drug therapy is used, instruct the patient regarding self-medication. Caution patients on estrogen to report any signs of circulatory disorders (numbness, pain in calf, shortness of breath) to the physician immediately. Additional information about drug therapy is summarized in the Drug Therapy table on pp. 1041 to 1043. The patient who cannot or chooses not to take hormone therapy needs additional assistance to cope with the symptoms of menopause. Women who wish to prevent "menopausal" pregnancy should utilize a reliable form of contraception for at least 1 year after cessation of menses.

Key Points

- The female reproductive system includes the external and internal genitalia and the breasts.
- Common therapeutic measures for the female reproductive system include douche, cauterization, heat application, and topical medications.
- Two common uterine bleeding disorders are metrorrhagia (bleeding or spotting between menstrual periods) and menorrhagia (menstrual periods characterized by profuse bleeding).
- The primary nursing diagnoses for the patient with a uterine bleeding disorder are Deficient Knowledge of condition and treatment and Anxiety related to unknown cause of bleeding.
- The effects of reproductive tract infections may include infertility, changes in relationships, feelings of distrust toward sexual partners, shame, embarrassment, and diminished self-esteem.
- Because most infections are treated on an outpatient basis, the nurse's primary role is to educate the patient in preventing and treating infections.
- Benign growths of the female reproductive system include cysts of the breasts and ovaries and endometriosis.

- The primary nursing diagnoses for the patient with endometriosis, a disorder marked by the growth of endometrial tissue outside the uterus, are Acute Pain and Deficient Knowledge.
- Cysts are saclike structures that contain fluid, semisolid, or solid material and are usually benign.
- Fibroid tumors (myomas, leiomyomas) are benign but may have to be removed because they can compress abdominal structures and lead to infertility, crowding, and malpositioning of the fetus during pregnancy and degenerative changes related to interruption of blood supply.
- Herniation of the bladder (called *cystocele*) or of the rectum (called rectocele) into the vagina can disrupt urinary and bowel function and is often corrected surgically.
- Nursing diagnoses after surgery for correction of a cystocele or rectocele may include Impaired Urinary Elimination, Risk for Injury, and Acute Pain.
- Uterine prolapse, the descent of the uterus into the vagina, may be treated with corrective surgery or vaginal hysterectomy.
- Abnormal uterine positions include retroversion (backward tilt), retroflexion (uterine body bends backward), anteversion (forward tilt), and anteflexion (uterine body bends forward); these conditions rarely require treatment.
- Breast cancer is the most prevalent form of cancer in American women. It has a 5-year survival rate of more than 90% when detected early.
- After mastectomy, nursing diagnoses may include Risk for Injury, Impaired Physical Mobility, Risk for Infection, Disturbed Body Image, and Ineffective Sexuality Pattern.
- Cervical cancer can be detected early by regular pelvic examinations and Papanicolaou smears. Prompt treatment is usually curative.
- Ovarian cancer has the highest mortality rate of all female reproductive system cancers because it is asymptomatic in the early stages.
- Nursing diagnoses for the patient with cancer of the reproductive system may include Anxiety, Fear, Disturbed Body Image, Ineffective Sexuality Pattern, Compromised Family Coping, and (if treated with radiotherapy) Risk for Injury.
- Infertility, the inability to produce viable offspring, can sometimes be treated medically or surgically.

 Go to your Companion CD-ROM for a Pharmacology Tutorial, Audio Glossary, and 3-D animations.

evolve Be sure to visit the companion Evolve site at http://evolve.elsevier.com/Linton/ for WebLinks and additional online resources.

REVIEW QUESTIONS *Choose the best answer.*

1. The site of fertilization is in the:
   1. Uterus
   2. Ovary
   3. Fallopian tube
   4. Vagina

2. Which question collects data about the patient's menarche?
   1. At what age did you begin menstruating?
   2. Would you describe your menstrual flow as light or heavy?
   3. What was your age when you first experienced hot flashes?
   4. Do you usually have any changes in mood before your menstrual period?

3. To prepare a patient for culdoscopy, the nurse should tell her:
   1. You will be positioned as if you were having a routine pelvic examination
   2. You will have no restrictions following the procedure
   3. You will need to return in a week to have your sutures removed
   4. You may have shoulder pain caused by air entering the pelvic cavity

4. You are teaching a class on breast self-examination (BSE) to women of various ages. What should you tell women who no longer menstruate about BSE?
   1. BSE is not necessary once a woman is menopausal.
   2. Perform BSE on the same day of each month.
   3. Older women should perform BSE every day.
   4. Mammograms are needed only if you discover a lump.

5. A young woman has come to the doctor's office for a routine pelvic examination. During the health history, she tells you that her mother says douching is an essential part of feminine hygiene. What is the best response?
   1. Your body has normal processes to cleanse the vagina so douching is unnecessary.
   2. Douching is not really necessary, but it is a harmless procedure.
   3. There are no medically appropriate reasons for douching.
   4. Douching is safe if sterile solution is used.

6. Which organism is most often associated with pelvic inflammatory disease?
   1. *Neisseria gonorrhoeae*
   2. *Chlamydia trachomatis*
   3. *Mycoplasma hominis*
   4. *Escherichia coli*

7. A patient completed a 6-month course of danazol (Danocrine) for treatment of endometriosis. She would like to become pregnant. It is important for her to understand that:
   1. She will begin menstrual bleeding within 1 week after stopping the danazol
   2. Her best chances of pregnancy are in the first month after completing danazol therapy
   3. She should not become pregnant for 1 month because danazol can cause birth defects
   4. She is unlikely to become pregnant for at least 1 year after taking danazol

8. An older woman with uterine prolapse is being fitted with a pessary. What information should be included in the teaching plan?
   1. The pessary permanently corrects the uterine prolapse.
   2. Once the pessary is in place, no further care is needed.
   3. There are no complications associated with pessaries.
   4. The position of the pessary must be checked in 24 hours.

9. Which palpable breast lump is most characteristic of breast cancer?
   1. A single painless lump in the upper, outer quadrant of one breast
   2. A firm, painful lump that feels oval-shaped and is freely movable
   3. Bilateral multiple small lumps that are tender just before menstruation
   4. Soft, painless, symmetric lumps in the lower outer quadrant of both breasts

10. A 30-year-old female who reports menarche at age 10, first sexual intercourse at age 14, a history of treatment for *Chlamydia* infection at age 15, and gonorrhea at age 17 is at increased risk for:
    1. Breast cancer
    2. Uterine prolapse
    3. Cervical cancer
    4. Fibroid tumors

CHAPTER 48

48 Male Reproductive Disorders

Objectives

After reading and studying this chapter, you should be able to:

1. Describe the major structures and functions of the normal male reproductive system.

2. Identify data to be collected when assessing a male patient with a reproductive system disorder.

3. Discuss commonly performed diagnostic tests and procedures and the nursing implications of each.

4. Identify common therapeutic measures used to treat disorders of the male reproductive system and the nursing implications of each.

5. For selected disorders of the male reproductive system, explain the pathophysiology, signs and symptoms, complications, medical diagnosis, and medical treatment.

6. Assist in developing a nursing care plan for a male patient with a reproductive system disorder.

Key Terms

Be sure to check out the bonus material on the Companion CD-ROM, including selected audio pronunciations.

corpus (*pl.* corpora) cavernosa (KŎR-pŭs, KŎR-pō-ră, p. 1080)

ejaculation (ē-jăk-ū-LĀ-shŭn, p. 1080)

emission (ē-MĬSH-ŭn, p. 1080)

epididymitis (ĕp-ĭ-dĭd-ē-MĪ-tĭs, p. 1087)

erectile dysfunction (ē-RĔK-tĭl dĭs-FŬNK-shŭn, p. 1081)

erection (ē-RĔK-shŭn, p. 1078)

hematocele (HĔM-ăh-tō-sēl, p. 1083)

hydrocele (HĬ-drō-sēl, p. 1085)

infertility (ĭn-fĕr-TĬL-ĭ-tē, p. 1097)

phimosis (fī-MŌ-sĭs, p. 1097)

prostatectomy (prŏs-tă-TĔK-tō-mē, p. 1088)

prostatitis (prŏs-tă-TĪ-tĭs, p. 1085)

smegma (SMĔG-mă, p. 1082)

sterile (STĔR-ĭl, p. 1088)

testis (*pl.* testes) (TĔS-tĭs, TĔS-tēz, p. 1077)

ANATOMY AND PHYSIOLOGY OF THE MALE REPRODUCTIVE SYSTEM

ANATOMY

The male reproductive system consists of the scrotum, testes, epididymis, vas deferens, seminal vesicles, prostate gland, ejaculatory duct, internal urethra, and penis (Fig. 48-1).

SCROTUM

The scrotum is a thin, pendulous sac on the outside of the body that encloses each of the two testicles in separate compartments. The scrotum contracts into thick folds during fear, anger, arousal, or cold, drawing the testes close to the body for protection and insulation. On warm days the scrotal muscles relax and allow the scrotum to hang free of the body. Sweat glands may be activated to cool the testes and maintain a testicular temperature that is below body temperature.

TESTES

The two **testes** (testicles) are the male reproductive organs. They lie within the scrotum, suspended from the spermatic cord (Fig. 48-2). They are composed of numerous highly coiled seminiferous tubules that produce spermatozoa and sex hormones. The testicles develop in the embryo at about the seventh week of gestation and begin producing small amounts of testosterone. Secretion of this male hormone results in the development of other male reproductive organs and causes the testes to descend into the scrotum during the last 2 months of gestation. At around 10 to 13 years of age, during puberty, the increased production of testosterone results in the production of sperm and the development of body hair, muscle mass, and other secondary sex characteristics.

EPIDIDYMIS

Newly developed sperm move from each testicle through the epididymis, a coiled tubule almost 20 feet long that rests along the top and side of the testes. This passage may take several days and allows the sperm to mature and develop the capability for motility (movement) and fertilization (see Fig. 48-2).

VAS DEFERENS

As mature sperm leave the epididymis, they enter the vasa deferentia (*sing.*, vas deferens), which are tubes of secretory ducts that serve as the primary storage sites for sperm, contribute to the fluid content of semen and contract to help propel the mature sperm into the urethra during ejaculation. The vas deferens is bundled together with the spermatic artery and veins, lymphatic vessels, and nerves by the spermatic cord; the bundle exits the scrotum and enters the pelvic cavity via the inguinal canal (see Figs. 48-1 and 48-2).

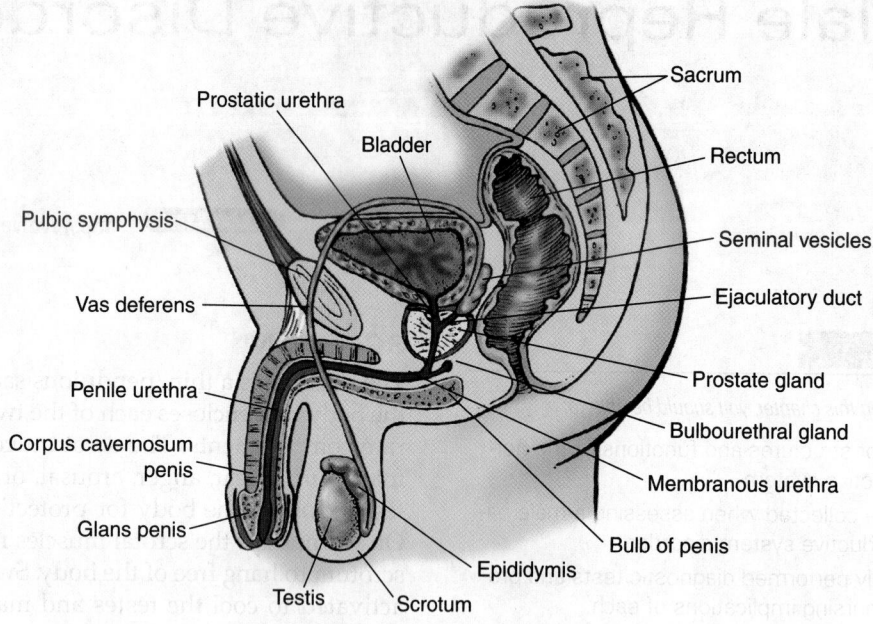

FIGURE **48-1** Male reproductive system.

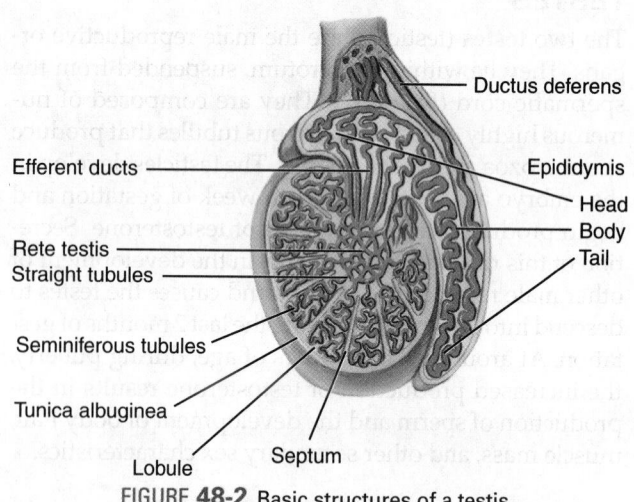

FIGURE **48-2** Basic structures of a testis.

SEMINAL VESICLES

The seminal vesicles are hollow, twisted, tubular secretory glands located on the posterior surface of the bladder. They produce a mucoid fluid that constitutes about 60% of the volume of the semen and provides nutrients and hormones important for motility and successful fertilization (Figs. 48-1 and 48-3).

PROSTATE GLAND

The prostate is a walnut-sized fibromuscular gland that surrounds the neck of the urinary bladder and the first inch of the internal urethra. The prostate produces a thin, milky, alkaline liquid that enhances the motility and fertility of the sperm and contracts to propel semen into the urethra during ejaculation (see Fig. 48-3).

COWPER'S GLANDS

Cowper's glands (bulbourethral glands) are pea-sized structures, located just below the prostate, that secrete a clear mucus into the urethra. The secretion contributes little to semen volume but provides lubrication during sexual arousal.

URETHRA

The urethra extends from the bladder to the urinary meatus at the end of the penis. The vas deferens and the seminal vesicles come together to form the ejaculatory duct, which passes through the prostate and empties into the internal urethra. The sperm and fluids from the vasa deferentia, seminal vesicles, and prostate are propelled through the ejaculatory duct into the penile urethra during ejaculation. Although the urethra serves to empty urine from the bladder and provide outflow for semen during ejaculation, urine and semen are never in the urethra at the same time.

PENIS

The external penis in its flaccid state is a soft, round cylinder of spongy tissue ending in an acorn-shaped tip known as the *glans*. The glans has a sensitive ridge at its base called the *corona* that gives rise to a hood or foreskin. In uncircumcised men, the foreskin can be rolled back to expose the glans. About one half of the penis extends within the body toward the anus and attaches to the pelvis. Two corpora cavernosa lie on the upper side of the penis. These erectile chambers provide a huge surface area for the inflow of blood and blood storage, which results in expansion of the penis during sexual arousal, called an **erection**. The corpus spongiosum on the underside of the penis

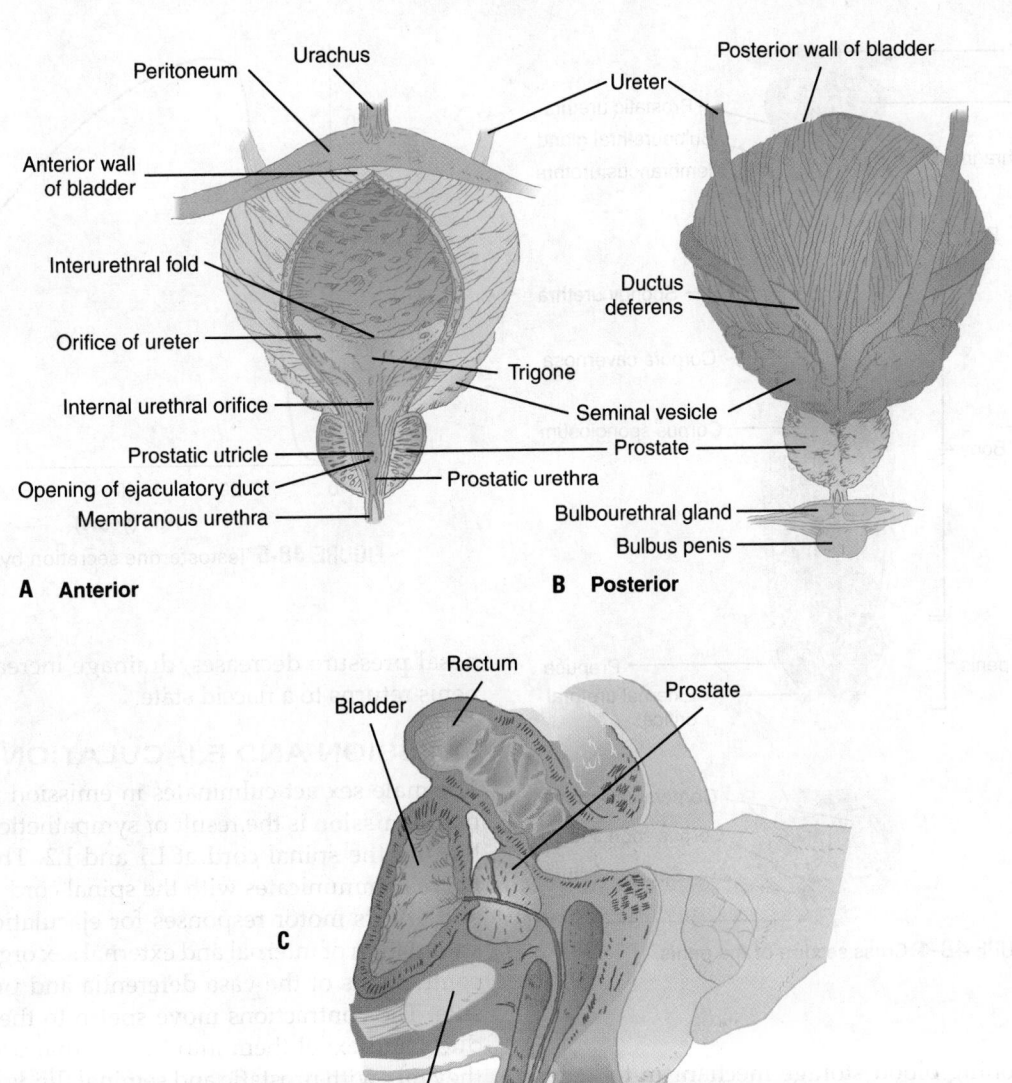

FIGURE 48-3 **A** and **B**, Anterior and posterior views of the prostate gland. **C**, Diagrammatic representation of the anatomic position of the prostate gland. It surrounds the urethra at the base of the bladder.

surrounds the urethra and supplies blood to the glans (Fig. 48-4).

PHYSIOLOGY

SPERMATOGENESIS

Sperm are produced in the seminiferous tubules of the testes from about age 13 years throughout the remainder of life. Testosterone is believed to set in motion the division of germinal cells into spermatocytes, which subsequently develop into sperm. The process may take 75 days.

The cooling function of the scrotum is essential for spermatogenesis. An increase in testicular temperature may cause degeneration of some of the cells of the seminiferous tubules and may contribute to sterility.

Cryptorchidism, or failure of the testicles to descend from the abdomen into the cooler scrotum, may result in sterility. Incomplete or partial descent of the testicles may be resolved by surgical assistance before maturity, but if fetal testes are abnormally formed and do not secrete enough testosterone to cause the testicles to descend into the scrotum, surgical intervention is unlikely to be successful. The tubular epithelium of testes that remain in the warm abdomen degenerates completely and is incapable of producing sperm.

ERECTION

For the penis to become erect, it must have a high-pressure supply of arterial blood, a means of relaxing the smooth muscle tissue of the cavernosal arterioles,

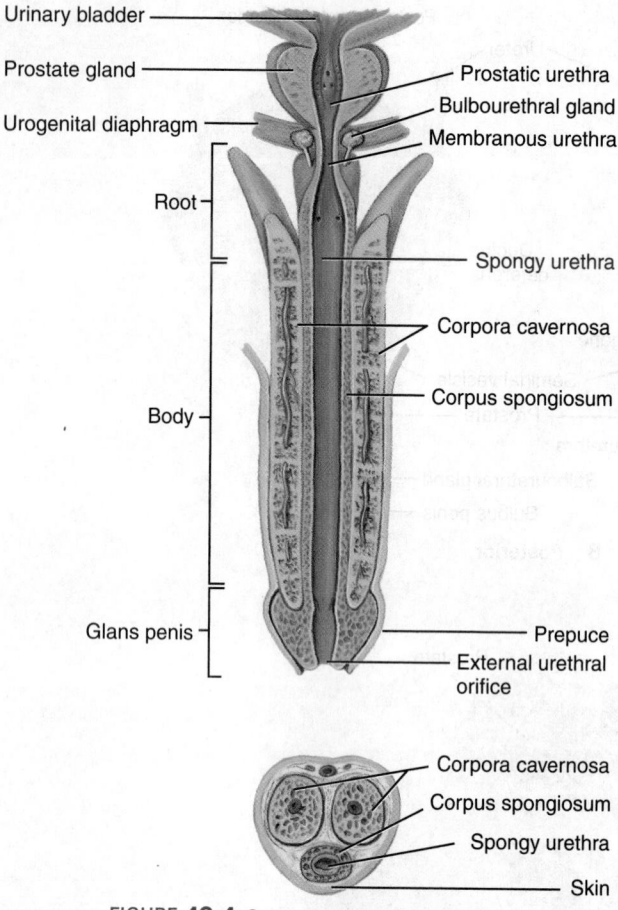

FIGURE **48-4** Cross section of the penis.

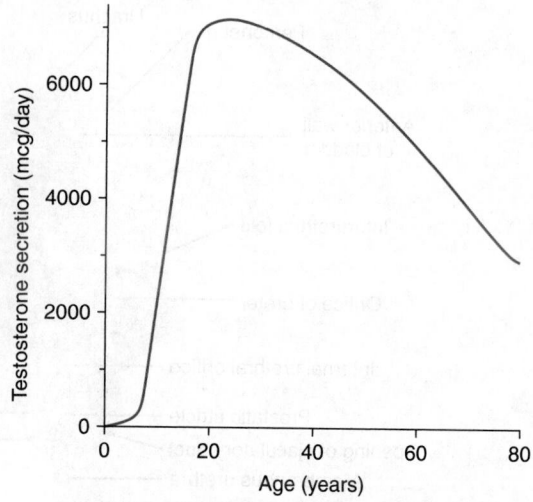

FIGURE **48-5** Testosterone secretion by age.

and a functioning blood storage mechanism to keep the blood in the penis long enough for sexual function. The blood pressure in the flaccid corpus cavernosa is about 6 to 8 mm Hg—very low when compared with the 120/90 mm Hg blood pressure in the arm or cavernosal artery.

During sexual arousal, parasympathetic nerves release neurotransmitters that cause the cavernosal arteriole walls to relax. This allows the relatively high-pressure arterial blood to flood the sinuses of the erectile chambers, increasing the blood volume of the penis to eight to ten times the flaccid volume and raising the cavernosal blood pressure to approximately the same as arterial blood pressure.

The blood storage mechanism for the penis is unique. The cavernosal artery is buried deep in the erectile chambers, causing them to fill from the inside. The venules that drain blood from the erectile chambers are near the surface and are compressed against the outer coat of the chambers during engorgement. The elastic limitations of this covering severely decrease the drainage of blood from the chamber sinuses and maintain the erection. After stimulation ceases or ejaculation occurs, sympathetic nerves release constricting neurotransmitters that narrow the arteriole walls and decrease the inflow of blood. As the caver-

nosal pressure decreases, drainage increases and the penis returns to a flaccid state.

EMISSION AND EJACULATION

The male sex act culminates in emission and ejaculation. Emission is the result of sympathetic stimulation leaving the spinal cord at L1 and L2. The pudendal nerve communicates with the spinal cord at S2 and S3 and affects motor responses for ejaculation. Physical stimulation of internal and external sex organs initiates contractions of the vasa deferentia and prostatic capsule. The contractions move sperm to the ejaculatory ducts and expel them into the internal urethra. There they mix with prostatic and seminal fluids and are propelled forward through the penile urethra. The filling of the urethra excites nerves in the sacral region of the spinal cord to initiate rhythmic muscular contractions of the internal genital organs, pelvis, and body trunk and results in ejaculation (expulsion) of semen.

Although psychic stimulation is not essential to the male sex act, it is an enhancing factor and should be considered in the physiology. Experience, culture, and self-development influence the impact of visual, fantasy, and dream stimulation on sexual sensation and nocturnal erections and emissions.

AGE-RELATED CHANGES IN THE MALE REPRODUCTIVE SYSTEM

Normal aging produces several changes in the male reproductive system. Testosterone production continues throughout life after puberty but decreases rapidly after the age of 50 (Fig. 48-5). This phenomenon has been called the *male climacteric* and may be associated with symptoms of hot flashes, feelings of suffocation, and psychic disorders similar to those of menopause. These symptoms may be relieved by the administration of testosterone and other androgens.

Many men believe they are too old for sex, and when this belief is supported by functional decline, they may lose interest or become depressed. Men in their late 40s and early 50s may be slower to arouse and have a longer refractory period between erections, but in a healthy man, spermatogenesis and the ability to have erections last a lifetime. Changes in lifestyle related to alcohol consumption, dietary habits, exercise, and the complexities of managing chronic conditions such as hypertension and diabetes and multiple medication therapies also contribute to loss of function and satisfactory sexual activities.

NURSING ASSESSMENT OF THE MALE REPRODUCTIVE SYSTEM

Assessment of the male reproductive system should include information on changes in the patient's health status, sexual function, and sexual relationships, as well as the patient's knowledge level and ability for self-care. The extent of the nursing assessment of the male reproductive system depends on the nurse's education, experience, and role in the setting. This section describes a complete nursing assessment, although some aspects may be performed only by an examiner with advanced training. The LPN/LVN contributes data for the overall assessment.

The interview and physical assessment may be particularly difficult for some male patients because of health beliefs, the need for privacy, or defensiveness about behaviors. It is important to allow the patient to tell his own story and maintain as much control over the environment and experience as possible. Establishing a comfortable relationship with the patient is most successful if open-ended questions are used. The examiner should avoid questions beginning with "why?" and leave sensitive questions until later in the interview. Although it is helpful to empathize with the patient and gently press for important details, comments on how he *should* feel or behave are inappropriate. The assessor should not jump to conclusions too early or bias the patient's story by adding his or her personal opinion.

HEALTH HISTORY
Present Illness
The health history begins with a detailed description of the current problem. Complaints may include pain, weight loss, infertility, erectile dysfunction (impotence), alteration in self-image, scrotal masses, penile discharge, or skin lesions. If the symptoms are acute, detailed information about the onset and development of the problem and about activities related to the symptoms should be documented. If the patient has pain, descriptors such as pain scales provide objective data. If the problem is a chronic one, the interviewer should determine what caused the patient to

seek help at this time and what his expectations are for care.

Past Medical History
The past medical history helps link the current problem with previous symptoms, injuries, diseases, operations, or allergies and the treatments or medications prescribed for them. The interviewer should question the patient about his management of chronic health problems such as diabetes, thyroid or pituitary dysfunction, cardiovascular disease, neurologic injury or disease, and addictive behavior. Because trauma to the groin or perineum may be related to disorders of the urethra and/or penile circulation, childhood injuries or accidents should be documented. Spinal cord injuries are significant because the level of the injury is associated with specific types of sexual dysfunctions.

Patients who are reluctant to discuss what many consider to be the most private part of their lives also may be unwilling to do regular self-examinations or follow recommended self-care regimens. Thoughtfully planned questioning provides clues about knowledge deficits and patient participation in health management. This information is important in developing plans for care that include the patient and his significant other and require their cooperation.

Family History
In the family history, the age and health or age at death of parents, grandparents, and siblings is noted. In addition, any family history of cancer, diabetes, hypertension, stroke, and blood disorders such as sickle cell anemia and hemophilia should be recorded.

Review of Systems
Review of all systems with a focus on male reproductive system disorders begins with an assessment of the patient's general health. Questions focus on changes in appetite, weight, exercise or activity level, and the management of daily self-care. These data may reveal general changes in health status that may affect the reproductive system.

Changes in the skin, including lesions, drainage, bleeding, itching, or pain, should be described. If the patient has itching or pain, note whether it is intermittent or continuous and whether it has any relationship to specific activities or time. The patient should be encouraged to use descriptive terms, such as "stinging" or "aching." When assessing pain, having the patient describe the intensity on a scale from 1 to 10 is helpful.

A review of the circulatory and pulmonary systems provides data about hypertension, cardiac or pulmonary disease, and exercise tolerance.

Symptoms of possible endocrine dysfunction are important because undiagnosed or poorly managed endocrine disorders may have a direct and devastating impact on sexual function, sterility, and self-image for the male patient. Questions about fatigue, nervousness, heat or cold intolerance, polyphagia, polydipsia, polyuria, and medications taken for pituitary or thyroid conditions may yield important clues.

Review of the musculoskeletal and nervous systems should include questions about weakness, paralysis, coordination problems, joint pain or stiffness, mood changes, and depression.

The health history should note medications the patient is taking because many drugs, including a number of antihypertensives, can impair sexual function.

Functional Assessment

The functional assessment elicits information about diet, usual activities, sleep and rest, medications, and the use of tobacco, alcohol, and illicit drugs. Record sources of stress and coping strategies. Once you establish a therapeutic relationship with the patient, you also should cover the interest level and satisfaction of sexual relationships. Questions may include the frequency of intercourse, the ability to have and maintain an erection, the desire and ability to have children, and the relationship of sexual function to self-image.

PHYSICAL EXAMINATION

The physical examination of the male reproductive system is usually done by the physician or nurse practitioner. The LPN/LVN may prepare the patient for the examination, collect some data, and see that specimens are processed properly. The patient is instructed to empty the bladder before the examination and to collect a urine specimen if needed. The patient should be properly draped for privacy. The examiner should allow adequate time for questions. Gloves always are worn to examine the genitals.

The patient's height, weight, and vital signs should be recorded and his general appearance noted. The skin is inspected for lesions or discolorations and the breasts for gynecomastia (enlargement). For the examination of the genitals, the patient may be standing or supine with the legs slightly spread. The skin of the external organs and perineum should be warm, dry, and free of lesions, edema, and odor. The pubic hair is normally distributed in a diamond-shaped area across the symphysis pubis, covering the base of the penis and spreading along the inner thighs. The lower abdomen and groin are palpated for masses.

Penis

The normal flaccid penis is semisoft and straight. The size, shape, and appearance are noted. The examiner palpates for nodules, swelling, and lesions. If the patient is uncircumcised, the foreskin is retracted to inspect the glans (Fig. 48-6). There may be a small amount of white, thick, odoriferous smegma (sebaceous secretion) between the glans and the foreskin. The urethral meatus should be at the tip of the penis. If there is any discharge from lesions or the urethra, a specimen may be collected for culture.

Scrotum

The skin of the scrotum should be slightly darker in color, wrinkled, and loose. Because the scrotum is close to the body and may not be well ventilated, it is susceptible to irritation from heat and moisture, fungal infections, abscesses, and parasites.

Each side of the scrotum should be palpated for the right and left testes, epididymis, and vasa deferentia. It is normal for the testes to retract temporarily when the scrotum is touched or cooled; they will reappear with relaxation or rewarming. The left testicle hangs lower than the right. Both should be oval in shape, smooth, firm, and without masses or tenderness. Older patients may have smaller, softer testes. It is important, especially in the young patient, to note that there are two testes.

The examiner proceeds to palpate the epididymis and the vas deferens. If scrotal thickening, nodules, masses, or asymmetric conditions are discovered, they can be further investigated by shining a light through the scrotum in a darkened room, a technique called

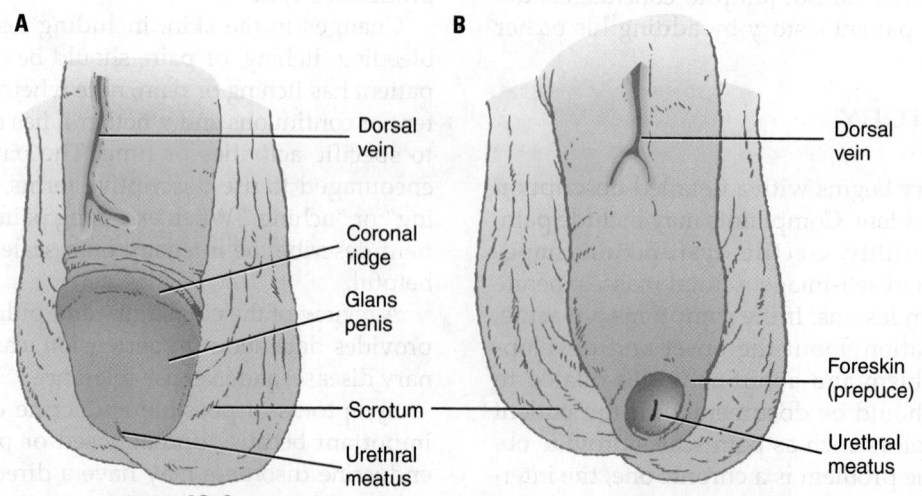

A

Dorsal vein

Coronal ridge

Glans penis

Scrotum

Urethral meatus

B

Dorsal vein

Foreskin (prepuce)

Urethral meatus

FIGURE **48-6** Appearance of the penis. **A,** Circumcised. **B,** Uncircumcised.

FIGURE **48-7** Transillumination of the scrotum.

transillumination (Fig. 48-7). Hydrocele, a mass filled with serous fluid, glows red in the light. If the mass is solid (e.g., a hematocele or tumor), no light passes through it, making it appear as a dark shadow.

The examiner inspects for hernias, which are protruding segments of the bowel through the abdominal wall. The most common sites for hernia are the lower abdomen, groin, and upper scrotal area. The examination is done first with the patient standing quietly and again when straining as if to have a bowel movement. The practitioner with advanced training is able to palpate inguinal hernias by reaching up through the scrotum into the inguinal canal. Abnormal findings should be noted and referred to a physician.

The advanced practitioner or physician also examines the prostate gland by inserting the examining finger through the anus toward the anterior wall of the rectum. Variations in the firmness and size of the prostate may be associated with benign hypertrophy, chronic prostatitis, or malignancy.

The skin of the perineum is darker than the skin on the buttocks and should be intact. The anal area has more coarse skin and is moist and without hair. Inspect the area for lesions, irritation, inflammation, fissures, abscesses, and dilated veins (hemorrhoids). With the patient bearing down, the examiner reinspects the anus for rectal prolapse or internal hemorrhoids. The advanced practitioner or physician examines the anal canal with an index finger to assess for resistance, bleeding, sphincter tone, nodules, or polyps. A stool specimen may be tested for occult blood when appropriate.

The assessment of the male reproductive system is summarized in Box 48-1.

DIAGNOSTIC TESTS AND PROCEDURES

Diagnostic tests and procedures for disorders of the male reproductive system include laboratory studies and radiologic imaging procedures.

LABORATORY STUDIES

Semen Analysis

Analysis of the semen may be done to assess male fertility or to document sterilization after a vasectomy. The analysis may include gross evaluation of semen for volume, thickness, color, and pH; and microscopic evaluation of the sperm for count, motility, shape, and ability to penetrate cervical mucus. The patient is instructed to abstain from sexual activity for 2 to 3 days and then collect a semen specimen in a clean container. Discourage patients from prolonged abstinence, because it may result in diminished quality and motility of the sperm. If the patient is unable to collect the specimen in the physician's office or laboratory by masturbating, it may be collected at home by using a plastic condom or coitus interruptus. Rubber condoms should not be used because the powders and lubricants used in their manufacture may be spermicidal. The specimen should be kept at room temperature, protected from heat or cold, and brought to the laboratory within 1 hour after collection.

Endocrinologic Studies

The endocrine system secretes hormones directly into the blood that regulate metabolism, growth, stress response, and reproduction (gonadotropins). The serum levels of these hormones can be determined from blood drawn from the patient without special preparation.

Testosterone is secreted by Leydig cells in the interstitium of the testes. Below-normal levels of testosterone may be the result of hypothalamic or pituitary dysfunction or seminiferous tubule destruction. Among the causes of increased levels of testosterone in the adult male are testicular tumor, adrenal tumor, adrenal dysfunction, and some drugs (anticonvulsants, barbiturates). Lower serum levels of testosterone may be related to gonad hypofunction, orchidectomy, hepatic cirrhosis, and some drugs (androgens, alcohol, phenothiazines, spironolactone, corticosteroids). Testosterone levels fall with age, beginning around the age of 30.

Follicle-stimulating hormone (FSH) is secreted by the anterior pituitary gland and causes stimulation of Sertoli cells in the testes to complete the formation and maturation of sperm. The negative feedback system prevents oversecretion of FSH and maintains a constant level of sperm production. Below-normal levels of sperm result in increased secretion of FSH from the pituitary gland and high serum levels of FSH. Spermatogenesis results in decreased excretion of FSH and normal serum levels.

Luteinizing hormone (LH) is secreted by the anterior pituitary gland and causes stimulation of special

| Box 48-1 | *ASSESSMENT of the Male Reproductive System* |

Health History

Present Illness:
Pain, weight loss, infertility, erectile dysfunction, scrotal mass, penile discharge, lesions

Past Medical History:
Previous injuries, diseases, or surgeries

Chronic Illnesses:
Diabetes mellitus, cardiovascular disease, addictive behavior

Allergies

Current Medications

Family History:
Diabetes, hypertension, stroke, blood disorders, cancer

Review of Systems:

General Health State:
Changes in appetite, weight, activity, self-care

Skin:
Lesions, drainage, bleeding, itching, pain

Cardiovascular:
Edema

Respiratory:
Cough, dyspnea

Endocrine:
Fatigue, heat or cold intolerance, nervousness

Nervous:
Paralysis

Genitourinary:
Changes in urination or urine characteristics

Sexual Function:
Interest in sexual relationship, frequency of intercourse, erectile dysfunction, desire to have children, effect of sexual function on self-image

Functional Assessment:

Usual Day:
Occupation, home roles and responsibilities, diet, rest

Use of Tobacco and Alcohol

Stressors and Coping Strategies

Sexual Relationships

Physical Examination
Vital Signs

General Appearance of Genitalia:
Skin lesions or discoloration, hair distribution

Penis:
Size, shape, skin lesions, discharge, position of urinary meatus, nodules, swelling

Scrotum:
Color, edema, irritation, presence of testicles, testicular tenderness or masses

Inguinal Hernia

Prostate:
Size, texture, masses

Perineum:
Color, lesions

Anus:
Lesions, irritation, inflammation, fissures, abscesses, hemorrhoids, prolapse

---

cells (Leydig cells) in the testes to produce testosterone. As testosterone is produced, a negative feedback system reduces the amount of LH secreted by the pituitary. Low levels of testosterone result in high levels of serum LH. This indicates an effort by the pituitary to stimulate Leydig cell function and return testosterone levels to normal.

Prolactin, another hormone secreted by the anterior pituitary gland, is closely related to LH. It has a potentiating effect on testosterone production. In some patients, when endocrine function is in question, serum prolactin levels may be tested. Secretion of prolactin is controlled by a negative feedback system. Abovenormal levels of prolactin may be caused by a benign pituitary tumor and may result in gynecomastia in the male patient.

Tumor Markers

Tumor markers are substances found in the serum of cancer patients. When used in conjunction with other diagnostic tools, they can be helpful in diagnosing cancer, estimating the degree of cancer development, predicting the effect of treatment, and monitoring the effect of treatment on the cancer or the return of cancer after treatment. Prostate-specific antigen (PSA) is used as a screening tool to detect prostate cancer. Annual PSA screening is recommended for all men after age 50. Men considered at high risk for prostate cancer may be advised to begin screening at age 40. There is no special preparation for these tests.

General Laboratory Studies

Urinalysis provides information about infection of the genitourinary tract as well as measures of kidney function. Clean-catch samples usually can be used unless the patient is unable to collect the urine without contamination. If appropriate instruction is given for collection, there is no need for other patient preparation. If the patient is unable to properly clean himself, cannot see well enough, or is not able to understand the instructions, it may be necessary to obtain a specimen by catheterization.

Blood studies may include a complete blood cell count to establish baseline data and provide information in forming a diagnosis when anemia or bone metastases are suspected. Alkaline phosphatase and serum calcium

| Table 48-1 | *Laboratory Tests for Male Reproductive Disorders* |

TEST	REFERENCE VALUES	CONDITION IN WHICH LEVELS ARE ALTERED
HEMATOLOGIC TESTS (CBC)		
Hemoglobin	14-18 gm/dL	↓ In anemia; nonspecific; may indicate malignancy
Hematocrit	40%-50%	↓ In anemia; nonspecific; may indicate malignancy
Leukocytes (WBCs)	4800-11,000/mm^3	↓ In metastatic bone disease
Neutrophils	54%-62%	↓ In bone marrow depression
Lymphocytes	25%-30%	↓ In bone marrow depression
Eosinophils	1%-3%	↓ In bone marrow depression
Platelets	150,000-300,000/mm^3	↓ In bone marrow depression
BLOOD/SERUM TESTS		
Acid phosphatase	0.11-0.60 mU/mL	↑ In metastatic prostate cancer
Alkaline phosphatase	20-90 mU/mL	↑ In cancer of bone or bone metastases, liver cancer
Calcium	9.0-11.0 mg/dL	↑ In bone metastasis
TESTS FOR TUMOR MARKERS		
AFP	<10 ng/mL	↑ In nonseminomatous testicular cancer
CEA	0-2.5 ng/mL nonsmokers	↑ In prostate cancer
hCG	0.5 IU/L	↑ In germ cell testicular cancer
Prostatic acid phosphatase	0.26-0.83 U/L	↑ In metastatic prostate cancer
PSA	0-4 ng/mL	↑ In prostate cancer

Modified from Black, J.M., & Matassarin-Jacobs, E. (1993). *Luckmann and Sorensen's medical-surgical nursing: A psychophysiologic approach* (4th ed., pp. 496-497). Philadelphia: Saunders.
CBC, Complete blood cell count; *WBCs,* white blood cells; *AFP,* alpha-fetoprotein; *CEA,* carcinoembryonic antigen; *hCG,* human chorionic gonadotropin; *PSA,* prostate-specific antigen.

levels also may be measured because they increase with metastasis to bone (Table 48-1). The acid phosphatase level also may be increased with prostate cancer and with bone metastasis. PSA levels, as just noted, may be increased with cancer of the prostate. Thyroid function studies and tests for diabetes mellitus may be done in patients with erectile dysfunctions. No special preparation for these tests is usually necessary. The venipuncture site should be observed for bleeding and dressed with a small pressure bandage on completion of sample collection.

RADIOLOGIC IMAGING STUDIES

Computed tomography (CT) may be used in assessing metastatic testicular and prostatic tumors. Ultrasound may be used to examine scrotal masses or define prostatic lesions. Examination of the prostate is done via the rectum.

Radionuclide imaging may be done to assess testicular abnormalities such as torsion, tumors, abscesses, epididymitis, or hydroceles. Radioactive substances are injected intravenously or given orally. After a waiting period to allow for distribution of the substance throughout the body, scans are done to locate organs and tissues that have increased concentrations of the isotopes due to abnormal tissue metabolism.

Diagnostic tests and procedures and related nursing care are summarized in the Diagnostic Tests and Procedures table on pp. 1086 to 1087.

DISORDERS OF THE MALE REPRODUCTIVE SYSTEM

INFECTIONS AND INFLAMMATORY CONDITIONS

Infections of the male reproductive system may be caused by bacteria, viruses, protozoa, fungi, and ectoparasites that can be acquired through sexual contact. Sexually transmitted infections are covered in Chapter 49. The most common inflammatory conditions are prostatitis and epididymitis. Orchitis is rare but important because it can cause sterility.

Prostatitis

Prostatitis is inflammation of the prostate gland. The four categories of prostatitis are acute bacterial prostatitis, chronic bacterial prostatitis, chronic prostatitis/chronic pelvic pain syndrome, and asymptomatic inflammatory prostatitis. Inflammation caused by bacterial infection can be acute or chronic. The patient who has prostate pain but no evidence of infection is said to have *chronic prostatitis/chronic pelvic pain syndrome.* When no pathogens can be detected, the condition is classified as *asymptomatic inflammatory prostatitis.* The cause of asymptomatic inflammatory prostatitis is uncertain.

Signs and symptoms of acute prostatitis are swelling, warmth, and tenderness. The patient also may have dysuria, frequency, hematuria, and foul-smelling urine. Patients with chronic inflammation may have

DIAGNOSTIC TESTS and PROCEDURES | *The Male Reproductive System*

TEST/PURPOSE	PATIENT PREPARATION	POSTPROCEDURE NURSING CARE
MUMPS TEST Determines whether a person is susceptible or resistant to the mumps virus. An antigen is injected intradermally; the site is marked with waterproof ink and examined after 48 hr to detect an immune response.	Inform the patient that an injection will be given under the skin to determine if he has resistance to mumps. He must not wash off the marking, and he must return in 48 hr to have the results read.	To read the test, examine the site for redness and swelling after 48 hr. A red area larger than 10 mm in diameter is a positive result and indicates susceptibility to mumps. A negative result indicates resistance.
URETHRAL SMEARS AND STAINS Prepares a small amount of material for microscopic study to detect sexually transmitted infections and identify pathogens. The physician may massage the prostate to increase the organisms in the urethra.	Tell patient a sterile swab will be inserted into the urethra to obtain a specimen. Specimens also may be obtained from the anal canal and pharynx. Use Standard Precautions to handle body fluids and contaminated instruments. Collect the specimen for culture before beginning prescribed antimicrobials.	Prepare specimens, and send them to the laboratory.
CULTURES OF ORGANISMS (obtained from a source being tested) Permit identification of pathogens and susceptibility to various antimicrobials.	Explain specimen collection process.	Prepare specimens according to laboratory protocol. Send to laboratory.
SERUM ACID PHOSPHATASE Detects elevations associated with metastatic prostate cancer and many other conditions. Used to assess effects of treatment for prostate cancer.	Inform patient that a venous blood sample will be drawn.	Assess venipuncture site for bleeding. Apply small dressing.
SEMEN ANALYSIS Examines a semen specimen to assess male fertility or to document sterilization after vasectomy.	Instruct patient to abstain from sexual activity for 3-5 days; then collect specimen in a clean container. Rubber condoms should not be used. Specimen should be kept at room temperature and brought to the laboratory within 1 hr.	No special care needed.
ENDOCRINOLOGIC STUDIES (luteinizing hormone, prolactin, follicle-stimulating hormone, testosterone) Assess level of hormones needed for sexual development and function.	Tell the patient that a venous blood sample will be drawn.	Assess the venipuncture site for bleeding. Apply small dressing.
TUMOR MARKERS (e.g., serum prostate-specific antigen) Detect increases that may be associated with prostatic cancer, prostatic hypertrophy, cirrhosis, osteoporosis, and a number of other conditions.	Patient should fast for 8 hr before the test. Tell patient a venous blood sample will be drawn.	Assess the venipuncture site for oozing or hematoma. Apply small dressing.
CYSTOSCOPY Uses a lighted instrument inserted through the urethra to visualize the urethra, bladder, and prostatic urethra. May detect prostatic hypertrophy, bladder tumors.	Routine preoperative measures are indicated (signed consent form, skin scrub, food restriction). Antibiotics may be prescribed. Inform the patient the procedure is done in a special room under sterile conditions. Local anesthetic is instilled in the urethra, and a sedative is given intravenously (IV).	Measure urine output for 24 hr. Urine will be pink tinged. Report excessive bleeding or inability to void promptly. Encourage fluid intake when patient is voiding well. Burning and hesitancy are common for several days. Give antibiotics as ordered.

DIAGNOSTIC TESTS and PROCEDURES   *The Male Reproductive System—cont'd*

TEST/PURPOSE	PATIENT PREPARATION	POSTPROCEDURE NURSING CARE
COMPUTED TOMOGRAPHY Creates images of internal structures to locate or assess testicular and prostatic tumors.	Assess allergy to iodine or previous contrast reactions if contrast dye will be injected. Report allergy to radiologist. Tell patient he will lie on a movable table while a machine moves around him. There are no sensations unless dye is injected. Some patients react to dye with nausea, vomiting, flushing, itching, or a bitter taste. Claustrophobic patients may need mild sedation.	No special postprocedure care is required. If dye is injected, the patient is encouraged to drink fluids to flush the dye from the body.
ULTRASONOGRAPHY Uses sound waves to create images of internal structures; used to study the prostate for enlargement or lesions.	Tell the patient an instrument will be inserted into the rectum to study the prostate. A full bladder is no longer required. Tell patient the procedure is uncomfortable.	No special care is needed.
RADIONUCLIDE IMAGING Uses radioactive substances injected IV or given orally followed by imaging to assess testicular abnormalities (torsion, tumors, abscesses, epididymitis, hydrocele).	Assess allergies to radioactive substance, and inform radiologist if allergic. Reassure patient that radiation dose is low and does not cause cell destruction.	Fluid intake is encouraged to promote elimination of the isotope.

minimal symptoms or malaise. Diagnosis is based on the patient's complaints confirmed by laboratory studies of prostatic secretions. Other diagnostic procedures may include urinalysis, white blood cell count, and PSA. Imaging studies using magnetic resonance imaging (MRI) or transabdominal ultrasound may be done to rule out prostate abscess.

Acute bacterial prostatitis and *chronic bacterial prostatitis* are treated with antibiotics, analgesics, and sitz baths. A 4-week course of antibiotics usually is prescribed for acute bacterial prostatitis, and up to 16 weeks of therapy for chronic bacterial prostatitis. Several antibiotics may be appropriate including trimethoprim-sulfamethoxazole (Bactrim) or ciprofloxacin (Cipro). Chronic prostatitis/chronic pelvic pain syndrome may be treated with a short course of antibiotics, but it often is ineffective. Depending on the severity of the pain, anti-inflammatory drugs or opioid analgesics may be used. However, opioids must be used cautiously with chronic pain because of the potential for abuse. The patient is advised to increase fluid intake and to rest. Stool softeners may be prescribed to prevent constipation, which is especially painful with prostatitis. Urethral catheterization is contraindicated with urethral inflammation, but suprapubic catheterization may be necessary if the patient has difficulty voiding.

Asymptomatic inflammatory prostatitis may be treated with a single daily dose of an alpha-adrenergic blocker to improve voiding by relaxing the bladder neck and prostate. Symptoms are managed with analgesics, anti-inflammatory agents, and sitz baths.

Most patients with prostatitis are treated as outpatients, but hospital admission may be indicated if a high fever is present, the patient has urinary retention, or intravenous antibiotic therapy is needed. Ask the patient about pain, and administer analgesics and other treatments as ordered. If the patient is discharged with medications, provide instructions and information about the drugs. Prostate massage and ejaculation may be helpful with some types of prostatitis because they drain excess prostatic secretions.

Epididymitis

Epididymitis, inflammation of the epididymis, may be caused by infections, trauma, or the reflux of urine from the urethra through the vas deferens. Signs and symptoms are painful scrotal edema, nausea, vomiting, chills, and fever. Epididymitis is treated with bed rest, ice packs, sitz baths, analgesics, antibiotics, anti-inflammatory drugs, and scrotal support. A bridge made of tape and gauze or a rolled towel can be placed across the patient's thighs while in bed to elevate the scrotum and reduce pain. If the condition is associated with a sexually transmitted infection, the patient's sexual partner is treated with antibiotic therapy as well. Nursing care involves monitoring temperature, edema, and comfort. Carry out prescribed treatments, and record their effects.

Orchitis

Orchitis is inflammation of one or both testes. It may be related to trauma or to infections such as mumps, pneumonia, or tuberculosis. Signs and symptoms of orchitis include fever, tenderness and swelling of the affected testicle, and scrotal redness. The inflammation can lead to reduced fertility or sterility. Orchitis is treated with analgesics, antipyretics, bed rest, scrotal support, and local heat to the scrotum. Nursing care includes pain management, assistance with activities of daily living, patient teaching, and anxiety reduction.

BENIGN PROSTATIC HYPERTROPHY (HYPERPLASIA)

Benign prostatic hypertrophy is enlargement of the prostate gland. Although, it is a common age-related change, the exact cause is unknown.

Signs and Symptoms

Signs and symptoms of benign prostatic hypertrophy are described as *obstructive* or *irritative*. Obstructive symptoms include decreasing size and force of the urinary stream, urine retention, and post-void dribbling. Irritative symptoms include urgency, frequency, dysuria, nocturia, hematuria, and sometimes urge incontinence. Factors that may trigger retention are alcohol, infections, delayed voiding, bed rest, opioids, antihistamines, and chilling.

Consider the Alternative

Saw palmetto is an extract from berries of a small tree. Like finasteride (Proscar), it effectively relieves urinary symptoms associated with benign prostatic hypertrophy (BPH) without reducing prostate size. It has few adverse effects but does reduce serum levels of PSA, which could give a false-negative result in patients with prostate cancer.

Medical Diagnosis

A diagnosis of benign prostatic hypertrophy is based on results of the rectal examination, laboratory and radiographic studies, endoscopy, ultrasound, catheterization for residual urine, and sometimes urodynamic testing (see Chapter 40). A urine specimen and prostatic secretions are obtained and examined for evidence of infection.

Medical Treatment

Conservative measures can decrease urinary retention. Drugs that may be prescribed to treat benign prostatic hypertrophy and related symptoms include 5-alpha reductase inhibitors and alpha 1 adrenergic receptor blocking agents. 5-alpha-reductase inhibitors suppress prostatic tissue growth by decreasing testosterone levels. Examples are Finasteride (Proscar) and dutasteride (Duagen). Alpha-adrenergic blocking agents like tamsulosin (Flomax), doxazosin (Cardura), and terazosin (Hytrin) are used to relax smooth muscle in the blad-

der neck and prostate, thereby reducing obstruction to urinary flow.

Surgical/Invasive Treatments

Surgical or other invasive intervention is usually advised if complete urinary obstruction develops, if evidence of existing or impending renal damage exists, if the patient has repeated urinary tract infections, or if significant bleeding occurs. In general, invasive procedures involve surgical removal of all or part of the prostate (prostatectomy) or ablation (destruction) of prostate tissue.

Types of Prostatectomy. The most widely used surgical procedure is the transurethral resection of the prostate, in which obstructing portions of the gland are cut away through a resectoscope inserted into the urethra. There is no external incision. A triple-lumen urinary catheter commonly is used to maintain continuous irrigation and bladder drainage. Continuous irrigation is intended to clear the bladder of blood and debris. If the catheter output is less than the irrigating fluid delivered, the catheter may be obstructed. Manual irrigation may be needed as ordered to clear the clots and restore drainage. If drainage cannot be restored, the physician should be notified immediately. Pressure in the bladder is one cause of painful bladder spasms. Because only part of the gland is removed, the remaining tissue can continue to grow and obstruction may recur.

A suprapubic prostatectomy is performed through the bladder by way of a low abdominal incision. It may be selected when the prostate is very large or when there are also bladder abnormalities that require surgical correction. Convalescence is longer than with a transurethral prostatectomy, and some patients develop incontinence or erectile dysfunction. A retropubic prostatectomy employs a low abdominal incision of the front of the prostate. The bladder is not cut. Although the risk is small, some men develop incontinence, erectile dysfunction, or both. A perineal prostatectomy requires an incision between the scrotum and the anus to gain access to the prostate. Radical prostatectomy is discussed on p. 1102 in the Prostatic Cancer section.

Complications. Depending on the type of prostatectomy, the patient is at risk for urinary infection and incontinence, hemorrhage, urinary leakage, inflammation of the pubic bone, and erectile dysfunction. Retrograde ejaculation may occur, meaning that semen enters the bladder instead of being ejected through the urethra. The semen is then voided later with urine. This is not harmful to the patient but does render him sterile (infertile).

Alternative Invasive Procedures. Alternative procedures employ heat (microwave thermotherapy or transurethral needle ablation) to destroy selected prostate tissue or laser incision and vaporization of prostate tissue. Stents can be placed to prevent obstruction of urine flow. Balloon dilation is controversial.

DRUG THERAPY   Disorders of the Male Reproductive System

DRUG	USE/ACTION	SIDE EFFECTS	NURSING INTERVENTIONS
TESTOSTERONE			
Methyltestosterone (Metandren) Fluoxymesterone (Halotestin) Testosterone cypionate in oil (Depo-Testosterone)	Treats hormone deficiency caused by developmental disorders, testicular diseases, or removal of testicles. Increases testosterone level.	Retention of water, sodium, potassium, and chloride. Jaundice. GI distress. Increased effects of anticoagulants and oral hypoglycemics.	Assess for hypertension and edema. Intramuscular injections should be given deeply into the gluteus muscle using the Z-track technique.
ESTROGEN PRODUCTS			
Chlorotrianisene (Tace) Estrone (Theelin Aqueous) Ethinyl estradiol (Estinyl)	Treats prostate cancer. Decreases testosterone level.	Fluid retention. Nausea and vomiting. Temporary breast enlargement (gynecomastia) and erectile dysfunction in males. Contraindicated with thrombophlebitis or clotting disorders.	Rotate vials of injectable suspension to mix. Inject into large muscle mass. Monitor blood pressure and weight.
Diethylstilbestrol (DES)	Palliative therapy for inoperable prostate cancer.	Anorexia, nausea, gynecomastia, hypertension.	Monitor blood pressure and weight. Monitor blood glucose, and be alert for signs of thrombosis.
TESTOSTERONE INHIBITORS			
Flutamide (Eulexin) Bicalutamide (Casodex) Nilutamide (Nilandron)	Decreases testosterone level. Used with LHRH to treat prostate cancer.	GI distress, hepatotoxicity, gynecomastia, erectile dysfunction, hot flashes, edema, hypertension, anxiety, confusion, mental depression.	Liver function must be monitored. Do not double up if a dose is missed. Be sure patient understands that drug must be taken with LHRH. Advise of effects on sexual function. Tell patient to report GI distress, pain in right side, dark urine, yellowish color of skin or sclera.
AGENTS USED TO TREAT ERECTILE DYSFUNCTION			
Sildenafil (Viagra) Vardenafil (Levitra) Tadalafil (Cialis)	Relaxes smooth muscle in corpus cavernosum, which increases blood flow with subsequent erection.	Headache, dizziness, abnormal vision, diarrhea, dyspepsia, priapism, urinary tract infection, flushing, rash. MI, *sudden death, cardiovascular collapse*, especially if taken with organic nitrate therapy. Numerous other contraindications including MAO inhibitors, severe hepatic or renal impairment, pregnancy or lactation (not recommended for women at this time), history of coronary artery disease, CHF, dysrhythmias, or stroke. Many interactions; refer to a drug handbook when administering.	Patient teaching: take 1 hr before sexual activity. Do not take more than once daily. *Do not take* if taking organic nitrates (e.g., nitroglycerin); combination can be fatal. Drug is only effective with sexual stimulation. Patients over age 65 may be started on the lowest dose (25 mg) and increased if necessary.
Alprostadil injection (Caverject) and intraurethral suppositories (MUSE)	Increases blood flow to penis.	Injection: priapism, fibrotic nodules. Suppository: urethral pain, inflammation.	Teach patient self-administration. Advise to seek treatment for persistent erection.

GI, Gastrointestinal; *LHRH*, luteinizing hormone–releasing hormone; *MI*, myocardial infarction; *MAO*, monoamine oxidase; *CHF*, congestive heart failure.

NURSING CARE *of the Patient with Benign Prostatic Hypertrophy*

Assessment

Data needed for assessment of the patient with benign prostatic hypertrophy include a complete description of urinary symptoms: frequency, urgency, hesitancy, a change in stream size or force, and nocturia. Record the presence of pain or hematuria. Palpate the lower abdomen to detect bladder distention. If ordered, the patient may be catheterized after voiding to measure residual urine.

**Nursing Diagnoses, Goals, and Outcome Criteria:
Benign Prostatic Hypertrophy**

NURSING DIAGNOSES	GOALS AND OUTCOME CRITERIA
Impaired Urinary Elimination related to obstruction	Normal bladder emptying: no distention on palpation, urine output approximately equal to fluid intake
Fear related to invasive diagnostic and therapeutic procedures	Reduced fear: patient states fear is reduced, appears calm
Ineffective Therapeutic Regimen Management of treatment and self-care related to lack of knowledge, limited resources	Patient understands condition and treatment and follows prescribed plan of care: patient correctly describes condition and treatment, demonstrates self-care

Interventions

Impaired Urinary Elimination

Instruct the patient to void promptly when the urge is felt and to space fluid intake throughout the day rather than consuming large amounts of liquids at one time. Fluid restriction is *not* recommended because it increases the risk of urinary tract infection. The patient should avoid alcohol and antihistamines.

If the patient is unable to void and the bladder becomes distended, notify the physician. Perform catheterization as ordered, but it may be difficult to pass the catheter because of the enlarged prostate. If the catheter does not pass easily, do not force it. Inform the physician. The procedure is usually done by a urologist using special instruments.

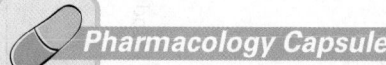
Pharmacology Capsule

Common nonprescription drugs, including many cold remedies, may cause urinary retention in the patient with prostatic hypertrophy.

Fear

Explore the patient's fears, and provide information about anticipated procedures and effects.

Ineffective Therapeutic Regimen Management

Because this condition requires long-term management, the patient or a caregiver must understand how to man-

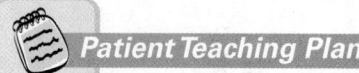
Patient Teaching Plan

Prostatic Hypertrophy

- An enlarged prostate constricts the urethra, which interferes with passage of urine.
- To prevent urinary retention, drink fluids throughout the day.
- Consult your physician or pharmacist about nonprescription drugs. Common drugs such as antihistamines can cause urinary retention.
- Report signs and symptoms of infection (burning on urination, foul urine odor, cloudy urine) and obstruction (feeling of bladder fullness, inability to empty bladder, lower abdominal pain).
- Take your medications as prescribed, and notify your physician of any adverse effects. (Provide the patient with information about specific drugs.)

age the condition. Advise the patient that over-the-counter drugs containing phenylephrine or pseudoephedrine, which are commonly found in cold remedies, can aggravate urinary symptoms. Some patients find that alcohol and caffeine also increase their symptoms.

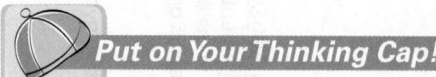
Put on Your Thinking Cap!

Draw an illustration that you could use to teach a patient the effects of prostate enlargement.

NURSING CARE *of the Prostatectomy Patient*

Detailed care of the surgical patient is presented in Chapter 17. This section addresses the specific needs of the postoperative prostatectomy patient (see Nursing Care Plan: The Patient with a Prostatectomy on p. 1092).

Assessment

When the patient returns to the nursing unit, measure his vital signs and compare them with preoperative measurements. Inspect urine, dressings, and wound drainage for excess bleeding. Maintain careful records of fluid intake and output to avoid overdistention of the bladder. Input and output should be balanced. Record the color of the urine and any clots present. Check intravenous fluids, and regulate rate of flow. Monitor the patient's level of comfort for incisional pain and bladder spasms.

Nursing Diagnoses, Goals, and Outcome Criteria: Prostatectomy

NURSING DIAGNOSES	GOALS AND OUTCOME CRITERIA
Risk for Deficient Fluid Volume related to hemorrhage	Normal fluid balance: balanced fluid intake and output, stable vital signs consistent with patient norms

Acute Pain related to tissue trauma and bladder spasms	Pain relief: patient states pain is relieved, relaxed expression
Risk for Infection related to invasive procedures of the urinary tract and surgical incision	Reduced risk of infection: freely flowing, clear urine
Risk for Injury related to obstructed urine flow, excessive absorption of irrigating fluids, trauma to the urinary sphincter	Absence of complications due to obstruction, water intoxication, or sphincter injury
Urge Urinary Incontinence related to poor sphincter control	Improved control of urine elimination: patient controls urine passage; has decreasing incidents of incontinence
Sexual Dysfunction related to removal of prostate, retrograde ejaculation, possible neurologic injury	Management of sexual dysfunction: patient states he understands sexual dysfunction and identifies appropriate adaptations and resources
Situational Low Self-Esteem related to anticipated alteration in sexual function	Improved self-esteem: patient makes positive statements about self
Deficient Knowledge of postoperative routines and self-care	Patient understands routines and self-care: patient correctly describes limitations and demonstrates self-care activities

Interventions

Risk for Deficient Fluid Volume

Restlessness and an increasing heart rate are early signs of fluid volume deficit. Blood in the urine is expected for several days after a prostatectomy; however, the drainage should be light pink within 24 hours. Bleeding with clots can signal hemorrhage and must be reported immediately to the physician. Bright red blood may indicate arterial bleeding that requires surgical intervention. Dark blood may require pressure on the surgical area at the neck of the bladder. To apply pressure, the physician may inject additional fluid into the balloon that anchors the indwelling catheter. The catheter is then pulled so that the balloon fits tightly against the neck of the bladder, and various forms of traction are used, including taping the catheter to the thigh. This traction may be maintained for several hours or more and then released by the physician.

Continuous bladder irrigation helps prevent clot formation and subsequent obstruction that can cause bladder spasms and infection. Hang irrigating fluids (usually normal saline), and regulate flow at the prescribed rate.

Acute Pain

Pain after prostatectomy may be associated with urinary obstruction, bladder spasms, and surgical trauma. If urine is not draining freely, reposition the tubing and irrigate according to agency policy. Antispasmodics such as oxybutynin chloride (Ditropan), belladonna and opium suppositories, or propantheline bromide (Pro-Banthine) are usually effective in relieving bladder spasms. Administer analgesics as ordered, and assess effectiveness.

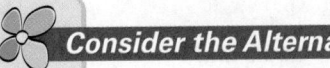

Consider the Alternative

In addition to analgesics, try nonpharmacologic interventions for postoperative pain such as repositioning, back rubs, and relaxation exercises.

Risk for Infection

To reduce the risk of infection, use strict aseptic technique when handling urinary drainage, wound drains, and dressings. Keep closed urinary drainage systems intact to prevent the introduction of pathogens. Provide wound care in accordance with the physician's orders or the agency's policy. Monitor for signs of infection, including temperature above 38.3° C (101° F), purulent wound drainage, and confusion in older patients.

Risk for Injury

Urinary obstruction and bladder distention can lead to renal complications (hydronephrosis), infection, and increased bleeding. Therefore it is critical to maintain urine flow. If urine flow ceases, assess the bladder for distention. If the bladder is distended, temporarily turn off the irrigating fluid and manually irrigate the bladder as ordered. If you cannot clear the tubing, notify the surgeon immediately. After the catheters are removed, you must continue to monitor output because edema or scarring may occur and obstruct the urethra.

Urge Urinary Incontinence

Urinary incontinence or dribbling is common immediately after the catheter is removed. In most cases, control can be improved with perineal exercises. Instruct patients to contract and relax the perineal muscles 10 to 20 times each hour. If control does not improve, the physician may recommend biofeedback, a penile clamp, a condom catheter, or incontinence briefs. In severe cases, an artificial sphincter may be surgically implanted. Some patients never regain full control of urination. For additional information, see Chapter 23 (Incontinence).

Sexual Dysfunction and Situational Low Self-Esteem

Alterations in sexual function that may distress the patient include sterility, retrograde ejaculation, and

NURSING CARE PLAN
The Patient with a Prostatectomy

ASSESSMENT

Health History: Patient is a 77-year-old retired radio announcer who underwent a transurethral prostatectomy this morning. He returned to the nursing unit 3 hours ago. He complains of genital pain and states that he feels like he needs to empty his bladder. He appears tense and is clenching the side rails.

Physical Assessment: Vital signs: temperature, 98° F orally; pulse, 84; respiration, 18; blood pressure, 122/70. Alert and oriented. Breath sounds clear on auscultation. Intravenous fluids infusing at 100 mL/hr. Three-way Foley catheter in place, taped to inner thigh, and draining freely into collection bag. Irrigation fluid set at the prescribed flow rate. Urine pink, not viscous. Several clots observed in bag.

Nursing Diagnosis	Goals and Outcome Criteria	Interventions
Risk for Deficient Fluid Volume related to hemorrhage	The patient will have balanced fluid intake and output without signs of hypovolemia (tachycardia, decreased urine output, hypotension, restlessness).	Monitor urine for excessive bleeding: thick, bright blood with clots. Assess for signs of hypovolemia. Be sure traction is maintained on catheter by keeping tape in place until surgeon removes it. Maintain flow of irrigating fluid as ordered. If urine flow decreases or bladder distention is detected, irrigate the catheter as ordered. Inform surgeon if unable to irrigate or urine output remains low.
Acute Pain related to tissue trauma and bladder spasms	The patient will verbalize relief from pain and will appear more relaxed.	Check tubing to be sure urine is draining freely. If not, reposition the tubing and milk or irrigate it as ordered or per agency policy. Notify surgeon immediately if unable to clear tubing. Administer analgesics and antispasmodics as ordered. Reposition patient. Give back rub. Use distraction. Assess effects of pain relief interventions.
Risk for Infection related to invasive procedures of the urinary tract or catheterization	The patient will remain free of infection, as evidenced by normal body temperature, normal white blood cell count, and absence of confusion or cloudy, foul urine.	Use strict aseptic techniques when handling the urinary drainage system. Keep closed system intact. Monitor temperature and urine characteristics. Report fever (greater than 101° F), confusion, cloudy or foul urine.
Risk for Injury related to obstructed urine flow or trauma to urinary sphincter	The patient will have no injuries, as evidenced by continuous urine flow.	Maintain flow of isotonic irrigating fluid as ordered. Monitor output, and assess bladder for distention. Monitor vital signs. Administer stool softeners as ordered to prevent constipation. Encourage fluid intake when able.
Sexual Dysfunction related to removal of prostate or retrograde ejaculation	The patient will correctly describe the physiologic effects of prostatectomy.	Be open to patient's questions about effects of surgery on sexual function. Reinforce preoperative teaching that erectile dysfunction is not common after transurethral prostate resection. Retrograde ejaculation may occur but is not harmful. Offer to include sex partner in teaching. Be sensitive to possible feelings about loss of masculinity. Patient may demonstrate some anger or sadness related to a sense of loss.
Deficient Knowledge of postoperative routines or self-care	The patient will demonstrate understanding of postoperative exercises and procedures.	Support and encourage patient to turn and deep breathe at least q 2 hr. Explain catheter and irrigation system. Tell him that some blood is normal the first few days after surgery. Encourage early ambulation as soon as permitted, and explain benefits of activity to recovery. Before discharge, advise to restrict strenuous activity and heavy lifting (no more than 10-20 lb as specified by physician) for 4-6 weeks. If he will go home with a catheter, discuss catheter care.

? **CRITICAL THINKING** QUESTIONS

■ Describe the application of strict aseptic technique in the care of this patient.

■ Why might this surgery affect sexual function?

erectile dysfunction. The patient should be encouraged to discuss these concerns with the physician before surgery. Erectile dysfunction is not common after surgical treatment of benign prostatic hypertrophy, but if it does occur, the patient may need counseling, as described on p. 1096 in the Erectile Dysfunction (Impotence) section. There is no treatment for retrograde ejaculation, but you can reassure the patient that it is not harmful. All of these alterations can threaten the patient's self-image and self-esteem. Be sensitive to the patient's feelings of loss and need to assert a masculine image. The patient may wish to include his sex partner in teaching and counseling sessions.

Deficient Knowledge

Teaching for postoperative care must begin in the preoperative period because patient hospitalizations are usually short and the patient may be discharged with a catheter. Verbal instructions should be accompanied by written material.

ERECTILE DYSFUNCTION (IMPOTENCE)

Erectile dysfunction, which is the inability to produce and maintain an erection for sexual intercourse, can be devastating for a man and his partner. An adequate erection requires intact neurologic function, sufficient inflow of blood to fill the corpus cavernosa, and a leak-proof storage mechanism for maintaining the erection (Table 48-2).

Contributing Factors

A number of vascular, neurologic, endocrine, and psychological factors may cause or contribute to erectile dysfunction.

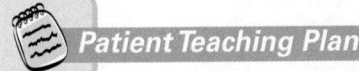

Patient Teaching Plan

Post-Prostatectomy

- After a prostatectomy, semen may be ejaculated into the bladder (retrograde ejaculation). This is not harmful.
- Signs and symptoms of complications that should be reported include inability to pass urine, bladder distention, renewed bleeding, fever, and cloudy or foul-smelling urine.
- Practice perineal exercises as instructed to reduce the risk of incontinence.
- Walking is encouraged, but avoid strenuous activity or heavy lifting as advised by physician.
- Drink at least eight glasses of fluids each day.
- To prevent constipation and straining, which could cause bleeding, take stool softeners as prescribed and consume a high-fiber diet.
- Keep your urinary drainage system closed except when emptying it. Wash your hands before and after handling the system.
- Do not resume driving or sexual intercourse until directed by the surgeon (usually about 6 weeks).

Vascular Disorders. Systemic or local changes in blood flow can impair the ability to achieve an erection. Generalized atherosclerosis may be a factor in inadequate filling of the corpus cavernosa. Many modifiable factors contribute to the development of atherosclerosis. These include high cholesterol levels, smoking, excessive alcohol consumption, illicit drug use, and inadequate exercise. The cavernosal artery in the perineum between the scrotum and the anus may be damaged by physical injury to the pelvis, falls on the crossbar of a bicycle, horseback riding, or other blows. Significant damage to the artery limits the inflow of blood to the corpus cavernosa.

Endocrine Disorders. Patients with diabetes mellitus are at risk for erectile dysfunction due to atherosclerosis and autonomic neuropathy. Autonomic neuropathy is the dysfunction of some aspect of the autonomic nervous system, which is essential to normal sexual response.

Approximately 50% of men who have diabetes, regardless of type of treatment, develop erectile dysfunction, making diabetes the most common cause of erectile dysfunction. Diabetes is believed to interfere with blood supply to the penis when arterial walls lose flexibility, or distensibility, as a result of hardening of the arteries (atherosclerosis). Atherosclerosis may be accelerated by diabetes.

Autonomic neuropathy in patients with diabetes affects the ability of nerves to relax the smooth muscle surrounding the tiny sinuses (lacunar spaces) of the erectile chambers. Without relaxed muscle tone and expansion of the sinuses, adequate filling with blood for an erection may not be possible.

Effective management of diabetes mellitus is always desirable for general good health, but maintenance of strict blood glucose levels has not been shown to reduce the incidence of erectile dysfunction. Although the primary cause of erectile dysfunction related to diabetes mellitus is physiologic, the psychological reaction to the problem is an important factor. Cognitive behavioral therapy may be used to teach the patient to manage negative thinking.

Vascular surgery to clear blocked arteries is not usually recommended for people with diabetes because they often have complicating problems with nerves, cells, erectile tissue, and blood vessels throughout the penis.

Penile implants (Fig. 48-8) may be recommended for patients with problems of failure to initiate (nerve damage) or failure to fill (artery damage), which are related to diabetes. As many as one third of penile implant patients have diabetes.

Phosphodiesterase type 5 inhibitors such as sildenafil (Viagra) are oral drugs that may be effective. Papaverine plus phentolamine self-injection is indicated as a treatment for failure to initiate or fill and has been widely accepted by patients. Alprostadil (prostaglandin E_1) is available in an injectable form and as a pellet

Table 48-2	*Symptoms, Causes, and Treatment of Erectile Dysfunction*		
TYPE OF ERECTILE DYSFUNCTION	**SYMPTOMS***	**CAUSES**	**TREATMENTS**
Failure to initiate	Inability to initiate (develop) an erection.	Nerve damage due to disease or injury; stress, anxiety, or other psychological problems; hormonal disorders.	Sex therapy, hormonal therapy, vacuum constriction device, penile injections, penile implant.
Failure to fill†	Erections develop slowly and may not be sufficiently rigid for intercourse or masturbation except sometimes after extended foreplay or stimulation; sleep erections or erections on awakening may appear more rigid.	Arterial blockage(s) due to atherosclerosis, aging, or injury.	Sex therapy, vacuum constriction device, revascularization surgery (arterial bypass surgery), penile implant, sildenafil.
Failure to store†	Erections poorly maintained and not rigid enough for intercourse or masturbation.	Abnormal storage due to stress, aging, injury, or any process that causes erectile tissue to stiffen and not expand enough to compress subtunical venules.	Sex therapy, vacuum constriction device, penile injections, sildenafil, venous ligation surgery, crural plication surgery, penile implant.

Reprinted by permission of the Putnam Publishing Group from Goldstein, I., & Rothstein, L. (1990). *The potent male* (p. 39). Los Angeles: The Body Press. Copyright 1990 by Price Stern Sloan, Inc., and Irwin Goldstein and Larry Rothstein.

*Changes in erections (in rigidity or sustaining capability, or both) must occur with morning erections, during masturbation, and during intercourse for a period of 6 months to a year before the patient is considered in need of treatment of erectile dysfunction.

†Failure-to-fill erectile dysfunction and failure-to-store erectile dysfunction often occur together as the result of a disease process, atherosclerosis, or aging.

A,

Bulbocavernous muscle

Small-Carrion rod prosthesis

Prosthesis inserted into ischiocavernous muscle and crus of penis

B, HINGE

C,

Reservoir

Silicone tubes

Inflatable cylinders

Bulb

D,

Pump

Reservoir

Inflatable cylinder

FIGURE **48-8** Penile prostheses. **A,** Small-Carrion prosthesis. **B,** Flexi-rod semirigid implant. **C,** Inflatable prosthesis. **D,** Self-contained prosthesis.

that is inserted into the urethra. Patients need training in self-injection and must have hand dexterity and adequate vision.

Neurologic Disorders. Spinal cord injuries and other neurologic disorders may cause erectile dysfunction. If communication between the spinal cord and the penis remains intact, the penis becomes erect with direct stimulation. For the penis to remain erect, smooth muscle relaxation is necessary and in some way relies on communication between the brain and the spinal cord. The more complete the injury and the lower the injury, the more likely it is that erection will be affected, even though higher injuries tend to cause more paralysis and loss of sensation.

Treatment of erectile dysfunction related to spinal cord injuries or neurologic disorders such as multiple sclerosis may include phosphodiesterase type 5 inhibitors, papaverine, or alprostadil; vacuum constriction devices; or penile implants.

Medication Side Effects. Medications used to treat a variety of conditions may cause or contribute to erectile dysfunction. Drugs used to reduce high blood pressure (antihypertensives) are the most likely to interfere with erection. If systemic hypertension is accompanied by blockages and stiffening in the arterial walls of the penis, antihypertensives that lower the blood pressure in all the arteries of the body may reduce the blood pressure in penile arteries to the extent that failure to fill occurs. Digoxin, which is used to treat heart conditions, may increase levels of estrogen and decrease levels of testosterone; medications for stomach ulcers, such as cimetidine, and anticancer may decrease libido; and anticholinergics and antihistamines may block neurotransmitters that cause relaxation of smooth muscle.

Treatment for erectile dysfunction related to these drugs' side effects may include changes in drugs or dosage, but such changes can be made only on a physician's order. Counseling or sex therapy, vacuum constriction devices, drug therapy, or penile implants may be appropriate for these patients.

Pharmacology Capsule

Antihypertensive drugs are among those most likely to interfere with erection.

Psychological Factors. The psychological aspects of erectile dysfunction are extremely important and should be included in the medical history. Psychogenic erectile dysfunction is often the result of anxiety about performance. Problems may arise with aging, sexual beliefs or behavior; communication patterns or relationships with sex partners; changes in lifestyle; changes in medications; or chronic or poorly managed disease processes. Anxiety may cause constriction of smooth muscle tissue in the penis and its arteries, reducing inflow and increas-

ing outflow of blood from the penis, leaving it flaccid. Sex therapy that includes behavior modification techniques may be able to restore potency.

Consider the Alternative

Siberian ginseng and *Ginkgo biloba* are herbs that some believe increase penile blood flow. Scientific validation is lacking at this time.

Consider the Alternative

Therapies that may be used alone or with traditional medication to treat erectile dysfunction include acupuncture, aromatherapy (with essential oils of sandalwood, rose, jasmine, and ylang ylang), imagery, biofeedback, and progressive relaxation.

Medical Treatment

Drug Therapy.

Phosphodiesterase Type 5 Inhibitors. Examples are sildenafil (Viagra), tadalafil (Cialis), and vardenafil (Levitra). These oral vasodilators may be prescribed for failure to fill or store. They must be prescribed with care in patients with cardiovascular disease because of the risk of myocardial infarction and sudden death. They are contraindicated for patients taking nitrate vasodilators or alpha-adrenergic antagonists due to the risk of hypotension and cardiovascular collapse.

Alprostadil. Alprostadil can be used for intracavernosal injection (Caverject) or urethral suppositories (MUSE). It has been successful for some men. They, too, are vasodilators but produce a more localized effect on arteriole filling and improved storage. Urethral pain and urethritis are possible complications.

Papaverine. Self-injection of intracavernosal papaverine may be recommended for failure to initiate, fill, or store or for psychogenic causes. Papaverine is injected with a small needle into the erectile chambers, with relatively little pain. Erection is achieved within 10 to 15 minutes and lasts 30 to 60 minutes. Papaverine acts on smooth muscle to relax arterial walls and erectile tissue, increasing blood flow into the penis. Papaverine is often mixed with phentolamine, which blocks the constriction of erectile tissue, making it possible to sustain the erection.

Testosterone. Testosterone replacement for men with low hormone levels may be recommended for decreased desire and failure to initiate (see the Drug Therapy table on p. 1089).

Vacuum Constriction Devices. Vacuum constriction devices may be prescribed for failure to initiate, fill, or store or for psychogenic causes. The flaccid penis is slipped into a cylinder, and then the patient squeezes a pump that removes all of the air from the space in the cylinder around the penis, creating a vacuum that draws blood into the penis. When the erection has been achieved, a rubber ring is slipped off the bottom of the cylinder onto the penis near the base, trapping the blood safely for up to about 30 minutes. When air is again allowed into the cylinder, the cylinder can be removed.

Revascularization. Revascularization is a surgical procedure that bypasses blocked arteries, removes or ties off incompetent veins, and tightens the surrounding tissue. This procedure is not commonly done.

Penile Implants. Penile implants (see Fig. 48-8) may be prescribed for patients with failure to initiate, failure to fill or store (if they are not candidates for revascularization), and for some patients with psychogenic problems that are not appropriate for or responsive to counseling or sex therapy. Semirigid implants are silicon cylinders placed in the erection chambers that keep the penis firm at all times but without increasing in circumference. Some models are inflexible and create problems concealing the erection, but others are flexible enough that they can be bent downward and the erection more easily concealed. Hydraulic implants have cylinders that can be inflated by squeezing a pump in the scrotum or at the end of the penis behind the glans. The pumping action causes the cylinders to fill with fluid from a reservoir in the abdomen or the scrotum. These implants more closely duplicate the natural states of flaccidity and erection.

NURSING CARE *of the Patient with Erectile Dysfunction*

Assessment

The nursing assessment of a man with erectile dysfunction includes a health history that elicits information about the frequency of intercourse and the ability to enjoy sexual relations. The LPN/LVN may collect data that contribute to the complete assessment. The interviewer should not assume that sexual activity is no longer important to older adults. Erectile dysfunction may be the first sign of diabetes mellitus, so a complete exploration of the patient's general health and family history to look for diabetes is important. Surgical procedures, injuries, illness, cancer, and medications used regularly should be recorded. The patient's habits and lifestyle including daily activities, diet, use of alcohol and illicit drugs, exercise habits, lifestyle, health care beliefs, interpersonal relationships, capability for self-care, age, physical condition, and educational needs should be explored.

Nursing Diagnoses, Goals, and Outcome Criteria: Erectile Dysfunction

Nursing Diagnoses	Goals and Outcome Criteria
Sexual Dysfunction related to erectile dysfunction	Improved sexual function or satisfying alternatives to sexual intercourse: patient states function has improved or he is satisfied with alternatives
Situational Low Self-Esteem related to impaired sexual function	Improved self-esteem: patient makes more positive comments about self
Ineffective Therapeutic Regimen Management related to lack of knowledge of factors contributing to erectile dysfunction and measures to improve sexual function, or related to reluctance to seek help	Patient understands factors contributing to erectile dysfunction and employs measures to improve sexual function: patient states management is satisfactory

Interventions

The management of erectile dysfunction requires sensitivity and knowledge. When you have a therapeutic relationship with the patient, he may choose to share his concerns with you. Listen and be careful not to dismiss the issue as unimportant. Provide factual information and resources. If you are not well-informed about erectile dysfunction, you should refer patients to the physician, advanced practice nurse, or a counselor with training in this area.

What Does Culture Have to Do with Erectile Dysfunction?

Beliefs and values in relation to sexual function, as well as acceptable forms of sexual expression, are largely learned in one's culture. If a cultural belief is that older adults lose interest in sex as their abilities decline, then older adults may try to act accordingly. That is, they may accept erectile dysfunction as "normal" and not seek treatment.

PEYRONIE'S DISEASE

Peyronie's disease is the development of a hard, nonelastic, fibrous tissue (plaque) just under the skin of the penis of men between 45 and 70 years of age. The plaque develops as a result of an injury that causes inflammation and scarring of the tunica surrounding the corpora cavernosa. Loss of elasticity of the tunica results in decreased ability to fill during an erection and failure to store because of low pressure on the veins against the covering of the erectile tissue. The plaque is usually located on the dorsal midline surface of the penis and results in an upward bending of the penis during erection that may be painful and interfere with successful vaginal penetration (Fig. 48-9).

Medical Treatment

Treatment of Peyronie's disease may include topical or oral medications with vitamin E, oral para-aminobenzoic acid, tamoxifen, and colchicine. Local

FIGURE 48-9 Peyronie's disease.

radiation, injections into the lesions, ultrasonography, and surgical correction are other options. The choice of treatment depends on the size of the plaque and the curvature and the resultant degree of dysfunction.

PRIAPISM

Priapism is a prolonged penile erection that is not related to sexual desire. Priapism may be caused by many factors including injury to the penis, sickle cell crisis, and neoplasms of the brain or spinal cord. Drugs that may be responsible include phenothiazines, alpha-adrenergic blockers, anticoagulants, alcohol, cocaine, marijuana, vardenafil (Levitra), and intracavernosal injections. Prolonged priapism can interfere with blood flow to the penis. It can also obstruct urine flow, causing hydronephrosis. This erection may be very painful and constitutes an emergency situation. Failure to resolve the problem within 12 to 24 hours may result in penile ischemia, gangrene, fibrosis, and erectile dysfunction.

Medical Treatment

Immediate removal of blood may be accomplished by aspirating blood from the erectile chambers or by injecting drugs that cause contraction of smooth muscle, inhibiting inflow of blood and allowing outflow. If these efforts fail, emergency surgery may be needed.

Nursing care must be particularly sensitive to the embarrassment the patient may experience. Understanding the condition and alleviating pain are important.

PHIMOSIS

Normally the penile foreskin can be retracted, exposing the glans. However, inflammation under the foreskin, often associated with poor hygiene, causes edema that may prevent retraction of the foreskin. This condition, called phimosis, is treated with antimicrobials and proper cleansing. Circumcision is sometimes recommended. Uncircumcised men need to retract the foreskin for cleaning as part of daily hygiene.

INFERTILITY

Infertile is a term used to describe couples who have had unprotected intercourse over a 12-month period and have been unable to become pregnant. Infertility may be caused by a reproductive problem in the male, the female, or both.

Etiology and Risk Factors

Male infertility may be related to endocrine disorders, testicular problems, or abnormalities of the ejaculatory system. Correction of endocrine disorders may restore fertility. Infections can affect both testicular and ejaculatory function. Structural factors that can affect testicular function are cryptorchidism, testicular torsion, and varicocele (dilation of the veins that drain the testes). Drug therapy, radiation, substance abuse, and environmental hazards also can affect the testes. In addition to infection, the ejaculatory mechanism can be disrupted by obstruction and some surgical procedures.

Infections. Destruction of the seminiferous tubular epithelium results in failure or reduced ability to produce sperm. Mumps may result in acute orchitis and epididymitis, accompanied by fever and debilitating pain, bilateral swelling, and redness of the testicles. If damage to seminiferous epithelium occurs, the size of the testes will be reduced. Other infections such as tuberculosis, pneumonia, and syphilis may affect the testes but less dramatically than mumps.

Genitourinary tract infections can cause infertility in males. *Chlamydia trachomatis* is sexually transmitted and is most prevalent in young adults with multiple sex partners. The infection is most commonly limited to the urethra and causes varying degrees of painful urination and discharge. Progressive infection may include the epididymis and prostate gland. *Neisseria gonorrhoeae* is a common urethral infection in the United States. It is sexually transmitted and may cause extremely painful urination and a purulent discharge. Infections that ascend to the epididymis may result in decreased fertility.

Cryptorchidism. Cryptorchidism is defined as any testis located in other than a dependent scrotal position. It is a common congenital condition, being found in approximately 30% of preterm male infants and in 1.0% to 3.4% of full-term male infants (Fig. 48-10). Although genetic disorders can cause cryptorchidism, the cause is usually unknown. Because the abdominal cavity is warmer than the scrotum, excessive warmth can damage the seminiferous epithelium of undescended testes and result in decreased spermatogenesis.

Medical Treatment. Cryptorchidism must be corrected within the first 18 months of life to give the best chance for fertility. Men with undescended testes have a 10 to 30 times higher incidence of testicular cancer than men whose testes descended normally. The risk remains higher even if the condition is subsequently corrected. If the testes are within the normal path but do not descend or cannot be pulled into the scrotum, they usually do not respond to hormonal therapy and surgery is needed. Whether medical or surgical therapy is indicated, it is performed after the first birthday and before the second birthday. Untreated bilateral cryptorchidism results in sterility. Unilateral cryptorchidism may result in a low sperm count, but spermatogenesis continues and pregnancies are sometimes initiated without difficulty.

Testicular Torsion. Testicular torsion occurs unilaterally when the testicle is mobile and the spermatic cord twists, cutting off the blood supply to the testicle (Fig. 48-11). It is an acute surgical emergency requiring immediate release of the torsion or removal of the testicle. It most commonly occurs in adolescents and usually occurs when the scrotum is warm and relaxed but may occur for no apparent reason. Symptoms are intense pain, often accompanied by nausea and vomiting. After testicular torsion is corrected, lowered sperm counts and infertility may follow. There is sometimes a collateral effect on the healthy testicle. After the testicle that underwent torsion is removed, sperm counts are normal.

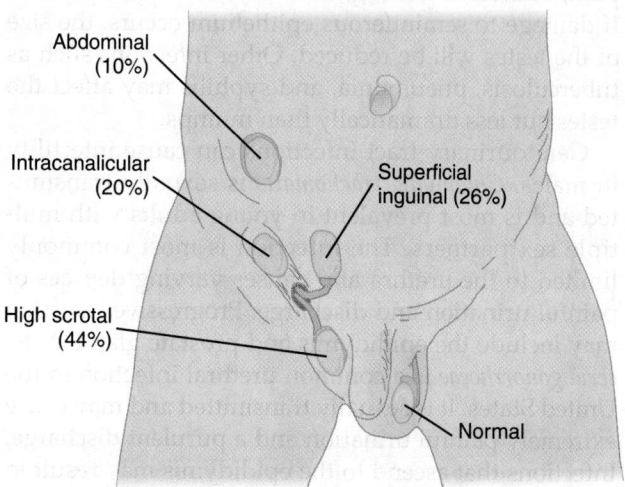

FIGURE **48-10** Common sites of undescended or mispositioned testicles.

Abdominal (10%)
Intracanalicular (20%)
Superficial inguinal (26%)
High scrotal (44%)
Normal

Varicocele. A varicocele is a lengthening and enlargement of the scrotal portion of the venous system that drains the testicle (see Fig. 48-11). Varicoceles are caused by incompetent or absent valves in the spermatic venous system, which allows pooled blood and the resulting increased pressure to dilate the veins. Most often, only the left testicle is affected. Affected testicles may be smaller and may have reduced spermatogenesis. The effect of a varicocele on fertility is debated. Treatment includes scrotal support or surgical ligation and is indicated when fertility is thought to be affected. Varicoceles may reappear after surgery, and fertility or the ability to conceive may or may not improve.

Vasectomy. Vasectomy is the surgical removal of a portion of the vasa deferentia (Fig. 48-12). Although sperm are no longer found in the semen after the procedure, erection, ejaculation, and intercourse are unaffected. Vasectomy is usually performed as an outpatient procedure in a physician's office or outpatient clinic. Postoperative pain or swelling can be managed with application of an ice bag, mild analgesics, and scrotal support. The patient can resume intercourse as soon as he feels comfortable, but it is important that he use other methods of birth control until analysis of the semen determines that there is a complete absence of sperm. The patient can expect the analysis to be done after about 15 ejaculations following the vasectomy.

Nursing care of the vasectomy patient should include preoperative teaching about the procedure itself

Put on Your Thinking Cap!

A couple visits the clinic seeking help for infertility. During the initial interview, one of them says, "My brother and his wife couldn't get pregnant either. Then he switched from briefs to boxer shorts. Within a few months, his wife was pregnant! Do you think his underwear could have had anything to do with that?" How would you reply appropriately and accurately?

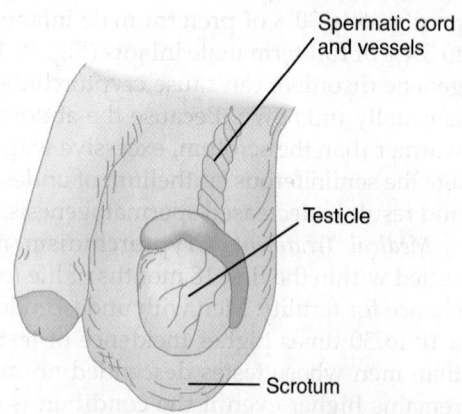

Spermatic cord and vessels
Testicle
Scrotum

A   Testicular torsion

Varicosed veins

B   Varicocele

FIGURE **48-11** Disturbances of the testes. **A,** Torsion of the testis. **B,** Varicocele.

and the resultant infertility. Although a vasectomy can sometimes be successfully reversed, it should be considered permanent. The nurse should be sensitive to the readiness of the male patient to undergo this procedure. Fears related to postoperative loss of sexual function and the development of cancer may cause anxiety in some men, even though they desire the procedure. Acceptance and reassurance are important.

PENILE CANCER

Cancer is a frightening diagnosis for any patient. Cancer of the male reproductive system may arouse the worst fears about sexual dysfunction, disfigurement, and diminished self-esteem. Penile cancer is relatively rare and occurs almost exclusively in uncircumcised men. Risk factors include chronic irritation, poor hygiene, a history of multiple sexual partners, sexually transmitted infection, and long-term tobacco use. Can-

cer may appear as a dry, wart-like, painless growth on the penis that does not respond to antibiotic therapy. It can be removed surgically if treated in early stages. Growths in advanced stages may ulcerate and involve the foreskin and penile shaft. Extensive resection or amputation as well as resection of nearby lymph nodes may be necessary.

TESTICULAR CANCER

Testicular germ cell carcinoma occurs most often in young men between the ages of 18 and 34 years. The three established risk factors for this type of cancer are cryptorchidism, white race, and previous testicular cancer. Other risk factors are a history of orchitis, human immunodeficiency virus (HIV) infection, and in utero exposure to diethylstilbestrol. Patients most often present with hard, painless tumors (Fig. 48-13). The diagnosis is often delayed because patients do not seek medical help.

What Does Culture Have to Do with Testicular Cancer?

White males, ages 10 to 34 years, are at highest risk for testicular cancer. Early detection needs to be targeted at young white males. Self-examination of the testicles should be taught to all young men, regardless of culture and ethnicity.

Early Detection

Self-examination and early diagnosis offer the highest chance of finding early-stage disease and subsequent cure. Therefore men need to be educated about the need for self-examination. Although men are used to touching their genitals, they may not feel comfortable examin-

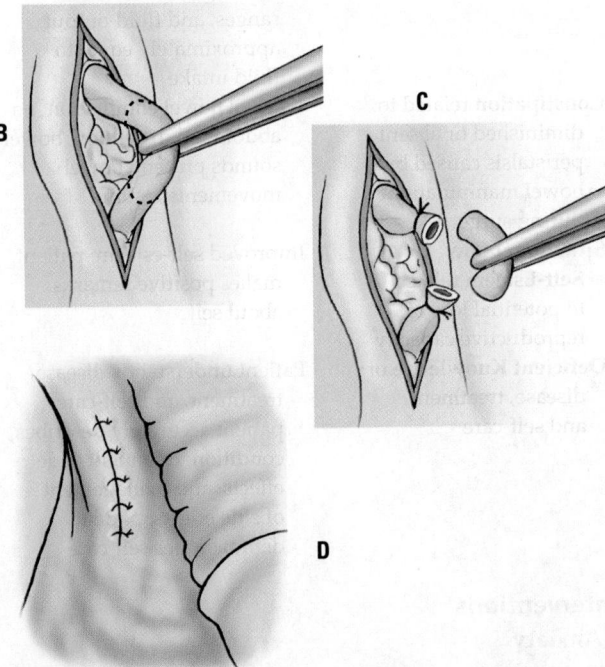

FIGURE **48-12** Vasectomy. **A,** Vas deferens located. **B,** Vas deferens exposed. **C,** Small segment of vas deferens removed and severed ends tied. **D,** Scrotal wound closed.

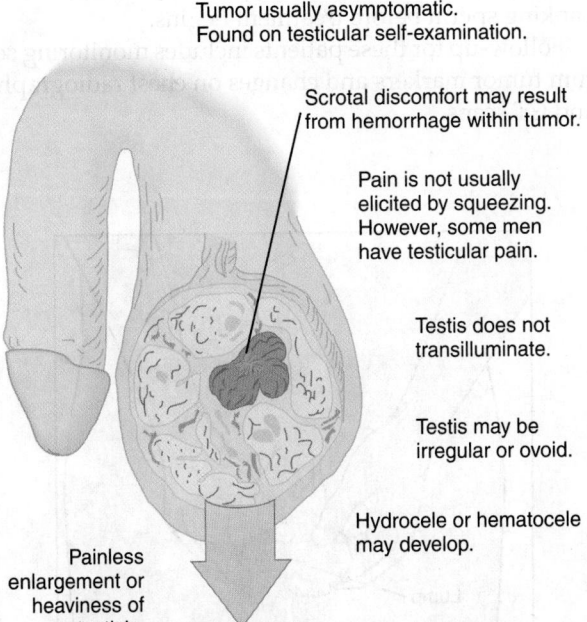

Tumor usually asymptomatic. Found on testicular self-examination.

Scrotal discomfort may result from hemorrhage within tumor.

Pain is not usually elicited by squeezing. However, some men have testicular pain.

Testis does not transilluminate.

Testis may be irregular or ovoid.

Hydrocele or hematocele may develop.

Painless enlargement or heaviness of testicle.

FIGURE **48-13** Characteristics of testicular tumors.

ing themselves. Self-examination includes monthly examination of the penis, scrotum, and perineal area. The individual should use a mirror to visualize areas that he cannot see and look for any changes from normal such as swelling, lumps, tenderness, lesions, asymmetry, discoloration, or discharge. The examination is best done after a warm bath or shower, when he is warm and the scrotum is relaxed. The scrotum is held in the palm of his hands with the index and middle fingers on the underside of the testicle and the thumb on top (Fig. 48-14). Each testicle is palpated between the thumbs and forefingers of both hands, with the testicle rolled gently between the fingers. The left testicle usually is lower than the right. The testicles are egg-shaped and should feel firm but not hard, and smooth without lumps. The epididymis, located on the top and posterior side of each testicle, feels soft and spongy. The spermatic cords are smooth, firm, tubular structures that run upward from the testicles on the back side.

Medical Diagnosis

Diagnostic procedures include ultrasound and blood studies to measure tumor markers: alpha-fetoprotein and human chorionic gonadotropic. If there is doubt about the diagnosis, surgical exploration is done. Radiographs and CT scans may be done to assess for metastasis.

Medical Treatment

Treatment for testicular cancer is designed according to the type of cancer and the stage. Treatment options are orchiectomy, radical orchiectomy, radiation, and chemotherapy. Follow-up includes monitoring tumor marker levels and radiographic examinations of lymph nodes for a period of 5 years from diagnosis. Treatment of testicular cancer may affect fertility and erections. The physician will inform the patient of the option of banking sperm before treatment begins.

Follow-up for these patients includes monitoring serum tumor markers and changes on chest radiographs and CT scans.

FIGURE **48-14** Testicular self-examination.

Lump

NURSING CARE *of the Patient with Testicular Cancer*

Nursing care of the surgical patient is covered in Chapter 17, and care of the patient who has cancer is discussed in Chapter 25. Therefore this discussion is limited to nursing care specific to the patient with testicular cancer.

Assessment

The nursing assessment of the male reproductive system is outlined in Box 48-1. When a patient has testicular cancer, fears or concerns related to the effects of surgery and other treatment must be assessed.

Nursing Diagnoses, Goals, and Outcome Criteria: Testicular Cancer, Postoperative	
NURSING DIAGNOSES	GOALS AND OUTCOME CRITERIA
Anxiety related to the diagnosis of cancer and the anticipation of side effects of treatments	Reduced anxiety: patient states anxiety is reduced, calm manner
Acute Pain related to surgical incision	Pain relief: patient states pain relieved, relaxed manner
Impaired Urinary Elimination related to the effects of anesthesia and abdominal surgery	Normal urine elimination: no bladder distention
Risk for Injury (shock, infection, fluid and electrolyte imbalances) related to surgery	Absence of excess bleeding or infection and normal fluid balance: vital signs consistent with patient norms, oral temperature less than 38.3° C (101° F), electrolytes within normal ranges, and fluid output approximately equal to fluid intake
Constipation related to diminished or absent peristalsis caused by bowel manipulation during surgery	Normal bowel elimination: no abdominal distention, bowel sounds present, bowel movements resume
Situational Low Self-Esteem related to potential loss of reproductive capacity	Improved self-esteem: patient makes positive remarks about self
Deficient Knowledge of disease, treatment, and self-care	Patient understands disease, treatment, and self-care: patient accurately describes condition, treatment, side effects, and management of side effects; patient demonstrates self-care

Interventions

Anxiety

From the time cancer is suspected, the patient faces anxiety-producing threats to self-image and self-esteem. You must be sensitive to the patient's fears of altered sexual function, loss of fertility, stressful treatments, and the threat of a potentially fatal disease. You can help the patient through active listening, providing information, and referring him for counseling if needed. The patient may wish to have a significant other included in interactions with you and other health professionals.

Acute Pain

There is no pain in the early stages of testicular cancer. If the disease is advanced or if the patient has undergone surgery or radiotherapy, pain may be a problem. If so, describe the pain and take steps to treat it promptly. Analgesics may be appropriate, but you can also employ other pain control techniques such as mental imagery and relaxation exercises (see Chapter 15).

Impaired Urinary Elimination

Radical orchiectomy usually requires a short hospitalization and has few complications. Nevertheless, monitor the patient's urinary status to confirm normal function before discharge. If the patient has a radical retroperitoneal lymph node dissection, he will probably have a catheter immediately after surgery.

Risk for Injury

Some patients with testicular cancer undergo radical retroperitoneal lymph node dissection. These patients have extensive surgical incisions and usually need intensive nursing care initially. As with any major abdominal surgery, the patient is at risk for shock, infection, bowel and bladder dysfunction, and fluid and electrolyte imbalances. Shock can result from fluid loss and the effects of anesthesia during the lengthy surgery. Measure and evaluate vital signs and fluid intake and output. Monitor the patient's electrolyte levels, and administer intravenous fluids as ordered to maintain fluid and electrolyte balance. He is likely to have a urinary catheter in place and a nasogastric tube attached to suction.

Constipation

Palpate the abdomen for bowel or bladder distention, and auscultate for bowel sounds. When permitted, encourage ambulation and a diet with adequate fiber to promote bowel elimination.

Situational Low Self-Esteem

The patient may or may not be rendered sterile as a result of the treatment employed. Radical orchiectomy results in sterility but does not impair erection and orgasm. After radiotherapy, the patient's sperm count typically declines at first but usually returns to normal by 2 to 3 years after treatment is completed. The effects of chemotherapy on fertility vary with the drug used. Retroperitoneal lymph node dissection often causes erectile dysfunction and problems with ejaculation. Help the patient formulate questions for the physician about the effects of specific treatments on sexual function and fertility. If sterility is anticipated, the patient should be counseled preoperatively about the possibility of banking sperm for future use. Because this type of cancer commonly affects young men, the potential to father a child at a later date may be very important to them.

Deficient Knowledge

Teaching is essential to prepare the patient for treatment and to provide the tools needed for him to cope with the diagnosis. The patient teaching plan will vary greatly with the extent of the cancer and the type of treatment given. Include the type of therapy prescribed, side effects, management of side effects, and available resources.

PROSTATIC CANCER

Cancer of the prostate is found on postmortem examination in 30% of men over the age of 50, and the incidence increases steadily with each decade to 100% of men in the tenth decade. Over 200,000 new cases were diagnosed in the United States in 2005, and more than 30,000 men died of prostate cancer that year. Although the cause is unknown, the risk factors include age over 50 years, African-American race, overweight, ingestion of a high-fat diet, and family history of prostate cancer.

 What Does Culture Have to Do with Prostate Cancer?

Rates of prostate cancer are much higher among African-American men than among white men. This group should be targeted to explain the importance of early evaluation of urinary symptoms.

Medical Diagnosis

Prostatic lesions are typically slow-growing and confined to the prostatic capsule. Younger men, however, tend to have very aggressive tumors. Prostatic tumors may go undetected until the disease is advanced and has metastasized to bone or liver. Large tumors may cause bladder outlet obstruction, rectal pressure, stool changes, painful defecation, or painful ejaculation. Because early diagnosis may improve treatment results, methods to permit early detection may be advised. The American Cancer Society recommends that all men over age 50 undergo annual digital rectal examinations and that PSA blood tests be done annually beginning at age 50. Men at higher risk may be advised to begin screening at age 40.

The diagnosis may be based on rectal examination, transrectal ultrasound, serum tumor markers, and needle aspiration/biopsy. If a diagnosis of prostate cancer is made, additional procedures may be done to identify the stage of the disease. These may include radiographs, radionuclide imaging, bone scans, excretory urography, transurethral ultrasound, CT, and MRI.

Medical Treatment

The treatment of prostatic cancer is controversial because of the difficulty in staging tumors and the unpredictable biologic behavior of the disease. However, the discovery of PSA as a tumor marker has allowed earlier identification and treatment of prostatic cancer. PSA is a product of prostatic tissue. It is extremely important to measure this antigen during the follow-up of patients who have undergone treatment. Persistent or rising PSA levels indicate advancing or recurrent tumor growth. PSA can be free or bound to plasma proteins. Prostate cancer cells produce more bound than free PSA.

Treatment options include "watchful waiting," conventional radiotherapy, brachytherapy, cryosurgery, and radical surgery. Chemotherapy is useful in limited cases. Sometimes "watchful waiting" is recommended for patients with a life expectancy of less than 10 years who have small cancers or who are not good surgical risks. The patient is monitored frequently, and treatment is initiated if the tumor begins to enlarge. Cryoablation, freezing of prostate tissue, is used mainly to treat prostate cancer. However, it is associated with a significant incidence of postoperative complications including necrosis.

Radical prostatectomy includes removal of the prostate gland, the outer capsule, the seminal vesicles, sections of the vas deferens, and sometimes a portion of the bladder neck. Most operations include removal of the pelvic lymph nodes to check for metastasis. The surgical approach usually is perineal or retropubic. The latter approach permits an autonomic nerve-sparing technique, which preserves erectile function in 70% of patients. The urinary incontinence that occurs in 10% to 15% of men who undergo radical prostatectomy subsides within 6 months in 85% to 90% of those affected. Minimally invasive radical prostatectomy using a laparoscope and robot-assisted technology is available in some settings. It is believed that less-invasive techniques will result in less blood loss and less postoperative pain.

Radiation alone often is effective when the cancer is confined to the prostate. Radiation can be delivered by external beam or by implanting seeds (brachytherapy) of radioactive gold, iodine, or iridium in the prostate through hollow needles inserted under anesthesia. External beam radiation requires only a few minutes, 5 days a week for 6 to 8 weeks. Side effects include skin dryness and irritation; diarrhea, cramping, GI bleeding; sexual dysfunction; fatigue; bone marrow suppression; and various urinary symptoms such as dysuria, frequency, hesitancy, urgency, and nocturia. The radioactive seeds affect surrounding tissues less than external beam radiation. Patients often have some urinary symptoms of irritation or obstruction after the seeds are implanted.

Prostate cancer growth is influenced by hormones. Therefore hormonal therapy is used to eliminate the androgenic effect by interfering with androgen production or blocking receptors for the androgens. Testosterone production also can be achieved by removing the testicles. Many men elect drug therapy over the surgical option. Types of drugs used in hormonal therapy include estrogen, luteinizing hormone–releasing hormone (LHRH) agonists, and androgen receptor blockers. Estrogen (i.e., diethylstilbestrol) decreases the production of testosterone, inhibits LH secretion, and blocks circulating testosterone. However, it is used less often now than in the past because of its adverse effects, including blood clots, heart failure, and breast enlargement. LHRH analogues include leuprolide (Lupron), goserelin acetate (Zoladex), buserelin (Suprefact), and triptorelin (Trelstar). These agents inhibit the release of pituitary hormones necessary for testosterone production. They are given intramuscularly or subcutaneously. One form is available in pellets that are implanted subcutaneously and deliver medication for a year. With initial therapy, patients may experience bone pain, which resolves over time. Drugs that inhibit the action of testosterone include flutamide (Eulexin), bicalutamide (Casodex), and nilutamide (Nilandron). They may be used in combination with LHRH agonists (see the Drug Therapy table on p. 1089).

The adverse effects of all of these agents can include hot flashes and erectile dysfunction. When these agents are no longer effective, other drugs may be used that reduce testosterone production in the adrenals. Examples are spironolactone (Aldactone), aminoglutethimide (Cytadren), and glucocorticoids. Hormonal therapy is usually effective for a limited period of time, generally 1 to 3 years. Bone pain and fractures are complications of prostate cancer. Bisphosphonates such as alendronate (Fosamax) may be ordered to help relieve bone symptoms.

Transurethral laser treatment works well but is used for benign prostatic hypertrophy only—not for cancer of the prostate.

NURSING CARE *of the Patient with Prostatic Cancer*

Details of the assessment of the male reproductive system are summarized in Box 48-1. Nursing care of male patients should include encouragement to have annual screening for prostate cancer. Stress the value of early diagnosis and treatment. If the patient has undergone surgery, nursing care is similar to that described in the Nursing Care of the Patient with Benign Prostatic Hypertrophy section on p. 1090. Nursing care of the patient with cancer is presented in Chapter 25, and the care of patients having urologic surgery is covered in Chapter 40. Specific problems that may require special interventions after prostate surgery are bladder spasms, erectile dysfunction, urinary incontinence, and body image disturbances associated with changes in the reproductive system.

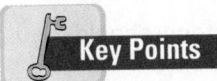
Key Points

- The male reproductive system consists of the scrotum, testes, epididymides, vasa deferentia, seminal vesicles, prostate gland, ejaculatory duct, Cowper's glands, internal urethra, and penis.
- Prostatitis is an inflammation of the prostate gland that is treated with antimicrobials, analgesics, and sitz baths.
- Epididymitis is an inflammation of the epididymis that is treated with bed rest, cold packs, sitz baths, analgesics, antibiotics, and scrotal support.
- Benign prostatic hypertrophy—enlargement of the prostate gland that may lead to obstruction of the urethra—may be treated with drugs or surgical intervention.
- Nursing care after prostatectomy addresses Risk for Deficient Fluid Volume, Acute Pain, Risk for Infection, Risk for Injury, Urge Urinary Incontinence, Sexual Dysfunction, Situational Low Self-Esteem, and Deficient Knowledge.
- Erectile dysfunction (impotence), the inability to achieve or maintain an erection adequate for sexual intercourse, may be treated with psychological intervention, oral drug therapy, vacuum constriction devices, self-injection therapy, intraurethral pellets, or penile implants.
- Nursing care of the patient with erectile dysfunction may focus on Sexual Dysfunction, Situational Low Self-Esteem, and Ineffective Therapeutic Regimen Management.
- Peyronie's disease is the formation of fibrous tissue in the penis that causes it to bend upward during erection, causing pain and interfering with vaginal penetration.
- Priapism is prolonged penile erection not related to sexual desire that requires emergency treatment to prevent ischemia, gangrene, fibrosis, and future erectile dysfunction.
- Infertility is the inability to impregnate despite unprotected intercourse over a 12-month period.
- Causes of infertility include endocrine or testicular dysfunction and disorders of the ejaculatory system.
- Cancer of the male reproductive system may affect the penis, testicles, or prostate gland.
- Nursing care of the patient with testicular cancer focuses on Anxiety, Acute Pain, Risk for Injury, Impaired Urine Elimination, Constipation, Situational Low Self-Esteem, and Deficient Knowledge.
- Other disorders affecting the male reproductive system are hydrocele, phimosis, and paraphimosis.

 Go to your Companion CD-ROM for a Pharmacology Tutorial, Audio Glossary, and 3-D animations.

evolve   Be sure to visit the companion Evolve site at http://evolve.elsevier.com/Linton/ for WebLinks and additional online resources.

REVIEW QUESTIONS *Choose the best answer.*

1. The hormone that is responsible for male sexual development is:
   1. Luteinizing hormone
   2. Testosterone
   3. Gonadotropin
   4. Progesterone

2. Normal age-related changes in the reproductive system of a healthy male include:
   1. Steady production of testosterone from puberty to death
   2. Longer refractory period between erections
   3. Loss of ability to maintain an erection by age 70 years
   4. Decreased time needed for sexual arousal

3. Which of the following should be included when teaching a patient about benign prostatic hypertrophy?
   1. Moderate use of alcohol will promote emptying of the bladder.
   2. Practice delaying voiding as long as you can to increase bladder capacity.
   3. Medications that contain antihistamines may cause you to retain urine.
   4. Prolonged exposure to warm temperatures promotes bladder spasms.

4. Bleeding after a transurethral prostatectomy is most likely to be detected by inspection of the:
   1. Abdominal dressing
   2. Perineal drainage
   3. Urine characteristics
   4. Suprapubic drain

5. A drug that reduces the size of the prostate without lowering circulating testosterone levels is:
   1. Tamsulosin (Flomax)
   2. Flutamide (Eulexin)
   3. Oxybutynin chloride (Ditropan)
   4. Finasteride (Proscar)

6. Normal saline is the preferred fluid used to irrigate urinary catheters after prostatectomy because:
   1. It is isotonic and will not cause water intoxication
   2. It is less expensive than sterile water for irrigation
   3. It is absorbed into the bloodstream to maintain blood volume
   4. Sterile water stings when it comes in contact with the surgical sites

7. A childhood disease that can cause infertility in males is:

   1. Measles
   2. Chickenpox
   3. Mumps
   4. Diphtheria

8. Cryptorchidism must be treated early in life to prevent:

   1. Testicular torsion
   2. Varicocele
   3. Chronic infection
   4. Sterility

9. Patient teaching related to vasectomy should include:

   1. You will be sterile immediately after the procedure.
   2. Vasectomy is easily reversible if you wish to father a child later.
   3. Postoperative problems with erection and ejaculation are common.
   4. You will need to have a semen analysis to determine if sperm are present.

10. After surgery for prostate cancer, how is treatment effectiveness monitored?

    1. Measurement of the PSA level
    2. Periodic biopsies of perineal tissue
    3. Studies of urine flow rates
    4. Radiographs of the abdomen

49 Sexually Transmitted Infections

 http://evolve.elsevier.com/Linton/

Objectives

After reading and studying this chapter, you should be able to:

1. List infectious diseases classified as sexually transmitted infections.
2. Explain the importance of the nurse's approach when dealing with patients who have sexually transmitted infections.
3. Describe tests used to diagnose sexually transmitted infections and the nursing considerations associated with each.
4. Explain why specific sexually transmitted infections must be reported to the health department.
5. Describe the pathophysiology, signs and symptoms, complications, and medical treatment for selected sexually transmitted infections.
6. Design a teaching plan on the prevention of sexually transmitted infections.
7. List nursing considerations when a patient is on drug therapy for a sexually transmitted infection.
8. Identify data to be collected when assessing a patient with a sexually transmitted infection.
9. Assist in developing a nursing care plan for a patient with a sexually transmitted infection.

Key Terms

Be sure to check out the bonus material on the Companion CD-ROM, including selected audio pronunciations.

chancre (SHĂNG-kěr, p. 1111)
latent (LĀ-těnt, p. 1112)
opportunistic infection (p. 1115)
pelvic inflammatory disease (p. 1110)
sexually transmitted infection (STI) (p. 1105)

Sexually transmitted infections (STIs) continue to be a serious public health problem in the United States despite medical advances. These diseases spread primarily through sexual contact and may have serious and permanent consequences. Worldwide the incidence of STIs increases every year. Each year, more than 100,000 women are left sterile by STIs. In the United States, an estimated 19 million new infections occur each year. Almost half of these are in persons ages 15 to 24. Although STIs are more common in peo-

ple of lower socioeconomic status and in those with less education and limited access to health care, all segments of the population are represented. Drug abuse and having multiple sexual partners also are risk factors. In the United States, STI rates are highest among African Americans, followed by Latinos, and then by non-Latino whites.

What Does Culture Have to Do with Sexually Transmitted Infections?

The incidence of STIs varies among races, but poverty, lack of education, and limited access to health care probably play a larger role than race/ethnicity. Also, cultural beliefs about sexual practices, use of condoms, and education of children about STI prevention may all affect the incidence of STIs in any given population.

Despite public education efforts, some people resist taking preventive measures. Infected people do not always inform their sexual partners, so the disease continues to be passed on. Also, symptoms are sometimes subtle; thus STIs that go undetected can spread and invade other parts of the body.

Nurses must be aware of their feelings about working with people who have STIs. There is a stigma associated with these infections, and we must ensure the same quality of care to these patients that is given to patients with any other diagnoses. Judgmental behavior on the part of health care providers discourages people from seeking appropriate medical care. In this chapter, specific diseases are explained, followed by a general discussion of nursing care appropriate for all patients with STIs.

DIAGNOSTIC TESTS AND PROCEDURES

The primary measures used to diagnose STIs are serologic tests and studies of smears and cultures.

SEROLOGIC TESTS

Serologic tests may be ordered to detect infections with hepatitis A, B, C, D, and E; syphilis; human immunodeficiency virus (HIV); herpes simplex; and cytomegalovirus. These tests are designed to detect infectious diseases by measuring antigens or antibodies in the blood. Many factors can cause inaccurate results, especially with older tests. Agency laboratory procedures specify the patient preparation for specific tests.

SMEARS AND CULTURES

Patients with gonococcal, chlamydial, herpes simplex, *Trichomonas,* or yeast infections often have discharge from the vagina or penis. In addition to this discharge, exudate from lesions can be collected and studied to determine the exact infecting organism. For females, the sample may be collected from the vagina or from the cervix. The procedure varies with the type of organism suspected. To collect a sample from a male patient, a swab or a special loop may be used. The person who collects the sample wears gloves and treats the sample as a potential source of infection. The sample may be submitted for microscopic examination or for culture and sensitivity tests.

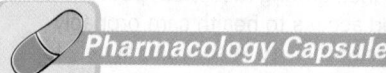
Pharmacology Capsule

When you have an order to obtain a specimen for culture and another order to administer anti-infectives, collect the specimen before giving the first dose of the anti-infective.

DRUG THERAPY

The drugs recommended by the Centers for Disease Control and Prevention (CDC) (2004) are noted with the discussion of each specific infection. The CDC also recommends alternate drugs for people who are allergic to the primary drugs, pregnant women, infants and children, and people who are being treated for multiple infections. Details are available at the CDC website: http://www.cdc.gov/mmwr/preview/mmwrhtml/rr5106al.htm. Examples of drugs used to treat sexually transmitted infections are presented in the Drug Therapy table on pp. 1107 to 1109.

REPORTING SEXUALLY TRANSMITTED INFECTIONS

Confirmed cases of HIV, acquired immunodeficiency syndrome (AIDS), gonorrhea, syphilis, chlamydia, chancroid, and viral hepatitis must be reported to the local health department. An investigator asks the patient to name sexual contacts. Those individuals are contacted and advised that they have been exposed to the disease and are encouraged to seek medical evaluation. The purpose of this process is to identify and treat infected individuals so that transmission of the disease can be slowed.

SPECIFIC SEXUALLY TRANSMITTED INFECTIONS

CHLAMYDIAL INFECTION

Chlamydial infection is thought to be the most common bacterial STI in the United States. An estimated 2.8 million people are diagnosed with chlamydia each year. The symptoms are similar to those of gonorrhea. The infecting organism is a virus-like bacterium called *Chlamydia trachomatis,* which infects both men and women. This disease is transmitted by contact with the mucous membranes in the mouth, eyes, urethra, vagina, or rectum.

Signs and Symptoms

One reason chlamydial infection is so common is that most people have no symptoms. Symptoms are more noticeable in men and include penile discharge, which is initially thin and then becomes creamy later. Symptoms, if any, are generally noted 1 to 3 weeks after infection. Another common complaint among males is painful or frequent urination. Females may experience vaginal discharge, painful urination, nausea, fever, painful intercourse, bleeding between menstrual periods, and lower abdominal pain.

Complications

If left untreated, chlamydial infection can result in sterility in both sexes. The sperm ducts can become inflamed and blocked. In females, pelvic inflammatory disease can block the fallopian tubes and damage the uterus. The risk of ectopic pregnancy (the fertilized ovum develops outside the uterus) is increased in the presence of chlamydial infection. Also, women with chlamydial infection are approximately 5 times more likely to become infected with HIV if exposed to it. Newborns of infected women may have eye infections or infant pneumonia. Therefore erythromycin ophthalmic ointment may be ordered for the newborn because it is effective against chlamydial infection as well as gonorrhea.

Medical Diagnosis and Treatment

The diagnosis is based on the individual's sexual history and the results of laboratory studies. A *Chlamydia* antigen test is used to screen for chlamydial infection. A urine test also is available. The most accurate test, however, is the cell tissue culture.

The infection usually is treated with a single dose of azithromycin (Zithromax) or a 7-day course of doxycycline (Vibramycin). Review the patient's complete drug profile because azithromycin (Zithromax) interacts with many other common drugs. Other antimicrobials also may be administered because patients with chlamydial infection may have gonorrhea as well. The culture should be repeated in 4 to 7 days after treatment to confirm successful treatment. The patient is advised to avoid all sexual contact (genital, oral, anal) until a cure has been achieved.

Text continued on p. 1110.

DRUG THERAPY | *Drugs Used to Treat Sexually Transmitted Infections*

GENERAL CONSIDERATIONS

Always assess for history of allergies before giving any anti-infective.
If patient reports being allergic to the prescribed drug, withhold it and notify the physician.
Observe all patients for possible allergic responses: rash, difficulty breathing, hypotension.
Obtain specimens for culture before administering first dose of anti-infective.
When giving intravenous anti-infectives through a secondary line, check compatibility with primary fluid.
Tell patient it is important to complete full course of treatment to prevent organisms from becoming resistant and to prevent relapse because all organisms had not been killed.
Tell patient that sexual partner(s) should be treated at the same time to prevent infection.
Assess for drug interactions.

DRUG	USE/ACTION	SIDE EFFECTS	NURSING INTERVENTIONS
ANTIBACTERIALS			
Beta-lactams Penicillin G (Benzathine, Bicillin, Pfizerpen, Crysticillin)	Effective against organisms that cause gonorrhea and syphilis.	Nausea, vomiting, diarrhea, pain at injection site, anaphylaxis. Jarisch-Herxheimer reaction: headache, fever, chills, diaphoresis, tachycardia, muscle and joint pain.	Scratch test may be ordered to assess allergy. Check drug insert for preparation of injection. Give by deep injection in large muscle. Do not pause during injection; needle may clog. Massage site. Have patient wait 30 min after injection in case there is allergic reaction. Tell patient Jarisch-Herxheimer reaction may occur 12-24 hr after injection. If allergic to cephalosporins, may also be allergic to penicillins.
Cefixime (Suprax)	Effective against gonorrhea.	Seizures, pseudomembranous colitis, diarrhea, nausea, vomiting, rash, blood dyscrasias, pain on injection, serum sickness, superinfection.	If allergic to penicillin, may also be allergic to cephalosporins. Monitor intravenous (IV) injection site for pain, red streak. Monitor stools for diarrhea; notify physician if bloody mucus is present. Report vaginal or anal itching. Assess for bruising, bleeding.
Ceftriaxone sodium (Rocephin)	Effective against organism that causes gonorrhea.	Nausea, vomiting, headache, dizziness, and (rarely) bleeding. Allergic reactions, including anaphylaxis, in patients allergic to cephalosporins or penicillin. Nephrotoxicity with high doses or renal disease. Superinfections: diarrhea, candidiasis. IV route: pain, thrombophlebitis. Intramuscular (IM) route: pain, induration at injection site.	
TETRACYCLINES			
Tetracycline hydrochloride (Achromycin, Panmycin, Tetracyn)	Effective against organisms that cause gonorrhea, syphilis, and chlamydial infections.	Nausea, vomiting, diarrhea, pain at injection site, allergic reactions, discoloration of developing teeth.	Contraindicated in pregnancy and lactation. Check patient's medication list for possible interactions. Oral form given with full glass of water. No milk, calcium, or antacids within an hour of tetracycline.
Doxycycline (Vibramycin)	Effective against organisms that cause gonorrhea, granuloma inguinale, syphilis, and lymphogranuloma venereum.	Anorexia, nausea, vomiting, diarrhea, dysphagia, fungal infections, anaphylaxis, increased intracranial pressure, photosensitivity. Rarely: rash, urticaria, hemolytic anemia.	Assess allergies to tetracycline and to sulfites. Monitor food intake and stools. Assess blood pressure and level of consciousness. Report genital or anal itching. Give with full glass of water.

Continued

DRUG THERAPY — Drugs Used to Treat Sexually Transmitted Infections—cont'd

DRUG	USE/ACTION	SIDE EFFECTS	NURSING INTERVENTIONS
MACROLIDES Erythromycin (E-Mycin, Ilosone, Erythrocin Stearate)	Effective against organisms that cause chlamydial infection, syphilis, and gonorrhea. Ophthalmic ointment used in newborn to prevent eye infection.	Nausea, vomiting, diarrhea, phlebitis at infusion site, allergic reactions, hepatitis, ototoxicity.	Report tinnitus or jaundice. Give oral drug on empty stomach with full glass of water—no fruit juice.
FLUOROQUINOLONES Ciprofloxacin (Cipro)	Effective against gonorrhea.	Dizziness, headache, drowsiness, seizures, hepatotoxicity, pseudomembranous colitis, tendon rupture, Stevens-Johnson syndrome, crystalluria.	Monitor liver function tests. Do not administer within 4 hr of magnesium, aluminum, zinc, or iron preparations. Can be given with food. Milk and yogurt decrease absorption.
Azithromycin (Zithromax)	Effective against *Chlamydia* (which causes urethritis and cervicitis).	Diarrhea, nausea, vomiting, abdominal pain, vaginitis.	Caution if patient has liver impairment. Do not give with antacids. Give 1 hr before meals or 2 hr after meals.
SULFONAMIDES Trimethoprim-sulfamethoxazole (Bactrim, Septra)	Used to treat urinary tract infections and *Pneumocystis jiroveci* infections.	Rash, pruritus, nausea, vomiting, unpleasant taste, epigastric distress, crystalluria, photosensitivity, thrombocytopenia, neutropenia, anemia, leukopenia. Rarely: anaphylaxis, elevated blood urea nitrogen and creatinine levels.	Assess for itching, rash, fever, sore throat, bleeding. Tell patient to avoid excessive sun exposure. Increased fluid intake is needed to prevent crystal formation in the urine that could harm kidneys. Can be taken with food if gastrointestinal (GI) upset occurs.
MISCELLANEOUS ANTI-INFECTIVES Metronidazole (Flagyl)	Effective against *Trichomonas.*	Headache, dizziness, nausea, vomiting, abdominal pain, anorexia, diarrhea, skin irritation, peripheral neuropathy, leukopenia.	Give with food or milk. Instruct patient not to take a double dose if a dose is missed. Tell patient to avoid alcohol. Advise patient to follow safety precautions if dizziness occurs. Monitor fluid status because drug contains sodium. Urine may be dark. Monitor blood cell counts. Severe reaction with alcohol.
Pentamidine isethionate (Pentam 300)	An antiprotozoal used to treat infection with *Pneumocystis jiroveci,* an opportunistic organism that often causes infection in people with acquired immunodeficiency syndrome (AIDS). Routes of administration include IM, IV, and inhalation.	Elevated serum creatinine levels, leukopenia, thrombocytopenia, hypoglycemia, nausea, anorexia, renal damage, bronchospasm. Pain and sterile abscess at IM injection site. Phlebitis with IV infusion.	Inhalation route contraindicated in patients with asthma or a history of anaphylactic reaction to any drug. Monitor blood pressure, pulse, blood glucose. Check IM and IV sites. Assess appetite and food intake. Watch for dyspnea.
Foscarnet sodium (Foscavir)	Treats cytomegalovirus retinitis in AIDS patients.	Fever, nausea, vomiting, diarrhea, abnormal kidney function, bone marrow suppression, changes in blood pressure, seizures, bronchospasm, urinary retention, and a number of other adverse side effects.	Monitor electrolytes. Record intake and output. Implement safety precautions if seizures occur. Monitor vital signs and blood cell counts. Encourage adequate fluid intake.

ANTIVIRALS

Acyclovir (Zovirax) — Decreases frequency and severity of genital herpes infections. Is not curative. — Dizziness, headache, diarrhea, nausea, vomiting, renal failure, seizures. — Apply ointment with gloved finger. Do not double up if an oral dose is missed. Tell patient drug is not curative. Condoms should be used during sexual contact, and sexual contact should be avoided when lesions are present.

Dermatologic Agents

Podophyllin — Topical agents used to remove genital warts. — Highly caustic; can be applied directly on warts. Excessive application can cause kidney damage, neuropathy, blood dyscrasias. Teratogenic; contraindicated during pregnancy. — Should be applied only by physician. Treated area must be washed with alcohol or soap and water within 1-4 hr.

Imiquimod (Aldara) — — Erythema, erosion, flaking. Local itching, burning, pain. No systemic effects. — Instruct patient to apply at bedtime and wash off in morning. Usual application is 3 times/wk for 16 wk or until warts are gone.

Podofilox (Condylox) — — Local inflammation, erosion, pain, itching, bleeding. Causes more discomfort than imiquimod, but costs less and treatment is shorter. — Instruct patient to apply twice daily for 3 consecutive days, then take 4 days off. The cycle can be repeated if needed for a maximum of 4 cycles until the warts are gone. Does not have to be washed off. Advise patient not to use more than 0.5 mg/day and apply only to warts, not to normal skin.

HAART (Highly Active Antiretroviral Therapy Agents)

A highly effective strategy to treat human immunodeficiency virus (HIV) infection by using various combinations of non-nucleoside reverse transcriptase inhibitors, nucleoside reverse transcriptase inhibitors, and protease inhibitors. Examples from each category are listed below.

Nucleoside Reverse Transcriptase Inhibitors

Didanosine (Videx) — Used in combination with or instead of zidovudine to treat HIV infection. — Rash, inflammation of oral mucous membranes, fever, and (rarely) pancreatitis. — Assess skin and mouth. Advise patient to practice good oral hygiene. Monitor temperature. Report nausea, vomiting, abdominal pain.

Protease Inhibitors

Indinavir (Crixivan), Ritonavir (Norvir), Saquinavir (Invirase) — Used to treat HIV infection. Are not curative. — Indinavir: gastrointestinal upset, risk of urinary calculi, agitation, headache, muscle pain, anemia, cough, body odor, skin disorders, blurred vision. Ritonavir: gastrointestinal upset, peripheral neuropathy, rash, muscle pain. Saquinavir: phototoxicity, bleeding in hemophiliacs, many other side effects when given with AZT or DDI. Interferes with metabolism of many other drugs. — Monitor results of liver function studies. Check drug profile for possible interactions. Stress need to take every day as ordered. Be sure patient understands that infection can still be transmitted. Indinavir: take at least 1500 mL of fluids daily. Ritonavir: chocolate milk masks taste. Saquinavir: take within 2 hr of full meal, avoid direct sunlight.

Non-nucleoside Reverse Transcriptase Inhibitors

Delavirdine (Rescriptor) — Used with other drugs to treat HIV infection. Not curative. — GI distress, fatigue, dizziness, nephrotoxicity, muscle pain, hepatitis, psychiatric symptoms. Many drug-drug interactions. — Monitor tests of liver and kidney function. Assess mental/emotional state. Help patient design schedule of multiple drugs.

Table 49-1 | *Chlamydial Infection*

SIGNS/SYMPTOMS	POSSIBLE COMPLICATIONS	MEDICAL TREATMENT	NURSING CONSIDERATIONS
Sometimes no signs or symptoms. *Males:* penile discharge (thin at first, then creamy); painful, frequent urination. *Females:* vaginal discharge, lower abdominal pain.	Sterility in both sexes. Transmission to newborn infants, causing eye infections or pneumonia.	Azithromycin (Zithromax) or doxycycline (Vibramycin).	Counsel about importance of treatment to prevent complications. Advise of need for follow-up to be sure infection has been treated successfully. Tell patient to avoid sexual contact until cured.

Nursing care of the patient with chlamydial infection and other STIs is discussed in the Nursing Care of the Patient with a Sexually Transmitted Infection section on p. 1116. Information about chlamydial infection is summarized in Table 49-1.

GONORRHEA

Gonorrhea is one of the most commonly reported STIs in the United States. According to the CDC, 339,593 new cases of gonorrhea were reported in 2005. In children between the ages of 10 and 14, more than 4000 cases are reported annually. Gonorrhea is transmitted most often through direct sexual contact. There have been cases of transmission to newborn infants by infected mothers and to medical personnel with skin lacerations who have come in contact with infected fluids. The infection is not picked up from toilet seats, doorknobs, or towels.

The bacterium that causes this disease is *Neisseria gonorrhoeae*. This organism lives in warm, moist areas of the body such as the cervix and the urethra. Areas affected by local gonorrhea infections may include the pharynx, rectum, urethra, prostate, epididymis, uterus, and fallopian tubes. There is a high incidence of rectal gonorrhea among homosexual and bisexual males. The presence of bacteria in the throat is common among individuals who perform oral sex (fellatio) on an infected partner. With systemic (disseminated) infection, the heart, joints, skin, and meninges may become involved.

Signs and Symptoms

Many people with gonorrhea have no symptoms. When present, symptoms typically occur 2 days to 3 weeks after exposure and are generally more apparent in males than in females. Males who do have symptoms often present with whitish or greenish discharge from the penis and often complain of a burning sensation during urination. Females may experience vaginal discharge, redness and swelling of the external genitalia, a burning sensation during urination, abdominal pain, or abnormal menstruation. A rectal infection may cause discharge, anal itching, soreness, bleeding, or painful bowel movements. Throat infections usually have no symptoms, but a sore throat may be present. Symptoms generally disappear after a few weeks, but if the infection is untreated, the bacteria remain in the body and the person remains highly infectious.

Complications

If untreated, gonorrhea can cause sterility in both sexes and infections that may lead to damage to heart tissue and joints. Males may develop epididymitis and prostatitis. Females may develop **pelvic inflammatory disease**, which is an infection of the ovaries, fallopian tubes, and pelvic area. People with gonorrhea are at increased risk for HIV; people with HIV and gonorrhea are more likely to transmit HIV to another person.

Medical Diagnosis

The diagnosis is based on the individual's health history and physical examination findings as well as on laboratory analysis of exudate from infected body parts or urinalysis.

Medical Treatment

Treatment employs a single dose of intramuscular (IM) ceftriaxone sodium (Rocephin) or oral cefixime (Suprax), ciprofloxacin (Cipro), or ofloxacin (Floxin). If concurrent chlamydial infection has not been ruled out, the initial drug is followed with 7 days of oral doxycycline calcium (Vibramycin). One of these regimens cures most cases of gonorrhea quickly and safely. Penicillin is not used as much as it once was because many organisms have developed resistance to it. Erythromycin ophthalmic ointment may be ordered for the newborn to prevent eye infection caused by exposure to gonococci during delivery.

Instruct patients to follow up with a physician to be sure the treatment was effective. Additional information about drug therapy for gonorrhea is provided in the Drug Therapy table on pp. 1107 to 1109.

Nursing care of the patient with gonorrhea and other STIs is covered in the Nursing Care of the Patient with a Sexually Transmitted Infection section on p. 1116. Table 49-2 summarizes information related to the signs and symptoms of gonorrhea, the possible complications, the medical treatment, and the nursing considerations.

Follow-up examination is essential after antimicrobial therapy for gonorrhea to be sure the infection has been eradicated.

Table 49-2 | *Gonorrhea*

SIGNS/SYMPTOMS	POSSIBLE COMPLICATIONS	MEDICAL TREATMENT	NURSING CONSIDERATIONS
Male: Thick urethral discharge (purulent green or yellow); swelling and redness of the meatus; urinary urgency and dribbling.	Epididymitis, urethritis, infections of Cowper's and Tyson's glands.	Collect specimen for culture. Treated with ceftriaxone (Rocephin), cefixime (Suprax), followed by Doxycycline (Vibramycin).	Instruct the patient that all sexual partners should also be treated. Instruct the patient to take complete prescription of the drug (if receiving ciprofloxacin [Cipro] or tetracycline for self-medication), even if symptoms have disappeared. Stress abstinence or condom use.
Female: Increased, foul-smelling vaginal discharge; dysuria (difficulty urinating); fever; abnormal or painful menstruation; vulval soreness; peritonitis; backache; lower back pain (usually involving only one side).	Infertility, urethral and labial infection, risk of tubal pregnancy, pelvic inflammatory disease, septicemia.	Same as for male patients.	Counsel about potential complications.

SYPHILIS

Syphilis is caused by a microscopic organism, a spirochete (coiled bacterium) called *Treponema pallidum*. The organism is generally transmitted by sexual contact but also can be spread through breaks in the skin. It also can be passed through the placenta, thus causing an infant to be born with the disease (congenital syphilis). In the United States, 8724 new cases of syphilis were reported in 2005.

Signs and Symptoms

Signs and symptoms change throughout the course of the disease. If untreated, syphilis progresses through four stages: primary, secondary, latent, and late.

Primary Stage. A typical lesion, called a chancre, is the first sign of syphilis. The chancre is generally first noticed 1 to 12 weeks after contact. During the primary stage, a reddish papule appears where the organism entered the body, usually on the genitals, anus, or mouth. Within a week, the papule becomes a painless red ulcer. Lymph nodes in the area of the chancre may be enlarged but are not tender. The chancre may last from 1 to 5 weeks. When it disappears, patients may assume they are cured when, in fact, the infecting organism has moved into the blood (Fig. 49-1).

Secondary Stage. The secondary stage occurs 1 to 6 months after contact. Symptoms may include a rash on the extremities, chest or back, palms of the hands, and soles of the feet. Pustules that contain highly contagious material often develop. Fever, sore throat, and generalized aching are also seen in this stage. The patient is contagious during the first and second stages.

A

B

FIGURE **49-1** Chancre typical of primary syphilis. **A,** Chancre typical of primary syphilis (female). **B,** Chancre typical of primary syphilis (male).

Latent Stage. The latent stage, in which there are no symptoms, follows the secondary stage. Although there are no symptoms, the organisms are invading the major organs. The disease is not spread by sexual contact during the latent stage but may be transmitted by blood exposure.

Late Stage. It is generally 3 years after contact before late syphilis develops, although it may be decades. Signs and symptoms of late syphilis include arthritis, numbness of the extremities, ulcers of the skin and internal organs, and pain due to damage to the heart, blood vessels (especially the aorta), spinal cord, or brain.

Complications

The patient with untreated syphilis may develop severe, potentially fatal complications, including blindness, mental illness, paralysis, and heart disease. The lesions also make it easier for a person to contract HIV infection.

Medical Diagnosis

The diagnosis is based on physical examination findings and a blood test to detect the presence of antibodies. Tests for syphilis include screening and confirma-

Pharmacology Capsule

Treatment of syphilis with penicillin commonly causes the Jarisch-Herxheimer reaction. Patients have headache, fever, and muscle aches that may persist for 24 hours after treatment.

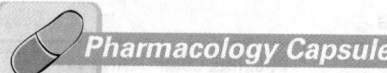

Pharmacology Capsule

Patients who do not complete the prescribed course of antibiotic therapy may not be cured of the infection.

tion tests. Two screening tests are the Venereal Disease Research Laboratory (VDRL) test and the rapid plasma reagin (RPR) test. Both detect a protein that appears in the blood when a person has syphilis. Screening tests can be inaccurate because other factors can cause false positive reactions. Also, the tests are not effective until antibodies for *T. pallidum* are present in the blood. This may not occur until 3 to 4 weeks after exposure.

Confirmation tests, those that specifically detect *T. pallidum*, are needed to confirm the disease. They are the fluorescent treponemal antibody absorption test (FTA-ABS) and the microhemagglutination test. Because patients with syphilis often have multiple infections, HIV testing is often recommended as well.

Medical Treatment

The treatment of choice for syphilis is parenteral penicillin G unless contraindicated. For an infection of less than 1 year's duration, a single dose is usually sufficient. For infections of a year's duration or longer, a longer course of therapy is indicated. Information about drug therapy for syphilis is presented in the Drug Therapy table on pp. 1107 to 1109. Advise the patient to make a follow-up appointment with a physician to see whether the treatment was effective. Also, advise the patient not

---

Table 49-3 | *Syphilis*

SIGNS/SYMPTOMS	POSSIBLE COMPLICATIONS	MEDICAL TREATMENT	NURSING CONSIDERATIONS
PRIMARY SYPHILIS			
Chancre (round ulcer with well-defined margin): lesion is thickened, rubbery, and painless. If untreated, lesion persists only 3-6 wk and then heals. Regional lymphadenopathy: enlarged lymph nodes only in the area of the chancre.	Prompt, effective treatment can result in complete recovery without complications. Otherwise, complications may include arthritis, bursitis, osteitis, liver enlargement, heart disease, meningitis, and central nervous system disorders.	Parenteral penicillin G given in a single dose for 8-12 days *Or* If patient is unable to take penicillin, PO tetracycline or doxycycline is used.	Ensure that ordered blood studies are done: VDRL, RPR, FTA-ABS. Assess for transient fever, flu-like symptoms, malaise. Provide rest periods. Wear gloves to assess the skin and mucous membranes. Inspect skin changes, lesions. Provide medications. After administration of parenteral antibiotics, observe patient for 30 min for allergic reactions such as rash, fever, or chills. Have emergency drugs on hand in the event of anaphylaxis.
SECONDARY SYPHILIS			
Sore throat, malaise, rash, fever, weight loss, headaches, musculoskeletal pain.			

FTA-ABS, Fluorescent treponemal antibody, absorbed (test); *RPR,* rapid plasmin reagin; *VDRL,* Venereal Disease Research Laboratory.

to engage in sexual activity until 1 month after completing treatment for primary or secondary syphilis.

Nursing care of the patient with syphilis and other STIs is covered in the Nursing Care of the Patient with a Sexually Transmitted Infection section on p. 1116. Table 49-3 summarizes the signs and symptoms of syphilis, possible complications, medical treatment, and nursing considerations.

HERPES SIMPLEX

The herpes virus has plagued humans for many centuries. Several different types of the virus are easily passed from person to person. The virus that causes cold sores (*herpes febrilis* or herpes simplex virus 1, HSV type 1) was first described in 100 AD and is transmitted through contact with open lesions, usually on the lips or inside the mouth. Prevention strategies generally focus on avoiding direct contact (kissing) and using good hand-washing technique when caring for infected persons.

The incidence of genital herpes (caused by herpes simplex virus 2, or HSV type 2) has been on the rise since the 1960s. HSV type 2 is generally transmitted by sexual contact. Vaginal or anal intercourse and oral-genital contact are the primary transmission modes, but HSV type 2 can be transferred by hand contact as well.

Although herpes simplex virus types 1 and 2 are similar, type 1 is *usually* nongenital, with lesions typically above the waist. Type 2 is considered an STI because it is *most often* below the waist and is transmitted by genital contact.

Signs and Symptoms

Symptoms of genital herpes infection include painful, itching sores on or around the genitals approximately 2 to 20 days after infection. These symptoms last about 2 to 3 weeks. A rash may appear first, followed by small blisters that eventually ulcerate. People often complain of flu-like symptoms and a burning sensation during urination. Episodes of active symptoms may recur and are frequently precipitated by anxiety (Fig. 49-2).

Complications

There is an increased risk of cervical cancer in women who have genital herpes. An infected woman should be taught to have a Papanicolaou smear done annually to detect cervical cancer early. If she is pregnant, she should be supervised closely by a physician. Obstetricians recommend cesarean sections for infected women who have active lesions to decrease the risk of transmission to the baby. New diagnostic procedures allow the physician to detect active disease more accurately than in the past.

Medical Diagnosis and Treatment

A diagnosis of HSV type 2 may be suspected based on the appearance of genital lesions. Laboratory tests are used to confirm the diagnosis. Exudate from lesions can

FIGURE **49-2** Genital herpes lesions on the vulva and inner thigh.

be examined under a microscope and cultured to reveal the virus. An antibody test called the *Herp-Check* can detect active herpes. The Herp-Check results are available in 4 hours. The test is used to assess for active infections during pregnancy. If negative results are obtained near the time of delivery, the physician may permit a vaginal delivery rather than requiring a cesarean section.

There is no cure for HSV infection, but the oral antiviral drugs acyclovir (Zovirax), valacyclovir (Valtrex), or famciclovir (Famvir) help by partially controlling the signs and symptoms during initial and recurrent episodes. Patients should know to start the drug when preliminary (prodromal) symptoms of recurrence are experienced or within 1 day of the outbreak of lesions. Some patients take one of these drugs continuously to reduce the frequency of outbreaks.

Nursing care of the patient with HSV and other STIs is discussed in the Nursing Care of the Patient with a Sexually Transmitted Infection section on p. 1116. Table 49-4 summarizes the signs and symptoms of HSV infections, possible complications, medical treatment, and nursing considerations.

TRICHOMONIASIS

Trichomoniasis is caused by the protozoan parasite *Trichomonas vaginalis* and is usually sexually transmitted. The parasite can survive for hours, however, on damp cloths and clothing. The CDC estimates that there are over 7 million new cases each year. This infection usually affects the vagina in women and the urethra in men.

Signs and Symptoms

Women complain of a frothy, yellowish vaginal discharge that has a foul odor. Vaginal irritation and

Table 49-4 | *Herpes Simplex Infections*

SIGNS/SYMPTOMS	POSSIBLE COMPLICATIONS	MEDICAL TREATMENT	NURSING CONSIDERATIONS
Painful genital lesions, burning during urination.	Localized infections; risk of infecting baby on delivery.	Treatment is basically symptomatic and includes sitz baths. Acyclovir may minimize symptoms; however, there is no cure for herpes. Recurrences may be treated with acyclovir, valacyclovir, or famciclovir.	Ensure that patient notifies sexual contacts. Inform the patient that virus can survive on objects such as towels. Assist in decreasing patient's anxiety by allowing him or her to verbalize feelings. Instruct patient to avoid sexual contact when lesions are present and to use condoms at other times.

FIGURE **49-3** Trichomoniasis vaginal discharge is profuse and watery and appears purulent.

itching may also be present. Urinary frequency and burning suggest that the infection has invaded the urethra (Fig. 49-3). If the infection becomes chronic, bladder and anal involvement are possible. Although the incidence of trichomoniasis is less common in males, it can certainly occur. Men usually have no symptoms although some have a mild discharge or slight burning after urination or ejaculation.

Medical Diagnosis and Treatment

The organism may be detected by microscopic study of vaginal discharge or urine (in males). The discharge also can be cultured to reveal the organism.

Metronidazole (Flagyl) is the drug of choice for treating trichomoniasis. It is important that the patient and any sexual partners be treated at the same time to avoid reinfection.

Nursing care of the patient with trichomoniasis and other STIs is covered in the Nursing Care of the Patient with a Sexually Transmitted Infection section on p. 1116.

CONDYLOMATA ACUMINATA

Condylomata acuminata, or venereal warts, are caused by the human papillomavirus. They generally affect the genital and anal regions of both men and women. Transmission of the virus is by vaginal, anal, or genital contact with an infected person. There have been incidents of transmission from persons who had no visible signs of infection. The incubation period usually ranges from 3 weeks to 8 months.

Signs and Symptoms

Males generally present with warts on the glans, foreskin, urethral opening, penile shaft, or scrotum. These lesions may be single or multiple. In females, warts generally appear in or around the vulva, vagina, cervix, perineum, anal canal, and urethra. Less often, the lesions are seen on the labia and deep within the vaginal canal and endocervix. In homosexual and bisexual men and women who engage in anal intercourse, warts are common in the anal area. Oral, pharyngeal, and laryngeal lesions occur as well.

Condylomata warts are generally pink or red and soft, with a cauliflower-like appearance. Multiple warts can become so large that they obstruct the vaginal opening or rectal canal. Genital warts tend to grow large if they are located in an area that is kept moist by vaginal or urethral discharge. Pregnancy can stimulate venereal warts to grow very large. The reason for this rapid growth is unknown (Fig. 49-4).

Medical Diagnosis

The diagnosis is usually made on the basis of a simple observation of the warts. A biopsy of the lesions is necessary to make a definitive diagnosis.

Medical Treatment

Although there is no cure for condylomata acuminata, removal of visible warts provides symptomatic relief. Some treatments such as the application of podofilox or imiquimod can be managed by the patient. Others must be administered by the physician. Other treatment provided by the physician may include cryotherapy, which uses liquid nitrogen or solid carbon dioxide to freeze the warts, topical trichloroacetic acid

FIGURE **49-4** Condylomata acuminata in a female patient.

or podophyllin resin, surgical removal, and the injection of interferon into the lesions. Note that the safety of podofilox and imiquimod and of podophyllin resin during pregnancy has not been established. None of these methods has proven totally effective in all cases. The recurrence rate is very high.

Nursing care of the patient with condyloma warts as well as other STIs is discussed in the Nursing Care of the Patient with a Sexually Transmitted Infection section on p. 1116.

BACTERIAL VAGINOSIS

Bacterial vaginosis is caused by *Gardnerella vaginalis* and other anaerobic bacteria. The infectious bacteria tend to emerge when the normal bacteria in the vagina are suppressed. It has been associated with having multiple sex partners and douching, but it is not clear whether it is actually transmitted sexually. The signs and symptoms are genital irritation and itching, a thin gray discharge, and a fishy odor; however, some women report no symptoms. The infection is diagnosed by microscopic examination of the discharge fluid and by culture. Some commercially available card tests are available also. The condition is treated with metronidazole (Flagyl) administered orally or vaginally or clindamycin vaginal cream. The patient is advised not to consume alcohol while taking metronidazole. The combination of alcohol and metronidazole may trigger a disulfiram-like reaction, with vomiting, tachycardia, and hypotension. When using clindamycin cream, the patient should know that the cream can weaken latex condoms and diaphragms. Treatment of sex partners has not been found to affect relapse or recurrence. See

Preventing Complications of Bacterial Vaginosis

In most cases, bacterial vaginosis causes no complications. However, an association has been documented between bacterial vaginosis and conditions such as pelvic inflammatory disease (PID), gonorrhea, and human immunodeficiency virus (HIV) infection. Bacterial vaginosis can also cause premature birth and low-birth-weight infants. Therefore some health experts recommend that all pregnant women be checked for bacterial vaginosis if they have previously delivered a premature baby. A pregnant woman who has not delivered a premature baby should be treated if she has symptoms and laboratory evidence of bacterial vaginosis.

In an effort to improve treatment and prevention of vaginosis and its complications, research into the pathophysiology of vaginal microbes is now under way. No longer considered merely a harmless annoyance, this condition is the object of serious study as research nurses and other scientists try to clarify its role in such conditions as PID and pregnancy-related complications.

Adapted from National Institute of Allergy and Infectious Diseases, National Institutes of Health: *Vaginitis due to vaginal infections,* www.niaid.nih.gov/factsheets/vaginitis.htm.

the Health Promotion Considerations box above for a discussion of the potential complications of bacterial vaginosis.

HUMAN IMMUNODEFICIENCY VIRUS INFECTION

Many diseases that cause illness or death have plagued Americans, but it is likely that none of these has had the profound medical, social, economic, and psychological effects as has the HIV infection known as AIDS. This syndrome is a disorder of the immune system caused by HIV. HIV gradually destroys T4 lymphocytes, which are essential for resisting pathogens. As the number of T4 lymphocytes declines, the patient becomes increasingly susceptible to opportunistic infections. An opportunistic infection is one that thrives when the immune system is impaired. When the immune system ceases to function effectively, the patient is said to have AIDS. Chapter 34 is devoted to a thorough discussion of HIV infection.

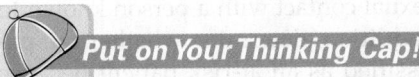
Put on Your Thinking Cap!

Consider this situation: A 30-year-old minister's wife is admitted after being injured in an auto accident. While hospitalized, she is diagnosed with gonorrhea. You recognize that staff are treating her differently since the gonorrhea was diagnosed. What behaviors would indicate lack of acceptance of the patient?

Do you think you would feel differently about her? What could you do to demonstrate acceptance and caring?

NURSING CARE *of the Patient with a Sexually Transmitted Infection*

Assessment

Assessment of the female and male reproductive systems is discussed in Chapters 47 and 48 and outlined in Boxes 47-1 and 48-1. When a patient has an STI, certain aspects of that assessment are especially important (see Nursing Care Plan: The Patient with Gonorrhea on p. 1117). The LPN/LVN may be responsible for collecting important data to contribute to the assessment.

Health History

A thorough history is necessary to identify high-risk behaviors. A discussion of sexual behavior can be awkward for the nurse and the patient. Before nurses can deal with patients' sexuality, they must be aware of their own feelings and values. Privacy is essential for the patient interview. Questions about sexuality should be addressed in a straightforward manner. The interviewer should keep in mind that many patients lack scientific knowledge about the reproductive system and sexual activity. The patient may use some words that are considered crude by professionals, but the nurse must be careful not to embarrass or shame the patient.

History of Present Illness. The history begins with exploration of the patient's reason for seeking medical care. With an STI, common reasons include pain, fever, lesions, or genital discharge. Obtain a thorough description of the signs and symptoms, including onset, duration, and severity.

Past Medical History. In the discussion of past health, document serious conditions or chronic illnesses. The obstetric history may be significant as well. If the patient is of childbearing age, record the date of the last menstrual period. Record recent and current medications, and note drug allergies.

Review of Systems. The review of systems elicits potentially significant signs and symptoms, including weight change; fever; weakness; fatigue; skin rashes or lesions; oral lesions; dysuria; whether the patient is sexually active; pain, lesions, or lumps in the genitals; vaginal or penile discharge; and altered sexual functioning. A history of blood transfusions is important to document.

Functional Assessment. Relevant aspects of the functional assessment include frequency and variety of sexual behaviors, intravenous drug use, past infections with STIs, and sexual contact with a person known to have an STI. In addition, determine whether the patient may be classified as an at-risk patient because age (e.g., an adolescent experimenting with sexuality), sexual preference (male homosexual or bisexual), or habits (drug use) place him or her at a higher risk for acquiring an STI. Victims of sexual abuse (of all ages) may have been exposed to STIs. Occupation may also be significant if the patient comes into contact with potentially infected body fluids. Health care providers at risk for exposure include nursing personnel, physi-

cians, emergency medical technicians, operating room technicians, housekeepers in health care facilities, and medical laboratory technicians.

Physical Examination

The physical examination begins with inspection of the patient's skin for rashes and lesions. During the head and neck examination, the mouth is inspected for lesions. The neck is palpated for enlarged lymph nodes. The abdomen is inspected for distention and palpated for tenderness. Depending on the setting and your specialized education, you may examine the genitals or assist the physician or nurse practitioner in the examination. The examiner wears gloves to examine the genitals. A good light source is essential for thorough inspection. In the male patient, the examiner notes the general appearance of the penis, scrotum, and anal area. Any skin breaks, rashes, or redness is noted.

The LPN/LVN may prepare the female patient for a pelvic examination. While the patient is on the examination table, the genitalia and the perianal area are inspected. The labia are separated and inspected for skin breaks, redness, or rashes. If a vaginal examination is to be done, ensure that the speculum and other supplies are ready. The speculum is warmed and lubricated before insertion into the vagina. Tissue and fluid specimens may be taken, including tissue scrapings for a Papanicolaou smear. You may be responsible for preparing the specimen and sending it to the laboratory.

In cases of sexual assault, it is especially important that the examiner be specially trained to deal with such situations. Not only does the patient need a great deal of support but also the examination may produce evidence that must be preserved for legal purposes.

If a discharge is present, its color, amount, and consistency are recorded. Specimens may be collected for laboratory study. The specimen is handled as infective material, prepared according to agency procedures, labeled, and sent to the laboratory.

Assessment of the patient with an STI is outlined in Box 49-1.

Nursing Diagnoses, Goals, and Outcome Criteria: Sexually Transmitted Infection	
NURSING DIAGNOSES	GOALS AND OUTCOME CRITERIA
Impaired Tissue Integrity related to lesions, rash	Restored tissue integrity: healed, intact skin and mucous membranes
Acute Pain related to lesions, inflammation	Pain relief: patient reports pain is relieved, relaxed manner
Risk for Injury related to disease process, potential adverse effects of drugs	Freedom from additional injury: absence of signs and symptoms of complications
Anxiety related to possible effects of STI, reaction of partner	Reduced anxiety: patient reports anxiety is reduced, calm manner

NURSING CARE PLAN

The Patient with Gonorrhea

ASSESSMENT

Health History: A 23-year-old woman comes to the physician's office because of painful urination, abdominal pain, and vaginal discharge of 3 days' duration. She has had no serious illnesses or injuries. She has had two sexual partners in the past 6 months, with her most recent contact 2 weeks ago, when a condom was not used. The patient expresses concern about sexually transmitted infections (STIs) and human immunodeficiency virus (HIV). She states that she cannot believe she was "so stupid" and is very embarrassed about these symptoms.

Physical Examination: The physical examination findings are all normal except the genital and pelvic examination. The vaginal tissues are red and edematous with a whitish discharge. A smear is taken for examination and reveals a gonococcal infection. Antimicrobial therapy is prescribed.

Nursing Diagnosis	Goals and Outcome Criteria	Interventions
Impaired Tissue Integrity and Acute Pain related to infection and inflammation	The patient will report decreased pain, and redness and discharge will diminish.	Tell the patient that the symptoms should improve with treatment. Mild analgesics may be needed as ordered. Sitz baths may be soothing.
Risk for Injury related to disease process	The patient will report for follow-up examination and remain free of signs and symptoms of complications.	Explain that persistent infection can lead to sterility and affect the heart and joints. Emphasize the importance of returning for an examination to ensure successful treatment.
Anxiety related to possible complications of gonorrhea or stigma of STI	The patient will express reduced anxiety and will be calm.	Provide opportunity to talk. Help her focus on the source of anxiety. For example, if she does not know what to expect, information is needed. If she is trying to decide how to discuss the condition with her sexual partners, help her solve the problem. Assure her that proper treatment is usually effective and prevents complications.
Situational Low Self-Esteem related to diagnosis	The patient's self-image will improve, as evidenced by positive comments about self.	Be accepting and nonjudgmental. Assure her that she has done the right thing by seeking medical attention.
Deficient Knowledge of disease process, treatment, or prevention of future infections	The patient will verbalize importance of treatment, complications of untreated infection, and measures to prevent future infections.	Explore her understanding of gonorrhea. Provide information as needed. Emphasize use of condoms in sexual contacts to reduce risk of future infections with gonorrhea or other STIs. Ask about drug allergies before giving antimicrobials. Explain self-medication dosage, side effects, and adverse effects.

? CRITICAL THINKING QUESTIONS

- How can you help this patient decide how to discuss this condition with her significant other?

- Describe the best approach in addressing the patient's embarrassment about her condition. How might you put her at ease?

Situational Low Self-Esteem related to diagnosis of STI	Improved self-esteem: increased positive comments about self, confident manner	**Ineffective Coping** related to stigma associated with STI, shame, anger	Effective coping: patient states is better able to deal with stress of condition
Impaired Social Interaction related to presence of communicable disease, social stigma	Resumption of satisfying social interactions: patient states is satisfied with socialization	**Ineffective Therapeutic Regimen Management** related to denial, embarrassment, lack of understanding of disease process, mode of transmission, treatment, and prevention	Effective management of therapeutic plan: patient seeks medical care and follow-up, accurately describes self-care measures, expresses intent to follow plan of care and preventive measures
Sexual Dysfunction related to fear of transmission, impaired tissue integrity	Practices safe sexual behaviors: patient accurately describes safe behaviors, indicates will not engage in unsafe behavior		

Interventions

Impaired Skin Integrity

If you have daily contact with the patient, assess the patient's skin on a daily basis. Record changes in lesions. Carry out orders for treatments including topical medications and sitz baths for patients in health care settings. Monitor the temperature at regular intervals to detect fever that may accompany acute infection. Handle soiled clothing and bed linens in accordance with agency policy. Be sure that patients who will treat themselves at home understand the prescribed therapy.

Acute Pain

Some STIs are painless, but patients may have pain associated with pelvic infection, oral lesions, or rectal lesions. The lesions of HSV are especially painful. Document the severity of the patient's pain, and provide analgesics as ordered. Apply topical medications, ice packs, or warm compresses as ordered, or teach the patient how to do so.

Risk for Injury

Untreated STIs can lead to serious complications such as pelvic inflammatory disease and sterility. The patient with AIDS is at high risk for secondary infections (called *opportunistic infections*) because of impaired immune function. Infected patients also pose a threat to their sexual partners. An STI may be passed to the fetus in utero or transmitted during delivery. Therefore it is important for the patient to receive the entire course of prescribed therapy. Also stress the importance of notifying sexual contacts so that they can be tested and treated as well if necessary.

Drug therapy itself has the potential for injury. Before administering medications, assess the patient's allergies. When injections are given to an outpatient, ask the patient to remain for 30 minutes afterward in case an allergic reaction occurs. Emergency drugs, including epinephrine, corticosteroids, and diphenhydramine hydrochloride (Benadryl), must be readily available. Information about drugs commonly used to treat STIs is presented in the Drug Therapy table on pp. 1107 to 1109.

Anxiety

People may be anxious about the outcome of treatment and the potential complications of the disease. Anxiety may be heightened by the stigma associated with having contracted an STI, and the patient may feel ashamed. Encourage the patient to verbalize fears and frustrations. Provide accurate information, and teach the patient how to avoid reinfection and infecting others. Patients with HIV infections also must deal with a life-threatening illness.

Situational Low Self-Esteem

The patient's self-esteem may suffer because of a diagnosed STI. Provide an opportunity for the patient to talk about the effects of the disease on self-concept. Try to guide the patient to focus on his or her positive attributes. If the patient's self-esteem remains low despite nursing intervention, a referral to a mental health counselor may be suggested.

Impaired Social Interaction

A diagnosis of STI can be very distressing to the patient, who may fear rejection by others. The patient may be angry at the person who transmitted the infection and may be concerned about infecting others. Because STIs must be reported to public health authorities who attempt to trace all sexual contacts, the patient may also fear reprisals. One way you can help is by demonstrating acceptance of the patient through kindness and touch.

| Box 49-1 | *ASSESSMENT of the Patient with a Sexually Transmitted Infection* |

Health History	**Physical Examination**
Present Illness:	**General Survey:**
Pain, fever, lesions, genital discharge	Distress, lethargy
Past Medical History:	**Skin:**
Serious conditions, chronic conditions, hemophilia, obstetric history, date of last menstrual period, recent and current medications	Rashes, lesions
	Mouth:
	Lesions
Review of Systems:	**Abdomen:**
Weight change, fever, weakness, fatigue, skin rashes or lesions, oral lesions, dysuria, whether sexually active, sexual contact with a person known to have a sexually transmitted infection, sexual dysfunction, history of blood transfusions	Distention, tenderness
	Genitals:
Functional Assessment:	General appearance; lesions; rashes; redness; color, amount, odor, and consistency of discharge
Frequency and variety of sexual behaviors, intravenous drug use, past sexually transmitted infections, sexual preference, occupational exposure to infective material	

Sexual Dysfunction

Patients with STIs may experience sexual dysfunction related to fear of transmission, the presence of lesions, or anxiety. In addition, precautions that should be taken to prevent transmission of the disease may require changes in sexual practices. In general, sexual activity should be avoided until the infection is cured. Chronic infections such as HSV and HIV require permanent alterations in sexual activity. Explore the importance of sexual activity to the patient. Accept the patient's feelings in a nonjudgmental way. Explain that emotions and sexual function are closely related and that dysfunction may be overcome by dealing with the emotional reactions to the disease. For persistent dysfunction, advise the patient to discuss the problem with the physician. Offer to make a referral to a therapist who specializes in sexual dysfunction. Encourage the patient to communicate openly with the sexual partner about the difficulties experienced. Alternative means of sexual expression (other than intercourse) may be suggested. Box 49-2 compares the relative safety of various sexual practices.

Ineffective Coping

Ineffective coping may be related to guilt, shame, anger, actual or anticipated rejection, or a combination of these. Behaviors associated with ineffective coping include failure to adhere to the prescribed treatment, failure to exercise precautions to prevent spread of the disease or reinfection, chronic anxiety or depression, and inability to cope. The patient with an HIV infection also must deal with the potential for developing AIDS, often with inadequate personal support. Show support for the patient by being sensitive, courteous, and nonjudgmental. Point out inappropriate behaviors. Encourage the patient to evaluate his or her lifestyle and to identify modifications that could reduce future risks. You may refer patients who have HSV and HIV infections to support groups. A spiritual counselor also may be contacted if the patient desires.

Ineffective Therapeutic Regimen Management

Patient teaching is essential for effective treatment and prevention of future infections. Explain to the patient what causes the infection, how it is transmitted, how it can be prevented, and why treatment and follow-up care are important. Key points to teach the patient with an STI shown in the Patient Teaching Plan below.

 Nutrition Concepts

1. Persons with oral lesions may require modified diets.
2. Patients taking antibiotics generally are advised to drink at least 2000 mL of fluids each day to prevent harm to the kidneys.

 Patient Teaching Plan

Sexually Transmitted Infections

- Be sure to complete the prescribed course of antibiotics and return so the physician can determine whether the treatment was effective.
- STIs are transmitted by sexual contact. Avoid sexual contact with high-risk individuals: people who have had multiple sex partners, prostitutes, and those with known human immunodeficiency virus (HIV) or hepatitis B infections.
- Avoid sexual activity until the condition is cured. If you engage in sexual activity, wear condoms.
- Wear condoms for all genital contact, not just intercourse.
- If you have sexual contact with high-risk individuals, people you do not know well, or persons who do not use condoms, you should have periodic medical examinations.
- Use condoms if you have condylomata.
- If you have herpes simplex virus (HSV) infection, you should abstain from sexual activity when lesions are present. Use condoms at other times. It is important to realize that although there are periods of remission, the condition is chronic.
- Females with HSV or condylomata are advised to have annual Papanicolaou smears, because they are at increased risk of cervical cancer.
- If you have HIV infection, medical treatment may delay the development of acquired immunodeficiency syndrome (AIDS). Precautions must be taken to prevent infecting sexual partners even though you may not have signs and symptoms of disease.
- Because HIV is transmitted through body fluids, you cannot donate blood if you are HIV positive.

Box 49-2 *Comparative Safety of Various Sexual Practices to Prevent Transmission of Infection*

Safe
- Mutual masturbation
- Closed-mouth kissing
- Body massage
- Use of own sex devices or toys

Possibly Safe
- Open-mouthed kissing
- Vaginal or anal intercourse with properly used condom
- Oral sex with properly used condom

Unsafe
- Vaginal or anal intercourse without condom
- Oral sex without condom
- Oral/anal contact
- Insertion of hand into vagina or rectum
- Ingestion of urine or semen
- Contact with blood

Modified from Lewis, S.M., & Rickert, B.D. (1992). Altered immune response. In S.M. Lewis & I.C. Collier (Eds.). *Medical-surgical nursing* (p.156). St. Louis: Mosby.

Knowledge does not guarantee compliance, but patients cannot comply unless they understand what they need to do to care for themselves. Provide information about the disease and its treatment in terms the patient can understand. If the patient can read, include supplementary written material. Stress the importance of completing the course of therapy and returning for follow-up to reduce the risk of complications associated with untreated disease. Evaluate the patient's understanding of the material covered, and explore any barriers that might prevent the patient from following the instructions.

CONDOM USE

Many people do not know how to use condoms correctly. At this time, only male condoms are in common use, although female condoms are available. Key points to stress about condom use are shown in the Patient Teaching Plan below.

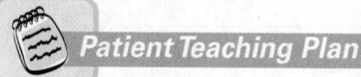

Use of a Condom

- Condoms do not provide 100% protection against disease transmission.
- Latex condoms are preferred because some pathogens can pass through natural membrane condoms.
- Protect condoms from heat and sunlight to keep them from deteriorating.
- Do not use condoms that are brittle, discolored, or in damaged packages.
- Use only water-based lubricants because other lubricants can cause the condom to break. Spermicides may be used.
- To put a condom on, hold it by the tip and unroll it onto the penis. Leave a space of about 1 inch at the tip for semen.
- Withdraw the penis carefully after ejaculation to keep the condom from slipping off and spilling the contents and to avoid unprotected contact.
- Always discard used condoms for sanitary disposal.

- Gonorrhea is one of the most commonly reported STIs in the United States, but it often has no symptoms.
- Gonorrhea can lead to damage to the heart and joints as well as to pelvic inflammatory disease.

- Chlamydial infection is diagnosed in more than 2 million people in the United States each year; it can result in sterility in both sexes.
- Syphilis, if untreated, progresses through four stages, with eventual damage to the cardiovascular and nervous systems, the skin, and the joints.
- Newborns of women with gonorrhea or chlamydial infection may acquire eye infections during birth.
- Herpes simplex virus (HSV) can be transmitted by sexual contact, but unlike most other STIs, it can also be transmitted by hand contact.
- Because HSV increases the risk of cervical cancer in infected women, they are advised to have annual Papanicolaou smears.
- Condylomata acuminata, or genital warts, are caused by a virus and have a high rate of recurrence despite drug therapy, cryotherapy, cautery, and surgical or laser excision.
- Infection with HIV causes AIDS; gradual destruction of T4 lymphocytes leaves the patient unable to resist opportunistic infections.
- Human immunodeficiency virus is transmitted through exposure to body fluids, and there is no cure for the infection although combination drug therapy can delay progress of the disease.
- Most STIs except HSV infection and HIV infection can be cured by antimicrobial agents.
- HSV infection is minimized but not cured by acyclovir sodium (Zovirax).
- Abstinence from sexual contact is the best way to prevent transmission of STIs, but use of condoms during sexual contact also reduces the risk. Standard Precautions prescribe specific protective measures to be taken when working with people who have infections that can be transmitted through body fluids.
- The nursing care of patients with STIs may address Impaired Skin Integrity, Acute Pain, Risk for Injury, Anxiety, Situational Low Self-Esteem, Impaired Social Interactions, Sexual Dysfunction, Ineffective Coping, and Ineffective Therapeutic Regimen Management.
- Patient teaching is essential for patients with STIs and should include information about drug therapy and other treatment options, disease transmission, abstinence during treatment, and preventive measures.

 Go to your Companion CD-ROM for a Pharmacology Tutorial, Audio Glossary, and 3-D animations.

evolve Be sure to visit the companion Evolve site at http://evolve.elsevier.com/Linton/ for WebLinks and additional online resources.

REVIEW QUESTIONS *Choose the best answer.*

1. The purpose of reporting sexually transmitted infections is to:
   1. Prosecute the individuals who are transmitting the disease to others
   2. Emphasize to infected persons the importance of practicing safe sex
   3. Treat all infected persons to reduce transmission of the infection
   4. Teach the general public about measures to prevent STIs

2. Erythromycin ophthalmic ointment may be ordered for the newborn because it is effective against:
   1. Genital warts
   2. Chlamydial infections
   3. Human immunodeficiency virus
   4. Hepatitis B virus

3. A patient who was diagnosed with gonorrhea did not return for treatment. When contacted, she reported that her symptoms had gone away so she thought she had recovered from the infection. The most appropriate response by the nurse would be which of the following?
   1. Without treatment, the bacteria remain in your body and you remain highly infectious.
   2. As long as your symptoms have cleared up, there is no reason to treat you now.
   3. If you have symptoms in the future, come to the clinic immediately.
   4. Fortunately, gonorrhea has no serious complications, but I must advise you to seek treatment anyway.

4. The primary stage of syphilis is usually characterized by:
   1. A rash on the extremities, chest or back, palms of the hands, and soles of the feet
   2. A reddish papule on the genitals, anus, or mouth that becomes a painless red ulcer
   3. Tender lymph nodes in the area of the skin lesion
   4. Fever, sore throat, and generalized aching

5. The patient with untreated syphilis may develop:
   1. Blindness, mental illness, paralysis, and heart disease
   2. Acquired immunodeficiency syndrome (AIDS)
   3. Cancer of the genitals
   4. Septicemia

6. Which statement is true regarding the herpes simplex virus types 1 and 2?
   1. Type 1 is most often transmitted by genital contact.
   2. The modes of transmission of both types 1 and 2 are the same.
   3. Type 1 *only* affects the genitals, and type 2 only affects the mouth.
   4. Type 1 is usually nongenital, with lesions typically above the waist.

7. The teaching plan for a woman with a type 2 genital herpes simplex virus infection should include which of the following statements?
   1. You should have yearly Pap smears because you are at increased risk for cervical cancer.
   2. You should not become pregnant because the herpes virus causes fetal deformities.
   3. Once you have finished taking your medicine, you will be cured of the herpes infection.
   4. Your partner must use a condom for intercourse until you are completely cured.

8. The teaching plan for a patient with genital warts should include which of the following?
   1. This condition cannot be transmitted to a sexual partner.
   2. Genital warts are caused by poor personal hygiene.
   3. A topical medication can remove the warts but is not curative.
   4. Once the warts are removed, they are unlikely to come back.

9. Information for effective use of condoms should include which of the following?
   1. Condoms provide 100% protection against disease transmission.
   2. Natural membrane condoms are preferred over latex condoms.
   3. Use only oil-based lubricants to prevent breakage of the condom.
   4. Leave a space of about 1 inch at the tip for semen.

10. Which of the following sexually transmitted infections can usually be cured with antibiotics? (Check all that apply)
    1. Gonorrhea
    2. Herpes simplex
    3. Syphilis
    4. Trichomoniasis

50 Skin Disorders

CHAPTER

ADRIANNE DILL LINTON AND MARY WALKER

evolve http://evolve.elsevier.com/Linton/

Objectives

After reading and studying this chapter, you should be able to:

1. Describe the structure and functions of the skin.
2. List the components of the nursing assessment of the skin.
3. Define terms used to describe the skin and skin lesions.
4. Explain the tests and procedures used to diagnose skin disorders.
5. Explain the nurse's responsibilities regarding the tests and procedures for diagnosing skin disorders.
6. Explain the therapeutic benefits and nursing considerations for patients who receive dressings, soaks and wet wraps, phototherapy, and drug therapy for skin problems.
7. Describe the pathophysiology, signs and symptoms, diagnostic tests, and medical treatment for selected skin disorders.
8. Assist in developing a nursing care plan for the patient with a skin disorder.

Key Terms

Be sure to check out the bonus material on the Companion CD-ROM, including selected audio pronunciations.

acne (ĂK-nē, p. 1138)
acrochordon (ăk-rō-KŌR-dŏn, p. 1124)
angioma (ăn-jē-Ō-mă, p. 1124)
débridement (dā-BRĒD-mĕnt, p. 1148)
dermatitis (dĕr-mă-TĪ-tĭs, p. 1132)
intertrigo (ĭn-tĕr-TRĪ-gō, p. 1135)
keratolytic (kĕr-ă-tō-LĬT-ĭk, p. 1129)
lentigo (*pl.* lentigines) (lĭn-TĒ-gō, lĭn-TĬ-jŭ-nēz, p. 1123)
nevus (*pl.* nevi) (NĒ-vŭs, NĒ-vī, p. 1125)
pemphigus (PĔM-fĭ-gŭs, p. 1142)
pruritus (proo-RĪ-tŭs, p. 1123)
psoriasis (sō-RĪ-ă-sĭs, p. 1134)

ANATOMY AND PHYSIOLOGY OF THE SKIN

The skin is an organ that covers the body surface. The anatomy of the skin is illustrated in Figure 50-1. It is composed of two distinct layers: the epidermis and the dermis. The epidermis is the outermost layer that covers the dermis. The base of the epidermis continu-ally produces new cells to replace those at the surface. Epidermal cells produce melanin, a dark pigment that helps determine the color of the skin. Strong ultraviolet light, such as in sunlight, stimulates the production of melanin.

The dermis is strong connective tissue that contains nerve endings, sweat glands, and hair roots. The dermis is well supplied with blood vessels, causing the skin to redden when surface vessels are dilated. Subcutaneous tissue lies beneath the dermis.

The hair, nails, and sebaceous glands are append-ages (or derivatives) of the skin. The hair root is located in a tube in the dermis called a *hair follicle*. The arrector muscles of the hair (arrectores pilorum), located around the hair follicles, can contract, causing the hairs to stand erect and the skin to take on a gooseflesh appearance. Also around the hair follicles are sebaceous glands that secrete an oily substance called *sebum*. Sweat glands, found in most parts of the skin, secrete through the skin surface water that contains salts, ammonia, amino acids, lactic acid, ascorbic acid, uric acid, and urea.

FUNCTIONS OF THE SKIN

The functions of the skin are protection, body temperature regulation, secretion, sensation, and synthesis of vitamin D. In addition, the blood vessels of the skin can serve as a blood reservoir.

Protection

The skin performs its protective function by shielding underlying tissues from trauma and pathogens and by preventing excess loss of fluids from those tissues. A second type of protective function is fulfilled by Langerhans' cells, which initiate an immune response when foreign substances invade the epidermis.

Temperature Regulation

The skin participates in temperature regulation by altering the diameter of surface blood vessels and through sweating. To dissipate heat, the blood vessels dilate. As the blood flows close to the body surface, heat is lost through the surface. To retain heat, blood vessels constrict and heat loss is minimized. Sweating helps cool the body because heat is lost as sweat evaporates from the skin.

Hair shaft
Rete ridges
Epidermis
Dermal papillae
Meissner's corpuscle
Sebaceous gland
Dermis
Arrector pili muscle
Dermis
Artery
Subcutaneous
Vein
Pacinian corpuscle
Adipose tissue

Stratum corneum
Stratum lucidum
Stratum granulosum
Stratum spinosum
Stratum basale
Sweat gland
Hair follicle

FIGURE 50-1 Anatomy of the skin.

Secretions

Sweat is one skin secretion; sebum is another. Sebum coats the skin, creating an oily barrier that holds in water. Sweat promotes loss of body heat through evaporation, as noted previously, and plays a role in excretion of wastes.

Sensation

The skin is heavily endowed with sensory receptors for touch, pressure, pain, and temperature. When these sensory receptors are stimulated, nerves convey messages to the brain for interpretation.

Synthesis of Vitamin D

Ultraviolet rays in sunlight activate a substance in the skin that eventually is converted into vitamin D.

Blood Reservoir

The skin contains an extensive blood vessel network that can store as much as 10% of the body's total blood volume. Constriction of these superficial blood vessels shunts blood to vital organs when needed.

AGE-RELATED CHANGES IN THE SKIN

Changes in the skin are probably the most readily recognized of all signs of physical aging. Wrinkling of the skin occurs as a result of thinning of the skin layers and degeneration of elastin fibers. There is a loss of elasticity and strength. Sweat glands decrease in size and

 Put on Your Thinking Cap!

A patient who has just returned from surgery complains of being cold. Your assessment reveals pale hands and feet, weak pedal pulses, and slight shivering. Both feet and ankles are cold to the touch. Her vital signs are normal, and her wound dressing is dry. Explain the basis of each of her symptoms noted.

You obtain an extra blanket and cover the patient snugly, turn up the heater in the room, and ask her to call you if she does not feel better soon. When you return in 15 minutes, her hands and feet are warm and pedal pulses are palpable. She is resting quietly with no shivering. Explain how her condition changed.

number, although sweat production changes little until advanced age. The production of sebum by sebaceous glands decreases with age, becoming apparent earlier in women than in men. Dryness and **pruritus** (itching) are common. Skin often becomes paler as people age because the number of cells that produce melanin decreases. Many skin lesions are more common in older adults. They include the following:

1. **Lentigines:** pigmented spots on sun-exposed areas; they are commonly called *liver spots*, although they have nothing to do with the liver (*sing.* lentigo).
2. **Senile purpura:** large, purplish bruises that resolve very slowly; they can result from minor trauma.

3. Senile angiomas: bright-red papules.
4. Seborrheic keratoses: waxy, raised lesions; they are flesh-colored to dark brown or black and variously sized from small and nearly flat to large and prominent.
5. Acrochordons (skin tags): small, soft, raised lesions; they are flesh-colored or pigmented.

Figure 50-2 illustrates some age-related changes in the skin.

The risk of premalignant and malignant skin lesions also increases with age. These are discussed along with other pathologic conditions in the Cancer section on p. 1142.

By age 50 years, approximately half of all people have some gray hair. Men commonly begin to lose some hair from the scalp in their fourth decade, and by the time they are 80 years of age, many men are almost bald. Scalp hair thins in women as well but usually is less obvious. Many older women and men have an increase in facial hair. Men also may have increased hair in the nares, eyebrows, or helix of the ear. In addition to aging changes in the skin and hair, the nails flatten and become dry, brittle, and discolored.

FIGURE **50-2** Common skin changes in the older adult. **A,** Lentigines. **B,** Seborrheic keratoses. **C,** Skin tags.

NURSING ASSESSMENT OF THE SKIN

HEALTH HISTORY

Chief Complaint and History of Present Illness

When a patient has a skin disorder, the chief complaint may be discomfort, pruritus, color changes, lesions, hair loss, or abnormal hair growth. The history of the present illness should describe the onset of the condition and any precipitating and alleviating factors. The progression of symptoms and changes in the distribution or appearance of lesions may be helpful in the diagnostic process.

Past Medical History

Document previously diagnosed skin diseases or problems, current and recent medications (including nonprescription drugs), and allergies. In addition to skin diseases, conditions that may have skin manifestations include diabetes mellitus, cancer, kidney failure, thyroid disease, liver disease, and anemia.

Review of Systems

The review of systems includes additional data that may be related to the skin problem: change in skin color or pigmentation, change in a mole, sores that have been slow to heal, itching, dryness or scaliness, excessive bruising, rashes, lesions, hair loss, unusual hair growth, changes in nails. The review of systems also may reveal other disorders that cause changes in the skin. Specific signs and symptoms may be associated with circulatory, respiratory, renal, hepatic, gastrointestinal, and endocrine conditions.

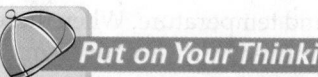 *Put on Your Thinking Cap!*

Can you think of one change in the skin that might occur with disorders of each of the following systems/organs: circulatory system, respiratory system, urinary system, and the liver?

Functional Assessment

Because the functional assessment can provide important clues to skin problems, record the patient's past and present occupations, exposure to chemicals or other irritants, skin care habits, and extent of sun exposure. Note recent changes in the work or living environment. Also inquire about current stresses and sources of anxiety.

PHYSICAL EXAMINATION

The LPN/LVN has many opportunities to collect data about the skin while providing care. When a complete physical examination is done, the examiner assesses the skin throughout the examination. The skin is inspected with attention to the color and variations in pigmentation. Sun-exposed areas are typically darker than protected areas. Dilated blood vessels and angiomas (benign tumors composed of blood vessels) should be documented. Table 50-1 describes variations in skin color and the significance of each. Nevi (moles) should be carefully inspected for irregularities in shape, pigmentation, and ulcerations or changes in surrounding skin. Nevi also are palpated for tenderness and measured in centimeters. If there is a rash, the location, distribution, and characteristics should be described. If there is any drainage,

the color, amount, and odor are noted. Terms used to describe skin lesions are defined in Table 50-2 and illustrated in Figure 50-3.

Palpating the skin is a way to collect data about the temperature, moisture, texture, thickness, edema, mobility, and turgor. Assessment of mobility and turgor is illustrated in Figure 50-4.

Some skin changes are less apparent in dark-skinned people than in light-skinned people. Healthy black skin has a reddish undertone. A grayish tone may reflect cyanosis, which is best seen around the mouth, over the

Table 50-1 | *Variations in Skin Color*

COLOR CHANGE	DESCRIPTION	CAUSES
Pallor	White or pale in light-skinned people. Yellowish-brown in brown-skinned people. Ashen in black-skinned people. May be evident in mucous membranes, lips, and nail beds, as well as skin.	Vasoconstriction due to acute anxiety or fear, cold, some drugs, cigarette smoking. Edema.
Erythema	Bright red.	Increased local blood flow due to inflammation, fever, or emotions such as embarrassment or anger.
Cyanosis	Bluish.	Excess deoxygenated blood in the tissue due to anemia, respiratory disorders, or cardiovascular disorders.
Jaundice	Golden or greenish-yellow.	Reflects increased bilirubin in the blood due to liver disease or destruction of red blood cells.

Table 50-2 | *Common Skin Lesions*

LESION	CHARACTERISTICS	EXAMPLES
Macule	Distinct flat area with color different from surrounding tissue	Freckle, petechiae, hypopigmentation
Papule	Any raised, solid lesion with clearly defined margins; <1 cm in diameter	Mole, wart
Vesicle	Raised, fluid-filled cavity, <1 cm in diameter	Herpes simplex, herpes zoster
Pustule	Raised, well-defined cavity that contains pus	Acne, impetigo
Patch	Macule >1 cm	Vitiligo
Plaque	Combined papules that form a raised area >1 cm in diameter	Psoriasis
Nodule	Raised, solid lesion >1 cm in diameter; may be hard or soft and may extend deeper into dermis than papule	Fibroma, xanthoma
Wheal	Superficial, irregular swelling caused by fluid accumulation	Allergic response, insect bite
Tumor	Firm or soft lesion that extends deep into dermis; may be firm or soft	Lipoma, hemangioma
Bulla	Thin-walled, fluid-filled chamber >1 cm in diameter	Blister
Crust	Thick, dried exudate remaining after vesicles rupture	Impetigo, weeping eczematous dermatitis
Scale	Dry or greasy skin flakes	Psoriasis, seborrheic dermatitis, eczema
Fissure	Distinct linear crack extending into dermis	Cheilosis, tinea pedis
Erosion	Shallow, superficial depression	
Ulcer	Depression deeper than erosion, may bleed	Pressure ulcer, chancre
Excoriation	Abrasion caused by scratching	Scratching with insect bites, scabies, dermatitis
Nevus (mole)	Flat or raised, color darker than surrounding skin	
Cyst	Fluid-filled cavity in dermis or subcutaneous tissue	Sebaceous cyst

Macule

Telangiectasia

Papule

Plaque

Nodule

Cyst

Pustule

Wheal

Vesicle

Bulla

Scales

Crust

Fissures

Erosion

Ulcer

Lichenification

FIGURE **50-3** Skin lesions.

FIGURE **50-4** Skin mobility is determined by assessing how easily a large fold of skin is pinched up. Skin turgor is evaluated by observing how quickly the fold returns to the previous position.

cheekbones, and on the earlobes. Inflammation may be better detected by areas of abnormal warmth and firmness than by color changes. Rashes are better seen by shining a light at an angle to reveal irregularities in skin surface.

The hair is inspected for color, distribution, and oiliness and palpated to determine the texture. The scalp is inspected for scaliness, infestations, and lesions.

The shape and contour of the fingernails and toenails should be inspected. The color of the nail bed is noted. Capillary refill is checked by applying pressure to the nail to cause blanching and then releasing the pressure. The color should return to normal within 3 to 5 seconds. The angle of the nail base reveals clubbing of the nails (see Fig. 30-5).

The nursing assessment of the patient with a skin disorder is outlined in Box 50-1. The link between nu-

Box 50-1   *ASSESSMENT of the Patient with a Skin Disorder*

Health History

Chief Complaint or History of Present Illness:
Pruritus, skin color changes, lesions, hair loss, abnormal hair growth

Past Medical History:
Skin diseases or problems, drug therapy, allergies, chronic illnesses: diabetes mellitus, cancer, kidney failure, thyroid disease, liver disease, anemia

Review of Systems:
Change in skin color or pigmentation, change in a mole, sores that heal slowly, itching, dryness or scaliness, excessive bruising, changes in nails

Functional Assessment:
Occupation, exposure to chemicals or other irritants, skin care habits, extent of sun exposure, dietary habits

Physical Examination

Skin:
Color, pigmentation, dilated blood vessels, angiomas, nevi, lesions, rash, drainage, temperature, texture, moisture, thickness, edema, mobility, turgor, scars

Hair:
Color, distribution, oiliness, texture, nits

Scalp:
Scaliness, lesions

Nails:
Shape, contour, color of nail bed, blanching with pressure, capillary refill, angle of nail base

---

What Does Culture Have to Do with Skin Assessment?

It may be more difficult to assess some skin characteristics in dark-skinned people. To inspect for cyanosis, jaundice, and pallor, check the oral mucous membranes, the conjunctivae, the palms of the hands, and the soles of the feet.

---

trition and skin health is discussed in the Nutrition Concepts box at right.

Nutrition Concepts

1. Vitamin A is essential for healthy skin.
2. Food sources of vitamin A are liver, pumpkin, sweet potatoes, carrots, spinach, broccoli, cantaloupe, and apricots.
3. Food allergies can cause atopic dermatitis.
4. Skin changes associated with malnutrition include cracked skin, dermatitis, xerosis (dry skin), purpura, and petechiae (purple or red spots).

DIAGNOSTIC TESTS AND PROCEDURES

MICROSCOPIC EXAMINATION OF SKIN SPECIMENS

Studies of skin specimens that are used to diagnose skin conditions include the following:

- A potassium hydroxide (or KOH) examination is done to diagnose fungal infections of the skin, hair, or nails by studying a skin specimen. For a culture, the skin scraping or a nail clipping is implanted in medium.
- A Tzanck smear is used to diagnose viral skin infections.
- A scabies scraping is used to detect scabies (mites), eggs, or feces excreted by mites.

WOOD'S LIGHT EXAMINATION

In a Wood's light examination, a black light is used to assess for pigmentation changes and superficial skin infections.

PATCH TESTING FOR ALLERGY

To identify allergens, very small amounts of common irritants are applied to the skin, covered, and later examined for allergic reactions. Assessment and treatment of allergies are explained in detail in Chapter 13.

BIOPSY

A biopsy is the removal of tissue for microscopic examination. The three types of skin biopsies (Fig. 50-5) are the following:

- *Shave biopsy:* a specimen no deeper than the dermis is obtained with a scalpel or other specialized instrument. Bleeding is usually minimal and controlled with pressure, cautery, or chemicals.
- *Punch biopsy:* a circular tool cuts around the lesion, which is then lifted up and severed. Pressure or chemicals usually control bleeding, but suturing may be needed to close the site. The excision is relatively shallow.
- *Surgical excision:* for deep specimens, surgical excision biopsy is indicated. Sutures are required to close the defect left by the procedure.

The Diagnostic Tests and Procedures table on p. 1129 presents additional details and nursing interventions for patients undergoing diagnostic procedures.

FIGURE **50-5** Types of biopsy procedures: **A,** Shave. **B,** Punch. **C,** Surgical excision.

COMMON THERAPEUTIC MEASURES

DRESSINGS

Dressings are used to protect healing wounds and to retain surface moisture to promote healing. There are many types of dressings, including wet, dry, absorptive, and occlusive dressings. Dry dressings protect wounds and absorb drainage. Wet dressings are used to decrease inflammation, soften crusts, and promote tissue granulation. Absorptive dressings are used to promote removal of excess exudate and are especially useful in wounds with necrotic tissue. Occlusive dressings protect wounds and maintain moisture to promote healing.

NEGATIVE PRESSURE WOUND THERAPY

Negative pressure wound therapy is a relatively recent development in wound care that appears to greatly reduce the time required for healing of traumatic wounds, dehisced surgical wounds, pressure ulcers, and chronic ulcers. To use this approach, the wound is first cleansed with normal saline. Then a skin preparation product is applied around the wound to receive the adhesive dressing. The wound is then filled with one of two types of sponges, depending on the wound characteristics. A tube in the sponges is used to exert negative pressure. A transparent adhesive dressing is applied over the sponges and around the tubing so that the wound closure is airtight. The tubing is connected to suction that is set at a prescribed negative pressure. Suction may be applied intermittently or continuously as ordered. Continuous suction is less painful than intermittent suction. Notify the enterostomal therapist or physician if the pain is distressing. The pressure may have to be reduced or converted from intermittent to continuous suction. Because dressing changes are painful, give the patient an analgesic about 1 hour before the procedure. If sponges adhere to the wound surface, they can be moistened with normal saline before removal.

SOAKS AND WET WRAPS

Soaks and wet wraps are used to soothe, soften, and remove crusts, debris, and necrotic tissue. Warm water is used, and various agents may be added for specific skin conditions. A wet wrap may be applied to a single affected area or to the entire body. It is usually covered by a dry dressing and left in place for 15 to 20 minutes. Unless débridement is intended, moisten the wet dressing again before removal. Otherwise, healthy tissue may adhere to the dry material and be traumatized. After a soak, gently dry the treated area. Then apply topical medications as ordered.

PHOTOTHERAPY

Phototherapy is the use of light in combination with photosensitive drugs to promote shedding of the epidermis. Types of ultraviolet light are A (UVA), B (UVB), and C (UVC). Phototherapy may be used in the treatment of psoriasis, vitiligo, and chronic eczema. It is contraindicated in patients with a history of herpes simplex infection, skin cancer, cataracts, and lupus erythematosus because it aggravates these conditions. After phototherapy, the patient may have pruritus and dry skin. Assess for signs and symptoms of phototoxicity (redness, vesicles, pain).

Phototherapy with a psoralen and ultraviolet A (PUVA) is a treatment that uses a combination of oral or topical 8-methoxypsoralen and ultraviolet A (long-wave ultraviolet light). It is used to treat vitiligo, psoriasis, and cutaneous T-cell lymphoma. For 8 hours before and after the treatment, the patient is instructed to wear sunscreen, protective clothing, and dark glasses to decrease exposure to other sources of ultraviolet light. The Goeckerman regimen is a type of phototherapy specifically used to treat psoriasis and atopic dermatitis. The patient first bathes in a tar emulsion bath. Then a topical tar product is applied, and the patient is exposed to ultraviolet light.

DIAGNOSTIC TESTS and PROCEDURES | *Skin Disorders and Related Nursing Implications*

TEST/PURPOSE	PATIENT PREPARATION	POSTPROCEDURE CARE
Potassium hydroxide (KOH) examination is used along with a culture to diagnose fungal infections of the skin and nails.	Inform patient that a small scraping of skin will be taken from the affected area for microscopic examination. The skin scrapings and a nail clipping are used for cultures to determine the exact cause of the lesion. Procedure is painless.	Inform patient when results will be available.
Tzanck smear is used to diagnose viral infections.	Tell the patient the lesion will be washed and opened to obtain a fluid sample, which will be examined microscopically. Procedure may cause mild discomfort. Results may be available immediately.	No special care.
Scabies scraping is used to assess skin lesions for the presence of scabies (mites), eggs, or feces excreted by the mites.	Inform the patient that the top of a lesion will be taken off for microscopic examination. The procedure is briefly uncomfortable but requires no anesthesia.	No special care.
Wood's light examination uses black light to reveal superficial skin infections and changes in pigmentation.	Tell the patient the procedure is done in a dark room. The skin will be carefully inspected under black light. The procedure is noninvasive and painless.	No special care.
Patch testing is used to identify substances to which patients are allergic.	Inform the patient that various common irritants are applied to the skin and covered with special patches or tape. The patches must be left in place and examined ("read") after 48, 72, 96 hours and sometimes after 1 week. Skin reactions that indicate allergy include redness, swelling, and blisters. Patch testing is painless.	No special care.
A *biopsy* is the removal of tissue for microscopic examination.	Tell the patient the physician will remove some tissue for diagnostic evaluation. Small, shallow biopsies usually require only a dressing. Deeper biopsies require sutures. Patients are usually advised to avoid aspirin or other NSAIDs for 48 hours before the biopsy to prevent excessive bleeding.	Inspect the site for bleeding. Apply direct pressure if necessary to control bleeding. If sutures are used, instruct the patient to return on a specified date for suture removal. Tell the patient how to care for the biopsy site (protocols vary) and when results are expected.

 Consider the Alternative

Topical herbal preparations that are used as emollients include balm of Gilead, coltsfoot, and comfrey.

DRUG THERAPY

A number of topical and oral drugs are used to treat skin disorders and skin manifestations of other conditions. Topical drugs include **keratolytics** (capable of dissolving keratin), antipruritics, emollients, lubricants, sunscreens, tars, anti-infectives, glucocorticoids, antimetabolites, antihistamines, antiseborrheic agents, and vitamin A derivatives. Examples of selected drug classifications and their actions, side effects, and nursing interventions are presented in the Drug Therapy table on pp. 1130 to 1131.

For topical application, drugs are combined with various substances in forms called *vehicles*. Topical medication vehicles include powders, lotions, aerosols, gels, creams, and ointments.

DISORDERS OF THE SKIN

PRURITUS

Pruritus is simply itching. It is a symptom rather than a disease but is very common with many skin and systemic disorders. Therefore an overview of pruritus is presented here.

Etiology and Risk Factors

The sensation of itching is not completely understood, but it may be triggered by touch, temperature changes, emotional stress, and chemical, mechanical, and electrical stimuli. The severity of the response to stimulation is enhanced by emotional stress, anxiety, and fear.

DRUG THERAPY *Disorders of the Skin*

DRUG	USE/ACTION	SIDE EFFECTS	NURSING INTERVENTIONS
KERATOLYTICS			
Benzoyl peroxide Salicylic acid Sulfur Coal tar	Dissolve keratin and slow bacterial growth. Used to treat acne and psoriasis.	Excessive dryness, irritation, scaling, edema, photosensitivity.	Advise patient to avoid excessive sun exposure. Assess effects.
TOPICAL ANTIBACTERIALS			
Bacitracin Polysporin	Destroy microorganisms. Used to treat skin infections.	Contact dermatitis. Allergy (rare): itching, burning, anaphylaxis.	Ask about allergies before applying. Apply as prescribed after allergy ruled out. Report itching, burning, rash, redness.
Silver sulfadiazine (Silvadene)	Bactericidal. Used to prevent and treat wound infection with serious burns.	Rash, pruritus, burning, pain. Rare: nephritis, anorexia. Can cause blood dyscrasias, hepatitis, nephrosis, hypoglycemia.	Apply to clean burn surface with gloved hand. Cover burn completely and continuously. Monitor renal and GI distress, headache, joint pain, hepatic function. Monitor vital signs, complete blood count, serum glucose.
ANTIVIRAL AGENTS			
Acyclovir (Zovirax) Famciclovir Valacyclovir Foscarnet	Interfere with viral replication. Used to treat infections caused by herpes simplex virus types 1 and 2 and herpes zoster. Not curative but may reduce severity and duration of symptoms.	*Topical form:* burning, stinging, pruritus. *Oral form:* nausea and vomiting. *IV form:* phlebitis, rash, urticaria, hypotension, hematuria, diaphoresis. Rare: confusion, agitation, seizures. Nephrotoxicity with high IV doses.	Ask about allergies. Monitor closely if patient has renal impairment. Measure intake and output. Monitor infusion site for redness. Monitor neurologic status. Use gloved finger to apply ointment. Encourage adequate fluid intake.
TOPICAL ANTIFUNGAL AGENTS			
Nystatin (Mycostatin) Clotrimazole (Mycelex) Oxiconazole (Oxistat) Naftifine (Naftin) Terbinafine (Lamisil)	Effective against fungi. Used to treat fungal infections.	Irritation, erythema, burning, rash. Abdominal cramps and cystitis with vaginal preparations.	Apply as directed. Do not apply occlusive dressings without order.
ORAL ANTIFUNGAL AGENTS			
Terbinafine (Lamisil) Griseofulvin (Fulvicin P/G) Ketoconazole (Nizoral)	Used to treat fungal infections that do not respond to topicals. Common use: nail infections.	Terbinafine: hepatotoxicity, headache, diarrhea, GI distress. Griseofulvin: headache, rash, insomnia, GI distress. Ketoconazole: hepatotoxicity.	Give ketoconazole with food or milk to minimize GI effects, and 2 hours apart from any drugs that reduce gastric acidity. Monitor liver function with ketoconazole and terbinafine. Griseofulvin decreases effects of warfarin.
TOPICAL ANTI-INFLAMMATORIES			
Hydrocortisone (Cortizone and others) Triamcinolone (Aristocort and others) Fluocinolone (Bio-Syn and others)	Reduce inflammation in various skin disorders.	Itching, erythema, irritation. Severe allergic reactions rare.	Do not apply occlusive dressing without order. Apply sparingly, and rub in thoroughly.
TOPICAL ANTI-INFECTIVE			
Azelaic acid (Azelex)	Antimicrobial against *Propionibacterium acnes* and *Staphylococcus epidermides*.	Pruritus, burning, stinging, tingling. Allergy: mild-moderate inflammatory acne vulgaris.	Avoid occlusive dressings. Keep away from mouth, eyes. Temporary skin irritation common.

GI, Gastrointestinal; *IV,* intravenous; *PUVA,* psoralen ultraviolet A-range.

DRUG THERAPY | *Disorders of the Skin—cont'd*

DRUG	USE/ACTION	SIDE EFFECTS	NURSING INTERVENTIONS
VITAMIN A DERIVATIVE Tretinoin (Retin-A) Isotretinoin (Accutane, Amnesteem, Roaccutane, Claravis, Isotane, Sotret, and Oratane)	Reduces formation of comedones. Increases mitosis of epithelial cells. Used to treat acne. Decreases size of sebaceous glands. Decreases sebum production. Used to treat severe acne. May decrease risk of skin cancer and PUVA.	Stinging, erythema, scaling expected. Allergy rare. Occasionally severe erythema, blistering. Excessive dryness of skin, nose, mouth. Conjunctivitis, vomiting, elevated serum triglycerides, bone or joint pain, muscle aches. Rare: hepatitis, inflammatory bowel disease, depression.	Tell patient not to use with keratolytics. Do not apply to eyes, mouth, angles of nose. Patient should avoid sun exposure, use sunscreen. If dryness excessive, decrease frequency of use. Tell patient to expect symptoms to worsen at first, then improve. Do not use topical acne drugs at same time. Report severe GI symptoms. Avoid sun exposure because of photosensitivity. Explain importance of preventing pregnancy 1 mo before, during, and 1 mo after therapy. Recommend two reliable forms of contraception to be used simultaneously.
Acitretin (Soriatane)	May decrease risk of skin cancer and PUVA.	Contraindicated during pregnancy: can cause major fetal deformities.	
Tazarotene (Tazorac) Adapalene (Differin)	Tazarotene and adapalene both are topical agents used to treat acne. Tazarotene is also used to treat psoriasis.	Both can cause itching, burning, and stinging. More serious skin reactions sometimes occur.	Advise patients to avoid direct sunlight and use sunscreens because of photosensitivity. Acne may worsen before beneficial results occur. Instruct patient in correct application (see instructions for each drug).
PEDICULICIDES AND SCABICIDES Crotamiton (Eurax) Permethrin (Nix)	Kill parasites and their eggs. Used to treat pediculosis (lice) and scabies (mite) infestations.	Skin and eye irritation. Systemic effects with excessive use.	Follow directions specifically. Avoid contact with eyes. Most products are effective with one application, but a repeat treatment may be recommended. Clothing and bed linens must be treated to prevent reinfestation.
ANTIPSORIATICS Anthralin Tar (Estar gel)	Used to treat psoriasis.	Anthralin: erythema, inflamed eyes, staining. Tar: skin irritation, photosensitivity, staining.	Protect skin and clothing from preparations that stain. Most have unpleasant odor.
RETINOID ANTIPSORIATIC Acitretin (Soriatane)	Decreases proliferation of epidermal cells; anti-inflammatory, immunomodulatory. For severe psoriasis only.	Hair loss, skin peeling, dry mouth, rhinitis, gingivitis, elevated liver enzymes and triglycerides. Many other side and adverse effects.	*Contraindicated during pregnancy!* Be sure patient understands risk to fetus and uses contraception if sexually active for at least 3 years after therapy completed. Should be taken with meals. Monitor for all side effects.
PHOTOSENSITIVITY DRUG Methoxsalen (Oxsoralen)	Decreases proliferation of epidermal cells in psoriasis.	Nausea, headache, vertigo, rash, pruritus, burning and peeling of skin. Can cause anemia, leukopenia, thrombocytopenia, ulcerative stomatitis, bleeding, alopecia, cystitis.	Encourage patient to return for periodic blood tests as ordered and to report easy bruising or excessive bleeding.
BIOLOGIC AGENTS Alefacept (Amevive)	Immune system suppressant. Used for chronic plaque psoriasis.	Pain at injection site, sore throat, infections, chills, lymphopenia, malignancies, hepatic injury.	12-week therapy, given once a week. Monitor T-lymphocyte levels every 2 weeks. Should not be used in patients whose T-lymphocyte counts are <250 μL. IV and IM only.

Pruritus is a prominent symptom with psoriasis, dermatitis, eczema, and insect bites. It may also be present with the following systemic conditions: urticaria, some cancers, renal failure, diabetes mellitus, thyroid disorders, liver disease, and anemia. Among the drugs that can cause pruritus are opiates and phenothiazines.

Medical Treatment

When the cause of pruritus is known, treatment is directed at correcting the cause. Measures that may help control the symptom include stress management and avoidance of known irritants, sudden temperature changes, and alcohol, tea, and coffee. Lubricants in the bath water and emollients applied after bathing also may help. Medications that often are ordered for pruritus include corticosteroids, antihistamines, and local anesthetics. In some situations, antidepressant and antiserotonin drugs may be ordered.

NURSING CARE *of the Patient with Pruritus*

Assessment

When a patient has pruritus, collect data about his or her symptoms that may help determine the cause. The history of the current illness is important because pruritus may be just one symptom of a condition that requires attention. Possible contributing factors to be documented include exposure to irritants, drug therapy, and past medical history.

Nursing Diagnoses, Goals, and Outcome Criteria: Pruritus

NURSING DIAGNOSES	GOALS AND OUTCOME CRITERIA
Impaired Skin Integrity related to scratching	Intact skin: absence of abrasions
Ineffective Therapeutic Regimen Management related to lack of understanding of prevention or management of pruritus	Patient adheres to prescribed measures to prevent or treat condition: patient correctly states correct measures, demonstrates self-care

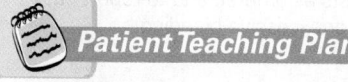

Patient Teaching Plan

Pruritus

- Avoid factors that aggravate itching such as temperature extremes, extremely dry air, irritating fabrics, chemicals, frequent hot baths, sweating, stress.
- To prevent itching, avoid extreme temperatures, humidify room air, take less frequent and cooler baths, apply emollients, avoid irritating fabrics and chemicals, and practice stress management.
- Use therapeutic measures as prescribed:
  - Topical agents: lotions, creams
  - Systemic agents: antihistamines—dosage, side effects
  - Treatment of underlying conditions

Interventions

The specific interventions vary with the cause of pruritus. If the patient has dry skin, application of lubricants or emollients may be helpful. The addition of oils to bath water is often recommended but could create an unsafe situation in the bathtub. Advise patients to avoid bathing in very hot water. Lotion can usually be applied to unbroken skin without a physician's order. If topical or systemic drugs are ordered, administer them or instruct the patient in their use. Inspect the skin daily to determine the effects of the treatments. Explain possible causes of pruritus, and encourage the patient to avoid them.

INFLAMMATORY CONDITIONS AND INFECTIONS

Atopic Dermatitis (Eczema)

Pathophysiology

Atopic dermatitis is one of several disorders referred to as *eczema*. Eczema has three stages. The acute stage is characterized by a red, oozing, crusty rash and intense pruritus. Manifestations of the subacute stage include redness, excoriations, and scaling plaques or pustules. Fine scales may give the patient's skin a silvery appearance. In the chronic stage, the skin becomes dry, thickened, scaly, and brownish-gray in color (Fig. 50-6). Open lesions invite infection, and scarring may occur. Multiple stages may be present at the same time.

Etiology and Risk Factors

Most patients with atopic dermatitis have a personal or family history of asthma, hay fever, eczema, or food allergies. People with atopic dermatitis have an immune dysfunction, but it is not known whether that dysfunction is a cause or an effect of the disorder.

Medical Diagnosis

A medical diagnosis of atopic dermatitis is based primarily on the health history and physical examination. Other procedures that might be done to confirm the diagnosis are skin biopsy, serum immunoglobulin E levels, and cultures to diagnose secondary infections. If allergy is suspected as a cause of dermatitis, the physician may perform allergy tests to identify allergens.

FIGURE **50-6** Atopic dermatitis.

Medical Treatment

Topical corticosteroids provide the best control of inflammation. Soaks, occlusive dressings, and emollients help keep the skin moist. Systemic antihistamines may be ordered to relieve itching and inflammation. In severe cases that do not respond to topical agents, a short course of systemic corticosteroids may be ordered. Research is in progress to determine the efficacy of the immunosuppressants *tacrolimus* and *cyclosporine*. Treatment of allergic disorders is detailed in Chapter 13

NURSING CARE *of the Patient with Atopic Dermatitis*

Assessment

Assessment of the patient with a skin disorder is summarized in Box 50-1. When the patient has atopic dermatitis, specifically inquire about known allergies, bathing practices (frequency, water temperature, use of soaps), and current medications to identify possible contributing factors. The physical examination includes inspection and palpation of the skin for lesions, moisture, and abrasions.

Nursing Diagnoses, Goals, and Outcome Criteria: Atopic Dermatitis

Nursing Diagnoses	Goals and Outcome Criteria
Impaired Skin Integrity related to excessive dryness, scratching	Improved skin integrity: intact, moist skin
Risk for Infection related to break in skin, decreased resistance to infection	Absence of infection: no fever, decreasing redness and drainage
Disturbed Body Image related to lesions	Improved body image: positive patient statements about self

Interventions

Impaired Skin Integrity

Measures that decrease itching and moisturize the skin help maintain skin integrity. Encourage the patient to maintain the room temperature at 68° F to 75° F with 45% to 55% humidity. Advise the patient to avoid possible irritants. New clothing should be washed before wearing. Mild detergent should be used for laundry, and clothes should be rinsed twice. Recommend open-weave fabrics and loose clothing. Advise the use of moisturizers and sunscreens. If drugs are ordered for pruritus, administer them or instruct the patient in self-medication. Evaluate skin integrity and hydration on an ongoing basis.

Risk for Infection

Any break in the skin presents a portal for pathogens. Inspect the skin, and report new lesions to the physician. Monitor the temperature for elevation that may reflect a systemic infection. Teach the patient the importance of protecting the skin from trauma. If scratching is a problem, the fingernails need to be cut short

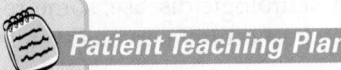

Patient Teaching Plan

Atopic Dermatitis

- Avoid known irritants and constrictive clothing.
- Use moisturizers and sunscreens.
- Take drugs as prescribed: name, dosage or application instructions, adverse effects.
- After swimming in chlorinated water, shampoo and bathe (or shower) using a mild soap. Then apply a moisturizer.

and kept smooth. Gloves or mittens may help prevent traumatic scratching during sleep or in the confused person. Administer antibiotics as ordered.

Disturbed Body Image

Demonstrate acceptance of the patient's appearance through attentive care and touch. Teach the patient and family that dermatitis is not contagious and is not caused by poor hygiene. Explore the patient's concerns about the skin disorder. If the patient is very stressed, the nurse can discuss coping strategies or request a referral for professional counseling.

Contact Dermatitis

Contact dermatitis is an inflammatory condition caused by contact with a substance that triggers an allergic response. Allergic and immune disorders are addressed in Chapter 13.

Consider the Alternative

When a patient has an allergic skin reaction, be sure to assess for topical use of herbal products. For example, aloe can cause allergic dermatitis in susceptible persons and angelica can cause a skin rash if a patient is exposed to sunlight.

Seborrheic Dermatitis

Pathophysiology

Seborrheic dermatitis is a chronic inflammatory disease of the skin. It usually affects the scalp, eyebrows, eyelids, lips, ears, sternal area, axillae, umbilicus, groin, gluteal crease, and the area under the breasts. Seborrheic dermatitis of the scalp is called *dandruff*. Areas affected by this condition may have fine, powdery scales, thick crusts, or oily patches. Scales may be white, yellowish, or reddish. Pruritus is common.

Etiology and Risk Factors

The cause of seborrheic dermatitis is unknown. It may be an inflammatory reaction to infection with the yeast *Malassezia*. Because the condition is aggravated by emotional stress and neurologic disease, some researchers think there may be a central nervous system influence.

Medical Diagnosis

Diagnosis of seborrheic dermatitis is based on the health history and physical examination.

Medical Treatment

Initial treatment of seborrheic dermatitis employs topical ketoconazole (Nizoral), sometimes with topical corticosteroids. Dandruff is treated with medicated shampoos used two or three times a week. Appropriate shampoos are those that contain selenium sulfide (Selsun), ketoconazole, tar, zinc pyrithione, salicylic acid, or resorcin. Some corticosteroid solutions also may be prescribed.

NURSING CARE *of the Patient with Seborrheic Dermatitis*

Although seborrheic dermatitis does not require inpatient treatment, it is a common condition encountered among patients hospitalized for other reasons.

Assessment

Relevant data include symptoms and identification of treatments being used. Inspect and describe the affected areas.

Nursing Diagnoses, Goals, and Outcome Criteria: Seborrheic Dermatitis

NURSING DIAGNOSES	GOALS AND OUTCOME CRITERIA
Ineffective Therapeutic Regimen Management related to lack of knowledge about treatment	Patient implements the prescribed treatment plan: correctly describes plan and self-care
Disturbed Body Image related to altered appearance (lesions)	Improved body image: decreasing signs of the condition, patient's statements reflect a positive view of self

Interventions

Explain the condition, and reinforce the physician's instructions for treatment. Suggest measures to relieve pruritus, as described on p. 1132. Discuss the patient's concerns about the condition, and emphasize that seborrheic dermatitis can be controlled with treatment. Demonstrate acceptance of the patient by genuine interest and use of touch.

Psoriasis

Pathophysiology

Psoriasis is an inflammatory disorder characterized by abnormal proliferation of skin cells. The classic sign of psoriasis is the appearance of bright-red lesions that may be covered with silvery scales (Fig. 50-7). Although

FIGURE **50-7** Psoriasis.

the onset is common in young adulthood, it can appear at any age. Psoriasis may affect a limited body area or may be extensive. Some people have systemic effects of the disease, such as psoriatic arthritis.

Etiology and Risk Factors

Psoriasis is a condition caused by rapid proliferation of epidermal cells. It is usually chronic with cycles of exacerbations and remissions. Multiple factors acting on a genetically predisposed person are thought to cause this disorder. Factors that aggravate psoriasis are stress, streptococcal infections, overuse of alcohol, and drugs such as lithium and beta-blockers.

Medical Diagnosis

Psoriasis is diagnosed based on the health history and the physical examination.

Medical Treatment

There is no cure for psoriasis, but it can be treated topically or systemically. Patients with mild psoriasis are usually treated with topical medications: corticosteroids, tazarotene, Estar, and vitamin D derivatives (calcipotriene [Dovonex]). Topical salicylic acid may be used with the corticosteroids. Tazarotene (Tazorac) is a topical retinoid that stays in the skin longer, leading to longer remissions. Anthralin (Anthra-Derm) may be used to remove heavy scales. With a gloved hand, it is applied only to the lesions. After a specified period of time, anthralin is removed with tissues. The patient removes the residue by showering or bathing. The medication must be handled carefully because it stains hair, skin, fingernails, furniture, and bathroom fixtures. Newer preparations that may not stain (e.g., Estar gel) are now available. UVB may be used to enhance topical therapy with tar and anthralin.

Moderate to severe psoriasis may be treated with PUVA—a combination of methotrexate and UVA. Other oral drugs include oral retinoids (acitretin [Soriatane]) and biologic agents (alefacept). Oral retinoids may reduce the risk of skin cancers associated with PUVA. Systemic corticosteroids may be used on a short-term basis. Patients on most forms of systemic therapy require periodic liver testing and blood studies because of the adverse effects. Methotrexate and oral retinoids both are contraindicated during pregnancy because of the risk of fetal harm.

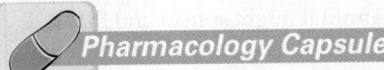

Pharmacology Capsule

If the patient of childbearing age is taking methotrexate or oral retinoids, be sure she understands that these drugs are harmful to a fetus.

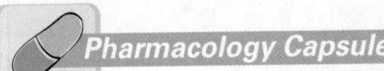

Pharmacology Capsule

Because of risks to the fetus, women should use reliable contraception during and for 3 years after therapy with Soriatane.

NURSING CARE *of the Patient with Psoriasis*

Assessment

Relevant data for the patient with psoriasis include a description of symptoms and identification of treatments being used (see Nursing Care Plan: The Patient with Psoriasis on p. 1136). Inspect the affected areas for lesions and scales. Document joint pain or stiffness because the condition may cause arthritis. Explore the impact of psoriasis on the patient's everyday life and the coping strategies used.

Nursing Diagnoses, Goals, and Outcome Criteria: Psoriasis	
NURSING DIAGNOSES	GOALS AND OUTCOME CRITERIA
Ineffective Therapeutic Regimen Management related to lack of knowledge	Effective management of treatment regimen: patient correctly describes and demonstrates self-care
Disturbed Body Image related to lesions and scales on skin	Improved body image: patient's efforts to improve appearance and positive remarks about self
Social Isolation related to embarrassment about skin lesions	Decreased social isolation: patient's continued involvement in social activities

Interventions

Ineffective Therapeutic Regimen Management

The focus of nursing care for the patient with psoriasis is patient education that enables the patient to manage the prescribed regimen. The patient and family need to know that the condition is chronic but not contagious and usually responds to treatment. Teach the patient about the prescribed medications and treatments. Tell the patient to report signs of secondary infection (fe-

ver, purulent discharge, increased redness) to the physician. Also encourage adequate rest, good nutrition, and stress management.

Disturbed Body Image

Give the patient the opportunity to express feelings about psoriasis and the effects on his or her life. Demonstrate acceptance of the patient's appearance and the feelings that are expressed. Learning to manage the condition can help the patient feel more hopeful, realizing that remission will occur.

Social Isolation

Encourage the patient to maintain social contacts and plan strategies to deal with exacerbations without undue stress.

Intertrigo

Pathophysiology

Intertrigo is inflammation of the skin where two skin surfaces touch: axillae, abdominal skinfolds, and the area under the breasts. The affected area is usually red and "weeping" with clear margins. The area may be surrounded by vesicles and pustules.

Etiology and Risk Factors

The inflammation of intertrigo results from heat, friction, and moisture between two touching body surfaces. These factors create the perfect environment for infection by *Candida albicans* (yeast) or bacteria.

Medical Diagnosis and Treatment

The medical diagnosis is based on the site and appearance of the inflamed skin and the presence of *C. albicans* as confirmed by potassium hydroxide examination and culture of skin scrapings. If the skin is not broken, it can be washed with water twice daily. The area is then rinsed and patted dry. Soft gauze may be used to separate layer of body tissue and absorb moisture. Cornstarch is contraindicated because it supports the growth of *C. albicans*. For severe inflammation or fungal infection, treatment may include a topical corticosteroid or antifungal agent. Examples of topical antifungal agents are nystatin, ketoconazole, clotrimazole, and terbinafine. Vytone 1% is a combination corticosteroid, antibacterial, and antifungal preparation. Wet soaks with tap water or Burow's solution are sometimes ordered to remove exudate if an infection is present.

NURSING CARE *of the Patient with Intertrigo*

Assessment

Intertrigo is fairly common among patients in long-term care facilities. Investigate complaints of pain, irritation, or redness in body folds. Monitor body temperature to detect possible infection. Inspect susceptible areas (axillae, groin, beneath breasts, abdominal skinfolds) on a daily basis.

NURSING CARE PLAN

The Patient with Psoriasis

ASSESSMENT

Health History: A 45-year-old police officer came to the physician's office because of a "rash" on his trunk. He reports that he is in good health and has had no major injuries or illnesses except a left knee injury sustained in a fall as a teenager. He is taking no medications but is allergic to penicillin. He is alarmed at the rash and is afraid it might spread and that it might be something serious. The physician diagnoses psoriasis. He is divorced and enjoys socializing, especially dancing. He is concerned about how people might react to his condition.

Physical Examination: Vital signs: temperature, 98.2° F orally; pulse, 84; respiration, 16; blood pressure, 144/88. Height, 5'10". Weight, 164 lb. He is alert and oriented but mildly anxious. The skin on the face and extremities is normal. Bright-red lesions with silvery scales are distributed over the anterior and posterior chest, abdomen, buttocks, and hands. Heart and breath sounds are normal. The abdomen is soft, with bowel sounds present in all four quadrants. There is full range of motion of all joints with crepitation in the left knee. Peripheral pulses are strong and symmetric. The extremities are warm and dry.

Nursing Diagnosis	Goals and Outcome Criteria	Interventions
Ineffective Therapeutic Regimen management related to lack of understanding of psoriasis and its treatment	The patient will correctly describe psoriasis and prescribed treatment measures.	Explain that psoriasis typically has periods of exacerbation and remission, that it is not contagious, and that symptoms can be improved with treatment. Explain the prescribed treatment, including proper application of topical medications and side and adverse effects of drug therapy. For oral drugs, provide information about schedule as well as adverse and side effects. Tell the patient signs of secondary infection (fever, purulent drainage, increased redness) that should be reported to the physician. Encourage patient to plan for adequate rest and to eat a balanced diet. Explore stress management strategies. Refer to mental health counselor if needed. Supplement verbal teaching with written material.
Disturbed Body Image related to lesions and scales on skin	The patient's body image will improve, as evidenced by positive statements about self.	Demonstrate acceptance of the patient by eye contact and touch. Be aware of personal reaction to lesions. Encourage patient to share feelings about condition. Help the patient feel "in control" by providing information about management of psoriasis.
Social Isolation related to embarrassment about skin lesions	The patient will continue social activities and identify strategies to deal with social situations.	Explore how the patient thinks others will react to his condition. Role-play strategies to use in social situations. Encourage continued activity. Emphasize expected improvement.

? CRITICAL THINKING QUESTIONS

- Why is stress management important in the treatment of psoriasis?

- What are the psychosocial effects of a diagnosis of psoriasis?

Nursing Diagnoses, Goals, and Outcome Criteria: Intertrigo

NURSING DIAGNOSES	GOALS AND OUTCOME CRITERIA
Impaired Skin Integrity related to inflammation	Improved skin integrity: intact skin without redness
Risk for Infection related to moist environment, broken skin	Absence of infection: no fever, pain, or edema

Interventions

Areas where skin surfaces are in close contact must be kept clean and dry. Apply topical medications (antifungals and corticosteroids) as ordered. Report increasing redness and tenderness, fever, and broken skin to the physician. Encourage women with pendulous breasts to wear a soft, supportive bra. If incontinence has contributed to perineal intertrigo, positioning the patient with the legs apart allows moisture to evaporate.

Fungal Infections

Pathophysiology

Humans are susceptible to a number of fungal infections. Superficial infections of the skin and mucous membranes caused by fungi include tinea pedis (athlete's foot), tinea manus (hand), tinea cruris (groin), tinea capitis (scalp), tinea corporis (body), tinea barbae (beard), and candidiasis, which can affect the skin, mouth, vagina, gastrointestinal tract, and lungs.

Etiology and Risk Factors

The organisms that cause tinea infections take advantage of trauma in moist, warm tissue. Some organisms can be spread through direct contact or by inanimate objects. Lesions vary but may be scaly patches with raised borders. The lay term *ringworm* is sometimes used to describe these circular lesions. Pruritus is a common symptom of tinea. Tinea capitis, tinea corporis, and tinea pedis are rather easily spread by sharing contaminated objects.

Candidiasis, commonly called a *yeast infection*, is caused by *C. albicans*. Patients at risk for candidiasis include those who are pregnant, malnourished, immunosuppressed, or taking antibiotics or oral contraceptives. People with diabetes mellitus are also at risk for this disease. Common sites affected are the mouth, vagina, and skin. The skin around an ostomy site also is susceptible to candidiasis because of the constant moisture there. Infections of the mucous membranes are manifested as red lesions with white plaques. Skin infections with *C. albicans* are seen as moist, red lesions (Fig. 50-8). The lesions often are found in folds of body tissue (see Intertrigo section on p. 1135).

Medical Diagnosis

Fungal infections are usually diagnosed on the basis of the history and physical examination but may be confirmed by microscopic examination of skin scrapings using a potassium hydroxide wet mount preparation.

Medical Treatment

Fungal infections are treated with antifungal powders and creams. Wet compresses and keratolytics may be ordered to soften scales with some tinea infections. Oral candidiasis is treated with clotrimazole troches, nystatin mouthwash or lozenges, or oral amphotericin B. For AIDS patients, clotrimazole is superior to nystatin.

NURSING CARE *of the Patient with a Fungal Infection*

Assessment

The nursing assessment identifies conditions that might make a person susceptible to fungal infections: diabetes mellitus, malnutrition, and immunosuppression. Note antibiotic therapy, another risk factor. During the physical examination, inspect the skin and mucous membranes for lesions. Creamy white lesions that can be scraped off easily are characteristic of oral candidiasis.

Nursing Diagnoses, Goals, and Outcome Criteria: Fungal Infection	
NURSING DIAGNOSES	GOALS AND OUTCOME CRITERIA
Disturbed Body Image related to skin lesions	Improved body image: absence of skin lesions, patient's positive statements about appearance
Impaired Oral Mucous Membrane related to oral candidiasis	Healthy oral mucous membranes: absence of oral lesions
Risk for Injury related to reinfection, spread of infection	Decreased risk of recurrent infection: patient correctly describes and demonstrates self-care

Interventions

Disturbed Body Image

Be sensitive to the patient's reaction to a skin infection. Visible lesions may be embarrassing to the patient. If the genitalia are affected, the patient may think the symptoms are due to a sexually transmitted infection. Explain the cause of the infection, how it is treated, whether it is contagious, and how transmission and reinfection can be avoided. If medication is prescribed, instruct the patient in proper use of the agent. Tell the patient to keep the affected areas of the skin as clean and dry as possible. A cool environment helps by reducing perspiration.

Eradication of candidiasis infections in bedridden patients can be especially challenging. Frequently reposition the patient to permit evaporation of moisture. The thighs can be separated by using a pillow between the knees, and a folded cloth may be placed beneath pendulous breasts.

Impaired Oral Mucous Membranes

Instruct the patient with oral candidiasis in the proper use of prescribed medications. Mouthwashes may be swished to coat all oral surfaces before swallowing. Lozenges should be dissolved in the mouth. If the patient wears dentures, they should be soaked in an antifungal solution.

Pharmacology Capsule

Antibiotic therapy eliminates the microorganisms that normally control fungal growth, making the patient susceptible to fungal infections.

FIGURE **50-8** Candidiasis.

Risk for Injury

Advise patients with tinea infections to avoid sharing personal items such as hairbrushes and clothing. They also should dry thoroughly after bathing and wear absorbent underwear and socks.

Acne

Pathophysiology

Acne is a skin condition that affects the hair follicles and sebaceous glands. It is characterized by comedones (whiteheads and blackheads), pustules, and cysts. These lesions most often develop on the face, neck, and upper trunk. Acne commonly begins in adolescence and may last into adulthood. Most cases are mild, but serious cases with extensive inflammation can cause permanent scarring.

Etiology and Risk Factors

Acne lesions develop when androgenic hormones cause increased sebum production and bacteria (*Propionibacterium acnes*) proliferate, causing sebaceous follicles to become blocked and inflamed. Despite popular opinion, acne is not caused by fatty foods, chocolate, or poor hygiene. In addition to androgenic hormones, exacerbations of acne can be triggered by high levels of progestin in birth control pills, oil-based cosmetics, high doses of systemic corticosteroids, hormonal changes associated with the menstrual period, and some endocrine disorders.

Medical Diagnosis

Acne is diagnosed on the basis of the health history and physical examination findings.

Medical Treatment

Treatment varies with the severity of the condition. Mild cases may respond very well to topical antimicrobials or retinoids (vitamin A preparations). Topical antimicrobials include azelaic acid (Azelex) and benzoyl peroxide; topical retinoids include tretinoin (Retin-A) or tazarotene (Tazorac). If these agents do not adequately control acne, oral antibiotics (tetracycline, azithromycin, erythromycin) may be given over a period of several months. Estrogen also may be prescribed to counteract the effects of androgenic hormones. Spironolactone may be used for its antiandrogenic effects. If acne is severe and unresponsive to all of these treatments, isotretinoin (Accutane) may be prescribed.

Pharmacology Capsule

Accutane can cause mental depression, possibly leading to suicidal ideation.

Nonpharmacologic treatment may include comedo extraction or cryotherapy. Dermabrasion may be used to reduce scarring.

Pharmacology Capsule

Isotretinoin (Accutane) can cause severe fetal deformities. Therefore females who take the drug must prevent pregnancy until at least 1 month after therapy has been completed.

NURSING CARE *of the Patient with Acne*

Assessment

Explore the patient's concerns and knowledge about acne. Document any treatments being used. Note all medical conditions and medications because some contribute to or aggravate acne. Inspect the skin to determine the extent and severity of the condition.

Nursing Diagnoses, Goals, and Outcome Criteria: Acne

Nursing Diagnoses	Goals and Outcome Criteria
Disturbed Body Image related to comedones, pustules, and cysts	Improved body image: decreased lesions and patient's expression of improved body image
Ineffective Therapeutic Regimen Management related to lack of understanding of causes and treatment of acne	Effective treatment management: patient correctly describes and demonstrates prescribed skin care and self-medication

Interventions

Disturbed Body Image

When working with a person who has acne, provide support and information. Because acne almost always affects the face, most patients with moderate or severe acne suffer body image disturbances. Be sensitive to this concern and encourage the patient to see a dermatologist for treatment. This condition can be very harmful to the patient's self-esteem and should not be dismissed as a minor problem.

Ineffective Therapeutic Regimen Management

Explain the causes of acne as well as the many myths about the disease. Assure the patient that acne does not reflect poor hygiene but that cleanliness does reduce the risk of infections. Dietary interventions are no longer thought to be useful. Discourage picking or squeezing lesions because it may force infected material deeper into the follicle. Advise the patient that harsh cleansers and vigorous scrubbing have no therapeutic value.

Explain prescribed drugs, and discuss any adverse effects. Patient teaching is especially important if isotretinoin is used. Isotretinoin is an oral medication that has a drying effect on the skin. Tell the patient to expect the condition to worsen initially and then begin to improve. Advise the patient that the drug is teratogenic, meaning it is harmful to a developing fetus. Therefore two forms of effective contraception must be used if the patient is sexually active while taking the drug.

Herpes Simplex

Etiology and Risk Factors

The herpes simplex virus (HSV) causes an infection that begins with itching and burning and progresses to the development of vesicles that rupture and form crusts (Fig. 50-9). Sites most often infected by the virus are the nose, lips, cheeks, ears, and genitalia. Oral HSV lesions are commonly called *cold sores* or *fever blisters*. There are two types of HSV. Infections on the face and upper body are usually caused by HSV type 1; genital infections are usually caused by HSV type 2. However, either type may cause oral or genital infections. Patients typically have repeated outbreaks and remissions. Herpes simplex virus can be transmitted by direct contact. Genital infection is therefore considered a sexually transmitted infection and is discussed in detail in Chapter 49.

Medical Diagnosis

Diagnostic tests used to identify herpes infections include laboratory studies of exudate from a lesion and blood studies to detect specific antibodies.

Medical Treatment

Herpes simplex infections are treated with acyclovir (Zovirax) or (for cold sores) docosanol (Abreva). Antiviral drugs are not curative but may hasten healing. Analgesics and topical anesthetics may be prescribed for pain.

NURSING CARE of the Patient with Herpes Simplex

Nursing care consists primarily of patient education about the nature of the herpes simplex infection and its treatment and prevention. Emphasize that the condition is contagious and tends to recur. Prevention of sexually transmitted herpes simplex is discussed in Chapter 49. This section focuses on HSV type 1.

FIGURE 50-9 Herpes simplex lesions.

Assessment

The health history describes the development of the herpetic lesions. Sexual contacts are documented so that those persons can be advised of the need for medical evaluation. A complete medical history is taken with particular attention to disorders or medications that might suppress the immune response. The physical examination includes a careful inspection of the lesions. The examiner should wear gloves to avoid direct contact with lesions.

Nursing Diagnoses, Goals, and Outcome Criteria: Herpes Simplex	
NURSING DIAGNOSES	GOALS AND OUTCOME CRITERIA
Acute Pain related to lesions	Pain relief: patient statement of pain relief, relaxed expression
Ineffective Coping related to anticipated recurrent lesions, embarrassment	Effective coping: patient statement of ability to cope with condition
Ineffective Therapeutic Regimen Management related to inadequate knowledge of disease, treatment, and risk of transmission	Effective Management: patient describes self-care, follows plan of care, takes precautions to protect partner

Interventions
Acute Pain

Document patient reports of pain. Administer analgesics and topical anesthetics as ordered, or instruct the patient in self-medication. Compresses saturated with astringent solutions such as Burow's solution are sometimes ordered.

Ineffective Coping

Explore the patient's knowledge and concerns about HSV type 1. Lesions on the face may be especially distressing because they are so obvious. Demonstrate acceptance of the patient's feelings, and provide factual information to enable the patient to cope with the condition.

Ineffective Therapeutic Regimen Management

Topical and oral drugs may be ordered. Instruct the patient in use of the drugs. Stress that HSV remains in a dormant state in the body after the initial infection. Periodic recurrences are expected and may be triggered by stresses, including emotional distress, fever, trauma, sunburn, or fatigue. The patient may be able to identify personal triggers and try to avoid or minimize them. Recurrent episodes are typically less severe than the initial one.

Pharmacology Capsule

Acyclovir (Zovirax) does not cure herpes simplex virus infections. Patients still can transmit the infection to others despite antiviral therapy.

To prevent transmission of the infection to others, advise the patient to avoid oral contact while the lesions are present. The patient should exercise good hand washing and avoid touching the lesions. Immunosuppressed patients are especially susceptible to herpes infections and must be protected from infected people.

Herpes Zoster

Etiology and Risk Factors

Herpes zoster infection is commonly called *shingles.* It is caused by the varicella-zoster virus, the same organism that causes chickenpox. In some people who have had chickenpox, the virus remains latent (alive but inactive) in nerve tissue until the infection is activated in the form of shingles. The first symptoms are pain, itching, and heightened sensitivity along a nerve pathway, followed by the formation of vesicles in the area. When the skin is affected, crusts form (Fig. 50-10). When the mucous membranes are affected, ulcers develop. The lesions typically last approximately 2 weeks. The infection is contagious to people who have not had previous exposure to the virus.

Older adults are especially susceptible to complications, which include postherpetic neuralgia, trigeminal herpes zoster (affecting the facial and acoustic nerves), and ophthalmic involvement. With postherpetic neuralgia, pain and itching may persist for years. Immunosuppressed people are at greater risk for herpes zoster infections and may have very serious systemic complications.

Medical Diagnosis

A diagnosis of herpes zoster infection usually can be made on the basis of the health history and physical examination findings. The diagnosis can be confirmed by a Tzanck smear or a viral culture of material from a lesion.

Medical Treatment

Herpes zoster infection is treated with antiviral agents. Available drugs include acyclovir, famciclovir, valacyclovir, and foscarnet. Oral treatment is effective for most patients. However, the intravenous route is used for persons who have impaired immune system function. Treatment is most effective

FIGURE **50-10** Herpes zoster lesions ("shingles").

if initiated within 72 hours of the onset of the rash. Wet dressings soaked in Burow's solution may be ordered to loosen crusts, decrease oozing, and soothe the affected areas. Pain may be treated with analgesics and sedatives. After crusts form, a topical antibiotic ointment may be ordered two or three times a day. Systemic corticosteroids seem to be helpful in reducing pain and may or may not decrease the risk of herpetic neuralgia.

Postherpetic neuralgia is treated with a variety of analgesics, anticonvulsant drugs, and antidepressants. Topical anti-inflammatory and anesthetic drugs may be applied. Other methods that may be tried to relieve pain are transcutaneous electrical nerve stimulation, nerve blocks, and acupuncture.

NURSING CARE *of the Patient with Herpes Zoster*

Assessment

The history of the patient's present illness should be described. A complete medical history is needed to identify conditions or treatments that might cause the patient to have a reduced immune response. The effect of the symptoms on the patient's life should be explored. If this is a recurrent infection, the patient's understanding of the condition should be evaluated. In the physical examination, the distribution and appearance of the lesions should be documented.

Nursing Diagnoses, Goals, and Outcome Criteria: Herpes Zoster	
NURSING DIAGNOSES	GOALS AND OUTCOME CRITERIA
Impaired Skin Integrity related to lesions	Improved skin integrity: absence of vesicles and pruritus
Acute Pain related to lesions, inflammation, or postherpetic neuralgia	Pain relief: patient statement of pain relief, relaxed manner
Ineffective Coping related to long-term pain associated with postherpetic neuralgia	Effective coping: patient uses strategies to cope with acute and chronic symptoms

Interventions

Impaired Skin Integrity

Inspect the lesions each day. Apply cool medicated compresses and administer antipruritic agents as ordered. Individuals who have not had chickenpox are susceptible to herpes simplex infection. They should avoid contact with the lesions.

Acute Pain

Administer prescribed analgesics and antiviral medications, or instruct the patient in self-medication. Follow up to determine the effectiveness of the drugs in relieving pain. Inform the physician if the patient's pain persists despite medication.

Ineffective Coping

Emotional support is especially important for the patient who has chronic pain. Management of chronic pain is discussed in detail in Chapter 15. To promote healing, prevent transmission, and support coping, provide information about herpes zoster: cause, course, treatment, and communicability. Advise the patient that the condition is communicable to people who have never been exposed to chickenpox.

Necrotizing Fasciitis

Necrotizing fasciitis is an infection of the deep fascial structures under the skin. Both aerobic and anaerobic organisms may be present, including *Streptococcus, Staphylococcus, Peptostreptococcus, Bacteroides,* and *Clostridium* species. The organisms excrete enzymes that destroy tissue, including blood vessels that supply the affected area. Deprived of blood flow, tissue necrosis occurs.

Necrotizing fasciitis should be suspected when a patient has a small external wound with evidence of larger underlying inflammation. The infection may progress rapidly with loss of large amounts of tissue and can result in death Treatment involves extensive débridement, intravenous and topical antibiotics, and eventual skin grafting.

Other Infections

A number of skin infections can occur in addition to those discussed in this chapter. Some of the more common conditions (impetigo, folliculitis, furuncles, carbuncles, erysipelas, cellulitis, warts) are presented in Figure 50-11 and Table 50-3.

INFESTATIONS

Lice and scabies infestations are described in Table 50-4. Pediculosis is illustrated in Figure 50-12.

FIGURE 50-11 **A,** Folliculitis. **B,** Furuncle and abscess. **C,** Tinea corporis.

Table 50-3 | *Additional Skin Infections*

INFECTION	CAUSE	SIGNS AND SYMPTOMS	TREATMENT
Impetigo	Group A streptococci	Vesicle or pustule that ruptures, leaving a thick crust	Antibiotic therapy: erythromycin or dicloxacillin
Folliculitis	*Staphylococcus aureus*	Inflamed hair follicles with white pustules	Warm compresses, topical antibiotics
Furuncle (boil)	*Staphylococcus aureus*	Inflamed skin and subcutaneous tissue with deep, inflamed nodules	Warm compresses, topical antibiotics
Carbuncle	*Staphylococcus aureus*	Clustered, interconnected furuncles	Systemic antibiotics, incision and drainage
Erysipelas	β-hemolytic group A streptococci	Round or oval patches that enlarge and spread; redness, swelling, tenderness, warmth	Systemic antibiotics, usually penicillin
Cellulitis	Usually *Streptococcus pyogenes*	Local tenderness and redness at first, then malaise, chills, and fever; site becomes more erythematous; nodules and vesicles may form; vesicles may rupture, releasing purulent material identified by culture	For *S. pyogenes*, penicillin, a cephalosporin, or vancomycin; other antibiotics for other organisms
Verruca (wart)	Human papillomavirus	At first, small shiny lesions; they enlarge and become rough	Electrical current to destroy lesion followed by removal with curette, cryotherapy (freezing), topical medications

Table 50-4 *Infestations of the Skin*

INFECTION	CAUSE	SIGNS AND SYMPTOMS	TREATMENT
Scabies	*Sarcoptes scabiei*, sometimes called "itch mite"	Thin, red lines on skin; itching	Topical scabicide applied and repeated 1 wk later; clothing and bed linens washed in hot water or dry cleaned
Lice	*Pediculus humanus* or *Phthirus pubis*	Itching of hairy areas of body (head, pubis); nits (eggs) seen as tiny white particles attached to hair shafts	Head lice: pediculicide shampoo applied to dry hair, then hair combed with fine-toothed comb to remove nits and dead lice; also treat brushes and combs Body or pubic lice: apply pediculicide lotion as directed For both sites: wash clothing and bed linens in hot water or have dry cleaned; usually need to treat all members of household Assure patient that infestations are common and not caused by unsanitary living

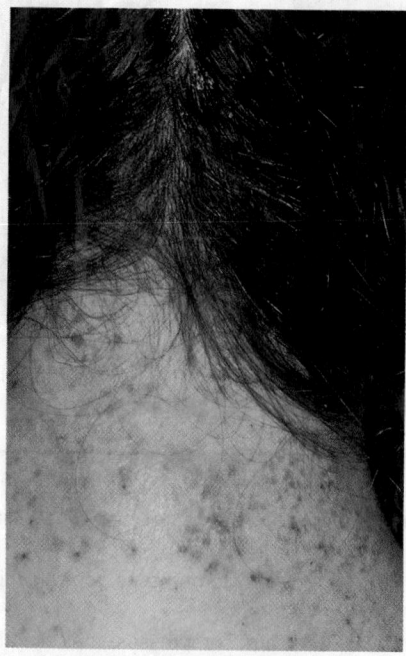

FIGURE **50-12** Pediculosis

PEMPHIGUS

Pemphigus is a chronic autoimmune condition in which bullae (blisters) develop on the face, back, chest, groin, and umbilicus. The blisters rupture easily, releasing a foul-smelling drainage. Potassium permanganate baths, Domeboro solution, and oatmeal products with oil may be ordered to soothe the affected areas, reduce odor, and decrease the risk of infection. Treatments may include corticosteroids, other immunosuppressants, and oral or topical antibiotics. Patients with extensive skin loss require the same care as burn patients (see the Nursing Care of the Patient with a Burn Injury section on p. 1149).

CANCER

Skin cancers are classified as nonmelanoma or melanoma. Nonmelanoma skin cancers include basal cell carcinoma and squamous cell carcinoma. Risk factors for skin cancer are sun exposure, fair skin with freckling, light-colored hair and eyes, male gender, cigarette smoking, and a tendency to sunburn easily. The risk of nonmelanoma skin cancers increases with the total amount of sun exposure. The risk of melanoma increases with the severity of sunburn. The role of tanning beds in skin cancer is still under study. However the U.S. Preventive Services Task Force recommends that they be avoided as one strategy to reduce the risk of skin cancer.

A discussion of skin cancers begins with actinic keratosis, which is actually considered a precancerous condition. Cutaneous T-cell lymphoma (Fig. 50-13) and Kaposi's sarcoma are mentioned here as well because they are manifested by skin lesions. The reader is referred to Chapter 25 for detailed nursing care of the patient with cancer.

Skin cancers may be suspected because of the lesion appearance and location. The diagnosis is confirmed by microscopic examination of cells obtained from the excised lesion or a tissue sample obtained by biopsy.

 What Does Culture Have to Do with Skin Cancer?

Whites have a higher incidence of skin cancer than either African Americans or American Indians. Patients with light skin who live in sunny climates should protect themselves from excessive exposure and routinely assess for skin changes.

FIGURE **50-13** Skin cancers. **A,** Actinic keratosis (a premalignant lesion). **B,** Basal cell carcinoma. **C,** Squamous cell carcinoma. **D,** Malignant melanoma.

Actinic Keratosis

Actinic keratoses are precancerous lesions most often found on the face, neck, forearms, and backs of the hands—all areas exposed to sunlight. They may become malignant if not treated. Actinic keratoses are most common among white older adults. They typically appear as papules or plaques of irregular shape. The hard scale on the lesion may shed and reappear (see Fig. 50-13).

A number of treatments for actinic keratosis exist, including drug therapy, cryotherapy, electrodesiccation, and surgical excision. Drugs used to treat actinic keratosis include topical 5-fluorouracil and diclofenac sodium. Another choice is topical aminolevulinic acid with blue light photoactivation after 14 to 18 hours. Topical treatments cause irritation and photosensitivity. Therefore patients should be cautioned to avoid direct sun exposure during treatment. Cryotherapy is the use of liquid nitrogen to freeze and destroy the lesion. The procedure may cause a blister to form but is only slightly painful. Electrodesiccation is the use of electrical current to destroy the lesion, which is then scraped off. The patient is given a local anesthetic. Surgical excision may be done in several ways, and the patient may or may not have sutures.

Nonmelanoma Skin Cancer

Basal Cell Carcinoma

Basal cell carcinomas usually begin as painless, nodular lesions that have a pearly appearance (see Fig. 50-13). They are thought to be related to sun exposure. Basal cell carcinomas grow slowly and rarely metastasize. Nevertheless, they should be removed because they can cause local tissue destruction. Basal cell carcinomas are treated with surgical excision, Mohs' micrographic excision, electrodissection and curettage, cryotherapy, radiation, or drugs that are applied topically or injected into the lesion. Mohs' surgery is a technique in which microscopic tissue samples are studied to determine the margins of the malignancy.

Squamous Cell Carcinoma

Squamous cell carcinomas may appear as scaly ulcers or raised lesions. There are usually no clear lesion margins (see Fig. 50-13). Like basal cell carcinomas, they most often develop on sun-exposed areas including the lips and in the oral cavity. Squamous cell carcinomas are most often caused by overuse of tobacco and alcohol. Unlike basal cell carcinomas, they grow rapidly and metastasize. Treatment may include surgical excision, cryotherapy, and radiation therapy.

Melanoma

A malignant melanoma arises from the pigment-producing cells in the skin. It is the most serious form of skin cancer because it can be fatal if it metastasizes. Melanomas can be found anywhere on the body, not just sun-exposed areas. Typical melanomas have irregular borders and uneven coloration (see Fig. 50-13). Many are very dark, but some are light in color. They usually begin as a tan macule that enlarges. Malignant melanomas are removed surgically with Mohs' technique often used. This approach is meant to avoid leaving malignant tissue around the excised lesion. A wide area around a melanoma is usually excised. Chemotherapy and immunotherapy also may be employed.

Cutaneous T-Cell Lymphoma

Cutaneous T-cell lymphoma is characterized by the migration of malignant T cells to the skin. There are several manifestations of cutaneous T-cell lymphoma including mycosis fungoides and Sézary syndrome. At first, cutaneous T-cell lymphoma may resemble eczema, with macular lesions appearing on areas protected from the sun. They form tumors, enlarge, and can spread to distant sites. When confined to the skin, this type of lymphoma can be cured with topical chemotherapy, systemic psoralens with UVA, and/or superficial radiotherapy.

Kaposi's Sarcoma

Kaposi's sarcoma is a malignancy of the blood vessels. It is manifested by red, blue, or purple macules accompanied by pain, itching, and swelling. The lesions appear first on the legs and then on the upper body, face, and mouth. They enlarge to form large plaques that may drain. Kaposi's sarcoma may be seen in patients with human immunodeficiency virus infection, but it is not confined to this group. Local lesions may be excised or injected with intralesional chemotherapy. Systemic lesions are treated with chemotherapy, immune therapy, and radiotherapy. Unfortunately, treatment results have been discouraging (see Chapter 34).

DISORDERS OF THE NAILS

The two major conditions affecting the nails are infections (fungal or bacterial) and inflammation caused by ingrown nails. Infections are usually indicated by redness, swelling, and pain around the margin of the nail. They are treated with warm soaks and topical or systemic anti-infectives. Incision and drainage may be necessary.

An ingrown toenail causes painful inflammation at the distal corner of the nail. It is usually caused by trimming the nail too short at the corners or wearing shoes that are too tight on the toes. The ingrown nail should be protected from pressure as it grows out. Warm soaks may be soothing. Sometimes surgical excision of the ingrown portion of the nail is needed.

NURSING CARE *of the Patient with a Nail Disorder*

Nail disorders do not often require inpatient care unless there are complications. However, nurses may be the first to detect nail problems and often teach patients how to prevent or treat them.

Assessment

The health history should document the diagnoses of diabetes mellitus or peripheral vascular disease. In the physical examination, inspect around the nails for redness, swelling, or pain. Inspect the extremities for lesions and abnormal color, and palpate for warmth and peripheral pulses.

Nursing Diagnoses, Goals, and Outcome Criteria:
Nail Disorder

NURSING DIAGNOSES	GOALS AND OUTCOME CRITERIA
Risk for Injury related to improper nail trimming, poor peripheral circulation	Decreased risk of injury: properly trimmed nails Absence of injury: no evidence of inflammation (redness, swelling, pain, excess warmth)
Ineffective Therapeutic Regimen Management related to lack of understanding of proper nail care and treatment of nail disorders	Effective management of therapeutic measures: patient demonstrates correct nail care and prescribed treatments

Interventions

Teach patients how to trim their nails correctly and the importance of properly fitting shoes. Toenails should be cut straight across and even with the end of the toe. Show patients with peripheral vascular disease or diabetes mellitus how to inspect their feet daily, and advise them to seek medical attention for any abnormality. A seemingly minor foot infection can have drastic consequences, including amputation, for

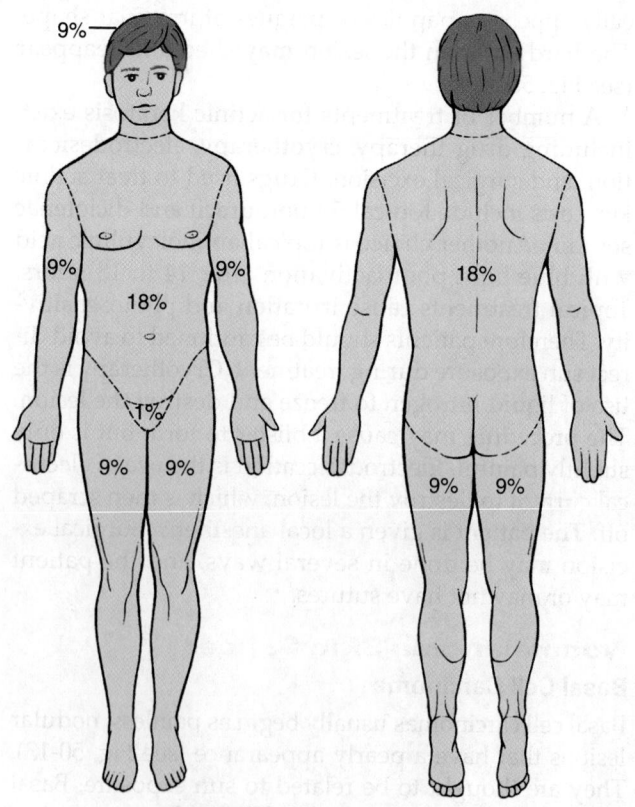

FIGURE 50-14 Rule of nines.

the patient with poor circulation. If the patient cannot care for the feet adequately, seek a referral to a podiatrist.

BURNS

Burns are tissue injuries caused by heat. Depending on the source of the injury, the burn is described as thermal (flame, flash, scalding liquids, hot objects), chemical, electrical, radiation, or inhalation. Burns are a leading cause of accidental death despite improved survival rates attributed to tremendous advances in the care of burn patients. Sadly, 75% of all burn injuries could have been prevented.

Emergency treatment of the burn patient is discussed in Chapter 16. Acute care of seriously burned patients is an advanced specialty that is beyond the scope of this book; therefore this section provides a limited discussion of nursing care of the patient after reaching a medical facility.

CLASSIFICATION OF BURNS

Burns are classified by the size and depth of the tissue injury. It is important periodically to reevaluate the burn because evidence of extent of injury can change over time. Extent is often defined as the percentage of body surface area affected. To describe depth, a burn is classified as *partial thickness* or *full thickness*, depending on the layers of tissue injured.

Burn Size

Burn size may be estimated using the *rule of nines* or the Lund and Browder method. The rule of nines estimates the percentage of body surface area burned. Areas of the body are assigned percentage values of nine or multiples of nine (Fig. 50-14). The percentages are totaled to estimate burn size. For example, in an adult, if one arm and hand are burned, the burn size is estimated as 9.5%.

The Lund and Browder method also estimates the percentage of body surface burned, but the body is divided into smaller segments. Different percentages are assigned to body parts depending on the patient's age. This is more accurate than the rule of nines because it accounts for differences in body proportions. For example, the head of an infant is 19% of the total body surface area, whereas the head of an adult is only 7% of the total body surface area. Figure 50-15 is an example of the Lund and Browder chart as modified by Berkow. A quick method of estimating percent of body surface burned is to use the patient's palm. The size of the palm represents one percent.

Burn Depth

Partial-thickness burns are sometimes called *first-* or *second-degree* burns. A burn affecting only the epidermis is a *superficial* (or *first-degree*) burn. A burn that affects the epidermis and the dermis is a *superficial* or *deep partial-thickness* (or *second-degree*) burn, depending on the tissues affected. Burns that extend into even

Body area	0-1 Years	1-4 Years	5-9 Years	10-14 Years	15 Years	Adult
Head	19	17	13	11	9	7
Neck	2	2	2	2	2	2
Ant. trunk	13	13	13	13	13	13
Post. trunk	13	13	13	13	13	13
R. buttock	2.5	2.5	2.5	2.5	2.5	2.5
L. buttock	2.5	2.5	2.5	2.5	2.5	2.5
Genitalia	1	1	1	1	1	1
R. u. arm	4	4	4	4	4	4
L. u. arm	4	4	4	4	4	4
R. l. arm	3	3	3	3	3	3
L. l. arm	3	3	3	3	3	3
R. hand	2.5	2.5	2.5	2.5	2.5	2.5
L. hand	2.5	2.5	2.5	2.5	2.5	2.5
R. thigh	5.5	6.5	8	8.5	9	9.5
L. thigh	5.5	6.5	8	8.5	9	9.5
R. l. leg	5	5	5.5	6	6.5	7
L. l. leg	5	5	5.5	6	6.5	7
R. foot	3.5	3.5	3.5	3.5	3.5	3.5
L. foot	3.5	3.5	3.5	3.5	3.5	3.5

FIGURE **50-15** Berkow's adaptation of Lund and Browder method of estimating body surface area burned.

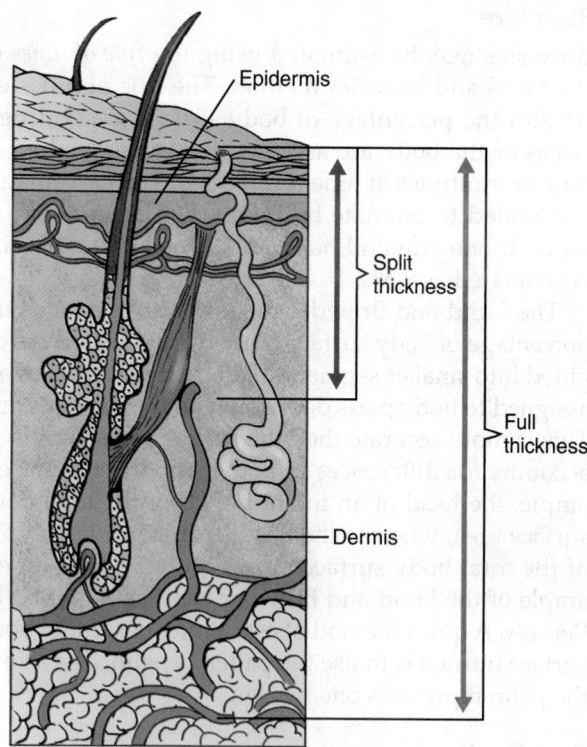

FIGURE **50-16** Burn classification by depth.

deeper tissue layers are called *full-thickness* (or *third-degree, fourth-degree*) burns (Figs. 50-16 and 50-17).

Superficial Burns. A superficial burn, like a sunburn, is pink to red and painful.

Superficial Partial-Thickness Burns. Superficial partial-thickness burns are painful and usually appear blistered or weepy and pale to red or pink. A severe sunburn can be a superficial partial-thickness burn.

Deep Partial-Thickness Burns. A deep partial-thickness burn is characterized by large, thick-walled blisters or by edema and weeping, cherry-red, exposed dermis. It is painful and sensitive to cold air.

Full-Thickness Burns. Full-thickness burns involve the epidermis, dermis, and underlying tissues, including fat, muscle, and bone. Full-thickness burns typically appear dry, feel leathery, and may be red, white, brown, or black. The burned tissue usually lacks sensation.

Burn Severity

Burn severity is based on size, depth, location, age, general health status, and mechanism of injury. Various criteria are used to define major burns. The American Burn Association criteria for a major burn in an adult are the following:

1. Burn size: 25% or more body surface area for people younger than 40 years; 20% or more body surface area for people older than 40 years
2. Disfiguring or disabling injuries to the face, eyes, ears, hands, feet, or perineum
3. High-voltage electrical burn injury
4. Inhalation injury
5. Major trauma in addition to the burn

PATHOPHYSIOLOGY OF BURN INJURY

Local Effects

Burn-injured tissue releases chemicals that cause increased capillary permeability, which permits plasma to leak into the tissues. Injury to cell membranes permits excess sodium to enter the cell and allows potassium to escape into the extracellular compartment. These shifts in fluids and electrolytes cause local edema and a decrease in cardiac output. Fluid evaporates through the wound surface, further contributing to the declining blood volume. Eighteen to 36 hours after a burn injury, capillary permeability begins to normalize and reabsorption of edema fluid begins. Cardiac output returns to normal and then increases to meet increased metabolic demands.

Systemic Effects

Fluid Balance. The shift of plasma proteins from the capillaries may result in hypoproteinemia, which causes fluid to shift from the bloodstream to the extracellular tissue. This shift decreases blood volume and causes generalized edema in the early post-burn period. Blood is shunted from the kidneys to compensate for the fluid volume deficit, and urine output falls. These fluid shifts, if not corrected, result in decreased tissue perfusion and decreased cardiac output that may lead to hypovolemic shock. Fluid resuscitation is critical during the first 24 to 48 hours. Intake and output should be strictly monitored to prevent shock.

As the capillaries recover and edema fluid is reabsorbed, the patient's blood volume increases. If kidney function is adequate, urine output increases to prevent hypervolemia.

Gastrointestinal Function. Blood flow to the intestines decreases, and an ileus may develop. Some patients have stress ulcers, sometimes called Curling's ulcers, after severe burns. They are, therefore, routinely treated with antacids to neutralize gastric acid and H_2-receptor blockers to reduce gastric acid secretion.

Immune System. Because immunity is depressed after a serious burn, the patient is less able to resist infection. The loss of the protective skin barrier also puts the patient at risk for life-threatening infection.

Respiratory System. The burn patient may suffer inhalation injuries, including carbon monoxide poisoning, smoke poisoning, and thermal damage. Inhalation injury occurs with flame burns or from being trapped in an enclosed space filled with smoke. Suspect inhalation injury if the patient has facial burns, redness and swelling of the pharynx, restlessness, cough, dyspnea, or sooty sputum. Carbon monoxide displaces oxygen on hemoglobin, so the blood is unable to transport oxygen to the tissues. The patient will show signs of hypoxia and die if the condition is not corrected. See Chapter 16 for additional discussion of carbon monoxide poisoning. Smoke poisoning is the result of inhaling combustion by-products. Thermal damage to the lower airway is rare but can

FIGURE 50-17 Burn depth. **A,** Partial thickness ("second degree"). **B,** Full thickness ("third degree"). **C,** Full thickness ("fourth degree").

happen if the patient was unconscious or inhaled live steam. With inhalation injury, pulmonary edema develops that may progress to adult respiratory distress syndrome.

Myocardial Depression. There is evidence of myocardial depression in the early post-burn period.

Psychological Effects. Psychological responses to burn injuries are highly individual. Four stages of psychological response have been identified: impact, retreat or withdrawal, acknowledgment, and reconstruction.

STAGES OF BURN INJURY

Care of the burn patient is often described in terms of three stages: emergent, acute, and rehabilitation. The emergent stage begins with the injury and ends when fluid shifts have stabilized. The acute stage begins with fluid stabilization. Some sources mark the end of the acute stage when all but 10% of the burn wounds are closed, but others define the acute stage as extending until all wounds are closed. The rehabilitation stage follows the acute stage and lasts as long as efforts continue to promote improvement or adjustment. There is some overlap between the acute and rehabilitation stages because nursing care in the acute stage can significantly affect the potential for rehabilitation. In reality, rehabilitation starts as soon as the patient stabilizes. Physical therapy and occupational therapy should be consulted immediately when the patient is admitted.

MEDICAL TREATMENT IN THE EMERGENT STAGE

In the emergency department, the staff first assesses airway, breathing, and circulation and then determines whether the patient has injuries in addition to the burn. If inhalation injury is suspected, oxygen therapy is started. The patient may require intubation if the airway is compromised. Intravenous lines are established to begin fluid resuscitation and to provide emergency vascular access. An indwelling urinary catheter and a nasogastric tube are usually inserted. Blood is drawn for baseline laboratory studies (hematocrit, electrolytes, and blood gases, if indicated). Tetanus prophylaxis may be administered. Pain is assessed, and analgesics are ordered. The wound is then cleaned, débrided, and inspected. Unless the patient is at a major burn center, the burns may not be débrided immediately. If the patient is to be transported, the burns are covered with clean sheets.

Once the initial care is completed, the patient with serious burns is transferred to a burn specialty care unit or a critical care unit. Intravenous fluid therapy is an essential aspect of care during the first few days of burn treatment. Several formulas are used to select the volumes and solutions to be administered. Volume is based on the patient's weight and extent of injury. For the first 24 hours, intravenous fluids may consist of various combinations of electrolyte, colloid, and dextrose solutions. However, specific formulas vary among specialty care units. For example, some formulas prescribe *only* electrolyte solutions in the first 24 hours.

For the second 24 hours, volume is usually decreased based on urine output. Fluids then consist of different combinations of electrolyte, colloid, and dextrose solutions. Some formulas omit electrolyte solutions in the second 24 hours.

In addition to fluids, medical care may include antibiotic therapy and surgical procedures.

WOUND CARE

Wound care after a burn injury is intended to promote healing, prevent infection, control heat loss, retain function, and minimize disfigurement. Burn wounds may be treated by the open or closed method. The method of wound care is based, in part, on the state of the wound. The open method involves the use of topical antimicrobials but no dressings. Open care is less restrictive and simpler than closed care but provides greater opportunity for loss of fluid and heat through the wound surface. Closed care uses topical medications covered by dressings. Because some areas of the wound may be deeper than other areas, it is not unusual to see open care for some of the patient's wounds and closed care for others. Examples of topical medications that may be used are silver sulfadiazine (Silvadene) and mafenide acetate (Sulfamylon). To prevent tetanus, a tetanus toxoid booster is usually given if the patient has not been immunized within the past 5 years. Patients who have never been immunized are given tetanus immune globulin and the first in a series of tetanus toxoid.

For clean partial-thickness wounds that will heal without grafting, temporary wound coverings often are used. Temporary wound coverings include amniotic membranes, grafts from cadavers or pigs, and a number of synthetic materials that promote wound healing or protect donor or graft sites. Grafted areas in need of protection are often covered by temporary wound coverings as well. Graft sites are also treated with negative pressure wound therapy. This assists grafts from shifting during the first 72 hours. Donor sites also are treated with a variety of products, including fine-mesh gauze and synthetic and biosynthetic products. Donor sites are more painful than graft sites due to the exposure of nerve endings.

Débridement

A partial-thickness burn may blister, peel, and heal with minimal long-term effects. A full-thickness burn, however, is often covered by a thick, leathery layer of burned tissue (eschar) that shelters microorganisms and inhibits healing. Eschar must be removed before healing can take place. Further, if eschar encircles a limb, it may need to be incised to permit tissue swelling without compromising circulation. Débridement is the removal of debris and necrotic (dead) tissue from a wound. In the case of a burn wound, débridement includes removal of eschar. Débridement may be ac-

complished by mechanical means (using scissors and forceps), surgical excision, or the use of enzymes. Enzymatic débridement is the use of topical medications containing enzymes capable of dissolving necrotic tissue. These substances are applied directly to the wound but should not be applied to wounds that communicate with major body cavities or to exposed nerves. Enzymatic agents may cause pain and bleeding.

Skin Grafting

A burn wound may be covered using the patient's own skin, called an *autograft*. The graft is usually taken from the thigh or buttocks using a tool called a *dermatome*. The thickness of the graft determines whether it is a split-thickness or a full-thickness graft. If a thin layer of skin is used, it is considered a split-thickness graft. A split-thickness graft may be a sheet graft (an intact section of skin) or a meshed graft. A meshed graft has multiple tiny slits that allow the skin to be stretched to cover a larger area. The slits also allow for wound exudate to be absorbed by the cover dressing. Grafts vary in size, with the smallest being pinch and postage stamp grafts. Larger grafts may be needed to cover all or part of the burn.

For very deep burns and burns of the face, neck, or hands, a full-thickness graft may be preferred. A full-thickness graft includes skin and subcutaneous tissue and provides better cosmetic results. Another type of full-thickness graft is a pedicle or flap graft, in which one end of a section or tube of donor tissue is sutured to the recipient site while another section remains attached to the donor site. This type of graft continues to receive blood from the donor site. Once the graft "takes" or attaches to the recipient site, the pedicle or flap is cut free from the donor site.

After grafting, the recipient site is inspected for bleeding under the graft that could interfere with survival of the graft. The area is immobilized for 3 to 7 days to permit attachment of the graft to the wound base. Splints, traction, and restraints may be used for immobilization. This will vary with the institution. In most burn centers, the grafts are inspected on day 3 to assess the degree of attachment. The graft is again inspected on day 5, and a determination is made about removal of staples. By day 7, all staples should be removed. After an autograft, the patient's donor site requires care as well. The donor site is usually covered with fine-mesh gauze or synthetic dressings and bandages. The dressings are usually removed 24 hours after surgery to allow the site to air dry. If the donor site is still wet, a heat lamp may be used to assist in the drying process. As the donor site dries, the fine-mesh gauze or xeroform will begin to lift off the skin. The excess material is trimmed as it lifts off.

Scarring

The formation of burn scars can be minimized by the use of pressure dressings in the early stages of care, hypoxia (restlessness, tachypnea), excess fluid volume (bounding pulse, hypertension), deficient fluid volume (tachycardia, hypotension), hypovolemia (hypotension, tachycardia), or infection (fever, tachycardia). Height and weight are measured if the patient is stable enough.

Throughout the examination, the skin is inspected for burn wounds and other lesions. Wound color and the presence of eschar should be noted. Intact skin should be palpated for temperature and turgor. Chest expansion should be observed, and the lungs should be auscultated for wheezing, stridor, or atelectasis. The apical pulse should be auscultated for rate and rhythm. The abdomen is assessed for active bowel sounds and distention. The extremities are inspected for injury and deformity. Range-of-motion assessment is delayed if an extremity is immobilized.

FIGURE **50-18** Antiscar pressure garment minimizes the hypertrophic scarring that is common after burn injuries.

followed by the use of custom-fitted garments that apply continuous pressure. These garments are worn 23 hours a day and may be prescribed for as long as 2 years (Fig. 50-18). Explain to the patient that the garments need to be tight. Massage of the area with battery-operated devices also helps reduce the appearance of scars.

NURSING CARE *of the Patient with Burn Injury*

Assessment

When the patient is stabilized, a complete assessment should be done. As priorities change, additional relevant data will be needed.

Health History

The history of the present illness describes the circumstances surrounding the burn injury. The past medical history documents any chronic diseases, surgeries, or hospitalizations. Identify medications and allergies. Take a family history even though it is not specific to burn injuries because it may alert the staff to other problems. The review of systems detects current problems with each body system. In the functional assessment, the patient's habits and lifestyle, roles and responsibilities, stressors, and coping strategies are described.

Physical Examination

The physical examination begins with vital signs. The examiner should be alert for abnormalities that suggest

Nursing Diagnoses, Goals, and Outcome Criteria: Burns

Depending on the severity and type of burn, nursing diagnoses for the patient with burns may include those listed in this table. The first two are most likely to occur in the emergent stage; the remaining diagnoses may be made in the emergent, acute, or rehabilitation stage.

Nursing Diagnoses	Goals and Outcome Criteria
Decreased Cardiac Output related to hypovolemia secondary to shift of fluid from vascular to extracellular compartment	Normal cardiac output: pulse and blood pressure consistent with patient norms
Excess Fluid Volume related to changes in capillary permeability and accumulation of fluid in body tissues	Normal fluid balance: edema decreasing or absent, increased urine output
Acute Pain related to tissue trauma of burn injury	Pain relief: patient statement of pain relief, more relaxed manner
Risk for Infection related to loss of protective skin barrier	Absence of infection: normal body temperature and white blood cell count, negative wound cultures
Hypothermia related to impaired heat-regulating ability of injured skin	Normal body temperature: temperature within patient norms
Imbalanced Nutrition: Less Than Body Requirements related to high metabolic demands	Adequate nutrition: stable body weight
Impaired Physical Mobility related to contractures, therapeutic immobilization, pain	Adaptation to physical limitations: minimal contractures, clear breath sounds, bowel movements at least every 2 to 3 days

Continued

Ineffective Coping related to possible disfigurement, dysfunction, fear of death

Effective patient coping: positive patient statements about future; participates in rehabilitation efforts

Compromised Family Coping related to uncertain outcome, fear of patient death, and altered family function

Effective family coping: positive family statements about the future; family interest in ways to help patient's recovery

Interventions

Decreased Cardiac Output

The risk of decreased cardiac output is greatest in the emergent stage when fluid has shifted from the blood to the extracellular compartment. If blood volume is not maintained, the patient's blood pressure falls and tissue perfusion is impaired. To monitor cardiac output, record the patient's vital signs and fluid intake and output. Signs of decreased cardiac output include hypotension, tachycardia, and decreased urine output. Inadequate tissue perfusion may be manifested by cool, pale or cyanotic skin, restlessness, and confusion. Administer intravenous fluids as ordered with close, continuous monitoring of fluid status. Strict monitoring of intake and output is essential. The patient may also need invasive lines, such as a pulmonary artery catheter, to monitor cardiac output.

Excess Fluid Volume

Excess fluid volume may result from the retention of fluid in the extracellular compartment. As capillary permeability returns to normal and fluid is reabsorbed, the patient's blood volume increases. If the patient's kidneys can eliminate the excess fluid efficiently, the patient suffers no ill effects from the increasing blood volume. There is a risk, however, that the patient's circulatory system may be unable to adapt to the increased volume. This puts the patient at risk for heart failure.

Monitor the patient's vital signs for hypertension, dyspnea, and full, bounding pulse. Measure urine output and compare with fluid intake. Administer intravenous fluids as ordered and monitor closely. Document data collected for the assessments.

Acute Pain

Partial-thickness wounds are typically very painful. Full-thickness burns lack sensation because of the destruction of the superficial nerves. However, burns are often uneven in depth, so patients with full-thickness burns often have pain as well. The burn patient is given opioid analgesics such as morphine as ordered. An opioid agonist such as fentanyl (Sublimaze) may be given intravenously or orally before performing painful wound care. If given orally, administer the medication 45 minutes before the procedure. If given intravenously, administer the drug 5 to 10 minutes ahead of time. The intramuscular route is not routinely used until fluid shifts have stabilized, because absorption is less reliable. Nonsteroidal anti-inflammatory drugs also may be prescribed. Pain is aggravated by anxiety, so use measures to reduce fear and anxiety in the management of pain. Document patient response to interventions. Additional nursing measures for pain are described in Chapter 15.

Risk for Infection

The burn patient, without protective skin, is at great risk for infection. Routinely monitor for signs of local infection (pus, foul odor, increased redness) and systemic infection (fever, increased white blood cell count). Infection can come from the staff, visitors, the environment, and the patient's own body. Specific infection control measures vary with the agency. Strict hand washing should be practiced by the patient and all who enter the room. Body hair around wounds is usually shaved or cut to prevent wound contamination. Do *not* shave the eyebrows because, if shaved, they tend to grow back in a disorganized pattern. Carry out wound care as ordered or according to routines of the specialty care unit.

Hypothermia

Loss of heat through the burn wound surface places the patient at risk for hypothermia (low body temperature). This is especially problematic for older adults whose ability to maintain body temperature is already compromised because of various age-related changes.

Monitor the patient's tympanic or rectal temperature to detect declining body temperature. Keep the room warm, and use external heat sources as needed. The room temperature should be above 76° F. In a burn intensive care unit, the temperature may be above 85° F. Attempt to limit body surface area exposure during wound care. Body heat loss may be greater if the patient is on an air-fluidized bed, so carefully monitor the temperature of the bed.

Imbalanced Nutrition: Less Than Body Requirements

Healing of a large burn wound requires considerable energy. It is, therefore, critical that adequate nutrition be provided to meet the increased metabolic demands. Consult with the dietitian about the patient's nutritional needs and preferences. Calorie needs may be as much as twice the patient's baseline needs. Regular meals may need to be supplemented with between-meal feedings. Stress to the patient the need for increased intake during the recovery period. Try to create an environment conducive to eating, and encourage the patient to eat all food served. Provide assistance with meals if needed. Some patients require tube feedings or total parenteral nutrition to meet their calorie needs. Encourage the patient to drink protein drinks rather than water. Calorie counts may be done at the bedside to ensure that the patient is consuming enough calories to meet the increased metabolic needs associated with burns.

Impaired Physical Mobility

Patients with burns may have mobility restrictions imposed by the injury or the treatment. The hazards of immobility, including pressure sores, joint contractures, pneumonia and atelectasis, constipation, and urinary infections, are covered in Chapter 21. Monitor range of motion in affected joints, and perform passive or active exercises unless contraindicated. Keep injured limbs in functional positions as much as possible (Fig. 50-19). Also, exercise unaffected joints to maintain flexibility and strength. Impaired mobility may interfere with the patient's ability to participate in his or her own care. Evaluate the ability to provide self-care, and provide assistance as needed. As the patient moves toward recovery, the rehabilitation team helps the patient adapt self-care activities for permanent injuries.

Ineffective Coping

Severe burns can result in disfigurement and loss of function. The patient faces a long and difficult recovery period. The emotional responses of the burn patient are often like those of any grieving person: shock, disbelief, withdrawal, denial, regression, depression, and anger. Demonstrate acceptance of the patient regardless of the emotional state. Provide opportunities for the patient to express his or her thoughts and feelings. The patient may find it helpful to talk to a clinical nurse specialist, counselor, or spiritual adviser. Some patients find support groups helpful in learning to live with their injuries. Encourage the patient to identify and use coping strategies that have been effective in

the past. If effective coping strategies are used, the patient eventually incorporates the physical and functional changes into a new body image.

Compromised Family Coping

A serious burn injury that may require months or years of therapy has a tremendous impact on the family. Significant others must be included in the patient's care. When the family arrives after the injury, the physician or clinical nurse specialist advises them of the patient's injuries, what to expect when they see the patient, and what is being done for the patient. The family should be offered an opportunity to talk with a social worker, clinical nurse specialist, counselor, or spiritual adviser. A social worker or case manager should be assigned to the patient soon after admission.

CONDITIONS TREATED WITH PLASTIC SURGERY

Plastic surgery includes aesthetic (cosmetic) and reconstructive procedures. Aesthetic surgical procedures are performed to improve appearance, whereas reconstructive procedures are done to correct abnormalities. In addition to usual surgical approaches, plastic surgery may include use of flaps and grafts, skin expansion, implants, liposuction, and microvascular surgery.

AESTHETIC SURGERY

In general, aesthetic surgery alters a body feature that is structurally normal but perceived by the patient as unattractive. Examples of aesthetic surgery are

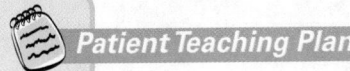

Patient Teaching Plan

Burns

When the patient is acutely ill, patient teaching consists of telling the patient what is being done, why, and what to expect. As the patient stabilizes, the teaching plan should include the following points:

- You can help prevent wound infection by practicing good hygiene and avoiding others with infections.
- Because your nutritional needs are greatly increased as a result of the healing that needs to occur, you need to eat all food provided, including meal supplements.
- Positioning, exercise, and splints help prevent stiffening of joints, skin breakdown, and blood clots in your legs.
- Pain management is possible, so tell the nurse or the physician if your pain is not controlled.
- Protect grafts from pressure and shearing force so they can heal.
- Clothing, makeup, hairpieces, and prostheses can be used to conceal scars and improve appearance.
- Adaptive devices are available to compensate for disabilities.
- Rehabilitation resources will be provided once the acute phase has passed.

FIGURE **50-19** Therapeutic positioning. This patient's arms are extended to prevent flexion contractures. Pressure dressings on legs prevent edema and minimize scarring.

rhytidectomy, blepharoplasty, chin implants, rhinoplasty, abdominoplasty, breast augmentation, and breast reduction. A rhytidectomy, commonly called *a face-lift,* is done to remove facial wrinkles and tighten sagging tissue. A blepharoplasty is the removal of excess tissue around the eyes. It is usually an aesthetic procedure but may be done to improve function if droopy eyelids impair vision. Chin implants are done by placing a prosthesis to correct a receding chin. A rhinoplasty alters the shape or size, or both, of the nose. In an abdominoplasty, excess skin and adipose tissue are removed and the abdominal muscles are tightened.

Breast augmentation is breast enlargement, which may be performed to increase the size of both breasts or to improve breast symmetry. A variety of techniques have been used for breast augmentation. The most common procedure has been to implant a silicone rubber implant filled with saline. Silicone implants are being used again after a 14-year ban because of concerns about possible adverse effects of silicone leakage. Breast reduction decreases breast size and may be requested to improve appearance or body proportion or to eliminate discomfort associated with excessively large breasts. Liposuction is the removal of excess adipose tissue with a suction device, most commonly used on the thighs, abdomen, arms, and buttocks.

RECONSTRUCTIVE SURGERY

A number of procedures may be classified as reconstructive. Reconstructive surgery may be done to repair disfiguring scars, restore body contours after radical surgery like mastectomy, eliminate benign lesions such as birthmarks, restore features damaged by trauma or disease, and correct developmental defects.

 What Does Culture Have to Do with Plastic Surgery?

Because attractiveness is culturally defined, people may seek various procedures that they perceive will increase their attractiveness. Be careful not to impose your views on the patient.

NURSING CARE *of the Patient Having Plastic Surgery*

When working with people who are having plastic surgery, you must be aware of your own biases and feelings. If you view cosmetic procedures as vain or frivolous, you may have difficulty being supportive of patients who choose to have these procedures done. Many factors may motivate people to have aesthetic surgery. Physical appearance is a component of body image and may affect self-esteem. Some people believe that a change in appearance will benefit their personal or professional lives. A person who is very self-conscious about a physical feature can benefit immensely from aesthetic surgery. It is important not to judge the patient's motivation for seeking surgery. It is also important to be alert to the patient's unrealistic expectations for the surgical outcome.

Although each procedure may require some specific nursing interventions, this section addresses general nursing care for the patient having plastic surgery. Some specific procedures are presented in Table 50-5.

PREOPERATIVE NURSING CARE

Many of these procedures may be done in day surgery or short-stay surgical units. Therefore patient preparation emphasizes teaching for self-care. Initial teaching may be done by the physician, office nurse, or staff nurse.

Assessment
Health History

The patient's description of the problem being treated with plastic surgery and what the patient expects the procedure to accomplish should be documented. The past medical history may elicit conditions that might affect wound healing, such as diabetes mellitus, circulatory disorders, and impaired blood coagulation. In the review of systems, the surgical area should receive special attention. For example, if a blepharoplasty is being done, visual acuity should be tested and documented. The functional assessment describes the patient's lifestyle and usual activities, which may require some temporary modification after plastic surgery.

Physical Examination

The routine preoperative physical examination is performed as described in Chapter 17. The condition that is being treated is described. Most plastic surgeons have preoperative photographs made to document the condition. If you take the photograph, be sensitive to the patient's discomfort or embarrassment.

Nursing Diagnoses, Goals, and Outcome Criteria: Plastic Surgery, Preoperative	
NURSING DIAGNOSES	GOALS AND OUTCOME CRITERIA
Anxiety related to uncertain outcome, anticipated change in appearance, surgical procedure	Reduced anxiety: patient's statement of less anxiety; absence of trembling or tachycardia; and relaxed expression
Deficient Knowledge related to unfamiliarity with surgical routines	Understanding of surgical routines: patient correctly describes routines, identifies any actions to be carried out before admission and postoperatively

Interventions
Anxiety

Note if the patient seems anxious by observing for nervousness, trembling, increased pulse, and difficulty

| Table 50-5 | *Complications of Common Plastic Surgery Procedures* |

PROCEDURE	DESCRIPTION	COMPLICATIONS
Rhytidectomy (face-lift)	Removal of excess skin and tissue from face	Hematoma, hemorrhage, temporary or permanent facial nerve damage, wound infection, bruising, edema, skin necrosis, hair loss
Blepharoplasty	Removal of bulging fat and excess skin around eye	Hematoma, ectropion, corneal injury, visual loss (rare), wound infection (rare)
Rhinoplasty	Removal of excess cartilage and tissue from nose with correction of septal defects if indicated	Hematoma, hemorrhage, temporary bruising and edema, wound infection, septal perforation, minor skin irritation
Augmentation mammoplasty	Insertion of breast-shaped synthetic implants	Hematoma, hemorrhage, wound infection, phlebitis Capsule formation and contraction
Reduction mammoplasty	Excision of excessive breast tissue and skin	Hematoma; hemorrhage; infection; fat necrosis; wound dehiscence; necrosis of nipple, areola, and skin flap

Modified from Ignatavicius, D.D., Workman, M.S., & Mishler, M.A. (Eds.), *Medical-surgical nursing across the health care continuum* (3rd ed., p. 1748). Philadelphia: Saunders.

concentrating. Share such observations, and ask how the patient feels about the planned surgery. Anxiety may be reduced by encouraging the patient to express concerns, acknowledging that these feelings are normal, and providing information about what to expect.

Deficient Knowledge

Determine the patient's perception of the procedure and its outcome. Discuss surgical preoperative and postoperative procedures and self-care. Advise the patient if swelling, bruising, and scars are expected in the immediate postoperative period. Usually, patients have been told not to take drugs that prolong bleeding time, including aspirin, before surgery. Smoking is discouraged because nicotine causes vasoconstriction, which can interfere with healing. The patient may be instructed to scrub the surgical area at intervals before the procedure. Specific teaching depends on the exact procedure and the surgeon's orders or agency's protocol.

POSTOPERATIVE NURSING CARE

Routine postoperative nursing care is detailed in Chapter 17. This section emphasizes special considerations when a patient has plastic surgery.

Assessment

The patient may have had general, regional, or local anesthesia. Monitor vital signs and level of consciousness. Inspect dressings for drainage or bleeding but do not remove them without specific orders. Some dressings, such as those used after rhinoplasty, may serve as splints, so they must not be disturbed. Observe flaps and grafts for color and evidence of fluid accumulation, and palpate for warmth. If drains are present, inspect and measure the contents each shift. The fluid should gradually lighten from sanguineous (red) to se-

rosanguineous (pink) to serous (pale yellow). Monitor the patient's comfort level also.

Nursing Diagnoses, Goals, and Outcome Criteria: Plastic Surgery, Postoperative

NURSING DIAGNOSES	GOALS AND OUTCOME CRITERIA
Acute Pain related to tissue trauma	Reduced pain: patient states pain relieved, relaxed manner
Risk for Infection related to surgical incision	Absence of infection: no fever or foul drainage; decreasing redness and edema
Risk for Injury related to inadequate circulation to grafted tissue, pressure created by edema or implants, nerve damage	Adequate tissue perfusion: normal tissue warmth and color; normal neuromuscular function: sensation, movement, and reflexes
Risk for Deficient Fluid Volume related to effects of liposuction	Normal fluid balance: vital signs consistent with patient norms, fluid intake equal to output
Disturbed Body Image related to altered appearance	Healthy body image: patient expresses understanding of temporary appearance; expresses satisfaction with outcome
Ineffective Therapeutic Regimen Management related to lack of information about postoperative care	Appropriate postoperative self-care: patient describes and demonstrates self-care correctly

Interventions

Acute Pain

Minor procedures such as blepharoplasty usually cause minimal pain, but major procedures such as grafting or abdominoplasty can be very painful. Pain is treated with analgesics as ordered. Aspirin usually is not ordered because it prolongs bleeding time. After surgery on the face or head, the head of the bed usually is elevated and cold compresses are ordered to decrease swelling. Document the effects of interventions. Notify the physician if the patient reports increasing pain or if pain is not responsive to treatment.

 Consider the Alternative

In addition to analgesics, recommend comfort measures, such as positioning, relaxation, and imagery, to decrease pain.

Risk for Infection

Monitor for signs and symptoms of infection, although these are unlikely to be seen during a brief hospitalization. Therefore instruct the patient to report increasing redness, swelling, drainage, or fever. The nurse and patient must exercise good hand washing before any contact with the incisions, flaps, or grafts. Give antimicrobial drugs as ordered. Some plastic surgeons order topical antimicrobials applied to the incisions. After rhytidectomy, the patient is usually not permitted to shampoo the hair for several days to avoid contamination of the incisions.

Risk for Injury

After plastic surgery, inspect the affected tissues for evidence of adequate circulation. Grafts rely on blood flow in underlying tissue to supply nutrients and oxygen and to remove wastes. Therefore grafts must be protected from trauma and pressure. Pallor, cyanosis, and coolness in a graft suggest inadequate circulation and must be reported to the surgeon immediately. If fluid accumulates under the graft, it separates the graft from the underlying tissue, depriving it of oxygen and nutrients. Therefore swelling or blisters must be reported to the surgeon, who may remove the accumulated fluid with a small-gauge needle and syringe.

Rhytidectomy poses a risk of injury to the facial nerve, which is manifested by facial asymmetry. If asymmetry is observed, notify the surgeon immediately. The patient may be returned to surgery in an effort to relieve the pressure on the nerve and prevent permanent damage.

After blepharoplasty, monitor the patient's visual status. Although the risk is slight, the eye could be injured during the procedure.

After abdominoplasty, the patient may be required to protect the operative site by remaining in a flexed position for a specified period of time. Familiarize yourself with specific postoperative orders of your patient's surgeon. Position the bed so that the head and knees are elevated to reduce stress on the suture line. When out of bed, the patient may be required to continue the flexed position. The patient is gradually permitted to straighten up. Again, such directions vary with different surgeons.

After breast augmentation, monitor the patient for bleeding, infection, and altered sensation. The patient is also at risk for capsule formation, in which scar tissue gradually encloses the implant, causing the breast to become hard and misshapen. The surgeon may advise the patient to massage the breast to reduce the risk of capsule formation. This procedure involves pushing each breast up, to the side, and toward the center of the chest, holding each position to the count of 10. For a period specified by the surgeon, the patient should avoid raising the arms above the head.

Risk for Deficient Fluid Volume

Patients who have liposuction are at risk for hypovolemia due to excessive fluid loss. Intravenous fluids may be ordered after surgery, and oral fluids are usually encouraged when the patient is fully alert. Monitor vital signs for tachycardia and hypotension associated with fluid volume deficit. Use caution when assisting patients out of bed. If the blood volume is low, the patient may feel dizzy or faint.

Disturbed Body Image

In the immediate postoperative period, the patient often has edema and bruising as well as visible incisions. Assure the patient that these effects will gradually resolve. You can explore measures to conceal the evidence of trauma, but no makeup should be applied to surgical incisions until they are well healed.

Ineffective Therapeutic Regimen Management

In preparing for discharge, provide verbal and written instructions for self-care. The following topics must be included: drug therapy (names of drugs ordered, schedule), wound care, signs and symptoms of infection, activity restrictions, and measures to prevent complications.

 Key Points

- The functions of the skin are protection, body temperature regulation, secretion, sensation, synthesis of vitamin D, and blood storage.
- The skin assessment may detect skin disorders and systemic disorders that affect the skin.
- Pruritus (itching) is a symptom rather than a disease. It is treated by correction or removal of the underlying cause, skin moisturizers, and drugs such as antihistamines, corticosteroids, and local anesthetics.
- Atopic dermatitis, one type of eczema, is abnormally dry, itchy skin that is treated with moisturizers, antihistamines, antibiotics, and corticosteroids.

- Seborrheic dermatitis is a chronic inflammatory disease of the skin caused by increased sebum production. It is treated with medicated shampoos for the scalp and topical corticosteroids and antibiotics for other body sites.
- Psoriasis, characterized by bright-red lesions with silvery scales, may require treatment with topical corticosteroids, keratolytics, vitamin A derivatives, antipsoriatics, oral retinoids, biologic agents, ultraviolet light, antipsoriatics, and vitamin D derivatives (calcipotriene [Dovonex]).
- Fungal infections, including tinea pedis, tinea manus, tinea cruris, tinea corporis, tinea barbae, and candidiasis, are usually treated with antifungal drugs.
- Necrotizing fasciitis, a very serious infection that affects the fascia under the skin, is treated with antibiotics, débridement, and skin grafting.
- Acne, which is characterized by comedones, pustules, and cysts primarily on the face, neck, and upper trunk, may be treated with topical medications, oral antibiotics, estrogen, spironolactone, and retinoids.
- The herpes simplex virus types 1 and 2, which cause outbreaks of vesicles that rupture and form crusts, is treated with antiviral drugs that hasten healing but are not curative.
- Herpes zoster infection (shingles) causes pain and itching along a nerve pathway and may respond to antiviral drugs such as acyclovir.
- Common nursing diagnoses for the patient with an infectious or inflammatory skin disorder include Impaired Skin Integrity, Acute Pain, Risk for (secondary) Infection, Disturbed Body Image, Social Isolation, and Ineffective Therapeutic Regimen Management.
- Lice and scabies are tiny parasites that may infest the hair and skin, causing intense itching.

- Pemphigus is a chronic autoimmune condition in which fragile bullae develop and rupture, spilling a foul drainage.
- Skin cancers include basal cell carcinoma, squamous cell carcinoma, melanoma, cutaneous T-cell lymphoma, and Kaposi's sarcoma; actinic keratosis is a premalignant lesion.
- The two major conditions affecting the nails are infections and inflammation caused by ingrown nails.
- Burns are classified by size and depth of the tissue injury.
- Serious burns affect not only the skin but also fluid balance, gastrointestinal function, respiratory function, and the immune system.
- The three stages of burn injury are emergent, acute, and rehabilitation.
- Wound care after burn injury is intended to promote healing, prevent infection, control heat loss, retain function, and minimize disfigurement.
- Nursing care of the burn patient may address Decreased Cardiac Output, Excess Fluid Volume, Acute Pain, Risk for Infection, Hypothermia, Imbalanced Nutrition: Less Than Body Requirements, Impaired Physical Mobility, Ineffective Coping, Compromised Family Coping, and Ineffective Therapeutic Regimen Management.

 Go to your Companion CD-ROM for a Pharmacology Tutorial, Audio Glossary, and 3-D animations.

evolve   Be sure to visit the companion Evolve site at http://evolve.elsevier.com/Linton/ for WebLinks and additional online resources.

REVIEW QUESTIONS *Choose the best answer.*

1. The skin regulates body temperature by:
   1. Reacting to foreign substances that invade the epidermis
   2. Dilating and constricting surface blood vessels
   3. Secreting sebum to insulate the outer layers of skin
   4. Reacting to sunlight by producing vitamin C

2. When inspecting the skin of an older adult, you observe flat, pigmented spots on the backs of both hands. You should recognize these as:
   1. Lentigines
   2. Angiomas
   3. Keratoses
   4. Purpura

3. Which interventions will help prevent scratching and skin injury in a patient with atopic dermatitis?
   1. Maintain the room temperature around 80° F.
   2. Apply keratolytics liberally to promote healing.
   3. Wash new clothing before wearing it.
   4. Encourage hot baths.

4. Contact dermatitis is caused by:
   1. Infestations of parasites
   2. Reactions to drugs
   3. Excessive skin dryness
   4. An allergic response

5. Patient teaching related to psoriasis should include:
   1. Psoriasis usually can be cured with drug therapy.
   2. Direct contact with others can transmit psoriasis.
   3. Anthralin must be kept on the skin continuously.
   4. In most people, psoriasis affects only the skin.

6. An obese older patient in a long-term care facility has had intertrigo in body folds (axilla, beneath the breasts) on several occasions. Which measure is most appropriate to reduce the risk of a recurrence?
   1. Keep body folds clean and dry.
   2. Reduce bathing to three times each week.
   3. Liberally sprinkle cornstarch on body creases.
   4. Scrub affected areas with topical antiseptics.

7. A female patient is being treated with isotretinoin (Accutane) at the clinic for severe acne after other treatments have failed. All of the following points should be included in the teaching plan. Which is *most* important?

   1. Your skin may become very dry and peel.
   2. It may take several months to see improvement.
   3. You will sunburn very easily while on this drug.
   4. If sexually active, you must use reliable contraception.

8. A drug used to treat herpes simplex type 1 is:

   1. Hydrocortisone (Cortizone)
   2. Isotretinoin (Accutane)
   3. Acyclovir (Zovirax)
   4. Methoxsalen (Oxsoralen)

9. The best way to prevent skin cancer is to:

   1. Maintain good skin hydration
   2. Avoid excessive sun exposure
   3. Take large doses of vitamin A
   4. Avoid use of tobacco products

10. Characteristics of melanomas include:

   1. Nodular lesion with a pearly appearance
   2. Irregular lesion with uneven coloration
   3. Scaly ulcer with no clear margins
   4. Painful red, blue, or purple macules

51 Eye and Vision Disorders

Objectives

After reading and studying this chapter, you should be able to:

1. Identify the data to be collected in the nursing assessment of the eye and vision.
2. Identify the nursing responsibilities for patients having diagnostic tests or procedures to diagnose eye disorders.
3. List measures to reduce the risk of eye injuries.
4. Describe the nursing care of patients who require common therapeutic measures for eye disorders: irrigation, application of ophthalmic drugs, and surgery.
5. Describe the pathophysiology, signs and symptoms, diagnosis, and treatment of selected eye conditions.
6. Assist in developing a nursing care plan for the patient with an eye disorder.

Key Terms

Be sure to check out the bonus material on the Companion CD-ROM, including selected audio pronunciations.

astigmatism (ă-STĬG-mă-tĭzm, p. 1175)
cataract (KĂT-ă-răkt, p. 1176)
conjunctivitis (kŏn-jŭnk-tĭ-VĪ-tĭs, p. 1172)
cycloplegic (sī-klō-PLĒ-jĭk, p. 1165)
ectropion (ĕk-TRŌ-pē-ŏn, p. 1172)
entropion (ĕn-TRŌ-pē-ŏn, p. 1172)
enucleation (ē-nŭ-klē-Ā-shŭn, p. 1185)
hyperopia (hī-pĕr-Ō-pē-ă, p. 1160)
keratitis (kĕr-ă-TĪ-tĭs, p. 1172)
miotic (mī-ŌT-ĭk, p. 1165)
mydriatic (mĭd-rē-ĂT-ĭk, p. 1165)
myopia (mī-Ō-pē-ă, p. 1174)
presbyopia (prĕz-bē-Ō-pē-ă, p. 1160)
refraction (rē-FRĂK-shŭn, p. 1162)
scotomata (skō-TŌ-mă-tă, p. 1160)
tonometry (tō-NŎM-ĕ-trē, p. 1162)

It has been said that the eye is the window to the world. Indeed, vision plays an extremely important part in everyday life. It enables people to move about freely, to avoid danger, and to appreciate physical beauty. The eyes also are credited with conveying (or betraying!) one's emotions and communicating trust. Romantics speak of gazing into the eyes of a loved one.

In the United States, more than 11 million people have some vision impairment. For most people, loss of vision is perceived as a most tragic event. Nurses can play important roles in the prevention of vision loss, treatment of disorders of the eye, and rehabilitation of people with vision disturbances.

ANATOMY AND PHYSIOLOGY OF THE EYE

The eyeball is the primary structure involved in seeing. Several structures in addition to the eyeball serve to make up the visual system. The external structures of the visual system include the eyelids, eyelashes, conjunctiva, cornea, sclera, and extraocular muscles.

EXTERNAL STRUCTURES

The external structures of the visual system serve to protect and move the eyeball. The eyelids and eyelashes protect the eye by keeping it moist and shielding it from foreign substances. The lids are lined with a mucous membrane called the *palpebral conjunctiva*. The membrane continues from the inner eyelid margins to form a pocket around the eye and then covers the sclera up to the margin of the iris. The portion of the membrane that covers the anterior sclera is the bulbar conjunctiva.

Lacrimal glands located above the eyes secrete tears into the eyes through lacrimal ducts in the upper eyelids. Spontaneous blinking (approximately 15 times a minute) bathes the eyeballs in tear fluid. Tear fluid provides oxygen and some nutrients to the cornea. Normally, the fluid drains from the eye through the lacrimal sac into the nose. With excessive tear production, tears run from the eyes. Increased tear production occurs with trauma, irritation, or emotional distress. Decreased tear production occurs to some extent with aging. It should be noted that the passage of tear fluid through the lacrimal sac is the route by which eye drops can be absorbed into the system. That is why eye drops can have systemic effects and explains the need to apply pressure to the lacrimal sac after instilling eye drops. Severe deficiencies in tear fluid cause dry eyes, making the cornea susceptible to injury (see Fig. 51-1).

Normal vision requires the eyes to move together. The simultaneous movement of both eyes in the same direction is called *conjugate movement*. Eye movements are coordinated by three cranial nerves and six extra-ocular muscles.

THE EYEBALL

The eyeball consists of three layers of tissue: the sclera, the choroid, and the retina (Fig. 51-2).

Sclera

The sclera is the tough outer layer of the eyeball. It is mostly white except for the clear cornea over the iris. The cornea is covered by a protective membrane called the *conjunctiva.*

Choroid

The choroid or middle layer makes up the iris and ciliary muscle at the front of the eye. The colored part of the eye, the iris, is actually a muscle. The hole in the center of the iris is the pupil. The iris contracts and relaxes to control the amount of light entering the eye through the pupil. Dim light or severe stress causes the iris to contract. This makes the pupil dilate, or enlarge. Bright light causes the iris to relax, leaving the pupil constricted. The

choroid is rich in blood vessels that deliver nourishment to the retina in the back of the eye.

Retina

The retina is the inner lining of the eyeball. It is composed of two layers. The pigmented layer is between the choroid and the sensory layer; it receives nutrients and oxygen from the choroid and supplies the sensory layer.

The area at the back of the eye contains light-sensitive receptors called *rods* and *cones.* Rods are most important for vision in dim light. Cones are used for daylight vision and color perception. The area of sharpest vision on the retina is the *macula.* Because the macula has no blood vessels, it depends on the choroid for nourishment.

Optic Nerve

The optic nerve enters the back of the eyeball. This nerve sends visual messages to the brain for interpretation. When the eye is examined with an ophthalmoscope, the part of the optic nerve that can be seen is referred to as the *optic disc.*

Fluid Chambers

Anterior Chamber. Within the eyeball are two chambers separated by the lens. The anterior chamber is located between the iris and the cornea. It is filled with aqueous humor, a clear, watery fluid. Aqueous humor is produced in the ciliary body. It flows over the lens, through the pupil, and out through the trabecular meshwork into the canal of Schlemm. The canal of Schlemm returns the fluid to the venous circulation. The flow of aqueous humor is illustrated in Figure 51-3.

The function of aqueous humor is to moisturize and nourish the lens and cornea. The production and

Lacrimal gland
Lacrimal sac
Lacrimal canal
Nasolacrimal duct
Maxillary sinus
Inferior nasal concha
Lacrimal fold

FIGURE **51-1** Lacrimal structures.

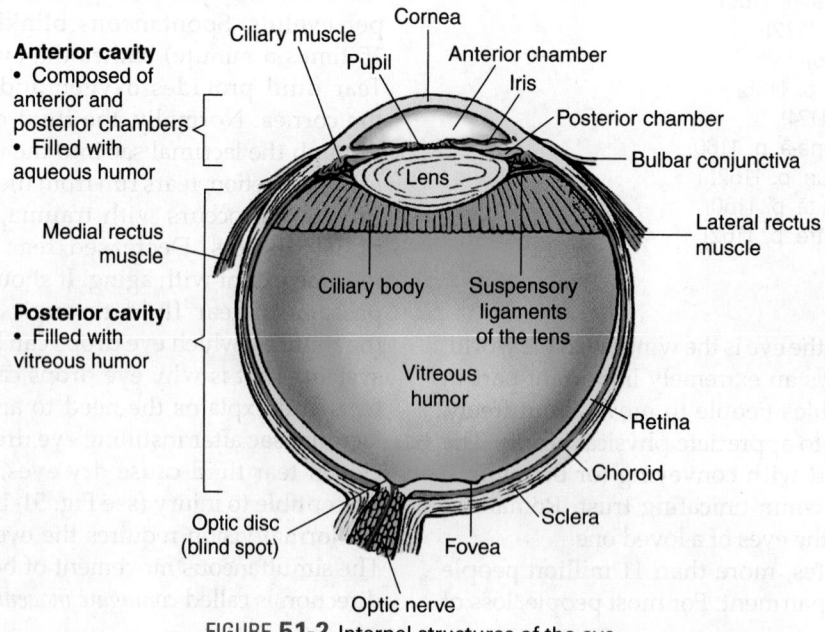

Anterior cavity
• Composed of anterior and posterior chambers
• Filled with aqueous humor

Posterior cavity
• Filled with vitreous humor

Medial rectus muscle

Ciliary muscle
Cornea
Pupil
Anterior chamber
Iris
Posterior chamber
Bulbar conjunctiva
Lens
Lateral rectus muscle
Ciliary body
Suspensory ligaments of the lens
Vitreous humor
Retina
Choroid
Optic disc (blind spot)
Sclera
Fovea
Optic nerve

FIGURE **51-2** Internal structures of the eye.

FIGURE 51-3 The flow of aqueous humor through the eye. Fluid is produced by the ciliary body. It flows through the pupil into the anterior chamber and out through the trabecular meshwork and the canal of Schlemm.

drainage of the fluid from the eye must be balanced to maintain normal pressure within the eye.

Posterior Chamber. The larger posterior chamber behind the lens is filled with vitreous humor. Vitreous humor is a clear, gelatinous material that helps hold the retina in place.

Lens

The lens is a transparent structure behind the iris. It is attached to the ciliary muscle. The ciliary muscle relaxes and contracts to change the shape of the lens. This process, called *accommodation*, permits the eye to focus on objects at different distances. To focus on a near object, the ciliary muscle contracts, making the lens curve. For distance, the muscle relaxes, making the lens flatter.

VISUAL PATHWAY

As light enters the eye, it passes through the transparent cornea, aqueous humor, lens, and vitreous humor. These structures are called *refractive media.* They refract (bend) horizontal and vertical light rays so that the light rays focus on the retina.

On the retina, the light rays reflected from the image are reversed and upside down. Images are carried as impulses through the optic nerve. At the optic chiasm, fibers from the left field from each eye join to form the left optic tract. Fibers from the right field of each eye join to form the right optic tract. Images are transmitted to the brain by way of the optic tracts (Fig. 51-4).

FIGURE 51-4 The visual pathway.

AGE-RELATED CHANGES IN THE EYE

As people age, typical changes occur in the structures and function of the eye. The skin around the eye becomes wrinkled and looser. The eyelids usually have some excess tissue; this is not important unless it interferes with vision. The amount of fat around the eye decreases, permitting the eyeball to sink deeper into the orbit. Tear secretion diminishes, and the cornea becomes less sensitive. A grayish ring may be seen around the outer margin of the iris. This ring is called the *arcus senilis.* There is some disagreement about the significance of the arcus senilis. It may be related to elevated serum lipid levels; it does not affect vision. The pupil is usually smaller in the older person and responds somewhat more slowly to light.

Vision changes associated with age are related to changes in the lens and the ciliary muscle. The lens becomes less elastic, more dense, opaque, and yellow. These changes have several significant effects. First, light passing through the lens scatters, causing the patient to be sensitive to glare. The second, more important, effect is that the ability to focus is impaired. This farsightedness (hyperopia) in older people is called presbyopia. This is the reason most older people have to wear glasses for reading or other close work. Some older people report seeing specks moving across the field of vision. These dark spots, called floaters, are actually bits of debris in the vitreous.

Despite the age-related changes in the eye, most older people retain adequate vision for daily activities.

NURSING ASSESSMENT OF THE EYE

HEALTH HISTORY
History of Present Illness

When collecting data for the assessment of specific eye complaints, record changes in vision, including blurring, diplopia (double vision), spots, floaters, flashes of light, tunnel vision, altered color perception, halos around lights, blind spots (scotomata), and loss of part of the visual fields. If the patient reports pain, inquire about its location and nature (sharp, stabbing, aching). Document sensitivity to light, called *photophobia*. Ask the patient to describe any discharge from the eyes. Drainage might be described as tears, purulent discharge, or crusting of the eyelids or eyelashes. Also note complaints that the eyes feel dry and irritated. Other complaints that might prompt the patient to seek medical attention are redness or swelling of the lids, eyes, or periorbital area (around the eyes).

Past Medical History

People tend to assume that changes in vision are caused by problems in the eye or related structures. Although this is often true, visual disturbances also can be associated with many other conditions. Therefore it is important to obtain a good history of past medical problems from the patient who reports with vision problems. Conditions to be alert for include the following:

- *Diabetes.* Elevated blood glucose can cause temporary blurring of vision. Permanent changes in the retina associated with diabetes can cause blindness.
- *Neurologic disorders.* Brain tumors, head injuries, and strokes are examples of conditions that may impair vision. Effects may be blurred vision, diplopia, inability to move eyes, or loss of part of the visual fields.
- *Thyroid disease.* Hyperthyroidism may cause exophthalmos (bulging eyes).
- *Hypertension.* Hypertension can cause changes in the blood vessels of the eye, eventually leading to vision loss.

Note any eye injury or previously diagnosed eye disease, including date of last examination and treatment.

A current medication history also is important in assessing vision problems. Some drugs can cause temporary or permanent changes in visual acuity and color vision. Others may contribute to the development of cataracts or glaucoma.

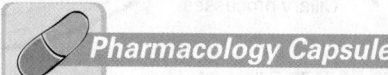
Pharmacology Capsule

Drugs that are especially likely to be related to vision disturbances are digitalis, corticosteroids, indomethacin, and sulfisoxazole. Patients taking thioridazine, chlorpromazine, or ethambutol also should be monitored for ocular toxicity.

Family History

The family history includes any known eye diseases as well as a history of arteriosclerosis, diabetes, and thyroid disease.

Functional Assessment

The functional assessment documents the patient's occupation, roles, and usual activities. Be alert for activities that might pose a risk to the eyes.

PHYSICAL EXAMINATION

The physician performs a complete examination, including inspection of the inner eye. The nurse, however, can inspect the external eye, assess response of the pupil to light, and evaluate gross visual acuity. If abnormalities are suspected, inform the physician or advise the patient to seek medical evaluation.

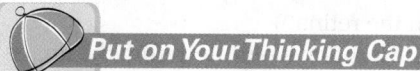
Put on Your Thinking Cap!

What are some ways you could assess gross visual acuity when diagnostic charts are not available or not practical?

In the eye examination, first inspect the eyelids for redness, drainage, and position. The lids should cover the eyeball completely when closed. When the eyes are open, the lower lid should be at the level of the iris. The upper lid should barely cover the upper margin of the iris. The lids should fit closely to the eyeball, and the eyelashes should not turn toward the eye. Describe any crusting or drainage on the lids or the lashes.

Inspect the eyeball for color and moisture. The sclera should be clear white. Excessive redness may be due to irritation or inflammation. A yellow color, called *icterus,* is associated with liver dysfunction.

Observe the pupils for size, equality, and reaction to light. Pupils that are unequal or dilated or do not respond to light suggest neurologic problems. Some medications also can affect pupil characteristics. Accommodation is tested by having the patient focus on the examiner's finger held at a distance and then having the patient watch the finger as it is slowly moved toward the patient's nose. The pupils should constrict and the eyes converge, meaning the pupils become smaller and both eyes move to fix on the same point.

Visual acuity is commonly tested using the Snellen chart (Fig. 51-5). The Snellen chart has rows of progressively smaller letters. From a distance of 20 feet, the patient is instructed to read down the chart until more than two mistakes are made on a single line. Each eye is tested separately and then together. The lines are numbered 20 over 200, 100, 70, 50, 40, 30, 25, 20, and 15. The findings are reported as the last line the person could read with no more than two errors. That is, if the person read the 20/30 line with one error but made three errors on the 20/25 line, the vision would be recorded as 20/30 in the eye tested. This means that the person could read at 20 feet what a person with normal vision could read at 30 feet. The Snellen chart may be used for vision screening in clinic and office settings. In the hospital, it may be more practical simply to ask the patient to read available print. This provides some practical measure of visual acuity.

Some nurses learn to assess visual fields, extraocular movements, and the corneal reflex. There are also several tests used to detect strabismus.

When assessing the eyes, be alert for the signs of trouble listed in Box 51-1. If any of these are present, refer the patient to the physician for evaluation. The nursing assessment of the patient with an eye disorder is summarized in Box 51-2.

FIGURE **51-5** The Snellen chart is used to measure visual acuity.

Box 51-1 *Signs of Possible Eye Problems*

- Particular trouble adjusting to a dark room
- Squinting or blinking due to unusual sensitivity to light or glare
- Change in color of iris
- Red-rimmed and crusted or swollen eyelids
- Inflamed or red eyes
- Recurrent pain in or around eyes
- Sudden loss of vision in one eye
- Sudden hazy or blurred vision
- Flashes of light or showers of black spots
- Halos or rainbows around light
- Curtain-like loss of vision
- Loss of peripheral or side vision

Data from The Texas Society to Prevent Blindness. *Signs of possible eye trouble in adults.*

Box 51-2 *ASSESSMENT of the Patient with an Eye Disorder*

Health History
Present Illness:
Changes in vision, symptoms of eye disorders: pain, photophobia, drainage, dryness, irritation, redness, swelling

Past Medical History:
Diabetes, neurologic disorders, thyroid disease, hypertension, previously diagnosed eye disease or injury, date of last eye examination, current medications (specifically, digitalis, corticosteroids, indomethacin, sulfonamides)

Family History:
Known eye diseases, arteriosclerosis, diabetes, thyroid disease, arthritis

Functional Assessment:
Occupation, roles, usual activities, changes required by eye problems

Physical Examination
Eyelids:
Redness, drainage, position, closure, crusting, inversion, or eversion

Eyeball:
Color, moisture

Sclera:
Color, redness, jaundice

Pupils:
Size, equality, reaction to light, accommodation

Visual Acuity:
Measured with Snellen chart, gross acuity

Visual Fields

Extraocular Movements

Corneal Reflex

Inner Eye:
Ophthalmoscopic examination of anterior chamber, lens, vitreous, and fundus (inner surface of retina)

FIGURE **51-6** An ophthalmoscope is used to examine the inner structure of the eye.

FIGURE **51-7** Assessment of visual fields.

DIAGNOSTIC TESTS AND PROCEDURES

Several professionals are trained to assess and treat conditions of the eye. An ophthalmologist is a physician with specialized training in diagnosing and treating eye conditions. The ophthalmologist prescribes corrective lenses for refractive errors and treats other eye conditions with medications and surgery. An optometrist is trained to diagnose errors of refraction and to prescribe corrective lenses. An optician fills prescriptions written by an ophthalmologist or optometrist and fits the prescribed lenses.

Nursing care related to diagnostic tests and procedures for disorders of the eye is described in the Diagnostic Tests and Procedures table on p. 1163.

OPHTHALMOSCOPIC EXAMINATION

The ophthalmoscopic examination involves using an ophthalmoscope (Fig. 51-6) to examine the lens, vitreous humor, retina, and optic disc. A solution such as phenylephrine ophthalmic preparation may be instilled in the eye first to dilate the pupil. This permits a better view of the inner eye. A darkened room also causes the pupil to dilate.

The examiner studies the cornea, lens, and vitreous for opacities. The blood vessels at the back of the eye (called the *fundus*) are inspected for evidence of disease. Degenerative changes of the retina may be observed.

REFRACTOMETRY

As light enters the eye, it passes through the aqueous humor, lens, and vitreous humor. The light rays bend so that they focus on the retina. This bending is called **refraction.** Refractive errors occur when the light does not bend properly. This causes alterations in vision, which sixre discussed on pp. 1174 to 1175 in the Errors of Refraction section. Refraction is assessed by dilating the pupil and having the patient read a chart through a series of lenses. The patient identifies which lens permits the clearest image. This procedure, called *refractometry,* enables the examiner to detect refractive errors. The procedure requires no special preparation or aftercare. In patients who cannot cooperate, retinoscopy may be done to measure refractive error.

VISUAL FIELDS

Visual fields include the area a person can see while looking straight ahead without moving the head. Some conditions, such as glaucoma, retinal detachment, and certain neurologic abnormalities, cause loss of parts of the visual fields. Visual fields are assessed by comparing the patient's field of vision with that of a normal examiner (Fig. 51-7). The patient and examiner sit facing each other. The examiner moves his or her hand out of line of vision and then brings it into expected line of vision in a specific pattern. The patient states when the examiner's fingers are seen. No special preparation, equipment, or postprocedure care is needed.

TONOMETRY

Tonometry is the measurement of pressure in the anterior chamber of the eye. Normal intraocular pressure is 10 to 21 mm Hg. Routine measurement of intraocular pressure is important to detect high pressures that damage the retina if untreated.

Several procedures are used to measure intraocular pressure. The Schiøtz tonometer, shown in Figure 51-8, may be used for this purpose. Another, more accurate procedure is called *applanation.* It is done with a slit-lamp microscope. A biomicroscope measures pressure even more accurately. Procedures in which the instrument touches the eye require that the cornea be anesthetized with eye drops such as proparacaine 0.5% (Ophthaine). The new Tonometer Diaton measures pressure through the closed eyelid.

DIAGNOSTIC TESTS and PROCEDURES The Eye

TEST/PURPOSE	PATIENT PREPARATION	POSTPROCEDURE NURSING CARE
Ophthalmologic examination Examines the inner eye through the pupil to diagnose abnormalities of retina, optic disc, and blood vessels.	Administer cycloplegic medication if ordered to dilate pupil and prevent accommodation. Room is darkened during examination.	If pupils are dilated, advise patient of need for sunglasses. Visual acuity may be reduced because of pupil dilation. Patient may need someone else to drive home.
Refractometry Identifies refractive errors and corrective lens needed.	No special preparation.	If pupils are dilated, advise patient of need for sunglasses until pupils return to normal.
Tonometry One of several instruments used to measure intraocular pressure.	For procedures in which an instrument touches cornea, anesthetic drops are ordered. Inform patient of need to remain still during procedure.	Advise patient not to rub eyes for 15 min after the procedure because injury could occur when eye is anesthetized.
Fluorescein angiography Pictures of blood vessels in the eye are taken after a dye is injected into a vein in the hand or arm. Permits diagnosis of abnormalities of vessels and retina.	Signed consent required. Administer mydriatic or cycloplegic medication as ordered to dilate the pupil. Assess allergies to iodine, seafood. Notify physician if patient is allergic. Diphenhydramine (Benadryl) may be ordered to reduce risk of allergic reaction to dye; have emergency supplies available in case of severe allergic reaction. Tell patient a dye will be given intravenously, then photographs taken through the pupil. A blue light that will flash when photos are taken may cause temporary vision disturbance. Flashing light can trigger seizure activity in patients with epilepsy.	Dye may cause a yellowish skin color for 6-24 hr. Urine may be greenish as dye is eliminated. Visual acuity may be reduced because of pupil dilation. Advise patient to wear sunglasses. May need someone to drive patient home.
Visual fields Identifies the area a person can see while looking straight ahead. Assessed by comparing the fields the patient can see with those of an examiner with normal visual fields. Patient and examiner sit facing each other. They cover opposite eyes. Examiner moves his or her hand out of line of vision and then brings it into expected line of vision in a specific pattern. Patient states when examiner's fingers are seen.	No preparation needed.	No postprocedure care needed.
Electroretinography Used to detect some retinal disorders. A contact lens electrode is placed and the eye exposed to flashes of light. The retinal response is recorded.	Anesthetic eye drops will be administered. The patient will need to remain still and focus on a target.	Advise patient not to rub eye because of risk for injury while anesthetized.

The pneumatonometer is a handheld instrument that directs a puff of air to the surface of the eye. It measures intraocular pressure by measuring resistance to the air.

MEASURE OF ELECTRICAL POTENTIAL

Because the retina is composed of nerve tissue, it has an electrical potential that can be measured. This is useful in detecting retinal disorders, including retini-tis pigmentosa, massive ischemia, widespread infection, and some chemical toxicities. One procedure used to measure electrical potential is electroretinography. For electroretinography, anesthetic drops are instilled. Then a contact lens electrode is placed on the eye and exposed to flashes of light at varying intensities and speeds. The response of the retina is recorded. The patient must fix his or her gaze on a target and remain very still.

FIGURE **51-8** Techniques for measuring intraocular pressure. **A,** Palpation (useful only when pressure difference between eyes is large). **B,** Schiøtz tonometry. **C,** Air puff tonometry. **D,** Goldman's applanation tonometer.

FLUORESCEIN ANGIOGRAPHY

To detect abnormal blood vessels or blood flow, fluorescein is injected intravenously and the retina is observed and photographed as the dye circulates (Fig. 51-9). Preparation for fluorescein angiography includes (1) the use of mydriatic drops to dilate the pupil and (2) initiation of intravenous access. The patient should be asked about allergies to dyes. A signed consent form is required. The dye will cause the patient's skin to appear yellow for several hours after the test. Encourage the patient to drink flu-

ids to promote elimination of the dye. As the dye is excreted, the urine will appear bright green. It is common for patients to feel nauseated after the procedure.

CORNEAL STAINING

Topical dyes can be applied to the eye to detect abrasions of the cornea. Fluorescein is applied and is followed by a saline rinse. The cornea is then examined through a blue filter. Dye permits scratches to be seen more readily.

FIGURE **51-9** Fluorescein angiography permits visualization of the blood vessels of the eye to examine the inner structure of the eye.

IMAGING PROCEDURES

To obtain images of the eye for diagnostic purposes, the physician may order computed tomography (CT) scanning, ultrasonography, radioisotope scanning, or magnetic resonance imaging (MRI).

COMMON THERAPEUTIC MEASURES

EYE IRRIGATION

Irrigations are done to remove irritating chemicals from the eye. Sterile normal saline is the best solution to use. Plain water also is acceptable, especially in emergencies. In the hospital or clinic setting, the physician sometimes orders irrigations with ophthalmic medications. Key points in irrigating the eye include the following:

1. Wearing gloves, cleanse the eyelids and eyelashes.
2. Position the patient with the affected eye down so that contaminated fluid does not run into the unaffected eye.
3. Place a basin and waterproof pad to collect the fluid.
4. Gently direct the fluid into the lower conjunctival sac from the inner canthus (corner of the eye) to the outer canthus.
5. Do not touch the eye with the tip of the irrigating syringe.
6. Have the patient blink occasionally to move particles toward the lower conjunctival sac.
7. If extended irrigation is needed, special irrigation systems may be used.

TOPICAL MEDICATIONS

A number of medications can be applied directly to the eye. These include miotics, mydriatics, anesthetics, cycloplegics, antibiotics, and anti-inflammatory drugs.

Mydriatics dilate the pupils; miotics constrict the pupils; and cycloplegics prevent accommodation. Some drug manufacturers color-code the caps and labels of topical ophthalmic drugs to help you select the correct drug. The caps and labels of mydriatics are red; miotics are green; nonsteroidal anti-inflammatory drugs are gray; anti-infectives are brown or tan; and beta-blockers are yellow or blue. Nevertheless, you must always read the drug label carefully and compare it to the physician's order. Some systemic drugs also may be ordered, such as diuretics to reduce pressure in the eye. Examples of ophthalmic drugs are included in the Drug Therapy table on pp. 1166 to 1167.

The following are key points to remember when administering topical eye medications:

1. Be *very* careful that only medications labeled for *ophthalmic* use are put in the eye!
2. Drops should be room temperature when administered. Rolling the bottle between the palms is a good way to warm the medication.
3. Tell the patient to tilt his or her head back and look at the ceiling. The head can be turned slightly so that excess medication runs out the outer canthus of the eyes and does not contaminate the opposite eye.
4. Place your finger below the lower lid and gently pull the eyelid down to expose the conjunctival sac and create a pouch.
5. Brace the hand holding the medication and then drop the medication into the conjunctival sac without touching the eyelid with the container to avoid contaminating the medication container.
6. Tell the patient to close his or her eyes and move them as if looking around. This distributes the medication over the eye.
7. You or the patient should apply gentle pressure to the lacrimal sac at the inner canthus of the eye for approximately 1 minute. This reduces the amount of the medication entering body fluids.
8. If more than one medication is being given, wait 5 minutes between each medication.

EYE SURGERY

A number of eye conditions are treated or corrected with surgery. Eye surgery may involve surgical incisions, the use of lasers, and the application of cold probes (cryotherapy). Individualized care plans must be developed based on the specific type of procedure done. Some general considerations, however, apply to most patients having eye surgery.

PREOPERATIVE NURSING CARE

Assessment

Preoperative assessment and care are discussed in detail in Chapter 17. The preoperative assessment specifically focuses on the patient's emotional state, ability to perform self-care, and knowledge of surgical routines and outcomes. Most patients awaiting eye surgery are

DRUG THERAPY | *Disorders of the Eye*

GENERAL NURSING CONSIDERATIONS

1. Advise patient to follow directions exactly.
2. If condition worsens or does not improve, notify the physician.
3. If multiple ophthalmic drugs are ordered, wait 5 minutes between them.
4. After administering ophthalmic solutions, apply gentle pressure to lacrimal sac for approximately 1 minute to decrease absorption and systemic effects.
5. Teach patient or family member correct technique for drug administration.
6. Emphasize that patients should never share eye medication.

DRUG	USE/ACTION	SIDE EFFECTS	NURSING INTERVENTIONS
ADRENERGICS			
Epinephrine bitartrate (Epitrate) Dipivefrin HCl (Propine) Phenylephrine (Neo-Synephrine)	Dilate pupil. Used in open-angle (chronic) glaucoma. Decrease corneal congestion. Control hemorrhage.	Cardiac stimulation, headache, brow pain, allergy, worsening of acute (narrow-angle) glaucoma.	Sunglasses needed for 6 hr. Tell patient to report eye pain immediately—may be caused by increased intraocular pressure.
ANTICHOLINERGICS (ANTIMUSCARINICS)			
Atropine (Isopto Atropine) Homatropine (Isopto Homatropine) Scopolamine (Isopto Hyoscine) Cyclopentolate (Cyclogyl) Tropicamide (Mydriacyl)	Dilate pupil. Used before eye examinations and for uveitis. Decrease lacrimal gland secretion. Cyclopentolate and tropicamide preferred for eye examination because of shorter duration of action.	Photophobia, inability to accommodate, corneal dryness and irritation.	Apply at ordered time before eye examination. If eye pain occurs, may indicate undetected glaucoma. Safety measures while pupils dilated, because vision is blurred. Artificial tears may be needed.

somewhat anxious. They may be fearful that the procedure will not be successful or that some complication will lead to further loss of vision. Determine whether there is now or will be any activity limitations. If the patient has poor vision, document the type of help needed. Also note the physician's orders for intravenous fluids or preoperative medications, or both. The patient's food and fluid intake is usually restricted from the evening before surgery to reduce the risk of nausea, vomiting, and aspiration after surgery. Because many procedures on the eye are done in day surgery facilities, be sure the patient understands the preoperative routine.

Nursing Diagnoses, Goals, and Outcome Criteria:
Eye Surgery, Preoperative

NURSING DIAGNOSES	GOALS AND OUTCOME CRITERIA
Anxiety related to uncertain outcome, lack of knowledge about surgery and surgical routines	Reduced anxiety: patient states anxiety is reduced, relaxed manner
Self-Care Deficit (feeding, hygiene, grooming) related to visual impairment	Achievement of activities of daily living: daily activities successfully completed

Interventions

Anxiety

Explore the patient's feelings about the surgery, and provide information. Refer specific questions about the surgical procedure, risks, complications, or outcomes to the physician. Explain general surgical and postoperative routines.

Self-Care Deficit

On admission, orient the visually impaired patient to the room. Keep objects in one place, and advise the patient of any new equipment or articles in the environment. Follow agency policy for obtaining consent for surgery. Offer to read any written material to the patient.

POSTOPERATIVE NURSING CARE

Assessment

After surgery, check the patient's vital signs and level of consciousness during recovery from anesthesia. Inspect the dressing or the operative eye for bleeding or drainage. Also ask about patient comfort, including pain and nausea. If vision is impaired, inspect the environment for safety hazards. Before discharge, determine the patient's understanding of and ability to administer prescribed medications by having the patient demonstrate self-medication.

DRUG THERAPY *Disorders of the Eye—cont'd*

DRUG	USE/ACTION	SIDE EFFECTS	NURSING INTERVENTIONS
ANTIBACTERIALS Gentamicin sulfate (Garamycin Ophthalmic) Erythromycin (Ilotycin) Polymyxin B sulfate (neomycin sulfate, bacitracin) Sulfonamides (Sulamyd Ophthalmic)	Treatment or prevention of eye infections.	Allergic reaction, conjunctivitis.	Screen for previous allergic reactions. Withhold drug and notify physician if allergic. Inspect eyes and lids for increasing redness.
ANTIFUNGALS Natamycin (Natacyn)	Effective against some fungal infections of eye.	Rarely: allergic reaction, conjunctival edema.	Advise patient to continue treatment as prescribed (usually 14-21 days). Notify physician if symptoms continue or if edema develops.
ANTIVIRALS Vidarabine (Vira-A)	Treatment of herpes simplex, keratitis.	Irritation, redness, edema, pain, itching, photophobia. Rarely: allergic reactions.	Advise sunglasses for sensitivity. Refrigerate.
TOPICAL ANESTHETICS Proparacaine HCl (Ophthaine, Ophthetic) Tetracaine HCl (Pontocaine)	Block sensation in external eye for tonometry, removal of sutures or foreign bodies, some surgical procedures.	Stinging, irritation. Allergic reactions rare.	Do not use discolored solution. Caution patient not to touch or rub eye or insert contact lens until sensation returns.
ANTI-INFLAMMATORY AGENTS Prednisolone acetate Prednisolone sodium phosphate Dexamethasone Fluorometholone	Prevent redness and swelling because of inflammation from causes other than bacterial infection.	Systemic effects possible if sufficient drug is absorbed, including fluid retention, nausea, mood swings, hypokalemia, and many others.	Apply pressure to lacrimal sac for 1-2 min after application to reduce absorption. Monitor blood studies.

Nursing Diagnoses, Goals, and Outcome Criteria: Eye Surgery, Postoperative

NURSING DIAGNOSES	GOALS AND OUTCOME CRITERIA
Risk for Injury related to pressure or trauma	Decreased risk of injury: patient avoids potentially harmful activities (e.g., rubbing eye, bending forward)
Disturbed Sensory Perception related to vision changes caused by disease process, trauma to the eye, patching	Adaptation to impaired vision: patient makes adjustments in lifestyle to accommodate vision change
Acute Pain related to tissue trauma	Pain relief: patient states pain reduced or absent, relaxed manner
Anxiety related to temporary vision impairment	Decreased anxiety: patient states is less anxious; calm demeanor
Ineffective Therapeutic Regimen Management related to lack of understanding of self-care measures and usual postoperative course	Patient adheres to plan of care: patient demonstrates appropriate self-care

Interventions
Risk for Injury

The physician may prescribe limitations on activity or position, or both. The head of the bed is usually elevated. The patient may be wearing a bulky dressing or a small eye patch. Either may be covered with a lightweight metal or plastic shield (Fig. 51-10). The dressing absorbs any drainage, and the shield protects the eye from rubbing. Instruct the patient not to rub the eye. Check the physician's orders to determine whether the dressing can be changed. Eye drops or ointments may be ordered. They may be different from those used

FIGURE **51-10** The shield protects the operative eye from pressure or rubbing.

before surgery. When an eye is patched, take safety precautions to prevent injury.

An important aspect of the postoperative care of patients having eye surgery is to prevent increased intraocular pressure. Caution the patient against straining, leaning forward, lifting, and lying on the affected side. Because vomiting and retching raise intraocular pressure, treat nausea promptly.

 Put on Your Thinking Cap!

After eye surgery, patients often go home the same day. Considering the usual restrictions imposed to prevent increased intraocular pressure, what are some obstacles the patient might encounter? What strategies might you suggest to the patient?

Disturbed Sensory Perception

Measures to assist the patient with visual impairment are discussed in detail on p. 1170 in the Nursing Care of the Visually Impaired Patient section.

Acute Pain

Although one might expect eye surgery to be painful, postoperative pain is usually mild to moderate. Give mild analgesics as ordered. If a patient reports severe pain, notify the physician.

Anxiety

To reduce anxiety, explain what is being done and why and encourage the patient to express concerns and ask questions.

Ineffective Therapeutic Regimen Management

Patients who have had eye surgery often are discharged with some medications. Provide careful directions and a written schedule for the medications. To determine the patient's ability to self-administer eye medications, have the patient demonstrate the procedure before discharge. If necessary, instruct a family member in administering the medications.

 Put on Your Thinking Cap!

An 80-year-old patient is being discharged after ocular surgery. He has several topical ophthalmic drugs that must be applied twice daily. One eye is to remain patched until he sees the physician in 1 week. What information would you want to gather to determine whether he will be able to manage at home?

PROTECTION OF THE EYES AND VISION

Maintaining adequate vision involves the prevention of injuries and the treatment of abnormalities. Nurses must be knowledgeable about the protection and care of the eyes.

PATIENT TEACHING

Nurses can teach people how to care for their eyes to protect vision. Adults younger than 40 years should have their eyes examined every 3 to 5 years. After the age of 40 years, eye examinations should be done every 2 years and should include testing for glaucoma. This permits early detection and treatment of eye disorders.

Tell patients to report sharp, stabbing eye pain or deep, throbbing eye pain. Other symptoms that should be reported to a physician are photophobia (sensitivity to light), blurred or double vision, loss of part of the visual fields, halos around lights, and floaters. Floaters are spots that appear to move across the field of vision. Some patients describe floaters as being like birds swooping past one's face. Other symptoms that require medical evaluation are burning sensations, itching, excessive tearing, and the presence of drainage from the eyes.

When there are symptoms of eye problems, patients should seek medical advice rather than try home remedies. First aid for eye injuries is explained in Chapter 16.

Sometimes nurses have the opportunity to correct misconceptions that people have about vision. The following are some examples of *misconceptions:*

- Watching too much television or sitting too close to the television injures the eyes.
- Eating foods that contain large amounts of vitamin A improves vision. However, it is true that vitamin A deficiency can cause vision impairment (see the Nutrition Concepts box on p. 1169).
- Eyes need to be rinsed regularly.

Prevention of Injuries

Injuries caused by foreign objects are a major cause of vision loss. Teach young children the danger of throw-

Nutrition Concepts

1. Vitamin A is essential for normal vision.
2. An early symptom of vitamin A deficiency is night blindness.
3. Severe vitamin A deficiency causes clinical eye disease that leads to blindness.

---

ing or poking objects at the faces of playmates. Assess toys for safety. Adult activities that produce sparks or cause fragments to be dispersed also cause injuries. Advise protective eyewear for such potentially dangerous activities.

Basic Eye Care

Gently cleanse the eyelids each time the face is washed. Use a clean cloth without soap. Wash the eye from the inner canthus (near the nose) toward the outer canthus. Dry crusts on the eyelids and eyelashes can usually be wiped off. If necessary, place a warm, damp cloth on the lids for several minutes to soften the crusts.

Routine eye rinses and drops are unnecessary for most people. Exceptions are people with inadequate tear production and those whose eyes do not close completely. Lubricating drops called *artificial tears* are available for those people. Sometimes, eye patches are applied or the lids are taped shut to prevent drying of the cornea.

IMPACT OF VISUAL IMPAIRMENT

Vision loss usually has significant impact on all areas of a person's life. Mild losses may require only some adaptations. More serious losses affect independence, mobility, employment, and interpersonal relationships. In addition, there is the loss of pleasure in seeing the people and things a person treasures.

The loss of vision triggers a grief response. People grieve for the lost function just as they might grieve after the death of a loved one. Reactions that are likely to follow loss of vision include shock, denial, anger, bargaining, and depression.

Factors that affect a person's response to this loss include personality, usual coping style, impact of vision loss on the person's life, and the circumstances of the loss. If grief is resolved in a healthy manner, adaptation and acceptance eventually occur. People who have progressive loss of vision may experience anticipatory grief. Nursing care to help the person who is grieving is discussed in Chapter 24.

NURSING CARE *of the Visually Impaired Patient*

When people hear the word *blind,* they think of someone who is unable to see. There are, however, degrees of

visual impairment. Although some visually impaired people are unable to see at all, many others have partial vision. Therefore medical literature is more likely to use terms such as *visual impairment* or *visually handicapped* rather than *blind.* Also, there may be a stigma attached to the word *blind.* Some people automatically associate blindness with helplessness.

Trauma, disease, and some congenital defects account for visual handicaps throughout the life span. Some types of visual disturbances are more common in older people.

To work with the visually impaired, you need to be aware of their thoughts and feelings about visual handicaps. You should assume that people with visual impairments can be independent and productive. Pity has no place in this situation because it encourages hopelessness and helplessness. The person needs help with some tasks but should still be treated as an adult.

The extent of vision loss determines the types of assistance that might be needed. Many people have visual problems that can be corrected with eyeglasses, drug therapy, or surgical treatment. Many products are available to enable visually impaired people to function more independently. When planning care, consider whether the patient's condition is temporary, permanent, correctable, treatable, or progressive.

Assessment

The nursing assessment of the patient with an eye disorder is summarized in Box 51-2.

Nursing Diagnoses, Goals, and Outcome Criteria: Impaired Vision

Nursing Diagnoses	Goals and Outcome Criteria
Disturbed Sensory Perception related to altered reception, transmission, interpretation of visual stimuli	Adaptation to vision impairment: patient has no falls or other traumatic injuries; uses assistive devices and techniques to maintain as much independence as possible
Ineffective Coping related to decreased independence, threat to body image, denial	Effective coping: patient makes efforts to adapt, participates in self-care to maximal degree possible
Self-Care Deficit (feeding, hygiene, grooming) related to visual impairment	Appropriate self-care: patient performs activities of daily living with minimal assistance
Ineffective Therapeutic Regimen Management related to lack of understanding of treatment of vision impairment	Effective regimen management: prescribed plan of care is managed appropriately: patient carries out plan of care; participates in rehabilitation programs if indicated

Interventions

Disturbed Sensory Perception

When a visually impaired person is admitted to a health care facility, provide an orientation to the environment. The fact that the patient has visual impairment should be reflected on the nursing care plan. In addition, a sign may be posted to alert other caregivers and employees. Safety is a primary consideration for these patients. Measures to support the patient with impaired vision and to prevent injury include the following:

1. When you enter the room, announce your presence and introduce yourself to avoid startling or embarrassing the patient.
2. Speak before touching the patient to avoid startling him or her.
3. Speak in a normal tone of voice. People tend to act as if those who cannot see cannot hear, so there is a tendency to raise one's voice when talking to the visually impaired.
4. Address the patient in the appropriate manner for his or her age and intellectual ability. Visual impairment is not associated with mental impairment.
5. Advise the patient what to expect during procedures.
6. Tell the patient when you leave the room.
7. Leave the bed in low position.
8. Place the call bell within reach, and be sure the patient knows how to use it.
9. Keep doors either open or closed so that the ambulatory patient does not run into a partially closed door.
10. Do not rearrange the room after orienting the patient.
11. Eliminate meaningless noise from the environment as much as possible.
12. To lead a blind person, have him or her take your arm (Fig. 51-11).

The environment significantly influences the visually impaired patient's ability to function. The environment should be safe and promote maximal independence. As mentioned, orientation to the setting is especially important. Make sure the patient can use the call system, locate personal items, and use the bathroom. Tell the patient if any new equipment or furniture is brought into the room. Keep pathways in the room free of clutter.

For patients who are partially sighted, lighting is very important. Glare must be reduced because it actually interferes with vision. Windows should have adjustable shades, blinds, or sheers. Floors should not be highly polished (Fig. 51-12). Color can provide important cues to enable the partially sighted person to function. This is especially true of the older person whose color perception often changes. Older people perceive warm colors (red, orange, yellow) more accurately than cool colors (blue, green). Furniture color should be distinctly different from the color of floors

FIGURE **51-11 A,** To escort a visually impaired person, allow the person to grasp your upper arm. **B,** To enter a narrow passage or doorway, bring your arm behind your back to alert the person.

and walls. Light switches, handrails, and steps marked with contrasting colors are easier to locate. Dishes and cups with colored rims facilitate self-feeding and reduce spills.

Ineffective Coping

People who have lived with vision impairment usually have developed routines and strategies to cope with the situation. Ask about such routines, and maintain them as much as possible. If the patient uses assistive devices such as eyeglasses or magnifying glasses, make sure they are available and encourage their use. The older person who becomes confused during hospitalization may show dramatic improvement when eyeglasses are provided.

Encourage diversional activities when appropriate. The patient with some vision may be able to enjoy reading with magnifiers or large-print reading material. Talking books are available without charge through the American Foundation for the Blind. Many bookstores stock books on tape. Braille reading material and typewriters can be used by those who have been trained in this method. Braille uses arrangements

FIGURE 51-12 Glare perceived by a person with normal vision **(A)** and an older person whose eyes have undergone age-related changes **(B)**.

of raised dots to represent letters. The reader reads the material by moving the fingertips over the characters. Not everyone is able to master reading Braille because of the sensitive touch needed. Special telescopic lens and magnifiers can enable patients to read, write, and use a computer. Canes and guide dogs permit independent ambulation. Voice recognition programs permit computer use without typing.

Self-Care Deficit

Ask the patient what assistance is required instead of assuming that help is needed. Many patients are quite independent despite impaired vision. Do not encourage dependence during hospitalization. To orient the patient to the location of foods, fluids, or other objects, think of their arrangement as a clock face (e.g., "your meat is at 3 o'clock"). A consistent environment enables the patient to be more independent with less risk of injury. Do not move furniture, personal effects, and equipment without patient consent.

Some visually impaired people have guide dogs that enable them to move about more independently. These dogs are trained to guide their owners both inside and outside the home. They usually can go anywhere their owners go. Laws that restrict pets in public places usually do not apply to guide dogs. When the dogs are wearing their harnesses, they are working and should not be distracted by friendly strangers.

Ineffective Therapeutic Regimen Management

Patients with severe impairment should be referred to specialists in rehabilitation. They need to learn self-care

activities, safe mobility, and strategies to carry out usual roles such as child care and occupational skills. Teach patients with diseases of the eye any prescribed measures to cure or slow the progression of the disease.

DISORDERS AFFECTING THE EYE OR VISION

EXTERNAL EYE DISORDERS
Inflammation and Infection

The eye is a potential site for infectious and inflammatory conditions. Because of the sensitivity of the eye, such disorders can cause considerable discomfort. Some may even threaten vision if not treated.

Blepharitis. Blepharitis is an inflammation of the hair follicles along the eyelid margin. It can be caused by bacteria, most often by staphylococci. Seborrheic blepharitis is often found with seborrhea of the scalp and eyebrows.

Symptoms include itching, burning, and photophobia. Scales or crusts may be seen on the lid margins. The patient may complain that the eyelids are sealed shut by dried crusts on awakening.

Untreated blepharitis could lead to inflammation of the cornea or hordeolum (stye). The physician may prescribe an antibiotic ointment for the condition. Be certain that any medication applied to the eye is an *ophthalmic* preparation. The eyelids also can be gently cleansed with baby shampoo solution.

Hordeolum. Hordeolum is commonly called a *stye*. It is a common acute staphylococcal infection of the eyelid margin that originates in a lash follicle. The affected area of the lid is red, swollen, and tender. The primary treatment is the application of warm, moist compresses several times a day. If a person has repeated infections, these may be related to staphylococcal infections at some other location on the body. The physician attempts to locate any other infections and may order the hordeolum treated with ophthalmic antibiotics.

Chalazion. Chalazion is an inflammation of the glands in the eyelids. Swelling prevents fluid from leaving the glands, causing them to become enlarged and tender. Warm compresses may bring some relief. The physician may order antibiotics if infection is present. Surgical removal of the gland is necessary if the condition persists.

Conjunctivitis. Conjunctivitis is an inflammation of the conjunctiva caused by microorganisms, allergy, or chemical irritants. Bacterial conjunctivitis is commonly called *pinkeye.* It is characterized by redness of the conjunctiva, mild irritation, and drainage. Warm or cool compresses and topical vasoconstrictors may be ordered.

If inflammation is caused by an infectious agent, the infection can be passed from one person to another. Infected people should practice good hand washing and should avoid sharing washcloths. The condition usually clears up spontaneously, but antibiotics may be prescribed.

Viral conjunctivitis can be caused by herpes simplex virus type 1, herpes zoster virus, or adenoviruses. Viral infections are characterized by redness and drainage. The drainage in viral infections is watery rather than purulent. Round, raised areas that are white or gray in color may be seen on the conjunctiva. These areas are called *follicles.*

Viral infections tend to persist longer than bacterial infections. They also are more likely to produce severe eye damage. The medical management varies with the causative organism. Infections caused by herpes simplex virus type 1 are treated with idoxuridine (Herpex) ointment or other topical medications. Corticosteroids are contraindicated with the herpes virus. If given in the presence of herpes simplex virus type 1, corticosteroids may contribute to deep corneal ulcers and other complications.

Other organisms that can cause conjunctivitis include chlamydia and fungi. These eye infections are more common in developing countries but are occasionally seen in the United States. They are treated with topical or systemic antimicrobial medications.

Keratitis. Keratitis is inflammation or infection, or both, of the cornea. The structure of the cornea makes it especially vulnerable to injury. The portion of the cornea in front of the pupil has no blood vessels because it must remain transparent. This means that it has no direct blood supply, making it vulnerable to infections.

Sources of infection include bacteria, viruses, and fungi. Also, chemical or mechanical injuries cause inflammation that may be followed by infection. If scar

FIGURE **51-13** Eversion of the eyelid for inspection of the sclera and conjunctiva.

tissue forms, that portion of the cornea becomes cloudy and vision is impaired. Also, the infection can extend to the inner structures of the eye. Serious lesions can rupture if the eye is rubbed. Prompt treatment of keratitis therefore is very important to preserve vision.

Keratitis does not produce noticeable drainage, but it causes considerable pain. Medical treatment includes topical antibiotics and topical corticosteroids. Systemic antibiotics also may be ordered after culture and sensitivity results are obtained. Sometimes the physician injects antibiotics directly into the conjunctiva. Topical anesthetics are not used because the patient might accidentally cause additional injury to the anesthetized cornea. Eye pads are not used with keratitis because they provide a dark, damp environment for microorganisms to grow.

Entropion and Ectropion

Proper closure of the eyelids is important to protect the eye and keep the cornea moist. Entropion is a condition in which the lower lid turns inward. Eyelashes rub against the eye, causing pain and possibly scratching the cornea. Surgical correction usually is recommended.

Ectropion is a condition in which the lower lid droops and turns outward. The eye does not close completely, causing it to become dry and irritated. The dry cornea is easily injured. Like entropion, ectropion requires surgical correction.

Foreign Body

Everyone has experienced the discomfort of having a foreign body in the eye. Blinking and tearing usually will wash small irritants from the eye. If the foreign body remains in the eye, evert the upper and lower lids as illustrated in Figure 51-13. If the object is clearly

FIGURE **51-14** Keratoplasty. The damaged cornea is removed and then replaced with a corneal graft from a donor eye.

visible and does not appear to be embedded in the eye, you may attempt to remove it. Use a sterile cotton swab to touch the object gently. If the object is not embedded, it usually clings to the swab and can be removed. Foreign bodies that are embedded in the eye should be removed only by a physician.

Chemical Spills and Splashes

Chemical spills and splashes are discussed in Chapter 16.

Corneal Opacity

A healthy cornea is clear, allowing light to enter the pupil. When the cornea is injured by infection or trauma, scar tissue may form. In some cases, a rigid contact lens can correct the uneven corneal surface. If scar tissue prevents light from entering the eye, varying degrees of vision impairment occur. The only treatment for corneal opacity is removal of the scarred cornea and replacement with a healthy cornea. The surgical procedure is called a *keratoplasty.*

Healthy corneas are obtained from donors shortly after death. This may be authorized by the donor before death or by the family. The entire donor eye is removed (enucleation) and preserved, preferably within 4 hours of death. Eye tissue is easier to preserve than other body tissues. This permits keratoplasty to be done as a scheduled procedure rather than as an emergency on-call procedure. It can be done under local anesthesia. Before surgery, eye drops may be ordered to either dilate or constrict the pupil. Usually, drops are used that constrict the pupil (miotics). Constriction of the pupil pulls the iris over the lens like a curtain and protects the lens during surgery. Sometimes, however, it is necessary to remove the lens as well as the cornea. Lens extraction is necessary if the lens is cloudy because of injury or age-related changes. In this case, preoperative mydriatic drops are ordered to allow access to the lens.

The types of grafts used in keratoplasty are *penetrating* and *lamellar.* A penetrating graft consists of all layers of the cornea. A lamellar graft is only the superficial tissue layers of the cornea. The type of graft used depends on the extent of injury to the recipient's cornea.

FIGURE **51-15** Keratoplasty. **A,** Appearance of the eye soon after keratoplasty. **B,** Acute corneal rejection.

During a keratoplasty, the surgeon first removes the patient's damaged cornea. An identically sized graft is then taken from the donor eye and secured to the recipient's eye with very fine sutures, as shown in Figures 51-14 and 51-15. When a penetrating keratoplasty is done, the aqueous humor is lost from the anterior chamber of the eye. The surgeon replaces the fluid with a saline solution.

NURSING CARE *of the Patient Having Keratoplasty*

Preoperative nursing care of the patient having eye surgery is on pp. 1165 to 1166 in the Preoperative Nursing Care section. After surgery, the keratoplasty patient has an eye pad and a metal shield over the operative eye. Sometimes the other eye is temporarily patched as well because the eyes normally track together. This reduces eye movement until the operative eye heals. Corticosteroid eye drops may be ordered to reduce inflammation. Unlike other tissue transplants, corneal transplants do not require immunosuppressant therapy to prevent tissue rejection.

Assessment

Inspect the dressing for drainage, and ask if the patient is having any pain or nausea. After the dressing is removed, inspect the eye for corneal opacity. Also evaluate the patient's visual acuity. It is common for vision to be blurry the first few weeks followed by gradual improvement. Complete healing may take as long as 6 months.

The normal appearance of the eye soon after keratoplasty is seen in Figure 51-15, *A*.

In addition to routine postoperative care after eye surgery, the following specific care may apply after keratoplasty:

Nursing Diagnoses, Goals, and Outcome Criteria: Keratoplasty, Postoperative

NURSING DIAGNOSES	GOALS AND OUTCOME CRITERIA
Risk for Injury related to activities that increase intraocular pressure	Decreased risk for injury: patient avoids activities that increase intraocular pressure (bending forward, lifting, straining)
Acute Pain related to tissue trauma	Pain relief: patient states pain relieved, relaxed manner
Disturbed Sensory Perception related to inflammation, rejection of transplanted tissue	Adaptation to temporary vision impairment: patient performs usual activities with minimal assistance Gradual improvement in visual acuity: patient report, improved visual acuity scores
Ineffective Therapeutic Regimen Management related to lack of understanding of usual postoperative course	Effective management of prescribed plan of care: patient correctly describes and demonstrates self-care measures

Interventions

Risk for Injury

Caution the patient to avoid any activities that increase pressure in the eye, including rubbing the eye, bending forward, lifting, straining at stool, and coughing. Report and promptly treat nausea because vomiting raises intraocular pressure. Administer stool softeners as ordered to prevent constipation. The patient probably will be instructed to wear the shield for several weeks while sleeping to prevent accidental trauma.

Acute Pain

Only mild to moderate pain is expected after keratoplasty. The physician usually orders analgesics such as acetaminophen to be given as needed. Notify the physician of severe or increasing pain because it suggests increased intraocular pressure or infection.

Disturbed Sensory Perception

Rejection of corneal grafts is not common, but it can happen. When rejection occurs, blood vessels appear in the cornea and the cornea becomes cloudy (see Fig. 51-15, *B*). Corticosteroid drops are ordered to reduce inflammation and the risk of rejection. Patients should know that symptoms of rejection include redness, swelling, decreased vision, and pain. Other topical medications that usually are ordered are antibiotics to prevent infection and mydriatics to dilate the pupil.

Ineffective Therapeutic Regimen Management

Nurses and patients should realize that the grafted eye must heal just like any other body part that has undergone surgery. In the movies, the physician removes the dressing dramatically. The patient blinks a few times, and the world comes into focus. In reality, it takes a while before the patient's vision clears. Reassure the patient that this is normal.

Before discharge, determine what medications the patient will be taking at home. Review the medications with the patient, demonstrate proper self-administration, and have the patient return the demonstration. Instruct the patient to promptly report symptoms of graft rejection, which include unusual redness in the eye, eye pain, sudden change in visual acuity, and increased light sensitivity.

ERRORS OF REFRACTION

Light must pass through the cornea, aqueous humor, lens, and vitreous humor to reach the retina. These structures through which light passes are called *refractive media*. The term *refraction* refers to the bending of light rays—in the case of the eye, so that they focus on the retina. Abnormalities, called *errors of refraction*, occur when refractive media do not bend light rays correctly. Myopia, hyperopia, and astigmatism are common problems caused by variations in the structure of the eyeball. Figure 51-16 illustrates these variations and the type of correction required.

Types of Errors of Refraction

Myopia and Hyperopia. Myopia is the medical term for *nearsightedness*. In myopia, the lens is situated too far from the retina. Light rays come together to focus in front of the retina. People with myopia have difficulty

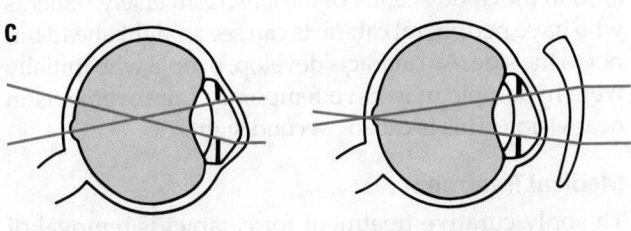

FIGURE **51-16** Refraction. **A,** Myopia: light rays converge before they reach the retina because the lens is too far from the retina. **B,** Hyperopia: light rays converge beyond the retina because the lens is too close to the retina. **C,** Astigmatism: uneven surfaces of the cornea bend light rays in a way that causes distortion of the image.

seeing distant images clearly. It is often recognized in the early school years. Typically, the condition slowly progresses until adolescence. New glasses usually are needed approximately every 2 years.

When the lens is too close to the retina, light rays come together behind the retina. This condition creates *hyperopia,* commonly known as *farsightedness.* The hyperopic person sees clearly in the distance but has difficulty focusing on close objects. Convex corrective lenses are needed for correction.

Astigmatism. When there are irregularities in the cornea or lens, astigmatism results. Most people have some degree of astigmatism. If the condition is mild, the natural lens can correct for the abnormality. If it is severe, however, vision is distorted, and corrective lenses are needed. A person can have astigmatism with myopia or hyperopia.

Presbyopia. Presbyopia is another disorder that is classified with errors of refraction. Presbyopia is poor accommodation that is due to loss of elasticity of the ciliary muscles. Accommodation is the adjustment of the lens for near and distant vision. It is accomplished by contraction or relaxation of the ciliary muscles, which causes the lens to change shape.

Presbyopia is usually considered a normal age-related change. It most often develops after age 40 years. As it progresses, people may be observed holding reading material at arm's length. People who are already hyperopic tend to have presbyopia at an earlier age than other people. Myopic people are usually able to read small print by holding it close.

Corrective lenses are needed when the visual changes become bothersome. Bifocal lenses are often prescribed. Bifocals have two different lenses. The upper part of the lens is used for distant vision, and the lower part is used for near vision. Trifocals have three lenses, for distant, closer, and near vision. Progressive lenses gradually blend the lens needed for seeing various distances. The wearer scans the lens to find the area needed for a particular task. Reading lenses must usually be changed every 2 to 3 years.

Medical Treatment

The primary treatment of errors of refraction is the prescription of corrective lenses. Eyeglasses are used most often. The obvious advantage of eyeglasses is that they require no special skills to use. Disadvantages are heavy frames and dirty lenses.

Contact lenses are tiny plastic disks made to fit over the patient's cornea. The lenses float on the tear film over the cornea. The primary advantages of contact lenses are convenience and appearance. Disadvantages include cost, the need for training and dexterity to insert and remove the lenses, and that they are easily lost. Another important disadvantage is the risk of corneal injury.

Several types of contact lenses are available. Hard lenses were developed first. They must be removed from the eye at the end of the day to prevent damage to the cornea. Soft lenses can be worn longer than hard lenses and require a shorter period of adjustment. Gas-permeable lenses are made of materials that allow oxygen and carbon dioxide to pass through them. This is important because the cornea exchanges gasses through the tear film beneath the contact lens. Extended-wear contact lenses can be worn for as long as 2 weeks. For this reason, they may be prescribed for older patients who have cataract surgery. Extended-wear contact lenses are more expensive than other lenses. The patient is cautioned to follow the prescribed cleaning schedule. Disposable contact lenses can be worn for up to 1 week and are then discarded.

Surgical Treatment

The past decade has seen several advancements in the surgical correction of refractive errors. *Photorefractive keratectomy* (PRK) uses an excimer laser to reshape the cornea for treatment of myopia or hyperopia. For the *laser in situ keratomileusis* (LASIK) procedure, a thin layer of the cornea is peeled back and the laser is used to reshape the middle layer of the cornea. These procedures are done under local anesthesia in outpatient facilities. The outcomes cannot be evaluated immediately because refraction stabilizes slowly after surgery. The newest surgical treatment for refractive errors uses plastic half rings called *Intacs.* The rings are inserted around the pupil between the layers of the cornea.

NURSING CARE *of the Patient with Errors of Refraction*

Nursing responsibilities for the patient with errors of refraction are limited except to encourage periodic examinations and to know if the patient uses corrective lenses. In emergency situations, the nurse may have to remove contact lenses for the patient. When caring for patients who have laser surgery, it may be your responsibility to teach postoperative care to the patient. You should include proper use of any prescribed eye drops (e.g., steroids), measures to protect the eye, and symptoms to be reported to the surgeon.

INTERNAL EYE DISORDERS
Cataract

The lens is a clear, flexible structure encased in an elastic capsule. It is located behind the iris and changes shape to focus on images of various sizes. When the lens becomes opaque (cloudy) so that it is no longer transparent, the condition is called a cataract.

Causes

Cataracts may be congenital, traumatic, or degenerative. Congenital cataracts are those that are present at birth. Traumatic cataracts are caused by chemical, mechanical, heat, or radiation injury. Degenerative cataracts are more common with aging, but they occur earlier in people with diabetes or Down syndrome.

Pathophysiology

The lens may become opaque (cloudy) quickly or slowly. Injuries tend to cause opacity rapidly, whereas age-related opacity progresses slowly. As opacity increases, light is unable to enter the eye and vision becomes cloudy. Blindness eventually results if a cataract is untreated. With age, both eyes are usually affected, although they may not change at the same rate.

Signs and Symptoms

Signs and symptoms of cataracts include cloudy vision, seeing spots or ghost images, and floaters. The pattern of vision changes depends on the location of the developing cataract. A central cataract is located in the center of the lens. Patients with central cataracts may have fairly good peripheral vision. They may actually see better in dim light because the pupil dilates, allowing them to see around the cloudy center of the lens. Conversely, patients who have peripheral cataracts can see straight ahead but not to the side. As cataracts develop, people who initially were hyperopic may have temporary improvements in near vision. This is called "second sight."

Medical Treatment

The only curative treatment for cataract is removal of the lens, although mydriatics may be helpful in the early stages. Cataract extraction is the most frequently performed eye operation in the United States. There are several types of cataract extraction, as illustrated in Figure 51-17. If the lens and capsule are removed, it is called an *intracapsular cataract extraction.* For the *extracapsular cataract extraction,* the lens is removed, leaving the capsule in place. The most common extracapsular

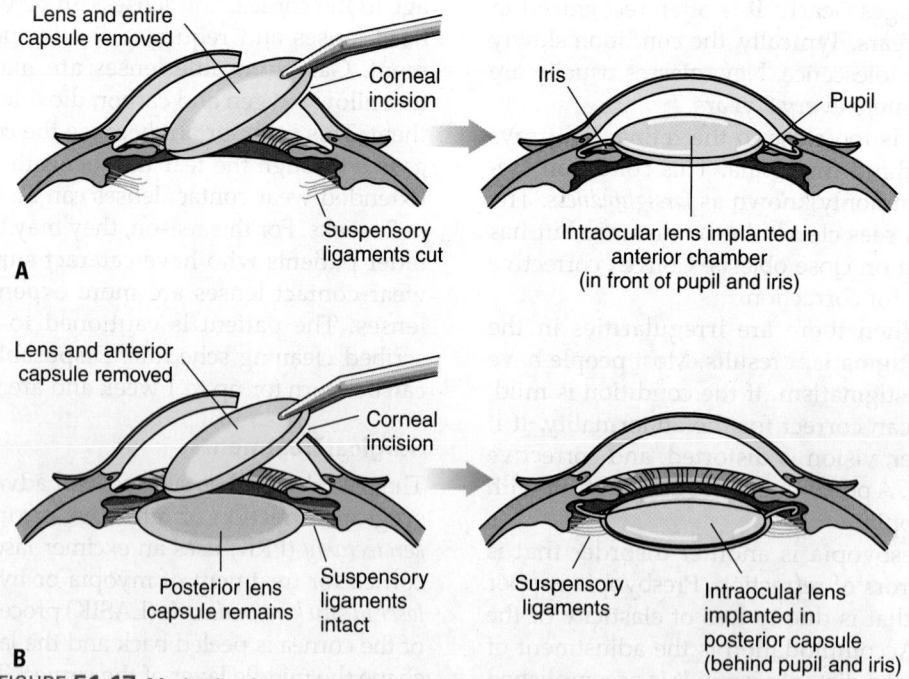

FIGURE 51-17 Methods of cataract extraction. **A,** Intracapsular cataract extraction with removal of entire lens and capsule. **B,** Extracapsular cataract extraction leaving posterior lens capsule intact.

procedure is phacoemulsification and aspiration, in which sound waves are used to break up the lens. The lens fragments are then suctioned out of the eye. The extracapsular cataract extraction is usually preferred. It typically is accompanied by placement of an artificial lens behind the iris. The remaining capsule can become cloudy, causing vision to become blurred again. This can usually be corrected easily with laser treatment.

Cataract extraction is commonly done on an outpatient basis. Most patients tolerate the procedure well with just a mild sedative and local anesthesia. In some cases, general anesthesia may be preferred. Cataract surgery is usually considered safe, even for those who are very old.

Complications

Complications that sometimes occur include leakage of vitreous humor, hemorrhage into the eye, and opening of the incision.

Lens Replacement

Once the lens has been removed, the eye is said to be *aphakic*. The patient is extra farsighted and unable to accommodate for changes in object size. Some type of artificial lens is needed for correction.

Cataract Eyeglasses. In the past, the only option for lens replacement was thick eyeglasses. They were heavy, unattractive, and left the patient with poor peripheral vision. Cataract eyeglasses magnified objects so much that the patient also had poor depth perception. The result was that patients misjudged distances. This caused difficulty in everything from eating to driving. Another disadvantage to the use of eyeglasses was that the patient either had to have the lenses removed from both eyes or be blind in the unoperated eye. Otherwise, the strong magnification caused double vision.

Contact Lenses. Contact lenses overcome many disadvantages of eyeglasses, but they have drawbacks as well. Considerable dexterity is required to insert, remove, and care for contact lenses. This makes them impractical for some older patients. The main complication of contact lens use is corneal injury.

Intraocular Lenses. The invention of plastic lenses (Fig. 51-17) that can be implanted in the eye has been a tremendous advance for many cataract patients. This type of lens is called an *intraocular lens*. The intraocular lens is almost always implanted immediately after removal of the natural lens. Complications of insertion include corneal edema, secondary glaucoma, lens displacement, and retinal detachment. Even with intraocular lenses, the patient may require reading glasses for close work.

NURSING CARE *of the Patient with Cataracts*

Cataract extractions often are done in day-surgery clinics. You may have limited opportunity for patient and family teaching. Care of the patient having eye surgery

is presented on pp. 1165 to 1168. This section emphasizes additional care specific to cataract surgery.

PREOPERATIVE CARE

Eye drops often are ordered at frequent intervals before cataract surgery. The orders must be followed exactly. Common drops used before cataract surgery are mydriatics, cycloplegics, antibiotics, and nonsteroidal anti-inflammatory agents. Mydriatics dilate the pupil, making it easier for the surgeon to access the lens. Cycloplegics temporarily paralyze the muscles of accommodation, keeping the eye still during the procedure. Antibiotics may be given to reduce the risk of infection, and anti-inflammatory drugs to reduce inflammation.

POSTOPERATIVE NURSING CARE

Assessment

After cataract surgery, ask about pain and nausea. The patient is likely to return from surgery wearing a patch and shield over the operative eye. Note the presence of the patch and any apparent drainage. Also note the patient's level of consciousness and orientation (see Nursing Care Plan: The Patient Having Cataract Surgery on p. 1178).

Nursing Diagnoses, Goals, and Outcome Criteria: Cataract Surgery: Postoperative	
NURSING DIAGNOSES	GOALS AND OUTCOME CRITERIA
Risk for Injury related to increased intraocular pressure	Reduced risk for injury: patient avoids activities that increase intraocular pressure; intraocular pressure remains 12-21 mm Hg
Disturbed Sensory Perception related to vision impairment	Adaptation to impaired vision: patient demonstrates self-care, maneuvers in environment without injury, performs activities of daily living, administers medications properly

Interventions

Risk for Injury

After cataract surgery, the most important thing is to prevent strain on the operative eye. Caution the patient not to rub the eye. Reinforce the physician's postoperative orders related to activity restrictions. Examples of restrictions intended to decrease strain are to sleep on the unaffected side, not to lift more than 5 pounds, and to avoid bending forward. Administer stool softeners as ordered to prevent straining at stool, or instruct the patient in self-medication. If nausea occurs, promptly administer an antiemetic as ordered.

Always be aware of safety precautions after cataract surgery. When one eye is patched, the patient has limited peripheral vision. The unoperated eye often

---

NURSING CARE PLAN

The Patient Having Cataract Surgery

ASSESSMENT

Health History: A 72-year-old retired welder is seeking medical care because of cloudy vision that has become increasingly worse. He reports spots moving across his field of vision. Cataracts were diagnosed, with the right lens affected more severely than the left. He had a right extracapsular cataract extraction under local anesthesia this morning in the outpatient surgery department. He says he has mild pain in the eye area at this time. His record reveals a history of myocardial infarction 5 years ago and surgery for prostate enlargement 6 months ago. Although he is retired, he works every day on his small farm. He lives with his wife and an adult daughter.

Physical Examination: He is alert and oriented. Vital signs: temperature, 98° F orally; pulse, 88; respirations, 18; blood pressure, 142/68. He is in semi-Fowler's position. An eye pad is in place over the right eye, protected with a metal shield. A small amount of clear drainage is noted seeping below the dressing.

Nursing Diagnosis	Goals and Outcome Criteria	Interventions
Risk for Injury related to increased intra-ocular pressure (IOP), trauma	Decreased risk for injury: patient avoids activities that increase IOP. Intra-ocular pressure remains 12-21 mm Hg.	Keep head of bed elevated. Instruct the patient not to impose stress on operative eye, rub the operative eye, strain, lean forward, or lie on the affected side. Administer antiemetics immediately as ordered for nausea and/or vomiting. Change damp pad as allowed. Administer eye drops (mydriatics, antimicrobials, and corticosteroids) as ordered. Encourage patient to take stool softeners as ordered to prevent constipation.
Disturbed Sensory Perception related to surgical trauma, lens removal, patching	The patient will adapt to visual impairment and function in environment without injury.	Keep the bed in low position. Approach the left side. Place the call bell on the left and instruct in use. Remove obstacles in the room. Assist with activities of daily living as needed.
Acute Pain related to tissue trauma	The patient will report that pain has decreased, will appear relaxed.	Assess pain. Notify the surgeon if severe (may indicate increased IOP). Administer analgesics as ordered, and evaluate effects.
Anxiety related to temporary vision impairment, activity restrictions	The patient will report decreased anxiety and will appear calm.	Explain what is being done and why. Explore feelings about surgery. Answer questions. Acknowledge fear of vision loss common with eye surgery. Respond promptly to needs.
Ineffective Therapeutic Regimen Management related to lack of understanding of condition, self-care, and limitations	Effective regimen management: the patient (and family member) will demonstrate instillation of medications and state activity limitations.	Explain postoperative limitations. No lifting over 5 lb, bending forward, or straining until cleared by physician. Review procedure for eye drops, and have patient or family member demonstrate instillation. Supplement verbal instructions with written information.

? CRITICAL THINKING QUESTIONS

- Why is it important to prevent constipation in a patient who has had cataract surgery?

- Explain why activities that increase intraocular pressure must be avoided postoperatively.

---

has some degree of impairment as well. Medications may be ordered that cause blurred vision. To prevent injury, make sure that the patient is familiar with the environment and knows how to use the call bell. Keep the bed in low position and the environment free of obstacles.

Impaired Sensory Perception

Confusion sometimes occurs in the postoperative period, especially in those who are very old. The confused person may fail to follow safety precautions or may place strain on the operative eye. Therefore moni-

tor mental status and ensure that a caregiver is readily available.

Medications prescribed after cataract surgery usually include antibiotics and corticosteroids. You may need to teach a family member or friend how to give the medications until the patient is able to administer them.

A mild analgesic is usually ordered as needed. Postoperative patients with cataract surgery should not have severe pain. If a patient complains of severe pain, notify the physician. Severe pain may indicate hemorrhage or rising pressure within the eye.

Glaucoma

Glaucoma is one of the leading causes of blindness in the United States. It occurs in infants, children, and adults. It is thought to affect 1% of Americans older than 60 years and to account for 10% of all cases of blindness in the United States. It is much more common in African Americans than whites.

Pathophysiology

Normally, aqueous humor enters and leaves the anterior chamber so that intraocular pressure is maintained between 10 and 21 mm Hg. Glaucoma is a condition in which intraocular pressure is increased above normal. It can be caused by a number of changes that affect the flow of aqueous humor in the anterior chamber of the eye. It most often is caused by some interference with the outflow of aqueous humor. Although glaucoma may follow trauma, the exact cause is often unknown.

Excess pressure damages the back portion of the eye. It impairs blood flow to the optic nerve and retina, resulting in vision impairment. Peripheral vision is lost first. The field of vision gradually narrows until the patient has tunnel vision. The patient who has tunnel vision can see only a small circle, as if looking through a tube or a tunnel. As the disease progresses, complete blindness eventually occurs. Vision may be restored if glaucoma is treated early; otherwise, vision loss is permanent.

Types of Glaucoma

The two most common types of glaucoma are open-angle glaucoma and angle-closure glaucoma. They are similar in that increased intraocular pressure is present in both, but they have some important differences. Both open-angle and angle-closure glaucoma are considered *primary glaucomas*. Increased intraocular pressure due to other conditions is called *secondary glaucoma*.

Open-Angle Glaucoma. Open-angle glaucoma also is called *chronic glaucoma*. It is more common than angle-closure glaucoma. Open-angle glaucoma results from some alteration that prevents the normal passage of aqueous humor through the trabecular meshwork. It is more common among African Americans on corticosteroid therapy and those with a parent or sibling who has the condition.

There usually are no signs and symptoms at first. Some patients complain of tired eyes, occasional blurred vision, and halos around lights. Another clue may be the need for frequent changes in eyeglass prescriptions.

Open-angle glaucoma usually is treated first with drug therapy. The types of medications used include beta–adrenergic blockers, adrenergics, cholinergics, carbonic anhydrase inhibitors, and hyperosmotic agents. Drugs work either by decreasing the production of aqueous humor or by improving the outflow of aqueous humor.

Beta-blockers often are the first drug used in the treatment of glaucoma. Timolol maleate (Timoptic), Betoptic (betaxolol), metipranolol (Optipranolol), carteolol (Ocupress), and levobunolol HCl (Betagan Liquifilm) are examples of beta-blockers used topically for glaucoma. These drugs probably lower intraocular pressure by decreasing the production of aqueous humor.

Examples of adrenergic drugs used for glaucoma are epinephrine HCl (Epifrin), apraclonidine (Iopidine), brimonidine (Alphagan), and dipivefrin (Propine) eye drops. Adrenergics decrease intraocular pressure by decreasing the formation of aqueous humor.

Cholinergic miotics such as pilocarpine (e.g., Akarpine, Isopto Carpine, Pilocar) and carbachol (Isopto Carbachol) and cholinesterase inhibitors such as echothiophate iodide (Phospholine Iodide) and physostigmine facilitate the outflow of aqueous humor. These drugs constrict the pupil, which permits fluid to flow more easily through the angle where the iris meets the cornea and into the trabecular meshwork. A disadvantage of many currently used miotics is that they must be administered frequently. Some new preparations, including ocular inserts, are effective for a longer period of time. These may eventually replace the preparations now in use.

Carbonic anhydrase inhibitors reduce intraocular pressure by decreasing the production of aqueous humor. Oral preparations include acetazolamide (Diamox), dichlorphenamide (Daranide), and methazolamide (Neptazane); topical forms are brinzolamide (Azopt) and dorzolamide (Trusopt). Some of these drugs can be given parenterally. Additional information about drugs used to treat glaucoma is provided in the Drug Therapy table on pp. 1180 and 1181. Hyperosmotic agents, including oral glycerin and intravenous mannitol (Osmitrol), promote movement of fluid from the intraocular structures.

Surgical intervention may be recommended when drugs do not reduce pressure adequately, the patient does not use prescribed drugs properly, or adverse reactions interfere with drug therapy. Surgical procedures for glaucoma include trabeculoplasty, trabeculectomy, and cyclocryotherapy. Trabeculoplasty may be tried first because it can be done under local anesthesia in an outpatient setting. The procedure involves the use of a laser to create multiple holes in the trabecular meshwork This is intended to improve drainage of aqueous humor from the anterior chamber. If the procedure is successful, intraocular pressure falls over a period of time. Meanwhile, the physician usually has the patient continue using glaucoma medications.

A trabeculectomy is one of several surgical procedures that create a channel to allow aqueous humor to drain under the conjunctiva. If this procedure is not effective, cyclocryotherapy may be done. A cold probe, called a *cryoprobe*, is used to freeze part of the ciliary body. Freezing destroys some of the tissue, resulting in decreased production of aqueous humor.

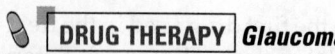

DRUG THERAPY | *Glaucoma*

GENERAL NURSING CONSIDERATIONS

1. Teach patient or caregivers, or both, proper way to administer eye drops.
2. Recognize that failure to control intraocular pressure can result in permanent blindness.
3. Avoid corticosteroids, succinylcholine, and anticholinergics in glaucoma patients.
4. Ophthalmic solutions should be tightly capped and protected from light.
5. Ophthalmic solutions should not be used if they change color or other characteristics.
6. Be alert for systemic effects of ophthalmic drugs.

DRUG	USE/ACTION	SIDE EFFECTS	NURSING INTERVENTIONS
BETA-ADRENERGIC BLOCKING AGENTS			

Timolol (Timoptic)
Metipranolol
  (OptiPranolol)
Carteolol (Ocupress)
Levobunolol
  (Betagan Liquifilm)
Betaxolol (Betoptic)
	Treatment of chronic (open-angle) glaucoma. Decreases aqueous formation. Does not affect pupil or visual acuity. Often used in combination with other drugs. Only betaxolol is beta-1 selective, so it is preferred with asthma and COPD.	Eye irritation.
		Possible systemic effects: bronchospasm, heart failure. Contraindicated with asthma.
			Monitor pulse, blood pressure, and respiration. Assess for wheezing, bronchospasm, bradycardia, hypotension, dysrhythmias.

CHOLINERGICS			
Pilocarpine (Isopto Carpine)	All cholinergics increase aqueous outflow.	Myopia. Poor vision in dim light. Lacrimation (tearing). Systemic effects: change in pulse rate or rhythm, bronchospasm, decreased blood pressure, gastric distress, diarrhea, headache.	Advise patient to use caution for tasks requiring distant vision or vision in dim light. Antidote: atropine. Minimize side effect by applying pressure over lacrimal duct.
Pilocarpine (Ocusert ocular system)		Few side effects.	Ocusert therapeutic system lasts 1 wk. More costly.
Carbachol (Isopto Carbachol)		Carbachol at first may cause aching of the eyes, brow pain, headache, light sensitivity, and blurred vision.	
Acetylcholine (Miochol)	Acetylcholine is used primarily in operating room because effect lasts only about 10 min.		Acetylcholine comes in a two-compartment vial. It is reconstituted immediately before use.
Echothiophate iodide (Phospholine Iodide)		Blurred vision, brow ache, eyelid twitching, watering eyes	
Physostigmine (Eserine)		Long-term use of Eserine causes conjunctivitis.	
ADRENERGICS			
Epinephrine HCl (Epifrin) Dipivefrin (Propine)	Decrease aqueous formation. For open-angle glaucoma.	Headache, brow ache, blurred vision, ocular irritation. Tachycardia and increased BP with systemic absorption.	Contraindicated with acute closed-angle glaucoma. Avoid concurrent use with MAOIs. Monitor heart rate and rhythm.
Apraclonidine (Iopidine)	Short-term use only.	Headache, dry mouth, conjunctivitis, ocular itching.	Monitor pulse and BP.
Brimonidine (Alphagan)	Long-term use with open-angle glaucoma or ocular hypertension.	Hypertension with Alphagan but not with Iopidine. Drowsiness.	Monitor BP.

BP, Blood pressure; *COPD,* chronic obstructive pulmonary disease; *MAOI,* monoamine oxidase inhibitor.

Angle-Closure Glaucoma. Angle-closure glaucoma is also called *acute glaucoma.* It accounts for only approximately 10% of all glaucomas. With angle-closure glaucoma, the flow of aqueous humor through the pupil is blocked. Pressure forces the iris forward, causing it to block the trabecular meshwork. There is a rapid rise in intraocular pressure. Pressure is often greater than 50 mm Hg. If the pressure is not lowered promptly, permanent blindness can result. Therefore angle-closure glaucoma is considered a medical emergency. Unlike open-angle glaucoma, angle-closure glaucoma causes sudden, acute pain.

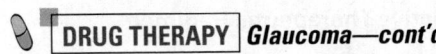 **DRUG THERAPY** *Glaucoma—cont'd*

DRUG	USE/ACTION	SIDE EFFECTS	NURSING INTERVENTIONS
PROSTAGLANDINS			
Latanoprost (Xalatan)	Increases aqueous outflow. Treats open-angle glaucoma and ocular hypertension.	Permanent darkening of green-brown, yellow-brown, and blue/gray/brown irides of the eyes. Also, blurred vision, burning, headache, conjunctival hyperemia.	
CARBONIC ANHYDRASE INHIBITORS			
Oral Acetazolamide (Diamox) Dichlorphenamide (Daranide) Methazolamide (Neptazane)	Treatment of acute and chronic glaucoma. Decreases aqueous formation.	Increased urinary output. Potential hypokalemia. Possible allergic response in people who are allergic to sulfonamides. Tingling of fingers and toes (paresthesia). Itching. Sore throat, skin rash, and fever may suggest serious blood disorders.	Monitor intake and output. Withhold and notify physician if patient is allergic. Assess for hypokalemia (pulse changes, mental status changes, muscle weakness, abdominal distention). Expect increased urine output. Provide access and assistance to toilet. Do not give at bedtime.
Topical Eyedrops Brinzolamide (Azopt)	Open-angle glaucoma	Irritation, bitter taste	Monitor for local and systemic allergic reactions.
OSMOTIC DIURETICS	Preoperative preparation for glaucoma surgery.	Increased urinary output. Potential hypokalemia. Elevated blood glucose. Headache. Tissue necrosis because of infiltration of intravenous solution.	Record intake and output. Assess for hypokalemia (pulse changes, muscle weakness, mental status changes, abdominal distention). Monitor patients with diabetes for elevated glucose. Monitor IV infusion. Stop infusion if infiltration is suspected, and notify RN.
Mannitol (Osmitrol)		Mannitol reserved for crisis situations because of risk of circulatory overload.	Mannitol may form crystals if cooled. If this happens, place vial in warm water until crystals dissolve. Cool to body temperature before administration.
Urea (Ureaphil)			Urea should be used within 24 hr after reconstitution.
Glycerin (Osmoglyn)			Synthetic glycerin available for people with diabetes to reduce effects on blood glucose.
COMBINATION AGENT			
Dorzolamide (Cosopt)	Combined action of beta-blocker and carbonic anhydrase inhibitors.	See each type.	See each type. Contraindicated with asthma.

Other signs and symptoms are blurred vision, halos around lights, nausea and vomiting, and headache on the affected side.

The goal of medical treatment is to reduce the intraocular pressure quickly. Drugs used initially to treat angle-closure glaucoma include miotics and oral or intravenous carbonic anhydrase inhibitors (see the Drug Therapy Table above and on p. 1180 for details). After the pressure has been lowered, iridotomy or iridectomy is usually recommended to prevent recurrence. These procedures create an opening in the iris to permit aqueous humor to flow through the pupil normally. The procedure may be done on both eyes because the healthy eye is likely to experience similar problems in the future. There are two types of iridotomy: peripheral and keyhole.

One other procedure is cyclodialysis, a procedure that involves opening the angle in the anterior chamber with a special instrument inserted through a small incision in the sclera.

NURSING CARE *of the Patient with Glaucoma*

Nurses who work in acute care settings are most concerned with drug therapy and patient teaching for self-care. Patients with chronic glaucoma who are hospitalized for other reasons still require management of their glaucoma.

Assessment

General assessment of the patient with an eye disorder is outlined in Box 51-2. Nurses who work in special clinics or units may also measure intraocular pressure as indicated. When a patient has glaucoma, you must collect data about patient knowledge of the disease and treatment and patient ability to carry out self-care.

If the patient has impaired vision, additional diagnoses may be appropriate. These are discussed in detail on pp. 1169 to 1171 in the Nursing Care of the Visually Impaired Patient section. General surgical care was also addressed on pp. 1165 to 1168.

Nursing Diagnoses, Goals, and Outcome Criteria: Glaucoma	
NURSING DIAGNOSES	GOALS AND OUTCOME CRITERIA
Risk for Injury related to increased intraocular pressure	Decreased risk for injury: adherence to prescribed measures to reduce intraocular pressure, normal intraocular pressure readings
Fear related to actual or potential loss of vision	Decreased fear: patient states feeling less fearful
Ineffective Therapeutic Regimen Management related to lack of understanding of disease, treatment, complications	Effective management of condition: patient correctly describes and adheres to prescribed drug therapy
Acute Pain related to acute increase in intraocular pressure, inflammation caused by corrective procedures	Pain relief: patient states reduced or relieved, relaxed manner

Interventions
Risk for Injury

One of the most important things you can do to keep intraocular pressure within normal limits is to administer prescribed medications. Be extremely cautious in selecting and administering ophthalmic medications. Different medications are often ordered for the affected and the unaffected eye. The procedure for applying eye drops and ointments is described on p. 1165 in the Topical Medications section.

Fear and Ineffective Therapeutic Regimen Management

You must be sensitive to the patient's fears about glaucoma leading to blindness. Emphasize that adherence to prescribed drug therapy can usually control intraocular pressure and reduce the risk of complications. Because open-angle glaucoma is painless, the patient may not appreciate the need for ongoing treatment. Stress the importance of keeping regular appointments for evaluation of intraocular pressure. Unfortunately, noncompliance with drug therapy is a frequent nursing diagnosis with glaucoma. Remember (and teach the patient) that any drugs that dilate the pupil are contraindicated. Patients may not be aware that many nonprescription cold and allergy remedies contain chemicals that dilate the pupil. The physician or pharmacist should be consulted before taking any additional drugs.

Patients who have glaucoma should wear a bracelet to alert health care providers to the condition. They should keep their medications on hand at all times. When traveling, the patient with glaucoma should keep spare medications in separate locations in case one is lost. It is helpful to have a wallet card stating the exact medication schedule in case the patient becomes ill and is unable to give this information.

Acute Pain

Pain in acute glaucoma attacks is treated with drugs that reduce intraocular pressure. Analgesics may be given as ordered. If the patient has surgery for glaucoma, postoperative care is similar to the general care after eye surgery, described on pp. 1166 to 1168 in the Postoperative Nursing Care section. Monitoring intraocular pressure is especially important after glaucoma surgery. Postoperative pain can usually be treated with nonopioid analgesics. Report increasing or unrelieved pain to the surgeon.

Many drugs are contraindicated with glaucoma. Caution patients not to take nonprescription drugs without consulting their pharmacist or physician.

Consider the Alternative

Caution patients not to take over-the-counter products containing ephedra (ma huang) because they can raise intraocular pressure.

Retinal Detachment
Pathophysiology

Retinal detachment is a separation of the sensory layer of the eyeball from the pigmented layer. It begins when a tear in the retina allows fluid to collect between the sensory and the pigmented layers. The fluid causes the two layers to separate. Separation deprives the sensory layers of nutrients and oxygen that normally are supplied by the blood vessels in the choroid. This leads to damage to the nerve tissue in the sensory layer and

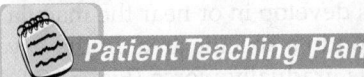

Patient Teaching Plan

Glaucoma

- Glaucoma usually responds to treatment, but it can lead to blindness if untreated.
- It is essential to have regular checkups to monitor intra-ocular pressure because glaucoma is usually painless.
- Consult with a pharmacist or physician before taking any new medication.
- Wear a medical alert tag.
- Take spare medication when traveling.
- Notify your physician if visual acuity or peripheral vision decreases.

---

resultant partial or complete loss of vision. Retinal tears may occur spontaneously or as a result of trauma. They are more common in older people and in people with myopia.

Signs and Symptoms

Signs and symptoms of retinal detachment depend on the location and extent of the detachment. Patients may report seeing flashes of light or floaters. Vision may be cloudy. If the area of detachment is large, vision may be lost completely. Some patients say it seems as if a curtain has come down or across the line of vision (Fig. 51-18). This is very frightening to the patient.

Medical and Surgical Treatment

Special procedures are required to repair retinal detachments. Most holes or tears must be sealed promptly. Laser photocoagulation is one method commonly used to do this. The intense light burns the detached portion of the retina. As the area heals, scar tissue forms that seals the tear. Cryotherapy also causes scar tissue to form, but it uses a cold probe applied to the eyeball behind the tear. The cold radiates through the layers of tissue, freezing the torn tissue. Another procedure that may be employed is retinopexy in which gas is injected into the eye to apply pressure to the tear.

Scleral buckling is often done along with laser treatment or cryotherapy. The scleral buckle is a Silastic band that is secured around the eyeball under the

Detached retina

FIGURE **51-18** Loss of partial field of vision due to retinal detachment.

sclera. Small silicone implants are sutured under the band opposite the area of detachment. This procedure brings the layers of tissue back together by pressing from the outside. The band is left in place permanently (Fig. 51-19). The physician may inject an air bubble or some normal saline into the vitreous humor after the surgical procedure. The purpose of this is to apply internal pressure to the detached portion of the retina.

Sometimes tears cause bleeding into the vitreous. Significant amounts of blood in the vitreous interfere with vision. When this occurs, the physician may do a vitrectomy to remove the bloody tissue. Vitrectomy also is indicated when the vitreous is creating traction on the retina.

NURSING CARE of the Patient with Retinal Detachment

Before corrective measures are taken, the patient usually is placed on strict bed rest with the head elevated. In the preoperative period, many patients are very anxious. Encourage them to talk about their fears and to ask questions. Even though the procedure may be done under local anesthesia, oral intake may be restricted to

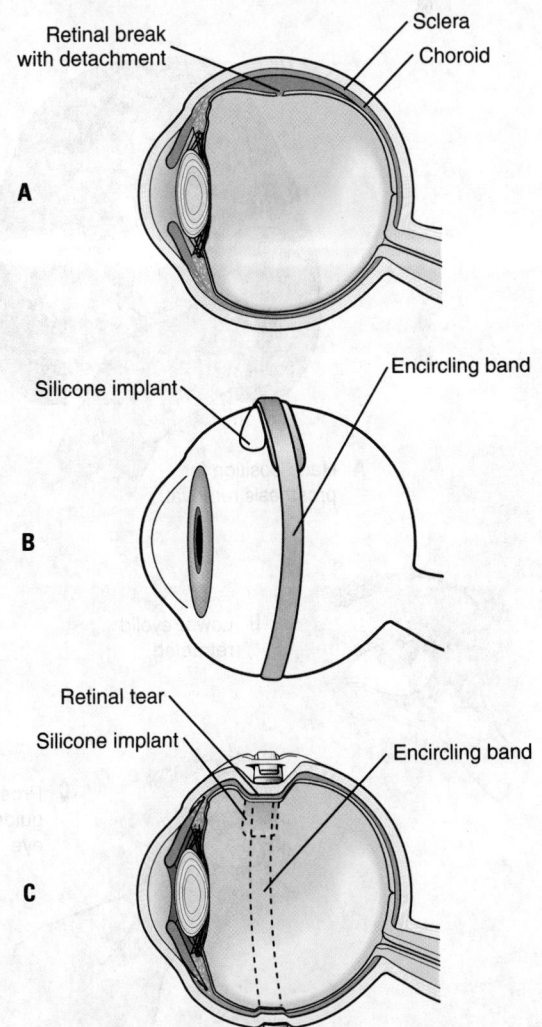

FIGURE **51-19** **A**, Retinal detachment. **B** and **C**, Scleral buckle and silicone implant in place to treat retinal detachment.

reduce the risk of postoperative vomiting. Intravenous fluids may be ordered.

Postoperative care is essentially the same as for other patients undergoing eye surgery, as described on pp. 1166 to 1168 in the Postoperative Nursing Care section. Positioning orders may be very specific for these patients. If an air bubble has been injected, it will rise to the top of the eye. If the patient's detachment is in the back of the eye, a face-down position is necessary to keep the bubble in the right place. Saline travels down rather than up, so the same patient would need to stay face up if saline had been injected. The surgeon prescribes any activity limitations. The length of hospitalization varies depending on the location and severity of the tear, the type of repair, and the surgeon's routines.

Senile Macular Degeneration

The macula is the part of the retina that is responsible for central vision. As people age, changes in the eye cause the macula to degenerate. Both eyes are usually affected. The two types of macular degeneration are dry (strophic) and wet (exudative). In the wet form,

abnormal blood vessels develop in or near the macula resulting in loss of vision in a specific area. In the dry form, central vision gets gradually worse (Fig. 51-20). Patients often report difficulty reading or doing close work. Both types are progressive. Peripheral vision remains intact. It is usually adequate to allow mobility in familiar settings.

Regular eyeglasses do not improve vision with macular degeneration. Special telescopic lenses may

Macular degeneration

FIGURE **51-20** Vision of the patient with macular degeneration.

A Hand position for prosthesis removal

B Lower eyelid retracted

C Prosthesis guided from eye

D Ocular prosthesis (note notched end)

E Upper eyelid retracted

F Notched end of prosthesis sliding under upper eyelid

G Prosthesis sliding under lower eyelid

FIGURE **51-21** Removal (**A-C**) and insertion (**D-G**) of an eye prosthesis.

be helpful. Laser treatments may offer hope to some patients with macular degeneration. The nurse needs to help the patient and family members learn to cope with declining vision. The nursing care is like that described on p. 1170 in the Nursing Care of the Visually Impaired Patient section.

Consider the Alternative

Some practitioners believe that antioxidants (vitamins C and E) may delay the onset and slow the progression of age-related macular degeneration. Research is in progress to determine if antioxidants are effective.

Enucleation

Some eye conditions are so serious that removal of the eyeball is the only treatment. **Enucleation** is the term used for removal of the eye. Conditions that may result in enucleation include injury, infection, sympathetic ophthalmia, and some glaucomas and malignancies.

During the surgical procedure, the eyeball is removed. A round device is placed in the cavity, and muscles are sutured over it. The conjunctiva is then sutured over the muscle. This procedure creates a foundation for the future placement of a prosthesis. The patient returns from surgery with a temporary shell called a *conformer* in the prosthesis base, which is covered with a pressure dressing. Observe for excessive bleeding or increasing pain. Report any temperature elevation. After the pressure dressing is removed, the physician may order wound care and topical medications.

Approximately 1 month after the enucleation, a prosthesis can be fitted by an optician. The prosthesis is carefully made to look like the patient's natural eye. The patient must learn to insert, remove, and clean the prosthesis. Nurses also should know how to care for an eye prosthesis as illustrated in Figure 51-21. The steps to remove and clean a prosthesis are the following:

1. Wash hands thoroughly.
2. Gently depress and pull the lower lid down.
3. Allow the prosthesis to slip out over the lower lid.
4. Wash the prosthesis under running water, using the fingers to remove any debris.

If the prosthesis is to be stored, it should be placed in a container with normal saline or water. To reinsert the prosthesis, do the following:

1. Raise the upper lid by pressing it up against the orbit.
2. Slip the top of the prosthesis under the orbit.
3. Pull the lower lid down so that the prosthesis can slip into place.

The patient's nursing care plan should always inform staff that the patient has a prosthesis.

Key Points

- Eleven million people in the United States have some vision impairment.
- After eye surgery, nursing care addresses Risk for Injury, Disturbed Sensory Perception, Acute Pain, Anxiety, and Ineffective Therapeutic Regimen Management.
- Increased intraocular pressure must be controlled to prevent permanent vision loss.
- Vision loss affects all aspects of a person's life: independence, mobility, employment, communication, and interpersonal relationships.
- Common nursing diagnoses for patients with impaired vision include Disturbed Sensory Perception, Ineffective Coping, Self-Care Deficit, and Ineffective Therapeutic Regimen Management.
- Infectious and inflammatory conditions of the eye include blepharitis, hordeolum, chalazion, conjunctivitis, and keratitis.
- Entropion is inversion of the lower lid; ectropion is eversion of the lower lid.
- A foreign body embedded in the eye should be removed only by a physician.
- Corneal opacity is treated with removal of the scarred cornea and replacement with a healthy donor cornea in a procedure called *keratoplasty*.
- Errors of refraction include myopia, hyperopia, and astigmatism and are often correctable with corrective lenses.
- An opaque lens, called a *cataract*, can be removed and vision restored with a lens replacement in the form of eyeglasses, contact lenses, or intraocular lenses.
- Glaucoma, increased intraocular pressure, is a leading cause of blindness and is treated with drug therapy or surgery, or both.
- Nursing care of the patient with glaucoma focuses on Risk for Injury, Fear, Ineffective Therapeutic Regimen Management, and Acute Pain.
- Retinal detachment is separation of the sensory layer of the eyeball from the pigmented layer and can result in partial or complete loss of vision.
- Treatments for retinal detachment include laser therapy, cryotherapy, retinopexy, scleral buckling, and vitrectomy.
- Senile macular degeneration causes progressive loss of central vision but may be improved by laser treatment.
- Enucleation is removal of the eyeball necessitated by injury, infection, sympathetic ophthalmia, and some glaucomas and malignancies.
- After enucleation, a prosthesis can be used to restore the patient's normal appearance.

Go to your Companion CD-ROM for a Pharmacology Tutorial, Audio Glossary, and 3-D animations.

evolve   Be sure to visit the companion Evolve site at http://evolve.elsevier.com/Linton/ for WebLinks and additional online resources.

REVIEW QUESTIONS *Choose the best answer.*

1. The fluid that fills the anterior chamber of the eye is:
    1. Aqueous humor
    2. Ciliary fluid
    3. Vitreous humor
    4. Refractive fluid

2. Your examination of the eyes of an older adult reveals eyeballs slightly sunken in the orbits, small pupils that do not respond to light, a grayish ring around the iris, and a complaint that the eyes feel dry sometimes. Which of these would you consider *abnormal* in an older adult?
    1. Eyeballs slightly sunken
    2. Small pupils
    3. Pupils not responsive to light
    4. Eyes that feel dry sometimes

3. You are assisting with a community vision screening project. A participant says, "The nurse says my vision is 20/40 in both eyes. What does that mean?" Your response should be which of the following?
    1. You see best at 20 to 40 feet from objects.
    2. You cannot see more than 40 feet in the distance.
    3. At 40 feet, you can read what most people can read at 20 feet.
    4. At 20 feet, you can read what a person with normal vision could read at 40 feet.

4. When a patient comes to the office for an eye examination, the ophthalmologist administers phenylephrine 2.5% eye drops to:
    1. Reveal any scratches on the cornea
    2. Dilate the pupil
    3. Anesthetize the cornea
    4. Dilate retinal blood vessels

5. A patient is being discharged after cataract surgery. Discharge instructions should include:
    1. Always lie on the affected side
    2. Avoid pressure on the operative eye
    3. Moderate to severe pain is expected
    4. Resume normal activities immediately

6. To guide a visually impaired person, you should:
    1. Stand side by side and hold the person's hand
    2. Let the person hold your upper arm
    3. Walk behind the patient and advise of obstacles
    4. Have the person walk behind you with hands on your shoulders

7. After keratoplasty, you observe that the patient's cornea is cloudy. You should:
    1. Reassure the patient that cloudiness is normal for several weeks after surgery
    2. Elevate the patient's head and encourage increased fluid intake
    3. Report signs of corneal rejection to the physician
    4. Prepare the patient for emergency surgery

8. Drugs used to treat open-angle glaucoma act by decreasing aqueous formation or:
    1. Increasing aqueous outflow
    2. Dilating the canal of Schlemm
    3. Relaxing the trabecular meshwork
    4. Dilating the pupil

9. The most serious complication of angle-closure glaucoma is:
    1. Rupture of the eyeball
    2. Permanent blindness
    3. Nausea and vomiting
    4. Increased intracranial pressure

10. Positioning after surgery for retinal detachment depends on:
    1. Patient preference
    2. Intraocular pressure
    3. Location of the repaired tear
    4. Amount of bleeding

Ear and Hearing Disorders

Objectives

After reading and studying this chapter, you should be able to:

1. Identify the data to be collected for the assessment of a patient with a disorder affecting the ear, hearing, or balance.
2. Describe the tests and procedures used to diagnose disorders of the ear, hearing, or balance.
3. Explain the nursing considerations for each of the tests and procedures.
4. Explain the nursing care for patients receiving common therapeutic measures for disorders of the ear, hearing, or balance.
5. Describe the pathophysiology, signs and symptoms, complications, and medical or surgical treatment for selected disorders.
6. Assist in the development of a nursing care plan for a patient with a disorder of the ear, hearing, or balance.
7. Identify measures the nurse can take to reduce the risk of hearing impairment and to detect problems early.

Key Terms

Be sure to check out the bonus material on the *Companion CD-ROM,* including selected audio pronunciations.

cerumen (sĕ-ROO-mĕn, p. 1187)
dizziness (p. 1196)
equilibrium (ē-kwĭ-LĬB-rē-ŭm, p. 1187)
otalgia (ō-TĂL-jē-ă, p. 1189)
otic (Ō-tĭk, p. 1193)
ototoxic (ō-tō-TŎK-sĭk, p. 1190)
presbycusis (prĕz-bē-KŪ-sĭs, p. 1188)
tinnitus (tĭ-NĪ-tĭs, p. 1189)
tympanic membrane (tĭm-PĂN-ĭk MĔM-brān, p. 1187)
vertigo (VĔR-tĭ-gō, p. 1196)

Approximately 1 in 1000 infants born in the United States has some hearing impairment. No one knows exactly how many adults are hard of hearing, but approximately half of those older than 75 years have some hearing loss. Regardless of the numbers of people affected, the impact of hearing loss is certainly significant. Health care providers can reduce disability by teaching people how to prevent hearing loss and by helping rehabilitate those who are impaired.

ANATOMY AND PHYSIOLOGY OF THE EAR

The ears are essential organs for hearing and for position sense. Position sense enables a person to know the position of body parts without looking. It is also necessary for **equilibrium** (state of balance needed for walking, standing, and sitting).

ANATOMY

The ear has three major sections: the external ear, the middle ear, and the inner ear (Fig. 52-1).

External Ear

Auricle. The external ear includes the auricle and the external auditory canal. The auricle, also called the *pinna,* is the visible part of the ear.

Innervation. Many nerves innervate the ear. This is the reason pain in the ear can sometimes be traced to disorders of the nose, mouth, or neck. Of special importance is the facial nerve (the seventh cranial nerve), which lies alongside the auditory canal. The facial nerve is protected in the canal by a thin bony covering. It exits from the skull just in front of the ear and branches across the face to control muscle movement.

Lymph Drainage. Lymph nodes located in front of, behind, and below the auricle drain the ear. In the presence of ear infections, they may become enlarged.

External Auditory Canal. The external auditory canal extends from the external opening of the ear to the tympanic membrane. The **tympanic membrane** is commonly called the *eardrum.* The canal is lined with cells that secrete **cerumen** (earwax). The waxy secretion coats and protects the canal.

Tympanic Membrane. The tympanic membrane at the end of the external auditory canal is shiny and pearl-gray. Sound waves entering the external auditory canal cause the membrane to vibrate.

Middle Ear

Bones. The middle ear is an air-filled space in the temporal bone. It contains three small bones (ossicles): the malleus (hammer), the incus (anvil), and the stapes (stirrup). The function of these bones is to forward the sound waves transmitted by the tympanic membrane to the inner ear.

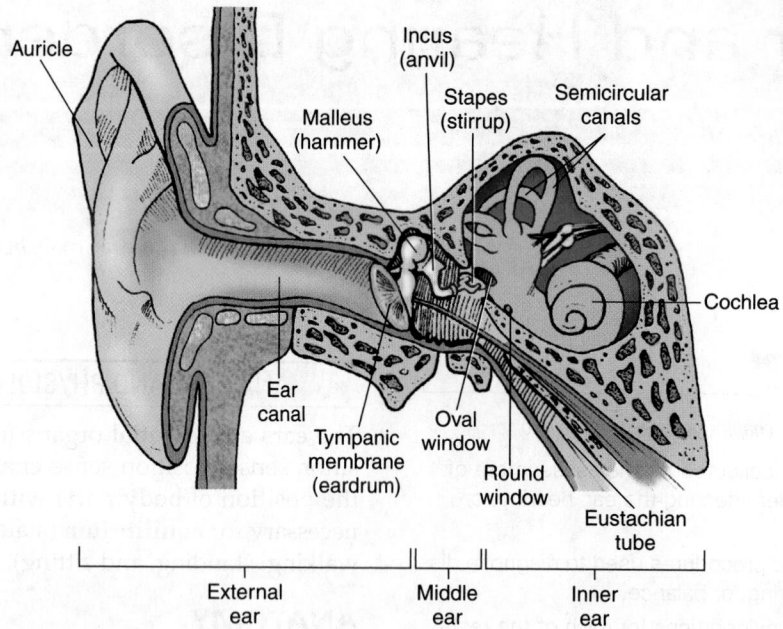

FIGURE **52-1** Anatomic structure of the ear illustrating the three major sections: the external ear, the middle ear, and the inner ear.

The malleus lies directly under the tympanic membrane. One portion of the malleus is attached to the membrane, and another portion is connected to the incus. The incus is connected to the stapes. The stapes has a footplate that fits into the oval window. The oval window, which opens into the vestibule, separates the middle ear from the inner ear. Sound waves are transmitted from the tympanic membrane to the malleus, the incus, the stapes, and then to the oval window.

Eustachian Tube. An important structure in the middle ear is the eustachian tube. The eustachian tube extends from the middle ear to the nasopharynx, as illustrated in Figure 52-2. It creates an air passage to the middle ear so that air pressure remains the same on both sides of the tympanic membrane.

Mastoid Process. The mastoid process is the bony structure behind the auricle. The interior is made up of air cells that are directly connected to the middle ear. The mastoid process is very close to the brain.

Inner Ear

The inner ear consists of the membranous labyrinth and the bony labyrinth. The membranous labyrinth contains fluid called *endolymph*. Endolymph moves with changes in body position.

The parts of the bony labyrinth are the vestibule, semicircular canals, and cochlea. The oval window opens into the vestibule. Receptors in the vestibule monitor the position of the head to maintain posture balance. Receptors in the semicircular canals monitor changes in rate or direction of movement to maintain balance during movement. The cochlea is a coiled tube that looks like a snail. It contains the organ of Corti, which is the receptor end-organ of hearing. The organ

of Corti transmits stimuli from the oval window to the acoustic (auditory) nerve.

PHYSIOLOGY OF HEARING

The perception and interpretation of sound depend on a complex series of steps. A malfunction at any step can result in some type of hearing impairment. Figure 52-3 illustrates the steps involved in the hearing process.

AGE-RELATED CHANGES IN THE EAR

Changes occur in the external, middle, and inner ear with aging. Some changes have no functional significance, but others can lead to serious problems with hearing or balance.

The skin of the auricle may become dry and wrinkled. Dryness of the external canal causes itching. Cerumen production declines, and the protective wax is drier. Hairs in the canal become coarser and longer, especially in men. The combination of dry cerumen and coarse hairs sometimes leads to obstruction of the canal. The eardrum thickens, and the bony joints in the middle ear degenerate somewhat. Surprisingly, these changes are not thought to impair hearing significantly.

Changes in the inner ear, however, affect sensitivity to sound, understanding of speech, and balance. Degenerative changes include atrophy of the cochlea, the cochlear nerve cells, and the organ of Corti. The result is that many older people have some degree of hearing loss and some have problems with balance. The type of hearing loss most often associated with age is called **presbycusis.** Presbycusis is discussed in the Presbycusis section on pp. 1205 and 1206.

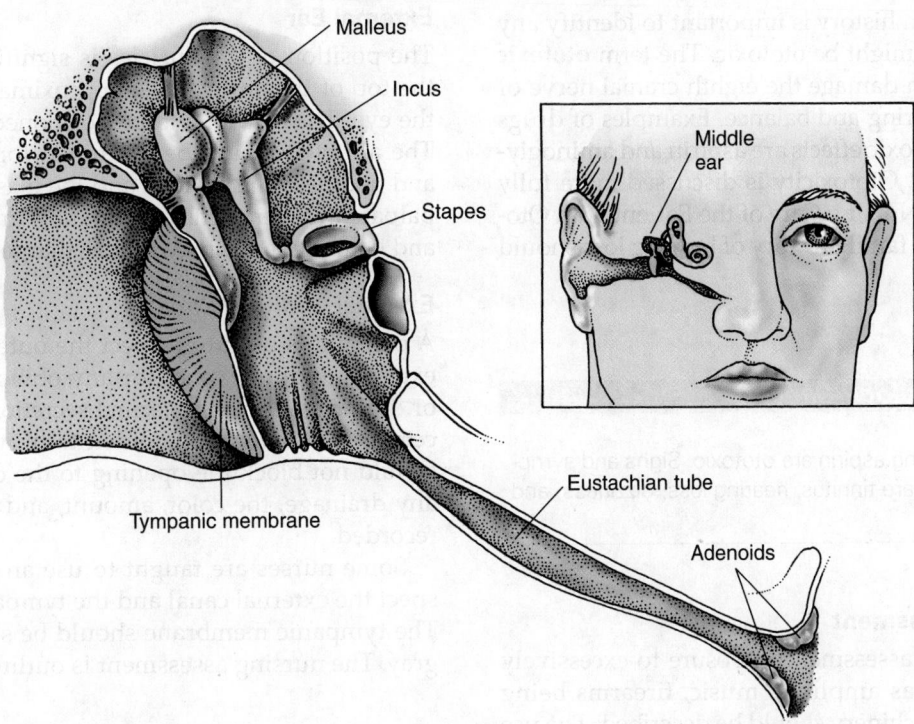

FIGURE **52-2** The eustachian tube extends from the middle ear to the nasopharynx.

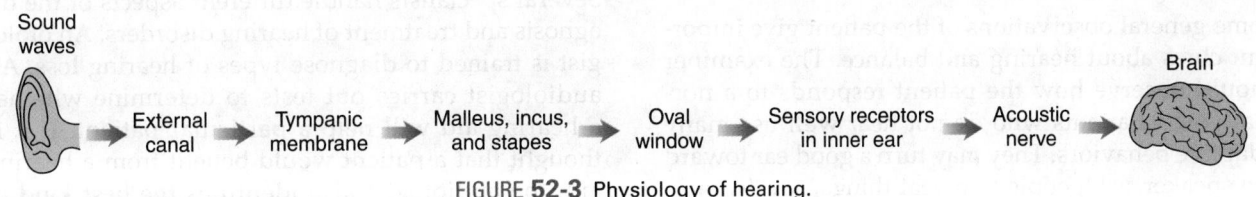

FIGURE **52-3** Physiology of hearing.

NURSING ASSESSMENT OF THE EXTERNAL EAR, HEARING, AND BALANCE

The nursing assessment of the ear includes inspection of the external ear and evaluation of hearing and balance. In addition to collecting data about the patient's hearing and balance, the LPN/LVN may be trained to perform some specific diagnostic procedures to evaluate hearing. To collect data from the patient, the assessor must first determine if the patient has a hearing impairment that interferes with verbal communication. If the patient's hearing impairment is severe, determine the usual means of communication. It may be necessary to call on a family member or a sign language interpreter or to use written communication during the assessment.

HEALTH HISTORY

History of Present Illness

The health history begins with a full description of any symptoms that may reflect problems with the ear, including changes in hearing acuity, pain, tinnitus, dizziness, vertigo, nausea, vomiting, and problems with balance. Changes in hearing acuity are described to include the kind of change that occurred and whether it was sudden or gradual. The patient is asked to describe the nature of the pain (e.g., sharp, throbbing, dull) and when it occurs. Pain in the ear is called otalgia. If tinnitus (ringing in the ears) is present, ask if the sound heard is continuous or intermittent. Dizziness, vertigo, nausea, vomiting, or problems with balance and the circumstances under which they occur should be documented.

Past Medical History

The interviewer should ask about any previous acute or chronic ear problems. Acute conditions that may affect hearing or balance include sinus infections, dental problems, allergies, and upper respiratory infections. Chronic conditions that may be significant are hypertension, diabetes mellitus, and hypothyroidism. Recent surgical procedures on the ear or throat or a recent head injury should be noted.

Hearing impairments are often congenital (present at birth). One cause of hearing loss in an infant is rubella during the mother's pregnancy. Therefore it should be noted whether female patients have had rubella or have been immunized for the infection.

The medication history is important to identify any drugs taken that might be ototoxic. The term ototoxic means a drug can damage the eighth cranial nerve or the organs of hearing and balance. Examples of drugs that can have ototoxic effects are aspirin and aminoglycoside antibiotics. Ototoxicity is discussed more fully on p. 1206 in the Nursing Care of the Patient with Ototoxicity section. A family history of hearing loss should be documented.

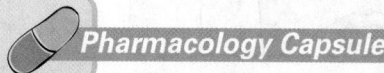
Pharmacology Capsule

Some drugs including aspirin are ototoxic. Signs and symptoms of ototoxicity are tinnitus, hearing loss, dizziness, and ataxia.

Functional Assessment

In the functional assessment, exposure to excessively loud noise such as amplified music, firearms being used, or noisy machinery should be described. The use of any assistive hearing devices should be noted.

PHYSICAL EXAMINATION

Some general observations of the patient give important clues about hearing and balance. The examiner should observe how the patient responds to a normal voice. Patients who do not hear well use many adaptive behaviors. They may turn a good ear toward the speaker, ask people to repeat things, say "what?" frequently, or watch the speaker's mouth closely. The presence of a visible hearing aid should be noted. The patient's posture and balance while walking and sitting alert the examiner to possible inner ear problems.

External Ear

The position of the auricles is significant. Normally, the top of the auricle is at approximately the level of the eye. The ears should be positioned symmetrically. The auricles should be examined for shape, lesions, and nodules. The auricles and the mastoid process are palpated for tenderness. Palpation in front of, below, and behind the ear may locate enlarged lymph nodes.

External Auditory Canal

A penlight is used to inspect the outer portion of the external auditory canal for any obvious obstructions or drainage. The only normal secretion in the canal is cerumen. It should be golden to brown in color and should not block the opening to the canal. If there is any drainage, the color, amount, and odor should be recorded.

Some nurses are taught to use an otoscope to inspect the external canal and the tympanic membrane. The tympanic membrane should be shiny and pearl-gray. The nursing assessment is outlined in Box 52-1.

DIAGNOSTIC TESTS AND PROCEDURES

Several specialists handle different aspects of the diagnosis and treatment of hearing disorders. An otologist is trained to diagnose types of hearing loss. An audiologist carries out tests to determine whether a hearing aid will help a particular patient. If it is thought that a patient would benefit from a hearing aid, the audiologist also identifies the best kind of hearing aid. An otolaryngologist is a physician who specializes in diseases of the ears and throat.

Procedures and tests commonly used to diagnose disorders of the ear, hearing, and balance include the otoscopic examination, audiometry, the caloric test,

---

Box 52-1 | **ASSESSMENT of Patients with Disorders of the Ear, Hearing, and Balance**

Health History

Present Illness:
Changes in the external ear, hearing acuity, or balance

Past Medical History:
Sinus infections, dental problems, allergies, upper respiratory infections, hypertension, diabetes mellitus, hypothyroidism, surgery on ear or throat, recent head injury, rubella and rubella immunization, recent and current medications

Family History:
Hearing impairments

Review of Systems:
Pain in ear or throat, tinnitus, dizziness, vertigo, nausea, vomiting

Functional Assessment:
Exposure to excessively loud noise, use of hearing aid

Physical Examination

General Survey:
Response to normal voice, gait, posture, and balance

External Ear:
Position of auricles; lesions, tenderness, or nodules

Lymph Nodes:
Enlargement of lymph nodes in front of or behind ear

Mastoid:
Tenderness

External Auditory Canal:
Obstruction, lesions, drainage

Tympanic Membrane:
Redness, bulging

electronystagmography, hearing acuity tests, and tuning fork tests. Radiographic examinations, especially the computed tomographic (CT) scan, may be used to study the mastoid bone, middle ear, and inner ear.

Diagnostic tests and procedures for patients with disorders of the ear, hearing, and balance are described in the Diagnostic Tests and Procedures table on p. 1192.

OTOSCOPIC EXAMINATION

The otoscope is the instrument used to examine the external auditory canal. The purpose of the otoscopic examination is to inspect the external auditory canal and tympanic membrane. The examination permits diagnosis of inflammatory and infectious processes as well as obstructions of the external canal.

When using an otoscope, you should:

1. Use the largest speculum that fits the ear canal easily.
2. For adult patients, pull the auricle up and back to straighten the canal and then guide the speculum gently into the canal.
3. Steady the otoscope by resting the little finger against the patient's cheek, as illustrated in Figure 52-4.
4. Never force the speculum into the ear.
5. If the patient is unable to cooperate, have someone hold the head still during the examination.
6. Clean the speculum between patients and between ears on each patient.

The appearance of the normal tympanic membrane is illustrated in Figure 52-5.

AUDIOMETRY

Audiometry is the assessment of the ability to hear simple sound waves. It requires a machine called an *audiometer.* Special training is needed to use the audiometer and to interpret test results. Nurses in some work settings learn to do these tests. The patient needs no special preparation for this test.

CALORIC TEST

The caloric test is used to diagnose disorders in the vestibular system or its central nervous system connections. The ear is irrigated with warm or cold water, and the patient is observed for reactions that suggest vestibular problems. A person with a labyrinth disorder responds with specific abnormal eye movements (nystagmus), vertigo, and nausea and vomiting. A person with vestibular disease has a decreased or absent response to the test.

Test results are altered by central nervous system depressants, barbiturates, and alcohol. Inform the examiner if the patient has had any of these drugs before the examination.

ELECTRONYSTAGMOGRAPHY

Electronystagmography is used to detect lesions in the vestibule. Electrodes are placed around the eyes, and eye movements are measured as the patient focuses on specific targets, as the ears are irrigated with water, as air is blown into the ears, and as the head position is changed.

The patient is usually allowed nothing by mouth for 3 hours before the test. No caffeine or alcoholic beverages should be consumed for 24 to 48 hours before the test. Medications may be withheld on the physician's directions. Patients who normally wear eyeglasses are instructed to bring them to the test. After the test, the patient may report nausea and may vomit. If the patient is dizzy, take appropriate safety precautions.

FIGURE **52-4** Correct technique for using an otoscope to examine the external auditory canal and the tympanic membrane. The adult auricle is pulled up and back; the examiner's hand is stabilized against the patient's face.

FIGURE **52-5** Normal appearance of the tympanic membrane through the otoscope.

DIAGNOSTIC TESTS and PROCEDURES | *Disorders of the Ear, Hearing, and Balance*

TEST/PURPOSE	PATIENT PREPARATION	POSTPROCEDURE NURSING CARE
AUDIOMETRY		
Pure tone audiometry tests Detect hearing impairment by assessing the patient's ability to hear a range of sounds.	Tell the patient test will be conducted in a sound-isolated room. The examiner will place earphones on the patient and introduce tones. The patient will be asked to identify when sounds are heard and when they disappear. A tuning fork will be placed near the patient's ear, and the patient is asked when vibrating sound is heard and when it ceases. No other preparation is needed.	No special postprocedure care.
Speech audiometry Measures the ability to hear spoken words.	The patient will listen to simple words through earphones and repeat the words that are understood. No special preparation.	No special postprocedure care.
VESTIBULAR TESTS		
Caloric test The ears are irrigated with warm or cool water to assess for dizziness. Dizziness is consistent with a diagnosis of Ménière's disease.	Tell the patient that the ears will be irrigated to assess for dizziness. Tell the examiner if the patient has had central nervous system depressants, alcohol, or barbiturates, because they alter test response. The examiner will then observe the patient for nystagmus, nausea, vomiting, or dizziness.	Assess for nausea. Offer small amounts of clear liquids at first. Safety measures if dizzy.
Electronystagmography Used to detect lesions in the vestibule.	Nothing by mouth for 3 hr before the test. No alcohol or caffeine for 24-48 hr before the test. Take eyeglasses to the test. Withhold medications as ordered. Tell the patient electrodes will be placed around the eyes, and he or she will be asked to focus on specific targets. The ears are irrigated and the patient is turned in various positions in a special chair.	Assess for nausea. Offer small amounts of clear fluids at first. Safety precautions if dizzy.

HEARING ACUITY TESTS

Audiometry gives a precise measurement of hearing acuity. Other simple tests can be done by the nurse for a gross assessment of hearing. The whisper test can easily be done in any setting. Stand 1 to 2 feet from the patient, facing away from him or her. Have the patient occlude the ear on the opposite side. Exhale, and then speak in a low whisper. Ask the patient to tell you what was whispered. The words can be repeated louder until the patient is able to hear them. After assessing one ear, change sides and assess the other ear. This simple test gives you an idea about the patient's general hearing ability.

TUNING FORK TESTS

Rinne and Weber tests use a tuning fork to assess the conduction of sound by air and by bone. These are useful in determining the nature of the hearing loss and in selecting the best treatment. Some nurses are taught to

perform these tests. The procedures are described here in case you need to be able to use these skills.

Rinne Test

For the Rinne test, tap the tuning fork on the hand to activate it. Then place the base of the tuning fork on the patient's mastoid bone. If the vibration is conducted through the bone, the patient hears a humming sound. When the sound is no longer heard, move the fork so that the tines of the tuning fork are near but not touching the ear canal. Ask the patient if he or she can hear the sound and, if so, to report when the sound disappears. This assesses the patient's ability to hear sound waves conducted through the air.

Normally, air conduction is better than bone conduction. Therefore the patient should be able to hear the sound transmitted through air even after it can no longer be heard through bone. This normal finding is recorded as "AC > BC" (air conduction is greater than bone conduction). If bone conduction is greater than air conduction, the patient has a conductive hearing loss.

Weber Test

In the Weber test, place the base of an activated tuning fork on the midline of the skull. Ask the patient to identify the side in which the sound is loudest. With normal hearing in both ears, the sound is heard equally on each side. The sound is louder in an ear with conductive hearing loss and softer in an ear with sensorineural hearing loss.

OTHER AUDITORY TESTS

Other tests that may be ordered to assess the auditory system are auditory evoked potential, auditory brainstem response, and electrocochleography. These tests are helpful in determining the origin of certain hearing losses. Additional tests of vestibular function are posturography and rotary chair testing.

COMMON THERAPEUTIC MEASURES

Problems of the ear and related structures sometimes require medications or surgery. Other therapeutic measures for problems of the ear include irrigations and the use of hearing aids. You may encounter patients who are being treated by any of these measures.

EAR DROPS

Medications intended to be placed directly into the external ear canal are called otic drops, or simply *ear drops*. Ear drops may be ordered to treat infection or inflammation, to reduce pain, or to soften earwax. When administering ear drops, keep the following points in mind:

1. Be sure to use an *otic* solution.
2. Warm the drops to body temperature by rolling the bottle between the palms.
3. Have the patient tilt the head so that the ear to be treated is positioned toward you.
4. Straighten the external auditory canal of an adult by pulling the auricle up and back. For a child, the auricle is pulled down and back.
5. Hold the dropper at the opening of the canal, but do not contaminate the tip by touching the skin.
6. Instruct the patient to keep the treated ear up for several minutes to keep the medication from leaking from the ear. Sometimes the physician orders a cotton ball to be placed loosely in the canal to keep the medicine in place.

Pharmacology Capsule

Medications intended to be administered into the external ear are called *otic drugs*.

Examples of commonly used otic medications are listed in the Drug Therapy table on p. 1194.

IRRIGATION

Irrigation is the use of a solution to cleanse the external ear canal or to remove something from the canal. A common indication for irrigation is impacted cerumen. Impacted cerumen is dried earwax that blocks the canal. The nurse may perform the irrigation, if agency policy permits, or may assist with the procedure. The following key points should be remembered when irrigating an ear:

1. Select the correct solution as ordered by the physician.
2. Warm the solution to body temperature (95° F to 105° F).
3. Have the patient sit up and hold an emesis basin under the ear to be irrigated.
4. Drape the shoulder under the basin.
5. Straighten the external canal of an adult by pulling the auricle up and back. For a child, pull the auricle down and back.
6. Select an irrigating syringe or bulb syringe with a tip that is smaller than the canal.
7. Direct the solution toward the top of the canal in a steady stream. The procedure can be repeated several times if needed.
8. Sometimes ear drops are ordered to soften impacted cerumen before irrigating.
9. Describe any substances rinsed out of the ear. If the impacted cerumen or foreign body does not wash out, inform the physician.
10. If the tympanic membrane (eardrum) is ruptured, the canal should *not* be irrigated because fluid could be forced into the middle ear.

HEARING AIDS

A hearing aid is a device that amplifies sound; that is, it makes sound louder. People with conductive hearing loss benefit the most from using a hearing aid. Those who have sensorineural or mixed losses may experience some benefit but often not as much.

All hearing aids have four components: (1) a microphone to receive sound waves and convert them to electrical signals, (2) an amplifier to strengthen the signals, (3) a receiver to convert signals to sound waves, and (4) a battery to power the device. Various aids are designed to be worn in the ear, behind the ear, or in the middle of the chest. The device worn in the middle of the chest ("body hearing aid") is the most powerful. It consists of a wire that connects the ear speaker to an amplifier and battery worn on the body (Fig. 52-6).

The two basic types of hearing aids are bone conduction receivers and air conduction receivers. Bone conduction receivers are worn behind the ear against the skull. Air conduction receivers are worn in the

DRUG THERAPY | *Otic Medications*

DRUG	USE/ACTION	SIDE EFFECTS	NURSING INTERVENTIONS
ANTIBIOTICS			
Chloramphenicol (Chloromycetin Otic)	Broad-spectrum antibiotic used to treat infections of lining of external auditory canal.	Hypersensitivity: redness, rash, swelling, burning, pain.	If patient shows signs of hypersensitivity, withhold drug and notify physician.
TOPICAL CORTICOSTEROIDS			
Hydrocortisone combined with neomycin sulfate and polymyxin B (Cortisporin Otic, Otocort) Polymyxin B (Otobiotic Otic) Neomycin and colistin (Coly-Mycin S Otic)	Treat inflammation, pruritus, and allergic response. Usually combined with antibacterial or antifungal drug.		Do not put in ear if tympanic membrane is perforated. Caution to avoid eye contact.
ANTIBACTERIAL AND SOFTENING AGENTS			
Carbamide peroxide with glycerin (Debrox, Murine Ear Drops)	Soften earwax. Treat aphthous ulcers.	Redness, irritation, superinfection.	Contraindications: ear surgery, perforated tympanic membrane; ear drainage, redness, pain, or tenderness. Teach patient not to clean ear with cotton swabs, which force wax deeper into ear.
DRYING AGENTS			
Boric acid in isopropyl alcohol (Ear-Dry, Swim-Ear)	Dry external canal after swimming or bathing. Decrease risk of infection.	Local irritation.	Instilled in external canal immediately after swimming or bathing. Contraindicated with perforated tympanic membrane.
ANTIEMETICS			
Scopolamine (Transderm Scop) Dimenhydrinate (Dramamine) Diphenhydramine (Benadryl) Meclizine (Antivert) Chlorpromazine (Thorazine)	Prevent or treat nausea, vomiting, motion sickness.	Sedation, drowsiness, tremor, fever, tachycardia, hypotension, constipation, dry mouth.	Safety precautions for drowsiness. Monitor pulse and blood pressure. Monitor stools and urinary output. Mouth care.

FIGURE 52-6 Types of hearing aids and components. **A,** In-the-canal aid. **B,** In-the-ear aid. **C,** Hearing aid components. **D,** Battery compartment.

external canal. An audiologist determines which type a patient needs.

Modern hearing aids use transistors, which allow the device to be very small. The hearing aid requires some care. Wash the ear mold (the part that fits into the ear) daily with soap and water and then dry it. When it is not being worn, turn the aid off and store it in a protective case with the battery compartment open. Keep extra batteries on hand.

If the hearing aid is not working, first check to be sure it is turned on. If it is on, check the ear mold to see if it needs cleaning. The next step is to check battery placement. If the battery is not inserted correctly, the hearing aid will not work. If the hearing aid has a cord, check it to see if it is broken or unplugged. If these checks fail to locate the problem, change the battery. If a new battery does not correct the problem, the cord can be changed. Should the hearing aid still not work, return it to the dealer for service.

Nurses and other health care providers need to be familiar with hearing aids and how they work. The patient's nursing care plan should indicate that the patient usually wears a hearing aid. Confusion in some older patients might be avoided if the hearing aid were kept in place. The cost of hearing aids can range from several hundred to several thousand dollars if both ears are involved. When patients are hospitalized, take care to prevent loss of these devices.

It may take considerable persuasion from family and health care providers to get a hearing-impaired person to try a hearing aid. It may be helpful to point out the benefits of improved hearing in the patient's everyday life.

Hearing aids amplify all sounds, including background noise. This is especially annoying when a person first tries to use an aid. Patients are advised to wear the aid first in quiet settings. Once they learn to adjust the volume and tone comfortably, they can try it in noisy settings. It may take several months before a hearing aid feels comfortable.

COCHLEAR IMPLANTS

A cochlear implant may be recommended for people who cannot benefit from regular hearing aids. A cochlear implant has variable results for the profoundly deaf. Some can hear well enough to understand speech on a telephone; others can hear only environmental sounds, such as sirens, doorbells, and telephones.

The cochlear implant consists of a microphone, a processor, a transmitter, and a receiver. The microphone, at ear level, picks up sounds that are amplified by the processor (Fig. 52-7). The sound, in the form of magnetic signals, is transmitted electronically to the receiver. The receiver is surgically implanted behind the ear. Electrodes attached to the receiver stimulate nerve fibers in the cochlea to produce sound. Several months of training are needed to learn to tell sounds apart.

Therefore candidates for the cochlear implant must be highly motivated and carefully screened.

TEMPORAL BONE STIMULATORS

Patients with conductive hearing loss may benefit from a temporal bone stimulator. A receiver is implanted into the skull. An external device, worn above the ear, transmits sound through the skin to the receiver. This device is not widely used.

SURGERY ON THE EAR AND RELATED STRUCTURES

Many ear disorders are treated surgically. Nursing care of patients having specific surgical procedures is discussed with the appropriate pathophysiologic process. However, some general measures apply to most patients after surgery on the ear.

NURSING CARE *of the Patient Having Ear Surgery*

Before surgery, determine what the patient understands about the procedure and surgical routine. Ask whether the patient is feeling nervous or anxious. Deficient Knowledge and Anxiety are typical nursing diagnoses. Supply needed information about the preoperative and postoperative routines. If the patient is anxious, explore the specific concerns. Sometimes patient teaching and reassurance are sufficient to reduce anxiety. Notify the physician if the patient is very anxious.

Immediate preoperative care usually includes having the patient remove any articles such as eyeglasses or hearing aids. The hearing-impaired person going to surgery may feel very helpless without the hearing aid. Notify the operating room staff and ask if the patient can wear the hearing aid to the surgical suite. Place a note on the front of the chart to alert caregivers of the patient's hearing impairment and to the presence of a hearing aid.

Assessment

In the postoperative period, monitor the patient for pain, nausea, dizziness, and fever. Inspect the wound dressing for drainage. Document drainage color, odor, and amount.

Nursing Diagnoses, Goals, and Outcome Criteria: Ear Surgery, Postoperative	
NURSING DIAGNOSES	GOALS AND OUTCOME CRITERIA
Acute Pain related to tissue trauma or edema	Pain relief: patient states pain is relieved, relaxed manner
Risk for Injury related to dizziness or vertigo, fluid accumulation, pressure in the ear	Decreased risk for injury: maintains prescribed position, avoids behavior that increases pressure
	Absence of injury: patient does not fall
Risk for Infection related to surgical incision	Healing without infection: normal body temperature and white blood cell count

Continued

1 Sound enters the system through a tiny microphone behind the ear.

7 The brain receives the signals and interprets them as sound.

5 The transmitting coil, a plastic covered ring about 1 inch in diameter, sends the codes across the skin to the receiver/stimulator.

Transmitter   Microphone

Receiver

Electrode

Cochlea

2 The sound is sent from the microphone to the speech processor through the thin cord that connects them.

4 These electronic codes are sent back up through the thin cable to the transmitter.

3 The speech processor selects and codes the elements of sound that are most useful for understanding speech.

Processor

6 The receiver/stimulator contains an integrated circuit that converts the codes into special electrical signals and sends them along the electrode array. The electrode array is a set of 22 tiny electrode bands arranged in a row around a piece of tapered flexible tubing. Each electrode has a wire connecting it to the receiver/stimulator. The coded electrical signals are sent to specific electrodes. Each electrode is programmed separately to deliver signals that can vary in loudness and pitch. These electrodes then stimulate different hearing nerve fibers, which send the messages on to the brain.

FIGURE **52-7** Cochlear implant to restore hearing.

Disturbed Sensory Perception related to packing and edema in affected ear

Effective communication: patient and nurse use effective strategies to facilitate verbal communication

Interventions

Acute Pain

Determine the nature of the patient's pain, and have the patient rate the pain on a scale from 1 to 10, with 10 being the worst pain imaginable. Surgical pain usually requires analgesics for several days. In addition, use measures such as positioning and massage to promote relaxation.

Risk for Injury

Dizziness and vertigo are common after surgery on the ear. Dizziness is a feeling of unsteadiness, whereas vertigo is the sensation that one's body or the room is spinning.

Vertigo is often triggered by sudden movements, so advise the patient to move slowly and carefully. Instruct the patient to call for help when getting up the

first few times. Assist as long as dizziness is a problem. Raise side rails, and leave the bed in low position.

The ear is commonly packed and covered with a dressing. A drain may be in place. The packing is removed only by the physician. A specific position may be ordered after surgery. If drainage is being encouraged, the patient is most likely positioned on the affected side. If the procedure includes a graft on the tympanic membrane, however, the patient is usually positioned on the unaffected side.

Straining is contraindicated because it increases pressure in the ear. The patient should avoid nose blowing, coughing, and sneezing; however, if these are unavoidable, the mouth should be kept open to relieve pressure. Stool softeners may be ordered to prevent constipation and straining. Ear surgery, like any other type of surgery, creates a wound that must heal. Healing requires a balanced diet with adequate protein and vitamin C.

Risk for Infection

Take measures to reduce the risk of postoperative infection. Advise the patient to avoid crowds and people with colds for several weeks. The ear canal should be kept dry for 2 to 4 weeks as instructed by the physician. Shampooing usually is not allowed for 2 weeks, although it is restricted longer in some cases.

Disturbed Sensory Perception

While the affected ear is packed, the patient's hearing in that ear is impaired. If the patient does not hear well in the unaffected ear, you must devise appropriate means of communication. It is best to plan this with the patient before surgery.

HEARING LOSS

TYPES OF HEARING LOSS

The term *hard of hearing* can describe any level of impairment, including the total inability to hear (deafness). Millions of Americans have some degree of hearing impairment. Hearing losses are classified into categories. The categories of hearing loss discussed here include conductive, sensorineural, mixed, and central.

Conductive Hearing Loss

Conductive hearing loss results from interference with the transmission of sound waves from the external or middle ear to the inner ear. Factors that may cause conductive hearing loss include obstruction of the external canal or eustachian tube and otosclerosis. Otosclerosis is a condition in which the stapes in the middle ear does not vibrate.

Patients who have conductive hearing loss hear better in noisy settings than in quiet settings. They do not speak loudly because bone conduction allows them to hear their own voices.

Most conditions that cause conductive hearing loss are treatable. Obstructions usually can be removed. Otosclerosis can be treated surgically with a procedure called a *stapedectomy*. This condition is discussed in more detail on p. 1201 in the Nursing Care of the Patient Having Stapedectomy section. Hearing aids are usually helpful for patients with conductive hearing loss.

Sensorineural Hearing Loss

Sensorineural hearing loss is sometimes called *nerve deafness*. It is a disturbance of the neural structures in the inner ear or the nerve pathways to the brain. Sensorineural hearing loss may be congenital, but it also can be caused by noise, trauma, aging, Ménière's disease, ototoxicity, diabetes, and syphilis.

Patients with sensorineural hearing loss can hear sounds but have difficulty understanding speech. They often complain that speech sounds muffled. This type of hearing loss is not as easily corrected. Hearing aids may help by amplifying the sound, but it still sounds muffled.

Mixed Hearing Loss

Mixed hearing loss is a combination of conductive and sensorineural losses. Treatment of any reversible problems often results in improvement of mixed hearing loss.

Central Hearing Loss

Central hearing loss is due to some problem in the central nervous system. The patient either cannot perceive or cannot interpret sounds that are heard.

SIGNS AND SYMPTOMS

Most hearing loss progresses over time. Patients may not readily recognize the losses. They may complain that their hearing is fine but that others are mumbling. There are many behaviors that should lead the nurse to suspect hearing loss. The patient may lean toward the speaker or turn one ear toward the speaker. The patient with a hearing loss may fail to follow directions, speak while others are speaking, or turn the radio or television up very loud. Irritability and even hostility are not unusual. Some people become very suspicious of others because they cannot hear what others are saying. Hearing loss often has no other symptoms. Otalgia (ear pain), dizziness, and tinnitus (ringing in the ears) may be present with certain types of disorders.

THE IMPACT OF HEARING IMPAIRMENT

People with obvious physical disabilities usually receive some consideration and understanding from strangers. People who have hearing impairments may not be treated as well.

Those who had impairments in early childhood usually have speech difficulties. If speech is not clear, others may assume the patient is intellectually impaired. Sadly, the phrase *deaf and dumb* has been used to refer to people who neither hear nor speak. This term is understandably offensive to the hearing-impaired person. The term *deaf* is not offensive but suggests a total inability to hear. *Hearing impairment*, on the other hand, implies a range of abilities.

It is interesting that most people accept the use of eyeglasses fairly easily but often are resistant to using a hearing aid. There is a tendency to deny one's hearing loss. When a person refuses to admit to a hearing loss, family members and others may stop trying to communicate. The hearing-impaired person may alienate those who would like to be close and supportive.

People with severe hearing impairment probably suffer the most severe social isolation of those with sensory disorders. Nurses can help by educating the public about hearing loss.

ADAPTATIONS TO HEARING LOSS

Some hearing impairments can be corrected. If not, the patient and family need to learn to cope with the loss. For many people, hearing aids produce at least some improvement in hearing. Many patients read lips and observe body language closely to enhance understanding of spoken messages.

Sign language uses a universal set of hand signals. It provides a very effective means of communicating as long as there are others who know how to use it. Unfortunately, most nurses are not trained in this skill.

Several electronic devices are available to serve the hard of hearing. Telephones can be adapted to send and receive written messages. Earphones are readily available for use with radios, stereos, and televisions. These allow the hearing-impaired person to adjust the volume as needed. They also reduce environmental noises. Some television channels provide closed-captioned programming, in which a written script is shown on the bottom of the screen. A portable tele-communication device for the deaf makes telephone communication possible. In the home, flashing lights can be used to alert the person to doorbells, telephone rings, and alarm clocks. For the person who does not speak, small handheld computers called *personal communicators* print out messages typed by the user.

For many years, guide dogs have been used to help people with visual impairments. A similar intervention is being used with dogs trained to assist the hard of hearing. These dogs are taught to recognize common sounds (doorbell, telephone, smoke alarm, crying baby) and to get the attention of the owner.

NURSING CARE *of the Patient with Impaired Hearing*

Assessment

Assessment of the patient with impaired hearing is summarized in Box 52-1.

Nursing Diagnoses, Goals, and Outcome Criteria: Hearing Impairments

Nursing Diagnoses	Goals and Outcome Criteria
Impaired Verbal Communication related to inability to hear	Effective communication: patient and others use alternative means of communication
Social Isolation related to inability to communicate verbally	Reduced social isolation: participation in social activities
Ineffective Coping related to change in social interaction, threat to body image, or denial	Effective coping with permanent hearing impairment: patient has satisfying social interactions, makes positive statements about self, plans realistically
Deficient Knowledge of prevention, diagnosis, and treatment of hearing impairment, and resources for adaptation	Patient knowledge of prevention and treatment: patient correctly practices preventive measures and describes treatments

Interventions

Impaired Verbal Communication

Many techniques are available to improve communication with the hard of hearing. You can use these approaches and teach others to use them as well. When working with a hearing-impaired patient, follow these guidelines:

1. Be sure the patient knows you are present. Try to move into the patient's line of vision before touching him or her.
2. Find out the patient's usual means of communication, and be sure he or she has access to any assistive devices.
3. Speak slowly and distinctly.
4. Be sure the patient can see your face clearly. Do not turn away while speaking.
5. Do not eat, smoke, or chew gum if the patient reads lips.
6. Provide adequate lighting directed *toward* your face. A strong light behind you creates a glare and makes it hard to see your features.
7. Lower your voice tone.
8. Assess the patient's ability to hear a normal voice tone. The volume can be increased a little if needed, but shouting simply distorts the message. People who wear hearing aids often complain that everyone shouts at them.
9. If the patient has a good ear, speak toward that side.
10. Amplify your voice, if necessary, by using a rolled-up sheet of paper or a stethoscope. To use the stethoscope, put the earpieces in the patient's ears and speak into the bell.
11. Help patients follow spoken messages by informing them of the topic to be addressed.
12. Use short sentences or phrases.
13. Use body language to support the verbal message.
14. Have a writing pad or Magic Slate available. Use it if the patient cannot understand you or if you do not understand the patient.
15. Try to validate patient understanding by encouraging feedback and assessing whether directions are followed.
16. When a hearing-impaired patient is hospitalized, be sure a call bell is provided but remind staff that the patient cannot use the intercom.

Social Isolation

The preceding guidelines may improve communication with the hearing-impaired person. The most important thing you can do, however, is to have a positive attitude toward trying to communicate with the patient. Genuine interest and attention encourage the patient to express himself or herself in whatever way is possible.

When other people seem hurried or annoyed, they discourage the patient's attempts to communicate. Some patients withdraw from social interactions. They may become isolated and depressed. Encourage the patient to learn new communication methods. Teach the patient how to use assistive devices. Provide information about community resources for the hard of hearing. Explore the type of activities that are satisfying to the patient, and encourage continued involvement. Advise the physician if the patient becomes increasingly sad or withdrawn. Counseling with a mental health professional may be suggested.

Ineffective Coping

The way people cope with hearing loss varies with the individual. Some deny the problem for as long as possible; others deliberately learn everything they can about treatments and adaptive strategies. Recognize that both of these behaviors are responses to a stressful situation. It is important to explore the patient's feelings about hearing loss. If the patient is anxious, you may use stress-reduction techniques (relaxation exercises, massage, meditation). The patient who denies hearing loss is often resistant to teaching, so he or she may not take advantage of opportunities to deal with the problem effectively.

Deficient Knowledge

Most people with hearing impairment have some hearing ability. Emphasize measures to reduce the risk of additional impairment. Advise the patient to seek prompt treatment of any symptoms of infection (fever, pain in the ear, drainage). Hearing protection is recommended in excessively noisy settings. Patients taking ototoxic drugs (e.g., aspirin) are told to contact the physician if hearing acuity worsens or tinnitus develops. If ear drops or irrigations are ordered, demonstrate the procedure and reinforce the physician's orders. Patients also need instruction in the use of hearing aids, as described in the Hearing Aids section on pp. 1193 to 1195.

Patient Teaching Plan

Hearing Impairments

- Many types of hearing loss are correctable or at least capable of being improved.
- Hearing is not related to intelligence.
- There is no reason to be ashamed of a hearing impairment.
- Some measures can be taken to reduce the risk of certain types of hearing loss.
- All women of childbearing age should be immunized for rubella to prevent one form of congenital hearing impairment.

DISORDERS AFFECTING HEARING AND BALANCE

EXTERNAL EAR AND CANAL
Foreign Bodies and Cerumen

Occasionally, foreign bodies get into the external ear canal. Most small objects can be flushed from the ear by gentle irrigation. Insects can be killed by instilling a small amount of mineral oil. They can then be flushed from the canal. An alternative method is to hold a flashlight near the auricle. Because insects are often attracted to light, they may move out of the canal.

One of the most common causes of obstruction of the external ear canal is impacted cerumen. The patient is not always aware of the obstruction but may complain of hearing loss or tinnitus. When a large amount of hardened cerumen is present, the physician may order ear drops to soften the cerumen before irrigation. It may be necessary to repeat the procedure several times before all cerumen is removed. If the foreign body or cerumen is not removed by irrigation, the physician can use ear forceps or a cerumen spoon to remove it.

NURSING CARE of the Patient with Impacted Cerumen

Nurses, especially in long-term care facilities, need to inspect the ear canal routinely for impacted cerumen. The dry cerumen may be gold to dark brown. Sometimes it fills the entire canal. If both ears are affected, the patient has some degree of hearing impairment.

In this situation, the primary nursing diagnosis is Disturbed Sensory Perception related to obstruction of the external auditory canal. The nursing goal is restored hearing. Report the findings to the physician, and carry out orders for ear drops. Irrigations may be done by the physician or the nurse if policy permits. Successful interventions are evaluated by examining the canal and documenting the absence of obstructions. Educate patients to avoid trying to remove cerumen with cotton-tipped applicators or other tools such as hairpins. These efforts can harm the ear canal or the tympanic membrane in addition to forcing cerumen or foreign bodies further into the canal.

Infection and Inflammation

Infection or inflammation of the lining of the external ear canal is called *external otitis* or *swimmer's ear*. It may be caused by scratching or cleaning the ear with sharp objects. Swimming can lead to otitis by washing out protective cerumen, which leaves the lining of the external canal susceptible to injury. When infection is present, it often is caused by staphylococci or streptococci but may also be fungal in origin.

Signs and Symptoms

The most characteristic symptom of external otitis is pain that increases when the auricle is pulled. Other symptoms can include dizziness, fever, and drainage. Drainage may be purulent or blood tinged.

Medical Treatment

Topical antibacterial or antifungal drugs are ordered to treat external otitis. Corticosteroid drops may be ordered to reduce inflammation unless the infection is caused by a fungus. In that case, corticosteroids are contraindicated. If the external canal is obstructed by edema, the physician may insert an ear wick through the blocked canal. An ear wick is a long piece of gauze that extends out of the ear canal. Medication placed on the external portion of the ear wick soaks the gauze and distributes the medication in the canal. Pain is treated with aspirin or codeine. Any drainage from the ear should be treated as infected material and handled carefully.

NURSING CARE *of the Patient with External Otitis*

External otitis is typically treated on an outpatient basis, so nursing care is limited. Assessment includes inspection of the external canal and evaluation of pain. Nursing diagnoses are Acute Pain related to inflammation and Deficient Knowledge of preventive practices and treatment of external otitis. Goals of nursing care are pain relief, patient knowledge of prevention, and patient management of treatment plan.

Oral analgesics and topical corticosteroids and antibiotics are given as ordered to treat pain and to reduce inflammation and infection. Administer the prescribed drops, or teach the patient to do so. Because it is awkward to put drops into one's own ear, you also may need to teach a family member how to do it. Teach patients to prevent external otitis by not using sharp instruments to clean the auditory canal and by avoiding suspected irritants such as hair spray and earphones. Advise the use of ear plugs while swimming. The physician may instruct the patient to use a drying agent (e.g., Ear-Dry) after swimming or bathing.

Criteria for effective nursing interventions are patient statement of pain relief and the patient's correct description of preventive measures and appropriate administration of prescribed medication.

Furuncle

A furuncle is an inflamed area in the external auditory canal caused by infection of a hair follicle. The area is very painful to the touch. Hearing may be impaired if swelling blocks the canal. A ruptured furuncle releases fluid that may drain from the canal. Treatment includes systemic and topical antibiotics (with an ear wick if needed). If the condition does not improve, the physician may incise and drain it. Nursing care of the patient with a furuncle is like that for external otitis.

MIDDLE EAR

Conditions of the middle ear are serious because of the risk of complications, including permanent hearing loss and involvement of the inner ear.

Otitis Media

Otitis media is an infection of the middle ear. There are several types of otitis media. Acute otitis media and chronic otitis media are sometimes called *suppurant* or *purulent otitis media* because of the presence of purulent material. In serous otitis media, sterile fluid accumulates behind the tympanic membrane. It can precede or follow acute otitis media. Adhesive otitis media may develop if fluid remains in the middle ear. It is characterized by thickening and scarring in the middle ear structures.

Acute Otitis Media

Acute otitis media usually develops with colds. Edema leads to blockage of the eustachian tubes. Fluid accumulates in the middle ear, causing painful pressure on the tympanic membrane. The tympanic membrane may rupture, resulting in scarring and subsequent hearing loss. The patient often has a fever and complains of headache. Acute otitis media is more common in children than in adults.

Medical Treatment. Oral antibiotics usually are prescribed for acute otitis media. Another option is topical ear drops, usually combinations of antibacterials and corticosteroids, that are given for 1 week. Before the drops are administered, the canal should be cleared of debris. Have the patient lie on the unaffected side for a few minutes after instilling the drops to promote flow of the medication into the canal. If a wick has been placed in the canal because of swelling, apply the ear drops directly to the wick. Antihistamines may be ordered if allergies are thought to be contributing to the problem. Sometimes myringotomy is performed. Myringotomy is the creation of a small opening in the tympanic membrane to reduce pressure and allow fluid to drain. If infection is eliminated, the tympanic membrane should heal without permanent damage. A tympanostomy tube may be placed to allow for continuous drainage.

Chronic Otitis Media

Chronic otitis media is characterized by hearing loss and continuous or intermittent drainage. The condition usually is not painful. On examination, the eardrum is usually perforated (ruptured) or shows signs of a healed perforation. An audiogram may detect some conductive hearing loss if the bones in the middle ear have been damaged by the chronic infection.

Possible complications of chronic otitis media include mastoiditis, meningitis, labyrinthitis, cholesteatoma, and hearing impairment.

Mastoiditis. Because the middle ear is directly connected to the air cells in the mastoid bone, infection in the middle ear can extend into the mastoid bone. And because the brain lies next to the mastoid bone, the infection can spread there as well. Signs and symptoms of mastoiditis include mastoid swelling (directly behind the ear) and soreness, headache, malaise, and an elevated white blood cell count. There may be thick, purulent drainage from the ear. Mastoiditis is very serious because it can lead to a brain abscess, meningitis (inflammation of the covering of the brain), or paralysis of the facial muscles.

Cholesteatoma. A cholesteatoma is a growth in the middle ear. When the tympanic membrane is perforated around the margin where it attaches to the ear canal, epithelial cells grow into the middle ear. The cells form a ball of tissue that grows and that may damage the facial nerve and the labyrinth. A cholesteatoma must be removed surgically.

Medical Treatment. Chronic otitis media is treated with systemic antibiotics and, if the eardrum is intact, irrigations to remove debris. If the tympanic membrane does not heal, tympanoplasty may be done to repair it. The procedure may be done through the ear canal or through an incision behind the auricle. Sometimes grafts of the patient's tissue are used to repair the tear. Tissue may be taken from the external canal or the temporalis muscle. After the graft is placed, the middle ear is filled with Gelfoam, and a cotton ball is put in the external ear to hold the graft in place. If the ossicles (bones) in the middle ear are diseased, they may be replaced with prostheses.

If the infection has extended to the mastoid bone, a mastoidectomy is often done at the same time. A mastoidectomy can be modified (simple) or radical. In a modified procedure, infected mastoid tissue is removed but the middle ear is left intact. In a radical mastoidectomy, all the structures in the middle ear are removed. The radical procedure is not done now as often as it was in the past.

NURSING CARE *of the Patient Having a Mastoidectomy*

General care of the patient having surgery on the ear is discussed on pp. 1195 to 1197 in the Nursing Care of the Patient Having Ear Surgery section. Before surgery, the emphasis is on patient teaching and reduction of anxiety. Primary considerations after surgery on the middle ear include comfort, safety, prevention of infection, and prevention of pressure on the tympanic membrane. Nausea is another common problem after middle ear surgery. Keep an emesis basin nearby. The physician usually orders antiemetics to be given as needed for nausea. If the patient vomits frequently, there is a risk of deficient fluid volume. Monitor intake and output and give intravenous fluids if ordered.

The type of dressing varies. It may be small and placed over the auricle. If the surgeon entered through the mastoid bone, however, expect a large head dressing with a drain. Inspect the dressing and describe any drainage, but do *not* disturb or remove the dressing. Assist the patient the first time out of bed in case dizziness is a problem. The patient should avoid any activity that creates pressure on the tympanic membrane (blowing the nose, coughing, sneezing, straining). If the patient needs to cough or sneeze, advise him or her to do so with the mouth open.

Otosclerosis

Otosclerosis is a hereditary condition in which an abnormal growth causes the footplate of the stapes to become fixed. The fixed stapes cannot vibrate, so sound waves cannot be transmitted to the inner ear. The effect of this abnormality is a conductive hearing loss. If the disease also involves the inner ear, the patient has sensorineural hearing loss as well. The condition affects both ears but may progress faster in one ear than in the other.

Otosclerosis is most common in young white women. The onset is usually in the late teens or early 20s. During pregnancy, it progresses at a faster rate.

Signs and Symptoms

The primary symptom of otosclerosis is slowly progressive hearing loss in the absence of infection. In the early stages, the patient may report tinnitus. The Rinne test reveals bone conduction to be greater than air conduction.

Medical Treatment

The most common treatment for otosclerosis is a surgical procedure called *stapedectomy*. The physician advises the patient of the surgical risks, including complete hearing loss, infection, prolonged vertigo, and damage to the facial nerve. Stapedectomy is done under local anesthesia. The stapes is removed and replaced with a prosthesis. A tissue graft taken from the patient is placed over the oval window. The physician puts packing in the ear canal at the completion of the stapedectomy. A small dressing is then placed over the ear. When the graft heals, hearing is restored in most patients (Fig. 52-8).

After surgery, bed rest may be ordered for several days and drugs prescribed to control nausea and vertigo. Usually, the patient is allowed to lie on the back or the unaffected side, but specific position restrictions may be ordered.

NURSING CARE *of the Patient Having Stapedectomy*

Care of the patient having ear surgery is detailed earlier in the Nursing Care of the Patient Having Ear Surgery section on pp. 1195 to 1197. In addition to the usual preoperative teaching, tell the patient that hearing usually is worse immediately after stapedectomy but gradually improves over approximately 6 weeks.

After surgery, you should be concerned with pain relief, safety, prevention of infection, and avoidance of pressure in the ear. Because pressure can cause the graft to separate, it is especially important that the patient not do anything that increases pressure in the ear.

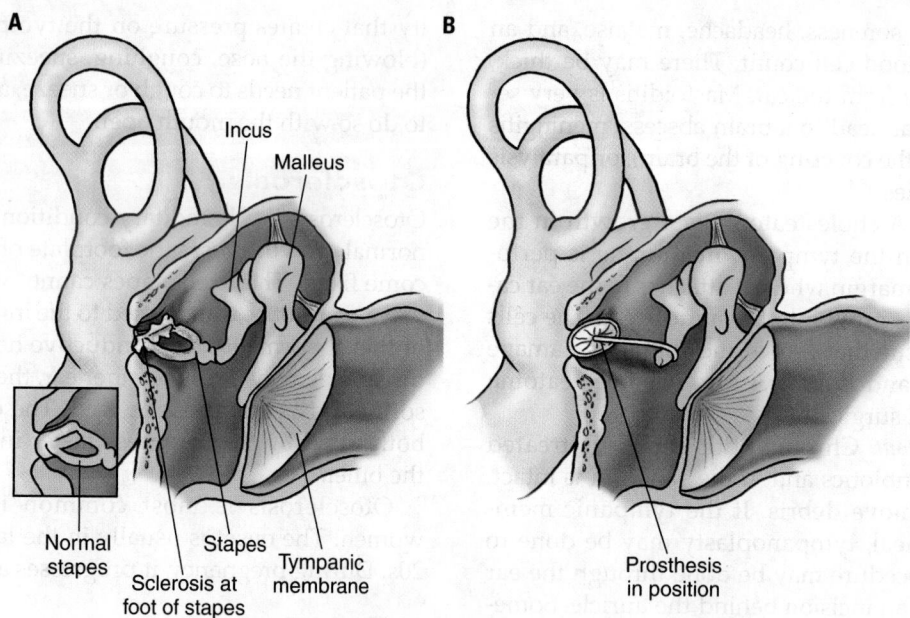

FIGURE **52-8** Otosclerosis: Before **(A)** and after **(B)** stapedectomy.

After stapedectomy, nausea, vomiting, and vertigo are common.

The packing in the ear should not be disturbed. The physician removes it approximately 1 week after the surgery. After the dressing and packing are removed, the patient usually is advised to keep the ear dry for at least 2 weeks. Swimming and showering usually are not permitted for approximately 6 weeks.

The patient should avoid contact with people who have colds. A balanced diet and adequate rest are needed for tissue healing and resistance to infection. Vertigo may persist after discharge, and you must help the patient plan for assistance with activities of daily living. It is important to reinforce that hearing improvement is gradual.

INNER EAR

Labyrinthitis

Labyrinthitis is inflammation of the labyrinth. It may be acute or chronic. Acute labyrinthitis usually follows an acute upper respiratory infection, acute otitis media, pneumonia, or influenza. It also can be an adverse effect of some drugs. One type of labyrinthitis is suppurative labyrinthitis. It is an inner ear infection that usually follows an upper respiratory infection, ear infection, or ear surgery. The effects can destroy the labyrinth and cochlea, causing permanent deafness.

Signs and Symptoms

Signs and symptoms of labyrinthitis include vertigo, nausea, vomiting, headache, anorexia, nystagmus, and sensorineural hearing loss on the affected side. A typical episode lasts 3 to 6 weeks. Nystagmus is an abnormal, rhythmic jerking movement of the eyes. Additional symptoms of suppurative labyrinthitis are tinnitus and hearing loss. A condition with some simi-larities is vestibular neuronitis. Vestibular neuronitis is caused by a viral infection and resolves within 10 days. Unlike labyrinthitis, it does not cause tinnitus or hearing loss.

Medical Treatment

Labyrinthitis is treated with antiemetics and support-ive care until it resolves. Antibiotics are prescribed if infection is present.

Consider the Alternative

Caution patients who have inner ear disorders that many herbal products can cause dizziness, nausea, and vomiting. Drowsiness is another side effect of many herbals, which may enhance the sedative effects of drugs used to manage vertigo.

NURSING CARE *of the Patient with Labyrinthitis*

Assessment

During an acute episode of labyrinthitis, describe the patient's symptoms. Monitor intake and output, daily weights if possible, and food intake if there is persis-tent vomiting.

Nursing Diagnoses, Goals, and Outcome Criteria: Labyrinthitis

Nursing Diagnoses	Goals and Outcome Criteria
Risk for Injury related to vertigo	Safety: absence of injury or falls
Imbalanced Nutrition: Less Than Body Requirements related to anorexia and nausea	Adequate nutrition: stable body weight

Risk for Deficient Fluid Volume related to vomiting	Adequate hydration: equal fluid intake and output, moist mucous membranes, vital signs consistent with patient norms
Anxiety related to acute illness	Reduced anxiety: patient states anxiety is reduced, calm manner

Interventions

Safety is a major concern for the patient with vertigo. Assist and supervise the patient when out of bed. Give antiemetics as prescribed for nausea and vomiting. If vomiting persists, the patient is at risk for development of fluid and electrolyte imbalances (hypokalemia, fluid volume deficit) and intravenous fluids may be needed. The patient needs reassurance that the condition resolves in time.

Ménière's Disease

Ménière's disease is a disorder of the labyrinth. More than 2 million Americans are thought to have attacks of Ménière's disease. The onset is usually in people ages 30 to 60 years. The cause is unknown, but the symptoms are related to an accumulation of fluid in the inner ear. Some things that have been found to trigger attacks include alcohol, nicotine, stress, and certain stimuli such as bright lights and sudden movements of the head.

Signs and Symptoms

Some patients with Ménière's disease have more serious symptoms than others. Acute attacks occur at intervals and last for hours to days. The frequency of attacks often can be reduced with medical treatment. During an acute attack, the classic symptoms are hearing loss and vertigo accompanied by pallor, sweating, nausea, and vomiting. The hearing loss is unilateral, meaning that only one ear is affected. Tinnitus accompanies acute attacks. It is heard as a low buzzing sound that sometimes becomes a roar. Hearing usually improves between attacks, but some loss of low-frequency sounds may remain. Patients who have had many attacks may eventually have permanent sensorineural hearing loss.

Vertigo is a sensation of movement that causes dizziness and nausea. Patients may say that the room seems to be spinning or that they feel like they are spinning. A feeling of fullness and pressure in the ear often precedes a vertigo attack. Attacks may last several minutes to several hours. Sudden movement during an attack of vertigo can cause vomiting.

Medical Diagnosis

Diagnosis of Ménière's disease is based on the history and physical findings. The patient describes hearing and balance disturbances as described earlier. An audiogram often reveals a loss of the ability to hear low-frequency sounds. If the caloric test or electronystagmography is done, the patient with Ménière's disease has a severe attack of vertigo. A glycerol test involves audiometry testing before and after giving the patient oral glycerol (a diuretic that draws fluid from the inner ear). Improved hearing after glycerol is given suggests Ménière's disease.

Ménière's disease is actually diagnosed by ruling out other conditions that can cause similar symptoms. Therefore the physician is likely to order a number of radiographs and other tests to detect any neurologic, allergic, or endocrine disorders.

Medical Treatment

Ménière's disease may be treated medically or surgically. Drugs prescribed during an acute attack include atropine, epinephrine, benzodiazepines such as diazepam (Valium), antihistamines, antiemetics, anticholinergics, vasodilators, and diuretics. Drugs also may be prescribed between attacks in an attempt to reduce their frequency and severity.

A low-sodium diet seems to increase the length of time between attacks by reducing edema in the inner ear. If moderate sodium restriction is not effective, the patient may be put on a strict sodium-free diet. (See the Nutrition Concepts box below.) Caffeine, nicotine, and alcohol are discouraged. Vestibular rehabilitation is a series of exercises performed to help the patient develop a tolerance for vertigo. It begins with moving the eyes and the head up and down and side to side and progresses to more vigorous activity. Vestibular rehabilitation usually is taught by the physical therapist. Most patients respond positively to conservative medical treatment.

Surgical Treatment

Surgery is usually advised only when all other measures have failed. Surgical procedures work by draining excess fluid from the inner ear (endolymphatic shunt) or by cutting the part of the acoustic nerve that controls balance (vestibular nerve section). The incision may be inside or behind the ear. In general, these surgical procedures pose some risk for permanent hearing loss. More destructive surgical procedures are labyrinthotomy and labyrinthectomy.

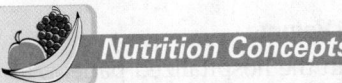

Consider the Alternative

Biofeedback, self-hypnosis, and relaxation techniques may be recommended to help the patient learn to live with Ménière's disease.

Nutrition Concepts

A low-salt diet is sometimes prescribed for people with Ménière's disease.

Potential complications of surgery for Ménière's disease include infection, hearing loss, loss of cerebrospinal fluid, and damage to the seventh cranial nerve. The leakage of cerebrospinal fluid may occur with procedures that require opening the skull. Cerebrospinal fluid is clear and thin in consistency. The seventh cranial nerve is the facial nerve that is located very close to the ear canal. It controls the movement of certain muscles of the face. Surgical procedures in and around the ear can result in trauma to the facial nerve.

NURSING CARE *of the Patient with Ménière's Disease*

Assessment

The pattern of acute attacks should be documented (see Nursing Care Plan: The Patient with Ménière's Disease on p. 1205). If you are collecting data for the assessment, note substances or stimuli that trigger the episodes. Document specific symptoms including nausea, vomiting, vertigo, and tinnitus. Determine how the condition affects the patient's life, what the patient knows about the disease, and what coping mechanisms are used.

Nursing Diagnoses, Goals, and Outcome Criteria: Ménière's Disease

NURSING DIAGNOSES	GOALS AND OUTCOME CRITERIA
Risk for Injury related to vertigo	Safety: absence of falls, injuries
Risk for Deficient Fluid Volume related to vomiting	Normal hydration: equal fluid intake and output, normal vital signs, moist mucous membranes
Anxiety related to acute illness or disruption of usual lifestyle	Reduced anxiety: patient states anxiety is reduced, calm manner
Ineffective Therapeutic Regimen Management related to lack of knowledge about management of Ménière's disease	Effective therapeutic regimen management: appropriate self-care, patient correctly describes and demonstrates self-care measures

Interventions

Risk for Injury

Safety is a major concern. Attacks come on suddenly and can be dangerous in many circumstances. Fortunately, many people can recognize an aura, or peculiar feeling, that precedes an attack. They should know to seek safety promptly when an aura occurs. If driving, the patient should pull over and stop the car as soon as possible.

Risk for Deficient Fluid Volume

During an acute attack in the hospitalized patient, allow the patient to remain still because movement may trigger vomiting. Keep the room dark and quiet. Postpone nonessential care such as bathing. Promptly give

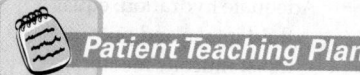

Ménière's Disease

- You need to know prescribed medications and how to manage their side effects (provide specifics).
- Avoid alcohol and tobacco because they affect fluid in the inner ear.

medications for nausea and vomiting, and keep an emesis basin close by. An intravenous infusion probably will be ordered to provide fluids or medications, or both. After the symptoms subside, assist the patient when getting up until dizziness goes away.

Anxiety

Patients with Ménière's disease may be anxious about the condition and the limitations it imposes. Encourage the patient to share concerns, and help the patient learn how to manage the condition.

Ineffective Therapeutic Regimen Management

Interventions involve patient teaching as presented in the Patient Teaching Plan above.

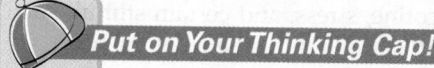
Put on Your Thinking Cap!

Think about a routine day. Consider how a person's life might be affected by frequent attacks of Ménière's disease.

POSTOPERATIVE CARE

If the patient has surgery for Ménière's disease, postoperative care depends on the exact procedure. Carefully check the physician's orders for position and activity limitations. General nursing care is concerned with safety, comfort, and detection of complications. The first few days after surgery, the patient's symptoms are usually severe. Antiemetics are ordered to control nausea and vomiting. Delay nonessential care until the patient tolerates movement. Assist patients when getting up and walking until they are able to walk steadily. The call bell should always be within reach. It is not unusual for these patients to be dizzy for several days and unsteady for several weeks.

Observe for facial nerve damage by having the patient smile and show his or her teeth. If the facial nerve is damaged, the muscles on the affected side do not respond and the patient's face is not symmetric. Im-

Put on Your Thinking Cap!

Explain why patients with inner ear disorders often have problems with balance as well as with hearing.

NURSING CARE PLAN

The Patient with Ménière's Disease

ASSESSMENT

Health History: A 62-year-old male has had repeated episodes of nausea, hearing loss, and vertigo over the past year. His attacks last 2 to 3 hours, during which he is completely incapacitated. His wife brought him to the emergency department after he vomited repeatedly and seemed very weak. His health history reveals repeated urinary tract infections but no other serious illness or injuries. He is an accountant who has his own business.

Physical Examination: Vital signs: Oral temperature, 98° F; pulse, 88; respiration, 16; blood pressure, 136/82. Mr. Riojas appears acutely ill and unable to sit or stand. Physical findings are normal except for mild hearing loss. The physician diagnosis is probable Ménière's disease.

Nursing Diagnosis	Goals and Outcome Criteria	Interventions
Risk for Injury related to vertigo	A safe environment is provided: The patient will have no injuries during acute episodes.	Assist the patient to bed, and allow him to remain still. Raise side rails, and put the bed in low position. Place the call bell within reach, and caution the patient not to try to get up unassisted. Darken the room, and keep it quiet. Postpone nonessential care. Provide a urinal for voiding. When the attack subsides, assist the patient out of bed until he is no longer dizzy.
Risk for Deficient Fluid Volume related to vomiting	The patient will be adequately hydrated, as evidenced by vital signs consistent with patient's norms, moist mucous membranes, and fluid intake equal to output.	Give antiemetics and antihistamines as ordered. Provide an emesis basin. If the patient vomits, promptly empty, clean, and return the emesis basin. Administer intravenous fluids as ordered.
Anxiety related to acute illness, disruption of usual lifestyle	The patient will state that anxiety is reduced and will appear more relaxed.	Be available, but let patient lie quietly. When the patient is able to talk, explore how the condition affects his life and how he can deal with it. Tell him that the condition can usually be improved with treatment.
Ineffective Therapeutic Regimen Management related to lack of knowledge of condition and treatment	The patient will describe measures to manage acute attacks and to reduce frequency of attacks.	Explain drugs to patient, including dosage, schedule, side and adverse effects, and information that should be reported to the physician. If sodium restriction is prescribed, explain that some patients benefit from the restriction. Request dietary consult if special diet ordered.

❓ CRITICAL THINKING QUESTIONS

■ Why is it important to let the patient lie still and remain undisturbed as much as possible?

■ Why do some patients with Ménière's disease benefit from sodium restriction?

---

mediately notify the surgeon of any evidence of facial nerve damage. Nerve damage may be reversible if treated promptly.

Presbycusis

Although many older people hear very well, approximately half of those older than 75 years have some difficulty hearing. *Presbycusis* is the term used to describe hearing loss associated with aging. It is the result of changes in one or more parts of the cochlea. The extent of the disability depends on the location of the changes in the cochlea.

Signs and Symptoms

People with presbycusis may hear well in quiet surroundings but hear poorly in noisy places. Some patients deny that they do not hear well. They may blame others for not speaking clearly.

Medical Diagnosis and Treatment

A thorough hearing evaluation is indicated for the older person whose hearing seems to be declining. Many people have the mistaken idea that hearing loss in older adults is inevitable and not treatable. In fact, many patients with presbycusis do benefit from hearing aids. If a hearing aid is recommended, the patient needs to learn how to use and care for it, as described in the Hearing Aids section on pp. 1193 to 1194. Hearing aids are helpful but are not the only way to improve communication. The patient needs to be willing to tell others how they can more easily be understood. The patient also can practice and improve listening skills.

| Box 52-2 | *Ototoxic Drugs* |

Antibiotics

Aminoglycosides
Amikacin sulfate (Amikin)
Gentamicin sulfate (Garamycin)
Kanamycin sulfate (Kantrex)
Neomycin sulfate
Streptomycin sulfate
Tobramycin sulfate (Nebcin)

Erythromycin
Erythromycin estolate (Ilosone)
Erythromycin ethylsuccinate (Pediamycin)
Erythromycin stearate (Erythrocin)
Erythromycin lactobionate (Erythrocin)

Tetracycline
Minocycline (Minocin)

Miscellaneous
Vancomycin

Diuretics
Furosemide (Lasix)
Ethacrynic acid (Edecrin)

Antidysrhythmics
Quinidine

Anti-Inflammatories/Analgesics
Aspirin
Ibuprofen (Motrin)
Indomethacin (Indocin)

Antineoplastics
Bleomycin (Blenoxane)
Cisplatin (Platinol, CDDP)
Dactinomycin (Cosmegen)
Mechlorethamine (nitrogen mustard, Mustargen)

In addition to hearing aids, other electronic devices are available to improve hearing. These are described in the Adaptations to Hearing Loss section on pp. 1197 to 1199 and include phone amplifiers and personal earphones for radios and televisions.

NURSING CARE *of the Patient with Presbycusis*

Nursing assessment, diagnosis, goals, and interventions for the patient with impaired hearing are described on pp. 1197 to 1199. In addition, nurses need to educate people about hearing loss and aging. They can also work to overcome the resistance that many people have to admitting hearing loss. Once the problem has been diagnosed, nurses can help the patient adapt and learn to use supportive devices.

Ototoxicity

Ototoxicity is damage to the ear or eighth cranial nerve caused by specific chemicals, including some drugs. Common ototoxic drugs are salicylates (aspirin) and aminoglycoside antibiotics. These and other ototoxic drugs that pose a threat to hearing are listed in Box 52-2. Ototoxicity can range from reversible tinnitus to permanent hearing loss. Hearing, balance, or both may be affected. The primary symptom of ototoxicity with salicylates is tinnitus, which disappears when the drug is discontinued. Aminoglycosides, on the other hand, can cause permanent hearing loss. The extent depends on the drug dosage and how long it was given. Patients who have poor renal function are at special risk for ototoxicity because drugs are excreted more slowly. This increases the likelihood of toxicity.

NURSING CARE *of the Patient with Ototoxicity*

The primary nursing responsibilities are early detection and prevention of progressive hearing loss caused by ototoxic drugs. To reduce the risk of ototoxicity,

be familiar with these drugs. Instruct patients to report hearing loss, tinnitus, or problems with balance. Promptly report such symptoms to the physician. Also teach patients that aspirin is not a harmless drug. Monitor the urine output of patients on ototoxic drugs, because low urine output may mean the potentially toxic drug is excreted slowly, increasing the risk of toxicity. Report low urine output to the physician. The nursing care plan should alert all staff to the potential for ototoxicity.

Disorders that impair hearing or balance can have a profound effect on a person's life and well-being. The nurse plays an important role in the prevention, early detection, and treatment of hearing and balance disturbances.

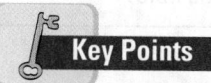

Key Points

- Approximately half of all adults older than 75 years have some hearing loss.
- Common nursing diagnoses after ear surgery include Acute Pain, Risk for Injury, Risk for Infection, and Disturbed Sensory Perception.
- Hearing losses are classified as conductive, sensorineural, mixed, or central.
- Adaptations for the hard of hearing include sign language, electronic devices, television closed captioning, personal communicators, telephones for the deaf, and trained dogs.
- Nursing care of the patient with hearing impairment addresses Impaired Verbal Communication, Social Isolation, Ineffective Coping, and Deficient Knowledge.
- Cerumen (earwax) can become impacted and obstruct the external ear canal, causing pain and hearing impairment.

- External otitis, infection and inflammation of the external ear canal, is treated with topical antibiotics and corticosteroids.
- Otitis media, infection of the middle ear, can cause permanent hearing loss and inner ear problems.
- Otosclerosis is a condition in which the stapes becomes fixed, causing a conductive and sometimes sensorineural hearing loss.
- Hearing aids are useful if the patient has only conductive hearing loss.
- The results of cochlear implants range from minimal to marked improvement.
- Labyrinthitis, which is inflammation of the labyrinth, causes vertigo and nausea and may be treated with antiemetics and antibiotics.
- Ménière's disease, characterized by attacks of hearing loss and vertigo, may be treated with drug therapy, low-sodium diet, or surgical intervention, or a combination of these.

- Nursing care of the patient with Ménière's disease may address Risk for Injury, Risk for Deficient Fluid Volume, Anxiety, and Ineffective Therapeutic Regimen Management.
- Presbycusis is hearing loss associated with aging that may be improved with a hearing aid.
- Ototoxicity is damage to the eighth cranial nerve producing effects that may range from tinnitus to permanent hearing loss.

 Go to your Companion CD-ROM for a Pharmacology Tutorial, Audio Glossary, and 3-D animations.

evolve Be sure to visit the companion Evolve site at http://evolve.elsevier.com/Linton/ for WebLinks and additional online resources.

REVIEW QUESTIONS *Choose the best answer.*

1. For an otoscopic examination of the external auditory canal of an adult, the examiner should:
   1. Pull the auricle straight up
   2. Pull the earlobe down
   3. Pull the auricle up and back
   4. Pull the auricle straight back

2. During the Rinne test, a patient reports hearing the tuning fork when it is placed on the mastoid bone and when the tines are then positioned near the ear canal. How should this information be interpreted?
   1. The patient probably has an obstruction in the ear canal.
   2. The patient probably has a conductive hearing loss.
   3. The patient's response to this test is normal.
   4. The patient probably has a sensorineural hearing loss.

3. Normal age-related changes in the ears of the older adult include:
   1. Increased cerumen secretion
   2. Hair in the ear canal is coarser
   3. Progressive hearing loss
   4. Increased risk of otitis media

4. A slightly confused patient in a long-term care facility points to her ear and loudly says "I can't hear!" The patient's hearing aid appears to be positioned correctly in her ear canal. What is the *first* thing you should do?
   1. Remove the aid and clean it.
   2. Replace the battery.
   3. Turn up the volume.
   4. See if it is turned on.

5. During report, it is noted that a new patient is severely hard of hearing. What is the most important question for you to ask about this patient initially?
   1. What means of communication does the patient use?
   2. Is the patient aware of the latest technology to assist the hard of hearing?
   3. Has the patient ever been hospitalized before?
   4. Why doesn't a family member stay with the patient to interpret?

6. You are preparing to administer otic drops when you notice the patient has gauze in the affected ear with a piece of narrow gauze extending from the ear. What should you do?
   1. Gently remove the packing, instill the drops, and replace the packing.
   2. Apply the drops to the narrow piece of gauze for transport into the ear.
   3. Trim the gauze so that the packing is not accidentally pulled out.
   4. Inform the registered nurse that the drops cannot be given at this time.

7. Which nursing measures are appropriate for the patient who is having an acute attack of Ménière's disease?
   1. Encourage the patient to ambulate.
   2. Advise the patient to drink additional fluids.
   3. Delay routine care until the patient is no longer dizzy.
   4. Monitor vitals every hour until stable and then every 4 hours.

8. When a patient is taking an aminoglycoside antibiotic, instructions should include:

   1. Let me know if you have any "ringing" in your ears.
   2. Check the white part of your eyes for a color change.
   3. Restrict your fluid intake to one liter each day.
   4. Change position slowly in case your blood pressure drops.

9. Stapedectomy is used to correct:

   1. Sensorineural hearing loss
   2. Ménière's disease
   3. Otosclerosis
   4. Otitis media

10. Patients who are considering having a cochlear implant should be told:

   1. This procedure restores perfect hearing in 99% of patients.
   2. Complications of cochlear implant are often disabling.
   3. Results vary from minimal to excellent improvement in hearing.
   4. Cochlear implants cannot enable you to discriminate speech.

CHAPTER 53

Nose, Sinus, and Throat Disorders

Objectives

After reading and studying this chapter, you should be able to:

1. Describe the nursing assessment of the nose, sinuses, and throat.
2. Identify nursing responsibilities for patients undergoing tests or procedures to diagnose disorders of the nose, sinuses, or throat.
3. Describe the nurse's role when the following common therapeutic measures are instituted: administration of topical medications, irrigations, humidification, suctioning, tracheostomy care, and surgery.
4. Explain the pathophysiology, signs and symptoms, complications, and medical or surgical treatment of selected disorders of the nose, sinuses, and throat.
5. Assist in developing nursing care plans for patients with disorders of the nose, sinuses, or throat.

Key Terms

Be sure to check out the bonus material on the Companion CD-ROM, including selected audio pronunciations.

aerosol (ĂR-ō-sŏl, p. 1213)
allergen (ĂL-ĕr-jĕn, p. 1219)
antihistamine (ăn-tĭ-HĬS-tă-mēn, p. 1218)
coryza (kŏ-RĪ-ză, p. 1219)
decongestant (dē-kŏn-JĔS-tănt, p. 1213)
epistaxis (ĕp-ĭ-STĂK-sĭs, p. 1220)
laryngectomy (lăr-ĭn-JĔK-tō-mē, p. 1229)
laryngitis (lăr-ĭn-JĪ-tĭs, p. 1226)
polyp (PŎL-ĭp, p. 1218)
rhinitis (rī-NĪ-tĭs, p. 1219)
sinusitis (sī-nŭ-SĪ-tĭs, p. 1217)
tonsillitis (tŏn-sĭ-LĪ-tĭs, p. 1223)

The nose and throat provide passageways to the respiratory and digestive tracts. In addition, they provide routes for drainage of the sinuses and are essential for normal voice production.

Many common conditions affect the nose, sinuses, and throat. Most are not life-threatening, but they can cause considerable aggravation and loss of productivity. The most serious conditions of the nose, sinuses, and throat are hemorrhage and malignancy.

ANATOMY AND PHYSIOLOGY OF THE NOSE, SINUSES, AND THROAT

NOSE

The nose can be divided into internal and external sections. The external nose is made up of bone, cartilage, and mucous membrane. Only the upper one third of the external nose has a bony skeleton. The remainder is shaped by cartilage.

The internal nose is divided by the nasal septum, a thin wall that creates two passages. The openings on each side of the septum are the nares. The outermost portion of the internal nose, called the *vestibule,* is covered by skin that contains nasal hairs. The rest of the interior is lined with mucous membrane. The internal nose is well supplied with blood by branches of the internal and external carotids.

A layer of mucus covers the membrane. The mucus traps inspired particles and moisturizes dry air. Mucus also protects the airway because it is acidic and contains an enzyme that destroys most bacteria. Cilia sweep particles that are trapped in the mucus toward the throat to be swallowed.

Olfactory cells line the roof of the nasal cavity. These are specialized sensory cells that detect odors and relay information about odors to the brain by way of the first cranial nerve (the olfactory nerve).

The side walls of the internal nose have folds of tissue called *turbinates.* Turbinates are projections that increase the surface area that inspired air crosses. As air swirls over the turbinates, it is quickly warmed to body temperature. The turbinates also contain openings through which secretions drain from the sinuses.

SINUSES

The sinuses are spaces in the bones of the skull. They are lined with mucous membrane and filled with air. The sinuses produce mucus that drains into the nasal cavity. They also act as sound chambers for the voice, and they reduce the weight of the skull. The sinuses around the nose are called the *paranasal sinuses.* They include the maxillary, frontal, ethmoid, and sphenoid sinuses. There are pairs of sinuses on either side of the face (Fig. 53-1).

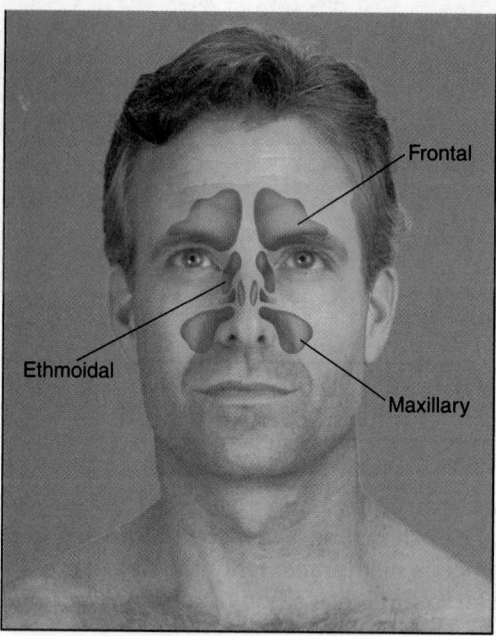

FIGURE **53-1** The paranasal sinuses.

THROAT

The throat, or pharynx, extends from the back of the nasal cavities to the esophagus. It provides passageways from the nose and mouth to the digestive and respiratory tracts. Figure 53-2 illustrates the structures in the throat.

The eustachian tubes that originate in the middle ear open into the nasopharynx. These tubes serve as pressure vents to prevent excessive pressure from building up in the middle ear.

Other important structures in the throat are the tonsils and adenoids. Tonsils and adenoids are masses of lymphatic tissue that guard against bacterial invasion of the respiratory and digestive tracts.

The larynx is the passageway between the throat and the trachea. The larynx is commonly referred to as the *voice box*. Two bands of tissue, the vocal cords, stretch across the interior of the larynx. The cords tighten and relax, producing different pitch sounds, as air moves through them. The sounds produced are modified and refined by the oral, nasal, and sinus cavities.

The epiglottis lies on top of the larynx. It is a flap that works like a trapdoor, closing during swallowing to prevent food and fluid from entering the airway.

NURSING ASSESSMENT OF THE NOSE, SINUSES, AND THROAT

HEALTH HISTORY
Chief Complaint and History of Present Illness

Patients often seek medical attention for symptoms that affect the nose, sinuses, and throat. Among the common complaints might be "runny nose," sore throat, hoarseness, and headache. You can assist by obtaining a detailed description of the patient's complaints.

Past Medical History

The past medical history should list previous streptococcal infections; sinus infections; surgery on the nose, sinuses, or throat; known allergies; and current and recent medications.

Review of Systems

The review of systems collects specific data such as the presence of nasal discharge (amount, color), obstruction, bleeding, sneezing, snoring, throat pain or soreness, hoarseness, aphonia (loss of voice), and earache. An altered sense of smell or the presence of facial pain should be noted.

PHYSICAL EXAMINATION

The nurse's examination of the nose and sinuses is usually confined to inspection of the external nose and palpation over the paranasal sinuses. The external nose is examined for size, shape, color, and lesions. If any drainage is present, the amount, color, and consistency should be noted. The examiner listens for any abnormal breath sounds and notes whether the patient is breathing through the nose or the mouth. The patency of the nostrils is determined by gently closing one naris at a time and instructing the patient to breathe through the other naris.

The sinuses are assessed indirectly. The examiner palpates over the frontal and maxillary sinuses for tenderness or pain. Transillumination is a procedure in which a special light is shone into the patient's mouth. The amount of light reflected through the sinuses reveals whether the cavities are filled with air, as they should be, or with fluid.

Examination of the throat is primarily an inspection of the throat at the back of the oral cavity. The mucous membranes and the tonsils are inspected for redness, swelling, drainage, and lesions. Inspection along with palpation of the neck may reveal enlarged lymph nodes.

Additional physical examination may be done by the physician or a nurse with advanced preparation. A nasal speculum and a lighted scope are used to observe the mucosa of the nasal cavity. Observations should include color, drainage, and the presence of foreign bodies. The sense of smell is assessed by asking the patient to identify common scents like coffee and rubbing alcohol. Assessment of the nose, sinuses, and throat is summarized in Box 53-1.

AGE-RELATED CHANGES IN THE NOSE, SINUSES, AND THROAT

As a person ages, the nose gets longer and tends to droop somewhat. Nasal obstruction is more common because of the softening of the cartilage of the external nose. The mucous membrane becomes thinner and produces less mucus. Some older people

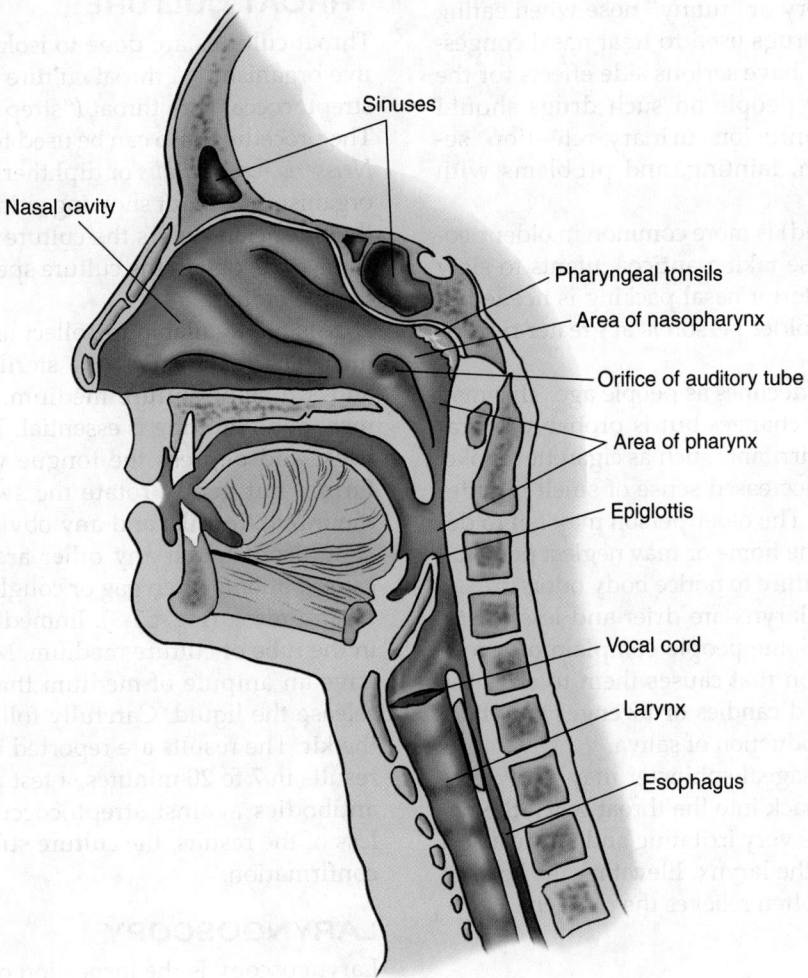

FIGURE **53-2** The nose and throat.

Labels on figure:
- Sinuses
- Nasal cavity
- Pharyngeal tonsils
- Area of nasopharynx
- Orifice of auditory tube
- Area of pharynx
- Epiglottis
- Vocal cord
- Larynx
- Esophagus

Box 53-1 | **ASSESSMENT of the Nose, Sinuses, and Throat**

Health History

Chief Complaint and History of Present Illness:
Nasal discharge, obstruction, bleeding; upper airway symptoms; sneezing, snoring; pain or soreness in the throat or face; change in voice; earache

Past Medical History:
Allergies, medications, history of streptococcal infections

Review of Systems:
Amount and color of nasal discharge; nasal obstruction; blood in nasal discharge or sputum; sneezing; snoring; throat pain or soreness; hoarseness; earache; altered sense of smell; facial pain

Physical Examination

External Nose:
Size, shape, lesions, drainage (color, amount, consistency)

Abnormal Breathing Sounds

Mouth Breathing

Palpation of Paranasal Sinuses:
Tenderness, pain

Patency of Nares

Nasal Mucosa:
Color, drainage, foreign bodies

Transillumination of Sinuses:
Air, fluid

Throat:
Inspection of mucous membranes and tonsils for redness, swelling, drainage, or lesions

Palpation of Neck for Enlarged Lymph Nodes

Ability to Recognize Common Odors

report having a watery or "runny" nose when eating spicy or hot foods. Drugs used to treat nasal congestion or discharge can have serious side effects for the older patient. Older people on such drugs should be monitored for confusion, urinary retention, sedation, hypertension, fainting, and problems with coordination.

Epistaxis (nosebleed) is more common in older people, especially in those taking anticoagulants to slow blood clotting. If posterior nasal packing is needed to control bleeding, the older person is at greater risk for airway obstruction.

The sense of smell declines as people age. This may be due to neurologic changes but is probably aggravated by exposure to irritants such as cigarette smoke. The implications of decreased sense of smell in older adults are significant. The older person may fail to detect smoke or gas in the home or may neglect personal hygiene because of failure to notice body odors.

The tissues of the larynx are drier and less elastic in the older person. Some people complain of a constant tickling sensation that causes them to clear the throat frequently. Hard candies or lozenges may help by stimulating the production of saliva.

A weakened esophageal sphincter may allow gastric contents to flow back into the throat when the patient lies down. This is very irritating and may cause a burning sensation in the larynx. Elevating the head of the bed during sleep often relieves the problem.

DIAGNOSTIC TESTS AND PROCEDURES

Conditions of the nose, sinuses, and throat are diagnosed by cultures, measures of antibodies, and procedures to visualize internal structures, as outlined in the Diagnostic Tests and Procedures table below.

THROAT CULTURE

Throat cultures are done to isolate and identify infective organisms. A throat culture usually is done when streptococcal sore throat ("strep throat") is suspected. The procedure also can be used to screen for carriers of *Neisseria meningitidis* or diphtheria. Carriers harbor the organisms without showing evidence of the disease. If the physician orders the culture and antibiotics at the same time, obtain the culture specimen before starting the antibiotics.

Kits are available to collect and contain the specimen. The kit consists of a sterile swab or applicator and a tube of culture medium. To obtain the specimen, good lighting is essential. Tilt the patient's head back, and depress the tongue with a tongue blade. Firmly but gently rotate the swab over the back of the throat, tonsils, and any obvious lesion. The swab should not touch any other area of the mouth. Because patients often gag or cough, stand to one side or wear a mask (Fig. 53-3). Immediately place the swab in the tube of culture medium. Many commercial kits have an ampule of medium that must be broken to release the liquid. Carefully follow the directions on the kit. The results are reported in 24 to 48 hours. For results in 7 to 20 minutes, a test can be done to detect antibodies against streptococcus antigens. Regardless of the results, the culture still should be done for confirmation.

LARYNGOSCOPY

Laryngoscopy is the inspection of the larynx to aid in diagnosis of abnormalities or to remove foreign bodies. A laryngoscopy may be either direct or indirect. In the direct procedure, the physician uses a fiberoptic laryngoscope (a flexible lighted tube). An indirect procedure uses mirrors to visualize the larynx. Contrast medium is sometimes instilled to outline the struc-

---

DIAGNOSTIC TESTS and PROCEDURES *Disorders of the Nose, Sinuses, and Throat*

COMMON NURSING IMPLICATIONS
1. Confirm orders, and check agency protocol.
2. Tell the patient what to expect.

TEST/PURPOSE	PATIENT PREPARATION	POSTPROCEDURE CARE
Throat culture is done to identify infective organisms.	Tell the patient a swab will be used to collect a specimen from the back of the throat. Analysis of the specimen will reveal the infecting organism, if any.	No special care.
Laryngoscopy permits visualization of the larynx.	NPO several hours before procedure. Administer drugs as ordered to decrease secretions and to relax the patient. Note allergies to local anesthetics on the patient's chart and identification band.	Nothing by mouth until the gag reflex returns. Monitor vital signs and respiratory status according to agency protocol. Provide lozenges or gargles as ordered for sore throat. Discourage the patient from talking, coughing, or clearing the throat for several hours after the procedure.

FIGURE 53-3 Throat culture technique.

tures in the larynx. A tissue specimen may be taken for examination.

COMMON THERAPEUTIC MEASURES

NOSE DROPS

Some drugs are given by the nasal route—primarily to decrease nasal congestion and obstruction. Many over-the-counter nasal **decongestants** are available. Occasional use is not thought to be harmful, but frequent use is believed to damage the protective mechanisms in the nose. This increases the likelihood of additional obstruction and infection.

Other drugs used to treat conditions of the nose, sinuses, and throat include sympathomimetics (adrenergics), anticholinergics, antihistamines, antipyretics, analgesics, anesthetics, and anti-infectives. Examples of these drugs, their uses and side effects, and nursing interventions are presented in the Drug Therapy table on pp. 1214 and 1215.

To administer nose drops, the patient may be sitting or lying down, but the head must be tilted back so that the solution flows into the back of the nose. Gently push the tip of the nose upward. Place the dropper at the opening of the nostril, and squeeze to deliver the prescribed amount of medication. The dropper should not touch the nose. The patient should keep his or her head tilted back for several minutes. The patient may

report feeling medication run down the throat. Provide a tissue for any nasal drainage or expectorated solution. Discard any unused solution that remains in the dropper rather than returning it to the bottle.

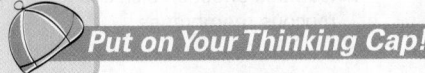

Put on Your Thinking Cap!

When instilling nose drops, why should the dropper *not* be allowed to touch the nose?

Some medications are available as sprays. Many sprays have pumps that administer metered doses. These require that the pump be depressed several times before using to fill the dose chamber. The drug is administered by holding the head upright, inserting the tip into the nostrils, and pumping two or three times. The patient then should inhale deeply through the nose.

Pharmacology Capsule

Chronic use of nasal decongestant sprays may damage the protective mechanisms of the nose and cause rebound congestion.

NASAL AND THROAT IRRIGATIONS

Nasal irrigation is the washing of secretions from the nasal cavity. The procedure is not common but may be done on occasion. A throat irrigation washes out the throat. It is done to treat congestion or pain. Like nasal irrigation, it is not commonly done. See a procedure manual for details.

HUMIDIFICATION

The inspiration of dry air is uncomfortable, causes loss of body fluid, and can contribute to upper airway infections. Mouth breathing, necessitated by nasal obstruction, bypasses the turbinates that normally moisturize inspired air. A variety of devices are available to increase the humidity of inspired air.

Room humidifiers work in one of two ways: by creating an **aerosol** or by creating steam. Aerosols dispense tiny droplets of water into the room. Steam humidifiers increase humidity by distributing vaporized water (steam).

Because steam production requires raising water to the boiling point, there is little danger of steam humidifiers becoming contaminated. Aerosol humidifiers, however, are easily contaminated. Therefore sterile distilled water should be used with aerosol units. Plain distilled water is acceptable with steam units.

With any type of room humidifier, the fluid reservoir should be checked and refilled regularly. Daily cleaning reduces the risk of bacterial contamination.

DRUG THERAPY *Nose, Sinuses, and Throat*

DRUG	USE/ACTION	SIDE EFFECTS	NURSING INTERVENTIONS
TOPICAL ANESTHETICS			
Benzocaine Cocaine Lidocaine	Anesthetic effect on skin and mucous membranes.	Allergy, sensitization, rash, burning, stinging. When sprayed on throat, can decrease gag reflex and cause dysphagia. If absorbed, lidocaine can cause drop in pulse and blood pressure. Cocaine can cause excitement and stimulation.	Inspect treated areas for side effects. Assess gag reflex before giving oral fluids or food. Monitor pulse, blood pressure, and mental status.
ANTI-INFECTIVES	Kill or suppress growth of microorganisms.	Nausea, vomiting, diarrhea, superinfections. Anaphylaxis if allergic.	Instruct patient to complete course of therapy as ordered. Report diarrhea or signs of new infections. Check allergies before giving drug.
ANTIPYRETICS			
Aspirin Ibuprofen	Reduce body temperature; used to treat fever. Analgesic effects.	Aspirin: high risk for allergy in patients with nasal polyps, asthma, or both; prolonged bleeding time, nephrotoxicity.	Aspirin: Assess for history of high risk for allergy. Watch for bleeding. Do not give with other anticoagulants. Report tinnitus, vertigo, hearing loss to physician. Tell patient not to use with possible viral infections. Ibuprofen: assess for bleeding, tinnitus, vertigo, hearing loss, gastric discomfort. Take with full glass of water. Do not take with other drugs that prolong bleeding time.
OPIOID ANALGESICS	Reduce pain.	Drowsiness; decreased pulse, blood pressure, respirations; constipation; urinary retention; nausea and vomiting; pupillary constriction.	Monitor vital signs and level of consciousness. Withhold if respirations are below 12/min. Assess elimination. Safety precautions.

Patients who use humidifiers at home should be shown how to care for the devices. Patients who use tap water in home units can clean them with a solution of one cup of white vinegar in one gallon of water. They also are advised not to inhale aerosol directly from units that do not contain sterile water.

After nasal or sinus surgery, a bedside room humidifier may be ordered. A more effective option is a face tent or aerosol mask.

Patients who have tracheostomies inspire air directly into the trachea. Until the airway adjusts to this situation, humidification is essential to prevent excessive drying of the mucosa and secretions. If a tracheostomy tube is in place, aerosol nebulizers are used. For patients who have open stomas with tubes, tracheostomy masks with adjustable oxygen are used.

TRACHEOSTOMY SUCTIONING

Suctioning is done to remove secretions from the upper airway. It is especially important for patients who cannot clear their upper airways effectively. Depending on the site of the secretions, you may need to suction the oral cavity, the oropharynx, the nasopharynx, and/or the trachea.

Suction *only* when there is evidence that it is necessary. Signs that indicate a need for suctioning include increased heart and respiratory rates, restlessness, and noisy expiration. Patients with tracheostomies also need suctioning when mucus is apparent in the tracheostomy tube. An indication for suctioning when a patient is on a ventilator is increased peak airway pressure.

Suctioning is not done unless indicated because it can cause complications, including hypoxia, tissue trauma, infection, vagal stimulation, and bronchospasm. The following are key points to remember when suctioning a patient:

1. Use sterile technique. Wear a face shield if secretions may be splashed.
2. Use water-soluble rather than oil-based lubricant to avoid getting oil into the respiratory tract.

DRUG THERAPY | Nose, Sinuses, and Throat—cont'd

DRUG	USE/ACTION	SIDE EFFECTS	NURSING INTERVENTIONS
SYMPATHOMIMETICS (ADRENERGICS)			
Phenylephrine	Decongestion, vasoconstriction.	Increased pulse and blood pressure, dysrhythmias, angina, nausea, vomiting, urinary retention. Contraindicated with monoamine oxidase inhibitors.	Monitor vital signs, especially in patients with heart disease, hypertension, urinary dysfunction, diabetes, and hyperthyroidism.
ANTICHOLINERGICS			
Atropine Scopolamine	Decrease salivary and respiratory secretions.	Side and adverse effects vary with dosage but may include dry mouth, constipation, drowsiness, blurred vision, mydriasis, urinary hesitancy, tachycardia. May cause dizziness in older adults.	Safety precautions if dizzy or drowsy. Contraindicated in narrow-angle glaucoma and acute hemorrhage. Monitor pulse, urine output, bowel elimination. Oral hygiene.
ANTIHISTAMINES			
Diphenhydramine (Benadryl) Clemastine fumarate (Tavist)	Block effects of histamine. Used to treat allergic reactions and prevent motion sickness.	Dry mouth, anorexia, tinnitus, urinary retention or frequency, drowsiness, increased or decreased pulse. Some patients experience nervousness, stimulation, sleep disturbances.	Oral hygiene. Assess pulse, appetite, voiding. Safety precautions if drowsy. Give with food if it causes gastric distress.
GLUCOCORTICOIDS			
Nasal inhalers: Beclomethasone (Beconase, Vancenase) Flunisolide (Nasalide) *Oral inhalers:* Beclomethasone (Beclovent, Vanceril) Flunisolide (Aerobid) Triamcinolone acetonide (Azmacort)	Decrease bronchial and nasal inflammation. Decrease mucus production.	Decreased resistance to infection. Burning and dryness of nose and throat with nasal inhaler. Oral fungal infection with oral inhaler. Tachycardia, dizziness, headache, cough, unpleasant taste in mouth.	Teach patient how to use inhaler, and stress prescribed frequency of use. Advise to take on schedule and not to make up missed doses. Rinse mouth after using oral inhaler.

3. Oxygenate the patient before suctioning:
   A. If able, the patient should take three deep breaths.
   B. Other patients should be ventilated with 100% oxygen for 30 seconds to 3 minutes by manual resuscitator or by oxygen mask.
4. During insertion of the catheter, the vent should be open so that suctioning does not occur.
5. Apply suction as the catheter is withdrawn. Current thinking is that continuous suction should be applied during withdrawal of the catheter because it is less traumatic. However, some sources still recommend intermittent suction.
6. Removal of the catheter and suctioning should not take more than 10 seconds. Holding your breath while suctioning the patient helps remind you not to suction too long.
7. Rinse the catheter by suctioning normal saline through it.

8. Suction the mouth and pharynx, if needed, *after* suctioning the trachea.
9. Oxygenate the patient again after suctioning.
10. With a cuffed tracheostomy tube, the oropharynx and trachea are suctioned before deflating the cuff.
11. Document respiratory status before and after suctioning.

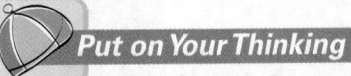 **Put on Your Thinking Cap!**

Why should you limit suctioning to 10 seconds?

TRACHEOSTOMY CARE

In addition to suctioning, the tracheostomy requires care to maintain cleanliness and protect the integrity of the surrounding skin. In the early postoperative phase, you will provide this care for the patient. The patient with a permanent tracheostomy should begin to participate as soon as he or she is able. Start the teaching process by placing a mirror so that the patient can see and by enlisting the patient's assistance.

A procedure manual should be consulted for details, but the following are key points to remember when doing tracheostomy care:

1. Use Standard Precautions.
2. Suction the tracheostomy before removing the old dressings.
3. Don sterile gloves to remove and clean the inner cannula.
4. Use a sterile solution of half hydrogen peroxide and half sterile water to clean the inner cannula.
5. Rinse and dry the inner cannula with normal saline or sterile water before reinserting it into the outer cannula.
6. Cleanse the stoma and surrounding skin with normal saline or sterile water, and pat dry.
7. Be careful not to get solution into the stoma.
8. Change tracheostomy ties if soiled. If an assistant is not available, leave the old ties in place until the new ties are secure.
9. Replace the tracheostomy dressing with a pre-cut pad or with a gauze pad folded as illustrated in Figure 53-4. Do not *cut* a pad because fibers will get into the stoma.
10. Tie the ties at the side of the neck in a square knot (not a bow).
11. Document the procedure and observations, including the appearance of the stoma, surrounding skin, and secretions.

NASAL SURGERY

Nasal surgery may be indicated for various obstructions, injuries, and chronic infections. Specific nursing care needs are discussed under individual disorders of the nose and sinuses, but general considerations are summarized here.

NURSING CARE *of the Patient Having Nasal Surgery*

General care of the surgical patient is discussed in Chapter 17. Specific nursing care after nasal surgery is added here. These procedures often are done in day surgery, so your contact with the patient may be limited.

Assessment

After nasal surgery, collect data related to pain, bleeding, anxiety, and dyspnea. Monitor the patient's vital signs to detect signs of excessive blood loss (tachycardia, restlessness, tachypnea, hypotension). Take the temperature to detect fever associated with infection. The patient with nasal packing will not be able to close the mouth for an oral temperature, so an alter-

nate route will be necessary. Patients often have nasal packing in place with a moustache dressing to absorb drainage. Note the number of dressings saturated and the frequency of changes. Remember that bleeding from the nasal cavity may flow into the throat and be swallowed while the dressing remains dry. Therefore check the back of the throat for bleeding. Also, be alert for frequent swallowing, which may be a response to bleeding into the throat. Inspect vomitus and stool for signs of blood (bright red or "coffee ground" emesis and red, maroon, or black stools).

Nursing Diagnoses, Goals, and Outcome Criteria: Nasal Surgery, Postoperative	
NURSING DIAGNOSES	GOALS AND OUTCOME CRITERIA
Decreased Cardiac Output related to blood loss from vascular nasal passageways	Normal cardiac output: pulse and blood pressure consistent with patient norms
Acute Pain related to tissue trauma, edema, or packing	Pain relief: patient states pain reduced, appears relaxed
Impaired Gas Exchange related to airway obstruction	Adequate gas exchange: respiratory rate and effort and heart rate consistent with patient norms
Disturbed Body Image related to facial bruising	Improved body image: patient accepts temporarily altered appearance: patient acknowledges that facial discoloration is temporary, resumes normal activities

Interventions

Decreased Cardiac Output

The nasal cavity has an extensive blood supply, so there is a risk of hemorrhage after nasal surgery. To reduce the risk of bleeding, advise the patient not to do anything that increases pressure in the nose. This includes blowing the nose and straining. Laxatives or stool softeners may be ordered to prevent straining due to constipation. The patient should not take any products containing aspirin because aspirin interferes with coagulation.

Notify the physician of indications of excessive bleeding: frequent, steady saturation of dressings with blood; increased pulse and respirations; restlessness; decreased blood pressure; frequent swallowing; hematemesis (blood in vomitus); and melena (dark stools associated with blood in stool).

Acute Pain

After nasal surgery, some nasal pain is expected because of the trauma and swelling. Semi-Fowler's to high-Fowler's position helps control swelling. Administer analgesics and apply ice packs as ordered. Cold

Purchased dressing with precut slit

Fold 4-inch gauze square in thirds

Fold corners down to midline

A

B

FIGURE **53-4** Tracheostomy dressings. **A,** Manufactured dressing with a precut slit has no fine threads that could enter the stoma. **B,** A 4 × 4 gauze pad folded for use as a tracheostomy dressing has no cut edges that could fray and permit fibers to enter the airway. The slit can be placed downward or upward.

decreases pain by decreasing swelling. Other sources of discomfort after nasal surgery are dry mouth and sore throat. Frequent mouth care and, when allowed, oral fluids are soothing.

Impaired Gas Exchange

Nasal packing is commonly used after nasal or sinus surgery, often with a moustache dressing in place on the upper lip to absorb drainage. Only the physician removes the packing, but nurses can change the moustache dressing as needed.

Nasal packing, especially posterior packing, can interfere with breathing. Position the patient in semi-Fowler's position with the head flat against the bed.

When the nasal cavity is packed, the patient breathes through the mouth. A humidifier helps decrease dryness of the mucous membranes. Frequent oral hygiene also is comforting. Because of the nasal packing, the patient will hear a sucking sound when swallowing. Reassure him or her that this is normal. It also is common for patients to have poor appetites when the packing is present.

Disturbed Body Image

Some types of nasal surgery tend to cause "black eyes." The application of cool compresses to both eyes may reduce or prevent this effect. Reassure the patient that this effect is temporary, but be sensitive to any patient distress about it.

DISORDERS OF THE NOSE, SINUSES, THROAT, AND LARYNX

DISORDERS OF THE NOSE AND SINUSES

Sinusitis

Sinusitis is inflammation of the sinuses, most often the maxillary and frontal sinuses. The most common causative organisms are *Staphylococcus pneumoniae, Haemophilus influenzae, Diplococcus* and *Bacteroides*. The infection usually spreads from the nasal passages into the sinuses.

Sinusitis can be acute or chronic. Acute sinusitis follows obstruction of the flow of secretions from the sinus. Causes of acute sinusitis include allergic rhinitis, deviated septum, nasal polyps, tumors, airborne pollutants, and inhaled drugs such as cocaine. Chronic sinusitis is a permanent thickening of the mucous membranes in the sinuses after repeated infections.

Signs and Symptoms

Patients with sinusitis usually report pain or a feeling of heaviness over the affected area. They may report purulent drainage from the nose. When the maxillary sinuses are affected, the pain may seem like a toothache. Headache is common, especially in the morning. Fever may be present, and the white blood cell count may be elevated.

Complications

Although most patients recover without serious effects, sinus infections can be dangerous. Chronic sinusitis may follow acute sinusitis. Other potential complications are meningitis, brain abscess, osteomyelitis, and orbital cellulitis. The possibility of brain infection exists because of the location of the sinuses in the skull. Suspect neurologic complications if the patient has a high fever, vomiting, chills, seizures, or blurred vision.

Medical Diagnosis and Treatment

Sinusitis usually is based on the findings of the history and physical examination. Sinus radiographs and computed tomography (CT) are useful; CT provides the best confirmation. Sinus aspiration or nasal endoscopy may be done to obtain a specimen for culture.

Antibiotics are prescribed for acute sinusitis. Other drugs that may be ordered to improve drainage or to relieve symptoms include decongestants, nasal corticosteroids, analgesics, and antipyretics. Antibiotic treatment for acute sinusitis usually is prescribed over 10 to 14 days. For chronic sinusitis, 4 to 6 weeks of treatment with broad-spectrum antibiotics may be necessary. First-generation antihistamines such as Benadryl are not recommended because they may dry secretions, making them more difficult to clear. However, second-generation antihistamines such as Allegra or Zyrtec may be helpful, especially if sinusitis is related to allergies. Warm, moist packs applied to the face can promote drainage and reduce pain. Other measures to promote drainage include twice-daily hot showers, increased fluid intake, and use of a humidifier. After hot showers or use of a humidifier, the patient is encouraged to blow the nose thoroughly. Sinus irrigation is sometimes ordered.

Surgical Treatment

Chronic sinusitis sometimes is treated surgically. Surgery may correct the underlying problem, remove the thickened membrane, or enlarge the opening through which secretions drain. Underlying problems that might be treated surgically include deviated septum, nasal polyps, and hypertrophy of turbinates.

Two types of surgery used for sinusitis that does not respond to medical treatment are functional funduscopic sinus surgery (FESS) and the Caldwell-Luc procedure. FESS is an outpatient procedure in which specialized instruments are passed into the sinuses through the nasal cavity. Diseased tissue can be removed, and the sinus ostia (the openings that drain the sinuses) can be enlarged. Nasal packing may be done to control bleeding. The packing usually is removed after a few hours. Complications of FESS can include nasal bleeding and scarring. Although rare, cerebrospinal fluid (CSF) leakage and injury to the optic nerve are possible.

The Caldwell-Luc procedure is used to treat chronic maxillary sinusitis. The procedure involves making an incision in the upper gum line above the teeth. An opening is made between the affected sinus and the nose. This allows secretions to drain, relieving the pressure. The cavity is packed, and the packing is left in place for 48 hours. It is removed only by the physician. After the Caldwell-Luc procedure, swelling, bruising, and numbness are normal. The numbness usually lasts several weeks.

NURSING CARE *of the Patient Having Sinus Surgery*

Nursing care after sinus surgery is essentially the same as that described earlier for nasal surgery. After FESS, the patient is usually able to return to work in 4 to 5 days. Saline nasal sprays may be ordered to prevent crusting and promote healing. After the Caldwell-Luc procedure, the semi-Fowler's position is recommended to prevent swelling and promote drainage. Apply cold compresses as ordered during the first 24 hours. Provide gentle oral care to avoid injury to the incision. Nasal packing is usually left in place until the first postoperative day. Antral packing is left in place for 36 to 72 hours. Caution the patient to avoid blowing the nose or straining, which could cause bleeding and tissue damage. The patient should not wear dentures or chew on the affected side until permitted by the physician (usually approximately 2 weeks). Three to 5 days after the Caldwell-Luc procedure, nasal saline sprays may be ordered to moisten the nasal mucosa. Temporary numbness of the upper teeth is common after the Caldwell-Luc procedure.

Nasal Polyps

Nasal polyps are swollen masses of sinus or nasal mucosa and connective tissue that extend into the nasal passages. They tend to grow, and they eventually obstruct the nasal airway. Polyps resemble white grapes in size and shape. Most patients have multiple polyps. The exact cause is unknown, but patients often have a history of allergic rhinitis or infections. Patients who have nasal polyps, asthma, and aspirin allergy are said to have *triad disease*.

The size of the polyps may be reduced by removing allergens or treating the allergic response. Corticosteroids inhaled nasally may be prescribed. Surgical removal under local anesthesia, however, is often necessary. Unfortunately, nasal polyps tend to recur.

NURSING CARE *of the Patient Having Nasal Polyp Surgery*

Nursing care after surgery for nasal polyps is like that described earlier for nasal surgery. This procedure is often done in an outpatient surgical facility, so patient teaching before discharge is especially important. Advise the patient not to take aspirin because it increases the risk of bleeding and because some of these patients are allergic to aspirin.

Allergic Rhinitis

Allergic rhinitis, or "hay fever," is a common condition. It is classified as acute (seasonal) or chronic (perennial).

Pathophysiology

Allergic rhinitis follows exposure to a substance, called an allergen, that causes an allergic response. An allergic response is a reaction to the release of chemicals, including histamine, that cause vasodilation and increased capillary permeability. Fluid leaks from the capillaries, causing swelling of the nasal mucosa. Occasionally, these changes are triggered by overuse of decongestant nose drops or sprays.

Acute allergic rhinitis most often is due to exposure to pollens. It typically lasts several weeks, resolves, and does not return until the offending pollens reappear. The chronic form is more likely due to allergens that are continuously in the environment, such as house dust and animal dander. Symptoms may be constant or intermittent, depending on the frequency of exposure.

Signs and Symptoms

Signs and symptoms of allergic rhinitis include nasal obstruction; sneezing; clear nasal discharge; frontal headache; and itchy, watery eyes. The nasal mucosa is often pale, but it can be red or bluish.

Medical Diagnosis

Diagnosis is made on the basis of a detailed history. With chronic symptoms, the patient may be instructed to keep a diary describing all episodes. This can help identify possible allergens.

Medical Treatment

The patient also may be referred to an allergist for further evaluation. The allergist applies solutions of common allergens to the skin. The allergens are applied in a specific pattern so that the patient's reaction to them can be assessed individually. Desensitizing injections may be advised to decrease the patient's reaction to the offending allergens. Patients often call these injections "allergy shots." The injections are composed of dilute solutions of the allergens to which the person reacts. The strength of the solution is gradually increased as the patient's tolerance grows. In a sense, this process causes the body to get used to the allergen so that it no longer reacts with an allergic response. Another outcome of allergy testing is that it identifies substances that the patient should avoid.

The drugs used to treat allergic rhinitis are primarily antihistamines and decongestants. Many such medications are available without a prescription. In general, these products should be used only on a short-term basis. Antihistamines should be used cautiously in older patients because they are sedating, which could lead to falls. Advise patients to consult with a physician or a pharmacist about the most appropriate over-the-counter drugs.

NURSING CARE *of the Patient with Allergic Rhinitis*

Patients with allergic rhinitis usually are treated as outpatients. The nurse who works in a clinic or physician's office may need to reinforce teaching about desensitization and drug therapy.

Acute Viral Coryza

Acute viral coryza, known as the *common cold,* can be caused by any of some 30 viruses. It is contagious and spread by droplet infection.

Signs and Symptoms

Signs and symptoms of the common cold are well-known to most people. They usually consist of fever, fatigue, nasal discharge, and sore throat.

Complications

The infection usually runs its course in approximately a week. Complications that sometimes develop include otitis media, sinusitis, bronchitis, and pneumonia. Complications are more common in people with poor resistance.

Medical Treatment

Medical management of the common cold is directed primarily at relief of symptoms. Drug therapy includes antihistamines, decongestants, and antipyretics. Patients often expect to receive antibiotics. The nurse can inform them that antibiotics are not effective against infections caused by viruses. Inappropriate use of antibiotics promotes the development of resistant strains of bacteria.

Prevention

Prevention of the common cold is best accomplished by avoidance of people with colds. People with colds are most contagious during the first 2 or 3 days after symptoms appear. The very young, the very old, and those with weakened immune systems especially should be protected from exposure.

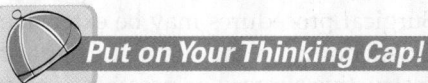

Put on Your Thinking Cap!

Design a short teaching plan on prevention of colds for first-grade children. Be creative!

NURSING CARE *of the Patient with Acute Viral Coryza*

Nursing intervention in relation to the common cold is primarily public education about prevention and about drugs prescribed for treatment. Encourage patients to rest and to drink plenty of fluids.

Consider the Alternative

Echinacea is an herb that is widely used to boost the immune system. Only recently have these claims come under study. Early evidence is that it may decrease the severity and duration of a cold but probably does not prevent it. Similar results have been found related to the value of vitamin C.

Tumors

Signs and Symptoms

Tumors sometimes develop in the nasal passages and sinuses. They can be benign or malignant. Sinus malignancies are more common among people in certain occupations—notably furniture makers. This suggests that the exposure to wood dust may be a factor. The primary symptom is nasal obstruction. Either one or both sides may be affected. Another sign suggestive of a tumor is a bloody discharge from one nasal passage.

Carcinomas of the external nose are more common than those of the nasopharynx. They are more common in men, usually between the ages of 50 and 70 years. The lesions typically begin as small, painless ulcers that do not heal. External nasal tumors are usually either basal cell or squamous cell carcinomas. Squamous cell carcinomas are more dangerous because they grow faster and tend to metastasize early. Basal cell carcinomas grow more slowly, but they still can be fatal if not removed.

Medical Diagnosis

A diagnosis is made by taking a biopsy sample of the tumor or removing the entire tumor for examination. The earlier a malignancy is detected and treated, the better the chances of survival. Unfortunately, carcinomas in the nasopharynx tend to metastasize to the neck, liver, and lungs fairly early. Therefore a patient with persistent nasal obstruction or bleeding should be examined by a physician.

Medical Treatment

Treatment of nasal malignancies usually consists of some combination of surgery, radiation therapy, and chemotherapy. Surgical procedures may be extensive and disfiguring, depending on the site and extent of the cancer. Reconstructive surgery or prostheses may be needed.

Benign tumors do not metastasize but are likely to require removal because they still can obstruct the nasal passages.

NURSING CARE *of the Patient with Nasal Cancer*

The general nursing care of patients undergoing nasal surgery is discussed in the Nursing Care of the Patient Having Nasal Surgery section on pp. 1216 and 1217. A diagnosis of cancer has special implications for the nurse. The patient may be especially anxious and fearful of disfigurement or even death. Be supportive, and encourage the patient to ask questions and express concerns. Nursing care of the patient with cancer is discussed in detail in Chapter 25.

Deviated Nasal Septum

The nose is divided into two passages by a cartilaginous wall called the *septum*. In most adults, the septum is slightly deviated, meaning it is off center. Minor deviations cause no symptoms and require no treatment. Major deviations, however, can obstruct the nasal passages and block sinus drainage. The patient may complain of headaches, sinusitis, and epistaxis (nosebleeds).

Treatment

Conservative treatment involves management of nasal allergies. Septal deviations can be corrected by a surgical procedure called a *submucosal resection* or *nasal septoplasty*. The procedure usually is done under local anesthesia. An incision is made in the nasal mucosa, and the displaced bone and cartilage are removed. The mucosa is repositioned, and the nasal passage is packed with petrolatum gauze. The physician removes the packing after 24 to 48 hours.

The two major complications of submucosal resection are tears of the septum and saddle deformity. Saddle deformity is collapse of the bridge of the nose caused by removal of excessive support tissue or by contraction of the surgical scar. Nursing care of the patient having nasal surgery was described on pp. 1216 and 1217.

Epistaxis

The nose has an abundant blood supply that permits it to bleed easily. The medical term for a nosebleed is epistaxis. Problems that may lead to bleeding include trauma, clotting disorders, dryness, inflammation, and hypertension.

First Aid

When epistaxis occurs, the patient should sit down and lean forward. Direct pressure should be applied for 3 to 5 minutes, as illustrated in Figure 16-7, unless the patient has had a traumatic injury to the face.

Facial trauma suggests a possible nasal fracture, and direct pressure may do more harm. An ice pack or a cold compress can be applied to the nose regardless of whether facial trauma has occurred. Once the bleeding stops, advise the patient not to blow the nose for several hours because this may trigger renewed bleeding.

Medical Treatment

If bleeding continues, medical attention is needed. The physician tries to identify the bleeding site and may treat it with a topical vasoconstrictor or electric cautery. If cautery is used, the patient is given a local anesthetic.

FIGURE **53-5** Placement of a posterior nasal pack used for emergency treatment of epistaxis.

If bleeding is not controlled, the next step is direct pressure to the nasal cavity. Two methods used to do this are placement of a nasal balloon catheter and placement of nasal packing.

Nasal Balloon Catheter. A nasal balloon catheter may be passed into the nasal cavity by the physician. The balloon then is inflated to apply pressure to the blood vessels. Smaller balloons anchor the catheter in place. Several different types of nasal catheters with single or double cuffs are available.

Nasal Packing. The physician may pack the anterior or posterior nasal cavity, or both. Posterior nasal packing is more complicated and requires close patient monitoring. One method of packing the posterior nasal cavity is described here. Catheters are passed into the nostrils and pulled out through the mouth. Two strings are tied to the catheters and to a rolled pad. A third string is attached to the pad. As the catheters are pulled back out the nostrils, the pad is pulled into place in the posterior nasal cavity. An anterior pack is placed over the nares and secured with the two strings that are tied to the catheter. The third string remains attached to the packing.

The loose end of the third string is brought out of the mouth and taped to the cheek. Figure 53-5 illustrates this procedure.

Complications. Complications related to posterior packing include infection, blockage of the eustachian tube, and airway obstruction. Posterior packing is usually left in place a minimum of 3 days. The bulky posterior pad can depress the soft palate, causing airway obstruction. If the packing should slip out of place, it could block the airway.

NURSING CARE *of the Patient with Epistaxis*

Assessment

Severe epistaxis is an emergency, so collect only priority data until the patient is stabilized. The priority data when a patient has severe epistaxis are evidence of uncontrolled bleeding and excessive blood loss. Inspect the nose and back of the throat for obvious bleeding, and observe for frequent swallowing. Monitor the patient's level of consciousness and vital signs to detect signs of hypovolemia (restlessness, tachycardia, tachypnea, hypotension). Document allergies and major illnesses.

Once a nasal balloon catheter or nasal packing is in place, monitor for early signs of infection and airway obstruction (dyspnea, anxiety, tachycardia). Also ask the patient about pain in the nose, pharynx, or ears.

Nursing Diagnoses, Goals, and Outcome Criteria: Epistaxis

NURSING DIAGNOSES	GOALS AND OUTCOME CRITERIA
Decreased Cardiac Output related to hypovolemia secondary to hemorrhage	Normal cardiac output: pulse and blood pressure consistent with patient's norms
Anxiety related to threat of excessive bleeding or unpleasant procedures	Reduced anxiety: patient calm, able to cooperate, states less anxious
Risk for Injury related to pressure (of packing, balloon) and possible airway obstruction	Absence of complications of balloon or packing: respiratory rate of 12 to 20/min without distress
Risk for Infection related to presence or nasal packing	Absence of infection: no fever

Interventions

Decreased Cardiac Output

Throughout the period of care for epistaxis, monitor for signs of continued and excessive blood loss. Immediately report signs and symptoms of hypovolemia (increased pulse, restlessness, decreased urine output) to the physician.

Anxiety

When a nasal balloon or packing is used, support the patient and assist the physician during placement of the device. The patient is probably frightened by the

Pharmacology Capsule

Patients who are prone to bleeding usually are advised to avoid aspirin because it inhibits blood clotting.

visible blood and needs calm reassurance. Because of the discomfort and anxiety associated with posterior nasal packing, a mild sedative may be ordered.

Risk for Injury and Risk for Infection

After the catheter is inserted and the balloon inflated, it is taped in place. Because the balloon can depress the soft palate and impair breathing, check the patient's respiratory status frequently. If a catheter is used instead of packing, the catheter placement also should be checked at least every 4 hours. Deflate anchor cuffs for 10 minutes every 24 hours as ordered or according to agency policy. Be careful to deflate the correct bulb.

Patients usually are hospitalized while nasal packing is in place. Frequent mouth care is needed because the patient must breathe through the mouth. It is also important to monitor the patient's temperature for elevation, which may indicate infection of the nasopharynx. If the posterior packing slips out of place, it could block the airway. If the airway is obstructed by the packing, the strings holding the anterior pad must be cut and the packing pulled out with the third string that is taped to the cheek.

Under normal circumstances, the physician removes the packing. You can assist by supporting the patient in a sitting position and providing an emesis basin to receive the packing. Drape the patient to protect the clothing. Once the packing is removed, the patient appreciates mouth care.

DISORDERS OF THE THROAT

Pharyngitis

Pharyngitis is inflammation of the mucous membranes of the throat or pharynx. It usually occurs along with acute rhinitis or sinusitis and is more common in late fall and spring. Pharyngitis usually is caused by a virus but sometimes is caused by bacteria. It also can follow exposure to irritating substances in the environment.

Signs and Symptoms

Signs and symptoms of pharyngitis are dryness, pain, dysphagia (difficulty swallowing), and fever. The throat appears red, and the tonsils may be enlarged. Viral and bacterial pharyngitis differ in several respects. Table 53-1 shows the key features of each. Compared with viral pharyngitis, bacterial pharyngitis has a more abrupt onset and is characterized by abnormal blood cell counts, fever greater than 101° F, and muscle and joint pain. Additional signs of infection associated with beta-hemolytic streptococci are a strawberry-red tongue, vomiting, and a rash.

Complications

Patients with bacterial pharyngitis are more likely to have serious complications than those with viral pharyngitis. The most important complications are acute glomerulonephritis and rheumatic fever. If acute glomerulonephritis develops, it usually appears 7 to 10 days after the throat infection. When rheumatic fever develops, it usually appears 3 to 5 weeks after the initial infection.

Medical Diagnosis

Pharyngitis is diagnosed on the basis of the patient history and physical examination. A more specific diagnosis of viral or bacterial pharyngitis is made after the results of a throat culture and a complete blood count are obtained.

Medical Treatment

Pharyngitis is treated with rest, fluids, analgesics, and throat gargles or irrigations. Bed rest may be recommended as long as the patient has a fever. If the patient's oral intake is low, intravenous fluids may be ordered. A soft or liquid diet may be ordered because of painful swallowing. A humidifier also may be ordered to increase moisture in the room air.

The physician often orders antibiotics, usually penicillin or erythromycin, while awaiting the results of

Table 53-1 | *Comparison of Viral and Bacterial Pharyngitis*

CHARACTERISTIC	VIRAL	BACTERIAL
Symptoms	Rhinorrhea Headache Mild hoarseness	Dysphagia Joint and muscle pain Malaise
Onset	Gradual	Abrupt
Temperature	Mild elevation	>101° F
Diagnosis	CBC: normal Culture: negative	CBC: abnormal Culture: positive
Complications	Rare	Occur in 1% to 3%; can be glomerulonephritis, rheumatic fever, otitis media, sinusitis, mastoiditis

the throat culture. Obtain the culture specimen before the antibiotics are started. When the culture results are reported, the antibiotic is discontinued if there is no evidence of bacterial growth. If bacterial infection is confirmed, the antibiotic is usually continued until 48 hours after all signs and symptoms disappear. A course of antibiotic therapy may be as long as 10 days.

Prevention

To reduce the risk of pharyngitis, people with poor resistance should avoid others with upper respiratory infections. Measures that help maintain resistance to throat infections include good nutrition, adequate rest, avoidance of chilling, and avoidance of inhaled irritants. People who have pharyngitis are contagious in the early stages and should avoid contact with susceptible people.

NURSING CARE *of the Patient with Pharyngitis*

Assessment

Mild pharyngitis usually is treated on an outpatient basis, so nursing interventions are limited. Relevant data include the presence of throat pain, dysphagia, muscle and joint pain, nausea and vomiting, and rash. Take the patient's temperature, and inspect the throat for redness and enlarged tonsils.

Nursing Diagnoses, Goals, and Outcome Criteria: Pharyngitis

The primary nursing diagnosis for the patient with pharyngitis is Ineffective Therapeutic Regimen Management related to lack of understanding of treatment and importance of follow-up care. The goal of nursing care is effective management of therapeutic regimen. The criteria for goal achievement are the patient correctly describing self-care measures—including drug therapy and symptoms that should be reported—and making and keeping a follow-up appointment.

Interventions

Reinforce the physician's directions for drug therapy, if ordered. Stress the importance of completing prescribed antibiotics. Encourage patients to take 2000 to 3000 mL of fluids daily unless contraindicated. Fluids must be increased cautiously in older adults because they do not adjust well to sudden changes in blood volume. Advise patients that they are contagious at first and should avoid people with poor resistance. Assist the patient to schedule a follow-up appointment, and advise the patient to contact the physician if a rash or strawberry-red tongue develops within the next 2 months.

Tonsillitis

Tonsillitis is inflammation of the tonsils and other lymphatic tissue in the throat. It is most common in children but often more severe in adults. Low resistance seems to invite tonsillitis.

Causes

Tonsillitis is usually a bacterial infection, but it is sometimes caused by a virus. Common causative organisms include streptococci, staphylococci, *H. influenzae,* and pneumococci. The infection is contagious and is spread by food or airborne routes. Most cases run their course in 7 to 10 days. A person may have repeated infections that respond to treatment or may have a chronic infection.

Signs and Symptoms

A patient with tonsillitis usually reports a sore throat, difficulty swallowing, fever, chills, muscle aches, and headache. If swollen tissue blocks the eustachian tubes, there may also be pain in the ears. Offensive breath odor is often present with chronic infection.

The tonsils typically are enlarged and red. Purulent drainage or yellowish or white patches may be seen on the tonsils. Lymph nodes in the neck may be tender and enlarged.

Medical Diagnosis

To diagnose tonsillitis, the physician will probably order a complete blood count, throat culture and sensitivity, and a test for infectious mononucleosis. An elevated white blood cell count suggests a bacterial infection. The culture and sensitivity identify the pathogenic organisms present and what antibiotics are likely to be effective. A chest radiograph also may be ordered to assess for respiratory complications.

Medical Treatment

The medical treatment of tonsillitis usually includes a course of antibiotic therapy for 7 to 10 days. Analgesics and anesthetic lozenges may be prescribed for pain and antipyretics for fever. Warm saline gargles or irrigations may be ordered to decrease swelling and remove drainage. Rest and adequate fluids promote recovery and decrease the risk of complications.

Complications

A peritonsillar abscess may develop with streptococcal tonsillitis. A peritonsillar abscess is an infection of the tissue surrounding the tonsil. The affected side is very painful, and the patient has difficulty swallowing, talking, and opening the mouth. The immediate treatment is drainage of the abscess. Once the acute infection has subsided, tonsillectomy is performed.

Surgical Treatment

Tonsillectomy, removal of the tonsils, was once considered routine childhood surgery. Current thinking is that the tonsils play an important protective role as part of the immune system and should be retained if possible.

Tonsillectomy is usually recommended under the following conditions:
- Repeated tonsillitis in a year, especially if caused by beta-hemolytic streptococci

- Presence of a peritonsillar abscess
- Malignancy of the tonsil
- Airway obstruction by enlarged tonsils or adenoids
- Evidence that the patient is a carrier of the diphtheria organism
- Hearing loss associated with otitis media due to enlarged tonsils

If surgery is indicated, it usually is delayed until the patient's temperature returns to normal. Even though tonsillectomy is a common procedure, it should not be considered minor. The usual procedure is a tonsillectomy and an adenoidectomy. The adenoids are usually removed because they are almost always infected when the tonsils are. If only the adenoids are infected, an adenoidectomy alone may be done. In adult patients, these procedures may be done under local or general anesthesia.

NURSING CARE of the Patient Having a Tonsillectomy

Preoperative nursing care is discussed in detail in Chapter 17. Postoperative nursing care is as follows (see also Nursing Care Plan: The Patient Having a Tonsillectomy on p. 1225).

Assessment

In the immediate postoperative phase, frequently monitor the patient's responsiveness and vital signs. They usually are checked every 5 minutes until stable, then every 15 minutes for an hour, and hourly for the remainder of the first 24 postoperative hours. Inspect drainage from the mouth or vomited fluid for blood. Blood-tinged drainage is normal at first but should gradually decrease. Note excessive swallowing, which may indicate bleeding. Monitor respiratory effort and skin color to evaluate oxygenation. Evaluate pain and dysphagia.

Nursing Diagnoses, Goals, and Outcome Criteria: Tonsillectomy

Nursing Diagnoses	Goals and Outcome Criteria
Decreased Cardiac Output related to excessive bleeding	Normal cardiac output and decreasing bleeding: pulse and blood pressure consistent with patient's norms, decreasing bloody drainage
Ineffective Airway Clearance related to bleeding, edema, or effects of anesthesia	Effective airway clearance and adequate oxygenation: no restlessness, normal skin color, no respiratory distress
Acute Pain related to tissue trauma	Pain relief: patient states pain relieved, relaxed manner
Deficient Knowledge of postoperative care	Knowledge of care: patient describes and carries out self-care as prescribed

Interventions

The two major problems that may develop in the postoperative phase are hemorrhage and respiratory distress.

Decreased Cardiac Output

Continually monitor for signs of excessive bleeding. Increased pulse rate and restlessness are early signs of hypovolemia. To reduce the risk of bleeding, remind the patient not to cough or clear the throat. If suctioning is needed, do so very gently because it may cause further bleeding. Once oral fluids are permitted, the patient should not use a straw. The sucking may dislodge the clots that form at the surgical site.

Ineffective Airway Clearance

A patient who has had local anesthesia is at less risk for respiratory complications than one who had general anesthesia. After local anesthesia, position the tonsillectomy patient with the head of the bed elevated at a 45-degree angle. After general anesthesia, the bed should be flat and the patient positioned on the side or semiprone. This promotes drainage of fluid from the mouth that might otherwise be aspirated. Once the patient is fully awake, he or she may prefer a semi-Fowler's position.

Increased pulse rate, restlessness, and confusion may be early signs and symptoms of inadequate oxygenation. Cyanosis (bluish discoloration of the nail beds or lips) is a late sign of inadequate oxygenation.

Acute Pain

Analgesics are ordered for pain. Ice collars may be applied to the neck as ordered to decrease swelling and pain. Intravenous fluids usually are prescribed until the patient is able to take oral fluids well. A clear liquid diet is ordered first. Cold or frozen liquids are especially soothing after tonsillectomy.

Deficient Knowledge

Before discharge, advise the patient of measures to promote healing and prevent complications. The diet should be soft and high in protein and calories for about 10 days. Fluid intake should be 8 to 12 8-ounce glasses daily. Citrus juices are not recommended because they irritate the healing throat tissues. Earaches are common and are not cause for alarm. It is also nor-

Patient Teaching Plan

Tonsillectomy

- Avoid strenuous activity for 2 weeks.
- Avoid aspirin, which interferes with blood clotting.
- Avoid smoking, which may disrupt healing.
- Drink 8 to 12 8-ounce glasses of fluid daily.
- Report bleeding to the physician.

NURSING CARE PLAN

The Patient Having a Tonsillectomy

ASSESSMENT

Health History: A 20-year-old college student has had tonsillitis three times this year that has resulted in absences from school. Her symptoms included sore throat, dysphagia, fever and chills, muscle aches, and headache. She has had no other serious illnesses but was hospitalized overnight after an automobile accident in 2001. She takes no medications except occasional acetaminophen for headache. She was admitted for tonsillectomy, which was performed under local anesthetic this morning. She expressed hope that it will relieve her recurrent illness. She clutches her throat and complains of throat pain.

Physical Examination: Patient is drowsy but responds appropriately. Vital signs: temperature, 98° F orally; pulse, 100; respiration, 18; blood pressure, 110/88. She has a small amount of sanguineous drainage. Respiratory effort and breath sounds are normal. Intravenous fluids are infusing into the antecubital space of the left arm.

Nursing Diagnosis	Goals and Outcome Criteria	Interventions
Decreased Cardiac Output related to excessive bleeding	The patient will maintain normal cardiac output, as evidenced by vital signs consistent with preoperative readings, minimal visible bleeding, and absence of restlessness.	Assess for signs of excessive bleeding: tachycardia and restlessness. Advise the patient not to cough or clear throat. Inspect drainage for bleeding. (Note frequent swallowing.) Report continued or excessive bleeding to surgeon. When oral fluids are permitted, have patient sip from a glass or cup rather than use a straw.
Ineffective Airway Clearance related to bleeding, edema, effects of anesthesia	The patient will maintain a patent airway, as evidenced by clear breath sounds and respiratory rate of 12 to 20.	Position on one side until fully alert. Elevate head of bed 45 degrees. Monitor for signs and symptoms of inadequate oxygenation: tachycardia, restlessness. Auscultate breath sounds. Have suction equipment in room.
Acute Pain related to tissue trauma	The patient will state that pain is relieved and will appear more relaxed.	Administer analgesics as ordered. Apply ice collar as ordered. Give cold or frozen liquids when permitted. Provide simple explanations and reassurance.
Deficient Knowledge of postoperative care	The patient will describe postoperative self-care.	Before discharge, teach the following: 1. Consume soft, high-protein, high-calorie diet for 10 days. Omit rough foods. 2. Drink 8 to 12 8-ounce glasses of fluids daily. No citrus juices. 3. Avoid strenuous activity or straining for 2 weeks. 4. No aspirin. 5. Earaches are common. 6. White patches naturally form over tonsillectomy sites. 7. Report any bleeding to the physician.

❔ CRITICAL THINKING QUESTIONS

- What is the significance of frequent swallowing?
- Why are patients *not* encouraged to cough after tonsillectomy?

- Why is it important for tonsillectomy patients to sip from a glass instead of using a straw while drinking liquids?

---

mal for white patches to form over the tonsillectomy sites. This tissue is like a scab, and it will slough off.

If any bleeding occurs after discharge, the physician should be informed. To reduce the risk of bleeding, the patient should avoid strenuous activity or straining for 2 weeks. Aspirin should not be used because it impairs blood clotting. Smoking also is discouraged.

Obstructive Sleep Apnea

Obstructive sleep apnea (OSA) is a condition marked by airway obstruction during sleep. The tongue and soft palate fall backward, partially or completely

blocking the airway and causing apnea (cessation of breathing) and hypopnea (abnormally slow, shallow breathing). The patient's blood oxygen level falls, and the carbon dioxide level rises. These changes stimulate ventilation and cause the patient to arouse. The patient startles, snorts, and gasps, causing the tongue and soft palate to move forward so the airway is open. These episodes occur repeatedly during sleep as depicted in Figure 53-6.

Symptoms of OSA are related to the disrupted sleep pattern. The patient often is irritable and sleepy during the day. The sleeping partner may report loud snoring

FIGURE **53-6** Sleep apnea. **A,** The patient predisposed to obstructive sleep apnea (OSA) has a small pharyngeal airway. **B,** During sleep, the pharyngeal muscles relax, allowing the airway to close. Lack of airflow results in repeated apneic episodes. **C,** With nasal continuous positive airway pressure (CPAP), positive pressure splints the airway open, preventing airflow obstruction.

FIGURE **53-7** Management of sleep apnea often involves sleeping with a nasal mask in place. The pressure supplied by air coming from the compressor opens the oropharynx and nasopharynx.

or episodes of apnea. The symptoms can dramatically affect many aspects of life. Concentration and memory may be impaired. Hypertension and cardiac dysrhythmias may occur. OSA is confirmed by polysomnography, which may be done in a sleep laboratory or in the patient's home.

Conservative treatment of OSA includes weight loss if obese and avoidance of sedatives and alcohol for 3 to 4 hours before bedtime. An oral appliance that shifts the mandible and tongue forward may be effective. More serious symptoms are treated with nasal continuous positive airway pressure (CPAP). For sleep, the patient wears a mask that is attached to a blower (Fig. 53-7). Airway closure is prevented because the device maintains a pressure of 5 to 15 cm H_2O in the airway. Some patients have trouble exhaling against the sustained high pressure. Bilevel positive airway pressure (BiPAP) is preferred by some patients because it adjusts to deliver higher pressure during inspiration and lower pressure during expiration.

Surgical procedures that may be used to correct OSA are uvulopalatopharyngoplasty (UPPP or UP3), genioglossal advancement and hyoid myotomy (GAHM), and laser-assisted uvulopalatoplasty (LAUP). For UPPP, obstructing tissues including the tonsillar pillars, uvula, and posterior soft palate are excised. For GAHM, the muscular attachment of the tongue to the mandible is moved forward. UPPP usually is done at the same time as GAHM. LAUP uses a laser to relieve the obstruction.

DISORDERS OF THE LARYNX

Laryngitis

Laryngitis is inflammation of the larynx. It may occur alone, or it may accompany other upper respiratory infections. A number of factors may lead to laryngitis. Upper respiratory infections, voice strain, smoking, alcohol ingestion, and inhalation of irritating fumes are all possible factors. Some patients have chronic laryngitis caused by prolonged exposure to irritants.

Signs and Symptoms

Symptoms of laryngitis include hoarseness, cough, and scratchy or painful throat. The patient may report "losing" his or her voice. This absence of sound production is called *aphonia,* and it occurs in varying degrees. Changes in the voice may be permanent after long periods of chronic inflammation.

Medical Diagnosis

Diagnosis of laryngitis is based primarily on the patient's history and symptoms. The physician may use a laryngeal mirror to examine the larynx for color, edema, and growths such as polyps and tumors. With laryngitis, the vocal cords appear red and swollen. If an upper respiratory infection is suspected, a throat culture may be done to determine the pathogen and best treatment.

Medical Treatment

Treatment of acute laryngitis is aimed primarily at reducing irritation of the larynx. Voice rest is advised, meaning that the patient is to rest the larynx by not talking. An important aspect of treatment for chronic laryngitis is removal of the irritant.

NURSING CARE *of the Patient with Laryngitis*

Patients with laryngitis rarely require hospitalization; however, it may occur in patients who have been hospitalized for other reasons.

Assessment

For the patient with laryngitis, collection of relevant data begins with a history of the problem. Document the severity of the condition, how long it has persisted, and any factors that seem to aggravate or precipitate it. Information about the patient's occupation and hobbies may provide some clues to the cause of the laryngitis. Take the patient's temperature and describe respiratory status to detect possible infection.

Nursing Diagnoses, Goals, and Outcome Criteria: Laryngitis

Nursing Diagnoses	Goals and Outcome Criteria
Impaired Verbal Communication related to aphonia or prescribed voice rest	Effective communication: patient uses nonverbal communication means
Ineffective Therapeutic Regimen Management related to lack of understanding of treatment and prevention of laryngitis	Effective management of therapeutic regimen: patient practices voice rest as ordered, avoids irritants

Interventions

When voice rest is prescribed, explain to the patient that it allows the larynx to heal. Meanwhile, an alternative means of communication must be established. Provide a pad and pencil or Magic Slate for written communication. For patients who cannot read or write, hand signals or pictures may be needed. A sign over the bed is needed to advise staff and visitors that the patient should not speak. It is also a good idea to put a notice on the intercom at the nurses' station that the patient cannot (or should not) speak. This alerts staff to go to the patient's room rather than asking what is needed on the intercom.

The teaching plan emphasizes measures to promote comfort and reduce future episodes of laryngitis. Discourage smoking. Advise the patient to remain in an environment with a constant temperature because sudden changes in temperature tend to aggravate laryngitis. If the air is very dry, a room humidifier reduces the discomfort of a dry nose and throat. Lozenges containing a topical anesthetic also may be ordered to soothe the irritation (see the Drug Therapy table on p. 1214).

When the patient has chronic laryngitis, the primary goal of treatment is to remove the irritant. Advise the patient who smokes that stopping smoking is likely to improve the symptoms. Changes in the voice may be permanent after long periods of chronic inflammation.

Teach patients that irritants can lead to laryngitis. Patients need to recognize irritants in the home and workplace and know how to protect themselves from harm. If the patient is inclined to stop smoking, information about resources in the community can be provided. The American Cancer Society is a good source of information on how to stop smoking.

Laryngeal Nodules

Laryngeal nodules are benign masses of fibrous tissue that result primarily from overuse of the voice, but they can also follow infections. Singers and public speakers are prone to development of nodules because of the strain they put on their voices. The only symptom is hoarseness.

Nodules are surgically removed under local or general anesthesia. The removal of nodules is usually fairly simple, but they may recur if the voice is again misused. After the procedure, the patient is placed on voice rest for several days. Explain voice rest as described in the Laryngitis section, and emphasize the need to avoid strain on the voice.

Laryngeal Polyps

A laryngeal polyp is a swollen mass of mucous membrane attached to the vocal cord. It can cause continuous or intermittent hoarseness, depending on its location and attachment.

In heavy smokers, flabby masses of tissue may develop on both vocal cords. A procedure called *stripping of the vocal cords* is necessary to treat this condition. Unless the patient continues smoking, the condition usually does not return. As with other vocal cord surgery, voice rest is prescribed for patients who have polyps removed.

Cancer of the Larynx

Cancer of the larynx accounts for more than 10,000 new cancers each year. It causes approximately 4000 deaths yearly and is increasing in frequency. Cancer of the larynx is most common in men ages 50 to 65 years. The higher incidence in men is thought to be related to greater alcohol and tobacco use.

Factors believed to predispose to laryngeal cancer are exposure to smoke or other noxious fumes, alcohol consumption, vocal strain, and chronic laryngitis. People who both smoke and use alcohol are at particularly high risk.

Malignant tumors can develop at various points throughout the larynx: above the glottis, on the vocal cords, or below the vocal cords. Most malignancies of the larynx are squamous cell carcinomas.

The cure rate is highest for patients with tumors that are confined to the vocal cords. Unfortunately, malignancies in the larynx tend to spread fairly early. The most common site of metastasis is the lung. The more widespread the cancer is, the more difficult it is to treat. Over recent years, the death rate among men has declined slightly but it has increased dramatically for women.

Signs and Symptoms

Early symptoms of cancer of the larynx include persistent hoarseness or sore throat and ear pain. Some patients report throat discomfort or a sensation that there is a "lump" in the throat. Later signs and symptoms of laryngeal cancer are hemoptysis (blood in sputum) and difficulty swallowing or breathing. Pain and anorexia leading to weight loss are usually late symptoms of the disease.

Prevention

The most important measures to reduce the risk of cancer of the larynx are for people to stop smoking and drinking alcohol. The public also should be educated to recognize the signs and symptoms of laryngeal cancer and seek prompt medical attention. Early treatment may be able to preserve the voice.

Medical Diagnosis

A diagnosis of cancer of the larynx is confirmed by study of a tissue sample obtained during a laryngoscopy. Radiographs, CT scans, and magnetic resonance imaging (MRI) are done to define the extent of the cancer. These studies give more detail about the primary site and help locate metastases. Laboratory findings often seen with malignancies include decreased hemoglobin and hematocrit and elevated alkaline phosphatase. Remember that these changes can be due to causes other than cancer.

Medical Treatment

Treatment involves the use of surgery, radiotherapy, chemotherapy, or some combination of these. The diagnostic tests just described aid the physician in selecting the treatment of the patient with laryngeal cancer. Another important consideration is the patient's overall health state and ability to cope with the effects of specific treatments.

Radiotherapy alone can cure some small cancers that have not spread to surrounding tissues. In addition, radiation may be used before and after surgery. Brachytherapy is a form of radiotherapy that involves placing thin, hollow needles into and around the tumor. Radioactive seeds are then placed in the needles to emit continuous radiation to the area.

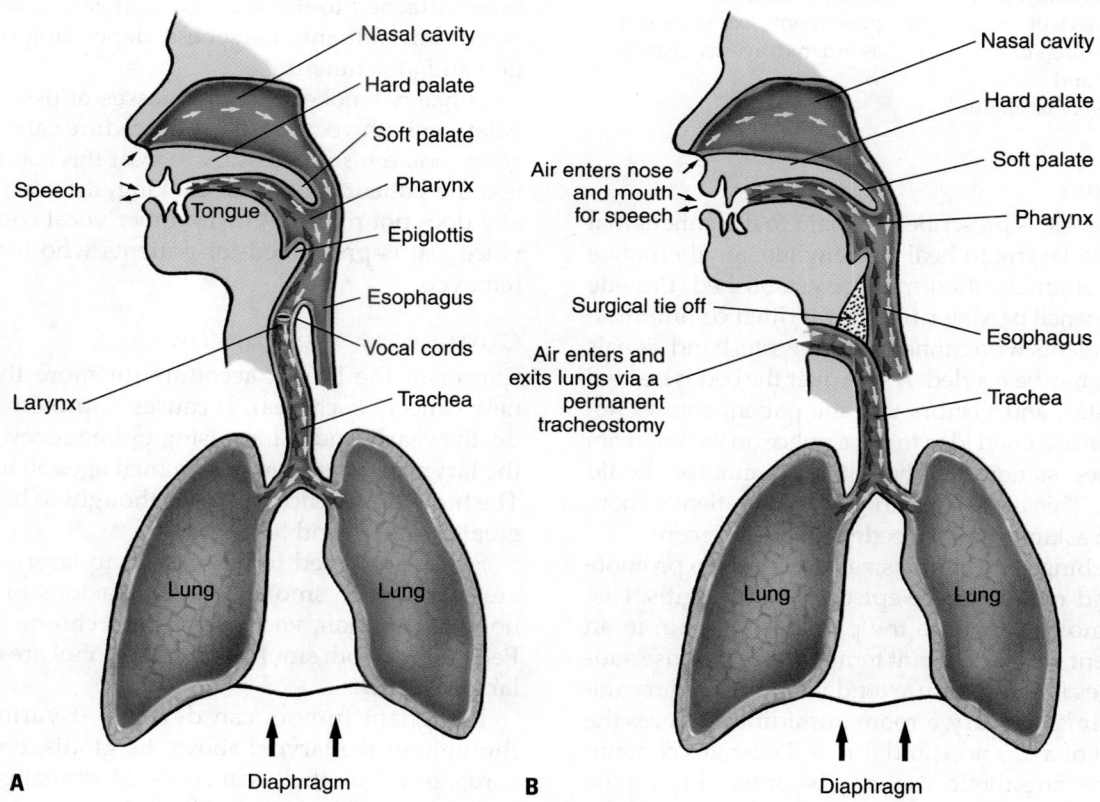

FIGURE 53-8 The throat before **(A)** and after **(B)** total laryngectomy. *Arrows* indicate the route of airflow.

Chemotherapy may be administered as palliative treatment, before surgery to reduce tumor size or postoperatively to reduce the risk of metastasis. Care of the patient undergoing radiotherapy or chemotherapy is discussed in Chapter 25.

Surgical Treatment

Surgical procedures for cancer of the larynx range from simple removal of the tumor to extensive procedures such as laryngectomy and modified or radical neck dissection. Laser surgery may be used alone or with radiation therapy for small tumors. A laryngectomy can be total or partial. The voice can be preserved with hemilaryngectomy or supraglottic laryngectomy. However, total laryngectomy causes permanent loss of the natural voice. Figure 53-8 illustrates airflow before and after laryngectomy.

Radical neck dissection often is done at the same time as laryngectomy, especially if lymph nodes are positive for cancer. Radical neck dissection is the excision of all nonessential structures on the affected side. The sternocleidomastoid muscle, jugular vein, submaxillary salivary gland, and surrounding soft tissue are removed. The spinal accessory nerve is cut, causing the shoulder to droop on the affected side. Figure 53-9 illustrates the appearance of the incisions after radical neck dissection. A modified radical neck dissection spares the internal jugular vein, the major cervical lymphatic vessels, and the sympathetic, vagus, and spinal accessory nerves.

NURSING CARE of the Patient Having a Total Laryngectomy

General preoperative nursing care is discussed in Chapter 17. This section addresses the specific needs of the patient facing surgery for laryngeal cancer. Try

FIGURE **53-9** A radical neck dissection incision with drain tubes in place.

to find out which procedure will be done so that preoperative teaching can be individualized.

If the patient will lose the ability to speak, information about other means of communication should be available. The physician and speech therapist can advise the patient about appropriate alternatives. The anticipated loss of the voice is very stressful to patients. The full impact may not actually hit them until later because the first concern is eliminating the cancer. Listen compassionately, and accept the patient's expressions of anger or despair. Some patients benefit from meeting a volunteer from an organization for people who have had laryngectomies. Consult the patient about this before inviting a volunteer.

The patient who will have a laryngectomy and radical neck dissection can expect to go to an intensive care unit for several days. This allows close monitoring and maintenance of a patent airway with the new tracheostomy. Advise the patient in advance that this is routine and does not mean that anything has gone wrong. You can also help prepare the patient to expect intravenous lines, wound drains, a feeding tube, and, perhaps for a short time, a ventilator.

Postoperative care varies with the exact procedure. Procedures include partial laryngectomy, supraglottic laryngectomy, and total laryngectomy. Nursing care of the patient with a total laryngectomy is presented in detail. The unique needs of the patient with a partial or supraglottic laryngectomy are identified.

A total laryngectomy involves removal of the entire larynx, vocal cords, and epiglottis as well as supportive tissues. The opening of the pharynx to the trachea is closed, and the tracheostomy is created by bringing the trachea to the opening in the neck. The upper airway is no longer connected to the lower airway. The patient breathes through the trachea. Figure 53-8 illustrates the changes with total laryngectomy. A radical neck dissection is often done because of the high risk of metastasis to the neck.

Complications

Complications of total laryngectomy with radical neck dissection include salivary fistula, carotid artery blowout, and tracheal stenosis. A salivary fistula is a drainage pathway that forms when saliva leaks through a defect in the suture line in the pharynx. It usually closes spontaneously but sometimes requires surgical closure. Until the fistula closes, the patient must be fed through a nasogastric tube. Otherwise, whatever the patient eats leaks out the fistula.

Patients at highest risk for carotid artery blowout (rupture) are those who had radiation therapy before surgery and acquired a salivary fistula after surgery. Carotid blowout is an emergency that must be corrected surgically.

Tracheal stenosis is narrowing of the trachea that develops weeks or months after surgery. If the airway becomes obstructed, surgical correction is necessary.

The general nursing care of the postoperative patient is discussed in Chapter 17. This section addresses the special needs of the patient with total laryngectomy.

Assessment

In the immediate postoperative period, the assessment focuses on oxygenation, circulation, and comfort. You assist by collecting relevant data. Document the patient's level of consciousness. Ask about pain, and observe for signs of discomfort. Measure vital signs at frequent intervals. Continuous electrocardiogram monitoring and pulse oximetry also may be used to assess oxygenation and circulation. Record fluid intake and output, and describe the characteristics of wound drainage.

Additional aspects of assessment after total laryngectomy are weight changes, ability to swallow, and effectiveness of alternate means of communication. The patient's response to the surgery, coping strategies used, and sources of support also are very important. During the rehabilitation phase, members of the health care team help the patient anticipate the effects of the surgery on everyday life and the adaptations that need to be made. Also collect data that indicate the patient's readiness and ability to participate in self-care.

Nursing Diagnoses, Goals, and Outcome Criteria: Total Laryngectomy, Postoperative

Nursing Diagnoses	Goals and Outcome Criteria
Ineffective Airway Clearance related to increased pulmonary secretions or weak cough	Patent airway: respiratory rate 12 to 20/min without dyspnea, breath sounds clear
Anxiety related to revised airway, uncertain outcome of cancer surgery, or threat to self-concept	Reduced anxiety: patient calm, states anxiety is reduced
Decreased Cardiac Output related to excessive blood loss	Adequate cardiac output: pulse and blood pressure consistent with patient norms, fluid intake and output equal Minimal blood loss: decreasing bleeding, drainage lightens in color
Acute Pain related to tissue trauma	Pain relief: patient states pain reduced, relaxed manner
Risk for Injury related to excision of muscles in the neck or altered upper airway	Reduced risk for injury: patient demonstrates protection of incision during movement, avoids introduction of harmful substances into trachea
Imbalanced Nutrition: Less Than Body Requirements related to dysphagia or diminished sense of smell	Adequate nutrition: stable body weight, maintenance of patient's admission weight if normal
Impaired Verbal Communication related to surgical excision of larynx	Effective communication: patient uses a means of communication that meets his or her needs
Ineffective Coping related to loss of verbal communication or altered appearance	Effective coping with body changes: patient makes realistic plans to adapt lifestyle to physical and functional changes
Risk for Infection related to altered airway or interrupted skin integrity	Absence of infection: normal body temperature and white blood cell count, no purulent drainage or secretions
Ineffective Therapeutic Regimen Management related to fear, lack of understanding of self-care	Patient assumes self-care: correctly demonstrates care of tracheostomy

Interventions

Ineffective Airway Clearance

As previously emphasized, oxygenation status must be monitored frequently. If the patient is on a ventilator, it usually is discontinued within a day after surgery. At first, the patient has a laryngectomy tube in the tracheostomy. The laryngectomy tube is shorter and wider than a tracheostomy tube, but care of the two is essentially the same.

Because the new tracheostomy bypasses the upper airway, the respiratory tract has to adjust to a dramatic change. The mucous membranes respond to the unexpected trauma and irritation by increasing secretions. Because normal humidification is absent, the secretions tend to be drier than normal, making it more difficult to remove them from the airway.

The trachea and laryngectomy tube must be kept open at all times, or the patient would suffocate. Data that indicate the need for suctioning include increased pulse, restlessness, and audible or visible mucus. Use sterile technique to clear the airway as needed. Tracheostomy suctioning is described on pp. 1214 to 1216 in the Tracheostomy Care section. Consult a procedure manual for additional details.

Factors that affect respiratory status are positioning, fluids, and humidification. Semi-Fowler's or Fowler's position permits maximal lung expansion. Turning, coughing, and deep breathing prevent pooling of secretions in the lungs. Intravenous fluids and enteral feedings maintain hydration and nutrition. Good hydration helps thin secretions. A tracheostomy collar is used to provide oxygen and humidification of inspired air.

Anxiety

Be sensitive to the patient's anxiety. A calm approach, attentive monitoring, and simple explanations help reduce anxiety. You must also remember to talk to the patient! There is a tendency to treat the patient who cannot speak as if he or she cannot hear either.

Decreased Cardiac Output

In the early postoperative period, the patient is at risk for excessive bleeding. Frequent monitoring of vital signs allows detection of indicators of hemorrhage, such as increasing pulse and respiratory rates and restlessness. Inspect secretions for excessive bleeding.

Drains usually are in place to remove excess fluid. Note the color and the amount of the drainage. Over the first few postoperative days, the color should change from bright red to pink to clear or straw-colored. The amount of drainage also should decrease steadily.

Acute Pain

Analgesics are given as ordered after surgery. You may be surprised that the patient who has had a radical neck dissection may not seem to have much pain. Because the procedure is so extensive, many nerves are cut, so sensation is impaired. Some areas of numbness are permanent.

Risk for Injury

The patient may be fearful of moving his or her head, especially after radical neck surgery. You can help at first by placing a hand behind the patient's head when he or she gets out of bed. The patient can also learn to roll on one side and support the head while rising up from the bed.

The tracheostomy is open to the environment and must be protected from foreign substances. Teach the patient to avoid dusty places and to cover the tracheostomy loosely during shaving or haircuts. The patient cannot submerge the neck or allow bath water to splash into the trachea because the water would go directly into the airway.

Imbalanced Nutrition: Less Than Body Requirements

Nutrition is often a problem after laryngectomy. The patient's sense of smell is impaired because inspired air no longer goes through the nose. The patient also may have some difficulty swallowing because of tissue trauma around the surgical site. Nasogastric tube feedings are given initially. Oral fluids and foods are reintroduced gradually. Nursing measures to improve appetite should be used, and the patient's weight should be monitored. Chapter 9 discusses nursing interventions for anorexia and for tube feedings. (See the Nutrition Concepts box below.)

Nutrition Concepts

1. Malignancies of the upper airway often lead to inadequate nutritional intake.
2. Patients who have had partial laryngectomies are at high risk for aspiration while learning to swallow again.
3. Gastrostomy or nasogastric (NG) tubes may be placed to maintain nutrition after partial laryngectomy.

Impaired Verbal Communication

A number of options exist for restoring some form of speech to the patient with laryngectomy. The speech therapist and the physician will recommend appropriate methods (Fig. 53-10).

Many patients are able to learn to use "esophageal speech." Air is swallowed and held in the upper esophagus. The patient then belches. The patient learns to control and use the air to produce sounds. The voice is deep but understandable. Considerable motivation and practice are needed to master esophageal speech. Patients and their families are likely to have periods of discouragement. You can help by acknowledging their feelings and demonstrating patience.

A second option is the use of an artificial larynx. Several types of electronic devices are available that produce sound. The "voice," however, has a mechanical, computerized sound that tends to attract attention.

Some patients are candidates for laryngoplasty, a procedure performed during total laryngectomy. It is done to create a connection between the pharynx and the trachea. The patient is able to speak by occluding the tracheostomy with a finger. This procedure is not an option for all patients and is not always successful.

Tracheostomy tubes and valves that facilitate speech are available.

One final option for speech is the tracheoesophageal prosthesis. The surgeon creates a fistula between the trachea and the esophagus. A catheter is placed in the fistula until it heals. When the catheter is removed, a prosthesis is inserted into the fistula. Two prostheses that may be used are the Blom-Singer trapdoor prosthesis and the Panje voice button. The patient occludes the stoma with a finger during speech. A one-way valve allows air to flow only from the trachea to the esophagus. These tubes are illustrated in Figure 53-10, *E* and *F*.

Those patients who are unable to use any form of speech must rely on written communication, gestures, or some assistive devices. A word board is a computerized device that enables the patient to select words that are "spoken" by the computer. A personal communicator produces a printed message that the patient enters on a keyboard.

It is especially important to direct the laryngectomy patient to community resources. Organizations such as the Lost Chord Club or New Voice Club are especially useful because the members have had personal experiences with laryngectomies. The American Cancer Society can provide information about resources in the local community.

Ineffective Coping

It has been said that language separates humans from animals. The permanent loss of the ability to communicate verbally is very traumatic. Patients who require laryngectomy usually have some time to prepare for this procedure in advance, but the actual event still evokes

FIGURE **53-10** Postlaryngectomy speech aids. **A** and **B**, Patient using the Electrolarynx Servox artificial larynx, which is held against the throat to detect vibrations from silently mouthed words and convert them to electronic sounds. **C** and **D**, The Cooper-Rand electronic speech aid allows the patient to adjust tone, pitch, and volume. **E**, Blom-Singer trapdoor tracheoesophageal prosthesis. **F**, Panje voice button.

Labels in figure E:
- Esophagus
- Voice prosthesis
- Housing
- Tracheostoma valve
- Voice prosthesis in stoma
- Trachea
- Air from lungs

Labels in figure F:
- The Panje voice button

a variety of emotional responses. Learning to live with a permanent tracheostomy and loss of the natural voice requires considerable adjustment. The patient may demonstrate behaviors typical of any loss situation: denial, anger, depression, bargaining, or acceptance. Depression may be reflected in withdrawal or refusal to learn about self-care and rehabilitative measures.

Acknowledge the patient's feelings, and gently urge participation in self-care and use of alternative means of communication. The patient who learns to care for the tracheostomy and to communicate effectively feels more confident of the ability to cope.

Support groups can be especially helpful because the patient sees potential role models of successful adaptation to tracheostomy. The family also requires support, encouragement, and teaching.

Risk for Infection

The tracheostomy permits unfiltered air to enter the respiratory tract. The effects are drying of the mucous membranes, increased secretions, and increased risk of infection. Use sterile technique during tracheostomy care. Protect the patient from people who have respiratory infections.

Ineffective Therapeutic Regimen Management

As soon as the patient is able, encourage participation in self-care. At first, just ask the patient to hold some supplies. Explain what is being done and why. Gradually, the patient should assume more responsibility for care of the tracheostomy. Even if the patient seems quite competent by discharge, a referral to a home health agency or visiting nurse association is recommended. The home care nurse helps the patient learn to adapt care to the home setting and to deal with various unanticipated problems. A family member or significant other should be taught tracheostomy care as well. Verbal teaching should be accompanied by written information for later use. Remember that people recall only a small percentage of what they hear.

NURSING CARE of the Patient Having a Supraglottic Laryngectomy

For patients whose cancer is located above the vocal cords, supraglottic laryngectomy and radical neck dissection are the usual procedures. These patients also have temporary tracheostomies. Cuffed tubes are used at first because of the danger of aspiration. These patients require oral and tracheal suctioning.

Nursing care of the patient having supraglottic laryngectomy is in many ways like that of the patient having total laryngectomy except that the tracheostomy is temporary, the voice is not lost, and swallowing is more problematic. Therefore additional nursing interventions are indicated to maintain good nutrition. Enteral feedings may be needed for a long time, so begin to instruct the patient in self-feeding. Some patients never regain the ability to swallow without aspirating, and total laryngectomy is recommended for them.

An example of the swallowing techniques taught to these patients is outlined in Box 53-2.

When the patient has a tracheostomy, any aspirated food or fluids may be ejected through the tracheostomy. The patient with a supraglottic laryngectomy is also at increased risk for aspiration pneumonia. Be alert for signs and symptoms of this complication: increased pulse and respiratory rates, dyspnea, cough, crackles and rhonchi, fever, wheezing, and frothy, pink sputum. Keep a suction machine readily available.

Box 53-2 | Steps for Performing the Supraglottic Swallow

1. Take a deep breath to aerate lungs.
2. Perform Valsalva maneuver to approximate cords.
3. Place food in the mouth and swallow. Some food will enter airway and remain on top of closed vocal cords.
4. Cough to remove food from top of the vocal cords.
5. Swallow so food is moved from top of vocal cords.
6. Breathe after cough-swallow sequence to prevent aspiration of food collected on top of vocal cords.

From Lewis, S.M., Heitkemper, M.M., & Dirksen, S.R. (2004). *Medical-surgical nursing* (6th ed.). St. Louis: Mosby.

NURSING CARE of the Patient Having a Partial Laryngectomy

If a patient has a partial laryngectomy, a temporary tracheostomy for 2 to 5 days can be expected. Intravenous fluids and enteral feedings usually are ordered at first. Like patients with supraglottic laryngectomies, these patients have considerable difficulty swallowing when oral nourishment is resumed. In general, the nursing care is similar to that of the patient having a supraglottic laryngectomy. To prevent aspiration, seat the patient upright, with the head flexed slightly forward. Semisolids are often easier to manage than thin liquids. A suction machine should be on hand in case it is needed.

Key Points

- Sinusitis is an acute or chronic inflammation of the sinuses that can lead to meningitis, brain abscess, osteomyelitis, and orbital cellulitis.
- Sinusitis is treated with drug therapy or with surgery to remove obstructions and to improve drainage.
- Nasal polyps are masses of tissue that extend from the sinuses into the nasal passage; they can be surgically excised.
- Allergic rhinitis, or "hay fever," is an allergic response to a substance that produces sneezing; nasal obstruction; clear nasal discharge; frontal headache; and itchy, watery eyes.
- Allergic rhinitis may be treated with antihistamines and decongestants or with desensitizing injections of identified allergens.
- Acute viral coryza, the common cold, is caused by a virus; is contagious; and is treated symptomatically with antihistamines, decongestants, and antipyretics.
- Tumors of the nasal passages typically cause nasal obstruction requiring surgical excision.
- Malignant tumors of the nasal passages and pharynx tend to metastasize early and may be treated with some combination of surgery, chemotherapy, and radiation therapy.
- The two kinds of carcinomas of the external nose are squamous cell carcinomas, which grow rapidly and tend to metastasize, and basal cell carcinomas, which grow more slowly and are less invasive.
- A deviated nasal septum may obstruct the nasal passages and interfere with sinus drainage.
- Surgical procedures for deviated nasal septum include nasal septoplasty and submucosal resection.
- Epistaxis (nosebleed) usually can be controlled with external pressure but sometimes requires placement of a nasal balloon catheter or packing.
- Tonsillitis is more common in children but is more often severe in adults.
- Tonsillitis may be treated with drug therapy, irrigations, or surgical excision.
- Nursing care after tonsillectomy focuses on Decreased Cardiac Output, Ineffective Airway Clearance, Acute Pain, and Ineffective Therapeutic Regimen Management.

- Cancer of the larynx may be treated with surgery, radiation therapy, chemotherapy, or a combination of these.
- After laryngectomy (removal of the larynx), the nurse addresses problems of Ineffective Airway Clearance, Anxiety, Decreased Cardiac Output, Acute Pain, Risk for Injury, Imbalanced Nutrition: Less Than Body Requirements, Impaired Verbal Communication, Ineffective Coping, Risk for Infection, and Ineffective Therapeutic Regimen Management.

 Go to your Companion CD-ROM for a Pharmacology Tutorial, Audio Glossary, and 3-D animations.

evolve   Be sure to visit the companion Evolve site at http://evolve.elsevier.com/Linton/ for WebLinks and additional online resources.

REVIEW QUESTIONS *Choose the best answer.*

1. The function of the turbinates in the internal nose is to:

   1. Trap inspired particles
   2. Destroy microorganisms
   3. Warm inspired air
   4. Detect odors

2. Age-related changes in the nose, sinuses, and throat include:

   1. Thickening of the mucous membrane
   2. Increased mucus production
   3. Decreased sense of smell
   4. Less risk of epistaxis

3. The maximum time that suction should be applied during nasotracheal suctioning is:

   1. 10 seconds
   2. 15 seconds
   3. 20 seconds
   4. 25 seconds

4. After nasal surgery, a patient has packing in place and a nasal drip ("moustache") dressing on the upper lip. When the moustache dressing has become saturated, you should:

   1. Replace the packing and the moustache dressing
   2. Notify the physician
   3. Reinforce the moustache dressing
   4. Change the moustache dressing

5. A patient who had nasal surgery is restless. His pulse rate has increased from 70 to 90 bpm, and his respiratory rate is 20. His nasal dressing has no fresh bleeding. What should you do *first*?

   1. Order one unit of blood
   2. Take his vital signs again
   3. Inspect the back of his throat
   4. Encourage increased fluid intake

6. The most serious complications of sinusitis include:

   1. Headache
   2. Pain
   3. Meningitis
   4. Rhinitis

7. A patient who has "triad disease" is allergic to aspirin, has asthma, and has:

   1. Elevated triglycerides
   2. Nasal polyps
   3. Tonsillitis
   4. Laryngeal nodules

8. Immediate treatment of epistaxis is to have the patient:

   1. Sit up, lean slightly forward, and pinch the nostrils
   2. Assume a semi-Fowler's position with the head tilted back
   3. Lie supine and apply a cold pack to the nose
   4. Sit up and lean forward to put the head between his knees

9. The priority nursing diagnosis after total laryngectomy is:

   1. Anxiety
   2. Acute Pain
   3. Ineffective Airway Clearance
   4. Impaired Verbal Communication

10. The primary advantage of supraglottic laryngectomy over total laryngectomy is that:

    1. Swallowing is easier
    2. The voice is preserved
    3. The tracheostomy is permanent
    4. There is less risk of aspiration pneumonia

CHAPTER

54 Psychological Responses to Illness

MARK D. SOUCY

evolve   http://evolve.elsevier.com/Lint

Objectives

After reading and studying this chapter, you should be able to:

1. Define mental health.
2. Discuss the concepts of stress, anxiety, adaptation, and homeostasis.
3. Discuss how age and cultural and spiritual beliefs affect an individual's ability to cope with illness.
4. Identify some basic coping strategies (defense mechanisms).
5. Discuss the concepts of anxiety, fear, stress, loss, grief, helplessness, and powerlessness in relation to illness.
6. Describe several factors that may precipitate adaptive or maladaptive coping behaviors in response to illness.
7. Discuss implementation of the nursing process to enhance a patient's mental health as the patient deals with the stresses of illness.

Key Terms

Be sure to check out the bonus material on the Companion CD-ROM, including selected audio pronunciations.

adaptation (p. 1236)
anxiety (ăng-ZĪ-ĭ-tē, p. 1239)
conflict (p. 1236)
coping (p. 1240)
crisis (p. 1236)
defense mechanism (p. 1240)
feelings (p. 1239)
helplessness (p. 1241)
maladaptive coping (măl-ă-DĂP-tĭv, p. 1240)
self-esteem (p. 1238)
stress (p. 1236)
stressor (p. 1236)

Part of being human is having to cope with different types of stressors at different times of life. Individual coping strategies are influenced by many factors, such as personal beliefs and values, the family, cultural practices, and community resources. Patients and their families may experience a wide range of feelings and emotions in response to illness. To promote adaptation to illness and to minimize maladaptive behaviors, you need to be well acquainted with the range of responses that individuals can experience during illness. The nursing process provides a systematic approach to individualized care based on careful assessment and understanding of human behavior.

DEFINITION OF MENTAL HEALTH

A person is a living being with physical, cognitive, affective, behavioral, and social dimensions who interacts with the environment to achieve a chosen life purpose. The *physical dimension* includes the biologic and physiologic aspects of a person, and it is integrated with cognitive, affective, behavioral, and social dimensions. The *cognitive dimension* involves an individual's ability to formulate thoughts, process information, and solve problems. The *affective dimension* involves an individual's ability to experience and express feelings and emotions. The *behavioral dimension* reflects a person's individuality and involves integration of the physical, cognitive, and affective dimensions. The *social dimension* involves an individual's skills in living as a member of a family and community. Together these dimensions form a holistic or total person.

Environment is everything outside a person. It includes the physical and social elements that are external to and interactive with an individual. In a health care setting, you are a part of the environment.

Mental health is a dynamic process in which a person's physical, cognitive, affective, behavioral, and social dimensions interact functionally with one another and the environment. Mentally healthy individuals are able to perceive reality accurately, manage the way that emotions are experienced and expressed, think clearly and logically, communicate effectively, anticipate events and solve problems, initiate and maintain meaningful relationships, develop a positive self-concept, and generally behave in ways that promote personal growth and development.

According to Maslow, healthy individuals possess several characteristics:

- An accurate perception of reality
- The ability to accept oneself and others
- The ability to be spontaneous
- The ability to solve problems

need for privacy
dependence or autonomy
he ability to express the self emotionally
A frequency of "peak experiences"—happy moments that produce a sense of worth, hope, and love of life
- Identification with humankind
- The ability to maintain satisfactory relationships
- A sense of ethics
- Some sense of resistance to conformity

STRESS

Stressors can originate in any or all of the dimensions of the self. At any given moment, individuals are adapting to a variety of stressors from each of the five dimensions. Thus a person's level of health is directly related to the ability to adjust to a variety of internal and external stressors.

Stress is caused by a stressor. A stressor can be anything, positive or negative, that necessitates an adaptive response on the part of the individual. Stress is necessary for growth and development. Mild stress produces mild anxiety and enables people to use energy focused exclusively on the problem. The result can be successful problem solving, which in turn promotes self-esteem. However, stress can also be perceived as harmful. Examples of potentially harmful stressors are the loss of a job or the death of a family member.

Adaptation to stress affects the whole organism. For example, a person who is immobilized lacks the stress of exercise, so the muscles begin to atrophy, joints become rigid and inflexible, and so on, until all the systems of the body are affected. With daily stress such as moderate exercise, muscles increase in mass, circulation improves, and joints become more flexible. So it is with mental health. The dimensions of the person—physical, cognitive, affective, behavioral, and social—are not separate entities. These dimensions interact, resulting in the development of a unique human being.

HOMEOSTASIS

Stress, response, and adaptation can be thought of as a process aimed at maintaining homeostasis or equilibrium. If stressors are relatively mild and the person is able to respond and adapt, mental health is maintained. If, however, the person is overwhelmed by many stressors or does not have sufficient coping behaviors or problem-solving strategies to maintain equilibrium, illness or crisis may ensue. A crisis results in inner tension and anxiety, which may affect an individual's ability to function.

GROWTH AND DEVELOPMENT

Growth refers to an individual's gradual process of evolution from conception until death. As human beings move through sequential stages of development, they become increasingly complex. Each individual is shaped throughout life by all of the events and perceived interactions with individuals, the community, and the environment. Growth, then, refers not only to a change in physical size and structure but also to an increasingly complex process of development.

Many theorists have attempted to explain how personality develops. Most believe that early human experiences provide the framework for all future references. Development is usually divided into stages that correspond to a specific age-group. Developmental tasks are a part of the work of moving through each of these stages. In part, successful development depends on how individuals negotiate through each stage. Individual experiences influence how people respond to illness.

Infancy and early childhood are times when nurturing is critical and exploration of the world begins. As children grow and progress through school, they must learn the rules of society. Preschoolers must learn to handle joint decision making and interpersonal conflicts. Middle childhood is a time for learning to deal with frustration and unfavorable events while also learning to celebrate good things and feeling pleasure. During adolescence, teenagers learn to develop as individuals, become independent, and begin to think for themselves. They have to learn how to delay gratification, relax, and interact with peers of both sexes. In early adulthood, most people find a life partner and life work and may begin a family. Adults progressing through middle age begin to look at the impact their lives have had or could have. Older age is often a time of introspection, when older adults look back on their lives, accept what has been, and attempt to face increasing frailty with grace. Throughout life, individuals strive to make sense of the world by searching for meaning.

BEHAVIORAL THEORY

Behavioral theory is based on the idea that all behaviors are learned responses. Conditioning is one type of learning. An example of a conditioned response was demonstrated by Pavlov, who would ring a bell (stimulus) when feeding (reinforcement) his dog. The dog would salivate when the food was presented. The reflex response of salivation eventually occurred with the ringing of the bell only. Theorists such as B.F. Skinner, Albert Bandura, and Joseph Wolpe have based their theories on the idea that all behavior is learned and is a series of habitual responses to familiar stimuli.

PSYCHOLOGICAL RESPONSES TO ILLNESS

Responses to illness are as unique as patients themselves. Individual responses to illness are related to the individual's life experiences, self-concept, perceptions, values, cultural perspectives, and spiritual beliefs, to name a few.

COPING WITH ILLNESS

Most people see illness as a distressing, abnormal state of being. This state of distress demands that individuals draw from their inner resources to cope. These resources may come from any or all of the following dimensions: physical, cognitive, affective, behavioral, social, and spiritual. For some, the inner strengths drawn from these various dimensions may be sufficient to cope effectively with illness. For others, however, attempts to cope may be ineffective or maladaptive. This is where effective nursing intervention becomes essential.

A caring attitude is basic to helping a patient cope with illness. Through the trust developed in a therapeutic nurse-patient relationship, the nurse can help the patient cope with stressors precipitated by illness (see the Patient Teaching Plan at right).

To assess an individual's potential for coping with an illness effectively, you need to understand that the ability to cope is affected by various factors. Among these factors are age, cultural beliefs, spirituality, self-concept, family and community resources, emotions, stress, fear, anxiety, loss, grief, and mourning.

Factors That Affect Coping with Illness

Age. Age affects the coping ability of children and adults alike. The developmental process continues throughout the life span. Illness can interfere with developmental progress, and the patient's developmental stage can influence how he or she responds to illness. Much stress may be experienced when illness interferes with development. Illness can interfere with a number of adult roles. New or existing relationships, careers, family responsibilities, and a host of other roles may be affected by the onset of illness. An illness can be especially traumatic if a family breadwinner is self-employed or has insufficient health insurance.

There also are differences in the way people of different ages respond to illness. For example, young children who do not understand the gravity of an illness may not experience much stress as long as they feel well and are not separated from their parents. Among adults, it has been found that cancer patients who were younger than 50 years experienced more frequent and more severe psychological problems than those older than 70 years (Hymovich and Hagopian, 1992).

When collecting data about the patient's ability to cope with illness, you need to understand that illness is a stressful, disruptive experience regardless of age.

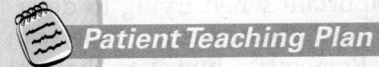

Patient Teaching Plan

Helping Patients and Their Families Cope with a Serious Diagnosis

Share with patients the following steps to help them deal effectively with the initial diagnosis and make the best possible decisions for themselves and their families:

- **Step 1: Take the time you need.** Do not rush important decisions about your health. In most cases, you will have time to carefully examine your options and decide what is best for you.
- **Step 2: Get the support you need.** Look for support from family and friends, people who are going through the same thing you are, and those who have "been there." They can help you cope with your situation and make informed decisions.
- **Step 3: Talk with members of your health care team.** Good communication with your health care team can help you feel more satisfied with the care you receive. Research shows it can even have a positive effect on things such as symptoms and pain. Getting a second opinion may help you feel more confident about your care.
- **Step 4: Seek out information.** When learning about your health problem and its treatment, look for information that is based on a careful review of the latest scientific findings published in medical journals. Be skeptical of websites and other sources that stand to make a profit by influencing your decision.
- **Step 5: Decide on a treatment plan.** Work with your physician and other members of the health care team to decide on a treatment plan that best meets your needs. Research shows that patients who are more involved in their health care tend to get better results and be more satisfied.

Adapted from Agency for Healthcare Research and Quality, Department of Health and Human Services. (July 2005). "Next steps after your diagnosis," www.ahrq.gov/consumer/ diaginfo.htm.

It not only disrupts the developmental process of the individual but also has a traumatic impact on spouses, children, and other loved ones. You will play an essential role in helping patients and their loved ones cope with an illness and the changes that result.

Cultural Beliefs. Culture is a system of symbols shared by a group of humans. Culture is transmitted from each generation to the next and is influenced by other social contexts as well. Culture brings organization and security to people's lives. It provides many of the underlying values and beliefs on which behavior is based. Culture can affect attitudes toward health and illness, diet and eating practices, reaction to pain, and values concerning death and dying. Ethnicity is a broader term that denotes a group's affiliation because of shared language, race, and cultural values.

For individuals to be seen as unique, their cultural and ethnic backgrounds must be considered. This becomes especially important when trying to determine whether patients need assistance in coping with the stresses of illness. Remember, however, that not all people who look as if they belong to a specific cultural or ethnic group because of language, surname, or physical characteristics necessarily identify with any specific group. Effective nursing interventions can be determined only when we understand the patient as a unique individual, not only as black or Latino, male or female, gay or straight.

When helping patients cope with illness, you need to recognize that your own racial and cultural background may affect your ability to intervene effectively. This is especially true if the patient's cultural values and your own values differ greatly. It is important to respect the patient, regardless of your own personal beliefs, values, and culture. A judgmental attitude on your part interferes with delivering the best nursing care possible.

In the nursing plan of care, you should consider whether the nursing approach being suggested is relevant to the patient's individual needs. Does the nursing care help patients deal with stress, or does it contribute to stress? Effective care is individualized according to the patient's needs, values, and beliefs.

What Does Culture Have to Do with Illness?

Culture shapes attitudes toward health and illness, nutrition, pain, and death and dying.

Spirituality. During the crisis of illness, patients often turn to their spiritual beliefs and values to find meaning in the experience. Patients who perhaps had not thought of themselves as being religious may suddenly have a need to visit with a spiritual counselor. Many patients experience spiritual distress when under the stress of an illness. They may feel that the illness is unfair and that God has betrayed and/or abandoned them. Sometimes people feel that the illness is a punishment from God for some transgression they believe they have made.

Spiritual distress can be characterized by the following: (1) patients question the meaning of suffering or existence; (2) patients experience a sense of conflict between their personal beliefs (or desires) and their relationship with their God; or (3) patients experience symptoms such as nightmares, sleep disturbances, and alterations in behavior and mood.

To determine whether spirituality is an asset or a liability to the patient's ability to cope with illness, you must understand that all individuals are experts about their own spiritual needs and paths. Patients need an opportunity to express their feelings in a therapeutic and nonjudgmental environment. Simply put, your role is to listen, support, and care. Effective therapeutic

nursing interventions enhance the healing process by supporting patients as they work through their spiritual distress and by shoring up their relationship with their spiritual connectedness.

Self-Concept. Self-concept refers to the notions, beliefs, and convictions persons hold about themselves. It is related to self-esteem and influences a person's relationship with others. Self-esteem develops from individuals' own evaluations of their competence and of the value others place on them. Body image refers to the combination of conscious and unconscious attitudes people have about their own bodies. Both past and present perceptions of the body and the person's feelings about their body's size, shape, function, appearance, and potential make up the body image.

Self-concept can be affected by changes in self-esteem as well as changes in body image. Patients' perception of these changes and their ability or inability to cope with the changes may result in stress, fear, and anxiety. Age and developmental levels may directly affect the patient's self-esteem and body image. Adolescents are especially vulnerable to changes in body image because they have a strong need to look like their peers. Certain changes in body image can be quite traumatic at this developmental stage. Adults also can be vulnerable.

People such as actors, models, or professional football players, who rely on their physical characteristics to make a living, may not be able to cope well with an illness or injury that affects body image. A disfiguring or disabling injury could have a devastating effect on body image and self-esteem. Their personal strengths and weaknesses would determine how well they are able to cope with the threat that illness imposes on the self-concept.

Some patients, through their life experiences, have developed coping styles that allow them to confront problems effectively. Others may require more external resources such as friends, family, and the community to cope with the stress of illness.

Family and Community Resources. The basic functions of the family include providing for physical needs, giving love, providing a sense of belonging, and strengthening the self-esteem of its members. Functional families may provide optimal support for a patient facing the stress of illness. However, the family's ability to provide support for the patient depends on many factors including the quality of relationships among family members and the family's ability to access needed resources.

Because of increasing stresses on the family unit, many families are not able to provide as much support as the patient may need. The stress of illness in a family member may overburden a family that was already only marginally coping. Illness may have precipitated such stressors as changes in family roles, economic pressures, and geographic isolation that may make it difficult to access medical and other needed resources.

Many of the functions once provided by families are increasingly being assumed by social institutions within the community. Like families, communities vary in their ability to assist their members. Some communities are well equipped to assist the family with many challenges that it may face (e.g., financial, physical, legal, spiritual, emotional). Other communities are less able to meet those same needs. This is especially true if the patient lives in an impoverished, underserved, and/or rural community. Your knowledge of available resources can be invaluable to patients and families. Throughout the hospital stay, you must anticipate the patient's needs before discharge. Providing contact information and creating links for patients in the community to help meet the needs of the patient outside the institution are essential parts of preparing the patient and his or her family for discharge. Local, state, and/or national organizations can be very helpful resources that may keep a family from succumbing to the pressures of a catastrophic illness.

Emotions. When a serious illness occurs, patients and their families must adapt to many changes. Some of these changes may involve permanent alterations in lifestyle, frequent visits to health care providers, frequent hospitalizations, financial problems, and increased social isolation. For those in crisis, coping can be difficult at best and seemingly impossible at worst.

This section discusses a broad range of feelings and emotions that people may experience. Many of these feelings are normal and to be anticipated. However, there are times when the coping methods being utilized by patients and families are maladaptive. It is important for you to differentiate adaptive from maladaptive coping mechanisms.

Stress. The term *stress* is derived from the Latin word *stringer*, which means "to draw tight." Stress is any physiologic or psychological tension that threatens a person's total equilibrium. Stress affects all dimensions of the individual. If prolonged or chronic, it poses a serious threat to physical and emotional health. As the duration or intensity of stress or the number of stressors increases, a person's ability to adapt effectively decreases.

Perceptions of stress and coping mechanisms are highly individualized. People subjected to prolonged stressors eventually became totally exhausted. Individuals who cannot cope adequately with stress may experience a threat to their emotional well-being. They may find their perceptions of reality skewed, their ability to solve problems considerably compromised, and their stress consequently increased. In other words, without effective coping strategies, individuals can be caught in a vicious cycle of ineffective coping and increased stress that will stop only at the point of total exhaustion and may result in death.

You must learn to recognize individuals whose coping skills are ineffective and who consequently are caught in a downward spiral of debilitating exhaustion. Without effective nursing interventions to reverse this downward spiral, serious impairment will result.

Fear. The words *fear* and *anxiety* often are used interchangeably. However, fear generally denotes a response to a specific threat, and anxiety is often a response to a nonspecific threat. The body's physiologic reaction to fear is similar to its response to anxiety. The person experiencing the crisis of illness has much to fear. There may be fear of pain, fear of financial ruin, fear of disfigurement, fear of the loss of self-esteem, and fear of not being able to return to a previous lifestyle.

Fears vary according to the developmental status and age of the individual. For example, toddlers may fear separation from their mothers, whereas adolescents may fear threats to their body image. Terminally ill patients may be struggling with fears of death and dying.

You can be very helpful in assisting patients and families to cope with fear. Sometimes just allowing an opportunity to express fear helps lessen the stress caused by fear. Providing information about tests or surgical procedures may empower clients to begin to cope with fear. However, too much information also can be very stressful. In deciding how much information to provide, you must assess the patient's current understanding of the situation and any anticipated procedures he or she may be about to face. Providing basic information and then following up by answering the patient's questions is usually best.

Anxiety. Anxiety is a vague and sometimes intense sense of impending doom or apprehension that may appear to have no clearly identifiable cause. Anxiety is often an early response to illness. The degree of anxiety may vary with the severity of the illness. Anxiety may lead to physical and psychological stress and may be caused by real or imagined fear resulting from loss. As people develop, they learn to cope with this painful emotion. The fight-or-flight response actually provides the physiologic ability for one to either fight or flee. Individuals continually regulate their behavior based on their level of perceived anxiety. When anxiety intensifies to an excessive level, the perception of reality becomes focused solely on the crisis.

Loss. Loss is an experience usually related to the involuntary separation of the self from someone or something loved or treasured. It may involve a separation from a person or object, relationship, personal attribute, hope, dream, desire, role, functional ability, or potential. Perceived loss of control, sense of worth, and loss of health are also types of loss.

Actual loss can be recognized by others as well as by the patients. Examples of actual loss include loss of a spouse or the loss of a limb. *Anticipatory loss* is a sense of loss experienced before the actual loss occurs. Families may experience anticipatory loss during the terminal stages of a loved one's illness.

Loss can be a significant stressor that precipitates feelings of fear and anxiety. The fears associated with loss can be stressful enough to compromise the ability of an individual to recover from illness. One of the first psychological steps that must be taken to begin the process of coping is to permit oneself to experience the full emotional impact of the loss. This emotional response is known as *grief* or *mourning.*

The experience of loss is related to the individual's self-concept. The extent of loss depends on how strongly the individual's sense of self was connected to that which was lost.

Grief and Mourning. Grief is the subjective, emotional response that evolves from a sense of loss. Mourning is the process through which grief is faced and ultimately resolved or altered over time. Mourning occurs when a person is forced to relinquish original hopes. The process of mourning prepares the individual to reappraise values and to accept substitutions for hope.

Individuals experiencing grief may be under a great deal of stress, and stress may make them even more vulnerable to disease. They may become irritable and difficult to get along with. Sometimes they may experience a sense of guilt. Some people blame themselves for whatever they have lost. They may perceive their illness and subsequent loss as a punishment from God for not having been a better person, a better parent, or a better spouse.

To alter the loss that grief causes, the self must change. The process of change is unique to each individual and each circumstance. One individual's need for change may require only a change in exercise and dietary habits. Another person's need for change may encompass a career, a lifestyle, or the development of better strategies to cope with stress. Most changes in a person's life are stressful. The greater the change, the greater the resulting stress. To cope with stress, the individual may mobilize psychological resources known as *coping mechanisms.* Adaptive coping mechanisms can be effective, therapeutic ways of dealing with stress. Maladaptive coping behaviors, however, can be detrimental and decrease the ability to cope with illness. Care of the patient who has suffered a loss is detailed in Chapter 24.

COPING MECHANISMS AND STRATEGIES

Coping is the process of responding to stress or a potential stressor. Coping with stress is a self-regulatory process by which people manage their responses to stress and thus relieve the tension related to the stressor. Coping strategies can be conscious or unconscious behaviors. Unconscious coping strategies are referred to as defense mechanisms.

Defense Mechanisms

According to Freud, the ego may devise strategies or defense mechanisms to cope with stress or anxiety. Defense mechanisms are used in an effort to diminish anxiety; however, when used excessively or inappropriately, they can hinder the developing personality. Defense mechanisms used to protect against anxiety include the following:

- *Compensation*—an attempt to make up for real or imagined weakness. For example, an adolescent perceived as unattractive becomes an outstanding athlete.
- *Denial*—a refusal to acknowledge a real situation. For example, a woman who finds a suspicious lump in her breast does not keep an appointment for a breast biopsy.
- *Displacement*—transferring the feelings associated from one source to another that is considered less threatening. For example, a boy who is angry with a teacher comes home and yells at his dog.
- *Identification*—the emulation of admirable qualities in another to enhance one's self-esteem. For example, a child dresses and uses mannerisms similar to those of a famous rock star.
- *Rationalization* or *intellectualization*—the use of logic, reasoning, and analysis to avoid unacceptable feelings. For example, a student fails to complete an assignment correctly and rationalizes subsequent feelings of incompetence by complaining about the teacher's expectations for the assignment.
- *Introjection*—internalizing or taking on the values and beliefs of another person. For example, a child takes on the values and beliefs of a parent.
- *Isolation*—the separation of emotion from an associated thought or memory. For example, a man appears apathetic as he discusses a fire fight in which he participated in Vietnam.
- *Projection*—transferring unacceptable feelings or impulses to another. For example, a partner who is jealous of her significant other accuses the partner of being jealous.
- *Reaction formation*—avoiding unacceptable thoughts and behaviors by expressing opposing thoughts or behaviors. For example, a patient who unconsciously hates his father continuously tells how great his father is.
- *Regression*—withdrawing to an earlier level of development to benefit from the associated comfort levels of the previous level. For example, a child starts sucking her thumb when her new baby brother comes home from the hospital.
- *Repression*—an unconscious defense mechanism in which unacceptable ideas, impulses, and memories are kept out of consciousness. For example, a woman cannot remember a sexual assault.
- *Somatization*—the transfer of painful feelings to body parts, thus the person's feelings are expressed in the form of a physical symptom. For example, a woman who has experienced intolerable internal conflict develops a physical complaint of pain in the wrist that cannot be explained by diagnostic means.

- *Sublimation*—the transformation of unacceptable impulses or drives (e.g., aggressiveness, anger, sexuality) into constructive or more acceptable behavior. For example, a person who has aggressive tendencies becomes a jackhammer operator.
- *Suppression*—(a conscious mechanism) a conscious or voluntary inhibition of unacceptable ideas, impulses, and memories. For example, a child who fails an algebra class puts that event out of his or her mind.
- *Undoing*—actually or symbolically attempting to cancel out an action that was unacceptable. An example is sprinkling salt over one's left shoulder to prevent bad luck after spilling salt on the table.
- *Substitution*—replacing a highly valued, unattainable object with a less-valued, attainable object. For example, the person who has a strong unconscious sexual attraction to a parent marries someone who resembles that parent.
- *Conversion*—turning an emotional conflict into a physical symptom, which provides the individual with some sort of benefit (secondary gain). For example, the individual who witnesses a murder then experiences sudden blindness without an organic cause.

Defense mechanisms are adapted by the individual as protective measures to allow the ego relief from anxiety. One factor that enhances the development of ego is an environment with experiences that match the child's capacity to adapt. Ideally, unhealthy defense mechanisms are shed and replaced by more realistic and efficient methods of adaptation as the individual matures.

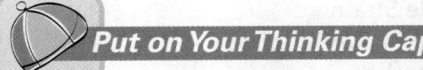
Put on Your Thinking Cap!

Recall two incidents when you recognized a defense mechanism being used to cope. Describe the behavior, label the mechanism, and indicate the positive and negative outcomes of the mechanism. Share and discuss with your classmates.

Conscious Coping Strategies

Conscious coping strategies are purposeful behaviors that are used to make an unfamiliar situation into one that is perceived as more controllable and predictable. Coping strategies and mechanisms vary from individual to individual. What all these behaviors have in common is that they are attempts to help people feel less stressed and anxious about their illness. Some of these methods provide only temporary relief, whereas others provide more permanent results. It is important for you to identify and evaluate the effectiveness of coping mechanisms used by the patient.

Some techniques that can be used to help patients cope are known as *relaxation techniques*. Relaxation techniques include interventions such as imagery, relaxation strategies, therapeutic touch, and music therapy. Relaxation techniques elicit the relaxation response that reduces the effects of stress and decreases anxiety. These techniques can provide clients with self-control during moments of stress. Relaxation techniques are taught only when patients are not in acute discomfort, because the exercise will be ineffective if the patient cannot concentrate. *Imagery* is the use of the imagination to develop sensory images that focus the mind away from the stressful experience and emphasize other sensory experiences and pleasant memories. *Relaxation strategies* include biofeedback, meditation, deep-breathing exercises, yoga, and Zen practices. *Therapeutic touch* is a process by which the therapist acts as a channel for environmental and universal energy through the therapist's mental concentration.

Music therapy is another relaxation technique that may help the patient cope by enhancing the relaxation response and facilitating positive imagery. Musical selections should match a patient's mood and musical taste. Earphones with audio CDs or cassettes help the patient avoid annoying others and allow concentration on the music. This coping method provides only temporary relief of stress; however, use of such techniques can help establish a therapeutic environment in which you can begin to discuss the real sources of the patient's concerns, fears, and anxieties.

Tapping into the spiritual dimension also can be a very effective way of coping with the stress of illness. You can talk with patients about their spiritual needs without relying on traditional religious language. The opportunity to discuss beliefs about a higher power or the search for meaning in suffering proves to be an effective way of coping for many patients.

MALADAPTIVE COPING MECHANISMS AND STRATEGIES

In an effort to reduce the stress and anxiety that is precipitated by the crisis of an illness, an individual may sometimes engage in thinking patterns or behaviors that are ineffective or even self-destructive. These ineffective coping mechanisms may evolve from a sense of helplessness or powerlessness.

Helplessness

Helplessness typically occurs when individuals have had repeated exposure to events they perceive as being uncontrollable. This leads to loss of motivation, feelings of despair or anxiety, and cognitive impairment. The individual may begin to express anger as a means of diminishing feelings of helplessness. This anger may take the form of a personal attack on you and other caregivers. The expression of anger is really not aimed at you but is simply an attempt to cope with feelings of loss of control. Helplessness can be prevented by allowing individuals to control as many events as possible within the constraints imposed by treatment and their energy level.

Powerlessness

Powerlessness is a feeling that one's actions cannot affect an outcome or that one lacks personal control over certain events or situations. Characteristics of powerlessness include (1) passivity; (2) nonparticipation in care and decision making; (3) dependence on others, which may lead to anger, resentment, or guilt; and (4) verbal expression of loss of control over situations or outcomes (Miller, 1992).

When people are not ready to cope with the threat of illness, unconscious defense mechanisms of avoidance, such as denial, may be used. These avoidance defense mechanisms protect individuals from having to confront and deal with the threat of illness.

Denial

Denial is the subconscious blocking out of emotional experiences. Denial can take several forms: (1) verbal denial, (2) minimizing the severity of the illness, (3) displacing symptoms onto another organ system, and (4) engaging in behaviors contrary to medical advice. The outcome of denial may be positive or negative. Denial can lead to negative consequences if people fail to engage in appropriate problem-focused behaviors. Patients who claim that they were never afraid or insist that there is nothing wrong with them are engaging in denial. Denial is maladaptive when the patient's behavior interferes significantly with obtaining appropriate care. Arguing with patients about their denial only reinforces the inappropriate behavior.

When working with people in denial, make a special effort to accept them even though it may be uncomfortable to care for individuals who deny their illnesses. You may need to allow the individual to deny the illness and at the same time ask for cooperation. Once an effective therapeutic nurse-patient relationship has been established, patients may be better able to lower unconscious defenses and begin to discuss true feelings of fear and anxiety.

THE NURSING PROCESS IN ILLNESS

In this section, the various steps of the nursing process are discussed to help you collect relevant data and help to plan nursing interventions that will facilitate the patient's task of dealing with the crisis of illness.

ASSESSMENT

An individual's ability to cope with an illness varies from moment to moment and from situation to situation. Therefore assessment must be an ongoing process. To determine the effectiveness of individual coping strategies, seek answers to the following questions:

- Do individuals see themselves as effective in coping with their illness?
- What efforts have individuals made to seek information about their situation?
- How skillful are individuals in caring for themselves?
- What resources do individuals believe are available to them in dealing with their illness?
- Do individuals effectively adhere to their medical regimen?
- Do individuals feel they have been able to keep a sense of normalcy in their life despite their illness?
- How have individuals and their families been able to cope with any role modification that the illness has brought about?
- Have individuals been able to maintain a sense of hope in spite of the demands of the illness?
- Do individuals feel that the important relationships in their life remain intact?

Data collected by the LPN/LVN can help answer these questions. After problem areas have been identified, meaningful nursing diagnoses can be formulated.

NURSING DIAGNOSIS

The purpose of a nursing diagnosis is to clearly identify and frame patient problems. The nursing diagnosis leads to the formulation of a plan of care that includes nursing interventions to help patients achieve their desired goals. Patients and their families must be included in the process so that nursing care plans are based on patients' values and perceptions of the problems. The following are a few nursing diagnoses often identified in persons with inadequate coping:

- Anxiety
- Caregiver Role Strain
- Compromised Family Coping
- Decisional Conflict
- Defensive Coping
- Delayed Growth and Development
- Disturbed Body Image
- Disturbed Personal Identity
- Disturbed Sleep Pattern
- Fatigue
- Fear
- Grieving
- Impaired Adjustment
- Ineffective Coping
- Ineffective Denial
- Ineffective Role Performance
- Ineffective Sexuality Pattern
- Interrupted Family Processes
- Powerlessness
- Risk for Loneliness
- Sexual Dysfunction
- Situational Low Self-Esteem
- Social Isolation
- Spiritual Distress

These serve only as examples of nursing diagnoses that could be identified for patients and their families. Appropriate nursing diagnoses follow a careful nursing assessment and are formulated once the patient and the family have had a chance to contribute by sharing their perception of the problem(s). Patients or family members need to agree that the identified problems are important ones if effective coping is to take place. This is especially true if a patient has a long-term or chronic illness.

NURSING GOALS, OUTCOME CRITERIA, AND INTERVENTIONS

The goal of nursing care is to help people manage and successfully cope with their illness. When effective coping strategies are used, patients can manage their illness and adapt to a new lifestyle that incorporates healthy behaviors and realistic goals. In addition, patients should emerge from the process with a positive self-concept and self-esteem.

People with chronic, debilitating illnesses may have difficulty acquiring and maintaining coping skills for long periods of time. Individuals may be able to cope with their illness today, but tomorrow may bring a whole new set of challenges. This is especially true in terminal stages of illness, when physical deterioration is on an accelerated course and every day brings new losses that need to be mourned and coped with.

Nursing interventions are based on identified nursing diagnoses. Box 54-1 provides a sample nursing care plan for a patient who is ineffectively coping with illness.

Box 54-1 | *A Sample Nursing Care Plan for a Patient Ineffectively Coping with Illness*

Nursing Diagnosis
Ineffective Coping related to feelings of powerlessness, as evidenced by patient's verbalization "I don't know if I can live through this."

Goal and Outcome Criteria
Patient will demonstrate more effective coping, as evidenced by verbalization that he or she feels more capable of dealing with the demands of the illness.

Interventions
1. Give patient an opportunity to verbalize feelings of powerlessness by approaching patient care in an unhurried manner.
2. Determine the patient's and family's current coping strategies and behaviors.
3. Conduct teaching sessions with the patient and family to enhance their coping skills and empower the patient to begin self-care.
4. Provide community resource information, and encourage the patient to ask for help from others.
5. Implement stress reduction strategies (e.g., music therapy) to help patient cope with stressful moments.

Key Points

- Individuals' level of health is directly related to their ability to adjust to a variety of internal and external stressors.
- Stress is necessary for growth and development.
- A stressor is anything that causes the individual stress, and adaptation to stress affects the entire organism.
- Illness or crisis may ensue if individuals are overwhelmed by many stressors or do not have the coping behaviors or problem-solving strategies necessary to maintain equilibrium.
- A crisis is the point at which the individual may move toward illness on the continuum between illness and health and can result in inner tension and anxiety, which may affect an individual's ability to function.
- Growth refers to a process of development that becomes increasingly complex.
- Anxiety is a painful emotion that results from one's perception of danger, and individuals continually regulate their behavior based on the level of perceived anxiety.
- Defense mechanisms are strategies used in an effort to diminish anxiety; however, when unconscious defense mechanisms are used excessively, they can hinder the developing personality.
- Behavioral theory is based on the idea that all behavior is a learned response.
- Each person's response to illness is unique and is based on such subjective experiences as self-concept, perception of threat to body image, and spiritual and cultural values.
- Illness produces a stressful state that requires individuals to draw on their innate resources or inner strengths.
- Some people have enough inner strength to cope effectively with illness; others, however, may have ineffective or maladaptive coping abilities.
- Factors that influence an individual's ability to cope with illness are age, cultural beliefs, spirituality, self-concept, family and community resources, and emotional responses to illness.
- Specific emotional responses to illness include stress, fear, anxiety, loss, and grief and mourning.
- Coping is the process of responding to stress or a potential stressor.
- Coping strategies are conscious, purposeful behaviors that are used to make an unfamiliar situation into one that is perceived as more controllable and predictable.
- Ineffective coping mechanisms may evolve from a sense of helplessness or powerlessness.
- A nurse's caring and nonjudgmental attitude is basic to helping a client cope with illness.

 Go to your Companion CD-ROM for a Pharmacology Tutorial, Audio Glossary, and 3-D animations.

evolve Be sure to visit the companion Evolve site at http://evolve.elsevier.com/Linton/ for WebLinks and additional online resources.

REVIEW QUESTIONS *Choose the best answer.*

1. The statement "Sometimes I feel so overwhelmed and sad" reflects which dimension of a human being?
   1. Cognitive
   2. Affective
   3. Behavioral
   4. Social

2. Which option best describes stress?
   1. Anything that requires the individual to adapt
   2. A negative or harmful experience
   3. A barrier to growth and development
   4. An emotional response to an unpleasant event

3. A developmental task of old age is to:
   1. Learn how to delay gratification
   2. Find a life partner and life work
   3. Become independent
   4. Accept what has been

4. The primary difference between fear and anxiety is that anxiety:
   1. Is much more disabling than fear
   2. Indicates that the patient has poor coping skills
   3. Interferes with effective problem solving more than fear
   4. Is evoked by a nonspecific threat rather than a specific threat

5. Which statement suggests that the patient is experiencing spiritual distress?
   1. "The medication that you gave me is not relieving my pain."
   2. "I think my cancer is punishment for the bad things I have done."
   3. "I will never be able to perform again with these terrible scars."
   4. "My family is too busy to come see me and do things for me."

6. Which data best support a nursing diagnosis of "Disturbed Body Image"?
   1. Patient states he is just glad to be alive despite some paralysis.
   2. Although burns have healed well, patient refuses to go out in public.
   3. Patient dresses every morning, brushes her hair, and applies makeup.
   4. During dressing change, patient carefully examines her incision.

7. The basic function of defense mechanisms is to:
   1. Enhance self-esteem
   2. Avoid reality
   3. Disguise true feelings
   4. Reduce anxiety

8. A 9-year-old girl likes to wear her 14-year-old sister's nail polish and tries to fix her hair like the older sister. This is an example of:
   1. Regression
   2. Introjection
   3. Identification
   4. Projection

9. The benefits of relaxation strategies include decreased anxiety and:
   1. Reduced stress
   2. Improved muscle tone
   3. Increased alertness
   4. Enhanced sensation

10. Mrs. A has been in a long-term care facility for 6 months. She has given up participation in group activities, rarely leaves her room, and is fretful and irritable. Her behavior is characteristic of:
    1. Denial
    2. Isolation
    3. Helplessness
    4. Regression

55 Psychiatric Disorders

MARK D. SOUCY

evolve   http://evolve.elsevier.com/Linton/

Objectives

After reading and studying this chapter, you should be able to:

1. Describe the differences between social relationships and therapeutic relationships.
2. Describe key strategies in communicating therapeutically.
3. Describe the components of the mental status examination.
4. Identify target symptoms, behaviors, and potential side effects for the following types of medications: anti-anxiety (anxiolytic), antipsychotic, and antidepressant drugs.
5. Summarize current thinking about the etiology of schizophrenia and the mood disorders.
6. Identify key features of the mental status examination and their relevance in anxiety disorders, schizophrenia, mood disorders, cognitive disorders, and personality disorders.
7. Identify common nursing diagnoses, goals, and interventions for persons with anxiety disorders, schizophrenia, mood disorders, cognitive disorders, and personality disorders.

Key Terms

Be sure to check out the bonus material on the Companion CD-ROM, including selected audio pronunciations.

biologic approach (bī-ō-LŌJ-ĭk, p. 1245)
denial (dē-NĪ-ăl, p. 1245)
depersonalization (dē-PĔR-sŭn-ŭl-ĭ-ZĀ-shŭn, p. 1251)
extrapyramidal side effects (EPS) (ĕks-tră-pī-RĂM-ĭ-dăl, p. 1253)
interpersonal approach (p. 1246)
parkinsonian syndrome (SĬN-drōm, p. 1253)
projection (p. 1245)
psychoanalytic approach (sī-kō-ăn-ă-LĬT-ĭk, p. 1245)
psychosis (sī-KŌ-sĭs, p. 1252)
sensorium (sĕn-SŌ-rē-ŭm, p. 1249)
tardive dyskinesia (TĂR-dĭv dĭs-kĭ-NĒ-zē-ă, p. 1253)

How people think about and explain mental health and mental illness has varied from one geographic location and culture to another and from one time period to another. In early cultures, people believed that supernatural forces were responsible for mental illness. People used rituals to appeal to these supernatural forces to cure mental illnesses. It is now understood that many factors contribute to the development of a mental illness and many strategies are available for helping people with psychiatric disorders. Treatment settings include outpatient, intensive outpatient, partial hospitalization, and inpatient hospitalization as well as residential settings. Within these settings, treatment methods include milieu therapy, individual therapy, group or family therapy, psychoeducational groups, and treatment with medications. With the advent of new medications, treatment is handled primarily on an outpatient basis. Nursing interventions are diverse and geared toward helping patients and families cope with the mental illness, manage their lives, and enhance quality of life. Mental illness and mental health exist along a continuum. People experiencing a psychiatric disorder may present with acute symptoms and require hospitalization. Others may have chronic and persistent mental illnesses. Therefore nursing interventions are delivered in many settings, including the hospital and the community.

Nurses who work with patients in other health care settings such as medical clinics, medical and surgical inpatient units, or intensive care units also see patients who have psychiatric difficulties along with their other health problems. Therefore the ability to provide quality nursing care to patients with mental illness in any work setting is important.

Nursing interventions are based on a number of theoretical approaches, which are described according to biologic, psychoanalytic, interpersonal, cognitive-behavioral, and other theories.

The biologic approach assumes that mental disorders are related to physiologic changes within the central nervous system. In this approach, mental illness is managed with medications, much as any other acute or chronic illness—such as diabetes—is managed. The biologic approach dominates much of the current thinking about psychiatric disorders.

The psychoanalytic approach is based on the theory that (1) humans function at different levels of awareness, ranging from conscious to unconscious; and (2) people use ego defense mechanisms to prevent anxiety. Some important defense mechanisms are repression, denial, and projection.

The **interpersonal approach** has three components: (1) anxiety is often communicated interpersonally; (2) the patient learns new ways of coping or maturing in a therapeutic relationship; and (3) the establishment of trust is an important first step in working with patients.

Key ideas from the cognitive-behavioral approach are (1) behavior is learned, (2) behavior increases as a result of a response to that behavior from the environment (reinforcement), and (3) the way a person thinks about things (their thoughts) influences emotional states and behavior.

 Put on Your Thinking Cap!

Four patients are receiving different treatments for mental illness. An aspect of each type of treatment is listed below. Can you identify the theoretical approach behind each of them?
1. A patient is helped to develop new coping skills through a therapeutic relationship.
2. A patient is guided to recall events that could be related to her present illness.
3. A patient is helped to understand the consequences of his behavioral patterns.
4. A patient is prescribed an antianxiety (anxiolytic) drug.

ESTABLISHING THERAPEUTIC RELATIONSHIPS

In caring for a patient with a psychiatric disorder, you must first establish a therapeutic (rather than a social) relationship (Table 55-1). A range of interpersonal strategies have been found to be particularly helpful in promoting the patient's level of comfort with the nurse. They include being available, listening, clarifying, sharing observations, and accepting silence. Therapeutic use of self is key to providing good care to patients with psychiatric illness, avoids advice giving, and assists patients at their level of comprehension.

BEING AVAILABLE

When you are working with a patient, direct all your attention completely toward that person. Avoid involvement in any other activity, such as reading a newspaper or watching television, which might be interpreted by the patient as lack of availability. Avoid interruptions in your conversation with the patient as much as possible.

LISTENING

Use empathy when you are listening to the patient. Concentrate on what the patient is saying, and remember that you are trying to hear how he or she experiences and describes his or her life. When listening therapeutically, make every effort to avoid cutting the patient off or jumping to conclusions. You are trying to get the essence of how the patient perceives his or her situation, experiences certain symptoms, and describes his or her circumstances.

To listen well, you must be aware of your own thoughts and feelings. These feelings are an important source of data for you because you may experience a wide range of feelings while interacting with patients. If you are aware of your own feelings, you will be able to manage your physical (body language) and verbal responses. Listening is done by concentrating on the patient and by refraining from thinking of responses while the patient is speaking.

CLARIFYING

Clarifying is one way of validating that you understand what the patient is saying. For example, you might ask, "So what you are saying is that you are feeling very sad right now?" Asking questions may also help patients clarify their thoughts. For example, if a patient says, "I have problems at home," you might ask, "What is happening at home that is troubling you?" If a patient states, "My world is falling apart," you might say, "Tell me more about what you mean when you say 'My world is falling apart.'" It is helpful to avoid the word "why" when asking questions. For example, instead of "Why do you feel that way?," try "How did you come to feel that way?"

SHARING OBSERVATIONS

Patients benefit from knowing what you see and hear while listening. For example, you might say, "You are saying that your life is falling apart, and I notice that

Table 55-1 *Therapeutic Relationships Versus Social Relationships*

THERAPEUTIC	SOCIAL
1. Purpose is to benefit the patient.	1. Purpose is to benefit both participants in the relationship.
2. Relationship develops purposefully.	2. Relationship develops spontaneously.
3. Focus is on personal and emotional needs of patient.	3. Focus is on personal and emotional needs of both participants.
4. Helper has responsibility for evaluating the interaction and the changing behavior.	4. Participants are not formally responsible for evaluating their interaction.
5. Relationship has some boundaries (purpose, place, time) and a clear ending.	5. Relationship may or may not have clear boundaries and a clear ending.

you are fidgeting and tapping your foot. It looks like this is really difficult for you." This statement provides the patient with input that he or she is heard and that you are really listening.

ACCEPTING SILENCE

Sometimes it is therapeutic to allow moments of silence between you and the patient. This is called *therapeutic silence*. It is important that you feel comfortable with silence, since silence enables patients to consider their own thoughts as well as what you are communicating to them. Although it may feel strange at first, silences allow patients to sort through their feelings and organize their thinking.

NURSING ASSESSMENT OF THE PSYCHIATRIC PATIENT

The nursing assessment of a patient with mental illness provides the foundation for nursing diagnoses and development of the plan of care. The observations of the LPN/LVN contribute important data to the assessment. In addition to the usual data for the physical assessment, you will want to understand what brings the patient to the care setting where you are practicing. This is often called the *chief complaint*. Ask the patient to tell you what has been happening recently that has caused him or her to seek treatment. After the patient has explained factors leading to seeking treatment, inquire about the person's past psychiatric history. This is done by asking the patient if they have ever felt like this before. You should also ask if the patient has been treated in the past for anxiety, depression, or other mental health problems. This information adds to the nursing assessment and will assist in developing the proper plan of care.

Another major feature of a complete health assessment of a psychiatric patient is the mental status examination. This examination is usually conducted as part of the admission process and is an ongoing assessment

tool throughout the course of treatment. It consists of observations regarding appearance, activity, mood and affect, speech and language, thought content, perceptual disturbances, insight and judgment, sensorium, memory, attention, and general intellectual level. Each of these components is evaluated by collecting the data detailed in Table 55-2.

Nursing diagnoses commonly identified in persons with major psychiatric disorders are derived from the health assessment. A partial list of these diagnoses is presented. Etiologies and/or related factors for each diagnosis are quite specific depending on the individual and his or her unique presentation. Therefore you should consult a text specific to nursing diagnoses common to psychiatric and mental health nursing.

 Consider the Alternative

Be aware of any herbal supplements the patient is taking. Some can interact with drugs used for mental illness.

MENTAL STATUS EXAMINATION

Appearance

The first step in a mental status examination is to observe how a person looks. Specific data include the following:

- Appearance in relation to stated age (does the patient look his or her stated age?)
- Appropriateness of clothing in relation to patient's particular peer group or subculture
- Personal grooming and hygiene
- Unique physical characteristics
- Motor activity

Note any recent change in the patient's activity level (increase or decrease). Other types of activity that are observed include the following:

- Hyperactivity or activity at a level considerably above average purposeful activity

---

| Table 55-2 | *Components of the Mental Status Examination* |

COMPONENT	RELEVANT DATA
Appearance	Age, clothing, personal hygiene, unusual physical characteristics
Activity	Recent change in activity level, hyperactivity, agitation, psychomotor retardation, repetitive mannerisms, stereotypes
Mood and affect	Happiness, sadness, worry; constricted or expanded feelings; intensity; lability; appropriateness
Speech and language	Mutism, paucity, pressured speech, tangential speech, blocking, loose associations, word salad
Thought content	Obsessions, compulsions, phobias, delusions
Perceptual disturbances	Illusions, hallucinations
Insight and judgment	Potential for suicide
Sensorium	Orientation to time, place, person; level of consciousness
Memory and attention	Remote and recent memory; attention; calculation
General intellectual level	Vocabulary; knowledge of current events; abstract thinking

- Agitation or purposeless activity, such as wringing of hands, pacing, picking at clothing, foot tapping
- Psychomotor retardation or a decrease in movement; slowness; delayed actions, thoughts, and speech
- Repetitive movements that are part of a purposeful activity (mannerisms)
- Repetitive movements that are not part of purposeful activity (stereotypy)

Mood and Affect

Mood is a sustained feeling state or emotion that a person experiences in several aspects of life. Mood is assessed in terms of its intensity, depth, duration, and fluctuation. Words that often are used to describe mood include *irritable, anxious, depressed, euphoric, labile* (up and down), and *despairing.*

Affect describes a person's external presentation of a feeling state and emotional responsiveness. Affect ranges from blunted, flat, and constricted to euphoric, expansive, and intense. A normal affect exists when the person's body language, mannerisms, and verbal responses are consistent with the person's mood and within an average range of emotional intensity. Affect is also described according to its appropriateness and congruence. Appropriate affect exists when the person's outward emotional expression matches what he or she is saying or doing. For example, a patient who is discussing sadness and despair may be tearful and look sad. An example of an inappropriate affect is when someone is telling you that they are sad and feeling guilty about something that happened but at the same time are smiling, laughing, and very animated. In the latter example, the affect is considered incongruent with mood.

The intensity of feelings may be increased or decreased (diminished). Feelings also may be stable or consistent rather than labile or rapidly changing.

Speech and Language

Assessment includes characteristics of speech and language. Normally, speech is of appropriate rate, rhythm, and volume. Unusual findings in the assessment of speech include mutism (not speaking), long pauses before responding, minimal or very little speech (paucity), and pressured speech (loud and insistent). Some clues to problems of thought are evidenced in a person's speech, which is described in the following section.

Thought Content

Tangential speech may be noted, which means that a patient starts out toward a particular point but veers away and never reaches the point. Tangential speech is commonly an indicator of disorganized thinking. When the person stops speaking before reaching the point, it is called *thought blocking.* Loose associations—continual shifting from topic to topic—and shifting between topics to the point of incoherence ("word salad") may also be noted. Tangentiality, thought blocking, looseness of associations, and "word salad" are all noteworthy findings that are related to thought content in speech. Further assessment of thought content includes identifying the following:

- Obsessions—repetitious, unwanted thoughts
- Compulsions—actions repeatedly carried out in a specific manner; they typically include washing, counting, or checking
- Phobias—unrealistic fears of specific objects or situations
- Delusions—false ideas not based on reality and not congruent with the patient's specific religious and cultural orientation
- Suicidal ideations—thoughts and/or plans of killing oneself
- Obsessions and compulsions are often closely related.

This area must be assessed with clear and direct questions such as asking, "Do you have any thoughts of harming yourself or killing yourself?" Further assessment includes determining whether the patient has constructed any plans to hurt himself or herself. If the patient endorses suicidal ideations, you must ask whether the patient has made any plans to do so. If so, ask him or her to describe the plans. This information is useful in assessing the lethality of the plans. Another part of the assessment includes determining whether the patient has any means available to carry out a suicide plan. For example, if a patient has planned to shoot himself or herself, is a gun available at home? If the patient has thoughts of overdosing on medication, does the patient have available supplies of medications?

Perceptual Disturbances

Perceptual disturbances may involve any one of the senses such as vision, hearing, taste, touch, and smell. One type of perceptual disturbance is an illusion, in which a specific stimulus, such as a spot on the wall, is misinterpreted (e.g., a spot is perceived as a bug). Another is hallucination, which is a sensory experience that occurs without an external stimulus (e.g., a person sees nonexistent bugs crawling on the floor or feels nonexistent bugs crawling on the skin). Sometimes this is referred to as *internal stimuli.* Evidence of this may include a person sitting alone, talking as if someone were present, or looking around as if someone is talking to or calling the patient.

Insight and Judgment

Insight is the ability of a person to understand the correct cause or meaning of a situation, and judgment is the ability to assess a situation accurately and determine the appropriate course of action. Insight and judgment are often considered in relation to suicide potential.

Sensorium

Data collection related to sensorium focuses on orientation in terms of time, place, person, and self. These data are obtained by asking the patient direct questions (e.g., "What time is it now?"; "What day is today?"; "Where are we now?"; or "Tell me your name"). The patient's level of consciousness also is noted. The four levels of consciousness are (1) comatose; (2) stuporous; (3) drowsy; and (4) alert.

Memory and Attention

Remote memory (distant past) is assessed by comparing the patient's memory of past events with what is recalled by other reliable historians. If you are collecting data related to recent memory, or the ability to recall new information, ask the patient to learn three unrelated words and to recall these words 5 minutes later. A quick way to determine recent memory is to ask what was eaten at the previous meal. Asking the patient to subtract 7's from 100 or 3's from 20 or to spell a word like "world" backwards can test attention as well as ability to calculate (as an aspect of general intellectual level).

General Intellectual Level

General intellectual level is estimated by determining the patient's vocabulary and knowledge of current events. For example, ask the patient to name the president of the United States and the name of the previous president. Abstract thinking is another area of general intellectual level. Data that provide evidence of the intellectual level can be collected by asking the patient to identify the common element of two objects such as a banana and an apple (e.g., "What do a banana and an apple have in common?") or asking the patient to interpret proverbs (e.g., "What does the phrase *a rolling stone gathers no moss* mean?").

TYPES OF PSYCHIATRIC DISORDERS

ANXIETY DISORDERS

A patient with an anxiety disorder either directly experiences the highly uncomfortable feeling of anxiety or experiences a symptom like compulsive hand washing that prevents or reduces the occurrence of anxiety. Common physical signs and symptoms of anxiety are increased heart rate, elevated blood pressure, sweaty palms, trembling, urinary frequency, diarrhea, a tight sensation in the chest, and difficulty breathing. Psychological manifestations often include irritability, restlessness, tearfulness, thought blocking, and lack of concentration.

Anxiety is experienced on various levels, ranging from mild to panic stages, depending on each person's subjective experience and ability to cope. Mild anxiety can be useful. It may motivate a person to take constructive action or focus attention on a particular task (e.g., concentrating on an examination). Moderate anxiety often is considered the optimal level for learning to take place. As anxiety progresses to severe or panic levels, however, an individual's ability to think clearly and to solve problems becomes progressively impaired. A person in a panic state may misperceive surrounding events altogether and may react impulsively by running or striking out. This may explain instances in which individuals jump from burning buildings despite imminent rescue.

All people experience anxiety. For most people, it is episodic and does not interfere greatly with day-to-day functioning. Even normally well-adjusted people can experience anxiety of panic proportions under significant stress. If anxiety persists at a high level for an extended period and causes significant interference with daily functioning, the person usually is determined to have an anxiety disorder. Examples of anxiety disorders are panic disorder, agoraphobia, obsessive-compulsive disorder, and post-traumatic stress disorder.

Panic Disorder

In panic disorder, the person experiences recurrent panic attacks, which are episodes of intense apprehension. Panic attacks vary in length, may progress to the point of terror, and are often accompanied by feelings of impending doom. Often no triggering event can be identified. Physical symptoms of severe anxiety, such as increased pulse, elevated blood pressure, trembling, diaphoresis, shortness of breath, chest pain, and nausea, also are present. This disorder tends to run in families.

Agoraphobia

The person with agoraphobia is extremely fearful of situations outside the home. This often includes fearfulness that the person may be in a place from which quick escape would be difficult (e.g., a grocery store) or a place where help may be unavailable. The person typically copes by avoiding the anxiety-producing place or situation, often becoming progressively reclusive and very dependent on family and friends. Agoraphobia may occur by itself or together with panic disorder.

Obsessive-Compulsive Disorder

Obsessive-compulsive disorder (OCD) consists of recurrent obsessions (thoughts) or compulsions (behaviors), or both, that produce distress, are time-consuming, and interfere with functioning. Obsessions frequently involve intrusive thoughts about unpleasant or even violent acts that a person cannot stop. For example, a person may be obsessed with the idea of being dirty and needing to wash. Compulsive behaviors typically evolve as a way to reduce the anxiety experienced as a result of obsessive thoughts. Examples of compulsions are hand washing, counting, and checking (e.g., repeated checking to see whether the door is locked). The person experiencing obsessions and compulsions knows these thoughts and behaviors are not "normal" and often is embarrassed by them. However, if the compulsion is resisted, the internal anxiety may become too overwhelming to handle.

Research has found that neurophysiology plays a role in the origin of this disorder. Some studies have shown that there are changes in electroencephalography (EEG) findings in people with OCD. Many people with obsessive-compulsive disorders have considerably reduced their symptoms with therapeutic levels of particular medications such as antidepressants (tricyclics and selective serotonin reuptake inhibitors [SSRIs]). This phenomenon also suggests that the etiology of this disorder may be physiologic rather than a response to some unresolved unconscious conflict as was previously proposed.

Post-Traumatic Stress Disorder

Post-traumatic stress disorder is a cluster of symptoms experienced after a distressing event that is outside the range of normal events (e.g., watching one's family being murdered) and one in which the person experienced intense fear, helplessness, and/or horror. Examples of symptoms include re-experiencing the trauma through repeated and intrusive recall of the event (at times as a flashback); avoiding situations that in some way remind the person of the event; feeling detached from other people; and having a heightened sense of arousal, which is experienced as difficulty falling asleep, hypervigilance, an exaggerated startle response, or a combination of these. The case of Patrick T. provides a clinical example of post-traumatic stress disorder:

Patrick T. was admitted to the psychiatric inpatient unit with the diagnosis of post-traumatic stress disorder. Two months before admission, he and his co-worker friend were in a truck accident on an overpass. Patrick watched in horror as his friend fell out of the truck, which was hanging over the edge. The fall killed his friend instantly. Patrick was able to climb out of the passenger side and sustained injuries to his back and legs. He received physical therapy for his injuries. For the past 2 weeks he has been continually preoccupied by the event, has had persistent insomnia and nightmares, repeatedly says that he should have been the one to die, becomes easily irritable, does not show feelings when with others, and jumps whenever he hears a loud noise or someone touches him unexpectedly. The nurse assigned to work with Patrick found him pacing. She remained with him as he paced. The following nursing diagnoses were immediately relevant: Anxiety, Disturbed Sleep Pattern, and Dysfunctional Grieving. Patrick and the nurse decided together that the priorities were to decrease his anxiety and to improve sleep. Patrick was willing to learn a progressive relaxation exercise (which involves relaxing one group of muscles at a time until the body is relaxed). After learning the exercise, Patrick worked on deep abdominal breathing and agreed to use this strategy when he found himself preoccupied with the accident. The nurse did not purposefully probe the details of the event, but if Patrick had brought it up, she would have listened attentively and offered support and empathy.

Acute Stress Disorder

As in post-traumatic stress disorder, the person with acute stress disorder has been exposed to a distressing event that is outside the range of normal events. The event or events have happened recently. This disorder is characterized by the following:

- Feeling a sense of detachment: having a reduced awareness of one's surroundings
- Derealization: a change in self-awareness (e.g., a person does not feel real or feels that what is happening around him or her is not real)
- Depersonalization: feeling of being detached from one's body or mental processes
- Dissociative amnesia: a type of amnesia caused by trauma or stress resulting in an inability to recall important personal information

SOMATOFORM DISORDERS

An individual with one of the somatoform disorders experiences physical symptoms without actual physiologic dysfunction or with physical cause(s) that are affected by psychological factors in terms of onset, severity, duration, or continuance of symptoms.

Conversion Disorder

In conversion disorder, symptoms may include blindness, deafness, or paralysis of the legs without a physiologic cause. Usually the symptoms are neurologic and occur in response to some threatening or traumatic event. The symptoms are real and not created; they can cause significant distress or impairment in social, occupational, or other important areas of functioning. In some cases a true physiologic cause for the symptoms has been discovered years later; therefore a diagnosis of conversion disorder is usually tentative and provisional.

Pain Disorder

In pain disorder, the patient experiences pain in one or more sites that causes significant distress or impairment in function. Psychological factors play a significant role in the experience of the pain; however, the pain is not intentionally produced or contrived. The pain may be related to a physiological problem; however, the psychological component is significant.

Hypochondriasis

In hypochondriasis, individuals are convinced that they have a serious medical problem in spite of the absence of any concrete medical findings. They will seek other opinions if one physician does not validate their concerns, and they often take multiple prescription medications from various health care providers. Concern about the feared illness often becomes a central part of people's lives and may impair social, occupational, or other important areas of functioning. In some cases of hypochondriasis, the person does not recognize that the concern about having a serious illness is excessive or unreasonable.

DISSOCIATIVE DISORDERS

Dissociative disorders involve a change in identity, memory, or consciousness. The change may be sudden or gradual, may be transient or occurring over a long period, and is thought to be an escape from anxiety. In a sense, persons unconsciously dissociate or remove themselves psychologically from anxiety-provoking situations because the situations are too much to bear. Even normal persons may experience depersonalization under severe stress. In this case, individuals feel they are outside of themselves or floating overhead watching what is happening, as if it were happening to someone else. Examples of dissociative disorders include amnesia or dissociative identity disorder (formerly multiple personality disorder).

Amnesia is characterized by a gap in memory, usually of a traumatic or stressful nature, that is too extensive to be explained by normal forgetfulness. There are five major types of amnesia: (1) localized amnesia, or difficulty remembering anything about the first few hours after a profoundly disturbing event; (2) selective amnesia, or the ability to remember some but not all of the events surrounding a traumatic experience; (3) generalized amnesia, or failure to remember one's entire life; (4) continuous amnesia, or inability to recall events after a specific time up to and including the present; and (5) systematized amnesia, or loss of memory for certain categories of information, such as all memories related to one's family or to a particular person.

Dissociative identity disorder is a relatively rare dissociative disorder in which two or more distinct personalities exist within the person and at least two personalities repeatedly take control of the person's behavior. Legal identity is retained by the "host personality." Other personalities within the body are called "alter personalities." Individuals with this disorder experience frequent gaps in memory for personal history, both remote and recent. Most patients with dissociative identity disorders report severe childhood abuse, including physical, sexual, or ritual cult abuse; however, these experiences are difficult to verify. Women are five times more likely to have the disorder than men are. There appears to be an inherited predisposition to the occurrence of dissociative identity disorder.

Medical Treatment

Drug Therapy. The primary anxiolytic (antianxiety) medications are the benzodiazepines (e.g., diazepam [Valium], chlordiazepoxide hydrochloride [Librium], lorazepam [Ativan], alprazolam [Xanax], and clonazepam [Klonopin]). (The nursing implications and patient teaching needs are described in the Drug Therapy table below.) They usually are prescribed for brief periods. Side effects are those associated with sedation, such as drowsiness, fatigue, dizziness, and confusion. Because physical and psychological dependence occur, withdrawal from these medications must be medically supervised. Abrupt cessation of benzodiazepines may result in withdrawal symptoms including seizures and even death.

Antidepressants are now used much more commonly to treat anxiety disorders, either alone or in combination with anxiolytics. Antidepressants, such as the SSRIs and some of the newer antidepressants such as venlafaxine (Effexor), nefazadone (Serzone) and duloxetine (Cymbalta), are often very useful in reducing anxiety, decreasing distress, and improving overall

---

💊 **DRUG THERAPY** | *Common Anxiolytics (Anti-Anxiety Medications) in the Benzodiazepine Class*

DRUG NAME	NURSING IMPLICATIONS	PATIENT TEACHING
Alprazolam (Xanax) Chlordiazepoxide (Librium) Clonazepam (Klonopin) Clorazepate (Tranxene) Diazepam (Valium) Halazepam (Paxipam) Lorazepam (Ativan) Oxazepam (Serax) Prazepam (Centrax)	Effective in treatment of anxiety and panic disorders. Sometimes used as preoperative sedatives and to treat certain side effects of other drugs (neuroleptics). Depress the central nervous system (CNS). May potentiate other CNS depressants; administer with caution with other CNS depressants. Administer with extreme caution in older adults and those who are frail, who may be more sensitive to the effects of these medications and be more prone to confusion or falls. Abrupt cessation after prolonged or excessive use may result in withdrawal, including seizures and death.	Avoid alcohol when taking medications in this class because alcohol will intensify their effects. Do not take more medication at one time than prescribed or use medication more frequently in a day than prescribed. Rebound anxiety may result when medication wears off, especially those with short half-lives. If this happens, report this to your practitioner. May impair driving, decrease attention and concentration, and cause drowsiness. Avoid driving or operating dangerous machinery until effects of the medicine on coordination, reaction time, motor control, and judgment are known. Do not abruptly stop taking this medication without consulting with your practitioner.

Pharmacology Capsule

Anxiolytic medications, which are given for anxiety disorders or as an adjunct medication for treating schizophrenia, may have side effects such as drowsiness, loss of coordination, fatigue, confusion, blurred vision, and psychological dependence.

functioning. This is especially true when the patient suffers from depression as well as anxiety.

NURSING CARE of the Patient with an Anxiety Disorder, Somatoform Disorder, or Dissociative Disorder

Assessment

The patient's self-report of symptoms as well as objective observations help determine the presence and level of anxiety (mild, moderate, severe, or panic). Particularly relevant mental status examination categories include motor activity, speech and language, and thought content.

Nursing Diagnoses, Goals, and Outcome Criteria: Anxiety, Somatoform, and Dissociative Disorders

Nursing Diagnoses	Goals and Outcome Criteria
Anxiety related to severe stress, as evidenced by patient's self-report, wringing and trembling of hands, and fearful appearance	Reduced anxiety: patient able to problem-solve, labels symptoms as those of anxiety, appears calm and relaxed
Ineffective Coping related to dissociation, amnesia in stressful situations	More effective coping with anxiety: patient recognizes ineffective ways of coping; identifies and implements new ways of coping with anxiety, stress, and their precipitants; learns and implements relaxation techniques, guided imagery, and other coping strategies

Interventions

Strategies to help patients reduce anxiety from a panic state or a severe level to a mild level center on remaining calm; speaking firmly with short, simple instructions (e.g., "sit down with me here"); and walking to a less-stimulating area of the unit. Once the anxiety is reduced to a manageable level, assist patients in exploring what happened, clarifying their usual ways of relieving anxiety (e.g., anger or somatic symptoms instead of experiencing more typical anxiety symptoms), and identifying what triggered the anxiety (e.g., feelings of self-doubt regarding finding employment after discharge). You can assist clients in problem-solving decisions and can teach ways to prevent and manage heightened anxiety in the future.

Consider the Alternative

Useful techniques to manage anxiety include relaxation techniques, warm baths, positive self-talk, and physical exercise.

SCHIZOPHRENIA

Schizophrenia is a term used to refer to a group of very serious, usually chronic thought disorders in which the affected person's ability to interpret the world accurately is impaired by psychotic symptoms. Psychosis is a state in which a person has distorted perceptions of reality. Psychotic symptoms include delusions, hallucinations, and impaired speech or behavioral patterns. The symptoms are characterized as either positive or negative. Positive symptoms appear to reflect an excess or distortion of normal functions and include delusions, hallucinations, problems with communication, and bizarre behavior. Negative symptoms appear to reflect a decrease or loss of normal functions and include diminished emotional expression (flattened affect), slowed thinking and speech, and difficulty initiating goal-directed behavior.

Typically, schizophrenic patients have functioned normally in early life; they often are very intelligent and well educated before the onset of the first symptoms. The symptoms usually begin in adolescence or early adulthood; however, some types of schizophrenic disorders are more often diagnosed in later life. The patient's ability to function in the areas of work, interpersonal relationships, or self-care deteriorates significantly during acute episodes and may not return to baseline after the first psychotic episode. With each subsequent episode, the ability to function independently continues to deteriorate; intelligence quotient (IQ) levels drop; and thinking becomes very concrete. Patients are unable to tolerate even the typical stressors of daily living. However, newer medications have been very successful in helping people return to their previous activities.

In one research study, the brains of persons with chronic schizophrenia were examined after death. The ventricles of the brain were found to be enlarged, whereas brain tissues that correlated with higher-level thinking had atrophied. This finding is consistent with the loss of capacity to think and function independently that is seen with most of the patients diagnosed with this disease.

Etiology and Risk Factors

The cause of schizophrenia is not certain. The model that integrates diverse potential causes states that patients who are most vulnerable to acquiring the disorder encounter factors (stress) that precipitate the disorder. The model is called the *stress-diathesis model*. Researchers have established that people with schizophrenia probably were genetically vulnerable to the disorder. The range of biologic factors being investigated includes (1) neurotransmitters (e.g., dopamine, norepinephrine, and gamma-aminobutyric acid) and their receptors; (2) structural abnormalities such as degeneration of the limbic system, enlargement of the lateral and third ventricles, and loss of neurons in the temporal lobe; (3) infectious agents; and (4) hormonal dysregulation.

In men, the disorder usually first occurs between 15 and 25 years of age. The usual age range for first occurrence in women is 25 to 35. There is no difference in rate by gender. The incidence worldwide is between 0.5% and 1%. Approximately 50% of all mental hospital beds are occupied by patients with schizophrenia, and 40% to 60% of people with schizophrenia are readmitted within a 2-year period after discharge from their first hospitalization. It has been estimated that two thirds of all homeless people have schizophrenia. Fifty percent of people with schizophrenia attempt suicide; 10% complete a suicide during a 20-year follow-up period.

Medical Treatment

Drug Therapy. The most commonly administered medications for people with schizophrenia are neuroleptic (antipsychotic) medications and antiparkinsonian medications, which are at times administered to prevent or relieve some of the side effects of the neuroleptics. (The nursing implications and patient teaching needs are described in the Drug Therapy table on p. 1254.) Anxiolytic medications also may be administered in conjunction with the neuroleptics to decrease agitation and akathisia (a potential side effect of neuroleptics in which the patient is restless and unable to sit still). There are two broad categories of neuroleptics: typical and atypical neuroleptics. The typical neuroleptics are the older neuroleptics that were very useful in treating the positive symptoms of schizophrenia such as auditory and visual hallucinations; however, they were not particularly useful in treating the negative symptoms, such as poverty of thought, delayed thinking, and decreased function. The atypical neuroleptics are known to help with both the positive and the negative symptoms and have a reduced incidence of side effects in comparison with the older, typical agents.

When working with patients who are receiving neuroleptics, you are responsible for observing and recording accurately all data relevant to the target behaviors and symptoms of the medications as well as the potential side effects. There are a variety of potential side effects, some of which have rapid onset and require immediate treatment.

One side effect that can be managed with nursing interventions and patient teaching is orthostatic hypotension (or postural hypotension), which is a drop in blood pressure when a person changes position from lying down to sitting or from sitting to standing. This problem, which creates a risk for falls, occurs most frequently in the early weeks of treatment and is more common in the morning, after the patient has been in bed during the night, as well as after a large meal. Older adults and those in poor physical health are at particular risk for this side effect. See Chapter 37 for details on the assessment and management of orthostatic hypotension.

Another group of side effects are referred to as extrapyramidal side effects (EPS), which stem from the impact of the antipsychotics on the extrapyramidal tracts of the central nervous system. These tracts play a role in the control of involuntary movements. Different EPS may occur at different periods in the course of medication therapy and are described as follows.

Acute dystonic reactions may occur after one dose of medication or during the first few days of treatment. The reactions consist of severe muscle contractions involving the tongue, face, neck (torticollis), and back (opisthotonos). The larynx also may be constricted (laryngospasm), which compromises the patient's airway. The reaction is reversed with benztropine mesylate (Cogentin) given intramuscularly or intravenously or with diphenhydramine hydrochloride (Benadryl), administered intravenously as ordered. Acute dystonia is a medical emergency and must be treated immediately. It is important to note that certain antiemetics such as promethazine (Phenergan) and prochlorperazine (Compazine) may also cause dystonic reactions.

After 1 to 2 weeks of treatment with antipsychotic medications, the parkinsonian syndrome—consisting of masklike face, rigid posture, shuffling gait, and resting tremor—may occur. Other extrapyramidal syndromes that may occur later in treatment are akathisia, a reversible restlessness manifested as an urge to pace and difficulty sitting still. Some references state that akathisia is the most common side effect of neuroleptic medications.

Tardive dyskinesia is usually an irreversible syndrome that may occur after prolonged use of neuroleptic drug therapy. It consists of persistent involuntary movements of the face, jaw, and tongue that lead to grimacing; jerky movements of the upper extremities; and tonic contractions of the neck and back. Treatment includes discontinuing the causative agent; however, the symptoms usually continue.

Neuroleptic malignant syndrome occurs in 1% of people receiving neuroleptics and certain antiemetics such as prochlorperazine (Compazine). Mortality rates reported for people with this condition range from 14% to 30%. The first symptom is usually muscular rigidity accompanied by akinesia (emotional unresponsiveness and blunted affect) and respiratory distress and may include involuntary muscle movements, but the cardinal sign is hyperthermia (101° to 103° F or higher).

Neuroleptic malignant syndrome is a medical emergency that requires immediate intervention and intensive care. Neuroleptic malignant syndrome may result in permanent impairment or even death.

DRUG THERAPY | *Selected Neuroleptics (Antipsychotics)*

DRUG NAME	NURSING IMPLICATIONS	PATIENT TEACHING
TYPICAL NEUROLEPTICS		
Chlorpromazine (Thorazine) Fluphenazine (Prolixin) Haloperidol (Haldol) Loxapine (Loxitane) Mesoridazine (Serentil) Perphenazine (Trilafon) Thioridazine (Mellaril) Thiothixene (Navane) Trifluoperazine (Stelazine)	These agents are helpful in the treatment of positive symptoms of schizophrenia and other psychotic processes. May cause drowsiness and sedation. May cause postural hypotension, dry mouth, and blurred vision, especially in frail and older people. Watch for extrapyramidal side effects (EPS) such as Parkinson syndrome–like movements, muscle rigidity, dystonia, akathisia, and oculogyric crisis. Long-term administration may result in tardive dyskinesia.	Caution the patient to rise slowly from a lying position to a sitting position and from sitting to standing to avoid a sudden drop in blood pressure. Caution patients to avoid driving or operating dangerous machinery until effects of the medicine on coordination, reaction time, motor control, and judgment are known. Assess the patient for abnormal, involuntary movements, and report these to the prescribing practitioner. Administer medications to treat motor movement side effects as ordered. Provide the patient with hard candy or sugarless chewing gum to help with dry mouth. Provide dietary teaching to help the patient avoid or manage weight gain and diabetes associated with these and other neuroleptics.
ATYPICAL NEUROLEPTICS		
Aripiprazole (Abilify) Clozapine (Clozaril) Olanzapine (Zyprexa) Quetiapine (Seroquel) Risperidone (Risperdal) Ziprasidone (Geodon)	Atypical neuroleptics treat both the positive and negative symptoms of schizophrenia and other psychotic disorders. May cause drowsiness and sedation. May cause postural hypotension, dry mouth, and blurred vision, especially in frail and older people. Watch for EPS such as Parkinson syndrome–like movements, muscle rigidity, dystonia, akathisia, and oculogyric crisis. Although these side effects are less common in the atypical class of neuroleptics, they are still seen in patients taking these drugs. Long-term administration may also result in tardive dyskinesia, although this may be less likely.	Caution the patient to rise slowly from a lying position to a sitting position and from sitting to standing to avoid a sudden drop in blood pressure. Caution patients to avoid driving or operating dangerous machinery until effects of the medicine on coordination, reaction time, motor control, and judgment are known. Assess the patient for abnormal, involuntary movements, and report these to the prescribing practitioner. Administer medications to treat motor movement side effects as ordered. Provide the patient with hard candy or sugarless chewing gum to help with dry mouth. Provide dietary teaching to help the patient avoid or manage weight gain and diabetes associated with these and other neuroleptics.
	In addition to the other side effects associated with atypical neuroleptics, clozapine may result in a significant drop in the white blood count. Routine blood count monitoring must be done to identify any drop in white blood cells, and the medication must be held and usually discontinued if this happens.	In addition to the above, teach the patient taking clozapine to watch for and report sore throat, fever, chills, and any other signs of infection immediately to the prescribing practitioner.

One neuroleptic, clozapine (Clozaril), presents a risk for the blood disorder known as *agranulocytosis,* an extreme decrease in granulated white blood cells, which frequently manifests as a sore throat and fever. Patients receiving this medication require close supervision and frequent white blood cell counts. If the white cell count drops significantly or if the patient presents with sore throat, fever, and/or flu symptoms, the medication must be held and the physician must be notified at once. Severe infection may result when the white blood cell counts drop below acceptable levels.

It is clear that in monitoring a patient for drug side effects, a wide range of data is relevant from vital signs to facial expression. Pay close attention to all patient descriptions of symptoms.

After a period of time, patients taking typical neuroleptic medications almost always experience extrapyramidal side effects such as akathisia and pseudoparkinsonism. Tardive dyskinesia also is a significant risk when patients are taking the typical neuroleptic medications; thus the atypical medications are now considered first-line agents.

Weight gain, hyperglycemia and onset of type 2 diabetes have all been associated with the use of atypical antipsychotics. Therefore it is important that you teach patients taking these medications about proper diet, exercise, and the need for regular checkups. A few of the atypical neuroleptics may cause an abnormal increase in serum progesterone (hyperprolactinemia), which can lead to an enlargement of the breasts (gynecomastia) and production of milk (galactorrhea) in both men and women.

NURSING CARE *of the Patient with Schizophrenia*

Assessment

The following data contribute to the mental status examination of the person with schizophrenia: (1) appearance: may have poor grooming and failure to bathe; (2) activity: may exhibit agitation, bizarre postures, catatonic excitement or stupor, mannerisms or stereotypes, or stiff body movements; (3) mood and affect: may have flat affect or inappropriate rage or happiness; (4) speech and language: mutism, tangential speech, blocking, or loose associations; (5) thought content: delusions that may include persecutory, grandiose, religious, or somatic; (6) perceptual disturbances: auditory hallucinations most commonly, visual hallucinations next most commonly; (7) insight and judgment: usually little insight into illness; (8) sensorium: oriented to person, place, and time; (9) memory: usually intact, but difficulties with attention make assessment difficult.

Nursing Diagnoses, Goals, and Outcome Criteria: Schizophrenia

Nursing Diagnoses	Goals and Outcome Criteria
Disturbed Thought Processes related to delusions (false beliefs), loose associations, concrete thinking, symbolism, as evidenced by patient statements such as that the president is out to get him or her	Improved thought processes: patient differentiates illusions from reality, fewer loose associations, more logical thinking
Disturbed Sensory Perception related to hallucinations, illusions, heightened response to irrelevant stimuli, as evidenced by patient's inability to tolerate group therapy, talking to herself, and looking for something when nothing is there	Improved sensory perceptual function: reduced frequency of hallucinations, less response to irrelevant environmental and other stimuli
Impaired Verbal Communication related to delayed thinking, as evidenced by very slow and delayed speech	Improved verbal communications: patient expresses thoughts clearly
Self-Care Deficit related to withdrawal and loss of motivation and judgment, as evidenced by poor hygiene, poor grooming, and avoiding others	Improved self-care: patient performs activities of daily living with maximum independence in relation to level of ability

Interventions

Disturbed Thought Processes

Nursing interventions include speaking in a gentle and non-confrontational manner, decreasing unwanted environmental stimuli, focusing on reality (real events, real people), letting the patient know that you do not share the delusion without directly confronting the delusion (do not argue or try to disprove the delusion), encouraging the patient to express feelings and anxiety, and connecting delusions with anxiety-provoking situations (see interventions for anxiety, discussed on p. 1252).

Disturbed Sensory Perception

Interventions include making brief, frequent contacts with the patient (to interrupt hallucinatory experiences), encouraging the patient to pay attention to what is occurring in the environment (instead of external stimuli), encouraging involvement in quiet activities, and informing patients that hallucinations are part of the disease process.

Impaired Verbal Communication

Interventions may include seeking clarification and verbalizing the implied, which may be useful if the patient is not speaking (e.g., "It must have been difficult for you when your father didn't come after he told you he would"). You will also want to provide regular contact with the patient and use gentle encouragement, understanding that the patient's thinking may be slowed.

Self-Care Deficit

Possible interventions include providing recognition for all constructive self-care actions (e.g., "I see you've bathed and washed your hair"), demonstrating how to perform an activity if necessary, intervening to assist when necessary, offering finger foods or cans of food for the patient to open, or serving family style if the patient believes food has been poisoned.

MOOD DISORDERS

People with mood disorders experience significantly elevated or depressed moods. Some people experience cycles of elevated mood and depressed mood. An episode of persistent depressed mood is referred to as *major depression.* An episode of elevated mood is called a *manic episode.* Alternation between significantly depressed mood and significantly elevated mood over time is termed *bipolar disorder.*

Major depression is one of the most common psychiatric disorders, with a lifetime prevalence of 6%. The mean age for the occurrence of depression is 40. About twice as many women as men are diagnosed with major depression. People who are single, divorced, or lacking in close relationships are more vulnerable. There is no association between major depression and race or between major depression and socioeconomic status.

For bipolar disorder, the lifetime prevalence is 1%, with the mean age at onset being 30. Rates are similar for men and women and are higher among single and divorced people than among married people. People in higher socioeconomic groups and those with lower levels of education have higher rates of bipolar disorder.

Etiology and Risk Factors

Definite causes of mood disorders have not been established. Probable causes include neurotransmitter dysregulation, neuroreceptor deficits, neuroendocrine dysfunctions, genetic factors, loss of significant others, learned helplessness, and negative thoughts about life experiences.

Medical Treatment

Drug Therapy. There are several types of antidepressant medications: SSRIs; newer agent antidepressants such as nefazadone (Serzone), venlafaxine (Effexor), and duloxetine (Cymbalta); tricyclic antidepressants (TCAs); and monoamine oxidase inhibitors (MAOIs). (Important considerations are listed in the Drug Therapy table on p. 1257.)

Pharmacology Capsule

The side effects of tricyclic antidepressant medications are drowsiness, fatigue, orthostatic hypotension, dry mouth, blurred vision, urinary retention, and constipation.

The manic phase of bipolar disease is usually treated with lithium or divalproex (Depakote). (Nursing implications and patient teaching needs are described in the Drug Therapy table on p. 1258.) When administering medications, you are responsible for ensuring that medication has been swallowed, as opposed to being held in the mouth and later discarded or saved for an overdose. As the patient responds to antidepressant medication and the energy level increases, the risk of suicide also increases.

MAOIs sometimes are prescribed for patients with a depression that is resistant to the SSRIs, TCAs, and other antidepressants. A 2-week period should elapse between ending most antidepressants and beginning an MAOI. The very serious side effect of a hypertensive crisis occurs if the patient taking an MAOI ingests tyramine-containing food or drink, such as avocados, bananas, beer, bologna, canned figs, chocolate, cheese (except cottage cheese), liver, papaya products, pâté, herring, fava beans, raisins, salami, sausage, sour cream, soy sauce, some wines, and yogurt. These foods also must be avoided for 3 weeks after stopping treatment with an MAOI. Symptoms of a hypertensive crisis, which requires immediate treatment, include headache, palpitations, visual changes, neck stiffness, nausea, vomiting, sweating, sensitivity to light, pupil changes, and bradycardia or tachycardia. A "washout" period of about 4 weeks must elapse when discontinuing a MAOI before starting most other antidepressants.

Consider the Alternative

Many people use the herbal preparation St. John's wort to relieve depression. However, additional study is needed before it can be recommended as a replacement for conventional drugs used to treat major mental illnesses.

Sexual dysfunction (anorgasmia, delayed or absent ejaculation, decreased libido) may occur with any antidepressant but seems to be more commonly related to the SSRI antidepressants. Some antidepressants such as nefazadone (Serzone) and bupropion (Wellbutrin) are much less likely to cause this troublesome side effect.

Put on Your Thinking Cap!

A patient with bipolar disorder is being treated for severe depression in an inpatient facility with bupropion (Wellbutrin) and divalproex sodium (Depakote). Identify the nursing implications related to these medications.

Electroconvulsive Therapy

Electroconvulsive therapy (ECT) is a form of therapy in which an electrical current is introduced to the brain through electrodes placed on the temples. The electrical current produces a grand mal seizure; however, drugs are administered to minimize the manifestations of a seizure. This type of therapy most often is prescribed when other forms of therapy have failed with people who are severely depressed. Its advantage is that it acts more quickly than medications, and in older people it may have fewer side effects.

💊 DRUG THERAPY | *Antidepressant Drugs*

DRUG	CONSIDERATIONS
SSRIs Citalopram (Celexa) Fluoxetine (Prozac) Fluvoxamine (Luvox) Paroxetine (Paxil) Sertraline (Zoloft)	SSRIs can be taken once a day, making adherence to a prescribed treatment easier for the patient. SSRIs are not considered cardiotoxic; thus an overdose is unlikely to cause life-threatening dysrhythmias. Besides depression, SSRIs may be useful in panic disorder and obsessive-compulsive disorder. Most patients tolerate the medications in the morning, whereas others may feel tired and thus should take the SSRI in the evening.
TRICYCLICS Amitriptyline (Elavil) Clomipramine (Anafranil) Desipramine (Norpramin) Doxepin (Sinequan) Imipramine (Tofranil) Nortriptyline (Pamelor) Trimipramine (Surmontil)	Tricyclics affect not only serotonin but also epinephrine/norepinephrine and as such may cause cardiac complications. Severe and life-threatening dysrhythmias may result from an overdose. Side effects may be more problematic in this group of medications than with SSRIs. Many of these medicines cannot be taken once a day; bid or tid dosing must be used to reach the total daily dose.
TETRACYCLICS Maprotiline (Ludiomil) Mirtazapine (Remeron)	At least as potentially dangerous as tricyclics; significant sedation may occur. May be given in single or divided doses.
OTHER AGENTS Bupropion (Wellbutrin) Nefazodone (Serzone) Trazodone (Desyrel) Venlafaxine (Effexor)	Divided doses (increase risk of seizures). Divided doses (sedating). Divided doses >100 mg (sedative). Divided doses.
MAOIs Phenelzine (Nardil) Tranylcypromine (Parnate)	Not first-line (first choice) drugs. Strict diet restrictions. Interactions with foods containing tyramine, other antidepressants, and many other drugs can lead to life-threatening hypertensive crisis. Must be given in divided doses.

MAOI, Monoamine oxidase inhibitor; *SSRI,* selective serotonin reuptake inhibitor.

Key nursing interventions include patient and family teaching, making certain that the patient takes nothing by mouth after midnight on the day of a treatment, asking the patient to void and to remove eyeglasses or contact lenses and dentures, administering atropine sulfate as ordered (to decrease secretions), positioning the patient on the side after the procedure to prevent aspiration, monitoring vital signs, remaining with the patient until the patient is awake, and providing orienting information as needed (e.g., "It's 10 AM Wednesday, and you just finished your treatment."). Temporary memory loss and confusion are common side effects of ECT, and instances of prolonged memory loss have occurred. You must take appropriate safety precautions and be patient with the person who has undergone this procedure.

NURSING CARE *of the Patient with Major Depression*

Assessment

Data that are relevant to the mental status assessment of a patient who has depression include the following:

- Activity: patient is likely to exhibit psychomotor retardation and possibly no spontaneous movements, with a downcast gaze, although the patient may exhibit agitation (e.g., hand wringing and hair pulling), especially if an older adult.
- Mood and affect: may or may not have depressed feelings and may not appear depressed.
- Speech and language: speech volume and rate may be decreased; response to questions may be delayed; and mutism may be present.
- Thought content: patient expresses generally negative view of self and world; may ruminate about loss, guilt, suicide, and depression; if psychotic, may have delusions of guilt, failure, worthlessness, or terminal illnesses.
- Insight and judgment: suicidal ideation occurs in two thirds of depressed patients, with 10% to 15% committing suicide; suicide risk increases as the patient gains the energy needed to commit suicide; insight into illness may be impaired due to negative perceptions of reality.
- Sensorium: patient is oriented but may not have energy to answer questions.
- Memory and attention: patients commonly complain of impaired concentration and forgetfulness.

DRUG THERAPY *Mood Stabilizers (Anti-Manic Agents)*

DRUG NAME	NURSING IMPLICATIONS	PATIENT TEACHING
Lithium (Lithium Carbonate, Lithobid, Lithium SR)	Used in the treatment of bipolar disorders; occasionally used as adjunct treatment for depression. Narrow therapeutic range of 0.5 to 1.5 mEq/L. Watch for signs of lithium toxicity (tremulousness, nausea, vomiting, diarrhea, changes in level of consciousness). Maintain adequate hydration. Monitor renal function (serum creatinine and BUN), and report abnormal findings. Monitor serum level of lithium. Do not change from immediate release to sustained release or vice versa unless directed by prescriber because this may alter serum levels unexpectedly.	Take exactly as prescribed. Drug must be taken regularly to achieve and maintain adequate blood level. Do not alter salt intake. Do not double up on doses if one is missed. Maintain adequate fluid intake, especially in hot weather. Avoid excessive use of caffeinated beverages. Keep follow-up appointments and have blood levels drawn as directed. Report signs of toxicity at once.
Valproic acid, divalproex sodium (Depakote, Depakene)	Used in the treatment of bipolar disorders. Serum levels must be monitored for therapeutic range (50 to 100 mcg/mL). Metabolized by the liver, thus periodic monitoring of liver enzymes is necessary. May cause some sedation. May cause hair loss; if moderate to severe, notify prescribing practitioner.	Take medication exactly as prescribed. Drug must be taken regularly to achieve and maintain adequate blood level. Do not double up on medication if a dose is missed. Avoid driving or operating dangerous machinery until exact effects of medication are known. Keep follow-up appointments and have blood levels drawn as directed.

BUN, Blood urea nitrogen.

Nursing Diagnoses, Goals, and Outcome Criteria: Depression

NURSING DIAGNOSES	GOALS AND OUTCOME CRITERIA
Risk for Self-Directed Violence related to hopelessness, increased energy level associated with treatment, as evidenced by patient endorsing suicidal ideations	Reduced risk of harm to self: patient seeks out staff member if an urge to harm self is experienced: develops coping skills to replace self-destructive behavior and acceptable ways of expressing anger, rage, and hostility; mobilizes social support systems
Chronic Low Self-Esteem or Situational Low Self-Esteem related to negative feelings about self	Improved self-esteem: patient accepts own body, has positive feelings about self, identifies aspects of self he or she likes; identifies thoughts about self
Imbalanced Nutrition: Less Than Body Requirements related to anorexia	Adequate nutrition: achieves and maintains ideal weight and has more energy
Disturbed Sleep Pattern related to anxiety	Improved sleep pattern: patient sleeps within 30 minutes of retiring and remains asleep for 6 to 8 uninterrupted hours

Interventions

Risk for Self-Directed Violence

Interventions may include establishing a no-harm contract; frequently assessing a patient's suicidal potential (see p. 1248 in the Nursing Assessment of the Psychiatric Patient section); taking necessary suicide precautions; removing dangerous objects such as pantyhose, belts, and any sharp objects; maintaining continuous one-to-one contact if indicated; encouraging honest expression of feelings; assisting in identifying symbols of hope in patient's life; identifying community resources for times of crisis; and communicating message that the patient is worthwhile.

Chronic Low Self-Esteem or Situational Low Self-Esteem

Interventions may include helping the patient identify positive aspects and limitations regarding his or her body; to like the body despite its imperfections; to improve hygiene, grooming, and posture, which makes positive affirmations about self; to limit self-criticism; to be aware of negative self-statements; to learn to give and receive compliments; and to develop social skills.

Imbalanced Nutrition: Less Than Body Requirements

Possible interventions include involving a dietitian in planning an adequate diet for the patient; directly assisting patients to make healthy choices regarding their menu and eating choices; documenting intake; determining food preferences and attempting to satisfy those preferences; and offering small, frequent meals.

Disturbed Sleep Pattern

For patients with sleep disturbances, discourage sleep during the day; provide sleep-producing measures like a light, small snack and warm bath; and teach relaxation exercises to be used before retiring. The patient should avoid exercising before bedtime, watching TV in bed, and ingesting caffeine after 2 PM. The patient may be asked to keep a sleep diary.

See the Nursing Care Plan: The Patient with Major Depression on p. 1260.

NURSING CARE of the Patient with Bipolar Disorder with Manic Episodes

Assessment

The nurse may observe the following:

- Appearance: dress is often inappropriate (e.g., bright, nonmatching colors, excessive makeup and jewelry).
- Activity: hyperactive.
- Mood, affect, and feelings: although frequently euphoric, the patient may also be very irritable, angry, and hostile, based on low frustration tolerance, and emotionally labile.
- Speech and language: talkative, pressured speech that is difficult to interrupt; flight of ideas (continuous, rapid shift from one topic to another); rate and volume increased.
- Thought content: themes of self-confidence and self-aggrandizement and possibly delusions of grandeur (e.g., false belief that one has great wealth or power) or delusions of persecution.
- Sensory perception: hallucinations may occur.
- Insight and judgment: patient often has little insight regarding illness; judgment impaired, as evidenced by actions such as large spending sprees, sexual activities incongruent with usual behavior, suicide attempts, and homicide attempts.

Nursing Diagnoses, Goals, and Outcome Criteria: Manic Episodes

Nursing Diagnoses	Goals and Outcome Criteria
Risk for Injury related to impaired judgment	Reduced risk for injury: patient does not exhibit potentially injurious activities
Risk for Other-Directed Violence related to impaired judgment, low frustration tolerance, and emotional lability	Reduced risk of violence toward others: patient does not harm others; patient verbalizes anger appropriately
Imbalanced Nutrition: Less Than Body Requirements related to hyperactivity	Balanced nutrition: patient consumes necessary daily nutrients in appropriate form for manic state; maintains body weight
Disturbed Sleep Pattern related to hyperactivity	Improved sleep pattern: patient sleeps at least 6 uninterrupted hours

Interventions

Risk for Injury

Interventions include decreasing environmental stimuli (e.g., providing a quiet, simply decorated room), discouraging group activities, encouraging a few one-to-one contacts, removing hazardous objects and substances from the environment, and providing a structure that includes physical activities such as brisk walks.

Risk for Other-Directed Violence

Interventions include decreasing environmental stimuli, observing the patient frequently, removing harmful objects, finding physical outlets, demonstrating a show of strength if necessary, administering prescribed medications, and restraining if other measures have failed to calm the patient. Restraints should be applied following an established protocol by staff who have been educated to restrain patients in a safe and humane manner. The patient in restraints should be checked at least every 15 minutes to make certain that circulation to extremities is satisfactory and to assess needs regarding nutrition and elimination.

Imbalanced Nutrition: Less Than Body Requirements

Interventions include providing foods that can be consumed on the run, attempting to have the patient's favorite foods and easy-to-eat and finger foods available, and educating the patient on the importance of satisfactory nutrition. See the Nutrition Concepts box below.

Disturbed Sleep Pattern

Interventions may include making sure the environment has low stimuli; observing closely for signs of

Nutrition Concepts

1. During manic episodes, patients may not meet nutritional needs because of increased physical activity and difficulty sitting down to complete a meal.
2. Anorexia may be a problem for depressed patients.

NURSING CARE PLAN

The Patient with Major Depression

ASSESSMENT

Health History: A 53-year-old woman is admitted to a psychiatric hospital with a diagnosis of major depression. During the past few weeks she has become increasingly listless, apathetic, and disinterested in anyone or anything. She cries frequently and says her life has not seemed to be worth living. She complains that she cannot sleep and has no appetite. She frequently talks about wanting to commit suicide. She was referred to a psychiatrist, who recommended that she be admitted to the hospital for treatment.

Physical Examination: Blood pressure, 110/70; pulse, 78; respiration, 22; temperature, 98.8° F orally. Height, 5'4". Weight, 120 lb. Appears apathetic and sad and cries frequently. Somewhat disheveled. Gaunt and tired-looking.

Nursing Diagnosis	Goals and Outcome Criteria	Interventions
Risk for Self-Directed Violence related to suicidal feelings	The patient will not harm herself, as evidenced by seeking out nursing staff if she experiences the urge to harm herself, developing coping skills to replace self-destructive behavior, and developing acceptable ways to express anger, rage, and hostility.	Establish a no-harm contract (e.g., ask her to state or write that she will not harm herself and will inform a nurse if she has thoughts of harming herself while in the hospital). Frequently assess patient's suicidal potential, and take necessary suicide precautions; remove dangerous objects from the environment; maintain continuous one-to-one contact; encourage honest expression of feelings; assist in identifying symbols of hope in patient's life, such as recognizing personal strengths or setting small, realistic goals.
Chronic Low Self-Esteem or Situational Low Self-Esteem related to depression	The patient will maintain or enhance self-esteem, as evidenced by acceptance of own body and sense of self, identification of negative thoughts about self, and identification of aspects of self she likes.	Help patient to identify positive aspects and limitations regarding her body and to accept her body regardless of limitations. Encourage patient to improve hygiene. Assist patient to accept compliments and to limit self-criticism.
Imbalanced Nutrition: Less Than Body Requirements related to anorexia or lack of interest in food	Patient will gain weight and experience higher energy level, as evidenced by more participation and interactions in activities with others.	Involve dietitian in planning adequate diet. Determine food preferences, and attempt to satisfy preferences. Offer small, frequent meals.
Disturbed Sleep Pattern related to depression relapse	Patient will sleep within 30 minutes of retiring and remain asleep for 6 to 8 uninterrupted hours.	Provide sleep-producing measures such as small snacks, warm baths, and relaxation exercises before patient retires.

? **CRITICAL THINKING** QUESTIONS

■ Explain why the patient requires close monitoring when she begins to feel more energetic.

■ What are some examples of symbols of hope in a person's life?

---

fatigue, such as fine tremor and puffy, dark circles below the eyes; and encouraging warm baths and soft music at bedtime.

The key medications for people with manic episodes are divalproex sodium (Depakote) or lithium carbonate. Because relief from symptoms may take up to 3 weeks, the patient also may receive an antipsychotic (neuroleptic) medication.

The therapeutic level of divalproex sodium in the blood is 50 to 100 mcg/mL (depending on the laboratory). The patient may develop toxicity if the blood level exceeds the therapeutic range. Therefore

a valproic acid level is done at intervals to assess blood levels. Divalproex is metabolized by the liver; thus patients with liver disorders may receive lower dosages.

Lithium is excreted by the kidneys and has a narrow therapeutic range. The therapeutic blood level for acute mania is 0.5 to 1.5 mEq/L (depending on the laboratory). If the level is above 1.5 mEq/L, symptoms of toxicity occur. It is critical for the patient taking lithium to stay well hydrated. If a patient taking lithium becomes dehydrated, he or she can easily become lithium-toxic. Signs and symptoms of lithium toxicity include tremor, nausea, vomiting, diarrhea, and changes in level of consciousness.

COGNITIVE DISORDERS

The key problems for people with cognitive disorders stem from impairments in cognition or memory. The term *cognitive disorders* replaced the term *organic mental disorders* because the latter incorrectly implied that "nonorganic" mental disorders do not have a biologic basis. Delirium and dementia are two different disorders that involve deficits in orientation, memory, language comprehension, and judgment. Delirium is potentially reversible, whereas dementia usually is not. Delirium is usually fairly rapid in onset. Dementia is slow in its onset.

Common causes of delirium are meningitis, neoplasms, drugs ranging from alcohol to steroids, electrolyte imbalance, endocrine dysfunction, liver abnormalities, renal failure, thiamine deficiency, and postoperative states. Common types of dementia are dementia of the Alzheimer's type, vascular dementia, Pick's disease, and Parkinson's disease. Delirium and dementia are discussed in greater detail in Chapter 22.

PERSONALITY DISORDERS

Every individual exhibits particular personality traits. A person may be shy, aggressive, dependent, or manipulative. When personality traits become inflexible and dysfunctional, a person may have a personality disorder. The essential features of a personality disorder are that it is pervasive (it concerns all aspects of one's life), chronic, and maladaptive. Examples of personality disorders are as follows:

1. Paranoid Personality Disorder—a pattern of distrust and suspiciousness such that others' motives are interpreted as hostile (individual suspects that others are out to harm or deceive, doubts loyalty of friends, does not confide in others, bears grudges, feels attacked by others).
2. Schizoid Personality Disorder—a pattern of detachment from social relationships and a restricted range of emotional expression (individual does not desire or enjoy close relationships, chooses solitary activities, lacks close friends, shows emotional coldness or detachment).
3. Schizotypal Personality Disorder—a pattern of difficulties in social and interpersonal relationships in which the person suffers from acute discomfort with close relationships and therefore

has a decreased capacity for such relationships. Persons with this disorder also have cognitive and perceptual distortions as well as eccentricities of behavior that make close relationships difficult. MNSD 9 People with paranoid, schizoid, and schizotypal personality disorders often appear odd or eccentric.

4. Antisocial Personality Disorder—a pattern of disregard for and violation of the rights of others (individual repeatedly breaks the law; lies; fails to plan ahead; shows a reckless disregard for the safety of self and others; is irresponsible; lacks remorse for having hurt, mistreated, or stolen from another).
5. Borderline Personality Disorder—a pattern of instability in interpersonal relationships, self-image, and affect and marked impulsivity (individual makes frantic efforts to avoid real or imagined abandonment; has chronic feelings of emptiness; shows inappropriate, intense anger or has difficulty controlling anger; has unstable self-image or sense of self; and exhibits recurrent suicidal behavior, gestures, or threats).
6. Histrionic Personality Disorder—a pattern of excessive emotionality and attention seeking (individual prefers to be the center of attention; is often sexually seductive or provocative; displays rapidly shifting and shallow expression of emotion; consistently uses physical appearance to draw attention to self; and shows self-dramatization, theatricality, and exaggerated expression of emotion).
7. Narcissistic Personality Disorder—a pattern of grandiosity, need for admiration, and lack of empathy (individual has an exaggerated sense of self-importance; requires excessive admiration; takes advantage of others to achieve own ends; is often envious of others; and exhibits arrogant, haughty behaviors or attitudes). MNSD 9 People with antisocial, borderline, histrionic, or narcissistic personality disorder often appear dramatic, emotional, or erratic.
8. Avoidant Personality Disorder—a pattern of social inhibition accompanied by feelings of inadequacy and hypersensitivity to negative evaluation (individual avoids occupational activities that involve interpersonal activities because of fear of criticism, disapproval, or rejection; is unwilling to get involved with people unless certain of being liked; is preoccupied with being criticized or rejected in social situations; views self as inferior to others; and is unusually reluctant to take personal risks).
9. Dependent Personality Disorder—a pattern of submissive and clinging behavior related to an excessive need to be taken care of (individual has difficulty making everyday decisions without an excessive amount of advice and reassurance

from others, needs others to assume responsibility for most major areas in life, has difficulty initiating projects because of lack of confidence in own judgment or abilities, and urgently seeks a relationship as a source of care and support).

10. Obsessive-Compulsive Personality Disorder—a pattern of preoccupation with orderliness, perfectionism, and control (individual is preoccupied with details, rules, lists, order, organization, or schedules to the extent that the major part of the activity is lost; shows perfectionism, rigidity, and stubbornness). MNSD 9

Individuals with avoidant, dependent, or obsessive-compulsive personality disorder often appear anxious or fearful.

BORDERLINE PERSONALITY DISORDER

The person with borderline personality disorder has patterns involving unstable relationships, unstable self-image, and unstable mood. Two theories offer explanations for the cause of this disorder. First, because families of patients with this disorder have a greater history of alcoholism, a genetic influence is thought to exist. The second explanation is related to particular developmental experiences. Some theorists view an essential component of psychosocial development as separation-individuation. Some feel that there are problems with attachment. It is thought that between 2 and 3 years of age, the child separates from the parents as a unique self. If the parents are nonaccepting or ambivalent of the child's increasing autonomy and if the parents reinforce dependent behavior, the child does not fully experience self as separate. This problem with separation-individuation is thought to form the basis of *splitting*, a frequently utilized mechanism in borderline personality disorder. Persons who are splitting view others as all good or all bad and may shift their views of a particular other from all good to all bad. A person who has a clearly developed sense of self and who does not split views others as having a mix of good qualities and negative qualities. The case of Bonnie P. provides a clinical example of borderline personality disorder.

Nora N., a licensed vocational nurse, worked part-time on a psychiatric unit. She reported to work at 11 PM one night after 5 days of not working to discover that Bonnie P. had been readmitted after opening the suture line on her wrists with a steak knife. One year ago Bonnie had cut this wrist, saying that she was trying to feel something. Bonnie told Nora that she had missed her terribly and that she hoped Nora would work with her that night. Nora said that Susan (the full-time registered nurse) would work with her that night. Bonnie swore and returned to her room. When Nora made rounds, Bonnie said she was sure something was wrong and began walking around the room with a staggering gait. Bonnie said that she had not taken anything to create this problem. Her vital signs were stable, and her pupils were normal in size and reaction to light. Nora reported the situation to Susan and reflected on her

responses to Bonnie. Initially she felt anger, telling herself that Bonnie was manipulative when she did not have her way. She thought about how Bonnie manipulates others when she feels helpless (she has no idea of how to meet her own needs). She also thought about Bonnie's splitting (seeing Nora as good nurse and Susan as bad nurse). Nora felt less angry as she considered the reasons for Bonnie's behavior. When Susan entered Bonnie's bedroom, Bonnie's gait was normal. Susan contracted with Bonnie for two 10-minute periods (at the beginning and end of shift) during which Bonnie could share whatever was on her mind and discuss her goals and plans for the following day.

NURSING CARE *of the Patient with Borderline Personality Disorder*

Assessment

The most relevant aspects of the mental status examination are the following:

- Mood, affect, feelings: patient may experience mood swings or chronic feelings of emptiness and boredom or intense anger.
- Insight and judgment: patient makes repeated suicidal threats and gestures and exhibits self-mutilating behavior.

Nursing Diagnoses, Goals, and Outcome Criteria: Borderline Personality Disorder

NURSING DIAGNOSES	GOALS AND OUTCOME CRITERIA
Risk for Self-Directed Violence or **Risk for Self-Mutilation** related to episodes of anger and impaired judgment	Absence of self-directed violence: patient does not harm self
Impaired Social Interaction related to unstable relationships	Improved social interaction: patient maintains relationships
Disturbed Personal Identity related to splitting	Improved sense of personal identity: patient clarifies own unique characteristics, differentiates thoughts and feelings of self and others; less splitting, clinging, and disturbing behaviors

Interventions

Risk for Self-Directed Violence and Risk for Self-Mutilation

In addition to the interventions identified on p. 1248 in the Mood Disorders section, various interventions are more specific to the issues of borderline personality disorder. It is important to be aware of your own feelings in order to refrain from any automatic responses that are not helpful (e.g., avoiding the patient who has cut himself). If patients mutilate themselves, it is important to care for wounds without acting in a way that might reinforce the self-mutilation (e.g., offering sympathy). Conversely, it is not appropriate to express disgust or in any way denigrate the patient. Ask patients to talk about feelings that occurred just before the self-mutilation. You can act as a role model for constructive expression of angry feelings and acknowledge the patient's positive expressions of negative feelings.

Impaired Social Interaction

Interventions include assisting patients in examining their own behaviors in relationships, communicating availability, acknowledging (reinforcing) independent behavior, and setting limits as appropriate.

Disturbed Personal Identity

Interventions include helping the patient discuss and take ownership of own thoughts and feelings; clarifying values while being cautious not to impose one's own values; and avoiding empathetic responses that may be viewed as mind reading (e.g., "I know how you feel.").

SUMMARY

Nurses work with patients with psychiatric disorders in a variety of settings, including psychiatric inpatient units. Treatment for psychiatric disorders is influenced by the particular culture, place, and historical time frame. You can use various strategies in communicating therapeutically with patients. The mental status examination is one aspect of the assessment of patients and is particularly relevant on a psychiatric unit. Systematically use the mental status examination with patients on admission and on an ongoing basis. For each of the major psychiatric disorders, possible observations for the relevant mental status examination categories are presented. Possible nursing diagnoses, goals, and interventions have been suggested for each disorder.

Key Points

- According to current thinking, mental illnesses are related to specific physiologic changes in the central nervous system.
- The psychoanalytic approach to mental illness is based on the theory that human beings function at different levels of awareness, ranging from conscious to unconscious, and that people use ego defense mechanisms to prevent anxiety.
- The interpersonal approach to mental illness has three components: (1) anxiety is often communicated interpersonally; (2) the patient learns new ways of coping or maturing in a therapeutic relationship; and (3) establishing trust is an important first step in the nurse's work with patients.
- Key ideas from the cognitive behavioral approach to mental illness are that behavior is learned, that behavior changes in response to positive consequences (positive reinforcement) or in response to the removal of negative stimuli (negative reinforcement), and that particular thoughts influence emotional states.
- In caring for a patient with a psychiatric disorder, nurses establish therapeutic (as opposed to social) relationships.
- The mental status examination consists of observations regarding appearance, mood and affect, speech and language, thought content, perceptual disturbances, insight and judgment, sensorium, and memory and attention.
- A patient with an anxiety disorder experiences either the highly uncomfortable feeling of anxiety directly or a symptom such as compulsive hand washing that prevents or reduces the occurrence of anxiety.
- In panic disorder, a patient experiences recurrent panic attacks, which are intense episodes of apprehension, at times to the point of terror, and often are accompanied by the feeling of impending doom.
- A person with agoraphobia is extremely fearful of situations outside the home from which escape may be difficult or in which help may be unavailable.
- Obsessive-compulsive disorder involves recurrent obsessions (thoughts), compulsions (behaviors), or both that produce distress and interfere with functioning.
- Post-traumatic stress disorder is a cluster of symptoms experienced after a distressing event that is outside the range of normal events (e.g., watching one's family being murdered).
- Individuals with a somatoform disorder, such as conversion disorder or hypochondriasis, are convinced that they have serious medical problems despite the absence of any concrete medical findings.
- Dissociative disorders involve a change in identity, memory, or consciousness, usually to escape from anxiety.
- Goals for the nursing care of patients with anxiety, somatoform, and dissociative disorders are to decrease anxiety to a point at which problem solving can occur and to teach methods such as relaxation techniques to interrupt anxiety as it escalates.
- The term *schizophrenia* refers to a highly problematic group of biologic disorders in which there are symptoms of psychosis, including delusions, hallucinations, marked loosening of associations, catatonia, and flat or inappropriate affect.
- People with mood disorders, such as major depression and bipolar depression, experience a significantly elevated mood, a significantly depressed mood, or both.
- Dementia is a group of disorders characterized by cognitive deficits sufficiently severe enough to impair social or occupational functioning.
- Personality disorders occur when personality traits become inflexible and dysfunctional and are pervasive (concern all aspects of one's life), chronic, and maladaptive.

 Go to your Companion CD-ROM for a Pharmacology Tutorial, Audio Glossary, and 3-D animations.

evolve Be sure to visit the companion Evolve site at http://evolve.elsevier.com/Linton/ for WebLinks and additional online resources.

REVIEW QUESTIONS *Choose the best answer.*

1. The primary focus of nursing care for patients with mental illness and their families is on:
   1. Helping them cope with and manage mental illness
   2. Administering medications
   3. Protecting other people from the patient
   4. Controlling the patient's behavior

2. Which of the following reflects an important characteristic of a therapeutic relationship?
   1. The relationship should benefit the patient and the nurse.
   2. The relationship has a clear purpose and ending.
   3. The relationship develops spontaneously.
   4. The relationship has no clear boundaries.

3. Which statement best illustrates the strategy of *clarifying* in a nurse-patient interaction?
   1. "When you mention your son, you look very sad."
   2. "What were you saying while I was on the telephone?"
   3. "Why do you get quiet when I ask about your husband?"
   4. "Are you saying that you are afraid of him?"

4. In the mental status examination, the nurse collects data on multiple areas, including:
   1. Thought content
   2. IQ
   3. Reflexes
   4. Reaction time

5. Mr. Brooks was hospitalized after a major automobile accident in which another person died. Mr. Brooks reports having no sensation in his legs and is unable to move them. Diagnostic studies reveal no physical basis for his symptoms. The patient's symptoms are typical of:
   1. Hypochondriasis
   2. Post-traumatic stress disorder
   3. Conversion disorder
   4. Panic disorder

6. John is a young college student who has just been diagnosed with schizophrenia. His concerned parents ask for information about his diagnosis. Which reply would be correct and appropriate?
   1. Schizophrenia is a mental illness that affects a person's thinking and distorts his view of reality.
   2. Most people with schizophrenia eventually require permanent care in a psychiatric facility.
   3. At this time there are no medications or treatments for schizophrenia.
   4. Most episodes of schizophrenia resolve within a week or two.

7. Nursing interventions to promote communication with the person who has schizophrenia include:
   1. Go along with delusions to avoid upsetting the patient
   2. Provide a variety of environmental stimuli
   3. Point out the flaws in the patient's illogical statements
   4. Do not argue or try to disprove his delusions

8. What are the nursing implications when a patient is taking phenelzine sulfate (Nardil)?
   1. Nardil is more effective if given with a tricyclic antidepressant.
   2. Patients should be taught to avoid foods that contain tyramine.
   3. Drugs that interact with Nardil can cause hypotensive crisis.
   4. Because Nardil has few interactions, it is often used in combination with other drugs.

9. People who are arrogant, need excessive admiration, and take advantage of others for their own gain may have which type of personality disorder?
   1. Borderline
   2. Obsessive-compulsive
   3. Narcissistic
   4. Histrionic

10. A patient taking divalproex (Depakote) is advised that blood samples will be taken periodically to monitor for:
    1. Liver damage
    2. Dystonic reactions
    3. Kidney damage
    4. Extrapyramidal syndromes

56 Substance-Related Disorders

MARK D. SOUCY

Objectives

After reading and studying this chapter, you should be able to:

1. Discuss the biologic, sociocultural, behavioral, and intrapersonal theories of the etiology of substance abuse or dependence.
2. Describe the data to be collected for the nursing assessment of a patient with substance abuse or dependence.
3. Describe alcohol dependence, alcohol withdrawal syndrome, medical complications of alcohol dependence, and treatment of alcohol abuse and dependence.
4. Discuss the pathophysiologic effects of frequently abused drugs.
5. Describe disorders associated with substance abuse and dependence.
6. Differentiate between drug abuse treatment and alcohol abuse treatment.
7. Describe the nursing diagnoses and interventions associated with substance abuse and dependence.
8. Discuss populations who present special problems in relation to drug abuse and dependency.

Key Terms

Be sure to check out the bonus material on the Companion CD-ROM, including selected audio pronunciations.

addiction (Ă-DĬK-shŭn, p. 1269)
co-dependent (p. 1270)
delirium tremens (p. 1269)
dual diagnosis (dī-ăg-NŌ-sĭs, p. 1283)
physical dependence (p. 1275)
psychological dependence (sī-kō-LŎJ-ĕ-kăl, p. 1274)
substance abuse (p. 1265)
substance dependence (p. 1265)
tolerance (TŎL-ŭr-ŭns, p. 1265)
12-Step Program (p. 1270)
withdrawal (p. 1269)

Substance abuse and dependence have become major problems in the United States and in other parts of the world over the past 40 years. These problems have reached the point of such significance that a great deal of energy and financial resources have been targeted toward a better understanding of them. Many researchers continue to try to discover the specific causes of substance abuse and dependence to combat these disorders more effectively. It appears that many factors contribute to the development of substance abuse and dependence.

The Diagnostic and Statistical Manual (4th ed.) (DSM-IV-TR) provides the criteria for understanding whether an individual has substance dependence or if the disorder is less severe—substance abuse. Alcohol and/or substance abuse, if not adequately treated, may progress to alcohol and/or substance dependence. Tolerance, a term used to describe the individual's need for more alcohol or other substance of choice to create the desired effect, is one of the criteria for the diagnosis of substance dependence. Another criterion is a diminished effect, resulting from using the same amount over time, the experience of physical withdrawal and/or substituting a similar substance in place of the usual one to treat discomfort associated with discontinuing the substance. In both abuse and dependence, there exists a significant degree of impairment or distress in the person's life.

ETIOLOGY AND RISK FACTORS

BIOLOGIC THEORY

Most experts in addictionology accept the biologic theory, often referred to as the *medical model*, which proposes that a faulty physiologic process that is not clearly understood contributes to dependence on a specific substance or substances (substance dependence). This theory is supported by the fact that children have been shown to be four times more likely to become alcoholic if their biologic parent or parents are alcoholic, even when the children are raised apart from the parents in homes where they are not exposed to the excessive use of alcohol. Widely publicized studies implicate a dopamine gene on human chromosome 11 for transmitting a predisposition for alcoholism from generation to generation. On the basis of these and many other studies, the medical community considers drug dependency to be a physical illness, like those that have the following characteristics: (1) incurability, (2) a genetic predisposition to develop under the right conditions, and (3) a potential to be treated effectively only by total abstinence from the substance that the body cannot handle.

SOCIOCULTURAL THEORY

Another theory suggests that sociocultural factors play a major role in the process of becoming dependent on a particular drug. Many people who live in poverty and in crime-ridden areas use drugs to relieve the stress inherent in these environments. In contrast, it can be observed that individuals with strong religious values prohibiting the excessive use of drugs have lower rates of addiction. Among certain subcultures, the use of certain drugs can be a rite of entry into a gang or a badge of honor proving that one has "made it." Even among middle-class Americans, the average person often parties to excess on New Year's Eve, for example. Certain cultural groups, such as the Irish, are commonly stereotyped as heavy drinkers. For country music fans, "crying in your beer" is often portrayed as the typical means of coping with loss and rejection.

BEHAVIORAL THEORY

Behavioral and learning theories look at the triggers for drinking and drug-using behaviors and how these patterns are reinforced. Substance abuse is believed to be a learned maladaptive way of coping with stress and anxiety. Family and peer group role models are studied closely for their use of substances, along with the beliefs and customs surrounding the use of drugs and alcohol. For example, if a shy teenage girl gets more attention and feels socially more comfortable when drinking with her friends, she is more likely to continue the use of alcohol to be accepted by her peers. See the Health Promotion Considerations box at right.

INTRAPERSONAL THEORY

The intrapersonal or psychological theory addresses those factors innate to the personality of the individual that may predispose him or her to substance abuse. These theorists believe that the quality of intrapersonal relationships during critical developmental stages of our lives affects us profoundly. Thus if children experience early childhood rejection, increased responsibility, unrealistic expectations, or overprotection, they may develop a dependent type of personality and consequently view themselves as inadequate or failures when attempts to get their needs met fail. Individuals may ultimately turn to alcohol or other drugs to numb the anxiety or frustration evoked by self-doubt and the daily stressors of reality.

Persons who abuse substances often have personality traits in common: many are very self-centered, have a strong need to be in control of others, seek attention, and have great difficulty delaying gratification of their needs. All of these characteristics are likely to increase the odds that they will resort to the use of drugs or alcohol to cope.

These types of intrapersonal theories originally supported the widespread acceptance of the perspective that alcoholism or drug addiction is a product of moral weakness. A more modern conclusion acknowledges

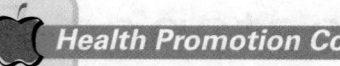

Health Promotion Considerations

Preventing Alcohol Use Among Children

- Alcohol use often begins at an early age, and the proportion of young people who drink frequently or heavily is alarming. The *Leadership to Keep Children Alcohol Free* initiative is a coalition of federal government agencies and private foundations dedicated to mobilizing resources to combat this public health problem.
- Research has shown that adolescents who abuse alcohol recall 10% less of what they have learned than those who don't drink. Alcohol use may also lead to increased sexual activity, unplanned pregnancy, exposure to sexually transmitted infection, criminal activity (including drunk driving), suicide attempts, and other destructive or violent behavior.
- The age at which a person first uses alcohol is a powerful predictor of lifetime alcohol abuse and dependence. An epidemiologic study published in the *Journal of Substance Abuse* found that more than 40% of those who begin drinking before age 15 will develop alcohol abuse or alcohol dependence at some time in their lives.
- As a health professional, talking to people about this issue will help to keep it high on the public agenda. Here are some suggestions:
  - Talk to children about the dangers of early alcohol use. As appropriate, encourage your patients, friends, and neighbors to talk to their children.
  - Ask other health care professionals, such as pediatric nurses, to discuss alcohol use during children's annual physicals.
  - Share literature about preventing alcohol abuse with members of your community.
  - Support recreational alternatives to drinking in your community.
  - Encourage parents to learn about their responsibilities regarding alcohol access and serving alcohol to minors in their homes.
  - Talk to teachers, counselors, school administrators, and school board members to make sure that school prevention programs put equal emphasis on alcohol and illicit drug use.
  - Place the issue of alcohol use by children on agendas for meetings of the PTA, the city council, faith groups, the Rotary Club, the chamber of commerce, and other community groups and organizations.
  - Involve young people in your community's prevention efforts.
  - Write letters to the editors of your local newspapers asking them to print articles about the dangers of early alcohol use.
  - Contact elected and appointed officials at local and state levels to inform them about the problem and what can be done to solve it.
  - Enlist support for immediate and consistent enforcement of underage alcohol-related drinking laws in your community.

Adapted from the National Institute on Alcohol Abuse and Alcoholism, National Institutes of Health: "Leadership to Keep Children Alcohol Free," in *Keep Kids Alcohol Free: Strategies for Action*, www.alcoholfreechildren.org.

that although the specific causes of misuse and addiction to various substances have not been established, they most likely involve a combination of biologic, social, cultural, behavioral, and psychological factors.

NURSING ASSESSMENT OF THE SUBSTANCE ABUSER

HEALTH HISTORY

Thorough data collection is essential to initiate the nursing process effectively when working with the substance-abusing patient. Information can be gathered from a variety of sources, including an interview with the patient, family members, and significant others; a social assessment; medical records; and school or military records. The LPN/LVN may participate in the collection of data from these sources. Many substance abusers have sustained major losses—of jobs, relationships, property, self-esteem, and health. They may face legal charges. Often they will not seek professional help until they have "hit bottom." Even then, they may seek help only when presented with an ultimatum of some type, often from their family, employer, or a court of law.

Questioning the patient produces the most reliable data when the questioning is nonjudgmental, direct, and specific and the answers are verified by more than one source when possible. For example, if the patient reports drinking a couple of beers after work each night, you should ask exactly how many were ingested, how many ounces each contained, or how big the bottle or glass used actually was. It also is important to know when the patient ingested the drug last and how much was taken to predict the possibility and timing of physical withdrawal symptoms. A nonjudgmental and matter-of-fact manner is the least likely to alienate an already defensive patient. At the same time, do not be so supportive and nurturing that clients can avoid facing the negative impact substance abuse has had on their lives. Finding the most appropriate balance of support and reality-based confrontation is a highly developed skill that increases the likelihood that patients will continue in the treatment process. Many team members who work in substance abuse treatment centers are recovering from addiction themselves, which often helps the client be more honest and less defensive and feel less hopeless and alone.

Patterns and Consequences of Abuse

The patient who has been abusing one or more substances will describe typical patterns of behavior and a combination of physical or psychological withdrawal symptoms characteristic of the substances abused. A few patients may not experience any physical withdrawal symptoms despite a history of prolonged, frequent, and heavy abuse, even of some substances that usually are physically addicting. Much depends on the stage of addiction, the habitual patterns of use, the pa-

tient's baseline physical status, and the combinations and interactions of the drug or drugs being misused.

Many substance abusers experience erratic and unprovoked mood swings. They may describe a lifestyle revolving almost totally around obtaining and using the substance of choice, starting early in the day, often alone, and requiring more of the substance over time to get the desired effects. Many substance abusers make efforts to hide the extent of their habit from others and, despite their best efforts to limit use of the substance, have been unsuccessful in doing so. Blackouts may have occurred when under the influence of a particular substance (especially alcohol). Blackouts are episodes of amnesia in which the individual does not remember what happened during a period of time. Patients often have significant work problems or damaged relationships as a result of being unable to meet the expectations placed on them.

Defense Mechanisms Employed

Typical defense mechanisms used by the substance abuser include denial, rationalization, intellectualization, and projection. Denial is readily apparent when patients state that they do not have a problem with drug use despite evidence to the contrary. Individuals also may initially minimize the problems they have had with using. Some deny that they need help in staying clean and sober. Some insist that they do not need to change friends or attend a 12-step program meeting such as Alcoholics Anonymous regularly.

The defense mechanism of rationalization is one in which abusers attempt to justify the reasons for their abuse of substances. This is an "excuse" for addiction. An example is the individual who insists he or she had to use heroin because there was no other way to cope with the pain of a physical injury: "The drugs my doctor gave me weren't working."

Intellectualization is closely related to rationalization but differs in that the person focuses only on objective facts as a way of avoiding dealing with unconscious conflicts and the emotions they evoke. For example, an alcoholic who killed someone while driving under the influence of alcohol would be intellectualizing if he or she stated that it was better that the victim die suddenly rather than have to live as a paraplegic.

Projection in substance abusers involves shifting the blame for their behavior onto someone or something else. Drug abusers using projection might insist that they became addicted to alcohol as a result of the pressure to drink at work-related social functions to keep colleagues from thinking they were prudes. They also may blame a spouse or loved one.

PHYSICAL EXAMINATION

On physical examination, many substance abusers appear malnourished and poorly cared for. Evidence of physical trauma from falls, abrasions, or fights may be present. Jaundice or discolored sclera of the eyes may

Nutrition Concepts

1. Heavy drug or alcohol intake has a negative effect on nutrition because it displaces foods in the diet that are more nutritious and impairs absorption and metabolism of nutrients in the body.
2. The nutritional goals for persons with alcoholism are to support them in avoiding alcohol and to correct nutritional deficits.
3. Individuals with chronic alcoholism may receive supplements of folate and vitamin B$_6$.
4. Stimulants may induce anorexia; however, as the effects of the stimulants subside, hunger develops.

suggest cirrhosis or other liver problems. Hypertension is a critical sign of withdrawal and is often accompanied by the physical signs of fluid retention in the legs or a protuberant abdomen swollen by liver ascites. Changes in mental status such as anxiety, confusion, irritability, memory loss, tremors, lack of coordination, and other neurologic signs are significant and may be associated with a number of causes including nutritional deficits (see the Nutrition Concepts box above). It is important for you to recognize and report these findings because they may indicate that the patient is entering physical withdrawal and may be at risk for delirium tremens and seizures if the drug of abuse is alcohol and/or a benzodiazepine. Be alert for needle tracks in unexpected parts of the body in an individual who is believed to have been abusing drugs intravenously. The atypical client may not have any obvious signs of physical problems, but abnormalities may be found on laboratory tests done when the client enters a treatment program.

DIAGNOSTIC TESTS

To assess the patient's physical status, a thorough physical examination is done on initiation of treatment, along with a basic laboratory screen chosen to identify problems in any of the major organ systems. Abnormalities are often seen on liver function tests, in electrolyte values, and on tests reflecting nutritional status and gastric function. Diseases such as hepatitis B and hepatitis C that can be spread through blood and body fluids may be identified, especially among intravenous drug users. Syphilis rates are increasing, and the escalating rate of human immunodeficiency virus (HIV) infection in this population is of national concern. Infections of various kinds are common. Special neurologic, neuropsychological, and imaging studies may disclose brain damage.

BLOOD ALCOHOL STUDY

A blood alcohol study is the most accurate type of test available to measure the degree of intoxication on ini-

tiation of treatment for alcohol abuse. A blood alcohol level above 0.3% requires treatment for overdose; at concentrations of over 0.4%, death is likely. Legal intoxication definitions vary from state to state but commonly are determined when a person's blood alcohol level is above 0.05%.

URINE DRUG SCREENING

Urine drug screening is the preferred way of screening for the recent use of an unknown drug and is commonly done along with the initial laboratory work. Drugs that are most likely to be identified in this way include amphetamines, barbiturates, benzodiazepines, cocaine, "crack," the opiates, marijuana, PCP, LSD, opioid analgesics, sedatives, and stimulants. With this test, drug metabolites can be identified for days or weeks after use, depending on the drug used. A special screen is necessary when looking for methadone. Typically, the collection of urine samples for this type of toxicology is witnessed by a staff member of the same sex to ensure that tampering with the specimens or substitution of another person's urine has not occurred. After collection, the sample is kept under "chain of custody": each person handling the sample signs a special document that accompanies the sample until it can be analyzed. Any temporary storage of the sample is maintained under secure conditions.

HAIR ANALYSIS

Hair analysis is a recent addition to the methods for the detection of abused substances. It requires sensitive technology but may be very helpful in monitoring patients for relapse. Depending on the length of the hair, substance use can be detected for up to 1 year after only 2 or 3 days of use. However, the presence of addiction or whether the person is currently under the influence of the substance cannot be inferred from a positive finding. The evidence this test provides regarding long-term substance use may prove to be a valuable tool in the diagnosis and follow-up of substance abusers in the future.

ALCOHOL AND ALCOHOLISM

Alcohol is the most commonly abused drug in the United States. According to the American Society of Addiction Medicine, alcoholism is:

a primary, chronic disease with psychosocial and environmental factors influencing its development and manifestations. The disease is often progressive and fatal. It is characterized by continuous or periodic impaired control over drinking, preoccupation with the drug alcohol, use of alcohol despite adverse consequences, and distortions in thinking, most notably denial.

It can be noted that alcohol is referred to as a "drug" in this definition, reflecting the thinking of most health care professionals that alcohol is indeed a drug with addictive qualities similar to those of other abused drugs.

Simple intoxication from alcohol usually lasts less than 12 hours and is followed by the unpleasant experience of a hangover beginning about 4 to 6 hours after the last drink. Typical symptoms include headache, upset stomach, vomiting, sweating, thirst, fatigue, and blurred vision or "seeing stars." The cause of these symptoms has not been pinpointed; however, it is believed to be a result of hypoglycemia, dehydration, and the buildup of acetaldehyde and lactic acid in the blood.

Chronic use involves the regular daily ingestion of large quantities of alcohol, regular heavy drinking only on weekends, or binges of heavy drinking followed by long periods of abstinence. Physical addiction occurs when alcohol becomes integrated into physiologic processes at the cellular level. The cell becomes dependent on the alcohol to carry on certain metabolic processes; if alcohol is no longer available, the cell goes into "shock" and is unable to compensate for the loss quickly. Thus alcohol withdrawal syndrome begins after the individual stops or decreases the amount ingested. Heavy chronic drinkers may experience the onset of withdrawal without actually stopping drinking simply because they are no longer able to ingest enough alcohol to meet the body's demands for the substance in order to function.

Alcohol withdrawal syndrome involves physiologic and behavioral symptoms that begin when the individual's blood alcohol level drops. It is divided into two stages, depending on the onset and severity of symptoms. The first stage usually occurs within 6 to 12 hours after the last drink and is called *early withdrawal.* Symptoms begin with anxiety, agitation, and irritability. If the patient does not drink, tremors may be observed. Blood pressure, pulse, and temperature all begin to rise. Sweating, nausea, vomiting, and diarrhea are typical.

The second stage, *major withdrawal,* begins with the onset of seizures and hallucinations and can advance to life-threatening delirium tremens (or "DTs"). This stage usually occurs after approximately 3 days (sometimes less) without alcohol or treatment and can be predicted from extreme elevations in temperature, pulse, and blood pressure. The patient typically becomes disoriented and confused. Hallucinations are often visual and "animal" in nature. Bugs, snakes, and rats are commonly described, sometimes perceived to be crawling on the person. Familiar jokes about seeing "pink elephants" probably evolved out of this type of withdrawal experience.

Alcohol withdrawal is the *most* life-threatening withdrawal syndrome compared with those associated with other types of commonly abused drugs, even heroin. (Withdrawal from barbiturates and benzodiazepines also can result in delirium tremens; both types of drugs have similar central nervous system [CNS] depressant effects.) Thus it is critical to counsel alcoholics never to attempt to withdraw on their own or "go cold turkey." They always should seek medical treatment. Most require inpatient hospitalization and administration of medications such as lorazepam (Ativan) or chlordiazepoxide (Librium) to prevent the severe consequences of withdrawal and to ensure early detection and treatment of symptoms.

MEDICAL COMPLICATIONS

Common medical complications of chronic alcoholism include cirrhosis of the liver, pancreatitis, gastrointestinal bleeding (often from esophageal varices), Wernicke's encephalopathy, Korsakoff's psychosis, and fetal alcohol syndrome.

Wernicke's Encephalopathy

Wernicke's encephalopathy is due to vitamin B_1 (thiamine) deficiency. Its symptoms include delirium, confabulation due to memory loss, unsteady gait, a sense of apprehension, and altered levels of consciousness that can proceed to coma. If it is not properly treated with vitamin supplementation, Korsakoff's psychosis may develop.

Korsakoff's Psychosis

In this disorder, both thiamine and niacin deficiencies contribute to the degeneration of the cerebrum and the peripheral nervous system. Symptoms include amnesia, confabulation, disorientation, and peripheral neuropathies. Despite treatment, some residual problems persist in both Wernicke's encephalopathy and Korsakoff's psychosis. However, dementia is permanent if the patient progresses to Korsakoff's psychosis. Both of these disorders are classified as *alcohol amnesic disorders.*

Fetal Alcohol Syndrome

Fetal alcohol syndrome is a medical complication that is of great concern in many countries. If a woman drinks to excess throughout pregnancy, the unborn child is at risk for symptoms such as low birth weight, mental retardation, growth deficiencies, heart defects, facial malformations, learning disabilities, and hyperactivity. Recent controversy has arisen over whether maternal alcoholism constitutes child abuse and is thus reportable under child protection statutes.

TREATMENT FOR ALCOHOL ABUSE

In recent years, active family involvement in the treatment of alcohol abuse has come to be seen as a critical factor in the effectiveness of treatment outcomes. It is accepted that the disease of alcoholism affects everyone in the family system. Alcoholism often produces predictable patterns of individual behavior or changes in roles that may significantly handicap various family members in getting their needs met. Examples of some of the labels given these atypical roles include the hero, the mascot, the lost child, and the scapegoat. Adult children of alcoholics may struggle with issues throughout their lives as a result of dysfunctional patterns of thoughts and behaviors learned in childhood through the enactment of these types of roles. Spouses of alcoholics frequently struggle with "enabling" behaviors. These are described as any behavior that "covers up" or protects alcoholics from the consequences of their drinking behaviors. For example, a woman might lie to her husband's boss as to the reasons why he will not be at work, when in reality the husband is too "hung over" to perform adequately. Those who enable are sometimes considered co-dependent in that their behavior is highly structured around managing and adapting to the substance abuser's dysfunctional behavior.

Family and peer pressure and confrontation can be critical factors in inducing the alcoholic to seek treatment. Through participation in a 12-step self-help support group for the significant others of substance abusers, called *Al-Anon* and *Al-Ateen*, spouses, children, friends, and co-workers can learn new ways of coping with issues and how to avoid enabling the alcoholic so that it becomes harder for him or her to continue the destructive pattern of drinking.

Intervention

An intervention is a planned, structured meeting by family and friends to confront the alcoholic with the effect that the person's alcohol abuse has on each member of the group. Often the alcoholic or substance abuser is brought into the meeting without prior notification about the intervention. The intervention is led by a specially trained interventionist who helps those involved in the process to prepare by writing down the ways that the person's alcohol abuse affects them personally. The interventionist offers suggestions on how to word ideas in ways less likely to evoke defensiveness and how to focus on the issues to reject the problem drinking but not the person. During the intervention, all of the participants have an opportunity to read their letters aloud to the alcohol abuser. At the end of each letter, the reader requests that the alcoholic go into treatment to get help. Usually, after hearing out a roomful of significant people confront them, the user will go unhappily, but voluntarily, directly from the intervention into a treatment program that has been arranged for in advance in the event of that outcome.

The use of this strategy has come under criticism because the user confronted in this way often feels co-

erced into treatment. After the intervention, the user may harbor angry feelings directed at members of the family for being critical, pushy, and having "tricked" him or her. Ideally, for treatment to be most effective, individuals should choose to go voluntarily. Proponents of the use of intervention respond that the user may die or suffer terrible consequences of the disease before seeking help on a totally voluntary basis and thus the end justifies the means.

Detoxification

Detoxification is usually done in an inpatient hospital. During detoxification, the patient's vital signs are monitored frequently. Initially, patients do not participate in group therapy because of their physical status. Rest and nutrition are emphasized. Drugs from the anxiolytic (benzodiazepine) group most often are used in detoxification of the alcoholic; however, hypnotics like phenobarbital or chloral hydrate are used occasionally. Intravenous magnesium sulfate may be used to prevent seizures in rare cases. Scheduled anticonvulsants are prescribed if seizures occur. Fluids are encouraged to combat dehydration, and vitamin replacement therapy is instituted.

Rehabilitation

Once patients are medically stable, they are referred to either an inpatient or an outpatient treatment program, depending on individual needs and resources. The traditional inpatient program, or Minnesota model, lasts about 28 days and includes highly structured scheduling of drug education films and presentations; increasingly confrontational individual, group, and family therapy; recreational and occupational therapy; milieu therapy; and introduction to Alcoholics Anonymous (AA), a self-help support group. However, the availability of third-party reimbursement for an inpatient rehabilitation stay has diminished significantly. More commonly, patients are referred to partial hospitalization programs (day treatment programs) and outpatient therapy as well as other community resources. Less common is an extended residential program that may last 1 to 2 years.

Alcoholics Anonymous. Alcoholics Anonymous is a nonprofit, worldwide organization of alcoholics who meet together anonymously in small groups at various times during the day throughout the year to assist each other in staying sober. The organization uses a strong spiritual base, which is controversial, and a 12-step program (Box 56-1) involving discussions and written exercises designed around each of the 12 steps as a means of keeping the alcoholic from relapsing. Members identify another participant of the same sex who is seasoned in the recovery process, and to whom they can relate, to act as their sponsor. The sponsor agrees to be available to the person for support and advice in staying sober. Service work in the community also is seen as integral to focusing outside oneself.

Box 56-1   *The 12 Steps of Alcoholics Anonymous*

1. We admit we were powerless over alcohol—our lives had become unmanageable.
2. Came to believe that a Power greater than ourselves could restore us to sanity.
3. Made a decision to turn our will and lives over to the care of God, as we understood Him.
4. Made a searching and fearless moral inventory of ourselves.
5. Admitted to God, to ourselves, and to another human being the exact nature of our wrongs.
6. Were entirely ready to have God remove all these defects of character.
7. Humbly asked Him to remove our shortcomings.
8. Listed all persons we had harmed and became willing to make amends to them all.
9. Made direct amends whenever possible except when to do so would injury them or others.
10. Continued to make personal inventory and when we were wrong promptly admitted it.
11. Sought through prayer and meditation to improve our conscious contact with God, as we understood Him, praying only for knowledge of His will for us and the power to carry it out.
12. Having had a spiritual awakening as the result of these steps, we tried to carry this message to alcoholics and to practice these principles in all our affairs.

The Twelve Steps are reprinted with permission of Alcoholics Anonymous World Services, Inc. Permission to reprint the Twelve Steps does not mean that AA has reviewed or approved the contents of this publication, nor that AA agrees with the views expressed herein. AA is a program of recovery from alcoholism—use of the Twelve Steps in connection with programs and activities that are patterned after AA, but which address other problems, does not imply otherwise.

Box 56-2   *The 12 Traditions of Alcoholics Anonymous*

1. Our common welfare should come first; personal recovery depends upon AA unity.
2. For our group purpose there is but one ultimate authority—a loving God as He may express Himself in our group conscience. Our leaders are but trusted servants; they do not govern.
3. The only requirement for AA membership is a desire to stop drinking.
4. Each group should be autonomous except in matters affecting other groups or AA as a whole.
5. Each group has but one primary purpose—to carry its message to the alcoholic who still suffers.
6. An AA group ought never endorse, finance, or lend the AA name to any related facility or outside enterprise, lest problems of money, property, and prestige divert us from our primary purpose.
7. Every AA group ought to be fully self-supporting, declining outside contributions.
8. Alcoholics Anonymous should remain forever nonprofessional, but our service centers may employ special workers.
9. AA, as such, ought never be organized; but we may create service boards or committees directly responsible to those they serve.
10. Alcoholics Anonymous has no opinion on outside issues; hence the AA name ought never be drawn into public controversy.
11. Our public relations policy is based on attraction rather than promotion; we need always maintain personal anonymity at the level of press, radio, and films.
12. Anonymity is the spiritual foundation of all our traditions, ever reminding us to place principles before personalities.

The Twelve Traditions are reprinted with permission of Alcoholics Anonymous World Services, Inc. Permission to reprint the Twelve Traditions does not mean that AA has reviewed or approved the contents of this publication, nor that AA agrees with the views expressed herein. AA is a program of recovery from alcoholism—use of the Twelve Traditions in connection with programs and activities that are patterned after AA, but which address other problems, does not imply otherwise.

Members use regular readings from the "Big Book" of AA, written by founding members to keep themselves on track. (Box 56-2 lists the 12 traditions of AA.) There are no dues; the organization relies on donations. There is no political involvement or endorsements of candidates or products. Everyone involved does so on a voluntary basis. Even group leaders are volunteers and are not professional counselors. Meetings may be advertised in the community using the title "Friends of Bill W." as a means of maintaining the anonymity of participants. (Bill W. was one of the two originators of the organization.) Before discharge from an inpatient treatment program, alcoholics have the opportunity to attend various community AA meetings to increase the odds of continued outpatient participation and to begin the process of finding a "home group" to which they can connect.

Recently, research has begun to question what actually works in alcohol rehabilitation. Actual outcomes of the traditional types of treatment approaches have not been clearly documented. As a result, many insurance companies no longer fund 28-day inpatient treatment. Many inpatient 28-day treatment programs have been forced to close because of a lack of clients able to afford the cost of this intensive treatment. Treatment facilities have been forced to provide brief and creative inpatient rehabilitation with rapid referral to an outpatient program and aftercare.

One trend is toward using more nontraditional treatment approaches that have produced successful outcomes. Some components of alcohol rehabilitation that have been shown to be very useful in maintaining continued sobriety are the teaching of stress management, social skills training, behavioral approaches, marital therapy, and matching clients with a therapist who uses a style most likely to benefit their personality type. A move also is underway in which treatment programs are attempting to group patients with similar lifestyles and characteristics together rather than to "lump" everyone together. Other factors being considered in developing more homogeneous small groups are styles of thinking (abstract vs. concrete thinkers), sex role–related issues, ethnicity, and age. The current trend is away from a "recipe card" approach to treatment that is expected to work for anyone who is an alcoholic (see Nursing Care Plan: The Patient Abusing Alcohol on p. 1273).

Cost-containment has stimulated the development of many new types of outpatient programs for the treatment of alcoholism. Most day treatment or partial hospitalization programs are very similar to the traditional inpatient milieu and offer similar types of therapies, but they allow patients to return to their own homes at night. In this case, the risk of relapse often requires the use of medication such as disulfiram (Antabuse) or metronidazole (Flagyl), which makes the user ill if mixed with alcohol. Usually, involvement in the program is intensive but does not last for the traditional 30 days.

Other individuals utilize active involvement in AA as the primary means for recovery by attending at least "90 meetings in 90 days." Other community programs also are available to assist the alcoholic in the recovery process and should not be overlooked. Some are church related; some are focused on getting the recovering user back to work by providing job placement or an opportunity to return to school. One example of a community recovery program that exists in various parts of the country is the Patrician Movement. In addition, halfway houses may be available in the local area as a service of community mental health organizations.

Relapse Prevention

Relapse prevention is a key component in the treatment of persons with substance abuse or dependence. Relapse prevention involves assisting patients to identify triggers to their substance use. For example, a person may identify friends who consistently use the abused substance or places where there is drinking or using; the person recognizes that being with those friends or in those places sets himself or herself up to drink or use. As part of the relapse prevention strategy, the person then actively avoids those people and places. Other coping strategies also are developed that can be used if the person encounters a trigger.

Aftercare and Recovery

One of the newer aspects of the recovery process involves various types of aftercare services to assist alcoholics who have completed a treatment program successfully to make a gradual transition back into the community with the support necessary to prevent relapses. Many inpatient substance abuse programs now provide aftercare groups to discharged patients as a supplement to continued involvement in AA and other 12-step support groups such as Adult Children of Alcoholics and Codependents Anonymous.

Medications

The treatment team may recommend the use of disulfiram (Antabuse) to assist the alcoholic who is highly

motivated to remain sober but recognizes that poor impulse control may increase the odds of relapse. This particular drug inhibits the metabolism of alcohol in the body, producing an uncomfortable, potentially life-threatening reaction to exposure to alcohol. Disulfiram is taken daily and lasts in the body for up to 2 weeks. Thus if the alcoholic gets the urge to drink, the presence of the drug in the system usually provides the necessary negative reinforcement to resist the impulse. Signs and symptoms of a disulfiram-alcohol reaction include flushing, headache, nausea, vomiting, dizziness, rapid heart rate, difficulty breathing, sweating, confusion, and hypotension that may lead to coma, convulsions, and death. The severity of the symptoms varies from person to person, and symptoms can last for 30 to 60 minutes or more.

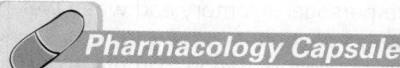
Pharmacology Capsule

Disulfiram (Antabuse) is sometimes used to assist a recovering alcoholic who is highly motivated to remain sober but recognizes that poor impulse control may increase odds of relapse.

The danger of giving disulfiram to a person who is poorly motivated to stop drinking is that he or she might either stop taking the medication in order to drink or drink in spite of taking the medication and become seriously ill. As a result, careful patient teaching is essential. The patient must be taught to avoid alcohol in foods (e.g., salad dressings, sauces, candies, or chocolate prepared with liqueurs), in topical preparations (e.g., cologne, aftershave, or liniments), in medications (e.g., over-the-counter cold preparations or cough syrups), and in mouthwashes containing alcohol. Alcohol wipes cannot be used by the nurse to cleanse the skin in preparation for an injection without a topical reaction. Because of the risks of accidental exposure to a substance containing alcohol, patients are encouraged to wear a medical alert bracelet or carry a card in their wallet to alert emergency care personnel to a possible disulfiram-alcohol reaction in the event they are found unconscious. Patients also are asked to sign a consent form for the use of the drug before it is prescribed to document that proper instructions about diet, risks, precautions, and type of emergency care needed in the event of exposure to alcohol have been offered and are understood. It is important for the nurse to be alert for

Pharmacology Capsule

Do not use alcohol to cleanse injection sites if the patient is taking disulfiram.

NURSING CARE PLAN

The Patient Who Is Abusing Alcohol

ASSESSMENT

Health History: A 37-year-old man was admitted for alcohol detoxification. He was found lying on the floor at home, passed out, and appeared to have vomited and been incontinent of urine and feces. He has a long history of alcohol abuse but claims he does not have a problem because he drinks only beer. He recently lost his job because he was not reporting for work on time, and his wife has threatened to leave him if he does not stop drinking. His two children, ages 8 and 10, are afraid of him when he drinks. His usual intake of alcohol is two six-packs of beer a day. He has been detoxified in the hospital and is now ready for the rehabilitation phase of his treatment.

Physical Examination: Vital signs: temperature, 97.6° F orally; pulse, 80; respiration, 20; blood pressure, 128/72. Height, 5'10". Weight, 160 lb. The patient's skin and eyes have a slightly yellowish tinge. A cast is on his left arm from below the elbow to the fingers. He appears thin and wasted.

Nursing Diagnosis	Goals and Outcome Criteria	Interventions
Ineffective Denial related to continued alcohol abuse	Patient will acknowledge that he has a problem, stop ingesting alcohol, and attend Alcoholics Anonymous (AA) meetings on a regular basis.	Use confrontational techniques to help patient accept the diagnosis of alcoholism, and support patient's 12-step program of rehabilitation.
Ineffective Coping related to alcohol ingestion as a means of coping with stressors	Patient will overcome his impulse to drink alcohol until intoxicated and to use alcohol as a coping mechanism, as evidenced by stopping ingestion of alcohol and substituting other coping mechanisms.	Help patient overcome cravings by introducing new coping mechanisms such as exercise and stress management skills; encourage patient to attend treatment program and AA meetings on a regular basis.
Chronic Low Self-Esteem related to loss of control, guilty feelings	Patient will maintain an adequate self-concept, as evidenced by lessened self-criticism, good hygiene, and positive interactions with others.	Help patient maintain self-esteem after confrontational therapy sessions by allowing him to vent his feelings and acting as a role model for dealing with others.
	Patient will develop a realistic sense of self, verbalize positive aspects of self and begin to forgive himself, and express his true feelings.	Allow patient to vent his feelings about his illness and to explore his feelings about his past behaviors; support patient in his 12-step program of rehabilitation.
Risk for Injury related to excessive use of alcohol and high risk for relapse	Patient will not injure himself or others as a result of excessive ingestion of alcohol.	Encourage patient to abstain from drinking by supporting his participation in rehabilitation activities. Intervene at the first signs of impending relapse.

❓ CRITICAL THINKING QUESTIONS

- Describe two techniques you might use to help the patient vent his feelings.

- Describe in detail two coping mechanisms that may help the patient overcome cravings for alcohol.

---

patient attempts to bypass the prohibitive effects of disulfiram by ingesting large doses of vitamin C in order to have a drink on occasion. Patients who are addicted are often very knowledgeable about drug treatment and can easily find out that massive doses of vitamin C

are given intravenously for the treatment of overdose or disulfiram-alcohol reactions.

The use of disulfiram is contraindicated in individuals with impaired liver function, heart problems, or significant debilitation. Obviously, safe use of the drug also requires that the person have no memory impairments, self-destructive intentions, or poor judgment.

Sometimes, metronidazole (Flagyl) is used for similar purposes because it also produces an uncomfortable reaction when combined with alcohol but does not produce the severe life-threatening reactions described for disulfiram. Also, it does not remain in the system for an extended period and it still can be given in the event of many medical problems in which disulfiram is contraindicated.

Research efforts continue to attempt to identify other types of drugs that could assist alcoholics to go through withdrawal more comfortably and avoid relapse. Medications currently under scrutiny for this purpose include naltrexone hydrochloride (Trexan), antidepressants such as amitriptyline hydrochloride (Elavil), desipramine hydrochloride (Norpramin), fluoxetine hydrochloride (Prozac), and angiotensin-converting enzyme (ACE) inhibitors such as enalapril maleate (Vasotec).

PSYCHOACTIVE SUBSTANCES OTHER THAN ALCOHOL

Six classes of psychoactive substances other than alcohol are often associated with substance abuse or, using the term that is currently popular, *chemical dependence*. These are the stimulants, depressants (barbiturates and benzodiazepines), hallucinogens, narcotics (opioids), inhalants, and designer drugs (Table 56-1). Each class is different in the types of symptoms produced and the way in which patients abusing them are managed.

STIMULANTS

Stimulants include amphetamines ("speed") and similar drugs, plus cocaine or "crack."

Amphetamines

Amphetamines usually are used orally or intravenously on a daily basis or on binges. They are very psychologically addictive (producing **psychological dependence**)—the dose is gradually increased over time to produce the euphoria (or "high") that is extremely pleasurable. Symptoms often include hyperactivity, irritability, combativeness, and after extended use, paranoia. A person intoxicated by amphetamines may be very dangerous. There are no physical with-

drawal symptoms, but the user typically experiences a profound depression and sense of exhaustion called "crashing." Selective serotonin reuptake inhibitors (SSRIs) and other types of antidepressants such as bupropion (Wellbutrin) are commonly used to treat the depression, which may persist in chronic users for up to 2 years after the last amphetamine use. Toxic psychosis may occur in approximately 90% of chronic users up to 1 year past the last use. Unfortunately, 5% to 15% of these individuals never fully recover. Neuroleptics may be used to treat toxic psychosis.

"Ice" is a form of methamphetamine ingested by smoking, with results similar to those produced by crack (a form of cocaine that is smoked). Effects last as long as 14 hours; the user often will do anything to obtain the drug and also is considered at risk for being very dangerous while under the influence.

Cocaine

Cocaine is a highly addictive alkaloid of the plant *Erythroxylon coca*, which grows in Peru and Bolivia. Cocaine produces an intense feeling of euphoria that usually lasts only 30 to 60 minutes; however, the substance remains in the brain for about 10 days after use. Pure forms of cocaine are quite expensive. It is typically inhaled nasally or mixed with other drugs, like heroin, and injected intravenously ("speedballs"). It is very psychologically addicting, which is thought to be due to overstimulation of the pleasure centers of the brain. Physical withdrawal symptoms have not traditionally been thought to occur; however, a physical syndrome has been hypothesized and is currently under debate.

Symptoms of chronic inhalation include runny nose, sniffles, frequent colds, weight loss, hyperactivity, and damage to the nasal mucosa or septum that may be severe enough to require surgical repair. Psychologically, cocaine abusers lose interest in their usual activities and demonstrate abrupt mood swings, poor judgment, impatience, and ultimately suspiciousness and hallucinations. Cocaine intoxication also can occur but usually lasts only about 24 hours after the last use. Cocaine is a very dangerous drug in that strokes, seizures, and heart attacks that are sometimes fatal can occur even in first-time users.

Treatment often employs diazepam (Valium) or phenobarbital for their sedative effects. Neuroleptics may be used in the event of psychosis. Many clients are severely depressed for up to 2 years after quitting. Studies have shown that damage to the brain may impair the patient's ability to experience pleasure. Antidepressants such as bupropion (Wellbutrin) and cardiac drugs such as propranolol hydrochloride (Inderal) or calcium channel blockers may be helpful in this event.

Crack

Crack is a hardened form of cocaine that is smoked. It presents major problems in many urban areas of the United States because it is readily available and inexpensive compared with other drugs. It produces a tremendously addicting, short-acting psychological euphoria that is quickly followed by "crashing," which stimulates continued cravings and use. The cravings are so intense that, as with "ice," the user will do almost anything to obtain more of the drug and often resorts to violence if thwarted. Overdose of this drug is life-threatening because no drug is available to counteract the overstimulation, which results in respiratory failure.

DEPRESSANTS

Drugs misused in this category include the sedatives, hypnotics, and anxiolytics. They are obtained by prescription for anxiety or insomnia or are purchased illegally. They are typically taken orally. Regular use results in physical dependency. Symptoms of overdose include oversedation, respiratory depression, impaired coordination, and brain damage. Intoxication with barbiturates is even more dangerous than with benzodiazepines. Although benzodiazepines and barbiturates are similar to alcohol in terms of dangerous physical withdrawal reactions (delirium tremens, seizures), barbiturate overdose induces an anesthesia-like state. Symptoms of barbiturate withdrawal usually occur somewhat later, sometimes days after the last use, depending on the half-life of the particular drug. Once a person is dependent, abruptly stopping any of these drugs also may trigger psychosis.

HALLUCINOGENS

Hallucinogens include LSD (lysergic acid diethylamide or "acid"), PCP (phencyclidine or "angel dust"), MDMA (3, 4-methylenedioxymethamphetamine, known as "ecstasy" or "Adam"), and marijuana.

LSD

LSD is not physically addicting but can produce physical symptoms of altered perceptions that are dreamlike, often with an altered sense of time and feelings that one has attained special insight. Emotions are intensified and labile. Individuals often experience depersonalization, in which they feel as if they are floating outside of themselves or in unreal surroundings. The drugs typically are used to enhance self-awareness and usually are taken episodically (approximately twice a week). Acute adverse reactions are most often described as a "bad trip" involving paranoia, depression, frightening hallucinations, and occasionally an acute confusional state. The person experiencing a bad trip is responsive to verbal support and reassurance. The primary danger of the use of these drugs is accidental death as a result of perceptual distortions (e.g., attempting to fly off a building) or seizures related to the cutting agent used. Cutting agents are chemicals that may be quite toxic, which are used in the manufacturing or dilution of the final drug product. Chronic long-term adverse reactions include psychosis, depression, paranoia, and flashbacks. LSD use is regaining popularity.

PCP

PCP differs from other hallucinogens in that abusers experience a psychotic state similar to that observed in schizophrenics. Brain reward areas are stimulated so that abusers can stimulate themselves mentally in a pleasurable way. Studies also suggest that this drug is strongly physically addictive, with a severe withdrawal reaction occurring after binge use. Unexpected sensory stimuli that interrupt the individual's internal experience may provoke unpredictable violence. The person may possess enormous strength and may feel no pain. The risks of use thus involve serious injury to oneself or others, in addition to severely elevated temperature, hypertensive crisis, and renal failure. Under acute intoxication, patients are best managed by reducing stimuli as much as possible, often by seclusion, even to the point of avoiding talking or performing routine treatments until the patient is stabilized. If violent, mechanical restraint is necessary.

Marijuana

Marijuana often is included in the hallucinogenic category of abused drugs because it produces an effect similar to that of LSD when smoked. The inner experience is altered so that individuals experience heightened awareness, distortion of space and time, heightened sensitivity to sound, and sometimes depersonalization. Although use may produce paranoia, the "bad trip" phenomenon of LSD is rare with marijuana. It also tends to have a sedative rather than stimulant effect and is unlikely to produce true hallucinations. Marijuana is psychologically addicting. Controversy persists about the negative effects of chronic use of this drug. It has been suggested that marijuana may produce psychosis in fragile individuals and a lack of motivation and a reduction in fertility and sexual performance in young men. However, the studies that suggest these conclusions can be challenged by others just as convincing that present the opposite findings. Chronic smoking of marijuana irritates the lungs and may contribute to the occurrence of lung cancer.

In the medical community, derivatives of marijuana show promise as medication for the treatment of glaucoma, asthma, nausea and vomiting as a result of chemotherapy, and as an appetite stimulant.

NARCOTICS (OPIOIDS)

The narcotic drugs often misused include the opioids heroin, morphine, oxycodone (OxyContin), hydrocodone, pentazocine (Talwin), methadone, and meperidine (Demerol).

Heroin

Heroin is a highly addictive narcotic that produces a euphoria on intravenous use. The person experiences a "rush" and then gradually nods off to sleep. On awakening, the person feels immune to stressors until the withdrawal symptoms begin to trigger the

Table 56-1 *Common Mood-Altering Chemicals*

DRUG NAME	EFFECTS	SITE OF ACTION	LENGTH OF EFFECT
HALLUCINOGENS			
Mushroom (psilocybin)	Altered body image	Central nervous system (CNS)	Onset: 40-60 min
LSD (lysergic acid diethylamide)	Euphoria		Duration: 6-12 hr
Mescaline (from peyote cactus)	Sharpened perceptions		
	Somatic effects: dizziness, tremors, weakness, nausea		
DOM (dimethoxy-methylamphetamine)	Psychosis-like symptoms		
	Emotional swings		
STP (no chemical name)	Suspiciousness		
	Bizarre behavior		
MDA, Ecstasy (methylenedioxy-amphetamine)	Increased blood pressure		
	Increased temperature		
	Objective signs: dilated pupils, flushing, tremors		
CANNABINOIDS			
Marijuana	Failure in judgment and memory	CNS	Administration and dose dependent
Hashish	Euphoria	Cardiovascular system	Onset: 20-30 min
	Mild intoxication	Respiratory system	Duration: 3-7 hr
	Relaxation		
	Sexual arousal		
	Panic states		
	Visual hallucinations		
	Objective signs: reddened eyes, dry mouth, incoordination; heart rate to 140/min		
OPIOIDS (OPIOIDS, SEMISYNTHETIC, AND SYNTHETIC ANALGESICS)			
Codeine	Analgesia	CNS (opioid receptors)	Onset: 20-30 min
Morphine	Euphoria	Respiratory system	Duration: 4-8 hr
Heroin	Escape		
Hydromorphone (Dilaudid)	Reduced sexual and aggressive drives		
Methadone	Respiratory depression		
Meperidine (Demerol)	Sedation, sleepiness		
Propoxyphene (Darvon)	Objective signs: hypertension, pupillary constriction, constipation		
Designer drugs			
SEDATIVE-HYPNOTICS AND ANXIOLYTICS			
Barbiturates	Drowsiness, sedation	CNS	Onset: 30-40 min
Secobarbital (Seconal)	Euphoria	Cardiovascular system	Duration: varies with each drug, barbiturates may have longer half-life than benzodiazepines depending on the agent
Phenobarbital (Nembutal)	Escape	Respiratory system	
Amobarbital (Amytal)	Loss of aggressive and sexual drives		
Amobarbital/Secobarbital (Tuinal)	Emotional lability		
	Poor judgment		
Barbiturate-like (methaqualone [Quaalude])			
Benzodiazepines (alprazolam [Xanax], chlordiazepoxide [Librium], diazepam [Valium], lorazepam [Ativan])			

Data from Naegle, M.A. (1997). Substance-related disorders. In J. Haber, B. Krainovich, A.L. McMahon, & P. Price-Hoskins (Eds.). *Comprehensive psychiatric nursing* (5th ed., pp. 513-515). St. Louis: Mosby.

need to "cop a fix" again. This usually occurs 8 to 12 hours after the last use. Risks of chronic use of heroin include overdose, malnutrition, and respiratory arrest as well as hepatitis B, hepatitis C, and HIV infections from shared needle use.

Symptoms of withdrawal include tearing of the eyes, runny nose, gooseflesh, sweating, alternating fever and chills, muscle and joint pain, upset stomach, diarrhea, loss of appetite, restlessness, and irritability. Individuals usually are in such subjective distress that

Table 56-1   *Common Mood-Altering Chemicals —cont'd*

DRUG NAME	EFFECTS	SITE OF ACTION	LENGTH OF EFFECT
STIMULANTS			
Amphetamine (methamphetamine, Dexedrine, Benzedrine) Methylphenidate (Ritalin) Cocaine, crack	Euphoria, grandiosity Wakefulness Relief of fatigue Stimulation, energy, anxiety Depression Suppression of appetite Aggressive feelings, paranoia Objective signs: sweating, dilated pupils, increased blood pressure, rapid heart and respiratory rates, tremors, seizures	CNS Peripheral nervous system Cardiovascular system	Onset: route related; 10-30 min Duration: drug related
PHENCYCLIDINES			
PCP (phencyclidine, "angel dust")	Detachment from surroundings Decreased sensory awareness Illusions of superhuman strength Acute intoxication Objective signs: flushing, fever, sweating, coma, agitation, confusion, hallucinations, paranoia, violence	CNS	Rapid onset: 2-3 min up to 45 min Duration: drug and dose related
INHALANTS			
Benzene (paint thinner, cleaning fluid, glue) Nitrites Nitrous oxide	Euphoria Giddiness, headache, fatigue, drowsiness Objective signs: dysrhythmias, damage to kidneys, liver abnormalities	CNS Cardiac effect	Onset: immediate Duration: 20-45 min
ALCOHOL			
Beverage alcohol, beer, wine	Relaxation, sedation, release of inhibitions Objective signs: incoordination, nausea, vomiting, slurred speech	CNS Respiratory system	Onset: 20 min-1 hr Duration: dose related
XANTHINES			
Caffeine	Stimulation Restlessness Anxiety Objective signs: increased heart and respiratory rates, diarrhea, gastric disorder, insomnia, tremors	CNS	Onset: 10-30 min Duration: 3-7 hr
NICOTINE			
Cigarettes Smokeless tobacco	Stimulation Enhanced performance	CNS Respiratory system Cardiovascular system Endocrine system	Onset: immediate Duration: 5-15 min

they inappropriately seek medications from the staff while in treatment. It is very challenging to work with these patients and is sometimes difficult to remain nonjudgmental.

To support their ever-increasing habit, many people addicted to heroin resort to crime, such as stealing. Sometimes they seek detoxification only to reduce the level of the dose needed to experience the pleasurable response to the drug—a lower dose is less expensive to obtain.

INHALANTS

A very dangerous type of substance abuse is that involving inhalant misuse. Examples of chemicals often inhaled for the mind-altering response include paint, glue, aerosol sprays, "whiteout," and gasoline. They are usually placed in a plastic bag or other container that is then placed over the nose and mouth and inhaled. This is known also as "huffing." Symptoms appearing in the individual under the influence of the drug depend on the substance inhaled and include nosebleeds, bloodshot eyes, infected lesions around the nose and mouth, and severe disorientation or unconsciousness. The risks include progressive brain damage, asphyxiation, seizures, depressed bone marrow leading to aplastic anemia, liver or kidney damage, or cardiac dysrhythmias. There is no physical withdrawal syndrome.

This particular group of drugs often is misused among teenagers because of its easy availability and low cost. The cumulative brain damage from chronic use is a very serious problem among poor and minority adolescents.

DESIGNER DRUGS

A new group of abused drugs on the illegal market includes synthetic drugs especially designed to sidestep categorization with any of the drugs identified as illegal in the United States. Although use of these drugs may not be technically illegal, their misuse presents unique hazards. "Ecstasy" is an example of a synthetic drug generally grouped with the hallucinogens; it is also called "Adam." A very similar second-generation designer drug is called "Eve." "China White" is an example of a synthetic type of heroin that acts in much the same way as heroin. Major risks are present when the abuser mixes these drugs with those from the other groups, because the results are unpredictable.

DISORDERS ASSOCIATED WITH SUBSTANCE ABUSE

The risk of human immunodeficiency virus disease (HIVD), the illness that precedes acquired immunodeficiency syndrome (AIDS), continues to present the greatest danger for patients who are abusing intravenous drugs because of the common practice of sharing needles. The Centers for Disease Control and Prevention indicates an alarming number of new cases of HIV-positive diagnoses among intravenous drug users and their sexual partners. Nursing care for these patients now includes teaching them how to clean their "works" with bleach and how to use condoms correctly.

Individuals who have or are predisposed to a serious psychiatric illness may present with an active case of the mental disorder. By altering levels of brain chemicals that control emotions, thought processes, and behavior, misuse of these chemicals can trigger an exacerbation of an existing illness.

Another major area of concern is the effect of intrauterine exposure to these chemicals on the fetus. Fetuses carried by mothers who are physically addicted to an opioid are born addicted and also may experience developmental delays and a prolonged lack of the capacity to feel pleasure even after they have been successfully weaned from the abused drug. "Cocaine babies" are currently being studied for clues to the consequences of prenatal exposure to the drug. Findings suggest that attention deficit disorder (with or without hyperactivity) occurs more often in this population, along with dyslexia, other neurologic problems, and learning disabilities.

Clients with chronic pain disorders also are very vulnerable to the abuse of drugs, especially those of the opioid and depressant groups, because of their frequent frustration over an inability to manage their pain effectively. Also, many lack knowledge of the risks of regular use of pain medication. They often feel betrayed by their physician and other caregivers because they were not informed about prescribed analgesics and pain management (e.g., the importance of temperate use along with the use of exercise and other types of supportive techniques to manage pain and avoid addiction).

TREATMENT FOR SUBSTANCE ABUSE

Substance abuse treatment is very similar to alcohol detoxification and rehabilitation. Narcotics Anonymous (NA) is structured much like AA but focuses on the abuse of drugs other than alcohol. Often, inpatient treatment programs place recovering addicts with alcoholics for educational and therapy groups. However, the rate of relapse is much higher for most drug abuse patients, especially those who use highly addicting intravenous drugs. A booming area of research is the identification of alternative treatments and medications that will help drug abusers detoxify more comfortably from the chemicals that they are addicted to and reduce the risks of relapse. Currently, there is some support for treating drug abuse separately from alcohol abuse.

As with alcohol abuse treatment, family involvement in the process is very important. Al-Anon is the support group for family members or significant others of a substance-abusing person. It is recommended that members of the family begin attending meetings as soon as they realize that the person is using some type of drug. The intervention process described on p. 1270 may be used in an attempt to get the person into treatment.

Many patients who use drugs have legal problems, which may provide the catalyst for seeking help. Sometimes they are mandated by the courts to go into treatment; at other times their attorney recommends treatment before the case goes to court in order to influence the judge favorably before sentencing. In the past, many individuals were involuntarily committed to state hospital drug treatment programs for 30 days. However, many state hospital systems across the country are closing their drug and alcohol treatment units because of the program expense and the need to provide additional services to the seriously mentally ill, which often is judged more of a priority.

DETOXIFICATION

Detoxification from physically addicting drugs is very complex because of the likelihood of polysubstance abuse and the uncertainty of what to expect when two or more drugs are mixed together. Usually, inpatient hospitalization is recommended for safety. However, some individuals who have been using drugs that are primarily psychologically addicting may not demonstrate many physical symptoms but, rather, experience intense psychological cravings. For example, if a conversation about past drug use occurs within the recovering addict's hearing or if something in the environment triggers memories of the "high" sensation that he or she experienced while using, the person may experience cravings that stimulate feelings of restlessness, itching, hives, flushing, and elevated blood pressure and pulse, which are believed to be psychogenic in origin. These patients need a great deal of support to help them overcome the profound urge to use. This experience puts the patient at very high risk for relapse.

MEDICATIONS
Methadone

Methadone is one drug used in the treatment of heroin addicts. There is, however, some controversy about using this medication because the drug is a synthetic opioid analgesic that also may be prescribed appropriately for chronic severe pain. Given orally (in diskette or liquid form), it is absorbed slowly and does not produce the "rush" normally experienced with the intravenous use of heroin. It also alleviates the cravings for more opioids for a short period of time, depending on the dose given. In detoxification, the dose of the drug is gradually reduced without telling patients exactly what dose they are getting. Although this process is one of substituting another addictive drug for the one misused by the client, some believe it to be justified in that withdrawal from methadone is less uncomfortable for the patient. The patient also risks severe respiratory depression in the event that heroin is injected while methadone is in the system. The most typical problematic side effects of methadone include severe constipation and profound sweating.

 Pharmacology Capsule

Methadone is a synthetic opioid analgesic that may be used in the detoxification of heroin-related opioid addiction.

Clonidine

Clonidine hydrochloride (Catapres) has become a more popular means of assisting the substance abuser through detoxification. It is a non-opiate antihypertensive drug that partially blocks withdrawal symptoms. Clonidine does not completely remove the unpleasant feelings that accompany heroin withdrawal. Unfortunately, some may leave treatment because of the inherent discomfort and unrealistic expectations that they should not feel sick at all while using the drug to withdraw.

Naloxone

Naloxone hydrochloride (Narcan) and nalmefene (Revex) green label are opioid antagonists that counteract the dangerous respiratory depressant effects of heroin or other opiate overdose. When Narcan is given to a person who is addicted and under the influence of an opiate, the person may experience acute withdrawal symptoms.

 Put on Your Thinking Cap!

Can you explain why Narcan would cause a person who is addicted to opioids to experience acute withdrawal symptoms?

Many other drugs are currently under investigation to determine whether they could assist the substance abuser by reducing the cravings for the drug abused or by counteracting the long-term psychological consequences of use of certain drugs. Examples of these include some of the antidepressants, anticonvulsants, and various herbal agents.

Still other medications may be used in the supportive treatment of those undergoing opiate withdrawal to control symptoms such as diarrhea, abdominal cramping, and generalized, diffuse pain.

 Consider the Alternative

Some herbal remedies are being studied for use as agents to reduce withdrawal symptoms.

REHABILITATION

In most cases, the process of rehabilitation for drug abuse is very similar to that for alcohol abuse. Instead of attendance at AA meetings, the client often participates in NA at least some of the time. This support group is based on the 12 steps of AA except that the word "alcohol" is replaced by "drugs" in all of the literature. Also, the case histories used for reading assignments are about other addicts in recovery related specifically to the use of drugs other than alcohol; this is to help the client identify with people with similar struggles. Relapse rates for individuals abusing drugs other than alcohol alone are much higher and present unique issues. Trends suggest that future treatment programs will be more likely to separate clients into small groups of people facing similar issues and having similar characteristics; this is to individualize the recovery process much more than is done in most settings today. Most current settings may advertise more than one "track" for substance abuse treatment. However, in reality, clients share the same facilities and participate in most of the traditional programming mixed together despite different learning styles and other issues. It has been suggested that this practice may actually place clients who do not fit the traditional mold at higher risk for relapse.

On an outpatient basis, these clients are encouraged to participate in NA on a regular basis (90 meetings in the first 90 days), just as those recovering from alcoholism do. Attempts are usually made to allow the client to experience different group locations and times before discharge from the inpatient setting to increase the likelihood that the client will participate as recommended. Various other community programs may be available, such as the Patrician Movement, which provides outpatient treatment on an ongoing basis for those who cannot afford more costly inpatient rehabilitation. Many private health care systems are opening day treatment programs for substance abusers as insurance reimbursement for long-term inpatient programs becomes less available.

AFTERCARE AND RECOVERY

Recovering substance abusers may be offered an opportunity to participate in a support group provided by the hospital at which they received treatment. Many of the same people who went through treatment at the same time participate together. Because the relationships built during this time of crisis are often intense, the groups can be very helpful in preventing relapse. It is hoped that clients also will continue regular participation in NA groups on an ongoing basis. Some individuals do well in halfway houses, which allow for a new living environment surrounded by other recovering addicts during the difficult transition back into the community. Sometimes it is recommended that patients do not return to work until their ability to cope with stress is more developed.

METHADONE MAINTENANCE

Some patients who have experienced multiple relapses into heroin abuse after treatment may have sustained permanent damage to chemical receptor sites in the brain, which decreases their ability to resist relapse. As a result, methadone maintenance is not uncommon. In this process, the person goes to a methadone clinic on a daily or three-times-a-week basis to receive a dose or doses of the medication to cover the next 24 to 72 hours. A single dose may be administered in liquid form or in a diskette dissolved in juice, and the person is carefully observed by clinic staff members to ensure that the medication is actually taken and not hoarded in any way. The patient may continue this process indefinitely, often for many years. Sometimes the dose of the methadone is maintained at the same level without attempts to reduce the dose, whereas at other times gradual titration is attempted.

Methadone maintenance programs have been criticized highly across the United States because the process is often viewed as exchanging one addiction for another without attempts to detoxify the patient. In addition, clinic records and security have been lax in many instances, resulting in clinic methadone thefts and illegal sales on the street. Supporters of the programs counter these arguments by pointing out that criteria for involvement in these programs require that patients have been unsuccessful in remaining "clean" after detoxification on more than one occasion and that they no longer are "forced" into crime to support their habit. In addition, methadone is administered in such a way that no rush is experienced, allowing the person to return to school or work and reintegrate into society without the risk of losing everything to relapse. Methadone maintenance programs also are more cost-effective than residential treatment or jail time.

The controversy over methadone maintenance has resulted in the frequent use of naltrexone (Trexan) as an alternative. This drug is related to naloxone (Narcan) and is a pure opioid antagonist. This means that the drug reduces or completely blocks the effects of any intravenous opioids in the patient's system. The detoxified patient is placed on this drug to help prevent use of heroin. If the patient takes small doses of heroin while on naltrexone, no effect is experienced; however, if the patient injects large doses, he or she will become very physically ill and may die or sustain serious injury such as a coma. An addicted person taking naltrexone soon after regular use of heroin will experience withdrawal symptoms due to the antagonist actions of the drug.

Research is underway to evaluate the use of various types of other psychotropic medications to stabilize neurochemical and neurophysiologic alterations in the brains of addicted persons. This may eventually provide an answer to the high rates of relapse in opioid abusers.

NURSING CARE *of the Person with a Substance Disorder*

Assessment

The initial step in developing a nursing plan of care for the substance abuser is always a thorough assessment. The data you collect on first contact with the patient can help identify and prioritize problems that must be addressed to maximize the likelihood that the patient will remain sober. Examples of the types of problems often seen in substance abusers of any kind include denial, poor impulse control, high risk for injury, high

Pharmacology Capsule

Methadone maintenance is used for patients who have experienced multiple relapses into heroin abuse following standard treatment and rehabilitation efforts.

risk for relapse, guilt, and low self-esteem. Detailed assessment of the person with a substance disorder is detailed on pp. 1267 and 1268.

Nursing Diagnoses, Goals, and Outcome Criteria: Substance Abuse

NURSING DIAGNOSES	GOALS AND OUTCOME CRITERIA
Ineffective Coping related to substance use, as evidenced by using substances to deal with anxiety, emotional discomfort, and stress	Improved coping: identifies and uses healthy alternative coping strategies to deal with anxiety, emotional discomfort, and stress; patient verbalizes strategies to prevent relapse
Ineffective Denial related to substance use and refusal to acknowledge actual consequences of substance use	Verbalizes an internalized sense that the substance use is unhealthy, out of control, and that the treatment is required
Risk for Injury related to excessive use of the drug and high risk for relapse, manifested by a history of falls; driving while under the influence and combining the substance abused with other substances; being aggressive while under the influence; reduced attendance at AA or NA meetings; frequent dreams of drug use; returning to places where one used drugs; not seeking relief for high stress.	Decreased risk for injury to self and others: patient does not engage in dangerous activities when under drug influence

Interventions

Nursing interventions for substance abusers in detoxification involve regular physical assessment (with the frequency determined by the severity of symptoms), administration of appropriate medications, and teaching the patients about their actions and consequences. Providing adequate nutrition is critical, because the patient may have been eating very irregularly and also may be quite dehydrated. High levels of anxiety during detoxification also require a great deal of reassurance and support, providing the opportunity to help

the patient begin to process the impending decision to continue in rehabilitation.

Once the patient has agreed to participate in rehabilitation, the focus of nursing care changes from one of primarily attending to the physical concerns of the patient to assisting the client in processing the meaning of his or her substance abuse and planning for a future without continued use of that substance. The biggest issue to be addressed at first is the heavily entrenched denial that most substance abusers possess. Often they minimize the severity of the abuse, perhaps lying outright about how much they actually were using. You must work toward penetrating this denial without further damaging the individual's self-esteem. This has traditionally demanded more confrontational techniques than appropriate in other types of psychiatric treatment. In many "substance use only" treatment programs, the style of confrontation used was often overly hostile and critical. This approach is no longer seen as the most helpful to the patient. Studies now show that patients who were treated in this way were far more likely to leave treatment early to return to their "drugging and drinking." This is of great concern because the person may never return to treatment and may die or be seriously injured as a result of the continued substance abuse.

You also can be very helpful in assisting the patient to work through the 12-step process. After intense, educational AA or NA meetings and group therapy sessions during most of the day, patients often want to ventilate feelings and process thoughts about what they are learning. Conflicts with family members, bosses, friends, or parents often are overwhelming. Patients usually lack the skills to handle these types of interpersonal stressors because of habitual avoidance of issues through past substance abuse. You can act as an ally in helping patients cope and begin to practice new ways of reacting. Teaching stress management and practicing these new skills with patients can greatly increase the odds that they will not relapse after discharge.

Relapse prevention is a critical area to attend to in dealing with each patient. The patient must be taught to recognize symptoms that often lead to relapse. Examples of these include overtiredness or poor health, being unnecessarily dishonest with others, impatience, argumentativeness, depression, self-pity, cockiness, forgetting or minimizing the risk of relapse, unreasonable expectations of self and others, decreased or irregular participation in AA or NA meetings or daily meditation and self-inventory, use of a chemical other than those previously abused, forgetting to be thankful that their lives are better, and feeling all-powerful.

Another effective means of intervention is to act as a good role model in handling feelings, participating appropriately in meetings, and communicating to the patient in a way that supports the program. For example, telling patients that participation in AA meetings is not necessary for recovery could undermine their struggle to initiate the profound changes in lifestyle necessary to stay drug-free.

POPULATIONS OF SUBSTANCE ABUSERS WITH SPECIAL PROBLEMS

The unique characteristics of many groups of individuals influence the process of recovery and contribute to a high risk for relapse into chronic use of whatever substance the person has abused. Recent research in addressing these problems has proved very promising to date. As mentioned earlier, the trend is to provide specially designed treatment approaches for groups of individuals who have common traits and problems that may contribute to their dependency on alcohol or other drugs.

OLDER ADULTS

Although older adults use approximately 25% of the medications used in the United States, only about 2% to 5% of men and fewer than 1% of women older than 65 years abuse alcohol. Older adults are more likely to abuse over-the-counter and prescription sleeping pills, pain medications, or tranquilizers than illegal drugs such as cocaine. Misuse is seldom for recreational purposes among this age-group.

Because of a decreased ability to metabolize and eliminate alcohol or drugs from the body, older adults who do abuse drugs over extended periods of time may experience significant medical problems as a result. The most typical physical consequences of chronic alcohol abuse among older adults include malnutrition, cirrhosis of the liver, bone thinning, gastritis, poor memory, and decreased cognitive ability to process new information. If the person combines alcohol with any other medication that has central nervous system depressant effects, the danger of oversedation, impaired responses, or respiratory depression is very great.

Most of the older adults who abuse alcohol have maintained a regular pattern of use over many years without obvious problems. As their bodies age, their ability to tolerate the same quantities decreases, putting them at risk for falls or other injuries as a result of intoxication. Others turn to first-time or heavier patterns of use to cope with anxiety produced by the typical stressors of aging such as retirement, losses of significant others, family conflict, health problems, social isolation, and loss of self-worth. Among the older adults who move to more affluent retirement communities, a rise in alcoholism has been noted. This may be due to involvement in cocktail parties, regular drinking with meals, and peer pressure to participate in order to be accepted.

Problems of abuse in the older population are usually diagnosed by the family physician as a result of complaints related to the psychological or physical

effects of alcohol abuse, such as memory impairment or insomnia. Older adults often deny that they have a substance abuse problem and may resist treatment without the support and pressure of their family.

Treatment of alcoholism in older adults is similar to that of younger individuals except that the period of withdrawal must be more closely monitored and occur more slowly because of the older person's physical frailty. Rehabilitation groups and educational programs should ideally be structured to permit processing information more slowly to allow for the cognitive slowing that is normal for this age-group. Also, cognitive changes may be more pronounced because of the neurologic effects of chronic use of alcohol or other drugs, or both. Involvement in AA is critical and can be difficult if patients do not have easy access to a "home group" with other older adults who can relate to their problems and issues.

ADOLESCENTS

Substance abuse among adolescents has received much attention in recent years. It is estimated that one in four adolescents becomes involved in substance abuse. It also has become apparent that children are experimenting with drugs at younger ages than ever before. The younger the age at onset of drug use, the greater is the risk for significant interference in the physical and psychological development of the individual.

The developmental issues of this age-group also contribute to the adolescent's vulnerability. This is a stage of establishing one's identity, experimenting with newly developed abilities to think abstractly, egocentricity, limited impulse control, and poor judgment. Identification with one's peer group is an important aspect of feeling accepted. Average adolescents view themselves as omnipotent and deny the likelihood of negative consequences of their behaviors. This is the age of rebellion.

Substance abuse in this population also is viewed as a symptom of family issues. The family is often dysfunctional—patterns of communication may be ineffective, and children in the family may be emotionally or physically neglected, abused, or subject to rigid, unrealistic expectations for their behavior. There may be a family history of substance abuse, or the adolescent may fall in with the "wrong crowd" of other young people who are already involved in the drug culture.

The progression of physical consequences of substance abuse in the adolescent population is correlated with the risks related to the substance abused and the likelihood of polysubstance abuse. The risks of accidental overdose or suicide are significant. Intravenous drug use and the likelihood of sexual activity without the use of precautions have been linked to an increased risk of HIV infection among adolescents.

Entry into treatment usually occurs as a result of a crisis situation revealing the severity of drug use and parental insistence. Breaking through adolescents' denial is the most difficult aspect of treatment, especially because they seldom want to be in treatment and do not see the potential negative consequences of their behaviors. It also may be difficult to distinguish the abuser from the adolescent who is still in the early stages of experimentation and unlikely to persist in chronic substance abuse. Most adolescents do not reach the point of believing it when saying, "Hi, I'm an alcoholic" (or drug abuser), at the beginning of each AA or NA meeting.

Rehabilitation of the adolescent substance abuser requires that the approach to treatment be modified to meet the needs of this age-group more effectively. It remains very controversial to mix adolescents with adults in treatment programs because of adolescents' vulnerability to being influenced by the more experienced and usually charismatic adult substance user. Obviously, careful supervision is necessary if mixing age-groups for treatment is the only option. In addition, many of the abstract concepts addressed in the 12 steps of AA may need to be adapted to the level of understanding of the individual adolescent.

Successful rehabilitation usually involves regular involvement in an AA group made up of younger people to whom the adolescent can relate; successful development of a new, non–drug-using peer group; and reentry into school with the support of other recovering classmates. AA group meetings may be held at high schools in some cities.

THE DUALLY DIAGNOSED

Patients who already have been diagnosed with a serious psychiatric illness and also have a substance abuse problem (dual diagnosis) have special concerns for rehabilitation. Dually diagnosed patients usually have psychiatric illnesses of depression, schizophrenia, or bipolar illness. Often, mental retardation and organic brain disease also are included in the group of medical problems identified as presenting special concerns in the event of a concurrent substance abuse problem. (Many times, substance abusers have a personality disorder, although this group of psychiatric disorders is generally not considered to be the result of some physiologic process and usually is not included under dual diagnosis.)

In some individuals, chronic drug or alcohol abuse may exacerbate an already fragile neurophysiology, producing psychiatric symptoms. This is seen in cases of young adolescents who use marijuana or some other type of drug before their first psychotic break in schizophrenia. Toxic psychosis may occur more frequently with the use of cocaine or amphetamines mixed with alcohol. In other cases, people may use a mind-altering drug to treat psychiatric symptoms without understanding the reason. They just know that they feel better.

People with chronic psychiatric problems require special teaching and supervision in the event of substance relapse. Antipsychotic medications do not mix with alcohol. If a bipolar patient is on lithium, the fluid losses as a result of drinking alcohol could precipitate lithium toxicity. Patients taking anxiolytic or antidepressant agents with alcohol could risk accidental overdose as a result of additive effects on the central nervous system or could be deliberately attempting to harm themselves.

The approach to rehabilitation must be modified to adapt to this special population. Each patient's ability to comprehend the abstract ideas from the 12-step process of AA will vary. In addition, traditionalists in the recovery process often frown upon the use of any mind-altering chemical and may subtly pressure dually diagnosed clients to stop their prescribed medications. This lack of knowledge and rigid approach to recovery could contribute to exacerbation of the underlying psychiatric illness.

PEER ASSISTANCE PROGRAMS

Substance abuse is expected to be one of the most widespread problems of the next 20 years. People from all walks of life are at risk, including health care professionals who are at high risk because of easier access to addictive drugs. As a result, many professional groups have developed peer assistance programs. These programs are designed to offer a supportive alternative to health professionals (physicians, dentists, nurses, and others) who become addicted to a substance instead of taking immediate disciplinary action against their licenses. Peer assistance programs for nurses exist in every state. Referrals are made by the individuals themselves or by their employers and peers who have reason to believe an individual's practice is impaired by the use of a substance. With the help of representatives of the program, usually volunteers, information is gathered to support an intervention in hopes of getting the nurse into treatment and recovery.

The goals of an intervention for a nurse whose practice is impaired are as follows:

- Assist the nurse whose practice is impaired to receive treatment.
- Protect the public from an untreated nurse.
- Help the recovering nurse reenter nursing in a systematic, planned, and safe way.
- Assist in monitoring the continued recovery of the nurse for a period of time.

Usually there is also at least a 2-year time period after diagnosis and onset of treatment in which the nurse is required to attend AA or NA groups regularly, to participate in peer support groups, to meet routinely with an identified support person representing the peer assistance program, and to undergo random urine drug screens to ensure that he or she has not relapsed. If nurses are unable to comply with the process, then information regarding their substance use and how that has impaired their practice can be turned over to the Board of Nurse Examiners for that state. Until that point, however, the information regarding each nurse involved is kept confidential and, if they successfully complete the requirements of the program, will never become part of the licensing board's records. Many peer assistance programs also work with nurses whose practices have become impaired as a result of mental illness.

Substance abuse will continue to be a major health care problem in the future. Nurses who work in this field are presented with difficult challenges and must be able to be nonjudgmental and supportive of the patients with whom they work. The knowledge base for this specialty area is growing quickly as a result of the widespread research being done. No matter where nurses work, they will come in contact with patients whose health status is compromised by substance abuse. The opportunity to play a powerful role in promoting healthier lifestyles is one that can be very fulfilling.

Key Points

- The majority of experts in substance abuse subscribe to the biologic theory that proposes that faulty physiologic processes contribute to dependence on a specific substance and that drug dependency is a physical illness.
- Some theorists contend that sociocultural factors contribute to the development of substance abuse.
- According to behavioral and learning theories, substance abuse is a learned maladaptive way of coping with stress and anxiety.
- The interpersonal or psychological theory states that innate personality factors may predispose individuals to substance abuse. Substance abusers have many common personality traits, including self-centeredness, a need to be in control of others, attention seeking, and difficulty delaying gratification of their needs.
- Although the specific causes of substance abuse have not been established, it is most likely that the true cause involves a combination of biologic, cultural, behavioral, and psychological factors.
- To obtain reliable data when questioning a person about substance abuse, the nurse must be nonjudgmental, direct, and specific. The information obtained should be verified by more than one person when possible.
- The lifestyle of substance abusers may focus entirely on obtaining and using the substance of choice, with an increasing need for more and more to get the desired effects.
- Substance abusers often have erratic and unprovoked mood swings, blackouts, significant work problems, and damaged relationships.
- Typical defense mechanisms used by substance abusers include denial, rationalization, intellectualization, and projection.
- Many alcohol abusers appear malnourished and poorly cared for, have evidence of physical trauma from falls or violence, appear jaundiced, and when in withdrawal, may be hypertensive with signs of fluid retention.
- Tests for detecting substance abuse include a blood alcohol study, a urine drug screen, and hair analysis.
- Chronic alcoholism involves the regular daily ingestion of large amounts of alcohol, regular heavy drinking only on weekends, or binges of heavy drinking followed by long periods of abstinence.
- Physical addiction occurs when the cells of the body are dependent on alcohol to carry out certain metabolic processes; without the alcohol, the cells go into shock.
- Alcohol withdrawal syndrome begins after an individual stops or decreases the amount of alcohol ingested and involves physiologic and behavioral symptoms that begin when the individual's blood alcohol level drops.
- Alcoholism has an impact on the entire family. Family and peer pressure can be critical factors in inducing an alcoholic to seek treatment.
- Strategies that have been successful in alcohol rehabilitation are 12-step programs, stress management, social skills training, behavioral approaches to marital therapy, and matching clients with therapists who use a style most likely to benefit their personality type.
- The six classes of psychoactive substances other than alcohol that are often associated with substance abuse are stimulants, depressants, hallucinogens, narcotics (opioids), inhalants, and designer drugs.
- Drug abuse treatment is similar to alcohol detoxification and rehabilitation; however, relapse rates are higher and treatment may need to be more individualized.
- Methadone maintenance may be used for long-term heroin abusers who have sustained permanent damage to chemical receptor sites in the brain and therefore have a decreased ability to resist relapses or who fail multiple attempts at rehabilitation.

 Go to your Companion CD-ROM for a Pharmacology Tutorial, Audio Glossary, and 3-D animations.

evolve Be sure to visit the companion Evolve site at http://evolve.elsevier.com/Linton/ for WebLinks and additional online resources.

REVIEW QUESTIONS *Choose the best answer.*

1. The theory that substance dependence is caused by faulty physiologic processes is the:
   1. Biologic theory
   2. Behavioral theory
   3. Sociocultural theory
   4. Intrapersonal theory

2. Mr. White was arrested for public intoxication and was advised by his attorney to enroll in an alcohol treatment program. A nurse interviews him when he comes to a mental health center. He tells the nurse he really doesn't have a problem with alcohol—he just had a few too many while celebrating with a friend. This is an example of which defense mechanism?
   1. Rationalization
   2. Projection
   3. Denial
   4. Intellectualization

3. What is the chief advantage of using hair analysis to detect drug use?
   1. Hair samples can be taken without patient permission.
   2. Hair samples will reveal drug use as long as a year later.
   3. It is not possible for a patient to substitute someone else's hair.
   4. The chain of custody is unnecessary with hair samples.

4. An alcoholic patient was injured in an automobile accident. She said she had her last drink 2 hours before the accident. About 8 hours after admission, she developed symptoms of early alcohol withdrawal. You should anticipate delirium tremens by:
   1. 12 hours after her last drink
   2. 24 hours after her last drink
   3. 48 hours after her last drink
   4. 72 hours after her last drink

5. Mr. Jones calls the hospital to report that his wife, a dietitian, cannot come to work because she has the "flu." In reality, she consumed a large amount of alcohol the previous evening and has a hangover. This has happened several times in the past. Mr. Jones' behavior is an example of:
   1. Support
   2. Enabling
   3. Rationalization
   4. Compensation

6. When a patient who is taking disulfiram (Antabuse) consumes alcohol, expected outcomes include:
   1. Hypertensive crisis
   2. Cardiac depression
   3. Nausea and vomiting
   4. Abdominal pain and diarrhea

7. Young people should be warned that inhalants can cause:
   1. Progressive brain damage
   2. Sexual dysfunction
   3. Schizophrenia
   4. Aggressive behavior

8. A patient being treated for an overdose of opioids is given Narcan. Narcan is given to:
   1. Stimulate the heart
   2. Raise the blood pressure
   3. Treat respiratory depression
   4. Sedate the patient and prevent seizures

9. The primary drug abused by older adults is/are:
   1. Cocaine
   2. Amphetamines
   3. Sedatives/sleeping aids
   4. Alcohol

10. Which statement most accurately describes drug use among adolescents?
    1. Only 1 in 10 adolescents has problems with substance abuse.
    2. Adolescents tend to deny any possible negative outcomes of drug use.
    3. Most adolescents seek treatment for substance abuse on their own.
    4. Adolescents should be treated with adults who can model mature behavior.

ACTH	Adrenocorticotropic hormone	ECF	Extracellular fluid	NSAID	Nonsteroidal anti-inflammatory drug
AD	Autonomic dysreflexia	ECG	Electrocardiogram		
ADH	Antidiuretic hormone	EEG	Electroencephalogram	NTG	Nitroglycerin
ADL	Activities of daily living	ESR	Erythrocyte sedimentation rate	OA	Osteoarthritis
AICD	Automatic implantable cardioverter-defibrillator	ET	Enterostomal therapist	OBRA	Omnibus Reconciliation Act (included nursing home regulations)
		ETT	Exercise tolerance test		
AIDS	Acquired immunodeficiency syndrome	FEV	Forced expiratory volume		
		FFP	Fresh frozen plasma	OOB	Out of bed
ALL	Acute lymphocytic leukemia	FRC	Functional residual capacity	PACU	Postanesthesia care unit (recovery room)
ALS	Amyotrophic lateral sclerosis	FVC	Forced vital capacity		
AMI	Acute myocardial infarction	GBS	Guillain-Barré syndrome	PCA	Patient-controlled analgesia
AML	Acute myelogenous leukemia	GI	Gastrointestinal	PCP	Phencyclidine
ARDS	Adult respiratory distress syndrome	HCT	Hematocrit	PE	Pulmonary embolism
		HDL	High-density lipoprotein	PET	Positron emission tomography
ATC	Around the clock	Hgb	Hemoglobin	PIC	Peripherally inserted catheter
bid	Twice a day	HIV	Human immunodeficiency virus	PID	Pelvic inflammatory disease
BMR	Basal metabolic rate			PO	By mouth
BPH	Benign prostatic hypertrophy	IADL	Instrumental activities of daily living	PRN	As needed
BRM	Biologic response modifier			PTT	Partial thromboplastin time
BSE	Breast self-examination	IBD	Inflammatory bowel disease	PVD	Peripheral vascular disease
BUN	Blood urea nitrogen	IC	Inspiratory capacity	q	Every (see Appendix B for cautions pertaining to this abbreviation)
CAD	Coronary artery disease	ICP	Intracranial pressure		
CAL	Chronic airflow limitation	IDDM	Insulin-dependent diabetes mellitus (outdated term)		
CBC	Complete blood count			RA	Rheumatoid arthritis
CHF	Congestive heart failure	IE	Infective endocarditis	RA	Right atrium
CLL	Chronic lymphocytic leukemia	IM	Intramuscular, intramuscularly	RAP	Right atrial pressure
CML	Chronic myelogenous leukemia	IV	Intravenous	RBC	Red blood (cell) count
		LA	Left atrium	RMR	Resting metabolic rate
CNS	Central nervous system	LDH	Lactic dehydrogenase	ROM	Range of motion
CO	Cardiac output	LDL	Low-density lipoprotein	RV	Right ventricle
COLD	Chronic obstructive lung disease	LES	Lower esophageal sphincter	SCD	Sudden cardiac death
		LOC	Level of consciousness	SLE	Systemic lupus erythematosus
COPD	Chronic obstructive pulmonary disease	LSD	Lysergic acid diethylamide (a hallucinogenic drug)	STI	Sexually transmitted infection
				SVR	Systemic vascular resistance
CP	Cerebral palsy	LV	Left ventricle	TENS	Transcutaneous electrical nerve stimulation
CPK	Creatine phosphokinase	MG	Myasthenia gravis		
CSF	Cerebrospinal fluid	MI	Myocardial infarction	V_{TG}	Thoracic gas volume
CT	Computed tomography	MRI	Magnetic resonance imaging	TIA	Transient ischemic attack
CVA	Cerebrovascular accident	MS	Multiple sclerosis	TLC	Total lung capacity
CVP	Central venous pressure	MV	Minute volume	TPN	Total parenteral nutrition
DC	Dilated cardiomyopathy	NG	Nasogastric	UTI	Urinary tract infection
D & C	Dilation and curettage	NIDDM	Non–insulin-dependent diabetes mellitus (outdated term)	VAS	Visual analog scale
DES	Diethylstilbestrol			VC	Vital capacity
DI	Diabetes insipidus			VLVD	Very low density lipoprotein
DM	Diabetes mellitus	NPO	Nothing by mouth	WBC	White blood (cell) count
DRG	Diagnosis-related group				

B ISMP's List of Error-Prone Abbreviations, Symbols, and Dose Designations

Please see the following pages for the ISMP's List of Error-Prone Abbreviations, Symbols, and Dose Designations.

ISMP's List of *Error-Prone Abbreviations, Symbols,* and *Dose Designations*

The abbreviations, symbols, and dose designations found in this table have been reported to ISMP through the USP-ISMP Medication Error Reporting Program as being frequently misinterpreted and involved in harmful medication errors. They should NEVER be used when communicating medical information. This includes internal communications, telephone/verbal prescriptions, computer-generated labels, labels for drug storage bins, medication administration records, as well as pharmacy and prescriber computer order entry screens.

The Joint Commission on Accreditation of Healthcare Organizations (JCAHO) has established a National Patient Safety Goal that specifies that certain abbreviations must appear on an accredited organization's do-not-use list; we have highlighted these items with a double asterisk (**). However, we hope that you will consider others beyond the minimum JCAHO requirements. By using and promoting safe practices and by educating one another about hazards, we can better protect our patients.

Abbreviations	Intended Meaning	Misinterpretation	Correction
μg	Microgram	Mistaken as "mg"	Use "mcg"
AD, AS, AU	Right ear, left ear, each ear	Mistaken as OD, OS, OU (right eye, left eye, each eye)	Use "right ear," "left ear," or "each ear"
OD, OS, OU	Right eye, left eye, each eye	Mistaken as AD, AS, AU (right ear, left ear, each ear)	Use "right eye," "left eye," or "each eye"
BT	Bedtime	Mistaken as "BID" (twice daily)	Use "bedtime"
cc	Cubic centimeters	Mistaken as "u" (units)	Use "mL"
D/C	Discharge or discontinue	Premature discontinuation of medications if D/C (intended to mean "discharge") has been misinterpreted as "discontinued" when followed by a list of discharge medications	Use "discharge" and "discontinue"
IJ	Injection	Mistaken as "IV" or "intrajugular"	Use "injection"
IN	Intranasal	Mistaken as "IM" or "IV"	Use "intranasal" or "NAS"
HS	Half-strength	Mistaken as bedtime	Use "half-strength" or "bedtime"
hs	At bedtime, hours of sleep	Mistaken as half-strength	
IU**	International unit	Mistaken as IV (intravenous) or 10 (ten)	Use "units"
o.d. or OD	Once daily	Mistaken as "right eye" (OD-oculus dexter), leading to oral liquid medications administered in the eye	Use "daily"
OJ	Orange juice	Mistaken as OD or OS (right or left eye); drugs meant to be diluted in orange juice may be given in the eye	Use "orange juice"
Per os	By mouth, orally	The "os" can be mistaken as "left eye" (OS-oculus sinister)	Use "PO," "by mouth," or "orally"
q.d. or QD**	Every day	Mistaken as q.i.d., especially if the period after the "q" or the tail of the "q" is misunderstood as an "i"	Use "daily"
qhs	Nightly at bedtime	Mistaken as "qhr" or every hour	Use "nightly"
qn	Nightly or at bedtime	Mistaken as "qh" (every hour)	Use "nightly" or "at bedtime"
q.o.d. or QOD**	Every other day	Mistaken as "q.d." (daily) or "q.i.d. (four times daily) if the "o" is poorly written	Use "every other day"
q1d	Daily	Mistaken as q.i.d. (four times daily)	Use "daily"
q6PM, etc.	Every evening at 6 PM	Mistaken as every 6 hours	Use "6 PM nightly" or "6 PM daily"
SC, SQ, sub q	Subcutaneous	SC mistaken as SL (sublingual); SQ mistaken as "5 every;" the "q" in "sub q" has been mistaken as "every" (e.g., a heparin dose ordered "sub q 2 hours before surgery" misunderstood as every 2 hours before surgery)	Use "subcut" or "subcutaneously"
ss	Sliding scale (insulin) or ½ (apothecary)	Mistaken as "55"	Spell out "sliding scale;" use "one-half" or "½"
SSRI	Sliding scale regular insulin	Mistaken as selective-serotonin reuptake inhibitor	Spell out "sliding scale (insulin)"
SSI	Sliding scale insulin	Mistaken as Strong Solution of Iodine (Lugol's)	
i/d	One daily	Mistaken as "tid"	Use "1 daily"
TIW or tiw	3 times a week	Mistaken as "3 times a day" or "twice in a week"	Use "3 times weekly"
U or u**	Unit	Mistaken as the number 0 or 4, causing a 10-fold overdose or greater (e.g., 4U seen as "40" or 4u seen as "44"); mistaken as "cc" so dose given in volume instead of units (e.g., 4u seen as 4cc)	Use "unit"

Dose Designations and Other Information	Intended Meaning	Misinterpretation	Correction
Trailing zero after decimal point (e.g., 1.0 mg)**	1 mg	Mistaken as 10 mg if the decimal point is not seen	Do not use trailing zeros for doses expressed in whole numbers"
"Naked" decimal point (e.g., .5 mg)**	0.5 mg	Mistaken as 5 mg if the decimal point is not seen	Use zero before a decimal point when the dose is less than a whole unit

ISMP's List of *Error-Prone Abbreviations, Symbols*, and *Dose Designations* (continued)

Dose Designations and Other Information	Intended Meaning	Misinterpretation	Correction
Drug name and dose run together (especially problematic for drug names that end in "l" such as Inderal40 mg; Tegretol300 mg)	Inderal 40 mg Tegretol 300 mg	Mistaken as Inderal 140 mg Mistaken as Tegretol 1300 mg	Place adequate space between the drug name, dose, and unit of measure
Numerical dose and unit of measure run together (e.g., 10mg, 100mL)	10 mg 100 mL	The "m" is sometimes mistaken as a zero or two zeros, risking a 10- to 100-fold overdose	Place adequate space between the dose and unit of measure
Abbreviations such as mg. or mL. with a period following the abbreviation	mg mL	The period is unnecessary and could be mistaken as the number 1 if written poorly	Use mg, mL, etc. without a terminal period
Large doses without properly placed commas (e.g., 100000 units; 1000000 units)	100,000 units 1,000,000 units	100000 has been mistaken as 10,000 or 1,000,000; 1000000 has been mistaken as 100,000	Use commas for dosing units at or above 1,000, or use words such as 100 "thousand" or 1 "million" to improve readability

Drug Name Abbreviations	Intended Meaning	Misinterpretation	Correction
ARA A	vidarabine	Mistaken as cytarabine (ARA C)	Use complete drug name
AZT	zidovudine (Retrovir)	Mistaken as azathioprine or aztreonam	Use complete drug name
CPZ	Compazine (prochlorperazine)	Mistaken as chlorpromazine	Use complete drug name
DPT	Demerol-Phenergan-Thorazine	Mistaken as diphtheria-pertussis-tetanus (vaccine)	Use complete drug name
DTO	Diluted tincture of opium, or deodorized tincture of opium (Paregoric)	Mistaken as tincture of opium	Use complete drug name
HCl	hydrochloric acid or hydrochloride	Mistaken as potassium chloride (The "H" is misinterpreted as "K")	Use complete drug name unless expressed as a salt of a drug
HCT	hydrocortisone	Mistaken as hydrochlorothiazide	Use complete drug name
HCTZ	hydrochlorothiazide	Mistaken as hydrocortisone (seen as HCT250 mg)	Use complete drug name
MgSO4**	magnesium sulfate	Mistaken as morphine sulfate	Use complete drug name
MS, MSO4**	morphine sulfate	Mistaken as magnesium sulfate	Use complete drug name
MTX	methotrexate	Mistaken as mitoxantrone	Use complete drug name
PCA	procainamide	Mistaken as patient controlled analgesia	Use complete drug name
PTU	propylthiouracil	Mistaken as mercaptopurine	Use complete drug name
T3	Tylenol with codeine No. 3	Mistaken as liothyronine	Use complete drug name
TAC	triamcinolone	Mistaken as tetracaine, Adrenalin, cocaine	Use complete drug name
TNK	TNKase	Mistaken as "TPA"	Use complete drug name
ZnSO4	zinc sulfate	Mistaken as morphine sulfate	Use complete drug name

Stemmed Drug Names	Intended Meaning	Misinterpretation	Correction
"Nitro" drip	nitroglycerin infusion	Mistaken as sodium nitroprusside infusion	Use complete drug name
"Norflox"	norfloxacin	Mistaken as Norflex	Use complete drug name
"IV Vanc"	intravenous vancomycin	Mistaken as Invanz	Use complete drug name

Symbols	Intended Meaning	Misinterpretation	Correction
ʒ	Dram	Symbol for dram mistaken as "3"	Use the metric system
ℳ	Minim	Symbol for minim mistaken as "mL"	
x3d	For three days	Mistaken as "3 doses"	Use "for three days"
> and <	Greater than and less than	Mistaken as opposite of intended; mistakenly use incorrect symbol; "< 10" mistaken as "40"	Use "greater than" or "less than"
/ (slash mark)	Separates two doses or indicates "per"	Mistaken as the number 1 (e.g., "25 units/10 units" misread as "25 units and 110 units)	Use "per" rather than a slash mark to separate doses
@	At	Mistaken as "2"	Use "at"
&	And	Mistaken as "2"	Use "and"
+	Plus or and	Mistaken as "4"	Use "and"
°	Hour	Mistaken as a zero (e.g., q2° seen as q 20)	Use "hr," "h," or "hour"

**These abbreviations are included on the JCAHO's "minimum list" of dangerous abbreviations, acronyms and symbols that must be included on an organization's "Do Not Use" list, effective January 1, 2004. Visit www.jcaho.org for more information about this JCAHO requirement.

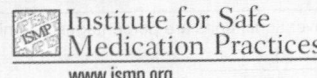
Institute for Safe Medication Practices
www.ismp.org

Laboratory Reference Values*

Reference Intervals for Hematology

TEST	CONVENTIONAL UNITS	SI UNITS
Acid hemolysis (Ham test)	No hemolysis	No hemolysis
Alkaline phosphatase, leukocyte	Total score, 14-100	Total score, 14-100
Cell counts		
Erythrocytes		
Males	4.6-6.2 million/mm³	4.6-6.2 × 10¹²/L
Females	4.2-5.4 million/mm³	4.2-5.4 × 10¹²/L
Children (varies with age)	4.5-5.1 million/mm³	4.5-5.1 × 10¹²/L
Leukocytes, total	4500-11,000/mm³	4.5-11.0 × 10⁹/L
Leukocytes, differential counts*		
Myelocytes	0%	0/L
Band neutrophils	3%-5%	150-400 × 10⁶/L
Segmented neutrophils	54%-62%	3000-5800 × 10⁶/L
Lymphocytes	25%-33%	1500-3000 × 10⁶/L
Monocytes	3%-7%	300-500 × 10⁶/L
Eosinophils	1%-3%	50-250 × 10⁶/L
Basophils	0%-1%	15-50 × 10⁶/L
Platelets	150,000-400,000/mm³	150-400 × 10⁹/L
Reticulocytes	25,000-75,000/mm³ (0.5%-1.5% of erythrocytes)	25-75 × 10⁹/L
Coagulation tests		
Bleeding time (template)	2.75-8.0 min	2.75-8.0 min
Coagulation time (glass tube)	5-15 min	5-15 min
D-Dimer	<0.5 mcg/mL	<0.5 mg/L
Factor VIII and other coagulation factors	50%-150% of normal	0.5-1.5 of normal
Fibrin split products (Thrombo-Welco test)	<10 mcg/mL	<10 mg/L
Fibrinogen	200-400 mg/dL	2.0-4.0 g/L
Partial thromboplastin time, activated (aPTT)	20-25 sec	20-35 sec
Prothrombin time (PT)	12.0-14.0 sec	12.0-14.0 sec
Coombs' test		
Direct	Negative	Negative
Indirect	Negative	Negative
Corpuscular values of erythrocytes		
Mean corpuscular hemoglobin (MCH)	26-34 pg/cell	26-34 pg/cell
Mean corpuscular volume (MCV)	80-96 μm³	80-96 fL
Mean corpuscular hemoglobin concentration (MCHC)	32-36 g/dL	320-360 g/L
Haptoglobin	20-165 mg/dL	0.20-1.65 g/L
Hematocrit		
Males	40-54 mL/dL	0.40-0.54
Females	37-47 mL/dL	0.37-0.47
Newborns	49-54 mL/dL	0.49-0.54
Children (varies with age)	35-49 mL/dL	0.35-0.49
Hemoglobin		
Males	13.0-18.0 g/dL	8.1-11.2 mmol/L
Females	12.0-16.0 g/dL	7.4-9.9 mmol/L
Newborns	16.5-19.5 g/dL	10.2-12.1 mmol/L
Children (varies with age)	11.2-16.5 g/dL	7.0-10.2 mmol/L

*Conventional units are percentages; SI units are absolute cell counts.

Continued

*From Rakel, R.E.; Bope, E.T. (2005). *Conn's current therapy* 2005. Philadelphia: Elsevier.

Reference Intervals for Hematology—cont'd

TEST	CONVENTIONAL UNITS	SI UNITS
Hemoglobin, fetal	<1.0% of total	<0.01 of total
Hemoglobin A$_{1C}$	3%-5% of total	0.03-0.05 of total
Hemoglobin A$_2$	1.5%-3.0% of total	0.015-0.03 of total
Hemoglobin, plasma	0.0-5.0 mg/dL	0.0-3.2 µmol/L
Methemoglobin	30-130 mg/dL	19-80 µmol/L
Erythrocyte sedimentation rate (ESR)		
Wintrobe		
Males	0-5 mm/hr	0-5 mm/hr
Females	0-15 mm/hr	0-15 mm/hr
Westergren		
Males	0-15 mm/hr	0-15 mm/hr
Females	0-20 mm/hr	0-20 mm/hr

Reference Intervals* for Clinical Chemistry (Blood, Serum, and Plasma)

ANALYTE	CONVENTIONAL UNITS	SI UNITS
Acetoacetate plus acetone		
Qualitative	Negative	Negative
Quantitative	0.3-2.0 mg/dL	30-200 µmol/L
Acid phosphatase, serum (thymolphthalein monophosphate substrate)	0.1-0.6 units/L	0.1-0.6 units/L
ACTH (see Corticotropin)		
Alanine aminotransferase (ALT, serum (SGPT)	1-45 units/L	1-45 units/L
Albumin, serum	3.3-5.2 g/dL	33-52 g/L
Aldolase, serum	0.0-7.0 units/L	0.0-7.0 units/L
Aldosterone, plasma		
Standing	5-30 ng/dL	140-830 pmol/L
Recumbent	3-10 ng/dL	80-275 pmol/L
Alkaline, phosphatase (ALP), serum		
Adult	35-150 units/L	35-150 units/L
Adolescent	100-500 units/L	100-500 units/L
Child	100-350 units/L	100-350 units/L
Ammonia nitrogen, plasma	10-50 µmol/L	10-50 µmol/L
Amylase, serum	25-125 units/L	25-125 units/L
Anion gap, serum calculated	8-16 mEq/L	8-16 mmol/L
Ascorbic acid, blood	0.4-1.5 mg/dL	23-85 µmol/L
Aspartate aminotransferase (AST), serum (SGOT)	1-36 units/L	1-36 units/L
Base excess, arterial blood, calculated	0 ±2 mEq/L	0 ±2 mmol/L
Bicarbonate		
Venous plasma	23-29 mEq/L	23-29 mmol/L
Arterial blood	21-27 mEq/L	21-27 mmol/L
Bile acids, serum	0.3-3.0 mg/dL	0.8-7.6 µmol/L
Bilirubin, serum		
Conjugated	0.1-0.4 mg/dL	1.7-6.8 µmol/L
Total	0.3-1.1 mg/dL	5.1-19.0 µmol/L
Calcium, serum	8.4-10.6 mg/dL	2.10-2.65 mmol/L
Calcium, ionized, serum	4.25-5.25 mg/dL	1.05-1.30 mmol/L
Carbon dioxide, total, serum or plasma	24-31 mEq/L	24-31 mmol/L
Carbon dioxide tension (Pco_2), blood	35-45 mm Hg	35-45 mm Hg
β-Carotene, serum	60-260 mcg/dL	1.1-8.6 µmol/L
Ceruloplasmin, serum	23-44 mg/dL	230-440 mg/L
Chloride, serum or plasma	96-106 mEq/L	96-106 mmol/L

*Reference values may vary, depending on the method and sample source used.

Continued

Reference Intervals for Clinical Chemistry (Blood, Serum, and Plasma)—cont'd

ANALYTE	CONVENTIONAL UNITS	SL UNITS
Cholesterol, serum or EDTA plasma		
Desirable range	<200 mg/dL	<5.20 mmol/L
Low-density lipoprotein (LDL) cholesterol	60-180 mg/dL	1.55-4.65 mmol/L
High-density lipoprotein (HDL) cholesterol	30-80 mg/dL	0.80-2.05 mmol/L
Copper	70-140 mcg/dL	11-22 µmol/L
Corticotropin (ACTH), plasma, 8 AM	10-80 pg/mL	2-18 pmol/L
Cortisol, plasma		
8:00 AM	6-23 mcg/dL	170-630 nmol/L
4:00 PM	3-15 mcg/dL	80-410 nmol/L
10:00 PM	<50% of 8:00 AM value	<50% of 8:00 AM value
Creatine, serum		
Males	0.2-0.5 mg/dL	15-40 µmol/L
Females	0.3-0.9 mg/dL	25-70 µmol/L
Creatine kinase (CK), serum		
Males	55-170 units/L	55-170 units/L
Females	30-135 units/L	30-135 units/L
Creatinine kinase MB isoenzyme, serum	<5% of total CK activity	<5% of total CK activity
	<5% of ng/mL by immunoassay	<5% of ng/mL by immunoassay
Creatinine, serum	0.6-1.2 mg/dL	50-110 µmol/L
Estradiol-17β, adult		
Males	10-65 pg/mL	35-240 pmol/L
Females		
Follicular	30-100 pg/mL	110-370 pmol/L
Ovulatory	200-400 pg/mL	730-1470 pmol/L
Luteal	50-140 pg/mL	180-510 pmol/L
Ferritin, serum	20-200 ng/mL	20-200 mcg/L
Fibrinogen, plasma	200-400 mg/dL	2.0-4.0 g/L
Folate, serum	3-18 ng/mL	6.8-41 nmol/L
Erythrocytes	145-540 ng/mL	330-120 nmol/L
Follicle-stimulating hormone (FSH), plasma		
Males	4-25 mU/mL	4-25 units/L
Females, premenopausal	4-30 mU/mL	4-30 units/L
Females, postmenopausal	40-250 mU/mL	40-250 units/L
Gastrin, fasting, serum	0-100 pg/mL	0-100 mg/L
Glucose, fasting, plasma or serum	70-115 mg/dL	3.9-6.4 nmol/L
γ-Glutamyltransferase (GGT), serum	5-40 units/L	5-40 units/L
Growth hormone (hGH), plasma, adult, fasting	0-6 ng/mL	0-6 mcg/L
Haptoglobin, serum	20-165 mg/dL	0.20-1.65 g/L
Immunoglobulins, serum (see table of Reference Intervals for Tests of Immunologic Function)		
Iron, serum	75-175 mcg/dL	13-31 µmol/L
Iron-binding capacity, serum		
Total	250-410 mcg/dL	45-73 µmol/L
Saturation	20%-55%	0.20-0.55
Lactate		
Venous whole blood	5.0-20.0 mg/dL	0.6-2.2 mmol/L
Arterial whole blood	5.0-15.0 mg/dL	0.6-1.7 mmol/L
Lactate dehydrogenase (LD), serum	110-220 units/L	110-220 units/L
Lipase, serum	10-140 units/L	10-140 units/L
Lutropin (LH), serum		
Males	1-9 units/L	1-9 units/L
Females		
Follicular phase	2-10 units/L	2-10 units/L
Midcycle peak	15-65 units/L	15-65 units/L
Luteal phase	1-12 units/L	1-12 units/L
Postmenopausal	12-65 units/L	12-65 units/L

Continued

Reference Intervals* for Clinical Chemistry (Blood, Serum, and Plasma)—cont'd

ANALYTE	CONVENTIONAL UNITS	SL UNITS
Magnesium, serum	1.3-2.1 mg/dL	0.65-1.05 mmol/L
Osmolality	275-295 mOsm/kg water	275-295 mOsm/kg water
Oxygen, blood, arterial, room air		
Partial pressure (PaO$_2$)	80-100 mm Hg	80-100 mm Hg
Saturation (SaO$_2$)	95%-98%	95%-98%
pH, arterial blood	7.35-7.45	7.35-7.45
Phosphate, inorganic, serum		
Adult	3.0-4.5 mg/dL	1.0-1.5 mmol/L
Child	4.0-7.0 mg/dL	1.3-2.3 mmol/L
Potassium		
Serum	3.5-5.0 mEq/L	3.5-5.0 mmol/L
Plasma	3.5-4.5 mEq/L	3.5-4.5 mmol/L
Progesterone, serum, adult		
Males	0.0-0.4 ng/mL	0.0-1.3 mmol/L
Females		
Follicular phase	0.1-1.5 ng/mL	0.3-4.8 mmol/L
Luteal phase	2.5-28.0 ng/mL	8.0-89.0 mmol/L
Prolactin, serum		
Males	1.0-15.0 ng/mL	1.0-15.0 mcg/L
Females	1.0-20.0 ng/mL	1.0-20.0 mcg/L
Protein, serum, electrophoresis		
Total	6.0-8.0 g/dL	60-80 g/L
Albumin	3.5-5.5 g/dL	35-55 g/L
Globulins		
α_1	0.2-0.4 g/dL	2.0-4.0 g/L
α_2	0.5-0.9 g/dL	5.0-9.0 g/L
β	0.6-1.1 g/dL	6.0-11.0 g/L
γ	0.7-1.7 g/dL	7.0-17.0 g/L
Pyruvate, blood	0.3-0.9 mg/dL	0.03-0.10 mmol/L
Rheumatoid factor	0.0-30.0 IU/mL	0.0-30.0 kIU/L
Sodium, serum or plasma	135-145 mEq/L	135-145 mmol/L
Testosterone, plasma		
Males, adult	300-1200 ng/dL	10.4-41.6 nmol/L
Females, adult	20-75 ng/dL	0.7-2.6 nmol/L
Pregnant females	40-200 ng/dL	1.4-6.9 nmol/L
Thyroglobulin	3-42 ng/mL	3-42 mcg/L
Thyrotropin (hTSH), serum	0.4-4.8 μIU/mL	0.4-4.8 mIU/L
Thyrotropin-releasing hormone (TRH)	5-60 pg/mL	5-60 ng/L
Thyroxine (FT$_4$), free, serum	0.9-2.1 ng/dL	12-27 pmol/L
Thyroxine (T$_4$), serum	4.5-12.0 mcg/mL	58-154 nmol/L
Thyroxine-binding globulin (TBG)	15.0-34.0 mcg/mL	15.0-34.0 mg/L
Transferrin	250-430 mg/dL	2.5-4.3 g/L
Triglycerides, serum, after 12-hr fast	40-150 mg/dL	0.4-1.5 g/L
Triiodothyronine (T$_3$), serum	70-190 ng/dL	1.1-2.9 nmol/L
Triiodothyronine uptake, resin (T$_3$RU)	25%-38%	0.25-0.38
Urate		
Males	2.5-8.0 mg/dL	150-480 μmol/L
Females	2.2-7.0 mg/dL	130-420 μmol/L
Urea, serum or plasma	24-49 mg/dL	4.0-8.2 nmol/L
Urea, nitrogen, serum or plasma	11-23 mg/dL	8.0-16.4 nmol/L
Viscosity, serum	1.4-1.8 × water	1.4-1.8 × water
Vitamin A, serum	20-80 mcg/dL	0.70-2.80 μmol/L
Vitamin B$_{12}$, serum	180-900 pg/mL	133-664 pmol/L

*JCAHO requires IU to be spelled out as International Units when written by hand.

Reference Intervals for Therapeutic Drug Monitoring (Serum or Plasma)*

ANALYTE	THERAPEUTIC RANGE	TOXIC CONCENTRATIONS	PROPRIETARY NAME(S)
ANALGESICS			
Acetaminophen	10-40 mcg/mL	>150 mcg/mL	Tylenol Datril
Salicylate	100-250 mcg/mL	>300 mcg/mL	Aspirin Bufferin
ANTIBIOTICS			
Amikacin	20-30 mcg/mL	Peak >35 mcg/mL Trough >10 mcg/mL	Amkin
Gentamicin	5-10 mcg/mL	Peak >10 mcg/mL Trough >2 mcg/mL	Garamycin
Tobramycin	5-10 mcg/mL	Peak >10 mcg/mL Trough >2 mcg/mL	Nebcin
Vancomycin	5-35 mcg/mL	Peak >40 mcg/mL Trough >10 mcg/mL	Vancocin
ANTICONVULSANTS			
Carbamazepine	5-12 mcg/mL	>15 mcg/mL	Tegretol
Ethosuximide	40-100 mcg/mL	>250 mcg/mL	Zarontin
Phenobarbital	15-40 mcg/mL	40-100 ng/mL (varies widely)	Luminal
Phenytoin	10-20 mcg/mL	>20 mcg/mL	Dilantin
Primidone	5-12 mcg/mL	>15 mcg/mL	Mysoline
Valproic acid	50-100 mcg/mL	>100 mcg/mL	Depakene
ANTINEOPLASTICS AND IMMUNOSUPPRESSIVES			
Cyclosporine	100-300 ng/mL	>400 ng/mL	Sandimmune
Methotrexate, high-dose, 48 hr	Variable	>1 μmol/L, 48 hr after dose	
Tacrolimus (FK-506), whole blood	3-20 mcg/L	>15 mcg/L	Prograf
BRONCHODILATORS AND RESPIRATORY STIMULANTS			
Caffeine	3-15 ng/mL	>30 mcg/mL	Elixophyllin
Theophylline (aminophylline)	10-20 mcg/mL	>30 mcg/mL	Quibron
CARDIOVASCULAR DRUGS			
Amiodarone (obtain specimen more than 8 hr after last dose)	1.0-2.0 mcg/mL	>2.0 mcg/mL	Cordarone
Digoxin (obtain specimen more than 6 hr after last dose)	0.8-2.0 mcg/mL	>2.4 ng/mL	Lanoxin
Disopyramide	2-5 mcg/mL	>7 mcg/mL	Norpace
Flecainide	0.2-1.0 mcg/mL	>1 mcg/mL	Tambocor
Lidocaine	1.5-5.0 mcg/mL	>6 mcg/mL	Xylocaine
Mexiletine	0.7-2.0 mcg/mL	>2 mcg/mL	Mexitil
Procainamide	4-10 mcg/mL	>12 mcg/mL	Pronestyl
Procainamide plus NAPA (N-acetyl procainamide)	8-30 mcg/mL	>30 mcg/mL	
Propranolol	50-100 ng/mL	Variable	Inderal
Quinidine	2-5 mcg/mL	>6 mcg/mL	Cardioquin Quinaglute
Tocainide	4-10 ng/mL	>10 ng/mL	Tonocard
PSYCHOPHARMACOLOGICAL DRUGS			
Amitriptyline	120-150 ng/mL	>500 ng/mL	Elavil Triavil
Bupropion	25-100 ng/mL	Not applicable	Wellbutrin
Desipramine	150-300 ng/mL	>500 ng/mL	Norpramin
Imipramine	125-250 ng/mL	>400 ng/mL	Tofranil
Lithium (obtain specimen 12 hr after last dose)	0.6-1.5 mEq/L	>1.5 mEq/L	Lithobid
Nortriptyline	50-150 ng/mL	>500 ng/mL	Aventyl Pamelor

*Values may vary depending on the method and sample collection device used. Always consult the reference values provided by the laboratory performing the analysis.

Reference Intervals* for Clinical Chemistry (Urine)

ANALYTE	CONVENTIONAL UNITS	SI UNITS
Acetone and acetoacetate, qualitative	Negative	Negative
Albumin		
Qualitative	Negative	Negative
Quantitative	10-100 mg/24 hr	0.15-1.5 μmol/day
Aldosterone	3-20 mcg/24 hr	8.3-55 nmol/day
δ-Aminolevulinic acid (δ-ALA)	1.3-7.0 mg/24 hr	10-53 μmol/day
Amylase	<17 units/h	<17 units/h
Amylase/creatinine clearance ratio	0.01-0.04	0.01-0.04
Bilirubin, qualitative	Negative	Negative
Calcium (regular diet)	<250 mg/24 hr	<6.3 nmol/day
Catecholamines		
Epinephrine	<10 mcg/24 hr	<55 nmol/day
Norepinephrine	<100 mcg/24 hr	<590 nmol/day
Total free catecholamines	4-126 mcg/24 hr	24-745 nmol/day
Total metanephrines	0.1-1.6 mg/24 hr	0.5-8.1 μmol/day
Chloride (varies with intake)	110-250 mEq/24 hr	110-250 mmol/day
Copper	0-50 mcg/24 hr	0.0-0.80 μmol/day
Cortisol, free	10-100 mcg/24 hr	27.6-276 nmol/day
Creatine		
Males	0-40 mg/24 hr	0.0-0.30 mmol/day
Females	0-80 mg/24 hr	0.0-0.60 mmol/day
Creatinine	15-25 mg/kg/24 hr	0.13-0.22 mmol/kg/day
Creatinine clearance (endogenous)		
Males	110-150 mL/min/1.73 m²	110-150 mL/min/1.73 m²
Females	105-132 mL/min/1.73 m²	105-132 mL/min/1.73 m²
Cystine or cysteine	Negative	Negative
Dehydroepiandrosterone		
Males	0.2-2.0 mg/24h	0.7-6.9 μmol/day
Females	0.2-1.8 mg/24h	0.7-6.2 μmol/day
Estrogens, total		
Males	4-25 mcg/24 hr	14-90 nmol/day
Females	5-100 mcg/24 hr	18-360 nmol/day
Glucose (as reducing substance)	<250 mg/24 hr	<250 mg/day
Hemoglobin and myoglobin, qualitative	Negative	Negative
Hemogentisic acid, qualitative	Negative	Negative
17-Hydroxycorticosteroids		
Males	3-9 mg/24 hr	8.3-25 μmol/day
Females	2-8 mg/24 hr	5.5-22 μmol/day
5-Hydroxyindoleacetic acid		
Qualitative	Negative	Negative
Quantitative	2-6 mg/24 hr	10-31 μmol/day
17-Ketogenic steroids		
Males	5-23 mg/24 hr	17-80 μmol/day
Females	3-15 mg/24 hr	10-52 μmol/day
17-Ketosteroids		
Males	8-22 mg/24 hr	28-76 μmol/day
Females	6-15 mg/24 hr	21-52 μmol/day
Magnesium	6-10 mEq/24 hr	3-5 mmol/day
Metanephrines	0.05-1.2 ng/mg creatinine	0.03-0.70 mmol/mmol creatinine
Osmolality	38-1400 mOsm/kg water	38-1400 mOsm/kg water
pH	4.6-8.0	4.6-8.0
Phenylpyruvic acid, qualitative	Negative	Negative
Phosphate	0.4-1.3 g/24 hr	13-42 mmol/day

*Values may vary, depending on the method used.

Reference Intervals* for Clinical Chemistry (Urine)—cont'd

ANALYTE	CONVENTIONAL UNITS	SI UNITS
Porphobilinogen		
Qualitative	Negative	Negative
Quantitative	<2 mg/24 hr	<9 µmol/day
Porphyrins		
Coproporphyrin	50-250 mcg/24 hr	77-380 nmol/day
Uroporphyrin	10-30 mcg/24 hr	12-36 nmol/day
Potassium	25-125 mEq/24 hr	25-125 mmol/day
Pregnanediol		
Males	0.0-1.9 mg/24 hr	0.0-6.0 µmol/day
Females		
Proliferative phase	0.0-2.6 mg/24 hr	0.0-8.0 µmol/day
Luteal phase	2.6-10.6 mg/24 hr	8-33 µmol/day
Postmenopausal	0.2-1.0 mg/24 hr	0.6-3.1 µmol/day
Pregnanetriol	0.0-2.5 mg/24 hr	0.0-7.4 µmol/day
Protein, total		
Qualitative	Negative	Negative
Quantitative	10-150 mg/24 hr	10-150 mg/day
Protein/creatinine ratio	<0.2	<0.2
Sodium (regular diet)	60-260 mEq/24 hr	60-260 mmol/day
Specific gravity		
Random specimen	1.003-1.030	1.003-1.030
24-hr collection	1.015-1.025	1.015-1.025
Urate (regular diet)	250-750 mg/24 hr	1.5-4.4 mmol/day
Urobilinogen	0.5-4.0 mg/24 hr	0.6-6.8 µmol/day
Vanillylmandelic acid (VMA)	1.0-8.0 mg/24 hr	5-40 µmol/day

*Values may vary, depending on the method used.

Reference Intervals for Toxic Substances

ANALYTE	CONVENTIONAL UNITS	SI UNITS
Arsenic, urine	<130 mcg/24 hr	<1.7 µmol/day
Bromides, serum, inorganic	<100 mg/dL	<10 mmol/L
Toxic symptoms	140-1000 mg/dL	14-100 mmol/L
Carboxyhemoglobin, blood	Saturation, percent	
Urban environment	<5%	<0.05
Smokers	<12%	<0.12
Symptoms		
Headache	>15%	>0.15
Nausea and vomiting	>25%	>0.25
Potentially lethal	>50%	>0.50
Ethanol, blood	<0.05 mg/dL	<1.0 mmol/L
	<0.005%	
Intoxication	>100 mg/dL	>22 mmol/L
	>0.1%	
Marked intoxication	300-400 mg/dL	65-87 mmol/L
	0.3%-0.4%	
Alcoholic stupor	400-500 mg/dL	87-109 mmol/L
	0.4%-0.5%	
Coma	>500 mg/dL	
	>0.5%	>109 mmol/L
Lead, blood		
Adults	<20 mcg/dL	<1.0 µmol/L
Children	<10 mcg/dL	<0.5 µmol/L
Lead, urine	<80 mcg/24 hr	<0.4 µmol/day
Mercury, urine	<10 mcg/24 hr	<150 nmol/day

Reference Intervals for Tests Performed on Cerebrospinal Fluid

TEST	CONVENTIONAL UNITS	SI UNITS
Cells	<5 mm³; all mononuclear	<5 × 10⁶/L, all mononuclear
Protein electrophoresis	Albumin predominant	Albumin predominant
Glucose	50-75 mg/dL (20 mg/dL less than in serum)	2.8-4.2 mmol/L (1.1 mmol/L less than in serum)
IgG		
Children <14 yr	<8% of total protein	<0.08 of total protein
Adults	<14% of total protein	<0.14 of total protein
IgG index		
$\left(\dfrac{\text{CSF/serum IgG ratio}}{\text{CSF/serum albumin ratio}}\right)$	0.3-0.6	0.3-0.6
Oligoclonal banding on electrophoresis	Absent	Absent
Pressure, opening	70-180 mm H₂O	70-180 mm H₂O
Protein, total	15-45 mg/dL	150-450 mg/L

Reference Intervals for Tests of Gastrointestinal Function

TEST	CONVENTIONAL UNITS
Bentiromide	6-hr urinary arylamine excretion >57% excludes pancreatic insufficiency
β-Carotene, serum	60-250 ng/dL
Fecal fat estimation	
Qualitative	No fat globules seen by high-power microscope
Quantitative	<6 g/24 hr (>95% coefficient of fat absorption)
Gastric acid output	
Basal	
Males	0.0-10.5 mmol/hr
Females	0.0-5.6 mmol/hr
Maximum (after histamine or pentagastrin)	
Males	9.0-48.0 mmol/hr
Females	6.0-31.0 mmol/hr
Ratio: basal/maximum	
Males	0.0-0.31
Females	0.0-0.29
Secretion test, pancreatic fluid	
Volume	>1.8 mL/kg/hr
Bicarbonate	>80 mEq/L
D-Xylose absorption test, urine	>20% of ingested dose excreted in 5 hr

Reference Intervals for Tests of Immunologic Function

TEST	CONVENTIONAL UNITS	SI UNITS
Complement, serum		
C3	85-175 mg/dL	0.85-1.75 g/L
C4	15-45 mg/dL	150-450 mg/L
Total hemolytic (CH$_{50}$)	150-250 units/mL	150-250 units/mL
Immunoglobulins, serum, adult		
IgG	640-1350 mg/dL	6.4-13.5 g/L
IgA	70-310 mg/dL	0.70-3.1 g/L
IgM	90-350 mg/dL	0.90-3.5 g/L
IgD	0.0-6.0 mg/dL	0.0-60 mg/L
IgE	0.0-430 ng/dL	0.0-430 mcg/L

Lymphocytes Subsets, Whole Blood, Heparinized

ANTIGEN(S) EXPRESSED	CELL TYPE	PERCENTAGE (%)	ABSOLUTE CELL COUNT
CD3	Total T cells	56-77	860-1880
CD19	Total B cells	7-17	140-370
CD3 and CD4	Helper-inducer cells	32-54	550-1190
CD3 and CD8	Suppressor-cytotoxic cells	24-37	430-1060
CD3 and DR	Activated T cells	5-14	70-310
CD2	E rosette T cells	73-87	1040-2160
CD16 and CD56	Natural killer (NK) cells	8-22	130-500
Helper/suppressor ratio: 0.8-1.8			

Reference Values for Semen Analysis

TEST	CONVENTIONAL UNITS	SI UNITS
Volume	2-5 mL	2-5 mL
Liquefaction	Complete in 15 min	Complete in 15 min
pH	7.2-8.0	7.2-8.0
Leukocytes	Occasional or absent	Occasional or absent
Spermatozoa		
Count	60-150 × 10^6 mL	60-150 × 10^6 mL
Motility	>80% motile	>0.80 motile
Morphology	80%-90% normal forms	>0.80-0.90 normal forms
Fructose	>150 mg/dL	>8.33 mmol/L

D Helpful Phrases for Communicating in Spanish

Useful Spanish Words

English	Spanish	Pronunciation
Abdomen	Abdomen	Ahb-doh-mehn
Abnormal	Anormal	Ah-nohr-mahl
Above	Arriba	Ah-ree-bah
Abuse	Abuso	Ah-boo-soh
Accident	Accidente	Ahk-see-dehn-teh
Activities	Actividades	Ahk-tee-bee-dah-dehs
Administration	Administracion	Ahd-meh-nees-trah-see-ohn
Adults	Adultos	Ah-dool-tohs
After	Después de	Dehs-poo-ehs deh
Aggressive	Agresivo	Ah-greh-see-boh
Air	Aire	Ah-ee-reh
Air conditioning	Aire acondicionado	Ah-ee-reh ah-kohn-dee-see-oh-nah-doh
Airway	Vía aérea	Bee-ah ah-eh-reh-ah
Alert	Avisele	Ah-bee-seh-leh
Allergies	Alergias	Ah-lehr-hee-ahs
Allergy	Alérgico	Ah-lher-hee-ahs
Allergy	Alergia	Ah-lher-hee-ah
Amputation	Amputación	Ahm-poo-tah-see-ohn
Amputee	Amputado	Ahm-poo-tah-doh
Analgesic	Analgésicos	Ah-nahl-heh-see-kohs
Anaphylactic shock	Choque anafilático	Choh-keh ah-nah-fee lah-tee-koh
Anemia	Anemia	Ah-neh-mee-ah
Anesthesia	Anestesia	Ah-nehs-teh-see-ah
Aneurysm	Aneurisma	Ah-neh-oo-rees-mah
Anger	Enojo	Eh-noh-hoh
Angina	Angina	Aahn-hee-nah
Ankle	Tobillo	Toh-bee-yoh
Anxiety	Ansiedad	Ahn-see-eh-dahd
Anxious axilla	Ansioso el sobaco	Ahn-see-oh-soh
Arrest	Arresto	Ah-rehs-toh
Arthritis	Arthritis	Ahr-tree-tees
Assessment	Avalúo	Ah-bah-loo-oh
Asthma	Asma	Ahs-mah
Baby	Bebé	Beh-beh
Bacteria	Bacteria	Bahk-teh-ree-ah
Bad	Mal	Mahl
Balanced	Balanceada	Bah-lahn-seh-ah-dah
Basin	Lavabo	Lah-bah-boh
English	Spanish	Pronunciation
Bathroom	Baño	Bah-nyoh
Bed	Cama	Kah-mah
Bed cover	Colcha	Kohl-chah
Bed rails	Barandal	Bah-rahn-dahl
Bedpan	Bacín	Bah-seen
Bedroom	Recamara	Reh-kahm-ah-rah
Bedspread	Colcha	Kohl-cha
Before	Antes de	Ahn-tehs deh
Behavior	Conducta	Kohn-dook-tah
Bell(s)	Campana/timbre	Kahm-pah-nah/teem-breh

English	Spanish	Pronunciation
Below	Abajo	Ah-bah-hoh
Bend	Doblar	Doh-blahr
Blanket	Frazada/covertor	Frah-sah-dah/koh-behr-tohr
Bleeding	Sangrado	Sahn-grah-doh
Blood	Sangre	Sahn-greh
Blood flow	Circulación sanguínea	Seer-koo-lah-see-ohn sahn-gee-neh-ah
Blouse	Blusa	Bloo-sah
Bottle	Botella	Boh-teh-yah
Bowel	Intestino	Een-tehs-tee-noh
Bradycardia	Bradicardia	Brah-dee-kahr-dee-ah
Breathe!	¡Respire!	Rehs-pee-reh
Broken bone	Hueso roto	Oo-eh-soh roh-toh
Bronchitis	Bronquitis	Brohn-kee-tees
Brother	Hermano	Ehr-mah-noh
Bruises/ecchymosis	Moretones/equimosis	Moh-reh-toh-nehs/eh-kee-moh-sees
Burns	Quemaduras	Keh-mah-doo-rahs
Burp	Repetir/eructar	Reh-peh-teer/eh-rook-tahr
Button	Botón	Boh-tohn
By mouth	Por la boca	Pohr lah boh-kah
Café (coffee)	Café	Kah-feh
Call (for/name)	Llamar	Yah-mahr
Call-bell	Campana/timbre	Kahm-pah-nah/teem-breh
Cancer	Cáncer	Kahn-sehr
Canes	Bastones	Bahs-toh-nehs
Cardiac	Cardíaco	Kahr-dee-ah-koh
Cardio-pulmonary	Cardio-pulmonar	Kahr-dee-oh-pool-moh-nahr
Care	Cuidado	Koo-ee-dah-doh
Carotid	Carótida	Kah-roh-tee-dah
Cast	Yeso	Yeh-soh
Cataract	Catarata	Kah-tah-rah-tah
Cavity	Cavidad	Kah-bee-dahd
Cereal (cooked)	Cereal/cocido	Seh-reh-ahl/koh-see-doh
Cereal (dry)	Cereal/seco	Seh-reh-ahl/ seh-koh
Chairs	Sillas	See-yahs
Chaplain/priest	Capellán/sacerdote/cura	Kah-peh-yahn/sah-sehr-doh-teh/koo-rah
Cheek	Mejilla	Meh-hee-yah
Chest	Pecho	Peh-choh
Chest pain	Dolor de pecho	Doh-lohr deh peh-choh
Chest/breast	Pecho/seno/la teta	Peh-choh
Child	Niño(a)	Nee-nyoh(-nyah)
Choking	Ahogar	Ah-oh-gahr
Clean	Limpiar	Leem-peahr

Translations taken from Joyce, E.V., Villanueva, M.E. (2000). *Say it in Spanish: A guide for health care professionals.* (2nd ed.). Philadelphia: W.B. Saunders. In Stassi, M. (2005). *Basic nurse assisting.* Philadelphia: W.B. Saunders.

English	Spanish	Pronunciation
Cognitive	Cognoscitivo	Kohg-noh-see-tee-boh
Cold	Frío	Free-oh
Cold water	Agua fría	Ah-goo-ah free-ah
Color	Color	Koh-lohr
Comatose	Comatose	Koh-mah-toh-soh
Comb	Peine	Peh-ee-neh
Communicate	Comunicar	Koh-moo-nee-kahr
Communication	Comunicación	Koh-moo-nee-kah-see-ohn
Complete	Completa	Kohm-pleh-tah
Complete dentures	Dentadura completa	Dehn-tah-doo-rah kohm-pleh-tah
Complications	Complicaciones	Kohm-plee-kah-see-ohn-ehs
Complications (major)	Complicaciones mayors	Kohm-plee-kah-see-oh-nes mah-yoh-rhes
Compound fractures	Fracturas compuestas	Frahk-too-rahs kohm-poo-ehs-tahs
Confuse	Confundir	Kohn-foon-deer
Consciousness	Conocimiento	Koh-noh-see-mee-ehn-toh
Constipation	Constipación/estreñimiento	Kohns-tee-pah-see-ohn/ehs- treh-nyee-mee-ehn-toh
Coping	Sobrellevando	Soh-breh-yeh-bahn-doh
Cough	Toser	Toh-sehr
Cry	Llorar	Yoh-rahr
Cubic centimeter	Centímetro cúbico	Sehn-tee-meh-troh koo-bee-koh
Cup	Tasa	Tah-sah
Cut	Cortar	Kohr-tahr
Dad	Papá	Pah-pah
Daughter	Hija	Ee-hah
Dehydrated	Deshidratado	Deh-see-drah-tah-doh
Dehydration	Deshidratación	Deh-see-drah-tah-see-ohn
Delirious	Delirio	Deh-lee-ree-oh
Demented	Demente	Deh-mehn-teh
Dementia	Demencia	Deh-mehn-see-ah
Dentist	Dentista	Dehn-tees-tah
Dentures	Dentadura	Dehn-tah-doo-rah
Deodorant	Desodorante	Deh-soh-doh-rahn-teh
Dependence	Dependencia	Deh-pehn-dehn-see-ah
Dependent	Dependiente	Deh-pehn-dehn-dee-ehn-teh
Depressed	Deprimido	Deh-pree-mee-doh
Develop	Desarrollar	Deh-sah-roh-yahr
Development	Desarrollo	Deh-sah-roh-yoh
Diabetes	Diabetes	Dee-ah-beh-tees
Diabetic	Diabética(o)	Dee-ah-beh-tee-kah
Diagnosis	Diagnóstico	Dee-ahg-nohs-tee-koh
Diaper	Pañal	Pah-nyahl
Diarrhea	Diarrea	Dee-ah-rreh-ah
Diet(s)	Dieta(s)	Dee-eh-tah(s)
Different	Diferente	Dee-feh-rehn-teh
Dizzy	Mareado	Mah-reh-ah-doh
Dizzy spell	Desmayo/mareo	Dehs-mah-yoh/mah-reh-oh
Doctor	Doctor(a)/medico(a)	Dohk-tohr(-toht-ah)/meh-dee-koh(-kah)
Doctor's office	Oficina/consultorio	Oh-fee-see-nah/kohn-sool-toh-ree-oh
Don't move!	¡No se mueva!	Noh seh moo-eh-bah
Door	Puerta	Poo-her-tah
Dress	Vestír	Behs-teer
Dress	Vestido	Behs-tee-doh
Dresser	Aparador	Ah-pah-rah-dohr
Drink	Beber/tomar	Beh-behr/toh-mahr
Drinking glass	Vidrio/vaso	Bee-dree-oh/bah-soh
Dry	Seca	Seh-kah
Ear	Oreja/el oído	Oh-reh-hah
Eat	Comer	Koh-mehr
Eat breakfast	Desayunar	Deh-sah-yoo-nahr
Eczema	Eczema	Ehk-seh-mah
Eight	Ocho	Oh-choh
Eighty	Ochenta	Oh-chehn-tah
Elbow	Codo	Koh-doh
Elder	Anciana (feminine)	Ahn-see-ah-nah
Elderly	Anciano	Ahn-see-ah-noh
Electrocardiogram	Electro cardiograma	Eh-lehk-troh-kahr-dee-oh-grah-mah
Embolism	Embolia	Ehm-boh-lee-ah
Embolism	Embolismo	Ehm-boh-lees-moh
Emergencies	Emergencias	Eh-mehr-hehn-see-ahs
Emergency	Emergencia	Eh-mehr-hehn-see-ah
Enema	Enema/sonda	Eh-neh-mah/sohn-dah
Epilepsy	Epilepsia	Eh-pee-lehp-see-ah
Examinations	Exámenes	Ehx-ah-meh-nehs
Exercise	Ejercicio	Eh-hehr-see-see-oh
Eye	Ojo	Oh-hoh
Facial	Facial	Fah-see-ahl
Familiar	Familiar	Fah-mee-lee-ahr
Family	Familia	Fah-mee-lee-ah
Father	Padre	Pah-dreh
Fear	Miedo	Mee-eh-doh
Feel	Sentír	Sehn-teer
Fever	Fiebre	Fee-eh-breh
Fifteen	Quince	Keen-she
Fifty	Cincuenta	Seen-koo-ehn-tah
Five	Cinco	Seen-koh
Fluid	Fluído	Floo-ee-doh
Foods	Comidas	Koh-mee-dahs
Fork	Tenedor	The-neh-dohr
Formula	Formula	Fohr-moo-lah
Forty	Cuarenta	Koo-ah-rehn-tah
Four	Cuatro	Koo-ah-troh
Fracture (pelvic)	Fractura pélvica	Frahk-too-rah pehl-bee-kah
Fractures	Fracturas	Frahk-too-rahs
Friday	Viernes	Bee-ehr-nehs
Fungus	Hongos	Ohn-gohs
Gallbladder	Vesicular biliar/hiel	Beh-see-koo-lah bee-lee ahr/ee-ehl
Gangrene	Gangrena	Gahn-greh-nah
Glass	Vaso	Bah-soh
Glaucoma	Glaucoma	Glah-oo-koh-mah
Gloves	Guantes	Goo-ahn-tehs
Goals	Metas	Meh-tahs
Gout	Gota	Goh-tah
Gown	Bata/vestido	Bah-tah/behs-tee-doh
Grandmother	Abuela	Ah-boo-eh-lah
Grief	Pena	Peh-nah
Grieve	Sufrir	Soo-freer
Grieving	Afligir	Ah-flee-heer
Groin	Ingle	Een-gleh
Growth	Crecimiento	Kreh-see-mee-ehn-toh

English	Spanish	Pronunciation
Guilt	Culpa	Kool-pah
Gynecologist	Ginecólogo	Hee-neh-koh-loh-goh
Hairbrush	Cepillo de pelo peh-loh	Seh-pee-yoh deh
Hazard	Peligro	Peh-lee-groh
Headache	Dolor de cabeza kah-beh-sah	Doh-lohr deh
Heal	Sano	Sah-noh
Healing	Curación	Koo-rah-see-ohn
Health	Salud	Sah-lood
Health (mental)	Salud mental	Sah-lood mehn-tahl
Heart(s)	Corazón (corazones)	Koh-rah-sohn/koh-rah-sohn-ehs
Hematoma	Hematoma	Eh-mah-toh-mah
Hemorrhage	Hemorragia	Eh-moh-rah-hee-ah
Hepatitis	Hepatitis	Eh-pah-tee-tees
Hernia	Hernia	Ehr-nee-ah
Hip	Cadera	Kah-deh-rah
Hip fracture	Fractura de cadera	Frahk-too-rah deh kah-deh-rah
Hope	Esperanza	Ehs-peh-rahn-sah
Hose/ stockings	Medias	Meh-dee-ahs
Hot water	Agua caliente	Ah-goo-ah kah-lee-ehn-teh
Hours (visiting)	Horas de visita	Oh-rahs deh bee-see-tah
Husband	Esposo	Ehs-poh-soh
Hypertension	Hipertensión	Ee-pehr-tehn-see-ohn
Hypertension (pulmonary)	Hipertensión pulmonar	Ee-pehr-tehn-see-ohn pool-moh-nahr
Hyperthermia	Hipertermia	Ee-pehr-tehr-mee-ah
Hypogly-cemia	Hipoglucemia	Ee-poh-gloo-seh-mee-ah
Identification	Identificacíon	Ee-dehn-tee-fee-kah-see-ohn
Illness	Enfermedad	Ehn-fehr-meh-dahd
Incision	Incisión	Een-see-see-ohn
Indepen-dence	Independencia	Een-deh-pehn-dehn-see-ah
Indigestion	Indigestión	Een-dee-hehs-tee-ohn
Infection	Infección	Een-fehk-see-ohn
Infections	Infecciones	Een-fehk-see-oh-nehs
Inflammation	Inflamación	Een-flah-mah-see-ohn
Internal	Interior	Een-teh-ree-ohr
Irritable	Irritable	Ee-ree-tah-bleh
Jacket	Chaqueta	Chah-keh-tah
Juice(s)	Jugo(s)	Hoo-goh(s)
Knee	La rodilla	Roh-dee-yah
Knife	Cuchillo	Koo-chee-yoh
Laboratory	Laboratorio	Lah-boh-rah-toh-ree-oh
Lamp	Lámpara	Lahm-pah-rah
Laxative(s)	Laxante(s)/ purgante(s)	Lahx-ahn-teh(s)/ poor-gahn-teh(s)
Left	Izquierda	Ees-kee-ehr-dah
Leg	Pierna	Pee-her-nah
Linen	Lino	Lee-noh
Liquid	Líquida	Lee-kee-dah
Loneliness	Soledad	Soh-leh-dahd
Lose	Perder	Pehr-dehr
Loss	Pérdida	Pehr-dee-dah
Love	Amor	Ah-mohr
Low cholesterol	Poco colesterol	Poh-koh koh-lehs-teh-rohl

English	Spanish	Pronunciation
Low cholesterol	Colesterol bajo	Koh-lehs-teh-rohl bah-hoh
Low fat	Poca grasa	Poh-kah grah-sah
Low sodium	Baja en sal/ poca sal	Bah-hah ehn sahl/ poh-kah sahl
Lunch	Comida	Koh-mee-dah
Lungs	Pulmones	Pool-moh-nehs
Management	Manejo	Mah-neh-hoh
Mattress	Colchón	Kohl-chohn
Measures	Medidas	Meh-dee-dahs
Mechanisms	Mecanismos	Meh-kah-nees-mohs
Medical	Médico	Meh-dee-koh
Memory	Memoria	Meh-moh-ree-ah
Meningitis	Meningitis	Meh-neen-hee-tees
Mental retardation	Retraso mental	Reh-trah-soh mehn-tahl
Milk	Leche	Leh-cheh
Minerals	Minerals	Mee-neh-rah-lees
Mirror	Espejo	Ehs-peh-hoh
Miss	Señorita	Seh-nyoh-ree-tah
Mom	Mamá	Mah-mah
Monday	Lunes	Loo-nehs
Monitor	Monitor	Moh-nee-tohr
Mother	Madre	Mah-dreh
Mouth	Boca/oral	Boh-kah/oh-rahl
Move!	¡Mueva!	Moo-eh-bah
Mr.	Señor	Seh-nyohr
Mrs.	Señora	Seh-nyoh-rah
Napkin	Servilleta	Sehr-bee-yeh-tah
Nasal	Nasal	Nah-sahl
Nausea	Náusea	Nah-oo-seh-ah
Navel	Ombligo	Ohm-blee-goh
Nervous	Nervioso	Nehr-bee-oh-soh
Nightgown/ gown	Camisa de dormir/bata	Kah-mee-sah deh dohr-meer/bah-tah
Nine	Nueve	Noo-eh-beh
Ninety	Noventa	Noh-behn-tah
No salt	Sin sal	Seen sahl
No smoking	No se permite fumar	Noh she pehr-mee-the foo-mahr
Normal	Normal	Nohr-mahl
Nose	Nariz	Nah-rees
Nurse	Enfermero(a)	Ehn-fehr-meh-roh(-rah)
Nutrition	Nutrición	Noo-tree-see-ohn
Obesity	Obesidad	Oh-beh-see-dahd
Observe	Observe	Ohb-sehr-beh
Obstruction	Obstrucción	Ohb-strook-see-ohn
Office	Oficina	Oh-fee-see-nah
Older	Mayors	Mah-yoh-rehs
One	Uno	Oo-noh
One hundred	Cien	See-ehn
Open!	¡Abra!	Ah-brah
Ophthalmic	Oftálmico	Ohf-tahl-mee-koh
Oral	Oral	Oh-rahl
Organ(s)	Órgano(s)	Ohr-gah-noh(s)
Ounces	Onzas	Ohn-sahs
Oxygen	Oxígeno	Ohx-ee-heh-noh
Pacemaker	Marcapasos	Mahr-kah-pah-sohs
Pain	Dolor	Doh-lohr
Pajama	Pijama	Pee-hah-mah
Pancreas	Páncreas	Pahn-kreh-ahs
Panic	Pánico	Pah-nee-koh
Pants/slacks	Pantalones	Pahn-tah-loh-nehs
Paralysis	Parálisis	Pah-rah-lee-sees
Pathogen	Patogénico	Pah-toh-heh-nee-koh

English	Spanish	Pronunciation
Patient (mental)	Enfermo mental	Eehn-fehr-moh mehn-tahl
Patient walkers	Pacientes con andadera	Pah-see-ehn- tehs kohn ahn-dah-deh-rah
Patient(s)	Paciente(s)	Pah-see-ehn-the(s)
Pelvis	Pelvis	Pehl-bees
People	Gente	Hehn-teh
Permission	Permiso	Pehr-mee-soh
Person	Persona(s)	Pehr-soh-nah(s)
Personal	Personales	Pehr-soh-nah-lehs
Personality	Personalidad	Pehr-soh-nah-lee-dahd
Phone	Teléfono	Teh-leh-foh-noh
Physician (f)	Médica-doctora	Meh-dee-kah/dohk-toh-rah
Physician (m)	Médico/doctor	Meh-dee-koh/dohk-tohr
Physicians	Los medicos	Lohs meh-dee-kohs
Pillow	Almohada	Ahl-moh-ah-dah
Pillowcase	Funda	Foon-dah
Plate	Platón	Plah-tohn
Pneumonia	Pulmonía/neumonía	Pool-moh-nee-ah/neh-oo-moh-nee-ah
Polydipsia	Polidipsia	Poh-lee-deep-see-ah
Polyphagia	Polifagia	Poh-lee-fah-hee-ah
Polyuria	Poliuria	Poh-lee-oo-ree-ah
Postoperative	Postoperatorio	Pohst-oh-peh-rah-toh-ree-oh
Potential	Posibles	Poh-see-blehs
Practice	Práctica	Prahk-tee-kah
Precaution	Precaución	Preh-kah-oo-see-ohn
Pregnant	Embarazada	Ehm-bah-rah-sah-dah
Preoperative	Preoperatorio	Preh-oh-peh-rah-toh-ree-oh
Preparation	Preparación	Preh-pah-rah-see-ohn
Prepare (to)	Preparar	Preh-pah-rahr
Priest	Sacerdote	Sah-sehr-doh-the
Problem	Problema(s)	Proh-bleh-mah(s)
Procedure(s)	Procedimiento(s)	Proh-seh-dee-mee-ehn-toh(s)
Psoriasis	Soriasis	Soh-ree-ah-sees
Pubic	Púbico	Poo-bee-koh
Pulse	Pulso	Pool-soh
Pureed	Puré	Poo-reh
Purpose	Propósito	Proh-poh-see-toh
Question(s)	Pregunta(s)	Preh-goon-tah(s)
Razor/shave	Navaja/máquina de afeitar	Nah-bah-hah/mah-kee-nah deh ah-feh-ee-tahr
Reach	Alcanzar	Ahl-kahn-sahr
Reassurance	Asegurar	Ah-seh-goo-rahr
Recognize	Reconocer	Reh-koh-noh-sehr
Recommen-dations	Recomen-daciones	Reh-koh-men-dah-see-ohn-es
Rectal	Rectal	Rehk-tahl
Rectum	El recto	Rehk-toh
Recuperating	Recuperando	Reh-koo-peh-rahn-doh
Regular	Regular	Reh-goo-lahr
Rehabilitation	Rehabilitación	Reh-ah-bee-lee-tah-see-ohn
Relation	Relación	Reh-lah-see-ohn
Relax	Descansa/relaja	Dehs-kahn-sah/reh-lah-hah
Remain	Quedese	Keh-deh-seh
Remember	Recordar/acordarse	Reh-kohr-dahr/ah-kohr-dahr-seh
Respiratory arrest	Paro respiratorio	Pah-roh rehs-pee-rah-toh-ree-oh
Response	Contestación	Kohn-tehs-tah-see-ohn
Respon-sibilities	Respon sabilidades	Rehs-pohn-sah-bee-lee-dah-dehs
Rest	Reposo	Reh-poh-soh
Restless	Inquieto	Een-kee-eh-toh
Restroom	Cuarto de baño	Koo-ahr-toh deh bah-nyoh
Rib(s)	Costilla(s)	Kohs-tee-yah(s)
Right	Derecha	Deh-reh-chah
Rigidity	Rigidez	Ree-hee-dehs
Room (operating)	Cuarto de cirugía quirófano	Koo-ahr-toh deh see-roo-hee-ah/kee-roh-fah-noh
Saliva	Saliva	Sah-lee-bah
Salt	Sal	Sahl
Sample	Muestra	Moo-ehs-trah
Saturday	Sábado	Sah-bah-doh
Scratch	Raspón	Rahs-pohn
Sebaceous	Sebásceo	She-bah-seh-oh
Semi-solid	Semisólido	Seh-mee-soh-lee-doh
Seven	Siete	See-eh-teh
Seventy	Setenta	Seh-tehn-tah
Sheets	Sábanas	Sah-bah-nahs
Shirt	Camisa	Kah-mee-sah
Shoes	Zapatos	Sah-pah-tohs
Shoulder	Hombro	Ohm-broh
Shower	Regadera/ducha	Reh-gah-deh-rah/doo-chah
Sign	Firme/letrero	Feer-meh/leh-treh-roh
Signs	Signos/señales	Seeg-nohs/seh-nyah-lehs
Similar	Similares	See-mee-lah-rhes
Sister	Hermana	Ehr-mah-nah
Sit!	¡Siéntese!	See-ehn-teh-seh
Six	Seis	Seh-ees
Sixty	Sesenta	Seh-sehn-tah
Skin	Piel	Pee-ehl
Skirt	Falda	Fahl-dah
Sleep	Sueño	Soo-eh-nyoh
Sneeze	Estornudo	Ehs-tohr-noo-doh
Soap	Jabón	Hah-bohn
Social	Social	Soh-see-ahl
Social worker	Trabajadora social	Trah-bah-hah-doh-rah soh-see-ahl
Sociocultural	Sociocultural	Soh-see-oh-kool-too-rahl
Socks	Calcetines/calcetas	Kahl-seh-tee-nehs/kahl-seh-tahs
Soft	Suave	Soo-ah-beh
Son	Hijo	Ee-hoh
Speak	Hablar	Ah-blahr
Specimen	Muestra	Moo-ehs-trah
Sternum	Esternón	Ehs-tehr-nohn
Stethoscope	Estetoscopio	Ehs-teh-tohs-koh-pee-oh
Stockings	Medias	Meh-dee-ahs
Subcutaneous	Subcutáneo	Soob-koo-tah-neh-oh
Sugar	Azúcar	Ah-soo-kahr
Sunday	Domingo	Doh-meen-goh

English	Spanish	Pronunciation
Suppository	Supositorio	Soo-poh-see-toh-ree-oh
Surgeon	Cirujano	See-roo-hah-noh
Surgery	Cirugía	See-roo-hee-ah
Surgical	Quirúrgico	Kee-roor-hee-koh
Sutures	Suturas/puntos	Soo-too-rahs/poon-tohs
Sweater	Chamarra/suéter	Chah-mah-rah/soo-eh-tehr
Swelling	Hinchazón	Een-chah-sohn
Swollen	Hinchado	Een-chah-doh
Symptoms	Síntomas	Seen-toh-mahs
Systole	Sístole	Sees-toh-leh
Table (overnight)	Mesa de noche	Meh-sah deh noh-cheh
Table(s)	Mesa(s)	Meh-sah(s)
Tablespoon	Cuchara/cucharada	Koo-chah-rah/koo-chah-rah-dah
Taste	Gusto	Goos-toh
Tea	Té	Teh
Teaspoon	Cucharita/cucharadita	Koo-chah-ree-tah/koo-chah-rah-dee-tah
Teeth	Dientes	Dee-ehn-tehs
Television	Televisor	The-leh-bee-sohr
Temperature	Temperatura	Tehm-peh-rah-too-rah
Temporal	Temporal	Tehm-poh-rahl
Ten	Diez	Dee-ehs
Tense	Tenso	Tehn-soh
Terminal	Terminal	Tehr-mee-nahl
Thank you	Gracias	Grah-see-ahs
The family	La familia	Lah fah-mee-lee-ah
Theories	Teorías	Teh-oh-ree-ahs
Thermometer	Termómetro	Tehr-muh-meh-troh
Thirty	Treinta	Treh-een-tah
Three	Tres	Trehs
Thrombus	Coágulo	Koh-ah-goo-loh
Thursday	Jueves	Hoo-eh-behs
Tissue (muscle)	Tejido	The-hee-doh
Tissues	Tisues	Tee-sooh(ehs)
Tissue damage	Daño del tejido	Dah-nyoh dehl teh-hee-doh
To bathe	Bañar	Bah-nyahr
To become ill	Enfermar	Ehn-fehr-mahr
To bleed	Sangrar	Sahn-grahr
To break	Romper	Rohm-pehr
To breathe	Respirar	Rehs pee-rahr
To change	Cambiar	Kahm-bee-ahr
To communicate	Comunicar	Koh-moo-nee-kahr
To complain	Quejar	Keh-hahr
To cure	Curar	Koo-rahr
To dress	Vestír	Behs-teer
To drink	Beber/tomar	Beh-behr/toh-mahr
To eat	Comer	Koh-mehr
To eat breakfast	Desayunar	Deh-sah-yoo-nahr
To examine	Examinar	Ex-ah-mee-nahr
To feel	Sentír	Sehn-teer
To get better	Mejorar	Meh-hoh-rahr
To get up/raise	Levanter	Leh-bahn-tahr
To go out	Salir	Sah-leer

English	Spanish	Pronunciation
To go to bed	Acostarse	Ah-kohs-tahr-she
To hear me	Oirme	Oh-eer-meh
To hear/listen	Escuchar/oír	Ehs-koo-chahr/oh-eer
To hurt	Doler	Doh-lehr
To lie down	Acostar/dormir	Ah-kohs-tahr/dorh-meer
To leave	Dejar	Deh-hahr
To listen	Oir	Oh-eer
To point	Señalar	She-nyah-lahr
To raise	Levanter	Leh-bahn-tahr
To reach	Alcanzar	Ahl-kahn-sahr
To remember	Acordar/recordar	Ah-kohr-dahr/reh-kohr-dahr
To sit	Sentar	Sehn-tahr
To sleep	Dormir	Dohr-meer
To speak	Hablar	Ah-blahr
To suffer	Sufrir	Soo-freer
To vomit	Vomitar	Boh-mee-tahr
To walk	Caminar	Kah-mee-nahr
To wash	Lavar	Lah-bahr
Toes	dedos	Deh-dos
Toilet	Excusado/inodoro	Ex-koo-sah-doh/ee-noh-doh-roh
Toothache	Dolor de muelas	Doh-lor deh moo-eh-lahs
Toothbrush	Cepillo de dientes	Seh-pee-yoh deh dee-ehn-tehs
Toothpaste	Pasta de dientes	Pahs-tah deh dee-ehn-tehs
Topical	Topical/tópico	Toh-pee-kahl/toh-pee-koh
Towel	Toalla	Too-ah-yah
Traumatic	Traumático	Trah-oo-mah-tee-koh
Treatment	Tratamiento	Trah-tah-mee-ehn-toh
Trust	Confianza	Kohn-fee-ahn-sah
Tuesday	Martes	Mahr-tehs
Tumor	Tumor	Too-mohr
Turn!	¡Voltée!	Bohl-the-eh
Twenty	Viente	Beh-een-teh
Two	Dos	Dohs
Ulcer(s)	Úlcera(s)	Ool-seh-rah(s)
Ultrasound	Ultrasonido	Ool-trah-soh-nee-doh
Underwear	Ropa interior	Roh-pah een-teh-ree-ohr
Universal	Universal	Oo-nee-behr-sahl
Urinal	Pato	Pah-toh
Urine	Orina	Oh-ree-nah
Use	Usar	Oo-sahr
Uterus	Útero	Oo-the-roh
Vaginal	Vaginal	Bah-hee-nahl
Vein	Vena	Beh-nah
Vitamins	Vitaminas	Bee-tah-mee-nahs
Vomit	Vómito	Boh-mee-toh
Vomiting	Vomitando	Boh-mee-tahn-doh
Warning	Advertencia	Ahd-behr-tehn-see-ah
Wednesday	Miércoles	Mee-ehr-koh-lehs
Wife	Esposa	Ehs-poh-sah
Worker	Trabajador	Trah-bah-hah-dohr
Wound	Herida	Eh-ree-dah
Wrist	Muñeca	Moo-nveh-kah
X-rays	Rayos-x	Rah-yohs eh-kiss
Young	Jovenes	Hoh-beh-nehs

Useful Spanish Phrases

English	Spanish	Pronunciation
A bowel movement.	Hacer del baño.	Ah-sehr dehl ban-nyoh
A glass of juice?	Un vaso de jugo?	Oon bah-soh deh hoo-goh
A heart.	Un corazón.	Oon koh-rah-sohn
About your baby.	En cuanto a su bebé.	Ehn koo-ahn-toh ah soo beh-beh
Activities are part of the plan while you are here.	Las actividades son parte del plan de su tratamiento minetras esté aquí.	Lahs ahk-tee-bee-dah-dehs sohn pahr-teh dehl plahn deh soo trah-tah-mee-ehn-toh mee-ehn-trahs ehs-teh ah-kee
After meals.	Después de las comidas.	Dehs-poo-ehs deh lahs koh-mee-dahs
Any questions?	¿Alguna pregunta?	Ahl-goo-nah preh-goon-tah
Are you allergic to anything?	¿Es alérgico a alguna cosa?	Ehs ah-lehr-hee-koh ah ahl-goo-nah koh-sah
Are you allergic to foods?	¿Es alérgico a comidas?	Ehs ah-lehr-hee-koh ah koh-mee-dahs
Are you cold?	¿Tiene frío?	Tee-eh-neh free-oh
Are you comfortable?	¿Está cómoda?	Ehs-tah koh-moh-dah
Are you constipated?	¿Está estreñido?	Ehs-tah ehs-treh-nyee-doh
Are you diabetic?	¿Es diabética?	Ehs dee-ah-beh-tee-kah
Are you dizzy?	¿Tiene mareos?	Tee-eh-neh mah-reh-ohs
Are you employed?	¿Trabaja usted?	Trah-bah-hah oos-tehd
Are you having problems breathing?	¿Tiene problemas al respirar?	Tee-eh-neh proh-bleh-mahs ahl rehs-pee-rahr
Are you hot?	¿Tiene calor?	Tee-eh-neh kah-lohr
Are you hungry?	¿Tiene hambre?	Tee-eh-neh ahm-breh
Are you hurting?	¿Tiene dolor?	Tee-eh-neh doh-lohr
Are you nauseated?	¿Tiene náuseas?	Tee-eh-neh nah-oo-seh-ahs
Are you okay?	¿Está bien/Se siente bien?	Ehs-tah bee-ehn/ seh see-ehn-the bee-ehn
Are you sleepy?	¿Tiene sueño?	Tee-eh-neh soo-eh-nyoh
Are you thirsty?	¿Tiene sed?	Tee-eh-neh sehd
At bedtime.	Al acostarse/ hora de dormir.	Ahl ah-kohs-tahr-seh/oh-rah deh dohr-meer
At eleven thirty.	A las once y media.	Ah lahs ohn-seh ee meh-dee-ah
At five PM.	A las cinco de la tarde.	Ah lahs seen-koh deh lah tahr-deh
At what time do you get up?	¿A qué hora se levanta?	Ah keh oh-rah seh leh-bahn-tah
At what time do you go to bed?	¿A qué hora se acuesta?	Ah keh oh-rah seh ah-koo-ehs-tah
Before/after meals.	Antes/después de las comidas.	Ahn-tehs/ dehs-poo-ehs deh lahs koh-mee-dahs
Bend the elbow.	Doble el codo.	Doh-bleh-ehl koh-doh
Bend the wrist.	Dobla la muñeca.	Doh-blah lah moo-nyeh-kah
Bend your hip.	Dobla su cadera.	Doh-bleh soo kah-deh-rah
Bend your knee!	¡Doble su rodilla!	Doh-bleh soo roh-dee-yah
Bend your shoulder.	Dobla tu hombro.	Doh-bleh too ohm-broh
Bend your toes.	Dobla tus dedos.	Doh-blah toos deh-dohs
Breast-feed or give a bottle every 3 hours.	Déle pecho o biberón cada tres horas.	Deh-leh peh-choh oh bee-beh-rohn kah-dah trehs oh-ras
Breast-feeding?	¿Tomando pecho?	Toh-mahn-doh peh-choh
Breathe deeply; let it out slowly.	Respira hondo; déjalo ir despacio.	Rehs-pee-rah oon-doh; deh-hah-loh eer dehs-pah-see-oh
Breathe deeply!	¡Respire hondo/ profundo!	Rehs-pee-reh ohn-doh/ proh-foon-doh
Breathe in.	Respire.	Rehs-pee-reh
Breathe out.	Saque el aire.	Sah-keh ehl ah-ee-reh
Brush your teeth!	¡Cepíllese los dientes!	Seh-pee-yeh-seh lohs dee-ehn-tehs
Call if you need help.	Llame sí necesita ayuda.	Yah-meh see neh-seh-see-tah ah-yoo-dah
Can you breathe?	¿Puede respirar?	Poo-eh-deh rehs-pee-rahr
Can you feed yourself?	¿Puede alimentarse?	Poo-eh-deh ah-lee-mehn-tahr-seh
Can you get out of bed?	¿Puede salir de la cama?	Poo-eh-deh sah-leer deh lah kah-mah
Can you hear me?	¿Puede oírme?	Poo-eh-deh oh-eer-meh
Can you move in bed?	¿Puede moverse en la cama?	Poo-eh-deh moh-behr-seh ehn lah kah-mah
Can you sit up?	¿Puede sentarse?	Poo-eh-deh sehn-tahr-seh
Can you talk?	¿Puede hablar?	Poo-eh-deh ah-blahr
Change into this gown.	Póngase esta bata.	Pohn-gah-seh ehs-tah bah-tah
Chest pain?	¿Dolor en el pecho?	Doh-lohr ehn ehl peh-choh

English	Spanish	Pronunciation
Close your mouth.	Cierre la boca.	See-eh-reh lah boh-kah
Cough deeply.	Tosa más fuerte.	Toh-sah mahs foo-her-teh
Cough!	¡Tosa!	Toh-sah
Daily.	Diariamente./Una por día./Cada día.	Dee-ah-ree-ah-mehn-teh/Oo-nah pohr dee-ah/Kah-dah dee-ah
Did you bring a hearing aid?	¿Trajo un aparato para oír?	Trah-hoh oon ah-pah-rah-toh pah-rah oh-eer
Did you bring an artificial eye?	¿Trajo un ojo artificial?	Trah-hoh oon oh-hoh ahr-tee-fee-see-ahl
Did you bring dentures?	¿Trajo una dentadura postiza?	Trah-hoh oon-ah dehn-tah-doo-rah pohs-tee-sah
Did you bring glasses?	¿Trajo anteojos/lentes?	Trah-hoh ahn-the-oh-hohs/lehn-tehs
Did you faint?	¿Se desmayó?	Seh dehs-mah-yoh
Did you have a bowel movement?	¿Hizo del baño/caca/evacuró?	Ee-soh dehl bah-nyoh/kah-kah/eh-bah-koo-oh
Did you see blood in the urine?	¿Vio sangre en la orina?	Bee-oh sahn-greh ehn lah oh-ree-nah
Difficulty in swallowing . . .	Dificultad al tragar . . .	Dee-fee-kool-tahd ahl trah-gahr
Do not smoke in the room when the oxygen is being used.	No fume en el cuarto donde se usa el oxígeno.	Noh foo-meh ehn ehl koo-ahr-toh dohn-deh seh oo-sah ehl ohx-ee-heh-noh
Do you dribble?	¿Se orina sin sentir?	Seh oh-ree-nah seen sehn-teer
Do you feel all right?	¿Se siente bien?	She see-ehn-the bee-ehn
Do you feel dizzy?	¿Se siente mareado?	Seh see-ehn-teh mah-reh-ah-doh
Do you feel nauseated?	¿Siente náuseas?	See-ehn-teh nah-oo-seh-ahs
Do you feel weak?	¿Se siente débil?	Seh see-ehn-teh deh-beel
Do you have a pacemaker?	¿Tiene marcapasos?	Tee-eh-neh mahr-kah-pah-sohs
Do you have allergies?	¿Tiene alergias?	Tee-eh-neh ah-lehr-ghee-ahs
Do you have any questions?	¿Tiene preguntas?	Tee-eh-neh preh-goon-tahs
Do you have any symptoms: nausea, dizziness, other unusual feelings?	¿Tiene algún síntoma como: náuseas, vértigo, otra sensación rara?	Tee-eh-neh ahl-goon seen-toh-mah koh-moh nah-oo-seh-ahs, behr-tee-goh, oh-trah sehn-sah-see-ohn rah-rah
Do you have chest pain?	¿Tiene dolor en el pecho?	Tee-eh-neh doh-lohr ehn ehl peh-choh
Do you have diarrhea?	¿Tiene diarrea?	Tee-eh-neh dee-ah-reh-ah

English	Spanish	Pronunciation
Do you have hesitancy (when urinating)?	¿Se corta el chorro de la orina?	She kohr-tah ehl choh-roh deh lah oh-ree-nah
Do you have problems with starting to urinate?	¿Tiene dificultad para empezar a orinar?	Tee-eh-neh dee-fee-kool-tahd pah-rah ehm-peh-sahr ah oh-ree-nahr
Do you have problems with your teeth?	¿Tiene(s) problemas con los dientes?	Tee-eh-neh(s) proh-bleh-mahs kohn lohs dee-ehn-tehs
Do you have questions?	¿Tiene dudas?	Tee-eh-neh doo-dahs
Do you have respiratory problems?	¿Tiene problemas respiratorios?	Tee-eh-neh proh-bleh-mahs rhes-pee-rah-toh-ree-ohs
Do you know the day of the week?	¿Sabe el día de la semana?	Sah-beh ehl dee-ah deh lah seh-mah-nah
Do you know the day?	¿Qué día es hoy?	Keh dee-ah ehs oh-ee
Do you know where you are?	¿Sabe dónde está?	Sah-beh dohn-deh ehs-tah
Do you need help?	¿Necesita ayuda?	Neh-she-see-tah ah-yoo-dah
Do you need more pillows?	¿Necesita más almohadas?	Neh-seh-see-tah mahs ahl-moh-ah-dahs
Do you speak English?	¿Habla ingles/Habla usted ingles?	Ah-blah een-glehs/Ah-blah oos-tehd een-glehs
Do you take a special diet?	¿Toma dieta especial?	Toh-mah dee-eh-tah ehs-peh-see-ahl
Do you understand?	¿Entiende?	Ehn-tee-ehn-deh
Do you use sugar in the coffee?	¿Usa azúcar en el café?	Oo-sah ah-soo-kahr ehn ehl kah-feh
Do you want the bedpan?	¿Quiere el pato/el bacín?	Kee-eh-reh ehl pah-toh/ehl bah-seen
Do you want the toast with butter?	¿Quiere el pan tostado con mantequilla?	Kee-eh-reh ehl pahn tohs-tah-doh kohn mahn-teh-kee-yah
Do you want water?	¿Quiére agua?	Kee-eh-reh ah-goo-ah
Do you want: A glass of water?	¿Quiere: Un vaso de agua?	Kee-eh-reh: Oon bah-soh deh ah-goo-ah
Do you want: Something to eat?	¿Quiere: Algo de comer?	Kee-eh-reh: Ahl-goh deh koh-mehr
Do you wear glasses?	¿Usas anteojos/lentes?	Oo-sahs ahn-teh-oh-hohs/lehn-tehs
Do you wish to have a bowel movement?	¿Quiere evacuar/hacer del baño?	Kee-eh-reh eh-bah-koo-ahr/ah-sehr dehl bah-nyoh
Do you wish to pass urine?	¿Quiére orinar?	Kee-eh-reh oh-ree-nahr

English	Spanish	Pronunciation	English	Spanish	Pronunciation
Do you wish/want something to eat?	¿Quiére algo de comer?	Kee-eh-reh ahl-goh deh koh-mehr	Hello. I need to take your temperature and blood pressure.	Hola. Necesito tomarle la temperatura y la presión de la sangre.	Oh-lah. Neh-seh-see-toh toh-mahr-leh lah tehm-peh-rah-too-rah ee lah preh-see-ohn deh lah sahn-greh
Do you wish/want to drink?	¿Quiére tomar/ beber?	Kee-eh-reh toh-mahr/ beh-behr	Here is the bell.	Aquí está la campana.	Ah-kee ehs-tah lah kahm-pah-nah
Does the pain move from one place to another?	¿El dolor se mueve de un lugar a otro?	Ehl doh-lohr seh moo-eh-beh deh oon loo-gahr ah oh-troh	How are you today?	¿Como está hoy?	Koh-moh ehs-tah oh-ee
Don't walk barefoot.	No camine descalzo.	Noh kah-mee-neh dehs-kahl-soh	How often do you feed the baby?	¿Qué tan a menudo alimenta al bebé?	Keh tahn ah meh-noo-doh ah-lee-mehn-tah ahl beh-beh
Don't worry!	¡No se preocupe!	Noh seh preh-oh-koo-peh	How often do you urinate?	¿Cuántas veces orina?	Koo-ahn-tahs beh-sehs oh-ree-nah
Drink.	Beba./Tome.	Beh-bah/Toh-meh	How old are you?	¿Cuántos años tiene?	Koo-ahn-tohs ah-nyohs tee-eh-neh
Eat!	¡Coma!	Koh-mah	How severe is the pain?	¿Qué tan severo es el dolor?	Keh tahn seh-beh-roh ehs ehl doh-lohr
Eight o'clock.	Las ocho.	Lahs oh-choh			
Eight o'clock (mil).	Las viente horas.	Lahs beh-een-teh oh-rahs	I also need a urine sample.	También necesito una muestra de orina.	Tahm-bee-ehn neh-seh-see-toh oo-nah moo-ehs-trah deh oh-ree-nah
Eleven o'clock.	Las once.	Lahs ohn-seh			
Eleven o'clock (mil).	Las veintitrés horas.	Lahs beh-een-tee-trehs oh-rahs	I am going to check the oxygen tank.	Voy a checar el tanque de oxígeno.	Boh-ee ah cheh-kahr ehl tahn-keh deh ohx-ee-heh-noh
Every time you go to the bathroom to void, you must place the urine in the container.	Cada vez que vaya al baño a orinar, debe poner la orina en el recipiente.	Kah-dah behs keh bah-yah ahl bah-nyoh ah oh-ree-nahr, deh-beh poh-nehr lah oh-ree-nah ehn ehl reh-see-pee-ehn-the	I am going to collect a stool sample.	Voy a recoger una muestra de excremento.	Boh-ee ah reh-koh-hehr oo-nah moo-ehs-trah deh ehx-kreh-mehn-toh
			I am going to cover you with a sheet.	Voy a cubrirlo con una sábana.	Boh-ee ah koo-breer-loh kohn oo-nah sah-bah-nah
Excuse me!	¡Perdón/ Excúseme/Con permiso!	Pehr-dohn/ Ehx-koo-seh-meh/ Kohn pher-mee-soh	I am going to cover you.	Lo voy a cubrir.	Loh boh-ee ah koo-breer
Extend your arm.	Extiende tu brazo.	Ehx-tee-ehn-deh too brah-soh	I am going to explain the collection of urine.	Le voy a explicar la colección de orina.	Leh boh-ee ah ehx-plee-kahr lah koh-lehk-see-ohn deh oh-ree-nah
Extend your leg and foot.	Extiende tu pierna y pie.	Ehx-tee-ehn-deh too pee-her-nah ee pee-eh			
Extend your wrist.	Extiende tu muñeca.	Ehx-tee-ehn-deh too moo-nyeh-kah	I am going to get a wheelchair.	Voy a traer una silla de ruedas.	Boh-ee ah trah-her oo-nah see-yah deh roo-eh-dahs
First, I want to brush your teeth.	Primero, quiero limpiarle los dientes.	Pree-meh-roh kee-eh-roh leem-pee-ahr-leh lohs dee-ehn-tehs	I am going to help you lie on the stretcher.	Voy a ayudarlo a acostarse en la camilla.	Boh-ee ah ah-yoo-dahr-loh ah ah-kohs-tahr-seh ehn lah kah-mee-yah
Five o'clock.	Las cinco.	Lahs seen-koh			
Five o'clock (mil).	Las diecisiete horas	Lahs dee-ehs-ee-see-eh-teh oh-rahs	I am going to help you.	Voy a ayudarlo.	Boh-ee ah ah-yoo-dahr-loh
Four o'clock.	Las cuatro	Lahs koo-ah-troh	I am going to insert your dentures.	Voy a ponerle la dentadura.	Boh-ee ah poh-nehr-leh lah dehn-tah-doo-rah
Four o'clock (mil).	Las dieciséis horas	Lahs dee-ehs-ee-seh-ees oh-rahs			
Good afternoon!	¡Buenas tardes!	Boo-eh-nahs tahr-dehs	I am going to take the radial pulse.	Voy a tomar tu pulso radial.	Boh-ee ah toh-mahr too pool-soh rah-dee-ahl
Good morning!	¡Buenos días!	Boo-eh-nohs dee-ahs			
Has the pain gotten worse or gotten better?	¿Se ha puesto el dolor peor o mejor?	Seh ah poo-ehs-toh ehl doh-lohr peh-ohr oh meh-hohr			
Have you been a patient before?	¿Ha sido paciente antes?	Ah see-doh pah-see-ehn-the ahn-tehs			
Have you eaten?	¿Ha comido?	Ah koh-mee-doh			

English	Spanish	Pronunciation	English	Spanish	Pronunciation
I am going to take your blood pressure and pulse.	Voy a tomar la presión y el pulso.	Boh-ee ah toh-mahr lah preh-see-ohn ee ehl pool-soh	Is there any pain?	¿Tiene algún dolor?	Tee-eh-neh ahl-goon doh-lohr
I am here to help you with exercises.	Estoy aquí para ayudarlo con ejercicios.	Ehs-toh-ee ah-kee pah-rah ah-yoo-dahr-loh kohn eh-hehr-see-see-ohs	Is there anything else bothering you?	¿Hay otra cosa que le moleste?	Ah-ee oh-trah koh-sah keh leh moh-lehs-teh
I am the nurse (female).	Yo soy la enfermera.	Yoh soh-ee lah ehn-fehr-meh-rah	Is your appetite bad?	¿Tiene mal apetito?	Tee-eh-neh mahl ah-peh-tee-toh
I am the nurse (male).	Yo soy el enfermero.	Yoh soh-ee ehl ehn-fehr-meh-roh	Keep moving.	Siga moviéndose.	See-gah moh-bee-ehn-doh-seh
I have the bedpan.	Tengo el bacín/pato.	Tehn-goh ehl bah-seen/ pah-toh	Keep the leg straight.	Antenga la pierna derecha.	Mahn-tehn-gah lah pee-her-nah deh-reh-chah
I need to take your temperature and blood pressure.	Necesito tomarle la temperatura y la presión de la sangre.	Neh-seh-see-toh toh-mahr-leh lah tehm-peh-rah-too-rah ee lah preh-see-ohn deh lah sahn-greh	Keep the side rails up at night.	Mantenga los barandales levantados durante la noche.	Mahn-tehn-gah lohs bah-rahn-dah-lehs leh-bahn-tah-dohs doo-rahn-the lah noh-cheh
I want to help you stand up.	Quiero ayudarlo a sentarse.	Kee-eh-roh ah-yoo-dahr-loh ah sehn-tahr-seh	Keep your feet together.	Mantenga los pies juntos.	Mahn-tehn-gah lah pee-ehr-nah eh-leh-bah-dah
I want you to use a cane.	Quiero que use un bastón.	Kee-eh-roh keh oo-seh oon bahs-tohn	Keep your leg elevated.	Mantenga la pierna elevada.	Mahn-tehn-gah lah pee-ehr-nah eh-leh-bah-dah
I will give you a bath.	Voy a bañarlo.	Boh-ee ah bah-nyahr-loh	Left . . .	Izquierdo . . .	Ees-kee-ehr-doh
I will help you sit.	Le ayudaré a sentarse.	Leh ah-yoo-dah-reh ah sehn-tahr-seh	Let me know how you feel.	Dígame cómo se siente.	Dee-gah-meh koh-moh seh see-ehn-teh
I will show you your room.	Le mostraré su cuarto.	Leh mohs-trah-reh soo koo-ahr-toh	Let's walk.	Vamos a caminar.	Bah-mohs ah kah-mee-nahr
I will start by taking vital signs.	Voy a empezar por tomar los signos vitals.	Boh-ee ah ehm-peh-sahr pohr toh-mahr lohs seeg-nohs bee-tah-lehs	Lie down (please)!	¡Acuéstese (por favor)!	Ah-koo-ehs-teh-seh (pohr fah-bohr)
I will start by taking vital signs.	Empezaré por tomar los signos vitales.	Ehm-peh-sah-reh pohr toh-mahr lohs seeg-nohs bee-tah-lehs	Lift the foot.	Levante el pie.	Leh-bahn-teh ehl pee-eh
			Lift your arm(s).	Levanta tu/los brazo(s).	Leh bahn-tah too/ lohs brah-soh(s)
			Lift your hand.	Levanta tu mano.	Leh bahn-tah too mah-noh
I will take your blood pressure.	Tomaré tu presión de sangre.	Toh-mah-reh too preh-see-ohn deh sahn-greh	Lift your head.	Levanta la cabeza.	Leh bahn-tah lah kah-beh-sah
			Lift your leg.	Levanta la pierna.	Leh bahn-tah lah pee-her-nah
If it hurts, tell me.	Si duele, avísame.	See doo-eh-leh, ah-bee-sah-meh	Lift your right arm.	Levente el brazo derecho.	Leh-bahn-teh ehl brah-soh deh-reh-choh
If you have questions, please let me know.	Si tiene preguntas, por favor avíseme.	See tee-eh-neh preh-goon-tahs, pohr fah-bohr ah-bee-seh-meh	Lift your right foot.	Levante el pie derecho.	Leh-bahn-teh ehl pee-eh deh-reh-choh
If you need more sheets, call the assistant.	Si necesita más sábanas, llame a la/al asistente.	See neh-seh-see-tah mahs sah-bah-nahs, yah-meh ah lah/ahl ah-sees-tehn-teh	Look straight ahead.	Mira hacia adelante.	Mee-rah ah-see-ah ah-deh-lahn-teh
			Lower the foot.	Baja el pie.	Bah-hah ehl pee-eh
Is that enough?	¿Es suficiente?	Ehs soo-fee-see-ehn-teh	Lower your head.	Baja la cabeza.	Bah-hah lah kah-beh-sah
Is that too much?	¿Es mucho?	Ehs moo-choh	Lower your legs.	Baje las piernas.	Bah-heh lahs pee-ehr-nahs
Is the pain there all the time, or does it come and go?	¿Está el dolor allí todo el tiempo, o va y viene?	Ehs-tah ehl doh-lohr ah-yee toh-doh ehl tee-ehm-poh, oh bah ee bee-ehn-eh?	Make a fist!	¡Cierre la mano/ Haga un puñto!	See-eh-reh lah mah-noh/ Ah-gah oon poo-nyoh
			May I help you?	¿Puedo ayudarlo?	¿Poo-eh-doh ah-yoo-dahr-loh?

English	Spanish	Pronunciation	English	Spanish	Pronunciation
Move it side to side.	Muévela de lado a lando.	Moo-eh-beh-lah deh lah-doh ah lah-doh	The bladder.	La vejiga.	Lah beh-hee-gah
Nine o'clock.	Las nueve.	Lahs noo-eh-beh	The doctor.	El doctor.	Ehl dohk-tohr
Nine o'clock (mil).	Las veintiuna horas.	Lahs beh-een-tee-oo-nah oh-rahs	The hospital.	El hospital.	Ehl ohs-pee-tahl
Noon/midnight.	Las doce.	Lahs doh-seh	The meals are served at 7 AM.	Los alimentos se sirven a las siete de la mañana.	Lohs ah-lee-mehn-tohs seh seer-behn ah lahs see-eh-teh deh lah mah-nyah-nah
Noon/midnight (mil).	Las cero horas.	Lahs seh-roh oh-rahs			
Now, stand up and walk.	Ahora, levántese y camine.	Ah-oh-rah, leh-bahn-teh-seh ee kah-mee-neh	The nurse.	El/la enfermero(a)	Ehl/lah ehn-fehr-meh-roh[ah]
Nursing care of the patient.	Cuidados del paciente.	Koo-ee-dah-dohs dehl pah-see-ehn-teh	The salt and pepper are in these packets.	La sal y la pimienta están en estos paquetes.	Lah sahl ee lah pee-mee-ehn-tah ehs-tahn ehn ehs-tohs pah-keh-tehs
On a scale from 1 (insignificant) to 10 (unbearable):	En una escala del uno (insignificante) al diez (intolerable):	Ehn oo-nah ehs-kah-lah dehl oo-noh (een-seeg-nee-fee-kahn-the) ahl dee-ehs (een-toh-leh-rah-bleh)	The water is in the glass/ pitcher.	El agua está en el vaso/la jarra.	Ehl ah-goo-ah ehs-tah ehn ehl bah-soh/ lah-hah-rah
One o'clock.	La una	Lah oo-nah	The water is warm. Can you feel?	El agua está tibia. ¿Puede sentir?	Ehl ah-goo-ah ehs-tah tee-bee-ah. Poo-eh-deh sehn-teer
One o'clock (mil).	Las trece horas	Lahs treh-seh oh-rahs			
Open your mouth.	Abra la boca.	Ah-brah lah boh-kah	There is an emergency light.	Hay una luz para emergencias.	Ah-ee oo-nah loos pah-rah eh-mehr-hehn-see-ahs
Open your mouth, please.	Abra la boca, por favor.	Ah-brah lah boh-kah, pohr fah-bohr	This is the call bell/buzzer.	Esta es la campana/el timbre.	Ehs-tah ehs lah kahm-pah-nah/ ehl teem-breh
Place the urine in the brown plastic bottle.	Ponga la orina en la botella de plástico café.	Pohn-gah lah oh-ree-nah ehn lah boh-teh-yah deh plahs-tee-koh kah-feh	Three o'clock.	Las tres	Lahs trehs
			Three o'clock (mil).	Las quince horas	Lahs keen-seh oh-rahs
Please, swallow.	Traga, por favor.	Trah-gah pohr fah-bohr	Three times a day.	Tres veces al día.	Trehs beh-sehs ahl dee-ah
Pull the cord in the bathroom.	Jale el cordón en el baño.	Hah-leh ehl kohr-dohn ehn ehl bah-nyoh	Tomorrow you are going to have your surgery.	Mañana le van a hacer la cirugía.	Mah-nyah-nah leh bahn ah ah-sehr lah see-roo-hee-ah
Put the spoon in your mouth.	Ponga la cuchara en la boca.	Pohn-gah lah koo-chah-rah ehn lah boh-kah			
Rest.	Descanse.	Des-kahn-seh	Try to calm down.	Trate de calmarse.	Trah-teh deh kahl-mahr-seh
Seven o'clock.	Las siete.	Lahs see-eh-teh	Twice a day.	Dos veces al día.	Dohs beh-sehs ahl dee-ah
Seven o'clock (mil)	Las diecinueve horas.	Lahs dee-ehs-ee-noo-eh-beh oh-rahs	Two o' clock.	Las dos.	Lahs dohs
			Two o' clock (mil).	Las catorce horas.	Lahs kah-tohr-seh oh-rahs
Sit down, please.	Siéntese, por favor.	See-ehn-teh-seh pohr fah-bohr	Void a little, then put urine in this cup.	Orine un poco, luego ponga la orina en esta taza.	Oh-ree-neh oon poh-koh, loo-eh-goh pohn-gah lah oh-ree-nah ehn ehs-tah tah-sah
Sit in the chair.	Siéntese en la silla.	See-ehn-teh-seh ehn lah see-yah			
Six o'clock.	Las seis	Lahs seh-ees			
Six o'clock (mil).	Las dieciocho horas	Lahs dee-ehs-ee-oh-choh oh-rahs	Wait!	¡Espere!	Ehs-peh-reh
Something to drink?	Algo de tomar/ beber?	Ahl-goh deh toh-mahr/ beh-behr	Wash your face!	¡Lávese la cara!	Lah-beh-seh lah kah-rah
Stay sitting.	Quédese sentado.	Keh-deh-seh sehn-tah-doh	Watch his navel.	Vigile su ombligo.	Bee-hee-leh soo ohm-blee-goh
Taking formula?	¿Tomando fórmula?	Toh-mahn-doh fohr-moo-lah	What can I help you with?	¿En que puedo ayudarlo?	Ehn keh poo-eh-doh ah-yoo-dahr-loh
Ten o'clock.	Las diez.	Lahs dee-ehs			
Ten o'clock (mil).	Las veintidós horas.	Lahs beh-een-tee-dohs oh-rahs	What caused the pain?	¿Qué causó el dolor?	Keh kah-oo-soh ehl doh-lohr
Thank you!	¡Gracias!	Grah-see-ahs	What did you eat?	¿Qué comió?	Keh koh-mee-oh
The bell will sound.	La campana sonará.	Lah kahm-pah-nah soh-nah-rah	What do you do?	¿Qué hace usted?	Keh ah-seh oos-tehd

English	Spanish	Pronunciation
What foods do you dislike?	¿Qué alimentos le disgustan?	Keh ah-lee-mehn-tohs leh dees-goos-tahn
What foods do you like?	¿Qué alimentos le gustan?	Keh ah-lee-mehn-tohs leh goos-tahn
What formula does he take?	¿Qué fórmula toma?	Keh fohr-moo-lah toh-mah
What is the color of the urine?	¿Cuál era el color de la orina?	Koo-ahl eh-rah ehl koh-lohr deh lah oh-ree-nah
What is the pain like?	¿Qué tipo de dolor tiene?	Keh tee-poh deh doh-lohr tee-eh-neh
What is this?	¿Qué es esto?	Keh ehs ehs-toh
What is wrong?	¿Qué pasa?	Keh pah-sah
What is your name?	¿Cómo se llama?	Koh-moh seh yah-mah
What makes the pain better?	¿Qué hace mejorar el dolor?	Keh ah-seh meh-hoh-rahr ehl doh-lohr
When was the last time you used the toilet?	¿Cuándo fue la última vez que hizo del baño/ que obró?	Koo-ahn-doh foo-eh lah ool-tee-mah behs keh ee-soh dehl bah-nyoh/ keh oh-broh
Where do you work?	¿Dónde trabaja?	Dohn-deh trah-bah-hah
Where does it hurt?	¿Dónde le duele?	Don-deh leh doo-eh-leh

English	Spanish	Pronunciation
You ate well.	Comió bien.	Koh-mee-oh bee-ehn
You can also ask for snacks.	También puede pedir aperitivos.	Tahm-bee-ehn poo-eh-deh peh-deer ah-peh-ree-tee-bohs
You can drink water.	Puede tomar agua.	Poo-eh-deh toh-mahr ah-goo-ah
You can smoke on the patio.	Puede fumar en el patio.	Poo-eh-deh foo-mahr ehn ehl pah-tee-oh
You cannot smoke here.	No puede fumar aquí.	Noh poo-eh-deh foo-mahr ah-kee
You have false teeth.	Tiene dentaduras postizas.	Tee-eh-neh dehn-tah-doo-rahs pohs-tee-sahs
You need to be admitted.	Necesita internarse al hospital.	Neh-seh-see-tah een-tehr-nahr-she ahl ohs-pee-tahl
You need to drink water.	Necesita tomar agua.	Neh-seh-see-tah toh-mahr ah-goo-ah
You will be all right!	¡Va a estar bien!	Bah ah ehs-tahr bee-ehn
Your appetite is good?	¿Tiene buen apetito?	Tee-eh-neh boo-ehn ah-peh-tee-toh
Your clothes go in the closet.	Su ropa va en el closet/ ropero.	Soo roh-pah bah ehn ehl kloh-seht/ roh-peh-roh

Answers to Review Questions

Chapter 1
1. 4
2. 3
3. 1
4. 2
5. 3

Chapter 2
1. 2
2. 2
3. 1
4. 3
5. 3
6. 4
7. 1

Chapter 3
1. 3
2. 2
3. 2
4. 3
5. 4
6. 1

Chapter 4
1. 4
2. 3
3. 3
4. 1
5. 4
6. 2

Chapter 5
1. 4
2. 4
3. 1
4. 3
5. 2
6. 2
7. 3

Chapter 6
1. 2
2. 1
3. 2
4. 4
5. 3

Chapter 7
1. 2
2. 3
3. 1

4. 4
5. 3

Chapter 8
1. 3
2. 2
3. 3
4. 4
5. 1
6. 4
7. 3
8. 2

Chapter 9
1. 2
2. 4
3. 1
4. 3
5. 4
6. 3
7. 3
8. 2
9. 4
10. 2
11. 1

Chapter 10
1. 3
2. 4
3. 2
4. 1
5. 2
6. 2

Chapter 11
1. 1
2. 1
3. 3
4. 3
5. 2
6. 2
7. 4
8. 3
9. 1
10. 4

Chapter 12
1. 4
2. 2
3. 1
4. 1

5. 1
6. 3
7. 4
8. 2
9. 1

Chapter 13
1. 3
2. 2
3. 1
4. 3
5. 4
6. 3
7. 1
8. 4
9. 2
10. 1
11. 2
12. 2
13. 3
14. 3
15. 4

Chapter 14
1. 4
2. 1
3. 3
4. 2
5. 4
6. 2
7. 2
8. 3
9. 1
10. 3
11. 2
12. 4

Chapter 15
1. 1
2. 2
3. 3
4. 4
5. 4
6. 2
7. 1
8. 4
9. 3
10. 3

Chapter 16
1. 1
2. 4

3. 2
4. 2
5. 1
6. 4
7. 3
8. 2
9. 4
10. 1

Chapter 17
1. 2
2. 2
3. 3
4. 3
5. 4
6. 4
7. 1
8. 2

Chapter 18
1. 1
2. 2
3. 4
4. 3
5. 1

Chapter 19
1. 4
2. 2
3. 1
4. 3
5. 3
6. 2
7. 2
8. 3
9. 4
10. 2

Chapter 20
1. 1
2. 1
3. 1
4. 3

Chapter 21
1. 3
2. 1
3. 2
4. 1
5. 4
6. 4
7. 2

Chapter 22
1. 1
2. 3
3. 1
4. 2
5. 3
6. 4

Chapter 23
1. 4
2. 2
3. 4
4. 1
5. 2
6. 1
7. 3
8. 3
9. 1
10. 2
11. 3

Chapter 24
1. 2
2. 4
3. 2
4. 3
5. 4
6. 4
7. 1
8. 2
9. 3
10. 1
11. 4

Chapter 25
1. 1
2. 3
3. 2
4. 3
5. 4
6. 4
7. 1
8. 3
9. 2
10. 4

Chapter 26
1. 2
2. 4
3. 1
4. 3
5. 4

6. 1
7. 3
8. 3
9. 3
10. 1

Chapter 27
1. 1
2. 3
3. 4
4. 4
5. 3
6. 2
7. 1
8. 4
9. 3

Chapter 28
1. 2
2. 3
3. 4
4. 4
5. 1
6. 2
7. 4
8. 3
9. 2

Chapter 29
1. 2
2. 1
3. 2
4. 3
5. 4
6. 4
7. 1
8. 3
9. 3
10. 1

Chapter 30
1. 3
2. 4
3. 1
4. 2
5. 2
6. 3
7. 4
8. 4
9. 1
10. 2

Chapter 31
1. 4
2. 1
3. 2
4. 3
5. 2
6. 4
7. 1
8. 2
9. 4
10. 2

Chapter 32
1. 4
2. 3
3. 3
4. 4
5. 2
6. 1
7. 3
8. 1
9. 1
10. 3

Chapter 33
1. 1
2. 3
3. 2
4. 4
5. 1
6. 3
7. 1
8. 2
9. 4

Chapter 34
1. 4
2. 1
3. 2
4. 1
5. 1
6. 1
7. 3
8. 2
9. 2
10. 3
11. 3

Chapter 35
1. 4
2. 1
3. 3
4. 2

5. 4
6. 1
7. 4
8. 3
9. 2
10. 4
11. 2
12. 3
13. 3
14. 1

Chapter 36
1. 2
2. 3
3. 1
4. 4
5. 3
6. 1
7. 4
8. 3
9. 2
10. 1

Chapter 37
1. 4
2. 3
3. 2
4. 3
5. 2
6. 2
7. 3
8. 1
9. 1

Chapter 38
1. 1
2. 3
3. 4
4. 2
5. 3
6. 1
7. 2
8. 4
9. 1
10. 4

Chapter 39
1. 2
2. 1
3. 2
4. 3
5. 4
6. 3

7. 1
8. 4
9. 2
10. 1

Chapter 40
1. 4
2. 1
3. 3
4. 2
5. 2
6. 4
7. 1
8. 2
9. 4
10. 2

Chapter 41
1. 1
2. 3
3. 1
4. 2
5. 4
6. 1
7. 4
8. 2
9. 3
10. 1

Chapter 42
1. 4
2. 3
3. 2
4. 4
5. 1
6. 4
7. 2
8. 1
9. 2
10. 3

Chapter 43
1. 2
2. 1
3. 4
4. 2
5. 4
6. 2
7. 2
8. 1
9. 4
10. 3

Chapter 44
1. 3
2. 1
3. 3
4. 4
5. 1
6. 2
7. 3
8. 2
9. 1
10. 2

Chapter 45
1. 1
2. 3
3. 2
4. 4
5. 2
6. 1
7. 2
8. 2
9. 3
10. 1

Chapter 46
1. 2
2. 1
3. 4
4. 3
5. 2
6. 4
7. 2
8. 1
9. 3
10. 4

Chapter 47
1. 3
2. 1
3. 4
4. 2
5. 1
6. 2
7. 3
8. 4
9. 1
10. 3

Chapter 48
1. 2
2. 2
3. 3

Chapter 44
1. 3
2. 1
3. 3
4. 4
5. 4
6. 1
7. 3
8. 4
9. 4
10. 1

Chapter 49
1. 3
2. 2
3. 1
4. 2
5. 1
6. 4
7. 1
8. 3
9. 4
10. 1, 3, 4

Chapter 50
1. 2
2. 1
3. 3
4. 4
5. 4
6. 1
7. 4
8. 3
9. 2
10. 2

Chapter 51
1. 1
2. 3
3. 4
4. 2
5. 2
6. 2
7. 3
8. 1
9. 2
10. 3

Chapter 52
1. 3
2. 3
3. 2
4. 4
5. 1
6. 2
7. 3

8. 1
9. 3
10. 3

Chapter 53
1. 3
2. 3
3. 1
4. 4
5. 3
6. 3
7. 2
8. 1
9. 3
10. 2

Chapter 54
1. 2
2. 1
3. 4
4. 4
5. 2
6. 2
7. 4
8. 3
9. 1
10. 3

Chapter 55
1. 1
2. 2
3. 4
4. 1
5. 3
6. 1
7. 4
8. 2
9. 3
10. 1

Chapter 56
1. 1
2. 3
3. 2
4. 4
5. 2
6. 3
7. 1
8. 3
9. 3
10. 2

Bibliography & Reader References

Chapter 1

AHRQ. (2005, Aug. 9). *Press Release: AHRQ issues new data on the uninsured.* Retrieved Sept. 28, 2005, from www.ahrq.gov/news/press/pr2005/mepstatspr.htm.

AHRQ. (2005). *HCUP Fact Book No. 6: Hospitalization in the United States, 2002.* Retrieved Oct. 1, 2005, from www.ahrq.gov/data/hcup/factbk6/factbk6b.htm.

Bodenheimer, T. (2005, May 17). High and rising health care costs. Part 1: Seeking an explanation. *Annals 2005, 142*(10), 847-854.

Hoffman, J.M., Shah, N.D., Vermeulen, L.C., Hunkler, R.J., & Hontz, K.M. (2004, Jan. 15). *American Journal of Health System Pharmacy, 61*, 145-158.

Rhoades, J.A. (2005, June). *The uninsured in America, 2004: Estimates for the U.S. civilian noninstitutionalized population under age 65.* MEPS Statistical Brief No. 83, Agency for Healthcare Research and Quality. Rockville, MD. Retrieved Sept. 25, 2005, from www.meps.ahrq.gov/papers/st83/stat83.pdf.

Strunk, B.C., & Ginsburg, P.B. (2004). Tracking health care costs: Trends turn downward in 2003. Health Affairs. Suppl. Web Exclusives: W4-354-62.

Tu, H.T. (2004, Sept.). Rising health costs, medical debt, and chronic conditions. *Issue Brief/Center for Studying Health System Change, 88,* 1-5.

United States Department of Health and Human Services. (2005). *Health care financing administration.* Retrieved Sept. 29, 2005, from www.os.dhhs.gov/about/opdivs/hcfa.html.

United States Department of Health and Human Services. (2005). *HHS: What we do.* Retrieved Sept. 28, 2005, from www.os.hhs.gov/about/whatwedo.html.

Medicare. (2005). *Your Medicare prescription drug coverage options.* Retrieved Oct. 1, 2005, from www.Medicare.gov.

Yu, W., Ravelo, A., Wagner, T.H., & Barnett, P.G. (2004). The relationship among age, chronic conditions, and healthcare costs. *American Journal of Managed Care, 10*(2), 909-916.

Additional Resources

American Association for Ambulatory Care Nursing: 1-800-262-6877; www.inurse.com/~AAACN.

Center for Patient Care Advocacy: www.patientadvocacy.org.

Home Health Care Nurse's Association: www.junior.apk.net/~nurse/.

Hospice Foundation of America: 1-800-854-3402; www.hospicefoundation.org.

Hospice Hands: http://hospice-cares.com.

National Committee for Quality Assurance: www.ncqa.org.

Chapter 2

Centers for Medicare and Medicaid Services. (2004, Aug.). *Medicare and home health care.* Baltimore, MD: Department of Health and Human Services.

Easton, K.L. (1999). *Gerontological rehabilitation nursing.* Philadelphia: Saunders.

Jackson, R. (2003). CMS describes nursing home trends. *Health Care Food Nutrition Focus, 20*(10), 4-5.

Matteson, M.A., McConnell, E.S., & Linton, A.D. (1997). *Gerontological nursing* (2nd ed.). Philadelphia: Saunders.

Monks, K.M. (2000). *Pocket guide to home health care.* Philadelphia: Saunders.

Stanhope, M., & Lancaster, J. (2004). *Community and public health nursing* (6th ed.). St. Louis: Mosby.

Chapter 3

Altman, W.M., Parmelee, P.A., & Smyer, M.A. (1999). The doctrine of informed consent. In L.A. Frolik (Ed.), *Aging and the law: An interdisciplinary reader* (pp. 297-311). Philadelphia: Temple University Press.

American Association of Colleges of Nursing. (1986). *Essentials of college and university education for professional nurses.* Washington, DC: Author.

Brooke, P.S. (2005). Understanding HIPAA compliance. *LPN2005, 1*(4), 37-39.

Brostron, J.C. (2001). Legal implications in nursing practice. In P.A. Potter & A.G. Perry (Eds.), *Fundamentals of nursing* (5th ed., pp. 422-443). St. Louis: Mosby.

Burkhardt, M.A., & Nathaniel, A.K. (2002). *Ethics and issues in contemporary nursing* (2nd ed.). Albany, NY: Delman.

Curtin, L., Flaherty, M.J. (1982). *Nursing ethics: Theories and pragmatics.* Bowie MD: Brady. Cited in Potter, P.A., & Perry, A.G. (2005). *Fundamentals of nursing,* 6th ed. St. Louis: Mosby.

Ecker, M. (2001). Ethics and values. In P.A. Potter & A.G. Perry (Eds.), *Fundamentals of nursing* (5th ed., pp. 401-422). St. Louis: Mosby.

Ham, K.L. (2002). *From LPN to RN role transitions.* Philadelphia: Saunders.

Hill, S.S., & Howlett, H.A. (1997). *Success in practical nursing* (3rd ed.). Philadelphia: Saunders.

Jameton, A. (1984). *Nursing practice: The ethical issues.* Englewood Cliffs, NJ: Prentice-Hall. Cited in Burkhardt, M.A., & Nathaniel, A.K. (2002). *Ethics and issues in contemporary nursing* (2nd ed.). Albany, NY: Delmar.

Model Nurse Practice Act. (2004). National Council of State Boards of Nursing. Retrieved Oct. 9, 2005, from www.ncsbn.org.

National Council of State Boards of Nursing. (2005). Model Nursing Act and Rules. Retrieved August 2, 2005 from http://ncsbn.org/regulation/nursingpractice_nursing_practice_model_act and _rules.asp.

National Council of State Boards of Nursing. (2006). National Council of State Boards of Nursing. (2006). *Working with others: A position paper.* Chicago: Author.

NAPNES Standards of Practice for Licensed Practical/Vocational Nurses. (2004). National Association for Practical Nurse Education and Service http://www.napnes.org/standards.pdf.

Potter, P.A., & Perry, A.G. (2005). *Fundamentals of nursing* (6th ed). St. Louis: Mosby.

Chapter 4

Anderson, M.A. (1997). *Nursing leadership, management, and professional practice for the LPN/LVN* (Chapters 5, 11). Philadelphia: Davis.

Boucher, M.A. (1998). Delegation alert. *American Journal of Nursing, 98*(2), 26-33.

NLN Council of Practical Nursing Programs. (1994). *Entry level competencies of graduates of educational programs in practical nursing.* New York: Author.

Hill, S., & Howlett, H. (1997). *Success in practical nursing: Personal and vocational issues* (Chapters 16, 18, 19). Philadelphia: Saunders.

National Council of State Boards of Nursing. (2006). *Working with others: A position paper.* Chicago: Author.

Spector, N. (2005). *Practical Nurse Scope of Practice White Paper.* Chicago: National Council of State Boards of Nursing. Retrieved January 29, 2007, from http://www.ncsbn.org/regulation/nursing.

Vicenzi, A.E. (1997). Chaos in nursing: Make it work for you. *American Journal of Nursing, 97*(10), 26-32.

Yoder-Wise, P.S. (1999). *Leading and managing in nursing* (Chapters 17, 19). St. Louis: Mosby.

Zerwekh, J., & Claborn, J. (Eds.). (2000). *Nursing today: Transition and trends* (3rd ed., Chapter 8). Philadelphia: Saunders.

Chapter 5

Alfaro-LeFevre, R. (1995). *Critical thinking in nursing: A practical approach*. Philadelphia: Saunders.

Anderson, M.A. (1997). Nursing leadership, management, and professional practice for the LPN/LVN. Philadelphia: Davis.

Curtin, L.L. (1996). The ethics of managed care: Part 1: Proposing a new ethos? *Nursing Management, 27*(8), 18-19.

Curtin, L.L. (1996). The ethics of managed care: Part 3: Toward a common vision. *Nursing Management, 27*(10), 71-74.

Ellis, J. (1995). *Nursing in today's world: Challenge, issues, and trends* (5th ed.). Philadelphia: Lippincott.

Heitman, K.K., & Robinson, B. (1997). Developing a nursing ethics roundtable. *American Journal of Nursing, 97*(1), 36-38.

Ignatavicius, D.D., Workman, M. L., & Mishler, M. (1995). *Medical-surgical nursing: A nursing process approach*. Philadelphia: Saunders.

Zerwekh, J., & Claborn, J. (Eds.). (1997). *Nursing today: Transition and trends*. Philadelphia: Saunders.

Chapter 6

American Nurses Association. (1998, Jan.-Feb.). ANA addressing cultural diversity in the profession. *American Nurse, 30*(1), 25.

Andrews, M.M., & Boyle, J.S. (Eds.). (1995). *Transcultural concepts in nursing care* (2nd ed.). Philadelphia: Lippincott.

Black, J.M., & Matassarin-Jacobs, E. (2001). *Medical-surgical nursing: Clinical management for continuity of care* (6th ed., Chapters 3, 4, 9). Philadelphia: Saunders.

Ellis, J.R. (1998). Cultural competence in nursing care. In F.D. Monahan, D.T. Drake, & M. Neighbors (Eds.). *Medical-surgical nursing: Foundations for clinical practice* (pp. 1230-1231). Philadelphia: Saunders.

Federwisch, A. (1998). Missing pieces: The puzzle of diversity in health care. *Health Week, 3*(16), 1.

Geissler, E.M. (1998). *Cultural assessment* (2nd ed.). St. Louis: Mosby.

Hill, S.S., & Howlett, H.A. (2005). *Success in practical nursing* (5th ed., Chapters 12, 13). Philadelphia: Saunders.

Ignatavicius, D.D., Workman, M.L., & Mishler, M. (1999). *Medical-surgical nursing: A nursing process approach* (3rd ed.). Philadelphia: Saunders.

Jarvis, C. (1996). *Physical examination and health assessment* (2nd ed., pp. 8-10, 50-57, 95-96, 217). Philadelphia: Saunders.

Keegan, L. (1998). Alternative and complementary therapies. *Nursing 98, 28*(4), 50-53.

Leininger, M.M. (1988). Transcultural eating patterns and nutrition: Transcultural nursing and anthropological perspectives. *Holistic Nursing Practice, 3*(1), 16-25.

Leininger, M.M. (1991). Transcultural nursing: The study and practice field. *Imprint, 38*(2), 55.

Luckmann, J. (1997). *Saunders manual of nursing care* (Chapter 2). Philadelphia: Saunders.

Meleis, A.I. (1996). Culturally competent scholarship: Substance and rigor. *Advances in Nursing Science, 19*(2), 1-16.

Spector, R. (1995). *Cultural diversity in health and illness* (4th ed., pp. 137-142). Norwalk, CT: Appleton & Lange.

White, L., & Duncan, G. (1998). *Medical-surgical nursing: An integrated approach* (Chapters 6, 7). Albany, NY: Delmar.

Chapter 7

De Montigny, F., Beaudet, L., & Dumas, L. (1996). The impact of a child's death on the family. *Canadian Nurse, 92*(10), 39-42.

Friedman, M.M. (1997). *Family nursing: Theory, research, and practice* (4th ed.). Stamford, CT: Appleton & Lange.

Hanson, S.M.H., & Boyd, S.T. (1996). *Family health care nursing: Theory, practice, and research*. Philadelphia: Davis.

Kahana, E., Biegel, D.E., & Wykle, M.L. (1994). *Family caregiving across the lifespan*. Thousand Oaks, CA: Sage.

Leahey, M., & Harper-Jaques, S. (1996). Family-nurse relationships: Core assumptions and clinical implications. *Journal of Family Nursing, 2*(2), 133-151.

Meckler, L. (2001, April 13). Traditional family seems to be making a comeback. *San Antonio Express News*, p. 10A.

Chapter 8

American heritage dictionary (3rd ed.). (1992). New York: Houghton Mifflin.

Black, J.M., Hawks, J.H., & Keene, A.M. (2001). *Medical-surgical nursing: Clinical management for continuity of care* (6th ed., Chapters 1, 2, 20). Philadelphia: Saunders.

Evans, B.M. (1999). Complementary therapies and HIV infection. *American Journal of Nursing, 99*(2), 42-45.

Henderson, V. (1964). The nature of nursing. *American Journal of Nursing, 64*, 64.

Ignatavicius, D.D., & Workman, M.L. (2002). *Medical-surgical nursing: A nursing process approach* (4th ed., Chapters. 1, 4). Philadelphia: Saunders.

Institute of Medicine. (1999). *Leading health indicators for Healthy People 2010. Second interim report*. Washington, DC: National Academy Press.

Potter, P., & Perry, A. (2001). Fundamentals of nursing (6th ed., Chapter 6). St. Louis: Mosby.

U.S. Department of Health and Human Services, Public Health Service. (2000). *Healthy People 2010*. Retrieved November 21, 2005, from www.healthypeople.gov/LHI/lhiwhat.htm.

Internet Resource

National Center for Complementary and Alternative Medicine: www.nccam.nih.gov.

Chapter 9

Cammon, S.A., & Hackshaw, H.S. (2000). Are we starving our patients? *American Journal of Nursing, 100*(5), 43-47.

Combs, G.F. (2005). The point of the new pyramid. *USDA Agricultural Research Service*. Retrieved November 29, 2005 from http://www.ars.usda.gov/News/docs.htm?docid=10819&pf=1&cg_id=0.

Dudek, S.G. (2000). Malnutrition in hospitals: Who's assessing what patients eat? *American Journal of Nursing, 100*(4), 36-43.

Hankins, J., Lonsway, R.A.W., Hedrick, C., & Perdue, M.B. (2001). *Infusion therapy in clinical practice* (2nd ed.). Philadelphia: Saunders.

Heitz, U.E., & Horne, M.M. (2001). *Fluid, electrolyte, and acid-base balance*. St. Louis: Mosby.

Institute of Medicine. (2004). Dietary reference intakes. Retrieved November 28, 2005 from http://www.iom.edu/CMS?3788/4574.aspx.

Mahan, L.K., & Escott-Stump, S. (2000). *Krause's food, nutrition, and diet therapy* (10th ed.). Philadelphia: Saunders.

Metheny, N., Wehrle, M.A., & Wiersema, L. (1998). Testing feeding tube placement: Auscultation vs. pH method. *American Journal of Nursing, 98*(5), 37-42.

Orbanic, S. (2001). Understanding bulimia. *American Journal of Nursing, 101*(3), 35-42.

Smith, R.M., & Myers, S.A. (2005). Two devices that unclog feeding tubes. *RN, 68*(1), 36-41.

U.S. Department of Agriculture. (2005). Dietary Guidelines for Americans 2005. Retrieved November 28, 2005 from http://www.health.gov/dietaryguidelines/dga2005/recommendations.htm.

Chapter 10

American Cancer Society (ACS). (2000). *Annual Pap smears may not be necessary*. Retrieved Dec 9, 2005, from www.cancer.org.

American Cancer Society (ACS). (2004). *ACS cancer detection guidelines*. Retrieved Dec. 10, 2005, from www.cancer.org.

Erikson, E. (1963). *Childhood and society* (2nd ed.). New York: Norton.

Ignatavicius, D.D., Workman, M.L., & Mishler, M. (1999). *Medical-surgical nursing: A nursing process approach* (3rd ed., Chapters 5, 6). Philadelphia: Saunders.

MMWR Weekly Quick Guide. (2005, Oct. 14). *Recommended adult immunization schedule—United States, Oct. 2005-Sept. 2006.*

Sheehy, G. (1995). *New passages*. New York: Random House.

Stobbe, M. (2005, Dec. 9). Life in the U.S. just got longer: Up to 77.6 years. *San Antonio Express News*, p. 3A.

U.S. Department of Health and Human Services, Centers for Disease Control and Prevention. *NCHS FASTATS—Leading causes of death*. Retrieved Dec. 7, 2005, from www.cdc.gov/nchs/fastats/1cod.htm.

U.S. Department of Health and Human Services, Public Health Service. (2000). *Healthy People 2010.* Retrieved Nov. 21, 2005, from www.healthypeople.gov.htm.

Chapter 11

Alzheimer's Association. (2001). *General statistics/demographics.* Retrieved Feb. 6, 2001, from www.alz.org/hc/overview/stats.htm.

Erikson, E. (1963). *Childhood and society.* New York: Norton.

Guay, D.R.P., Artz, M.B., Hanlon, J.T., & Schmader, K. (2003). The pharmacology of aging. In R.C. Tallis & H.M. Fillit (Eds.), *Brocklehurst's textbook of geriatric medicine and gerontology* (6th ed., pp. 155-161). London: Churchill Livingstone.

Gunter, L., & Estes, C. (1979). *Education for gerontologic nursing.* New York: Springer.

Lehne, R.A. (2004). *Pharmacology for nursing care* (5th ed.). Philadelphia: Saunders.

Masters, W.H., & Johnson, V.E. (1966). *Human sexual response* (p. 233). Boston: Little, Brown.

Matteson, M.A., McConnell, E., & Linton, A.D. (1997). *Gerontological nursing: Concepts and practice* (2nd ed.). Philadelphia: Saunders.

Chapter 12

Aquilino, M.L., & Keenan, G. (2000). Having our say: Nursing's standardized nomenclatures. *American Journal of Nursing, 100*(7), 33-38.

Alfaro-LeFevre, R. (1998). *Applying nursing process: A step by step guide* (4th ed.). Philadelphia: Lippincott.

Carpenito, L. (1997). *Nursing diagnosis: Application to clinical practice* (7th ed.). Philadelphia: Lippincott-Raven.

Cirone, N. (1998). Charting tips: Correcting charting errors. *Nursing, 28*(4), 65.

Ennis, R. (1985). A logical basis for measuring critical thinking skills. *Educational Leadership, 43*(2), 44-48. Cited in P.R. Cook (1995). Using critical thinking skills to improve medication administration. *MEDSURG Nursing 4*(4), 309-313.

Facione, N.C., & Facione, P.A. (1996). Externalizing the critical thinking in knowledge development and clinical judgment. *Nursing Outlook, 44,* 129-136.

Hill, S.S., & Howlett, H.A. (2005). *Success in practical nursing: Personal and vocational issues* (5th ed.). Philadelphia: Saunders.

Ignatavicius, D., & Hausman, K.A. (1995). *Clinical pathways for collaborative practice.* Philadelphia: Saunders.

Ignatavicius, D., Workman, M., & Mishler, M. (2002). *Medical-surgical nursing: A nursing process approach* (4th ed., Chapter 1). Philadelphia: Saunders.

Jarvis, C. (2004). *Physical examination and health assessment* (4th ed.). Philadelphia: Saunders.

Johnson, M., Bulechek, G., Dochterman, J.M., Maas, M., & Moorhead, S. (Eds.). (2001). *Nursing diagnoses, outcomes, and interventions: NANDA, NOC, and NIC linkages.* St. Louis: Mosby.

Luckmann, J. (Ed.). (1997). *Saunders manual of nursing care* (Chapters 1, 4, 5). Philadelphia: Saunders.

National Council of State Boards of Nursing (NCSBN). (2006). *Working with others: A Position Paper.* Chicago: NCSBN.

North American Nursing Diagnosis Association. (2005). *Nursing diagnoses: Definitions and classification 2005-2006.* Philadelphia: Author.

Internet Resource

NurseCom: www.nursecominc.com.

Chapter 13

Black, J.M., Hawks, J.H., & Keene, A.M. (2001). *Medical-surgical nursing: Clinical management for continuity of care* (6th ed., Chapters 16, 17). Philadelphia: Saunders.

Centers for Disease Control and Prevention. (2005). *Contact precautions.* Retrieved Dec. 8, 2005, from www.cdc.gov/ncidod/dhqp/gl_isolation_contact.html.

Guyton, A.C., & Hall, J.E. (2006). *Textbook of medical physiology* (11th ed., Chapter 34). Philadelphia: Saunders.

Herlihy, B., & Maebius, N.K. (2000). *The human body in health and illness.* Philadelphia: Saunders.

HICPAC. (1995). *Recommendations for preventing the spread of vancomycin resistance. Recommendations of the Hospital Infection Control Practices Advisory Committee.* Retrieved Dec. 8, 2005, from www.cdc.gov.

Jones, L., & Hannum, D. (1998). Playing it safe with a particulate respirator. *Nursing, 28*(1), 50-51.

Lehne, R.A. (2004). *Pharmacology for nursing care* (5th ed.). Philadelphia: Saunders.

Phillips, J.K. (2004). Nursing management: Shock and multiple organ dysfunction syndrome. In S.M. Lewis, M.M. Hietkemper, & S.R. Dirksen, *Medical surgical nursing: Assessment and management of clinical problems* (6th ed., pp. 1796-1823). St. Louis: Mosby.

Potter, P.A., & Perry, A.G. (2005). *Fundamentals of nursing* (6th ed.). St. Louis: Mosby.

Sheff, B. (1998). VRE and MRSA: Putting bad bugs out of business. *Nursing, 28*(3), 40-44.

The Bioterrorism Institute, Ltd. (2005). *Bioterrorism basics for nurses* (Vol 1). Columbus, OH: Author.

Internet Resources

The Centers for Disease Control and Prevention: www.cdc.gov.

Information about infectious diseases and immunization: www.healthtouch.com.

The Agency on Health Care Research and Quality Guidelines for Clinical Practice: www.ahrq.gov.

Chapter 14

Abrams, A.C. (2005). *Clinical drug therapy: Rationales for nursing practice* (7th ed.). Philadelphia: Lippincott.

Black, J.M., Hawks, J.H., & Keene, A.M. (2001). *Medical-surgical nursing: Clinical management for continuity of care* (6th ed.). Philadelphia: Saunders.

DeJong, M.J. (1998). Emergency! Hyponatremia. *American Journal of Nursing, 98*(12), 36.

Guyton, A.C., & Hall, J.E. (2006). *Textbook of medical physiology* (11th ed.). Philadelphia: Saunders.

Heitz, U.E., & Horne, M.M. (2001). *Fluid, electrolyte, and acid-base balance.* St. Louis: Mosby.

Herlihy, B., & Maebius, N.K. (2000). *The human body in health and illness.* Philadelphia: Saunders.

Horne, C., & Derrico, D. (1999). Mastering ABGs. *American Journal of Nursing, 99*(8), 26-33.

Ignatavicius, D.D., Workman, M.L., & Mishler, M.A. (1999). *Medical-surgical nursing: A nursing process approach* (3rd ed.). Philadelphia: Saunders.

Jacobs, D.S., DeMott, W.R., Grady, H.J., Horvat, R.T., Huestis, D.W., & Kasten, B.L. (1996). *Laboratory test handbook.* Hudson (Cleveland): Lexi-Comp, Inc.

Jaffe, H.S., & McVan, B.F. (1997). *Davis's laboratory and diagnostic test handbook.* Philadelphia: Davis.

Jarvis, C. (1999). *Physical examination and health assessment* (3rd ed.). Philadelphia: Saunders.

Luckmann, J. (1997). *Saunders manual of nursing care.* Philadelphia: Saunders.

Phillips, L.D. (1997). *Manual of I.V. therapeutics* (2nd ed.). Philadelphia: Davis.

Wong, F.W.H. (1999). A new approach to ABG interpretation. *American Journal of Nursing, 99*(8), 34-36.

Chapter 15

Acute Pain Management Guidelines Panel. (1992). *Acute pain management: Operative and medical procedures and trauma. Clinical practice guidelines* (AHCPR Publication No. 92-0032). Rockville, MD: Agency for Health Care Policy and Research, Public Health Service, U.S. Department of Health and Human Services.

American Pain Society. (1999). *Principles of analgesic use in the treatment of acute pain and chronic cancer pain* (4th ed.). Skokie, IL: Author.

Deglin, J., & Vallerand, A. (2000). *Davis' drug guide for nurses* (7th ed.). Philadelphia: Davis.

Dossey, B. (1995). Using imagery to help your patient heal. *American Journal of Nursing, 95*(6), 40-47.

International Association for the Study of Pain. (1994). *IASP pain terminology, 1994.* Retrieved February 8, 2002, from www.iasp_pain/org/terms=p.html.

Jacox, A., Carr, C.B., Payne, R. et al. (1994, March). *Management of cancer pain: Clinical practice guideline No. 9* (AHCPR Publication No. 94-0592). Rockville, MD: Agency for Health Care Policy and Research, U.S. Department of Health and Human Services, Public Health Service.

Joint Commission on Accreditation of Healthcare Organizations. (2000). *Pain assessment and management.* Oakbrook Terrace, IL: Author.

Loeb, J. (1999). Pain management in long-term care. *American Journal of Nursing, 99*(2), 48-52.

Loeser, J.D. (Ed.). (2000). *Bonica's management of pain* (3rd ed.). Philadelphia: Lippincott Williams & Wilkins.

McCaffery, M., & Pasero, C. (1999). *Pain: Clinical manual.* St. Louis: Mosby.

Mersky, H. & Bugduk, N. (1994). Classification of chronic pain descriptions of chronic pain syndromes and definitions of pain terms. (2nd ed.). Seattle: IASP Press.

Pasero, C. (1998). Teaching patients how to use PCA. *American Journal of Nursing, 98*(9), 14-15.

Strevy, S. (1998). Myths and facts about pain. *RN, 61*(2), 42-47.

Waitman, J., & McCaffery, M. (2000). Meperidine—liability. *American Journal of Nursing, 100*(2), 57-58.

Internet Resources

Agency for Healthcare Research and Quality: www.ahrq.org.

American Cancer Society: www.cancer.org.

American Pain Society: www.ampainsoc.org.

Arthritis Foundation: www.arthritis.org.

Hospice Foundation of America: www.hospicefoundation.org.

Joint Commission on Accreditation of Healthcare Organizations: www.jcaho.org.

North American Chronic Pain Association: www.chronicpaincanada.org.

Chapter 16

Adam, R.D., & Sullivan, J.B. (2000). Venomous snake bites. In L. Goldman & J.C. Bennett (Eds.), *Cecil textbook of medicine* (21st ed., pp. 2001-2003). Philadelphia: Saunders.

American Association of Poison Control Centers. (2006). *Frequently asked questions.* Retrieved February 19, 2007 from www.aapcc.org.

American Heart Association. (2006). *BLS for healthcare providers.* Dallas: Author.

American Heart Association. (2000). *International CPR and ECC guidelines 2000: Major changes and revisions.* Retrieved April 21, 2002, from www.cpr-exx.org/Whats_new/Whats_menu.htm.

Barbarito, C. (1998). Emergency! Hypertension-induced epistaxis. *American Journal of Nursing, 98*(2), 48.

Huston, C.J. (1998). Emergency! Cervical spine injury. *American Journal of Nursing, 98*(6), 33.

Ignatavicius, D.D., Workman, M.L., & Mishler, M.A. (1999). *Medical-surgical nursing: A nursing process approach* (3rd ed.). Philadelphia: Saunders.

Wade, C.F. (2000). Keeping Lyme disease at bay. *American Journal of Nursing, 100*(7), 26-32.

Chapter 17

Abrams, A.C. (2004). *Clinical drug therapy* (7th ed.). Philadelphia: Lippincott.

Black, J.M., Hawks, J.H., & Keene, A.M. (2001). *Medical-surgical nursing: Clinical management for continuity of care* (6th ed.). Philadelphia: Saunders.

Faries, J. (1998). Easing your patient's postoperative pain. *Nursing 98, 28*(6), 58-60.

Hodge, D. (Ed.). (1999). *Day surgery: A nursing approach.* Edinburgh: Churchill Livingstone.

Ignatavicius, D.D., Workman, M.L., & Mishler, M.A. (1999). *Medical-surgical nursing: A nursing process approach* (3rd ed.). Philadelphia: Saunders.

Jarvis, C. (1999). *Physical examination and health assessment* (3rd ed.). Philadelphia: Saunders.

King, M.E., & Kinney, A.Y. (2001). Tissue adhesives: A sticky solution to wound repair. *Nursing, 31*(3), 52-53.

Kingsley, C. (2001). Epidural analgesia: Your role. *RN, 64*(3), 53-58.

Mahan, L.K., & Escott-Stump, S. (2000). *Krause's food, nutrition, and diet therapy* (10th ed.). Philadelphia: Saunders.

Messinger, J.A., Hoffman, L.A., O'Donnell, J.M., & Dunworth, B.A. (1999). Getting conscious sedation right. *American Journal of Nursing, 99*(12), 44-50.

Phillips, J.K. (1998). Actionstat: Wound dehiscence. *Nursing, 28*(3), 33.

Walton, J. (2001). Helping high-risk surgical patients beat the odds. *Nursing, 31*(3), 54-60.

Chapter 18

Ignatavicius, D.D., Workman, M.L., & Mishler, M.A. (1999). *Medical-surgical nursing: A nursing process approach* (3rd ed.). Philadelphia: Saunders.

Love, G. (1998). Controlling pain: Easing the discomfort of venipuncture. *Nursing, 28*(3), 30.

Masoorli, S. (1998). Removing a PICC? Proceed with caution. *Nursing, 28*(3), 56-57.

Perucca, R. (2001). Changing and discontinuing infusion therapy. In J. Hankins, R.A.W. Lonsway, C. Hedrick, & M.B. Perdue, *Infusion therapy in clinical practice* (2nd ed., pp. 398-403). Philadelphia: Saunders.

Perucca, R. (2001). Infusion monitoring and catheter care. In J. Hankins, R.A.W. Lonsway, C. Hedrick, & M.B. Perdue, *Infusion therapy in clinical practice* (2nd ed., pp. 389-397). Philadelphia: Saunders.

Perucca, R. (2001). Infusion therapy equipment: Types of infusion therapy equipment. In J. Hankins, R.A.W. Lonsway, C. Hedrick, & M.B. Perdue, *Infusion therapy in clinical practice* (2nd ed., pp. 300-333). Philadelphia: Saunders.

Perucca, R. (2001). Obtaining vascular access. In J. Hankins, R.A.W. Lonsway, C. Hedrick, & M.B. Perdue, *Infusion therapy in clinical practice* (2nd ed., pp. 375-388). Philadelphia: Saunders.

Walther, K. (2001). Intravenous therapy in the older adult. In J. Hankins, R.A.W. Lonsway, C. Hedrick, & M.B. Perdue, *Infusion therapy in clinical practice* (2nd ed., pp. 592-603). Philadelphia: Saunders.

Internet Resources

Intravenous Nurses Society: www.ins1.org.

SpringNet: www.springnet.com.

Chapter 19

Abrams, A.C. (2004). *Clinical drug therapy* (7th ed.). Philadelphia: Lippincott.

Atassi, K.A., & Harris, M.L. (2001). Disseminated intravascular coagulation. *Nursing, 31*(3), 64.

LaFramboise, L.N. (2001). Management of clients with shock and multisystem disorders. In J.M. Black, J.H. Hawks, & A.M. Keene (Eds.), *Medical-surgical nursing: Clinical management for positive outcomes* (6th ed., pp. 2231-2259). Philadelphia: Saunders.

Marshall, J. (2001). Inflammation, coagulopathy, and the pathogenesis of multiple organ dysfunction syndrome. *Critical Care Medicine, 29*(7), S99-S105.

McKinley, M. (2005). Shock and sepsis. In M.L. Sole, D. Klein, & M. Moseley (Eds.). *Introduction to critical care nursing* (4th ed., pp. 249-289). Philadelphia: Saunders.

Phillips, J.K. (2004). Nursing management: Shock and multiple organ dysfunction syndrome. In S.M. Lewis, M.M Heitkemper, & S.R Dirksen (Eds.), *Medical-surgical nursing: Assessment and management of clinical problems* (6th ed., pp. 1796-1823). St. Louis: Mosby.

Tierney, L. & Messina, L. (2003). Blood vessels and lymphatics. In L. Tierney, S. McPhee, & M. Papadakis (Eds.). *Current medical diagnosis and treatment* (pp. 465-468). 42nd edition. New York: Lange Medical Books/McGraw-Hill.

U.S. Department of Health and Human Services (USDHHS). (2000). *Healthy people 2010.* Rockville, MD: Author.

Chapter 20

Capezuti, E., Talerico, K.A., Cochran, I., Becker, H., Strumpf, N., & Evans, L. (1999). Individualized interventions to prevent bed-related falls and reduce siderail use. *Journal of Gerontological Nursing, 25*(11), 26-33.

Matteson, M.A., McConnell, E.S., & Linton, A.D. (1997). *Gerontological nursing.* Philadelphia: Saunders.

Meiner, S.E., & Miceli, D.G. (2000). Safety. In A.G. Lueckenotte (Ed.), *Gerontologic nursing* (2nd ed., pp. 232-255). St. Louis: Mosby.

Rogers, P.D., & Bocchino, N.L. (1999). Restraint-free care: Is it possible? *American Journal of Nursing, 99*(10), 26-33.

Stone, J.T., & Wyman, J.F. (1999). Falls. In J.T. Stone, J.F. Wyman, & S.A. Salisbury (Eds.), *Clinical gerontological nursing* (2nd ed., pp. 341-366). Philadelphia: Saunders.

Walker, B.L. (1998). Preventing falls. *RN, 61*(5), 40-43.

Chapter 21

Agency for Health Care Policy and Research. (1992). *How to predict and prevent pressure ulcers . . . clinical practice guidelines released by the Agency for Health Care Policy and Research.* Retrieved May 28, 2001, from www.ahcpr.gov.

Agency for Health Care Policy and Research. (1994). *Pressure ulcer treatment . . . clinical practice guidelines released by the Agency for Health Care Policy and Research.* Retrieved May 28, 2001, from www.ahcpr.gov.

Lueckenotte, A.G. (2000). *Gerontologic nursing* (2nd ed.). St. Louis: Mosby.

Matteson, M.A., McConnell, E.S., & Linton, A.D. (1997). *Gerontological nursing* (2nd ed.). Philadelphia: Saunders.

National Pressure Ulcer Advisory Panel. (1996). Pressure ulcer research: Etiology, assessment, and early intervention. *Dermatology Nursing, 8*(1), 41-47.

National Pressure Ulcer Advisory Panel. (2007). Pressure ulcer stages revised by NPUAP. Press Release, February 2007.

Stone, J.T., Wyman, J.F., & Salisbury, S.A. (1999). *Clinical gerontological nursing: A guide to advanced practice* (2nd ed.). Philadelphia: Saunders.

Chapter 22

Adams, T., & Clarke, C.L. (1999). *Dementia care.* London: Baillière Tindall.

Lancaster, M.M., Abusamra, L.C., & Clark, W.G. (1998). Management of difficult behaviors. In R.C. Hamdy, J.M. Turnbull, J. Edwards, & M.M. Lancaster (Eds.), *Alzheimer's disease: A handbook for caregivers* (3rd ed., pp. 150-170). St. Louis: Mosby.

Matteson, M.A., Linton, A.D., & Barnes, S.J. (1996). Cognitive developmental approach to dementia. *Image: Journal of Nursing Scholarship, 28*(3), 233-240.

Matteson, M.A., Linton, A.D., Barnes, S.J., Cleary, B.L., & Lichtenstein, M.J. (1996). The relationship between Piaget and cognitive levels in persons with Alzheimer's disease and related disorders. *Aging: Clinical and Experimental Research, 8*(1), 61-69.

Matteson, M.A., McConnell, E.S., & Linton, A.D. (1997). *Gerontological nursing: Concepts and practice* (2nd ed.). Philadelphia: Saunders.

Chapter 23

Ahronheim, J.C. (2000). Special problems in the geriatric patient. In L. Goldman & J.C. Bennett (Eds.), *Cecil textbook of medicine* (21st ed., pp. 22-25). Philadelphia: Saunders.

American Society of Colon and Rectal Surgeons. (2000). *Bowel incontinence.* Retrieved Sept. 21, 2000, from www.fascrs.org/brochures/bowel-incontinence.html.

Engelberg, S.J.H., McDowell, B.J., & Lovell, A. (2000). In A.G. Lueckenotte, *Gerontologic nursing* (2nd ed., pp. 586-614). St. Louis: Mosby.

Fantl, J.A., Newman, D.K., Colling, J. et al. (1996, Jan.). Managing acute and chronic urinary incontinence. In Clinical Practice Guideline. Quick Reference Guide for Clinicians, No. 2, 1996 Update (AHCPR Publication No. 96-0686). Rockville, MD: U.S. DHHS, Public Health Service, Agency for Health Care Policy and Research.

Fillingham, S., & Douglas, J. (1997). *Urological nursing* (2nd ed.). London: Baillière Tindall.

Gray, M. (2004). Nursing management: Renal and urologic problems. In S.M. Lewis, M.J. Heitkemper, & S.R. Dirksen (Eds.), *Medical-surgical nursing: Assessment and management of clinical problems* (6th ed., pp. 1172-1209). Philadelphia: Saunders.

Gray, M. (2000). Urinary retention: Management in the acute care setting, Part 1. *American Journal of Nursing, 100*(7), 40-48.

Gray, M. (2000). Urinary retention: Management in the acute care setting, Part 2. *American Journal of Nursing, 100*(8), 36-44.

Johnson, S.T. (2000). From incontinence to confidence. *American Journal of Nursing, 100*(2), 69-76.

Miller, J.B. (2000). Urinary incontinence: A classification system and treatment protocol for the primary care provider. *Journal of the American Academy of Nurse Practicners, 12*(9), 374-379.

Ouslander, J.G. (2000). Urinary incontinence. In L. Goldman & J.C. Bennett (Eds.), *Cecil textbook of medicine* (21st ed., pp. 640-642). Philadelphia: Saunders.

Potter, P.A., & Perry, A.G. (2001). *Fundamentals of nursing* (5th ed.). St. Louis: Mosby.

Roberts, R.G. (2001). Current management strategies for overactive bladder. *A Supplement to Patient Care for the Nurse Practitioner, Spring 2001,* 22-33.

Smith, M. (1998). Gynecologic disorders. In E.H. Duthie & P.R. Katz (Eds.), *Practice of geriatrics* (3rd ed., pp. 524-534). Philadelphia: Saunders.

U.S. Department of Health and Human Services. (1992). *Urinary incontinence in adults* (AHCPR Publication No. 92-0038). Rockville, MD: Author.

Chapter 24

Ad Hoc Committee of the Harvard Medical School to Examine the Definition of Brain Death. (1968). A definition of irreversible coma. *Journal of the American Medical Association, 205*(6), 337-340.

American Medical Association's Institute for Ethics, EPEC (Education for Physicians on End of Life Care). (1999). *Trainer's and participant's handbooks.* Princeton: The Robert Wood Johnson Foundation.

Banks, G. (2000). Verifying a death. *Nursing Standard, 14*(33), 22-23.

Capron, A.M. (2001). Brain death—Well settled yet still unresolved. *New England Journal of Medicine, 344,* 1244-1246.

Carpenito, L.J. (2004). *Handbook of nursing diagnoses.* (10th ed.). Philadelphia: Lippincott.

Davitz, L., Sameshima, Y., Davitz, J. et al. (1976). Suffering as viewed in six different cultures. *American Journal of Nursing, 76*(8), 1296-1297.

DeSpelder, L.A., & Strickland, A.L. (2005). The *last dance: Encountering death and dying* (7th ed.). Boston: McGraw-Hill.

Ebersole, P., & Hess, P. (1998). *Toward healthy aging* (5th ed.). St. Louis: Mosby.

Geissler, E.M. (1998). *Mosby's pocket guide: Cultural assessment.* St. Louis: Mosby.

King, C.R., & Hinds, P.S. (2003). *Quality of life: From nursing and patient perspectives* (2nd ed.). Boston, Jones & Bartlett.

Kübler-Ross, E. (1974). *Questions and answers on death and dying.* New York: Macmillan.

Kübler-Ross, E. (1975). *Death, the final stage of growth.* Englewood Cliffs, NJ: Prentice-Hall.

Kübler-Ross, E. (1978). *To live until we say goodbye.* Englewood Cliffs, NJ: Prentice-Hall.

Kübler-Ross, E. (1981). *Living with death and dying.* New York: Macmillan.

Kübler-Ross, E. (1983). *On children and death.* New York: Macmillan.

Lugton, J., & Kindlin, M. (Eds.). (1999). *Palliative care: The nursing role.* Edinburgh: Churchill Livingstone.

Lynn, J., & Harrold, J. (1999). *Handbook for mortals: Guidance for people facing serious illness.* New York: Oxford University Press.

Lynn, J., Schuster, J.L., & Kabcenell, A. (2000). *Improving care for the end of life.* New York: Oxford University Press.

Martocchio, B.C. (1985). Grief and bereavement: Healing through hurt. *Nursing Clinics of North America, 20*(6), 327-341.

Matteson, M.A., McConnell, E.S., & Linton, A.D. (1997). *Gerontological nursing: Concepts and practice* (2nd ed.). Philadelphia: Saunders.

National Council of Hospice Professionals. (1997). *Guidelines for curriculum development on end-of-life and palliative care in nursing education.* Arlington, VA: Author.

Rando, T.A. (1993). *Treatment of complicated mourning.* Champaign, IL: Research Press.

Roark, D.C. (2000). Overhauling the organ donation system. *American Journal of Nursing, 200*(6), 44-49.

Schonwetter, R.S., Hawke, W., & Knight, C.F. (Eds.). (1999). *Hospice and palliative medicine core: Curriculum and review syllabus,* American Academy of Hospice and Palliative Medicine. Dubuque, IA: Kendall/Hunt Publishing Co.

Strauss, A.L., & Glaser, B.G. (1970). Awareness of dying. In B. Schoenberg et al. (Eds.), *Loss and grief: Psychosocial management in medical practice.* New York: Columbia University Press.

The Quality Standards Subcommittee of the American Academy of Neurology. (1995). Practice parameters for determining brain death in adults (summary statement). *Neurology, 45,* 275-287.

Wijdicks, E.F.M. (2001). Current concepts: The diagnosis of brain death. *New England Journal of Medicine, 344,* 1215-1221.

Internet Resources

Aging with Dignity: www. AgingwithDignity.org.

Association for Death Education and Counseling: www.adec.org.

Caring Connections: www.caringinfo.org.

Center for Practical Bioethics: www.practicalbioethics.org.

Coalition of Donation: www.shareyourlife.org.

Last Acts—a national coalition to improve care at end of life: www .lastacts.org.

Online Information on Palliative and End-of-Life Care: www .palliativecarenursing.net.

On our own terms: Moyers on Dying: www.PBS.org.

Project on Death in America: www.soros.org.

The Task Force to Improve the Care of Terminally Ill OREGONIANS: www.OHSO.edu.

United Network for Organ Sharing: www.unos.org.

Chapter 25

Abebe, W. (2002). Herbal medication: Potential for adverse interactions with analgesic drugs. *Journal of Clinical Pharmacy and Therapeutics, 27*(6), 391-401.

Abrams, A.C. (2004). *Clinical drug therapy* (7th ed.). Philadelphia: Lippincott Williams & Wilkins.

American Cancer Society. (2006). *Cancer facts and figures.* Retrieved Feb. 9, 2006, from www.cancer.org.

American Cancer Society. (2001). *Cancer in minorities.* Retrieved June 7, 2001, from www.americancancersociety.org.

American Cancer Society. (2001). *Complementary and alternative methods.* Retrieved June 7, 2001, from www.cancer.org/alt_therapy/index.htm.

Black, J.M., Hawks, J., & Keene, A.M. (2001). *Medical-surgical nursing: Clinical management for continuity of care* (6th ed.). Philadelphia: Saunders.

Brenner, M.K. (2000). Stem cell transplantation. In L. Goldman & J.C. Bennett (Eds.), *Cecil textbook of medicine* (21st ed., pp. 987-991). Philadelphia: Saunders.

Concus, A.P., & Singer, M.I. (2000). Head and neck cancer. In L. Goldman & J.C. Bennett (Eds.), *Cecil textbook of medicine* (21st ed., pp. 2257-2262). Philadelphia: Saunders.

Dodd, M.J., Dibble, S.L., & Thomas, M.L. (1993). Predictors of concerns and coping strategies of cancer chemotherapy outpatients. *Applied Nursing Research, 6*(1), 2-7.

Held-Warmkessel, J. (1998). Chemotherapy complications. *Nursing, 28*(4), 41-45.

Ignatavicius, D.D., Workman, M.L., & Mishler, M.A. (2003). *Medical-surgical nursing: A nursing process approach* (4th ed.). Philadelphia: Saunders.

Keegan, L. (1998). Alternative and complementary therapies. *Nursing, 28*(4), 50-53.

Lewis, S.M., Heitkemper, M.M., & Dirksen, S.R. (Eds.). (2004). *Medical-surgical nursing: Assessment and management of clinical problems* (6th ed.). St. Louis: Mosby.

Mahan, L.K., & Escott-Stump, S. (2000). *Krause's food, nutrition, and diet therapy* (10th ed.). Philadelphia: Saunders.

Moldawer, N., & Carr, E. (2000). The promise of recombinant interleukin-2. *American Journal of Nursing, 100*(5), 35-40.

Pagana, K.D., & Pagana, T.J. (2003). *Mosby's diagnostic and laboratory test reference* (6th ed.). St. Louis: Mosby.

Sexton, S.M. (2003). Complementary and alternative medicine: Examining the evidence. *American Family Physician, 67*(1), 36-38.

Society of Interventional Radiology (n.d.). *Treatments: Chemoembolization.* Retrieved March 3, 2007, from http://www.sirweb.org/patPub/cancerTreatments.shtml.

Sorensen, J.M. (2002). Herb-drug, food-drug, nutrient-drug, and drug-drug interactions: Mechanisms involved and their medical implications. *Journal of Alternative and Complementary Medicine, 8*(3), 293-308.

Wu, K., Farrelly, J., Birnkrant, D., Chen, S., Dou, J., Atrakchi, A., Bigger, A., Chen, C., Chen, Z., Freed, L., Ghantous, H., Goheer, A., Hausner, E., Osterberg, R., Rhee, H., & Zhang, K. (2004). Regulatory toxicology perspective on the development of botanical drug products in the United States. *American Journal of Therapeutics, 11*(3), 213-217.

Internet Resources

American Cancer Society: www.cancer.org.

National Cancer Institute—International Cancer Information Center: www.nci.nih.gov.

Oncology Nursing Society: www.ons.org.

Additional Resources

The following resources are old but offer many good, practical tips for the patient:

American Cancer Society. (1997). *A cancer source book for nurses* (7th ed.). Atlanta, GA: Author.

National Cancer Institute. (1987). *Chemotherapy and you* (NIH Publication No. 88-1136). Bethesda, MD: National Institutes of Health.

National Cancer Institute. (1987). *Radiation therapy and you.* Bethesda, MD: Author.

National Cancer Institute. (1992). *Eating hints: Recipes and tips for better nutrition during cancer treatment.* Bethesda, MD: Author.

Chapter 26

Black, P. (2000). Practical stoma care. *Nursing Standard, 14*(41), 47-55.

Colwell, J.C., Goldberg, M., & Carmel, J. (2001). The state of the standard diversion. *The Journal of Wound, Ostomy, and Continence Nursing, 28*(1), 6-17.

Erwin-Toth, P. (2001). Caring for a stoma is more than skin deep. *Nursing, 31*(5), 36-41.

Lewis, S.M., Heitkemper, M.M., & Dirksen, S.R. (2004). *Medical-surgical nursing: Assessment and management of clinical problems* (6th ed.). St. Louis: Mosby.

Ringhofer, J. (2005). Meeting the needs of your ostomy patient. *RN, 68*(8), 37-42.

Wound Ostomy Continence Nursing Certification Board. (n.d.). *Entry level wound ostomy continence practice.* Retrieved Feb. 18, 2006, from www.wocncb.org/position/.

Internet Resources

American Cancer Society: www.cancer.org.

Crohn's & Colitis Foundation of America: www.ccfa.org.

United Ostomy Associations of America: www.uoaa.org.

Wound, Ostomy and Continence Nurses Society: www.wocn.org.

Additional Resource

Ostomy Quarterly lists mail order houses that sell discount ostomy supplies: 1-800-826-0826.

Chapter 27

Amella, E.J. (2004). Presentation of illness in older adults. *American Journal of Nursing, 104*(10), 40-52.

Bader, M.K. & Littlejohns, L.R. (2004). *AANN core curriculum for neuroscience nursing* (4th ed.). Philadelphia: Saunders.

Barker, E. (2002). *Neuroscience nursing: A spectrum of care.* St. Louis. Mosby.

Carson, P. (1993). Investing in the comeback: Parent's experience following traumatic brain injury. *Journal of Neuroscience Nursing, 25*(3), 165-173.

Chasen, E.R., & Umlauf, M.G. (2000). Post-polio syndrome. *American Journal of Nursing, 100*(12), 60-63.

Costello, K., & Harris, C. (2003) Differential diagnosis and management of fatigue in multiple sclerosis: Considerations for the nurse. *Journal of Neuroscience Nursing, 35*(3), 139-148.

Finlayson, M., Denend, T.V., & Hudson, E. (2004). Aging with multiple sclerosis. *Journal of Neuroscience Nursing, 36*(5), 245-251, 259.

Frohman, E.M. (2003). Multiple sclerosis. *Medical Clinics of North America, 87,* 867-897.

Halper, J., Kennedy, P., Miller, C.M., Morgante, L., Namey, M., & Ross, A.P. (2003). Rethinking cognitive function in multiple sclerosis: A nursing perspective. *Journal of Neuroscience Nursing, 35*(2), 70-81,

Hendrickson, S.G. (2003). Broadening the understanding of injury prevention: A case study. *Journal of Neuroscience Nursing, 35*(1), 30-39.

Kerr, M., & Crago, E.A. (2004). Nursing management: Acute intracranial problems. In S.M. Lewis, M.M. Heitkemper, & S.R. Dirksen (Eds.), *Medical-surgical nursing: Assessment and management of clinical problems* (6th ed., pp. 1491-1524). St. Louis: Mosby.

Lehman, C.A., Hayes, J.M., LaCroix, M., Owen, S.V., & Nauta, J.W. (2003). Development and implementation of a problem-focused neurological assessment system. *Journal of Neuroscience Nursing, 35*(4), 185-192.

Ozuna, J.M. (2004). Nursing assessment: Nervous system. In S.M. Lewis, M.M. Heitkemper, & S.R. Dirksen (Eds.), *Medical-surgical nursing: Assessment and management of clinical problems* (6th ed., pp. 1464-1490). St. Louis: Mosby.

Ozuna, J.M. (2004). Nursing management: Chronic neurologic problems. In S.M. Lewis, M.M. Heitkemper, & S.R. Dirksen (Eds.), *Medical-surgical nursing: Assessment and management of clinical problems* (6th ed., pp. 1549-1580). St. Louis: Mosby.

Sinclair, V.G., & Scroggie, J. (2005). Effects of a cognitive-behavioral program for women with multiple sclerosis. *Journal of Neuroscience Nursing, 37*(5), 249-257.

Skidmore-Roth, L. (2003). *Mosby's drug guide for nurses* (5th ed.). St. Louis: Mosby.

Stewart, R.M., Desaloms, J.M., & Sanghera, M.K. (2005). Stimulation of the subthalamic nucleus for the treatment of Parkinson's disease: Postoperative management, programming, and rehabilitation. *Journal of Neuroscience Nursing, 37*(2), 108-114.

Tornquest, A. (2001). Neurosurgery for movement disorders. *Journal of Neuroscience Nursing, 33*, 79-82.

Chapter 28

Adams, H.P., Adams, R.J., Brott, T. et al. (2000). Guidelines for the early management of patients with ischemic stroke. *Stroke, 3*, 1056-1083.

Albers, G.W., Caplan, L.R., Easton, J.D., et al. (2002). Transient ischemic attack: Proposal for a new definition. *New England Journal of Medicine, 347*(21), 1713-1716.

Alberts, M.J., Hademenos, G., Latchaw, R.E. et al. (2000). Recommendations for the establishment of primary stroke centers. Brain Attack Coalition. *JAMA, 283*, 3102-3109.

American Heart Association (AHA). (2004). *Heart disease and stroke statistics—2005 update.* Dallas, TX: Author.

Bahouth, M.N., & LaMonte, M.P. (2005). Acute ischemic stroke: Evaluation and management strategies. *Topics in Advanced Practice Nursing eJournal, 5*, 4. Medscape.

Frizzell, J.P., Argour, R., & March, K. (2005). Acute stroke: Pathophysiology, diagnosis, and treatment. *AACN clinical issues: Advance practice in acute and critical care, 16*(4), 421-440.

Solenski, M.J. (2004). Transient ischemic attacks. Part 1. Diagnosis and evaluation. *American Family Physician, 69*(7), 1665-1674.

Internet Resource

National Stroke Association: www.stroke.org.

Chapter 29

Bader, M.K., & Littlejohns, L.R. (2004). *AANN core curriculum for neuroscience nursing* (4th ed.). Philadelphia: Saunders.

Barker, E. (2002). *Neuroscience nursing: A spectrum of care.* St. Louis: Mosby.

French, J.K., & Phillips, J.A. (1991). Shattered images: Recovery for the SCI client. *Rehabilitation Nursing, 16*(13), 134-136.

Hulsebosh, C.E. (2002). Recent advances in pathophysiology and treatment of spinal cord injury. *Advances in Physiology Education, 26*(4), 238-255.

Skidmore-Roth, L. (2003). *Mosby's drug guide for nurses* (5th ed.). St. Louis: Mosby.

Warms, C. (2004). Nursing management: Peripheral nerve and spinal cord problems. In S.M. Lewis, M.M. Heitkemper, & S.R. Dirksen (Eds.). *Medical-surgical nursing: Assessment and management of clinical problems* (6th ed., pp. 1610-1631). St. Louis: Mosby.

Zigler, J.E., Anderson, P.A., Boden, S.D., Birdwell, K.H., & Vaccaro, A.R. (2003). Specialty update: What's new in spine surgery. *The Journal of Bone and Joint Surgery, 85-A*(8), 1626-1636.

Chapter 30

Abrams, A.C. (2004). *Clinical drug therapy* (7th ed.). Philadelphia: Lippincott-Raven.

Black, J.M., Hawks, J.H., & Keene, A.M. (2001). *Medical-surgical nursing: Clinical management for positive outcomes* (6th ed.). Philadelphia: Saunders.

Carroll, P. (1998). Closing in on safer suctioning. *RN, 61*(5), 22-27.

Crimlisk, J.T. (2004). Nursing management: Lower respiratory problems. In S.M. Lewis, M.M. Heitkemper, & S.R. Dirksen (Eds.). *Medical-surgical nursing: Assessment and management of clinical problems* (6th ed., pp. 592-636). St. Louis: Mosby.

Gibbar-Clements, T., Shirrell, D., Dooley, R., & Smiley, B. (2000). The challenge of warfarin therapy. *American Journal of Nursing, 100*(3), 38-40.

Hagler, D.A. (2004). Nursing assessment: Respiratory system. In S.M. Lewis, M.M. Heitkemper, & S.R. Dirksen (Eds.). *Medical-surgical nursing: Assessment and management of clinical problems* (6th ed., pp. 542-563). St. Louis: Mosby.

Hagler, D.A. (2004). Nursing management: Upper respiratory problems. In S.M. Lewis, M.M. Heitkemper, & S.R. Dirksen (Eds.). *Medical-surgical nursing: Assessment and management of clinical problems* (6th ed., pp. 566-591). St. Louis: Mosby.

Horne, C., & Derrico, D. (1999). Mastering ABGs. *American Journal of Nursing, 99*(8), 26-33.

Jarvis, C. (2004). *Physical examination and health assessment* (4th ed.). Philadelphia: Saunders.

Lehne, R.A. (2005). *Pharmacology for nursing care* (5th ed.). Philadelphia: Saunders.

Minino, A., Heron, M., Murphy, S.L., et al. (2005). Deaths: Final data for 2004. *NCHS Health and Statistics.* Retrieved March 3, 2007, from http://www.cdc.gov/nchs.

Owen, A. (1998). Respiratory assessment revisited. *Nursing, 28*(4), 48-49.

Skidmore-Roth, L. (2002). *Mosby's nursing drug reference.* St. Louis: Mosby.

Wong, F.W.H. (1999). A new approach to ABG interpretation. *American Journal of Nursing, 99*(8), 34-36.

Chapter 31

American Cancer Society. (2006). *Cancer facts and figures—2006.* Atlanta, GA: Author.

Benowitz, N.L. (2000). Tobacco. In L. Goldman & J.C. Bennett (Eds.), *Cecil textbook of medicine* (21st ed., pp. 33-37). Philadelphia: Saunders.

Centers for Disease Control and Prevention. (2003). *Treatment of tuberculosis.* Retrieved Feb. 20, 2006, from www.cdc.gov/mmwr/preview/mmwrhtml/rr5211a1.htm.

Drazen, J.M. (2000). Asthma. In L. Goldman & J.C. Bennett (Eds.), *Cecil textbook of medicine* (21st ed., pp. 387-393). Philadelphia: Saunders.

Heuther, S.E., & McCance, K.L. (2000). *Understanding pathophysiology.* St. Louis: Mosby.

Lewis, S.M., Heitkemper, M.M., & Dirksen, S.R. (Eds.). (2004). *Medical-surgical nursing: Assessment and management of clinical problems* (6th ed., Chapters 27, 28). St. Louis: Mosby.

Miller, Y.E. (2000). Pulmonary neoplasms. In L. Goldman & J.C. Bennett (Eds.), *Cecil textbook of medicine* (21st ed., pp. 449-454). Philadelphia: Saunders.

Reilly, J.J., & Mentzer, S.J. (2000). Surgical approach to lung disease. In L. Goldman & J.C. Bennett (Eds.), *Cecil textbook of medicine* (21st ed., pp. 475-479). Philadelphia: Saunders.

Rodarte, J.R. (2000). Chronic bronchitis and emphysema. In L. Goldman & J.C. Bennett (Eds.), *Cecil textbook of medicine* (21st ed., pp. 393-401). Philadelphia: Saunders.

Skidmore-Roth, L. (2002). *Mosby's nursing drug reference.* St. Louis: Mosby.

Weinberger, S.E. (2000). Sarcoidosis. In L. Goldman & J.C. Bennett (Eds.), *Cecil textbook of medicine* (21st ed., pp. 433-436). Philadelphia: Saunders.

Welsh, M.J. (2000). Cystic fibrosis. In L. Goldman & J.C. Bennett (Eds.), *Cecil textbook of medicine* (21st ed., pp. 401-405). Philadelphia: Saunders.

Chapter 32

American Association of Blood Banks, America's Blood Centers, and the American Red Cross. (2005). *Circular of information for the use of human blood and blood components.* Retrieved Sept. 2, 2005, from www.fda.gov/cber/gdlns/crclr.pdf.

Chernecky, C.C, & Berger, B.J. (2001). *Laboratory tests and diagnostic procedures* (3rd ed.). Philadelphia: Saunders.

DeVita Jr., V.T., Hellman, S., & Rosenberg, S.A. (2004). *Cancer: Principles and practice of oncology* (6th ed.). Philadelphia: Lippincott Williams & Wilkins.

Fischbach, F.T. (2004). *A manual of laboratory and diagnostic tests* (7th ed.). Philadelphia: Williams & Wilkins.

Key, J.L. (2004). *Handbook of laboratory and diagnostic tests with nursing implications* (5th ed.). Upper Saddle River, NJ: Pearson Prentice Hall.

Mannucci, P.M., & Tuddenham, E.G.D. (2001). Medical progress: The hemophilias—From royal genes to gene therapy. *New England Journal of Medicine, 344*(23), 1773-1779.

Skidmore-Roth, L. (2005). *Mosby's 2005 nursing drug reference.* St. Louis: Mosby.

Slaster, S., & Vichinsky, E.P. (2003). Managing sickle cell disease. *British Journal of Medicine, 327,* 1151-1155.

Yarbro, C.H., Frogge, M.H., Goodman, M., & Groenwald, S.L. (2000). *Cancer nursing: Principles and practice.* (5th ed.). Sudbury, MA: Jones & Bartlett.

Chapter 33

Abbas, A.K., & Lichtman, A.H. (2005). *Basic immunology: Functions and disorders of the immune system.* Philadelphia: Saunders.

American Cancer Society. (2006). *Cancer facts and figures—2006.* Atlanta, GA: Author.

Casciato, D.A. (2004). *Manual of clinical oncology* (5th ed.). Philadelphia: Lippincott Williams & Wilkins.

Chernecky, C.C, & Berger, B.J. (2001). *Laboratory tests and diagnostic procedures* (3rd ed.). Philadelphia: Saunders.

DeVita Jr., V.T., Hellman, S., & Rosenberg, S.A. (2004). *Cancer: Principles and practice of oncology* (6th ed.). Philadelphia: Lippincott Williams & Wilkins.

Durham, J.D., & Lashley, F.R. (2000). *The person with HIV/AIDS: Nursing perspectives* (3rd ed.). New York: Springer Publishing.

Fischbach, F.T. (2004). *A manual of laboratory and diagnostic tests* (7th ed.). Philadelphia: Williams & Wilkins.

Goldman, L., & Ausiello, D. (2004). *Cecil textbook of medicine* (22nd ed.). Philadelphia: Saunders.

Key, J.L. (2004). *Handbook of laboratory and diagnostic tests with nursing implications* (5th ed.). Upper Saddle River, NJ: Pearson Prentice Hall.

Skidmore-Roth, L. (2005). *Mosby's 2005 nursing drug reference.* St. Louis: Mosby.

Ungvarski, P.J., & Flaskerud, J.H. (1999). *HIV/AIDS: A guide to primary care management* (4th ed.). Philadelphia: Saunders.

Yarbro, C.H., Frogge, M.H., Goodman, M., & Groenwald, S.L. (2000). *Cancer nursing: Principles and practice* (5th ed.). Sudbury, MA: Jones & Bartlett.

Chapter 34

Avila, E. (2005). *A curandera's concept of medicine and wellness.* Retrieved June 12, 2005, from www.elena-curandera.com.

Bennett, J. (2003). Historical overview of the HIV pandemic. In C. Kirton (Ed.), *ANAC's core curriculum for HIV/AIDS nursing* (2nd ed., pp. 1-29). Thousand Oaks, CA: Sage Publications.

Carpenito, L.J. (2002). *Handbook of nursing diagnosis* (9th ed.). Philadelphia: Lippincott.

Centers for Disease Control and Prevention. (2004a). *HIV/AIDS surveillance report 2004, 14.*

Centers for Disease Control and Prevention. (2004b). *HIV/AIDS surveillance report 2004, 16.*

Colagreco, J. (2003). Pathophysiology of HIV infection. In C. Kirton (Ed.), *ANAC's core curriculum for HIV/AIDS nursing* (2nd ed., pp. 22-29). Thousand Oaks, CA: Sage Publications.

Diaz, R., Ayala, G., Bein, E., Henne, J., & Marin, B. (2001). The impact of homophobia, poverty, and racism on mental health of gay and bisexual Latino men: Findings from 3 U.S. cities. *American Journal of Public Health, 91*(6), 927-932.

Fugate, K. (2003). Pneumocystosis. In C. Kirton (Ed.), *ANAC's core curriculum for HIV/AIDS nursing* (2nd ed., pp. 86-87). Thousand Oaks, CA: Sage Publications.

Hughes, V. (2003). Prevention of HIV infection. In C. Kirton (Ed.), *ANAC's core curriculum for HIV/AIDS nursing* (2nd ed., pp. 18-22). Thousand Oaks, CA: Sage Publications.

Jaffe, M.S. (1996). *Medical-surgical nursing care plans* (3rd ed.). Stamford, CT: Appleton & Lange.

Keithley, J. (2003). Oral hairy leukoplakia. In C. Kirton (Ed.), *ANAC's core curriculum for HIV/AIDS nursing* (2nd ed., p. 66). Thousand Oaks, CA: Sage Publications.

Kirton, C. (Ed.). (2003). *ANAC's core curriculum for HIV/AIDS nursing* (2nd ed.). Thousand Oaks, CA: Sage Publications.

Kirton, C. (2001). Guidelines for the initiation of antiretroviral therapy. In C. Kirton, D. Talotta, & K. Zwolski (Eds.), *HIV/AIDS nursing handbook.* (pp. 65-79). St. Louis: Mosby.

Kirton, C. (Ed.). (2003). *ANAC's core curriculum for HIV/AIDS nursing* (2nd ed.). Thousand Oaks, CA: Sage Publications.

Moran, T. (2003). Kaposi's sarcoma. In C. Kirton (Ed.), *ANAC's core curriculum for HIV/AIDS nursing* (2nd ed., pp. 94-96). Thousand Oaks, CA: Sage Publications.

Ownby, K. (2003). Cryptosporidiosis. In C. Kirton (Ed.), *ANAC's core curriculum for HIV/AIDS nursing* (2nd ed., pp. 85-86). Thousand Oaks, CA: Sage Publications.

Ownby, K. (2003). Isosporiasis. In C. Kirton (Ed.), *ANAC's core curriculum for HIV/AIDS nursing* (2nd ed., p. 86). Thousand Oaks, CA: Sage Publications.

Porche, D. (2003). *Mycobacterium avium* complex. In C. Kirton (Ed.), *ANAC's core curriculum for HIV/AIDS nursing* (2nd ed., p. 76). Thousand Oaks, CA: Sage Publications.

Porche, D. (2003). *Mycobacterium tuberculosis.* In C. Kirton (Ed.), *ANAC's core curriculum for HIV/AIDS nursing* (2nd ed., p. 77). Thousand Oaks, CA: Sage Publications.

Robinson, P. (2003). Herpes Simplex virus. In C. Kirton (Ed.), *ANAC's core curriculum for HIV/AIDS nursing* (2nd ed., pp. 90-91). Thousand Oaks, CA: Sage Publications

Schulta, J. (2003). HIV testing. In C. Kirton (Ed.), *ANAC's core curriculum for HIV/AIDS nursing* (2nd ed., pp. 29-35). Thousand Oaks, CA: Sage Publications.

Sellers, C. (2003). Progressive multifocal leukoencephalopathy (PML). In C. Kirton (Ed.), *ANAC's core curriculum for HIV/AIDS nursing* (2nd ed., p. 77). Thousand Oaks, CA: Sage Publications.

Stanley, H.D., Marsco, L., & McNicholl, I. (2003). Bartonellosis. In C. Kirton (Ed.), *ANAC's core curriculum for HIV/AIDS nursing* (2nd ed., p. 66). Thousand Oaks, CA: Sage Publications.

Stanley, H.D., Marsco, L., & McNicholl, I. (2003). Toxoplasmosis. In C. Kirton (Ed.), *ANAC's core curriculum for HIV/AIDS nursing* (2nd ed., pp. 87-89). Thousand Oaks, CA: Sage Publications.

Vista Community Clinic. (2004). *Cultural facts.* Retrieved June 12, 2005, from Vista Community Clinic Cultural Awareness Program website: www.clas-sd.org/culturalfacts.htm.

Winson, G. (2001). HIV/AIDS nutritional management. In C. Kirton, D. Talotta, & K. Zwolski (Eds.), *HIV/AIDS nursing handbook* (pp. 344-361). St. Louis: Mosby.

Young, T. (2003). Baseline assessment. In C. Kirton (Ed.), *ANAC's core curriculum for HIV/AIDS nursing* (2nd ed., p. 66). Thousand Oaks, CA: Sage Publications.

Zwolski, K. (2001). HIV immunopathogenesis. In C. Kirton, D. Talotta, & K. Zwolski (Eds.), *HIV/AIDS nursing handbook* (pp. 3-23). St. Louis: Mosby.

Zwolski, K. (2001). Fungal infections. In C. Kirton, D. Talotta, & K. Zwolski (Eds.), *HIV/AIDS nursing handbook* (pp. 254-265). St. Louis: Mosby.

Chapter 35

Albert, N.M., Eastwood, C.A., & Edwards, M.L. (2004). Evidence-based practice for acute decompensated heart failure. *Critical Care Nurse, 24* (6), 14-29.

American Heart Association. (2001). *ACLS provider manual.*

American Heart Association. (2005). *Cholesterol levels.* Retrieved June 2005, from www.americanheart.org/presenter.jhtml?identifier=987.

American Heart Association. (2005). *Exercise (physical activity) for older people and those with disabilities.* Retrieved June 2005, from www.americanheart.org/presenter.jhtml?identifier=4557.

American Heart Association. (2005). *Heart attack, stroke & cardiac arrest warning signs.* Retrieved June 2005, from www.americanheart.org/presenter.jhtml?identifier=3053#Heart_Attack.

American Heart Association. (2005). *Inflammation, heart disease and stroke: The role of C-Reactive protein.* Retrieved June 2005, from www.americanheart.org/presenter.jhtml?identifier=4648.

American Heart Association. (2005). *Risk factors and coronary heart disease.* Retrieved June 2005, from www.americanheart.org/presenter.jhtml?identifier=500.

American Heart Association. (2007). *Heart disease and stroke statistics-2007 update.* Retrieved January 2007 from www.americanheart.org/presenter.jhtml?identifier=1928.

Ante, D.T. et al. (2004). ACC/AHA guideline for the management of patients with ST elevation myocardial infarction (Electronic version). *Circulation, 110,* 588-636.

Apple, M.S. (2005). Common cardiovascular disorders. In P.G. Morton, D.K. Fontaine, C.M. Hudak, & B.M. Gallo (Eds.), *Critical care nursing—A holistic approach* (8th ed., pp. 378-394). Philadelphia: Lippincott Williams & Wilkins.

Artinian, N.T. (2003). The psychosocial aspects of heart failure. *American Journal of Nursing, 103*(12), 32-42.

Baker, D.W. et al. (2002). *ACC/AHA guideline for the evaluation and management of chronic heart failure in the adult.* Retrieved June 2005, from www.americanheart.org/presenter.jhtml?identifier=11841.

Blum, K. (2005). Heart failure. In P.G. Morton, D.K. Fontaine, C.M. Hudak, & B.M. Gallo (Eds.), *Critical care nursing—A holistic approach* (8th ed., pp. 393-421). Philadelphia: Lippincott Williams & Wilkins.

Brashers, V.L. (2002). Alterations of cardiovascular function. In K.L. McCance & S.E. Huether (Eds.), *Pathophysiology: The biological basis for disease in adults and children* (4th ed., pp. 980-984, 1000-1025, 1027-1039). St. Louis: Mosby.

Braunwald, E. et al. (2002). *ACC/AHA guideline update management of patients with unstable angina and non-ST-segment elevation myocardial infarction.* Retrieved June 2005, from www.acc.org/clinical/guidelines/unstable/incorporated/index.htm.

Centers for Disease Control and Prevention & National Institutes of Health. *Healthy People 2010.* Retrieved June 2005, from www.healthypeople.gov/document/HTML/Volume1/12Heart.htm.

Chen-Scarabelli, C. (2002). Beating-heart coronary artery bypass graft surgery: Indications, advantages, and limitations. *Critical Care Nurse, 22*(5), 44-58.

Colbert, K., & Greene, M.H. (2003). Nesiritide (Natrecor): A new treatment for acutely decompensated congestive heart failure. *Critical Care Nurse Quarterly, 26*(1), 40-44.

Deglin, J.H., & Vallerand, A.H. (2005). *Davis's drug guide for nurses* (9th ed.). Philadelphia: Davis.

DeJong, M., Coombs, V. Rempher, K., Obias-Mann, D., & Gordon, C. (2005). Patient management: Cardiovascular system. In P.G. Morton, D.K. Fontaine, C.M. Hudak, & B.M. Gallo (Eds.) *Critical care nursing: A holistic approach* (8th ed., pp. 292-377). Philadelphia: Lippincott Williams & Wilkins.

Diehl-Oplinger, L. & Begliomini, R. (2005). Using glycoprotein inhibitors for acute coronary syndrome. *Nursing, 34*(9), 32cc1-32cc4.

Eagle, K.A. et al. (2004). ACC/AHA guideline for coronary artery bypass graft surgery: Summary article (Electronic version). *Circulation, 110.*

Futterman, L.G., & Lemberg, L. (2002). High-sensitivity C-reactive protein is the most effective prognostic measurement of acute coronary events. *American Journal of Critical Care, 11*(5), 482-486.

Gibbons, R.J. et al. (2002). *ACC/AHA 2002 update: Management of patients with chronic stable angina.* Retrieved June 2005, from www.americanheart.org/presenter.jhtml?identifier=3006769.

Hamner, J.B., Dubois, E.J., & Rice, T.P. (2005). Predictors of complications associated with closure devices after transfemoral percutaneous coronary procedures. *Critical Care Nurse, 25*(3), 30-37.

Hyett, J.M. (2004). Caring for a patient after CABG surgery. *Nursing, 34*(7), 48-49.

Lagrotteria, J.M. (2003). Biventricular pacing for congestive heart failure. *Critical Care Nursing Quarterly, 26*(1), 50-58.

Lindsey, M.R. (2003). Transmyocardial laser revascularization revisited. *Critical Care Nursing Quarterly, 26*(1), 69-75.

Loyola, S. (2005). Dysrhythmia interpretation. In M.L. Sole, D.G. Klein, & M.J. Moseley, (Eds.), *Introduction to critical care nursing* (4th ed., pp. 85-126). Philadelphia: Saunders.

Morton, P.G. (2005). Acute myocardial infarction. In P.G. Morton, D.K. Fontaine, C.M. Hudak, & B.M. Gallo (Eds.), *Critical care nursing: A holistic approach* (8th ed., pp. 422-447). Philadelphia: Lippincott Williams & Wilkins.

Morton, P.G., Tucker, T., & VanRoeden, K. (2005). Patient assessment: Cardiovascular system. In P.G. Morton, D.K. Fontaine, C.M. Hudak, & B.M. Gallo (Eds.), *Critical care nursing: A holistic approach* (8th ed., pp. 211-291). Philadelphia: Lippincott Williams & Wilkins.

Moseley, M., Czekaj, L.A., & Abbott, M.E. (2005). Hemodynamic monitoring. In M.L. Sole, D.G. Klein, & M.J. Moseley (Eds.), *Introduction to critical care nursing* (4th ed., pp. 127-158). Philadelphia: Saunders.

Munro, N. (2005). Cardiac surgery. In P.G. Morton, D.K. Fontaine, C.M. Hudak, & B.M. Gallo (Eds.), *Critical care nursing: A holistic approach* (8th ed., pp. 448-470). Philadelphia: Lippincott Williams & Wilkins.

Overbay, D., & Criddle, L. (2004). Mastering temporary invasive cardiac pacing. *Critical Care Nurse, 24*(3), 25-32.

Saul, L., & Shatzer, M. (2003). B-type natriuretic peptide testing for detection of heart failure. *Critical Care Nursing Quarterly, 26*(1), 35-39.

Sneed, N.V., & Paul, S.C. (2003). Readiness for behavioral changes in patients with heart failure. *American Journal of Critical Care, 12*(5), 444-453.

Steinbis, S. (2003). Hypertrophic obstructive cardiomyopathy and septal ablation. *Critical Care Nurse, 23*(3), 47-50.

Tarolli, K.A. (2003). Left ventricular systolic dysfunction and nonischemic cardiomyopathy. *Critical Care Nursing Quarterly, 26*(1), 3-15.

Timothy, P.R., & Rodeman, B.J. (2004). Temporary pacemakers in critically ill patients: Assessment and management strategies. *AACN Clinical Issues in Critical Care Nursing, 15*(3), 305-325.

Wade, C.R., Keith, K.K., Sikora, J.H., & Augustine, S.M. (2004). Postoperative nursing care of the cardiac transplant recipient. *Critical Care Nursing Quarterly, 27*(1), 17-28.

Weigand, D.L. (2003). Advances in cardiac surgery: Valve repair. *Critical Care Nurse, 23*(2), 72-89.

Whitman, G.R. (2004). Nursing-sensitive outcomes in cardiac surgery patients. *The Journal of Cardiovascular Nursing, 19*(5), 293-298.

Williams, J., Oenning, V., & Tuomala, B. (2005). Cardiovascular alterations. In M.L. Sole, D.G. Klein, & M.J. Moseley (Eds.), *Introduction to critical care nursing* (4th ed., pp. 291-341). Philadelphia: Saunders.

Zhang, J. (2003). Sudden cardiac death: Implantable cardioverter defibrillators and pharmacological treatments. *Critical Care Nursing Quarterly, 26*(1), 45-49.

Internet Resources

American College of Cardiology: www.acc.org

American Heart Association: www.americanheart.org

Cardiology: www.theheart.org

Heart Failure Society of America: www.hfsa.org

National Guideline Clearinghouse: www.guidelines.gov

Patient Education: www.heartcenteronline.com; also: www.heartinfo.org

Women's Heart Foundation: www.womensheart.org

Chapter 36

Boin, F., & Wigley, F.M. (2005). Understanding, assessing and treating Raynaud's phenomenon. *Current Opinion in Rheumatology, 17*(6), 752-760.

Davies, M.G., Waldman, D.L., & Pearson, T.A. (2005). Comprehensive endovascular therapy for femoropopliteal arterial atherosclerotic occlusive disease. *Journal of the American College of Surgeons, 201*(2), 275-296.

Lilley, L.L., & Aucker, R.S. (2001). *Pharmacology and the nursing process* (3rd ed.). St. Louis: Mosby.

Pagana, K.D., & Pagana, T.J. (2003). *Mosby's diagnostic and laboratory test reference* (6th ed.). St. Louis: Mosby.

Reilly, A., & Snyder, B. (2005). Raynaud phenomenon. *American Journal of Nursing, 105*(8), 56-66.

Wipke-Tevis, D.D., & Rich, K. (2004). Vascular disorders: Nursing management. In S.M. Lewis, M.M. Heitkemper, & S.D. Dirksen (Eds.), *Medical-surgical nursing: Assessment and management of clinical problems* (6th ed., pp. 912-945). St. Louis: Mosby.

Chapter 37

Abrams, A.C. (2004). *Clinical drug therapy* (7th ed.). Philadelphia: Lippincott.

Levine, B.S. (2004). Nursing management: Hypertension. In S.M. Lewis, M.M. Heitkemper, & S.R. Dirksen (Eds.). *Medical-surgical nursing* (6th ed., pp. 777-798). St. Louis: Mosby.

National Institutes of Health. (2003). *The seventh report of the Joint National Committee on Prevention, Detection, Evaluation, and Treatment of High Blood Pressure* (NIH Publication No. 03-5233). Bethesda, MD: Author.

National Institutes of Health. (2003). *Your guide to lowering blood pressure* (NIH Publication No. 03-5232). Bethesda, MD: Author.

Skidmore-Roth, L. (2002). *Mosby's nursing drug reference*. St. Louis: Mosby.

Chapter 38

Abrams, A.C. (2004). *Clinical drug therapy* (7th ed.). Philadelphia: Lippincott.

American Cancer Society. (2006). *Esophagus cancer.* Retrieved March 16, 2006, from www.cancer.org.

American Cancer Society. (2006). *Stomach cancer.* Retrieved March 16, 2006, from www.cancer.org.

Black, J.M., Hawks, J.H., & Keene, A.M. (2001). *Medical-surgical nursing: Clinical management for continuity of care* (6th ed.). Philadelphia: Saunders.

Blackwood, H.S. (2005, Fall). Help your patient downsize with bariatric surgery. *Med/Surg Insider,* pp. 4-9.

Bren, L. (2005, March 1). Incredible journey through the digestive system. *FDA Consumer,* 0362-1332, *39*(2). Retrieved March 17, 2006, from Academic Search Premier.

Cohen, S., & Parkman, H.P. (2000). Diseases of the esophagus. In L. Goldman & J.C. Bennett (Eds.), *Cecil textbook of medicine* (21st ed., pp. 658-668). Philadelphia: Saunders.

Croghan, A. (2004). Nursing assessment: Gastrointestinal system. In S.M. Lewis, M.M. Heitkemper, & S.R. Dirksen (Eds.). *Medical-surgical nursing* (6th ed., pp. 946-968). St. Louis: Mosby.

Graham, D.Y. (2000). Peptic ulcer disease: Therapy. In L. Goldman & J.C. Bennett (Eds.), *Cecil textbook of medicine* (21st ed., pp. 675-678). Philadelphia: Saunders.

Heitkemper, M.M. (2004). Nursing management: Upper gastrointestinal problems. In S.M. Lewis, M.M. Heitkemper, & S.R. Dirksen (Eds.). *Medical-surgical nursing* (6th ed., pp. 1003-1051). St. Louis: Mosby.

Jarvis, C. (2000). *Physical examination and health assessment* (3rd ed.). Philadelphia: Saunders.

Lehne, R.A. (2001). *Pharmacology for nursing care* (4th ed.). Philadelphia: Saunders.

Maher, L.K., & Escott-Stump, S. (2000). *Krause's food, nutrition, and diet therapy* (10th ed.). Philadelphia: Saunders.

National Institute of Diabetes and Digestive and Kidney Diseases. (2006). *Crohn's disease.* Retrieved March 16, 2006, from www.digestive.niddk.nih.gov.

National Institute of Diabetes and Digestive and Kidney Diseases. (2006). *Ulcerative colitis.* Retrieved March 16, 2006, from www.digestive.niddk.nih.gov.

Remedios, M.L., & Appleyard, M. (2005). Capsule endoscopy: Current indications and future prospects. *Internal Medicine Journal, 35*(4), 234-239.

Rustgi, A.K. (2000). Neoplasms of the stomach. In L. Goldman & J.C. Bennett (Eds.), *Cecil textbook of medicine* (21st ed., pp. 738-741). Philadelphia: Saunders.

Semrad, C.E., & Chang, E.B. (2000). Malabsorption syndromes. In L. Goldman & J.C. Bennett (Eds.), *Cecil textbook of medicine* (21st ed., pp. 712-722). Philadelphia: Saunders.

Snape, W.J. (2000). Disorders of gastrointestinal motility. In L. Goldman & J.C. Bennett (Eds.), *Cecil textbook of medicine* (21st ed., pp. 694-702). Philadelphia: Saunders.

Soll, A.H. (2000). Gastritis and *Helicobacter pylori.* In L. Goldman & J.C. Bennett (Eds.), *Cecil textbook of medicine* (21st ed., pp. 694-702). Philadelphia: Saunders.

Soll, A.H. (2000). Peptic ulcer disease: Epidemiology, pathophysiology, clinical manifestations, and diagnosis. In L. Goldman & J.C. Bennett (Eds.), *Cecil textbook of medicine* (21st ed., pp. 671-675). Philadelphia: Saunders.

Stenson, W.F. (2000). Inflammatory bowel disease. In L. Goldman & J.C. Bennett (Eds.), *Cecil textbook of medicine* (21st ed., pp. 722-729). Philadelphia: Saunders.

Wilcox, C.M. (2000). Miscellaneous inflammatory diseases of the intestine. In L. Goldman & J.C. Bennett (Eds.), *Cecil textbook of medicine* (21st ed., pp. 729-732). Philadelphia: Saunders.

Chapter 39

American Cancer Society. (2005). *Cancer facts and figures.* Retrieved Dec. 15, 2005, from www.acs.org.

Centers for Disease Control and Prevention. (2003, Sept.). *Hepatitis surveillance* (Report No. 58). Bethesda, MD: USDHHS.

Centers for Disease Control and Prevention. (2006). *Viral hepatitis.* Retrieved March 18, 2006, from www.cdc.gov/ncidod/diseases/hepatitis/common_faqs.htm.

Diehl, A.M. (2000). Acute and chronic failure and hepatic encephalopathy. In L. Goldman & J.C. Bennett (Eds.), *Cecil textbook of medicine* (21st ed., pp. 813-816). Philadelphia: Saunders.

DiMagno, E.P. (2000). Carcinoma of the pancreas. In L. Goldman & J.C. Bennett (Eds.), *Cecil textbook of medicine* (21st ed., pp. 750-752). Philadelphia: Saunders.

Durston, S. (2005). What you need to know about hepatitis. *Nursing, 35*(8), 36-42.

Fallon, M. (2000). Hepatic tumors. In L. Goldman & J.C. Bennett (Eds.), *Cecil textbook of medicine* (21st ed., pp. 819-821). Philadelphia: Saunders.

Friedman, S.L. (2000). Alcoholic liver disease, cirrhosis, and its major sequelae. In L. Goldman & J.C. Bennett (Eds.), *Cecil textbook of medicine* (21st ed., pp. 804-812). Philadelphia: Saunders.

Guyton, A.C., & Hall, J.E. (2006). *Textbook of medical physiology* (11th ed.). Philadelphia: Saunders.

Heitkemper, M.M. (2004). Nursing management: Liver, biliary tract, and pancreas problems. In S.M. Lewis, M.M. Heitkemper, & S.R. Dirksen (Eds.), *Medical-surgical nursing: Assessment and management of clinical problems* (6th ed., pp. 1104-1151). Philadelphia: Saunders.

Hoofnagle, J.H., & Lindsay, K.L. (2000). Acute viral hepatitis. In L. Goldman & J.C. Bennett (Eds.), *Cecil textbook of medicine* (21st ed., pp. 783-790). Philadelphia: Saunders.

Jarvis, C. (2004). *Physical examination and health assessment* (4th ed.). Philadelphia: Saunders.

Mahan, L.K., & Escott-Stump, S. (2000). *Krause's food, nutrition, and diet therapy* (10th ed.). Philadelphia: Saunders.

Pagana, K.D., & Pagana, T.J. (2003). *Mosby's diagnostic and laboratory test reference* (6th ed.). St. Louis: Mosby.

Parini, S. (2001). Hepatitis C. *Nursing, 31*(3), 36-43.

Roberts, J.P. (2000). Liver transplantation. In L. Goldman & J.C. Bennett (Eds.), *Cecil textbook of medicine* (21st ed., pp. 816-817). Philadelphia: Saunders.

Soergel, K.H. (2000). Pancreatitis. In L. Goldman & J.C. Bennett (Eds.), *Cecil textbook of medicine* (21st ed., pp. 752-759). Philadelphia: Saunders.

Whiteman, K. (2005). When your patient is in liver failure. *Nursing, 35*(4), 58-64.

Internet Resource

Division of Gastroenterology at the University of California, San Francisco: ww.sadieo.ucsf.edu.

Chapter 40

Bates, P. (2000). Nursing management: Renal and urologic problems: In S. M. Lewis, M.M. Heitkemper, & S.R. Dirksen (Eds.),

Medical-surgical nursing: Assessment and management of clinical problems (5th ed., pp. 1261-1298). Philadelphia: Saunders.

Brunier, G., & Bartucci, M. (2000). Nursing management: Acute and chronic renal failure. In S.M. Lewis, M.M. Heitkemper, & S.R. Dirksen (Eds.), *Medical-surgical nursing: Assessment and management of clinical problems* (5th ed., pp. 1299-1341). Philadelphia: Saunders.

Curtis, J.J. (2000). Treatment of irreversible renal failure. In L. Goldman & J.C. Bennett (Eds.), *Cecil textbook of medicine* (21st ed., pp. 578-586). Philadelphia: Saunders.

Eliopoulos, C. (1999). *Integrating conventional and alternative therapies.* St. Louis: Mosby.

Ignatavicius, D.D., Workman, M.L., & Mishler, M.A. (1999). *Medical-surgical nursing across the health care continuum* (3rd ed.). Philadelphia: Saunders.

Jarvis, C. (2000). *Physical examination and health assessment* (3rd ed.). Philadelphia: Saunders.

Lehne, R.A. (2001). *Pharmacology for nursing care* (4th ed.). Philadelphia: Saunders.

Luke, R.G. (2000). Chronic renal failure. In L. Goldman & J.C. Bennett (Eds.), *Cecil textbook of medicine* (21st ed., pp. 571-578). Philadelphia: Saunders.

Mitch, W.E. (2000). Acute renal failure. In L. Goldman & J.C. Bennett (Eds.), *Cecil textbook of medicine* (21st ed., pp. 567-571). Philadelphia: Saunders.

Shapiro, C.L., Garnick, M.B., & Kantoff, P.W. (2000). Tumors of the kidneys, ureter, and bladder. In L. Goldman & J.C. Bennett (Eds.), *Cecil textbook of medicine* (21st ed., pp. 631-635). Philadelphia: Saunders.

Chapter 41

Arnett, F.C. (2001). Rheumatoid arthritis. In L. Goldman & J.C. Bennett (Eds.), *Cecil textbook of medicine* (21st ed., pp. 1492-1499). Philadelphia: Saunders.

Ball, E.V. (2001). Behçet's disease. In L. Goldman & J.C. Bennett (Eds.), *Cecil textbook of medicine* (21st ed., pp. 1540-1541). Philadelphia: Saunders.

Ball, E.V. (2001). Nonarticular rheumatism. In L. Goldman & J.C. Bennett (Eds.), *Cecil textbook of medicine* (21st ed., pp. 1559-1560). Philadelphia: Saunders.

Black, J.M., Hawks, J.H., & Keene, A.M. (2001). *Medical-surgical nursing: Clinical management for positive outcomes* (6th ed.). Philadelphia: Saunders.

Calkins, E., & Vladutiu, A.O. (1998). Musculoskeletal disorders. In E.H. Duthie & P.R. Katz (Eds.), *Practice of geriatrics* (3rd ed., pp. 421-435). Philadelphia: Saunders.

Chernecky, C.C., & Berger, B.J. (2001). *Laboratory tests and diagnostic procedures* (3rd ed.). Philadelphia: Saunders.

Cush, J.J., & Lipsky, P.E. (2001). The spondyloarthropathies. In L. Goldman & J.C. Bennett (Eds.), *Cecil textbook of medicine* (21st ed., pp. 1499-1507). Philadelphia: Saunders.

Geissler, E. (1998). *Mosby's pocket guide to cultural assessment* (2nd ed.). St. Louis: Mosby.

Goldman, L., & Bennett, J.C. (2001). *Cecil textbook of medicine* (21st ed.). Philadelphia: Saunders.

Hershfield, M.S. (2001). Gout and uric acid metabolism. In L. Goldman & J.C. Bennett (Eds.), *Cecil textbook of medicine* (21st ed., pp. 1541-1548). Philadelphia: Saunders.

Hochberg, M.C. (2001). Sjögren's syndrome. In L. Goldman & J.C. Bennett (Eds.), *Cecil textbook of medicine* (21st ed., pp. 1522-1524). Philadelphia: Saunders.

Hodgson, B.B., & Kizior, R.J. (2000). *Saunders nursing drug handbook 2000.* Philadelphia: Saunders.

Jacob, S.W., & Francone, C.A. (1989). *Elements of anatomy and physiology* (2nd ed.). Philadelphia: Saunders.

Jarvis, C. (2000). *Health assessment and physical examination* (3rd ed.). Philadelphia: Saunders.

Lehne, R.A. (2001). *Pharmacology for nursing care* (4th ed.). Philadelphia: Saunders.

Mahan, L.K., & Escott-Stump, S. (2000). *Krause's food, nutrition and diet therapy* (10th ed.). Philadelphia: Saunders.

Monahan, F.D., & Neighbors, M. (1998). *Medical-surgical nursing* (2nd ed.). Philadelphia: Saunders.

Roberts, D. (2004). Nursing management: Arthritis and connective tissue diseases. In S.M. Lewis, M.M. Heitkemper, & S.D. Dirksen (Eds.), *Medical-surgical nursing: Assessment and management of clinical problems* (6th ed., pp. 1715-1755). Philadelphia: Saunders.

Ruddy, S., Harris Jr., E., & Sledge, C.B. (2001) *Kelley's textbook of rheumatology* (6th ed.). Philadelphia: Saunders.

Schnitzer, T.J. (2001). Osteoarthritis (degenerative bone disease). In L. Goldman & J.C. Bennett (Eds.), *Cecil textbook of medicine* (21st ed., pp. 1550-1554). Philadelphia: Saunders.

Sculco, T.P. (1998). Orthopedic disorders. In E.H. Duthie & P.R. Katz (Eds.), *Practice of geriatrics* (3rd ed., pp. 436-447). Philadelphia: Saunders.

Seton. (2001). New applications of technology relieve back pain without surgery. *Good Health* (pp. 28-29). Austin, TX: Author.

Wortman, R.L. (2001). Idiopathic inflammatory myopathies. In L. Goldman & J.C. Bennett (Eds.), *Cecil textbook of medicine* (21st ed., pp. 1534-1538). Philadelphia: Saunders.

Chapter 42

Centers for Disease Control and Prevention. (n.d.). *Falls and hip fractures among older adults.* Retrieved Feb. 25, 2006, from www.cdc .gov/ncipc/factsheets/falls/htm.

Kunkler, C.E. (2004). Nursing management: Musculoskeletal disorders. In S.M. Lewis, M.M. Heitkemper, & S.D. Dirksen (Eds.) *Medical-surgical nursing: Assessment and management of clinical problems* (6th ed., pp. 1692-1714). Philadelphia: Saunders.

Quisel, A., Gill, J.M., & Witherell, P. (2005). Complex regional pain syndrome underdiagnosed: CRPS type 1 is underrecognized problem in limbs recovering from fracture or immobilized post-stroke. *Journal of Family Practice,* 54(6), 524-529.

Tapson, V.F. (2000). Pulmonary embolism. In L. Goldman & J.C. Bennett (Eds.), *Cecil textbook of medicine* (21st ed., pp. 441-448). Philadelphia: Saunders.

Chapter 43

Kunkler, C.E. (2004). Nursing management: Musculoskeletal trauma and orthopedic surgery. In S.M. Lewis, M.M. Heitkemper, & S.D. Dirksen (Eds.), *Medical-surgical nursing: Assessment and management of clinical problems* (6th ed., pp. 1650-1691). Philadelphia: Saunders.

Monahan, F.D., & Neighbors, M.A. (1998). *Medical-surgical nursing: Foundations for clinical practice* (2nd ed., pp. 837-886). Philadelphia: Saunders.

Nunnelee, J.D. (2001). Management of clients with vascular disorders. In J.M. Black, J.H. Hawks, & A.M. Keene (Eds.), *Medical-surgical nursing: Clinical management for positive outcomes* (6th ed., pp. 1399-1432). Philadelphia: Saunders.

Williamson, V. (1998). Amputation. In A.B. Maher, S.W. Salmond, & T.A. Pellino (Eds.), *Orthopaedic nursing* (2nd ed., pp. 718-745). Philadelphia: Saunders.

Chapter 44

Abrams, A.C. (2004). *Clinical drug therapy* (7th ed.). Philadelphia: Lippincott.

Giddens, J.F. (2004). Nursing assessment: Endocrine problems. In S.M. Lewis, M.M. Heitkemper, & S.R. Dirksen (Eds.), *Medical-surgical nursing: Assessment and management of clinical problems* (6th ed., pp. 1248-1267). Philadelphia: Saunders.

Giddens, J.F. (2004). Nursing management: Endocrine problems. In S.M. Lewis, M.M. Heitkemper, & S.R. Dirksen (Eds.), *Medical-surgical nursing: Assessment and management of clinical problems* (6th ed., pp. 1303-1337). Philadelphia: Saunders.

Loriaux, D.L. (2000). The adrenal cortex. In L. Goldman & J.C. Bennett (Eds.), *Cecil textbook of medicine* (21st ed., pp. 1250-1257). Philadelphia: Saunders.

Mahan, L.K., & Escott-Stump, S. (2000). *Krause's food, nutrition and diet therapy* (10th ed.). Philadelphia: Saunders.

Molitch, M.E. (2000). Anterior pituitary. In L. Goldman & J.C. Bennett (Eds.), *Cecil textbook of medicine* (21st ed., pp. 1208-1225) Philadelphia: Saunders.

O'Connor, D.T. (2000). The adrenal medulla, catecholamines, and pheochromocytoma. In L. Goldman & J.C. Bennett (Eds.), *Cecil textbook of medicine* (21st ed., pp. 1257-1262). Philadelphia: Saunders.

Chapter 45

Abrams, A.C. (2004). *Clinical drug therapy* (7th ed.). Philadelphia: Lippincott.

Dillman, W.H. (2000). The thyroid. In L. Goldman & J.C. Bennett (Eds.), *Cecil textbook of medicine* (21st ed., pp. 1231-1250). Philadelphia: Saunders.

Giddens, J.F. (2004). Nursing assessment: Endocrine problems. In S.M. Lewis, M.M. Heitkemper, & S.R. Dirksen (Eds.), *Medical-surgical nursing: Assessment and management of clinical problems* (6th ed., pp. 1248-1267). Philadelphia: Saunders.

Giddens, J.F. (2004). Nursing management: Endocrine problems. In S.M. Lewis, M.M. Heitkemper, & S.R. Dirksen (Eds.), *Medical-surgical nursing: Assessment and management of clinical problems* (6th ed., pp. 1303-1337). Philadelphia: Saunders.

Skidmore-Roth, L. (2005). *Mosby's drug guide for nurses* (6th ed.). St. Louis: Mosby.

Spiegel, A.M. (2000). The parathyroid glands, hypercalcemia, and hypocalcemia. In L. Goldman & J.C. Bennett (Eds.), *Cecil textbook of medicine* (21st ed., pp. 1398-1406). Philadelphia: Saunders.

Chapter 46

American Diabetes Association. (2006). Diagnosis and classification of diabetes mellitus. *Diabetes Care 29*(Suppl. 1), S43-S48.

American Diabetes Association. (2005). Insulin: There are many different insulins for many different situations and lifestyles. *Diabetes Forecast 59*(1): RG10-15.

American Diabetes Association. (2006). Standards of medical care in diabetes. *Diabetes Care 29*(Suppl. 1): S4-S42.

Brenner, Z.R. (2006). Management of hyperglycemic emergencies. *AACN Clinical Issues 17*(1): 56-65.

Capriotti, T. (2005, Oct.). Type 2 diabetes epidemic increases use of oral anti-diabetic agents. *MedSurg Nursing 14*(5), 341-347.

Centers for Disease Control and Prevention. (2005). *Leading causes of death and number of deaths according to age: U.S. 1980-2002.* Atlanta, GA: U.S. Department of Health and Human Services. Retrieved Oct. 21, 2005, from cdc.gov/nchs/hus.htm.

Diabetes & Cardiovascular Disease Review. American Diabetes Association & American College of Cardiology. Issue 1, 2002.

Holcomb, S.S. (2005). Diabetes update: 2005 ACE guidelines. *The Nurse Practitioner 30*(5), 12-14.

National Institute of Diabetes and Digestive and Kidney Diseases. (2006). *National Diabetes Statistics fact sheet: general information and national estimates on diabetes in the United States, 2005.* Bethesda, MD: U.S. Department of Health and Human Services, National Institutes of Health. Retrieved Feb. 2, 2006, from diabetes.niddk .nih.gov/dm/pubs/statistics.

Pramlintide acetate: (2006). Adjunct therapy for both types of diabetes. *Nursing, 36*(2), 56.

Shamoon, H. (2001). Hypoglycemia. In P. Felig, J.D. Baxter, A.E. Broadus, & L. Frohman (Eds), *Endocrinology and metabolism* (4th ed.). New York: McGraw Hill.

Smith, W.D. (2005). Causes of hyperglycemia and hypoglycemia in adult inpatients. *American Journal of Health-System Pharmacy, 62*(7), 714-719.

Valenine, V. (2000). Patients with diabetes mellitus. In S.M. Lewis, M.M. Heitkemper, & S.R. Dirksen (Eds.), *Medical-surgical nursing* (5th ed.). St. Louis: Mosby.

Chapter 47

American Cancer Society. (2006). *Cancer facts and figures—2006.* Atlanta, GA: Author.

American Cancer Society. (2003). *Cancer facts for women.* Retrieved Oct. 28, 2005, from www.cancer.org.

Dell, D. (2001). Regaining range of motion after breast surgery. *Nursing, 31*(10), 50-52.

Dirksen, S.R. (2004). Nursing management: Breast disorders. In S.M. Lewis, M.M. Heitkemper, & S.R. Dirksen (Eds.), *Medical-surgical nursing: Assessment and management of clinical problems* (6th ed., pp. 1360-1383). St. Louis: Mosby.

Eliopoulos, C. (1999). *Conventional and alternative therapies.* St. Louis: Mosby.

Giddens, J.F. (2004). Nursing assessment: Reproductive system. In S.M. Lewis, M.M. Heitkemper, & S.R. Dirksen (Eds.), *Medical-surgical nursing: Assessment and management of clinical problems* (6th ed., pp. 1339-1359). St. Louis: Mosby.

Hoskins, C.N., & Haber, J. (2000). Adjusting to breast cancer. *The American Journal of Nursing, 100*(4), 26-33.

Jones, H.W. (2000). Ovarian carcinoma. In L. Goldman & J.C. Bennett (Eds.), *Cecil textbook of medicine* (21st ed., pp. 1381-1382). Philadelphia: Saunders.

Machia, J. (2001). Breast cancer: Risk, prevention, and tamoxifen. *American Journal of Nursing, 101*(4), 26-35.

Macmullen, N.J., & Dulski, L. (2004). Nursing management: Female reproductive problems. In S.M. Lewis, M.M. Heitkemper, & S.R. Dirksen (Eds.), *Medical-surgical nursing: Assessment and management of clinical problems* (6th ed., pp. 1339-1359). St. Louis: Mosby.

Muss, H.B. (2000). Breast cancer and differential diagnosis of benign nodules. In L. Goldman & J.C. Bennett (Eds.), *Cecil textbook of medicine* (21st ed., pp. 1373-1380). Philadelphia: Saunders.

Nichols, A., & Ignatavicius, D.D. (2002). Interventions for clients with breast disorders. In D.D. Ignatavicius & M.L. Workman (Eds.), *Medical-surgical nursing,* (4th ed., pp. 1730-1750). Philadelphia: Saunders.

Nichols, A., & Ignatavicius, D.D. (2002). Interventions for clients with gynecologic problems. In D.D. Ignatavicius & M.L. Workman (Eds.), *Medical-surgical nursing,* (4th ed., pp. 1751-1781). Philadelphia: Saunders.

Rebar, R.W. (2000). Menstrual cycle and fertility. In L. Goldman & J.C. Bennett (Eds.), *Cecil textbook of medicine* (21st ed., pp. 1327-1340). Philadelphia: Saunders.

Risks and benefits of estrogen plus progestin in healthy postmenopausal women. Retrieved Aug. 6, 2002, from www.jama.ama-assn.org/ issuesv288n3/ joc21036.html.

Writing group for the Women's Health Initiative investigators. *JAMA* (online) *288*(3), July 17, 2002.

Chapter 48

Allan, C.A., & MacLachlan, R.I. (2004). Age-related changes in testosterone and the role of replacement therapy in older men. *Clinical Endocrinology, 60*, 653-670.

American Cancer Society. (2006). *Cancer facts and figures—2006.* Atlanta, GA: Author.

Bates, P.M. (2001). Management of men with reproductive disorders. In J.M. Black, J. H. Hawks, & A.M. Keene (Eds.), *Medical-surgical nursing: Clinical management for positive outcomes* (6th ed., pp. 945-977). Philadelphia: Saunders.

Eliopoulos, C. (1999). *Integrating conventional and alternative therapies.* St. Louis: Mosby.

Giddens, J.F. (2004). Nursing assessment: Reproductive system. In S.M. Lewis, M.M. Heitkemper, & S.R. Dirksen (Eds.), *Medical-surgical nursing: Assessment and management of clinical problems* (6th ed., pp. 1339-1359). St. Louis: Mosby.

Giddens, J.F. (2004). Nursing management: Male reproductive disorders. In S.M. Lewis, M.M. Heitkemper, & S.R. Dirksen (Eds.), *Medical- surgical nursing: Assessment and management of clinical problems* (6th ed., pp. 1435-1461). St. Louis: Mosby.

Partin, A.W. (2000). Diseases of the prostate. In L. Goldman & J.C. Bennett (Eds.), *Cecil textbook of medicine* (21st ed., pp. 635-642). Philadelphia: Saunders.

Swerdloff, R.S., & Wang, C. (2000). The testis and male sexual function. In L. Goldman & J.C. Bennett (Eds.), *Cecil textbook of medicine* (21st ed., pp. 1306-1317). Philadelphia: Saunders.

Chapter 49

Blair, M. (2001). Management of clients with sexually transmitted diseases. In J.M. Black, J.H. Hawks, & AM. Keene (Eds.), *Medical-surgical nursing: Clinical management for positive outcomes* (6th ed., pp. 1041-1057). Philadelphia: Saunders.

Centers for Disease Control and Prevention. (2004). *Chlamydia.* Retrieved April 17, 2006, from www.cdc.gov/std/Chlamydia/ STDFact-Chlamydia.htm.

Centers for Disease Control and Prevention. (2004). *Genital herpes.* Retrieved April 17, 2006, from www.cdc.gov/std/Herpes/STDFact-Herpes.htm.

Centers for Disease Control and Prevention. (2004). *Genital HPV infection.* Retrieved April 17, 2006, from www.cdc.gov/std/HPV/STDFact-HPV.htm.

Centers for Disease Control and Prevention. (2004). *Gonorrhea.* Retrieved April 17, 2006, from www.cdc.gov/std/Gonorrhea/STDFact-Gonorrhea.htm.

Centers for Disease Control and Prevention. (2004). *HPV and men.* Retrieved April 17, 2006, from www.cdc.gov/std/HPV/STDFact-HPV.htm.

Centers for Disease Control and Prevention. (2004). *Sexually transmitted diseases treatment guidelines—2002.* Retrieved April 18, 2006, from www.cdc.gov/mmwr/preview/mmwrhtml/rr510a1.htm.

Centers for Disease Control and Prevention. (2004). *STDs surveillance 2004.* Retrieved April 17, 2006, from www.cdc.gov/std/stats/trends2004.htm.

Centers for Disease Control and Prevention. (2004). *Syphilis.* Retrieved April 17, 2006, from www.cdc.gov/std/Syphilis/STDFact-Syphilis.htm.

Centers for Disease Control and Prevention. (2004). *Trichomoniasis.* Retrieved April 17, 2006, from www.cdc.gov/std/Trichomonas/STDFact-Trichomoniasis.htm.

National Center for Health Statistics. (2005). *Sexually transmitted diseases/STD.* Retrieved April 29, 2006, from www.ckc.gov/nchs/fastats/stds.htm.

Skidmore-Roth, L. (2005). *Mosby's drug guide for nurses* (6th ed.). St Louis: Mosby.

Internet Resources

AIDSLINE, National Library of Medicine: www.healthgate.com/AMA/ search.html.

Centers for Disease Control and Prevention: www.cdc.gov.

University of California, San Francisco Library: www.library.ucsf.edu.

Chapter 50

Brooke, R.C.C., & Griffiths, C.E.M. (2003). Aging of the skin. In R.C. Tillis & H.M. Fillit (Eds.). *Brocklehurst's textbook of geriatric medicine and gerontology* (6th ed.). London: Churchill Livingstone.

Dirksen, S.R. (2004). Nursing assessment: Integumentary system. In S.M. Lewis, M.M. Heitkemper, & S.R. Dirksen (Eds.), *Medical-surgical nursing: Assessment and management of clinical problems* (6th ed., pp. 476-486). St. Louis: Mosby.

Dirksen, S.R., & Hill, M.J. (2004). Nursing management: Integumentary problems. In S.M. Lewis, M.M. Heitkemper, & S.R. Dirksen (Eds.), *Medical-surgical nursing: Assessment and management of clinical problems* (6th ed., pp. 487-514). St. Louis: Mosby.

Evans, E.C., & Gray, M. (2003). What interventions are effective for the prevention and treatment of cutaneous candidiasis? *Journal of Wound, Ostomy, and Continence Nursing 30,* 11-16.

Geilen, C.C., & Orfanos, C.E. (2002). Standard and innovative therapy of psoriasis. *Clinical and Experimental Rheumatology, 20*(6 Suppl. 28), S81-S87.

Hornung, R.L., Magee, K.H., Lee, W.J., Hansen, L.A., & Hsieh, Y.C. (2003). Tanning facility use: Are we exceeding Food and Drug Administration limits? *Journal of the American Academy of Dermatology, 49*(4), 655-661.

Leone, G., Rolston, K., & Spaulding, G. (2003). Alefacept for chronic plaque psoriasis: A selective therapy with long-lasting disease remissions and an encouraging safety profile. *Dermatology Nursing, 15*(3), 216-220.

Mosby's drug consult. (2004). St. Louis: Mosby.

Nickkels, A.F., & Pierard, G.E. (2002). Oral antivirals revisited in the treatment of herpes zoster: What do they accomplish? *American Journal of Clinical Dermatology, 3*(9), 591-598.

Parker, F. (2000). Skin diseases of general importance. In L. Goldman & J.C. Bennett (Eds.), *Cecil textbook of medicine* (21st ed., pp. 2276-2298). Philadelphia: Saunders.

Shipp, M.A., & Harris, N.L. (2000). Non-Hodgkin's lymphomas. In L. Goldman & J.C. Bennett (Eds.), *Cecil textbook of medicine* (21st ed., pp. 962-969). Philadelphia: Saunders.

Skidmore-Roth, L. (2005). *Mosby's drug guide for nurses* (6th ed.). St Louis: Mosby.

Chapter 51

Black, J.M., & Matassarin-Jacobs, E. (2001). *Medical-surgical nursing: Clinical management for continuity of care* (5th ed.). Philadelphia: Saunders.

Fay, A., & Jakobiec, F.A. (2000). Diseases of the visual system. In L. Goldman & J.C. Bennett (Eds.), *Cecil textbook of medicine* (21st ed., pp. 2224-2235). Philadelphia: Saunders.

Skidmore-Roth, L. (2005). *Mosby's drug guide for nurses* (6th ed.). St Louis: Mosby.

Smith, S.C., & Wilbur, M.E. (2004). Nursing assessment: Visual and auditory systems. In S.M. Lewis, M.M. Heitkemper, & S.R. Dirksen (Eds.), *Medical-surgical nursing: Assessment and management of clinical problems* (6th ed., pp. 416-438). St. Louis: Mosby.

Smith, S.C., & Wilbur, M.E. (2004). Nursing management: Visual and auditory problems. In S.M. Lewis, M.M. Heitkemper, & S.R. Dirksen (Eds.), *Medical-surgical nursing: Assessment and management of clinical problems* (6th ed., pp. 439-475). St. Louis: Mosby.

Internet Resources

American Foundation for the Blind: www.igc.apc.org/afb/index.html.

Guide Dogs for the Blind: www.guidedogs.com.

Talking Books: National Library Service for the Blind and Visually Handicapped: www.lcweb.loc.gov/nls.html.

Chapter 52

Baloh, R.W. (2000). Hearing and equilibrium. In L. Goldman & J.C. Bennett (Eds.), *Cecil textbook of medicine* (21st ed., pp. 2250-2257). Philadelphia: Saunders.

Skidmore-Roth, L. (2005). *Mosby's drug guide for nurses* (6th ed.). St Louis: Mosby.

Smith, S.C., & Wilbur, M.E. (2004). Nursing assessment: Visual and auditory systems. In S.M. Lewis, M.M. Heitkemper, & S.R. Dirksen (Eds.), *Medical-surgical nursing: Assessment and management of clinical problems* (6th ed., pp. 416-438). St. Louis: Mosby.

Smith, S.C., & Wilbur, M.E. (2004). Nursing management: Visual and auditory problems. In S.M. Lewis, M.M. Heitkemper, & S.R. Dirksen (Eds.), *Medical-surgical nursing: Assessment and management of clinical problems* (6th ed., pp. 439-475). St. Louis: Mosby.

Chapter 53

Clark, L.K. (2001). Management of clients with upper airway disorders. In J.M. Black, J.H. Hawks, & A.M. Keene (Eds.), *Medical-surgical nursing: Clinical management for positive outcomes* (6th ed., pp. 1651-1684). Philadelphia: Saunders.

Deglin, J.H., & Vallerand, A.H. (2001). *Davis's drug guide for nurses* (7th ed.). Philadelphia: Davis.

Hagler, D.A. (2004). Nursing assessment: Respiratory system. In S.M. Lewis, M.M. Heitkemper, & S.R. Dirksen (Eds.), *Medical-surgical nursing: Assessment and management of clinical problems* (6th ed., pp. 542-563). St. Louis: Mosby.

Hagler, D.A. (2004). Nursing management: Upper respiratory problems. In S.M. Lewis, M.M. Heitkemper, & S.R. Dirksen (Eds.), *Medical-surgical nursing: Assessment and management of clinical problems* (6th ed., pp. 566-591). St. Louis: Mosby.

Jarvis, C. (2004). *Physical examination and health assessment* (4th ed.). Philadelphia: Saunders.

Pagana, K.D., & Pagana, T.J. (2003). *Mosby's diagnostic and laboratory reference* (6th ed.). St. Louis: Mosby.

Potter, P.A., & Perry, A.G. (2001). *Fundamentals of nursing* (5th ed.). St. Louis: Mosby.

Skidmore-Roth, L. (2005). *Mosby's drug guide for nurses* (6th ed.). St. Louis: Mosby.

Strohl, K.P. (2000). Upper airway diseases. In L. Goldman & J.C. Bennett (Eds.), *Cecil textbook of medicine* (21st ed., pp. 2246-2249). Philadelphia: Saunders.

Chapter 54

Caunt, H. (1992). Preoperative nursing intervention to relieve stress. *British Journal of Nursing, 1*(4), 171-172.

Dossey, B.M., Guzzetta, C.E., & Kenner, C.V. (1992). *Critical care nursing: Body-mind-spirit*. Philadelphia: Lippincott.

Fortinash, K.M., & Holoday-Worret, P.A. (2000). *Psychiatric mental health nursing*. St. Louis: Mosby.

Fortinash, K.M., & Holoday-Worret, P.A. (1999). *Psychiatric nursing care plans*. St. Louis: Mosby.

Houldin, A.D., & Hogan-Quigley, B. (1995). Psychological intervention for older hip fracture patients. *Journal of Gerontological Nursing, 21*(12), 20-26, 48-49.

Hymovich, D.P., & Hagopian, G.A. (1992). *Chronic illness in children and adults: A psychosocial approach*. Philadelphia: Saunders.

Keltner, N.L., Schwecke, L.H., & Bostrom, C.E. (Eds.). (1999). *Psychiatric nursing* (3rd ed.). St. Louis: Mosby.

Maslow, A.H. (1968). *Toward a psychology of being*. New York: Van Nostrand Reinhold.

Miller, J.F. (2000). *Coping with chronic illness: Overcoming powerlessness* (3rd ed.). Philadelphia: Davis.

Milliken, M.E. (1998). *Understanding human behavior: A guide for health care providers*. Albany, NY: Delmar.

Oakland, S., Ostell, A., Herrmann, M., Britz, A., Bartels, C., & Wallesch, C. (1995). The impact of aphasia on the patient and family in the first year poststroke. *Topics in Stroke Rehabilitation, 2*(3), 5-19.

Pennock, B.E., Crawshaw, L., Maher, T., Price, T., & Kaplan, P.D. (1994). Distressful events in the ICU as perceived by patients recovering from coronary artery bypass surgery. *Heart & Lung: Journal of Critical Care, 23*(4), 323-327.

Selye, H. (1978). *The stress of life* (2nd ed.). New York: McGraw-Hill.

Stuart, G.W., & Laraia, M.T. (2001). *Principles and practice of psychiatric nursing*. St. Louis: Mosby.

Swan, B.A. (1996). Assessing symptom distress in ambulatory surgery patients. *MEDSURG Nursing, 5*(5), 348-354.

Townsend, M.C. (2000). *Psychiatric mental health nursing: Concepts of care* (3rd ed.). Philadelphia: Davis.

Varcarolis, E.M. (2002). *Foundations of psychiatric mental health nursing: A clinical approach*. Philadelphia: Saunders.

Chapter 55

Abrams, A.C. (1998). *Clinical drug therapy: Rationales for nursing practice* (5th ed.). Philadelphia: Lippincott-Raven Publishers.

American Psychiatric Association. (1994). *Diagnostic and statistical manual of mental disorders* (4th ed.). Washington, DC: Author.

Bendik, M.F. (2000). The schizophrenias. In K.M. Fortinash & P.A. Holoday-Worret (Eds.), *Psychiatric-mental health nursing*. St. Louis: Mosby.

Benjamin, L.S. (1996). *Interpersonal diagnosis and treatment of personality disorders* (2nd ed.). New York: Guilford Press.

Brandt, B., & Ugarriza, D.N. (1996). Electroconvulsive therapy and the elderly client. *Journal of Gerontological Nursing, 22*(12), 14-20.

Dawber, N. (1997). Current approaches and interventions for schizophrenia. *Nursing Standard, 11*(49), 49-56.

Haber, J., Krainovich-Miller, B., McMahon, A.L., & Price-Hoskins, P. (1997). *Comprehensive psychiatric nursing*. St. Louis: Mosby.

Lee, F. (1997). Understanding schizophrenia. *Nursing Standard, 11*(36), 26-27.

Legge, A. (1997). Care of the older person. Depression: It's not inevitable and it is treatable. *Community Nurse, 2*(11), 16-17.

Linton, A.D., & Harris, J.A. (2000). *Pharmacology companion for introductory nursing care of adults*. Philadelphia: Saunders.

Marston, T. (1997). Mental health: In search of the right balance—schizophrenia. *Nursing Times, 93*(22), 30.

Montgomery, S.A. (1995). Managing depression in the community. *Professional Nurse, 10*(12), 805-807.

Stuart, G.W., & Laraia, M.T. (2001). *Principles and practice of psychiatric nursing* (7th ed.). St. Louis: Mosby.

Tinklenberg, M. (1997). Healthwatch: Options for treatment of schizophrenia expanding. *Nurseweek* (California Statewide Edition), *10*(7), 19.

Chapter 56

Campbell, J. (1995). Making sense of the effects of alcohol. *Nursing Times, 91*(5), 38-39.

Castledine, G. (1995). Don't drink and nurse: Alcohol abuse in nursing. *British Journal of Nursing, 4*(2), 102.

Catanzarite, A.M. (1992). *Managing the chemically dependent nurse: A guide to identification, intervention, and retention*. Chicago: American Hospital Publishing.

Clement, M. (1995). Continuing education: Recognizing dependence on alcohol in the elderly. *Nurseweek* (California Statewide Edition), *8*(20), 8.

Cook, J.S. (1991). Drug abuse. In J.S. Cook & K.L. Fontaine (Eds.), *Essentials of mental health nursing* (2nd ed., pp. 484-528). Redwood City, CA: Addison-Wesley Nursing.

Cooper, D.B. (1994). Problem drinking. *Nursing Times, 90*(14), 36-39.

Cooper, D.B. (1994). Use of chlormethiazole in alcohol home detoxification. *Professional Nurse, 10*(3), 146.

Cooper, D.B. (1993). Substance abuse: Withdrawing gracefully. *Nursing Times, 89*(17), 42-44.

Dryfoos, J.G. (1993). Preventing substance use: Rethinking strategies. *American Journal of Public Health, 83*(6), 793-795.

Fishbain, D.A., Rosomoff, H.L., & Rosomoff, R.S. (1992). Drug abuse, dependence, and addiction in chronic pain patients. *The Clinical Journal of Pain, 8*(2), 77-85.

Gorman, M. (1996). Substance abuse: Alcoholic patients: Keeping hope alive. *American Journal of Nursing, 96*(1), 20.

Gorman, M. (1996). Substance abuse: Starting recovery. *American Journal of Nursing, 96*(9), 15.

Hepple, J. (1996). Alcohol and older people. *Elderly Care, 8*(6), 34-35.

Knowlton, L. (1995). Dual diagnosis: The challenge. *Journal of the American Psychiatric Nurses Association, 1*(3), 102-104.

Kupkowski, M.J., & Robinette, A.L. (1996). Intervention for a homeless alcoholic—PCLNs: Who are they? How can they help you? *American Journal of Nursing, 96*(11), 15.

Merritt, P. (1997). Guilt and shame in recovering addicts: A personal account. *Journal of Psychosocial Nursing and Mental Health Services, 35*(7), 46.

Moos, R.H., King, M.J., & Patterson, M.A. (1996). Outcomes of residential treatment of substance abuse in hospital- and community-based programs. *Psychiatric Services, 47*(1), 68-74.

Navarra, T. (1995). Enabling behavior: The tender trap. *American Journal of Nursing, 95*(1), 50-52.

Pizzi, C.L., & Mion, L.C. (1993). Alcoholism in the elderly: Implications for hospital nurses. *MEDSURG Nursing, 2*(6), 453-458.

Riggin, O.Z., & Redding, B.A. (2000). Substance related disorders. In K.M. Fortinash & P.A. Holoday-Worret (Eds.), *Psychiatric-mental health nursing*. St. Louis: Mosby.

Watson, H.E. (1996). Minimal interventions for problem drinkers. *Journal of Substance Misuse for Nursing, Health and Social Care, 1*(2), 107-110.

Wilson, S. (1994). Can you spot an alcoholic patient? *RN, 57*(1), 46-51.

Illustration Credits

Chapter 1

Figure 1–1 from Monahan, F.D., & Neighbors, M. (1998). *Medical-surgical nursing: Foundations for clinical practice* (2nd ed.). Philadelphia: Saunders.

Figures 1–2, 1–3 from Potter, P.A., & Perry, A.G. (2001). *Fundamentals of nursing* (5th ed.). St. Louis: Mosby.

Figure 1–4 from Ignatavicius, D.D., Workman, M.L., & Mishler, M.A. (1999). *Medical-surgical nursing across the health care continuum* (3rd ed.). Philadelphia: Saunders.

Chapter 2

Figure 2–1 courtesy Edwards Lifesciences, Irvine, CA.

Figure 2–2 from Potter, P.A., & Perry, A.G. (2001). *Fundamentals of nursing* (5th ed.). St. Louis: Mosby.

Figure 2–3 from Lindeman, C.A., & McAthie, M. (1999). *Fundamentals of contemporary nursing practice.* Philadelphia: Saunders.

Chapter 4

Figure 4–1 from Potter, P.A., & Perry, A.G. (2001). *Fundamentals of nursing* (5th ed.). St. Louis: Mosby.

Figure 4–2 modified from Tappen, R.M. (1989). *Nursing leadership and management: Concepts and practice* (2nd ed.). Philadelphia: Davis.

Chapter 5

Figures 5–2, 5–3 from Potter, P.A., & Perry, A.G. (2001). *Fundamentals of nursing* (5th ed.). St. Louis: Mosby.

Chapter 6

Figure 6–1 from Monahan, F.D., & Neighbors, M. (1998). *Medical-surgical nursing: Foundations for clinical practice* (2nd ed.). Philadelphia: Saunders.

Figure 6–2 from Potter, P.A., & Perry, A.G. (2001). *Fundamentals of nursing* (5th ed.). St. Louis: Mosby.

Chapter 7

Figure 7–1 from Potter, P.A., & Perry, A.G. (2001). *Fundamentals of nursing* (5th ed.). St. Louis: Mosby.

Chapter 8

Figure 8–1 from Ignatavicius, D.D., Workman, M.L., & Mishler, M.A. (1999). *Medical-surgical nursing across the health care continuum* (3rd ed.). Philadelphia: Saunders.

Figure 8–2 redrawn from Maslow, A.H. (1970). *Motivation and personality* (3rd ed.), reprinted by permission of Pearson Education, Inc., Upper Saddle River, NJ.

Chapter 9

Figure 9–1A-C from U.S. Department of Agriculture. (2006). Center for Nutrition Policy and Promotion, Washington, DC, www.mypyramid.gov.

Figure 9–2 from Food and Drug Administration. (1995). *Daily values for food labels.* Washington, DC: U.S. Government Printing Office.

Figure 9–3 from Monahan, F.D., & Neighbors, M. (1998). *Medical-surgical nursing: Foundations for clinical practice* (2nd ed.). Philadelphia: Saunders.

Figure 9–4 from Mahan, L.K., & Escott-Stump, S. (2000). *Krause's food, nutrition, and diet therapy* (10th ed.). Philadelphia: Saunders.

Chapter 10

Figure 10–1 from Ignatavicius, D.D., Workman, M.L., & Mishler, M.A. (1999). *Medical-surgical nursing across the health care continuum* (3rd ed.). Philadelphia: Saunders.

Chapter 11

Figure 11–1 from Ignatavicius, D.D., Workman, M.L., & Mishler, M.A. (1999). *Medical-surgical nursing across the health care continuum* (3rd ed.). Philadelphia: Saunders.

Figure 11–2 from CLG Photographics, St. Louis.

Chapter 12

Figures 12–1, 12–2, 12–3, 12–4, 12–5 from Jarvis, C. (2000). *Physical examination and health assessment* (3rd ed.). Philadelphia: Saunders.

Figure 12–6 Concept Map by Elaine Bishop Kennedy, RN, EdD.

Chapter 13

Figures 13–1, 13–2 from Monahan, F.D., & Neighbors, M. (1998). *Medical-surgical nursing: Foundations for clinical practice* (2nd ed.). Philadelphia: Saunders.

Figure 13–3 from Elkin, M.K., Perry, A.G., & Potter, P.A. (2000). *Nursing interventions and clinical skills* (2nd ed.). St. Louis: Mosby.

Figure 13–4 from Black, J.M., Hawks, J.H., & Keene, A.M. (2001). *Medical-surgical nursing: Clinical management for positive outcomes* (6th ed.). Philadelphia: Saunders.

Chapter 14

Figure 14–1 from Black, J.M., Hawks, J.H., & Keene, A.M. (2001). *Medical-surgical nursing: Clinical management for positive outcomes* (6th ed.). Philadelphia: Saunders.

Chapter 15

Figures 15–1, 15–4, 15–6 from Ignatavicius, D.D., Workman, M.L., & Mishler, M.A. (1999). *Medical-surgical nursing across the health care continuum* (3rd ed.). Philadelphia: Saunders.

Figure 15–3 from Acute Pain Management Guidelines Panel. (1992). *Acute pain management* (DHHS Publication No. 92-0052). Rockville, MD: Agency for Health Care Policy and Research, Public Health Service, U.S. Department of Health and Human Services.

Figure 15–7 from Lewis, S.M., Heitkemper, M.M., & Dirksen, S.R. (Eds.). (2000). *Medical-surgical nursing: Assessment and management of clinical problems* (5th ed.). St. Louis: Mosby.

Chapter 16

Figures 16–1, 16–3, 16–5 from Lewis, S.M., Heitkemper, M.M., & Dirksen, S.R. (Eds.). (2000). *Medical-surgical nursing: Assessment and management of clinical problems* (5th ed.). St. Louis: Mosby.

Figure 16–2 from Potter, P.A., & Perry, A.G. (2001). *Fundamentals of nursing* (5th ed.). St. Louis: Mosby.

Figures 16–8A and B from Jarvis, C. (2000). *Physical examination and health assessment* (3rd ed.). Philadelphia: Saunders.

Figure 16–9 from Monahan, F.D., & Neighbors, M. (1998). *Medical-surgical nursing: Foundations for clinical practice* (2nd ed.). Philadelphia: Saunders.

Chapter 17

Figures 17–1, 17–2, 17–6 from Harkreader, H., & Hogan, M.A. (2004): *Fundamentals of nursing* (2nd ed.). Philadelphia: Saunders.

Figures 17–3, 17–5 courtesy Northwest Hospital Center, Randallstown, MD.

Figures 17–4, 17–7, 17–8, 17–9, 17–10, 17–12A and B, 17–15 from Ignatavicius, D.D., Workman, M.L., & Mishler, M.A. (1999). *Medical-surgical nursing across the health care continuum* (3rd ed.). Philadelphia: Saunders.

Figures 17–11, 17–13 from Monahan, F.D., & Neighbors, M. (1998). *Medical-surgical nursing: Foundations for clinical practice* (2nd ed.). Philadelphia: Saunders.

Figure 17–12C and D courtesy C.R. Bard, Inc., Covington, GA.

Figure 17–4 courtesy DHD Healthcare, Wampsville, NY.

Chapter 18

Figure 18–1B from Potter, P.A., & Perry, A.G. (2001). *Fundamentals of nursing* (5th ed.). St. Louis: Mosby.

Figure 18–3 redrawn from Winters, B. (1984). *Oncology Nursing Forum, 11*(6), 25-30.

Figure 18–4A courtesy B. Braun Medical, Inc., Bethlehem, PA.

Figure 18–4B courtesy ICU Medical, Inc., San Clemente, CA.

Figure 18–5 from Lewis, S.M., Heitkemper, M.M., & Dirksen, S.R. (Eds.). (2000). *Medical-surgical nursing: Assessment and management of clinical problems* (5th ed.). St. Louis: Mosby.

Figure 18–7 from Perry, A.G., & Potter, P.A. (2006). *Clinical nursing skills and techniques* (6th ed.). St. Louis: Mosby.

Chapter 19

Figure 19–1 from Black, J.M., Hawks, J.H., & Keene, A.M. (2001). *Medical-surgical nursing: Clinical management for positive outcomes* (6th ed.). Philadelphia: Saunders.

Figure 19–2 from Ignatavicius, D.D., Workman, M.L., & Mishler, M.A. (1999). *Medical-surgical nursing across the health care continuum* (3rd ed.). Philadelphia: Saunders.

Chapter 20

Figure 20–1 courtesy National Aeronautics and Space Administration.

Chapter 21

Figure 21–2 from Ignatavicius, D.D., Workman, M.L., & Mishler, M.A. (1999). *Medical-surgical nursing across the health care continuum* (3rd ed.). Philadelphia: Saunders.

Figure 21–3 from Norton, D., McLaren, R., & Eston-Smith, A.N. (1962). *An investigation of geriatric nursing problems in the hospital.* London: National Corporation for the Care of Old People (now the Centre for Policy on Ageing).

Figure 21–4 courtesy Kinetic Concepts, Inc., San Antonio, TX.

Figure 21–5 from Black, J.M., Hawks, J.H., & Keene, A.M. (2001). *Medical-surgical nursing: Clinical management for positive outcomes* (6th ed.). Philadelphia: Saunders.

Chapter 22

Figures 22–1, 22–2, 22–3 from Leahy, J.M., & Kizilay, P.E. (1998). *Foundations of nursing practice: A nursing process approach.* Philadelphia: Saunders.

Chapter 23

Figure 23–1 modified from Jacob, S.W., & Francone, C.A. (1982). *Structure and function in man* (5th ed.). Philadelphia: Saunders.

Figure 23–2 from Black, J.M., Hawks, J.H., & Keene, A.M. (2001). *Medical-surgical nursing: Clinical management for positive outcomes* (6th ed.). Philadelphia: Saunders.

Figure 23–3 from Monahan, F.D., & Neighbors, M. (1998). *Medical-surgical nursing: Foundations for clinical practice* (2nd ed.). Philadelphia: Saunders.

Figure 23–4 from Greengold, B.A., & Ouslander, J. (1986). *Journal of Gerontological Nursing, 12*(6), 31-35.

Figure 23–5 from Thibodeau, G.A., & Patton, K.P. (1999). *Anatomy & physiology* (4th ed.). St. Louis: Mosby.

Chapter 24

Figure 24–1 reprinted by permission of the National Hospice and Palliative Care Organization, 1700 Diagonal Road, Suite 625, Alexandria, VA 22314 (703-837-1500), www.nhpco.org or www.caringinfo.org.

Figure 24–2 reprinted by permission of Aging with Dignity, 820 East Park Avenue, Suite D100, Tallahassee, FL 32301-2600 (888-5WISHES), www.agingwithdignity.org.

Chapter 25

Figure 25–1 from American Cancer Society, Inc. (2006). *Surveillance research;* used by permission.

Figure 25–2 courtesy National Institutes of Health.

Figure 25–3 from Monahan, F.D., & Neighbors, M. (1998). *Medical-surgical nursing: Foundations for clinical practice* (2nd ed.). Philadelphia: Saunders.

Figure 25–4 photograph by Stephen Matteson, Jr.

Figure 25–5 from Lindeman, C.A., & McAthie, M. (1999). *Fundamentals of contemporary nursing practice.* Philadelphia: Saunders.

Chapter 26

Figure 26–1A from Potter, P.A., & Perry, A.G. (2001). *Fundamentals of nursing* (5th ed.). St. Louis: Mosby.

Figure 26–1B permission to use and/or reproduce this copyrighted material has been granted by the owner, Hollister, Inc., Libertyville, IL.

Figures 26–2, 26–3, 26–5 from Monahan, F.D., & Neighbors, M. (1998). *Medical-surgical nursing: Foundations for clinical practice* (2nd ed.). Philadelphia: Saunders.

Figure 26–4 from Ignatavicius, D.D., Workman, M.L., & Mishler, M.A. (1999). *Medical-surgical nursing across the health care continuum* (3rd ed.). Philadelphia: Saunders.

Figure 26–6 from Black, J.M., & Matassarin-Jacobs, E. (1997). *Medical-surgical nursing: Clinical management for continuity of care* (5th ed.). Philadelphia: Saunders.

Chapter 27

Figures 27–1, 27–3, 27–4, 27–8, 27–12, 27–15, 27–17, 27–18 from Monahan, F.D., & Neighbors, M. (1998). *Medical-surgical nursing: Foundations for clinical practice* (2nd ed.). Philadelphia: Saunders.

Figures 27–2, 27–7, 27–9, 27–10, 27–13, 27–14, 27–19 from Black, J.M., Hawks, J.H., & Keene, A.M. (2001). *Medical-surgical nursing: Clinical management for positive outcomes* (6th ed.). Philadelphia: Saunders.

Figure 27–5 courtesy Linda R. Littlejohn, RN, BSN, CCRN, CNRN, Neuro Clinician, and Mission Hospital Regional Center, Mission Viejo, CA.

Figure 27–6 from Thibodeau, G.A., & Patton, K.P. (1999). *Anatomy & physiology* (4th ed.). St. Louis: Mosby.

Figure 27–11 from Black, J.M., & Matassarin-Jacobs, E. (1993). *Luckmann and Sorensen's medical-surgical nursing: A psychophysiologic approach* (4th ed.). Philadelphia: Saunders.

Figure 27–15 from Black, J.M., & Matassarin-Jacobs, E. (1997). *Medical-surgical nursing: Clinical management for continuity of care* (5th ed.). Philadelphia: Saunders.

Figure 27–20 from Ignatavicius, D.D., Workman, M.L., & Mishler, M.A. (1999). *Medical-surgical nursing across the health care continuum* (3rd ed.). Philadelphia: Saunders.

Chapter 28

Figures 28–1, 28–5 from Monahan, F.D., & Neighbors, M. (1998). *Medical-surgical nursing: Foundations for clinical practice* (2nd ed.). Philadelphia: Saunders.

Figures 28–2, 28–4 from Ignatavicius, D.D., Workman, M.L., & Mishler, M.A. (1999). *Medical-surgical nursing across the health care continuum* (3rd ed.). Philadelphia: Saunders.

Figures 28–3, 28–8 from Black, J.M., Hawks, J.H., & Keene, A.M. (2001). *Medical-surgical nursing: Clinical management for positive outcomes* (6th ed.). Philadelphia: Saunders.

Figures 28–6, 28–9 from Potter, P.A., & Perry, A.G. (2001). *Fundamentals of nursing* (5th ed.). St. Louis: Mosby.

Figure 28–7A, B, and C from Sammons Preston.

Figure 28–7D from Lewis, S.M., Heitkemper, M.M., & Dirksen, S.R. (Eds.). (2000). *Medical-surgical nursing: Assessment and management of clinical problems* (5th ed.). St. Louis: Mosby.

Chapter 29

Figures 29–1, 29–2 redrawn from Jarvis, C. (1996). *Physical examination and health assessment* (2nd ed.). Philadelphia: Saunders.

Figure 29–3 adapted from Jacob, W.W., & Francone, C.A. (1989). *Elements of anatomy and physiology* (2nd ed.). Philadelphia: Saunders.

Figures 29–4, 29–10 from Monahan, F.D., & Neighbors, M. (1998). *Medical-surgical nursing: Foundations for clinical practice* (2nd ed.). Philadelphia: Saunders.

Figures 29–5, 29–6, 29–7 from Ignatavicius, D.D., Workman, M.L., & Mishler, M.A. (1999). *Medical-surgical nursing across the health care continuum* (3rd ed.). Philadelphia: Saunders.

Figures 29–8, 29–9 from Black, J.M., & Matassarin-Jacobs, E. (1993). *Luckmann and Sorensen's medical-surgical nursing: A psychophysiologic approach* (4th ed.). Philadelphia: Saunders.

Chapter 30

Figures 30–1, 30–2 from Monahan, F.D., & Neighbors, M. (1998). *Medical-surgical nursing: Foundations for clinical practice* (2nd ed.). Philadelphia: Saunders.

Figures 30–3, 30–4, 30–5, 30–7, 30–8, 30–13, 30–14, 30–15 from Black, J.M., Hawks, J.H., & Keene, A.M. (2001). *Medical-surgical nursing: Clinical management for positive outcomes* (6th ed.). Philadelphia: Saunders.

Figure 30–6 from Black, J.M., & Matassarin-Jacobs, E. (1997). *Medical-surgical nursing: Clinical management for continuity of care* (5th ed.). Philadelphia: Saunders.

Figure 30–9 from Potter, P.A., & Perry, A.G. (2001). *Fundamentals of nursing* (5th ed.). St. Louis: Mosby.

Figures 30–10, 30–11, 30–12B from Ignatavicius, D.D., Workman, M.L., & Mishler, M.A. (1999). *Medical-surgical nursing across the health care continuum* (3rd ed.). Philadelphia: Saunders.

Figure 30–12A courtesy Genzyme Biosurgery, Fall River, MA.

Chapter 31

Figures 31–1, 31–3, 31–4, 31–10 from Black, J.M., & Matassarin-Jacobs, E. (1993). *Luckmann and Sorensen's medical-surgical nursing: A psychophysiologic approach* (4th ed.). Philadelphia: Saunders.

Figure 31–2 from Monahan, F.D., & Neighbors, M. (1998). *Medical-surgical nursing: Foundations for clinical practice* (2nd ed.). Philadelphia: Saunders.

Figures 31–5, 31–6, 31–7, 31–9 from Black, J.M., Hawks, J.H., & Keene, A.M. (2001). *Medical-surgical nursing: Clinical management for positive outcomes* (6th ed.). Philadelphia: Saunders.

Figure 31–8 from Ignatavicius, D.D., Workman, M.L., & Mishler, M.A. (1999). *Medical-surgical nursing across the health care continuum* (3rd ed.). Philadelphia: Saunders.

Chapter 32

Figure 32–1A from Thibodeau, G.A., & Patton, K.P. (1999). *Anatomy & physiology* (4th ed.). St. Louis: Mosby.

Figures 32–1B, 32–4 from Rodak, B.F. (1995). *Diagnostic hematology,* Philadelphia: Saunders.

Figure 32–2 from Monahan, F.D., & Neighbors, M. (1998). *Medical-surgical nursing: Foundations for clinical practice* (2nd ed.). Philadelphia: Saunders.

Figure 32–3 from Pagana, K.D., & Pagana, T.J. (2002). *Mosby's manual of diagnostic and laboratory tests* (2nd ed.). St. Louis: Mosby.

Chapter 33

Figure 33–1 from Monahan, F.D., & Neighbors, M. (1998). *Medical-surgical nursing: Foundations for clinical practice* (2nd ed.). Philadelphia: Saunders.

Figures 33–2, 33–3 from Young-McCaughan, S., & Jennings, B.M. (1998). Hematologic and immunologic systems. In I.G. Alspach (Ed.), *Core curriculum for critical care nursing* (5th ed.). Philadelphia: Saunders.

Chapter 34

Figure 34–2A from Taylor, P.K. (1995). *Diagnostic picture tests in sexually transmitted disease.* St. Louis: Mosby.

Figures 34–2B and C from Morse, S.A., Ballard, R., Holmes, K., & Moreland, A. (Eds.). (2003). *Atlas of sexually transmitted diseases and AIDS* (3rd ed.). St. Louis: Mosby.

Figure 34–2D from Friedman-Kien, A.E. (1989). *Color atlas of AIDS.* Philadelphia: Saunders.

Figure 34–3 from Phipps, W.J., Monahan, F.D., Sands, J.K., Marek, J.F., & Neighbors, M. (2003). *Medical-surgical nursing: Health and illness perspectives* (7th ed.). St. Louis: Mosby.

Chapter 35

Figures 35–1, 35–2, 35–3, 35–4, 35–5, 35–9, 35–10, 35–12, 35–15 from Monahan, F.D., & Neighbors, M. (1998). *Medical-surgical nursing: Foundations for clinical practice* (2nd ed.). Philadelphia: Saunders.

Figures 35–7, 35–13, 35–16 from Ignatavicius, D.D., Workman, M.L., & Mishler, M.A. (1999). *Medical-surgical nursing across the health care continuum* (3rd ed.). Philadelphia: Saunders.

Figure 35–11 from Ballard, J.C., Wood, I.I., & Lansing, A. (1997). Reprinted with permission. *Critical Care Nurse,* 17(1):42-49.

Figure 35–14A courtesy St. Jude Medical, Inc., St. Paul, MN. All rights reserved.

Figure 35–14B courtesy Medtronic, Inc., Minneapolis, MN.

Figure 35–14C courtesy American Red Cross Tissue Services and Baxter Healthcare Corporation, CardioVascular Group, Santa Ana, CA.

Figure 35–17 from Ignatavicius, D.D., Workman, M.L., & Mishler, M.A. (1995). *Medical-surgical nursing: A nursing process approach* (2nd ed.). Philadelphia: Saunders.

Figures 35–18, 35–19, 35–20, 35–21, 35–22, 35–23, 35–25, 35–26, 35–27, 35–28, 35–29, 35–30 from Ignatavicius, D.D., & Bayne, M.V. (1991). *Medical-surgical nursing: A nursing process approach.* Philadelphia: Saunders.

Figure 35–24 from Black, J.M., & Matassarin-Jacobs, E. (1993). *Luckmann and Sorensen's medical-surgical nursing: A psychophysiologic approach* (4th ed.). Philadelphia: Saunders.

Chapter 36

Figures 36–1, 36–2, 36–3, 36–4, 36–5, 36–8 from Monahan, F.D., & Neighbors, M. (1998). *Medical-surgical nursing: Foundations for clinical practice* (2nd ed.). Philadelphia: Saunders.

Figure 36–7 from Ignatavicius, D.D., Workman, M.L., & Mishler, M.A. (1999). *Medical-surgical nursing across the health care continuum* (3rd ed.). Philadelphia: Saunders.

Chapter 37

Figure 37–2 from Monahan, F.D., & Neighbors, M. (1998). *Medical-surgical nursing: Foundations for clinical practice* (2nd ed.). Philadelphia: Saunders.

Figure 37–3 courtesy National Heart, Lung, and Blood Institute, National Institutes of Health.

Chapter 38

Figures 38–1, 38–5, 38–8, 38–9, 38–11B, 38–13, 38–14, 38–16, 38–17, 38–18, 38–19 from Monahan, F.D., & Neighbors, M. (1998). *Medical-surgical nursing: Foundations for clinical practice* (2nd ed.). Philadelphia: Saunders.

Figures 38–2, 38–15 from Black, J.M., Hawks, J.H., & Keene, A.M. (2001). *Medical-surgical nursing: Clinical management for positive outcomes* (6th ed.). Philadelphia: Saunders.

Figure 38–3 from Laufer, I., & Levine, M.C. (1992). *Double contrast gastrointestinal radiology* (2nd ed.). Philadelphia: Saunders.

Figure 38–4 from Jacob, S.W., & Francone, C.A. (1998). *Elements of anatomy and physiology* (2nd ed.). Philadelphia: Saunders.

Figures 38–6, 38–20, 38–21, 38–22 from Lewis, S.M., Heitkemper, M.M., & Dirksen, S.R. (Eds.). (2000). *Medical-surgical nursing: Assessment and management of clinical problems* (5th ed.). St. Louis: Mosby.

Figures 38–7, 38–11A, 38–12 from Ignatavicius, D.D., Workman, M.L., & Mishler, M.A. (1999). *Medical-surgical nursing across the health care continuum* (3rd ed.). Philadelphia: Saunders.

Figure 38–10 from Shafer, W.G., Hine, M.K., & Levy, B.M. (1983). *A textbook of oral pathology* (4th ed.). Philadelphia: Saunders.

Chapter 39

Figures 39–1, 39–7, 39–10, 39–12 from Monahan, F.D., & Neighbors, M. (1998). *Medical-surgical nursing: Foundations for clinical practice* (2nd ed.). Philadelphia: Saunders.

Figure 39–5 from Lewis, S.M., Heitkemper, M.M., & Dirksen, S.R. (Eds.). (2000). *Medical-surgical nursing: Assessment and management of clinical problems* (5th ed.). St. Louis: Mosby.

Figures 39–6, 39–8, 39–9 from Ignatavicius, D.D., Workman, M.L., & Mishler, M.A. (1999). *Medical-surgical nursing across the health care continuum* (3rd ed.). Philadelphia: Saunders.

Figures 39–11, 39–13 from Black, J.M., Hawks, J.H., & Keene, A.M. (2001). *Medical-surgical nursing: Clinical management for positive outcomes* (6th ed.). Philadelphia: Saunders.

Chapter 40

Figures 40–1, 40–2, 40–3, 40–4, 40–5, 40–8, 40–10, 40–11, 40–15, 40–16 from Monahan, F.D., & Neighbors, M. (1998). *Medical-surgical nursing: Foundations for clinical practice* (2nd ed.). Philadelphia: Saunders.

Figure 40–6 from Jacob, S.W., & Francone, C.A. (1998). *Elements of anatomy and physiology* (2nd ed.). Philadelphia: Saunders.

Figures 40–7, 40–9, 40–14 from Black, J.M., Hawks, J.H., & Keene, A.M. (2001). *Medical-surgical nursing: Clinical management for positive outcomes* (6th ed.). Philadelphia: Saunders.

Figure 40–12 from Lewis, S.M., Heitkemper, M.M., & Dirksen, S.R. (Eds.). (2004). *Medical-surgical nursing: Assessment and management of clinical problems* (6th ed.). St. Louis: Mosby.

Chapter 41

Figures 41–1, 41–4, 41–8, 41–9A from Ignatavicius, D.D., Workman, M.L., & Mishler, M.A. (1999). *Medical-surgical nursing across the health care continuum* (3rd ed.). Philadelphia: Saunders.

Figures 41–2, 41–9B from the AHPA Arthritis Teaching Slide Collection, 1980; used with permission of the American College of Rheumatology.

Figure 41–3 from Black, J.M., & Matassarin-Jacobs, E. (1993). *Luckmann and Sorensen's medical-surgical nursing: A psychophysiologic approach* (4th ed.). Philadelphia: Saunders.

Figure 41–5 courtesy the Chattanooga Group, Hixson, TN.

Figure 41–6 from Stevens, A., & Lowe, J. (2000). *Pathology: Illustrated review in color* (2nd ed.). St. Louis: Mosby.

Figure 41–7 from Black, J.M., Hawks, J.H., & Keene, A.M. (2001). *Medical-surgical nursing: Clinical management for positive outcomes* (6th ed.). Philadelphia: Saunders.

Chapter 42

Figure 42–1 from Lewis, S.M., Heitkemper, M.M., & Dirksen, S.R. (Eds.). (2000). *Medical-surgical nursing: Assessment and management of clinical problems* (5th ed.). St. Louis: Mosby.

Figure 42–2 from Ignatavicius, D.D., Workman, M.L., & Mishler, M.A. (1999). *Medical-surgical nursing across the health care continuum* (3rd ed.). Philadelphia: Saunders.

Figures 42–3, 42–4, 42–10 from Black, J.M., Hawks, J.H., & Keene, A.M. (2001). *Medical-surgical nursing: Clinical management for positive outcomes* (6th ed.). Philadelphia: Saunders.

Figure 42–5 courtesy Stryker, Howmedica Osteonics, Inc. (Stryker Orthopaedics).

Figure 42–6 courtesy Smith & Nephew, Inc., Orthopaedic Division, Memphis, TN.

Figure 42–7 redrawn from Polaski, A.K., & Tatro, S.E. (1996). *Luckmann's core principles and practice of medical-surgical nursing,* Philadelphia: Saunders.

Figure 42–8, 42–9 from Potter, P.A., & Perry, A.G. (2001). *Fundamentals of nursing* (5th ed.). St. Louis: Mosby.

Chapter 43

Figure 43–1 from Monahan, F.D., & Neighbors, M. (1998). *Medical-surgical nursing: Foundations for clinical practice* (2nd ed.). Philadelphia: Saunders.

Figures 43–2, 43–3 courtesy Otto Bock Orthopedic Industry, Inc., Minneapolis, MN.

Figure 43–4 from Black, J.M., Hawks, J.H., & Keene, A.M. (2001). *Medical-surgical nursing: Clinical management for positive outcomes* (6th ed.). Philadelphia: Saunders.

Chapter 44

Figures 44–1, 44–2, 44–5, 44–6 from Ignatavicius, D.D., Workman, M.L., & Mishler, M.A. (1999). *Medical-surgical nursing across the health care continuum* (3rd ed.). Philadelphia: Saunders.

Figure 44–3 courtesy C.M. Charles & C.M. MacBryde.

Figure 44–4 from Mendelof, A., & Smith, D.E. (Eds.). (1956). Acromegaly, diabetes, hypermetabolism, proteinuria and heart failure, Clinical Pathological Conference, *American Journal of Medicine, 20,* 133.

Chapter 45

Figures 45–1, 45–7 from Monahan, F.D., & Neighbors, M. (1998). *Medical-surgical nursing: Foundations for clinical practice* (2nd ed.). Philadelphia: Saunders.

Figure 45–2 from Seidel, H.S., Ball, J.W., Dains, J.E., & Benedict, G.W. (1999). *Mosby's guide to physical examination* (4th ed.). St. Louis: Mosby.

Figure 45–3 from Ignatavicius, D.D., Workman, M.L., & Mishler, M.A. (1999). *Medical-surgical nursing across the health care continuum* (3rd ed.). Philadelphia: Saunders.

Figure 45–4 from Ignatavicius, D.D., & Bayne, M.V. (1991). *Medical-surgical nursing: A nursing process approach,* Philadelphia: Saunders.

Figure 45–5 from Jacob, W.W., & Francone, C.A. (1989). *Elements of anatomy and physiology* (2nd ed.). Philadelphia: Saunders.

Figure 45–6 from Wilson, J., & Foster, I. (1985). *Williams textbook of endocrinology* (7th ed.). Philadelphia: Saunders.

Chapter 46

Figure 46–2 adapted from American Diabetes Association. (1992). *Teaching standards for diabetes mellitus* (5th ed.). Austin, TX: American Diabetes Association, Texas Affiliate, Inc.

Figure 46–3 from Black, J.M., Hawks, J.H., & Keene, A.M. (2001). *Medical-surgical nursing: Clinical management for positive outcomes* (6th ed.). Philadelphia: Saunders.

Figures 46–4A and B courtesy Medtronic MiniMed, Northridge, CA.

Chapter 47

Figures 47–1, 47–2, 47–3, 47–4, 47–5, 47–7, 47–9, 47–10, 47–15 from Monahan, F.D., & Neighbors, M. (1998). *Medical-surgical nursing: Foundations for clinical practice* (2nd ed.). Philadelphia: Saunders.

Figure 47–6 from Ignatavicius, D.D., Workman, M.L., & Mishler, M.A. (1995). *Medical-surgical nursing: A nursing process approach* (2nd ed.). Philadelphia: Saunders.

Figures 47–8, 47–11, 47–12, 47–13, 47–14 from Ignatavicius, D.D., Workman, M.L., & Mishler, M.A. (1999). *Medical-surgical nursing across the health care continuum* (3rd ed.). Philadelphia: Saunders.

Chapter 48

Figures 48–1, 48–12, 48–14 from Monahan, F.D., & Neighbors, M. (1998). *Medical-surgical nursing: Foundations for clinical practice* (2nd ed.). Philadelphia: Saunders.

Figures 48–2, 48–4 from Applegate, E.J. (2000). *The anatomy and physiology learning system textbook* (2nd ed.). Philadelphia: Saunders.

Figures 48–3, 48–6, 48–7, 48–10, 48–11, 48–13 from Black, J.M., Hawks, J.H., & Keene, A.M. (2001). *Medical-surgical nursing: Clinical management for positive outcomes* (6th ed.). Philadelphia: Saunders.

Figure 48–5 from Guyton, A.C., & Hall, J.C. (1996). *Textbook of medical physiology* (9th ed.). Philadelphia: Saunders.

Figure 48–8 from Black, J.M., & Matassarin-Jacobs, E. (1997). *Medical-surgical nursing: Clinical management for continuity of care* (5th ed.). Philadelphia: Saunders.

Figure 48–9 courtesy Dr. Hans Stricker, Department of Urology, Henry Ford Hospital, Detroit, MI.

Chapter 49

Figures 49–1A, 49–2, 49–3 courtesy Leonard Wolf, MD, New York, NY.

Figure 49–1B, 49–4 courtesy New York City Heath Department.

Chapter 50

Figures 50–1, 50–3, 50–14, 50–15, 50–16 from Monahan, F.D., & Neighbors, M. (1998). *Medical-surgical nursing: Foundations for clinical practice* (2nd ed.). Philadelphia: Saunders.

Figures 50–2, 50–8, 50–9, 50–10, 50–11, 50–13A, B, and C from Lookingbill, D.P., & Marks, J.G. Jr. (1993). *Principles of dermatology* (2nd ed.). Philadelphia: Saunders.

Figures 50–4, 50–13D from Jarvis, C. (2000). *Physical examination and health assessment* (3rd ed.). Philadelphia: Saunders.

Figures 50–5, 50–19 from Black, J.M., & Matassarin-Jacobs, E. (1993). *Luckmann and Sorensen's medical-surgical nursing: A psychophysiologic approach* (4th ed.). Philadelphia: Saunders.

Figure 50–6 from Hurwitz, S. (1993). *Clinical pediatric dermatology: A textbook of skin disorders of childhood and adolescence* (2nd ed.). Philadelphia: Saunders.

Figure 50–7 courtesy Columbia-Presbyterian Dermatology Associates, New York, NY.

Figure 50–12 from Callen, J.P., Greer, K.E., Hood, A.F., et al. (1993). *Color atlas of dermatology.* Philadelphia: Saunders.

Figure 50–17 from Black, J.M., Hawks, J.H., & Keene, A.M. (2001). *Medical-surgical nursing: Clinical management for positive outcomes* (6th ed.). Philadelphia: Saunders.

Figure 50–18 courtesy Smith & Nephew, Inc., San Antonio, TX.

Chapter 51

Figures 51–1, 51–2, 51–3, 51–4, 51–21 from Monahan, F.D., & Neighbors, M. (1998). *Medical-surgical nursing: Foundations for clinical practice* (2nd ed.). Philadelphia: Saunders.

Figures 51–5, 51–7, 51–13 from Jarvis, C. (2000). *Physical examination and health assessment* (3rd ed.). Philadelphia: Saunders.

Figures 51–6, 51–8, 51–10 from Ignatavicius, D.D., Workman, M.L., & Mishler, M.A. (1999). *Medical-surgical nursing across the health care continuum* (3rd ed.). Philadelphia: Saunders.

Figures 51–9, 51–16 from Black, J.M., Hawks, J.H., & Keene, A.M. (2001). *Medical-surgical nursing: Clinical management for positive outcomes* (6th ed.). Philadelphia: Saunders.

Figure 51–11 courtesy Cleveland Society for the Blind.

Figure 51–12 from Linton, A.D. (2007). *Matteson & McConnell's gerontological nursing* (3rd ed.). Philadelphia: Saunders.

Figure 51–15A and B courtesy Ophthalmic Photography at the University of Michigan W.K. Kellogg Eye Center, Ann Arbor, MI.

Figure 51–17 courtesy Phipps, W.J., Monahan, F.D., Sands, J.K., Marek, J.F., & Neighbors, M. (2003): *Medical-surgical nursing: Health and illness perspectives* (7th ed.). St. Louis: Mosby.

Figures 51–18, 51–20 courtesy National Industries for the Blind, Wayne, NJ.

Figure 51–19 from Lewis, S.M., Heitkemper, M.M., & Dirksen, S.R. (Eds.). (2000). *Medical-surgical nursing: Assessment and management of clinical problems* (5th ed.). St. Louis: Mosby.

Chapter 52

Figures 52–1, 52–8 from Monahan, F.D., & Neighbors, M. (1998). *Medical-surgical nursing: Foundations for clinical practice* (2nd ed.). Philadelphia: Saunders.

Figure 52–2, 52–5 from Ignatavicius, D.D., Workman, M.L., & Mishler, M.A. (1999). *Medical-surgical nursing across the health care continuum* (3rd ed.). Philadelphia: Saunders.

Figure 52–4 from Seidel, H.S., Ball, J.W., Dains, J.E., & Benedict, G.W. (1999). *Mosby's guide to physical examination* (4th ed.). St. Louis: Mosby.

Figure 52–6 courtesy Arnold G. Schuring, MD.

Figure 52–7 from Black, J.M., Hawks, J.H., & Keene, A.M. (2001). *Medical-surgical nursing: Clinical management for positive outcomes* (6th ed.). Philadelphia: Saunders.

Chapter 53

Figures 53–1, 53–2, 53–3, 53–8 from Monahan, F.D., & Neighbors, M. (1998). *Medical-surgical nursing: Foundations for clinical practice* (2nd ed.). Philadelphia: Saunders.

Figures 53–4, 53–5, 53–10A and C from Black, J.M., Hawks, J.H., & Keene, A.M. (2001). *Medical-surgical nursing: Clinical management for positive outcomes* (6th ed.). Philadelphia: Saunders.

Figure 53–6 courtesy Robert Margulies, Miami, FL. In Smolley, L.A. (1990). How to help patients with obstructive sleep apnea, *The Journal of Respiratory Diseases 11*:723.

Figure 53–7 courtesy Respironics, Inc., Murrysville, PA.

Figures 53–9, 53–10E from Lewis, S.M., Heitkemper, M.M., & Dirksen, S.R. (Eds.). (2000). *Medical-surgical nursing: Assessment and management of clinical problems* (5th ed.). St. Louis: Mosby.

Figure 53–10B courtesy Servox AG, Germany.

Figure 53–10D courtesy Luminaud, Inc., Mentor, OH.

Figure 53–10F from Ignatavicius, D.D., Workman, M.L., & Mishler, M.A. (1999). *Medical-surgical nursing across the health care continuum* (3rd ed.). Philadelphia: Saunders.

Glossary

A

Acid A solution containing a high number of hydrogen ions.

Acid–base balance The homeostasis of the hydrogen ion (H+) concentration in body fluids.

Acidosis Abnormal pH of body fluids caused by excess acid in relation to bicarbonate.

Acne Inflammatory skin disorder characterized by comedones, pustules, and cysts.

Acquired immunity Antibody-mediated or cell-mediated response that is specific to a particular pathogen and is activated when needed.

Acrochordon Small, soft, raised lesion (skin tag).

Acromegaly Disease of middle-aged adults resulting from overproduction of growth hormone by the anterior pituitary.

Action Ability to respond to others with genuineness, compassion, sensitivity, and self-disclosure to promote their well-being.

Active acquired immunity Immunity developed after direct contact with an antigen through illness or vaccination.

Active exercise Exercise carried out by the patient.

Active transport Movement of solutes across membranes; requires the expenditure of energy.

Acute illness Illness or disease that has a relatively rapid onset and a short duration.

Acute pain Pain that occurs after injury to tissues from surgery, trauma, or disease. It is usually sudden in onset, temporary, easily localized, and decreases as healing takes place.

Adaptation The organism's attempts to return to homeostasis.

Addiction Behavioral pattern of compulsive drug use characterized by craving for an opioid and obtaining and using the drug for effects other than pain relief.

Addison's disease Disease resulting from a deficiency of adrenocorticotropic hormone caused by destruction or dysfunction of the adrenal glands.

Adrenaline Epinephrine; a powerful vasoactive substance produced by the adrenal medulla in times of stress or danger.

Adrenocorticotropic hormone (ACTH) A pituitary hormone that stimulates the cortex of the adrenal glands to produce adrenal hormones.

Advance directive Written statement of a person's wishes regarding medical treatment.

Advanced cardiac life support Use of drugs and equipment to provide continuing care for a person who has suffered cardiac or respiratory arrest.

Aerosol Solid or liquid particles suspended in a gas.

Affect Feelings such as happiness, sadness, or worry. Inappropriate affect is incongruence between the thought and the feeling expressed.

Afterload The amount of resistance the left ventricle must overcome to open the aortic valve.

Ageism A process of systematic stereotyping and discrimination against people because of their age; usually directed against older people.

Aging The process of growing older or more mature.

Agoraphobia Fear of situations outside the home.

AIDS Acquired immunodeficiency syndrome. Advanced HIV (human immunodeficiency virus) infection that weakens the body's immune system, progressively destroying the body's ability to fight pathogens and certain cancers. The condition is clinically diagnosed in HIV-positive individuals who have a T-cell count below 200 and one or more of the opportunistic viral, fungal, or bacterial infections associated with the disease.

Akathisia A reversible condition of restlessness manifested as an urge to pace.

Algor mortis Cooling of the body after death.

Alkaline (base) A solution containing a low number of hydrogen ions.

Alkalosis Abnormal pH of body fluids caused by excess bicarbonate in relation to acid.

Allergen An antigen that causes a hypersensitive reaction.

Alopecia Loss of hair.

Amino acids A group of 22 substances that can be bonded in different ways to make a variety of proteins. The body can manufacture sufficient amounts of these if the nine essential amino acids are provided in the diet.

Amputation Removal of a limb, part of a limb, or an organ; may be done by surgical means or through an accident.

Amputee Individual who has undergone an amputation.

Amyopathy (amyotonia) Loss of muscle tone.

Analgesia A state of not feeling pain.

Analgesic Drug that acts on the nervous system to relieve or reduce the suffering or intensity of pain.

Anaphylactic shock A severe, potentially fatal, allergic reaction characterized by hypotension and bronchial constriction.

Anastomosis Communication or connection between two organs or parts of organs.

Androgens Hormones produced by the adrenal cortex, the testes, and the ovaries that stimulate the development of male characteristics.

Anemia A reduction in the number of red blood cells or in the quantity of hemoglobin in the blood.

Anesthesia Partial or complete loss of sensation with or without loss of consciousness.

Anesthesiologist A physician who specializes in the administration of anesthetics and monitors the patient while the patient is under anesthesia.

Anesthetic An agent that abolishes the pain sensation.

Angioma Benign tumor composed of blood vessels.

Ankylosis Joint immobility.

Anorectal incontinence Fecal incontinence caused by weak perineal muscles, loss of anal reflexes, loss of anal sphincter tone, or rectal prolapse.

Anorexia Loss of appetite for food.

Anteflexion Bending forward of the top of an organ.

Anteversion Bending forward of an entire organ.

Antibody A protein that is created in response to a specific antigen.

Antibody-mediated acquired immunity Defensive response by B cells assisted by TH cells, aimed at invading microorganisms such as bacteria.

Antidiuretic hormone (ADH) A hormone released by the posterior pituitary gland that causes the reabsorption of water in the distal tubules and collecting ducts of the kidney.

Antigen A substance, usually a protein, that is capable of stimulating a response from the immune system.

Antihistamine Drug that blocks the effects of histamine, which is a body chemical that causes allergic symptoms.

Antineoplastic An agent that inhibits the maturation or reproduction of malignant cells.

Antithrombotic Capable of preventing the formation of blood clots.

Anuria Absence of urine production.

Anxiety A vague sense of impending doom or apprehension that appears to have no clearly identifiable cause.

Aphasia Inability to understand words or to respond with words, or both.

Apical Referring to the pointed end of a structure.

Apnea Cessation of breathing.

Arteriosclerosis Abnormal thickening, hardening, and loss of elasticity of the arterial walls.

Arthralgia Pain in a joint.

Arthritis Inflammation of a joint.

Arthroplasty Plastic repair of a joint.

Asbestosis Interstitial fibrosis of the lungs caused by inhalation of asbestos fibers.

Ascites Accumulation of excess fluid in the peritoneal cavity.

Assessment Collection of data about the health status of a patient or client.

Assignment Identification and delegation of specific tasks to a specific person who is hired and paid to perform these tasks.

Assimilation Process of replacing or giving up values, beliefs, and practices for those of another culture.

Asthma A condition characterized by episodes of bronchospasm that causes wheezing and dyspnea.

Astigmatism Error of refraction caused by uneven curvature of the cornea or lens; causes visual distortion.

Atelectasis Collapsed lung or part of a lung.

Atherosclerosis Abnormal thickening and hardening of the arterial walls caused by fat and fibrin deposits.

Aura A peculiar sensation that precedes a set of symptoms.

Auscultation Listening to sounds produced by the body, such as heart, lung, and intestinal sounds.

Autocratic leadership Authoritative, directive, or bureaucratic type of leadership.

Autoimmunity A condition in which the body is unable to distinguish self from nonself, causing the immune system to react and destroy its own tissues.

Automaticity Ability of a cell to generate an impulse without external stimulation.

Automatism Aimless behavior performed without conscious control or knowledge.

Autonomic dysreflexia Abnormally exaggerated response of the autonomic nervous system to a stimulus.

Autonomy Freedom from external authority to make decisions about one's own health and health care.

Autopsy Examination of a body after death to determine or confirm the cause of death.

Avulsion Tearing away of tissue.

Azotemia Accumulation of nitrogenous compounds in the blood.

B

Bacteria Several classifications of one-celled microorganisms that are capable of multiplying rapidly and causing illness.

Basal metabolic rate Energy expended in the resting state; measured with the body at complete mental and physical rest, but not asleep.

Basic life support Immediate care given to prevent cardiac or respiratory arrest or to support circulation and respiration of a victim of cardiac arrest until advanced medical support is available.

Behçet's disease Chronic syndrome with oral, gastrointestinal, and genital ulcerations and uveitis; arthritis, vasculitis, synovitis, meningitis, and phlebitis.

Beneficence The act of doing good; a health care provider's behaving in the patient's best interest.

Benign Not malignant.

Bioethics The ethics of biologic science, medicine, and health care.

Biologic age The functional capabilities of various organ systems in the body.

Biologic approach Assumes that mental disorders are related to physiologic changes within the central nervous system.

Biopsy Excision of a small piece of tissue for microscopic examination; usually done to determine a specific diagnosis.

Bipolar disorder Disorder characterized by alternating periods of elevated mood (manic episodes) and depression.

Blepharitis Inflammation of the hair follicles and glands on the margins of the eyelids.

Body image One's physical and psychological experiences that influence the perception of one's own body.

Bone marrow Spongy center of bones where the white blood cells, red blood cells, and platelets are made.

Bone remodeling Process in which immature bone cells are gradually replaced by mature bone cells.

Borderline personality disorder Disorder characterized by exhibition of unstable relationships, unstable self-image, and unstable mood.

Botulism Food poisoning caused by *Clostridium botulinum*.

Bouchard's nodes Enlarged proximal interphalangeal joints of the fingers.

Brachytherapy Placement of a radiation source in the body to treat a malignancy.

Bradycardia Slow heart rate, usually defined as fewer than 60 beats per minute.

Bronchiectasis Permanent dilation of a portion of the bronchi or bronchioles.

Bronchitis Bronchial inflammation.

Bruit A murmur detected by auscultation.

Bulla Blister.

C

Cachexia Profound wasting, loss of body mass, usually related to malnutrition.

Calculus (pl. calculi) Abnormal concentration, commonly called a stone, that is formed of mineral salts and is found in hollow organs or their passages.

Calorie Standard unit for measuring energy; the amount of heat needed to raise the temperature of 1 gm of water at a standard temperature by 1° C.

Cannula A tube that can be inserted into a body cavity or duct; needle or catheter employed for intravenous therapy.

Capitation Accepting a fixed amount of money to provide health care services to all health care plan members with no additional billing.

Carcinogen A substance that can cause cancer.

Cardiac output Liters of blood ejected by either ventricle per minute.

Cardiac tamponade The presence of blood in the pericardial sac that causes decreased cardiac output.

Cardiopulmonary arrest Absence of heartbeat and breathing.

Cardioversion Delivery of an electrical shock to the myocardium to restore normal sinus rhythm.

Caries Destructive process of tooth decay.

Caring A process characterized by understanding, action, and concern.

Cataract Clouding or opacity of the normally transparent lens within the eye; causes blurred vision and objects to take on a yellowish hue.

Catecholamines Chemicals (dopamine, epinephrine, norepinephrine) released at sympathetic nerve endings in response to stress.

Cathartic Agent that stimulates bowel evacuation; usually rapid in effect and producing a watery stool.

Cell-mediated acquired immunity Defensive response by Tc cells aimed at intracellular defects such as viruses and cancer.

Cerebral death Absence of cerebral cortex functioning.

Cerumen Waxy secretion in the external auditory canal; earwax.

Cervicitis Inflammation of the cervix (narrow, lower end of the uterus).

Chalazion An inflamed, enlarged meibomian gland on the eyelid.

Chancre A papule that breaks down into a painless ulcer at the site of entry of the organism that causes syphilis.

Cheilitis Inflammation of the lips.

Cheilosis Cracking of the lips and corners of the mouth.

Chemical restraints Psychotropic medications given to subdue agitated or confused patients.

Chemotherapy Use of chemicals to treat illness.

Choking Airway obstruction caused by a foreign body in the airway.

Cholangitis Inflammation of the biliary ducts.

Cholecystectomy Removal of the gallbladder.

Cholecystitis Inflammation of the gallbladder.

Choledocholithiasis Obstruction of the common bile duct by a gallstone.

Cholelithiasis Presence of gallstones in the gallbladder.

Chronic illness Permanent impairment or disability that requires long-term rehabilitation and medical or nursing treatment.

Chronic pain Pain that lasts longer than 3 to 6 months and is associated with nerve or tissue damage. It usually continues after the normal time for healing or it may occur spontaneously. It is difficult to localize, may not be detectable with current diagnostic techniques, and may not respond to usual treatments.

Chvostek's sign Spasm of the facial muscles when the facial nerve is tapped; indicative of hypocalcemia.

Cirrhosis Chronic, progressive liver disease.

Client Recipient of nursing care in situations; denotes a feeling of partnership or working with someone.

Closed amputation Amputation in which a limb or part of a limb is removed and the wound is surgically closed.

Closed or simple fracture Fracture in which the broken bone does not break through the skin.

Closed reduction or manipulation Nonsurgical realignment of the bones to their previous anatomic position using traction, angulation, or rotation or a combination of these.

Clotting factors Substances in the blood that help the blood to clot, numbered I through XII.

Co-dependency Exaggerated dependent pattern of self-defeating behaviors, beliefs, and feelings learned as a result of pathologic relationship to a chemically dependent, or otherwise dysfunctional, person.

Cognition Workings of the mind; language, memory, intellect, and reasoning.

Cognitive behavioral approach Approach to therapy that uses behavior modification (positive and negative reinforcement) and recognizes that particular thoughts influence emotional states.

Cognitive developmental approach Approach to management of behavioral symptoms of dementia in which the environment and interactions are adapted to the patient's cognitive abilities.

Collateral Accessory; side branch.

Colostomy Surgically created opening in the colon.

Colporrhaphy Operative technique that narrows the vagina by suturing the vaginal wall.

Comminuted fracture Fracture in which the bone is broken or crushed into small pieces.

Communicable disease Illness, caused by infectious organisms or their toxins, that can be transmitted, either directly or indirectly, from one person to another.

Community-acquired infections Infections that are acquired in day-to-day contact with the public.

Compartment syndrome Serious complication of a fracture caused by internal or external pressure on the affected area, resulting in decreased blood flow, pain, and tissue damage.

Compensation Adaptations made by the heart and circulation to maintain normal cardiac output.

Complement One of a series of proteins that enhance the inflammatory process and immune response.

Complementary proteins Combination of incomplete proteins that provide all nine essential amino acids when consumed together.

Complete fracture Fracture in which the break extends across the entire bone, dividing it into two separate pieces.

Complete protein Protein containing all nine essential amino acids; usually of animal origin (e.g., meat, eggs).

Compliance Elasticity.

Compromised host precautions Actions taken to help protect patients with low white blood cell counts from infection.

Compulsions Incessant behaviors such as hand washing that interfere with normal functioning.

Conduction deafness A hearing impairment due to a blockage of the ear canal caused by excessive wax buildup, abnormal structures, or infection.

Conductivity Ability of the cell to transmit electrical impulses rapidly and efficiently to distant regions of the heart.

Confidentiality The assurance that private information is accessible only to authorized parties for specific, limited, clearly defined purposes.

Conflict Psychological struggle that results when two incompatible possibilities occur at the same time.

Confusion Disordered consciousness; lack of orientation in relation to person, place, and/or time.

Congenital amputation Deformity or absence of a limb or limbs occurring during fetal development.

Conjunctivitis Inflammation of the membrane lining the eyelids and the eyeball.

Constipation Condition characterized by infrequent bowel movements with hard stools that are passed with difficulty.

Contamination Presence of an infectious organism on a body surface or an object.

Continent Capable of controlling natural impulses; in relation to an ostomy, able to retain feces or urine.

Contractility Capacity for shortening in response to stimuli.

Contracture Shortening of the muscles and tendons.

Contralateral Opposite side.

Conversion disorder Loss of body function (such as paralysis) without physiologic cause.

Coping Any behavioral or cognitive activity used to deal with stress.

Coping strategy An adaptive or maladaptive mental attitude, behavior, or both that is consciously or unconsciously perceived as helping to reduce stress, anxiety, or fear.

Cor pulmonale Right-sided heart failure associated with pulmonary disease.

Corpus cavernosum (pl. corpora cavernosa) Erectile chamber of the penis.

Coryza Discharge from the nasal mucous membranes.

Crackles Abnormal lung sounds heard on auscultation; discrete single sounds heard on inspiration, occur in brief bursts; may be fine (high pitched and soft) or coarse (low pitched and loud); "rales."

Crede's technique Expression of urine from the bladder by applying pressure over the lower abdomen.

Crepitus Crackling sound or sensation.

Crest syndrome A form of a systemic scleroderma less severe than other forms, consisting of calcinosis cutis, Raynaud's phenomenon, esophageal dysfunction, sclerodactyly, and telangiectasia.

Cretinism Permanent mental and physical retardation caused by congenital deficiency of thyroid hormones.

Crisis The point at which the individual moves toward illness and disequilibrium.

Cultural diversity The existence of many cultures in a society.

Culture Integrated system of learned values, beliefs, and practices that is characteristic of a society and that guides individual behavior.

Cushing's disease Disease caused by the hypersecretion of glucocorticoids due to excessive release of adrenocorticotropic hormone by the pituitary.

Cushing's syndrome Disorder resulting from excessive glucocorticoids in the body as a result of tumor or hypersecretion of the pituitary or by prolonged administration of large doses of exogenous steroids.

Cusp Cup-shaped structure; semilunar heart valves have three cusps.

Cycloplegic Agent that paralyzes the ciliary muscle so that the eye does not accommodate.

Cystectomy Removal or resection of the urinary bladder or of a cyst.

Cystocele Herniation of the urinary bladder into the vagina.

Cystotomy Creation of a surgical opening into the bladder.

Cytologic Related to cells or the study of cells.

D

Débride To remove debris, including necrotic tissue.

Decerebrate posturing Abnormal extension of the upper extremities with extension of the lower extremities; accompanies increased pressure on the entire cerebrum and the motor tract structures of the brain stem.

Decongestant Agent that reduces swelling, especially of the nasal mucous membranes

Decorticate posturing Abnormal flexion of the upper extremities with extension of the lower extremities; accompanies increased pressure on the frontal lobes.

Deep partial thickness burn A burn that involves the epidermis and the dermis.

Defense mechanism A mechanism, usually unconscious, used to relieve or diminish anxiety.

Defibrillation Termination of cardiac fibrillation, usually by electric shock.

Dehiscence Separation of previously joined edges; reopening of a surgical wound.

Delayed union Fracture healing that does not occur in the normally expected time.

Delegation Turning over part of one person's responsibility to another person, with that person's consent.

Delirium A disturbance of consciousness and a change in cognition that develop over a short period of time.

Dementia A clinical syndrome or collection of symptoms that is chronic in nature and is characterized by impairment of intellectual function, problem-solving ability, judgment, memory, orientation, and appropriate behavior.

Democratic leadership Achievement of goals through participation by all group members.

Denial A defense mechanism in which the individual thinks and behaves as if not aware of an unpleasant reality.

Deontology A theory that defines right and wrong based on *how* a person accomplishes goals rather than on *what* is accomplished; the idea that an act (the means) can be wrong even if it produces a result (an end) that is the best possible outcome.

Depersonalization A state of feeling outside of oneself, watching what is happening as if it were happening to someone else.

Depression A mood of sadness; a withdrawal from usual commitments.

Dermatitis Inflammation of the skin.

Dermatome Area of skin supplied by sensory nerve fibers from a single posterior spinal root.

Dermatomyositis An acute, subacute, or chronic disease marked by nonsuppurative inflammation of the skin, subcutaneous tissue, and muscles, with necrosis of muscle fibers.

Diabetes insipidus Disease caused by inadequate secretion of antidiuretic hormone by the posterior portion of the pituitary.

Diagnosis-related group (DRG) System of reimbursement standards for care in hospitals. The reimbursement is based on a fixed fee for a diagnostic category, regardless of cost.

Dialysis Passage of molecules through a semipermeable membrane into a special solution.

Diaphoresis Excessive perspiration.

Diaphoretic Wet with excessive perspiration.

Diarrhea The passage of frequent watery stools.

Diffusion The random movement of particles in all directions through a solution.

Diplopia Double vision.

Disability Measurable loss of function, usually delineated to indicate a diminished capacity for work (*see* Handicap).

Discoid lupus Circular, scaly lesions with erythematous raised rims; occurs over scalp, ears, face, and areas exposed to sun.

Disorder A term used when a definite organic cause is established for behaviors and symptoms (*see* Syndrome).

Dissociative disorder Change in identity, memory, or consciousness that allows persons to remove themselves from anxiety-provoking situations, for example, multiple personality disorder and amnesias.

Distress Stress that is perceived as harmful.

Diuresis Increased production of urine.

Dizziness Feeling of unsteadiness.

DNR order Do Not Resuscitate order; a written order from a patient or primary decision maker, in consultation with the health care team, that resuscitation is not to be attempted in the event of cardiac or respiratory arrest.

Dual diagnosis Simultaneous existence of a major psychiatric condition and a medical condition.

Dysarthria Inability to speak clearly because of neurologic damage that impairs normal muscle control.

Dysfunctional communication An unclear transmission of a message or information that prohibits the receiver from understanding the intent or meaning of what the sender transmits.

Dysmenorrhea Painful menstruation.

Dyspareunia Difficult or painful sexual intercourse in women.

Dyspepsia Epigastric discomfort after meals, caused by impaired digestion.

Dysphagia Difficulty swallowing.

Dysphasia Difficulty speaking.

Dysplasia Abnormal cells.

Dyspnea Difficulty breathing.

Dyspraxia Partial inability to initiate coordinated voluntary motor acts.

Dysreflexia Disordered response to stimuli; NANDA diagnosis for person with spinal cord injury at or above the seventh thoracic vertebra who experiences or is at risk for experiencing autonomic dysreflexia.

Dysrhythmia Disturbance of rhythm; arrhythmia.

Dysuria Difficult or painful urination.

E

Ecchymosis Purplish skin lesions resulting from blood leaking out of the blood vessels.

Ectropion In relation to the eyelid, outward turning of the lid.

Ego In psychoanalytic theory, the "rational self" or "reality" principle of personality; mediates between id and superego.

Egocentric Belief that one is the center of the universe.

Eicosanoid A class of fatty acids that regulate blood vessel vasodilation, temperature elevation, white blood cell activation, and other physiologic processes involved in immunity.

Ejaculation Reflexive expulsion of semen from the male urethra.

Ejection fraction Percentage of ventricular end-diastolic volume ejected with each contraction of the left ventricle.

Electroconvulsive therapy Controversial therapy that uses electrical current to the brain to evoke a grand mal seizure.

Electrolyte A substance that develops an electrical charge when dissolved in water.

Electromyography Diagnostic procedure in which needle electrodes are used to detect electrical impulses in muscle tissue; impulses are recorded and provide information about function of the nerves that supply muscles.

Embolism Sudden obstruction of an artery by a floating clot or foreign material.

Embolus (pl. emboli) An unattached blood clot or other substance in the circulatory system.

Emesis Vomiting.

Emission Delivery of semen into the internal urethra by rhythmic smooth muscle contractions of the epididymis, vas deferens, seminal vesicles, and prostate.

Emotional lability Instability; episodes of unexplained and uncontrollable happiness and sadness.

Empathy The ability to identify with and understand another person's situation, feelings, and motives.

Emphysema Abnormal accumulation of air in body tissue; in the lung, a disorder characterized by loss of lung elasticity with trapping of air, retained carbon dioxide, and dyspnea.

Empowerment Giving patients the information they need to be active participants in their care.

Encephalitis Inflammation of brain tissue.

Enculturation The process of learning to be part of a culture.

Endocrine gland Gland that secretes a substance directly into the blood.

Endogenous Internally produced or caused by internal factors.

Endometriosis A condition in which endometrial tissue is located outside the uterus.

Energy Capacity to do work; the way the body uses nutrients received through food consumption.

Entropion In relation to the eyelid, inward turning of the lid.

Enucleation Removal of an intact organ, such as the eyeball.

Enuresis Involuntary passage of urine, usually during sleep.

Epididymitis Inflammation of the epididymis.

Epidural Situated within the spinal canal or on the outside of the dura mater; opioids may be administered epidurally for pain relief.

Epistaxis Nosebleed.

Equianalgesic Having approximately the same degree of pain relief effect.

Equilibrium State of balance needed for walking, standing, and sitting.

Erection Swelling and rigidity of the penis.

Eructation Expulsion of gas from the stomach through the mouth; belching.

Erythema Redness of the skin; usually a sign that capillaries have become congested because of impaired blood flow.

Estrogens Hormones produced by the ovaries, adrenal glands, and fetoplacental unit in women that are responsible for the sexual development and maturation of women.

Ethics Values, codes, and principles related to what is right that influence decisions in nursing practice.

Ethnic group Group of individuals with a unique identity based on shared traditions, national origin, physical characteristics, and customs.

Ethics of care A theory that sees care as a "central activity of human behavior"; it places emphasis on relationships.

Ethical dilemma A situation in which there is an apparent conflict between moral imperatives and in which obeying one results in transgressing another.

Ethnocentrism A tendency to view the world from the perspective of one's own culture or ethnicity.

Euglycemia Normal blood glucose level.

Eustress Stress that is perceived as helpful (e.g., graduation, vacation).

Evisceration Protrusion of internal organs through a wound.

Excitability Ability of a cell to respond to an electrochemical stimulus.

Exocrine gland Gland that secretes substances externally through ducts.

Exogenous Developed outside the organism.

Exophthalmos Protrusion of the eyeballs associated with hyperthyroidism.

Expressive aphasia Difficulty speaking, reading, and writing; characterized as nonfluent; caused by lesion in Broca's area.

External fixation Use of rods, pins, nails, screws, or metal plates to align bone fragments and keep them in place for healing; similar to internal fixation, but the devices in the bone are attached to an external frame.

Extracellular fluid Fluid outside the cell.

Extrapyramidal effects Side effects of antipsychotic drugs on the portion of the central nervous system controlling involuntary movements.

Extravasation Escape of fluid or blood from a blood vessel into body tissue.

Extrinsic factors Factors in the environment.

F

Fall Circumstance in which one unintentionally falls to the ground or hits an object such as a chair or stair.

Family Two or more persons who are joined together by bonds of sharing and emotional closeness and who identify themselves as being part of a family.

Fasciculation Small involuntary muscle contraction.

Fat embolism Condition in which fat globules are released from the marrow of the broken bone into the bloodstream, migrate to the lungs, and cause pulmonary hypertension.

Fat-soluble vitamins Vitamins that are soluble in fat solvents, are absorbed into the body with other lipids, and build up in fat cells; includes vitamins A, D, E, and K.

Fear Analogous to anxiety, but related to dread of a specific or real occurrence.

Fecal incontinence The inability to control the passage of feces.

Fee for service An established fee set by physicians or health care providers for services or procedures actually provided.

Feelings All emotional and physical responses and sensations.

Feminist ethics A branch of ethical study that focuses on gender inequalities and other disparities between and among individuals and groups of people. Feminist ethics places a particularly high value on relationships.

Filtration Transfer of water and solutes through a membrane from a region of high pressure to a region of low pressure.

Fixation Procedure done during the open reduction surgical procedure to attach the fragments of the broken bone together when reduction alone is not feasible.

Flaccid Soft; in relation to muscles, lacking tone.

Flaccidity Diminished muscle tone.

Flail chest Loss of support in the chest wall where several adjacent ribs are broken in more than one place.

Flatulence Formation of excessive gas in the stomach or intestines.

Flatus Gas in the digestive tract that is expelled through the rectum.

Fluent aphasia Ability to speak clearly but without meaning.

Fluid Any liquid or gas.

Fluid volume deficit An abnormally decreased volume of extracellular fluid.

Fluid volume excess An abnormally increased volume of extracellular water and electrolytes or intracellular water.

Fracture Break or disruption in the continuity of a bone.

Frostbite Serious tissue damage caused by cold.

Frostnip Mild tissue damage caused by cold.

Full thickness burn Burn involving the epidermis, dermis, and underlying tissues such as fat, muscle, and bone.

Functional communication The clear transmission of a message or information that enables the receiver to understand the intent or meaning of what the sender transmits.

Functional incontinence Inappropriate voiding in the presence of normal bladder and urethral function.

Fungi Vegetable-like organisms that feed on organic matter and are capable of producing disease.

G

Gangrene Necrosis or death of tissue, usually due to a deficient or absent blood supply; may result from inflammatory processes, injury, arteriosclerosis, frostbite, or diabetes mellitus.

Gastrectomy Removal of all or part of the stomach.

Gastritis Inflammation of the stomach.

Gastrostomy A surgically created opening in the stomach.

Gerontological nurses Professional nurses and advanced level practitioners such as nurse practitioners, clinical specialists, and nurses holding national certification in the specialty of gerontological nursing.

Gerontology The study of aging.

Gigantism Disease caused by excessive growth hormone in children and young adolescents resulting in excessive proportional growth.

Gingivitis Inflammation of the gums.

Gland Organ or structure that secretes substances used in other areas of the body.

Glaucoma Condition in which high pressure of the fluid in the eye causes damage to the optic nerve.

Glucocorticoid Class of adrenocortical hormones that affect protein and carbohydrate metabolism and help protect the body against stress.

Glucometer Electronic device used to measure blood glucose.

Gluconeogenesis Synthesis of glucose from sources other than carbohydrates.

Glycogenesis Formation of glycogen from glucose.

Glycogenolysis Splitting of glycogen into glucose.

Glycosuria Presence of glucose in the urine.

Goiter Enlargement of the thyroid gland.

Goitrogen Substance that suppresses thyroid function.

Goniometer Instrument used to measure joint range of motion.

Granuloma A collection of inflammatory cells commonly surrounded by fibrotic tissue that represents a chronic inflammatory response to infectious or noninfectious agents.

Gratification Sense of comfort and satisfaction derived from the fulfillment of one's needs.

Gravidity Describes state of a woman with respect to the total number of pregnancies.

Greenstick fracture Fracture in which the bone is broken on one side but only bent on the other; most common in children.

Grief An emotional response to a loss.

Growth and development Physical, cognitive, and psychological development that is predictable and sequential.

Guillotine amputation Type of amputation in which a limb or portion of a limb is severed from the body and the wound is left open; a type of open amputation.

H

HAART Highly active antiretroviral therapy. A combination of three or four antiretroviral drugs that may be prescribed when the HIV viral load reaches certain levels.

Handicap Inability to perform one or more normal daily activities because of mental or physical disability (*see* Disability).

Health maintenance organization (HMO) Health care organization responsible for both financing and delivering comprehensive health services to an enrolled population for a prepaid fixed fee.

Heartburn (pyrosis) Burning or tight sensation rising from the lower sternum to the throat.

Heat stroke Body core temperature of 106° F or more.

Heberden's nodes Protrusions of the distal interphalangeal finger joints associated with osteoarthritis.

Heimlich maneuver Technique for ejecting a foreign body from the airway by using abdominal thrusts.

Helminths Worms that are parasites found in the soil and water and are transmitted to humans from hand to mouth.

Hematocele Accumulation of blood in the scrotum, usually as a result of blunt trauma.

Hematocrit Percentage of red blood cells in whole blood.

Hematuria Blood in the urine.

Hemiparesis Weakness on one side of the body.

Hemiplegia Paralysis on one side of the body.

Hemoconcentration Concentration of the blood.

Hemodynamics Study of the movement of blood and the forces that affect it.

Hemoglobin Protein of the red blood cell that carries oxygen.

Hemorrhage Loss of a large amount of blood.

Hemostasis The control of bleeding.

Hemothorax Presence of blood in the pleural cavity causing the lung on the affected side to collapse.

Hepatic Pertaining to the liver.

Hepatitis Inflammation of the liver.

Hepatomegaly Enlargement of the liver.

HIV Human immunodeficiency virus.

HIV-positive A condition in which the blood has antibodies for the human immunodeficiency virus (HIV), meaning the individual has been infected with this virus.

Holism A way of viewing people as whole individuals.

Homeostasis A tendency of the biologic system to maintain stability of the internal environment while continuously adjusting to changes necessary for survival.

Homonymous hemianopsia Loss of half the field of vision; loss is on the side opposite the brain lesion.

Hopelessness A condition of lack of hope, which may hinder action.

Hordeolum Inflammation of a sebaceous gland of the eyelid; commonly called a "sty."

Humoral immunity An immediate response to specific antigens involving B lymphocytes and the production of antibodies.

Hydrocele Accumulation of clear fluid in the tunica vaginalis of the testicle or along the spermatic cord.

Hypercalcemia Abnormally high serum calcium.

Hypercapnia Excess carbon dioxide in the blood.

Hyperglycemia Abnormally high serum glucose.

Hyperkalemia Abnormally high serum potassium.

Hyperlipidemia Excess insoluble fats in the blood.

Hypernatremia Abnormally high serum sodium.

Hyperopia Farsightedness; ability to see distant objects better than near objects.

Hypertension Persistent elevation of arterial blood pressure of 140/90 mm Hg or greater.

Hyperthermia Elevation of body core temperature above 99° F.

Hypertonic solution A solution that has a higher concentration of electrolytes than normal body fluids.

Hypertrophy Enlargement of existing cells resulting in increased size of an organ or tissue.

Hyperuricemia Elevated level of uric acid in the blood.

Hyperventilation Abnormally prolonged and deep breathing.

Hypervolemia Increased circulating blood volume.

Hypocalcemia Abnormally low serum calcium.

Hypochondriasis Belief that a serious medical condition exists when medical findings are absent.

Hypoglycemia Abnormally low level of glucose in the blood.

Hypokalemia Abnormally low serum potassium.

Hyponatremia Abnormally low serum sodium.

Hypophysectomy Surgical removal of all or part of the pituitary gland.

Hypotension Abnormally low blood pressure.

Hypothermia Decrease in body core temperature below 95° F.

Hypotonic solution A solution that has a lower concentration of electrolytes than normal body fluids.

Hypovolemia Reduced circulating blood volume.

Hypoxemia Low level of oxygen in the blood.

Hypoventilation Reduced movement of air into the alveoli.

Hypoxia Low oxygen level; decreased availability of oxygen to body tissues.

Hysterectomy Surgical removal of the uterus.

I

Iatrogenic infections Infections transmitted in the care-giving process.

Icterus Jaundice; golden yellow skin color caused by deposition of bile pigments.

Id In psychoanalytic theory, the "pleasure principle" of the personality.

Ileostomy Surgically created opening in the ileum.

Immobility The inability to move; imposed restriction on entire body.

Immunity Resistance to or protection from a disease.

Immunodeficiency A condition in which the immune system is unable to defend the body against a foreign invasion of antigens.

Immunoglobulin Membrane-bound, Y-shaped binding proteins produced by B lymphocytes; when immunoglobulins are released from the cell membrane, they are called antibodies.

Immunosuppressant Agent that reduces immune response.

Impaction (fecal) Accumulation of stool in the intestines that is not readily eliminated.

Impairment Physical or psychological disturbance in functioning.

Impotence (erectile dysfunction) Inability to achieve and maintain an erection for sexual intercourse.

Incomplete fracture Fracture in which the bone breaks only part way across, leaving some portion of the bone intact.

Incomplete protein Protein lacking one or more essential amino acids.

Incontinence Inability to hold urine.

Infarct An area of ischemic necrosis caused by disruption of circulation.

Infection Condition in which the body is invaded by infectious organisms that multiply, causing injury and a local inflammatory response that may progress to a systemic response.

Infertility Inability to conceive and produce viable offspring.

Infiltration A collection of infused fluid in tissues surrounding a cannula inserted for intravenous therapy.

Inflammation Nonspecific immune response that occurs in response to bodily injury.

Informed consent A patient's ability to make an independent health care decision after being given sufficient information and advice regarding the risks, benefits, alternatives, and consequences of accepting or refusing treatment.

Innate immunity Defensive system that is operational at all times, consisting of anatomic and physiologic barriers, the inflammatory response, and the ability of certain cells to phagocytose invaders.

Insoluble fiber Indigestible roughage found in plant cells; aids in stool formation and elimination.

Isotonic A solution that has the same concentration of electrolytes as normal body fluids.

Inspection Purposeful observation or scrutiny of the person as a whole and then of each body system.

Inspissated Thickened and dried; often used to describe pulmonary secretions.

Instinct Inborn source of bodily need or impulse.

Interferon A substance produced in viral infections that inhibits the replication of viruses.

Intermediate care facility Nursing homes that provide custodial care for people who are unable to care for themselves because of mental or physical infirmity.

Internal fixation Use of rods, pins, nails, screws, or metal plates to align bone fragments and keep them in place for healing.

Interpersonal approach Approach to therapy whereby the patient learns new ways to behave in a therapeutic relationship built on trust.

Intertrigo Skin inflammation where two skin surfaces touch.

Intracellular fluid Fluid within the cell.

Intracerebral Within the cerebrum.

Intracranial Within the skull.

Intracranial pressure Pressure within the cranium/skull.

Intrinsic factors Factors related to the internal functioning of an individual, such as the aging process or physical illness.

Ipsilateral Same side.

Ischemia Deficient blood flow due to obstruction or constriction of blood vessels.

Isolation technique Isolation of infected patients from other patients and health care workers.

Isometric exercise Muscle contraction without movement used to maintain muscle tone.

Isotonic solution A term used to describe a solution that has the same concentration of electrolytes as normal body fluids.

J

Jaundice Golden yellow color of the skin, sclerae, and mucous membranes caused by deposition of bile pigments; associated with liver dysfunction or bile obstruction causing hyperbilirubinemia.

Justice The concept of fairness, equity, and appropriateness of treatment.

K

Keratitis Inflammation of the cornea.

Keratolytic Capable of dissolving keratin, the outer surface of the epidermis.

Ketoacidosis Metabolic acidosis related to accumulated ketone bodies in the blood.

Ketone bodies Products of fatty acid metabolism.

Kyphosis Abnormal curvature of the thoracic spine as viewed from the side.

L

Laissez-faire leadership Nondirective type of leadership.

Laryngectomy Surgical removal of the larynx.

Laryngitis Inflammation of the larynx.

Laryngospasm Spasmodic closure of the larynx.

Latent Dormant; during the latency period of a disease, there are no signs or symptoms of the disease.

Lavage Irrigation.

Laxative Agent that softens stool and promotes bowel evacuation.

Leadership Guidance or showing the way to others.

Lentigo (pl. lentigines) Pigmented spot on sun-exposed skin.

Leukemia Cancer of the white blood cells in which the bone marrow produces too many immature white blood cells.

Leukocytes White blood cells that play a key role in immune responses to infectious organisms and other antigens.

Leukocytosis Part of the inflammatory process that causes an increase in white blood cells.

Leukopenia Reduced number of leukocytes (white blood cells) in the blood.

Leukoplakia Hard white patches on the gums, oral mucosa, or tongue that tend to become malignant.

Libido In psychoanalytic theory, psychic energy used to operate the id, ego, and superego.

Lipids Fats in solid or liquid form; store energy, carry fat-soluble vitamins, maintain healthy skin and hair; supply essential fatty acids; and promote a feeling of fullness (satiety).

Lipoatrophy Decreased subcutaneous fat mass.

Lipohypertrophy Increased subcutaneous fat mass.

Lipoproteins Lipid-wrapped proteins carried into the bloodstream; they include high-density and low-density lipoproteins, which carry cholesterol.

Lithotomy Removal of calculi through an incision in a duct or organ.

Lithotripsy Crushing or disintegration of calculi.

Livor mortis Discoloration of the body after death.

Long-term care facility Nursing home that provides intermediate and nonskilled or custodial care for people who are unable to care for themselves because of mental or physical disabilities.

Loss A real or potential absence of someone or something that is valued.

Lymphocytopenia Reduced number of lymphocytes in the blood; also called lymphopenia.

Lymphoma Cancer of the lymph system.

Lymphopenia Lymphocytopenia; reduced number of lymphocytes in the blood.

M

Macrovascular Pertaining to the large blood vessels.

Macule A flat, colored lesion such as a freckle.

Maladaptive Attempts to cope using strategies that ultimately do not return the individual to homeostasis.

Malaise Vague feeling of discomfort.

Malignant Tending to progress in virulence; has the characteristics of becoming increasingly undifferentiated, invasive of surrounding tissues, and colonizing distant sites.

Malpractice Professional negligence by a health care provider that causes patient injury.

Managed health care The provision of comprehensive health care at a reasonable cost through enrollment in an HMO, PPO, or similar plan with incentives to save costs.

Management Effective use of selected methods to achieve desired outcomes.

Metastasis Process by which cancer spreads to distant sites.

Mastitis Inflammation of breast tissue.

Matrix Intercellular substance of a tissue.

Medicaid Program that provides health care services for needy, lower-income, and disabled individuals through funds distributed at the state level.

Medical asepsis Limiting the spread of microorganisms; often called clean technique.

Medicare Health insurance program administered by the federal government that is funded by Social Security payments.

Menarche Onset of menstrual function.

Menopause Cessation of menstruation.

Menorrhagia Menstrual periods characterized by profuse or prolonged bleeding.

Menstruation Vaginal discharge of a mixture of blood and other fluids and tissue that is formed in the uterus to receive a fertilized ovum.

Mental health continuum A model used to demonstrate the range of mental health on a line between health at one end and illness at the opposite extreme.

Mental status examination Observations and descriptions regarding appearance, mood and affect, speech and language, thought content, perceptual disturbances, insight and judgment, sensorium and memory, and attention.

Metastasis Process by which cancer spreads to distant sites.

Metrorrhagia Bleeding or spotting between menstrual periods.

Microvascular Pertaining to the small blood vessels (i.e., arterioles, capillaries, and venules).

Micturition Urination.

Mineralocorticoid Type of hormone secreted by the adrenal cortex and involved in the regulation of fluid and electrolyte levels in the body.

Minerals Small amounts of metals (calcium, sodium, potassium) and nonmetals (chloride, phosphate) that are essential to the body; can build up.

Miotic agent Agent that causes the pupil to constrict.

Monoamine oxidase inhibitor (MAOI) Class of antidepressant drugs; patients on MAO inhibitors must be carefully monitored to avoid life-threatening food and drug interactions.

Mood Feeling state experienced by the patient over a period of time; can be constricted (not experiencing a variety of feelings) or expanded (experiencing more than usual feelings).

Moral distress A feeling of powerlessness that occurs when institutional barriers prevent a health care provider from acting in accordance with his or her own moral beliefs.

Moral outrage A feeling of being powerless to intervene after witnessing an immoral act by another health care provider.

Morality A shared concept in society of what is right or wrong.

Morals Ethical habits of a person.

Multiple personality disorder Exhibition by one person of two or more distinct personalities.

Murmur A sound heard on auscultation of the heart that usually indicates turbulent blood flow across heart valves.

Myalgia Muscle pain.

Mycoplasmas Gram-negative organisms usually causing infections in the respiratory tract.

Mydriatic agent Agent that causes the pupil to dilate.

Myelinated Surrounded with a sheath.

Myopathy Muscle disease; *adj.* myopathic.

Myopia Nearsightedness; ability to see near objects better than distant objects.

Myxedema Facial edema that develops with severe, long-term hypothyroidism; sometimes used as a synonym for hypothyroidism.

N

Natural immunity Immunity that is present at birth.

Necrotizing vasculitis Any of a group of disorders characterized by inflammation and necrosis of blood vessels occurring in a broad spectrum of cutaneous and systemic disorders.

Neoplasm Tumor; may be benign or malignant.

Nephropathy Kidney disease.

Nephrostomy Surgically created opening in the kidney to drain urine.

Nephrotoxic Having a harmful effect on kidney tissue.

Neuralgia Pain in a nerve or along the course of a nerve.

Neurogenic bladder Condition in which the bladder does not function normally because of some disorder affecting the nerves of the bladder.

Neurogenic (bowel) incontinence Reflexive uncontrolled bowel movement, usually seen with dementia.

Neurohypophysis Posterior portion of the pituitary gland.

Neuroleptic malignant syndrome Effect of medication that can develop after one dose or after years of drug therapy; the first symptoms usually are muscular rigidity, accompanied by akinesia and respiratory distress; the cardinal sign is hyperthermia (body temperature 101–103° F or higher).

Neuropathic pain Pain that arises from a damaged nerve.

Neuropathy Pathologic changes in the peripheral nervous system.

Neurotoxin Substance that poisons or impairs nerve tissue.

Neurotransmitter Biochemical messenger at nerve endings that stimulates an excitatory or inhibitory response.

Nevus (pl. nevi) Mole.

Nociception Process of pain transmission; usually related to pain sensation resulting from stimulation of pain receptors and transmission of stimuli to the pain fibers, spinal cord, and brain.

Nocturia Urination during the night.

Nodule Small mass of tissue that can be palpated.

Nonfluent aphasia Difficulty initiating speech.

Nonmaleficence The concept in health care of first doing no harm; in end-of-life issues, this involves providing treatment to control pain and not necessarily to heal.

Nonsteroidal anti-inflammatory drug (NSAID) Nonopioid drug that reduces pain and inflammation.

Nonunion Failure of a fracture to heal.

Nosocomial infections Hospital-acquired infections that were not present at the time of admission.

Nurse anesthetist A registered nurse who specializes in the administration of anesthetics and monitors the condition of patients receiving anesthetics.

Nursing diagnosis Actual or potential health problems derived from data gathered during the assessment of a patient or client.

Nursing process Systematic, problem-solving approach to providing nursing care in an organized, scientific manner.

O

Object permanence Idea that an object or person continues to exist even though no longer in sight; object permanence does not develop until about 2 years of age, according to Piaget.

Objective data Information about the patient that can be detected with the senses.

Obsessions Recurrent intrusive thoughts that interfere with normal functioning.

Obsessive-compulsive disorder Recurrent obsessions, compulsions, or both that produce distress and interfere with daily functions.

Oedipus complex Occurs during the phallic stage in psychoanalytic theory; the child unconsciously desires the parent of the opposite sex; this conflict is resolved when the child identifies with the parent of the same sex.

Older Americans Act Act passed in 1965 to ensure that elderly persons have an adequate income and suitable housing, physical and mental health services, community services, and the opportunity to pursue meaningful activities.

Oliguria Decreased urine output.

Omnibus Reconciliation Act (OBRA) Law enacted in 1987 to protect patients in long-term care facilities.

Oncofetal antigen A gene product that normally is suppressed in adult tissues but reappears in the presence of some types of cancer.

Open amputation Amputation that is left open; usually done in cases of infection or necrosis.

Open or compound fracture Fracture in which the fragments of the broken bone break through the skin.

Open reduction Surgical procedure in which an incision is made at the fracture site, usually on patients with open (compound) or comminuted fractures, to cleanse the area of fragments and debris.

Opioid agonist Any morphine-like drug that produces bodily effects including pain relief.

Opportunistic infection An infection caused by an organism that usually does not cause a disease but becomes pathogenic when body defenses are impaired.

Orthopnea Difficulty breathing when lying down.

Orthostatic hypotension Sudden drop in systolic blood pressure when changing from a lying or sitting position to a standing position.

Orthostatic vital sign changes Changes in the vital signs as a person moves from lying to sitting to standing positions in which the pulse increases by 20 points and the blood pressure decreases by 20 points, indicating that the patient is hypovolemic.

Osmolality The concentration of a solution; measured as the number of dissolved particles per kilogram of water.

Osmolarity The concentration of a solution; measured as the number of dissolved particles per liter of solution.

Osmosis Movement of water across a membrane from a less concentrated solution to a more concentrated solution.

Osteoarthritis A noninflammatory degenerative joint disease marked by degeneration of the articular cartilage, hypertrophy of bone at the margins, and changes in the synovial membrane.

Osteomyelitis Infection of the bone.

Osteoporosis Decreased bone mass.

Ostomy Surgical procedure that creates an opening into a body structure.

Otalgia Pain in the ear.

Otic Pertaining to the ear.

Ototoxic Capable of injuring the eighth cranial (acoustic) nerve or other structures involved in hearing and balance.

Overflow incontinence (fecal) Uncontrolled passage of stool associated with constipation.

Overflow incontinence (urine) Involuntary loss of urine associated with a full bladder.

Oximeter A device that uses a photoelectric sensor to measure the oxygen saturation of the blood.

Oxygenation The transport of oxygen from the lungs to the tissues.

P

Pain Unpleasant sensory and emotional experience associated with actual or potential tissue damage existing whenever the person says it does; a unique, private experience involving the whole person in a time dimension of past, present, and future and influenced by internal and external environments.

Pain threshold Level of intensity that causes the sensation or feeling of pain.

Pain tolerance Amount of pain a person is willing to endure before taking action to relieve pain.

Palliative Relieves symptoms or improves function without correcting the basic problem.

Palpation Method of physical examination that uses touch to assess various parts of the body.

Palpitation A heartbeat that is strong, rapid, or irregular enough that the person is aware of it.

Pancreatitis Inflammation of the pancreas.

Panic disorder Experience of intense episodes of apprehension to the point of terror.

Papule A raised area on the skin that is less than 1 cm in diameter.

Paracentesis Removal of ascitic fluid from the peritoneal cavity.

Paraphimosis Retraction of phimotic foreskin, causing painful swelling of the glans.

Paraplegia Loss of motor and sensory function due to damage to the spinal cord that spares the upper extremities but, depending on the level of the damage, affects the trunk, pelvis, and lower extremities.

Paresthesia An abnormal sensation.

Parity Describes state of a woman with respect to the number of pregnancies carried 20 or more weeks.

Parkinsonian syndrome Adverse effect of long-term antipsychotic drug therapy; patient exhibits mask-like face, shuffling gait, resting tremor, and rigid posture.

Parotiditis Inflammation of the parotid (salivary) gland; most commonly called parotitis.

Parotitis Inflammation of the parotid gland.

Paroxysmal nocturnal dyspnea Sudden difficulty breathing when asleep.

Participative leadership A mixture of autocratic and democratic leadership; feedback from group members is used by the leader to make a final decision.

Passive acquired immunity Temporary immunity acquired after receiving antibodies or lymphocytes produced by another individual.

Passive exercise Exercise of the patient that is carried out by the therapist or nurse without the assistance of the patient.

Pathogen Disease-causing microorganism.

Pathologic fracture Fracture that occurs because of a pathologic condition in the bone, such as a tumor or disease process, that causes a spontaneous break.

Patient A person for whom the nurse provides care; denotes a feeling of doing to or for.

Patient-controlled analgesia Self-administration of an analgesic by a patient instructed in doing so; usually refers to self-dosing with intravenous opioids through a programmable pump.

Patient's Bill of Rights Document issued by the American Hospital Association in 1973 that addresses the quality of care for patients.

Peer group Group of people with which the individual identifies and derives a sense of belonging.

Pelvic inflammatory disease An infection of the ovaries, fallopian tubes, and pelvic area.

Pemphigus Chronic autoimmune condition characterized by blisters on the face, back, chest, groin, and umbilicus.

Percussion Tapping on the skin to assess the underlying tissues.

Perforation Hole or break in a structure.

Perfusion Passage of blood through the vessels of an organ.

Periarteritis nodosa An inflammatory disease of the outer coats of small and medium-sized arteries, marked by a variety of systemic symptoms.

Periarticular Around the joint.

Periorbital edema Accumulation of excess fluid around the eye.

Peritoneum Membrane that lines the walls of the abdominal and pelvic cavities.

Peritonitis Inflammation of the peritoneum.

Personality Deeply ingrained patterns of behavior that include the way one relates to, perceives, and thinks about the environment and self.

Personality disorders Pervasive, chronic, and maladaptive personality characteristics that interfere with normal functioning; examples are paranoid, schizoid, antisocial, borderline, avoidant, obsessive-compulsive, and passive-aggressive.

Pessary A device inserted into the vagina to support the uterus.

Petechiae Small (1 to 3 mm) red or reddish purple spots on the skin resulting from capillaries breaking and leaking small amounts of blood into the tissues.

pH The symbol used to indicate hydrogen ion concentration. A solution with a low pH (<7) is an acid; a solution with a high pH (>7) is alkaline or base. A pH of 7 is neutral. The normal pH of body fluids is between 7.35 and 7.45.

Phagocytes Certain white blood cells (neutrophils, monocytes, and macrophages) that engulf and destroy invading pathogens, dead cells, and cellular debris.

Phantom limb Sensation that a limb still exists following amputation; the perception that pain exists in a removed limb is called phantom limb pain.

Phimosis Constriction of the opening in the prepuce so the prepuce cannot be retracted back over the glans.

Phlebitis Inflammation of a vein.

Phlebothrombosis Development of venous thrombi without venous inflammation.

Photophobia Excessive sensitivity to light.

Physical assessment Physical examination that is a systematic, thorough way of obtaining objective data.

Physical dependence Physical need for the substance on which one is dependent in order to avoid unpleasant physical withdrawal symptoms.

Physical restraint Anything that restricts movement, and cannot be removed by the individual.

Plasma Clear, straw-colored fluid that carries the red blood cells, white blood cells, and platelets through the circulatory system.

Platelet Small, disk-shaped blood component responsible for activating the blood clotting system.

Pneumoconiosis One of many occupational diseases caused by inhalation of particles of industrial substances.

Pneumonitis Inflammation of the lung.

Pneumothorax Presence of air in the pleural cavity that causes the lung on the affected side to collapse.

Poikilothermy Coolness in an area of the body due to decreased blood flow.

Poison Any substance that, in small quantities, is capable of causing harm following ingestion, inhalation, injection, or contact with the skin.

Polydipsia Excessive thirst.

Polymyalgia rheumatica A connective tissue disorder characterized by stiffness and pain in the shoulders and hips.

Polymyositis A chronic, progressive inflammatory disease of skeletal muscle.

Polyp Growth that protrudes from a mucous membrane.

Polyphagia Excessive hunger, food ingestion.

Polyuria Excessive urine output.

Postictal After a seizure.

Posttraumatic stress disorder Symptoms experienced following a traumatic event; examples are flashbacks, detachment, and sleep difficulties.

Powerlessness Feeling that one's action will not affect an outcome or that one lacks personal control over certain events or situations.

Preferred provider organization (PPO) System that uses a network of independent physicians, hospitals, and other providers who provide services to a pool of patients for a discounted fee.

Preload The amount of blood in the left ventricle at the end of diastole; the pressure generated at the end of diastole.

Presbycusis The term for hearing loss associated with old age.

Presbyopia A visual impairment associated with older age in which the lens becomes more rigid and less able to change shape, resulting in a decreased ability to focus on near objects.

Pressure ulcer An open wound caused by pressure on a bony prominence; also called a "pressure sore."

Primary prevention The first level of prevention; includes steps taken to improve health and prevent disease and injury.

Problem-oriented medical record Method of record keeping that focuses on patient problems rather than on medical diagnoses.

Progressive systemic sclerosis (PSS) Scleroderma; multisystem autoimmune disorder characterized by hardening of the skin and affecting blood vessels, gastrointestinal tract, lungs, heart, and kidneys.

Projection A defense mechanism in which one sees others as a source of one's own unacceptable thoughts, feelings, or impulses.

Prolapse Downward displacement.

Prostatectomy Removal of all or part of the prostate gland.

Prostatitis Inflammation of the prostate gland.

Prostatodynia Prostatic and pelvic pain in the absence of infection or inflammation.

Protease inhibitor A class of medications used to treat or prevent such viral infections as HIV and hepatitis C. These medications prevent viral replication by inhibiting the activity of protease.

Proteins Large organic compounds made of various combinations of amino acids; found in meat, milk, fish, and eggs.

Protozoa One-celled organisms capable of producing disease that usually is spread by contaminated food and water.

Pruritus Itching.

Psoriasis Skin condition characterized by scaly lesions and caused by rapid proliferation of epidermal cells.

Psychoanalytic approach Based on the theory that people function at different levels of awareness (conscious to unconscious) and that ego defense mechanisms such as denial and repression are used to prevent anxiety.

Psychological age The behavioral capacity of a person to adapt to changing environmental demands.

Psychological dependence Intense craving for the substance on which one is dependent without physical withdrawal symptoms.

Psychosis A state in which a person's perception of reality is impaired, thereby interfering with the capacity to function and to relate to others.

Ptosis Drooping of the upper eyelid.

Public Health Service Branch of the Department of Health and Human Services of the U.S. government whose chief purpose is to provide better health services for the American people.

Purpura Red or reddish purple skin lesions 3 mm or more in size, resulting from blood leaking outside the blood vessels.

Pyrogen A substance released in inflammation that causes body temperature to increase.

Q

Quadriplegia Loss of motor and sensory function in all four extremities due to damage to the spinal cord.

R

Radiotherapy The use of radiation in the treatment of cancer and other diseases.

Range-of-motion exercise Exercise in which each joint is moved in various directions to the farthest possible extreme without producing pain.

Receptive aphasia Inability to comprehend words; characterized as fluent; lesion in Wernicke's area.

Recovery Lifelong process of maintaining abstinence from the substance to which one is addicted; a return to moderate substance use is never the end result of recovery.

Rectocele Herniation of part of the rectum into the vagina.

Red blood cell Biconcave, disk-shaped blood component responsible for carrying oxygen to the tissues and removing waste carbon dioxide from the tissues.

Red blood cell count Total number of red blood cells found in one cubic millimeter of blood.

Reduction Process of bringing the ends of the broken bone into proper alignment.

Reflex training Technique to stimulate defecation using the Valsalva maneuver and rectal stretching.

Reflux Backward flow.

Refraction Bending of light rays.

Regeneration Replacement of damaged cells by cells of their own kind during the wound healing process.

Regurgitation Backward flow (cardiovascular system); gentle ejection of the stomach contents into the mouth without nausea or retching (digestive tract).

Rehabilitation Process of restoring individuals to best possible health and functioning following physical or mental impairment.

Reiter's syndrome A connective tissue disease characterized by a triad of arthritis, urethritis, and conjunctivitis.

Relaxation State of decreased anxiety and muscle tension.

Repair Replacement of damaged cells by connective tissue and then eventually by scar tissue during the wound healing process.

Replantation Surgical reattachment of a limb to its original site.

Residual limb Stump; partial limb remaining after amputation.

Resources Persons, items, concepts, or organizations that can be drawn on for a sense of support (e.g., family, money, skills, beliefs).

Respiration Exchange of oxygen and carbon dioxide in the alveoli (external respiration) and in the tissues and cells (internal respiration).

Respiratory arrest Absence of breathing.

Resting metabolic rate Measurement of energy expenditure made at any time of the day and 3 to 4 hours after the last meal.

Retinopathy Disease of the retina of the eye.

Retroflexion Bending backward of the upper portion of an organ.

Retroversion Bending backward of an entire organ.

Reverse isolation Protection of severely compromised clients from other patients and health care workers.

Reversible ischemic neurologic deficit Neurologic deficit that lasts more then 24 hours but resolves completely; caused by diminished cerebral blood flow.

Rheumatoid arthritis A chronic systemic disease characterized by inflammatory changes occurring throughout the body's connective tissues; most apparent in diarthroses (synovial joints).

Rhinitis Inflammation of the nasal mucous membrane.

Rhonchus (pl. rhonchi) Dry, rattling sound caused by partial bronchial obstruction.

Rickettsiae Microorganisms that usually are transmitted to humans through flea and tick bites.

Rigor mortis Stiffening of the body after death.

Role How a person is expected to behave in a situation or what is expected of a person in a certain position.

S

Salpingo-oophorectomy Surgical excision of a fallopian tube and ovary.

Sanguineous Bloody.

Saturated fatty acids Compounds that come chiefly from animal sources and are usually solid at room temperature; also coconut and palm oils.

Scheduled toileting Encouraging patients to use the toilet at specific times based on their usual patterns.

Schizophrenia Very serious group of usually chronic thought disorders in which patients' ability to interpret the world around them is severely impaired; symptoms include impaired thinking patterns, hallucinations, bizarre behavior, delusions, and emotional responses that do not coincide with events.

Sclerodactyly Hardening and shrinking of connective tissue of fingers and toes; scleroderma of fingers and toes.

Scleroderma Chronic multisystem autoimmune disease characterized by hardening of the skin and affecting the blood vessels, gastrointestinal tract, lungs, heart, and kidneys.

Sclerotherapy Injection of hardening agents into blood vessels.

Scotoma Blind spots.

Secondary prevention The second level of prevention; includes steps taken to detect disease early and begin treatment as soon as possible.

Seizure Convulsion; series of involuntary contractions of voluntary muscles.

Selectively permeable membranes Membranes that separate fluid compartments of the body and regulate movement of water and certain solutes from one compartment to another.

Self A term to describe one's personhood.

Self-concept One's mental image or picture of oneself.

Self-esteem The perception of self as having worth.

Sensorineural deafness A hearing impairment resulting from damage to the nerve centers within the brain as a result of exposure to loud noises, disease, and certain drugs.

Sensorium Level of consciousness and orientation to time, place, person, and self.

Septum A wall that divides a body cavity.

Serosanguineous Made up of blood and serum.

Serous Containing serum.

Sexually transmitted infection A disease that can be transmitted by intimate genital, oral, or rectal contact.

Shearing forces Caused by two contacting parts sliding on each other.

Shock Acute circulatory failure that can lead to death; caused by blood loss, heart failure, overwhelming infection, severe allergic reactions, or extreme pain or fright.

Shroud A wrap in which the body is placed after death for transport to the morgue or mortuary.

Sinusitis Inflammation of the paranasal sinuses.

Sjögren's syndrome A symptom complex of unknown etiology marked by the triad of keratoconjunctivitis, xerostomia, and the presence of a connective tissue disease.

Skilled nursing facility Type of long-term care facility that provides rehabilitative care for people who need nursing care that consists of observation during illness, administration of medications and treatments, bowel or bladder retraining, and changing of sterile dressings.

Skilled observation and assessment Used to determine adequacy of home environment, knowledge level of the patient and family regarding care procedures, side effects of treatment, and family's level of comfort in performing specific procedures.

Skilled procedures Certain nursing procedures, such as dressing changes, Foley catheter insertions, and venipuncture.

Smegma Sebaceous secretion found beneath the foreskin.

Social age The roles and habits of a person in relation to other members of society.

Soluble fiber Partially digestible roughage found in plant cells; aids in stool softening and works chemically to reduce absorption of certain substances in the bloodstream.

Solution A liquid containing one or more dissolved substances.

Somatoform disorder Characterized by vague, multiple, recurring physical complaints that are not caused by real physical illness.

Somogyi effect Rebound response to excess insulin, causing hyperglycemia.

Spastic Increased muscle tone, characterized by sudden, involuntary muscle spasms.

Spasticity Abnormally increased muscle tone.

Spermatocele A cystic mass on the epididymis.

Sprain An injury to a ligament.

Sputum Mucus secretion from the respiratory tract.

Staged amputation Amputation that is done over the course of several operations, usually to control the spread of infection or necrosis.

Statutory law Written laws (statutes) legislated by government in response to a perceived need to clarify the functioning of government, improve civil order, provide for a public need, or codify existing law.

Steatorrhea Excess fat in the stools.

Stenosis Narrowing of a passage or opening.

Sterile Free of microorganisms; infertile.

Sterility State of being free of microorganisms; unable to reproduce.

Stoma Opening created to drain contents of an organ.

Stomatitis Inflammation of the oral mucosa.

Strain An injury to muscle tissues or the tendons that attach them to bones, or both.

Stress A physical and emotional state always present in individuals that is intensified when an internal or external environmental change or threat occurs to which they must respond.

Stress fracture Fracture caused by either sudden force or prolonged stress.

Stress incontinence Involuntary loss of urine during physical exertion.

Stressor A factor that causes stress.

Stump The distal portion of an amputated limb.

Subarachnoid Between the arachnoid and pia mater layers of the membranes covering the brain.

Subculture A group of individuals within a culture whose members share different beliefs, values, and attitudes from those of the dominant culture.

Subjective data Information reported by patients or family members.

Substance abuse Maladaptive pattern of substance use that differs from generally accepted cultural norms; sometimes referred to as chemical abuse or drug abuse.

Substance dependence Ingestion of substances in gradually increasing amounts due to a physical need; used interchangeably with the terms chemical dependence and drug dependence.

Superficial partial thickness burn Burn that affects the epidermis.

Support system Resources that are used to cope with stress.

Surgical asepsis Elimination of microorganisms from any object that comes in contact with the patient; often called sterile technique.

Symptomatic incontinence Fecal incontinence associated with colorectal disease.

Syncope Fainting.

Syndrome Refers to behaviors and symptoms.

Syndrome of inappropriate antidiuretic hormone Disorder caused by excess antidiuretic hormone production; symptoms include decreased urination, edema, and fluid overload.

Systemic Related to the body as a whole.

Systole Contraction phase of the cardiac cycle.

T

Tachycardia Rapid heart rate, usually defined as greater than 100 beats per minute.

Tachypnea Rapid respiratory rate.

Tardive dyskinesia Frequently irreversible side effect of antipsychotic medication that develops after years of use; symptoms include involuntary movements of face, jaw, and tongue, leading to grimacing, jerky movements of upper extremities, and tonic contractions of neck and back.

Telangiectasis Vascular lesion created by dilation of a group of small blood vessels.

Tertiary prevention The third level of prevention; includes steps taken to prevent disease recurrence or complications of diagnosed disease or injury.

Testis (pl. testes) The male reproductive organs.

Tetany Steady muscle contraction; caused by hypocalcemia.

Theory X Management by autocratic rule with little participation in decision making by workers.

Theory Y Democratic style of management with some participation in decision making by workers.

Theory Z Management with full participation in decision making by workers.

Thoracentesis Insertion of a needle through the chest wall into the pleural space to remove fluid, blood, or air or to instill medication.

Thoracotomy Surgical opening of the chest wall.

Thrombocytopenia Abnormally reduced number of platelets in the blood.

Thromboembolism Obstruction of a blood vessel with a blood clot transported through the bloodstream.

Thrombophlebitis Development of venous thrombi in the presence of venous inflammation.

Thrombosis Development or presence of a thrombus.

Thrombus (pl. thrombi) Stationary blood clot.

Thyroiditis Inflammation of the thyroid gland.

Thyrotoxicosis Excessive metabolic stimulation caused by elevated thyroid hormone level.

Tinnitus Ringing, buzzing, or roaring noise in the ears.

Tissue perfusion Blood flow through the blood vessels of tissue.

Tolerance Physiologic result of repeated doses of an opioid where the same dose is no longer effective in achieving the same analgesic effect; a larger dose of the opioid is required to achieve the same analgesic effect.

Tonicity A measure of the concentration of electrolytes in a fluid.

Tonometry Measurement of pressure such as intraocular pressure.

Tonsillitis Inflammation of the tonsils.

Tophus (pl. tophi) Deposit of sodium urate crystals under the skin.

Tort A civil wrong against a person that is recognized as grounds for a lawsuit.

Transcultural nursing Integration of cultural considerations into all aspects of nursing care.

Transcutaneous electrical nerve stimulation (TENS) Method of producing analgesia through electrical impulses applied to the skin.

Transient incontinence Temporary loss of control over voiding.

Transient ischemic attack Diminished cerebral blood flow producing neurologic deficits that last less than 24 hours.

Triglycerides Lipids composed of three fatty acid chains and a glycerol molecule.

Trousseau's sign Carpopedal spasm after compression of the nerves in the upper arm; a sign of hypocalcemia.

12-step program Self-help support process outlining 12 steps to overcoming a physical or psychological dependence on something outside oneself that has a destructive impact on one's life.

Tympanic membrane Eardrum; the membrane that separates the external and middle portions of the ear.

U

Understanding Ability to listen to and relate to others in order to perceive their feelings and the meaning of their words.

Unipolar depression Depressed mood.

Universal donor Person with type O-negative blood who can donate blood to anyone because the person does not have any of the common antigens present in the blood.

Universal recipient Person with type AB-positive blood who can receive transfusions with any type of blood because the person has all the common antigens (A, B, and Rh) present in the blood.

Unsaturated fatty acids Compounds that come from plants or fish and are generally liquid at room temperature; can be monounsaturated (olive, peanut, canola, and avocado oils) or polyunsaturated (corn, safflower, and sesame oils).

Uremia Azotemia; the signs and symptoms typical of chronic renal failure.

Ureterostomy Surgically created opening in the ureter.

Urethritis Inflammation of the urethra.

Urge incontinence Involuntary loss of urine, usually shortly after a strong urge to void.

Urinary incontinence The inability to control the passage of urine.

Utilitarianism An ethical doctrine that holds that the moral worth of an action is determined by its contribution to overall utility in society—that is, the best course of action is the one that will produce the greatest good for the greatest number of individuals.

Uveitis Usually refers to inflammation of the iris, ciliary body, and/or choroid of the eye; also used to indicate inflammation of sclera, cornea, and/or retina.

V

Vaginitis Inflammation of the vagina.

Values Principles or standards that determine the worth you give to an idea or action.

Value system Personal standards for decision making.

Values clarification The process by which a person learns to make choices from alternatives that may be morally ambiguous.

Varices Enlarged, tortuous blood or lymphatic vessels.

Vasculitis Inflammation of blood vessels.

Vasoconstriction Decrease in blood vessel diameter.

Vasodilation Increase in blood vessel diameter.

Ventilation Movement of air in and out of the lungs.

Veracity In the health care setting, truth and honesty in discussions with patients, in documentation of care, and in communication with colleagues.

Vertigo Sensation that one's body or one's surroundings are rotating.

Vesicle Small fluid-filled bladder or sac; blister.

Vesicostomy Surgically created opening into the urinary bladder.

Viruses Infectious microorganisms that can live and reproduce only within living cells; capable of causing illness, inflammation, and cell destruction.

Viscosity Resistance to flow related to the friction between two components; thickness.

Vitamins Organic compounds supplied by food that the body needs for normal growth and development.

Void Urinate.

Vulvitis Inflammation of the vulva.

W

Water-soluble vitamins Vitamins that are soluble in water; not as potentially toxic as fat-soluble vitamins and readily excreted by the body; includes vitamins *except* A, D, E, and K.

Wheeze High-pitched sound heard as air passes through constricted airways.

Withdrawal Unpleasant and sometimes life-threatening physical substance-specific syndrome occurring after stopping or reducing the habitual dose or frequency of an abused drug.

X

Xerostomia Dry mouth caused by inadequate production of saliva.

Index

b indicates boxed material, *f* indicates illustrations, and *t* indicates tables.

I-1